ALEXANDER'S
CARE OF THE PATIENT
IN SURGERY

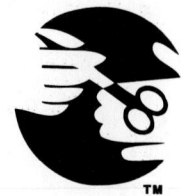

The material contained in this book is endorsed by AORN as a useful component in the ongoing education process of perioperative nurses.

™

ALEXANDER'S
CARE OF THE PATIENT IN SURGERY

MARGARET HUTH MEEKER, RN, BSN, CNOR

Director of Perioperative Nursing
The Ohio State University Hospitals
Columbus, Ohio

JANE C. ROTHROCK, RN, DNSC, CNOR

Professor and Program Coordinator, Perioperative Nursing
Delaware County Community College
Media, Pennsylvania

TENTH EDITION

with illustrations

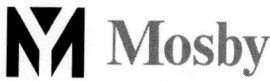 Mosby

St. Louis Baltimore Berlin Boston Carlsbad Chicago London Madrid
Naples New York Philadelphia Sydney Tokyo Toronto

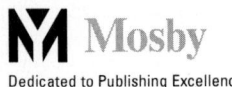
Mosby
Dedicated to Publishing Excellence

Publisher: Nancy L. Coon
Editor: Michael S. Ledbetter
Senior Developmental Editor: Teri Merchant
Associate Developmental Editor: Cecily Barolak
Project Manager: Karen Edwards
Production Editor: Rich Barber
Designer: Elizabeth Fett
Manufacturing Supervisor: Theresa Fuchs
Original art: Jack Reuter

Great care has been used in compiling and checking the information in this book to ensure its accuracy. However, because of changing technology, recent discoveries, and research and individualization of prescriptions according to patient needs, the uses, effects, and dosages of drugs may vary from those given here. Neither the publisher nor the authors shall be responsible for such variations or other inaccuracies. We urge that before you administer any drug you check the manufacturer's dosage recommendations as given in the package insert provided with each product.

Cover photograph courtesy of Carle Foundation Hospital, Urbana, Illinois.

TENTH EDITION

Printed in the United States of America
Composition by The Clarinda Company
Printing/binding by Maple Vail–Binghamton

Mosby-Year Book, Inc.
11830 Westline Industrial Drive
St. Louis, Missouri 63146

International Standard Book Number 0-8016-7924-9

96 97 98 99 / 9 8 7 6 5 4 3 2

CONTRIBUTORS

Kay A. Ball, RN, BSN, MSA, CNOR
Director of Education
United Medical Network
Dublin, Ohio
Ch. 31-Lasers

Cynthia A. Bray, RN, MS, CNOR
Director, Operating Rooms
Hahnemann University
Philadelphia, Pennsylvania
Ch. 32-Endoscopic Surgery

Patricia S. Coutellier, RN, BSN, CNOR
Nurse Manager-Perioperative Nursing
The Ohio State University Hospitals
Columbus, Ohio
Ch. 18-Otologic Surgery

Brenda Gregory Dawes, RN, BSN, CNOR
Director Surgical Services
Texas Orthopedic Hospital
Houston, Texas
Ch. 21-Orthopedic Surgery
Ch. 24-Thoracic Surgery

Katherine J. Donahoe, RN, CNOR
Perioperative Specialist
Crozer-Chester Medical Center
Upland, Pennsylvania
Ch. 23-Plastic and Reconstructive Surgery

Nancye Rae Feistritzer, RN, MSN, CNOR
Director of Operating Room Services
University of Kentucky Hospital
Lexington, Kentucky
Ch. 7-Mechanics of Wound Healing

Vicki J. Fox, RN, MSN, CRNFA
Clinical Nurse Specialist
Specialty Nursing Services, PC
Tyler, Texas
Ch. 9-Patient Education and Discharge Planning

Barbara D. Garner, MS, RN, CNOR
Clinical Nurse Specialist-Perioperative Nursing
Charleston Area Medical Center
Charleston, West Virginia
Ch. 3-Infection Control

Lynn S. Harkins, RN
Staff Nurse
Children's Hospital of Philadelphia
Philadelphia, Pennsylvania
Ch. 28-Pediatric Surgery

Jane Hershey Johnson, RN, MSN, CNOR
Perioperative Faculty
Delaware County Community College
Media, Pennsylvania
Ch. 15-Thyroid and Parathyroid Surgery

John Lee Hoffer, PhD, MD
Professor of Anesthesiology
Texas A & M University Health Science Center
Professor of Engineering
Texas A & M University
Temple, Texas
Ch. 6-Anesthesia

Brenda C. Kersten, RN, BSN
Operating Room Staff Nurse
Otolaryngology Head and Neck Surgery
The Ohio State University Hospitals
Columbus, Ohio
Ch. 19-Rhinologic and Sinus Surgery

Carol Slusarz Ladden, RN, MSN, CNOR
Lecturer
University of Pennsylvania School of Nursing
Philadelphia, Pennsylvania
Ch. 1-Concepts Basic to Perioperative Nursing

Antoinette K. Ledbetter, RN, MS, CNOR
Trauma Coordinator
St. John's Mercy Medical Center
St. Louis, Missouri
Ch. 30-Trauma Surgery

Beth Ann MacVittie, RN, MS, CNOR
Head Nurse, Vascular Operating Room
Strong Memorial Hospital
University of Rochester
Rochester, New York
Ch. 25-Vascular Surgery

Patricia Felice Meckes, RN, MN, CNOR
Assistant Director of Education
Kaiser Permanente Medical Center
Bellflower, California
Ch. 29-Geriatric Surgery

Gratia M. Nagle, RN, BA, CNOR, CRNFA
Senior Staff Nurse-Urology
Paoli Memorial Hospital
Paoli, Pennsylvania
Ch. 14-Genitourinary Surgery

Gwen Lynn Nelson, RN, BSN, CNOR
Clinical Product Specialist
Valleylab, Inc.
Boulder, Colorado
Ch. 13-Gynecologic Surgery and Cesarean Birth

Cheryl Nygren, RN, CNOR, RNFA
Staff Nurse-Cardiothoracic Surgery
Children's Hospital of Philadelphia
Philadelphia, Pennsylvania
Ch. 28-Pediatric Surgery

Jan Odom, MS, RN,CPAN
Clinical Nurse Specialist-Surgical Services
Forrest General Hospital
Hattiesburg, Mississippi
Ch. 8-Postoperative Care and Complications

Claire Olsen, MS, RN, CNOR
Program Director/Professor-Surgical Technology
Nassau Community College
Garden City, New Jersey
Ch. 5-Sutures, Needles and Instruments

Lynda Petty, RN, BSN, CNOR
Perioperative Educator
Arthur G. James Cancer Hospital and Research Institute
Columbus, Ohio
Ch. 10-Gastrointestinal Surgery
Ch. 11-Surgery of the Liver, Biliary Tract, Pancreas & Spleen

Merry Anne Pierson, RN, MSN
Director, Surgical Services
Middle Tennessee Medical Center
Murfreesboro, Tennessee
Ch. 2-Patient and Environmental Safety

Leslie Eileen Ricker, BSN, CNOR
Staff Nurse, Clinic Operating Room
The Ohio State University Hospitals
Columbus, Ohio
Ch. 4-Positioning the Patient for Surgery

Rosemary Ann Roth, RN, MSN, CNOR
ICU/Surgical Suite Nursing Director
The Genesee Hospital
Rochester, New York
Ch. 16-Breast Surgery

Cheryl A. Sangermano, RN, BSN, CNOR, CNA
Manager-OR, PACU, and Ambulatory Surgery Center
Grant Medical Center
Columbus, Ohio
Ch. 27-Ambulatory Surgery

Patricia C. Seifert, RN, MSN, CRNFA, CNOR
Operating Room Coordinator, Cardiac Surgery
The Arlington Hospital
Arlington, Virginia
Ch. 26-Cardiac Surgery

Amy B. Shannon, RN, BSN, MHA
Staff Nurse
The Ohio State University Hospitals
Columbus, Ohio
Ch. 12-Repair of Hernias

Sue Silcox, RN, CORLN
Head Nurse, ORL Operating Room
The Methodist Hospital
Neurosensory Center
Houston, Texas
Ch. 20-Laryngologic and Head and Neck Surgery

David M. Sileo, BSN, RN, CNOR
Level III Staff Nurse-Perioperative Nursing
Hospital of the University of Pennsylvania
Philadelphia, Pennsylvania
Ch. 21-Orthopedic Surgery

Elaine Thomson-Keith, RN, BSN, CNOR
Health Care Consultant
Houston, Texas
Ch. 17-Ophthalmic Surgery

Ruth E. Vaiden, RN, CNOR, CRNFA
Director Surgical Services
Healthsouth Medical Center
Richmond, Virginia
Ch. 22-Neurosurgery

Donna S. Watson, RN, MSN, CNOR
Managing Partner
Nursing Link
Fort Smith, Arkansas
Ch. 27-Ambulatory Surgery
Ch. 33-Contemporary Issues

CLINICAL CONSULTANTS

Teresa Abercrombie, MS, RN, CNOR
Perioperative Clinical Nurse Specialist
The Ohio State University Hospitals
Columbus, Ohio

Joyce Ackley, RN, CNOR
Clinical Educator
Memorial Medical Center
Springfield, Illinois

Mark W. Arnold, MD
Assistant Professor of Surgery
The Ohio State University College of Medicine
Columbus, Ohio

Larry Lee Asplin, RN, CNOR, RT
Day Charge
Northway Day Surgery-Division of St. Cloud Hospital
St. Cloud, Minnesota

Bart Beecher, RN, BS, CNOR
Staff Nurse
Sonoma Valley Hospital
Sonoma, California

Sally Betz, MS, RN, CCRN, CEN, EMT-A
Clinical Nurse Specialist
The Ohio State University Hospitals
Columbus, Ohio

James R. Bollinger, MD, FACS
Chief-Urology Section
Paoli Memorial Hospital
Paoli, Pennsylvania

Nelda Britton, RN, MEd, CNOR
Clinical Nurse Specialist-Perioperative Nursing
University of South Alabama Medical Center
Adjunct Faculty
University of South Alabama
Mobile, Alabama

Nancy T. Brooks, RN, BSN, CNOR
Assistant Head Nurse-Ophthalmology Operating Room
The Methodist Hospital
Houston, Texas

Nancy Burden, RN, BS, CPAN
Surgery Team Leader
Morton Plant East Lake Surgery Center
Palm Harbor, Florida

Christopher Caldwell, MD
Assistant Attending, Surgery
The Genesee Hospital
Rochester, New York

Joanne D. Cimorelli, RN, BS, CNOR, RNFA
Supervisor, Operating Room
Scheie Eye Institute
Department of Ophthalmology
University of Pennsylvania
Philadelphia, Pennsylvania

Mary Ann Coble, RN, CNOR
Educator
Surgical Services Department
Swedish Medical Center/Seattle Campus
Seattle, Washington

Laura Alice Cohen, CRNA, BS
PACU Coordinator, Senior Staff Nurse Anesthetist
Anesthesiology Service
VA Medical Center
New Orleans, Louisiana

Gloria Cole, RN, BA, CNOR
Operating Room Instructor
Gateway Community College
Phoenix, Arizona

Deborah A. Cruz, MSN, RNC
Clinical Nurse Specialist-Labor and Delivery
Pennsylvania Hospital
Philadelphia, Pennsylvania

Wanda Lou Dunkel, BSN, RN, CNOR
Clinical Nurse III
Memorial Medical Center
Springfield, Illinois

Sandra L. Dunn, RN, BSEd, CNOR
Director Education/CQI, Operating Room
St. Luke's Hospital Medical Center
Phoenix, Arizona

Delores Everts, RN, BA, BS, CNOR
Otorhinolaryngology Laser Safety Officer/Clinical III
Children's Hospital
Los Angeles, California

Susan J. Fetzer-Fowler, RN, MSN, MBA, CCRN
Assistant Professor
School of Health & Human Services
University of New Hampshire
Staff Nurse, PACU
Elliot Hospital
Manchester, New Hampshire

Nancymarie Fortunato, RN, BSN, BA, CNOR
Perioperative Instructor, Lakeland Community College
Perioperative Clinical Nurse, Cleveland Clinic
Cleveland, Ohio

John R. Garrett, MD, FACS
Chairman, Department of Surgery
Director of Cardiovascular Surgery
The Arlington Hospital
Arlington, Virginia

Sandra G. Gaylor, RN, BS, CNOR
Staff Nurse
Eastside Medical Center
Snellville, Georgia

Terri Goodman, BSN, MA, CNOR
Nurse Educator
Doctor's Hospital
Dallas, Texas

Virginia G. Hicks, BSN, MS
Assistant Professor
Northeast Louisianna State School of Nursing
Monroe, Louisianna

Megan E. Higgins, RN, BSN
Transplant Coordinator
Delaware Valley Transplant Program
Philadelphia, Pennsylvania

Sylvia Huie, PhD, RN
Nurse Clinician
Loyola University Medical Center
Maywood, Illinois

Marilyn A. Hunter, RN, PhD, CNOR
Program Director-Surgical Technologies
Daytona Beach Community College
Daytona Beach, Florida

Gloria B. Jimenea, RN
Head Nurse-Ophthalmology Operating Room
The Methodist Hospital
Houston, Texas

Kevin C. Kauffman, RN, ASN
Director of Endoscopy Training
Nevada Ob/Gyn Educational Foundation
Las Vegas, Nevada

David R. Kelly, MD
Assistant Professor-Department of Otolaryngology
The Ohio State University College of Medicine
Columbus, Ohio

Rosemary Kesler, RN, BS, MA, CNOR
Program Director
Perioperative Nursing/Surgical Technology
Gateway Community College
Phoenix, Arizona

Cecil King, RN, CNOR
Perioperative Consultant
Baltimore, Maryland

Joseph J. Kryc, MD
Vice Chairman and Clinical Associate Professor
Department of Anesthesiology
Clinical Associate Professor-Department of Obstetrics and Gynecology
University of Arizona Maricopa Medical Center
Phoenix, Arizona

Joann V. Lally, RN, CNOR
Perioperative Faculty
Delaware County Community College
Media, PA

Antoinette K. Ledbetter, RN, MS, CNOR
Trauma Coordinator
St. John's Mercy Medical Center
St. Louis, Missouri

Mary G. Martin, RN, BS, CNOR
Healthcare Consultant
Charleston, South Carolina

Ann T. McKennis, RN, CNOR, CORLN
Staff Nurse-Clinical Level III
Otorhinolaryngology Operating Rooms
The Methodist Hospital
Houston, Texas

Mary "Dee" Miller, RN, MS, CC
Manager, Infection Control
St. Joseph's Hospital and Medical Center
Faculty-Nursing and Business Colleges
University of Phoenix
Phoenix, Arizona

Dan Milloy, CRNA
Forrest General Hospital
Hattiesburg, Mississippi

Shirley Moore, PhD, RN
Assistant Professor
Barnes College at University of Missouri-St. Louis
St. Louis, Missouri

Elaine Neel, RN, MSN
Perioperative Nursing Instructor
Methodist Medical Center of Illinois
School of Nursing
Peoria, Illinois

Lillian H. Nicolette, RN, MSN, CNOR
Clinical Educator
Advanced Sterilization Products
Philadelphia, PA

Victoria U. Nugent, MS, RN, ANP
Nurse Practitioner
Private Surgical Oncology Practice
Rochester, New York

John O'Connell, BS, CCP
Cardiovascular Perfusionist
The Arlington Hospital
Arlington, Virginia

Kenneth Ouriel, MD
Assoiciate Professor of Surgery
University of Rochester College of Medicine
Rochester, New York

Sue Paquette, RN, BSN, CCRN
Trauma Coordinator
The Ohio State University Hospitals
Columbus, Ohio

Brian T. Pelczar, MD
Chief Resident, Otolaryngology
The Ohio State University Medical Center
Columbus, Ohio

Catherine C. Powers, MSN, RN, CCRN
Clinical Specialist-Pulmonary
Barnes Hospital at Washington University Medical Center
St. Louis, Missouri

Donna Prentice, MSN(R), RN, CCRN, TNS
Critical Care Clinical Nurse Specialist
Barnes Hospital at Washington University
St. Louis, Missouri

Donna DeFazio Quinn, BSN, MBA, RN, CPAN
Manager
Elliot 1-Day Surgery Center
Manchester, New Hampshire

Elaine Rak, RN
Laser Safety Officer
Shady Grove Adventist Hospital
Rockville, Maryland

Dr. Jean Reese, RN, PhD
Associate Professor, College of Nursing
University of Iowa
Iowa City, Iowa

Wyveda Rodriguez, RN, MSN, CNOR
Coordinator, Education and Research
Surgery and Outpatient Services
Harris Methodist Hospital
Fort Worth, Texas

Jess Salinas, RN, BA, ADN
Staff Nurse
Children's Hospital Medical Center
Seattle, Washington

Jacqueline Saunders, RN, BSN, CNOR
Nurse Educator-Perioperative Services
Hahnemann University Hospital

Jacqueline R. Schmitt, RN, CNOR
Laparoscopic Coordinator
The Bryn Mawr Hospital
Bryn Mawr, Pennsylvania

Schlomo Schneebaum, MD
Assistant Professor-Department of Surgery
The Ohio State University College of Medicine
Columbus, Ohio

Janet K. Schultz, RN, MSN
Vice President, Perioperative Products and Services
AMSCO Healthcare
Pittsburgh, Pennsylvania

Christine E. Smith, RN, MSN, CNOR
Perioperative Nursing Clinical Specialist
Delaware County Community College
Media, Pennsylvania

Maurice M. Smith, MD
Clinical Instructor-Division of Neurosurgery
Medical College of Virginia
Richmond, Virginia

Sandra Smyth, RN, CPSN, CNOR
Staff Nurse, Surgical Services
Williamsburg Community Hospital
Williamsburg, Virginia

Victoria M. Steelman, MA, RN, CNOR
Clinical Nurse Specialist II
Perioperative Nursing
The University of Iowa Hospitals and Clinics
Iowa City, Iowa

Mary L. Sweeney, RN, MN, CNOR
Staff Nurse
Providence Medical Center
Seattle, Washington

Annette Taube, RN, MS, BSN
Program Director
Surgical Technology
Columbus State Community College
Columbus, Ohio

Dorothy Thomas, RN, MSN
Assistant Professor
St. Louis Community College at Florissant Valley
St. Louis, Missouri

Allan R. Thomes, RN, CNOR
Central Minnesota Neurosciences, LTD.
St. Cloud, Minnesota

Gregory M. Thompson, MS, MD, FACS
Adult and Pediatric-Urologist
Paoli Memorial Hospital
Paoli, Pennsylvania

Patricia A. Timmins, AB, RN, CNOR
Perioperative Staff Nurse
Pennsylvania Hospital
Philadelphia, Pennsylvania

James C. Torraco, MBA
National Sales Manager
MP Video Inc.
Hopkinton, Massachusetts

Michael C. Townsend, MD
Assistant Professor of Surgery and Anesthesia
The Ohio State University College of Medicine
Columbus, Ohio

Carol Tyler, RN, BS, CNOR
Cardiovascular-Thoracic Team Leader-Operating Room
Evanston Hospital
Evanston, Illinois

Beth Van Camp, RN, CNOR
Specialty Nurse-Ophthalmology
Swedish Hospital Medical Center
Seattle, Washington

Carolyn Waddington, BSN, RN, CORLN
Staff Nurse
Methodist Hospital
Houston, Texas

Carolyn Webster, RN
Nurse Executive
The Fresno Surgery Center
Fresno, California

Anne P. Weiland, RN, MSN, ANP
Assistant Vice President-Clinical Services
The Washington Hospital Center
Washington, DC

D. Bradley Welling, MD
Assistant Professor-Department of Otolaryngology
The Ohio State University College of Medicine
Columbus, Ohio

Jane Wellmaker, RN
Genitourinary Coordinator
Missouri Baptist Hospital
St. Louis, Missouri

Laurel Wiersema, MSN, RN, CS
Clinical Nurse Specialist, Surgery/Wound
Barnes Hospital at Washington University Medical Center
St. Louis, Missouri

William Yorde, BS, CCP
Cardiovascular Perfusionist
The Arlington Hospital
Arlington, Virginia

Alexander's Care of the Patient in Surgery celebrated its 50th anniversary in 1993. The tenth edition marks another sentinel event for this textbook. For the first time, it is published with the endorsement of the Association of Operating Room Nurses, Inc. The AORN Logo is proudly displayed along with the acclamation that this book is recognized as a useful component in the ongoing education process of perioperative nurses. In recognition of that endorsement, this edition is dedicated to AORN's current and past leaders, who have invested their talent and infinite wisdom in underpinning the relationship between the contributions of science and the clinical practice of perioperative nursing. It is through their commitment to the profession that, while the place of surgery is constantly changing in society, the art and science of perioperative nursing remains as the unparalleled hallmark of quality nursing care for the recipients of surgery.

PREFACE

The tenth edition of *Alexander's Care of the Patient in Surgery* has been extensively updated to reflect new concepts in perioperative nursing practice and the increased sophistication and complexity of surgical procedures in the 1990s. However, the goal of this text remains essentially the same: to provide a comprehensive basic reference that will help perioperative personnel meet the needs of patients during surgical interventions safely, cost-effectively, and efficiently.

The standard in perioperative nursing for over 50 years, *Alexander's Care of the Patient in Surgery* is written primarily for professional perioperative nurses, but is also useful for nursing students, surgical technologists, health care industry representatives, medical students, interns, residents, and government officials concerned with health care issues. Practitioners of perioperative nursing, clinical nurse specialists, and educators from many geographic areas of the United States have served as contributors to this text, providing a broad range of perioperative nursing knowledge and procedural information.

This thoroughly revised edition highlights the most current techniques and innovations in surgery. Hundreds of illustrations, including many new photographs and drawings, help familiarize the reader with new methods and equipment. Classic illustrations, particularly of surgical anatomy, have been preserved to enhance the text.

Overall, the text imparts state-of-the-art information that reflects quality contemporary practice and promotes the delivery of comprehensive perioperative patient care.

Unit I, Foundations for Practice, provides information on basic principles and patient care requisites essential to the care of all recipients of perioperative patient care. The nursing process, a model for developing therapeutic nursing interventional knowledge, has been expanded to a six-step process with a clear identification of desired patient outcomes. Interest in patient outcomes and their improvement is an essential element of nursing in a reformed delivery system. As the country gears up for health data collection in an information age that requires clear identification of contributions to patient outcomes and quantification

of these in data-driven improvement of quality patient care, perioperative nurses must begin linking their interventions to clearly identified outcomes. This relationship is presented in Chapter 1 and explicated in each sample care plan throughout the text. Also beginning with Chapter 1, the reader will discover a new addition to the tenth edition—Research Highlights. The amount and quality of research relevant to perioperative patient care have steadily increased. Because the findings of research are often not effectively used in clinical practice, the editors and authors of *Alexander's* are committed to closing this research-practice gap. The research highlights will help perioperative nurses use the findings of research in their practice. A new chapter, Infection Control, emphasizes the important contributions of the perioperative nurse to the prevention of infection in surgical patients. Also new for Unit I is a chapter on Postoperative Care and Complications to help the perioperative nurse anticipate and obviate common problems that can occur during recovery from anesthesia. This vital information will help the perioperative nurse collaborate with the PACU nurse in the assessment of patients during the postoperative period and initiation of early intervention therapy. The reader will also find a new chapter, Patient Education and Discharge Planning, as the concluding chapter in Unit I. As the responsibilities of perioperative nurses become greater with regard to these important care components, it is imperative that we educate patients effectively. This chapter presents patient education in the framework of the nursing process, covering important principles and models of patient education, assessment, and instructional techniques, and case studies that explicate the provision of patient education.

The care and procedures involved with nearly 400 general and specialty surgical interventions arè included in Unit II, Surgical Interventions. Each chapter provides an overview of pertinent anatomy and details the steps of each procedure. Perioperative nursing considerations continue to be presented within the nursing process framework. Related NANDA-approved nursing diagnoses and Sample Care Plans for each surgical specialty are intended to help the perioperative nurse plan, implement, and evaluate individualized perioperative patient care. Increased emphasis on minimally invasive approaches to surgical intervention have been expanded to help the reader prepare for patient care in these technologic alternatives to traditional surgical approaches.

Unit III, Special Considerations, discusses the unique needs of ambulatory, pediatric, geriatric, and trauma surgery patients. In the new chapter, Trauma Surgery, the reader will find information on mechanisms of injury, pathophysiology, assessment, and resuscitative surgical intervention. The reader will also find in this unit a chapter on lasers and a new chapter, Endoscopic Surgery. This chapter includes information on theory as well as practical information on equipment, instrumentation, suturing techniques, and special considerations related to anesthesia and perioperative nursing care of patients undergoing endoscopic procedures. Important issues of cost-management

and educating the perioperative nursing team for competent care delivery are included. The final new addition to Unit III is a chapter, Contemporary Issues. Here the reader will find a lucid and relevant discussion of health care policy and research agendas, nursing issues related to a reformed delivery system, reimbursement, the nurse supply, the environment and its protection, as well as ethical dilemmas and the management of risk.

Many expert practitioners have contributed to this tenth edition, and we owe a debt of gratitude to each of them. We also acknowledge the valuable assitance of editors, reviewers, photographers, and illustrators who have contributed their time and expertise to the revision of this text.

Alexander's Care of the Patient in Surgery is written by and for perioperative nurses, and is dedicated to excellence in perioperative nursing practice.

MARGARET HUTH MEEKER
JANE C. ROTHROCK

BRIEF CONTENTS

DETAILED CONTENTS

UNIT TWO
SURGICAL INTERVENTIONS

UNIT THREE

SPECIAL CONSIDERATIONS

PART ONE

FOUNDATIONS FOR PRACTICE

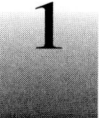

CONCEPTS BASIC TO PERIOPERATIVE NURSING

CAROL SLUSARZ LADDEN

T he specialty of perioperative nursing has come of age in both image and practice. In the few years since the last edition of this text was published, perioperative nurses have continued to expand their practice patterns and responsibilities, continued to enhance their self-concepts, and firmly established perioperative nursing as a professional nursing specialty, all with vibrant commitment to the profession and enduring commitment to the patient.

The term *perioperative nursing* is now used in both nursing and medical circles. Perioperative nursing is recognized and practiced in surgical suites, ambulatory surgery centers, endoscopy suites, laser centers, and physician's offices across the United States. Historically, the term *operating room nursing* was used to describe the care of patients in the immediate preoperative, intraoperative, and postoperative phases of the surgical experience. Such a term, however, intimated that nursing care activities were circumscribed to the geographic limits of the surgical suite. The term may have contributed to stereotypic images of a nurse who took care of the operating room and had little interface or nursing responsibility for medicated and anesthetized patients in the surgical suite. In this perspective, nursing practitioners outside the operating room had difficulty ascribing important elements of the nursing process and patient care accountability to the nurse who practiced behind the doors of the surgical suite.

Perioperative nursing includes the preoperative, intraoperative, and postoperative periods of the patient's surgical experience. It connotes, however, the delivery of nursing care through the framework of the nursing process. In such a framework, the perioperative nurse engages in patient assessment; collects, organizes, and prioritizes patient data; establishes nursing diagnoses; identifies desired patient outcomes; develops and implements a plan of nursing care; and evaluates that care in terms of outcomes achieved by the patient. In these activities the perioperative nurse functions dependently, independently, and interdependently. The pe-

rioperative nurse collaborates with other health care professionals, makes appropriate nursing referrals, and delegates and supervises nursing care. When perioperative nursing is practiced in its broadest scope, nursing care may begin in the patient's home, a clinic, a physician's office, the patient care unit, the presurgical care unit or the holding area (Research Highlight 1-1). Following the surgical intervention, nursing care may continue in postanesthesia care or in patient evaluation on the patient care unit, in the physician's office, in the patient's home, in a clinic, or through written or telephone patient surveys. Perioperative nursing may be practiced in diverse settings. When perioperative nursing is practiced in the narrower sense, patient care activities may be confined to the common areas of the surgical suite. Assessment and data collection may take place in the holding area; evaluation may take place on discharge from the operating room to the postanesthesia care unit. Despite the way perioperative nursing is operationalized in a health care setting, it is underscored by the nursing process and all the care activities inherent in that process.

CONSIDERATIONS

The various perioperative nursing roles all subsume elements of the behaviors and technical practices that characterize professional nursing. Probably no other area of nursing requires the broad knowledge base, the instant recall of nursing science, the need to be intuitively guided by past nursing experience, the diversity of thought and action, the stamina, and the flexibility needed in perioperative nursing endeavors. Whether a generalist or specialist, the perioperative nurse depends on stored knowledge pertinent to surgical anatomy, physiologic alterations and their consequences for the patient, intraoperative risk factors, potentials for patient injury and the means of preventing them, and psychosocial implications of surgery for the patient and significant others, as well as on clues to the needs of the

---

RESEARCH HIGHLIGHT 1-1

In this historical review four periods were analyzed to identify the changing focus of preoperative patient preparation. From 1900 to 1919 preparation of the patient for surgery took place primarily in the patient's home, as did much of surgery. The patient took light, nourishing food; baths; and frequent rest periods to build up the body. The nurse arrived at the home a few hours before surgery, choosing and preparing a room, emptying it of furniture, boiling sheets and instruments, and preventing excitement on the patient's part. The nurse also obtained a personal and family history from the patient, although little patient teaching took place.

Between 1920 and 1939, physicians became affiliated with hospitals, and minimum standards of preoperative patient preparation began to evolve. Both physical and mental preparation of the patient was stressed, the concept of patient consent for surgery was initiated, and preparation of the OR and instruments was addressed. Nursing manuals on care of the surgical patient included normal anatomy and physiology, pathophysiology, medical and surgical treatments, and nursing interventions.

The years between 1940 and 1959 witnessed enormous scientific medical discoveries; nursing care of surgical patients became more complex to accommodate rapid changes in surgical care. Patient teaching became part of preoperative patient preparation, individual patient needs were emphasized, and the psychologic preparation of the patient was increasingly recognized as important.

During 1960 to 1979 nursing research was being conducted and emphasized; early research linked preoperative preparation and postoperative recovery. Patients' emotional needs were recognized as they related to individual patients, and concepts of structured preoperative instruction were introduced and validated by nursing research.

Oetker-Black, S. L. (1993). Preoperative preparation: Historical development. *AORN Journal, 57*(6), 1402-1410.

---

members of the health care team, as an integral team member, truly an expert!

Perioperative nursing is a purposeful, dynamic, professional process. Through the process of planning patient care and identifying required nursing interventions and actions, perioperative nurses assure surgical patients of scientific, professional nursing care. Perioperative nurses historically have assumed responsibility for providing a safe, efficient, and caring environment for surgical patients, one in which the surgical team can function smoothly and efficiently to achieve positive patient outcomes. Such mutuality between nursing and other health care disciplines and the role of patient advocacy continue to be part of the essence of perioperative nursing in the 1990s.

A significant part of perioperative nursing is the delivery of scientifically based care: understanding the necessity for certain techniques of care; knowing how and when to initiate them; being creative in maintaining a technique when the situation calls for flexibility; and evaluating the safety, cost, and outcomes of the technical aspects of nursing science. Knowledge of nursing skills, procedures, setups, instruments, and equipment is essential during the implementation phase of nursing care. Without such knowledge, the perioperative nurse is unable to prepare for or anticipate the steps in the surgical procedure, with their concomitant implications for the patient and for the surgical team. Nurses who are well versed in the detailed nursing techniques contained in this text can best foresee the needs of both the patient and the surgical team during care plan implementation. Scientific nursing techniques are at the heart of perioperative nursing. In the many chapters of this text that focus on surgical interventions common to patients in the 1990s, these nursing techniques have clearly and deliberately been incorporated as part of the care plan. Such conceptualization integrates them as important elements of nursing care.

In this chapter, perioperative nursing is considered as an entity. The purpose is to place it in perspective by spelling out the place for and details of some of the behavioral and conceptual components. It sets the scene for the remainder of the text. A fundamental assumption is that perioperative nursing is a blend of the technical and behavioral; it is thinking as well as doing, caring for patients as well as handling instruments.

patient or surgical team. This stored knowledge enables the perioperative nurse to initiate nursing actions on a minute's notice. Such excellence in practice is the hallmark of perioperative nursing.

The size of this mental repertoire is staggering and points out the constant discipline, attention, ongoing education, and presence of mind demanded in perioperative nursing. However, the greater the requirements, the more satisfactory and indelible are the joys that come to the perioperative nurse who practices at this level of excellence. The perioperative nurse recognizes self, and is recognized by other

DESCRIPTION OF PERIOPERATIVE NURSING

Perioperative nursing, a term describing the scope and practice of nursing in surgical settings, has gained wide acceptance. Emanating from the work and influence of the Association of Operating Room Nurses (AORN), the term has helped to define and elucidate the activities of the professional nurse during three patient care phases: preoperative, intraoperative, and postoperative. A model depicting perioperative practice would illustrate a continuum on which the nurse functions from beginning competency to excellence.

Such a perioperative practice concept brings together both traditional and expanded nursing activities during intraoperative care, preoperative and postoperative patient education, counseling, assessment, planning, and evaluation functions. Perioperative nursing practice revolves around an individual patient who is undergoing a surgical intervention. The perioperative nurse's activities reflect the psychologic, social and physiologic problems that may result. Perioperative nurses scrub, circulate, assist the surgeon (RN first assistant), manage, teach, and conduct research. Because of an increased concern with containment of costs associated with the delivery of health care services, surgical procedures are now performed not only in traditional hospital operating rooms but also in freestanding surgical centers, ambulatory care or short-stay units, emergency departments, and physicians' offices. In these settings the professional nurse is a primary caregiver. From admission through discharge and home follow-up, the perioperative nurse plays a significant role in overseeing the patient's care. Such practice has helped to popularize and confirm the nature of a broad foundation for perioperative nursing roles. In the 1990s research will continue to test and validate the contribution of perioperative nursing to patient care outcomes in all settings where it is practiced. (See Chapter 33 for a full discussion of research and other contemporary issues in perioperative nursing.)

Within such a conceptual framework for the practice of perioperative nursing, a description of a comprehensive combination of head and hand skills emerges. A schema is provided whereby such nursing is viewed in a professional perspective and the nursing process is a pervasive thread.

NURSING PROCESS

Perioperative nursing is a systematic planned process, a series of integrated steps. If viewed only as setting up cases, perioperative nursing becomes nothing more than rote equipment preparation and paper shuffling. If, rather, it is viewed as patient care, it becomes a scientific process and stimulates the nurse to perform optimally.

The nursing process is a way of looking at nursing and bringing it into perspective as *a methodical thought process that guides actions,* which contrasts with considering nursing as only a set of cookbook rituals and procedures to be learned. The focus of the nursing process is on the patient, and the nursing interventions prescribed are those which meet patient needs. Because of the setting and the nature of the work, perioperative nursing is particularly vulnerable to being considered only a conglomeration of mechanical techniques and a carrying out of surgeons' orders. By using the nursing process, perioperative nurses can focus on the patient and, at the same time, put skills and know-how in proper perspective in dealing with patients and implementing procedures.

Use of the nursing process and nursing care plans has become an integral part of patient care in hospital nursing units. Their use in the perioperative setting has been less evident, in part because the perioperative setting is sufficiently different to require some alterations from the formal processes implemented on other nursing units. Because of these differences, including the short time the nurse has contact with the conscious patient and the movement through three different areas in the operative process, the perioperative nurse must adapt the process to the setting.

In its simplest form the nursing process defined by the ANA consists of six steps: assessment, nursing diagnosis, outcome identification, planning, intervention, and evaluation (Fig. 1-1). The process is circular and continuous.

Assessment is the collection of relevant data about the patient. Sources of data may be a preoperative interview with the patient and the patient's family by a perioperative or unit nurse; review of the nursing care plans, Kardex, and patient's chart; examination of the results of presurgical diagnostic studies; and consultation with the surgeon and anesthesiologist, unit nurses, or other personnel.

The format this assessment takes may vary from institu-

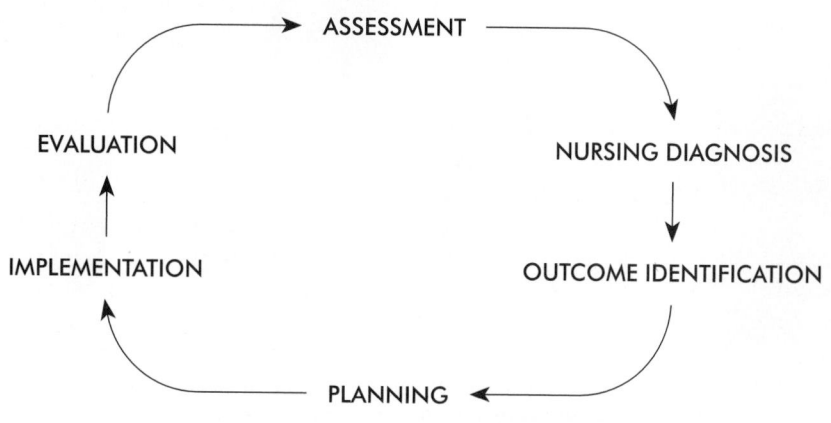

FIG. 1-1 Six phases of nursing process.

tion to institution but always includes both the physiologic and the psychosocial aspects of the patient. For a perioperative nurse, assessment may mean a thoughtful, quick scan of the patient and chart; a review of the surgical procedure; and a mental rehearsal of the resources and knowledge necessary to direct the patient through an operative course. At other times the perioperative nurse must thoroughly assess all aspects of the patient and the patient's condition, along with preoperative and postoperative reviews.

In a discussion of assessment the question of whether perioperative nurses should perform preoperative interviews invariably arises. Preoperative interviews or visits are standard procedure in many institutions. These interviews may be performed by a perioperative nurse in the presurgical care unit, or by telephone prior to the day of surgical admission. When data cannot be collected directly by a perioperative nurse, another information source, such as a nursing unit admission assessment, is reviewed to obtain baseline assessment information.

Preoperative visits by perioperative nurses are neither an end in themselves nor a means of getting nurses in touch with their patients. Also, preoperative patient contact alone does not mean that true perioperative practice exists; the perioperative nurse should beware of this fallacy. However, if planned properly to fill the needs of both patients and nurses, preoperative (and postoperative) interviews can be extremely beneficial (Fig. 1-2).

When thinking about preoperative interviewing and teaching, the nurse should consider the following: Is relevant, concise patient information already being transmitted to the perioperative nursing staff? Is enough information available to allow perioperative nurses to consider patient care needs when setting up the room (special equipment, supports, instruments, sutures)? Is sufficient time available to initiate a meaningful nurse-patient interaction before induction? Are surgical patients satisfied with their perioperative nursing care (do they express feelings of comfort and satisfaction regarding their care in the surgical setting), and do they have knowledge of the perioperative nurse's role? Is there continuity of care between the operating room and other nursing care units?

Being able to exchange information about their patients in face-to-face meetings (Fig. 1-3) or by telephone or written messages is helpful for unit and perioperative nurses. A thorough assessment, made and recorded by the unit nurses, can accompany patients to the operating room and serve as a guide to perioperative nursing personnel. Then the perioperative nurse has the responsibility to do a more in-depth and focused preoperative patient assessment.

Individual sessions with patients may be the answer to the issue of preoperative assessment. In some hospitals, group preoperative classes not only help nurses get to know the patients but also permit nurses to impart information on common routines, reactions, sensations, and nursing procedures that will take place preoperatively, intraoperatively, and postoperatively. The perioperative setting may dictate the type of interaction which may occur. The use of preoperative phone calls and questionnaires has gained acceptance. Soliciting information prior to the patient's arrival in the perioperative setting and this one-on-one contact from

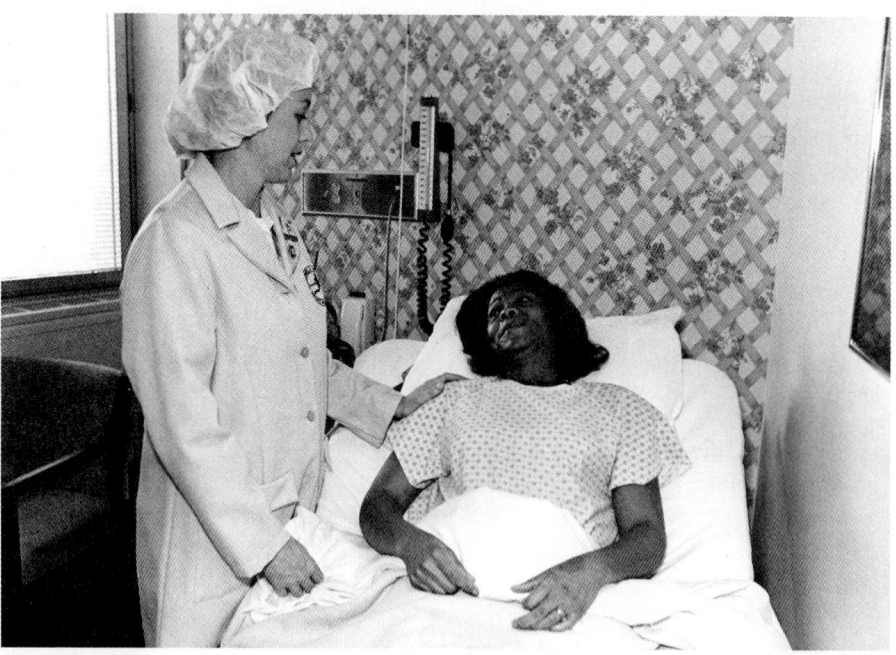

FIG. 1-2 Perioperative nurse interviews surgical patient. Purpose of visit is to assess patient needs, to obtain information about patient and family, and to teach patient regarding common perioperative routines, sensations, and nursing care.

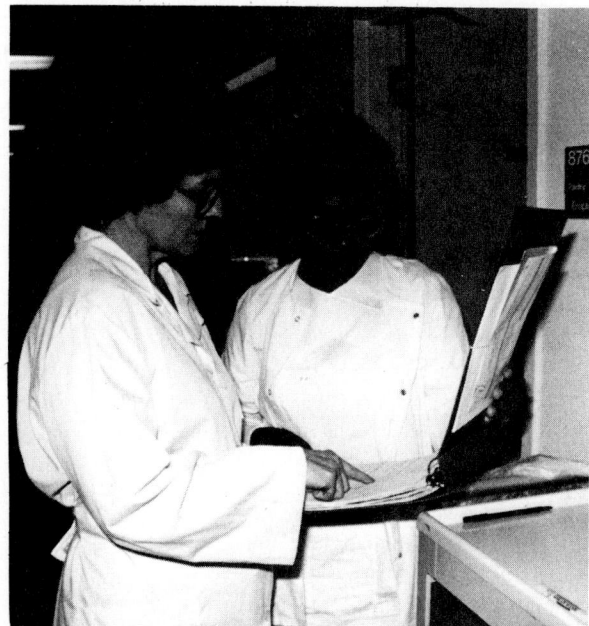

FIG. 1-3 Perioperative nurse and unit nurse discuss and plan patient care and preparation for surgery by sharing findings and relevant data.

RESEARCH HIGHLIGHT 1-2

This study was designed to quantify, through description, "good nursing care" by surgical patients undergoing back operations. Structured interviews of 30 patients yielded information about satisfaction with care during preoperative, intraoperative, and postoperative phases of care. Data indicated that patients had a strong need for information regarding the surgery, its risks and prognosis, and anesthesia. The majority of patients preferred this information 1 or 2 days before surgery, and the surgeon was identified as the preferred information giver. For the intraoperative phase, patients identified friendly, competent staff members who provided reassurance and protection for the patient; patients expressed confidence in the perioperative nurse's ability to care for them during anesthesia. Patients had vague recall of PACU care, but were able to identify close monitoring by a nurse and pain control as important to satisfaction with care provided.

Based on interview results, four areas for nursing research were noted: development and evaluation of perioperative information delivery systems; descriptions of nurse-patient roles and relationships; quantification of ways patients are respected during care episodes; and an analysis of the concept of loneliness during perioperative care phases.

Leino-Kilpi, H., & Vuorenheimo, J. (1993). Perioperative nursing care quality: Patient's opinions. *AORN Journal 57*(5), 1061-1071.

the perioperative nurse can affect patient outcomes. The important point is that some form of assessment and teaching should be done. How it is accomplished is up to the particular facility and nursing staff.

Assessment, then, is knowing and understanding the patient as a feeling, thinking, and responsible person and as a candidate for a surgical procedure (Research Highlight 1-2).

Data identified through assessment and determination of nursing diagnoses will help the perioperative nurse meet unique patient needs throughout the surgical intervention. Based on the data collected and interpreted during patient assessment, nursing diagnoses are formulated and pertinent patient information is recorded.

NURSING DIAGNOSIS

Diagnosis is the process of identifying and classifying the data collected in the assessment in a way that will yield a focus for the planning of nursing care. Nursing diagnoses have been evolving since they were first introduced in the 1950s. They have now reached the stage of development of being identified, named, and classified according to human response patterns and functional health patterns. The group responsible for delineating the accepted list of nursing diagnoses is the North American Nursing Diagnosis Association (NANDA) (Box 1-1). Each NANDA-approved nursing diagnosis has a set of components: definition (meaning of the diagnostic term), defining characteristics (pattern of cues that operationalize the meaning of the di-

agnosis), and related/risk/contextual factors (patient behaviors and factors in the environment that interact to place the individual at high risk of developing a particular diagnosis).

Not all patient problems encountered in the perioperative setting can be described by the list of accepted nursing diagnoses. Perioperative nurses must assist in the description and naming of new nursing diagnoses that describe unique perioperative patient problems. NANDA has established a "to be developed" category to designate nursing diagnoses that are partially developed and deemed useful to the nursing profession; perioperative nurses may develop unique diagnostic labels and definitions, then work to further develop and validate them through this process (Kim, McFarlane, & McLane, 1993).

Outcome identification is a statement that describes the desired or favorable patient condition that can be achieved through nursing interventions. Patient outcomes are derived from nursing diagnoses and direct the interventions to correct, alter, or maintain the nursing diagnoses. They are the standards or criteria by which the effectiveness of the interventions is measured. Outcomes should be stated in terms of expected or desired patient behavior; they should be specific and measurable in time (Gettrust and Brabec, 1992).

BOX 1-1

NANDA-Approved Nursing Diagnoses*

Activity intolerance
Activity intolerance, high risk for
Adjustment, impaired
Airway clearance, ineffective
Anxiety
Aspiration, high risk for
Body image disturbance
Body temperature, altered, high risk for
Breastfeeding, effective
Breastfeeding, ineffective
Breastfeeding, interrupted
Breathing pattern, ineffective
Cardiac output, decreased
Caregiver role strain
Caregiver role strain, high risk for
Communication, impaired verbal
Constipation
Constipation, colonic
Constipation, perceived
Coping, defensive
Coping, family: potential for growth
Coping, ineffective family: compromised
Coping, ineffective family: disabling
Coping, ineffective individual
Decisional conflict (specify)
Denial, ineffective
Diarrhea
Disuse syndrome, high risk for

Diversional activity deficit
Dysreflexia
Family processes, altered
Fatigue
Fear
Fluid volume deficit (1)
Fluid volume deficit (2)
Fluid volume deficit, high risk for
Fluid volume excess
Gas exchange, impaired
Grieving, anticipatory
Grieving, dysfunctional
Growth and development, altered
Health maintenance, altered
Health-seeking behaviors (specify)
Home maintenance management, impaired
Hopelessness
Hyperthermia
Hypothermia
Incontinence, bowel
Incontinence, functional
Incontinence, reflex
Incontinence, stress
Incontinence, total
Incontinence, urge
Infant feeding pattern, ineffective
Infection, high risk for
Injury, high risk for

*Includes those approved in 1992.

The perioperative nurse's identification of expected outcomes unique to the surgical patient provides the opportunity to prioritize care and direction for evaluation and continuity of care.

Having collected and interpreted the patient data and arrived at appropriate nursing diagnoses and desired outcomes, the perioperative nurse is prepared to plan the nursing care for the patient. Viewing the patient as an individual and not as a case allows the nurse to gain more satisfaction because the person having the surgery is now considered as well as the tools, setups, and environmental controls needed to perform the surgery. When perioperative nursing care puts its emphasis on the person having the operation, it validates its label "professional nursing."

Planning, in this process, means that perioperative nurses use their nursing knowledge and information about the patient to prepare the operating room environment. They check equipment, have usual and unusual supplies ready, and use their knowledge of anatomy to have proper instruments and sutures on hand for the procedure to be per-

formed. They know the usual steps in a procedure and use the surgeon's preference cards and nursing care guides to have the room and equipment ready for the patient.

Planning is knowing ahead of time what will happen and being prepared. Planning requires the perioperative nurse to determine the priorities for care. Planning is based on patient assessment that results in knowing the patient and the patient's unique needs so that alterations in positioning or in the surgical process are readily made. Planning also requires some knowledge of the patient's psychosocial state and feelings about the proposed operation so an extra, needed explanation or emotional support can be provided during the critical preinduction period (Fig. 1-4).

Planning requires a broad understanding of operating room routines and perioperative nursing. It requires participating in continuing education programs (Fig. 1-5), reading journals, reviewing and participating in research, and keeping up to date in the rapidly advancing world of perioperative nursing. Education is discussed in more detail later in this chapter.

BOX 1-1

NANDA-Approved Nursing Diagnoses—cont'd.

Knowledge deficit (specify)
Mobility, impaired physical
Noncompliance (specify)
Nutrition, altered: less than body requirements
Nutrition, altered: more than body requirements
Nutrition, altered: high risk for more than body requirements
Oral mucous membrane, altered
Pain
Pain, chronic
Parental role conflict
Parenting, altered
Parenting, altered, high risk for
Peripheral neurovascular dysfunction, high risk for
Personal identity disturbance
Poisoning, high risk for
Posttrauma response
Powerlessness
Protection, altered
Rape-trauma syndrome
Rape-trauma syndrome: compound reaction
Rape-trauma syndrome: silent reaction
Role performance, altered
Self-care deficit, bathing/hygiene
Self-care deficit, dressing/grooming
Self-care deficit, feeding
Self-care deficit, toileting
Self-esteem chronic low
Self-esteem disturbance

Self-esteem, situational low
Self-mutation, high risk for
Sensory/perceptual alterations (specify) (visual, auditory, kinesthetic, gustatory, tactile, olfactory)
Sexual dysfunction
Sexuality patterns, altered
Skin integrity, impaired
Skin integrity, impaired, high risk for
Sleep pattern disturbance
Social interaction, impaired
Social isolation
Spiritual distress (distress of the human spirit)
Stress syndrome, relocation
Suffocation, high risk for
Swallowing, impaired
Therapeutic regimen (individual), ineffective management of
Thermoregulation, ineffective
Thought processes, altered
Tissue integrity, impaired
Tissue perfusion, altered (specify type) (renal, cerebral, cardiopulmonary, gastrointestinal, peripheral)
Trauma, high risk for
Unilateral neglect
Urinary elimination, altered patterns
Urinary retention
Ventilation, spontaneous, inability to sustain
Ventilatory weaning response, dysfunctional
Violence, high risk for: self-directed or directed at others

Implementation is performing the nursing care interventions that were planned and responding to changes in surgical routine or to emergencies with calmness and orderly thinking. It is employing established standards of nursing care, recommended practices, and other guidelines developed and maintained by the nursing profession. During this phase, the perioperative nurse continues to assess the patient to determine the appropriateness of selected interventions and to alter the intervention as necessary to achieve the desired outcomes of care (Ackley & Ladwig, 1993). Intervention also means being the patient's advocate by carrying out nursing care as part of a team whose individual responsibilities in the operating room are well defined. The role of the patient advocate is especially important in the operating room, where patients are usually unconscious and unable to speak for themselves.

Accurate documentation of nursing care is an integral part of all phases of the nursing process, especially implementation and initiation of the plan of care. A description of the patient, the nursing diagnoses and desired patient outcomes, the nursing care given, and the patient's response to care (outcomes) should be included in the patient's record. Documentation of the nursing care given should include more than the technical aspects of care, such as the sponge count or the application of the electrosurgical dispersive pad. Nursing care documentation should be related to assessment and nursing diagnoses, with preestablished outcomes against which the appropriateness and effectiveness of care may be judged.

The form for this documentation may include both standardized protocols and interventions; space should be provided to write in interventions that are unique to individual patients. Documentation should require little time to complete, be specific to the perioperative setting, and provide continuity across the various areas in surgery from presurgery holding areas to the postanesthesia care units. Implicit in implementation of a perioperative plan of care is teamwork. Nowhere is a smoothly functioning team of more importance to the patient than in the operating room. Respect for others' expertise, the ability to work harmoniously, and the art of communicating effectively are necessary ingredients for a well-functioning team (Fig. 1-6).

Evaluation is checking, observing, and appraising the results of what was done. Although evaluation is traditionally listed as the last phase of the nursing process, it is an integral component of each step in planning and providing perioperative patient care. Evaluation of perioperative nursing care can be performed through on-the-spot correction of deficiencies. It is also accomplished through quality assessment and improvement activities, notably monitoring of

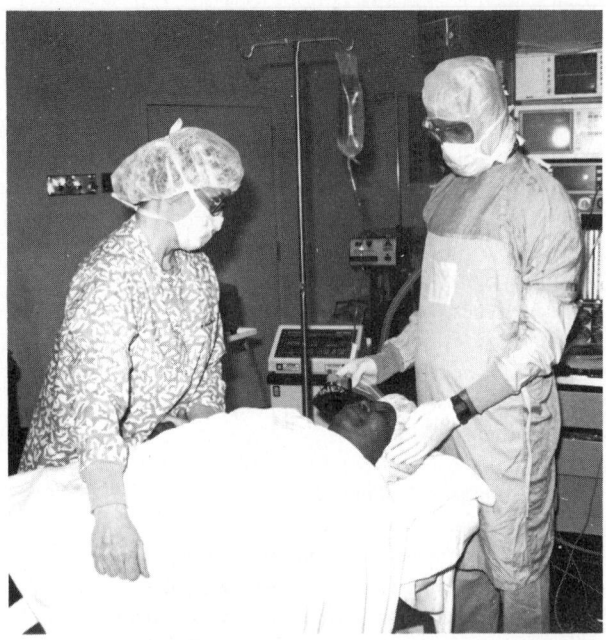

FIG. 1-4   Critical time for each surgical patient is preinduction phase.

important aspects of care, problem identification, problem solving, and peer review. Resources such as conferences, workshops, textbooks, and journal articles are available to assist in the initiation of these processes.

Hospital quality assessment and improvement programs demonstrate many ways of evaluating and improving care, including that given to surgical patients. Quality assurance programs identify problems in patient care, propose solutions, and monitor and evaluate specific actions in solving the problems.

Evaluation must also include reassessment of patients to determine outcomes and reactions to their surgical experiences. The emphasis is always on outcomes. The nursing process is continuous in that evaluation may lead back to assessment. Changes in patient care patterns may require new assessments and plans. The nursing process is never a dead end; it is continuous and always leads to a higher level of care (Fig. 1-7).

PHILOSOPHY, MISSION, AND OBJECTIVES OF PERIOPERATIVE NURSING

An organization's mission statement describes its purpose. That purpose is often grounded in the philosophy of the institution about patient care, and that philosophy should be reflected "down" and vertically integrated in each department of the institution, as is the mission statement. In the 1990s work has also evolved on the institution's vision, which is a realistic and credible model for the future. Philosophies, missions, and visions should be clearly articulated and well understood within the institution. They reflect the organization's history as well as its culture and values.

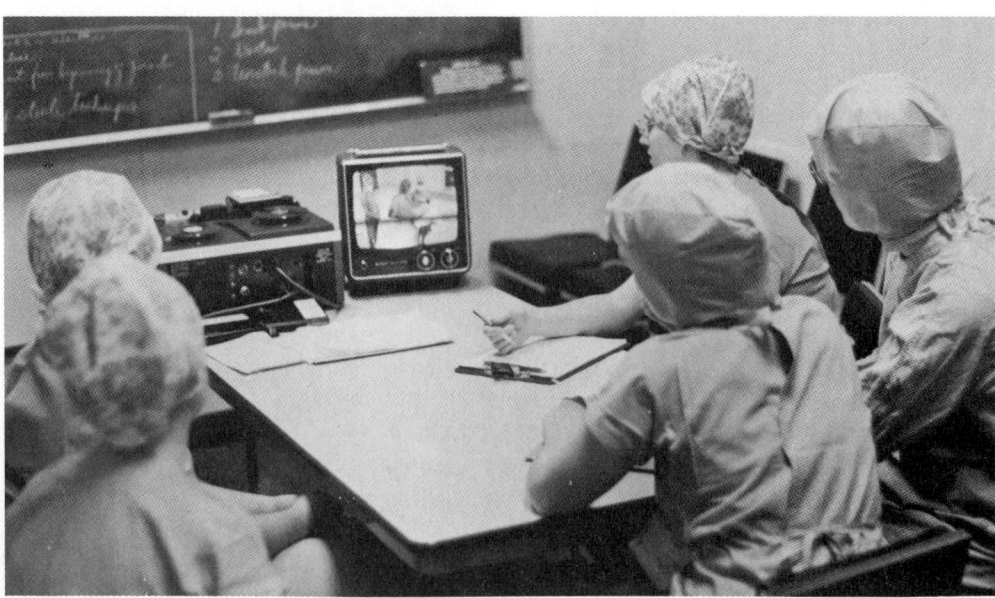

FIG. 1-5   Continuing education is necessary for all perioperative nurses. Self-instruction, use of literature, conferences, and informal discussions are examples.

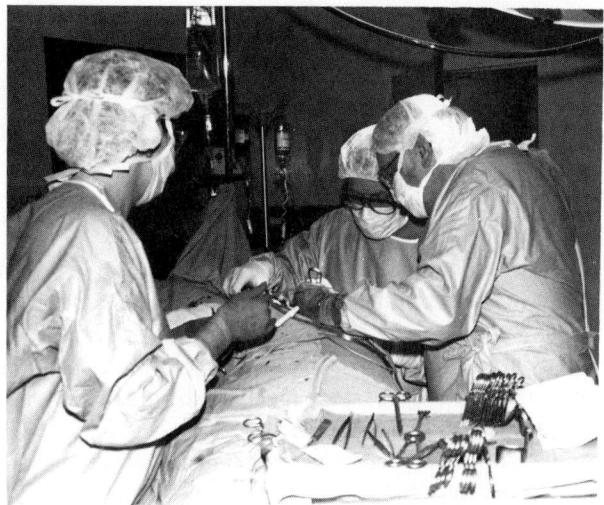

FIG. 1-6 Teamwork in the operating room implies collegial relationships, efficient use of skills and knowledge, and effective, respectful communication among team members (surgeons, anesthesia providers, and perioperative nurses).

Assessment . . .	Review medical record, validate important findings, corroborate with patient. Formulate nursing diagnoses based on analysis, interpretation, and prioritization of patient information.
Nursing . . . Diagnosis	Identifying and classifying the data collected. Can be actual or high risk. Based on nurse's clinical judgement.
Outcome . . . Identification	Achievable based on diagnosis. Ideally are mutually formulated by the nurse and patient and are congruent with medical regime. Allow implementation of nursing intervention. Measurable in terms of patient, not nursing, accomplishments.
Plan . . .	Incorporate information into a plan for the patient's care. Identify nursing interventions to achieve identified outcomes.
Implementation . . .	Carry out nursing plan. Gather equipment and supplies; participate in/guide/supervise patient preparation, transfer to OR bed, anesthesia induction, antimicrobial skin preparation, draping, patient positioning, monitoring of physiologic alterations during surgery, and patient discharge (transfer from OR bed, discharge to postanesthesia or postoperative unit).
Evaluation . . .	Determine whether outcomes were met; use outcome statements. Incorporate outcomes that have been met and those that are pending in report to nurse in postanesthesia care unit/discharge area.

FIG. 1-7 The nursing process is continuous, leading to a higher level of care.

PHILOSOPHY

A written statement of perioperative nursing philosophy describes values and beliefs that pertain to nursing practice in the surgical services department and serves as the basis for choosing the means to accomplish objectives. It formalizes nursings' vision of what practice is believed to be. Philosophy statements are value statements about people as patients or employees, about work that will be performed by nurses for patients, about nursing as a profession, about education as it pertains to nurses' competence, and about the setting in which nursing services are provided. The philosophy of perioperative nursing should blend with those of the hospital and the department of nursing, the general and specialty surgical programs, and appropriate educational and research programs.

One philosophy of perioperative nursing service may be summarized as follows:

1. Perioperative nursing is a dynamic, cognitive, behavioral, and technical process directed toward provision of quality patient care before, during, and after surgical intervention.
2. Perioperative nursing service comprises distinct functions concerned with a safe physical environment, protection of patients from high-risk events, and the achievement of optimal outcomes with continuous awareness of the dignity of persons and their physical, emotional, cultural, ethnic, and spiritual needs.
3. Perioperative nursing service promotes the knowledge and skills of its personnel to facilitate implementation of cost-effective, research-based scientific and technologic advances in health care.

The philosophy defined by the professional perioperative nursing staff should be consistent with that of the department of nursing.

MISSION

Every nursing department exists for a reason. The reason for existence is the purpose or mission of the department. Just as the nursing department has a mission statement, so should surgical services. This mission statement should be based on the philosophy, written in realistic terms and developed or revised with the participation of the perioperative nursing personnel who are governed by it. They should know and understand it. A meaningful mission statement indicates the relationships between the perioperative nursing personnel and patients, other personnel, the nursing department, and the hospital.

A mission statement for perioperative nursing might include the following:

1. To plan and provide perioperative nursing care that is consistent with standards for professional nursing practice as defined by the professional nurses of the staff and by the *Standards of Perioperative Nursing Practice*.
2. To collaborate and cooperate with other members of the health care team in meeting the preventive, emergency, and restorative health needs of patients in a safe, comfortable and therapeutic environment.

OBJECTIVES

The objectives of perioperative nursing should be practical, specific, and measurable for the persons performing nursing functions. They should be detailed statements supporting the defined philosophy. Well-stated objectives serve as criteria by which personnel can measure achievement of the mission. Effective objectives are developed and revised in accordance with the overall institutional mission through the cooperative efforts of the director, supervisors, and other staff members. In the absence of unified objectives, difficulties frequently arise in the delegation, coordination, and establishment of standards.

In developing objectives the professional perioperative nursing staff should consider the following factors:

1. Overall objectives of the department of nursing should be the core around which the perioperative nursing staff members work.
2. Objectives should be written in terms of the process to be used or the results to be achieved. The objectives should clearly reflect the overall functions of the personnel concerned, the limits of authority, and the managerial and training functions of the various staff members.
3. Objectives should provide for assignment of duties to permit staff members to perform at the highest potential and provide a means for them to broaden their knowledge base.
4. Objectives should be reasonable, attainable, behavioral, and measurable in the light of existing and foreseeable conditions, such as availability of trained personnel and facilities, operating time scheduled, and operational costs.
5. Overlapping objectives within the institution should promote cooperation among group members and collaboration and coordination among departments.
6. Objectives should be written for, freely available to, and understood by all personnel. A positive attitude on the part of the director, supervisors, head nurses, and staff members is essential to the fulfill-

ment of objectives. The nursing staff should be encouraged through daily conferences and training programs to help set measurable goals to meet the objectives.
7. Objectives should be reviewed and revised periodically.

Following are sample objectives for perioperative nursing:

1. Quality intraoperative nursing care that is professionally planned, implemented, and evaluated will be administered in an efficient, cost-effective manner.
2. Knowledgeable and skilled nursing personnel will be provided to meet the patient's individual needs during surgical intervention.
3. A safe and therapeutic environment will be provided for patients and personnel.
4. Proper equipment and supplies will be provided for all operative procedures.
5. Perioperative nursing standards will be evaluated and revised in accordance with current nursing practice.
6. Educational opportunities that encourage individual motivation and growth will be provided for personnel.

PERIOPERATIVE NURSING PRACTICE STANDARDS

Perioperative nurses are responsible for identifying, interpreting, and implementing contemporary professional standards. The provision of perioperative nursing services should be based on these standards. The AORN has established standards for perioperative nursing practice that can serve as guidelines for measuring the quality of patient care. These sound principles are broad in scope, attainable, definitive, and relevant for perioperative nurses. The standards represent a comprehensive approach to meeting the health care needs of surgical patients.

Nursing care standards consist of three elements: structure, process, and outcome. Structure standards describe organizational characteristics, administrative and fiscal accountabilities, personnel qualifications, and facilities and environmental requirements. The *AORN Standards of Perioperative Administrative Practice* provide structure standards and guidance for evaluating operational systems.

Process standards relate to nursing activities, interventions, and interactions and are used to explicate clinical, professional, and quality objectives in perioperative nursing. Examples of process standards are the AORN *Standards of Perioperative Clinical Practice, Standards of Perioperative Professional Performance,* and *Quality Improvement Standards for Perioperative Nursing.* These standards pertain to nursing during the perioperative period and are based on the nursing process.

Outcome standards identify desirable and measurable physiologic and physiologic responses of patients to nursing interventions. Patient outcomes are an essential indicator of the quality of care. *Patient Outcomes: Standards of Perioperative Care,* published by the AORN, provides guidelines for judging patient responses. The common goal of standards is quality care for the surgical patient. They should be used in conjunction with the AORN recommended practices, which are optimum goals that perioperative nursing personnel should strive to achieve.

POLICIES AND PROCEDURES

Perioperative departments have delegated responsibility, through the governing board of the institution, for the development of policies and procedures. Often referred to jointly as Surgical Services Standards of Care, these policies and procedures serve as the referent framework for delivering quality care and meeting the objectives of the department.

Policies are written statements which clearly outline responsibilities and appropriate actions for specific circumstances. Falkenhagen (1993) suggests that five criteria must be met for an effective policy: the policy must be consistent with both national and state practice standards; it needs to be realistic and achievable; it should be consistently followed, except where prior approval has been obtained; the policy should be based on reasoned and rational thinking; it should be related to the long-term intent of the surgical services department.

Procedures are the guides to implementing a policy; they set forth the detailed chronologic sequence of activities as they relate to a particular policy. Policies and procedures are usually combined into a manual that is kept readily available as a perioperative care resource in the surgical services department.

Written policies and procedures must be available to all personnel who provide patient care in the surgical setting. This information should be maintained in a readily accessible manual to facilitate uniform interpretation and administration of policies and procedures. The manual should be reviewed annually and revised as often as needed to meet the changing standards of practice. Policies and procedures affecting perioperative personnel should be formulated by representatives of the groups concerned with the delivery of patient care in this area.

A perioperative nursing policy and procedure committee comprising nursing personnel from all levels and specialties is an effective vehicle for drafting realistic new or revised policies and procedures. Participation of staff members in policy and procedure development increases their knowledge of the subject matter and generates a sense of ownership of the drafts. These effects usually result in meaningful interpretation of the approved policy or procedure to peers and successful implementation.

The surgical committee recommends policies and procedures relating to therapeutic aspects of patient care.

The surgical services manual should address but not be limited to the following:

1. Safety of patients and personnel
   a. Fire and disaster plans
   b. Risk management program requirements, such as unusual incident reports
   c. Emergency procedures, such as cardiopulmonary resuscitation
   d. Radiologic safety and monitoring
   e. Care and handling of hazardous materials/waste
   f. Electrosurgical unit use and safety
   g. Laser safety
2. Infection control
   a. Principles of asepsis
   b. Sterilization and disinfection
   c. Maintenance and surveillance of sterilization equipment
   d. Environmental sanitation
   e. Selection of draping and gowning materials.
   f. Surgical attire
   g. Traffic patterns in the surgical suite
3. Equipment
   a. Emergency power system
   b. Electrical and power equipment testing and maintenance
4. Perioperative patient care planning, including preoperative assessment
   a. Documentation of perioperative patient care
   b. Monitoring the patient receiving local anesthesia
   c. Communication and documentation of patient status during transfer from one patient care area to another
5. Sponge, sharp, and instrument counts
6. Care and disposition of surgical specimens
7. Handling and storage of blood and blood components
8. Patient positioning
9. Preoperative skin preparation of patients
10. Scheduling of patients for surgical procedures
11. Master staffing plan
12. Quality assessment and improvement program

Most surgical departments have separate procedure manuals, cards or computer-generated lists that enumerate surgeons' preferences for instruments, sutures, supplies, and equipment for each type of operation.

AUTOMATED INFORMATION SYSTEMS APPLICATIONS FOR PERIOPERATIVE NURSING

Pressures for more efficient management of fiscal, material, and human resources have stimulated many surgical services managers to pursue automated information systems for diverse management functions. Prompt access to accurate data is essential to maintain and improve the management and functioning of a surgical suite. A well-designed management information system can efficiently synthesize large volumes of data into meaningful reports. Ad hoc reporting capabilities are a vital component that can enhance the surgical services manager's decision making.

In many hospitals integrated surgical services management information systems are entered on a mainframe computer. This linkage to other systems in the hospital reduces data redundancy and paper flow. The availability of programmers and sufficient room on the mainframe to accommodate extensive surgical services applications are critical factors in determining whether to pursue this route or to purchase a microcomputer and appropriate software for use in the surgical services department.

The commercial development of surgical services management information systems has skyrocketed during the past few years and yielded a wide variety of software systems. Available applications include the following:

1. Scheduling of patients and surgical procedures
2. Recording of patient information (surgical services log)
3. Production of management reports, such as procedural hours, room use, volume and productivity statistics, and procedure-specific costs
4. Preparation of surgeons' preference cards
5. Inventory control
6. Capturing of patient charges
7. Equipment usage
8. Revenue by surgical service
9. Tracking of wound classifications for infection control purposes
10. Registry of implants
11. Staffing
12. Case cart ordering
13. Nursing care plans
14. Intraoperative documentation
15. Quality assessment and performance improvement measures

Weekly, monthly, year-to-date, and ad hoc reports are possible with most systems. When a management information system is chosen, the software must be adaptable to the specific needs of the surgical services manager and have the capacity for future enhancement to meet changing needs. A detailed user's manual should accompany the software and enable the user to adapt quickly to the system.

QUALITY ASSESSMENT AND PERFORMANCE IMPROVEMENT

Trends in health care payment reimbursement have mandated increased control of costs, efficient use of resources and supplies, decreased length of stay for surgical patients, and shifting of many surgical procedures from the inpatient to an ambulatory care setting. Along with this shift has come an increasing awareness of the need for continued quality assessment in the provision of perioperative patient care. The Joint Commission on the Accreditation of Healthcare Organizations (JCAHO) has taken a strong position on the need for continuously monitoring and evaluating the quality and appropriateness of care delivery to resolve any identified problems while striving to constantly improve delivery systems and processes. In 1994 the JCAHO instituted performance improvement as the core of its standards. This represented an evolution from quality assurance, to continuous quality improvement, to performance improvement. Such a transition was underscored by the belief that measuring outcomes and improving care are the essential purposes of health care delivery. Performance improvement efforts encompass measuring on a continuous basis to validate that systems and processes are stable. This is often accomplished by the use of statistical quality tools and techniques. As outcomes are measured, priority is assigned for improvement opportunity. Individual competence and performance are assessed when appropriate. Such performance improvement includes five activities: plan, design, measure, assess, and improve (*OR Manager,* 1993).

The surgical services quality assessment and performance improvement program should be based on established standards of care. The intent of each standard should be reflected in realistic and measurable outcomes. A plan to monitor and improve care should be in place, which includes both the scope of care and the important aspects of care. Specific indicators should be identified that reflect these important aspects of care. Thresholds are then established that identify the level of acceptability of variance for each indicator. Measurement methods include retrospective review, review of incident reports, utilization review, patient surveys and interviews, and peer review. Emphasis has evolved from process auditing to the current emphasis on structure, process, and outcome indicators.

A process improvement approach facilitates measurement of perioperative patient care. When processes are understood, they can be improved through a systematic plan of action. Following identification of improvement opportunities, they should be given priority according to impact on patient care, and solutions should be planned, studied, implemented, and standardized. Ongoing monitoring, on a scheduled basis with documented follow-up indicates if the standardized solutions were successful in reducing variance and process or system problems. Concepts and methods of performance measurement must be integrated into the surgical services department's philosophy and standards (Box 1-2).

Involvement in the development and implementation of a surgical services quality assessment and performance improvement can strengthen the staff's commitment to meeting standards and enhance program effectiveness. Staff members must be informed of how quality assessment and performance improvement findings will be used. Documentation of improvement activities is channeled through the

BOX 1-2

Concepts and Methods of Performance Measurement and Improvement

1. Effective performance measurement systems should provide accurate, complete, and relevant quality-of-care data that can be used in quality improvement efforts.
2. Both process and outcome measurement are essential to performance improvement.
3. Health care professionals and organizations must understand and believe in the benefits of performance measurement.
4. Potential barriers to performance measurement must be identified and resolved.
5. The organization's performance can be correlated with a variety of attributes such as outcomes of care, cost of care, quality, and perceived value.
6. Performance improvement requires the ability to measure specific functions and dimensions of performance such as appropriateness, availability, continuity, effectiveness, efficacy, efficiency, respect and caring, safety, and timeliness.
7. Organizational functions, structures, and key processes can be elucidated through common quality improvement tools such as flowcharting, cause-and-effect diagraming, brainstorming, and charting performance to understand and identify common and special cause variations.
8. Steps to establish a performance measurement system include establishing units of measure, developing instruments and tools that can quantify the units of measure, and using these instruments and tools to collect and analyze data for performance improvement.

appropriate reporting mechanisms to the institution-wide quality assessment and performance improvement committee (Fig. 1-8).

CONTINUING EDUCATION

The pace and complexity of advances in surgical procedures, minimally invasive surgery, newly developed technology with surgical applications, professional nursing issues, ongoing health care reform measures, changes in recommended practices, and the burgeoning body of nursing research and practice guidelines demand constant attention to professional education and development. Perioperative professionals must continue to tenaciously search for new research on patient outcomes, link nursing interventions to outcomes, and seek to determine the most cost-effective

method of implementing the intervention. Performance improvement initiatives require monitoring and evaluating the actual performance of health care practitioners and health care organizations in the application of healthcare's art and science. Performance improvement activities direct specific attention to the resulting outcomes of patient care activities (JCAHO, 1993).

Performance improvement also implicitly requires an assessment of resources and goals, participation in and high regard for continuing education, use of learning tools and resources (Fig. 1-8), and evaluation of professional goal achievement. Standards for professional performance posit that perioperative nurses are responsible for acquiring and maintaining current knowledge, for evaluating their own practice, and for using research findings (AORN, 1993). Rigorous professional credentialing is familiar to perioperative nurses. Credentialing is verification and evaluation of education and experience according to professional and institutional standards and practices. The voluntary seeking and certification as a perioperative nurse (CNOR) or RN first assistant (CRNFA) recognizes the professional achievement demonstrated when a perioperative nurse's performance exceeds that which is required for competency in practice. Thus certification recognizes proficiency and enhances professional growth through continued learning.

NURSING ROLES IN THE FUTURE

The profession of nursing is in a state of self-evaluation, renewal, and emergence as a strong force in health care. Nurses, as well as many others outside the profession, are questioning the profession's identity, status, and reward system. The triad of nurse-physician-administrator is under scrutiny. New roles, new definitions, and new parameters of practice are being proposed and tested. Regardless of title and function, every nurse working in a perioperative practice setting is assuming greater responsibility and is becoming a colleague of other health care professionals in patient care.

The role of the perioperative nurse as assistant at surgery is a good example of an evolving new role. In 1984 the AORN approved an official statement on the RN first assistant (RNFA); the statement was revised in 1993. The RNFA, who must have formal education for role preparation, works collaboratively with the surgeon (and the patient and surgical team) by handling tissue and instruments, providing exposure and hemostasis, and suturing. Many experienced perioperative nurses have obtained additional education to prepare themselves for this role. Performing as an RNFA allows the experienced perioperative nurse to advance in clinical knowledge and skill while still remaining directly involved with the provision of perioperative nursing care. This new role, which has gained wide acceptance and value in operating rooms across the country, is just one of the ways perioperative nurses are developing themselves

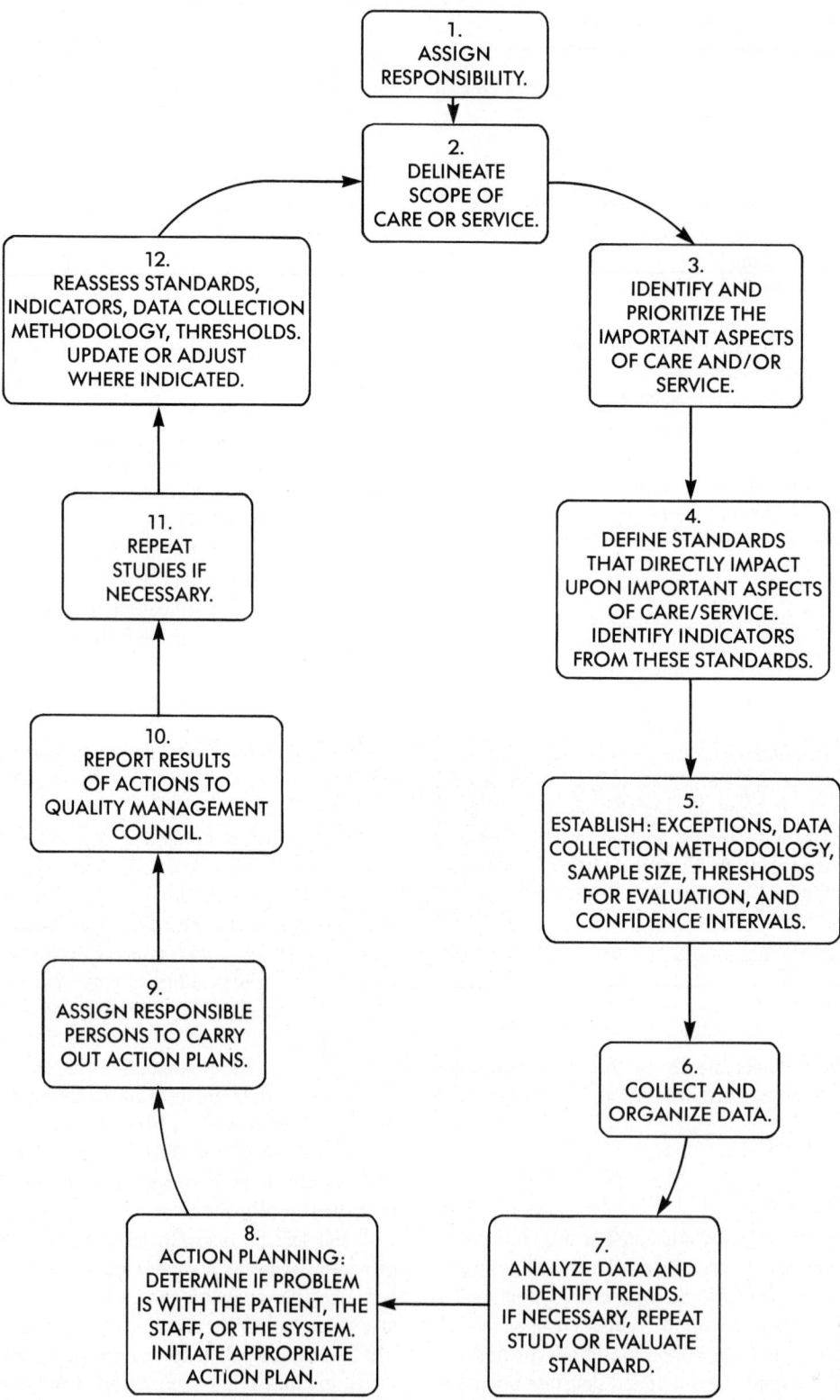

FIG. 1-8   The quality improvement cycle.

to meet the changing needs of health care delivery.

In addition to the role of practitioner-caregiver, the professional nurse is also teacher, advocate, and researcher. The perioperative nurse teaches staff and patients and counsels patients and their families/significant others who need assistance in adjusting to a new diagnosis or a changed body image. The nurse monitors the care given to the patient in the operating room and serves as patient advocate to ensure its high quality. Perioperative nurses should help nurse researchers delineate problems in the perioperative setting that need study, participate in those studies, and utilize the research findings in clinical practice.

Practice settings are engaging in work redesign efforts, and computerization is an increasingly vital component of operational restructuring (Tonges & Lawrenz, 1993). Perioperative nurses need to collaborate with one another to develop computerized patient care records, which have enormous potential for improving the quality and efficiency of patient care. They allow health care facilities and practitioners to connect to an electronic data network via their own computer-based record system. Such an effort requires developing national standards for documentation, sharing, and protecting the confidentiality of the patient record. As the technology link to work redesign and reengineering of work processes takes a preeminent role in the institution, the emerging role of the perioperative nurse in information systems management is increasingly important.

Finally, the perioperative nurse works in collaboration with surgeons, anesthesiologists, and other health care providers to plan the best course of action for each patient. To ensure the highest quality of care, input from each of the health care disciplines represented in the perioperative practice setting is crucial. Because the education of the professional nurse has more breadth than that of many other health care providers, the nurse is often in the best position to serve in a leadership role in fostering collegiality and collaboration among a variety of disciplines.

Perioperative nurses are accountable to their patients and demonstrate it by using standards, recommended practices, and quality assessment and performance improvement activities and by constantly strengthening their professional skills through education.

As perioperative nursing progresses, new roles will emerge. Each of these roles, whether staff nurse, clinician, manager, educator, or researcher, will make use of the nursing process and will demonstrate humanized care for surgical patients and their families. Perhaps a perioperative practitioner's role will include greater consultation with patients' families as an advanced practice perioperative clinical nurse specialist (Research Highlight 1-3). Perioperative nurses can also be excellent teachers of health promotion, disease prevention, and wellness regimens. Each new function must be tested with time and should be integrated into the profession only if it enhances overall care and wellness of people, especially those who require surgical interventions.

RESEARCH HIGHLIGHT 1-3

Surgery is usually a source of anxiety to both patients and their families. Perioperative nurses have well-developed interventions to assist patients with anxiety; these interventions can be found in many of the sample care plans in this book. However, perioperative nursing interventions for families are less well defined. This study was designed to answer two questions: What are reported anxiety levels of family members of elective surgery patients? What is the relationship of family member characteristics and length of waiting period to report anxiety levels?

Fifty family members of patients undergoing elective surgery which lasted for more than 30 minutes were included in the study. State anxiety levels were measured using a written tool; a portable monitor was used to measure blood pressure and heart rate. Results confirmed findings that family members waiting during elective surgery experience higher mean anxiety levels. Perioperative nurses need not only recognize this anxiety, but also develop nursing interventions designed to reduce it in family members during the intraoperative waiting period.

Lesky, J.S. (1993). Anxiety of elective surgical patient's family members: Relationship between anxiety levels, family characteristics. *AORN Journal, 57*(5), 1091-1101.

Scrubbing and *circulating* may become obsolete terms; already we know that they define circumscribed functions that are only a part of the perioperative nurse's sphere of responsibility. The future may bring new titles and functions but will never erase the critical function in surgical patient care that every perioperative nurse fulfills. The future of perioperative nursing is directly related to the sophistication of its practitioners. Sophistication means that perioperative nurses must be superior thinkers *and* doers. If either knowledge or practice is neglected, perioperative nursing as a profession will decline and give way to rote tasks.

The nature of nurse-physician working relationships will continue to be scrutinized. This relationship is critical to good patient outcomes but often is contaminated by power struggles and turf battles. Physician-nurse conflicts are not only professional-technical and master-servant in nature but have status and socioeconomic roots as well. That physicians are often in independent practice whereas nurses usually have employee status enlarges the gap between the two groups. However, true peer respect is emerging and must be nurtured, although it is not yet reality in many perioperative practice settings.

Outcomes of surgical interventions are directly related to the quality of perioperative nursing care provided, which in turn reflects the aptitudes and motivations of perioperative practitioners. With this perspective, the reader should consider the remainder of this book as one part of a perioperative nurse's knowledge bank. The remaining chapters contain vital information related to nursing practices and care processes that are needed to function in perioperative practice settings.

REFERENCES

Ackley, B.J., & Ladwig, G.B. (1993). *Nursing diagnosis handbook: A guide to planning care*. St. Louis: Mosby.

AORN Standards and Recommended Practices for Perioperative Nursing. (1993). Denver: The Association.

Falkenhagen, K. (1993). Policies/procedures. In *Optimizing resources: A manager's guide to success*. Denver: AORN.

Gettrust, K.V., & Brabec, P.D. (1992). *Nursing diagnosis in clinical practice: Guides for care planning*. New York: Delmar Publishers.

Joint Commission on Accreditation of Healthcare Organizations. New manual has major changes for 1994 surveys. *OR Manager, 9*(10), 1, 6-7.

Joint Commission on Accreditation of Healthcare Organizations. (1993). *The measurement mandate*. Chicago: The Commission.

Kim, M.J., McFarland, G.K., & McLane, A.M. (1993). *Pocket guide to nursing diagnosis*. St. Louis: Mosby.

Tonges, M.C., & Lawrenz, E. (1993). *Reengineering: The work redesign-technology link*. JONA, 23(10), 15-22.

BIBLIOGRAPHY

Andreola, N.M. (1993). Nursing certification: Evidence of expertise, or a "C" without substance. *The Nursing Spectrum, 1*(7), 6-7.

AORN official statement on RN first assistants. (1993). *AORN Journal, 57*(6), 1319-1321.

Atkinson, L.J. (1992). *Berry and Kohn's operating room technique*, (7th Ed.) St. Louis: Mosby.

Brazen, L. (1992, November/December). Perioperative nursing: A special nursing specialty. *NSNA/IMPRINT,* 47-49, 86.

Brown, S.M. (1991). The ambulatory surgery setting: Adding the caring touch. *Journal of Advanced Nursing, 15,* 1078.

Carmody, S., Hickey, P., & Bookbinder, M. (1991). Perioperative needs of families: Results of a survey. *AORN Journal, 54*(3), 561-567.

Chana, C.H. (1992). Documenting the nursing process: A perioperative nursing care plan. *AORN Journal 55*(5), 1231-1235.

Cunningham, L. (1991). *The quality connection in health care*. San Francisco: Jossey-Bass.

Goldfield, N., & Nash, D.B. (1989). *Providing quality care: The challenge to clinicians*. Philadelphia: The American College of Physicians.

Groah, L.K., & Girard, N. (1993). Professional nursing care delivery model: Implications for perioperative nursing. *AORN Journal, 57*(6), 1416-1424.

Joint Commission on Accreditation of Healthcare Organizations. (1991). *An introduction to quality improvement in health care*. Chicago: The Commission.

Joint Commission on Accreditation of Healthcare Organizations. (1991). *Development and application of indicators for continuous improvement in surgical and anesthesia care*. Chicago: The Commission.

Katz, J., & Green, E. (1992). *Managing quality: A guide to monitoring and evaluation nursing services*. St. Louis: Mosby.

Koch, M.W., & Fairly, T.M. (1993). *Integrated quality management: The key to improving nursing care quality*. St. Louis: Mosby.

Koerner, J. (1992). Differentiated practice: The evolution of professional nursing. *Journal of Professional Nursing, 8*(6), 335-341.

McCloskey, J.C., & Bulecheck, G.M. (1992). *Nursing interventions classification*. St. Louis: Mosby.

Omachonu, V.K. (1991). *Total quality and productivity management in health care organizations*. Milwaukee: American Society for Quality Control.

Palmer, R.H., Donabedian, A., & Povar, G.J. (1991). *Striving for quality in health care: An inquiry into policy and practice*. Ann Arbor, MI: Health Administration Press.

Parsons, E.C., Kee, C.C., & Gray, P. (1993). Perioperative nursing caring behaviors: Perceptions of surgical patients. *AORN Journal 57*(5), 1106-1114.

Pica-Furey, W. (1993). Ambulatory surgery—Hospital based vs. free-standing: A comparative study of patient satisfaction. *AORN Journal, 57*(5), 1119-1127.

Raffel, M.W., & Raffel, N.K. (1989). *The U.S. health system: Origins and functions*. New York: John Wiley & Sons.

Shirley, M.A. (1993). Perioperative documentation: A generic OR care plan. *AORN Journal, 57*(6), 1427-1440.

Smith, C.A. (1992). Solving the mystery of perioperative nursing: An OR nurse week program. *AORN Journal, 56*(5), 846-856.

Stone, E.M. (1990). The future of health care: Public concerns and policy trends. Waltham, Mass: Massachusetts Health Data Consortium.

Yale, E. (1993). Preoperative teaching strategy: Videotapes for home teaching. *AORN Journal, 57*(4), 901-908.

2

PATIENT AND ENVIRONMENTAL SAFETY

MERRY ANNE PIERSON

The safety and welfare of patients during surgical interventions are primary concerns of perioperative nurses. Hospital liability problems occurring in the operating room are increasing, necessitating a clear understanding of risk management by perioperative nursing personnel. Described as a systematic way of detecting potential problems and ensuring safe patient care, risk management has become increasingly important in the health care environment. Numerous intrinsic hazards can be prevented, reduced, or controlled by adherence to sound policies, procedures, and regulations, thereby managing risk. Patients entering the operating room are at risk for infection, impaired skin integrity, altered body temperature, fluid volume deficit, and injury related to positioning and chemical, electrical, and physical hazards (Sample Care Plan).

Policies and procedures are designed to ensure the safety of patients and personnel and to provide a setting in which all activities of the surgical team and ancillary personnel fit together to result in an efficient course of action for the benefit of each patient.

Regulations are usually mandated activities that the institution must be in compliance with to meet certain standards set by outside agencies.

SAFE ENVIRONMENT

SAFETY DESIGN FEATURES

Safety design incorporates features that prevent or control the potential of infection, flame, explosion, and chemical and electrical hazards. Well-devised traffic patterns, material-handling systems, and disposal systems; positive pressure and well-dispersed clean ventilation; and high-flow unidirectional ventilation systems for special applications all contribute to a safe surgical environment. In addition, a reliable and adequate emergency power source must be available for use during electrical interruptions and be tested regularly to ensure working order. Emergency shutoffs for piped medical gases must be clearly labeled and readily available. Education designed to familiarize staff with all safety and hazard prevention programs is required at least annually by the Joint Commission on Accreditation of Healthcare Organizations (JCAHO) (JCAHO, Plant technology and safety management, PL.4.2, 1994). Flame and explosion hazards have decreased significantly in recent years as a result of the use of nonflammable anesthetics and skin prepping solutions. Electrical hazards continue to be of concern and are discussed at length later in this chapter.

TRAFFIC FLOW

Perioperative patient care requires movement of patients, personnel, and materials within and through the surgical suite. Development and implementation of appropriate traffic patterns, based on the design of the surgical suite, help contain contamination. According to the Association of Operating Room Nurses (AORN) Recommended Practices for Traffic Patterns in the Surgical Suite, a three-zone designation of areas within the surgical suite facilitates appropriate movement of patients and personnel. *Unrestricted* areas are those in which personnel may wear street clothes, and traffic is not limited. In *semirestricted* areas, such as processing and storage areas for instruments and supplies, as well as corridors leading to the restricted areas of the surgical suite, personnel must wear surgical attire and patients must wear gowns and hair coverings. *Restricted* areas include operating rooms and clean core and scrub sink areas. Surgical attire and masks are required in these areas.

The flow of supplies should be from the clean core area through the operating rooms to the peripheral corridor. Soiled materials should not reenter the clean core area. Soiled linen and trash collection areas should be separated from personnel and patient traffic areas, if possible, for infection control purposes. If instruments and other supplies are partially or totally reprocessed within the surgical suite, a unidirectional traffic pattern should ensure movement of items from the decontamination area to processing and storage areas. Work areas for each task should be clearly identified to eliminate crossover or mixing of these soiled and cleaned instruments or supplies. These practices decrease the risk of infection by separating the clean from the contaminated (AORN, 1994).

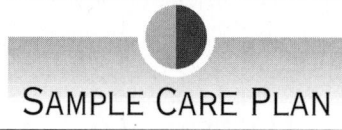

SAMPLE CARE PLAN

NURSING DIAGNOSIS: High risk for infection
OUTCOME: Patient will be free from infection.
INTERVENTIONS:
Assess and document patient's risk status preoperatively for preexisting conditions (such as nutritional status, skin integrity, or tissue trauma) and systems to be transsected that may increase susceptibility for infection.
Administer antibiotics as ordered preoperatively.
Follow policy and procedure for skin preparation.
Monitor traffic in the OR throughout the procedure.
Monitor and maintain surgical team's aseptic technique; correct any breaks in technique as they happen.
Record any medications administered by the perioperative nurse or at the sterile field.
Document classification of wound.
Ensure sterile dressing placement, if appropriate, before patient is moved from the OR bed.

NURSING DIAGNOSIS: High risk for impaired skin integrity
OUTCOME: The patient's skin integrity is maintained.
INTERVENTIONS:
Note and document the presence of any skin rashes, bruises, lesions, reddened areas, or lacerations.
Assess the patient record for any medical conditions that might predispose the patient to compromised skin integrity and document them.
Verify that patient has no known allergies to antimicrobial skin preparation agents.
Implement skin preparation according to institutional procedure.
Evaluate and document the status of skin integrity postoperatively.

NURSING DIAGNOSIS: High risk for injury
OUTCOME: Patient is free from injury related to positioning and electrical, chemical, or physical hazards.
INTERVENTIONS:
Note and document presence of any preexisting patient conditions (such as weight, limitations in mobility or range of motion, neurovascular impairment, and nutritional status) that place patient at risk for positional or other injury.
Position patient anatomically for surgical procedure.
Accomplish all positioning and positional changes slowly, gently, and gradually.
Utilize positioning devices, such as bean bags and rolls, where appropriate.

Place safety strap 2 in. above knees or where appropriate for procedure.
Pad all bony prominences, pressure sites, and vulnerable nerves to protect.
Check all electrical equipment and their cords prior to use.
Place electrosurgical dispersive pad (patient return electrode) as close to the surgical site as possible, on clean, dry, nonhairy skin, and on a major muscle group.
Assess pad site at end of procedure and document findings.

NURSING DIAGNOSIS: High risk for fluid volume deficit
OUTCOME: Patient's fluid volume and electrolyte balance are maintained.
INTERVENTIONS:
Obtain baseline data from medical record.
Assess patient's nutritional status preoperatively and use of medications affecting fluid balance.
Assess skin condition.
Alert surgical team periodically to blood loss volume and urine output.
Monitor and record all irrigation solutions being used on the surgical field.
Determine availability of replacement blood and/or blood products.
Initiate autotransfusion as required.
Monitor vital signs and oxygen saturation.

NURSING DIAGNOSIS: High risk for altered body temperature
OUTCOME: Patient will maintain a body temperature measured at 96° F or above.
INTERVENTIONS:
Provide temperature measuring device.
Monitor operating room temperature to ensure it stays in ideal range of 70° to 75° F.
Provide warm blankets for patient on entering and leaving the OR.
Cover all areas of patient not in surgical field to prevent heat loss.
Consider use of warming device that blows warm air over patient to prevent heat loss.
Warm all blood products while administering the infusion.
Use warm irrigation solutions.

PHYSICAL DESIGN ELEMENTS

Physical and structural elements influencing patient and environmental safety include surface materials used in suite design, airflow exchanges, and temperature and humidity control devices. The interior of the operating room has specific requirements for environmental control. Ceilings and walls should be nonporous, smooth, easy to clean, waterproof, and fire resistant. High-impact vinyl materials and flexible wall coverings, together with new adhesives, permit completely sealed wall, ceiling, and floor joints so that the surfaces may be washed effectively with microbicidal cleaning solutions. Tile walls are not desirable because most grout lines are porous and can harbor microorganisms.

Floor coverings have the same requirements as the wall coverings but, in addition to being highly wear resistant, they must also be made of slip-proof materials to prevent injuries to personnel.

Sliding doors should be used in the operating room to eliminate the air turbulence caused by swinging doors. A marked increase in microbial counts has been noted when swinging doors are opened or closed. Doors should be made of the surface sliding type, if possible, to facilitate cleaning of all surfaces. Fire regulations require that the doors be capable of being swung open if necessary.

ENVIRONMENTAL CONDITIONS

Appropriate environmental design aids in control of infection. Temperature should be maintained between 70 and 75° F to reduce metabolic demands on patients, and relative humidity should be 50% to 60% to reduce bacterial growth and suppress static electricity (Bartley, 1993). Each operating room should have individual temperature controls to accommodate patient safety, for example, when increased warmth is required for severely compromised patients during operative procedures. The nursing diagnosis of high risk for altered body temperature should always be considered when adjusting the operating room temperature. Newer operating rooms should have at least 15 room air exchanges per hour, three of which should be fresh air. High-efficiency particulate air (HEPA) filters used in many conventional operating room ventilation systems aid in controlling infection risk.

Positive pressure inside the operating room is created to prevent potentially contaminated air from entering through adjacent areas. This objective mandates keeping the doors to the operating room closed at all times other than during patient and personnel entry and exit. Without the use of HEPA filters, conventional operating room air may contain as many as 10 to 15 bacteria per cubic foot and as many as 250,000 particles per cubic foot. The cause and effect of infectious microorganisms and the basic principles of sterilization, disinfection, and aseptic technique are described in Chapter 3.

PERSONNEL IMPACT

People, rather than design or equipment, are frequently the real obstacles to the creation and maintenance of a safe environment.

PREVENTION OF ACCIDENTS AND INFECTIONS

All personnel should be instructed in the use of good body mechanics to avert common falls and strains when reaching, stretching, lifting, or moving heavy patients or other articles. Good body mechanics and application of work simplification principles conserve human energy, protect the worker, and thereby promote good performance.

Personnel should also be instructed and supervised in proper use of equipment to prevent injury such as burns from autoclaves and electrical equipment, abrasions from contact with metal accessory levers, injuries from swinging doors, cuts from knife blades, needle sticks, and splash exposures.

In accordance with the Department of Labor's Occupational Safety and Health Administration (OSHA) final rule on exposure to bloodborne pathogens (Dec. 6, 1991), personnel must be cognizant of what protective apparel is required in the surgical suite. Eye protection, face masks, head and shoe covers, gowns, gloves, and any other protective wear must be used whenever the potential for blood and body fluid contact exists (Research Highlight 2-1). Universal precautions, that is, all patients are considered to be infectious, should be practiced. An exposure control plan for the hospital and each potential area of high risk should be developed.

RESEARCH HIGHLIGHT 2-1

With the implementation of the OSHA rule, operating room personnel have had to choose adequate barrier methods of preventing blood and body fluids from contacting their skin and clothing. A new standardized test has been developed to determine the barrier effectiveness of surgical gowns to bloodborne pathogens. These tests, developed by the American Society for Testing and Materials (ASTM), are the first to provide uniform, scientific definitions for liquid and viral barriers.

The first test simulates the pressure from contact during surgery and measures strike-through. Materials that fail this test are not considered a liquid barrier and do not go on to the second step—viral barrier testing.

The viral challenge requires that material be tested with a bloodlike solution containing a noninfectious virus of similar size to HIV, hepatitis B, and hepatitis C. The test measures the fabrics at variable pressures for 1 hour. If any of the viral solution passes through fabric, the material fails the test.

These tests provide definitions for what types of materials provide an impervious barrier and should assist OR personnel in choosing such a fabric.

American Society for Testing and Materials (1993). Tests evaluate barrier effectiveness of gowns, *OR Manager*, May.

The exposure control plan for the operating room should be well documented and contain these key elements:

1. A determination of exposure
2. Methods for complying with the OSHA guidelines
3. A procedure to evaluate exposures when they happen
4. A list of job classifications or tasks that have exposure potential
5. A plan for offering hepatitis vaccine
6. A definition of universal precautions, including a clear plan of compliance

Steam, electrical, vacuum, hydraulic, ventilation, plumbing, and emergency generator systems should be inspected by the maintenance or engineering departments according to an established schedule.

The maintenance and cleaning program should be clearly defined and understood by the nursing staff. Prompt attention to spills, prompt drying of wet floors, use of warning signs in danger areas, and keeping the corridors and all traffic areas clear of obstacles are important housekeeping duties.

Cleaning, disinfection, and sterilization of equipment, control of contaminants, and application of aseptic techniques are basic to an effective infection control program. Breaks in asepsis may also result from the intrusion of pests, vermin, insects, noxious substances, chemicals, gases, and infectious body fluids and wastes into the protected areas.

Effective disposal procedures for soiled materials and hazardous waste are essential to render the area safe for patients and personnel. AORN has proposed a definition of regulated medical waste (the part of medical waste with the potential to transmit infectious disease) as being one of four categories: sharps, cultures and stocks of infectious waste, animal waste, and selected isolation waste. Also included in regulated medical waste (due to esthetic concerns of the public) are pathological waste, human blood, blood products, and body fluids. Some method for reducing the microbiological content for items falling in these four categories is recommended (AORN, 1993). In addition, all surgical procedures are treated as potentially contaminated (universal precautions); the outmoded dirty case rituals have been eliminated and a safe environment ensured.

The professional nursing staff has a responsibility to work with the infection control committee in establishing appropriate policies and reporting occurrences.

ADMINISTRATIVE CONTROL MEASURES

The perioperative nursing staff actively participates with the hospital administrative and medical staffs in creating and maintaining standards, usually through scheduled meetings with the surgical, infection control, and safety or disaster committees.

Each nurse should understand the professional, legal, and ethical responsibilities to each patient as established by the Nurse Practice Act of each state.

RECORDS AND FORMS

The operating room policy and procedure manual should contain current and accurate directions to protect patients and personnel. Protection of patients' personal, moral, and legal rights begins at the time of admission. The course of action involves correctly identifying patients, safeguarding their right to privacy and their right to make choices regarding their care, and keeping confidential all records and reports (JCAHO, 1994). Conditions of admission to the hospital, consent forms for treatment or surgical procedures, and advance directives are important records that protect both the patient and the persons who render care to them.

The hospital administration provides appropriate forms that are legally acceptable. Personnel who obtain consents or witness them should be aware of the conditions that ensure validity and their personal responsibility to appear in a court of law if necessary. A signed consent must also be an informed consent, which implies adequate communication with the patient regarding the procedure for which the consent is being signed. No surgical procedure should be performed without a signed and witnessed informed consent. The surgeon is responsible for informing the patient about the proposed operation, inherent risks, and complications. The ultimate responsibility for obtaining consent is the surgeon's. In some states consent forms must be signed before the administration of preoperative medications. On the patient's arrival in the operating room, the circulating nurse and the anesthesiologist are responsible for ensuring that the consent is on the chart, correct, and properly signed and witnessed.

Special permits for anesthesia administration, specific operations, such as sterilization, therapeutic abortion, disposal of severed body parts, and autopsy provide additional safeguards for the patient, staff, and hospital. In case of a death in the operating room or postanesthesia care unit (PACU), the nursing policy manual should state the course of action to be carried out in regard to informing the hospital authorities, notifying physicians, family, and clergy, referring to the medical examiner, and obtaining consent for organ donation.

DOCUMENTATION

The JCAHO requires that a record be kept of each operation, including the preoperative diagnosis, the surgery performed, a description of findings, the specimens removed, the postoperative diagnosis, and the names of all persons participating in intraoperative care. The AORN recommended practices for documentation of perioperative nursing care (1994) suggest that the intraoperative patient care record should also include, but not be limited to, the following:

1. Evidence of a patient assessment upon arrival at the operating room, as well as an assessment of the patient's skin condition immediately before and after the procedure
2. Evidence of a plan of care individualized for each patient
3. Any sensory aids or prosthetic devices worn by the patient on admission to the operating room and their subsequent disposition
4. Patient position, including supports or restraints used
5. Location of dispersive electrode pad placement and identification of electrosurgical unit and settings used
6. Location of temperature control device placement with identification of unit used and recording of time and temperature
7. Placement of monitoring electrodes
8. Medications administered or dispensed by the registered nurse
9. Presence of catheters, drains, packing, and dressings
10. Location of tourniquet cuff placement, identification of unit, pressure setting, and inflation and deflation times
11. Fluid output, including blood loss estimates, as appropriate
12. Type, size, and appropriate identifying information (for example, serial number) of implants
13. Skin preparation solutions used, areas prepped, and any reactions to prep
14. Known allergies to medications, prep solutions, tape, etc.
15. Sponge, sharp, and instrument counts taken and results obtained
16. Wound classification
17. Time of discharge and disposition of patient from operating room, including mode of transfer and patient status

Using the AORN recommended practices as guidelines, perioperative nurses can achieve objective documentation that accurately reflects assessment and planning, perioperative care given, and evaluation of outcomes. The operative record becomes a permanent part of the patient's chart.

ADMISSION OF THE PATIENT TO THE OPERATING ROOM

The operating room policy and procedure manual should contain the procedure and delegation of responsibilities for patient admittance. The admission procedure should include the following steps.

1. The perioperative nurse should verify the patient's identification verbally with the patient (if feasible), by the patient's armband, and by reviewing the chart. Information on the patient's identification band, the chart, and the tag on the stretcher or bed should be accurate and identical with the patient's name, hospital number, room number, and the physician's name.
2. The operative consent form, history and physical examination record, laboratory results, and other examination results should be complete (JCAHO, 1994). The governing body of the facility determines which examinations are mandatory as part of the patient's preoperative preparation. These may include completed records for physical examination, health history, recent determinations of blood and urine testing, and chest x-ray and ECG examinations. A preoperative checklist is frequently used to prevent oversights and omissions and is designed to protect patients and staff. Any allergies, previous unfavorable reactions to anesthesia or blood transfusions, previous reactions to latex, and religious preferences must be carefully noted (Young, 1992).
3. The patient should be examined for personal effects, including clothing, money, jewelry, wigs, religious symbols, and prostheses such as dentures, lenses, glass eyes, and hearing aids. The nurse is responsible for ensuring their safe handling and proper disposition.
4. The perioperative nurse should review the orders and results concerning nutrition and elimination, such as enema results and the amount of urine voided or collected through the catheter. Determining whether preoperative dietary and fluid restrictions (NPO status) have been maintained is important. Aspiration of gastric contents during anesthesia induction is a danger. Every precaution should be taken to prevent such an accident by ensuring that the suctioning apparatus is functional and by having personnel present to assist the anesthesiologist as necessary during induction.
5. The nurse should meticulously document any medications, fluids, blood, or plasma administered as ordered during the immediate preoperative period.
6. The nursing staff should apply siderails, locking devices, and restraint straps on stretchers and operating room beds, to prevent falls and injury to the patient during transport, transfer, and positioning.
7. Nursing personnel can bestow peace of mind and reassurance in their care of and concern for the patient. By judicious use of *directions* and *self*—assuming a calm, confident manner and a quiet voice, using gentle, precise movements in execution of activities, giving clear explanations, and providing spiritual assistance as requested—perioperative nursing personnel can help the patient face surgery with equanimity.

SAFETY MEASURES

All perioperative nursing personnel must adhere to the hospital safety program. A representative of the surgical services department should serve on the hospital safety committee. Each staff member should be prepared to carry out special duties in the care of patients in emergencies and disasters. Periodic review of duties, fire and disaster drills, chemical hazards, and safety education programs should be initiated. All personnel should be aware of the hazards peculiar to operating room activities and working conditions.

Minimizing human error helps to eliminate hazardous conditions. In the operating room, where the patient is relatively helpless, nursing personnel must always be alert.

Failure to communicate vital medical information to the surgical team members could be dangerous to the patient. An allergy identification band can prevent the administration of drugs or the use of materials that would evoke a sensitive reaction in the patient.

Preoperative medication errors can occur if both the surgeon and the anesthesiologist write orders; therefore orders should be written by only one of them and should be timed and dated.

All medications must be checked three times before administration: (1) when removed from the drug cabinet, (2) before being drawn up in the syringe, and (3) before being given to the patient.

The patient's hearing tends to become more acute after the administration of the preoperative medication and in the induction stage of anesthesia. A quiet environment is essential for all patients awaiting surgery. Recent studies indicate that some patients' hearing is acute throughout the surgical procedure. Even with the use of amnesia-invoking drugs, a small percentage of the population has recall of noise and events that occurred during their surgery (Kelly, 1992).

In addition, high noise levels interfere with accurate communication among members of the surgical team and may increase the likelihood of error. Noise in the operating room can be controlled and should be kept to a minimum.

Stretchers and operating room beds must be stabilized by locking the wheels and by personnel actions when a patient is moving from one to the other. The patient should be instructed and assisted to prevent an injury or fall. One person should stabilize the stretcher while another stands on the opposite side of the operating room bed to receive the patient. All safety devices on stretchers and operating room beds must be in proper working order. Locking mechanisms, side rails, knee straps, intravenous standards, hydraulic controls, and armboards should be used whenever necessary.

ELECTRICAL AND FIRE HAZARDS

Electrical and fire safety regulations pertinent to the operating room should be approved by the operating room committee and hospital administration. Perioperative nursing management should be delegated the responsibility and authority to see that regulations are put into effect by all operating room staff members. The regulations include the following:

1. Neither smoking nor the use of any apparatus or device producing open flame is permitted.
2. Preliminary evaluation and testing of all new equipment should ensure optimum safety and performance.
3. All electrical equipment, regardless of source, should be inspected for safety and proper functioning before use and be labeled with an inspection sticker according to hospital procedure.
4. The biomedical technician or electrical safety officer should determine whether electrical equipment, cameras, lights, and electrosurgical units are safe for use in a given situation.
5. Inventory control, regular inspection, preventive maintenance, and safety approval systems should be established.
6. Personnel must receive instruction in the safe use of all equipment and must demonstrate their proficiency in return. A standard procedure for care and use of electrical equipment should include the following:
   a. The plug, cord, and connections of electrical equipment must be checked before each use.
   b. All electrical cords should be of adequate length and flexibility to reach an outlet without stress and without the use of extension cords. Kinks and curls should be removed from electrical cords before they are plugged into wall outlets.
   c. The plug, not the cord, should be handled when electrical cords are plugged into or removed from an outlet. Pulling on the cord may cause it to break at the point where the wire is attached to the plug.
   d. Cords and connections should be handled in accordance with their delicacy. They cannot withstand pulling or rough treatment. Cord breakage is inconvenient and dangerous, and replacing broken cords is extremely expensive.
   e. Cords should not be wrapped tightly around equipment, which causes the protective covering to wear and breaks the wires inside the covering.
   f. Cords should always be removed from pathways before equipment such as a bed or a machine is moved. If the position of electrical equipment necessitates cords lying on the floor where persons will be walking during surgery, the cords should be taped down to prevent tripping (AORN, 1994).
7. All personnel must be familiar with the procedure for prompt removal from use and expeditious repair of defective equipment.
8. A qualified electrician should inspect electrical outlets and equipment at designated intervals or as requested and should file written reports with the director of surgical services.

Most hazardous situations in surgical suites are caused by the combination of electrical equipment and combustible materials found there. Because flammable anesthetics are rarely used today, environmental safety precautions associated with their use are not presented in this chapter.

For surgery areas in which only nonflammable inhalation anesthetic agents are used, signs indicating this practice must be posted at all entrances to the area. Conductive flooring and footwear are not required in the area. However, if conductive flooring exists, annual testing of the conductivity must be performed and test reports kept on file.

ISOLATED POWER SYSTEM

An isolated power system, although no longer required in nonflammable anesthetizing locations by the National Fire Protection Agency, may be provided in some operating rooms. These systems may reduce the hazard of shock or burn from electrical current flowing through the body to ground. Each isolated power system must have a continually operating line isolation monitor that indicates possible leakage or fault currents to ground (Spooner, 1983).

Most monitors have a green signal lamp that remains lighted when the system is isolated from ground. A red signal lamp and an audible warning signal are energized when a ground fault is detected. All operating room personnel must know the procedure to follow when this occurs:

1. The last electrical device to be plugged in must be shut off and unplugged.
2. If the red signal remains lighted, each piece of nonessential equipment must be systematically unplugged until the defective device is found.
3. A replacement must be obtained and the defective device removed from service, properly labeled as to the problem, and sent to the appropriate department for inspection and repair.
4. If a defective device cannot be identified and the red lamp remains lighted, the operating room must be shut down following the completion of that patient's surgery until the situation is corrected.
5. Individuals responsible for ensuring electrical safety must be notified.

VOLATILE LIQUIDS

Flammable liquids must be properly stored. Volatile liquids such as acetone and aerosol sprays are prohibited for cleaning and incidental use in hazardous locations. Skin prep solutions should be applied with care to prevent pooling, which can lead to a chemical burn. In addition, the solution may be ignited by a spark from an active electrode of the electrosurgical unit or from a charge of static electricity. Ignition of the vapors can occur as the solution evaporates. All solutions used for skin prepping should be nonflammable whenever an electrosurgical unit is used.

Personnel should be aware of the location and contents of the **materials safety data sheets** (MSDSs) (Fig. 2-1) for chemicals and solutions used in the operating room. The **Right to Know** directive published by OSHA in 1983 sets the standard for providing MSDS information. Each manufacturer of a chemical or solution should readily provide this safety information. MSDSs provide valuable patient and personnel safety information.

ELECTROSURGERY

High-frequency current from an electrosurgical unit (ESU) is frequently used to cut tissue and to coagulate blood vessels. Advanced technology has dramatically improved electrosurgical capabilities with the development of solid state generators and isolated systems (Fig. 2-2). These units significantly decrease the burn potential and the shock hazards that were inherent in the original spark gap units. Personnel must demonstrate competence in the proper use of electrosurgical equipment.

Before each use the ESU and associated safety features should be inspected for signs of damage and tested to ensure that they are functioning properly. The patient's skin integrity must be assessed before and after ESU use, particularly at positional pressure points and in the area under the dispersive pad (inactive electrode).

After the patient has been positioned, the desired connection between the patient and the ESU is established by placing the dispersive pad on a nonhairy area of clean, dry skin. The pad should be placed as close to the operative site as possible, on the same side of the patient's body as the operative site, and over a large muscle mass if possible; bony prominences, skin over metal prostheses, pressure points, and scar tissue should be avoided. If a dispersive pad requiring gel is used, the pad must be checked prior to placement to identify any dry spots on its surface. Placement should ensure that the pad's entire surface area maintains uniform body contact, without tenting or gapping. The ESU power settings should be as low as possible for each procedure, as determined by the surgeon in conjunction with the manufacturer's recommendations, and confirmed orally by the circulating nurse before activation. The ESU active electrode should be placed in a clean, well-insulated, safety container (holster) in a visible area when not in use to prevent accidental activation and injury (AORN, 1994).

The current supplied by the ESU is dispersed by the active electrode (for example, the electrosurgical pencil) through the body and is directed back to the generator by the dispersive electrode. In a nonisolated system, failure of this electrical pathway can result in current traveling in alternate pathways and causing burns in the area of contact. A faulty return pathway should be suspected if the surgeon requests higher settings because of inadequate cutting or coagulation. The connection from the patient to the machine should be examined immediately. A faulty return pathway may result from (1) inadequate patient contact with the dis-

Material Safety Data Sheet

May be used to comply with
OSHA's Hazard Communication Standard,
29 CFR 1910.1200. Standard must be
consulted for specific requirements.

U.S. Department of Labor

Occupational Safety and Health Administration
(Non-Mandatory Form)
Form Approved
OMB No. 1218-0072

IDENTITY *(As Used on Label and List)*

Note: *Blank spaces are not permitted. If any item is not applicable, or no information is available, the space must be marked to indicate that.*

Section I

Manufacturer's Name	Emergency Telephone Number
Address *(Number, Street, City, State, and ZIP Code)*	Telephone Number for Information
	Date Prepared
	Signature of Preparer *(optional)*

Section II — Hazardous Ingredients/Identity Information

Hazardous Components (Specific Chemical Identity; Common Name(s))	OSHA PEL	ACGIH TLV	Other Limits Recommended	% *(optional)*

Section III — Physical/Chemical Characteristics

Boiling Point		Specific Gravity (H$_2$O = 1)	
Vapor Pressure (mm Hg.)		Melting Point	
Vapor Density (AIR = 1)		Evaporation Rate (Butyl Acetate = 1)	

Solubility in Water

Appearance and Odor

Section IV — Fire and Explosion Hazard Data

Flash Point (Method Used)		Flammable Limits	LEL	UEL

Extinguishing Media

Special Fire Fighting Procedures

Unusual Fire and Explosion Hazards

(Reproduce locally)

OSHA 174, Sept. 1985

FIG. 2-1   Material safety data sheet (MSDS).

Medication information reprinted with permission of Johnson and Johnson.

Section V — Reactivity Data

Stability	Unstable		Conditions to Avoid
	Stable		

Incompatibility (*Materials to Avoid*)

Hazardous Decomposition or Byproducts

Hazardous Polymerization	May Occur		Conditions to Avoid
	Will Not Occur		

Section VI — Health Hazard Data

Route(s) of Entry:	Inhalation?	Skin?	Ingestion?

Health Hazards (*Acute and Chronic*)

Carcinogenicity:	NTP?	IARC Monographs?	OSHA Regulated?

Signs and Symptoms of Exposure

Medical Conditions
Generally Aggravated by Exposure

Emergency and First Aid Procedures

Section VII — Precautions for Safe Handling and Use

Steps to Be Taken in Case Material Is Released or Spilled

Waste Disposal Method

Precautions to Be Taken in Handling and Storing

Other Precautions

Section VIII — Control Measures

Respiratory Protection (*Specify Type*)

Ventilation	Local Exhaust		Special
	Mechanical (*General*)		Other

Protective Gloves	Eye Protection

Other Protective Clothing or Equipment

Work/Hygienic Practices

☆ USGPO 1986-491-529/43775

FIG. 2-1 CONT'D

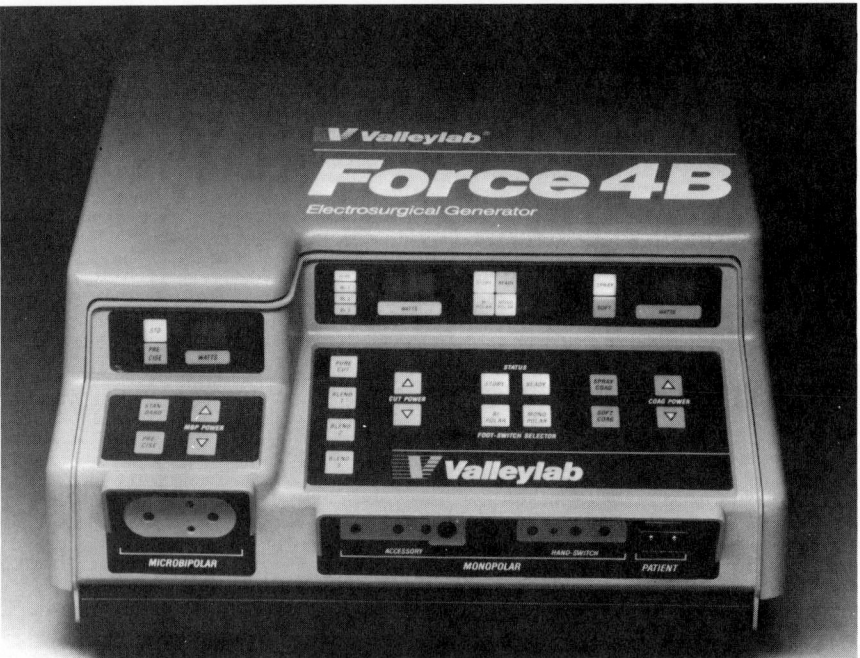

FIG. 2-2 Microprocessor-based electrosurgical unit includes the REM Contact quality monitoring system, providing safety against electrosurgical burns under the return electrode; dual independent simultaneous hand-switching monopolar outputs, allowing two surgeons to coagulate simultaneously yet independently, all from one unit; independent settings for monopolar and micropolar power, allowing for alternative bipolar and monopolar applications without repeated adjustments of power levels; and precise digital wattage controls and displays, offering exact power adjustments.

Courtesy Valleylab, Inc., Boulder, Colo.

persive pad, (2) poor placement of the pad, (3) inadequate connection of the cable to the pad, or (4) inadequate connection at the unit itself.

Electrosurgical burns may result from the unit's action on other electrical equipment. When an ECG monitor is used, the electrodes should be placed on the patient's shoulders and upper chest. The placement of ECG electrodes should always be as far as possible from the operative site. Distant positioning minimizes the alternate flow of electrosurgical current through the electrodes and monitor to ground.

Some contemporary ESUs possess a patient return electrode monitoring system. Current flowing from the active electrode is measured and compared with current returning from the patient return electrode. If the currents are not balanced, the circuit determines that the patient return electrode is not functioning properly, and the unit is deactivated. A significant safety feature is the capability of the return electrode monitoring system to measure the potential current concentration that may result in a burn at the return electrode site. It identifies inadequate electrode application or reduction of electrode contact area. It also measures the continuity of the entire electrical circuit (patient-pad-cord) for safe current flow. This capability represents a vital patient safety feature.

RADIATION SAFETY

Numerous sources of radiation exposure, such as x-ray machines (ionizing) and lasers (nonionizing), are used in the operating room. Members of the surgical team should avoid unnecessary exposure to these sources and be cognizant of the practices that reduce potential for exposure. Personnel present in the operating room must maintain the greatest practical distance from the radiation source when ionizing radiation is used during surgery. Nonessential personnel should leave the room, and members of the scrubbed team should move as far from the radiation source as is aseptically safe.

When feasible, appropriate devices should be used to hold patients or x-ray cassettes during radiography procedures to limit exposure of the surgical team. Otherwise leaded shields, aprons, and gloves should be used to reduce the intensity of radiation exposure. Careful handling and periodic examination of leaded garments can ensure the integrity of shielding. Because a fetus is particularly susceptible to injury from radiation exposure, women in the childbearing years should protect their reproductive organs from excessive exposure.

Radiation monitoring devices should be used in accordance with radiation safety standards and as deemed appropriate in the policies of individual facilities. Radiation safety devices include, but are not limited to, special eye-wear, lead gloves, aprons, and thyroid shields. Periodic staff development programs on radiation safety serve to correct misconceptions or unrealistic practices relating to radiation exposure and monitoring. Nonionizing radiation (laser) safety is discussed in Chapter 31.

ROUTINE PROCEDURES

ADMINISTERING LOCAL ANESTHETICS

Local anesthesia refers to the administration of an anesthetic agent to one part of the body by topical application, local infiltration, or subcutaneous injection (see also Chapter 6). It is usually administered by the surgeon. Local anesthesia is preferred if the patient's cooperation is necessary or the patient's physical condition warrants its use. The patient does not lose consciousness and may be aware of the surroundings if no supplemental sedation is given. Local anesthesia is economical and eliminates the undesirable effects of general anesthesia. However, adverse reactions may occur from large amounts of local agents. If the agent enters the bloodstream directly, convulsion, circulatory and respiratory distress, cardiovascular collapse, or even death can result.

The topical agent may be cocaine hydrochloride, tetracaine, or lidocaine applied to mucous membranes of the nose, throat, trachea, or urethra, or it may be ethyl chloride sprayed onto a specific area of the skin. Lidocaine 0.5% to 2%, with or without epinephrine, is the drug most commonly used for infiltration and local injection anesthesia, although bupivacaine (Marcaine) has seen increased use in recent years. Epinephrine, a vasoconstrictor, acts to control bleeding and prolong the local anesthetic effects. It should be used with caution in patients with hypertension, diabetes, or heart disease. All local anesthetic containers or syringes should be labeled when on the sterile table.

Patients should be carefully assessed preoperatively to determine if any allergies exist, and must be carefully observed intraoperatively for drug reactions; emergency drugs, suction apparatus, and resuscitation equipment should be readily available. Symptoms of adverse drug reactions include restlessness, unexplained anxiety or fearfulness, diaphoresis, complaints of nausea, palpitations, disturbed respiration, pallor or flushing, syncope, and convulsive movements. The nurse should also be aware of symptoms of allergic reaction such as urticaria, tachycardia, laryngeal edema resulting in breathing difficulties, nausea, vomiting, and elevated temperature. In some instances anaphylactoid symptoms, including severe hypotension, can occur. Emergency equipment should always be available to ensure safe patient resuscitation in the event of an allergic reaction.

Setup

Anesthetic drugs as ordered
The sterile local anesthesia tray includes the following items:

2 Luer-Lok syringes, 10 ml
1 Luer-Lok syringe, 2 ml
1 Needle, 25 gauge, 5/8 inch
1 Needle, 25 gauge, 1½ inches
1 Needle, 22 gauge, 1½ inches
1 Medicine cup, graduated, 2 oz
1 Cup, 6 oz
1 Basin, 4-inch diameter
Medication labels
Marking pen

Procedure

The patient should be monitored by a registered nurse or an anesthesiologist when a local anesthetic is used. A general recommendation is that no more than 50 ml of a 1% solution or 100 ml of a 0.5% solution of an anesthetic drug such as lidocaine be injected per hour for local anesthesia. For usual adult dosages see Table 2-1.

In the absence of an anesthesiologist or anesthetist, the circulating nurse or an additional monitor nurse is respon-

---

TABLE 2-1

Local Anesthetic Agents

Agent	Duration/potency	Route of administration	Concentration (%)	Recommended dose	Max. dose
Lidocaine	Intermediate/ intermediate	Infiltration/nerve block	0.5-2.0	1-60 ml	300 mg or 4.5mg/ kg body weight
Lidocaine with epinephrine 1:200,000	Same	Same	Same	1-225 ml	500 mg or 7 mg/kg body weight
Bupivicaine	Long/high	Infiltration	0.25-0.75	1-175 ml	150 mg
Bupivacaine with epinephrine 1:200,000	Same	Same	Same	1-225 ml	200 mg or 2 mg/kg body weight
Cocaine	Intermediate/ intermediate	Topical	4%/4 ml	Topical only	Topical only

sible for monitoring the patient's vital signs, cardiac readings, oxygen saturation, respiratory rate, and intravenous infusion. These data as well as the total amount of anesthetic and supplementary drugs administered to the patient should be documented. Psychologic support must be given to the patient throughout the operation (AORN, 1994).

HANDLING BLOOD AND BLOOD PRODUCTS

Maintenance of circulating blood volume is imperative during surgical procedures in which excessive blood loss may occur. In some instances synthetic volume expanders such as hetastarch (hydroxylethyl starch) and dextran may be used. These chemical solutions have colloidal properties similar to those of human albumin and act to expand plasma volume. Although not a replacement for blood or blood products, in some circumstances volume expanders are used to avoid the risks associated with blood and blood products. When blood must be given, appropriate precautions must be taken to reduce the hazards of administration.

When requesting blood or blood components, the appropriate institutional blood grouping Rh requisition should be sent to the blood bank. Included on or with this requisition should be the number of units desired. If the patient is sent to the operating room directly from the emergency department without a chart, all patient information must be plainly printed on a piece of paper. Many institutions have computerized ordering; the same information is required when requesting blood by computer. The blood bank should be contacted by the nurse in charge to explain the situation. Proper communication facilitates release of the needed units.

Before the administration of blood, the circulating nurse and the anesthesiologist or anesthetist should confirm the following:

1. Number on the unit of blood corresponds with the number on the blood requisition.
2. Name and number on the patient's identification band agree with the name and number on the unit of blood.
3. Patient's name on the unit of blood corresponds with the name on the requisition.
4. Blood group indicated on the unit of blood corresponds with that of the patient.
5. Date of expiration has not been reached.

When it becomes apparent that more blood will be needed than was originally anticipated, the blood bank should be requested to stay ahead a specific number of units. This procedure allows the blood bank to crossmatch the units on a routine basis without jeopardizing the patient. Crossmatch requisitions should be sent for the additional units requested. A new, properly labeled sample with a blood grouping requisition may also be needed to have adequate serum for crossmatching.

The need for rapid blood transfusion necessitates the warming of blood to prevent hypothermia, which may induce cardiac arrest. Blood should be warmed during its passage through the transfusion set. The warming device should incorporate a temperature monitor and, ideally, an audible warning system. Blood should never be warmed above 38° C (American Association of Blood Banks, 1993). The probability of a transfusion reaction increases in direct proportion to the number of units transfused. The circulating nurse should be alert to any signs of reaction. If any suspicious reactions occur, the circulating nurse should assist the anesthesiologist with the following:

1. Stopping the transfusion
2. Reporting the reaction to the surgeon and the blood bank
3. Returning the unused portion of the blood and a sample of the patient's blood to the blood bank
4. Sending a urine sample to the lab as soon as possible
5. Completing an incident report covering the details of the reaction

Unused blood should be returned as soon as the patient leaves the operating room suite. Returned blood can be reissued if it has not been allowed to warm above 10° C. New external blood thermometers (Hemo Temp II), much like the skin contact tape thermometer, are being used on blood bags by many blood banks to quickly identify blood that has become too warm. Autotransfusion—the reinfusion of a patient's own blood—is being used with increasing frequency (see Chapter 30). The blood may be collected days or weeks before surgery. Intraoperative autotransfusion facilitates recovery of blood as it is lost during the surgical procedure and retransfusion to the patient. Special sterile equipment simultaneously suctions, filters, anticoagulates, defoams, and returns blood from the operative site to the patient. This technique can be lifesaving in emergency situations such as major trauma.

ESTIMATING BLOOD LOSS

Measurement of blood loss is a vital procedure in the surgical management of infants, critically ill or elderly patients, and patients undergoing complex, extensive surgery. The gravimetric method of weighing sponges provides a reliable means of judging the amount of blood to be replaced. The weight of the unit of dry sponges and the plastic bag for soiled sponges must be known. Grams are converted to milliliters on a one-to-one basis.

Setup

Blood loss record
Gram scale
Plastic bags and twist ties to hold soiled sponges

Procedure

1. Allowing for the weight of the unit of dry sponges and the plastic bag, the scale is adjusted to register at zero.

2. Bagged sponges are placed on the scale.
3. The scale reading is recorded: 1 g equals 1 ml of blood loss.
4. The blood loss is noted on the record.
5. The new weight is added to the preceding weight each time sponges are weighed so that a current total blood loss from sponges is available.
6. Blood in the suction bottles is measured at regular intervals, and the amount of blood loss is added to the total recorded from sponges. Allowances must be made for any irrigating solutions that may have been used. The scrub person should announce the amount used so that the circulator can subtract the irrigating solution volume from the suction canister amount to obtain accurate blood loss estimates.

CARE AND HANDLING OF SPECIMENS

It is the responsibility of the circulating nurse to identify, document, and properly care for specimens collected in the operating room. Blood, soft tissue, bone, body fluids, and foreign bodies are examples of specimens commonly handled.

Each specimen is cared for according to the specific protocol established by the laboratory that will receive the specimen. Generally all tissue should be kept moist and transported to the laboratory as soon as possible.

Formalin (formaldehyde) is frequently used to preserve specimens if they cannot be taken to the laboratory immediately. Exposure to formaldehyde fumes should be monitored at least quarterly, and an MSDS sheet should be available to staff in case of spills.

When immediate diagnosis is needed, specimens are quick-frozen, sliced, and stained—a method of tissue examination known as frozen section. The extent or direction of surgery can be determined by frozen-section reports as they are communicated to the surgeon intraoperatively.

All specimens are considered a potential source of infection. The outside of specimen containers must be kept clean or placed in an impervious plastic bag to prevent contamination of the individuals transporting or receiving specimens. Gloves should always be worn when handling specimens.

A mislabeled specimen could result in misdiagnosis and subsequent inappropriate treatment of the patient. The circulating nurse must ensure each specimen is labeled with the proper patient name and origin of the specimen (example: Jane Doe, 100001, Right breast biopsy). The surgeon should provide descriptive information about the specimen (for example, suture tag at 6 o'clock). All specimens are documented on the operating room record.

SPONGE, SHARP, AND INSTRUMENT COUNTS

Every operating room should have established written policies and procedures for sponge, sharp, and instrument counts that define materials to be counted, the times when counts must be done, and the documentation required (AORN, 1994).

Certain general guidelines pertain to counting all three types of items. The scrub nurse and the circulating nurse should count all items in unison and aloud, quietly, as the scrub nurse touches each item. Counting should not be interrupted. If any uncertainty exists about a count, it should be repeated. The circulating nurse should immediately record the count for each type of item on the count record or worksheet. If additional items are dispensed during the procedure, the circulating nurse should record the number and initial it. The names of the circulating nurse and the scrub nurse should be recorded as soon as each count is completed. Linen or waste containers should neither be emptied nor their contents removed from the operating room until the procedure is completed and the patient has been taken out of the room. Extreme patient emergencies sometimes necessitate omission of counts, the occurrence of which should be documented on the operative record.

Sponge counts

All types of sponges should be counted in all procedures. The scrub nurse and the circulating nurse should count them before the beginning of the operation, before closure begins, and when skin closure is begun. Additional counts may be indicated according to individual hospital policy and circumstance. Additional counts should always be taken before a cavity within a cavity is closed, for example, when the uterus is closed during a cesarean section. Types and sizes of sponges used should be kept to a minimum. All soft goods that are used within a wound and that are not intended to be left in the wound after closure must contain an element detectable by x-ray examination. Radiopacity facilitates finding any item that may be presumed lost or left in the cavity when an incorrect count occurs. Along the same line, x-ray–detectable sponges should never be used for dressings to eliminate the possibility of a seemingly foreign body appearing on postoperative x-ray studies that may be done.

Each type and size of sponge should be kept separate from the other types. Sponges must be kept away from other supplies such as towels and drapes to prevent a sponge from being carried inadvertently into the wound or misplaced. Counted sponges should never be taken from the operating room for any reason during surgery to eliminate the possibility of an incorrect count.

If an incorrectly numbered package of sponges is dispensed to the field, it should be handed off the field, marked as not included in the count, and placed in an isolated spot. This practice reduces the potential for error by using only standard multiples of sponges.

During surgery the scrub nurse should discard soiled sponges into a plastic-lined bucket or receptacle. The circulating nurse transfers the discarded sponges into impermeable plastic bags or other appropriate containers, according to type and prescribed number after counting with the scrub nurse. The bag is then closed, secured, and labeled with the type and number of sponges and the initials of the persons who counted them. The bag can be set aside, and unless a discrepancy occurs, the sponges need not be taken out and counted again at the time of the closure sponge counts. Bagging of sponges reduces the possibility of airborne contamination arising from the sponges as they become dry and enables the anesthesiologist to make a visual assessment of the patient's blood loss.

The circulating nurse should tally the numbers of each type of sponge dispensed, as recorded on the count worksheet before the closure counts are taken. As the first layer of closure is begun, the scrub nurse and the circulating nurse should count all sponges consecutively, proceeding from the sterile field to the back table and off the field. The circulating nurse should inform the surgeon of the results of the count. The procedure should be repeated as skin closure is begun.

Sharp counts

Sharps should be counted in all procedures by the scrub nurse and the circulating nurse at the same time as sponges are counted. In addition to suture needles, sharps may include scalpel and electrosurgical blades, hypodermic needles, and safety pins. When needles are counted before surgery begins, opening every package of suture dispensed onto the field is not necessary. The needles may be counted according to the number indicated on the package. If a package indicates that five needled sutures are contained within, five needles should be documented on the worksheet. The scrub nurse is responsible for verifying the number of needles at the time the package is opened. The scrub nurse should continually count needles during the procedure and hand them to the surgeon on an exchange basis. Hands-free transfer of sharps by using an emesis basin or magnetic pad is recommended to prevent staff and surgeon needlestick injuries.

Collecting used needles on a needle pad or container helps to ensure their containment on the table. In procedures that may require use of a high volume of needles, the scrub nurse can count any filled needle pads with the circulating nurse and hand them off the field. The circulating nurse should then bag them and label them with the number of needles contained and the initials of the individuals who counted them.

Needles broken during the procedure must be accounted for in their entirety. Like sponges, needles should never be taken from the room for any reason during a procedure. Closure counts are conducted in the same format as that for sponges.

Instrument counts

Instrument counts for all procedures are recommended. However, the policy of some hospitals specifies that instrument counts be taken only when a major body cavity is entered or when the depth and location of the wound are such that an instrument could accidentally be left in the patient. Individual hospital policy must be followed without deviation. Instrument sets should be standardized for ease in counting, with the minimum number and type of instruments in each set. Instruments should be counted in the instrument room as sets are being assembled, in the operating room by the scrub nurse and the circulating nurse before the beginning of the operation, and before closure begins. Additional counts may be indicated according to hospital policy or individual circumstance. Instruments that are broken or disassembled during the procedure must be accounted for in their entirety. No instruments should be taken from the operating room during a procedure. Printed instrument count sheets with the names of all items to be counted help expedite the count procedure.

Incorrect counts

Any incorrect closure count should be repeated immediately. If it remains incorrect, the circulating nurse should notify the surgeon, and a search should be made for the missing item. All personnel should direct their immediate attention to locating the missing item. If it is not found, an x-ray film is taken. If the x-ray study is negative, the count is recorded as incorrect, and the x-ray results noted on the operating room record. An incident report should be initiated according to hospital policy. Accurate counting and recording of sponges, sharps, and instruments are essential for the protection of the patient, personnel, and the hospital.

EMERGENCY SIGNALS

Every surgical suite should have an emergency signal system that can be activated within each operating room proper. A light should appear outside the door of the room involved, and a buzzer or bell should sound in a central nursing or anesthesia area. The signals should remain on until the alarm is turned off at the source. All personnel should be familiar with the system and should know both how to send a signal and how to respond to it. Such a system, restricted to use in life-threatening emergencies, saves invaluable time in bringing additional assistance.

CARDIOPULMONARY RESUSCITATION

Cardiopulmonary resuscitation (CPR) is the immediate restoration of circulatory and respiratory functions by means of manual and mechanical methods and the administration of drugs to provide for ventilation and conversion of the heartbeat to normal sinus rhythm.

Cardiac arrest, standstill, or fibrillation may occur in patients undergoing surgery because of the hazards of surgery, such as blood loss and shock, or because of unfavorable reactions to anesthesia, such as hypoxia and poor ventilation.

For survival of the patient, all body organs and tissues must receive sufficient oxygen through the circulatory system. The circulating blood must carry the oxygen supplied by pulmonary ventilation. Ventilation may be reestablished by mouth-to-mouth breathing or by other means of artificial respiration, such as oxygen apparatus, face mask, and intubation (artificial airway and endotracheal tube). Cardiac compression is directed toward reestablishment of circulation.

A well-defined written protocol should be posted in a designated area in each operating room and should be clearly understood by all personnel. Periodic practice sessions for delegated duties should be scheduled as part of the safety program. Basic life support training should be provided for all perioperative nurses.

Setup

A movable emergency cardiopulmonary arrest cart (crash cart) containing all items that may be needed should be immediately available. A separate box for malignant hyperthermia and anaphylactic reaction is also a good practice. The surgical committee, the perioperative nursing staff, and the anesthesiology staff should determine the equipment needed and the plan of treatment to be initiated stressing the team approach. The following items should be included on or with the emergency cart:

Emergency thoracotomy kit
  1 Knife handle no. 4 with blade no. 20
  1 Mallet
  1 Lebsche knife
  1 Rib retractor
  1 Finochietto or Harken self-retaining retractor

Ventilation and resuscitation equipment
  Ambu resuscitator (bag), anesthesia machine, or mechanical ventilator
  Airways—oral and nasal
  Endotracheal tubes
  Laryngoscope and endotracheal forceps or stylets
  Suctioning devices

Syringes (Luer-Lok) and needles
  3 Syringes, 3 ml
  4 Syringes, 5 ml
  4 Syringes, 10 ml
  2 Syringes, 20 ml
  2 Syringes, 50 ml
  5 Needles, 25 gauge, ⅝ inch
  5 Needles, 20 gauge, 1½ inches
  5 Needles, 18 gauge, 1½ inches
  2 Needles, 20 gauge, 3 inches (intracardiac)

Emergency drugs
  Where available, commercially prefilled syringes should be used
  Sodium bicarbonate
  Lidocaine
  Epinephrine
  Calcium chloride
  Dopamine
  Dobutamine
  Isoproterenol hydrochloride (Isuprel)

Methylprednisolone sodium succinate (Solu-Medrol)
Magnesium sulfate
Adenosine
Atropine
Propranolol hydrochloride (Inderal)
Levarterenol bitartrate (Levophed)
Procainamide (Pronestyl)
Cedilanid-D (Deslanoside)
Aminophylline
Bretylium
Naloxone hydrochloride (Narcan)
Dextrose 50%
Flumazenil (Mazecon)
Sodium chloride for injection
Water for injection

Infusion equipment
  Fluids for intravenous infusion
  Venesection tray
  Infusion administration sets
  Cutdown tray and intracatheters
  Stopcocks
  Alcohol wipes (sponges)
  Prep swabs
  Tourniquets
  Infusion pump
  Blood sampling kit
  Blood tubes
  Heparinized syringes

Cardiac support equipment
  Defibrillator
  External paddles
  Sterile internal paddles
  Pediatric paddles, if indicated
  Cardiac monitoring equipment

Cardiac arrest board
  (for use if patient is in a bed)

A *thoracotomy setup* (Chapter 24) should be available in case open heart massage is attempted. Open heart massage is rarely performed today unless the chest is already open and a thoracic surgeon is present. Closed chest massage is considered equally effective with fewer inherent hazards.

Procedure

1. The emergency alarm should be activated to alert the operating room supervisor and appropriate surgical and anesthesia personnel. The exact time of arrest is recorded, and additional assistance procured as required.
2. In the absence of an anesthesiologist or resuscitative equipment, an airway should be established and ventilation of the patient begun by means of mouth-to-mouth resuscitation or other artificial respiration to restore and maintain oxygenation.
3. Closed chest massage is applied to maintain circulation and provision of oxygen to vital tissues.

4. Nursing personnel responding to the alarm should bring the cardiopulmonary arrest cart to the room.

5. As soon as additional personnel arrive, one person should be designated as the charge person (usually the anesthesiologist) and another as recorder. The recorder should maintain ongoing documentation of all medications given and procedures performed.

6. Medications are prepared and administered as ordered.

7. Infusions or transfusions are procured and prepared as ordered.

8. The surgeon and anesthesiologist are assisted as needed.

9. At the conclusion of the procedure, the event, care given, and disposition (outcome) of the patient are documented.

10. Appropriate administrative services are notified as the situation requires. Included would be a request to the service supplying religious rites and notification to the proper services of the change in the patient's condition and the need to inform the patient's family.

REFERENCES

American Association of Blood Banks. (1993). *Standards for blood banks and transfusion services,* ed 14, Arlington, Va: The Association.

American Society for Testing and Materials. (1993).

Association of Operating Room Nurses. (1994). *AORN standards and recommended practices for perioperative nursing,* Denver: The Association.

Bartley, JM. (1993, Sept/Oct): Environmental control: operating room air quality, *Today's O.R. Nurse.*

Doering EM (1992). Memory during anesthesia, *Anesthesiology* 77 (5):1052.

Ghoneim MM & Block RI. (1992). Learning and consciousness during general anesthesia, *Anesthesiology* 76(2):279.

Joint Commission on Accreditation of Healthcare Organizations (1994). *Accreditation manual for hospitals,* Chicago: The Commission.

Kelly JS & Roy RC. (1992). Intraoperative awareness with propolfol, oxygen total intravenous anesthesia for microlaryngeal surgery, *Anesthesiology* 77(1):207.

Occupational Safety and Health Administration. (1991). Occupational exposure to bloodborne pathogens, *Federal Register,* 56, 29CFR Part 1910.1030.

Occupational Safety and Health Administration. (Nov. 25, 1983). Toxic and hazardous substances, hazard communication standard, *Code of Federal Regulations,* title 29, chapter xvii, section 1910.7200, 48 FR 53280, Washington, DC: US Government Printing Office.

Regulated medical waste definition and treatment: a collaborative document. (1993). *AORN J* 58(1):110.

Spooner RB. (1983). Hospital electrical safety simplified, Research Triangle Park, NC: Instrument Society of America.

Tests evaluate barrier effectiveness of gowns, *OR Manager* 9(5):1.

Young MA, Meyers M & McCulloch LD et al. (1992). Latex allergy: a guideline for perioperative nurses, *AORN J* 56(3):488.

BIBLIOGRAPHY

Adult advanced cardiac life support. (1992). *JAMA* 268,

Bruning, LM (1993). The bloodborne pathogens final rule: understanding the regulation, AORN J 57(2):439.

Fox, V. (1992). Passing surgical instruments, sharps without injury, *AORN J* 55(1):264.

Lewis, SM & Collier, IC. (1992). Medical surgical nursing: assessment and management of clinical problems, ed 3, St Louis, Mosby.

Marriner, A: *Guide to nursing management,* ed 4, St Louis, Mosby.

Mathias, J (1992). Advanced technology in the operating room, *OR Manager* 8(5):10.

National Fire Protection Association. (1993). *National electric code,* NFPA no. 70, Boston, The Association.

National Fire Protection Association. (1989). *Standard for health care facilities,* NFPA no. 99, Quincy, Mass, The Association.

Owens MO & Zellers-Jacob L. (1992). *Adenosine: the newest drug for PSVT, RN* 55(38):38.

Patterson, P. (1997). OR Construction challenges for managers, *OR Manager* 8(4):1.

Patterson, P. (1992). Shift to OP surgery key issue in redesign, *OR Manager* 8(4):8.

Patterson, P. (1992). Early decisions crucial to successful building project, *OR Manager* 8(5):1.

Patterson, P. (1992). OR design: floor plans establish traffic plans for people and supplies, *OR Manager* 8(6):10.

Rowland, HS & Rowland, BL. (1990). *Operating room administration manual,* vol 1, Gaithersburg, Md, 1990.

Rupke, G. (1993). Fire safety in the operating room, *J Nurs Manage* 24(4):96i.

Walsh, J. (1993). Postoperative effects of OR positioning, *RN* 56:50.

3

INFECTION CONTROL

BARBARA D. GARNER

*A*sepsis, which means the absence of germs, infection, and septic matter, is directed toward cleanliness and the elimination of infectious agents; for perioperative personnel aseptic principles and techniques are a cornerstone of infection control efforts. Surgical asepsis facilitates healing by preventing infectious organisms from reaching a vulnerable body surface. Surgical asepsis is designed to exclude all microbes, whereas medical asepsis is designed to exclude microbes associated with communicable diseases. Practices that restrict microorganisms in the environment and on equipment and supplies and that prevent normal body flora from contaminating the surgical wound are termed *aseptic techniques*. The goal of each aseptic technique is to optimize primary wound healing, prevent surgical infection, and minimize the length of recovery from surgery. *Antisepsis* refers to the chemical disinfection of the skin, mucous membranes, and other living tissues.

Envisioning contemporary surgery without the complex foundation of science is difficult. However, the principles of asepsis as we know them today began during the middle of the nineteenth century. The rudiments of aseptic techniques and infection control were described as early as 450 BC. Hippocrates, the father of surgery, used wine or boiled water to irrigate wounds. Galen, a Roman who lived during the second century AD, is reported to have boiled his instruments before use.

Although various forms of surgery were practiced throughout the centuries, the first period of surgical prominence occurred during the 1500s, when Ambröise Paré developed the use of ligatures to control bleeding. In that same era, Fracastorius, the world's first epidemiologist, proclaimed that diseases were spread in three ways: by direct contact, by handling articles that infected people had handled previously, and by transmission from a distance.

In the middle of the nineteenth century a new era began that greatly expanded the horizons of surgery. Anesthesia became a beneficial tool of the surgeon, permitting pain-free operations and decreasing the need for speed during surgery. Interest in surgical techniques and the development of new operations flourished. The preservation of life, how-

ever, was still not being fulfilled. Wound infections were so common that they were considered normal. When pus appeared in the incision, it was thought to be a healthy sign, signaling the beginning of clinical improvement. *Hospitalism* was a term coined by Sir James Simpson to describe the array of infections that developed among hospitalized patients. Today these are referred to as nosocomial infections. Unfortunately, infected wounds often ruined the surgical procedure, lengthened the patient's hospital stay, and frequently threatened the patient's life (Larson, 1989).

During the mid-1800s three individuals developed concepts of hygiene and antisepsis within the health care community, but apparently independent of each other. Ignaz Semmelweis made a simple but momentous contribution to infection control by advocating that hands be washed between examinations of patients. Joseph Lister was applying principles of antisepsis to wound care in an effort to make surgery a safe practice. The third individual, Florence Nightingale, was instigating radical changes in sanitation, resulting in reductions in mortality from contagious diseases. The interventions of these leaders provided the structure of infection control practice today (Larson, 1989).

In the 1850s Louis Pasteur, founder of the science of microbiology, theorized that fermentation was caused by particles of living matter so small that they could not be seen but could be carried freely in the air. He referred to these microorganisms as *germs* and found that heat killed them. The relationship between the fermentation process and the putrefaction of tissue was not understood at that time. In 1860 Joseph Lister learned about Pasteur's work, recognized the analogous relationship between the two processes, and set out to investigate the relationship of the germ theory to the process of infection. By 1867 Lister was advocating carbolic soaks and sprays for hands, wounds, dressings, sutures, and the operating room itself. Even though Lister's antiseptic methods and principles were crude and undeveloped, their use resulted in a drop in surgical mortality from 45% to 15%. The antiseptic era and the modern age of surgery had begun.

CAUSE AND PREVENTION OF INFECTIONS

Infectious disease currently ranks as the fifth common cause of death in the United States (Grimes, 1991). How can the patient be protected from a hospital-acquired infection? How is surgical asepsis maintained? The answers to these and similar questions are derived from the principles of microbiology and bacteriology, the foundation for infection control.

Effective hospital and operating room infection control programs must be carried out by everyone who cares for patients. Infection control programs involve methods of environmental sanitation and maintenance of facilities; cleanliness of the air in the suite and of the skin and apparel of patients, surgeons, and personnel; sterility of surgical equipment; strict aseptic technique; and careful observance of well-defined written procedures, rules, and regulations.

The human body has three lines of defense to combat infection. The first line of defense consists of external barriers such as the skin and mucous membranes, which are usually impervious to most pathogenic organisms. The second line of defense is the inflammatory response, which prevents an invading pathogen from reproducing and possibly involving other tissue. The third line of defense, or the immune response, is triggered after the inflammatory response. When there is a break in this defense mechanism, the possibility for infection increases.

An infection control program is based on a knowledge of the nature and characteristics of microorganisms that are capable of producing infection in the surgical patient and an understanding of their transmission in the environment and wound. An ongoing and up-to-date program requires study and critical analysis of the latest accepted information to provide methods that destroy or inhibit specific microorganisms in particular situations.

Definitions of terms should be agreed on and clarified by the hospital epidemiologist as necessary. Each member of the surgical team must have some understanding of the nature and characteristics of pathogenic and nonpathogenic microorganisms.

TERMS RELATED TO INFECTION AND INFECTING AGENTS

Pathogens are microorganisms that are capable of producing tissue damage or disease under favorable conditions. In humans a satisfactory balance may be reached between the invading pathogens and the host, resulting in no noticeable ill effects. The aggressiveness and virulence of pathogens, the size and composition of the microbial population, the physical environment, and the susceptibility of the host determine the occurrence of an infection. *Virulence* refers to the potency of a pathogen and the ability to produce disease. The higher the virulence, the greater potential for disease.

Primary pathogens refer to highly virulent organisms that are capable of producing disease in low numbers. *Op-portunists* are of low virulence and require large numbers to produce infection.

Most pathogenic bacteria are capable of leading a parasitic or saprophytic existence. The more viable a pathogen, the more able it is to resist adverse conditions. Some pathogens reside naturally on or within humans without producing disease until the opportunity arises. For example, the enteric microorganisms are a large group of gram-negative, non–spore-forming bacilli whose natural habitat is within the lumen of the intestine of humans and animals. *Escherichia coli,* one of the enteric bacilli, is capable of producing infection on entrance into the peritoneal cavity.

Parasites are microorganisms that reside on or within the bodies of living organisms called *hosts* to find the environment and food they require for life and reproduction. Some microorganisms are obligatory parasites, meaning that they depend on their hosts for survival and reproduction. Other microorganisms are facultative parasites, meaning that they normally reside on dead matter but may receive nourishment from living matter. All disease-producing microorganisms are parasites; however, not all parasites are disease producing.

Saprophytes are microorganisms that reside on dead or decaying organic matter. They are found in water, soil, and debris—wherever the process of decay occurs. They reduce decaying matter to simple soluble compounds, which in turn become available to bacteria. For example, *Clostridium tetani,* which causes tetanus (lockjaw), cannot survive in healthy tissue but requires dead (necrotic) material.

Certain bacteria, members of the genera *Bacillus, Clostridium,* and *Sporozoa,* form and develop specialized structures called *spores* (endospores) within the cell under specific conditions. One cell generally produces one spore. The specific environment that starts sporulation is still unknown. When conditions are again favorable for growth, the spore germinates to produce one vegetative cell. The spore appears to possess a large number of active enzymes and is especially resistant to heat, chemicals, and drying.

Transient microorganisms are those having a very short life span, such as the normal flora present on the skin surface of humans. Gram-negative bacteria are transient on the hands of hospital personnel and account for 60% of infections.

Resident microorganisms are those which habitually live in the epidermis, deep in the crevices and folds of the skin.

Most bacteria produce one or more poisonous materials known as *toxins*. *Exotoxins* are specific injurious toxins that diffuse freely from the microorganisms into the environment. *Clostridium tetani, C. botulinum,* the sporulating anaerobes isolated from gas gangrene such as *C. perfringens, Streptococcus pyogenes,* and *Staphylococcus aureus* are microorganisms with this property. Diseases associated with exotoxins are tetanus, botulism, and diphtheria.

Endotoxins are toxins that are part of the cell wall. Endotoxic substances are not secreted to a significant degree into the parasites' environment but are released after death and dissolution of the microorganisms. Their poisonous effect depends on the species. *Salmonella typhosa* and *Neisseria meningitidis* are endotoxic pathogens. Diseases associated with endotoxins include staphylococcal food poisoning and cholera.

Bacteria differ from one another in their relationship to molecular oxygen. The strictly *aerobic* (obligatory-type) bacteria are unable to live and produce without access to free atmospheric oxygen. *Mycobacterium tuberculosis, Vibrio cholerae* (agent of Asiatic cholera), *Bacillus subtilis,* and *Corynebacterium diphtheriae* are aerobic bacteria. The strictly *anaerobic* bacteria can live only in the absence of air; atmospheric oxygen is poisonous to them. *Clostridium tetani, C. botulinum,* and *C. perfringens* are anaerobic bacteria. However, many facultative bacteria have enzyme systems that permit them to live and produce with, without, or with only a small amount of free oxygen.

An *infectious agent* is a parasite (bacterium, spirochete, fungus, virus, or any other type of organism) that is capable of producing infection. *Infection* is the process by which living pathogenic microorganisms enter the host's body under conditions favorable for their growth and, by the production of toxins, may act injuriously on the host's tissues. The potential of bacteria to produce infection is related to their ability to attach to the tissue or host cell.

A *source* is the object, substance, or individual from which an infectious agent passes to a host. In some cases transfer is direct from the reservoir, or source, to the host. The source may be at any point in the chain of transmission. For example, the nose of an individual may be the reservoir, or source; hands, clothing, or a mask may become the intermediate mechanism for the transfer of the agent to the host.

Nosocomial infections are acquired by patients during hospitalization, with confirmation of diagnosis by clinical or laboratory evidence. The infective agents may originate from endogenous sources, as from one tissue to another within the patient (self-infection), or from exogenous sources, as acquired from objects or other patients within the hospital (cross-infection). Nosocomial infections, which are often referred to as hospital-acquired infections, may not become apparent until after the patient has left the hospital. Factors that influence the development of nosocomial infections are the source of infection, the microbial agent, the route of transmission, the susceptibility of the host, and the environment.

The known incubation period of the disease is used to determine if the infection that developed is hospital or community acquired. The incubation period for surgical wound infections is 3 to 8 days postoperatively. Variables considered in determining the degree of risk for nosocomial infections are based on *wound classifications.* The four classifications for surgical wounds include the following: *class I* (clean wound)—no break in sterile technique, no inflammation, and the gastrointestinal (GI), respiratory, urinary, and genital tracts are not entered; class I wounds include surgeries such as herniorrhaphy, breast biopsy, and orthopedic procedures; *class II* (clean, contaminated wound)—

alimentary, genitourinary, or respiratory tracts are entered with no spillage of contents; class II wounds include surgeries of the biliary tract, appendix, vagina and oropharynx; *class III* (contaminated wound)—acute inflammation with pus encountered or trauma from a clean source; *class IV* (dirty)—pus or perforated viscus encountered, trauma from dirty source, or pathogenic organisms present prior to surgery.

The Centers for Disease Control and Prevention (CDC) have modified the definitions of surgical wound infections by eliminating the use of the word *wound* in describing postoperative infections. The term *incisional surgical site infection* (SSI) is used for infections involving the incision. *Superficial incisional SSI* involves the skin and subcutaneous tissue. *Deep incisional SSI* involves deep soft tissue, fascia, and muscle. *Organ/space SSI* involves any part of the anatomy other than the incision (Horan et al., 1992).

Typically the hospital epidemiology department holds the main responsibility for tracking nosocomial infections in surgical patients. The effectiveness of lowering surgical site infections has been difficult because there has been no consensus on which surveillance method is best for collecting data. Several surveillance methods that have been used include, but are not limited to, selective surveillance, sentinel surveillance, high-risk area surveillance, and rotating surveillance (Brachman, 1993) (Research Highlight 3-1).

With the increasing numbers of ambulatory surgical procedures performed, it becomes more difficult to accurately follow up on postoperative infections. Perioperative nurses must therefore work in conjunction with the epidemiologist to monitor trends and effect positive outcomes (Research Highlight 3-2).

A *carrier* is a person who harbors one or more specific pathogens in the absence of discernible clinical disease. Carriers may be classified into three groups: convalescent carriers who continue to harbor or shed microorganisms for variable periods during recovery from the disease; chronic or permanent carriers who harbor microorganisms usually for the duration of life; and transitory or temporary carriers who, without a recognized attack of the disease, harbor microorganisms for short periods.

Contamination is the presence of pathogenic microorganisms on or in an animate or inanimate vector. This term generally is used in reference to a specific object, substance, or tissue that contains microorganisms, especially disease-producing microorganisms. For example, a person's skin or an instrument may be contaminated by contact with pathogenic microorganisms, but it is not infected. Contamination is merely the presence of a microorganism, whereas infection is the implantation and successful reproduction of a microorganism on or in a susceptible human host.

Inflammation is a defense reaction by the body to an injury or abnormal stimulation caused by a physical, chemical, thermal, or biologic agent. Frequently the tissue of the host cells, assisted by phagocytes, localizes and destroys the pathogenic invader. This reaction is observed as a local

⚜
RESEARCH HIGHLIGHT 3-1

Postoperative wound infections may add from 7.4 to 10.1 days to the hospitalization of a surgical patient and increase the cost. Surveillance of surgical site infections has been studied at several institutions in an effort to identify a strategy to prevent nosocomial infections after surgical intervention. The purpose of this prospective study was to determine the sensitivity and specificity of standard infection control surveillance techniques for identifying surgical site infections.

This study used the surveillance components of the CDC's National Nosocomial Infection Surveillance System. Data were collected by infection control practitioners (ICP) by review of the medical records and discussion with patients' nurses and physicians. Simultaneously the hospital epidemiologist collected data and examined each patient's wound daily. There were 925 surgical procedures included in the first validation period, and 110 procedures were observed during the second validation period. Data collected during the first period by the ICPs identified 67 surgical site infections, and the hospital epidemiologist identified 80 surgical site infections. Overall sensitivity was 83.8% and specificity was 99.8%. (Three of the patients were discharged prior to observation by the ICP). Data collected during the second period identified 12 surgical site infections by the ICPs and 13 surgical site infections by the hospital epidemiologist. Overall sensitivity and specificity were 92.3% and 99%, respectively.

In comparison of the two groups of data collection, accuracy of surveillance appeared to be related to experience. Data also were analyzed according to incisional and deep surgical site infections. The ICPs had more difficulty identifying incisional infections than deep infections. During the second validation period the ICP correctly identified 100% of the deep infections and 80% of incisional infections. The authors note the accuracy of identifying surgical site infections without direct wound observation. With experience ICPs can achieve efficiency in identifying surgical site infections with a high level of sensitivity.

Cardo, M., Falk, P.S., & Mayhall, C.G. (1993, April). Validation of surgical wound surveillance. *Infection Control and Hospital Epidemiology*, 211-215.

⚜
RESEARCH HIGHLIGHT 3-2

With an increase in outpatient surgery, the traditional in-hospital surveillance of surgical site infections is not feasible. Shorter hospital stay limits the ability of the infection control practitioners to accurately detect surgical site infections. This prospective study evaluated the use of patient telephone surveys in addition to monthly physician surveys to determine postdischarge surgical site infections. There were 501 patients selected for the telephone contact, of whom 189 were successfully contacted. Data collected included information about the following wound complications: (1) presence of pus or yellowish discharge, (2) persistence of pain or redness around the incision, (3) poor wound healing, and (4) persistent or intermittent fever. Additional data collected included patient information received from the physician, follow-up office visits, rehospitalization, or antibiotic therapy.

Eighteen patients had one or more complaints related to their surgical wound. Of the 18 patients identified, 16 surveys were returned by physicians. Of the 16 surveys returned, one of the physicians reported a surgical site infection, none of the patients required antibiotics, and no patient was rehospitalized with the diagnosis of surgical site infections. Based on the results of this study, the authors note that patient telephone surveys were inefficient in the detection of surgical site infections where traditional surveillance or monthly physician questionnaires are already operational. Health care professionals are encouraged to complete similar studies to identify usefulness of patient telephone surveys to improve the accuracy of surgical site infection surveillance.

Manian, F.A., & Meyer, L. (1993, April). Comparison of patient telephone survey with traditional surveillance and monthly physician questionnaires in monitoring surgical wound infections. *Infection Control and Hospital Epidemiology*, 216-218.

inflammation (Fig. 3-1). Nature provides many barriers for protection against disease-producing microorganisms, such as intact skin and mucous membranes.

Normally the leukocytes (white blood cells) remove debris, including bacteria, from the blood by devouring these foreign particles. This process is called *phagocytosis,* and the devouring cells are called *phagocytes*. Neutrophils and monocytes act as phagocytes in the devouring process (Fig. 3-2). In some cases the white cells are killed in the process

and accumulate at the site of the infection. This accumulation of decayed cells and serum is called *exudate*. The inflammatory response is an overall reaction of the body to injury. The action of the phagocytes, the bactericidal substances in the blood, and the action of the tissues to localize the infection result in the cardinal signs of inflammation: redness, heat, swelling, pain, and loss of function (Table 3-1).

When tissue injury or the body's response to the implantation and successful reproduction of a microorganism results in symptoms of illness, an infection occurs. The stages that lead to overt symptoms of an infection are definable but vary in duration according to the infectious agent. The *latent stage* follows invasion of the cells by a microorganism and lasts until the infection is evident (patent) and the organism can be shed. The *incubation stage,* the phase in

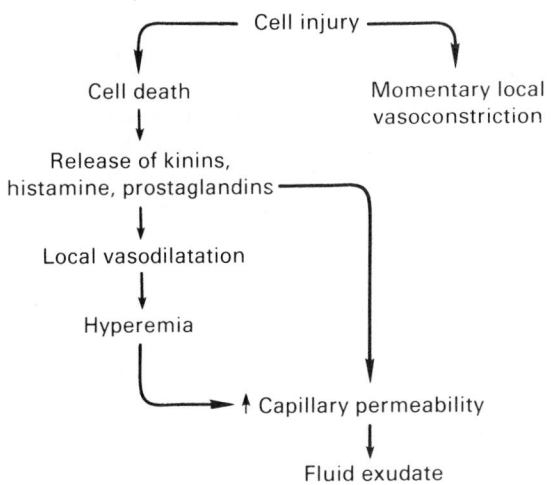

FIG. 3-1 Cellular response in inflammation.

From Lewis, S., & Collier, I. (1992). *Medical surgical nursing: Assessment and management of clinical problems* (3rd Ed.). St. Louis: Mosby.

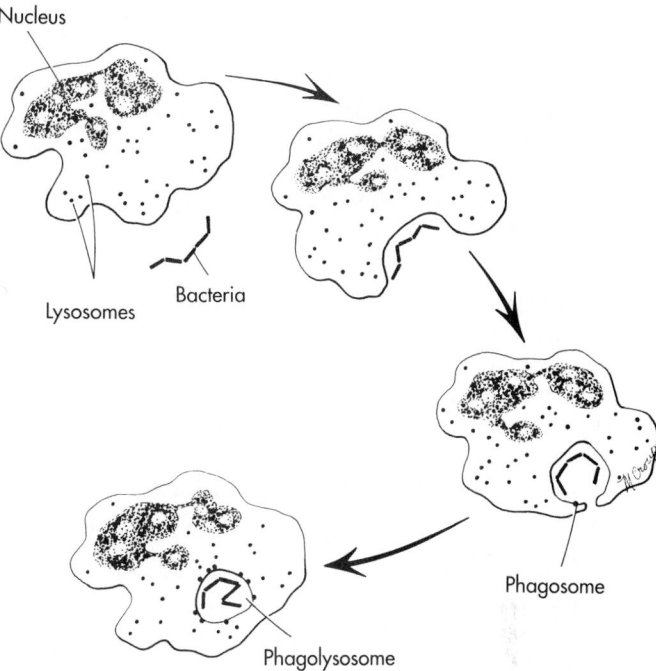

FIG. 3-2 Diagram of phagocytosis. Neutrophils and monocytes ingest particles by flowing their cytoplasm around the objects and internalizing them in an envelope of cell membrane, the phagosome. The digestive enzymes of the lysosomes are then released into the phagolysosome.

From Price, S.A., & Wilson, L. (1992). *Pathophysiology: Clinical concepts of disease processes* (4th Ed.). St. Louis: Mosby.

which the organism is multiplying, also starts with microorganism invasion and persists until the disease process is present. The *communicability period* begins when the latent period ends and continues as long as the agent is present. The *disease stage* may be asymptomatic (subclinical) or have observable presenting symptoms. This stage may resolve completely or become latent.

A *local* infection is one in which the causative agent is limited to one locality of the body and becomes circumscribed in a boil or abscess. *Primary* infection is the first infection that develops after microbial invasion. In *secondary* infection the microorganisms invade tissues in which there is an existing primary infection. When the infectious agents spread throughout the body tissues, the condition is termed a *systemic* infection. A *bacteremia* is the result of a singular or intermittent dissemination of microorganisms from a primary focus of infection into the bloodstream. In *septicemia* the microorganisms or their toxins are distributed more or less constantly and are continually present in the blood.

Sepsis is a generalized reaction to pathogenic microorganisms, their poisons, or both. The septic condition may be evident clinically by the signs of inflammation and the systemic manifestations of the patient.

An *antigen* is a foreign substance in the body that encourages specific immunity by production of specific substances called *antibodies*. General antibodies, which are proteins, appear to be produced mainly in the spleen, lymph glands, and bone marrow.

MICROORGANISMS THAT CAUSE INFECTION

Microorganisms are living organisms that are too small to be seen with the naked eye. These organisms include bacteria, fungi, protozoans, algae, and viruses. Microorganisms are classified to determine appropriate treatment for

TABLE 3-1

Local Manifestations of Inflammation

Manifestations	Cause
Redness (rubor)	Hyperemia from vasodilatation
Heat (calor)	Increased metabolism at inflammatory site
Pain (dolor)	Change in pH; change in local ionic concentration; nerve stimulation by chemicals (such as histamine, prostaglandins); pressure from fluid exudate
Swelling (tumor)	Fluid shift to interstitial spaces; fluid exudate accumulation
Loss of function (function laesa)	Swelling and pain

an infection. Each organism is assigned two names: genus is the first name, and the specific epithet (species) is the second. Scientific names can be assigned to organisms in various ways. For example, *Staphylococcus aureus* is a microorganism commonly found on the skin. *Staphylo* describes the clustered arrangement of the cells; *coccus* indicates they are shaped like spheres. The specific epithet *aureus* is Latin for golden, the color of the colonies of the bacterium.

Gram staining is one method used in identification of bacteria. Gram-positive bacteria have a thicker cell wall, whereas gram-negative bacteria have a thinner cell wall. The Gram stain of bacteria is necessary to determine which drug will be most effective against the disease. Gram-positive bacteria can usually be killed with penicillin and sulfonamide drugs. Gram-negative bacteria are resistant to penicillin, but sensitive to streptomycin, chloramphenicol, and tetracycline.

Staphylococci

Staphylococci are gram-positive cocci; they are facultative anaerobes, but grow best under aerobic conditions. Staphylococci are commensal constituents of the normal indigenous flora of the skin and mucous membranes of the nasopharynx, urethra, and vagina. They are very resistant to drying, heat, and high salt concentrations. This organism acts as an opportunist, usually as a result of trauma or foreign bodies.

Numerous disease processes are associated with *S. aureus*. The portals of entry are the skin, the respiratory tract, and the genitourinary tract. Staphylococci survive for long periods in the air, dust, debris, bedding, and clothing. Pathogenic staphylococci grow in the sweat, urine, tissue, and skin of humans. They are more difficult to destroy than many other non–spore-forming microorganisms.

The two most well known species of staphylococci are *Staphylococcus aureus* and *Staphylococcus epidermidis*. Coagulase-positive staphylococci produce coagulase and are considered more virulent or pathogenic. Coagulase-negative staphylococci (usually nonpathogenic) do not produce coagulase and are not as virulent. *S. aureus* is hemolytic, parasitic, pathogenic, and coagulase positive; *S. epidermidis* is parasitic, less pathogenic, and coagulase negative.

S. aureus, the most virulent species, produces invasive diseases such as endocarditis following open heart surgery. Toxigenic diseases produced as a result of *S. aureus* are toxic shock syndrome and food poisoning. *S. epidermidis,* the paradigm of the opportunistic pathogen, is involved in infections of the central nervous system, central venous catheters, peritoneal dialysis catheters, and orthopedic prostheses.

Studies of the response of staphylococci to various bacteriophages indicate that certain strains have epidemic potentials and that some are particularly virulent and drug resistant. Staphylococci are grouped in strains I, II, III, and miscellaneous. Two strains classified in this manner that are known to be highly virulent are 80/81 type and 77 type. In the past there were only one or two epidemic strains, whereas today there are several. Staphylococci vary in their resistance to antibiotics. For example, resistance of staphylococci to penicillin differs from their resistance to other antibiotics. Many formerly nonpathogenic strains are now disease-producing microorganisms (Ellner & Neu, 1992).

The emergence of methicillin-resistant *Staphylococcus aureus* (MRSA) requires antibiotic sensitivity testing. MRSA was first reported in hospitals in England around 1959, and in the United States around 1968. MRSA is highly virulent and resistant to many antibiotics. MRSA and other *aureus* strains have become one of the most frequent causes of hospital- and community-acquired infections. Isolation precautions to minimize the spread of MRSA in the hospital environment include basic measures such as handwashing between examination of patients, use of gloves (in addition to handwashing), masks, and infection control education to patients and health care personnel. Some hospitals have attempted to assign MRSA-positive staff members to MRSA-positive patients to decrease the number of patients and staff who might become exposed. The choice of whether to test, and if so whom to test, must be made by each hospital. The epidemiology department should establish a threshold of MRSA infections at which time further investigation, testing, and treatment would occur. The best means to control transmission of MRSA is following strict infection control guidelines (Shovein & Young, 1992).

Pathogenic staphylococci are capable of causing rapid suppuration. In many cases the staphylococci have a tendency to remain localized as an abscess and then break through to the outside. Eventually healing occurs. Wound sepsis is not the only manifestation of staphylococcal infection. Patients may suffer staphylococcal pneumonia, enterocolitis, urinary tract infection, or skin infection. Patients who undergo operations on the heart and great vessels seem to be particularly susceptible to coagulase-negative staphylococci.

Staphylococcal pneumonia may develop in patients who contract influenza in the hospital, especially surgical patients with advanced chronic bronchitis, uremia, or some other type of debilitating disease. If the pneumonia has been classified as caused by an epidemic strain of staphylococci, the patient may become a potent source of infection for other people. A patient with enterocolitis may suffer an acute onset of tachycardia, fever, and profuse diarrhea after surgery. For this reason terminal disinfection and zoning environmental principles, including adequate air changes, are important factors in an infection control program.

The skin surface is the most common site of staphylococci. Studies indicate that 30% to 70% of people carry staphylococci on their skin, which may lead to contamination of clothing and dispersal of the microorganisms. For no known reason, people who are skin carriers of staphylococci differ in their ability to shed the microorganisms. There is no obvious difference in hygiene and skin condition between light and heavy shedders, and no other contributing factor is apparent. Heavy shedders appear to be in normal good health.

The nasal and throat cavities are the most important reservoirs that continually replenish the external environment. *S. aureus* has been found in the nasal passages of 30% to 50% of the adult population (Malangoni & Hiram, 1989). Among operating suite personnel, *S. aureus* has been found in the respiratory passages 21% of the time (Grimes, 1991). The potential for patient infection increases greatly as the personnel carrier rate increases. Nasal carriers may also be skin carriers. Carriers usually harbor either coagulase-positive (pathogenic) or coagulase-negative (nonpathogenic) staphylococci—seldom both types—and rarely more than one strain. Because an individual may be a carrier of staphylococci one day and a noncarrier the next, frequent swab testing of the nose as a check to the spread of the microorganisms is impractical. Cleanliness of the environment, proper handling and sterilization of linens and equipment, and adherence to adequate washing techniques are important controls to prevent transmission of infection.

The severity of a staphylococcal infection in human beings is determined by many factors: type and size of the invading population, route of transmission, properties of the toxic products, and previous exposure and susceptibility of the host. Other contributing factors are the amount of physical trauma, the general health and nutritional state of the patient, the possibility of allergic states, and the presence of uncontrollable diabetes or toxemia.

Streptococci

Most streptococci are gram-positive, nonmotile, non–spore-forming microorganisms normally found in the indigenous flora of the upper respiratory, genitourinary, and gastrointestinal tracts. Streptococci can exist in either aerobic or anaerobic environments. Streptococci are classified according to their action on red blood cells (alpha, beta, or gamma hemolysis), their resistance to physical and chemical factors (for example, growth at 45° C, growth in 6.5% NaCl), and biochemical tests (for example, group-specific C carbohydrates). Alpha-hemolytic streptococci produce a number of toxic substances resulting in partial hemolysis of red blood cells. When alpha-hemolytic streptococci are present, a greenish discoloration surrounds the colony. Beta-hemolytic streptococci produce toxins that completely hemolyze red blood cells; when their cultures are grown on blood agar plates (preferably containing sheep blood), a colorless, clear zone surrounds the colony. Gamma-hemolytic streptococci do not hemolyze blood.

According to the immunologic differentiation proposed by Lancefield, group A hemolytic streptococci are primarily pathogens of humans, whereas group C hemolytic microorganisms are occasionally pathogens of humans. Other species are entirely saprophytic for humans. Group A streptococci account for most streptococcal infections in hu-

mans. An example is *S. pyogenes,* which is responsible for most soft tissue infections, otitis media, pharyngitis, impetigo, septicemia, and surgical site infections. Virulent streptococci are more serious invaders than are staphylococci because the former tend to involve wide areas of tissue and to cause necrosis without localization. However, this tendency is partially counterbalanced by the fact that, whereas these virulent streptococci are usually sensitive to penicillin, staphylococci may not be. Streptococci also occur in mixed infections with other pathogens.

In wounds a streptococcal infection is introduced through the skin, spreads by way of the lymph vessels and nodes, and results in inflammation, cellulitis, and sometimes suppuration. Alpha-hemolytic, or *viridans* type, streptococci, which normally reside in the respiratory tract or throat of humans, may produce a localized infection such as an abscess in the gums or teeth or subacute bacterial endocarditis. Alpha-hemolytic streptococci may also produce meningitis, although they are not very virulent, in contrast to pyogenic beta-hemolytic streptococci. Nonhemolytic streptococci or enterococci occasionally produce atypical pneumonia, endocarditis, or urinary tract infection.

Transmission of streptococci from the infected person to the susceptible host is accomplished by direct contact and by contamination of the environment. Direct contact may occur by inhalation of infectious droplets expelled from the nose and mouth or by hand-to-hand contact. Indirect contact is by means of infected air and dust in the environment. Most upper respiratory tract infections are caused by airborne microorganisms. The most dangerous carrier by far is the nasal carrier, who contributes large numbers of streptococci to the environment.

Prevention of streptococcal infections, via persons and via wounds, can be accomplished by adherence to aseptic techniques, including proper handling of contaminated clothing and masks, adequate ventilation with frequent air changes, exclusion from patient contact of personnel with acute sinusitis, and sterilization of supplies and instruments.

Streptococcus (Diplococcus) pneumoniae is a nonmotile, generally gram-positive, non–spore-forming diplococcus that produces no toxins of real significance. Pneumococci are the normal inhabitants of the upper respiratory tract of humans. Between 20% and 70% of people are at some time carriers of pneumococci. The carrier state is not permanent, but sporadic and intermittent. Most carriers tend to harbor the less virulent types of microorganisms. An individual may carry two or more types simultaneously. A healthy carrier is more important in dissemination of infection than is an infected patient.

Pneumococci are the primary cause of lobar pneumonia in humans. In this disease pneumococci do not remain in the lung but migrate from the source of infection through the nasal passages or are distributed by means of the vascular system to other parts of the body and then appear as a localized infection. Sinusitis, parotitis, conjunctivitis, peritonitis, and pyogenic infection such as arthritis are frequently caused by pneumococci.

Pneumococci are transmitted primarily by direct contact with and inhalation of droplets expelled into the air from the throat of the infected person or the carrier. Indirect transmission by way of contaminated objects is also possible. Prevention of pneumococcal infection is accomplished through environmental sanitation, exclusion of carriers from the operating room, effective care of patients, strict adherence to principles of asepsis, and use of chemotherapy.

Neisseria

Neisseria species are gram-negative, nonmotile, non–spore-forming diplococci. *N. catarrhalis* is found frequently in the nasopharynx of healthy people and in people with colds and other respiratory tract infections; *N. sicca* is present on the mucous membrane of the respiratory tract and may be a causative agent of kidney infection.

N. gonorrhoeae usually gains entrance to tissues after being deposited on and by burrowing through the mucous membranes, from which it is spread by the lymphatic or blood vessels. It may invade the bloodstream by means of local lesions. Gonorrheal vulvovaginitis is transmitted by bedding, clothing, and other inanimate vectors, whereas gonorrhea is spread by direct contact. Prophylaxis and control are accomplished by environmental sanitation and chemotherapy.

N. meningitidis, the meningococcus, is a pathogenic organism capable of producing acute meningitis in humans. Meningococci may gain access to the central nervous system via the nasopharynx. The method by which the meningococci leave the nasopharynx, invade the bloodstream, and reach the central nervous system is not known. Meningococcal meningitis is disseminated by direct contact and by droplet infection from secretions of the mouth, nose, and throat. Some persons are temporary carriers, whereas others are chronic meningococcal carriers.

Clostridium

Members of the genus *Clostridium* are gram-positive, anaerobic, spore-forming bacilli, many of which are pathogenic for humans. Clostridia are widely distributed in nature and are present in soil and the intestinal tract. The species include *C. tetani, C. perfringens, C. novyi, C. histolyticum, C. septicum,* and *C. botulinum; C. sporogenes* is one of the nonpathogenic species.

C. tetani produces tetanus (lockjaw) in humans. The bacilli normally reside in the soil and in the intestinal contents of some animals and humans. Tetanus toxin is a potent poisonous substance to humans. Tetanus is characterized by spasms of the voluntary muscles, particularly those of the jaw and neck—hence the name lockjaw. The bacilli gain entrance to the tissues by way of a deep, dirty wound and set up a localized infection. The toxin is disseminated throughout the body; when it reaches the nervous system, lockjaw occurs. Surgical tetanus may occur postoperatively and usually results from faulty sterilization of equipment or dressings. Puncture wounds provide anaerobic conditions that facilitate multiplication of tetanus bacilli. Injection-related tetanus in intravenous drug abusers is a contemporary public health problem. Tetanus of the newborn (tetanus neonatorum) may follow infection of the umbilicus. Treatment includes the use of antitoxin and an active immunization program.

Clostridial myonecrosis (gaseous gangrene) is produced by spores of *Clostridium* species present in contaminated wounds, especially those involving fracture or extensive tissue necrosis. Although usually associated with traumatic injuries, it sometimes develops in hospitalized patients in situations in which necrosis, vascular insufficiency, and possible fecal contamination occur. Accidental injuries, puerperal sepsis, and ruptured appendix may be accompanied by gaseous gangrene, which is usually caused by anaerobic, toxin-producing, spore-forming bacilli. The gangrenous process results from the activity of the sporulating obligate anaerobes and the exotoxins they produce. Several species of *Clostridium* may infect wounds and produce gaseous gangrene. The most common are *C. perfringens, C. novyi,* and *C. septicum; C. sporogenes,* although considered nonpathogenic, is found in many cases.

C. perfringens, an anaerobic pathogen, produces 80% of gaseous gangrene infections alone or with other anaerobic microorganisms in a closed abscess in uterine, gastrointestinal, genitourinary, or biliary infections. This microorganism is a normal inhabitant of the intestinal tract of humans. Entrance of *C. perfringens* into a wound does not always produce gaseous gangrene. The pathogenicity of a *Clostridium* species depends on the amount of powerful exotoxins it produces either within the body or in circumscribed tissues. In gaseous gangrene the gas in the tissues causes them to expand. This expansion creates pressure, thereby decreasing the flow of blood to the tissues, and necrosis results. The powerful exotoxins also weaken the general condition of the patient.

Clostridium difficile is the most common cause of antibiotic-related colitis. *C. difficile* is a gram-positive, spore-forming, anaerobic bacillus. This organism is widespread in the hospital environment. It can be found on toilets, bedpans, floors, or on the hands and in stool of asymptomatic hospital personnel. About 3% of healthy adults have *C. difficile* in their stool.

Pseudomonas

The best-known pathogenic, aerobic species of *Pseudomonas* for humans is *P. aeruginosa*. It thrives in moist environments and is frequently found in soil, water, sewage, debris, and air, and occasionally in the normal flora of the skin and intestines. Its incidence increases in the intestine when the coliform microorganisms are suppressed. Until recently it was considered a harmless saprophyte or possibly a microorganism of slight pathogenic power. *P. aeruginosa* has been found growing in intravenous fluids and soap solutions. Aqueous solutions such as benzalkonium chloride support the growth of *Pseudomonas*. It is now known to be associated with a great many suppurative infections in humans. *P. aeruginosa* appears to be a pathogen only when it is introduced into areas devoid of normal defenses, when it is superimposed on staphylococcal infection, or when it is present in a mixed infection. It may attack a debilitated patient who has extensive burns or traumatic injuries. *P. aeruginosa* is predominant in critical care and burn units.

P. aeruginosa is resistant to most antimicrobial agents. *P. maltophilia* and *P. cepacia* have been associated with intravascular cannula infections such as the use of pressure transducers. Environmental sanitation and strict adherence to aseptic techniques are important preventive measures.

Salmonella

Salmonella species are members of a large general classification of microorganisms that are often called *enteric* (or *coliform*) bacilli because they inhabit the intestinal tract of humans. These microorganisms are gram-negative, non–spore-forming, aerobic bacteria. Other well-known members are *Shigella* species (the dysentery bacilli), *Escherichia* species, and *Proteus* species (the paracolon bacilli).

Salmonella species are all pathogenic to a greater or lesser degree and are non–spore-forming, gram-negative, motile bacteria. They do not form exotoxins, but all of them possess endotoxins. *Salmonella* infection in humans is acquired by ingestion of the microorganism, usually in contaminated food or water. These bacteria may produce either clinical or subclinical infection. The three major diseases for which *Salmonella* are causative microorganisms are enteric fever, gastroenteritis, and septicemia. Other complications of *Salmonella* include endocarditis, meningitis, hepatitis, and intestinal perforation.

S. typhosa is the causative agent of typhoid fever. About 3% of patients with typhoid fever become carriers for some time. The bacteria remain in the gallbladder and intestine and occasionally in the urinary tract.

Escherichia

Escherichia coli, a gram-negative facultative bacillus, is the etiologic agent for 90% of community-acquired urinary tract infections (Ellner & Neu, 1992). *E. coli* is one of the most common causes of septicemia, inflammation of the liver, and infections of the gallbladder and urinary tract, especially when the host's defenses are inadequate, as in infants or elderly patients with terminal diseases. *E. coli* accounts for 40% of all nosocomial infections (Ellner & Neu, 1992). These microorganisms may also cause infection after radiation treatment and may escape through the wall of the bowel to cause secondary peritonitis. However, most strains of *E. coli* are nonpathogenic in the normal, healthy host.

Proteus

Proteus microorganisms are gram-negative, highly motile, aerobic bacilli, usually found free living in water, soil, dust, and sewage. *Proteus vulgaris* is often associated with *Pseudomonas aeruginosa*.

P. vulgaris is frequently found in the normal fecal flora of the intestinal tract. These bacilli also produce infection in humans only when they leave the intestinal tract. *Proteus* is a frequent cause of nosocomial infections of the urinary and respiratory tracts. This species may become the causative agent of cystitis and is most resistant to heat and antimicrobial agents. Specific antibiotics are active agents against *Proteus*.

Mycobacterium

Mycobacterium tuberculosis is a non–spore-forming, nonmotile, aerobic bacillus. *M. tuberculosis* multiplies best in an oxygen-rich environment. Disease is produced by establishment and proliferation of virulent microorganisms and interactions with the host. Tubercle bacilli spread in the host by direct extension through the lymphatic channels and bloodstream and by way of the bronchi and gastrointestinal tract. These bacilli can infect almost any tissue, including skin, bones, kidney, lymph nodes, intestinal tract, and fallopian tubes.

Tubercle bacilli are transmitted directly by means of discharge from the respiratory tract, less frequently through the digestive tract, by inhalation of droplets expelled during coughing, or by kissing. They are transmitted indirectly by means of contaminated articles and dust floating through the air. *M. tuberculosis* is carried by way of airborne particles when infected persons sneeze, cough, or speak. These particles are very small (1 to 5 μm) so that normal air current can keep them airborne (CDC, 1990). Once droplets are expelled, most will travel 3 to 4 feet and fall to the floor, while some will evaporate, leaving particles suspended in the air. When one or more mycobacteria enter an alveolus, they are promptly ingested by alveolar macrophages.

M. tuberculosis can be manifested in two ways. Tuberculosis infection is the presence of the mycobacteria in the tissue of a host, without clinical symptoms. Tuberculosis disease is a pathologic manifestation indicating destructive activity of mycobacteria in host tissue.

Recent outbreaks of tuberculosis have heightened concern about nosocomial transmission. Transmission is most likely to occur from patients with unrecognized pulmonary or laryngeal tuberculosis. The incidence of drug-resistant tuberculosis (DRTB) is rising in this country. Populations at greatest risk of developing TB or DRTB are the elderly, indigent, minorities, immigrants from countries where TB and DRTB are prevalent, and HIV-infected persons (Elpern & Girzadas, 1993). Transmission also occurs as a result of procedures such as bronchoscopy, endotracheal intubation and suctioning, and open abscess irrigation. Prevention of transmission includes the following practices:

1. Acid-fast bacilli isolation until antimicrobial therapy is successfully initiated for sputum-positive patients
2. Secretion precautions until wounds stop draining for patients with external TB lesions
3. Surgical intervention for massive hemoptysis, spontaneous pneumothorax, abscess drainage, or intestinal obstruction

4. Respiratory protection that provides a tight face seal and filters contaminants. In October, 1993 the Centers for Disease Control and Prevention presented draft guidelines for preventing the transmission of tuberculosis in health care facilities (Federal Register, Vol 58, No 195). Included in the guidelines are criteria for respiratory protection. The OSHA respiratory protection standard requires that all respirators:
   1. Have the ability to filter particles 1 micron in size, unloaded (without dust build-up) with a filter efficiency ≳ 95%.
   2. Must be fit tested to provide a face-seal leakage no greater than 10%.
   3. Be certified by the National Institute for Occupational Safety and Health (NIOSH).
   4. Are worn by persons potentially exposed to mycobacterium tuberculosis where engineering controls may not provide adequate protection (CDC, 1993).

The OSHA/CDC prevention and control guidelines include rigid environmental hygiene, disinfection and sterilization of contaminated equipment, and isolation of people with active infections as well as prompt identification, isolation and treatment of active TB patients, respiratory protection, training, testing of potentially exposed healthcare workers, and follow-up for those infected.

Chlamydia

Chlamydia is a gram-negative, anaerobic, nonmotile, coccoid bacteria. *Chlamydia* is highly infectious, easily transferred to new hosts, and is possibly the most successful parasite of all the microbial pathogens. Chlamydiae are transmitted by interpersonal contact or airborne respiratory routes. *Chlamydia* is found in 4% to 10% of pregnant women. Of the two species, *C. trachomatis* produces localized infection in mucous membranes and is the causative agent of trachoma, the most common cause of blindness in humans. This organism is also the major cause of sexually transmitted disease in the United States today. *C. psittaci* is the causative agent of ornithosis.

Viruses

Virus is the latin word for poison. The smallest infectious agents of humans are categorized as viruses. They are classified as small particles, rather than living cells, because viruses have no metabolic activity and must receive all sustenance for survival from a host cell. Viral pathogens are transmitted via the oral and respiratory tracts (for example, pox virus and rhinovirus), the intestinal and urinary tracts (such as poliovirus and hepatitis A virus [HAV]), the genital tract (including herpes simplex 2 and human immunodeficiency virus [HIV]), and through blood and some blood products (for instance, HIV, hepatitis B virus [HBV], and hepatitis C virus, formerly designated non-A, non-B hepatitis virus [NANB]). Some viruses have multiple routes of transmission. For example, HIV may be acquired through contact with blood, semen, or mother's milk or across the placenta.

Once a virus invades a host cell, it combines with the host cell's nucleic acid (DNA or RNA) and reprograms the host cell metabolism to accommodate virus replication. If the host cell dies, all the viruses are released; if the host cell lives, one virus at a time is released. This process approximates the latent stage of infection. Virus replication stimulates antibody defense in the host. Testing for the presence of the virus, in increasing order of difficulty and expense, may be by detecting virus-specific antibodies that are produced by the infected person's immune system, by detecting the antigens elaborated by the virus and present in the blood, or by growing a culture of the virus itself. Detection of virus-specific antibodies or antigens is termed *seropositivity* or *seroconversion*. Viruses are susceptible to destruction by high-level disinfection, a process that destroys most disease-producing microorganisms.

Viral hepatitis is one of the most frequently reported infectious diseases in the United States. The hepatitis virus invades, replicates, and produces damage only in the liver. Hepatitis A is the causative agent of infectious hepatitis. There is no specific treatment for the disease, but the incidence can be decreased by passive immunization. Persons at high risk can receive immune globulin (HBIG), which provides protection for several months.

Hepatitis B is the causative agent for serum hepatitis. The CDC estimate that 12,000 health care workers whose jobs place them at risk for exposure to blood or body fluid become infected with HBV each year. Of those infected, approximately 250 will die. Hepatitis B can be transmitted by virus-carrying blood (percutaneous) or any secretion of infective body fluid, (permucosal), such as blood, serum, saliva, semen, and vaginal fluids. The hepatitis B vaccine is recommended for health care workers regularly exposed to blood and body fluids. In 1987 the Department of Health and Human Services and the Department of Labor stated that hepatitis B vaccine should be available to all such workers without cost to the employee. Currently available hepatitis B vaccines provide over 90% protection against hepatitis B for 7 or more years after vaccination. Postexposure vaccination with hepatitis B vaccine has been 70% to 88% effective if given within 1 week of the exposure (CDC, 1989).

Hepatitis immune globulin provides passive protection after exposure. Postexposure prophylaxis for the unvaccinated person usually includes administration of HBIG and initiation of HB vaccine. Treatment for the vaccinated exposed person depends on the response of the hepatitis B surface antigen (HBsAg). When the source is found to be HBsAg negative, there is usually no treatment. If the source is found to be HBsAg positive, treatment varies from no treatment to administering HBIG followed by an HB vaccine booster dose.

HIV is the causative agent for acquired immune deficiency syndrome (AIDS). HIV has been isolated from blood, semen, vaginal secretions, saliva, tears, breast milk, cerebrospinal fluid, amniotic fluid, and urine of infected persons. Almost 180,000 cases of AIDS were reported in the United States as of May 1991. The World Health Organization predicts that by the year 2000 more than 40 million people may be infected with HIV. Transmission of HIV can occur by way of percutaneous or permucosal exposure to blood or other body fluids.

According to the CDC, postexposure treatment depends on hospital policy but should include the following measures:

1. The source patient is informed of the incident, and serology testing is done after consent is obtained. Policies should be established for instances when consent cannot be obtained.
2. The health care worker is counseled in regard to the risk of infection and evaluated clinically and serologically for evidence of HIV infection as soon as possible after exposure. The health care worker should be advised to seek medical evaluation for any acute febrile illness that occurs within 12 weeks of the exposure.
3. Seronegative health care workers should be retested after exposure at 6 weeks and then periodically, such as at 12 weeks and 6 months. Serologic testing should be available to all health care workers with concern of HIV exposure.

If a patient has parenteral or permucosal exposure to blood or other body fluid of a health care worker, the patient should be informed of the incident. The aforementioned procedure should apply for the management of exposure of the source health care worker and the exposed patient (CDC, 1987).

UNIVERSAL PRECAUTIONS

Universal precautions are not exclusively directed at the control of AIDS; rather, they are intended to control cross-infection of any pathogen, virus, or microorganism. The concept of universal precautions assumes that all recipients of health care are infectious. Universal precautions should be used for all invasive procedures to protect the health care worker and the patient. The CDC state that the blood and body fluids of all humans be considered contaminated and that the same safety precautions be followed whether or not the patient has a medically confirmed contagious disease. The difficulty in identifying patients with bloodborne HIV is the impetus for this recommendation. All patients who receive care might not have been tested for the virus; for those who have been tested, the reliability of the laboratory results may be questionable. The National Institutes of Health report that false positive results are possible when individuals do not have HIV, and false negative results may occur when persons possess all other criteria for AIDS. Further research is necessary before nursing actions can be selected based on the laboratory denial or confirmation of the presence of HIV.

Another influencing factor may perpetuate universal precautions indefinitely, even when testing is reliable. The latent phase of these HIV infections, shortly after exposure, is likely characterized by a lack of antibodies and low levels of virus proteins that fall below the threshold of detection. This information would dictate that health care professionals in the 1990s, as a safety measure, continue to presume all patients infectious. Although the national focus has been on HIV, the risk of acquiring the HBV is statistically greater than that for any of the other bloodborne viruses because the incidence of the disease is higher and it is more readily transmitted between hosts. The likelihood of HIV transmission by way of a needle-stick exposure is approximately 0.4%; the risk of transmission of HBV transmission by way of a needle stick exposure is 10% to 15%. HBV is preventable by using the vaccine, which provides protection in over 90% of individuals who receive all three injections (Bartlett, 1991).

The Occupational Safety and Health Administration (OSHA) published the final rule on exposure to bloodborne pathogens, which became effective March 6, 1992. OSHA determined that, in the case of bloodborne pathogens, the best way to reduce transmission is to reduce the risk. Universal precaution standards formed the basis of the bloodborne pathogen standard and are incorporated into this rule. This standard includes the following procedures:

1. An exposure control plan is the facility's overall plan for defining exposure and implementing the provisions set forth by the standard. This plan is to be reviewed and revised annually with this information provided to all employees.
2. Engineering and work practice controls shall be used to eliminate or minimize employee exposure. Provisions of this rule include the following. (a) The employer will provide everything necessary for proper handwashing. (b) Contaminated needles shall not be recapped or removed unless such action is required by a specific medical procedure. Such recapping or removal must be accomplished by the use of a mechanical device or one-handed technique. A clamp or other mechanical device should be used to disassemble a knife blade and handle. (Though the issue is not addressed in the bloodborne pathogen standard, the AORN recommends that a no-touch technique or neutral zone be established for all invasive procedures. This technique, also referred to as defensive scrubbing, was established to minimize health care workers touching the same instrument at the same time by placing the instrument in a neutral zone. All needles or sharp instruments should be returned to the neutral zone designated by the scrub nurse and surgeon, such as a basin or instrument magnet.) (c) Sharps are to be placed in labeled or color-coded, puncture-resistant, leakproof containers for disposal. (d) Specimens of blood or body fluids must be placed

in containers that prevent leakage and are labeled or color coded. (e) Food and drink are not to be kept in the same storage area where blood or other potential infectious materials are present.

3. Personal protective equipment (PPE) shall be provided by the employer at no cost to the employee. Appropriate equipment shall include, but is not limited to, gloves, gowns, masks, face shields or masks, and eye protection. Protective eyewear must have solid side shields. Gloves are to be worn when contact with blood or body fluids is anticipated. Single-use gloves are to be replaced as soon as possible after contamination occurs. Disposable gloves are not to be washed or decontaminated for reuse.

4. Housekeeping provisions are made to ensure that the workplace is maintained in a clean and sanitary condition. A written schedule for cleaning and a method of decontamination shall be established. All equipment and working surfaces shall be cleaned and decontaminated after contact with blood or other potentially infectious materials. Contaminated laundry must be placed in a labeled or color-coded container that is recognized by all affected employees.

5. All employees are to receive education and training about safe handling of hazardous substances and materials. Information must be provided to all occupationally exposed employees at no cost to them. OSHA requires that individuals receive training at the time of employment and annually thereafter. Individual employee training records are to be maintained by the employer for the duration of employment plus 30 years. Some institutions may have educational signs posted to assist employees in recognition of appropriate personal protective equipment (Fig. 3-3).

6. Warning labels shall be affixed to containers of regulated waste, refrigerators and freezers containing blood or potentially infectious material, and other containers used to transport blood or potentially infectious material (Fig. 3-4). The labels shall be fluorescent orange or orange-red. Signs shall be posted at the entrance to work areas of potential contamination and bear the biohazard legend with the following information: name of infectious agent; special requirements for entering the area; and name and telephone number of the responsible person.

7. The health care worker is highly encouraged to receive the hepatitis B vaccine after receiving the required information about the risk of exposure and about the vaccine. If the employee chooses not to accept the vaccination, the employer must have the employee sign a declination statement. Employees are to report all exposures to blood and body fluids for postexposure evaluation.

The bloodborne pathogen standard (BBPS) will be enforced by the Federal and State Occupational Safety and Health Administration by completion of on-site visits to health care facilities. OSHA may visit any site where an employee is exposed without notification to the employer. The visit may be a result of an employee concern, referral from another regulatory agency, or random inspections of facilities. The inspector requests an opening conference with management and outlines the extent of the inspection. Compliance will be determined by reviewing recordkeeping, the exposure control plan, and accident investigation records. A walk-through of the workplace with employee

BODY SUBSTANCE ISOLATION IS FOR ALL PATIENT CARE | **BODY SUBSTANCES INCLUDE ORAL SECRETIONS, BLOOD, URINE AND FECES, WOUND OR OTHER DRAINAGE.**

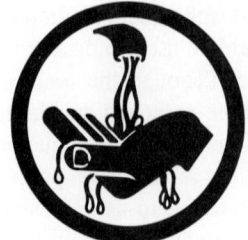 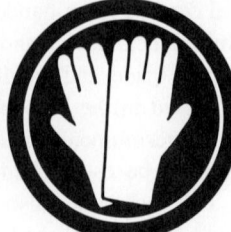  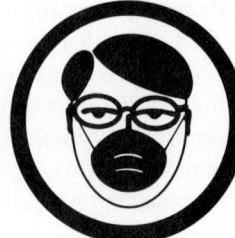 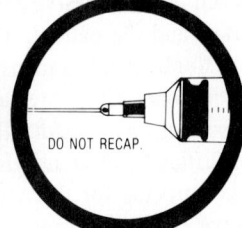

Wash hands.

Wear gloves when likely to touch body substances, mucous membranes or nonintact skin.

Wear plastic apron when clothing is likely to be soiled.

Wear mask/eye protection when likely to be splashed.

DO NOT RECAP.

Place intact needle/syringe units and sharps in designated disposal container. **Do not** break or bend needles.

© 1987 San Diego Forms

FIG. 3-3 Example of universal symbols for blood and body fluid protection.
From Whaley, L., & Wong, D. (1991). *Nursing care of infants and children* (4th Ed.). St Louis: Mosby.

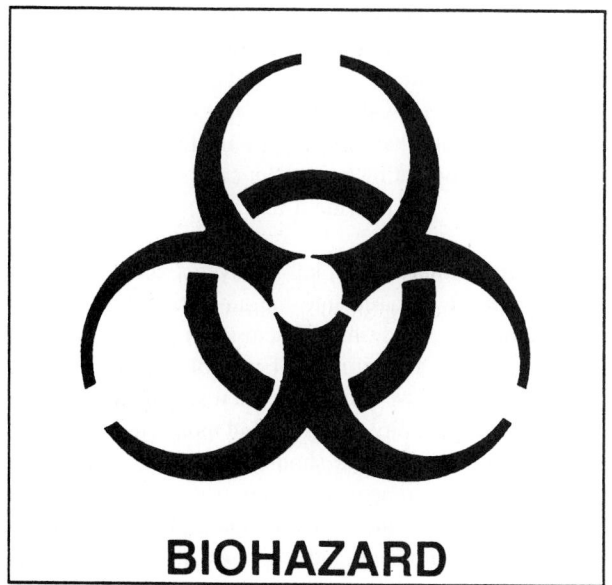

FIG. 3-4   Biohazard label.
Courtesy Charleston Area Medical Center.

INFECTION CONTROL PRACTICES FOR PERIOPERATIVE PERSONNEL

Large quantities of bacteria are present in the nose and mouth, on the skin, and on the attire of personnel who enter the restricted areas of the surgical setting. Proper design of facilities and regulations for use of surgical attire are important ways of preventing transportation of microorganisms into surgical settings, where they may infect patients' open wounds.

Infection control practices should focus on prevention. Transmission of infection involves a chain of events, which include a pathogenic agent, reservoir, portal of exit, transmission, portal of entry, and host susceptibility. Prevention occurs when there is a break in the chain of transmission.

Infection control practices also involve personal and administrative measures. Personal measures include personal fitness for work, skin disinfection (patient and personnel), preparation of personnel hands, surgical attire, and personnel technique (surgical conscience). Administrative measures include provision of adequate physical facilities, appropriate surgical supplies, and operational controls.

Areas should be provided where staff members may remove personal clothing, don surgical attire, and enter the semirestricted area of the surgical setting directly, without passing through a contaminated area. Daily body cleanliness and clean, dandruff-free hair help prevent superficial wound infections. Hair is a fertile source of bacteria. The hair of the head and of other areas of the body may shed debris and dead cells that can be transported to an open wound. The person who is well rested and healthy is less subject to infectious diseases. Personnel who have nose or throat infections, are known to be carriers, or have open sores should not be permitted in surgical settings.

PROPER SURGICAL ATTIRE

Every surgical department should have a written policy and procedure regarding proper attire in the surgical suite. Many points should be considered in establishing regulations for proper surgical apparel. Personal protective equipment (PPE), which includes protective eyewear, gloves,

interviews will also be done. A closing conference will be held to determine the extent of compliance to the bloodborne standard. OSHA will levy fines on facilities where violations have not been corrected (Jacobs, 1993).

Universal precautions serve to protect the health care provider and to minimize cross-infection of pathogens between patients (Table 3-2). Thus the circulating nurse should not wear the same pair of gloves during the entire surgical procedure, touching first the patient and then the sterile supply cart. All equipment and supplies, as well as all laundry and trash, that have been in contact with the patient are considered contaminated and should be considered infectious. Local health codes for trash and waste disposal should be consulted; all waste and trash should be confined in readily identifiable plastic bags. The implementation of universal precautions in surgical settings requires perioperative nursing judgment.

TABLE 3-2

Universal Precautions: Intraoperative Examples Applicable to Circulating Nurses

Nursing action	Potential contaminant	Precaution
Changing the refuse receptacle for pulsatile irrigation	Irrigation splashes out of container	Goggles, nonsterile gloves
Positioning of a multiple trauma patient with active bleeding	Direct contact with blood or excreta on the skin or scrub attire	Goggles, nonsterile gloves, waterproof apron or nonsterile gown
Removing drapes following a surgery with an estimated blood loss of 50 ml	Direct contact with contaminated drape	Nonsterile gown and gloves, impervious container

and fluid-resistant gowns, aprons, and shoe covers, should be included as part of the surgical attire regulations.

Street clothes should never be worn within semirestricted or restricted areas of the surgical suite. There should be a point of demarcation between unrestricted and semirestricted areas past which no one may go, unless properly attired. All persons who enter semirestricted or restricted surgical areas should be required to wear clean surgical apparel made of materials that meet the National Fire Protection Association standards. This apparel should include hat or hood, one- or two-piece pantsuit, shoe covers, and face mask (Fig. 3-5). Apparel should cover as much skin as possible to protect against shedding and should be flame resistant, lint free, cool, and comfortable.

When visibly soiled or wet, surgical attire should be changed to reduce the potential of cross-infection. All reusable attire should be laundered after each use in a laundry facility approved and monitored by the hospital, and it should be protected from contamination during transfer and storage.

The first item of apparel donned should be a clean, lint-free surgical hat or hood that completely covers all head and facial hair. It eliminates the possibility of hair or dandruff being shed on the scrub suit. The design and composition of the hat or hood should minimize dispersal of bacteria and be comfortable to wear. All hair must be confined as well as covered. Skullcaps that fail to cover the side hair above the ears and hair at the nape of the neck should not be worn in the operating room. Net caps should not be used because they do not provide a barrier to dandruff and hair fallout.

Hair acts as a filter when left uncovered and collects bacteria, which are released into the air during activity. Hair attracts, harbors, and sheds bacteria in proportion to its length, curliness, and oiliness. If reusable hats or hoods are worn, they should be laundered when soiled, or after each use in a laundry facility approved and monitored by the hospital. Disposable headgear should be discarded in a designated receptacle immediately after use. Headgear should not be worn outside the suite. It should always be worn in areas where equipment and supplies are processed and stored.

Scrub suits should be made of a closely woven fabric that minimizes bacterial shedding. They should fit well for comfort and appearance. Care must be taken when donning scrub pants to avoid dragging the pant legs on the floor.

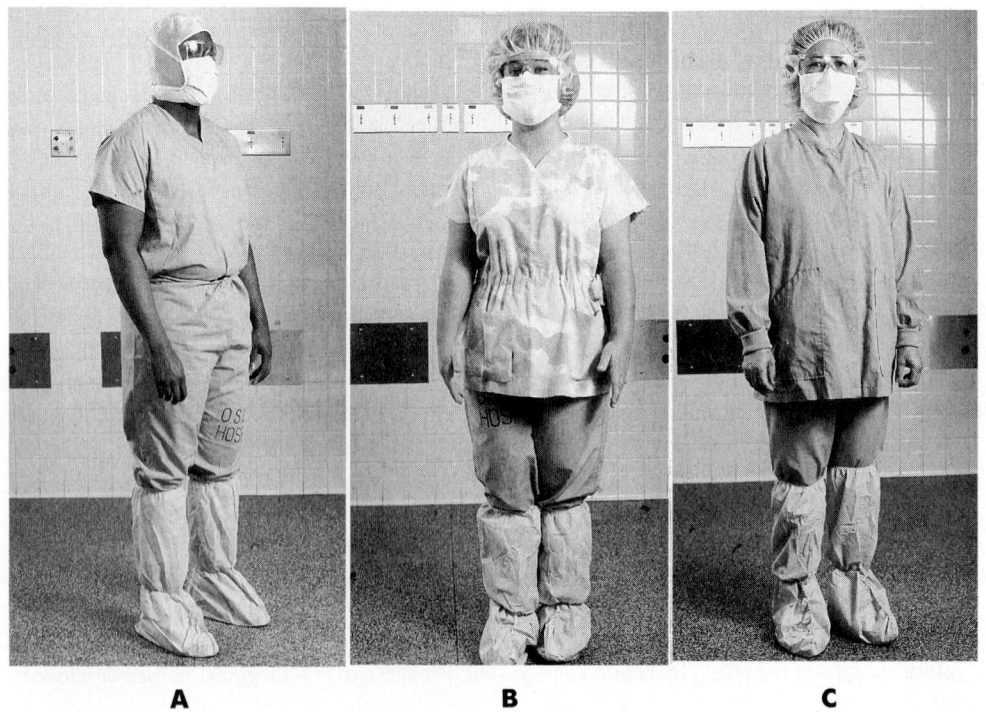

A   **B**   **C**

FIG. 3-5 Proper surgical attire consists of a two-piece pant suit or a one-piece coverall suit. Shoe covers may be worn; they should be changed whenever they become wet, torn, or soiled. All head and facial hair should be covered in the semirestricted and restricted areas. In the restricted area, all personnel should wear masks. Jewelry should be removed or totally confined. Nail polish or artificial nails should not be worn. When a two-piece scrub suit is worn, loose fitting scrub tops should be tucked into pants **(A)**, or tunic tops that fit close to the body may be worn outside of pants **(B). C,** Nonscrubbed personnel should wear long-sleeved jackets that are buttoned or snapped closed.

The top of a scrub suit should be secured at the waist, or tucked into the pants, or fit close to the body. Scrub pants may be designed with close-fitting cuffs or ankle closures to decrease dispersal of bacteria. Loose, flapping folds or shirttails and baggy trousers are sources of possible contamination as personnel move; bacteria are freed by friction. One-piece coverall suits may be worn as alternatives to two-piece suits. Scrub attire should be changed when soiled, and home laundering is not recommended.

Nonscrubbed personnel should wear warm-up jackets to prevent shedding from bare arms. Jackets should be snapped at all times in the operating room to eliminate the possibility of the material brushing against a sterile field.

Shoe covers may be worn by personnel entering the semirestricted or restricted areas of the surgical suite. The primary reason for the use of shoe covers is sanitation, because even the most conscientious person has difficulty keeping shoes clean all the time in a busy operating room. Knee-high shoe covers are recommended for use as PPE in surgical procedures where a large amount of fluid or blood is anticipated. They should be removed when leaving the operating room. Shoe covers should be worn only within the semirestricted or restricted areas; shoe covers should be changed when they are soiled, wet, or torn, which will reduce tracking and facilitate good housekeeping.

Shoe covers should be kept in an area adjacent to the semirestricted area entrance. They should be removed on leaving the semirestricted area, and clean shoe covers should be put on when returning to that area. Cross-contamination from the surgical suite to other areas of the hospital must be prevented. Footwear should provide support and protection for the feet and should be easy to clean. Clogs, sandals, and soft shoes present a safety hazard and are unacceptable footwear for use in surgical settings.

The use of specially designed masks in surgical settings is vital to prevention of infection. Masks are also vital in the protection of health care workers due to aerosolization caused by pathogenic organisms and aerosol particles from the high-technology surgical environment. Everyone should wear high-filtration/fluid-resistant masks at all times in the operating room and other designated areas where open sterile supplies or scrubbed people may be located. One mask is worn. Double masking provides a barrier rather than a filter and therefore is unacceptable.

Cloth or gauze masks are not acceptable for use in surgical settings. They have a very low filtration efficiency and may become ineffective as a bacterial barrier within 30 minutes of wear. The wearer who breathes through a face mask that is thickly inoculated with expired bacteria may expel a higher number of microorganisms into the atmosphere than does the individual who breathes normally and quietly without a mask. Forceful expulsion of the breath during talking, laughing, or sneezing propels large concentrations of microorganisms into the air.

When choosing a mask, one with a microbial filtration efficiency of 95% or above should be selected. Aerosol particles generated by the surgical team, sometimes visible to the naked eye, are most likely 10 μm or larger. The plume of lasers or the electrosurgical unit has been found to contain particles with a mass of 0.31 μm, smaller than that expelled by the surgical staff. Therefore the filtration efficiency of masks should ensure protection against aerosol particles as small as 0.1 μm (Chen & Willeke, 1992). However, the most effective filter mask is relatively useless if worn incorrectly and can be dangerous if handled improperly.

Before handling or donning a mask, the person should wash the hands to prevent contamination of the mask. Fig. 3-6 describes the proper application and removal of the surgical mask. The mask must cover the mouth and nose entirely, have facial compliance, and be tied securely to prevent venting. The strings should not be crossed when tied because the sides of the mask will gap and permit nonfiltered air to escape through venting. A pliable metal strip in the top hem of most masks provides a firm, contoured fit over the bridge of the nose. This strip also helps prevent fogging of eyeglasses.

Air should pass only through the filtering system of the mask. Masks should be either on (properly) or off. They should not be saved from one operation to the next by being left hanging around the neck or being tucked into a pocket. Bacteria that have been filtered by the mask will become dry and airborne if the mask is worn necklace fashion. Touching only the strings when removing the mask reduces contamination of the hands. Masks should be changed between procedures and sometimes during a procedure, depending on the length of the operation and the amount of talking done by the team.

To remove a mask, the wearer should handle only the ties. The facepiece, which is highly contaminated with droplet nuclei, should not come in contact with the hands of personnel. Immediately after removal, masks should be discarded directly into a designated, covered waste receptable. After discarding the mask, the wearer must wash and dry the hands thoroughly.

All jewelry should be confined within scrub attire or removed when personnel enter the semirestricted or restricted areas of the surgical suite. Before handwashing, rings, watches, and bracelets should be removed to eliminate harboring organisms. Total confinement of jewelry reduces the potential of it falling into a sterile field or wound.

Because nail polish may crack or chip during performance of intraoperative functions and subsequently harbor organisms, it should be removed before handwashing. Perioperative personnel should not wear acrylic or artificial nails because they may also harbor organisms and prevent effective handwashing (Research Highlight 3-3). Numerous state boards of cosmetology report that fungal growth occurs frequently under artificial nails.

Surgical attire should not be worn outside the operating room department. However, if this practice is not feasible, the scrub suit should be covered by a single-use cover gown with a back closure when a person leaves the department. Upon return to the unit the cover gown should be discarded.

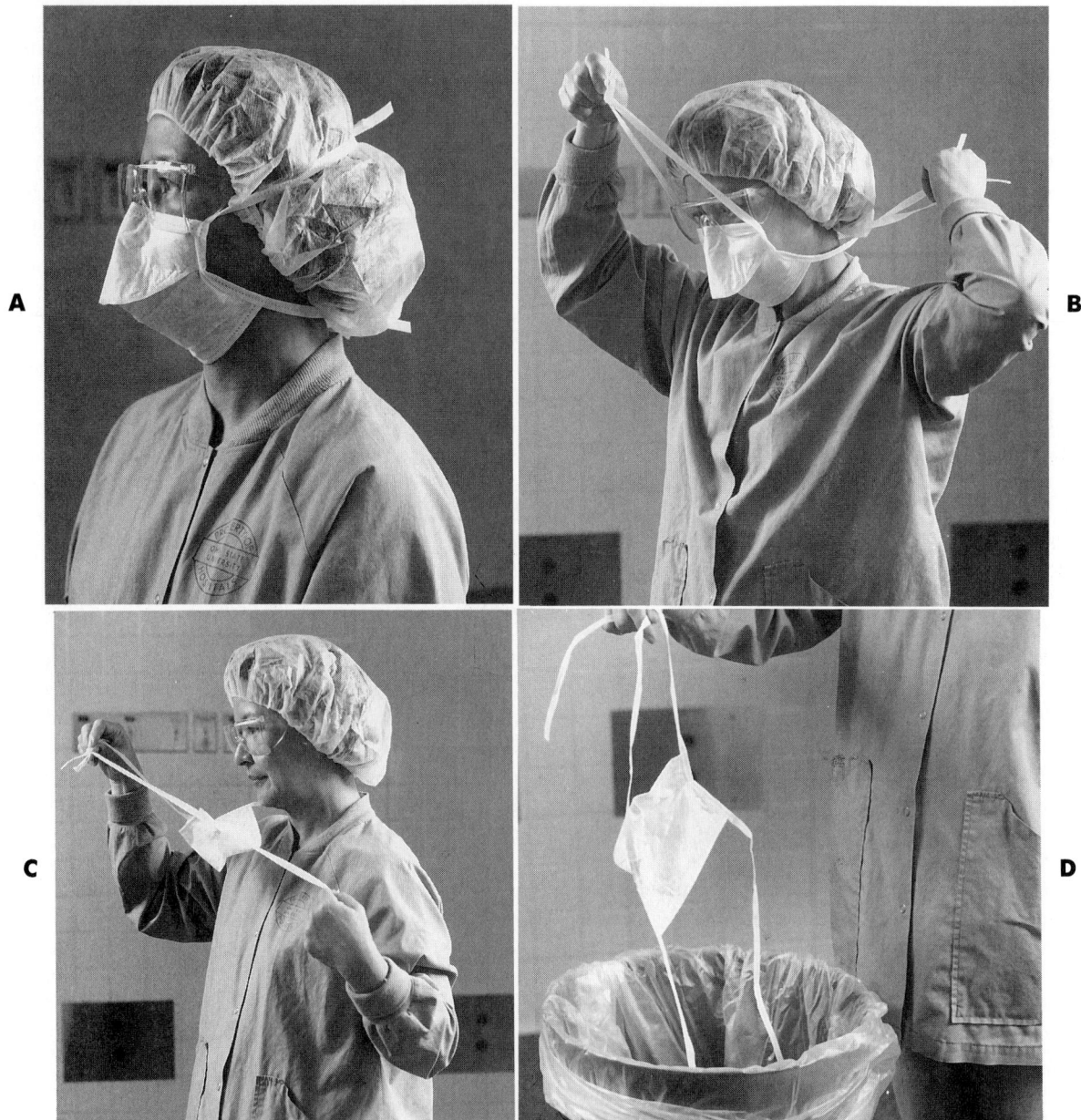

FIG. 3-6 Proper handling of mask. **A,** Edges of properly worn mask conform to facial contours when mask is applied and tied correctly. `**B** and **C,** Personnel should avoid touching filter portion of mask when removing it. **D,** Masks should be discarded upon removal.

If the cover gown is not disposable, it should be placed in the laundry. A front-opening lab coat is less suitable for protecting scrub attire outside the department. Head and shoe coverings should always be removed. When the person returns to the department, the scrub suit should be changed because the cover gown or lab coat is not an effective barrier to bacteria and other potential external contaminants. With the recent mandate for no smoking within health care facilities, individual institutional policies should be established to address the wearing of surgical attire outside of the facility.

BASIC ASEPTIC TECHNIQUE

An object or substance is considered sterile when it is completely free from living microorganisms and is incapable of producing any form of life. The basic principles of aseptic technique prevent contamination of the open wound, isolate the operative site from the surrounding unsterile physical environment, and create and maintain a sterile field in which surgery can be performed safely.

The surgical team is composed of scrubbed and circulating persons. Those who scrub their hands and arms and don sterile gowns and gloves are referred to as the *scrubbed*

RESEARCH HIGHLIGHT 3-3

As fashion trends support the wearing of artificial nails, the implications of these nails for infection control purposes among health care workers needs to be considered. This study was done to compare the number of bacterial organisms found on the fingertips of nursing personnel with artificial nails and the fingertips of nursing personnel with natural nails. A second purpose was to determine the effect of handwashing on the number of bacterial organisms on artificial versus natural nails. The sample size included 56 nurses with artificial nails and 56 nurses with natural nails. The study included nurses selected from five different hospitals. Organisms were classified into three categories: normal flora, gram-negative rods, and gram-positive cocci.

Results of this study found no significant difference when the following variables were compared with those of artificial and natural nail groups: the type of soap used, the number of handwashings, and the length of time between handwashing and the collection of cultures. Seven nurses had more than 500 colony forming units (CFU) after handwashing, and five nurses had more than 100 CFUs after handwashing. A pure culture of more than 500 CFUs of *Pseudomonas* was grown from samples taken before and after handwashing from a nurse with artificial nails. In the nurses with natural nails three had 3 to 14 CFUs of gram-negative rods before handwashing and 0 to 4 CFUs of gram-negative rods after handwashing. Gram-negative rods have been identified as a cause of nosocomial infections in the hospital setting. The gram-negative rod cultures grown from nurses with artificial nails were *Serratia, Acinetobacter,* and *Pseudomonas*. The study reported that nurses with artificial nails harbored greater numbers of gram-negative rods before and after handwashing than nurses with natural nails. This finding suggests a potential impact on bacterial transmission that influences the development of infection. Further epidemiologic investigation suggestive of person-to-person bacterial transmission would be reason to restrict health care workers who wear artificial nails from working in high-risk areas or have them remove the artificial nails.

Pottinger, J., Burns, S., & Manske, C. (1989). Bacterial carriage by artificial versus natural nails. *American Journal of Infection Control*, 340-344.

persons; those who supply the needs of the scrubbed team members, coordinate room activities, and attend to patient needs are referred to as *circulators* who are registered nurses.

Proper adherence to aseptic technique eliminates or minimizes modes and sources of contamination. Certain basic principles must be observed during surgery to provide a well-defined margin of safety for the patient.

1. All materials in contact with the wound and used within the sterile field must be sterile. The inadvertent use of unsterile items may introduce contaminants into the wound. When using or dispensing a sterile item, personnel must be assured that the item is sterile and will remain sterile until used. Items of doubtful sterility must be considered unsterile. Any item that falls on the floor or into any area of questionable cleanliness must be considered unsterile. The circulating nurse should check the package integrity, the expiration date, and the chemical process indicator before dispensing a sterile item.

2. Gowns of the surgical team are considered sterile in front from chest to the level of the sterile field. The sleeves are also considered sterile from 2 inches above the elbow to the stockinette cuff. The cuff should be considered unsterile because it tends to collect moisture and is not an effective bacterial barrier. Therefore the sleeve cuffs should always be covered by sterile gloves. Other areas of the gown that must be considered unsterile are the neckline, shoulders, areas under the arms, and back. These areas may become contaminated by perspiration or by collar and shoulder surfaces rubbing together during head and neck movements. Wraparound gowns that completely cover the back may be sterile when first put on. The back of the gown, however, *must not* be considered sterile because it cannot be observed by the scrubbed person and protected from contamination.

   The sterile area of the front of the gown extends to the level of the sterile field because most scrubbed personnel work adjacent to a sterile table. For this reason the scrubbed person should avoid changing levels, as would occur while moving from footstool to floor. To maintain sterility, scrubbed persons should not allow their hands or any sterile item to fall below the level of the sterile field. Scrubbed persons should neither sit nor lean against unsterile surfaces because the threat of contamination is great. The only time scrubbed persons may be seated is when the entire surgical procedure will be performed at that level.

3. Sterile drapes are used to create a sterile field. Only the top surface of a draped table is considered sterile. Although a bacterial barrier may be draped over the sides of a table, the sides cannot be considered sterile. Any item that extends beyond the sterile boundary is considered contaminated and cannot be brought back onto the sterile field. A contaminated item must be lifted clear of the operative field without contacting the sterile surface and must be dropped with minimum handling to an unsterile person, area, or receptacle. Interpretation of sterile areas versus unsterile areas on a draped patient requires astute observation and use of good judgment.

4. Items should be dispensed to a sterile field by methods that preserve the sterility of the items and the integrity of the sterile field. Good judgment must be used when dispensing items either by presenting them to the

scrubbed person or by placing them securely on the sterile field. Items should not be tossed onto a sterile field because they may roll off the edge and become contaminated, displace other items, or penetrate the drape.

After a sterile package or container is opened, the edges are considered unsterile. Sterile and unsterile boundaries are often intangible. A 1-inch safety margin is usually considered standard on package wrappers, whereas the sterile boundary on a wrapper used to drape a table is at the table edge. On peel-back packages, the inner edge of the heat seal is the line of demarcation. Being hypothetical, these boundaries may not apply to every situation.

The edge of a bottle cap is considered contaminated once the cap has been removed from the bottle. The sterility of the bottle contents cannot be ensured if the cap is replaced on the bottle. Therefore, when sterile liquids are dispensed, the entire contents of a bottle must be poured or the remainder discarded. Interpreting sterile boundaries requires good judgment based on an understanding of aseptic principles.

5. Motions of the surgical team are from sterile to sterile areas and from unsterile to unsterile areas. Scrubbed persons and sterile items contact only sterile areas; circulating nurses and unsterile items contact only unsterile areas. All members of the surgical team must understand which areas are considered sterile and which are con-

sidered unsterile. All must maintain a continual awareness of these areas. Scrubbed persons must guard their sterile fields to prevent any unsterile item from contaminating the fields or them. Circulating nurses must not touch or reach over a sterile field or allow any unsterile item to contaminate the field. When a circulating nurse opens a package, hand and arm motions are always from unsterile to unsterile objects. The circulating nurse avoids contact with the sterile area by placing the hands under the cuff to provide a protected wide margin of safety between the inside of the pack (sterile) and the hands (unsterile) (Fig. 3-7). As the circulating nurse opens a sterile article that is wrapped sequentially in two wrappers with the corners folded toward the center of the article, the corner farthest from the body is opened first, and the corner nearest the body last (Fig. 3-8).

When a scrub nurse opens a sterile wrapper, the side nearest the body is opened first. This portion of the wrapper then protects the gown and enables the individual to move closer to the table to open the opposite side (Fig. 3-9).

If a solution must be poured into a sterile receptacle on a sterile table, the scrub nurse holds the receptacle away from the table or sets it near the edge of a waterproof-draped table (Fig. 3-10). This procedure eliminates the need for the circulating nurse to reach over the sterile field. Maintaining a safe margin of space can reduce accidental contamination in passing items between sterile and unsterile fields. An instrument may be used as an extension of a team member's hands to ensure a safe margin between fields. The use of transfer forceps, however, is unacceptable. Maintaining the sterility of these forceps is questionable because of the many variables, such as sterilization method, type of container, and type and amount of soaking solution used. Incorrect handling of soaked forceps is always a problem. Transfer forceps have been replaced by a packaged sterile instrument that is used once and then considered contaminated.

6. Movement around a sterile field must not cause contamination of that sterile field. The patient is the center of the sterile field during an operation; additional sterile areas are grouped around the patient. If contamination is to be prevented, patterns of movement within or around this sterile grouping must be established and rigidly practiced. Scrubbed persons stay close to the sterile field. If they change positions, they turn face to face or back to back while maintaining a safe distance between. Accidental contamination is a threat to any scrubbed person who wanders into a traffic pathway or out of the clean area of the operating room. Circulating nurses approach sterile areas facing them and never walk between two sterile fields. Keeping sterile areas in view during movement around the area and maintaining at least a 1-foot distance from sterile fields help to prevent accidental contamination. Bacterial fallout from the body or

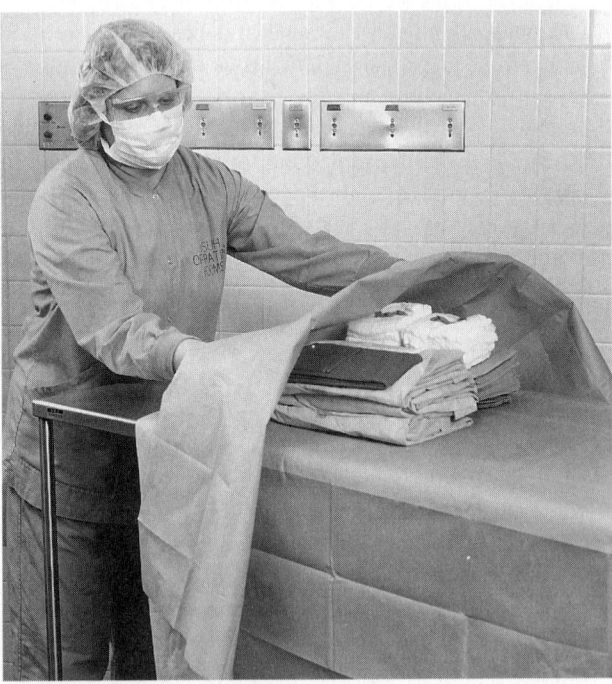

FIG. 3-7 Circulating nurse is shown opening outer cover of pack containing sterile drapes for surgery. Cover is cuffed to provide protection for sterile contents. Circulating nurse avoids contact with sterile area by keeping all fingers under cuff as cover is drawn back over table to expose inner pack.

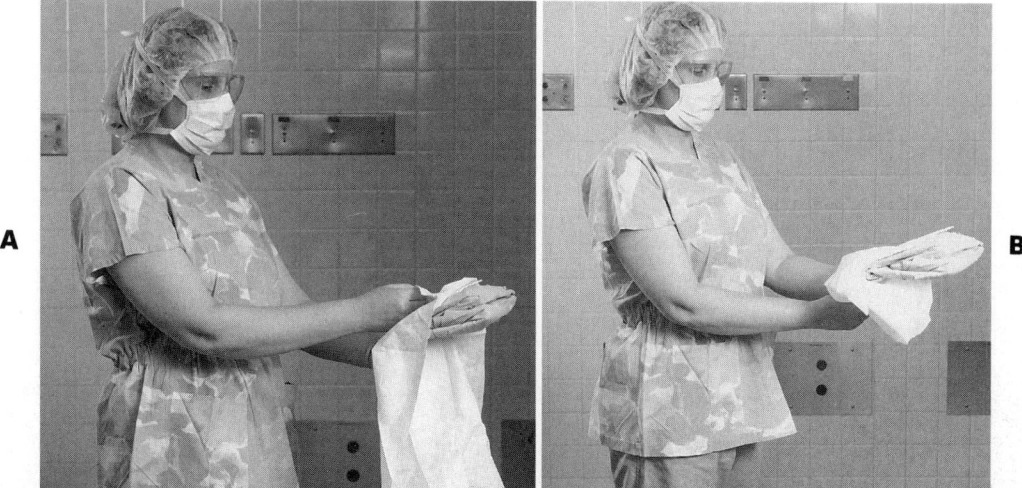

FIG. 3-8 **A,** When opening sterile package, circulating nurse opens corner nearest body last to avoid potential contamination of inner pack. **B,** To prevent unsterile corners of outer wrapper from touching scrub nurse or sterile field, circulating nurse draws back corners of opened wrapper when presenting inner package.

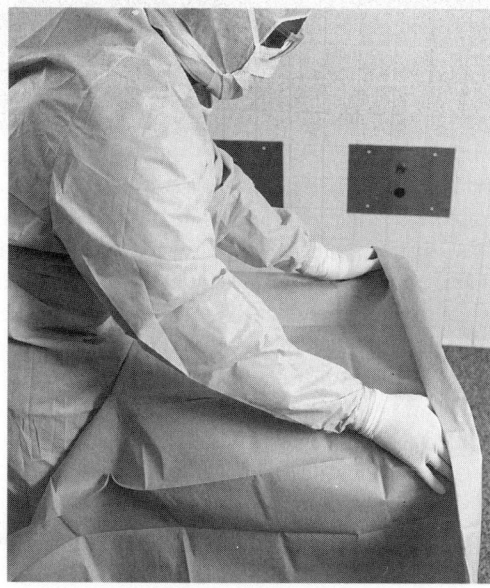

FIG. 3-9 Scrub nurse protects gloves with cuff of drape when opening inner wrapper of pack, which will serve as sterile table cover.

clothing is a source of contamination when a circulating nurse leans over a sterile field. All perioperative personnel must maintain a vigilant watch over sterile areas and point out any contamination immediately.
7. Whenever a sterile barrier is permeated, it must be considered contaminated. This principle applies to packaging materials as well as to draping and gowning materials. Obvious contamination occurs from direct contact between sterile and unsterile objects. Other less apparent modes of contamination are the filtration of airborne microorganisms through materials, the passage of liq-

uids through materials, and the undetected perforations in materials. When moisture soaks through a drape, gown, or package, *strike-through* occurs, and the item must be considered contaminated. Potential contaminants can be curtailed by the use of effective barrier materials, the characteristics of which are discussed later in this chapter.
8. Every sterile field should be constantly monitored and maintained. Sterility cannot be ensured without direct observation of the sterile field.

Preparation of sterile setups hours before needed and the subsequent covering of these setups with sterile sheets are not recommended for two reasons: the setups are usually left unguarded and thus become prey to sources of contamination, and removal of the cover sheets without contaminating the sterile setups is extremely difficult. Therefore sterile fields should be prepared as close as possible to the scheduled time of use.

Close adherence to principles of asepsis and consistent observance of the boundaries established in the principles provide protection against infection. Application of the basic principles of aseptic technique depends primarily on the individual's understanding and conscience. Every person on the surgical team must share the responsibility for monitoring aseptic practice and initiating corrective action when a sterile field is compromised.

INSTRUMENT DECONTAMINATION METHODS FOR PREVENTION OF INFECTION

To prevent infection, all items that come in contact with the patient or sterile field should be systematically decontaminated after a surgical procedure. Handling, transport,

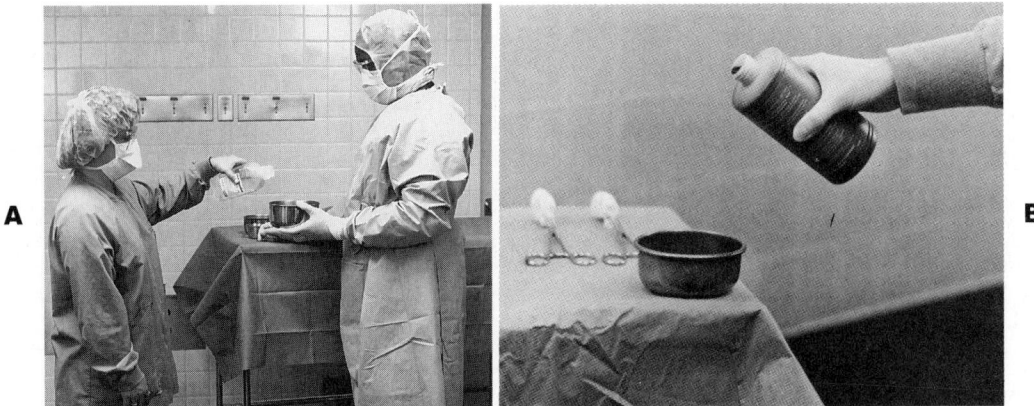

FIG. 3-10 **A,** When pouring solution into receptacle held by scrub nurse, circulating nurse maintains safe margin of space to avoid contamination of sterile surfaces. **B,** Care must be used when pouring solution into receptacle on sterile field to avoid splashing fluids onto sterile field. Placement of receptacle near edge of table permits circulating nurse to pour solution without reaching over any portion of sterile field.

and cleaning methods must be selected to prevent cross-contamination to other patients, exposure of personnel to bloodborne pathogens, and damage to instruments.

The cleaning and decontamination methods chosen should be economical and of demonstrated effectiveness. There are several choices for decontamination of surgical instruments. All methods begin with thorough cleaning to remove all visible debris. This is followed by a process that will kill or inactivate potentially pathogenic organisms that may remain after cleaning. Next, the instruments are inspected, reassembled into sets, placed in containers or wrapped, terminally sterilized, and stored for future use.

MANUAL AND MECHANICAL CLEANING

All workers handling soiled surgical instruments, whether in the operating room, substerile room, or a central decontamination area, must wear personal protective attire sufficient to prevent contact with any blood or fluid containing blood. This generally means scrub attire covered with a liquid-proof gown, coverall, or sleeved apron; hair-covering; surgical face mask and eye protection; rubber or latex gloves suitable to the task; and, if fluids may pool on the floor, liquid-proof boots or shoe covers.

During the surgical procedure instruments should be kept as free from body substances and other debris as possible, since debris contain microorganisms (bioburden). Instruments should be wiped with a sterile water-moistened sponge as frequently as required. Sterile water is selected because saline causes corrosion of the instrument surfaces. When the procedure is completed, all instruments that can be immersed are disassembled, or box locks are opened to allow contact with all soiled surfaces, and placed in a basin, solid-bottom container system, or bin with lid. They may be covered with a water-moistened surgical towel to prevent drying of debris.

An exception is made for instruments that have sharp or pointed edges, such as scissors, forceps with teeth, perforating towel clamps, curettes, and rongeurs. These items can penetrate the gloves and skin, creating a portal of entry for infectious organisms. They must not be placed in a basin or tray in such a way that a worker would have to reach into the container to retrieve the instrument, thus risking injury. Instead, they can be placed points down in a basin small enough so that the handles are outside the basin, thus allowing individual instruments to be grasped. An alternative to this is to place all instruments together and not handle them until after they have been through a mechanical cleaning process.

All soiled instruments should be transported from the actual operating room for cleaning and decontamination. They should be contained in leakproof containers or trays inside plastic bags. If sharps are being transported, the container should be puncture resistant. Means of containing instruments include plastic, rubber or metal bins with lids, solid-bottom sterilization container systems with the lids in place and filters in place, or simply placing the instrument tray in a plastic bag. All soiled containment packages should be labeled with the biohazard symbol to warn handlers as to the nature of the contents. Transporting instruments while they are soaking in water is discouraged because of the possibility of a liquid spill with the associated cleanup problems, and the difficulty of safely disposing of the contaminated liquid unless a flushing hopper is available. An exception may be made if instruments are not going to be cleaned within 2 to 3 hours, such as might occur on the late evening or night shift if the decontamination area is not staffed 24 hours each day. In this case the instruments can be left soaking in properly prepared enzymatic detergent solution and placed in a bin with lid to avoid spillage. This will prevent the blood and tissue from drying on the instruments and not only being hard to remove, but also damaging to the instrument surfaces because of the chloride in blood and most body fluids.

Mechanical, hands-off cleaning is the preferred method of processing instruments. Over the past several years a number of types of mechanical instrument washers and washer-decontaminators have been introduced to the market. In many hospitals they have replaced both hand washing of instruments and the use of washer-sterilizers. These units may have a single chamber where several phases of a rinsing, cleaning, rinsing, and drying process occur. Or they may have multiple chambers, each specialized for a specific function in the cleaning process, including initial cool water rinse to remove protein debris, enzymatic solution soak, washing with detergent, ultrasonic cleaning, sustained hot water (80° to 95° C) rinse, perhaps a liquid chemical germicide rinse (such as sodium hypochlorite solution), and drying. Contact with hot water for 1 minute at 80° C has been shown in some studies to be effective in sufficiently reducing the microbial population on clean instruments to allow handling by workers not wearing protective attire.

Not all instrumentation will tolerate this process and not all hospitals have access to mechanical washers that incorporate hot water or chemical decontamination as part of the cleaning cycle. For immersible instruments, washer-sterilizers offer a second option, although the cleaning function is not generally as good as with mechanical washers. If a washer-sterilizer is to be used, gross debris should be removed with a cold water rinse before placing the instruments in the washer-sterilizer, being careful to minimize splashing. Instruments are placed in perforated or mesh bottom trays or baskets and positioned so that the cleaning portion of the washer-sterilizer cycle can reach all parts of the instrument. This generally means placing the ring-handled instruments on racks or stringers with the tips up into the spray or agitating water.

There are two types of washer-sterilizers: those configured like a tunnel, with doors at each end and rotating spray arms on the sides, top, and bottom of the chamber; and those which cover the instruments with water and then blow steam and air through the water to cause agitation that produces the cleaning effect (Fig. 3-11). The former machines are generally found in central decontamination areas and may be connected to an automatic or manual conveyer. The second type of machine is generally small (about 16 to 20 inches in diameter) and located in the substerile room or instrument processing room of the surgery or obstetric suite.

After cleaning the instruments with detergent and water, then rinsing them, the washer-sterilizer begins a steam sterilization cycle. The exposure time for this cycle depends on the temperature at which the cycle is run. Some washer-sterilizers of the tunnel type operate at 285° F, for less than 1 minute. Others, including all of the second type of washer-sterilizers, operate at 270° F for 10 minutes. All rely on gravity air displacement to remove air from the chamber. Instruments processed through a single cycle of a washer-sterilizer are safe to handle and may indeed be sterile, depending on presterilization bioburden. They are not suitable for immediate use in another surgical procedure. They must be inspected, arranged in a manner convenient for the surgical team to use, and steam sterilized again. Debris remaining on the instruments because of possible inefficiencies of the cleaning process will be baked on by the sterilization portion of the process and may be difficult to remove.

Some instrumentation will not tolerate immersion in water or cannot take the heat or pressures involved in mechanical processes. These items must be hand washed using an appropriate detergent for the type of material and the type of soil on the item. If protein or other organic soil is present, then the detergent should have an alkaline pH (greater than 7). If inorganic soil is present, the detergent should have an acid pH (less than 7). The degree of alkalinity or acidity should be selected so that the instrument or item itself will not be damaged in the cleaning process. For example, stainless steel instrumentation with organic soil is best cleaned by alkaline detergents with a pH range of 7 to 10, according to most United States surgical instrument manufacturers. Using acidic or harshly alkaline solutions can remove the protective passivation layer from the instrument and allow pitting and other corrosive activity, which cannot be repaired, once present. This advice regarding detergent selection applies to mechanical washing also. The instrument manufacturer should be consulted to determine appropriate cleaning products and procedures.

During manual cleaning of instrumentation, debris may be removed by wiping the item with a detergent-soaked cloth or by using a brush or similar instrument. If any friction is used that could cause splash or aerosolization of debris, this should be accomplished while holding the portion of the item being cleaned under water in a basin or sink.

Items that were soiled with blood or body fluids and that have been manually cleaned only have not been sufficiently decontaminated to allow handling by workers not wearing protective attire. If such an item will tolerate steam sterilization, it can be further decontaminated by processing through an unwrapped steam sterilization cycle (flash sterilized). It is then safe to handle. The item can also be soaked in a liquid chemical germicide such as 2% alkaline glutaraldehyde for 20 minutes to disinfect it. If none of these methods is suitable for the item, either because of damage to the item, cost, or unavailability, workers in the preparation area can wear rubber or latex gloves when handling, inspecting, assembling and packaging these few items for terminal sterilization.

ULTRASONIC CLEANING

The ultrasonic cleaning process is designed to remove fine soil from cervices and box lock areas of instrumentation. It should be used only after instruments have had gross

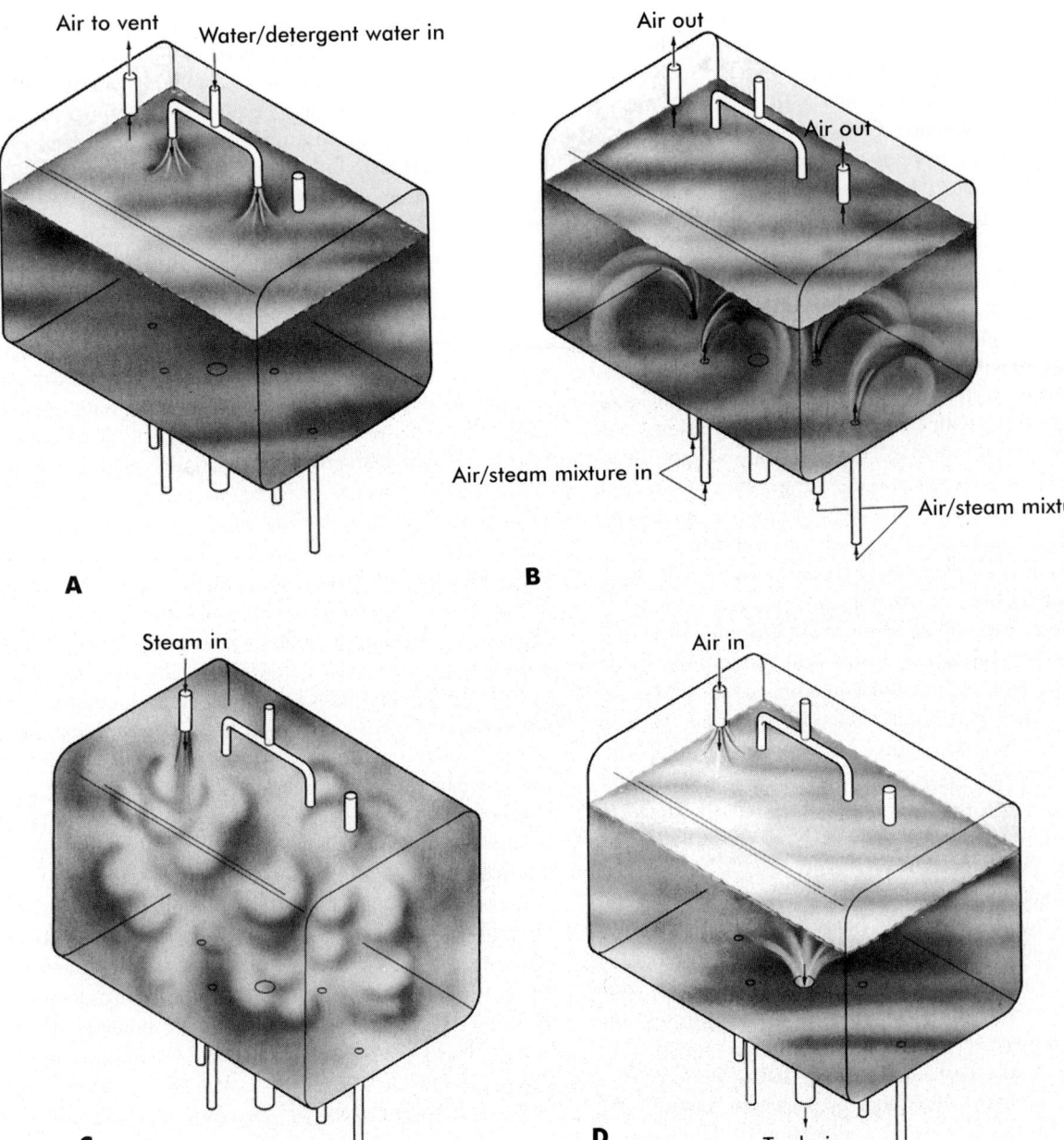

FIG. 3-11 Automatic washer-sterilizer. **A,** The cycle in this machine begins with a cold water rinse, entering through the top of the chamber, to loosen and remove gross soil such as blood and tissue without coagulating proteinaceous material, which would cause it to adhere to instruments. Then warm water and detergent enter the chamber to a level to cover the instruments. **B,** Next, jets of steam and air are injected into the filled chamber through ports in the floor of the chamber. Violent turbulence in the detergent-water solution removes any debris remaining on the instruments after the initial rinse. **C,** At the conclusion of the wash time, the water drains out of the chamber. Newer model washer-sterilizers may have microprocessor controls that allow the user to set the duration of wash time based on the nature of soil on the instruments. A final water rinse, coming in through the top of the chamber, carries any detergent residues and soil away from the instruments and out the drain. **D,** Finally, saturated steam begins to fill the chamber. Air in the chamber and load is heavier than the steam and, because of gravity, is displaced downward and out the drain. As pressure builds in the chamber from the incoming steam, the temperature rises to 132° C (270° F), the chamber drain closes, and that temperature is held for the duration of the sterilization exposure time selected by the user. Then steam is exhausted through the automatic condenser exhaust. Some machines have the capability of selecting drying times for the instruments. At the conclusion of the cycle, an audible signal indicates the unit is ready for unloading. Instruments and the inside of the sterilizer are very hot and, if no dry time was used, the instruments and trays are also wet. Use extreme caution in handling.

Courtesy American Sterilizer Company (AMSCO), Erie, Pa.

debris removed. Ultrasonic energy occurs in wave form and is generated by transducers on the sides or bottom of a specially constructed chamber that is filled with water or a water and detergent solution. The ultrasonic waves pass through the water and any solid objects, especially metal, are placed in the chamber. These energy waves create tiny bubbles in the water, which then collapse or implode, creating a negative pressure that pulls debris away from surfaces. This process is known as *cavitation*. Once the cleaning process is accomplished, the instruments should be rinsed to remove the loose debris. Some ultrasonic consoles have chambers for rinsing and drying instruments.

Effective ultrasonic cleaning requires that most of the dissolved gases be removed from the water in the chamber before cleaning begins. Otherwise, the bubbles formed are too large to produce effective cavitation. Degassing should be done each time the chamber is refilled with clean solution. It simply means running the ultrasonic machine without a load in the chamber for 5 to 10 minutes, as directed by the manufacturer.

The ultrasonic cleaner should always be used with the lid down. The fine aerosols created by the process can spread over greater distances than larger water splashes. Also, personnel working in the area of the ultrasonic should be wearing a surgical face mask and eye protection to protect the mucous membranes. The ultrasonic cleaner can be used in the cleaning process anytime after gross debris is removed from the instruments. It is most effective if used before fine debris is baked on, such as in the steam sterilization process. The ultrasonic machine should be placed in the soiled or decontamination area, not in the clean area, no matter at what stage it is used in the process. Previous prohibitions about using the ultrasonic machine only after cleaning and sterilization of instruments resulted from the concerns over the fine aerosols created by the process, and arose in a time when personal protective attire was neither routinely worn nor required by federal regulation.

Not all items will tolerate the energy waves of the ultrasonic process. Chrome-plated instruments should not be cleaned ultrasonically because it can loosen the chrome from the base metal underneath. Dissimilar metals such as stainless steel, titanium, copper, and lead should not be ultrasonically processed at the same time. The energy waves, combined with the heat and detergent solution, can cause electrolysis to occur, which plates one metal onto others, potentially ruining the instruments. Some manufacturers recommend that microsurgery instruments not be placed in the ultrasonic cleaner, both because of their delicate design and the fact that they may contain several types of metal. The detergent or enzyme cleaner used in the ultrasonic machine should be very carefully selected. The corrosiveness and overall effectiveness of some solutions can be dramatically affected by the combination of heat and ultrasonic energy in such a machine.

PREPARATION AND PACKAGING

Preparation and packaging of instruments is the final step before terminal sterilization as preparation for reuse. This occurs in a clean area, separate from the area where decontamination occurred. Instruments are carefully inspected for cleanliness and functionality. Soiled instruments are returned for further cleaning. Instruments with movable parts are treated with a water-soluble instrument lubricant solution that contains an antimicrobial agent to retard growth in the lubricant solution. Broken or worn instruments are set aside for repair. Instruments are assembled into sets according to set content lists prepared in consultation with the surgeons and perioperative nursing staff. These sets are then placed in reusable rigid sterilization container systems or wrapped, and sterilized or stored unsterile for future use.

STERILIZATION METHODS FOR PREVENTION OF INFECTION

Modern surgery demands increasingly intricate and delicate instruments and more effective supplies and equipment. Methods of sterilization of surgical items must result in complete destruction of microbial life, including spores, and the absence of toxic residue on the objects, as well as little or no deterioration or damage to heat- and moisture-sensitive instruments and other items. Sterilization is designed with a safety margin to allow for the killing of the odd survivor.

STEAM STERILIZATION

Saturated steam under pressure is recognized as the safest, most practical means of sterilizing surgical supplies, fluids, the majority of instruments, and other inanimate objects. Steam under pressure permits permeation of moist heat to porous substances by condensation and results in destruction of all microbial life. Saturated steam exerts the maximum pressure for water vapor at a given temperature and pressure.

Theory of microbial destruction

Microorganisms are believed to be destroyed by moist heat through a process of denaturation and coagulation of the enzyme-protein system within the bacterial cell. Microorganisms are killed at a lower temperature when moist heat is used than when dry heat is used. This fact is based on the theory that all chemical reactions, including coagulation of proteins, are catalyzed by the presence of water.

Compressed steam results in effective sterilization because moisture and heat are always present. When steam comes in contact with a cold object, condensation takes place immediately. As the steam condenses, it gives off latent heat that warms and wets the object; in other words, both moisture and heat are provided.

Principles and mechanism

Pure steam at sea level atmospheric pressure has a temperature of 100° C (212° F). When water is boiled in a vessel from which the steam cannot escape, a higher temperature is reached. To attain steam under pressure, a vessel that can be closed tightly must be used. A home pressure cooker generates steam from the water inside the tightly closed vessel when it is placed over a gas flame or electric plate. In the hospital autoclave, the steam coming from the boilers is compressed and gives off latent heat.

The higher the steam pressure, the higher the temperature. The steam is the sterilizing agent, not the compressed hot air. If steam is mixed with air at the same pressure, the temperature will be lower than pure steam at atmospheric pressure. For example, if the mixture is two-thirds steam and one-third air, the temperature at 15 pounds pressure per square inch (psi) will be 115° C (240° F) instead of 121° C (250° F). The air acts as a barrier to steam penetration.

Generally, the autoclave consists of two metal cylinders (the chamber and the shell), one within the other. Between the cylinders is an enclosed space (the jacket) in which steam and heat can be maintained. This steam jacket facilitates fast, efficient, and effective drying of the load following sterilization.

In the conventional steam sterilizer the sterilization process may be divided into five distinct phases:

1. Loading phase, in which the objects are packaged and loaded in the sterilizer
2. Heating phase, in which the steam is brought to the proper temperature and allowed to penetrate around and through the objects in the chamber
3. Destroying phase, or the time-temperature cycle, in which all microbial life is exposed to the killing effects of the steam
4. Drying and cooling phase, in which the objects are dried and cooled, filtered air is introduced into the chamber, the door is opened, and the objects are removed and stored
5. Testing phase, in which the efficiency of the sterilization process is checked

Phase 1—loading

Preparation of supplies. Packaging of surgical supplies and their arrangement in loads in the sterilizer are factors that govern the effectiveness of steam sterilization.

The prime function of a package containing a surgical item is to permit sterilization of the contents and to ensure the sterility of the contents up to the time the package is opened. Provision must be made for the contents to be removed without contamination. Numerous factors should be considered in selecting an effective packaging material. It must be suitable for the method of sterilization used, that is, permit adequate air removal and steam penetration when steam sterilization is used, and adequate penetration and release of sterilant gas and moisture when gas sterilization is used. It should be durable enough to resist tearing or puncture and be free from pinholes. It also should be moisture resistant. An effective wrapper should be flexible and memory free to allow easy aseptic presentation with assurance of no particulate contamination when the package is opened. It should establish a barrier to microorganisms or their vehicles.

Sterilization container systems are one way of packaging instruments. As rigid packaging systems that can be sterilized, stacked, and stored, they offer a simple yet effective method. Because they are rigid, they cannot be punctured, abraded, or easily contaminated by environmental microbes. Studies have indicated that, properly initiated, container systems are a cost-effective packaging method. Recommendations for sterilizing containers in various sterilizers should be obtained from the manufacturer. Performance testing should be carried out in the sterile processing department of the health care facility to ensure that all conditions essential for both sterilization and drying are effectively achieved. Before opening a container, the perioperative nurse should check for evidence of integrity and sterility. The lid should be removed with care. The scrub nurse should maintain a margin of safety between self and the unsterile outer container when removing the inner basket.

If textile wrappers are used, they must be laundered between sterilization exposures to ensure sufficient moisture content of the fibers, which prevents superheating and absorption of the sterilizing agent. By rehydrating woven materials, laundering also reduces their deterioration rate. All wrappers must be checked for torn areas and holes before they are used.

Many in-hospital packaging materials—woven and nonwoven, reusable and disposable—are marketed today. Available materials should be carefully evaluated before a product is chosen. The present standards for steam sterilization are based on a 140-thread-count woven fabric. Manufacturers of all packaging materials should be able to show that sterilization can be achieved with practical sterilizer operating cycles.

The size and density of woven textile packs must be restricted to ensure uniform steam penetration. The pack should not exceed 12 × 12 × 20 inches (30 × 30 × 50 cm) and should not weigh more than 12 pounds (5.4 kg). When the items in the pack are being assembled, the lighter materials should be placed near the center of the pack. Each succeeding layer of dry goods should be placed crosswise on the layer below to promote free circulation of steam and removal of air. Pack density should not exceed 7.2 pounds per cubic foot. A chemical indicator that accurately reflects one or more of the physical parameters of sterilization should be inserted in the center of each pack. The parameters for steam sterilization include time, temperature, and steam saturation and purity.

The pack should be wrapped sequentially in two barrier-type wrappers, which may be disposable or reusable. A single textile reusable wrapper is defined as one layer of 270- to 280-thread-count woven fabric. Cross-stitching and raw edges are not acceptable. Sequential double wrapping creates a package within a package, providing a better bacterial barrier and ease in presenting the wrapped item to the sterile field. Wrappers are made in suitable dimensions for the various items that must be packaged. The familiar envelope wrap is made by placing the article diagonally in the center of the wrapper. The near corner, which should point toward the worker, is brought over the item, and the triangular tip is folded back to form a cuff. The two side flaps are folded to the center in like manner. The far corner of the wrapper is then folded on top of the other three. The process is repeated with the second wrapper, and the package secured with autoclave indicator tape. When the pack is opened for use, the flaps at the corners are used to form a protective cuff over the nurse's hands during dispensing of the sterile contents. When the items are wrapped, the wrappers should not be folded tightly about the contents, but the package should be firm and sealed securely to prevent contamination in handling and storage.

Before being wrapped and sterilized, instruments should be placed in trays that have mesh or perforated bottoms. Tubes, needles, and drains must have moisture in the lumens that can turn to steam and prevent trapping of air, which creates a barrier against effective sterilization. Their containers must be covered with a material that permits penetration of steam to all inside surfaces of the containers.

Sterilization process (chemical) indicator tape should be used to hold wrappers in place on packages and to indicate that the packages have been exposed to the physical conditions of a sterilization cycle. When packages are opened, these tapes should be removed from reusable wrappers because they create laundry problems, such as stopping up screens and filters. In some cases the tapes leave a dye on the wrappers that may cause deterioration of the material.

Every package intended for sterile use should be imprinted or labeled with a load control number that identifies the date of sterilization, the sterilizer used, the cycle or load number, and the date of expiration. Load control numbers facilitate identification and retrieval of supplies, inventory control, and appropriate rotation to ensure that older packages are used first.

Loading the sterilizer. When the chamber of the sterilizer is loaded, the bundles and packages should be arranged to allow little resistance to the passage of steam through the load from the top of the chamber toward the bottom of the sterilizer. All packages should be placed in the sterilizer on edge in a vertical, loose-contact position to allow free circulation and penetration of steam, enhance air elimination, prevent entrapment of air or water, and preclude excessive condensation. A second or upper layer may be placed crosswise on the first or lower layer.

All jars, tubes, canisters, and other nonporous objects should be arranged on their sides with their covers or lids removed to provide a horizontal path for the escape of air and the free flow of steam and heat.

To guard against superheating, surgical packs and supplies should not be subjected to preheating in the sterilizer with steam in the jacket before sterilization.

Phase 2 — heating

When the steam enters the autoclave, it is at the same pressure as the atmosphere. With closure of the valves and doors to the outside, the pressure of the steam inside rises, increasing the temperature of the steam.

Gauges on traditional autoclaves register the pressure in both the jacket and the chamber. Most vacuums are designated in terms of inches of mercury. A perfect vacuum is represented by a column of mercury 29.92 inches high. Standard gauges indicate vacuum starting with 0 (at room or normal atmospheric pressure). As the air is removed, the gauge registers down to 30 inches.

Evacuation of air from the conventional sterilizer is necessary to permit proper permeation of steam. A common method for removal of air is the downward, or gravity displacement, method. This method is based on the principle that air is heavier than steam. The steam that is piped into the sterilizer through a multiport valve is introduced into the chamber. The steam forces the heavier air ahead of it, down and forward, until all the air is discharged from a line at the front of the sterilizer. If a sterilizer is improperly loaded, mixing of air with steam acts as a barrier to steam penetration and prevents attainment of the sterilization temperature.

Phase 3 — destroying

The destruction period is based on the known time-temperature cycle necessary to accomplish sterilization in saturated steam. Authorities have shown that the order of death in a given bacterial population subjected to a sterilizing process is determined by definite laws. If the temperature is increased, the time may be decreased. *The minimum time-temperature relationships in terms of sterilizing efficiency are as follows:*

2 minutes at 132° C (270° F)
8 minutes at 125° C (257° F)
18 minutes at 118° C (245° F)

To provide a safety margin, the minimum estimated exposure is extended to cover the lag between the attainment of the selected temperature in the chamber and the temperature of the load. The length of exposure varies with the type of sterilizer, cycle design, altitude, bioburden, packaging, and size and composition of items to be sterilized.

In a gravity-displacement sterilizer, instruments (metal only) in an unwrapped, perforated tray should be exposed for 3 minutes at 132° C (270° F) or 15 minutes at 121° C (250° F). When metal instruments are combined with porous instruments or materials in an unwrapped perforated tray, they must be exposed for 10 minutes at 132° C or 20 minutes at 121° C. Instruments wrapped in four thicknesses of muslin should be exposed for 15 minutes at 132° C or 30 minutes at 121° C. All types of linen packs should be exposed for 30 minutes at 121° C. Bulk loads of supplies, with the exception of rubber gloves and solutions, can be sterilized safely and practically at 121° C for 30 minutes.

In a prevacuum sterilizer, supplies should be exposed for 4 minutes after the temperature reaches at least 132° C at the center of the pack.

The recording thermometer, not the pressure gauge, is the important guide to the sterilizing phase. The recording clock on the sterilizer gives information about the run of the load and to what temperature the goods were exposed.

The temperature inside the chamber must be maintained throughout the determined time of exposure.

Phase 4—drying/cooling

Completion of sterilization cycle. At completion of the sterilization cycle the steam inside the chamber is removed immediately so that it will not condense and wet the packs. To assist in the drying process, the jacket pressure should be maintained to keep the walls of the chamber hot as the steam from the chamber is exhausted to 0 gauge pressure. When chamber pressure has been exhausted, the door may be opened slightly to permit vapor to escape. Another method is to introduce clean, filtered air by means of a vacuum dryer (ejector) device in conjunction with the operating valve on the sterilizer. The minimum drying time for all methods is approximately 15 to 20 minutes.

Following removal from the sterilizer, freshly sterilized packs should be left untouched on the loading carriage until adequately cooled. If a loading carriage has not been used, the packs should be placed on edge on wire mesh surfaces that are covered with several layers of woven material to prevent condensation and subsequent contamination. Likewise, fresh sterilized packages should not be placed on cold surfaces such as metal tabletops. Because bacteria are capable of passing through layers of wet material, any packages that are wet must be considered unsterile.

A written record of existing conditions during each sterilization cycle should be maintained. It should include the sterilizer number, the cycle or load number, the time and temperature of the cycle, the date of sterilization, the contents of the load, and the initials of the operator. These records should be retained for the length of time designated by the statute of limitations in each state.

Care of sterile packages. Sterile packages must be handled with care and only as necessary. They should be stored in clean, dry, dustproof, verminproof, limited-access areas that are well ventilated and have controlled temperature and humidity. Closed cabinets are preferred to open shelves for sterile storage. If open shelves must be used, the lowest shelf should be 8 to 10 inches from the floor and the highest should be at least 18 inches from the ceiling. All shelves should be at least 2 inches from outside walls. Shelving should be smooth and well spaced, with no projections or sharp corners that might damage the wrappers. Sterilized packs should never be stacked in close contact with each other. Their arrangement on the shelves should provide for air circulation on all sides of each package. Excessive handling, crowding, dropping, and pummeling of sterile packs tend to force particles through the mesh or matrix of the wrapping material, which might contaminate the contents. For proper rotation, the most recently dated sterile packages should be placed behind those already on the shelves. Sterile packages should not be stored in the same area as nonsterile items.

Shelf life refers to the length of time a pack may be considered sterile. It is actually event related, not time related.

Variables that must be considered in determining shelf life are the type and number of layers of packaging material used, the presence or absence of impervious protective covers, the number of times a package is handled before use, and the conditions of storage. Double-wrapped, 140-thread-count woven fabric, nonwoven fabric, and paper-wrapped items may be considered sterile for 21 to 30 days. Plastic or plastic-paper combination wraps that are heat sealed maintain sterility for 6 months to a year. Impervious protective covers may extend shelf life to 6 months or more, depending on the sealing method used. When used to protect sterilized items, impervious covers should be designated as such to prevent their being mistaken for a sterile wrap. They should be applied only to thoroughly cooled, dry packs at the time of removal from the sterilizer cart, following the required cooling period.

Many commercially prepared sterile disposable drapes, packs, and materials are sealed in nonwoven envelopes that are encased in plastic, sealed wrappers with set expiration dates. Theoretically sterility is maintained for indefinite periods; their sterility, however, depends on their exposure during storage, the amount of handling, and the kind and condition of the wrapper.

Supply standards should be planned to maintain adequate stock with prompt turnover. Appropriate volume and proper rotation of supplies reduce the need for concern about shelf life. The longer an item is stored, the greater the chances of contamination.

Phase 5—testing

All mechanical parts of sterilizers, including gauges, steam lines, and drains, should be periodically checked by a competent engineer. Reports of these inspections should be kept by the person responsible for the sterilizers. Temperature, humidity, and vacuum should be measured with control equipment, independent of the fixed gauges. There are several methods of keeping a constant check on the proper functioning of a sterilizer and ensuring the efficiency of the sterilizing process.

Mechanical controls such as thermometers and automatic controls assist in identifying and preventing malfunction of the sterilizing equipment and operational errors made by personnel. Indicating thermometers, located on the discharge line of the sterilizer, show the temperature throughout the sterilizing cycle on a dial on the front of the sterilizer. The device indicates a drop in temperature when and if it occurs and can act as a warning of sterilizer failure. Because lowering of the temperature may be intermittent and is not recorded permanently, it must be seen by those responsible for operating the sterilizer. This device cannot detect air pockets within the load or pack. Air is a poor conductor of heat; therefore, it is one of the most common causes, other than human error, of sterilization failure.

Recording thermometers indicate and record the same temperature as the indicating thermometers. They record the time the sterilizer reaches the desired temperature and the duration of each exposure. The recording thermometer can be helpful if several individuals are using the sterilizer or if the operator should forget to time the load. Its recordings are proof that the exposure time of loads has been correct and proper temperature limits have been maintained. The daily record should show the number of the sterilizer, the number of cycles run, the time, and the date. This evidence can be used to correct discrepancies, should error occur. Like the indicating thermometer, the recording thermometer does not detect cool air pockets; therefore additional controls are necessary for complete safety.

Automatic controls are devices that, by a predetermined plan, control all phases of the sterilizing process. The controls allow the steam to enter, time the sterilizing cycle, exhaust the steam, and initiate drying. Some lock the door so that it cannot be opened until the cycle is complete. A thermocouple may be placed within the pack or load to indicate whether the required temperature has been reached and maintained within the contents throughout the sterilizing cycle.

Chemical controls or sterilizer indicators, such as sealed glass tubes, sterilizer indicating tape, and color-change cards or strips, can be used to detect cool air pockets inside the sterilizing chamber. They can be useful in checking packaging and loading techniques on a package-by-package or load-by-load basis, as well as the mechanical functioning of the sterilizer. One chemical control is a sealed glass tube which contains a pellet that melts when favorable time and temperature conditions for sterilization are achieved. These tubes are placed in the center of each linen pack. Chemical indicator cards and strips are impregnated with a dye that changes color when steam initiates a chemical reaction. Indicators that are sensitive to ethylene oxide are also available.

Because chemical indicators vary in their abilities to monitor the parameters of sterilization, their inclusion in all packages to be sterilized is questionable on a cost-effectiveness basis. Every facility must formulate its own policy on the use of internal chemical indicators by considering the cost-benefit ratio, performance limitations, and personnel knowledge of sterilization principles. Tapes, labels, and legends printed on packaging materials may have lines, squares, or words that change color when exposed to the sterilizing agent for a certain time and temperature and identify packages that have been exposed to the physical conditions of a sterilization cycle.

An external chemical indicator should be clearly visible on every package to be sterilized. However, these indicators do not *prove* sterilization, because some of them react even when the temperature is inadequate for sterilization. The sensitivity of chemical indicators to temperature can be checked by exposing them to steam in a sterilizer set at 115° C (240° F) for 30 minutes. Because this temperature is inadequate for sterilization, the indicators should not react.

A biologic indicator is the most accurate method of checking sterilization effectiveness. Commercially prepared biologic indicators (manufactured in accordance with minimum performance criteria of the *United States Pharmacopeia*) should be stored and used according to the manufacturer's written instructions. They contain a known population of *Bacillus stearothemophilus,* a highly heat-resistant, spore-forming microorganism that does not produce toxins and is nonpathogenic.

Biologic testing for steam sterilizer loads should be conducted at least weekly on the first run of the day. The biologic indicator should be placed in a test pack that is positioned on edge in the front bottom section of a routinely loaded steam sterilizer, the area of the sterilizer that will most challenge all sterilization parameters. The test pack for gravity displacement and prevacuum steam sterilizers should consist of three muslin gowns, 12 towels, thirty 4 × 4 gauze sponges, five 12 × 4 laparotomy sponges, and one muslin drape sheet. Two biologic indicators and an internal chemical indicator are placed in the center of the pack, separated by towels. Commercially prepared test packs are available.

After the sterilization cycle the biologic indicators are removed from the pack and incubated according to the manufacturer's instructions. Negative reports indicate that wrapping techniques, loading procedures, and sterilizing conditions are correct and that the sterilizer is functioning properly. Results of these tests should be filed as a permanent record. A positive report does not necessarily indicate sterilizer failure because false positives sometimes occur. However, the sterilizer should immediately be retested and taken out of service until it is operationally inspected and the results of retesting are negative. If a sterilizer malfunction is found, all items prepared in the suspect load should be considered unsterile. They should be retrieved if possible and washed, repackaged, and resterilized in another sterilizer. Biologic indicators should also be used after a major sterilizer repair, when evaluating sterilization of a new product, and when sterilizing implantable materials.

Spore control ampules containing *B. stearothemophilus* are used for steam sterilization only and cannot be used in hot air (dry heat) sterilizers, because 121° C (250° F) would also sterilize them without sterilizing the load itself. In general, hot air sterilization is not as good as either steam or ethylene oxide and should be avoided whenever possible. Spore strips containing *B. subtilis* should not be used to check steam sterilizers because they are not sufficiently heat resistant. They may be used, however, to check ethylene oxide and dry heat sterilizers.

High-speed (flash) sterilization

The high-speed steam sterilizer, commonly referred to as a flash sterilizer, is adjusted to operate at 132° C (270° F) and 27 psi (Fig. 3-12). Although it can be used for sterilizing packs and solutions, it is most frequently used in the operating room for the sterilization of urgently needed unwrapped instruments. It should be used only when time does not permit sterilization of wrapped sets. Implantable devices should not be flash sterilized because the reliability of sterilization is reduced by the speed of the cycle. If, in an emergent situation, an implantable must be flash sterilized, a biologic indicator should be included in the tray.

The operational process consists of the following steps:

1. Steam is maintained in the jacket of the sterilizer before and during the daily operating schedule.
2. Soiled instruments are cleaned with warm tap water and detergent and then rinsed thoroughly in a fat-solvent solution.
3. The opened instruments are placed in a perforated metal tray or flash sterilization container with a chemical indicator, the tray positioned in the sterilizer, and the door of the sterilizer closed and locked. The chemical indicator is not considered porous material.
4. The chamber steam supply valve is opened, and the operating valve is turned to the sterilizing setting. Time exposure begins when the thermometer records 132° C (270° F). If the sterilizer is a gravity displacement type and automatic, the timer is set for a 3- or 10-minute exposure period (based on the composition of the instruments), and the selector switch is turned to the fast exhaust setting. Air-powered drills and other specialty instruments require different exposure times, as directed by the manufacturer.
5. On completion of the exposure period, the chamber steam valve is closed and the operating valve turned to exhaust. The exposure time and temperature of the cycle as recorded on the sterilizer recording device should be checked before opening the sterilizer door.
6. The door is opened when the exhaust valve registers zero.
7. The instruments are removed and delivered to the surgical field by aseptic technique.

Prevacuum, high-temperature sterilization

The automatic, prevacuum, high-temperature sterilization method has replaced, in many instances, the downward displacement method of sterilization. Prevacuum, high-temperature sterilization (Fig. 3-13) is usually accomplished by means of an air-blasted, oil-sealed rotary pump, protected by a condenser and coupled with an automatic control mechanism.

Air removal is accomplished by means of a powerful vacuum pump that draws a near-absolute vacuum in the chamber in the first 5 minutes of the cycle, before the steam is introduced. This mechanism reduces the time necessary to accomplish all phases of the sterilizing process. As steam is admitted, it rushes into every part of the load since air has been removed and cannot interfere. Steam penetrates into containers such as cardboard boxes, which cannot be accomplished in the gravity displacement sterilizer.

The prevacuum, high-temperature steam sterilizer provides a system that is automatically controlled and reduces the total cycle time to as little as 20 minutes. The cycle time varies with the size of the sterilizer, the adequacy of

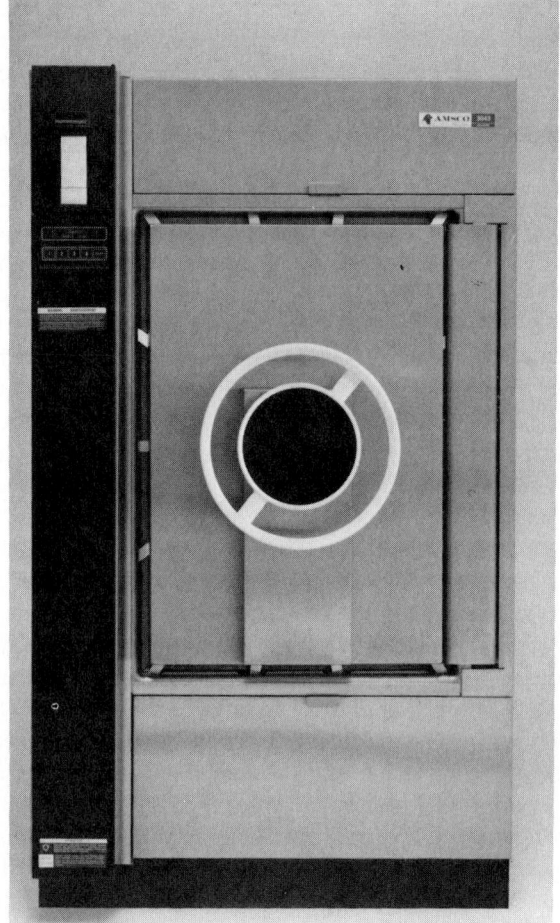

A

FIG. 3-12   For legend see opposite page.

the steam, and the supply of water. Faulty packaging and overloading or incorrect placement of objects in the chamber is not likely to interfere with air removal, and full heating of the load takes place more rapidly than with the downward displacement method. The prevacuum, high-temperature steam sterilizer permits more supplies to be sterilized within a given time.

The Bowie-Dick test should be used to evaluate the effectiveness of a prevacuum steam sterilizer in reducing air residuals from the chamber, preventing air reentrainment into the load, and detecting the presence of air pockets, which would result in the absence of sterilizing conditions. It should be used daily before the first sterilization cycle or at a designated time each day if sterilizers are used 24 hours a day. The test pack consists of hydrated surgical towels that are folded no smaller than 9 × 12 inches and are stacked to a height of 10 to 11 inches. A commercially prepared Bowie-Dick–type test sheet is placed in the center of the stack, and a single wrapper is loosely applied. Disposable test packs and devices are also available. The pack is placed horizontally in the bottom front of the sterilizer rack near the door in an otherwise empty chamber. The cycle is then run according to the sterilizer manufacturer's di-

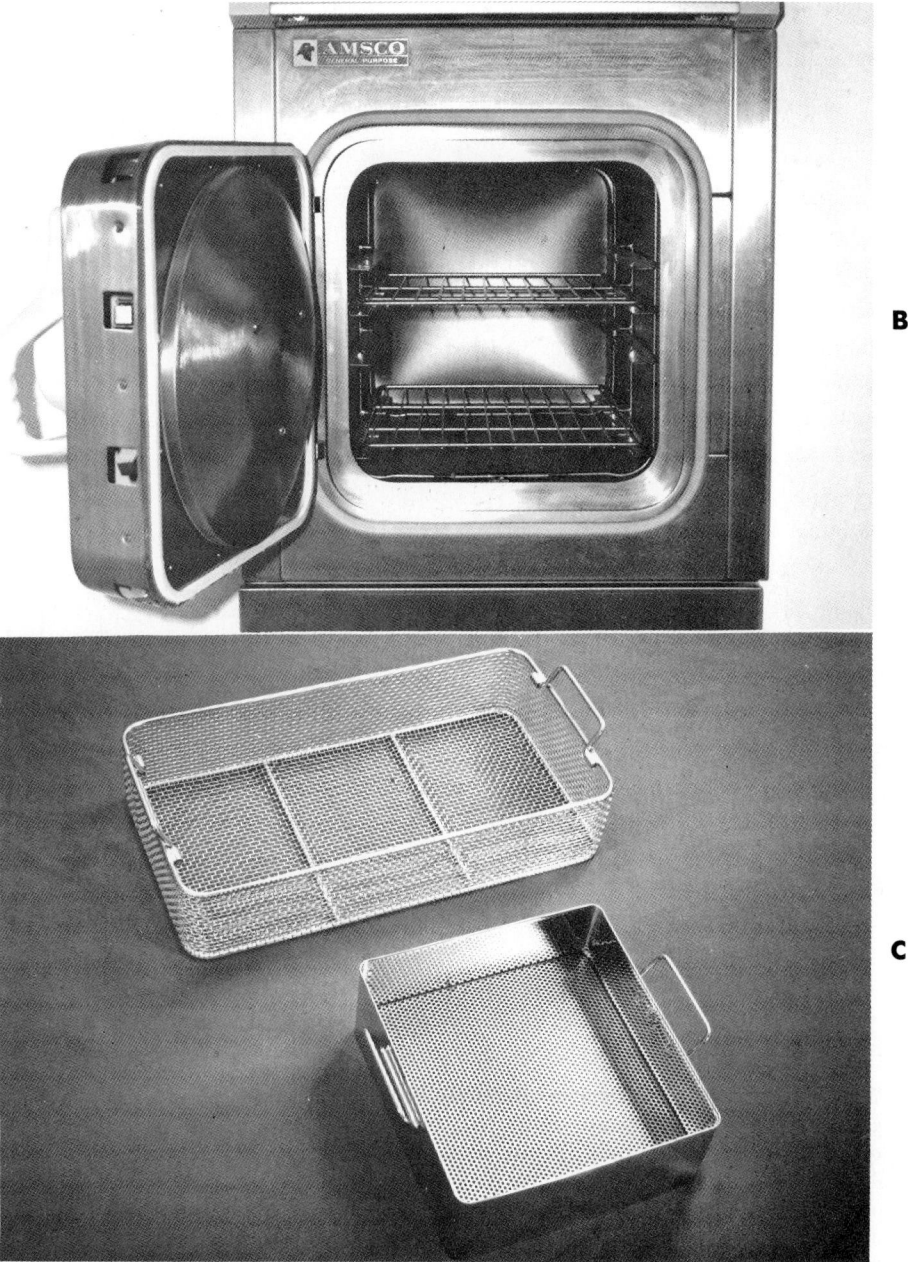

FIG. 3-12   General-purpose gravity air displacement steam sterilizer. This type of sterilizer can be used to sterilize wrapped or unwrapped instruments and utensils, linen packs, and solutions in specially designed vented flasks. **A,** These units come in several sizes, from the small unit similar in size to the washer-sterilizer in Fig. 3-11 to large floor-loading units. A medium size unit is pictured here. Newer units have sophisticated microprocessor controls that allow maximum flexibility in selecting sterilization and drying times and help in troubleshooting, should a problem occur during a cycle. Digital readouts and heat-sensitive paper printouts have replaced the round chart and pen found on older models. These changes have helped the operator more easily determine and document that the conditions needed for proper sterilization were met. **B,** Adjustable racks and loading cars with adjustable shelves are designed to permit maximum loading efficiency. **C,** Instrument baskets or trays should have either wire mesh bottoms or a sufficient number of perforations in sheet metal to allow for air removal and drainage of condensate during the sterilization cycle.

Courtesy American Sterilizer Company (AMSCO), Erie, Pa.

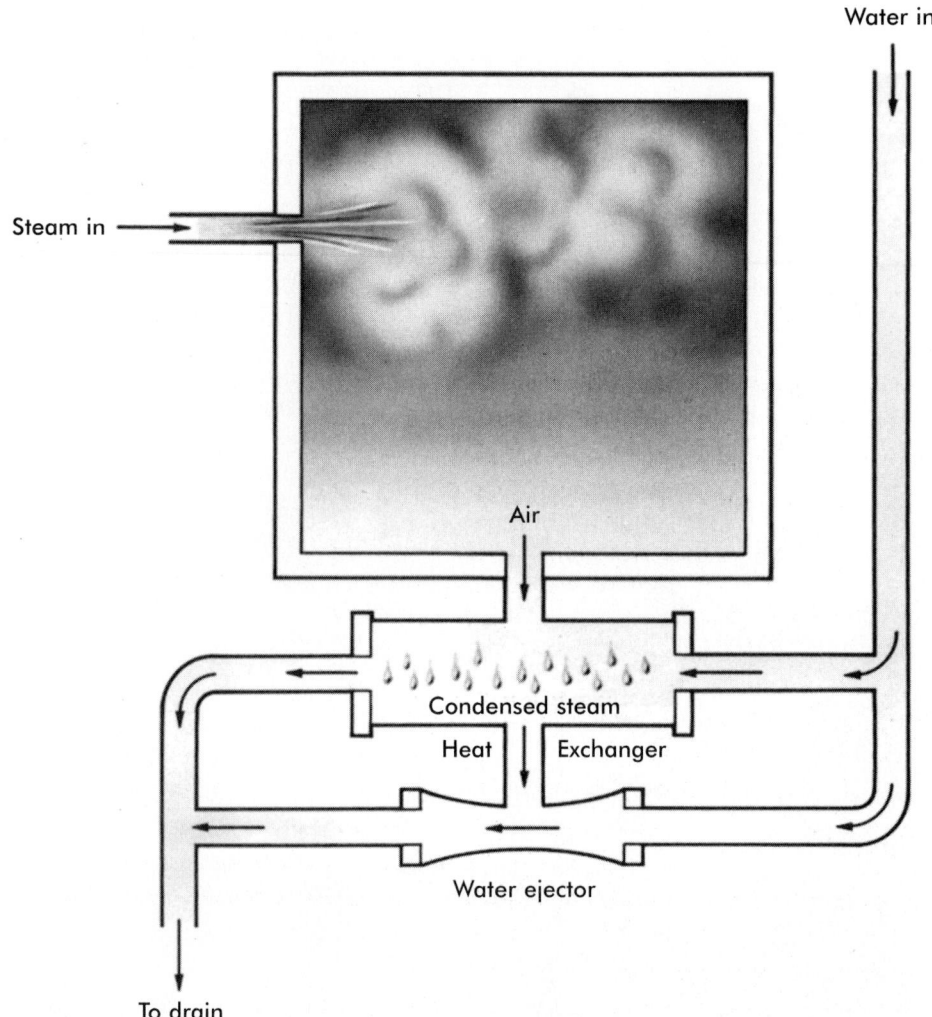

Water in

Steam in

Air

Condensed steam

Heat | Exchanger

Water ejector

To drain

FIG. 3-13 Prevacuum steam sterilizer. This type of sterilizer features active, aggressive removal of air, rather than relying on the passive action of gravity. The process has undergone several stages of development; therefore several cycle designs are in use. Newer models have the cycle characteristics described here. Steam flows into the chamber for a brief time and then rapidly drains, producing a partial vacuum. This process is repeated several times and deepens the level of vacuum drawn with each pulse. The effect of this pulsing cycle is to displace any air in the load and rapidly increase the chamber and load temperatures. At the conclusion of this conditioning phase, steam flows into the chamber and raises the temperature to sterilization levels, usually 132° C (270° F). The temperature is maintained for at least 3 minutes for unwrapped, nonporous materials and 4 minutes for wrapped or porous items. Steam is then removed from the chamber to draw a partial vacuum once again. Heated, filtered air is introduced into the chamber to dry the load. Drying times are selected and set by the user, depending on the nature of the load. Some newer units have a special cycle designed for rapid sterilization of an instrument tray in a single wrapper. This express cycle has fewer conditioning pulses, a 4-minute exposure time, and 1 or 2 minutes of dry time, for a total cycle time of approximately 12 minutes. Although the wrapper feels warm and dry to the touch, the contents may not be totally dry. Thus this package should be handled by persons wearing sterile gloves and using sterile towels for protection from burns. The instruments sterilized in this express cycle must be used immediately. Because the contents are not dry, the package is not suitable for any length of storage.

Courtesy American Sterilizer Company (AMSCO), Erie, Pa.

rections. At the completion of the cycle, the test sheet is removed from the pack and examined by a person trained in its interpretation. A uniform color change throughout the test sheet indicates a satisfactory test. The Bowie-Dick test does not measure the efficacy of the sterilization process.

PLASMA STERILIZATION

One of the most recent technological advances in sterilization technology is low temperature plasma sterilization. This process utilizes low temperature hydrogen peroxide gas plasma to achieve rapid, low temperature, low moisture sterilization of medical and surgical items (Fig 3-14, A). Low temperature gas plasma consists of a reactive cloud of ions, electrons, and neutral atomic particles; this state of matter can be produced through the action of either a strong electric or magnetic field.

Peroxide plasma sterilization has the potential of displacing many uses of both steam and ethylene oxide sterilization. It is designed to provide non-toxic, dry, low temperature sterilization in about one hour. This gas plasma process rapidly destroys a broad spectrum of microorganisms, including gram-negative and gram-positive vegetative bacteria, mycobacteria, yeasts, fungi, lipophilic and hydrophilic viruses, as well as highly resistant aerobic and anaerobic bacterial spores (Jacobs, 1989, 1993; AORN, 1994). At the completion of the sterilization process, no toxic residues remain on the sterilized items, making it a safe process for both patients and health care workers. Preparation of instrumentation for sterilization includes cleaning and decontamination procedures, reassembly, and wrapping with nonwoven polypropylene wraps or Tyvek-mylar pouches (Fig. 3-14, B); cellulosic based products like paper and linen cannot be used. Biological and chemical indicators for process verification are used in the same manner as those for steam and ethylene oxide sterilization procedures.

CHEMICAL STERILIZATION

New materials that cannot be heat sterilized are continually being introduced for use in hospitals. They require the use of other methods of sterilization. An effective alternative method is to use chemical agents.

Sterilization can be achieved by many agents when only vegetative cells are present. If the microbial population is unknown, however, a sporicidal agent must be employed to ensure sterilization. An antimicrobial agent must exhibit a wide microbiologic spectrum and sporicidal activity to qualify as a chemosterilizer. The use of chemosterilizers is governed by the U.S. Environmental Protection Agency (EPA) and has been restricted to ethylene oxide (a gaseous chemosterilizer), aqueous glutaraldehyde, and peroxyacetic acid (liquid chemosterilizers).

Chemical sterilization is frequently referred to as *cold sterilization*. This term refers to the maximum temperature of 54° C (130° F) to 60° C (140° F) of gaseous sterilization as compared with the 121° C (250° F) to 132° C (270° F) temperatures of steam sterilization.

Gaseous chemical sterilization

In recent years gaseous chemical sterilization has had considerable application for heat-labile and moisture-sensitive items, such as intricate, delicate surgical instruments, large pieces of equipment used in the hospital, plastic and porous materials, and electrical instruments—all of which are difficult to steam sterilize without deterioration and damage.

Ethylene oxide is the most frequently used gas. It is colorless at ordinary temperatures, has an odor similar to that of ether, and has an inhalation toxicity similar to that of ammonia gas. It is easily kept as a liquid that will boil at 10.73° C (51.3° F) and freeze at −111.3° C (−168.3° F).

Ethylene oxide is highly explosive and very flammable in the presence of air. These hazards are greatly reduced by diluting the ethylene oxide with inert gases such as carbon dioxide and fluorinated hydrocarbons (Freon). Neither of these two inert gases appears to affect the bactericidal activity of the ethylene oxide but serves only as an inert diluent that prevents the flammability hazard.

Several theories on how ethylene oxide kills bacteria have been proposed. The killing rate of bacteria is generally believed to be relative to the rate of diffusion of the gas through their cell walls and the availability or accessibility of one of the chemical groups in the bacterial cell walls to react with the ethylene oxide. The killing rate also depends on whether the bacterial cell is in a vegetative or spore state. Destruction takes place by alkylation through chemical interference and probably inactivation of the reproductive process of the cell.

The automatic control cycle of the sterilizing process consists of air evacuation, humidification, sterilization, gas evacuation, and admission of filtered air to relieve the vacuum.

In general, ethylene oxide sterilization should be used only if the materials are heat sensitive and unable to withstand sterilization by saturated steam under pressure. Any item that can be steam sterilized should never be gas sterilized.

Ethylene oxide's advantages are that it is easily available; is effective against all types of microorganisms; easily penetrates through masses of dry material; does not require high temperatures, humidity, or pressure; and is noncorrosive and nondamaging to items.

Sterilization with ethylene oxide also has numerous disadvantages. The long exposure and aeration periods make it a lengthy process. When compared with steam sterilization, ethylene oxide sterilization is expensive. Liquid ethylene oxide may produce serious burns on exposed skin if not immediately removed; insufficiently aerated materials can cause skin irritation, burns of body tissue, and hemolysis of blood; and diluents used with ethylene oxide cause damage to some plastics. Human error and mechanical breakdown can enhance these disadvantages.

Factors affecting sterilization with ethylene oxide are time of exposure, gas concentration, temperature, humid-

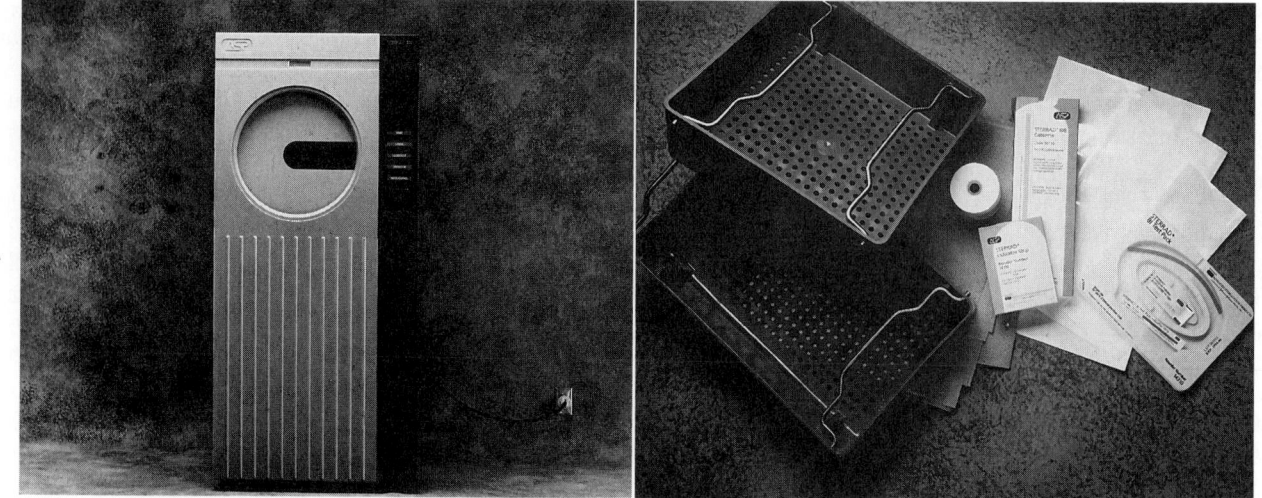

FIG. 3-14 **A,** STERRAD™ low temperature sterilization system has a front panel indicating cycle stage and elapsed time which also provides a paper printout for process confirmation and documentation. **B,** Supplies for use during the sterilization process include trays, pouches, and biological and chemical process indicators for process verification.

ity, and penetration. The time exposure required depends on temperature, humidity, gas concentration, the ease of penetrating the articles to be sterilized, and the type of microorganisms to be destroyed. Manufacturers of gas sterilizers have developed recommended exposure periods for various ethylene oxide concentrations in relation to the material to be sterilized. In general, an exposure period of 3 to 7 hours is necessary for complete sterilization. Exposure time is set for absolute destruction of the most resistant microorganisms, which is a very slow process.

Gas concentration is affected by the temperature and humidity inside the sterilizing chamber, which also affect the exposure period. Concentration is considered effective within the margin of 450 to 1000 mg/L of chamber space. If the concentration of gas is doubled, the exposure time may be shortened. The concentration and pressure of the ethylene oxide gas vary with types of sterilizers used; therefore the manufacturer's instructions should be followed.

Temperature has a marked influence on the destruction of microorganisms. It is important in gaseous sterilization with ethylene oxide because it affects the penetration of the gas through bacterial cell walls, as well as through wrappings and packaging material. The temperature for sterilizing is 21° to 60° C (70° to 140° F), and automatically controlled ethylene oxide sterilizers are usually preheated to 54° C (130° F).

Humidity of 35% to 70% is recommended with ethylene oxide to ensure enough moisture to kill microorganisms. Dry spores are most difficult to kill, but when moistened their resistance to gas penetration is lowered. Dehydration makes some microorganisms nearly immune to ethylene oxide sterilization, whereas droplets of moisture can inhibit the action of the gas by protecting the organism. Ethylene oxide sterilizers with automatic controls provide for moisture injection to raise the relative humidity within the chamber.

Items to be sterilized must be thoroughly cleaned and towel or air dried so that no visible droplets remain. Drying inhibits the formation of ethylene glycol during the sterilization cycle. Lumens of tubing, needles, and the like should be dry and open at both ends. Caps, plugs, valves, and stylettes should be removed from instruments or equipment to permit the gas to circulate through the items. The packaging material used should possess the characteristics described previously in this chapter. An ethylene oxide–sensitive chemical indicator should be used with each package to indicate only that the package was exposed to the gas; it does not indicate achievement of sterilization.

Specific instructions from the manufacturer of items to be sterilized should be followed closely. Penetration of gas throughout the load is essential. Care must be taken to avoid overloading the sterilizer. Compression of packages prevents penetration of the gas; if packages are wrapped in plastic, compression hinders evacuation of air and causes packages to open during the decrease in chamber pressure when a vacuum is drawn.

The sterilizer manufacturer's recommendations relating to opening the sterilizer door after completion of the sterilization cycle and subsequent transferring of items to the aerator must be closely followed. Excessive exposure to ethylene oxide represents a health hazard to personnel, since it has been linked to cancer, reproductive problems, and other disorders in animals. Therefore inhalation of ethylene oxide should be avoided or minimized, and direct contact with items sterilized by ethylene oxide should be avoided during transfer to the aerator. Various safety features such as a purge system, an audible alarm at the end of the sterilization cycle, and automatic door locking and sealing mechanisms are used on ethylene oxide sterilizers to protect personnel.

OSHA has issued standards relating to ethylene oxide. The ethylene oxide action level is the level of concentration of airborne ethylene oxide within the employee breathing zone. The standard reduces the permissible exposure to 0.5 part per million (ppm) averaged over 8 hours (AORN, 1993). An emergency plan should be established in the event that an ethylene oxide leak would occur. It requires that routine monitoring and surveillance be performed if the exposure exceeds a 0.5 ppm "action level" over 8 hours. Ethylene oxide monitoring badges are available. Adherence to these guidelines will help protect patients and hospital personnel from problems associated with ethylene oxide sterilization.

Smoking is prohibited in the sterilizer and aerator area. Because ethylene oxide is highly explosive and flammable, the sterilizer and aerator should be installed in a well-ventilated room and should be vented to the outside atmosphere as recommended by the manufacturer and required by the National Institute for Occupational Safety and Health.

The adequacy of every ethylene oxide cycle should be verified by the use of biologic monitors that contain *Bacillus subtilis*. Where feasible, implantable or intravascular items should not be used until the results of the test are known.

When items are removed from the sterilizer, they should be transferred immediately to the aerator or aeration area. The length of aeration required depends on the composition and porosity of the items, the sterilization wrap, the concentration of the diluent used with ethylene oxide for the sterilization process, and the airflow rate and temperature during aeration. Materials aerated in a mechanical aerator that provides a minimum of four air changes per hour and elevates the temperature within the cabinet to 50° to 60° C (122° to 140° F) require 8 to 12 hours of aeration based on the composition of the sterilized items and the aerator manufacturer's instructions. If a mechanical aerator is not available, items should be aerated at ambient room temperature for 7 days. Ambient aeration should be carried out in a limited access, well-ventilated room with controlled temperature between 18° and 22° C (65° and 72° F) and vented to the outside. Intravenous or irrigation fluids packaged in plastic bags should not be stored in this area.

Liquid chemical sterilization

When used properly, liquid chemosterilizers can destroy all forms of microbial life, including bacterial and fungal spores, tubercle bacilli, and viruses. Three liquid chemosterilizers used in hospitals are capable of causing sterilization: aqueous glutaraldehyde, aqueous formaldehyde, and peroxyacetic acid. Although formaldehyde is one of the oldest chemosterilizers known to destroy spores, it is rarely used because it takes from 12 to 24 hours to be effective, its pungent odor is objectionable, and controversy regarding its potential carcinogenic effect is ongoing. Glutaraldehyde is more rapid and less irritating than formaldehyde solutions.

Activated aqueous glutaraldehyde 2% is recognized as an effective liquid chemosterilizer. It is most useful in the disinfection of lensed instruments such as cystoscopes and bronchoscopes because it has minimal deleterious effects on the lens cement and is noncorrosive. Its low surface tension permits easy penetration and rinsing. Glutaraldehyde is not inactivated by organic matter and will not coagulate blood or protein. This agent does not affect the sharpness of delicate instruments.

Instruments must be free from bioburden and completely immersed in activated aqueous glutaraldehyde solution for 10 hours to achieve sterilization. Any period of immersion less than 10 hours will not kill spores that may be present and must be considered as only a disinfection procedure. During immersion, all surfaces of the instrument must be contacted by the liquid chemosterilizer. Following immersion, instruments must be rinsed *thoroughly* with sterile distilled water before being used.

In recent years, low concentrations (<0.1%) of peracetic acid combined with low concentrations (<1.0%) of hydrogen peroxide have been used as sterilants. The combination of these two oxidizing chemicals has offered the possibility of rapid sterilization of endoscopic equipment.

DISINFECTION

PROCESS

Disinfection is the process of destroying or inhibiting disease-producing microorganisms outside the body. It is most frequently achieved by chemicals in solution. The disinfection process may destroy tubercle bacilli and inactivate hepatitis viruses and enteroviruses but usually does not kill resistant bacterial spores.

Disinfection is brought about by various types of reactions or by combinations of them. These include denaturation and coagulation of proteins in the cell, halogenation, poisoning of vital enzymes, hydrolysis, oxidation, and combination with proteins to form salts. The microbial destruction depends on the concentration of the chemical and the effects on the microorganism.

Disinfection in health care settings is divided into two segments. When chemicals are used to disinfect inanimate materials, the chemical is called a disinfectant; when used to disinfect body surfaces, the chemical is called an antiseptic. Some chemicals can be used for both purposes. A germicide is any solution that will destroy germs, or microorganisms. Many germicides can be employed on living tissue as well as on inanimate objects.

Concurrent disinfection refers to the immediate disinfection process following discharge of infectious materials from the body of an infected person or after contamination of articles by an infectious agent. Terminal disinfection is the process of rendering all articles, materials, and their immediate physical environment incapable of conveying infectious agents to other persons after the patient has left the room.

Personnel in health care settings can choose from an array of germicides, many of which are claimed to be ideal for diverse purposes. A survey conducted by the American

Society for Microbiology of 16 U.S. hospitals showed the average number of different germicidal preparations used per hospital was 14.5, with a range of 8 to 22. Chemical germicides are regulated by the EPA and the Food and Drug Administration (FDA). Since 1982 the registration of germicidal products has been based solely on the manufacturer-supplied test data. Currently approximately 14,000 products are registered with the EPA. Research data do not support the efficacy of all claimed results; therefore health care professionals responsible for the purchase of such products must be reminded of the competitive market in regard to potential exaggerated claims of germicidal activity (Favero & Bond, 1991).

SELECTION OF A DISINFECTANT

Selection of a disinfectant depends on the type and population of microorganisms to be killed and the nature of the application. For disinfection purposes microorganisms may be grouped into three classes: nonsporulating, vegetative bacteria, which possess the least resistance; tubercle bacilli, which have more resistance than the vegetative microorganisms; and spores, which are extremely resistant to any disinfectant.

Most disinfectants are capable of destroying vegetative bacteria and tubercle bacilli but not spores. The vegetative forms of molds and yeast, as well as animal parasites, are susceptible to disinfectants. Some fungi and antibiotic-resistant staphylococci have been shown to be as resistant as bacterial spores. Viruses vary in their resistance to disinfectants. At present, prolonged time frames are required to deactivate the hepatitis virus. However, several liquid germicides commonly used in hospitals have been shown to kill HIV at concentrations much lower than are used in practice.

Instrumentation has been classified as critical, semicritical, and noncritical based on the risk of infection for the patient. The level of disinfectant required is based on the nature of the item and the manner in which it is to be used. Critical instruments are those which enter sterile tissue and should be presterilized commercially or steam sterilized by the user. Semicritical instruments are those which come in contact with mucous membranes but do not ordinarily penetrate the blood barrier. Examples of semicritical items include anesthesia breathing circuits, fiberoptic endoscopes, and laryngoscopes. Semicritical instruments require high-level disinfection. Noncritical instruments come in contact with intact skin and include items such as blood pressure cuffs, stethoscopes, linens, and furniture. Noncritical items require intermediate-level or low-level disinfection (Favero & Bond, 1991).

Further classification has been made between medical equipment surfaces and housekeeping surfaces. Medical equipment surfaces include items such as knobs, handles, buttons, and levers on x-ray machines, instrument trays and carts, and dental units. These surfaces should be cleaned with an intermediate-level disinfectant. Housekeeping surfaces include floors, walls, sinks, and tabletops. These environmental surfaces have not been associated with transmission of infections, but general cleaning or removal of visible soil should be done. Low-level disinfectants should be used for routine cleaning.

Disinfectants are categorized as high, intermediate, and low level. High-level disinfectants can kill bacteria and viruses if contact time is sufficient. Intermediate-level agents kill the more resistant bacteria and viruses. Low-level disinfectants kill only the less resistant bacteria and viruses. Neither intermediate- nor low-level disinfectants kill spores.

A strong concentration kills more rapidly than a weak one. A disinfectant is primarily bacteriostatic when the range of concentration over which inhibition of growth occurs is relatively wide; it is primarily bactericidal when the range is narrow. When the microorganisms are killed within a short time, the antimicrobial activity is termed *lethal*. When the rate of microbial death is slow, some microorganisms survive for a considerable time without multiplication. For those surviving, the antimicrobial activity is termed *growth inhibiting,* or *bacteriostatic*.

Products selected for use as surgical disinfectants are registered with the EPA and should be used according to the manufacturer's instructions. A disinfectant should be used at the lowest effective bactericidal concentration, because a concentration rapidly lethal for microorganisms may corrode and dull the blades of delicate instruments. However, the disinfecting power of a weak concentration is ineffective.

The larger the number of microorganisms present, the longer the disinfection time required to kill the resistant cells. According to genetic principles, when the population is large, the proportion of highly resistant bacteria is correspondingly greater than when the population is small. However, when the size of the population is extremely large, it may contain fewer highly resistant cells.

TEMPERATURE AND SURFACE TENSION OF DISINFECTANTS

Increased temperature accelerates the rate of disinfection. The only practical value of this fact is in disinfection of inanimate objects. With some disinfectants antimicrobial activity is increased when the chemical agent is added to warm water. The surface tension (wetness) of a disinfectant or antiseptic promotes contact between the agent and the microorganisms. A tension-reducing disinfectant, when combined with other chemicals, enhances the disinfecting power of that solution, thus decreasing the time-exposure rate.

PROCEDURE FOR DISINFECTION

An object must be thoroughly clean and as dry as possible to provide for effective disinfection and to avoid dilution of the disinfectant. A high-level disinfectant should be used for disinfection of surgical instruments when sterilization is not possible. All surfaces of an item must be in contact with the disinfectant solution for the recommended exposure time. Construction and composition of the object influence the disinfection time. A hard, flat, smooth-surfaced object requires less disinfection time than an uneven-surfaced object or a porous material. The disinfectant coagulates the proteins in blood and other organic debris present on the object. Thus organic material creates a barrier on the object against the disinfecting solution.

High-level disinfection of instruments and equipment should be carried out immediately before use of the items and after terminal cleaning prior to storage. Before use, disinfected items should be aseptically removed from the disinfectant solution, rinsed thoroughly, and dried sufficiently to minimize the risk of significant contamination. Because some disinfectant solutions can be irritating to skin and eyes, personnel should use caution when handling solution containers and disinfected items to avoid potential injury. Disinfectant solutions should be kept covered and used only in a well-ventilated area. The expiration date of an activated disinfectant should be determined according to the manufacturer's recommendations and marked on the container. Disinfectants become ineffective after multiple uses because of dilution, inactivation, or instability.

DISINFECTION OF ENDOSCOPIC EQUIPMENT

During recent years endoscopic surgery has increased in frequency and complexity. Because these instruments penetrate normally sterile areas of the body, they are classified as critical instruments. CDC guidelines state that sterilization of endoscopes such as laparoscopes and arthroscopes is preferable. If sterilization is not feasible, then a high-level disinfection is the minimum treatment that should be used. Some endoscopes are destroyed with repeated exposure to steam or gas sterilization; therefore these are cleaned and disinfected with a high-level disinfectant.

Endoscopes should be disassembled and thoroughly cleaned manually or with a processor. Following disinfection the endoscopes should be thoroughly rinsed, dried, and preferably stored in an enclosed area (see Chapter 32).

TYPES OF DISINFECTANTS

The various disinfectants on the market may be divided into the following major groups.

Halogens and halogen compounds

Of the halogen compounds, the hypochlorites and iodines are widely used in hospitals. The hypochlorites are available as powders containing calcium hypochlorite and sodium hypochlorite, in combination with hydrated trisodium phosphate, and as liquids containing sodium hypochlorite. Because of their unstable characteristics, preparations containing calcium hypochlorite (chlorinated lime) have been replaced by other detergents for cleaning purposes. Sodium hypochlorite 5% (household bleach) is effective in deactivation of HIV (the AIDS virus) and the hepatitis B virus.

Chlorine acts primarily by oxidation, and its odor may therefore be objectionable. The many organic chlorine compounds that liberate their chlorine more slowly (such as chloride of lime) are effective as mild disinfecting or intermediate agents. Inorganic chlorine is valuable in the disinfection of water.

Iodine acts directly by iodination and oxidation reactions. It is the most active antimicrobial of the halogens and combines readily with organic material. Because of its insolubility in water, it is prepared in various ways; the tinctures, or alcoholic solutions, are the most common forms.

Several syntheses of many organic iodine compounds in which iodine is held in dissociant complexes are available. The iodophors are iodine-detergent combinations capable of killing vegetative bacteria and tubercle bacilli if used in sufficient concentration (450 ppm of available iodine). Iodophors are not good sporicides.

Heavy metals

All metallic ions inhibit microorganisms if applied in sufficiently high concentrations. These compounds provide intermediate to low disinfectant qualities.

The ions of the heavy metals have such a strong affinity for proteins that the bacterial cells absorb them out of the solution. However, the property that makes these ions appear lethal limits their usefulness because their activity is reduced in the presence of organic matter. The ions are also irritating to tissues and are poisonous.

Attempts have been made to decrease the toxic, corrosive, and irritating qualities of mercuric disinfectants by incorporating mercury in complex organic molecules in preparations such as merbromin (Mercurochrome), thimerosal (Merthiolate), and nitromersol (Metaphen). Data indicate that aqueous solutions of both inorganic and organic mercurials don't reduce cutaneous flora. Mercurials are poor disinfectants and have no place in modern surgical disinfection.

Phenols and phenol derivatives

Phenol in the pure state (carbolic acid) is not used as a disinfectant because many of its derivatives are more effective. Like phenol, its derivatives act mainly by coagulation and partly by lytic and toxic effects that are not clearly understood. Because phenols appear to have a greater affinity for nonaqueous than for aqueous media, their action is believed to depend on their selective concentration at cell surfaces, resulting in the denaturation of proteins and an increase in permeability.

The aliphatic homologues of phenol have greater antimicrobial power than does phenol itself. Of this group, the methyl phenols—orthocresol, metacresol, and paracresol—and the halogenated phenols have phenol coefficients of three or more, but they are poorly soluble in water. The bisphenols have become the most useful of the phenolic disinfectants. The most important of these compounds are orthohydroxydiphenyl and chlorinated methylene and sulfur compounds. Of the chlorophenes, hexachlorophene is commonly used in soap. The bisphenols are relatively insoluble in water but are soluble in dilute alkali and in many organic solvents.

Synthetic detergent disinfectants

The quaternary ammonium compounds (often called *quats*) are among many surface-active detergents; they provide low-level disinfectant properties. These compounds are amines that contain pentavalent nitrogen and may be considered derivatives of ammonium chloride in which certain radicals are substituted for the hydrogen. The three types of surface-active detergent substances are those in which the organic radical is a cation, those in which the organic group is the anion, and those which do not ionize (nonionic).

These compounds possess bacteriostatic power in high dilutions and are not highly irritating or toxic. They are effective surface-tension reductants. Their antimicrobial activity is affected by the kind of water (acid or alkaline, hard or soft) used and the material or substance involved. In the presence of hard, acid, or iron-rich waters, the antimicrobial activity is lowered, especially for the cationic compounds. Quaternary ammonium compounds may be mixed with nonionic detergents that have good solubilizing activity to provide effective cleansing agents.

Alcohols

Ethyl (grain) alcohol and isopropyl (rubbing) alcohol are much more useful as antiseptics than as disinfectants. Alcohol, an intermediate-level disinfectant, is an active germicide against tubercle bacilli in concentrations of 70% to 90%, but it is not sporicidal.

Frequently alcoholic solutions are prepared by volume instead of by weight. The latter is the more accurate method of preparation. Alcohol is lighter than water and expands in the presence of heat.

Ethyl alcohol is nontoxic, colorless, tasteless, and nearly odorless and acts by denaturation of proteins. It may precipitate a protein covering around bacterial cells present in blood, pus, and mucus. Ethyl alcohol is less effective as a fat solvent than is isopropyl alcohol. A 70% solution of ethyl alcohol by weight is a satisfactory disinfectant for ordinary vegetative bacteria. It is more expensive than isopropyl alcohol.

Formaldehyde

An aqueous solution of formaldehyde (formalin) is highly germicidal and sporicidal in a strong concentration and provides high- to low-level disinfectant activity depending on concentration. When a combination of 8% formaldehyde and 70% isopropyl alcohol is used, the action is even greater. Tubercle bacilli and viruses (except the hepatitis virus, whose destruction with certainty is not known) are promptly killed.

Irritating fumes limit formaldehyde's usefulness. It is also toxic to tissues; therefore materials treated with formaldehyde must be thoroughly rinsed before use.

Glutaraldehyde

Glutaraldehyde is related to formaldehyde but is more active. An aqueous solution of 2% is equivalent to an 8% solution of formaldehyde and alcohol. It is a high-level disinfectant that is useful in disinfecting lensed instruments. Manufacturers' recommendations should be consulted for length of immersion time in glutaraldehyde. OSHA has established a permissible ceiling exposure limit of 0.2 ppm, as a result of reports on worker sensitivity (Vesley et al., 1992).

SKIN CLEANSING AND DISINFECTION

To prevent bacteria on the skin surfaces from entering the surgical wound, the skin area of and around the proposed incision, as well as the hands and forearms of the members of the operating team, must be cleansed and disinfected. Proper skin cleansing and disinfection depend on knowledge of the physiology and bacteriology of the skin and of the action of soaps, detergents, and antiseptic agents.

OBJECTIVES AND INFLUENCING FACTORS

Skin preparation methods vary, but all are based on the same principles and share the same objectives: to remove dirt and transient microbes from the skin, to reduce the resident microbial count as much as possible in the shortest time and with the least amount of tissue irritation, and to prevent rapid rebound growth of microbes.

The same general principles of skin cleansing apply whether the situation is preparation of the patient's skin at the operative site or preparation of the hands and arms of the members of the operating team. In either case, factors to be considered in skin disinfection are (1) the condition of the involved area, (2) the number and kinds of contaminants, (3) the characteristics of the skin to be disinfected, and (4) the general physical condition of the individual.

STRUCTURE AND PHYSIOLOGY OF THE SKIN

The skin consists of two distinct layers: the epidermis, which is a stratified squamous epithelium, and the true skin, or dermis (Fig. 3-15). The outer layer, or epidermis, is the tissue to be treated by cleansing and disinfecting procedures.

The epidermis constantly sheds the cells that form its horny outer layer, which are replaced by the multiplication and upward movement of cells from the lower levels. It has no blood vessels, although hair shafts, glandular ducts, and fine nerves reach through it. The dermis is a connective tissue containing blood and lymph vessels, sweat and sebaceous glands, nerves, and hair follicles.

Bacteria are found in all levels of the skin and comprise two groups, the transient and resident flora. Transient bacteria are usually limited to exposed areas of skin. They may be free on the skin or be loosely attached by grease or dirt, especially in the subungual areas. The transient flora are easily removed by mechanical cleansing of the skin.

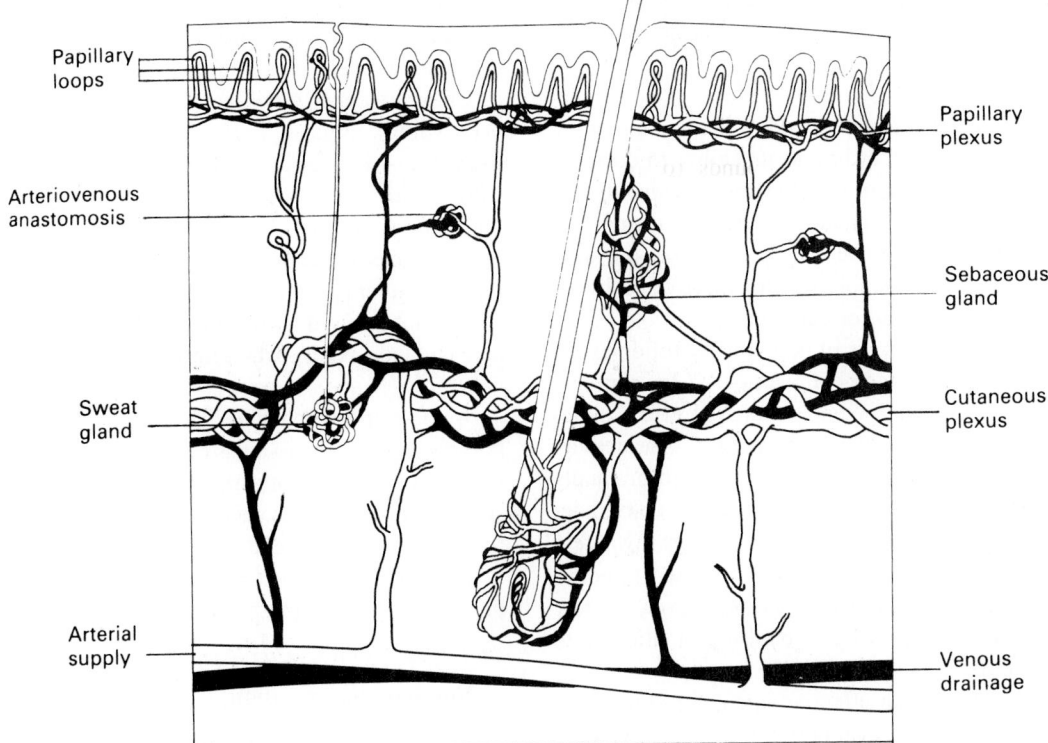

FIG. 3-15   The skin layers include the epidermis, the outermost layer, composed of stratified squamous epithelial cells. The basement membrane zone (BMZ) is the area that separates the epidermis from the dermis. The dermis contains the major proteins collagen and elastin. The hypodermis, or superficial fascia, forms a subcutaneous layer below the dermis. As shown in this figure, the hypodermis is an adipose layer containing a subdermal plexus of blood vessels that give rise to the cutaneous plexus in the dermis, which in turn gives rise to the papillary plexus and loops in the papillary dermis.

From Bryant, RA. (1992). *Acute and chronic wounds: Nursing management.* St. Louis, Mosby.

Bacteria that inhabit the deep structures of the dermis, the glands, and the hair follicles are considered the resident flora. They tend to move out and are shed with the old cells and skin secretions. The epidermal layers contain this debris from the dermis as well as soil and bacteria picked up by contact with various objects.

The resident flora of the skin are forced to the surface with perspiration and other secretions. This action is one way in which the skin disinfects and reconditions itself. The bacteria accompanying these secretions from the deep layers may, however, become a source of infection. The activity of sweat glands is increased by external heat, emotional stress, and certain diaphoretic drugs.

Generally, the acidity of perspiration acts as a protective barrier against the growth of certain microorganisms. However, the perspiration in axillary and pubic regions has a higher pH and may permit more bacterial growth. Bacteria are also protected by the folds, ridges, and crevices of the skin from which detritus is not as readily shed as from smoother surfaces.

AGENTS FOR SKIN CLEANSING AND DISINFECTION

Many soaps and detergents are available for skin cleansing. Although most of them produce similar results in the immediate removal of soil and microorganisms, certain factors need further consideration in selecting a product for surgical use. Equally important, an effective antimicrobial agent should be used to achieve appropriate disinfection of skin.

Soaps and detergents

Most soaps and detergents emulsify and peptize other waste products and oils that are absorbed in surface soil and permit the detritus to be rinsed off the skin with running water. The product selected should hydrolyze in the presence of water and yield a pH that corresponds to that of average, normal skin. An odorless agent that produces a good lather for easy, comfortable use is usually preferred. It should not irritate the skin or in any way interfere with normal functioning. Careful rinsing and drying help to minimize skin irritation resulting from frequent scrubbing.

Hexachlorophene added to agents used for cleansing the skin has been found to suppress bacterial growth on the skin. Hexachlorophene retains its antibacterial power in the presence of soap and is combined with it in numerous liquid and solid forms. However, it has known toxic effects that make it less popular today.

Sterilizing the skin is impossible because chemicals that have the power to destroy bacteria are also injurious to the living tissues of the skin. Thus new bacterial populations are constantly being brought to the surface of normal skin.

Antiseptic agents

The antimicrobial agent employed for disinfection of the skin should be selected according to its ability to decrease rapidly the microbial count of the skin and its capability of being applied quickly and remaining effective throughout the operation. It should not cause irritation or sensitization and should not be imcompatible with or inactivated by alcohol, organic matter, soap, or detergent.

Povidone-iodine, a complex of polyvinylpyrrolidone and iodine, is a common antimicrobial agent used for skin disinfection. It possesses the potent germicidal effect of iodine without many of its irritating properties. The activity of this agent is prolonged because it is released gradually from the binding polymer as the brownish iodine color fades from the skin. It is effective in the presence of pus, whereas the activity of the iodine complex is of somewhat shorter duration in the presence of blood or serum. It can be safely used on mucous membranes but should not be allowed to pool on the skin or in body cavities.

Tincture of iodine is an effective agent for skin disinfection, although not as commonly used as povidone-iodine. The modern iodine tincture *(USP XVIII)* contains 2% iodine, 2.4% potassium iodide, and 44% to 50% alcohol by volume. Iodine is a good bactericide but stains fabric and tissue. In combination with alcohol, iodine is tuberculocidal and appears to increase the efficiency of the alcohol as a skin antiseptic. Iodine has the disadvantage of potentially causing tissue irritation and sensitization.

The effectiveness of alcohol as an antiseptic is probably derived from the solution of lipoidal secretions of the skin and consequent mechanical removal of microorganisms. Absolute alcohol has little or no germicidal activity. For skin disinfection, 70% alcohol is the concentration typically used. Because of flammability, it is used in small quantities, applied with sponges or applicators, and not allowed to pool. A 70% alcohol solution is relatively safe and is a cost-effective skin-defatting agent and antiseptic.

Hexachlorophene is a bacteriostatic agent that is active against gram-positive microorganisms but only minimally active against gram-negative microorganisms. If the skin surface is washed frequently each day with hexachlorophene, a relatively low flora population may gradually be achieved and maintained. Hexachlorophene forms a long-lasting, imperceptible bacteriostatic film on the skin and develops a cumulative suppressive action with routine use. With the increasing problem of *Pseudomonas* and other gram-negative microorganisms as sources of wound infection, and because of studies demonstrating the toxicity of hexachlorophene, its use should be carefully evaluated.

Quarternary ammonium compounds (quats) such as benzalkonium chloride are surface-active agents that are bactericidal against gram-positive bacteria but less active against gram-negative bacteria and fungi. Quats do not kill endospores or tuberculosis bacteria and should not be considered a satisfactory antiseptic. The *Pseudomonas* microorganism actively grows in quats.

Chlorhexidene, a halogenated aromatic compound, has been widely used as a skin disinfectant. It has also been used in a 4% cleansing solution for a preoperative scrub. Chlorhexidene is effective against most vegetative bacteria but is not sporicidal. It works more rapidly than hexachlorophene, has fewer irritating qualities, and has been used more frequently than hexachlorophene. Chlorhexidene should not be used above the neck due to potential corneal damage and toxicity when introduced into the auditory canal.

A one-step iodophor (0.5% iodine, 70% isopropyl alcohol) has been tested to be as effective as the traditional two-step method (iodophor scrub and paint solutions) in patient skin preparation. This technique takes less time, provides for easy application, and has proven to be equally effective in infection prevention compared to the traditional two-step prep (Research Highlight 3-4).

PREOPERATIVE SKIN PREPARATION
Nursing considerations

Preoperative skin preparation of a surgical patient is the first step in the prevention of wound infection. Because the procedure may be alarming, embarrassing, or uncomfortable for the patient, every effort should be made to minimize these features by proceeding in a considerate, methodical, and professional manner.

If the preoperative skin preparation is done when the patient is awake, the nurse should explain the purpose and method of the procedure. Every effort should be made to allay any fears the patient may express and to answer questions in a reassuring manner. During the procedure, the nurse should observe the patient's general condition, particularly the condition of the skin under treatment. Any contraindication to the procedure because of an abnormal skin condition or an adverse reaction by or injury to the patient should be documented and reported to the physician.

In carrying out the procedure, the nurse should provide for the comfort, safety, and privacy of the patient. Good alignment of the patient's body should be maintained, and special supports for positioning should be used, as indicated.

Initial preparation of operative area

In the immediate preoperative period the skin of the involved part of the body is prepared by special cleansing. Hair should be removed from the operative site only as necessary. Three alternatives for hair removal are clipping, use of a depilatory, and wet shaving. Studies show that the wound infection rate is considerably higher for patients who are shaved preoperatively than for patients who have no preoperative shave preparation or a small amount of hair clipped, or for patients on whom a depilatory is used. If a shave is ordered by the surgeon, the patient should be

※
RESEARCH HIGHLIGHT 3-4

Preoperative preparation of the patient's skin at the surgical site can be accomplished with a number of agents. Depending on the agent selected and the technique of application, the skin preparation procedure varies in both length and efficacy. This study compared a 10-minute scrub with an iodophor detergent, followed by an application of an aqueous iodophor solution to skin antisepsis with application of a water-soluble iodophor in 70% isopropyl alcohol. There were 240 general surgery patients in the study who were randomly assigned to one of the skin preparation groups. Most patients did not complete a preoperative shower with an antimicrobial agent. If shaving of hair from the operative site was required, it was completed in the OR.

To compare the results of the two groups, a number of measures were used. Skin contact culture specimens, immediately before the skin prep and just after skin closure, were obtained from the first 30 patients in each group. All patients were followed for 30 days postoperatively to determine the presence of wound infection. Between-group comparisons indicated that there were no statistically significant differences in bacterial counts or wound infection. The authors noted the advantage of a shorter preparation time in terms of convenience, cost, and ease of use.

Howard, R.J. (1991, July). Comparison of a 10-minute aqueous iodophor and 2-minute water-insoluble iodophor in alcohol preoperative skin preparation. *Complications in Surgery*, 43-45.

shaved as close to the time of surgery as possible. The shave should be performed in an area within the surgical suite that affords privacy and is equipped with good lighting facilities. The amount of time between the preoperative shave and the operation has a direct effect on the wound infection rate. Hair removal should be performed by skillful personnel with great care taken to avoid scratching, nicking, or cutting the skin because cutaneous bacteria will proliferate in these areas and increase the chances of infection. The decision of where and by whom the procedure is performed depends on when it is to be done, the facilities and personnel available, the patient's reactions, and the philosophy and policies that have been determined and established by the surgical committee.

Although specific orders for the skin preparation are written by the surgeon, a manual with diagrams and instructions concerning the preoperative skin shave is useful for the guidance and information of the personnel to whom the task is delegated. The extent of the area to be shaved is determined by the site of the incision and the nature of the operation.

Shaving the face and neck of children or female patients is rarely necessary. The eyebrows are not shaved unless specifically ordered by the physician. The head and neck are not generally prone to wound infection because of the generous blood supply to this area. For cosmetic and psychologic reasons, preparation for head and neck surgery may be done in the operating room after the induction of anesthesia.

For orthopedic surgery on the extremities, the shave preparation usually extends from one joint above to one joint below the area of incision. If a pneumatic tourniquet will be used during surgery, the entire extremity may be prepared to facilitate proper draping technique. Preparation and draping of the entire extremity also permit manipulation of the limb during surgery.

Great care should be exercised in the skin preparations for orthopedic surgery because wound infections resulting from improper cleansing may cause an osteomyelitis that leads to crippling disfigurement and permanent dysfunction. The skin may be difficult to clean if it has been affected by casts, splints, or braces that interfere with normal skin care or cause skin damage. Daily soaking may help to clean badly soiled feet in preparation for surgery, just as daily washing is advisable in preparation for general elective surgery.

Patients with traumatic injuries that may be excessively painful, such as fractures, burns, and soft tissue lacerations, may require anesthesia for skin preparation. Traumatic wounds usually require copious irrigation to flush out foreign matter. In cleansing the injured area, the surrounding skin is first carefully washed with an antimicrobial detergent. The open wound is irrigated with an isotonic solution, and the area is treated with an antimicrobial solution.

If a patient must be shaved in the operating room, a heavy lather should be used on the skin to control hair clippings and epithelium removed by the razor. Skin preparation in the operating room has the disadvantages that the patient's anesthesia time is prolonged, optimum use of the operating room is infringed on, loose hair remaining on the surrounding linen may get into the wound, and water used to wash the skin can result in sterile drapes becoming wet.

Procedure for preoperative shave

Individual supplies are used for each patient. Commercially prepared kits that contain the basic essentials for shaving the site of incision are available. The use of disposable prep trays and razors can help ensure a safe, personal technique. The use of disposable gloves is a safeguard for the patient and for the worker. Blankets and supports for the patient's position, as well as the necessary lighting and handwashing facilities, should be provided in the area where shaving is performed. Basic equipment includes gloves, basins for warm water and soap, a disposable razor, sponges for washing, and towels or waterproof pads for draping. Solvent solution may also be required to remove adhesives or nail polish. Volatile liquids such as alcohol and acetone should be strictly regulated because of the danger of fire or burns.

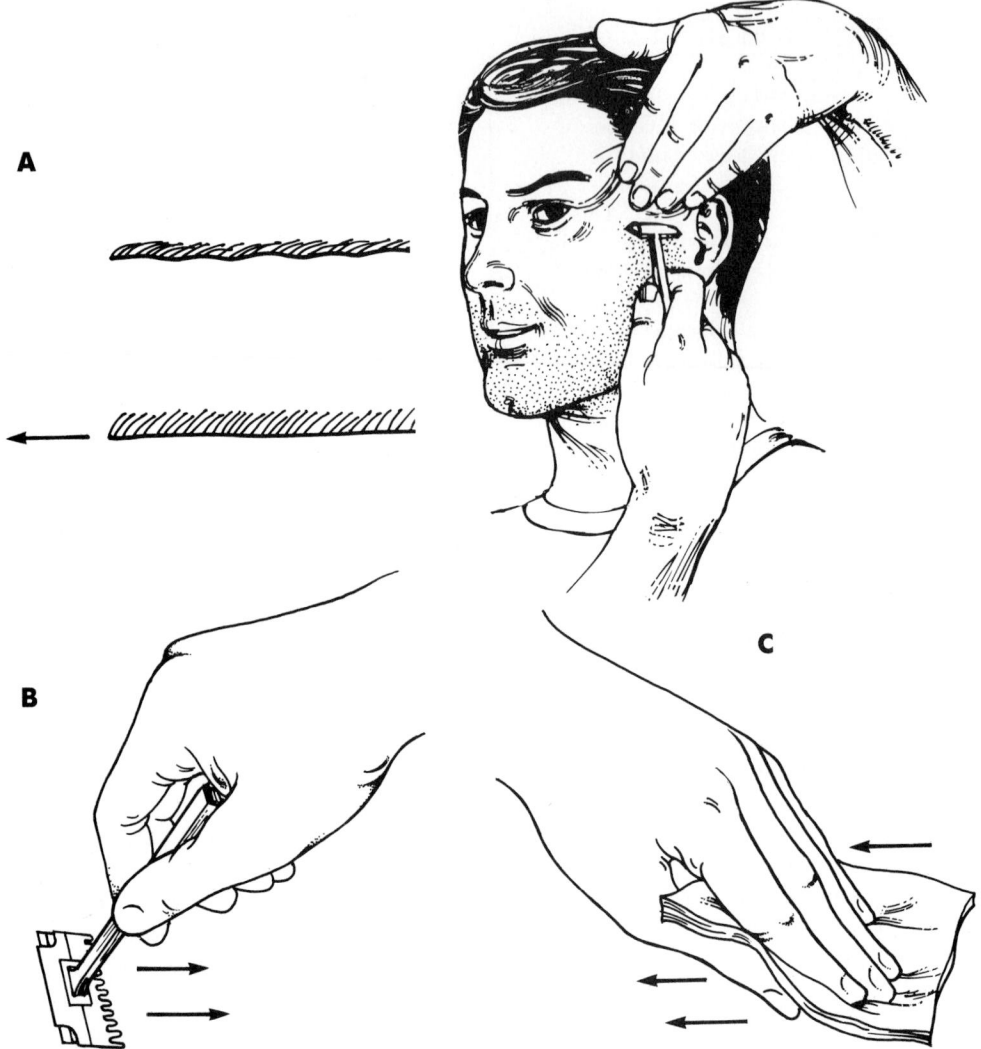

FIG. 3-16   Skin shaving. **A,** Skin traction is provided with free hand in direct opposition to slant of hair to tighten and smooth skin and raise hairs in more upright position. **B,** Hair and horny layer of skin are shaved off. **C,** Traction is applied with sponge, and hoe-type razor head is held against skin, as shown in **B.**

From Pate, M.O. *The preparation manual.* Long Island City, N.Y.: Edward Weck.

Antimicrobial soap or detergent should be applied to the skin area using sponges moistened with water. A lather is created by using a circular motion and light friction. Application of lather to skin hair for several minutes before shaving enables the keratin of the hair to absorb three to four times its weight in water. The water absorbtion makes the hair softer and easier to shave.

When using a standard razor for the wet method, a disposable razor with a sharp blade is used to shave off the lathered hair. Holding the soft areas and loose skin taut with the free hand raises the hair and permits easier access to the area. A clean shave can be obtained without injury to the skin by gently stroking in the direction of the hair growth (Fig. 3-16). The razor should be kept in contact with the patient's skin for each stroke. Nicks or cuts resulting from the shave should be reported as incidents, and the surgeon should be notified.

Depilatory cream is another mechanism for the removal of hair preoperatively. Before use of this cream the patient should be tested for sensitivity with a skin patch test. The manufacturer's recommendations for application of the depilatory cream should be followed.

Use of an electric clipper, with a disposable head, is another mechanism for hair removal. The patient's hair should be clean, and a wet or dry method may be used to clip the hair. The clipper blade is moved against the direction of hair growth while the nurse holds the skin taut.

The surgeon may order a 5-minute scrub of the prepared

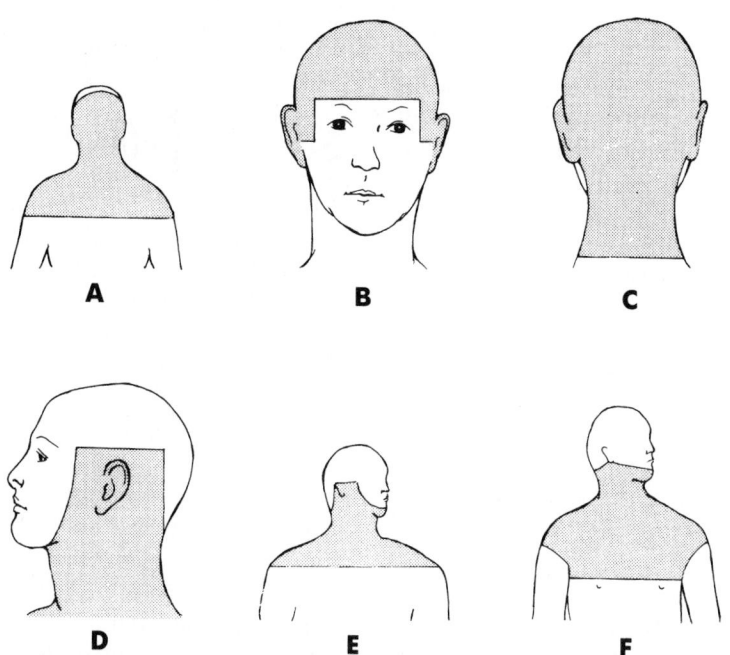

FIG. 3-17 Preparation for head, major neck, and upper thorax surgery. **A,** For posterior craniotomy. **B** and **C,** For craniotomy, frontal tumor excision. **D,** For major otologic operations. **E,** For removal of lesions of neck and glands. **F,** For esophageal diverticulectomy, esophagotomy, scalenectomy, cervicothoracic anterior approach, thyroidectomy, and laryngectomy.

Modified from Pate, M.O. *The preparation manual.* Long Island City, N.Y.: Edward Weck.

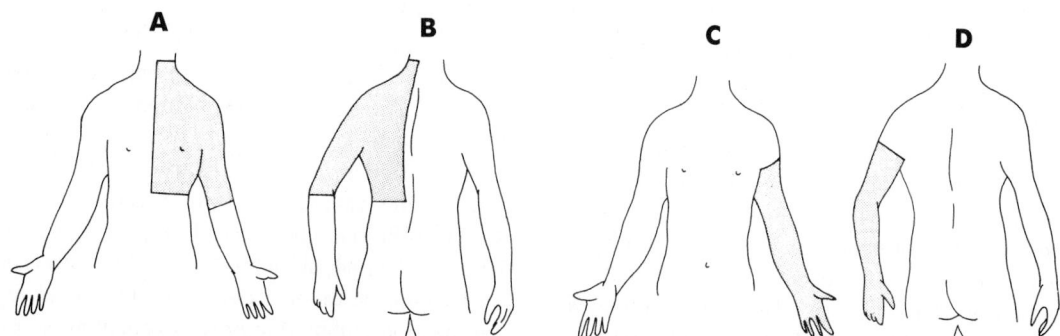

FIG. 3-18 Preparation for surgery of upper extremity. **A** and **B,** For major operations on shoulder and uppermost part of extremity, skin area is prepared from neckline to elbow line and axilla to midline anteriorly and posteriorly. **C** and **D,** For operations on forearm, preparation includes entire arm from fingertips to and including axilla.

Modified from Pate, M.O. *The preparation manual.* Long Island City, N.Y.: Edward Weck.

area with an antimicrobial soap or detergent after the area has been shaved. If so, the shaved area is scrubbed and rinsed carefully, and the skin is blotted dry to prevent chapping and irritation.

At the conclusion of the preparation, the patient should be made comfortable, the unit left in order, and the equipment disposed of or cleaned. Reusable items should be washed and sterilized. Expendable materials should be disposed of according to procedure. The worker should follow the principles of aseptic technique for the removal of gloves and for terminal handwashing before proceeding to the care of other patients.

Final skin disinfection of operative area

After the patient has been positioned on the operating room bed, final skin cleansing and disinfection are performed. If the patient has not showered with an antimicrobial detergent or soap immediately before leaving for the operating room, the operative area may be prepared with an antimicrobial scrub solution. While this is being carried out, the shave can be inspected and touched up or extended, as needed. Skin cleansing is followed by prepping with an antimicrobial solution.

Procedure for final skin prepping

The supplies required for the final skin prepping may be arranged on a separate sterile prepping table. The items should include stainless steel cups for the cleansing agent and the selected antimicrobial agent, sterile sponges, and sponge-holding forceps, if desired. Cotton-tipped applicators are needed to clean the umbilicus thoroughly, and a scrub brush may be required for nails, callused skin, or traumatic injuries of the hands and feet. Final skin disinfection may be done by the circulating nurse or the surgeon.

The skin scrub begins at the line of the proposed incision and proceeds to the periphery of the area (Figs. 3-17 to 3-24). The antimicrobial agent is applied by sponges held in sponge forceps or in the gloved hand. The gloved-hand method requires that the glove be sterile at the beginning of the skin scrub and that the surface of the patient's skin not be permitted to come into contact with the gloved hand. The sponges used in scrubbing are discarded as they become soiled, and fresh ones are taken. A soiled sponge is never brought back over a scrubbed surface. The lather is wiped off with dry, sterile sponges. Depending on the surgeon's preference, an antimicrobial tincture or "paint" may be carefully applied, avoiding any pooling beneath the patient. All wet drapes should be removed from the patient area after the skin scrub is complete.

When a stoma or other contaminated area is involved in the prep procedure, a prep sponge (4 × 4) soaked in the antimicrobial agent of choice is placed over the stoma when the prep is initiated. At the completion of the prep the sponge is discarded.

Sponges used to cleanse or disinfect a wound, sinus, ulcer, intestinal stoma, the vagina, or the anus are applied once to that area. After prep of the area, intestinal fistulas are generally walled off with one of the plastic transparent adhesive drapes. In contrast to the principle of working from the proposed incision to the periphery, open wounds and body orifices are potentially contaminated areas and as such are prepped after the peripheral intact skin is cleansed. The surgical principle is always to scrub the cleanest area first.

SURGICAL HAND SCRUB
GENERAL CONSIDERATIONS

The objectives of the surgical hand scrub are to remove dirt, skin oil, and microbes from hands and lower arms; to reduce the microbial count to as near zero as possible; and to leave an antimicrobial residue on the skin to prevent growth of microbes for several hours. The skin can never be rendered sterile, but it can be made surgically clean by reducing the number of microorganisms present. A lengthy mechanical scrub, even with strong antiseptics, will fail to remove all microorganisms. Friction and rinsing significantly decrease the number of bacteria on the epidermis, but their numbers are constantly replenished by the continuous secretory activity of the skin glands.

Only persons who feel well and are free from upper respiratory tract infections and skin problems should scrub. Cuts, abrasions, and hangnails tend to ooze serum, which is a medium for prolific bacterial growth and can endanger the patient by increasing the hazards of infection.

Hospital procedures govern the selection of materials and the methods used for the surgical handscrub. The selection of a reusable or disposable brush for scrubbing should be based on realistic considerations of effectiveness and economy. Studies show no significant difference in scrub effectiveness between reusable brushes and disposable brushes or sponges.

Individually packaged disposable brushes and sponges provide a cost-effective, labor-saving alternative to reusable brushes. The use of synthetic sponges in place of brushes has gained wide acceptance, especially where long and repeated scrubbing may be traumatic to the skin. Disposable brushes are available with several antimicrobial soap or detergent solutions impregnated in the sponge. If a reusable brush is desired, it should be easy to clean and maintain and should be durable enough to withstand repeated heat sterilization without the bristles becoming soft or brittle.

The antimicrobial soap or detergent used for the surgical hand scrub should act rapidly, have a broad spectrum, not depend on cumulative action, have a minimally harsh effect on skin, and inhibit rapid growth of microbes.

Two popular antimicrobial agents used for surgical hand scrubs are povidone-iodine and chlorhexidine gluconate. Both are rapid-acting, broad-spectrum antimicrobials that are effective against gram-positive and gram-negative microorganisms. For individuals who have demonstrated skin sensitivity to these agents, another broad-spectrum antimi-

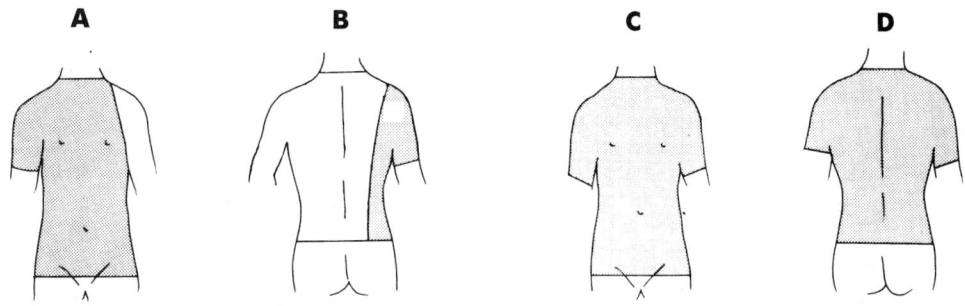

FIG. 3-19 **A** and **B,** For unilateral chest operations and radical mastectomies, affected chest, shoulder, and upper arm are prepared, from nipple on unaffected side to bedline on affected side. **C** and **D,** For combined thoracoabdominal operations, chest and shoulder are prepared bilaterally, anteriorly, and posteriorly. For cardiac surgery, this preparation may be extended to include legs.

Modified from Pate, M.O. *The preparation manual.* Long Island City, N.Y.: Edward Weck.

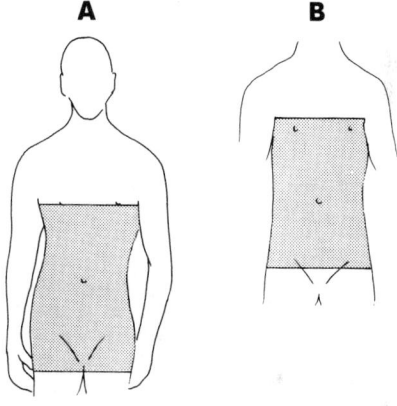

FIG. 3-20 Preparation for abdominal surgery. **A,** Skin area is cleansed and disinfected from nipple line to 3 inches below symphysis pubis, including external genitals, and from bedline to bedline. This preparation is done for gastrointestinal, biliary, and liver operations; splenectomy; herniorrhaphy; appendectomy; and surgery on great vessels of trunk. **B,** Skin prepared from above nipple line to above symphysis pubis. This preparation is done for gastrointestinal, biliary, and liver operations.

Modified from Pate, M.O. *The preparation manual.* Long Island City, N.Y.: Edward Weck.

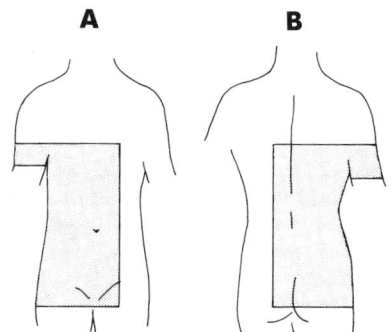

FIG. 3-21 Lateral preparation for operations on kidney and upper ureter. **A,** Anterior view. **B,** Posterior view.

Modified from Pate, M.O. *The preparation manual.* Long Island City, N.Y.: Edward Weck.

FIG. 3-22 **A,** Preparation for cervical laminectomy. **B,** Preparation for lumbar laminectomy. Preparation includes hairline to fold of buttocks and to bedlines laterally.

Modified from Pate, M.O. *The preparation manual.* Long Island City, N.Y.: Edward Weck.

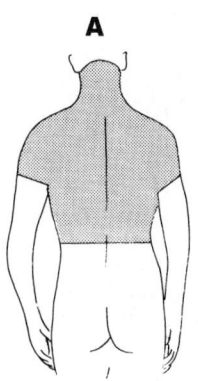
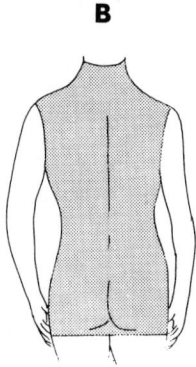

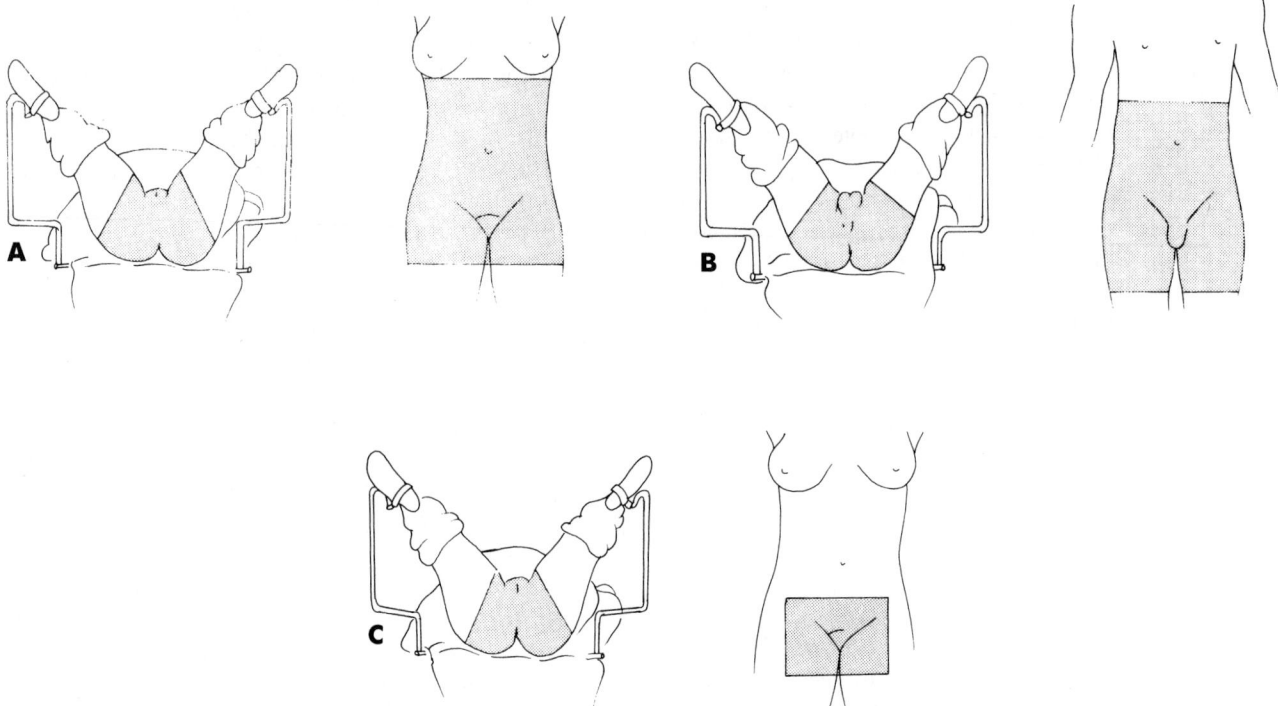

FIG. 3-23 Pelvic and perineal preparation for gynecologic and genitourinary operations. **A,** Preparation for combined vaginal and abdominal operations. **B,** Preparation for suprapubic prostatectomy and bladder operations. **C,** Preparation for minor vaginal and rectal operations.

Modified from Pate, M.O. *The preparation manual.* Long Island City, N.Y.: Edward Weck.

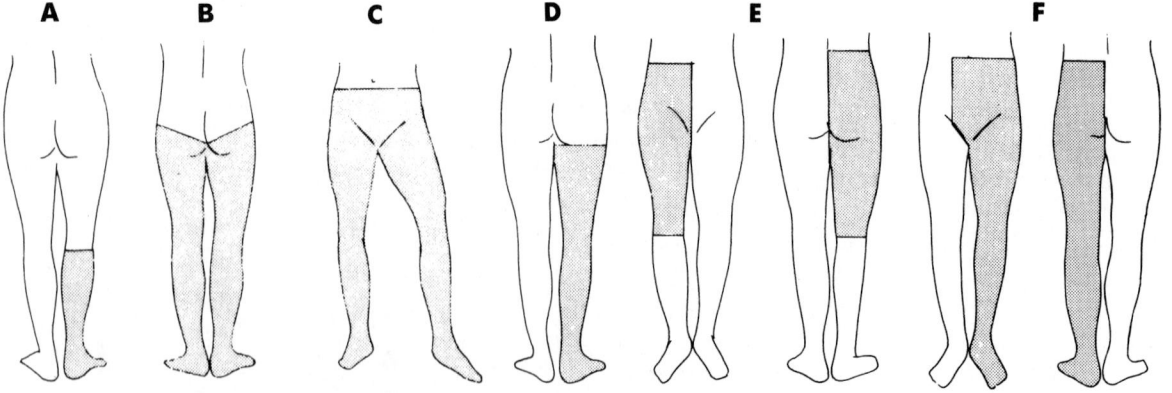

FIG. 3-24 Preparation for surgery of lower extremity. **A,** For operations on ankle, foot, or toes, lower leg is prepared anteriorly and posteriorly. **B** and **C,** For bilateral leg operations such as varicose vein ligation and skin and bone grafts. **D,** For operations on foot and lower leg, entire leg is prepared anteriorly and posteriorly. **E,** For unilateral hip operations. **F,** For unilateral operations involving hip and thigh.

Modified from Pate, M.O. *The preparation manual.* Long Island City, N.Y.: Edward Weck.

crobial agent, parachlorometaxylenol (PCMX), is being used as an effective alternative agent for surgical scrubbing. Many persons who previously were unable to use any surgical hand scrub other than hexachlorophene (which is ineffective against gram-negative microorganisms) are now safely using PCMX. It significantly reduces skin flora with an antibacterial effect that persists even after prolonged surgery. Moisturizing agents are now being incorporated into various surgical scrubs to reduce the potential of skin irritation resulting from multiple scrubs.

In scrubbing, light friction is effective in removing the detritus of the epithelium. The friction produces heat, dilatation of the blood vessels, and better circulation, which help to recondition the skin. Hard scrubbing and harsh bristles tend to cause desquamation, leaving a bleeding or weeping dermis that is painful and predisposes to infection. It also may massage bacteria into the deeper dermal layers.

An anatomic scrub using a prescribed amount of time or number of strokes plus friction is employed for effective cleansing of the skin. A properly executed surgical hand scrub, using the anatomic counted brush stroke method, usually takes approximately 5 minutes. Studies indicate no significant difference in microbial reduction between scrubs of 5 minutes' duration and those of 10 minutes' duration. Individual attention to detail is essential. The same scrub procedure should be used for every scrub, whether it is the first or last scrub of the day.

The prescribed number of strokes with a brush is usually 30 strokes to the nails and 20 strokes to each area of the skin. When scrubbing, the fingers, hands, and arms should be visualized as having four sides; *each* side must be scrubbed effectively.

The number of deep-resident flora is reduced by frequent scrubbing, but the number is increased when the surgical scrub is done only occasionally.

PROCEDURE

Surgical hand scrub techniques that personnel must observe should be defined in writing. Before beginning the surgical hand scrub, members of the surgical team inspect their hands to ensure their nails are short and free from polish, their cuticles are in good condition, and no cuts or skin problems exist. All jewelry is removed from the hands and forearms. The cap or hood is adjusted to cover and contain all hair. A fresh mask is carefully placed over the nose and mouth and tied securely to prevent venting. Goggles or protective eyewear is comfortably adjusted to ensure clear vision and to avoid lens fogging. Personnel confirm that the scrub shirt is fitted, tied, or tucked into the trousers to prevent potential contamination of the scrubbed hands and arms from brushing against loose garments.

The basic steps of the procedure follow:

1. The faucet is turned on, and the water brought to a comfortable temperature. Most scrub sinks have automatic or knee controls for the faucets.

2. The hands and forearms are dampened.

3. By a foot control, a few drops of the antimicrobial soap or detergent are dispensed into the palms. Small amounts of water are added to make a lather.

4. The hands and forearms are washed using an approved surgical scrub agent and rinsed prior to beginning the surgical hand scrub. The amount of time needed varies with the amount of soil and the effectiveness of the cleansing agent.

5. If a packaged scrub brush or sponge is used, the package is opened, the brush and nail cleaner removed, and the package discarded. The brush is held in one hand to clean the nails on the other hand. All nails and subungual spaces are cleaned. If a disposable nail cleaner is not available, a metal nail file can be used. Orangewood sticks are prohibited because they cannot be sterilized after use.

6. The hands and arms are rinsed thoroughly; care is taken to hold the hands higher than the elbows. Splashing water onto the scrub suit should be avoided because this moisture may cause subsequent contamination of the sterile gown.

7. If the brush or sponge is impregnated with antimicrobial soap, it should be moistened and scrubbing begun. If the brush or sponge is not impregnated with soap, antimicrobial soap or detergent solution is applied to hands. Starting at the fingertips, the nails are scrubbed vigorously while the brush is held perpendicular to them. All sides of each digit are scrubbed, including the web spaces between them. The palm and back of the hand are then scrubbed.

8. Each side of the forearm is scrubbed with a circular motion (Fig. 3-25).

9. The hands are held above the level of the elbows while scrubbing to allow the water and detritus to flow away from the first-scrubbed and cleanest area. The hands and arms are also held away from the body. Small amounts of water are added during the scrub to develop suds and remove detritus.

10. The hands and arms are rinsed thoroughly. The brush is discarded in a proper receptacle.

11. If the sink is not automatically timed, the faucet is turned off by using the knee control or by using the edge of the brush on a hand control.

12. The hands and arms are held up in front of the body with elbows slightly flexed while the nurse enters the operating room.

DRYING THE CLEANSED AREA

Moisture remaining on the cleansed skin after the scrub procedure is dried with a sterile towel before a sterile gown and gloves are donned. The gown and gloves should be opened on a flat surface prior to doing the surgical scrub. The gown and gloves should not be opened on the sterile back table because of the increased chance of contamination to the field. The towel must be used with care to avoid

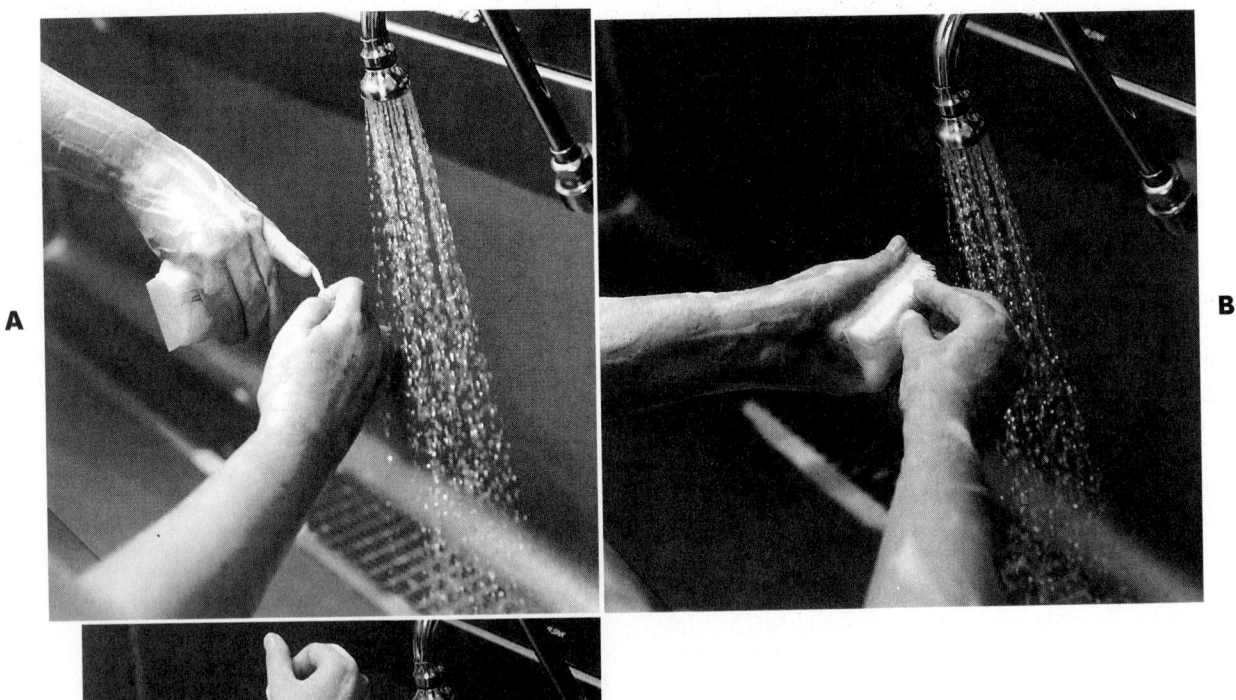

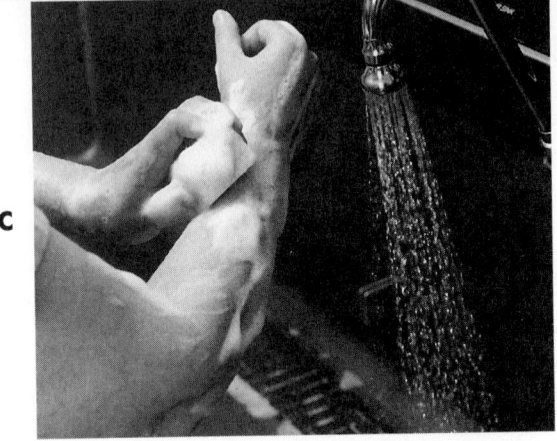

FIG. 3-25 Surgical scrub technique. **A,** Cleaning nails with plastic nail cleaner. **B,** Holding brush perpendicular to nails facilitates thorough scrubbing of undersides of nails. **C,** Holding brush lengthwise along arm covers maximum area with each stroke.

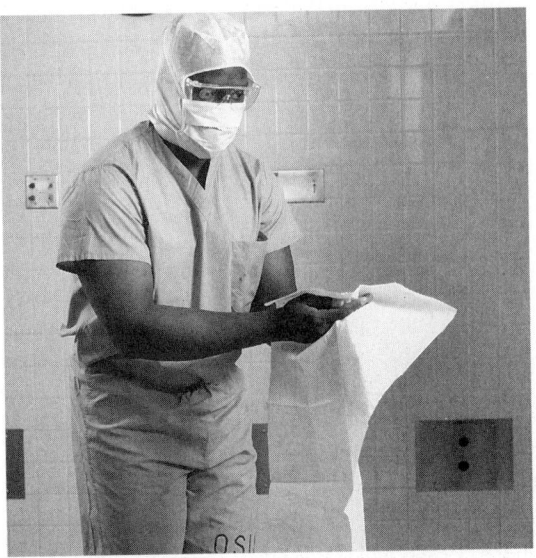

FIG. 3-26 Drying hands and forearms. Fingers and hand are dried thoroughly before forearm is dried. Extending arms reduces possibility of contaminating towel or hands.

contaminating the cleansed skin. The procedure for opening the sterile towel to dry the hands and forearms will vary, depending on the method used in folding the towel before sterilization.

The folded towel is grasped firmly near the open corner and lifted straight up and away from the sterile field without dripping contaminated water from the skin onto the sterile field. The person steps away from the sterile field and bends forward slightly from the waist, holding the hands and elbows above the waist and away from the body. The towel is allowed to unfold downward to its full length and width (Fig. 3-26).

The top half of the towel is held securely with one hand, and the opposite fingers and hand are blotted dry; the nurse ensures they are thoroughly dry before moving to the forearm. To avoid contamination, a rotating motion is used while moving up the arm, and an area is not retraced. The lower end of the towel is grasped with the dried hand, and the same procedure is used for drying the second hand and forearm. Care must be taken to prevent contamination of towel and hands. The towel is discarded.

GOWNING AND GLOVING PROCEDURES

Before scrubbed personnel can touch sterile equipment or the sterile field, they must put on sterile gowns and sterile surgical gloves to prevent microorganisms on their hands and clothing from being transferred to the patient's wound during surgery. The sterile gowns and gloves also protect the hands and clothing of personnel from microorganisms present in the patient or in the atmosphere.

DESIGN AND PACKAGING OF THE GOWN

The gown should be made of a material that establishes an effective barrier, minimizing the passage of microorganisms between unsterile and sterile areas. Reusable fabrics must allow complete penetration of steam during the sterilization process and should withstand multiple in-house processes and multiple launderings. Tests indicate that 280-count, water-repellent materials lose their barrier quality after laundering and sterilizing 75 times. Reusable materials should be checked for barrier effectiveness by examining for holes or fraying; if this occurs, the material should be removed from service. A mechanism should be established to monitor the number of launderings. The material should be resistant to tearing and puncture and as lint free as possible to reduce the dissemination of particles into the wound and the environment. It should facilitate aseptic technique and avoid excessive heat buildup. Regardless of the gown's material, the shape and size should fit the wearer and allow freedom of movement. To provide extra protection, the gown's front from the waist upward and the forearms of the sleeves are made of a water-repellent material. Each sleeve should be finished with a tight-fitting wristlet that

prevents the inner side of the sleeve from slipping down onto the outer side of the sterile glove. Cotton tapes, snaps, or Velcro fasteners are attached to the back of the gown to hold it closed. A wraparound gown should be used to achieve better coverage of the back.

Because the outer side of the front and sleeves of the gown come in contact with the sterile field during surgery, the gown must be folded so that the scrubbed person can put it on without touching the outer side with bare hands. For in-house wrapping and sterilization, the gown is folded with the inner side out and the back edges together. The sleeves are not turned inside out; consequently, they remain within the folded gown. The side folds of the gown are folded lengthwise toward the center back opening, overlapping slightly at the center. With the open edges of the gown remaining on the inside, the bottom third of the gown is folded upward and the top third of the gown is folded over the bottom portion. The gown is then folded in half widthwise so that the inside front neckline of the gown is visible on top.

Gowns with wraparound backs are prepared in the same manner, with care taken to tie the tape securely on the wraparound back flap to the external side tie of the gown before initial folding. A folded hand towel with its free corners facing up is usually placed on top of the folded gown before the gown is wrapped and sterilized.

PROCEDURE FOR DONNING THE STERILE WRAPAROUND GOWN

Scrubbed personnel use the following procedure for donning the sterile wraparound gown (Figs. 3-27 and 3-28).

1. The sterile gown is grasped at the neckline with both hands and lifted from the sterile gown wrapper; the

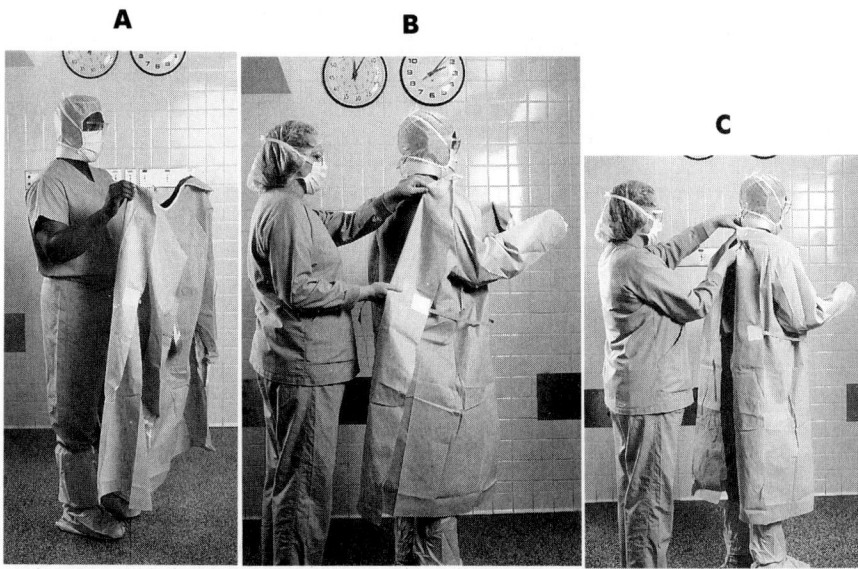

FIG. 3-27 Gowning procedure. **A,** Scrub nurse keeps hands on inside of gown while unfolding it at arm's length. **B,** Circulating nurse reaches under flap of gown to pull sleeves on scrub nurse. **C,** Circulating nurse snaps neckline of gown, touching only snap section of neckline.

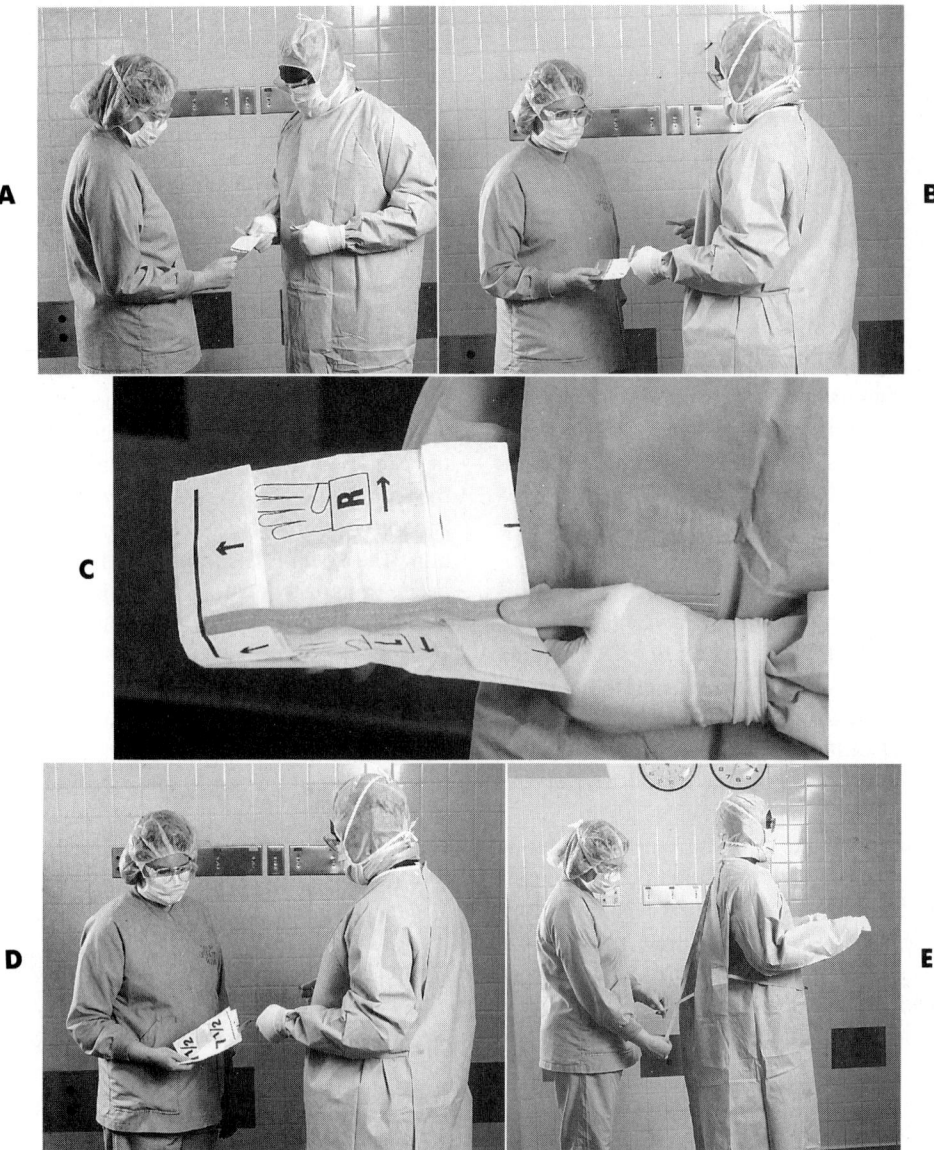

FIG. 3-28 Methods of tying wraparound gown. **A,** After handing tab on back tie of gown to circulating nurse, scrub nurse makes three-quarter turn toward left. **B,** Sterile back panel now covers previously tied unsterile ties; scrub nurse retrieves back tie by carefully pulling it out of tab held by circulating nurse and ties it securely with other tie. **C,** Using sterile inner glove wrapper, scrub nurse places end of back tie in crease of wrapper. **D,** After closing wrapper, scrub nurse hands it to circulating nurse, who grasps it carefully, touching neither tie nor gloved hand. **E,** After making three-quarter turn to left, scrub nurse carefully pulls back tie from wrapper.

scrub nurse steps into an area where the gown may be opened without risk of contamination.

2. The gown is held away from the body and allowed to unfold with the inside toward the wearer.
3. The gown is completely unfolded while the hands are kept on the inside of the gown.
4. Both hands are slipped into the open armholes at the

same time, keeping the hands at shoulder level and away from the body.

5. The hands and forearms are pushed into the sleeves of the gown, the hands advanced only to the proximal edge of the cuff if the closed gloving technique is used. If the open gloving technique is employed, the hands are advanced completely through the cuffs of the gown.

6. The circulating nurse pulls the gown over the shoulders and touches only the inner shoulder and side seams.

7. The circulating nurse ties or clasps the neckline and ties the inner waist ties of the gown by touching only the inner aspect of the gown. The gown should be completely fastened by the circulator before the scrub nurse dons gloves to prevent contamination from the gown flapping.

8. After gloving, the scrub nurse hands the tab attached to the back tie of the gown to the circulating nurse. The scrub nurse then makes a three-quarter turn to the left while the circulating nurse extends the back tie to its full length. This action effectively wraps the back panel of the gown around the scrub nurse and covers the previously tied inner waist ties. The scrub nurse retrieves the back tie by carefully pulling it out of the tab held by the circulating nurse and ties it with the other tie, which had been secured to the front top of the gown.

   a. If another scrubbed person is gowned and gloved, that individual, instead of the circulating nurse, may assist with the wraparound procedure. The assisting person must extend the back tie to its fullest length before the scrub nurse turns to avoid any potential contamination.

   b. When a reusable gown is utilized, an alternative method of tying a gown that does not have snaps should be used by the scrub nurse. If the closed gloving technique and commercially prepared, double-wrapped gloves are employed, the inner wrap can be used as a protective extension for the gown tie when the circulating nurse assists with tying a wraparound gown. After gloving, the scrub nurse unties the exterior gown ties (which were tied at the front of the gown before it was folded, wrapped, and sterilized) and holds both in the hands. The end of the back tie is placed in the center crease of the empty glove wrapper, approximately two thirds the way up to the edge of the opened wrapper. The glove wrapper is then closed so that the tie is concealed. The closed wrapper is handed to the circulating nurse, who firmly grasps the folded edge of the wrapper without touching the tie. The scrub nurse then pivots in the opposite direction from the circulating nurse, who extends the back tie to its full length. The scrub nurse grasps the exposed portion of the back tie, pulls it out of the glove wrapper while taking care to avoid touching the glove wrapper or the circulating nurse, and ties both ties. If a sterile glove wrapper is not available, a sterile hemostat may be clamped to the back tie and used in the same manner as a glove wrapper. After the gowning procedure has been completed, the circulating nurse retains the hemostat in the room to

avoid problems with the subsequent instrument count.

USE OF GLOVE LUBRICANTS

The use of powder as a glove lubricant is not recommended because of two primary hazards: the postoperative complication of powder granulomas is an ever-present danger, and powder fallout from hands and gloves provides a convenient vehicle for dissemination of microorganisms throughout the hospital. To remove any glove film or powder, the gloves must be wiped thoroughly after they are put on and before the surgical team member approaches the sterile field.

Cream or liquid lubricants of various types have been developed. Some of these contain antiseptic or bacteriostatic agents that assist in keeping the gloved hands relatively free from bacterial growth. Manufacturers of surgical gloves have also used silicone films to eliminate stickiness. Little or no lubrication of the hands is needed to don these gloves easily. Assessing these new products and practices requires determining their effectiveness for the purpose and their harmlessness to the skin and other body tissues of both patients and personnel.

The increased reporting of latex sensitivity has created concern among operating room personnel. Appropriate latex-free gloves should be provided for health care workers with known latex sensitivity or for procedures in which patients have known sensitivity or allergy. It is estimated that 7.9% of surgeons and 10% of operating room nurses exhibit signs of latex sensitivity (Fay, 1992). Nursing care policies for the care of patients with latex sensitivity should be developed. The irritation from latex products interferes with the integument's first line of defense against the transmission of most bloodborne pathogens.

PROCEDURE FOR DONNING STERILE GLOVES
Closed method

The closed method of gloving (Fig. 3-29) has the advantage of preventing the bare hands from coming in contact with the outside of the glove, which must remain sterile. The closed glove technique should be the technique of choice when donning sterile gloves. The gloves are handled through the fabric of the gown sleeves. The hands are not extended from the sleeves and wristlets when the gown is put on. Instead, the hands are pushed through the cuff openings as the gloves are pulled in place. Double gloving is recommended to decrease risk of percutaneous blood exposures.

Open method

With the open glove method the everted cuff of each glove permits a gowned person to touch the glove's inner side with ungloved fingers and to touch the glove's outer side with gloved fingers (Fig. 3-30). Keeping the hands in direct view, no lower than waist level, the gowned person flexes the elbows. Exerting a light, even pull on the glove

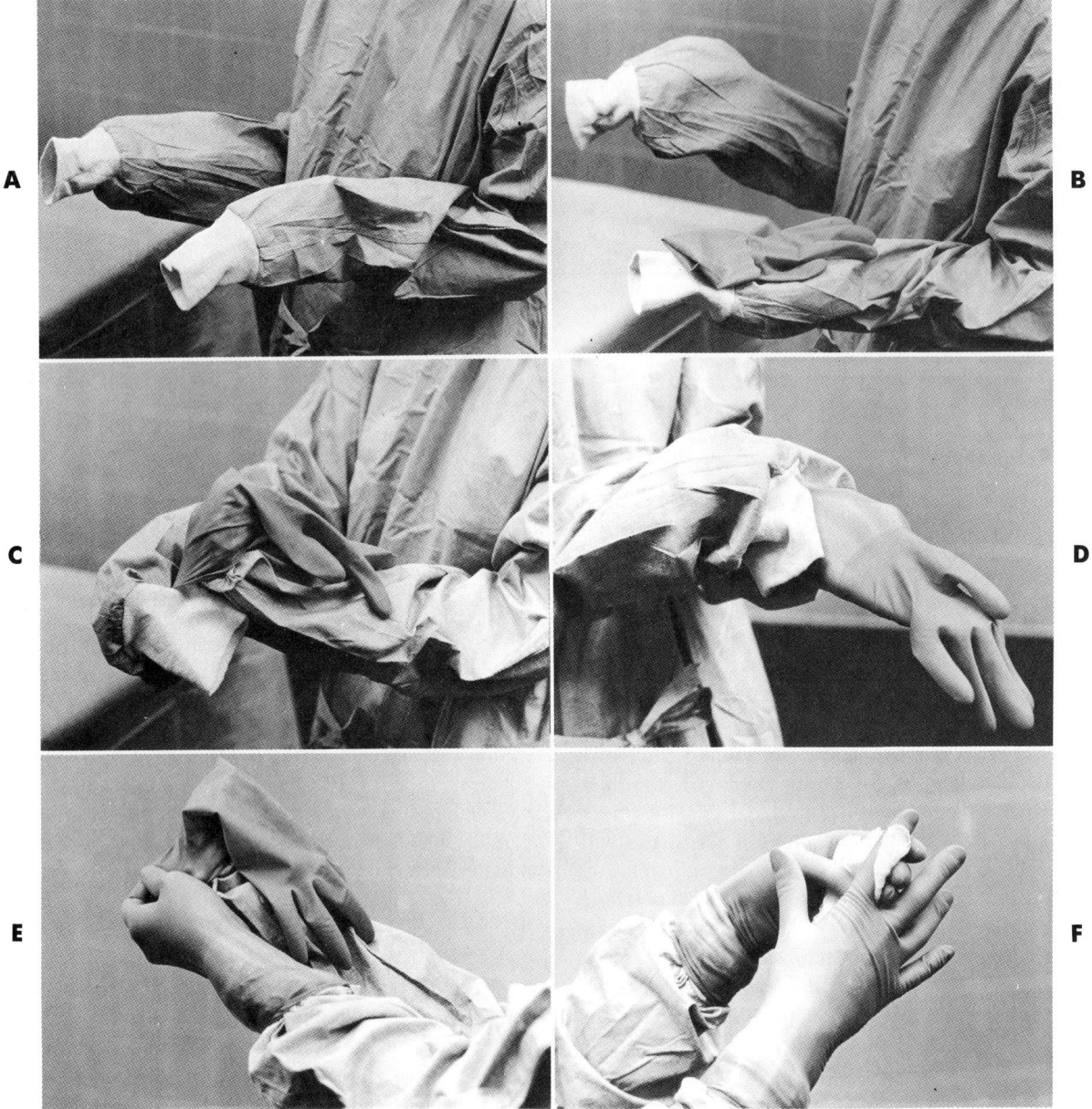

FIG. 3-29 Closed gloving procedure. **A,** When donning gown, scrub nurse does not slip hands through wristlets. Hands are not extended from sleeves. **B,** First glove is lifted by grasping it through fabric or sleeve. Cuff on glove facilitates easier handling of glove. Glove is placed palm down along forearm of matching hand, with thumb and fingers pointing toward elbow. Glove cuff lies over gown wristlet. **C,** Glove cuff is held securely by hand on which it is placed, and, with other hand, cuff is stretched over opening of sleeve to cover gown wristlet entirely. **D,** As cuff is drawn back onto wrist, fingers are directed into their cots in glove, and glove is adjusted to hand. **E,** Gloved hand is then used to position remaining glove on opposite sleeve in same fashion. Glove cuff is placed around gown cuff. Second glove is drawn onto hand, and cuff is pulled into place. **F,** Fingers of gloves are adjusted, and gloves are wiped with wet gauze sponge or commercially prepared sterile disposable glove wipe to remove any powder that may be on them.

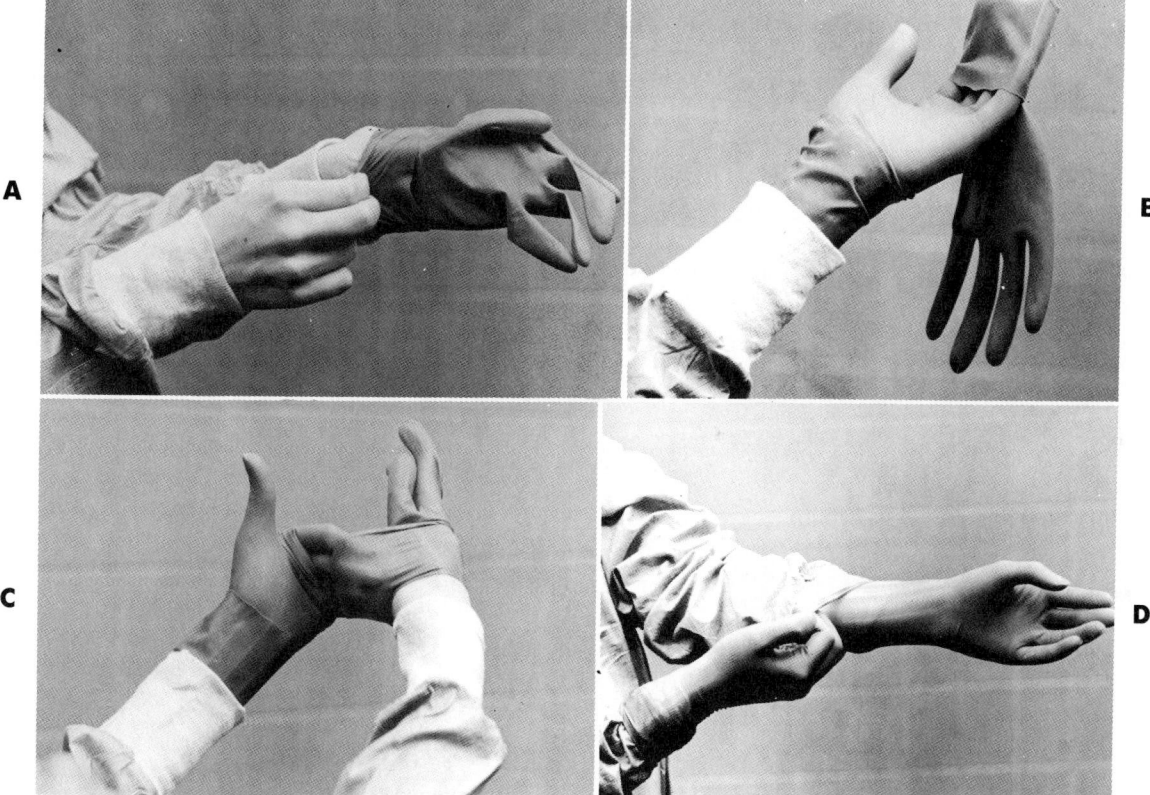

FIG. 3-30 Open gloving procedure. **A,** Scrub nurse takes one glove from inner glove wrapper by placing thumb and index finger of opposite hand on fold of everted cuff at a point in line with glove's palm and pulls glove over hand, leaving cuff turned back. **B,** Scrub nurse takes second glove from inner glove wrapper by placing gloved fingers under everted cuff. **C,** Scrub nurse, with arms extended and elbows slightly flexed, introduces free hand into glove and draws it over cuff of gown and upper part of wristlet by slightly rotating arm externally and internally. **D,** To bring turned-back cuff on other hand over wristlet of gown, scrub nurse repeats **C.**

brings it over the hand, and using a rotating movement brings the cuff over the wristlet. Extreme caution is necessary when using the open method to prevent contamination by the exposed hands.

ASSISTING OTHERS WITH GOWNING

A gowned and gloved scrub nurse may assist another person in donning a sterile gown (Fig. 3-31). The gown is opened in the manner previously described. The inner side with the open armholes is turned toward the individual who is to be gowned. A cuff is made of the neck and shoulder area of the gown to protect the gloved hands. The gown is held until the person's hand and forearms are in the sleeves of the gown. The circulating nurse assists in pulling the gown onto the shoulders, adjusting the back, and tying the tapes. The wraparound back on the gown is fixed into position by the scrubbed person after gloving is completed.

ASSISTING OTHERS WITH GLOVING

A gowned and gloved scrub nurse may assist another gowned individual with gloving according to the following procedure (Fig. 3-32):

1. The glove is grasped under the everted cuff.
2. The palm of the glove is turned toward the other individual's hand; the thumb of the other glove is opposed to the thumb of the person's hand.
3. The cuff is stretched to open the glove.
4. The gowned person exerts a slight upward pressure on the cuff while inserting the hand into the glove.
5. The gowned person brings the cuff over the wristlet of the gown while slipping the hand well into the glove.
6. The procedure is repeated to done the other glove.

REMOVING SOILED GOWN, GLOVES, AND MASK

To protect the forearms, hands, and clothing from contacting bacteria on the outer side of the used gown and gloves, members of the scrubbed surgical team should follow these steps to remove soiled gowns, gloves, and masks (Fig. 3-33):

1. The gloves are wiped with a clean, wet, sterile towel.
2. If a wraparound gown is worn, the front or side ex-

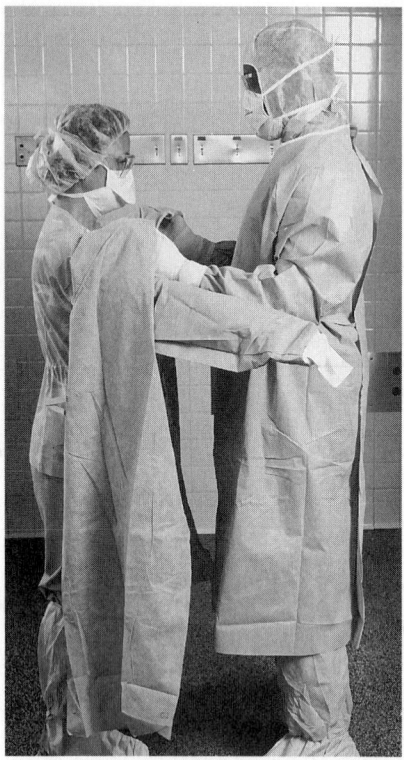

FIG. 3-31 Gowning another person. Gowned and gloved scrub nurse cuffs neck and shoulder area of gown over gloved hands to prevent contamination as scrubbed person puts hands and forearms into sleeves.

ternal waist tie is untied.

3. The circulating nurse unfastens the back closures of the gown.
4. The gown is grasped at one shoulder seam without touching the scrub clothes.
5. The neck of the gown and sleeve are brought forward and over and off the gloved hand, turning the gown inside out and everting the cuff of the glove.
6. Touching only the outside of the gown, step 5 is repeated for the other side, and the gown is pulled off completely.
7. The arms and soiled gown are kept away from the body while the gown is folded inside out and discarded carefully inside the appropriate receptacle.
8. The gloved fingers of one hand are placed under the everted cuff of the other glove, and care is taken not to touch skin with the soiled surface of either glove.
9. The glove is inverted as it is pulled off and then discarded in the appropriate receptacle.
10. The fold of the everted cuff on the remaining glove is grasped with the bare fingers of the ungloved hand; the glove is pulled off in the same way and discarded.

After leaving the restricted area, the person removes the mask by touching only the strings and discards it in the designated receptacle. The hands and forearms are washed. If

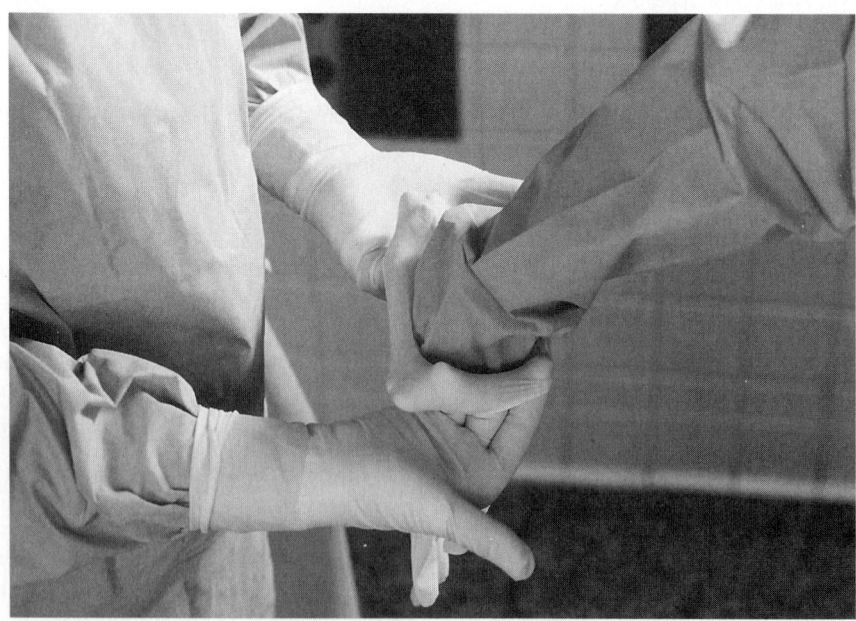

FIG. 3-32 Gloving another person. Gowned and gloved scrub nurse places fingers of each hand beneath everted cuff, keeping thumbs turned outward and stretching cuff as gowned person slips hand into sterile glove, using firm downward thrust.

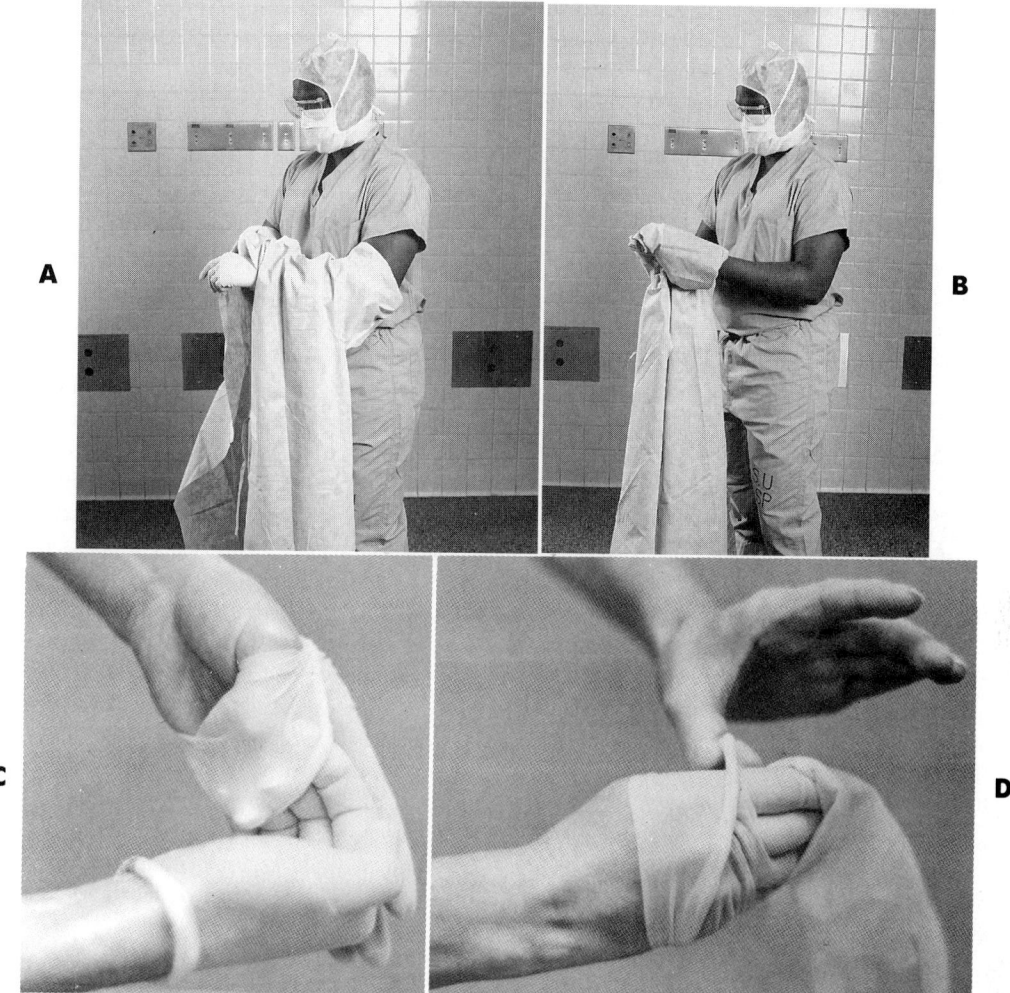

FIG. 3-33 Removing soiled gown and gloves. **A,** To protect scrub suit and arms from bacteria that are present on outer side of soiled gown, the gown is grasped without touching the scrub clothes. **B,** Scrub nurse turns outer side of soiled gown away from body, keeping elbows flexed and arms away from body, so that soiled gown will not touch arms or scrub suit. **C,** To prevent outer side of soiled gloves from touching skin surfaces of hands, scrub nurse places gloved fingers of one hand under everted cuff of other glove and pulls it off hand and fingers. **D,** To prevent ungloved hand from touching outer side of soiled glove, scrub nurse hooks bare thumb on inner side of glove and pulls glove off.

immediate scrubbing for another operation is necessary, the individual dons a fresh mask and repeats the prescribed scrub procedure.

SURGICAL DRAPING

Draping procedures create an area of asepsis called a *sterile field*. All sterile items that come in contact with the wound must be restricted within the defined area of safety to prevent transportation of microorganisms into the open wound.

The sterile field is created by placement of sterile sheets and towels in a specific position to maintain the sterility of surfaces on which sterile instruments and gloved hands may be placed. The patient and operating room bed are covered with sterile drapes in a manner that exposes the prepared site of incision and isolates the area of the surgical wound. Objects draped include instrument tables, basin and Mayo stands, trays, and some surgical equipment.

DRAPING MATERIALS

Draping materials are selected to create and maintain an effective barrier that minimizes the passage of microorganisms between nonsterile and sterile areas. To be effective, a barrier material is resistant to blood, aqueous fluid, and abrasion, as lint free as possible, and drapable. It should maintain an isothermic environment that is appropriate to body temperature. It should meet or exceed the requirements of the current National Fire Protection Association standards so that no risk from a static charge exists. Fabric draping materials must be penetrable by steam under pressure or by gas to achieve sterilization within hospital facilities.

Several reusable and numerous disposable materials that are currently available exhibit barrier qualities. However, they do not remain equally impermeable to moist contaminants for given periods of time. Barrier properties vary, depending on the stresses applied to the draping materials during actual use.

Reusable drapes

The performance characteristic of primary concern for drapes (or gowns) to be used repeatedly is fluid impermeability under the conditions of use.

Chemically treated cotton cloth and tightly woven 100% cotton with an approximate thread count of 280 per square inch provide a barrier to liquids and are abrasion resistant. Quantitative data verifying the impervious quality of a textile drape should be furnished by the manufacturer. Care should be taken with reusable drapes to eliminate pinholes caused by towel clamps, needles, or sharp objects. Should breaks in the fabric occur, a heat-sealed patch may be used for repair. Reusable materials with heat-applied vulcanized patches can be effectively sterilized. The limit to the percentage of exposed surface that can be patched depends on the mode of sterilizing, positioning in the sterilizer, and the number of layers of patched fabric.

As in the case of reusable gowns, laundering eventually impairs the barrier quality of the drape. Most manufacturers report a loss of barrier quality after 75 laundry or sterilization cycles. The process of steam sterilizing and laundering swells the fabric, whereas drying and ironing shrink the fibers. This cycle increases the propensity for loosened fibers that alter the fabric structure. A system to monitor the number of times an item has been laundered is essential for barrier quality control.

Several manufacturers offer services for sterilization and reprocessing of custom packs of reusable drapes and gowns. Increasing numbers of hospitals are choosing to contract with agencies or manufacturers that provide these options to eliminate handling, processing, and disposal costs.

Disposable drapes

Numerous synthetic disposable drapes prevent bacterial penetration and fluid breakthrough. These versatile materials can be manufactured to meet different specifications in both absorbent and nonabsorbent forms. The successful disposable drapes currently on the market are soft, lint free, lightweight, compact, moisture resistant, nonirritating, and static free. These products are available, packaged and sterilized, from commercial sources. White and colored drapes are available. Lightness and compactness of synthetic

drapes prevent heat retention by patients, contribute to ease in handling and storage, and conserve storage space and personnel time.

Disposable drapes reduce the hazards of contamination in the presence of known infectious microorganisms in body fluids and excretions and in situations in which laundering of grossly contaminated textiles is a problem. The danger inherent in the use of synthetic drapes is that solvents, volatile liquids, and sharp instruments tend to penetrate the barrier. Loss of effectiveness may be caused by cracking at the folds or by pinholes from the use of regular towel clamps. Manufacturers are continually improving disposable flat sheets, fenestrated drapes, and towels to permit easy handling and adaptability to the body.

When considering the purchase of disposable drapes, the buyer must determine whether they will satisfy the needs of surgery, be acceptable to the users, and be cheaper than the cost of laundering reusable drapes. If the cost is not lower, other significant advantages may warrant the purchase of disposable drapes. Availability of items, storage facilities, and disposal method must be analyzed.

Preassembled, sterile, disposable custom packs are now used in many operating rooms. Advantages of these packs include shorter setup and reduced turnover times, less risk of contaminated waste because fewer individually wrapped items are dispensed, improved inventory control, and fewer lost charges. Although custom packs may be more expensive than multiple separate items, indirect savings related to increased efficiency can offset those costs.

Disposal of drapes

Compactors provide a relatively inexpensive method of discarding disposable drapes. They accept any material and reduce the volume by at least a 4:1 ratio. Collection, transportation, and storage of waste materials can be a problem. Hospital engineers must establish methods of controlling odor and maintaining sanitation in the compactor area. Because a portion of the compacted material may be grossly contaminated, city or county codes may prohibit transporting this potentially infectious material through city streets or dumping it at landfills.

Incineration is an alternative method for destroying waste disposables. If incinerators are used, they must be properly managed to prevent environmental contamination. Many hospital incinerators do not meet federal pollution standards; therefore their use is prohibited.

The ecologic impact of disposable items can be only roughly estimated. Each hospital must carefully evaluate its capabilities and restrictions in the handling of disposable drapes before a conversion is implemented.

Plastic incisional drapes

Several types of impermeable polyvinyl sheeting are available in the form of sterile, prepacked surgical drapes. Plastic incisional drapes are available as a plain impermeable drape or impregnated with iodophor.

These plastic drapes are useful adjuncts to the conventional draping procedure. They can be applied after the fabric drape, alleviating the need for towel clamps. They obviate the need for skin towels and sponges to separate the surgeon's gloves from contact with the patient's skin. Skin color and anatomic landmarks are readily visible, and the incision is made directly through the adherent plastic drape. These materials facilitate draping of irregular body surfaces, such as neck and ear regions, extremities, and joints (Fig. 3-34).

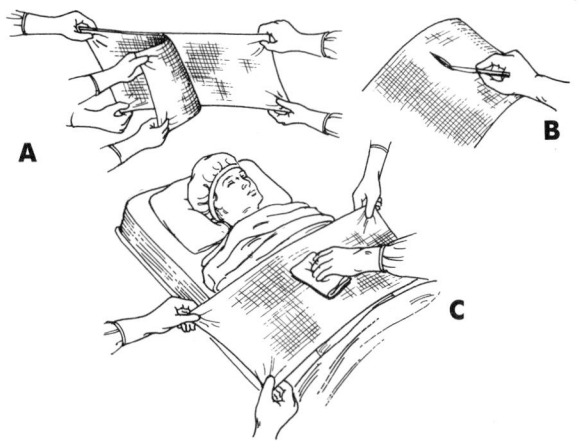

FIG. 3-34 Sterile impermeable adhesive drape. For maximum sealing to prevent wound contamination, prepped skin must be dry and drape applied carefully, preventing wrinkles and air bubbles. **A,** Surgeon and assistant hold plastic drape taut while another assistant peels off back paper. **B,** Surgeon and assistant apply plastic drape to operative site, and, using folded towel, apply slight pressure to eliminate air bubbles and wrinkles. **C,** Surgeon makes incision through plastic drape.

STANDARD DRAPES

Careful planning by nursing and surgical departments helps to determine the desired types and sizes of sheets and towels required for surgery. The variety of drapes should be kept to a minimum. The most effective sheets and towels are simple and economic in terms of time, body motions, and materials. Standard methods provide management control that ensures the safety of patients, simplifies teaching of staff, and conserves human and material resources.

A whole, or plain, sheet is used to cover instrument tables, operating tables, and body regions. The sheet should be large enough to provide an adequate margin of safety between the surrounding physical environment and the prepared operative field. Usually two sizes of sheets suffice.

Surgical towels should be available in several sizes to drape the operative site. Four surgical towels of woven or nonwoven material are usually sufficient (Fig. 3-35).

Fenestrated, or slit, sheets are used for draping patients. They leave the operative site exposed. A typical fenestrated (laparotomy) sheet is large enough to cover the patient and operating bed in any position and to extend over the anesthesia screen at the head of the bed and over the foot of the bed (Figs. 3-36 to 3-38). In some cases it may incorporate the Mayo stand that has been placed over the patient.

The typical fenestrated laparotomy sheet can be used for most procedures on the abdomen, chest, flank, and back. This type of sheet for adults should measure 9 to 10 feet long and 6 feet wide. A rectangular slit 10 inches long by 4 inches wide beginning 4 feet from the uppermost end of the sheet at a point in the center line of the sheet is usually suitable for a routine laparotomy sheet.

Other types of fenestrated sheets similar in length and width but with smaller or split fenestration may be used for

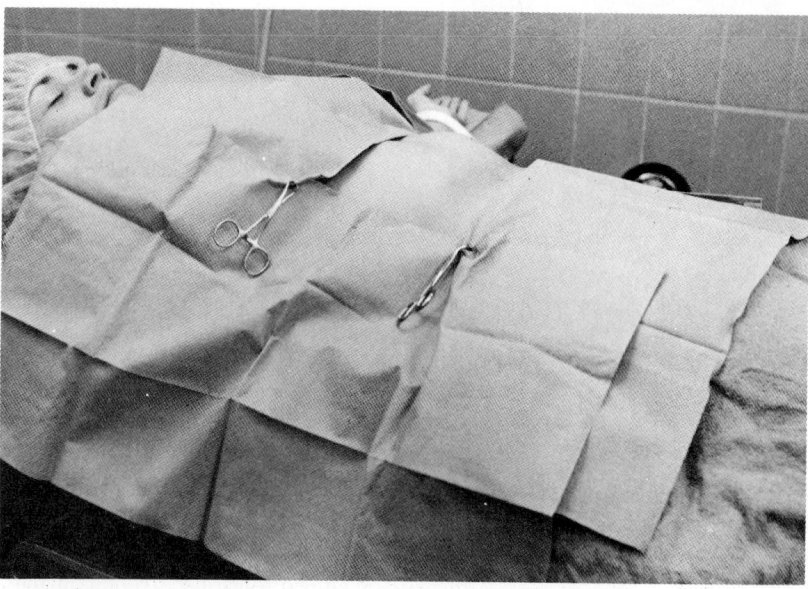

FIG. 3-35 Abdomen may be draped with four sterile towels, which are secured with nonperforating towel clamps. Standard method of placement of disposable towels is used.

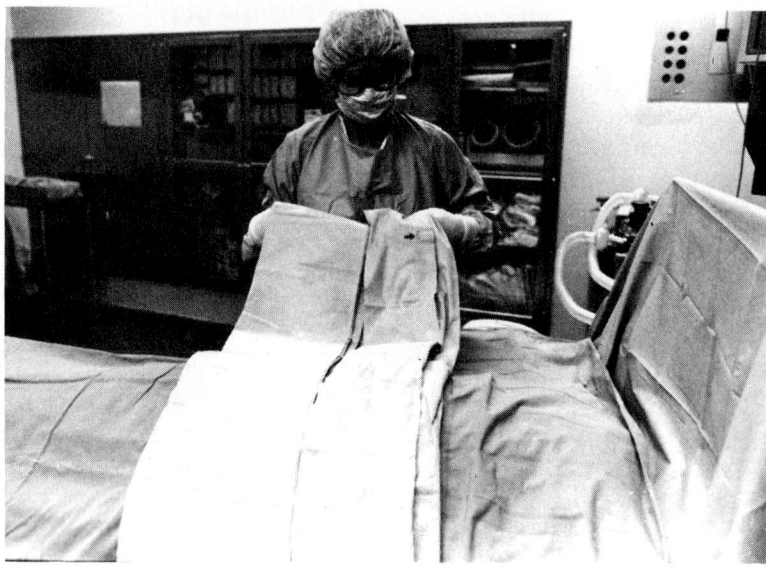

FIG. 3-36 Placement of laparotomy sheet. Identification of top portion of laparotomy sheet assists scrub nurse in readily determining correct placement of drape. After placing folded laparotomy sheet on patient, with fenestration of sheet directly over site of incision outlined by sterile towels, scrub nurse unfolds drape over sides of patient and bed.

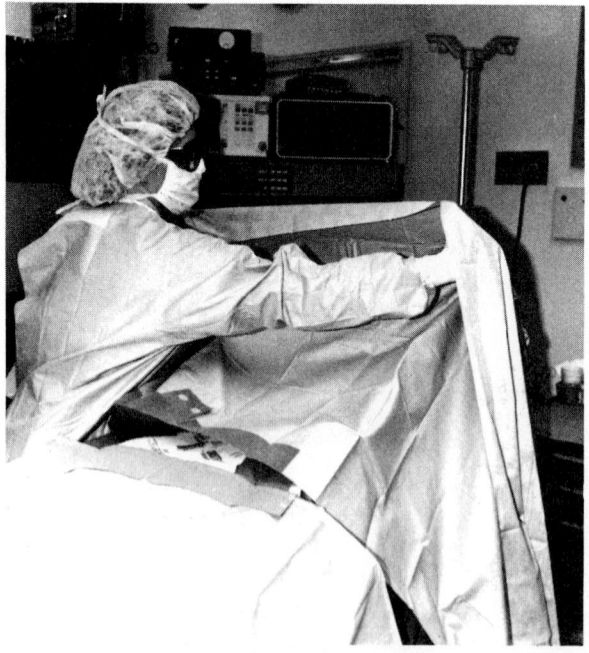

FIG. 3-37 Laparotomy draping continued. Scrub nurse protects gloved hands under cuff of fanfolded laparotomy sheet and draws upper section above fenestration toward head of bed, draping it over anesthesia screen. Bottom portion of fanfolded sheet is then extended over foot of bed in similar manner.

the limbs, head, and neck with the patient supine or prone. The size of the fenestration is determined by the use for which the sheet is intended. The fenestrated sheet is fanfolded and handled as a typical laparotomy sheet.

A perineal drape is needed for operations on the perineum and genitalia with the patient in lithotomy position. A lithotomy drape consists of a fenestrated sheet and two triangular leggings. The leggings may be attached to the sides of the sheet. The three-piece drape is less costly and is easier to handle and launder. A commercial, disposable lithotomy drape pack, including fenestration sheet, two leggings, absorbent and nonaborbent towels, and a small sheet, is suitable for childbirth, cystoscopy, hemorrhoidectomy, and vaginal procedures.

FOLDING DRAPES FOR USE

Drapes should be folded so that the gowned and gloved members of the team can handle them with ease and safety. The larger, regular sheet is usually fanfolded from bottom to top. The bottom folds may be 4 inches wider than the upper ones. The small sheet is folded in half and then quartered, and the top corners of the sheet may be turned back or marked for easy identification and handling.

To provide for safe, easy handling and a wide margin of safety between the unsterile item and the scrub nurse's gloved hands, the open end of the Mayo stand cover should be folded back on itself (Fig. 3-39).

Most fenestrated sheets are fanfolded to the opening from the top and the bottom, and then the folds are rolled or fanned toward the center of the opening. The edges of the top and bottom folds of the sheet are fanned to provide

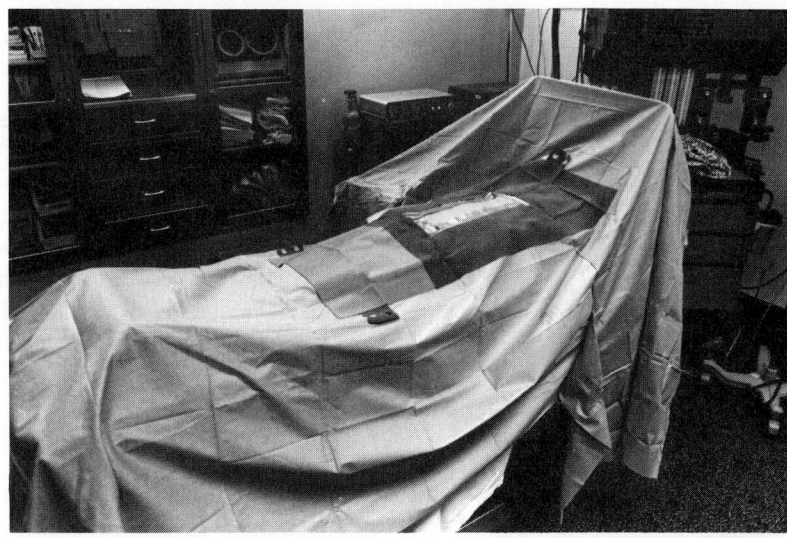

FIG. 3-38   Laparotomy draping completed. Fenestration provides exposure of prepped operative site. Special fabric surrounding fenestration is both absorbent and impermeable. Built-in instrument pad prevents instrument slippage. Perforated tabs provide means of controlling position of cords and suction tubes.

a cuff under which the scrub nurse may place gloved hands. The top and lower sections should be identified by a marking to facilitate easy handling.

DRAPING PROCEDURE

If a sterile field is to be created and maintained, numerous important points must be remembered when draping for a surgical procedure:

1. Allow sufficient time and space to permit careful draping of the patient and proper aseptic technique.
2. Handle sterile drapes as little as possible.
3. Carry the folded drape to the operative site, where the drape is carefully unfolded and placed in proper position. After a drape has been placed, it should not be moved.
4. Hold sterile drapes above waist level until properly placed on the patient or object being draped. If the end of a drape falls below waist level, it should not be retrieved because the area below the waist is considered unsterile.
5. Immediately discard a drape that becomes contaminated during the draping procedure without contaminating the gloves or other sterile items.
6. Protect the gown by distance and the gloved hands by cuffing drapes over them (Fig. 3-40). The scrub nurse should have all parts of the drape under positive control at all times during placement and should use precise and direct motions. Draping is always done from a sterile area to an unsterile area and by draping nearest first. The scrub nurse should

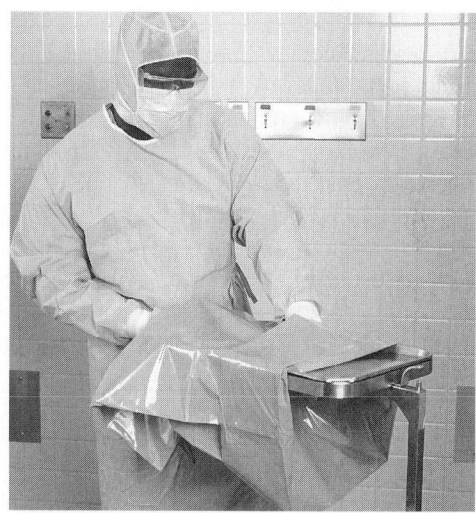

FIG. 3-39   Draping Mayo stand. Folded cover is slipped over frame. Scrub nurse's gloved hands are protected by cuff of drape. Cover is unfolded to extend over upright support of stand.

never reach across an unsterile area to drape. When the opposite side of the operating room bed must be draped, the scrub nurse must go around the bed to drape.

7. Do not flip, fan, or shake drapes. Rapid movement of drapes creates air currents on which dust, lint, and droplet nuclei may migrate. Shaking a drape also causes uncontrolled motion of the drape, which may cause it to come in contact with an unsterile

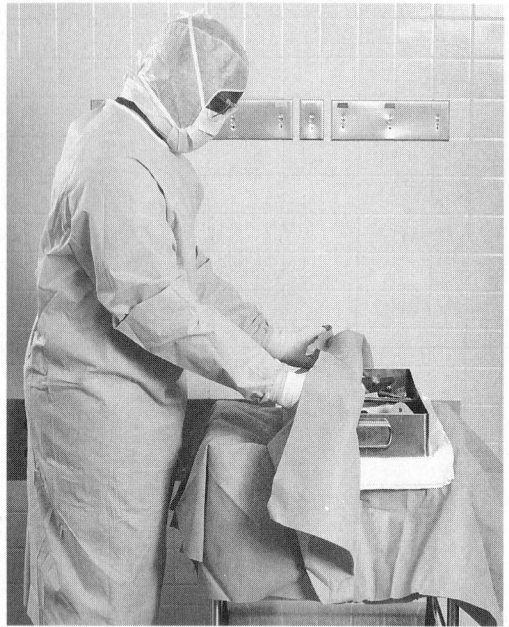

FIG. 3-40 When placing sterile drape on unsterile surface, scrub nurse rolls corners of drape over hands to avoid contamination.

surface or object. A drape should be carefully unfolded and allowed to fall gently into position by gravity. The low portion of a sheet that falls below the safe working level should never be raised or lifted back onto the sterile area.

8. Drape the incisional area first and then the periphery.
9. Use nonperforating towel clamps or devices to secure tubing and other items on the sterile field.
10. When sterility of a drape is questionable, consider it contaminated.

ARRANGEMENT OF ITEMS ON STERILE TABLES

The standard arrangement of instruments, drapes, sutures, and other items on sterile tables for particular operations should be determined by nursing personnel. Factors to be considered include the surgeon's method of working; ease in handling, preparing, and transporting items; and reduction in human energy. Methods of work are based on work simplification and aseptic principles.

The arrangement of the various setups should be clearly defined and understood by operating room personnel. Visual aids are excellent tools for teaching personnel proper procedural methods.

OPERATING ROOM ENVIRONMENTAL SANITATION

Effective sanitation techniques should be established to control and reduce the possibility of cross-infection of patients in the operating room. Blood and tissue fluids from any patient may contain microorganisms that are pathogenic to other persons. Operating room practices should be developed to provide complete isolation for each patient. This isolation is accomplished by considering every surgical wound to be potentially contaminated.

PRINCIPLE OF CONFINE AND CONTAIN

The principle of confine and contain was originally introduced to perioperative nurses in the early 1970s. This principle recommends that personnel restrict all patient microorganisms to an area of 3 feet around the patient and that, when patient microorganisms leave that limited area, they should be either confined to an impervious container or destroyed. Establishment of procedures to implement this principle prevents the transfer of microorganisms and protects patients and personnel. Adherence to this principle also eliminates the costly practice of special decontamination procedures for "dirty" cases.

PROCEDURE

Contamination in the operating room can occur from various sources. The patient, health care workers, and inanimate objects are all capable of introducing potentially infectious material to the surgical field. Techniques have been established to prevent some of the transmission of microorganisms in the surgical area. Proper surgical attire is one such mechanism already discussed. Designation of traffic patterns is essential to distinguish unrestricted, semirestricted, and restricted areas. Unrestricted areas allow entry of all authorized personnel and permit the wearing of street clothes. Semirestricted areas are designated for personnel in proper surgical attire and the patient undergoing surgical intervention. Restricted areas should be open only to the patient and surgical team. Proper surgical attire is required in addition to the proper wearing of surgical masks.

During the surgical procedure, traffic within and through the room should be kept to a minimum to reduce air turbulence and to minimize human shedding. All doors in and out of the operating room should be kept closed to decrease the air turbulence and the potential for contamination. High-efficiency particulate air filters (HEPA) placed between outside air processing and the operating room vents are used in some institutions. The HEPA filters are capable of screening out particles larger than 0.3 μm. Air exchanges in an operating room should occur at a minimum of 20-25 exchanges per hour with at least five exchanges from outside air. Fresh air is air that enters the system from the outside, free from gaseous pollutants. Total air is the sum of fresh air and the recirculated air from the room. Although total air may help to conserve energy, filters are necessary to remove gaseous pollutants (Everett & Kipp, 1991).

Efforts should be made to confine contamination to as small an area as possible around the patient. Sponges should be discarded in plastic-lined containers. As they are counted, they should be contained in an impervious receptacle. The circulating nurse must use protective eyewear and gloves, instruments, or both when collecting and counting sponges or handling contaminated items. Spills should be cleaned up immediately with a broad-spectrum detergent/germicide.

Specimens of blood or other potentially infectious material are placed in a container that prevents leakage. The container must be color coded or labeled using the biohazard symbol. If the outside of the container becomes contaminated, the primary container must be placed within a second container that prevents leakage and is labeled or color coded. Some facilities use biohazard-labeled impervious bags to transport blood or other potentially infectious material.

Between surgical procedures, personnel must remove their gowns and gloves and place them in the proper receptacles before leaving the operating room. All linens from open packs, whether soiled or not, should be discarded in fluid-impervious bags. The use of fluid-impervious bags eliminates potential contamination from wet linen soaking through to the outside of the bag. Used disposable and expendable items should be discarded in plastic bags and placed in containers for disposal.

The scrub nurse should place all instruments directly in wire mesh-bottom trays for processing in a washer-sterilizer. Basins, cups, and trays should also be washed and terminally sterilized. If a washer-sterilizer is not adjacent to the operating room, all these items should be contained for transportation to a central cleanup area, either in the surgical suite or in central service, for terminal sterilization or high-level disinfection. The contaminated instruments should be handled as little as possible. Personnel should avoid reaching into containers to retrieve contaminated instruments.

Identifying wastes for which special precautions are necessary is largely a matter of judgment. Bulk blood or suctioned fluid may be carefully poured down a drain connected to a sanitary sewer. Local and state environmental regulations may exist and should be consulted before establishing guidelines for waste disposal. Wall suction units should be disconnected by the circulating nurse to eliminate contamination of the wall outlet. Suction contents should be disposed of by the scrub nurse during the flushing of a hopper by the circulating nurse. Spills that occur during transport should be prevented. Depending on local and state regulations, powder treatments of a chlorine compound are available to solidify liquid material prior to transport. This chemical may also be tuberculocidal, virucidal, and bactericidal. Glass suction containers should be rinsed and terminally sterilized with basins and trays. Disposable suction tubing should be discarded. Reusable suction tubing should be avoided because of difficulties in cleaning the lumen properly.

Surgical lights and the horizontal surfaces of furniture and equipment that have been involved in the surgical procedure should be cleaned with a hospital-grade disinfectant/detergent. The floor should be cleaned with a disinfectant/detergent solution using the wet vacuum method. If a wet vacuum is not available, a clean mophead and clean solution should be used after each patient. The wheels and casters of furniture used during the surgical procedure should be pushed through the solution used for floor cleaning. All reusable bins, pails, cans and similar receptacles with the likelihood of becoming contaminated with blood or other potentially infectious materials must be inspected and decontaminated regularly.

At the end of each day's operative schedule, a complete housekeeping program should be initiated to ensure that every operating room, scrub room, and service room is properly cleaned. The decontamination process should begin at the highest level and progress downward. For example, the light tracks, air filters, and other ceiling fixtures should be disinfected prior to shelves, tables, kick buckets, and the floor. When items with removable parts, such as the operating room bed are cleaned, all removable parts should be disassembled and cleaned with disinfectant solution. A schedule should be established to specify when the cleaning of walls, ceilings, offices, and furniture occurs. Personnel should wear personal protective equipment when cleaning for protection against potentially infectious material.

The last part of sanitation takes place after all cleaning is completed and the cleaning equipment is sanitized. The wet vac is disassembled and thoroughly washed with a disinfectant. All mop heads are properly removed and if reusable sent to the laundry; mop handles are also cleaned with a disinfectant. Proper sanitation can provide a first line of defense to protect the patient and health care workers in the prevention of transmission of pathogenic microorganisms.

REFERENCES

Association of Operating Room Nurses. (1994). *Standards and recommended practices for perioperative nursing.* Denver: The Association.

Barlow, R., & Handleman, E. (1993). OSHA's final bloodborne pathogens standard. *American Association of Occupational Health Nursing, 41*(1), 8-15.

Bartlett, J.G. (1991). Needle stick injury. In *Decision making in surgical sepsis.* Philadelphia: B.C. Decker.

Brachman, P.S. (1993). Nosocomial infections surveillance. *Nosocomial Infections Surveillance, 14*(4), 194-196.

Cardo, D.M., Falk, P.S., & Mayhall, C.G. (1993). Validation of surgical wound surveillance. *Infection Control and Hospital Epidemiology, 14*(4), 211-215.

Centers for Disease Control. (1987). Recommendations for prevention of HIV transmission in healthcare settings, *MMWR, 36*(2S).

Centers for Disease Control. (1989). *Guidelines for prevention of transmission of human immunodeficiency virus and hepatitis B virus to health-care and public-safety workers.* U.S. Department of Health and Human Services, P.L. 100-607.

Centers for Disease Control. (1990). Guidelines for preventing the transmission of tuberculosis in health-care settings, with special focus on HIV related issues. *MMWR, 39,* No. RR-17.

Centers for Disease Control. (1991). Recommendations for preventing transmission of human immunodeficiency virus and hepatitis B virus to patients during exposure-prone invasive procedures. *MMWR, 40* No. RR-8.

Centers for Disease Control and Prevention. (1993). *Draft guidelines for preventing the transmission of tuberculosis in health-care facilities.* U.S. Department of Health and Human Services, Vol 5B, No. 195.

Chen, C.C., & Willeke, K. (1992). Aerosol penetration through surgical masks. *American Journal of Infection Control, 20*(4), 177-184.

Ellner, P.D., & Neu, H.C. (1992). *Understanding infectious disease.* St. Louis: Mosby.

Elpern, E.H., & Girzadas, A.M. (1993). Tuberculosis update: New challenges of an old disease. *MEDSURG Nursing, 2*(3), 176-183.

Everett, W.D., & Kipp, H. (1991). Epidemiologic observations of operating room infections resulting from variations in ventilation and temperature. *American Journal of Infection Control, 19*(6), 277-282.

Favero, M.S., & Bond, W.W. (1991). Sterilization, disinfection, and antisepsis in the hospital. In *Manual of clinical microbiology.* Washington, D.C.: American Society for Microbiology.

Fay, M.F. (1992). Safety issues of latex products. *Journal of the American Association of Nurse Anesthetists, 60*(3), 214-216.

Grimes, D.E. (1991). *Infectious disease: Clinical nursing series.* St. Louis: Mosby.

Horan, T.C., Gaynes, R.P., Martone, W.J., & Emori, T.G. (1992). CDC definitions of nosocomial surgical site infections, 1992: A modification of CDC definitions of surgical wound infections. *American Journal of Infection Control, 20*(5), 271-274.

Jacobs, P.T. (1989). Plasma sterilization. *Journal of Health Care Materials Management, 7*(5), 49.

Jacobs, P.T. (1993). *Sterrad™ sterilization system—A new technology for instrument sterilization.* (White Paper) Arlington, Tex.: Johnson & Johnson Medical, Inc.

Larson, E. (1989). Innovations in health care: Antisepsis as a case study. *American Journal of Public Health, 79*(1), 92-99.

Malangoni, M.A., & Hiram, C.P. (1989). Surgical infection, microbiology and antimicrobial agents. In *Scientific foundations of surgery* (4th Ed.). Chicago: Year Book Medical.

Manian, F.A., & Meyer, L. (1993). Comparison of patient telephone survey with traditional surveillance and monthly physician questionnaires in monitoring surgical wound infections. *Infection Control and Hospital Epidemiology, 14*(4), 216-218.

National Institutes of Health. (1989). The impact of routine HTLV-III antibody testing on public health. In *The NIH Consensus Development Conference Statement* (Vol. 6). New Fairfield, CT: National Organization for Rare Disorders.

Occupational Safety and Health Administration. (1991). *Occupational exposure to bloodborne pathogens; Final rule*, 29 CFR Part 1910.1030.

Pottinger, J., Burns, S., & Manske, C. (1989). Bacterial carriage by artificial versus natural nails. *American Journal of Infection Control, 17*(6), 340-344.

Proposed Recommended Practices for Sterilization in the Practice Setting. (1994). *AORN Journal, 60*(4).

Shovein, J., & Young, M.S. (1992). MRSA: Pandora's box for hospitals. *American Journal of Nursing, 92*(2), 48-52.

Vesley, D., Norilen, K.G., Nelson, B., Ott, B., & Streifel, A.J. (1992). Significant factors in the disinfection and sterilization of flexible endoscopes. *American Journal of Infection Control, 20*(6), 291-300.

BIBLIOGRAPHY

Association for the Advancement of Medical Instrumentation. (1988). *National standards and recommended practices for sterilization* (2nd Ed.). Arlington, VA: The Association.

Atkinson, L.J. (1992). *Berry and Kohn's operating room technique* (7th Ed.). St. Louis: Mosby.

Brown, J.F., Brumm, J.A., & Crim, B.J. (1993). *Infection prevention: Environmental sanitation*. Dallas: Baylor Surgical Services Institute.

Brumm, J.A. (1993). *Preparing skin for surgery*. Dallas: Baylor Surgical Services Institute.

Bruning, L.M. (1993). The bloodborne pathogens final rule. *AORN Journal, 57*(2), 439-460.

Burns, S. (1988). A multiple evaluation study on artificial nails. *Journal of Nursing Quality Assurance, 2*(4), 77-79.

Copp, G., et al. (1987). Footwear practices and operating room contamination. *Nursing Research, 36*(6), 366-369.

Curry, J.L., & Douglas, S.D. (1992). HIV/AIDS and HBV: A universal precautions update. *The Nursing Spectrum, 1*(2), 12-13.

Gilliam, D.L., & Nelson, C.L. (1990). Comparison of a one-step iodophor skin preparation versus traditional preparation in total joint surgery. *Clinical Orthopaedics and Related Research, 250* 258-260.

Girard, N. (1992). *Infection prevention: Aseptic practices*. Dallas: Baylor Surgical Services Institute.

Have OR blood exposures been neglected by hospitals? (1992). *Hospital Infection Control, 19*(11), 141-145.

Establishing a "neutral zone" may combat OR sharps injuries. (1992). *Hospital Infection Control, 19*(11), 149-150.

Kyle, J., & Carey, L. (1989). *Scientific Foundations of Surgery* (4th Ed.). Chicago: Year Book Medical.

Larson, E.L., Butz, A.M., Gullette, D.L., & Laughon, B.A. (1990). Alcohol for surgical scrubbing? *Infection Control and Hospital Epidemiology, 11*(3), 139-143.

Nichols, R.L., Hyslop, N.E., & Bartlett, J.G. (1991). *Decision making in surgical sepsis*. Philadelphia: B.C. Decker.

O'Neal, M. (1989). Contain and confine technique for OR cleanup. *AORN Journal, 45*, 979.

Pereira, L.J., Lee, G.M., & Wade, K.J. (1990). The effect of surgical handwashing on the microbial counts of operating room nurses. *American Journal of Infection Control, 18*(6), 354-364.

Quebbeman, E.J., Telford, G.L., Hubbard, S., Wadsworth, K., Hardman, B., Goodman, H., & Gottlieb, M.S. (1991). Risk of blood contamination and injury to operating room personnel. *Annals of Surgery, 214*(5), 614-620.

Roup, B.J. (1993). OSHA's new standard: Exposure to bloodborne pathogens. *American Association of Occupational Health Nursing Journal, 41*(3), 136-142.

Roy, C.A., & Barton, C.R. (1991). Intraoperative latex anaphylaxis compounded by atracurium sensitivity: A case report. *Journal of the American Association of Nurse Anesthetists, 59*(5), 399-404.

Sheretz, R.J., et al. (1992). Consensus paper on the surveillance of surgical wound infections. *American Journal of Infection Control, 20*(5), 263-270.

Tortora, G.J., Funke, B.R., & Case, C.L. (1989). *Microbiology: An introduction*. Redwood, CA: Benjamin/Cummings.

Young, M.A., Meyers, M., McCulloch, L.D., & Brown, L.J. (1992). Latex allergy. *AORN Journal, 45*(3), 488-50.

4

POSITIONING THE PATIENT FOR SURGERY

L E S L I E   E I L E E N   R I C K E R

OVERVIEW

Surgery is performed on all parts of the human anatomy. The body has to be positioned into multiple configurations so that the procedure can be done with accuracy and with the desired outcomes. Positioning the surgical patient is both an art and a science and is as well a key factor in the performance of a safe and efficient surgical procedure. All members of the surgical team have a duty to protect the patient from any harmful effects of the surgical position. Knowledge of anatomy and physiology is imperative to provide the patient safe and comfortable positioning in surgery.

The patient's position should provide optimum exposure and access to the operative site; should sustain body alignments and circulatory and respiratory function; must provide access to the patient for administration of intravenous fluids, drugs, and anesthetic agents; should not compromise neuromuscular structures and skin integrity; and should afford as much comfort to the patient as possible. Good positioning promotes patient well-being and safety while meeting these needs.

Although the choice of patient position is usually determined by the surgical approach, the responsibility for overall patient well-being rests with the surgeon, the anesthesiologist, and the nurse, who constantly monitor the patient's physiologic status. The circulating nurse may coordinate the details of restraints, support to the extremities, and safe transfers. In collaboration with the patient, the surgeon and the circulating nurse determine the position for patients who receive local anesthetics.

SURGICAL ANATOMY

The perioperative nurse must be aware of the anatomic and physiologic changes associated with anesthesia, positioning of the patient, and the operative procedure. These changes most frequently involve (1) the musculoskeletal system, (2) the nervous system, (3) the cardiovascular system, and (4) the respiratory system.

The *musculoskeletal system* of the patient may be subjected to unusual and exaggerated stress during operative positioning. Normal range of motion is maintained in the alert patient by pain and pressure receptors that warn against stretching and twisting of ligaments, tendons, and muscles. The tone of opposing muscle groups also acts to prevent strain and stress to the muscle fibers. When pharmacologic agents such as anesthetics and muscle relaxants depress the pain and pressure receptors and loss of tone causes muscular relaxation, the normal defense mechanisms cannot guard against joint damage and muscle stretch and strain. Obvious resistance to unusual range of motion is often noted only in patients whose arthritic changes prevent even slight exaggeration of the position. Bony prominences of the human anatomy are particularly vulnerable to injury by rubbing and sustained pressure. The position chosen should provide physiologic alignment while protecting the patient from pressure, abrasion, and other injuries.

Nervous system depression accompanies the administration of anesthetic agents and many other drugs. The degree of depression depends on the type of regional anesthesia or the level of general anesthesia. Pain and pressure receptors may be affected either regionally or systemically. The most important factor for the nurse to remember is that when nervous system depression occurs, the body's communication and command system becomes totally or partially ineffective. Changes in physical status and compensatory actions are no longer possible. Lifesaving, physiologic adaptive mechanisms do not function; the stresses of operative positioning are not automatically compensated. Pressure on superficial nerves must be prevented. The patient with poor cardiac status, hypovolemia, arteriosclerosis or obesity will be at greater risk for cardiovascular changes during anesthesia and positioning.

The *cardiovascular system* is most dramatically affected by anesthesia and change in position. Many patients are repositioned shortly after induction of general anesthesia. Except for physical injury, the major hazard patients can experience during repositioning is hypotension. Due to the effects of the anesthetics used, normal cardiovascular compensatory mechanisms are disrupted. This lack of self regulatory control of vascular dilatation and constriction to stabilize blood pressure requires frequent monitoring of vital signs by the anesthesiologist during repositioning. If hypotension occurs, the perioperative nurse should be available to assist the anesthesiologist as needed, and any position change should be delayed until blood pressure stabilizes.

The *respiratory system* can be compromised during positioning. Movement of the diaphragm may be impeded by abdominal viscera, adversely affecting pulmonary function. Obese patients and those with respiratory insufficiency may have difficulty breathing when lying supine. Any patients who experience dyspnea should be propped on pillows during local, regional, or spinal anesthesia. During general anesthesia these patients will be placed on mechanical ventilation by the anesthesiologist.

PERIOPERATIVE NURSING CONSIDERATIONS

ASSESSMENT

Nursing assessment begins with the preoperative interview. During this interview the circulating nurse reviews the patient's record and determines the patient's height, weight, and general physical condition. Skin integrity and range of motion of all extremities are assessed. Any reddened or ecchymotic areas, lesions, or decubiti will affect positioning and must be documented. Limitations in mobility should be noted, as should any preexisting neurovascular problems and complaints of discomfort. Positioning of the patient is dependent upon this assessment and on the planned procedure.

The important aspects of care during patient positioning are prevention of injury and patient comfort. Nursing assessment therefore involves recognition of the patient's risk factors affecting positioning and potential patient problems (vulnerable situations and patients).

Vulnerable situations include the following:

1. Long surgical procedures (2 hours or greater of direct skin pressure may result in disruption of skin integrity).
2. Vascular surgery (optimal blood perfusion may already be compromised due to the patient's disease process and by the effects of anesthesia).
3. Demineralizing bone conditions such as malignant metastasis or osteoporosis put the patient at higher risk for skeletal fractures.
4. Excessive sustained pressure to certain body areas because of the surgical procedure or retraction increases the potential for damage to skin integrity.

Vulnerable patients include the following:

1. Geriatric patients, whose thin skin layer and circulatory system make them more prone to skin breakdown due to pressure.
2. Pediatric patients, whose size and weight must be taken into consideration when selecting positioning aids.
3. Patients who are malnourished, anemic, obese, hypovolemic, paralyzed, arteriosclerotic, or diabetic are also prone to skin breakdown due to pressure.
4. Patients with prosthetic or arthritic joints require special attention.
5. Patients with edema, infection, cancer, or conditions of lowered cardiac or respiratory reserves.

NURSING DIAGNOSIS

Nursing diagnoses are formulated from the data collected during the preoperative assessment. The primary nursing diagnosis concerned with patient positioning is *high risk for injury* related to sustained pressure and misalignment of specific body areas during surgery.

OUTCOME IDENTIFICATION

The outcome identified for the nursing diagnosis concerned with patient positioning could be stated as: The patient will be free from injury related to positioning.

PLANNING

Specific nursing care is planned to address the preferred positioning for the procedure and to prevent individual patient problems. The care plan should be individualized for specific patient problems, such as diabetes, malnutrition, or paralysis. The care plan may include nursing interventions of determining the appropriate mode of patient transport and transfer, equipment and positioning aids, or the need for ancillary personnel to accomplish the positioning.

IMPLEMENTATION

The perioperative nurse must be familiar with the normal functions, maintenance, various uses, and potential hazards of operating room beds, their attachments, and other mechanical adjuncts to both patient position and the operative procedure (such as electrosurgical devices, drills, and radiologic procedures). Mechanical malfunctions must be recognized and corrected for the patient's safety.

Ensuring patient safety encompasses more than overseeing mechanical functions of equipment; it also includes direct patient care. Patients often comment on the cool temperatures in the operating room. The circulating nurse should provide the patient with a blanket heated in the warming cabinet. This is one measure to provide a warm, comfortable environment for the patient. If possible, patient transfers should be made when the patient is awake. When the patient is anesthetized or unable to assist, a four-person lift or a patient roller device should be used to provide support to the torso, head, and all extremities. A pillow may be placed under the knees to relieve pressure on the lower

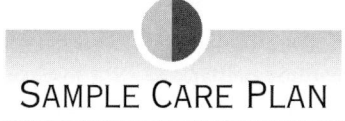

SAMPLE CARE PLAN

NURSING DIAGNOSIS: High risk for injury related to sustained pressure and misalignment of specific body areas during surgery.
OUTCOME: Patient will be free from injury related to positioning.
INTERVENTIONS:
Check operating room bed for proper functioning.
Gather positioning aids.
Assist in positioning, maintaining proper body alignment.
Place safety strap 2 inches above the knees with buckle at patient's side.

Pad and protect bony prominences, pressure sites, and vulnerable nerves.
Document in detail patient position, including:
• Type and placement of restraints
• Position of extremities
• Type and placement of positioning aids
• Site of electrosurgical dispersive pad
• Positional changes made during the procedure (for example, supine to lithotomy to supine)
• Use of warming or cooling blankets

---

lumbar region. The restraint strap should be placed 2 inches above the knees and should be snug, but should not compromise venous circulation or exert pressure on bony prominences or nerves. It should never be placed directly on the patient's skin but rather over the blanket covering the patient.

Mayo tables should be positioned high enough to prevent pressure on the patient's toes, knees, and legs. Pressure may also occur if a member of a surgical team leans or rests on the patient. This pressure in addition to the patient's weight could result in the development of a dermal pressure ulcer. The surgical team should be reminded not to lean on the patient's trunk or extremities because pressure may compromise anatomic and physiologic functions.

Focal alopecia can result from prolonged pressure to the occipital region following surgical intervention. Edema seroma formation occurs early in the postoperative phase followed by temporary hair loss. The anesthesiologist should turn the patient's head every 30 minutes to prevent alopecia (Poma, 1979).

Shearing and friction can also damage skin integrity. It is important to lift a patient into position rather than slide or pull to avoid shearing forces and friction. Shearing forces can cause small subcutaneous capillaries to stretch or tear when two or more layers of tissue slide on each other. This disruption in blood flow contributes to development of dermal pressure ulcers. In changing the position of the operating room bed while the patient is anesthetized, the weight of the patient's body slides in that direction and creates shear forces. Shearing is created by a parallel force, whereas pressure is created by a perpendicular force, such as a bony prominence.

Skin integrity should be assessed before, during, and after the operation for any unusual findings, such as redness, ecchymosis, lesions, blisters, or ulcers. Pressure ulcers are any lesions caused from unrelieved pressure resulting in skin damage to underlying tissue. These ulcers generally

occur over bony prominences and are staged according to the degree of assessed tissue damage, as follows:

1. Nonblanchable erythema of intact skin: Note that normal reactive hyperemia can be expected to be present for one half to three fourths as long as pressure was unrelieved to the area and should not be confused with a stage 1 pressure ulcer.
2. Partial-thickness skin loss involving epidermis or dermis: Although the ulcer is superficial, it appears as an abrasion, blister, or shallow crater.
3. Full-thickness skin loss involving damage or necrosis of subcutaneous tissue that may extend to fascia layer: These ulcers appear as a deep crater and may or may not involve adjacent tissue.
4. Full-thickness skin loss with extensive damage to muscle, bone, or supporting structures, such as tendon or joint capsule: Note that undermining and sinus tracts may also be associated with stage 4 pressure ulcers (Agency for Health Care Policy and Research, 1992).

Two to 3 hours of unrelieved pressure on tissues can result in dermal pressure ulcers and focal alopecia. Necrosis involved with pressure ulcers looks very similar to burns and is often mislabeled as such (Gendron, 1988). Clinical practice guidelines state that 2-hour patient turning can protect against the adverse effects of pressure, friction, and shear (Agency for Health Care Policy and Research, 1992). No positioning device can replace good nursing care of routine relief of pressure. The circulator should relieve pressure on critical contact areas (sacrum and coccyx, elbows and scapula, and heels) thereby restoring circulation and oxygenation of these tissues (Research Highlight 4-1).

EVALUATION

The evaluation of the nursing care plan should be ongoing during the procedure and conclude with a written and

⚹
────────────────
RESEARCH HIGHLIGHT 4-1

Garner studied pressure ulcer development in surgical patients at a midwestern university level I trauma center. The retrospective medical record study described risk factors associated with pressure ulcer development in surgical patients and compared the documented preoperative and postoperative dermal pressure ulcer risk assessment scores. Of the 107 medical records reviewed, 9.47% of the patients developed a stage 1 or stage 2 pressure ulcer following coronary artery bypass graft surgery. Garner found females to have a 7% greater chance of developing dermal pressure ulcers than males, and patients scoring a 4 or greater preoperatively were at greater risk for developing dermal pressure ulcers postoperatively.

The findings of the study support the importance of accurately assessing surgical patients' risk for pressure ulcer development. In addition, communication of the assessment, plan, interventions, and evaluation is essential in preventing postoperative dermal pressure ulcer development. Garner suggests that future research related to the operating room as a contributing factor to dermal pressure ulcer development will provide more information on the incidence of surgical patients' development of dermal pressure ulcers.

Garner, B. (1993). Pressure ulcer development in surgical patients, Unpublished master's thesis, Wright State University, Dayton, Ohio.

verbal report to the postanesthesia care unit nurse. The outcome of successful implementation of the care plan is the patient is free from injury related to positioning, as evidenced by the following:

· No redness or change in skin integrity at bony prominences, pressure areas, and the electrosurgical dispersive pad site
· No patient complaints of strained muscles or liga-

ments, altered range of motion, or compressed or injured nerves postoperatively
· Circulation in extremities consistent with preoperative status
· No adverse change in hemodynamics related to positioning

Any abnormalities noted should be documented on the postoperative assessment and reported to the surgeon and the postanesthesia care unit nurse.

Proper patient positioning is essential for safe, successful surgical procedures. Perioperative nurses play a significant role in ensuring uncompromised and physiologically satisfactory patient positioning.

OPERATING ROOM BEDS

Operating room beds are specifically designed to meet the peculiar and highly specialized requirements of surgical therapy. Modern manufacturing and design have done much to facilitate safe and effective positioning of the patient while providing the surgeon with anatomic accessibility (Fig. 4-1). Potential hazards of the operating room bed and its controls should be kept foremost in the perioperative nurse's mind to prevent any injury.

Perioperative nursing personnel have the responsibility of being well versed in the use of all types of operating room beds available in the institution. Nurses should keep informed of new developments and evaluate their usefulness in actual practice.

General operating room beds can be adjusted for height and length and can be tilted laterally to either side and horizontally at the head and foot (Fig. 4-2). They are divided into three or more sections that support the major body parts and permit their placement in flexion or extension. The head section is usually removable, and foot extensions may be added. Headrests of various designs enable the general operating room bed to be used for cranial and eye surgery.

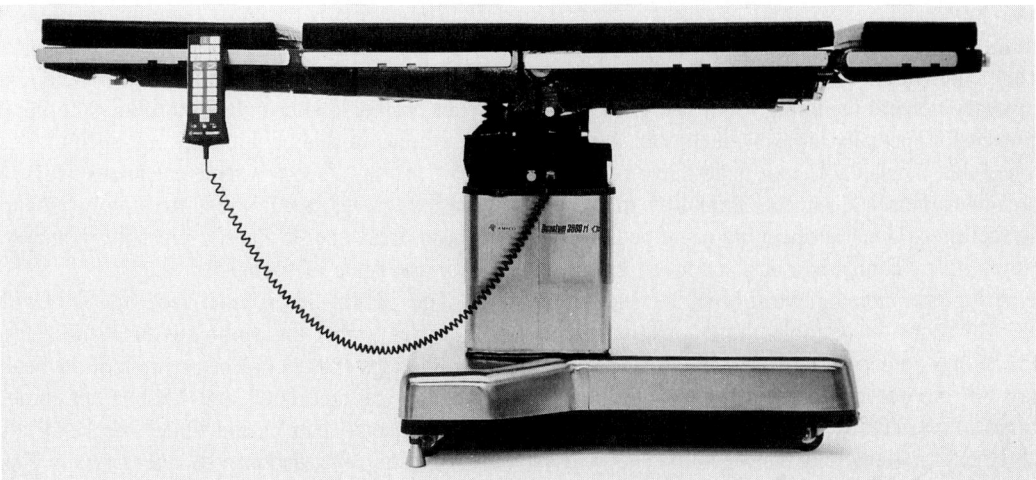

FIG. 4-1 Surgical OR bed adaptable to a wide range of surgical and fluoroscopic procedures.
Courtesy AMSCO/American Sterilizer Co., Erie, Pa.

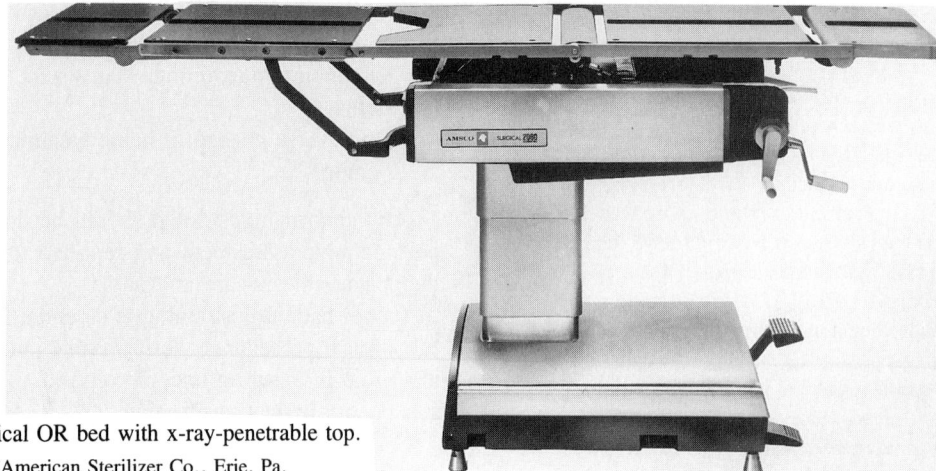

FIG. 4-2 Surgical OR bed with x-ray-penetrable top.
Courtesy AMSCO/American Sterilizer Co., Erie, Pa.

The mattress and armboards are covered with conductive rubber for comfort and ease in cleaning. Any covers with cracks found in the rubber should be replaced. A dual density mattress covered with a pliable liquidproof cover is a significant improvement from the traditional mattress; it relieves pressure and reduces skin shear.

Controls and accessories may be used to maintain the patient in standard or modified supine, lateral, or prone positions. All operating room beds are operated manually or electrically and have a brake for stabilization. Accessory equipment (such as stirrups, leg holders, armboards and footboards) is designed to stabilize the patient in a desired position and to provide flexibility in positioning. Armboards attach flush with the bed pad and lock within a 90-degree radius. These can be placed parallel to the operating room bed to provide extra width for obese patients.

Additional accessories for operating room beds include pillows, pads, and bolsters of various sizes and shapes. They are made to fit the different anatomic structures of patients and thereby facilitate physiologic functions and operative accessibility. All positioning devices should perform three functions: absorb compressive forces, redistribute pressure, and prevent excessive stretching.

In common surgical use are the general operating room bed, the orthopedic (fracture) table, and the urology table. The contemporary general operating room bed is so versatile that the need for specialty tables is declining. An operating room bed that is adaptable to a wide range of uses is an economic investment and permits flexibility in the use of operating facilities. General operating room beds can be purchased fluoroscopy compatible or can convert by placement of the radiopaque tabletop. Most operating room beds are available with x-ray–penetrable tunnel tops that permit insertion of cassette holders at any position along the bed.

The x-ray– or fluoroscopy-compatible table is utilized during orthopedic procedures, cholecystectomy with common bile duct exploration, and intraoperative angiogram during vascular surgery. The orthopedic table, with its multiple movable and removable parts and suspension frames, remains one of few specialty tables required (Fig. 4-3).

The urology table, designed for cystoscopic procedures, has radiologic equipment attached that facilitates intraoperative x-rays of the genitourinary system. Perineal cutouts and drainage trays fitted to the lumbar section adapt the general operating room bed for the perineal approaches used in gynecologic, urologic, and proctologic surgery.

STANDARD POSITIONS AND PHYSIOLOGIC CONSIDERATIONS

Because operative procedures are performed with the patient resting on either the back, abdomen, or side, three basic positions are described: supine, prone, and lateral. These basic positions can be modified in many ways to meet specific patient needs or surgeon preferences.

SUPINE POSITIONS

In the supine position the patient's back and spinal column are resting on the surface of the operating room bed mattress. Modifications of the position allow approach to the major body cavities (cranial, thoracic, and peritoneal), the four extremities, and the perineum.

The supine is the most common position. It is the most natural position of the body at rest. The patient is usually anesthetized in this position (Fig. 4-4, *A*), and modifications are made after induction of anesthesia. Potential pressure areas in this position are the occiput, scapula, olecranon, sacrum, coccyx, and calcaneus (Fig. 4-4, *B*). Skin pressure areas occur most frequently in supine position. These areas should have a pressure-reducing device, such as those made of foam, air, or gel.

The patient lies supine (face upward) with the arms at the sides (either on armboards or at the sides of the body) and the legs extended. The position of the head should place the cervical, thoracic, and lumbar vertebrae in a straight line. A small pad placed under the head allows the strap muscles to relax and prevents neck strain. Flexion or twisting may cause contracture in the neck and may interfere with a clear airway. Small, soft pillows may be placed under the small of the back and under the knees to maintain

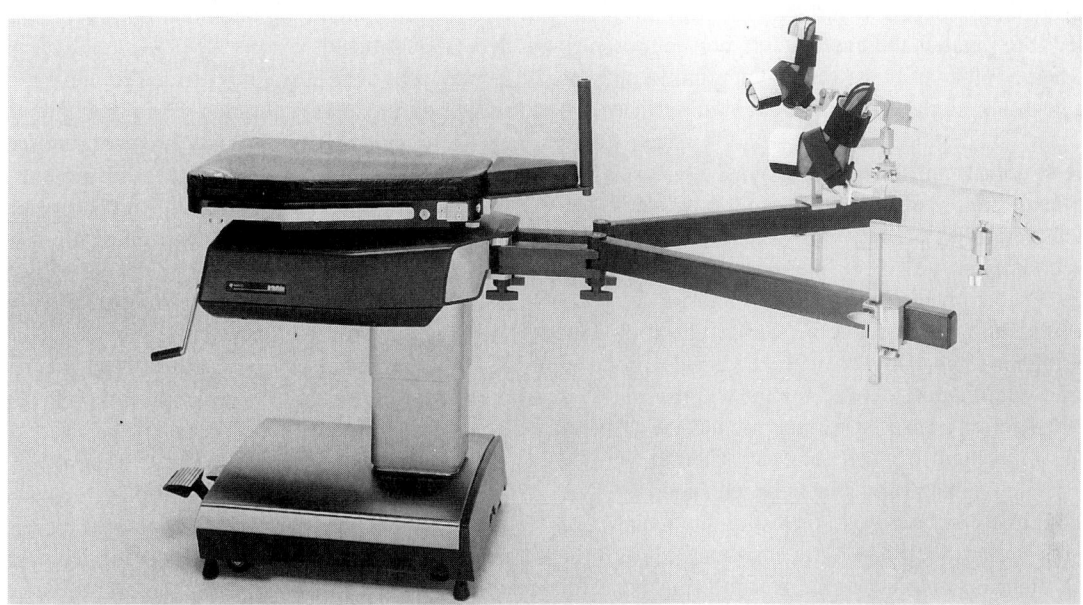

FIG. 4-3 Orthopedic fracture table.
Courtesy AMSCO/American Sterilizer Co., Erie, Pa.

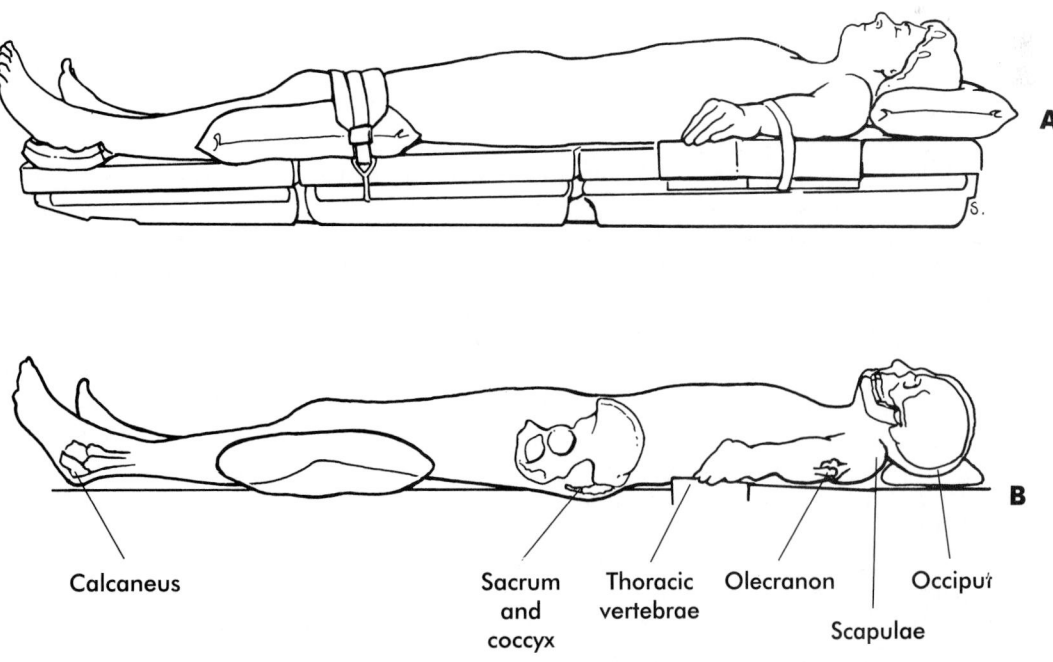

Calcaneus   Sacrum   Thoracic Olecranon   Occiput
             and   vertebrae
             coccyx   Scapulae

FIG. 4-4 **A,** Supine position. **B,** Potential pressure points noted.
David Schumick, The Ohio State University Biomedical Communications, Columbus, Ohio.

normal lumbar concavity and to prevent strain on the back muscles and ligaments; such strain may occur if the muscles and ligaments are allowed to assume the configuration of the flat operating room bed surface. The hips are parallel. The legs are parallel and uncrossed to prevent peroneal and tibial nerve injury, rubbing, and compromised circulation. The legs are slightly separated so skin surfaces are not in contact. The leg restraint (bed strap) is placed across the middle to upper thighs, 2 inches above the knees to prevent their flexion, so that the patient is secured but superficial venous return is not impaired. Heel prominences also need protection from prolonged pressure. Foam cushions, ankle rolls, or foam heel protectors may be used.

The arms should rest easily at the sides of the body with the palms against the body or with the hands pronated (palms down and fingers extended) on the mattress surface. A broad liftsheet can be used to tuck around the arms to support the full length of each arm. The elbows may be protected with eggcrate padding or sleds with padding. The elbows should neither be flexed nor rest on the metal edge of the bed. An elbow resting on the edge may cause pressure to the ulnar nerve as it passes over the epicondyle of the humerus. If the hands are placed under the buttocks, the fingers may be compressed. Wrist restraints can endanger the nerves and the blood supply to the hands. Leather restraints also may chafe and abrade the skin. When wrist restraints are necessary, the padded cloth clove hitch produces the least trauma.

Frequently, one or both arms rest on armboards. Abduction, extension, and external rotation may stretch the brachial plexus. Hyperabduction of the arm must be avoided to prevent stretching of the subclavian and axillary vessels under the coracoid process of the scapula, or compression between the clavicle and the first two ribs. To avoid potential injury, the arm should always be placed at less than a 90-degree angle to the body, with palms up to diminish the pressure on the median and ulnar nerves. The mattress and armboard pad should be of the same height. The armboard should lock into position on the bed to prevent inadvertent angle changes or sudden loss of support to the arm.

When the head is turned to one side or the other, it should be supported to keep the spine in alignment and secured in the desired position with a sandbag or special headrest. Pressure on the ear and other bony prominences where nerves and blood vessels lie superficially must be prevented. The eyes must be protected to prevent corneal irritation from textiles, solutions, and other foreign objects.

The circulatory system may be compromised in the supine position, not only by a tight restraint but also by the overall effect of the horizontal body posture and the changed effects of gravity. Depending on the degree of medullary and autonomic nervous system depression by general anesthesia, homeostatic compensatory mechanisms may not function to dilate and constrict blood vessels in response to cardiac or blood volume changes. The increased pressure of abdominal viscera or masses on the inferior vena cava may decrease blood return to the heart; blood pressure would then be lowered. Whenever possible, patient position should encourage venous drainage and avoid obstruction to the major veins. An example is tilting the supine cesarean section patient slightly to the left to prevent excessive pressure on the inferior vena cava before the baby is delivered, particularly with spinal anesthesia.

Respiratory function is also compromised in the supine position because the vital capacity is less than in the erect posture, excluding the effects of anesthesia. Although anterior and upward excursion of the chest during inspiration is not greatly impeded, diaphragmatic excursion may be lessened by the abdominal viscera. The supine position does allow a more even distribution of ventilation from apex to base of the lungs.

Trendelenburg's position

Trendelenburg's position is a variation of the supine position where the upper torso is lowered and the feet are raised (Fig. 4-5). Trendelenburg's position provides better visualization of the pelvic organs during open or laparoscopic surgeries on the lower abdomen or pelvis. Trendelenburg's position can be utilized to improve circulation to the cerebral cortex and basal ganglia when blood pressure

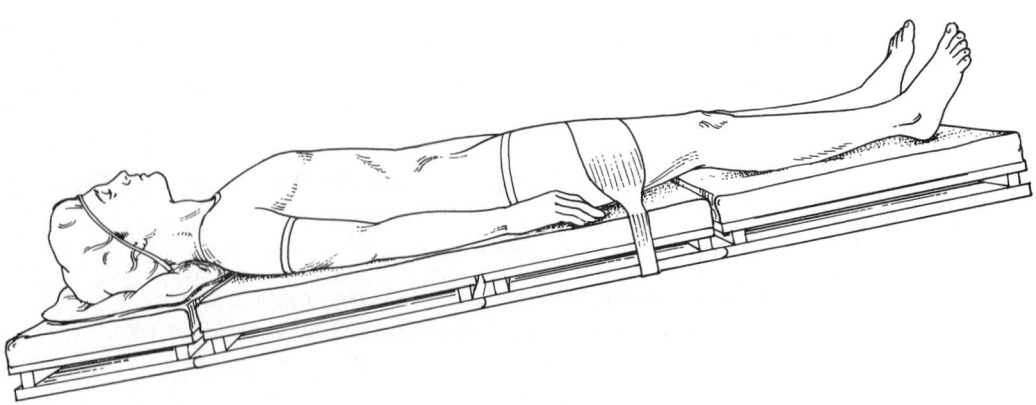

FIG. 4-5   Trendelenburg's position.

is suddenly lowered, and it increases arterial blood flow to the cranium. Occasionally in this position the knees are flexed by "breaking" the lower section of the bed, and the patient must have the knees over the break in the bed to maintain safe anatomic positioning. Another modification is that of keeping the trunk level and elevating only the legs by raising the lower section of the bed.

Any variation of Trendelenburg's position should be maintained only as long as necessary. In this position blood pools in the upper torso, increasing blood pressure. Although the head-downward position facilitates drainage of secretions from the bases of the lungs and the oropharyngeal passages, the weight of the abdominal viscera further impedes diaphragmatic movement. The patient should be returned slowly to the supine position to avoid hypotension. Slow, smooth postural transitions allow sufficient time for the body to adjust to physiologic changes.

Reverse Trendelenburg's position

Reverse Trendelenburg's position is described as the head-up, feet-down position. It is frequently used to provide access to the head and neck and to facilitate gravitational pull on the viscera away from the diaphragm and toward the feet. When the foot of the bed is tilted toward the floor, the patient's body must be supported by a padded footboard, by nonconstrictive body restraints, and by a lift-sheet that supports the arms from above the elbows to the fingers. Lumbar and popliteal pads also tend to prevent the body from slipping. In this position the tilted, head-up bed is usually in a straight line, the opposite of that shown in Fig. 4-5.

When a modification of this position is used for thyroid or parathyroid surgery (Fig. 4-6), the neck may be hyperextended by raising the patient's shoulders (using an inflatable pillow, bolster, foam roll, or sandbag), by lowering the headpiece of the bed, or both. There should be no gaps in the support of the neck in this position. When this position is used for biliary surgery, the right side of the patient may be elevated in the horizontal plane by a lengthwise bolster. To prevent twisting of the spine, the full length of the trunk needs support. The hips and shoulders are kept in the same plane.

In the reverse Trendelenburg's position respiratory function is more like that in the erect position. Venous circula-

tion may be compromised by extended time in the legs-downward position. When this situation is anticipated, the superficial venous return can be aided by the preoperative application of support hose, elastic bandages, or inflatable stockings. If the legs are wrapped, compression of the common peroneal nerve at the head of the fibula must be avoided. Return to the supine position from the reverse Trendelenburg's position should be accomplished slowly and smoothly to avoid overload to the cardiovascular system.

Lithotomy position

The lithotomy position is the most extreme variation of the supine posture (Fig. 4-7). With the patient supine, the legs are raised and abducted to expose the perineal region for procedures involving the pelvic organs and genitals. If the patient will be in this position for greater than 2 hours, ace bandages or antiembolitic stockings should be applied to the patient's legs.

This unnatural posture has great potential for injury to the patient. The hazards increase as the position is exaggerated for radical surgery of the groin, vulva, or prostate. Extreme flexion of the thighs impairs respiratory function by increasing intraabdominal pressure against the diaphragm and therefore decreasing the tidal volume. Gravity flow of blood from the elevated legs causes pooling in the splanchnic region during the operative procedure. Blood loss during surgery may not be immediately manifested because of this increased splanchnic volume. However, when the legs are lowered and 500 ml or more of blood is diverted to more total leg circulation, the circulating volume is depleted, and the blood pressure may decrease. Normal compensatory mechanisms are depressed by the effect of anesthesia on the nervous system, and homeostasis may not be achieved easily.

By placing the patient's anterior iliac spine on a line with the leg holder and the buttocks level and on a line with the edge of the break in the operating room bed, a good position can be achieved with a minimum of effort. A small lumbar pad helps to maintain the physiologic concavity of this area.

Supports for the legs must be carefully chosen and applied. Modern leg holders provide secure support for the legs without the popliteal pressure of knee crutches and

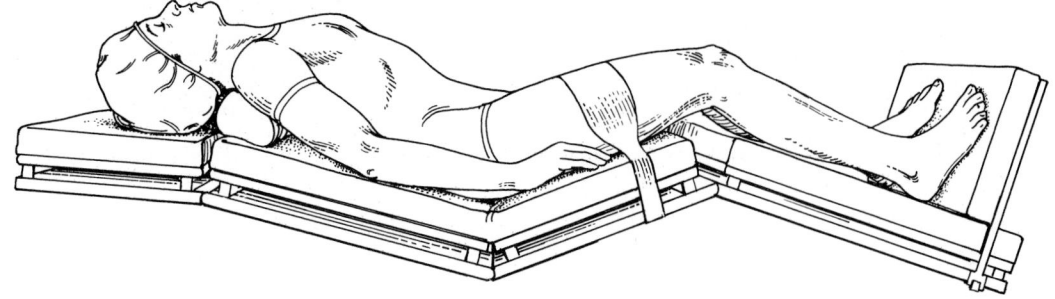

FIG. 4-6 Position for operations on thyroid and neck area.

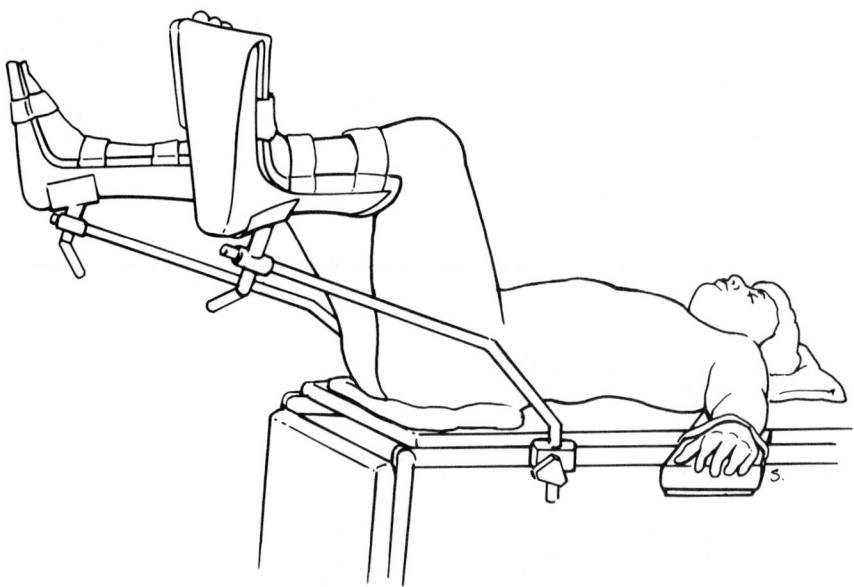

FIG. 4-7 Lithotomy position utilizing padded stirrups for vaginal and rectal operations. Care must be taken in positioning legs to assure that padding adequately protects them.

David Schumick, The Ohio State University Biomedical Communications, Columbus, Ohio.

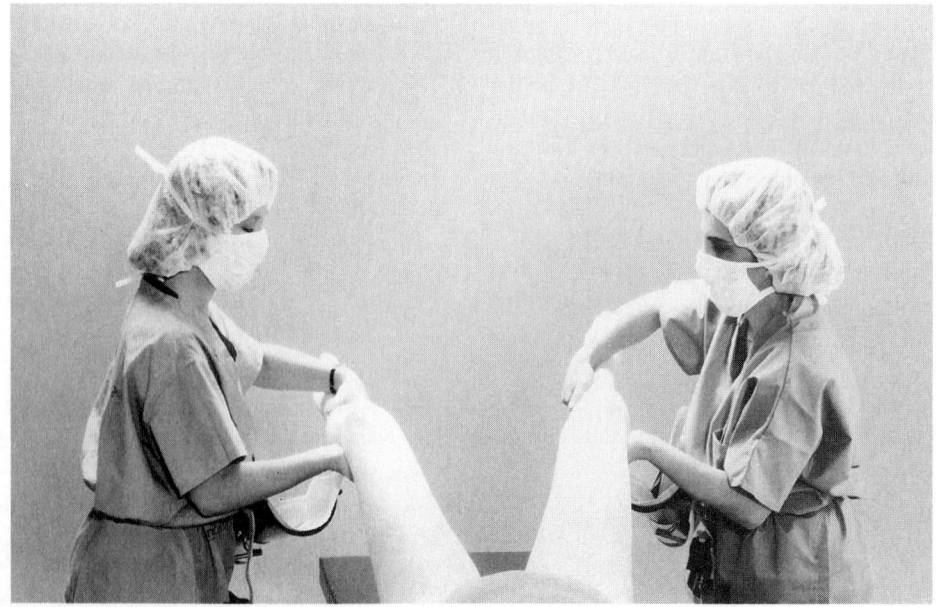

FIG. 4-8 Lithotomy position is achieved with the supine patient whose legs are raised simultaneously and abducted to expose the perineal area.

Courtesy Allen Medical Systems, Cleveland, Ohio.

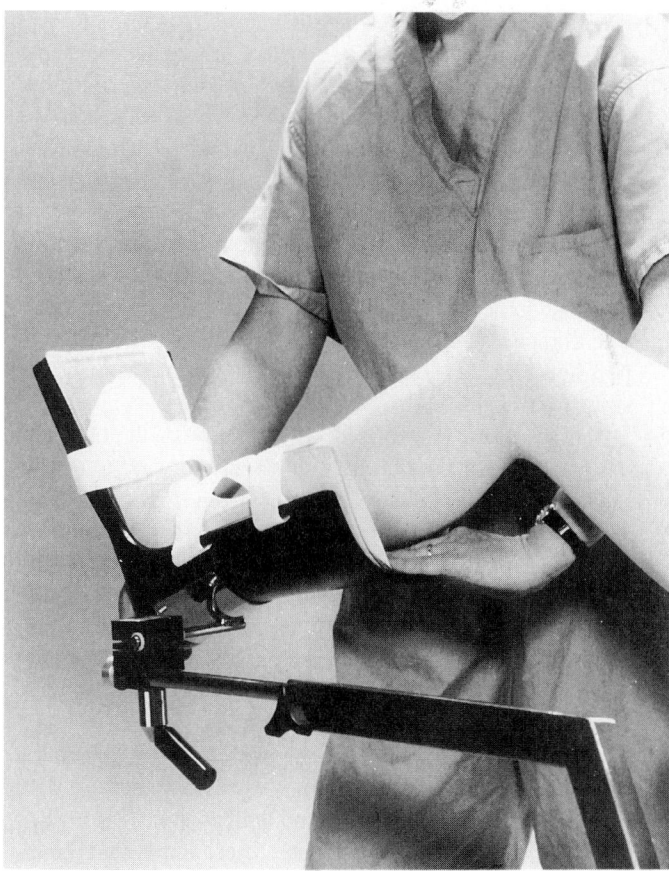

FIG. 4-9 Lower legs should be free from pressure against the leg holder to prevent patient injury. Damage can occur to the peroneal or femoral obturator nerves in lithotomy position.

Courtesy Allen Medical Systems, Cleveland, Ohio.

without undue external rotation and abduction, which stretch the abductor muscles and capsule of the hip joint.

The stirrups must be level. The height is adjusted to the length of the patient's legs. This adjustment prevents pressure at the knee and the lumbar spine. The patient's position must be symmetric. The perineum is in line with the longitudinal axis of the bed; the pelvis is level, and the head and trunk are in a straight line. This position aids the surgeon in identifying anatomic landmarks.

When positioning a patient in the lithotomy position, two members of the surgical team should raise the patient's legs simultaneously to avoid back strain and hip dislocation (Fig. 4-8). Each leg is raised by grasping the sole of the foot in one hand and supporting the leg near the knee in the other. The leg is raised, and the knee is flexed slowly. The padded foot is secured in the stirrup. The lower part of the leg should be free from pressure against the leg holder to prevent pressure on the peroneal nerve (Fig. 4-9). Damage to the peroneal nerve on the lateral aspect of the knee can cause footdrop. Pressure on the femoral obturator nerves on the medial aspect of the thigh may cause inner thigh sensory deficits. Proper position and padding of the stirrups will prevent pressure against the soft tissues of the leg which can predispose the patient to venous thrombosis.

Special care is needed for the patient who has limited range of motion due to hip prosthesis, arthritis, contractures, casts, amputations, or obesity. Severe hip flexion, as well as adduction of the joint, must be avoided in the lithotomy position. The stirrups should be as low as possible and tilted slightly outward, if appropriate. Again, slow and smooth movements are required. The patient can be placed in the lithotomy position before anesthesia induction. The patient then has a chance to voice any discomfort or pain, especially of the back, before the procedure begins, and appropriate therapeutic measures can be taken. Because of the exaggeration of this position, any changes in circulatory status or blood pressure can be monitored and treated by the anesthesiologist before induction. With proper explanation regarding this maneuver and adequate covering of the patient's perineal area, the nurse can facilitate the procedure and ease the patient's anxiety.

Arms require special care in the lithotomy position. They may be folded loosely across the abdomen and supported by the folded gown or a cover sheet, or they may be extended on armboards. They should not lie along the sides of the operating room bed because the hands will extend beyond the break of the foot section of the bed and be in danger of injury when the foot section is lowered and raised. Arms must not impede chest movement and respiration. The weight of the limbs on the chest, especially in infants and children, may fatigue the muscles used in respiration and induce respiratory problems.

As stated earlier, adequate assistance must be available for placing the patient in the lithotomy position and for releasing the patient from the position. The legs must be lowered or taken out of stirrups simultaneously, with support given to the joints above and below to prevent strain on the lumbosacral musculature, which can stretch and tilt, thereby placing the pelvis and limbs in imbalance.

Modified Fowler's position

Modified Fowler's (sitting) position causes most of the patient's weight to be on the dorsum of the body. Extra padding should be placed under the buttocks and the small of the back. A potential problem with prolonged pressure on the dorsum is sciatic nerve damage. The position of the body in relation to the breaks in the operating room bed must be carefully adjusted to prevent abnormal pressures. The backrest is elevated, the knees are flexed, and the footboard is set in place (Fig. 4-10, A). The more erect the patient's posture, the greater the need to support the shoulders and torso. Such support requires adequate padding to protect the axilla and brachial plexus. Other pressure areas requiring padding are the bony prominences of the scapula, ischial tuberosities, and calcaneus (Fig. 4-10, B). Frequently a special headrest is used for cranial ventricular procedures and for posterior fossa craniotomy (see Chapter 22). Air embolism is a potential threat in this position due to negative venous pressure in the patient's head and neck area. A Doppler ultrasound flowmeter and a central venous

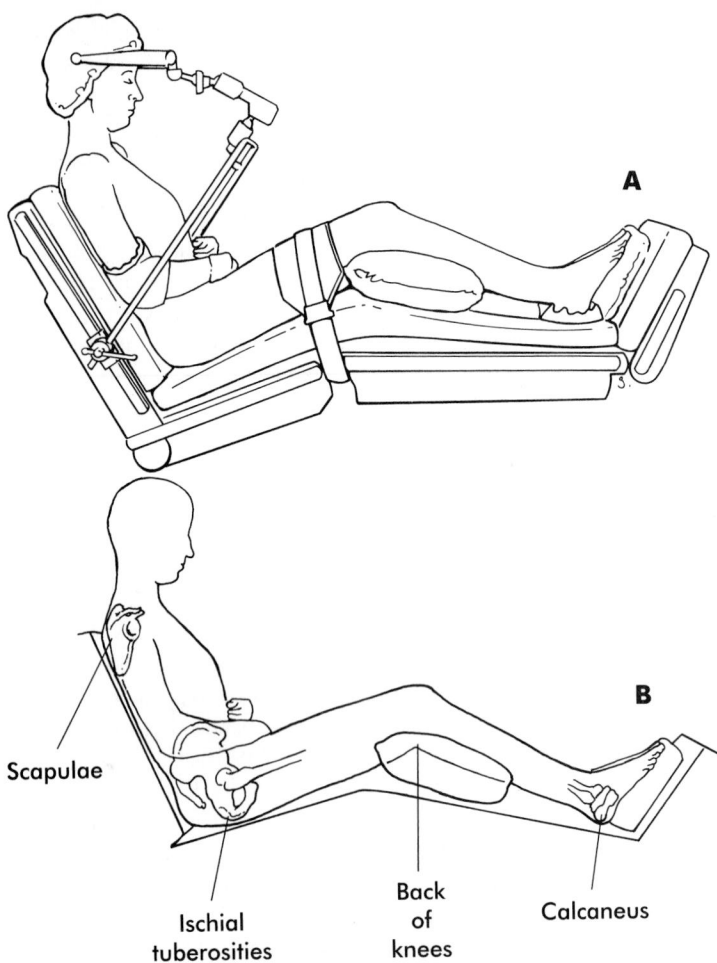

Scapulae

Ischial
tuberosities

Back
of
knees

Calcaneus

FIG. 4-10 **A,** Modified Fowler's or sitting position. **B,** Potential pressure areas shown.

David Schumick, The Ohio State University Biomedical Communications, Columbus, Ohio.

pressure line are usually used to monitor the patient during neurosurgical procedures.

The sitting position requires special attention for the arms. Depending on the surgery, the arms may be flexed across the abdomen, resting on a large pillow in the lap, or placed in front of the patient on a padded stand. Hyperextension of the shoulder region must be prevented, and the arms must be secure from falling or pressing against hard surfaces. To promote venous return in the lower extremities, support hose may be used.

PRONE POSITIONS

In the prone position the patient is lying with the abdomen on the surface of the operating room bed mattress (Fig. 4-11, *A*). Modifications of the position allow approaches to the cervical spine, back, rectal area, and lower extremities.

Induction of anesthesia is performed with the patient in the supine position. Before the patient is turned, the anesthesiologist secures the endotracheal tube with tape, applies

eye ointment in each eye, and then tapes the closed eyelids to prevent corneal abrasions. Scapula turning the supine patient to prone position can be accomplished safely, smoothly, and gently by four persons. The anesthesiologist supports the head and neck during the turn. One assistant stands at the side of the stretcher with hands at the patient's shoulders and buttocks to initiate the roll of the patient. A second assistant stands at the opposite side of the operating room bed, with arms extended to support the chest and lower abdomen as the patient is rolled forward and over. The third assistant stands at the foot of the stretcher to support and turn the legs. At the completion of the turn, the stretcher is removed.

An armboard is provided on each side of the bed, and the patient's arms are brought down and forward to rest on the armboards with elbows flexed and hands pronated. This movement is done to prevent shoulder dislocation and brachial plexus injury. Elbows should be padded and carefully checked for pressure areas. Other pressure areas that require special attention are the cheek, ear, patella, and toes (Fig. 4-11, *B*). The head is positioned on a foam pillow or towels, with the neck kept in alignment with the spinal column. The eyes are carefully protected.

The patient is placed in prone position on a laminectomy frame or premade body rolls. A Wilson frame may be used for procedures on the thoracic and lumbar spine (Fig. 4-12). These positioning devices raise the chest and permit the diaphragm to move freely and the lungs to expand. Supports must not press against the female breasts or male genitalia. These areas should be checked after final positioning to ensure that they are free from pressure. A bolster or pillow under the pelvis will decrease abdominal pressure on the inferior vena cava. A cushion or pillow is placed under the ankles to prevent pressure on the toes and plantar flexion of the feet. The restraining strap is again placed across the thighs and blanket so that the patient is secured but superficial venous return is not impaired.

The prone posture is initially hazardous as the anesthetized patient is turned from the supine position to the prone position. Normal compensatory mechanisms are depressed, and the patient cannot readily adjust to imposed hemodynamic changes.

The radial nerve may be compressed against the humerus if the forearm is allowed to hang over the side of the bed. The shoulders may be overextended unless the elbows are flexed and the palms pronated. The venous return may be compromised by a tight leg restraint, dependent lower extremities, and visceral compression of the inferior vena cava.

The respiratory system is most vulnerable in the prone position because normal anterolateral respiratory movement is restricted and normal diaphragmatic movement is inhibited by the compressed abdominal wall.

For spinal operations the prone position may be modified to flex the affected part of the spine, for example, the knee-chest position. The hips also may be flexed at one

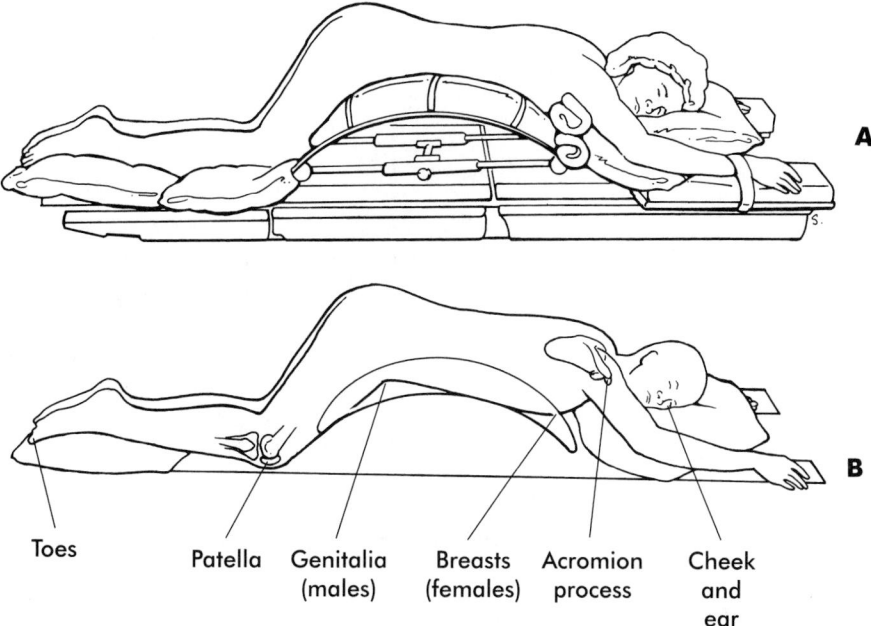

Toes   Patella   Genitalia   Breasts   Acromion   Cheek
                   (males)   (females) process   and
                                                       ear

FIG. 4-11 **A,** Prone position for procedures on the cervical spine, back, rectal area, and posterior lower extremities. **B,** Potential pressure areas for prone position are shown.

David Schumick, The Ohio State University Biomedical Communications, Columbus, Ohio.

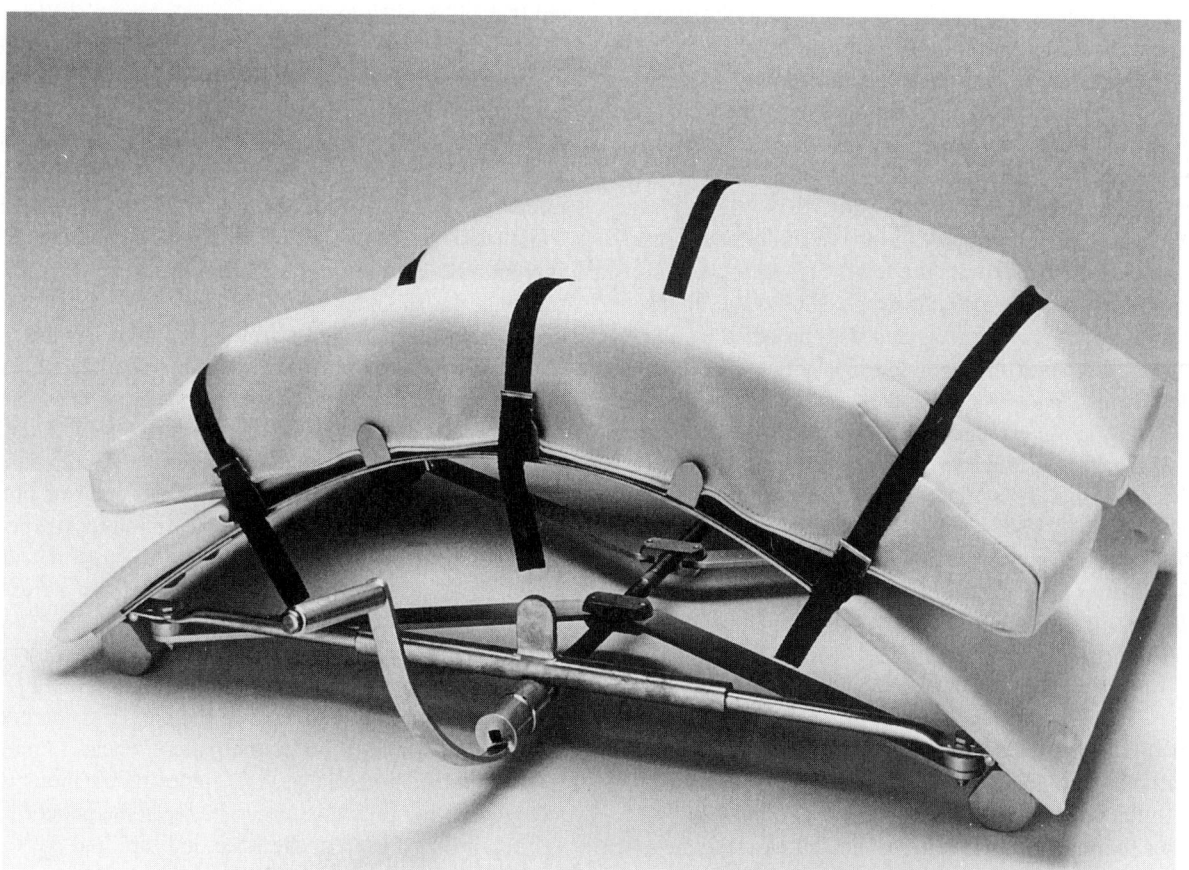

FIG. 4-12 The Wilson frame may be utilized for prone position during thoracic and lumbar spinal procedures.

Courtesy Zimmer, Dover, Ohio.

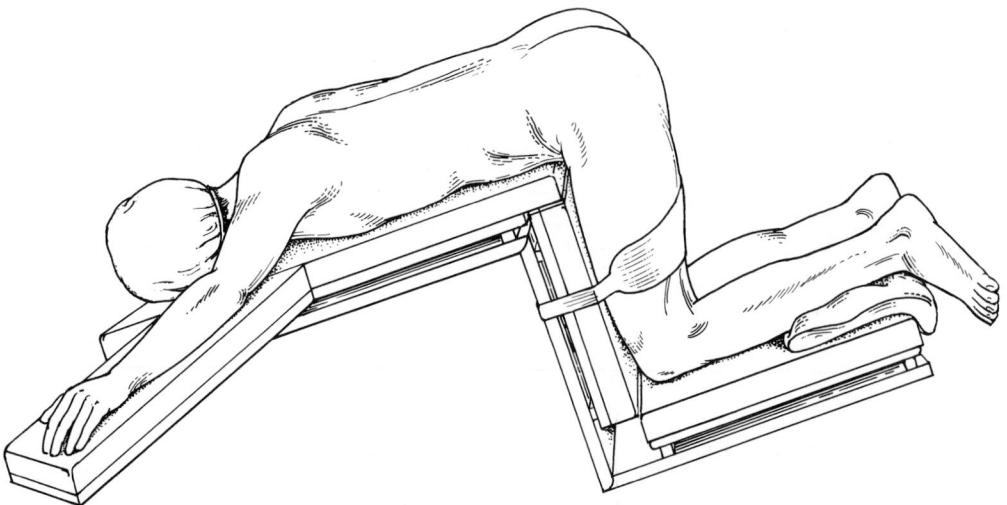

FIG. 4-13 Jackknife position for proctologic operations.

break in the operating room bed and the leg section raised to facilitate a "kneeling" position. The surgeon specifies the modifications preferred.

Jackknife (Kraske's) position

The jackknife, or Kraske's, position is a modification of the prone position that is used for proctologic procedures (Fig. 4-13). The patient's hips are placed on a bolster or pillow over the break in the operating room bed, and the bed is flexed at a 90-degree angle, raising the hips and lowering the head and body. The patient's head, chest, and feet need the usual supports in this position. A small roll placed under each shoulder will protect the brachial plexus. A pillow should be placed under the lower legs to prevent pressure on the toes. The restraint strap is across the thighs.

The buttocks may be separated with broad straps of adhesive tape secured firmly at the level of the anus a few inches from the midline on either side. These straps are pulled tight simultaneously and are fastened to the underside of the bed surface. The straps are released at the end of the procedure to facilitate approximation of the wound edges.

If the patient is to be placed on the recovery stretcher in the supine position, the operating room bed is first straightened, and the patient is turned by four people using a "log roll" technique.

LATERAL POSITIONS

In the lateral position the patient is lying on the unaffected side, providing access to the upper chest, the kidney, or the upper section of the ureter (Figs. 4-14 and 4-15, A). Positioning of the extremities and trunk facilitates the desired exposure.

In lateral positioning a special pad or beanbag device may be utilized on the operating room bed. The beanbag device or evacuatable mattress is made up of granules enclosed in a heavy duty, airtight, flexible material. Air can

be evacuated through a port or stopper valve. When air is removed, the granules firm up and the mattress holds its shape. Pressure on the skin is more evenly and widely distributed. This device increases the surface area supporting the patient's weight. The pad is placed prior to the patient's transfer and is to be under the patient's torso. The head and foot portions of the bed are padded to a height equal to the bag to prevent hyperextension of the body when the patient is supine on the bag.

After induction of anesthesia with the patient in the supine position on the operating room bed, the patient is turned to the side. A four-person team is necessary to accomplish a safe, smooth, gentle turn. The anesthesiologist supports the head and neck during the turn. One assistant stands at the shoulder of the operative side facing the patient's head; the assistant's arm and hand nearer the patient cross the chest and grasp the patient's shoulder; the other hand is placed under the nearer shoulder. The second assistant stands at the hips of the operative side, facing the patient's head; the assistant's arm and hand nearer the patient cross the hips and grasp the patient's opposite buttock; the other hand is placed under the nearer buttock. The third assistant stands at the foot of the bed to support and turn the legs. A lifting sheet under the patient can be used by the team to facilitate the turn. At a signal from the anesthesiologist, the first and second assistants lift and bring the patient to his or her side at their edge of the operating room bed; the patient is then placed in the center of the bed.

A pillow is placed under the patient's head to maintain good alignment with the cervical spine and the thoracic vertebrae. Another pillow is placed between the patient's legs, the bottom leg flexed at the knee and hip, and the top leg straight or slightly flexed. The lateral aspect of the bottom knee must be padded to prevent pressure on the peroneal nerve, located superficially at the head of the fibula. One assistant should remain at the patient's back to steady and support the torso during positioning of the extremities.

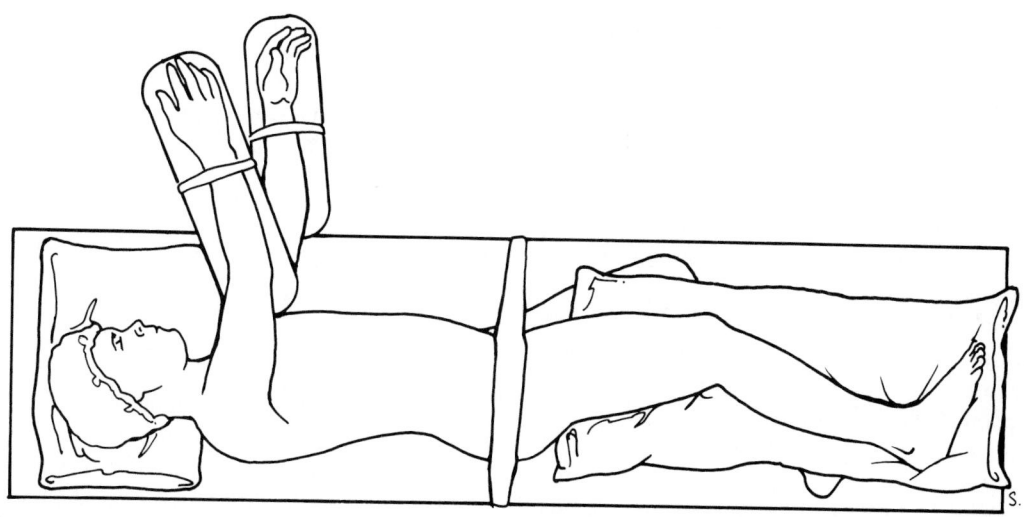

FIG. 4-14 Lateral position for chest procedures. In some instances the upper arm may be slightly flexed at the elbow, raised above the head, and supported on a special raised armboard.

David Schumick, The Ohio State University Biomedical Communications, Columbus, Ohio.

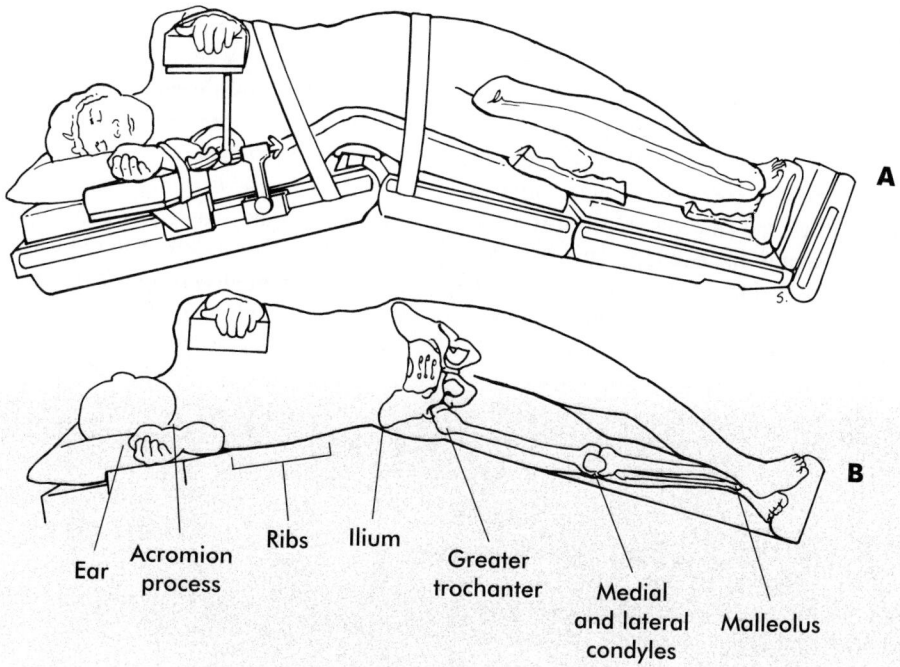

A

B

Ear   Acromion   Ribs   Ilium   Greater   Medial   Malleolus
       process   trochanter and lateral
                                                condyles

FIG. 4-15 Lateral position for kidney operations with potential pressures areas noted.

David Schumick, The Ohio State University Biomedical Communications, Columbus, Ohio.

Lateral chest position

The lateral chest position (Fig. 4-14) allows operative approach to the uppermost part of the thoracic cavity. The upper arm is flexed slightly at the elbow and raised above the head to elevate the scapula, provide access to the underlying ribs, and widen the intercostal spaces. This arm may be supported on a special raised armboard. The lower shoulder is brought slightly forward to prevent pressure on the brachial plexus and is flexed at the elbow. The lower shoulder may rest on a thin foam pad to prevent tissue pressure from the bony prominence. In chest surgery, infusion and monitoring lines may be placed in the upper or lower arm. Care must be taken to prevent compression of venous return in that arm.

The torso may be stabilized on the bed by well-padded body braces, sandbags, or beanbags. Some surgeons prefer to secure the arms, hips, and legs with wide tape and not use torso supports, which may impede respiratory expansion and decrease the surface area for the surgical approach. A soft roll may be placed at the apex of the scapula immediately adjacent to the axillary space to relieve pressure on the arm and allow more chest movement with respirations. True axillary rolls are controversial and seldom used. Slanting the upper section of the bed downward places the trachea and mouth at a lower level than the lungs. This slanting of the bed enables bronchial secretions and fluids from the lung bases to drain into the mouth and not pass into the unaffected side of the chest.

For torso stabilization the legs may be positioned in several ways, according to the surgeon's preference: (1) both legs may be flexed at a 90-degree angle at the hips and knees, a pillow placed between the legs, and adhesive tape placed across the hip area to both sides of the top of the bed; (2) the lower leg may be extended straight on the bed, the upper hip and knee flexed at a 90-degree angle with two pillows supporting the thigh and calf, the uppermost ankle secured in a padded restraint to the bed top at the patient's back, and adhesive tape placed across the hip area to both sides of the top of the bed; or (3) the lower hip and knee may be flexed at a 90-degree angle, two or more pillows supporting the extended upper leg, the uppermost ankle secured in a padded restraint to the bed top at the patient's back, and adhesive tape placed across the upper hip, between the iliac crest and greater trochanter, to both sides of the bed top.

Lateral kidney position

The lateral kidney position (Fig. 4-15, A) allows approach to the retroperitoneal area of the flank. After being turned from the dorsal to the lateral position, the anesthetized patient is moved so that the lower iliac crest is just below the kidney elevator. To render the kidney region readily accessible, the bridge (kidney rest) of the operating room bed is raised and the bed is flexed, so that the area between the twelfth rib and the iliac crest is elevated. A well-padded kidney brace may be placed against the iliac

crest. Elevating the kidney rest depends on the cardiovascular response of the body to the increased pressure transmitted from this area. The kidney rest is slowly raised; blood pressure is monitored frequently by the anesthesiologist. The bed is then flexed to lower the patient's head and legs. In this position the patient's affected side presents a straight horizontal line from shoulder to hip.

The upper arm is placed on a special raised armboard. The lower shoulder is brought slightly forward, and the arm is flexed to rest on an armboard or near the head on the mattress. A small bolster is placed under the lower axilla to facilitate chest expansion. The lower extremity is flexed and supported by a sandbag or pillow. Two or more pillows support the extended upper leg. The feet should be protected against plantar flexion and the ankles or heels protected from undue pressure (Fig. 4-15, B). In this position the gravitational force on the head and torso opposes that on the extended limb to facilitate operative exposure. To stabilize the body, a restraining belt or adhesive strap is placed across the shoulder and hip areas and is secured to the bed top. Before wound closure, the adhesive strap is released, the kidney rest lowered, and the bed straightened to facilitate approximation of the wound edges.

Physiologic changes in the lateral position occur in the healthy, alert person but may be more dramatic and stressful in the anesthetized patient. Normally, systolic and diastolic pressures decrease when the lateral position is assumed. Because normal compensatory mechanisms are depressed by pharmacologic agents and pathophysiologic processes, the patient may not readily compensate for abrupt postural changes. The acute angulation of the body in the lateral kidney posture and the effect of gravity may also decrease blood return to the right side of the heart.

Respiratory function is compromised by the weight of the body on the lower chest; chest movements are limited, and chest size may be decreased. Diaphragmatic movement is limited by the flexion of the lower limbs toward the abdomen. Another disadvantage of this position is that the weight of the body must rest on the unaffected side, which makes controlling the patient's aspiration of secretions from the lung on this side more difficult. In the lateral kidney position, pressure on the lower thorax and increased tension on the upper intercostal and lumbar musculature interfere with intercostal breathing.

The hazards of neuromuscular damage can largely be prevented through careful manipulation and adequate protective padding. Again, the brachial plexus and common peroneal nerve deserve thoughtful consideration.

ORTHOPEDIC FRACTURE TABLE POSITION

The orthopedic fracture table allows the patient to be positioned for hip fracture surgery or closed femoral nailing. The patient may be brought into the operating room in the hospital bed with traction applied. Prior to transfer the patient can be anesthetized. During transfer to the fracture table manual traction to the injured leg can be applied.

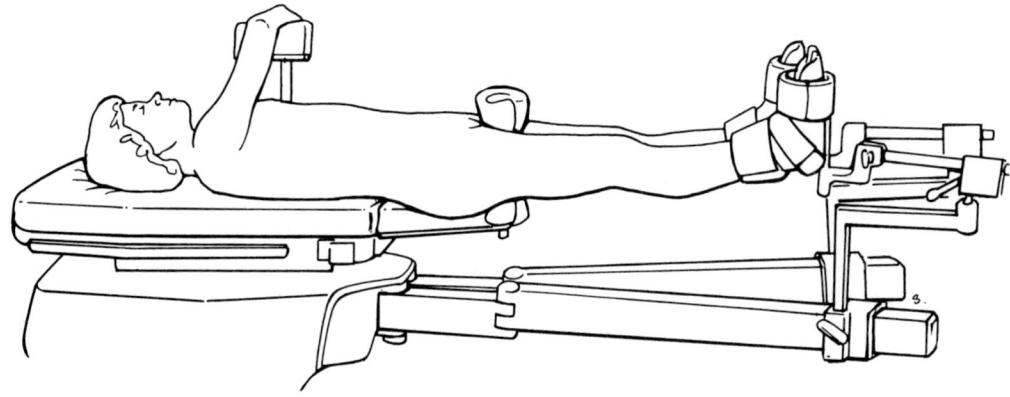

FIG. 4-16   Fracture table positioning.

The patient is positioned supine with the pelvis stabilized against a well-padded vertical perineal post (Fig. 4-16). Pressure on the genitalia from the perineal post can injure the pudendal nerves. Traction is achieved by restraining the injured leg in a well-padded bootlike device to protect the foot and ankle. The leg may be rotated, pulled into traction, or released, as the surgery requires. The unaffected leg rests on a well-padded elevated leg holder or secured in a well-padded bootlike device. C-arm or fluoroscopy x-rays can be taken during surgery because the unaffected leg is positioned well out of the field of the radiograph.

SUMMARY

Careful, planned positioning results in maximum patient safety and maximum surgical site exposure, as well as provides the anesthesiologist access to the head and neck to administer anesthesia care. All members of the surgical team have the responsibility to protect the patient from injury during positioning. Therefore all members should be familiar with possible risks to maintain patient safety. The following is a summary of important nursing interventions when positioning patients:

1. Check with anesthesia before moving the patient.
2. Determine number of personnel needed to safely and effectively position the patient.
3. Pad all bony prominences to prevent disruption to skin integrity (occiput, scapula, olecranon, sacrum, calcaneus).
4. Protect the brachial plexus, located in the axillary area, from strain or pressure.
5. Ensure that legs are not crossed to prevent pressure on nerves and blood vessels.
6. Support and secure extremities to prevent them from falling from the operating room bed.
7. Ensure that no part of the patient's body touches metal on the operating room bed.
8. Maintain patient privacy and dignity by avoiding unnecessary exposure.
9. Make certain no equipment, Mayo stand, or personnel are resting on the patient.
10. Protect self by using good body mechanics.

REFERENCES

Agency for Health Care Policy and Research (1992, May). *Clinical practice guideline number 3, Pressure ulcers in adults*, Publication no. 92-0047, p. 8. Rockville, Md.

Agency for Health Care Policy and Research. (1992, May). *Clinical practice guideline number 3, Pressure ulcers in adults: Prediction and prevention*. Publication no. 92-0050. Rockville, Md.

Garner B. (1993). Pressure ulcer development in surgical patients. Unpublished master's thesis. Wright State University, Dayton, Ohio.

Gendron, F. (1988). *Unexplained patient burns: Investigating iatrogenic injuries*, Brea: Quest. pp. 170, 173, 238.

Poma, P.A. (1979). Pressure-induced alopecia: report of a case after gynecologic surgery, *Journal of Reproductive Medicine*, 22(4), 220.

BIBLIOGRAPHY

Agency for Health Care Policy and Research. (1992, May). *Clinical practice guideline number 3, Preventing pressure ulcers a patient's guide*, Publication no. 92-0048. Rockville, Md.

Anderton, J.M., Keen, R.I., & Neave, R.: *Positioning the surgical patients*, London, 1988, Butterworths.

Groah, L. (1990). *Operating room nursing perioperative practice* ed 2, Norwalk: Appleton and Lange.

Gruendemann, B.J. (1987). *Positioning plus: a clinical handbook on patient positioning for perioperative nurses*. Chatsworth: Education Department of Devon Industries, Inc.

Kneedler, J.A., & Dodge, G.H. (1994). *Perioperative patient care: the nursing perspective*, ed 3, Boston: Jones and Bartlett Publishers.

Long, B.C., & Phipps, W.J. (1993). *Medical-surgical nursing: a nursing process approach*, ed 3, St. Louis: Mosby.

Martin, J.T. (1987). *Positioning in anesthesia and surgery*, ed 2, Philadelphia: WB Saunders.

Schmaus, D., Nelson, S., & Davis, D.: (1987). *Positioning the surgical patient*, Denver: The Association of Operating Room Nurses, Inc.

Thibodeau, G.A., & Patton, K.T. (1993). *Textbook of anatomy and physiology*, ed 13, St. Louis: Mosby.

5

SUTURES, NEEDLES, AND INSTRUMENTS

CLAIRE C. OLSEN

HISTORY AND EVOLUTION OF SURGICAL SUTURES (2000 BC TO PRESENT)

The development of surgical sutures has been closely allied with the development of the art of surgery. Medical writing of ancient Egyptian and Assyrian cultures dating back to 2000 BC mentions the various materials used, to a limited extent, for suturing and ligating. *Suture* is a generic term for all materials used to sew severed body tissue together and to hold these tissues in their normal position until healing takes place. A *ligature* is a strand of suture material used to tie off (seal) blood vessels to prevent hemorrhage and simple bleeding or to isolate a mass of tissue to be excised (cut out).

The concept of suturing and ligating is also recorded in the writings of the father of medicine, Hippocrates, born in 460 BC. Gut of sheep intestines was first mentioned as suture material in the writings of Galen, about AD 200. The Arabian surgeon Rhazes is credited with employing surgical gut, or catgut, in AD 900 for suturing abdominal wounds. The word *catgut* is a misnomer and its use is inappropriate. It has no relation to a cat but instead originated from the word *kitgut*. The Arabic word *kit* means a dancing master's fiddle, and kit strings were originally used for sutures.

Despite these promising early beginnings, the science of surgery, including suturing and ligating, progressed and then regressed, with several cultures never advancing much beyond the rudimentary stages. The principal reasons surgery and its allied practices did not progress in early times were the critical problems of hemorrhage, pain, and infection. Even Ambroise Paré, the famous French army surgeon of the middle 1500s who developed the technique for ligating to replace cautery in treatment of traumatic war injuries, was confronted with the grim fact that severe pain and subsequent infection markedly curtailed the advancements made possible by surgical repair and correction.

Surgery offered little promise of developing as a truly effective healing science until the nineteenth century, when an American surgeon, Crawford W. Long of Georgia, demonstrated the use of ether as an anesthetic (1842) and Joseph Lister of England first used carbolic acid solution to attempt antiseptic surgery (1865). Lister also experimented with surgical gut as an absorbable suture material and recognized the need for sterile surgical sutures.

Progress in the development of surgical sutures was rapid after the middle 1800s. By 1901 surgical gut and kangaroo gut were available to the surgeon in sterile glass tubes. Since then, numerous materials have been employed as sutures and ligatures. Gold, silver, metallic wire, silkworm gut, silk, cotton, linen, tendon, and intestinal tissue from virtually every creature that walks, swims, or flies have been used at one time or another throughout the evolution of surgery. During the early twentieth century surgical gut, silk, and cotton emerged as the most commonly used suture materials. The last half of this century saw the introduction and increased use of synthetic fibers such as nylon, polyester, polypropylene, and other polymer combinations.

As late as the 1930s the sterility of sutures commercially prepared and sterilized by manufacturers was subject to question. In addition, sutures varied considerably in their physical properties, such as diameter and strength. From the 1940s to the present, great strides have been made in the uniform preparation and sterilization of suture materials. Today the surgical team is assured of sterility, relatively uniform physical properties, and predictable performance in the sutures received in the operating room.

Since the early 1950s the trend has been toward individually packaged and presterilized suture materials, many with preattached (swaged) needles, delivered to the surgical suite in a ready-to-use form. This trend has relieved perioperative nurses of the time-consuming and consequently expensive tasks of preparing sutures and needles for sterilization and then sterilizing them.

SUTURE MATERIALS

A variety of suture materials is available for ligating, suturing, and closing the wound. The appropriate suture is selected according to a number of characteristics: whether it is absorbable or nonabsorbable, its breaking (tensile) strength, whether it is monofilament or multifilament, its knot-tying facility, and its tissue reactivity. An understanding of these characteristics of suture materials is essential for the perioperative nurse.

CHARACTERISTICS OF SUTURE MATERIAL

The three main ways to evaluate the general properties of suture material are: (1) physical characteristics, (2) handling characteristics, and (3) tissue reaction characteristics (see Box 5-1).

Physical characteristics

Physical characteristics of suture are officially defined and described by the United States Pharmacopeia (USP). They can be measured or visually determined and include the following properties:

- *Physical configuration:* single-stranded (monofilament) or multistranded (multifilament) containing a number of fibers rendered into a single thread by twisting or braiding (Fig. 5-1)
- *Capillarity:* ability to soak up fluid along the strand

- *Diameter:* determined in millimeters, and expressed in USP sizes with zeroes; the smaller the cross-sectional diameter, the more zeroes; sizes range from #7, the largest, to 11-0, the smallest; sizes 0 to 4-0 are the most commonly used sutures in general surgery. (The surgeon will usually select the finest suture possible for the tissue being closed. The finer diameter provides better handling qualities and small knots. Improved suturing techniques are possible with sutures of finer diameter.)
- *Tensile strength:* the amount of weight (breaking load) necessary to break a suture (breaking strength); varies with type of suture material (Table 5-1)
- *Knot strength:* the force necessary to cause a given type of knot to slip, either partially or completely
- *Elasticity:* inherent ability to regain original form and length after having been stretched
- *Memory:* capacity of a suture to return to its former shape after being re-formed, such as when tied; high memory yields less knot security

Handling characteristics

Handling characteristics of suture material are related both to pliability (how easily the material bends), and coefficient of friction (how easily the suture slips through tissue and ties). A suture with a high friction coefficient tends to drag through tissue. It is more difficult to tie because its knots do not set easily. Some suture materials are coated to reduce their coefficient of friction. This coating not only improves the way they pull through tissue on insertion, but also affects the force needed to remove the suture after the wound is healed. The coefficient of friction should not be too low, however, because knots come undone more easily.

BOX 5-1

Characteristics of Suture Material

I. Physical characteristics
  Physical configuration
  Capillarity
  Fluid absorption ability
  Diameter (caliber)
  Tensile strength
  Knot strength
  Elasticity
  Plasticity
  Memory
II. Handling characteristics
  Pliability
  Tissue drag   Related to coefficient of
  Knot tying   friction
  Knot slippage
III. Tissue reaction characteristics
  Inflammatory and fibrous cell reaction
  Absorption
  Potentiation of infection
  Allergic reaction

From Bennett, R.G.: Selection of wound closure materials, J. Am. Acad. Dermatol. 18:619, 1988.

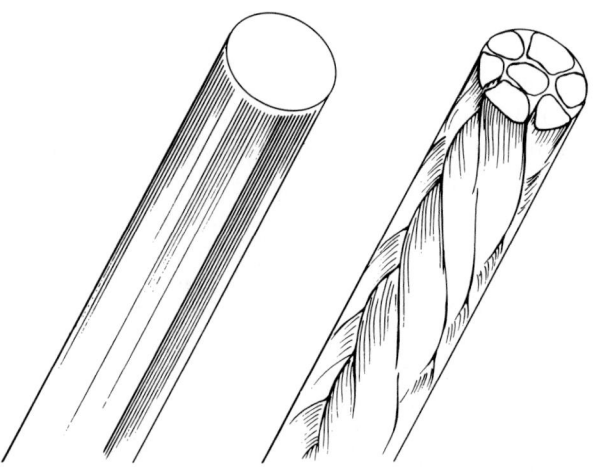

FIG. 5-1 *Left,* Monofilament suture; *right,* multifilament (braided) suture.

TABLE 5-1

Relative Straight Pull Tensile Strength of Suture Materials

	Nonabsorbable	Absorbable
G ↑	Steel	
R	Polyester	Polyglycolic acid
E	Nylon (monofilamen-	Polyglactin 910
A	tous)	
T	Nylon (braided)	
E	Polypropylene	Polydioxanone
R	Silk	Polyglecaprone
R		Catgut

Modified from Bennett, R.G. (1988). Selection of wound closure materials. *J Am Acad Dermatol* 18:619.

TABLE 5-2

Relative Tissue Reactivity to Sutures

	Nonabsorbable	Absorbable
M ↑		Catgut
O	Silk, cotton	
S	Polyester coated	Polyglactin 910
T	Polyester uncoated	Polyglycolic acid
	Nylon	Poliglecaprone
	Polypropylene	

Modified from Bennett R.G. (1988). Selection of wound closure materials. *J Am Acad Dermatol* 18:619.

Tissue reaction characteristics

Because it is a foreign substance, all suture material causes some tissue reaction. Tissue reaction begins when the suture inflicts injury to the tissue during insertion. In addition, tissue reaction to the suture material itself occurs (Table 5-2). This reaction begins with an infiltration of white blood cells into the area; macrophages and fibroblasts then appear; by about the seventh day fibrous tissue with chronic inflammation is present. The reaction persists until the suture is encapsulated (nonabsorbable material) or absorbed (absorbable material) by the body.

TYPES OF SUTURE MATERIAL

Suture materials are classified into two broad groups: absorbable and nonabsorbable.

Absorbable suture

The USP (1990) defines an absorbable surgical suture as follows:

. . . sterile, flexible strand prepared from collagen derived from healthy mammals, or from a synthetic polymer. . . . It is capable of being absorbed by living mammalian tissue, but may be treated to modify its resistance to absorption. . . . It may be modified with respect to body or texture. It may be impregnated with a suitable coating, softening, or antimicrobial agent. It may be colored by a color additive approved by the federal Food and Drug Administration.

Absorbable suture can be digested (by enzyme activity) or hydrolyzed (react with water in tissue fluids to breakdown) and assimilated by the tissues during the healing process. Absorbable sutures vary in treatment, color, size, packaging, and resistance to absorption, according to their purpose. Types of absorbable suture include plain or chromic surgical gut, collagen, and glycolic acid polymers (Table 5-3).

Surgical gut

Surgical gut is obtained from the collagen of the submucosal layer of the small intestine of sheep or the intestinal serosa of cattle or hogs. The processed strands or ribbons of collagen are either untreated (plain, type A) or treated with chromium salts (chromic, type C).

Chromatization delays absorption of the suture in living mammalian tissue. The strength of the chromium salt content and the duration of the chromatizing process are accurately controlled and tested. Proper chromatizing of gut ensures the integrity of the suture and maintenance of its strength during the early stages of wound healing. It enables a wound with slow healing power to heal sufficiently before the suture is entirely absorbed.

The elaborate processes of mechanical and chemical cleaning of the raw gut are followed by sterilization, usually with ionizing radiation, and storage in hermetically sealed packages. Modern manufacturing processes also ensure tensile strength, more controlled absorption, and more predictable results.

Absorption takes place via digestion of the gut by tissue enzymes. The absorption rate of surgical gut is influenced by the type of body tissue it contacts and, to some extent, by the patient's general physical condition. Studies also show that surgical gut is absorbed faster in serous or mucous membranes than in muscular tissues. When fine chromic gut is properly buried in successive layers of the gastrointestinal tract, for example, it retains its strength long enough for primary union to take place.

Surgical gut suture is wet-packed in an alcohol solution to provide maximum pliability and should be used immediately after removal from the packet. When a gut suture is removed from its packet and is not used at once, the alcohol evaporates, which causes the strand to lose its pliability. If required, the strand's pliability may be restored just before use by immersing it in sterile water or normal saline solution, preferably at body temperature, for only a few seconds. However, this is recommended only for eye sutures,

— TABLE 5-3 —

Comparison of Absorbable Sutures

Trade name	Company	Material	Configuration	Tensile strength	Tissue reactivity
Collagen (plain)	Davis & Geck	Beef flexor tendon	Twisted	Poor (0% at 2-3 weeks)	Moderate
Collagen (chromic)	Davis & Geck	Beef flexor tendon	Twisted	Poor (0% at 2-3 weeks)	Moderate
Surgical gut (plain)	Ethicon; Davis & Geck; U.S. Surgical	Animal collagen	Twisted	Poor (0% at 2-3 weeks)	High
Surgical gut (chromic)	Ethicon; Davis & Geck; U.S. Surgical	Animal collagen	Twisted	Poor (0% at 2-3 weeks)	Moderately high
Monocryl	Ethicon	Poliglecaprone	Monofilament	Fair (20% at 2-3 weeks)	Low
Coated Vicryl	Ethicon	Polyglactin 910 (coated with calcium stearate & polyglactin 370)	Braided	Good (50% at 2-3 weeks)	Low
Dexon S	Davis & Geck	Polyglycolic acid	Braided	Good (50% at 2-3 weeks)	Low
Dexon Plus	Davis & Geck	Polyglycolic acid (coated with poloxamer 188)	Braided	Good (50% at 2-3 weeks)	Low
Polysorb	U.S. Surgical	Glycolide colactide	Braided	Fair (20% at 3 weeks)	Low
PDS	Ethicon	Polydioxanone	Monofilamentous	Good (50% at 2-3 weeks)	Low
Maxon	Davis & Geck	Polyglyconate	Monofilament	Good (50% at 4 weeks)	Low

Modified from Bennett R.G. (1988). *Fundamentals of cutaneous surgery.* St Louis: Mosby.

since in other areas tissue fluids will moisten the gut sufficiently as it passes through the tissue when the surgeon sews. Excessive moisture will reduce tensile strength.

Collagen sutures

Collagen sutures are derived from the tendon of cattle. They are chemically treated to remove noncollagenous material, purified, and processed into strands that have physical properties superior to surgical gut. Collagen suture is most often used as a fine suture material for the eye.

Synthetic absorbable sutures

To produce synthetic absorbable sutures, specific polymers are extruded into suture strands. The base material for the synthetic absorbables is a combination of lactic and glycolic acid polymers (Vicryl, Dexon, Polysorb). The molecular structure of these products has a tensile strength sufficient for approximation of tissues for 2 to 3 weeks, followed by rapid absorption.

The newer synthetic polymers (PDS, Maxon, Monocryl), provide wound support for longer periods, up to 3 months. They are used when prolonged support for wound healing is desired, as with fascial closure, or for elderly or oncologic patients. Thus they combine the desirable qualities of extended wound support and eventual absorbability.

Synthetic absorbable sutures are absorbed by slow hydrolysis in the presence of tissue fluids. Hydrolysis is the chemical process whereby the polymer reacts with water to cause an alteration of breakdown of the molecular structure. These sutures are degraded in tissue by this process at a more predictable rate than surgical gut (or collagen) and with less tissue reaction.

These sutures are dry packaged in sizes 10-0 to #3. They should not be dipped in solutions because moisture reduces tensile strength. Some polymers have additional coatings to reduce drag in tissue.

Nonabsorbable sutures

Nonabsorbable sutures are strands of material that effectively resist enzymatic digestion in living animal tissue. The USP classifies nonabsorbable surgical suture as follows:

TABLE 5-3
Comparison of Absorbable Sutures—cont'd.

Handling	Knot security	Memory	Absorption	Degradation	Comments
Fair	Poor	Low	Unpredictable (12 weeks)	Proteolytic	Less impure than surgical gut
Fair	Poor	Low	Unpredictable (12 weeks)	Proteolytic	Less impure than surgical gut
Fair	Poor	Low	Unpredictable (12 weeks)	Proteolytic	May be ordered as fast-absorbing gut (Ethicon) for percutaneous sutures
Fair	Fair	Low	Unpredictable (14-80 days)	Proteolytic	Darker, more visible (Davis & Geck); mild or extra chromatization (Davis & Geck)
Good	Fair	Low	Predictable (90 days)	Hydrolytic	Clear
Good	Fair	Low	Predictable (80 days)	Hydrolytic	Clear, violet, coated
Fair	Good	Low	Predictable (90 days)	Hydrolytic	Uncoated
Good	Fair	Low	Predictable (90 days)	Hydrolytic	Clear, green, coated
Good	Fair	Low	Predictable (90 days)	Hydrolytic	Clear, violet
Poor	Poor	High	Predictable (180 days)	Hydrolytic	Violet, clear
Good	Good	Low	Predictable (180 days)	Hydrolytic	Green, clear

1. Class I suture is composed of silk or synthetic fibers of monofilament, twisted, or braided construction.
2. Class II suture is composed of cotton or linen fibers or coated natural or synthetic fibers where the coating significantly affects thickness but does not contribute significantly to strength.
3. Class III suture is composed of monofilament or multifilament metal wire.

The strand may be uncoated or coated with a substance to reduce capillarity and friction when passing through the tissue. There are a number of products used for coating, including silicone, Teflon, and various polymers. Fibers may be uncolored, naturally colored, or impregnated with a suitable dye.

Nonabsorbable suture materials are encapsulated or walled off by the tissues around it during the process of wound healing. In suturing skin, for which nonabsorbable materials are often the choice, the sutures are removed before healing is complete.

The most common nonabsorbable suture materials are silk, cotton, nylon, polyester fiber, polypropylene, and stainless steel wire (Table 5-4).

Silk

Silk is prepared from thread spun by the silkworm larva in making its cocoon. Top-grade raw silk is processed to remove the natural waxes and gum, manufactured into threads, and colored with a vegetable dye. The strands of silk are either twisted or braided to form the suture, which gives it high tensile strength and better handling qualities. Silk handles well, is soft, and forms secure knots.

Untreated silk has a capillary action through which body fluids may transmit infection along the length of the suture strand. For this reason surgical silk is treated to render it noncapillary (able to resist the absorption of body fluids and moisture). It is available in sizes 9-0 to 5, in sterile packets or precut lengths, and with or without attached needles. Silk should be kept dry by the scrub person. Wet silk loses up to 20% in strength.

In the strict sense, silk is not a true nonabsorbable material. When buried in tissue it loses its tensile strength after about a year and may disappear after several years. Silk sutures occasionally migrate gradually to a wound's exterior surface. This migration is called spitting. Spitting is

---

TABLE 5-4

Comparison of Nonabsorbable Sutures

Generic or trade name	Company	Material	Configuration	Tensile strength
Cotton	—	Cotton	Twisted	Good
Silk	Ethicon; Davis & Geck; US Surgical	Silk	Braided	Good
Ethilon	Ethicon	Polyamide (nylon)	Monofilament	High
Dermalon	Davis & Geck	Polyamide (nylon)	Monofilament	High
Surgamid	Look	Polyamide (nylon)	Monofilament or braided	High
Nurolon	Ethicon	Polyamide (nylon)	Braided	High
Surgilon	Davis & Geck	Polyamide (nylon) (coated with silicone)	Braided	High
Monosof	US Surgical	Polyamide (nylon)	Monofilament	High
Bralon	US Surgical	Polyamide (nylon)	Braided	High
Prolene	Ethicon	Polyolefin (polypropylene)	Monofilament	Fair
Surgilene	Davis & Geck	Polyolefin (polypropylene)	Monofilament	Good
Demalene	Davis & Geck	Polyolefin (polypropylene)	Monofilament	Good
Surgipro	US Surgical	Polyolefin (polypropylene)	Monofilament	Good
Novafil	Davis & Geck	Polybutester	Monifilament	High
Mersilene	Ethicon	Polyester	Braided	High
Dacron	Deknatel; Davis & Geck	Polyester	Braided	High
Polyviolence	Look	Polyester	Braided	High
Ethibond	Ethicon	Polyester (coated with polybutilate)	Braided	High
Ti-Con	Davis & Geck	Polyester (coated with silocone)	Braided	High
Polydek	Deknatel	Polyester (coated with Teflon-light)	Braided	High
Tevdek	Deknatel	Polyester (coated with Teflon-heavy)	Braided	High
Surgidac	US Surgical	Polyester (coated with silicone)	Braided	High
Stainless steel	Ethicon	Stainless steel	Monofilament, twisted, or braided	High

Modified from Bennett, R.G. (1988). Selection of wound closure materials. *J Am Acad Dermatol* 18:04.

annoying and sometimes frightening to the patient but has no deleterious effect on wound healing.

Cotton

Surgical cotton sutures are made from individual cotton fibers that are combed, aligned, and twisted to form a finished strand. They differ from other sutures in that twisted cotton gains 10% in tensile strength when wet. Therefore cotton sutures should be moistened before use. Fine cotton suture, when buried in tissue, produces minimum tissue reaction but, due to its capillary action, should not be used in the presence of infection. Cotton is used much like silk but is not as strong. It is more difficult to handle, known to stick to the surgeon's gloves. As newer fibers have been introduced, use of cotton suture appears to be declining. Some companies no longer manufacture it.

Umbilical tape, although not actually used for suturing, is produced by suture manufacturers and packaged the same

TABLE 5-4
Comparison of Nonabsorbable Sutures—cont'd

Tissue reactivity	Handling	Knot security	Memory	Comments
High	Good	Good	Low	Obsolete, use declining
High	Good	Good	Low	Predisposes to infection; does not tear tissue; D & G suture is silicone treated; Ethicon is coated
Low	Poor	Poor	High	Cuts tissue; nylon; black, clear, or green
Low	Poor	Poor	High	Nylon
Low	Poor	Poor	High	Nylon
Moderate	Good	Fair	Medium	May predispose to infection; black or white; waxed; nylon
Moderate	Fair	Fair	Medium	Nylon
Low	Fair	Fair	Medium	Clear, black
Low	Fair	Fair	Medium	Clear, black, coated
Low	Poor	Poor	High	Very low coefficient of friction; cuts tissue; blue or clear
Low	Poor	Poor	High	—
Low	Poor	Poor	High	—
Low	Poor	Poor	High	Clear or blue
Low	Fair	Poor	Medium	Blue or clear
Moderate	Good	Good	Medium	Green or white
Moderate	Good	Good	Medium	—
Moderate	Good	Good	Medium	Green or white
Moderate	Good	Good	Medium	Green or white
Moderate	Poor	Poor	Medium	—
Moderate	Good	Good	Medium	—
Moderate	Poor	Poor	Medium	—
Moderate	Good	Good	Medium	Green or white
Low	Poor	Good	Low	May kink

as suture. It consists of long woven ribbons of cotton $\frac{1}{16}$ to $\frac{1}{8}$ inch wide and is used for retraction of tissue or as a marker.

Nylon

Surgical nylon (Dermalon, Ethilon, Surgilon, Nurolon, Bralon, Monosof) is a synthetic polyamide material. It is available in two forms: multifilament (braided) and monofilament strands. Multifilament nylon is relatively inert in tissues and has a high tensile strength. It is used in conditions similar to those in which silk and cotton are used. Monofilament nylon is a smooth material particularly well suited for closing skin edges and also for tension sutures. Because of its poor knot security, the surgeon usually ties three knots in small sutures and a double square knot in large sutures. It is frequently used in ophthalmology and microsurgery because it can be manufactured in fine sizes. Size 11-0 nylon is one of the smallest suture materials available.

Polyester fiber

Surgical polyester fiber (TiCron, Dacron, Mersilene, Tevdek, Polydek, Ethibond, Surgidac) is available in two forms: a nontreated polyester fiber suture and a polyester fiber suture that has been specifically coated or impregnated with a lubricant to allow smooth passage through the tissue. Polyester fiber is available in fine filaments that can be braided into various suture sizes to provide good handling properties.

Polybutester (Novafil) is a special type of polyester suture that possesses many of the advantages of both polyester and polypropylene. Because it is a monofilament, it induces little tissue reaction.

Polyester material has many advantages over other braided, nonabsorbable sutures. It has greater tensile strength, minimum tissue reaction, maximum visibility, and does not absorb tissue fluids. It is frequently used as a general closure fascia suture, as well as in cardiovascular surgery for valve replacements, graft-to-tissue anastomoses, and revascularization procedures.

Polypropylene

Polypropylene is a clear or pigmented polymer. This monofilament suture material (Prolene, Surgilene, Surgipro, Deklene) is used for cardiovascular, general, and plastic surgery. Because polypropylene is monofilament and is extremely inert in tissue, it may be used in the presence of infection. It has high tensile strength and causes minimal tissue reaction. Sizes range from 10-0 to 2.

Stainless steel

Surgical stainless steel is formulated to be compatible with stainless steel implants and prostheses. This formula, 316L (L for low carbon), ensures absence of toxic elements, optimal strength, flexibility, and uniform size.

Monofilament and multifilament surgical stainless steel is known for its strength, inertness, and low tissue reaction. However, stainless steel suturing technique is very exacting. Steel can pull or tear out of tissue, and necrosis can result from too tight a suture. Barbs on the end of steel can tear gloves, thus breaking sterile technique, or they can traumatize surrounding tissue. Kinks in the wire can render it practically useless. For this reason, packaging has played an important part in the development of surgical stainless steel sutures. Surgical stainless steel is available in packets on spools or in packages of straight, precut, sterile lengths, with or without swaged needles. This packaging affords protection to the strands and delivery in straight, unkinked lengths.

Before surgical stainless steel's availability from suture manufacturers, it was purchased by weight with the Brown and Sharp (B&S) scale for diameter variations. Today the B&S gauge, along with USP size classifications, is used to distinguish diameter size ranges. Table 5-5 gives comparisons of steel suture sizes.

TABLE 5-5

Steel Suture Comparison

Size (USP)	B&S gauge	Size (USP)	B&S gauge
6-0	40	0	26
6-0	38	1	25
5-0	35	2	24
4-0	34	3	23
4-0	32	4	22
000	30	5	20
00	28	7	18

PACKAGING, STORAGE, AND SELECTION OF SUTURES

Manufacturers now supply suture materials in some form of sterile package ready for immediate use. The USP specifies, "Preserve . . . dry or in fluid, in containers so designed that sterility is maintained until the container is opened."

TYPES OF PACKAGING

In the dry packaging method the suture material is sealed in a primary inner packet, which may or may not contain fluid; then inside a dry, outer, peel-back packet; then sterilized. This method permits easy dispensing onto the sterile field. Various forms of foil, plastic, and special paper are used for both the inner and outer packets.

Each primary suture packet is self-contained, and its sterility for each patient is ensured as long as the integrity of the packet is maintained. Some suture packets have expiration dates that relate to stability and sterility. Packages should be stored in moistureproof and dustproof containers in units of one size and type.

Suture packets may contain single or multiple strands, with or without a needle attached to the strand. The needle may be permanently attached (swaged) to the suture and need to be cut off for removal, or it may be designed to separate easily from the suture with a quick tug of the needle holder (Controlled Release, D-Tach, Pop-off). Some sutures may be double-armed, with a needle at each end of the strand.

COLOR CODES

Color-coded packaging based on suture fiber is used by most companies to make identification quicker and easier (Table 5-6). Each individual packet is color coded, as is the dispenser box. Although most color codes are universal across companies, there are some exceptions. Ethibond, a coated polyester, is coded orange, whereas most polyesters are coded in shades of green. Dexon, a glycolic acid polymer, is gold, whereas Vicryl, a comparable polymer, is coded violet.

TABLE 5-6

Suture Packaging Color Codes

Fiber	Color code
Plain gut	Yellow
Chromic gut	Tan
Glycolic acid polymers	Violet*
Silk	Medium blue
Cotton	Pink
Polypropylene	Royal blue
Polyester	Medium green*
Nylon	Light green
Stainless steel	Mustard*

*These color codes may change from one manufacturer to another.

SELECTION OF SUTURE

Choice of suture depends on the procedure, the tissue being sutured, the general condition of the patient, and the surgeon's preferences.

An operating room committee or project team may be responsible for establishing standard suture uses for various operations. Current guides published by suture manufacturers should be consulted. These guides list the specific suture materials recommended for various wounds and are based on current clinical practices and research.

To make delivery of sutures to the field more efficient, one can arrange to have custom packets of mixed sutures for specific procedures or surgeons prepared in advance by suture companies.

HEMOSTASIS

Hemostasis is an ongoing process during surgery. In addition to the damaging physiologic effects of blood loss for the patient, bleeding from cut vessels obscures visualization of the operative site for the surgeon and must be controlled.

Hemostasis may be accomplished with suture materials, electrosurgical devices, lasers, and chemical agents. Prior to wound closure the surgeon carefully checks the operative site to ensure all active bleeding has been stopped.

METHODS OF LIGATING VESSELS

A *ligature* is a strand of suture material used to encircle and close off the lumen of a vessel to effect hemostasis, close off a structure, or prevent leakage of materials. Ties may be on a reel—a spool or disk containing a long length of suture that the surgeon may use to ligate several superficial vessels. Or they may be free ties—precut lengths of suture handed to the surgeon one at a time, usually for bleeders in deeper tissues.

Following are several techniques used to secure a ligature in deep tissues:

1. A hemostat is placed on the end of the structure; the ligature is then placed around the vessel. The knot is tied and tightened with the surgeon's fingers or with the aid of forceps.
2. A slipknot is made, and its loop is placed over the involved structure by means of a forceps or clamp.
3. In deeper cavities ties are often placed on clamps with the long end extending from the tip. These are sometimes called *ties on a pass or bow ties.* The extending long end is held tightly against the rings by the surgeon (creating the bow), who then passes the tip of the clamp under the vessel or duct to be ligated. The first assistant grasps the extending tie with a forcep; the surgeon releases it, and the tie is pulled under and up to the wound surface and tied.
4. A forceps or a clamp is applied to the structure; then transfixion sutures are applied and tied. A *suture ligature, stick tie,* or *transfixion ligature* is a strand of suture material threaded or swaged on a needle. This is usually placed through the vessel, then around it, to prevent the ligature from slipping off the end.

When two ligatures are used to ligate a large vessel, usually a free ligature is placed on the vessel and then a suture ligature is placed distal to the first ligature. To ligate a blood vessel situated in deep tissues, the strand must be of sufficient strength and length to allow the surgeon to tighten the first knot.

The preparation of ligatures and suture ligatures is discussed in a later section of this chapter.

LIGATING CLIPS

Ligating clips are small, V-shaped, staplelike devices, which are placed around the lumen of a vessel or structure to close it off. They may be made of one of several metals, such as stainless steel, tantalum, or titanium. Stainless steel clips are the most economical to use. Although more expensive, titanium clips are used frequently in specific surgical procedures because the starburst reflection on postoperative radiographic scans is less with titanium than with other metals. Absorbable clips made of PDS (synthetic absorbable suture material) are also available.

Ligating clips are available in several sizes; each size requires its own applier, which must be loaded by the scrub person (Fig. 5-2). These clips are available in disposable, prepackaged units. Preloaded, disposable clip appliers that can be used in open wounds, or through endoscope trocar cannulas, are available. Ligating clips afford a rapid and secure method of achieving hemostasis or of ligating arteries, veins, nerves, and other small structures.

Metal Cushing or Frazier clips are made of small diameter pieces of stainless steel or silver wire and are heat sterilized. They must be hand loaded onto special rack dispensers. Frazier clips are applied to the ends of severed nerves and blood vessels by means of a forceps designed for the purpose. They are used in neurosurgery and orthopedic pro-

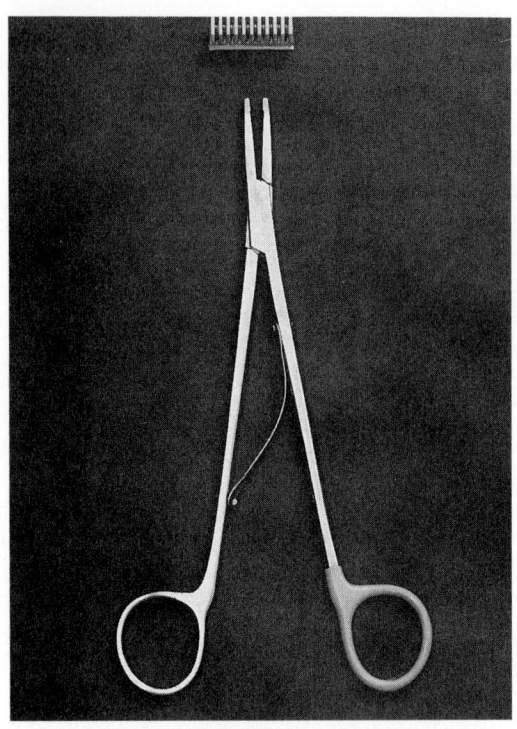

FIG. 5-2 Ligating clip applier.

cedures. Since the introduction of prepackaged ligating clips, their use is declining.

SKIN STAPLES

Skin staples are one of the most frequently chosen methods of skin closure. They can be used on many types of surgical incisions. The staple appliers are easy to use, and many are disposable. They reduce both operating time and tissue trauma, allowing uniform tension along the suture line and less distortion from the stress of individual suture points. When properly applied (Fig. 5-3) they provide excellent cosmetic results. They are usually removed within 5 to 7 days. An extractor is required for their removal.

Most staplers employ a similar anvil-type mechanism for forming the staple, but the applying device varies from company to company. Surgeon's choice is usually determined by the applier's weight, handling characteristics, ease of application, and unobstructed view of the site during application. They are packaged in various assortments of numbers and types of staples, depending on the length of the incision and the type of tissue encountered.

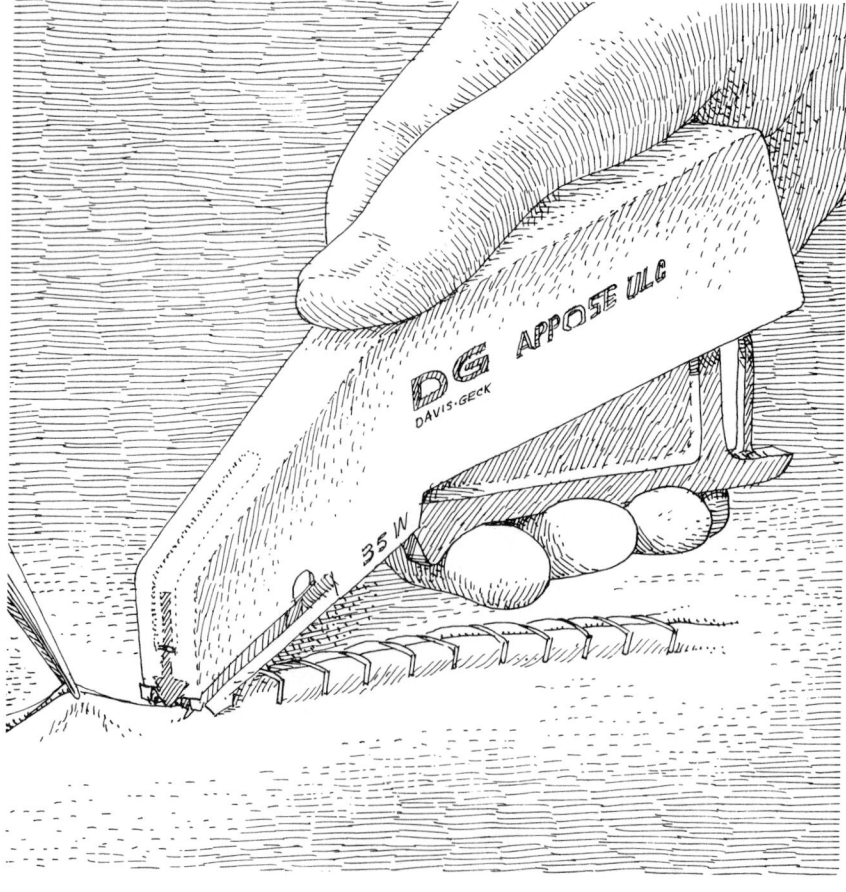

FIG. 5-3 Application of Skin Staples. The stapler is lightly positioned over everted skin edges. It is not necessary to press the staple, or stapler anvil, into the skin in order to get a proper "bite," (just "kiss" the skin). Staples are centered over the incision line, using the locating arrow or guideline, and placed approximately one-quarter inch apart.

Courtesy Davis & Geck.

SKIN TAPES

Wounds that are subjected to minimal static and dynamic tension are easily approximated with skin tape. The selection of surgical tape for skin closure is based on the tape's adhesive ability, tensile strength, and porosity. The tape must provide a firm tape-to-skin bond to keep the wound edges closely adherent. The tensile strength must be sufficient to maintain wound approximation. A tape that is too occlusive limits moisture vapor transmission; fluid may accumulate under the tape and lead to maceration and bacterial growth. Microporous tapes prevent this. The tape must be applied to dry skin; an adhesive adjunct (for example, tincture of benzoin) may be applied in a thin film to the skin at the wound edges prior to tape application. Tapes are applied perpendicular to the wound edge, first on one side and then the other, so that the edges can be pulled together (Fig. 5-4).

A. Perforated
tab is
removed

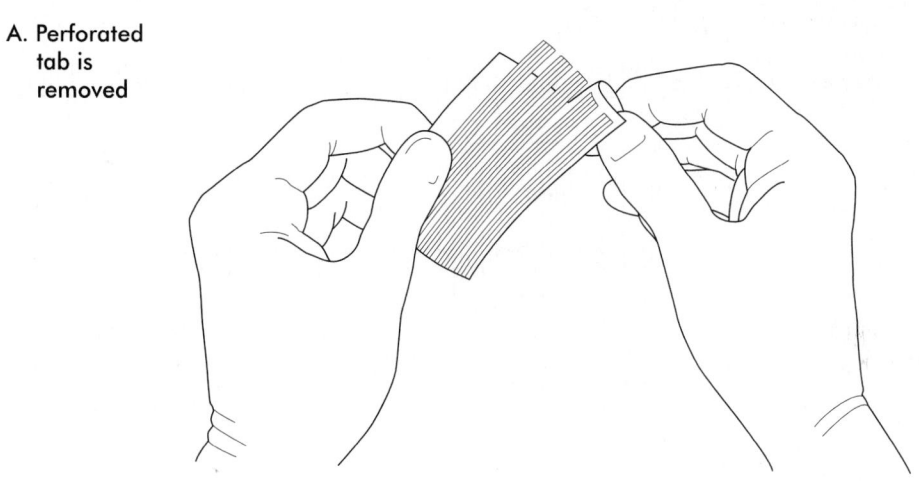

B. Tape is
peeled
from card

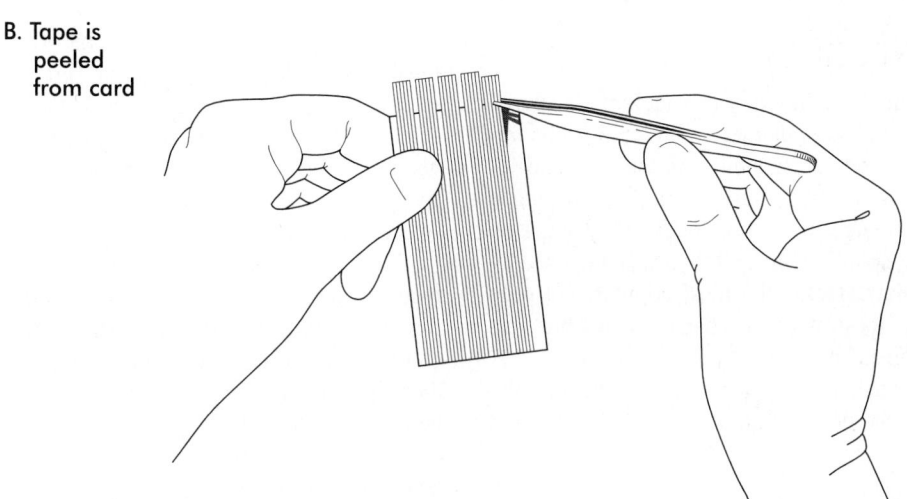

FIG. 5-4   Application of Skin Tapes. **A,** Perforated tab is bent and removed. **B,** Tape is peeled from the card.   *Continued.*

Courtesy of 3M.

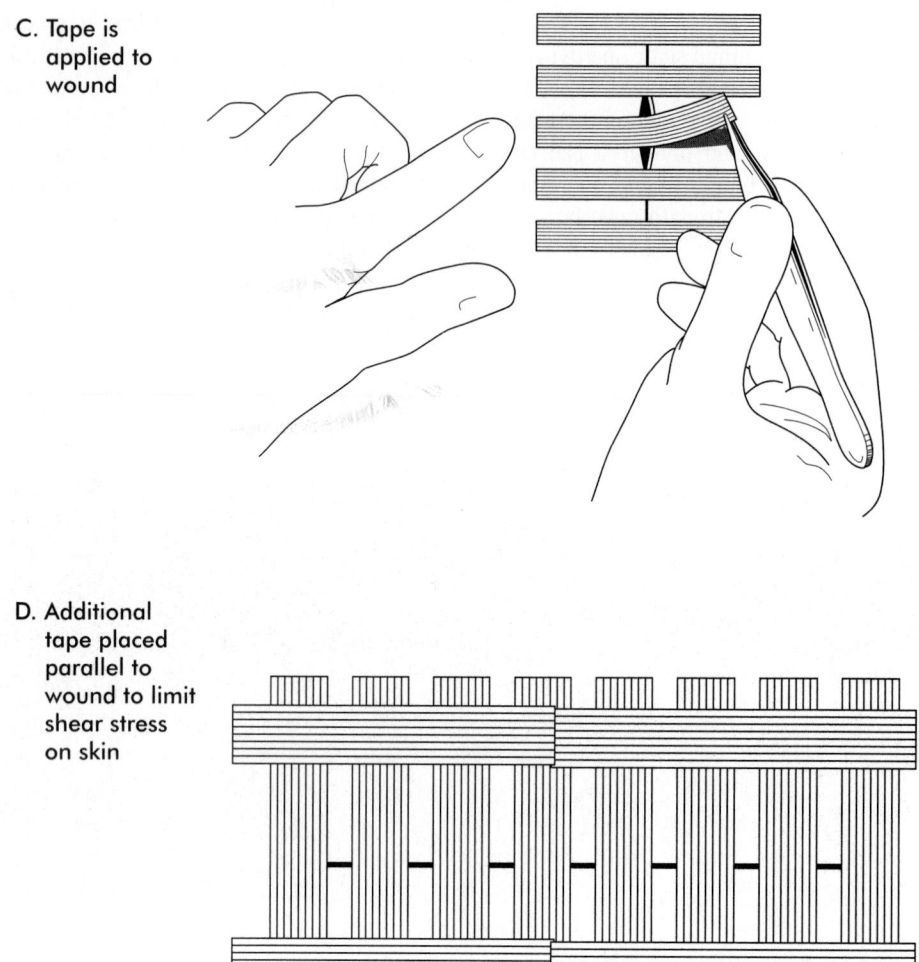

C. Tape is
applied to
wound

D. Additional
tape placed
parallel to
wound to limit
shear stress
on skin

FIG. 5-4, CONT'D **C,** Tape is applied to wound. **D,** Additional tape placed parallel to wound to limit shear stress on the skin.

SURGICAL NEEDLES

Surgical (surgeon's) needles vary considerably in shape, size, point design, and wire diameter (Fig. 5-5). The appropriate needle is selected depending on the type and location of tissue being sutured. Surgical needles are made from either stainless steel or carbon steel. They must be strong, ductile, and able to withstand the stress imposed by tough tissue. Stainless steel is the most popular, not only because it provides these physical characteristics but also because it is noncorrosive.

There are three basic parts to the surgeon's needle: the eye, the body, and the point or tip.

EYE

The eye of the surgical needle falls into three general categories: (1) eyed needles, in which the needle must be threaded with the suture strand, and two strands of suture must be pulled through the tissue (Fig. 5-6, *A*); (2) spring, or French eyed needles, in which the suture is placed or snapped through the spring (Fig. 5-6, *B*); and (3) eyeless needles, a needle-suture combination in which a needle is swaged (permanently attached) onto one or both ends of the suture material (Fig. 5-6, *C*).

The swaged needle is the most universally used needle type. Swaged needles eliminate threading eyed needles before and during surgery. The surgeon draws a single strand of suture material through the tissue, and tissue damage is thereby minimized (atraumatic). The swaged needle must be cut off with scissors.

A needle swaged for controlled release of the suture (semiswaged) facilitates interrupted suturing techniques. The needle remains attached until the surgeon releases it with a straight tug of the needle holder.

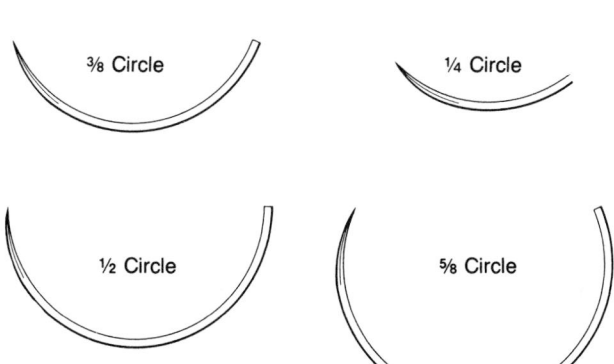

FIG. 5-5 Surgical needles vary in shape, size, type of point and body, and how the suture is attached.

Courtesy Davis & Geck.

BODY

The body, or shaft, of the needle may be round, triangular, or flattened (Table 5-7). Surgical needles may also be straight or curved; the curve is described as part of an imaginary circle (Fig. 5-5). As the radius of the imaginary circle increases, the size of the needle also increases. The body of a round needle gradually tapers to a point.

POINT

Choice of needle point relates to density of the tissue to be penetrated. Delicate tissue, such as bowel or kidney, requires a taper or blunted point, whereas skin, which is dense in structure, requires a cutting edge. Taper points tend to tear tissue less than cutting needles and leave a smaller hole in the tissue. Recently introduced blunt Protect-point needles are being recommended as an alternative to taper point needles (Research Highlight 5-1). Table 5-7 illustrates the type of points available for various tissues.

Triangular needles have cutting edges along three sides. The cutting action may be conventional or reverse. The conventional cutting needle has its cutting edge directed along the inner curve of the needle, facing the wound edge when suturing.

The reverse cutting needle is preferred for cutaneous suturing. When it transsects the skin lateral to the wound, the outside edge is pointed away from the wound edge, and the inside flat edge is parallel to the edge of the wound. This cutting action creates less of a tendency for suture to tear through tissue.

For certain types of delicate surgery, needles with exceptionally sharp points and cutting edges are used. Microsurgery, ophthalmology, and plastic surgery require needles of this type; special honing wheels provide needles of

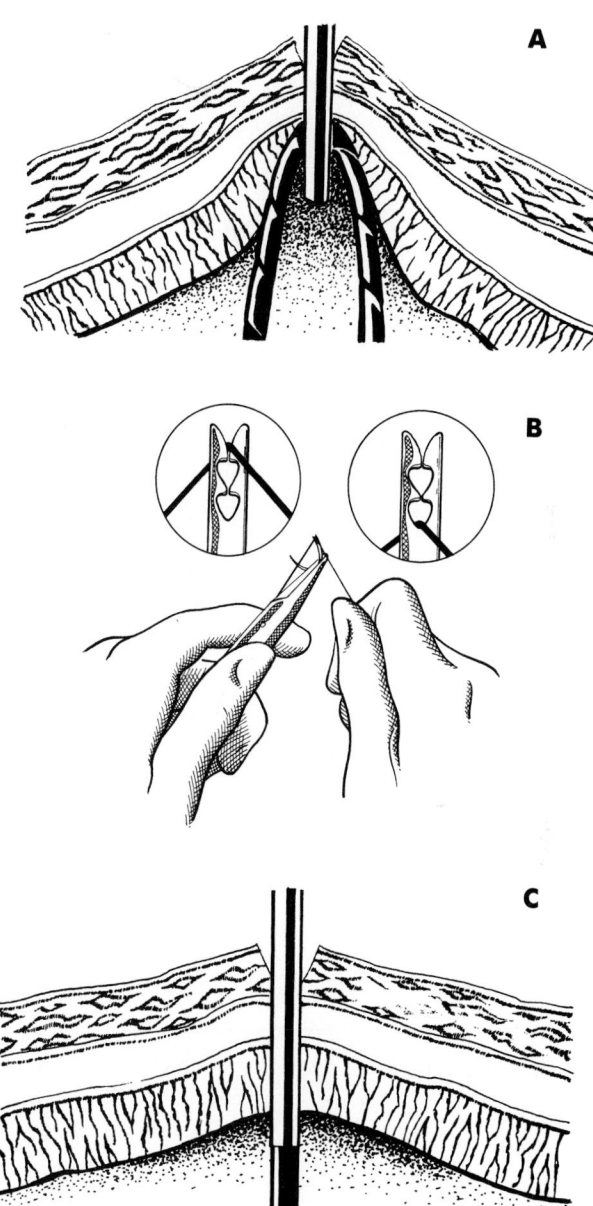

FIG. 5-6 Types of Needles. **A,** Eyed needle—greater tissue trauma is caused by the double suture strand threaded through eyed needles. **B,** Spring Eye—holding suture strand taut with left hand, bring strand down over top and spring into eye. **C,** Atraumatic needle—causes minimum tissue trauma by eliminating the double suture strand.

Courtesy Davis & Geck.

TABLE 5-7

Atraumatic Needles

Needle type	Point geometry	Description of body	Use
Taper point		Round shaft, straight or curved, tapered point, no cutting edge	Soft tissue closure such as gastrointestinal, fascia, vascular, and most soft tissues below the skin surface
Penetrating point		Taper body with finely sharpened point. Optimum penetration with less tissue wound	Ligaments, tendons, calcified, fibrous and cuticular tissue; mostly used for vascular, thoracic, plastic, OB/GYN and orthopedic surgery; excellent penetration through synthetic grafts and scar tissue during repeat surgeries
Blunt point		Taper body with a rounded point, no cutting edge	Primarily for liver repair or other friable tissues where neither cutting nor piercing properties are desirable; also used in parasternal closures
Protect-point		Taper body with a blunted point, no cutting edge	Used primarily in fascia and mass closure to minimize the potential of needle sticks
Reverse cutting		Triangular point with cutting edge on the outer curvature	Skin closure, retention sutures, subcutaneous, ligamentous, or fibrous tissues
Cutting taper		Reverse cutting tip with taper shaft	Used in microsurgery for excellent penetration through tough tissue, such as vasovasostomy, tuboplasty
Hand-honed reverse cutting		Same as reverse cutting, but hand-honed for added sharpness	Primarily used in plastic surgery for delicate work and where a good cosmetic result is a concern
Spatula side cutting		Two cutting edges in a horizontal plane	Ophthalmic surgery for muscle and retinal repair. Also used for delicate eyelid and/or plastic surgery; cutting edges "ride" along scleral layers
Regular cutting		Triangular point with cutting edge on the inner curvature	General skin closure, subcutaneous tissue, sometimes for ophthalmic surgery, plastic or reconstructive surgery
Lancet Inverted lancet		Spatula needle with the cutting edge on the inner (lancet) or outer (inverted lancet) curvature	Ophthalmic and microsurgery

From Davis & Geck: *Surgical atlas and suture selection guide,* ed 2, Wayne, NJ, 1992, American Cyanamid.

precision-point quality for surgeons in these specialties.

In some instances the application of a microthin layer of plastic to the needle surface provides for easier penetration and a reduction in drag of the needle through the tissue.

Most operating rooms have instituted standardization programs to control the variety of needle-suture combinations available for surgical procedures.

SUTURING METHODS

CLOSURE OF WOUNDS

The *primary suture line* refers to the sutures that obliterate dead space, prevent serum from accumulating in the wound, and hold the wound edges in approximation until healing takes place (Fig. 5-7). The *secondary suture line* refers to sutures that supplement the primary suture line. They are placed on each side of the primary suture line passing through several layers of tissue at once. They help eliminate tension on the primary sutures and reduce the risk of evisceration or dehiscence. Retention sutures are a type of secondary suture line.

An *interrupted suture* is inserted in tissues or vessels in such a way that each stitch is placed and tied individually. This type of suture is widely used and generally considered the strongest and most secure (Fig. 5-8, *A*). The various techniques used for the insertion of interrupted sutures in the tissue are designed to alter the angle of pull and the relationship of the wound's edges to each other. Such maneuvers cause the edges of the wound either to invert or to evert and aid in wound healing because fewer sutures are used. This type of stitch is usually used on skin and may be used on any underlying tissue layer.

A *continuous suture* consists of a series of stitches, of which only the first and last are tied (Fig. 5-8, *B*). With this type of suture a break at any point may mean a disruption of the entire suture line. It is used to close tissue layers where there is little tension but tight closure is required, such as the peritoneum, to prevent the intestinal loops from protruding, or on blood vessels to prevent leakage.

Retention, or stay, sutures placed at a distance from the primary suture line provide a secondary suture line (Fig. 5-8, *C*), relieve undue strain, and help obliterate dead

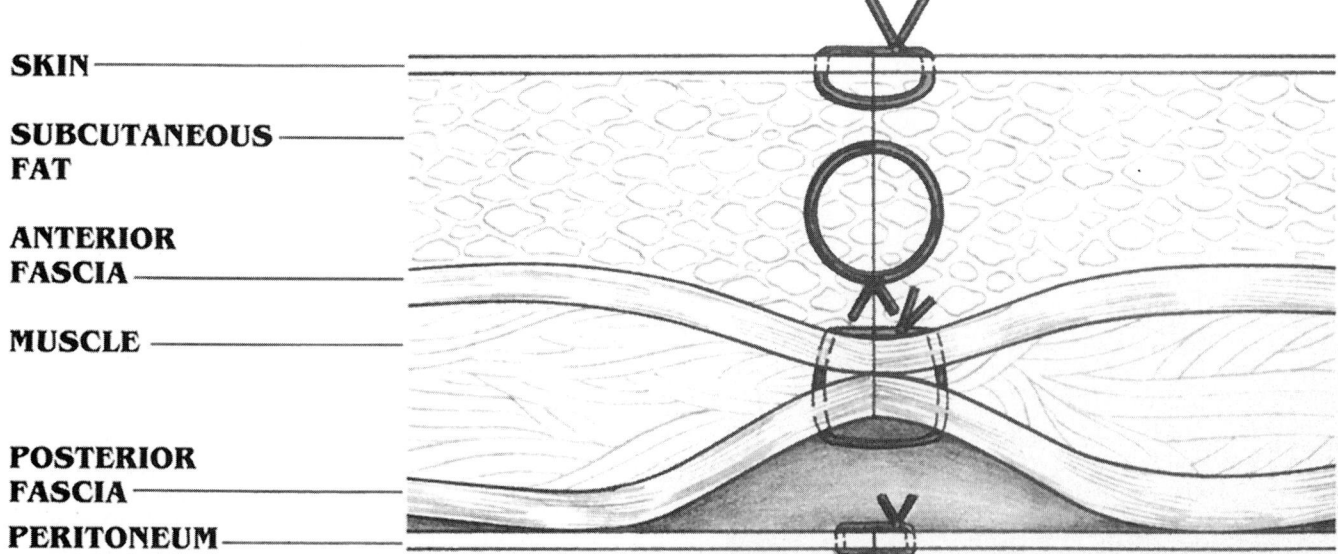

FIG. 5-7 Primary suture line on the abdominal wall, midline incision.
Courtesy Davis & Geck.

SKIN

SUBCUTANEOUS FAT

ANTERIOR FASCIA

MUSCLE

POSTERIOR FASCIA

PERITONEUM

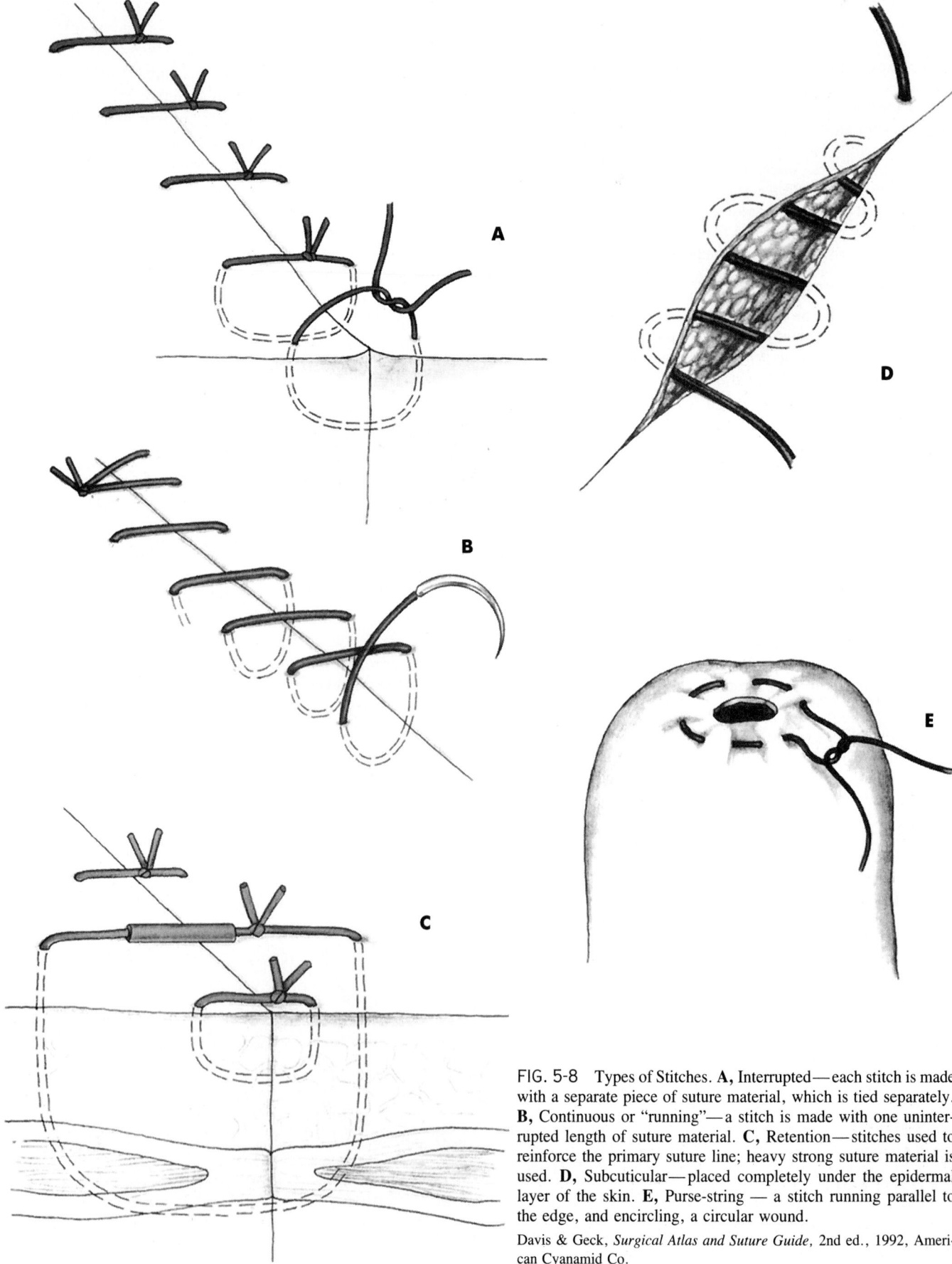

FIG. 5-8 Types of Stitches. **A,** Interrupted—each stitch is made with a separate piece of suture material, which is tied separately. **B,** Continuous or "running"—a stitch is made with one uninterrupted length of suture material. **C,** Retention—stitches used to reinforce the primary suture line; heavy strong suture material is used. **D,** Subcuticular—placed completely under the epidermal layer of the skin. **E,** Purse-string — a stitch running parallel to the edge, and encircling, a circular wound.

Davis & Geck, *Surgical Atlas and Suture Guide,* 2nd ed., 1992, American Cyanamid Co.

space. They are placed in such a way that they include most if not all layers of the wound. A simple interrupted or figure-of-eight stitch is used. Usually heavy, nonabsorbable suture materials such as silk, nylon, polyester fiber, or wire are used to close long, vertical abdominal wounds and lacerated or infected wounds. To prevent the suture from cutting into the skin surface, a small piece of rubber tubing (bumper, bolster, bootie) or other type of device (bridge, button) is passed over or through the exposed portion of the suture. The bridge device allows the surgeon to adjust tension over the wound postoperatively.

Subcuticular sutures, sometimes referred to as buried, are those placed completely under the epidermal layer of the skin (Fig. 5-8, *D*).

A *purse-string suture* is a continuous circular suture placed to surround an opening in a structure and cause it to close (Fig. 5-8, *E*). This type of suture may be placed around the appendix before its removal or in an organ such as the cecum, gallbladder, or urinary bladder before opening it so that a drainage tube can be inserted, followed by tightening of the purse-string suture around the tube.

HOLDING A DRAIN IN PLACE

If a drainage tube is inserted in a wound, the tube may be anchored to the skin with a nonabsorbable suture so that it will not slip in or out. A tube left in a hollow viscus, such as the gallbladder or common duct, may be secured to the wall of that organ with an absorbable suture.

KNOT-TYING TECHNIQUE

The successful use of the many varieties of suture materials depends, in final analysis, on the skill with which the surgeon or first assistant ties the knot. The completed knot should be firm, to prevent slipping, and small, with ends cut short, to minimize the bulk of suture material in the wound.

The suture may be weakened by inappropriate handling. One should avoid excessive tension, sawing, friction between the strands, and inadvertent crushing with clamps or hemostats.

PERIOPERATIVE NURSING CONSIDERATIONS
General considerations

In the preparation and use of sutures in surgery, every precaution must be taken to keep the sutures sterile, to prevent prolonged exposure and unnecessary handling, and to avoid waste. Before the room staff prepare the sutures, they should review the sutures listed in the card file for a particular procedure and surgeon. The scrub person should prepare only one or two sutures during the preliminary preparation, but the circulator should have an adequate supply of sutures available for immediate dispensing to the sterile instrument table. Use of suture materials in dry packages provides sterile sutures ready for use, reduces the time previously needed to prepare them, and decreases wasted motion.

Customized suture kits that contain a designated number and variety of sutures for particular procedures, surgeons, or both are available for use when suture preferences are consistently the same. These kits may be more economical than individually packaged sutures because of reduced packaging costs, decreased gathering and dispensing times, and less capital outlay for inventory.

Opening primary packets

The scrub person tears the foil packet across the notch near the hermetically sealed edge and removes the suture (Fig. 5-9). Some sutures are now packaged for delivery to the field in their inner folders, ready to load, with no foil wrapper.

Handling suture materials

To remove suture strands to be used for ties, the loose end is pulled out with one hand while the folder is grasped with the other hand. To straighten a long suture, the free end is grasped (using the thumb and forefinger of the free hand) and the kinks, caused by package memory, are removed by pulling gently with the free end secured, one in each hand, then the arms are slowly abducted to straighten the strands.

Kinks should never be removed by running gloved fingers over the strand because this action causes fraying. The tensile strength of a gut suture should not be tested before it is handed to the surgeon. Sudden pulls or jerks used to test the tensile strength may damage the suture so that it will break when in use.

To prepare individual lengths of ligature or suture, the strand is folded in equal parts and held between the fingers, then divided. Standard 54-inch lengths of suture may be cut in quarters, thirds, or halves by the scrub person to meet most procedure needs. For general surgery a continuous suture threaded on a needle is usually about 24 inches long, and its short end is 3 to 4 inches long (half lengths). An interrupted suture is 12 to 14 inches long, with 2 or 3 inches threaded through the needle (quarter lengths). To ligate a vessel in the epidermal and subcutaneous layers, the ligature may be 12 to 14 inches long (quarter lengths). However, vessels or structures deep in the wound are ligated with a suture or ligature that is 24 to 30 inches long (third to half lengths). Sutures are also provided in 12- to 60-inch precut lengths by the manufacturer.

Also supplied are labyrinth packs, where precut strands may be removed one at a time from the package, rather than all at once, and 54-inch lengths on reels or disks (discussed earlier).

To remove a suture-needle combination from the package, the scrub person grasps the needle of the suture with a needle holder and gently pulls the strand to remove it. To straighten the suture in a suture-needle combination, the scrub person grasps the suture 1 to 2 inches distal to the needle and pulls gently on the other end of the strand with the other hand, to remove kinks. The jaws of the needle

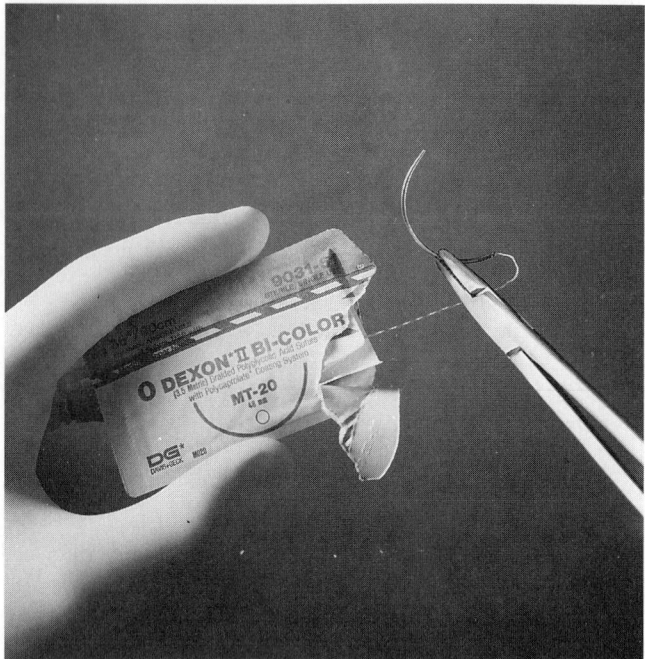

FIG. 5-9   Loading a suture directly from packet.
Courtesy Davis & Geck.

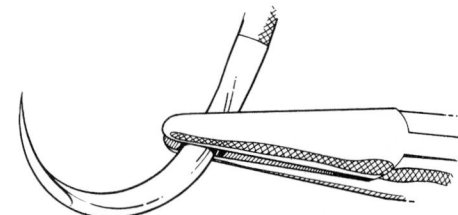

FIG. 5-10   Loading a needle holder. Clamp needle holder approximately ⅓ the distance from the swage or eye to point of needle.
Courtesy Davis & Geck.

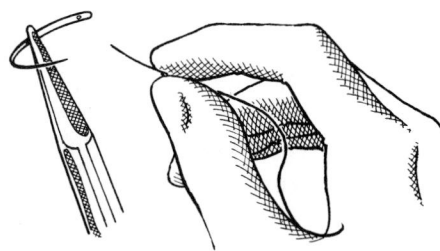

FIG. 5-11   Eyed needle is threaded from inside curvature. Take care to avoid pricking glove on sharp needle point.
Courtesy Davis & Geck.

holder grasp the flattened surface of the needle to prevent breakage and bending. To facilitate suturing, the needle is secured about ⅛-inch down from the tip of the needle holder (Fig. 5-10). The holder is placed on the needle about a third of the distance in from the eye or swaged end.

A suture or free ligature should not be too long or too short. A long suture is difficult to handle and increases the possibility of contamination because it may be dragged across the sterile field or fall below it. A short suture makes tying difficult and, if threaded on a needle, it may slip out of the eye.

The depth and distance to the site of tying or suturing guide the scrub person in preparing ties or sutures of the correct length.

Threading surgical needles

Free needles, those which come packaged separately from the suture, must be threaded by the scrub person for the surgeon. A curved needle is threaded from within its curvature so the short end falls away from the outside curvature (Fig. 5-11). This practice helps to prevent accidental pullout. The scrub person pulls the suture about 4 inches through the eye of the needle to prevent the suture from being pulled out of the eye during suturing.

Counting needles

Institutions vary in their policies regarding needle and sharp counts during operative procedures, but most follow procedure based on *AORN Recommended Practices on Sponge, Sharp, and Instrument Counts*. Initial counts, prior to the start of the procedure, provide the basis for subse-

quent counts. Items added during the procedure should be counted and documented. The count should be performed audibly and with each sharp visualized by the scrub person and circulator.

During the procedure, needles should be accounted for by the scrub person as they are handed to the surgeon on a one-for-one exchange basis. Subsequent counts should be performed by the scrub person and circulator prior to closure of a body cavity or deep, large incision, after closure of a body cavity, when scrub or circulator is relieved by other personnel, and immediately before completion of the surgical intervention. It is imperative that two persons be involved in the count—one counting and the other witnessing that the count is correct.

Many institutions have printed forms to keep track of routinely counted items. Others use erasable count boards visible to all personnel. Recording the count is the responsibility of the circulator. The count sheet may become part of the patient's record. To facilitate counting, used needles should be kept on a needle pad or counter on the scrub person's table. Broken or missing needles must be reported to the surgeon and accounted for in their entirety. Each institution should have established policies for dealing with incorrect counts.

Sharps no-touch technique

Based on OSHA regulations, institutions should have written policies regarding the handling of contaminated equipment, including handling contaminated sharp instruments and needles at the surgical field. OSHA recommends passing only clean sharps/needles to the surgeon. After use, the surgeon places the contaminated object in a predesignated basin, tray, collection device, or safe zone on the field, from which the scrub person will retrieve it. This technique eliminates hand-to-hand passing of contaminated sharps between the surgeon and the scrub person, reducing the chance of accidental needle punctures and cuts (Research Highlight 5-2). All sharps should be accounted for and properly disposed of prior to preparing the room for the next patient.

INSTRUMENTS

HISTORICAL PERSPECTIVE

The history of surgical instruments dates back to 2500 BC. The first instruments were sharpened flints and fine animal teeth. Ancient Greek, Egyptian, and Hindu instruments are amazing in their resemblance to contemporary instruments.

In the late 1700s, to be equipped for the practice of surgery, the surgeon had to employ various skilled artisans such as coppersmiths, steelworkers, needle grinders, turners of wood, bone, and ivory, and silk and hemp spinners. The surgeon had to explain the mechanisms of the instruments and supervise their manufacture. The resulting instruments were crude, expensive, and time-consuming to make. Each artisan used hand labor exclusively, devoted time to making only one type of instrument, and thereby gained proficiency. For example, a cutter would keep a small supply of surgical knives. Thus began physician's supply houses and surgical instrument making.

In the mid-1800s, physicians' principal tools were their eyes and ears. Official records show that amputation, the trademark of the Civil War, was the result in three of four operations. Surgeons were scarce and medical instruments almost nonexistent. Kitchen knives and penknives, carpenter saws, and table forks did the job. After the Civil War the advent of the administration of ether and chloroform brought a demand for new ideas and methods in surgery and instruments.

The division of general surgery into specialties took place in the late 1800s and early 1900s. Delicate instruments were seen as more useful than the force of crude and heavy instruments. So that instruments could withstand repeated sterilization, handles of wood, ivory, and rubber were discontinued.

The development of stainless steel in Germany ensured a better material for surgical instruments and other equipment. Today, surgeons and perioperative nurses assist manufacturers in research for new and better instrumentation. Most instrument companies will design an instrument to a physician's specifications.

COMPOSITION OF SURGICAL INSTRUMENTS

Perioperative nurses are responsible for the use, handling, and care of hundreds of surgical instruments a day. A basic knowledge of how these instruments are manufactured can help in their selection and maintenance. Surgical instruments are expensive and represent a major investment for every hospital.

Instruments used today are made in the United States and in other countries such as Germany, France, and Pakistan. The United States does not have an agency that reviews or sets standards for surgical instruments. The quality is set by the individual manufacturer. A reputable company stands behind its product. A properly cared for instrument should last 10 years or more.

Most instruments are manufactured from stainless steel. Stainless steel is a compound of iron, carbon, and chromium, which means that stainless steel can have varying qualities. These qualities are designated by grading the steel into series by the American Iron and Steel Institute (AISI). For example, the 400 series stainless steel has some noncorrosive characteristics and good tensile strength. It resists rust, produces a fine point, and retains a keen edge. Handheld ringed instruments, such as scissors and clamps, should be 400 series stainless steel.

For ringed instruments the raw steel is converted into instrument blanks by a machinist making an impression of the piece in a stainless steel blank. These blanks are then die forged into specific pieces, male and female halves. The excess metal is trimmed away, and the instrument parts are ready for the final steps.

The two halves are then milled to prepare the box lock fittings, jaw serrations, and ratchets; and the jaws and

---

✼

RESEARCH HIGHLIGHT 5-2

Diseases associated with blood exposure include HIV, hepatitis viruses, and others related to bloodborne pathogens. Operating room–related exposure rates vary from 4% to 50% in reported studies. To better quantify exposure rates in the operating room, the Collaborative Operative Blood Exposure (COBEX) project involved over 8500 surgical procedures at nine different hospitals. Although the authors caution that results are usually hospital-specific, there were some generalizable findings. The surgical specialities of thoracic surgery, orthopedics, and neurosurgery had the highest parenteral exposure rates from punctures. The no-tough technique of passing sharps was recommended by the authors as one way of preventing blood exposures.

Patterson P (1993). Targeting prevention programs to OR blood exposure patterns, *OR Manager, 9*(8):1.

shanks are properly aligned. After this step is done, the halves are assembled by hand. A hole is drilled through the box lock, and a pin/rivet is inserted through the hole. Final grinding and hardening accomplished by heat treating bring the object to proper size, weight, spring temper, and balance.

The last part of the process is called *passivation*. The instruments are put in nitric acid to remove any residue of carbon steel. The nitric acid also produces a surface coating of chromium oxide. Chromium oxide is important because it produces a resistance to corrosion in the stainless steel instrument. The instrument is then polished.

There are three types of instrument finishes. The first is the bright, highly polished mirror finish, which tends to reflect light and may interfere with the vision of the surgeon. The second is the satin or dull finish, which tends to eliminate glare and lessen eyestrain for the surgeon. The third finish is ebonizing, which produces a black finish. Ebonized instruments are used during laser surgery to prevent deflection of the laser beam. The final inspection and testing are for hardness, proper jaw closure, and smooth lock and ratchet action. The instrument is then ready for sale.

INSTRUMENT CATEGORIES

Although there is no standard nomenclature for specific instruments, there are four main categories: dissectors, clamps, retractors, and accessory/ancillary instruments.

Dissectors

Dissectors, which may be sharp or blunt, are instruments used to cut or separate tissue. The largest categories of sharps are scalpels and scissors. Scalpels are probably the oldest of all surgical instruments (Fig. 5-12). Most scalpels are handles with one end suited to the attachment of disposable blades. During an operation the blades may be conveniently changed by the scrub person as often as necessary. The blades come prepackaged and sterile and are passed onto the sterile field as needed by the circulator. Careful handling of blades during the procedure and disposal of blades at the end of a procedure are important in the implementation of universal precautions.

Scissors are designed in various shapes and sizes for different purposes in cutting body tissues and surgical materials (Fig. 5-13). The basic design consists of two blades, each having a chisel-shaped edge with the bevel consistent with the structure or material it has to cut. Scissor tips may be blunt or sharp and the blades straight or curved. Conventional scissors require two movements in use: one to open and another to close the jaws. Other scissors may have a spring action in the body design that holds the jaws in an open position. A single movement pressing the spring together closes the jaws to cut. Scissors designed for delicate plastic and eye surgery are often of the latter type. A basic instrument set usually includes a curved Mayo scissors for dissection of heavy tissues, a Metzenbaum scissors for dis-

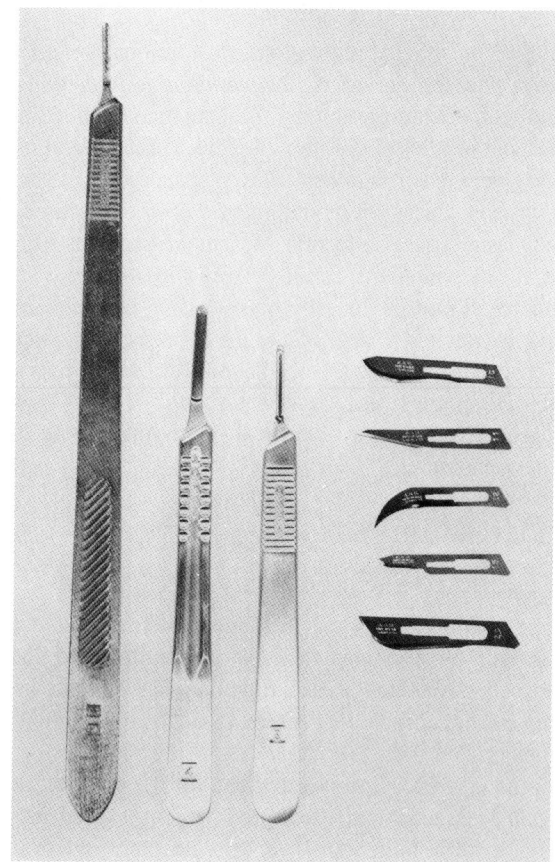

FIG. 5-12 Long and regular-length knife handles with assortment of blades. Blades, *top to bottom,* nos. 10, 11, 12, 15, and 20.

section of delicate tissues, and a straight scissors for cutting suture. For surgery in deep areas of the body scissors with long handles and short blades are used for better control and easier use.

Other sharp dissectors include drills, saws, osteotomes, rongeurs, and other instruments such as adenotomes and dermatomes.

Some instruments in the dissecting category are produced in sharp or blunt form, for example, curettes and periosteal elevators.

Instruments or devices used for blunt dissection include peanuts, a sponge on a stick, the back of a knife handle, and the surgeon's finger or hand.

Clamps

Clamps are instruments specifically designed for holding tissue or other materials, and most have an easily recognizable design. They have finger rings, for ease of holding; shanks whose length is appropriate to the wound depth; ratchets, on the shanks near the rings, which allow for the distal tip to be locked on the tissue or object grasped; a joint, usually a box lock (described later), which joins the

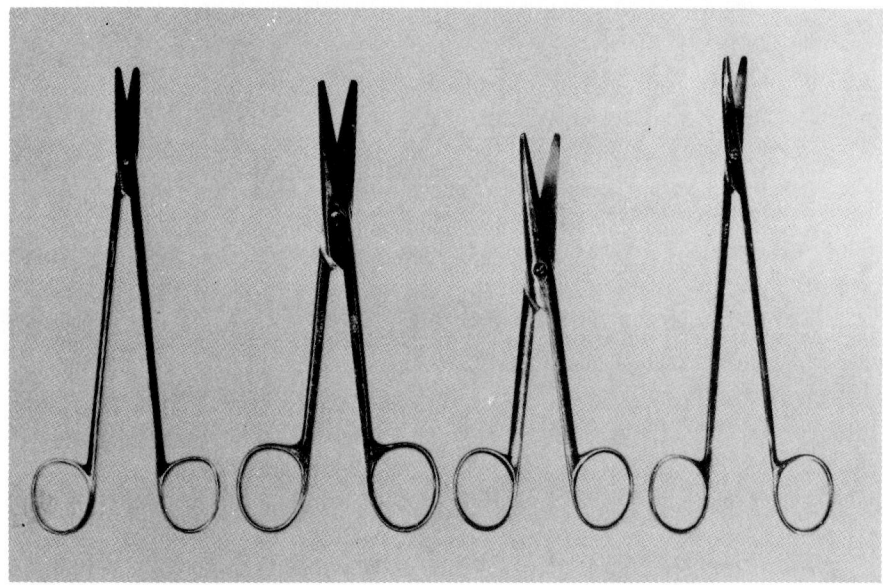

FIG. 5-13 Commonly used scissors. *Left to right,* Straight, blunt dissecting scissors; heavy or suture scissors; Mayo scissors; Metzenbaum scissors.

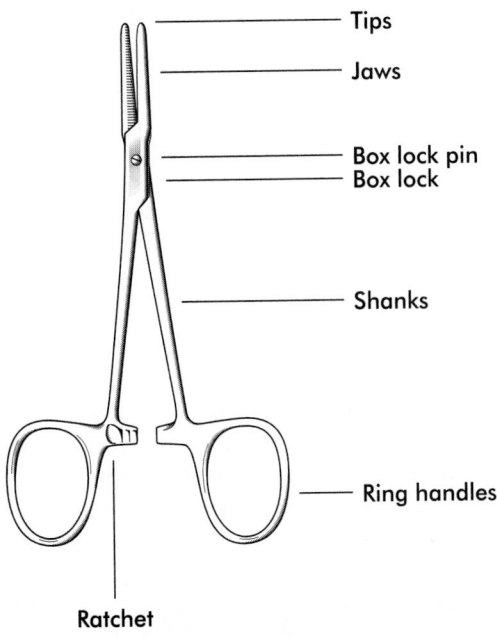

FIG. 5-14 Anatomy of a clamp.
Courtesy Miltex Instrument Co.

two halves of the instrument and allows opening and closing of the instrument; and a jaw, which is the working portion of the instrument and defines its use (Fig. 5-14). Clamps are divided into the following categories.

Hemostats are used to close the severed ends of a vessel with a minimum of tissue damage. They prevent the excessive loss of blood in the course of dissection. The jaws must have deep transverse cuts so that the bleeding vessels may be compressed with sufficient force to stop bleeding. The serrations must be cleanly cut and perfectly meshed to prevent the tissue from slipping free from the jaws of the clamp (Fig. 5-15).

Occluding clamps usually have vertical serrations or special jaws that have finely meshed, multiple rows of longitudinally arranged teeth to prevent leakage and to minimize trauma when clamping bowel, vessels, or ducts that are to

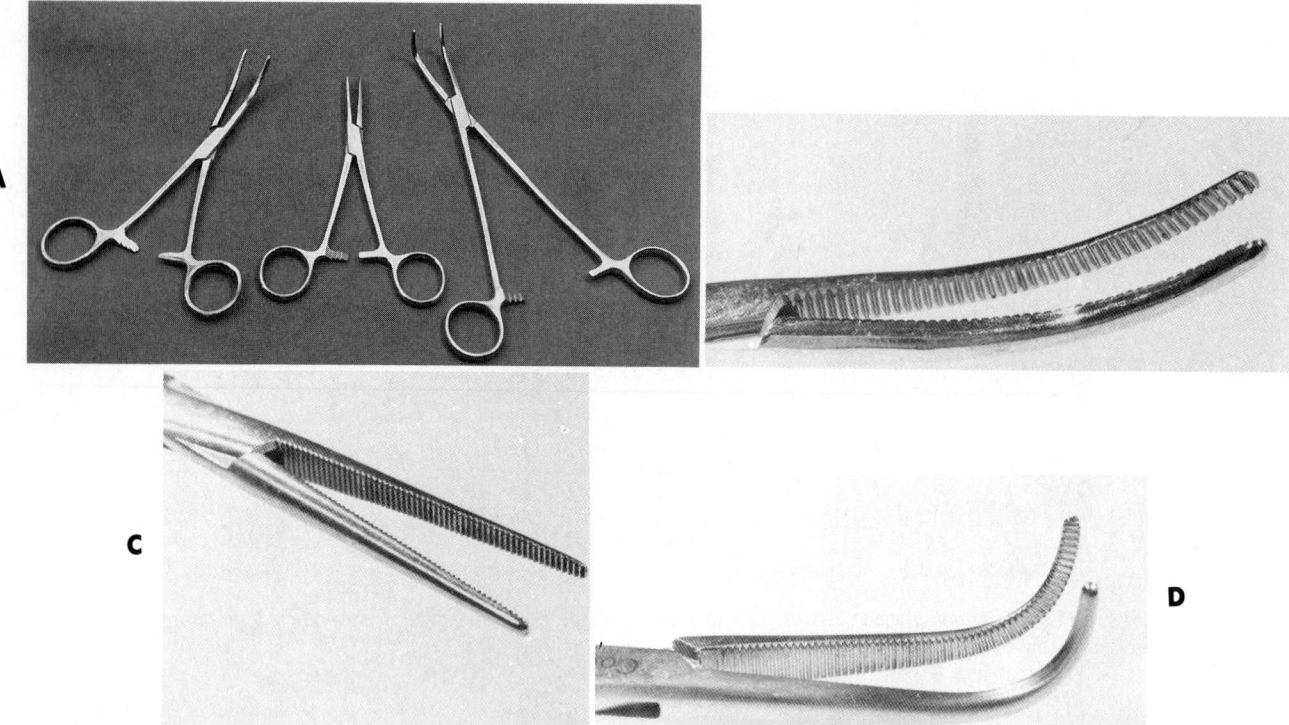

FIG. 5-15 **A,** Commonly used hemostatic clamps. **B,** Curved Kelly. **C,** Straight Kelly. **D,** Right-angle.

be reanastomosed. The surgical service usually selects a hemostat or clamp design according to the surgeons' preferences.

Graspers and holders are used for tissue retraction and generally have jaws of specific design based on their use. The Kocher clamp has transverse serrations as well as large teeth (1 × 2) at its tip to grasp tightly on tough, slippery tissue such as fascia (Fig. 5-16, *A*). The Allis clamp has multiple, fine teeth on the tip so as not to crush or damage tissue (Fig. 5-16, *B*). The Babcock clamp has curved, fenestrated tips with no teeth, and it grips or encloses delicate structures such as bowel, ureters, or fallopian tubes (Fig. 5-16, *C*). Other holding forceps have handles like clamps with specialized tips or jaws. These jaws may be triangular, straight, angular, or T-shaped.

Nonclamp graspers and holders are known as forceps or pickups because they are used to lift and hold tissue. Often, while the surgeon is cutting with scissors or sewing with a needle, forceps are used in the other hand. The most common kinds are the various two-arm spring forceps (Fig. 5-17). Tweezerlike, they vary in length and thickness and are available with and without teeth. Nontoothed forceps create minimal damage and hold delicate, thin tissues. Toothed forceps hold thick or slippery tissues that need extra grip.

Grasper and holder clamps may hold objects as well. Sponge-holding forceps with ring-shaped jaws are available in 7- and 9-inch lengths. They can be used to grasp or handle tissue but are usually used as sponge holders. A gauze sponge is folded and placed in the jaws and is then used to retract tissue, to absorb blood in the field, and occasionally for blunt dissection.

Needle holders (Fig. 5-18), because they must grasp metal rather than soft tissues, are subject to greater damage. As a result, needle holders must be repaired and replaced regularly.

For maximum usage, needle holders must retain a firm grip on the needle. Many types of jaws have been designed to meet this need. The so-called diamond jaw needle holder has a tungsten carbide insert designed to prevent rotation of the needle. In needle holders of standard design a longitudinal groove or pit in the jaw releases tension, prevents flattening of the needle, and holds the needle firmly. Needle holders may have a ratchet similar to that of a hemostat, or they may be of a spring action that may or may not lock.

Towel clamps are also considered holding instruments. Of the two basic types, one is a nonpenetrating towel clamp used for holding in place barrier draping materials. The other has sharp tips used to penetrate drapes and tissues, but it is damaging to both. The use of sharp towel clamps to penetrate drapes is highly discouraged, since they penetrate the sterile field and can be sources of contamination if removed.

Inspection and care

The apposition of the clamp tips is necessary for its functioning and must be periodically checked. When a hemostat is held up to the light and the handles are fully closed, no light should be visible between the jaws. These instru-

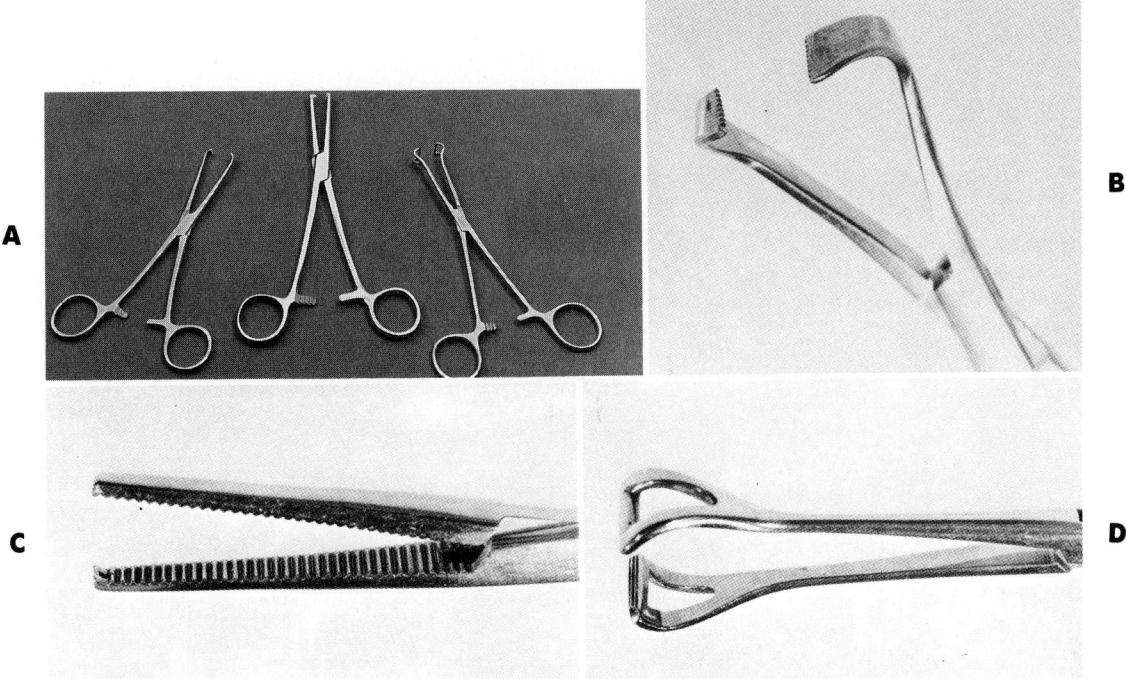

FIG. 5-16   **A,** Holding forceps with special jaws. **B,** Allis. **C,** Kocher or Ochsner. **D,** Babcock.

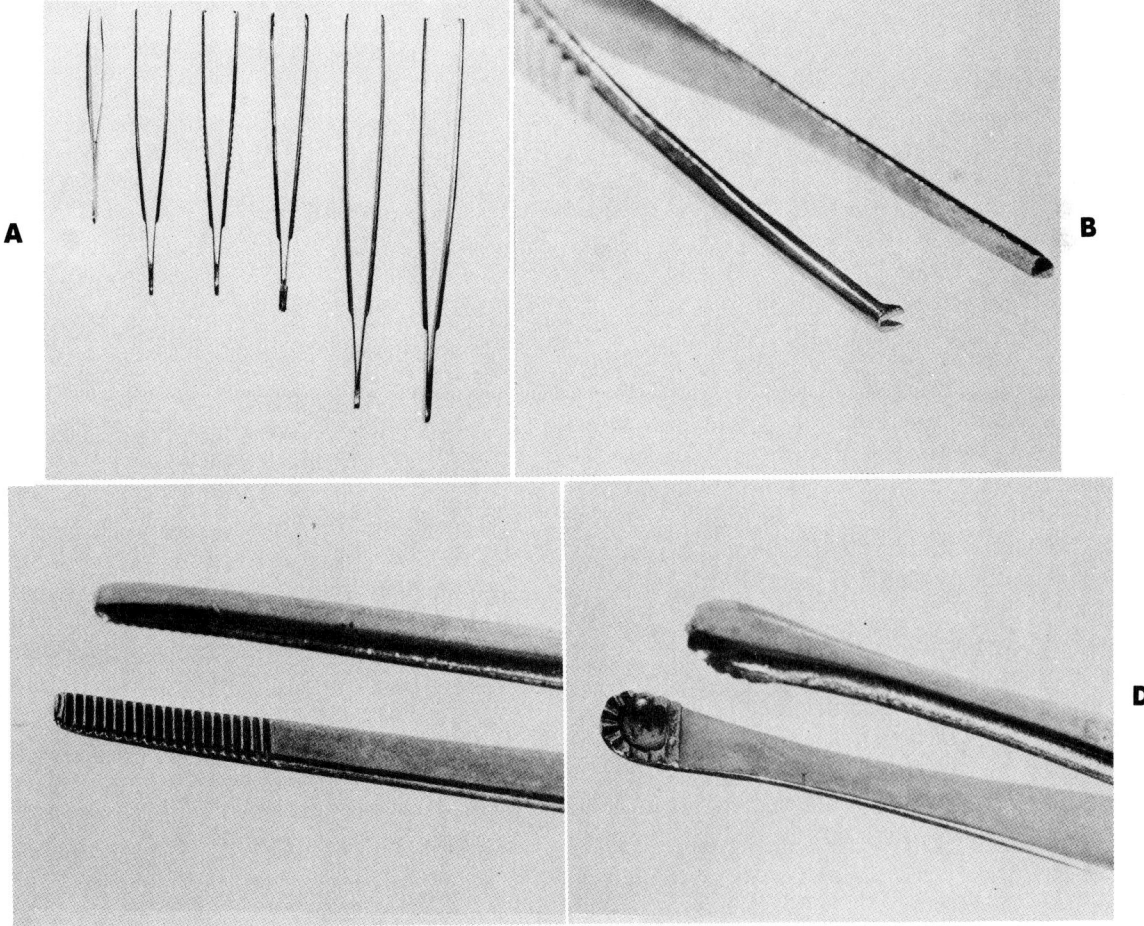

FIG. 5-17   **A,** Various types of tissue forceps or "pickups," ranging from those with very fine tips to heavy tips. **B,** Tips with teeth. **C,** Smooth tip. **D,** Tips of Russian forceps.

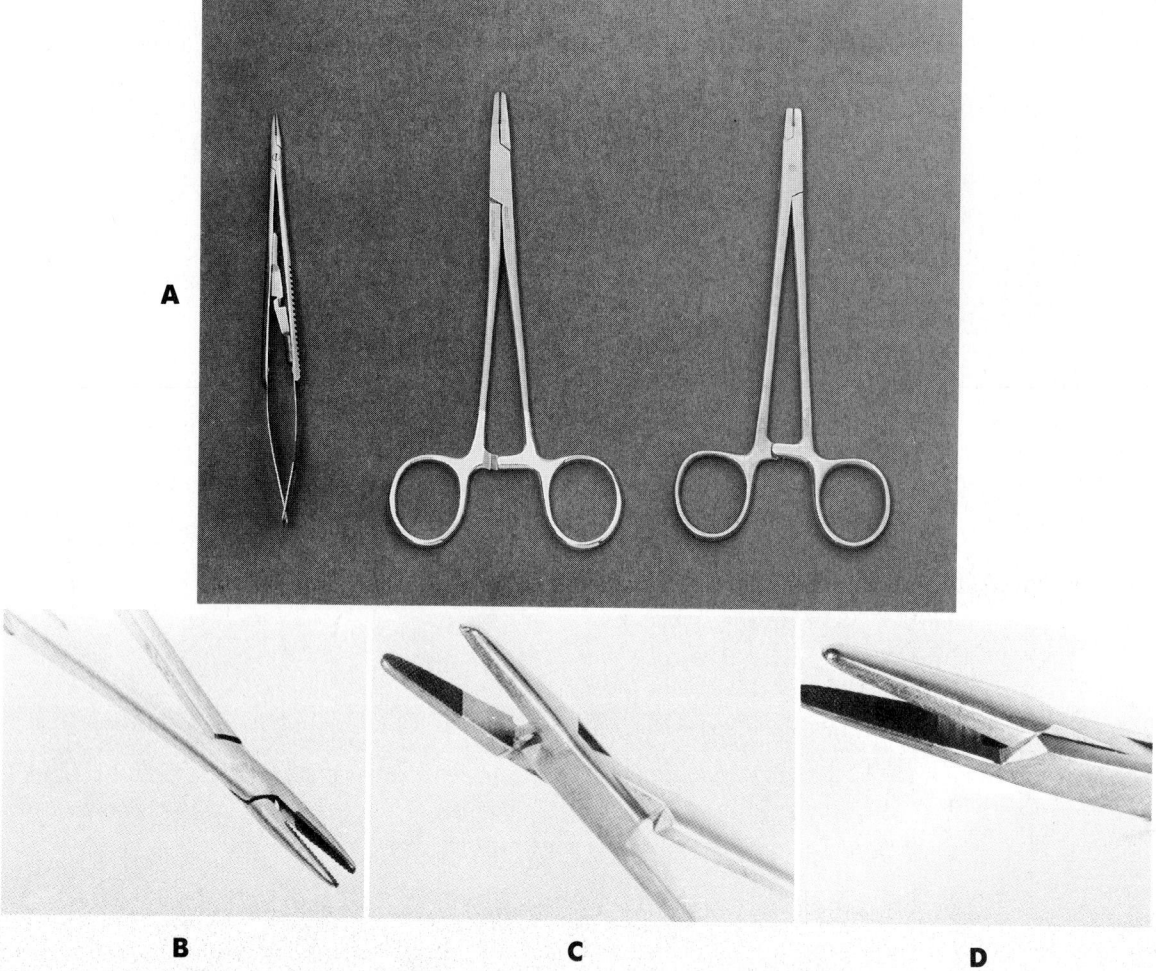

FIG. 5-18 **A,** Needle holders. **B,** Fine. **C,** Regular. **D,** Heavy.

ments, if used for purposes other than that for which they are intended, can be damaged and need to be repaired.

The instrument's joint must also be checked. Instruments made up of two halves may have three types of joints. The most common joint is the box lock, where one arm has been passed through a slot in the other arm and is riveted or pinned. This joint is needed where accurate approximation of the tips is necessary, and it is basic to most ringed instruments.

The second type is the screw joint. The two halves are placed one on top of the other, connected only by a screw. The joint must be checked and tightened periodically because the screw may work itself loose. Screw joint instruments are easy to make and comparatively inexpensive.

The final and least common type is the semibox, or aseptic, joint. It has the advantage that the two halves can be separated for easy cleaning.

All types of joints must be cleaned regularly, and any protein deposits or rust collecting at the site must be removed to ensure proper functioning.

Retractors

Retractors are used to hold back the wound edges to provide exposure of the operative site. A surgeon needs the best exposure possible that inflicts a minimum of trauma to the surrounding tissue. Retractors are either self-retaining (Fig. 5-19) or manually held in place by a member of the surgical team. The two types of self-retaining retractors are those with frames to which various blades may be attached and those with two blades held apart with a ratchet. An example of the latter is a Weitlaner retractor. With hand-held retractors (Fig. 5-20), the handles may be notched, hook shaped, or ring shaped to give the holder a firm grip without tiring. The blade is usually at a right angle to the shaft and may be a smooth blade, rake, or hook. A malleable (ribbon) retractor is a flat metal ribbon that may be shaped by the surgeon at the field.

Accessory/ancillary instruments

Accessory/ancillary instruments are designed to enhance the use of basic instrumentation or facilitate the procedure.

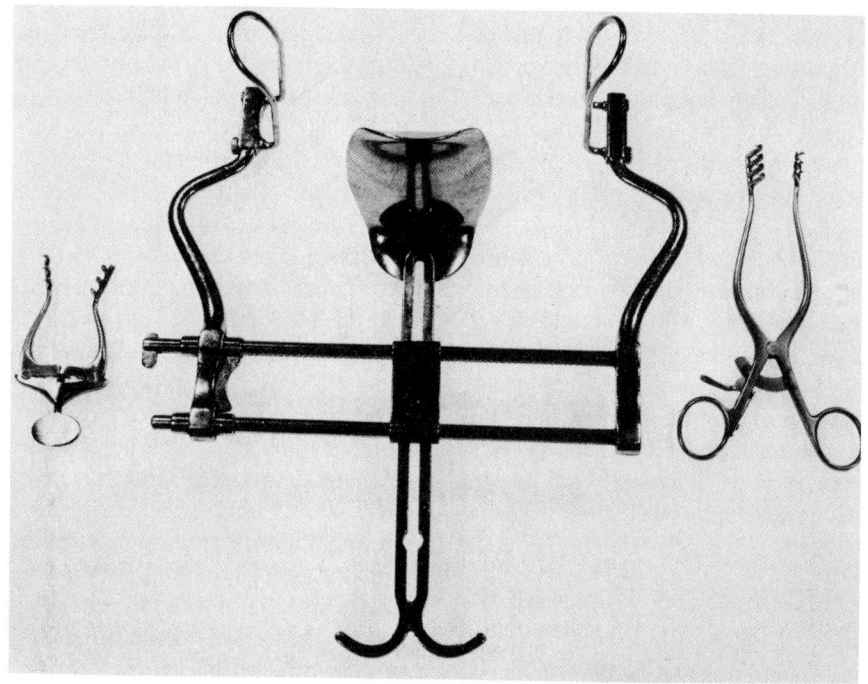

FIG. 5-19   Self-retaining retractors. *Left to right*, Mastoid, Balfour, and Weitlaner.

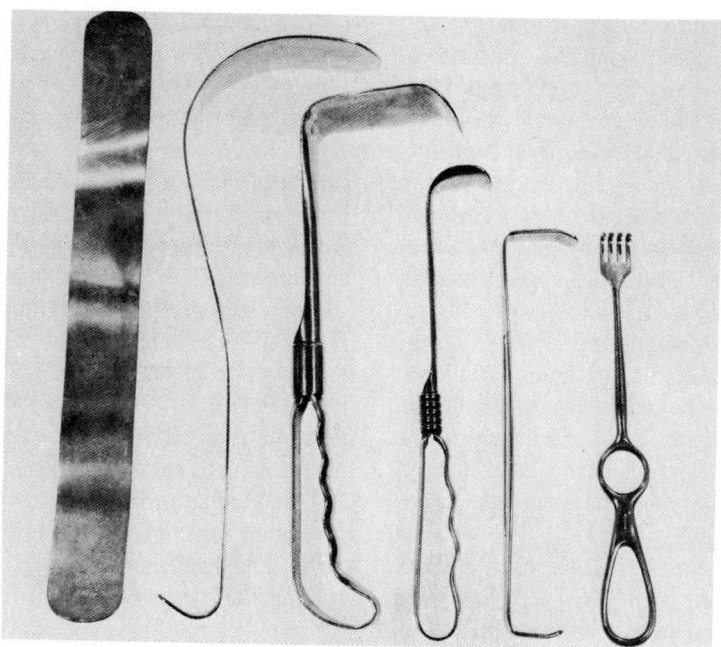

FIG. 5-20   Handheld retractors. *Left to right*, Ribbon, or malleable; Deaver; Kelly; Richardsons; Army-Navy, or USA; and rake.

These include suction tips and tubing, irrigator/aspirators, electrosurgical devices, and special use devices such as probes, dilators, mallets, and screwdrivers.

Many miscellaneous instruments or specialty items are particular to a certain service but generally fall into one of the above categories. Microsurgical instruments are delicate and expensive. They are extremely fine and should be handled separately from other instruments. Instruments used in specialty surgery and the instruments that compose various instrument sets are discussed in the chapters on surgical interventions in Part II.

When nursing team members can analyze the planned surgical procedure and approach and identify each instrument and its specific function, they will be able to select instrument sets without omitting necessary items and without including items that will not be used. This intelligent, planned approach ensures economy of time and motion, protects instruments from misuse, and prevents unnecessary handling. During the operation the informed scrub person who anticipates instrument needs becomes a more valuable member of the surgical team.

SELECTING AND PREPARING INSTRUMENTS FOR PATIENT USE

Designated operating room or central supply personnel arrange the various instruments in trays or sets. The trays are named according to their functions. Three basic operating room instrument sets are the basic laparotomy, the minor/plastic, and the D&C. For example, a minor (or plastic surgery) set includes instruments needed for a simple superficial incision, excision, and suturing. A basic laparotomy set includes instruments to open and close the abdominal cavity and repair any gross defects in the major body musculature. A D&C set, in addition to its use for dilatation and curettage, is often used as the basic instrumentation for vaginal surgery.

According to each procedure's needs, more individualized instruments, specialty sets such as an intestinal set or a vascular set, may be added. In the same way, basic instrument sets may be selected for opening other body cavities, such as the skull, chest, and pelvis.

Instruments are selected according to the size of the patient's body structures and the nature of the organs involved. Proper selection requires a general understanding of surgical procedures and approaches and knowledge of anatomy, possible pathologic conditions, and the design and purpose of instruments.

This knowledge is reinforced during the orientation of new personnel to the operating room. New personnel learn basic technique first in general surgery and then proceed to the specialty services, where different instruments and devices are added but the same basic principles of perioperative practice are applied.

BASIC TABLE SETUPS

In most operating rooms the instruments are set up on Mayo stands and back tables in a planned, standardized, organized, functional manner to maintain continuity when the original scrub person is replaced by another. The teaching manual should have illustrations or diagrams to which all personnel may refer. Each item used by the scrub person should have its own placement on the table to prevent the mass clutter that would occur if instruments and supplies were placed randomly.

A proficient scrub person must know the instrument inventory of the department, the routine instruments needed for each type of operation, the individual surgeon's preferences, correct use and handling, method of preparation, and aftercare of the instruments. A file of preference cards may list the procedures each physician performs, the physician's glove size, the preferred skin preparation solution, specific draping instructions, and instruments required for the procedure.

Before an operative procedure, the scrub person may assist the circulator in gathering the needed supplies, equipment, and sutures. The scrub person scrubs, dons gown and gloves (see Chapter 3), and begins to set up the sterile tables with drapes, instruments, supplies, and sutures. Instruments are arranged with those most frequently used on the Mayo stand (Fig. 5-21). Once the patient is on the operating room bed and is draped, the Mayo stand, set up for instrument use at the immediate operative site, is brought across the lower part of the patient's legs.

One or two back tables, according to the number of instruments and supplies, are also set up. The scrub person prepares the sutures and ligatures and places the knife blades on the handles. Other supplies needed are suction tubing and tips, electrosurgical cord and tip, drains, basins, gowns, gloves, drapes, sponges, and needles, all of which are sterile and set up on the back table according to standardized hospital policy (Fig. 5-22).

The scrub person must be attentive to the sterile field to anticipate the surgeon's needs. Instruments should be passed in a positive and decisive manner. Each instrument is placed or slapped firmly into the surgeon's palm in such a manner that it is ready for immediate use with no wasted motion. For example, when a needle holder with a needle is passed to the surgeon, the needle should be pointing in the direction of the surgeon's thumb; there should be no need for readjustment. Knowing if a surgeon or the assistant is left- or right-handed is necessary to load and pass a needle holder correctly.

Often the surgeon or assistant uses hand signals for the type of instrument desired to eliminate unnecessary talking. Scrub persons should become familiar with the basic signals for knife, scissor, suture, forceps, and clamp.

CARE AND HANDLING OF INSTRUMENTS

An instrument should be used only for the purpose for which it is designed. Proper use and reasonable care prolong its life and protect its quality. Scissors and clamps, which are most frequently misused, can be forced out of alignment, cracked, or broken when used improperly. Tissue scissors should not be used to cut suture or gauze dress-

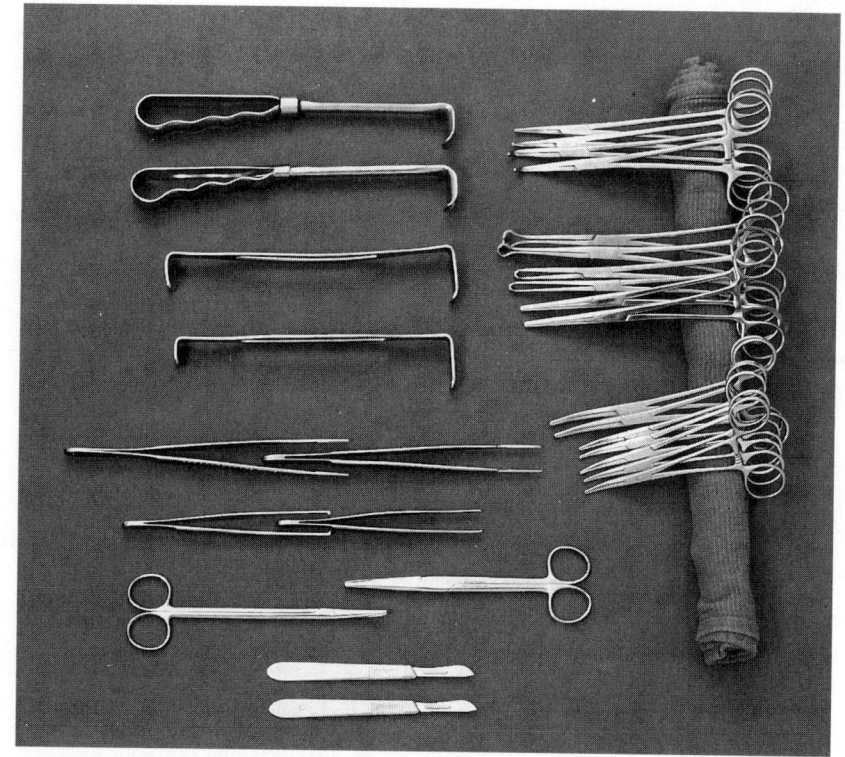

FIG. 5-21   Mayo stand setup.

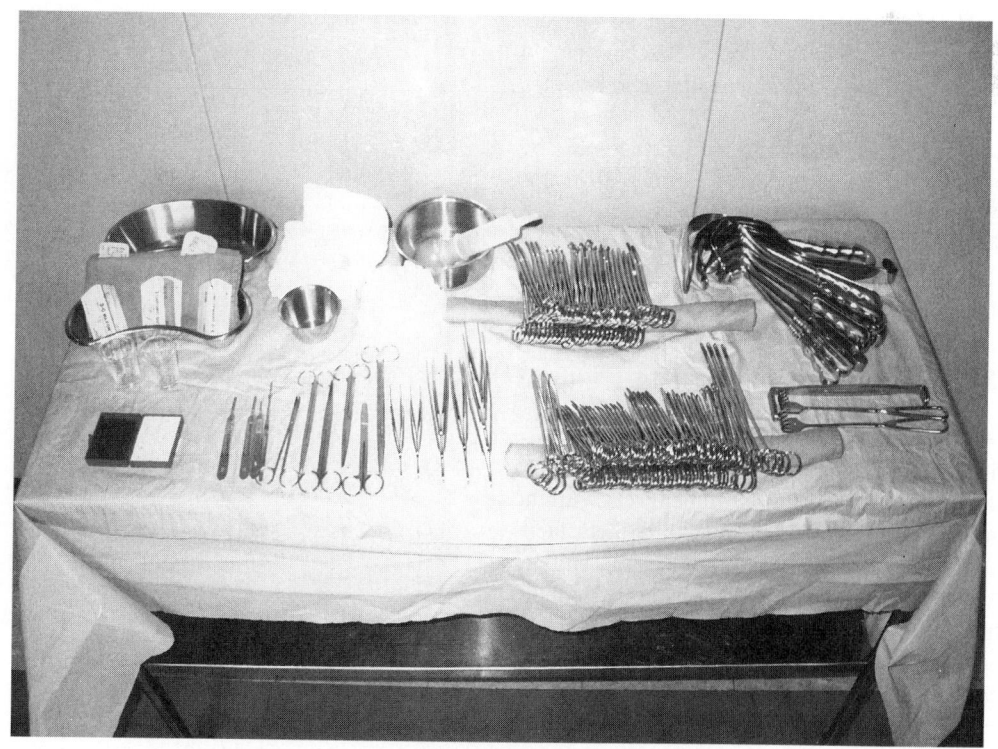

FIG. 5-22   Back table setup.

ings. Hemostatic clamps should not be used as towel clamps or to clamp suction tubing.

Instruments must be handled gently. Bouncing, dropping, and setting heavy equipment on top of them must be avoided. During the procedure, used instruments should be wiped with a damp sponge, or placed in a basin of sterile distilled water to prevent blood from drying on the instruments. Saline should never be used on instruments, as its salt content is corroding, and increases the rusting or deterioration of the metal. As time allows during the procedure, the scrub person should rinse and dry the used instruments, and replace them on the back table to facilitate closing counts.

At the end of a procedure, the instruments should not be thrown together in a tangled heap. They should be handled individually or in small groups. Sharp and delicate instruments should be set aside for individual handling and cleaning to avoid damage and accidental injury. Principles of universal precautions should be applied as dictated by institutional policy. All instruments set up for the procedure should be terminally sterilized or disinfected prior to reassembly. Instruments must be completely clean to ensure effective sterilization.

Each instrument should be inspected before and after each use to detect imperfections. An instrument should function perfectly to prevent needlessly endangering a patient's safety and increasing operative time because of instrument failure.

Forceps, clamps, and other hinged instruments must be inspected for alignment of jaws and teeth. Instrument jaws and teeth should meet perfectly so that blood flow is occluded without damaging the vein or artery. Ratchets should hold firmly yet release easily. Instrument joints should work smoothly.

The edges of scissors should be tested for sharpness by cutting smoothly through four layers of gauze. All instruments should be checked for worn spots, chips, dents, cracks, or sharp edges.

Damaged instruments should be set aside and sent for repair or replacement. An instrument repair service should be selected carefully and used for regular maintenance, such as sharpening and realignment.

INSTRUMENT COUNTS

Most institutions perform instrument counts as standard practice. Establishing standardized instrument sets with the minimum numbers and types of instruments in them facilitates instrument counts, as well as minimizes the amount of time and space required for set up. Initial counts should be carried out concurrently by the circulator and scrub person before the procedure. Items added during the procedure are counted and documented. Subsequent counts should be taken before closure of a cavity or large, deep incision, when the scrub person or circulator is relieved by other personnel, and at the completion of the procedure. Instruments that are disassembled during surgery, such as certain retrac-

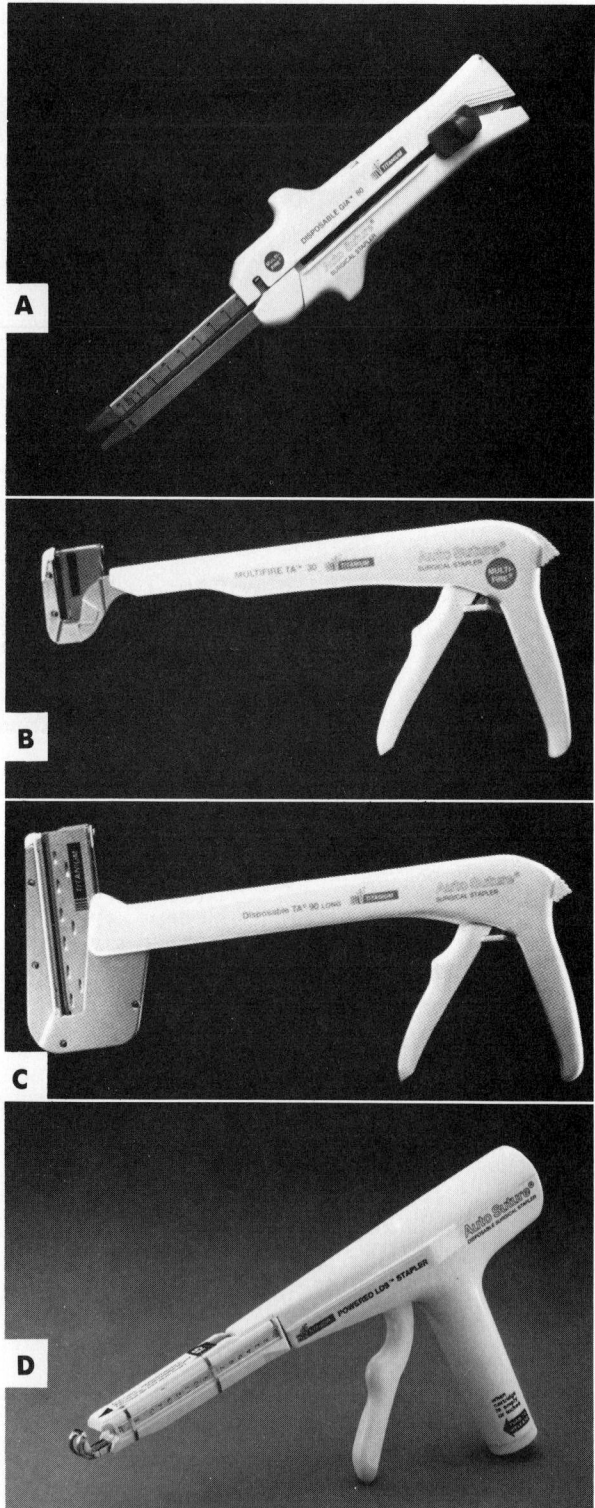

FIG. 5-23   Set of Auto Suture instruments. **A,** GIA instrument. **B,** TA-30 instrument. (TA-55 size instrument is also available.) **C,** TA-90 instrument. **D,** LDS instrument.

Courtesy United States Surgical Corp., Norwalk, Conn.

tors, must be accounted for in their entirety. All counts are documented by the circulator on the appropriate record.

STORING INSTRUMENTS

Instruments should be stored safely. Cabinet shelving should be adjustable and properly spaced for storage of various sizes and types of instruments. Most hospitals today store instruments in presterilized trays or containers. Attached labels and diagrams in cabinets assist personnel. An inventory of all instruments should be taken at periodic intervals.

STAPLING INSTRUMENTS

Instrumentation for internal stapling has been refined and is now widely used (Fig. 5-23). Various instruments to suture tissue mechanically are used for ligation and division, resection, anastomoses, and skin and fascia closure (Figs. 5-24 to 5-26). They may be employed in almost every specialty of surgery. Because of the mechanical application of these instruments, tissue manipulation and handling are reduced. The edema and inflammation that usually accompany anastomoses are minimized because the noncrushing B shape of the staples allows nutrients to pass through the staple line to the cut edge of the tissue. This characteristic reduces the possibility of necrosis and promotes healing.

Mechanical staplers (nondisposable and disposable) utilize cartridges of tiny stainless steel, or absorbable, nonmetallic staples that are commercially preloaded, prepackaged, and presterilized. The staples are essentially nonreactive; metal staples will remain permanently in the tissue. They may fire individually or lay down multiple rows in a straight or circular pattern. Devices to cut or anastamose bowel and other structures are available for open wound use or through endoscopic cannulas. The use of staplers significantly decreases operating time and may shorten postoperative stays.

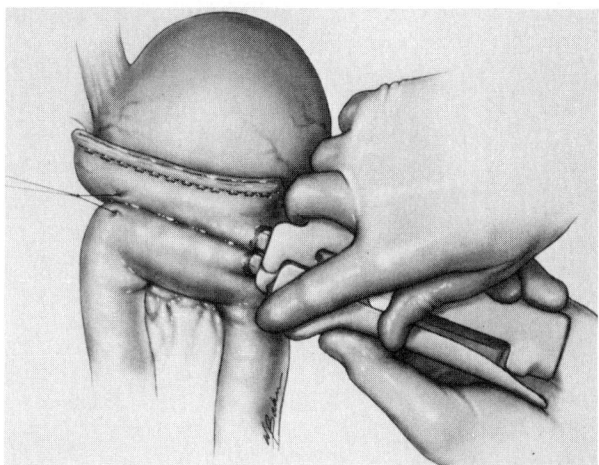

FIG. 5-25   Using GIA to staple and join stomach and jejunum. At same time, blade in GIA cuts between double staple lines, creating stoma for gastrojejunostomy.

Courtesy United States Surgical Corp., Norwalk, Conn.

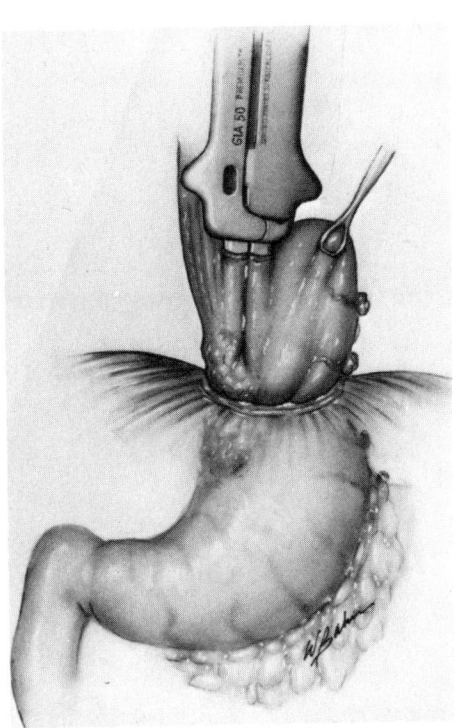

FIG. 5-24   GIA instrument used to perform esophagogastrostomy. Forks of the instrument are inserted into stab wounds made in the lateral wall of the esophagus and the medial wall of the gastric fundus. The instrument is closed and staples are fired.

Courtesy United States Surgical Corp., Norwalk, Conn.

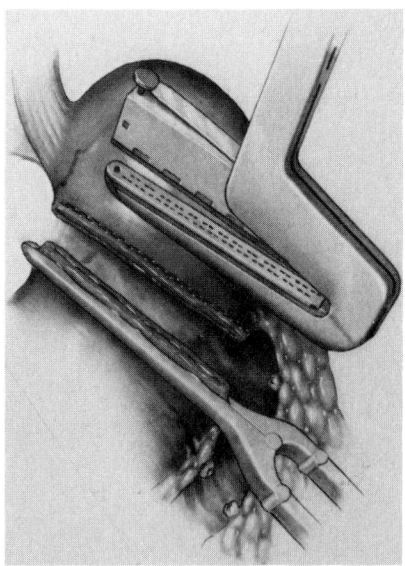

FIG. 5-26   Using TA-90 to close gastric pouch. Jaws of TA-90 are slipped around stomach at level of transection, the instrument is closed, and staples are fired.

Courtesy United States Surgical Corp., Norwalk, Conn.

BIBLIOGRAPHY

Abernathy, C.M. & Harken A.H. (1992). *Surgical secrets,* ed 2, St Louis, Mosby.

Association of Operating Room Nurses (1994). Recommended practices for sponge, sharp, and instrument counts. In *AORN standards and recommended practices for perioperative nursing,* Denver, The Association.

Brooks Tighe, S.M. (1989). *Instrumentation for the operating room,* ed 3, St Louis, Mosby.

Codman & Shurtleff. (1991). *Care and handling of surgical instruments* Randolph, Mass, Johnson & Johnson.

Davis, C.V. et al (1987). *Clinical surgery,* St Louis, Mosby.

Davis, J.A. & Forster, R.J. (1991). *Essentials of clinical surgery,* St Louis, Mosby.

Davis and Geck (1992). *Surgical atlas and suture selection guide,* ed 2, Wayne, NJ, American Cyanamid.

Fairchild, S (1993). *Perioperative nursing: principles and practice* Boston, Jones & Bartlett.

Fernsebner, B (1993). *Core curriculum for perioperative nurses,* Boulder, OR Manager.

Montz, F.J. & Fowler, J.M. et al (1991). Blunt needles in fascial closure, *Surg Gynecol Obstet* 173:147.

Patterson, P (1993). Targeting prevention programs to OR blood exposure patterns, *OR Manager* 9(8):6.

Vaiden, R & Fox, V & Rothrock, J (1990). *Core curriculum for the first assistant,* Denver, Association of Operating Room Nurses.

6

ANESTHESIA

JOHN LEE HOFFER

Without anesthesia, most modern surgical procedures would not be feasible. Therefore, the perioperative nurse should be familiar with the principles and practices of anesthesia and the perioperative functions of the anesthesiologist. This chapter presents an overview of the modern practice of anesthesia, the factors involved, and the interrelationship with the perioperative nurse. Included are discussions of the major types of anesthesia, an introduction to the more commonly used drugs, a review of the standards of anesthesia care, and an overview of some of the problems that can occur during the perioperative period. Descriptions of the anesthesia machines and monitoring equipment are also included so that the perioperative nurse can become familiar with their basic functions since minor procedures are done without anesthesia services.

The sections are organized so that they can be referred to independently without reading the entire chapter. For those with an interest in a specific topic, more detailed information is provided in the bibliography.

Many perioperative nurses are familiar with the commonly used abbreviations employed in this chapter. However, to provide a single reference source, all abbreviations are defined in Box 6-1.

HISTORY OF ANESTHESIA

The early history of modern anesthesia was fraught with controversy. Surgeons in the early nineteenth century frequently used alcohol or opium to intoxicate the patient for procedures involving intense pain or when muscle relaxation was needed. In some cases, hypnotism was also employed. Successful surgery was directly related to the speed of the surgeon.

In March 1842, Crawford W. Long, a physician in Danielsville, Georgia, using ether as an anesthetic, removed a cystic tumor from the neck of James Venable. As confirmed by other physicians in the area, Dr. Long subsequently used ether for other procedures but did not publish reports of his experiences.

In 1844, Horace Wells, a dentist in Hartford, Connecticut, began to use nitrous oxide for anesthesia and communicated his results to his former partner, William T.G. Morton. However, following a fatality with nitrous oxide, Wells quit the practice of dentistry and later committed suicide. Morton subsequently studied medicine and learned of the anesthetic effects of chloric ether from his preceptor, Charles T. Jackson, a chemist. In 1846, while employing this new drug, Morton was able to fill a tooth without the patient experiencing pain. He later learned from Jackson that sulfuric ether had similar properties and utilized it while extracting a deeply rooted bicuspid tooth from another patient.

Morton then contacted John C. Warren, a surgeon at the Massachusetts General Hospital, and persuaded him to give the new anesthetic a trial during a surgical procedure. With Morton as the anesthetist, this historic operation took place in the amphitheater (subsequently renamed The Ether Dome) of Massachusetts General Hospital on October 16, 1846. In 5 minutes, Warren operated on an unconscious, still patient and dissected "a congenital but superficial vascular tumor just below the jaw on the left side of the neck." As the patient regained consciousness, Warren exclaimed "Gentlemen, this is no humbug." The next day, a large fatty tumor on the shoulder of another patient was removed by Haywood with Morton as the anesthetist.

Based on these events, the first medical report of anesthesia was announced to the world on November 18, 1846, by Henry J. Bigelow in the *Boston Medical and Surgical Journal.* An era had ended in which successful surgery was largely predicated on the lightning speed of the surgeon while working on a struggling, distressed patient. Anesthetic techniques gave the surgeon more time to operate and permitted new procedures to be undertaken that would have been impossible before. Thus, many modern surgical techniques have become feasible due to the advances in the art and science of anesthesia.

The word *anesthesia* is derived from the Greek word *anaisthesis,* which literally means "not sensation." Anes-

BOX 6-1

Abbreviations Used in this Chapter

AA	Anesthesia Assistant(s): a physician assistant trained in anesthesia. See section on anesthesia providers.
ASA	American Society of Anesthesiologists
ACLS	Advanced Cardiac Life Support. A protocol for resuscitation from the American Heart Association.
ANSI	American National Standards Institute
APL	Adjustable Pressure Limiting valve. An adjustable pressure relief valve on anesthesia machines that limits the maximum pressure in the patient breathing circuit. Frequently referred to as the "pop-off valve."
BS	Bachelor of Science degree
CD	Computer disk. In this chapter, a 3.5 inch disk on which vital signs are recorded.
cm	centimeter, 1×10^{-3} meters
CO_2	Carbon dioxide
CRNA	Certified Registered Nurse Anesthetist. See section on anesthesia providers.
CSF	Cerebral Spinal Fluid. The fluid surrounding the brain and spinal cord. For spinal anesthesia, local anesthetics are injected into the CSF.
°C	Degrees centigrade.
ECG	Electrocardiograph. The older German term was EKG.
e.g.	Latin for *exempli gratia*. For example.
EGTA	Esophageal (Gastric Tube) Airway. A cuffed tube that is blindly inserted into the esophagus and connected to a mask. This permits ventilation via the mask and gastric suctioning through the cuffed tube.
$ETCO_2$	End Tidal Carbon Dioxide reported as a partial pressure. See section on capnography.
ETT	Endotracheal tube
F_IO_2	Fraction of Inspired Oxygen. This is a fraction (0.00-1.00) and it corresponds to the percent (0%-100%) of inspired oxygen.
FO	Fiberoptic
GRE	Graduate Record Examination
Hg	Mercury
HIV	human immunodeficiency virus
ICU	Intensive Care Unit
i.e.	Latin for *id est*, that is.
IM	Intramuscular, intramuscularly
IV	Intravenous, intravenously
JCAHO	Joint Commission on Accreditation of Healthcare Organizations
L	Liter(s).
LED	Light-emitting Diode. An electronic device that emits light at a predetermined frequency.
LMA	Laryngeal Mask Airway. See section on typical sequence of general anesthesia.
M	Molar
MAC	Monitored Anesthesia Care. See section under types of anesthesia care.
MCAT	Medical College Admission Test
mg	milligram(s)
MH	Malignant Hyperthermia. See section on malignant hyperthermia
MHAUS	Malignant Hyperthermia Association of the United States
ml	milliliter(s)
mm	millimeter(s)
MMS	Master of Medical Science degree
MS	Master of Science degree
NIOSH	National Institute for Occupational Safety and Health
N_2O	Nitrous Oxide
nm	Nanometers, 1×10^{-9} meters
NMS	Neuroleptic Malignant Syndrome. See section on malignant hyperthermia.
NPO	Latin for *nil per os*, nothing by mouth
NSAID	Non-Steroidal Anti-Inflammatory Drugs
OR	Operating Room
O_2	Oxygen
PA	Pulmonary Artery
$PaCO_2$	Partial pressure of Arterial Carbon Dioxide. The lower case *a* is arterial. An uppercase *A* is alveolar.

BOX 6-1

Abbreviations Used in this Chapter—cont'd

PACU	PostAnesthesia Care Unit (Recovery Room)
PaO_2	Partial pressure of Arterial Oxygen
PARS	PostAnesthesia Recovery Score. See section on postanesthesia recovery.
PCA	Patient Controlled Analgesia. See section on pain management.
PO	Latin *per os,* by mouth, orally
ppm	parts per million (1 ppm = 1×10^{-6})
psi	Pounds per Square Inch. A measurement of pressure.
RGV	Residual Gastric Volume
SICU	Surgical Intensive Care Unit
SpO_2	Saturation (pulse) of Oxygen in percent. See section on pulse oximetry.
$S\overline{v}O_2$	Saturation of mixed venous oxygen in percent. This measurement is made from a pulmonary artery catheter.

thesia was listed in *Bailey's English Dictionary* in 1721. When the effects of ether were discovered, Oliver Wendell Holmes suggested "anesthesia" be used as a name for the new phenomenon. Some believed that he coined this term; others thought that he knew of the Greek word that Plato had employed. In any case, anesthesia was, in the memorable phrase of Werr Mitchell, the "death of pain."

From these early beginnings, anesthesia has developed into a very precise and sophisticated science that interfaces with many other medical specialties.

ANESTHESIA PROVIDERS

In the United States, anesthesia care is usually provided by: (1) an anesthesiologist; (2) a Certified Registered Nurse Anesthetist (CRNA) working under the direction of an anesthesiologist or a physician; or (3) an Anesthesiologist's Assistant (i.e., Physician's Assistant in anesthesia) working under the direction of an anesthesiologist. An anesthesiologist is a physician with 4 or more years of specialty training in anesthesiology after medical school.

Nurse anesthesia programs are now a minimum of 2 years in length. They require a Bachelor of Science (BS) in Nursing or other appropriate field plus 1 year of acute nursing care experience before acceptance. Many nurse anesthesia programs are at the Masters degree level in the School of Nursing or Allied Health, although a number of programs are based in community hospitals.

In recent years, Anesthesiologist's Assistants (AA) have also been trained. These are physician's assistants to anesthesiologists. Acceptance into an AA program requires a BS degree including a college level "pre-med" education and a satisfactory score on the Medical College Admission Test (MCAT) and/or the Graduate Record Examination (GRE). These AA programs are offered only in medical schools with an approved residency program in anesthesiology. The two-year training program is based upon the classical pre-med education. The basic science courses are

taught by the regular medical school faculty. The AA are graduate students within the medical school and typically receive a Master of Medical Science (MMS) degree from the medical school. They also take a national certification examination administered by the National Commission on certification of AAs under the supervision of the National Board of Medical Examiners.

In this chapter, the term *anesthesia provider* will denote the person ***providing*** the continuous anesthesia care for the patient. Depending on the practice in a given hospital, this may be an anesthesiologist, a nurse anesthetist, or an anesthesiologist's assistant. In many hospitals, an *Anesthesia Care Team* includes nurse anesthetists and/or anesthesiologist's assistants supervised by an anesthesiologist. In small rural hospitals in some states, there may not be an anesthesiologist, and a CRNA may be the anesthesia provider.

The anesthesia provider is frequently said to be the patient's advocate in the perioperative period; as such, they must be concerned with many divergent factors when the patient's own sensory and cerebral functions are obtunded by anesthesia. The field of anesthesia has become so complex that in many large hospitals an anesthesia provider may further specialize in such areas as obstetric, neurosurgical, pediatric, cardiovascular, or ambulatory anesthesia. Anesthesiologists may also subspecialize in acute and chronic pain management or in critical care medicine.

PATIENT SAFETY

Patient safety is always a concern during surgery and anesthesia. Approximately 25 million anesthetics are administered each year in the United States. Of these, an anesthetic misadventure is the primary cause of death in about 2000 cases. For healthy individuals, the risk is only about 0.01%. Data from several studies indicate a death rate ranging from 1 per 20,000 to 1 per 35,000. These rates represent approximately a fourfold decline during the past 30 years, despite surgical procedures being performed on increasingly sicker and much higher risk patients than in the past. However, the general public still considers anesthesia to be a major risk of surgery. This is due to sensationalized reports in the news media and in magazine articles. In addition, anesthesia-related deaths often occur acutely in the perioperative period, whereas surgical or medical problems may not result in mortality until days after the procedure. Also, the American Society of Anesthesiologists (ASA) has been willing to report, analyze, and study anesthetic misadventures in an effort to improve the overall quality of patient care. Awareness of potential problems and constant vigilance are crucial to good patient care.

PREOPERATIVE PREPARATION

PATIENT EVALUATION

It is now common to perform the preoperative evaluation in advance of the scheduled surgical procedure. One or more days before the procedure, a patient will visit a preadmission clinic. (This may also be called pre-admission testing, pre-anesthesia clinic, or anesthesia assessment unit.) All of the admission and appropriate consent forms are processed, a preoperative history and physical examination may be done, a preanesthesia evaluation and examination are completed, and appropriate diagnostic and laboratory tests are processed. The patient's physical status is assessed, and the most appropriate anesthetic technique is

selected. The patient's questions and concerns are resolved and instructions are given to expedite admission on the day of surgery. This pre-admission processing has become very popular in the last two decades since third-party payers have agreed to reimbursement for outpatient testing. In addition, the patient is usually more relaxed and rested after sleeping at home rather than adapting to a strange hospital environment before surgery.

Before elective surgery the patient should be in optimal medical condition. Occasionally, it is felt that a patient's physical status could be improved to reduce the risks involved. In such cases, this is discussed with the patient's primary physician, and if necessary, elective surgery is deferred until the patient's condition is optimized. If, however, the intended surgery is emergent, any benefits gained from a delay must be carefully compared with the hazards of waiting.

The assignment of a physical status classification is based upon the patient's physiologic condition independent of the proposed surgical procedure. The physical status classification was developed by the American Society of Anesthesiologists (ASA) to provide uniform guidelines. It is an evaluation of the severity of systemic diseases, physiologic dysfunction, and anatomic abnormalities. Intraoperative difficulties occur more frequently with patients who have a poor physical status classification. The ASA classification is given in Table 6-1.

TABLE 6-1

Physical (P) Status Classification of the American Society of Anesthesiologists

Status*†	Definition	Description and examples
P1	A normal healthy patient.	No physiologic, psychologic, biochemical, or organic disturbance.
P2	A patient with a mild systemic disease.	Cardiovascular disease with minimal restriction on activity. Hypertension, asthma, chronic bronchitis, obesity, or diabetes mellitus.
P3	A patient with a severe systemic disease that limits activity, but is not incapacitating.	Cardiovascular or pulmonary disease that limits activity. Severe diabetes with systemic complications. History of myocardial infarction, angina pectoris, or poorly controlled hypertension.
P4	A patient with severe systemic disease that is a constant threat to life.	Severe cardiac, pulmonary, renal, hepatic, or endocrine dysfunction.
P5	A moribund patient who is not expected to survive 24 hours with or without the operation.	Surgery is done as last recourse or resuscitative effort. Major multisystem or cerebral trauma, ruptured aneurysm, or large pulmonary embolus.
P6	A patient declared brain dead whose organs are being removed for donor purposes.	

*In status 2, 3, and 4, the systemic disease may or may not be related to the cause for surgery.
†For any patient (P1 through P5) requiring emergency surgery, an E is added to the physical status, for example, P1E, P2E. ASA 1 through ASA 6 is often used for physical status.
Reprinted with permission from the American Society of Anesthesiologists, ASA, 520 N. Northwest Parkway, Park Ridge, IL 60068.

Preadmission clinics are widely used by many hospitals and ambulatory surgery centers. However, in some metropolitan areas where travel and congestion are problems, nurses may conduct preoperative telephone interviews with patients before the day of surgery. Then, on the day of surgery, patients arrive 1 or 2 hours before the scheduled surgery time to complete the other preoperative processes. In summary, this preadmission process has reduced the cost of health care, decreased the risk of nosocomial infections associated with longer hospital admissions, increased the utilization and efficiency of health care resources, improved patient relations, and enhanced the chances of having a well-informed patient in optimal health status.

In larger hospitals, the anesthesia provider for the surgical procedure is often not the individual who evaluated the patient in the pre-anesthesia clinic. Therefore, immediately before surgery, the anesthesia provider: (1) reviews the patient's chart, the laboratory data, and the diagnostic studies such as the electrocardiogram and chest x-ray; (2) identifies the patient; (3) verifies the surgical procedure; (4) confirms that the appropriate consents (surgery, anesthesia, use of blood products) have been signed; (5) verifies the choice of anesthesia; (6) examines the patient; and (7) gives preoperative medications if appropriate.

CHOICE OF ANESTHESIA

The choice of anesthesia for a given surgical procedure is primarily made by the patient and the anesthesiologist. A variety of factors influence this decision including: (1) the patient's wishes and understanding of the types of anesthesia that could be used; (2) the patient's physiologic status; (3) the presence and severity of coexisting diseases; (4) the patient's mental and psychologic status; (5) the postoperative recovery from various kinds of anesthesia; (6) options for management of postoperative pain; (7) the type and duration of the surgical procedure; (8) the patient's position during surgery; and (9) any particular requirements of the surgeon. It is often said that there is major and minor surgery, but only major anesthesia.

PREMEDICATIONS

The primary purpose of premedication before anesthesia is to sedate the patient and reduce anxiety. Premedications may be classified as sedatives and hypnotics, anxiolytics, amnestics, tranquilizers, analgesics or narcotics, antiemetics, and anticholinergics. A single drug may possess the properties of several classes. Midazolam (Versed) is frequently administered to relieve apprehension and provide amnesia. An analgesic or narcotic may be ordered if preoperative discomfort is anticipated during invasive procedures or during the administration of a regional anesthetic. An anticholinergic such as atropine or glycopyrrolate may be used to prevent bradycardia in pediatric patients, for controlling secretions in patients undergoing oropharyngeal procedures, or when a cardiac reflex may cause bradycardia such as during ophthalmic procedures.

To decrease the risk of aspiration, metoclopramide (Reglan) may be given to empty the stomach and to reduce nausea and vomiting. In addition, an antacid or an H_2 receptor-blocking drug such as cimetidine (Tagamet) or ranitidine (Zantac) may be included to decrease gastric acid production and the acidity of the gastric contents. Should aspiration occur, a pH above 2.5 decreases the resultant pulmonary damage.

Premedications may be administered either intramuscularly, intravenously, or orally with 15 to 30 ml of water. Oral premedication is less painful for the patient; the absorption and uptake are more predictable than with an IM injection; and the small amount of water is readily absorbed directly across the gastric mucosa.

Before a premedication is given, any last-minute questions from the patient concerning surgery and anesthesia should be answered and proper execution of all consent forms should be verified. Premedications are usually given 30 to 90 minutes before surgery but may be given IV after the patient arrives in the surgical suite. Except for the small amount of water needed to swallow any medications, adult patients have traditionally been kept NPO (nothing by mouth) for a minimum 4 to 6 hours before elective surgery. However, new studies indicate a shorter fasting period for clear liquids may be acceptable (Research Highlight 6-1).

Although premedications are commonly used, studies have shown that visits before surgery by the anesthesiologist and the perioperative nurse are far more important in relieving patient anxiety and concern. Major concerns include fear of the unknown, relinquishing control of one's life to someone else, being awake during surgery, and never awakening from anesthesia. Often premedication is not given to older patients because their anxiety levels are lower, their responses to medications are unpredictable, and additional sedation can be given IV in the operating room if required. Preoperative sedation is usually not given to ambulatory patients because residual effects of these drugs may persist for extended periods of time.

TYPES OF ANESTHESIA CARE

A frequently used classification of anesthesia care is the following:

1. *General anesthesia* is a reversible, unconscious state characterized by amnesia (sleep, hypnosis, or basal narcosis), analgesia (freedom from pain), depression of reflexes, muscle relaxation, and homeostasis or manipulation of physiologic systems and functions. Most patients think of general anesthesia when they are scheduled to have a surgical procedure; that is, they expect to be "put to sleep."
2. *Regional anesthesia* is broadly defined as a reversible loss of sensation when a local anesthetic is injected to block or anesthetize nerve fibers. Common regional anesthesia techniques include spinals, epidurals, caudals, and major peripheral nerve blocks.

3. *Monitored anesthesia care* (MAC) is provided when infiltration of the surgical site with a local anesthetic is performed by the surgeon and the anesthesia provider supplements the local anesthesia with IV drugs that provide sedation and systemic analgesia. The anesthesia provider also monitors the patient's vital functions and may use additional medication to optimize the patient's physiologic status. This technique can be used for some procedures in critically ill patients who may poorly tolerate a general anesthetic without extensive invasive monitoring and pharmacological support. Monitored anesthesia care is often used for healthy patients undergoing relatively minor surgical procedures. *Local standby* or *anesthesia standby* are older, less accurate terms frequently used interchangeably with monitored anesthesia care.

4. *Local anesthesia* is usually employed for minor procedures in which the surgical site is infiltrated with a local anesthetic such as lidocaine or bupivacaine. An anesthesia provider is not involved in the patient's care. A perioperative nurse usually monitors the patient's vital signs and may inject sedative or analgesic drugs as the surgeon directs. *Conscious sedation* during minor procedures without an anesthesia provider is a controversial topic. It is often used very effectively by nonsurgeon physicians for invasive procedures. Unfortunately, these procedures are often performed at "odd hours" or when anesthesia personnel are not available. Adequate discussion of this issue is beyond the scope of an overview on anesthesia practice. However, it should be noted that according to the JCAHO, the Department of Anesthesiology is responsible for anesthesia care throughout the hospital. It therefore seems appropriate that the OR supervisor in conjunction with the Chairman of Anesthesiology at each institution establish a policy for the administration of medications in this clinical setting. It seems reasonable that the perioperative nurse monitoring the patient in this situation should not have other responsibilities such as circulating for the procedure, and should be certified or skilled in *Advanced Cardiac Life Support (ACLS)*.

PERIOPERATIVE MONITORING

Significant advances in perioperative monitoring have occurred in the last few years. Among the medical specialties, anesthesiology has been a pioneer in the review and analysis of perioperative mishaps and the implementation of improved monitoring techniques and guidelines. These advances have resulted in significant decreases in mortality and morbidity. In several states malpractice insurance carriers have recognized the significance of these improvements and have decreased their premiums if certain monitors such as pulse oximetry (SpO_2) and end tidal carbon dioxide ($ETCO_2$) are routinely employed.

RESEARCH HIGHLIGHT 6-1

Shevde and Trivedi examined the effects of clear liquids on gastric volume and pH in 30 healthy volunteers. Subjects with any history of gastrointestinal problems, pregnancy, smoking, alcoholism, or taking any medications were excluded. After overnight fasting, a Salem-sump nasogastric tube was placed and the gastric fluid aspirated for measurement of volume and pH, and then reinserted into the stomach. The volunteers were randomly assigned to three groups ($n = 10$).

Each group orally ingested 240 ml of liquid over 5 minutes; Group I (water), Group II (black coffee) and Group III (pulp-free orange juice). The gastric contents were aspirated, the volume and pH measured, and reinserted through the nasogastric tube every half hour until the gastric volume was less than 25 ml. All volunteers had gastric volumes less than 20 ml in 2 hours with a slight decrease in the pH.

These data suggest that if healthy patients have ingested a moderate amount of clear liquids, general anesthesia may be safely induced after a 2-hour period of fasting.

Maltby and colleagues studied the correlation between the ingestion interval and the volume of clear fluid ingested with the volume and pH of residual gastric fluid at induction of anesthesia. Pregnant patients, those with gastric disorders, or those taking medications that affected gastric motility or secretions were excluded. Patients were instructed to eat no solid food after midnight. Either no premedication was given or diazepam 5-15 mg was given 90 minutes preoperatively.

Following induction of anesthesia, gastric fluid was aspirated and the volume and pH were measured. Results from the 199 healthy inpatients aged 18-70 years showed: (1) 12 patients fasted 1.3-3.0 hours after ingesting 244 ± 109 ml, and had a residual gastric volume (RGV) of 22 ± 19 ml with a pH of 1.5 ± 0.3; (2) 62 patients fasted 3.1-5.0 hours after ingesting 241 ± 177 ml and had a RGV of 32 ± 26 ml with a pH of 1.7 ± 1.3; (3) 31 patients fasted 5.1-8.0 hours after ingesting 230 ± 111 ml and had a RGV of 28 ± 19 ml with a pH of 1.6 ± 1.1; and (4) 94 patients fasted more than 8 hours and had an RGV of 25 ± 19 ml with a pH of 1.6 ± 0.9.

They concluded that healthy inpatients could ingest unrestricted volumes of clear liquids until 3 hours before the scheduled time of surgery.

Shevde, K., & Trivedi, N. (1991). Effects of clear liquids on gastric volume and pH in healthy volunteers. *Anesthesia and Analgesia*, 72:528-531.

Maltby, J.R., Lewis, P., Martin, A., & Sutherland, L.R. (1991). Gastric fluid volume and pH in elective patients following unrestricted oral fluid until three hours before surgery. *Canadian Journal of Anaesthesia*, 38(4):425-529.

BOX 6-2

Standards for Basic Intraoperative Monitoring

These standards apply to all anesthesia care although, in emergency circumstances, appropriate life support measures take precedence. These standards may be exceeded at any time based on the judgment of the responsible anesthesiologist. They are intended to encourage quality patient care, but observing them cannot guarantee any specific patient outcome. They are subject to revision from time to time, as warranted by the evolution of technology and practice. They apply to all general anesthetics, regional anesthetics and monitored anesthesia care. This set of standards addresses only the issue of basic anesthetic monitoring, which is one component of anesthesia care. In certain rare or unusual circumstances, (1) some of these methods of monitoring may be clinically impractical, and (2) appropriate use of the described monitoring methods may fail to detect untoward clinical developments. Brief interruptions of continual[†] monitoring may be unavoidable. *Under extenuating circumstances, the responsible anesthesiologist may waive the requirements marked with an asterisk (*); it is recommended that when this is done, it should be so stated (including the reasons) in a note in the patient's medical record.* These standards are not intended for application to the care of the obstetrical patient in labor or in the conduct of pain management.

STANDARD I

Qualified anesthesia personnel shall be present in the room throughout the conduct of all general anesthetics, regional anesthetics and monitored anesthesia care.

Objective

Because of the rapid changes in patient status during anesthesia, qualified anesthesia personnel shall be continuously present to monitor the patient and provide anesthesia care. In the event there is a direct known hazard, e.g., radiation, to the anesthesia personnel which might require intermittent remote observation of the patient, some provision for monitoring the patient must be made. In the event that an emergency requires the temporary absence of the person primarily responsible for the anesthetic, the best judgment of the anesthesiologist will be exercised in comparing the emergency with the anesthetized patient's condition and in the selection of the person left responsible for the anesthetic during the temporary absence.

STANDARD II

During all anesthetics, the patient's oxygenation, ventilation, circulation and temperature shall be continually evaluated.

OXYGENATION
Objective

To ensure adequate oxygen concentration in the inspired gas and the blood during all anesthetics.

Methods

(1) Inspired gas: During every administration of general anesthesia using an anesthesia machine, the concentration of oxygen in the patient breathing system shall be measured by an oxygen analyzer with a low oxygen concentration limit alarm in use.*

(2) Blood oxygenation: During all anesthetics, a quantitative method of assessing oxygenation such as pulse oximetry shall be employed.* Adequate illumination and exposure of the patient is necessary to assess color.*

VENTILATION
Objective

To ensure adequate ventilation of the patient during all anesthetics.

Methods

(1) Every patient receiving general anesthesia shall have the adequacy of ventilation continually evaluated. While qualitative clinical signs such as chest excursion, observation of the reservoir breathing bag and auscultation of breath sounds may be adequate, quantitative monitoring of the CO_2 content and/or volume of expired gas is encouraged.

(2) When an endotracheal tube is inserted, its correct positioning in the trachea must be verified by clinical assessment and by identification of carbon dioxide in the expired gas.* End-tidal CO_2 analysis, in use from the time of endotracheal tube placement, is strongly encouraged.

(3) When ventilation is controlled by a mechanical ventilator, there shall be in continuous use a device that is capable of detecting disconnection of components of the breathing system. The device must give an audible signal when its alarm threshold is exceeded.

(4) During regional anesthesia and monitored anesthesia care, the adequacy of ventilation shall be evaluated, at least, by continual observation of qualitative clinical signs.

†Note that "continual" is defined as "repeated regularly and frequently in steady rapid succession" whereas "continuous" means "prolonged without any interruption at any time."
(Reprinted with permission from the American Society of Anesthesiologists, ASA, 520 North Northwest Highway, Park Ridge, IL 60068-2573. Approved by ASA House of Delegates on October 21, 1986 and last amended on October 13, 1993.)

BOX 6-2

Standards for Basic Intraoperative Monitoring—cont'd

CIRCULATION
Objective

To ensure the adequacy of the patient's circulatory function during all anesthetics.

Methods

(1) Every patient receiving anesthesia shall have the electrocardiogram continuously displayed from the beginning of anesthesia until preparing to leave the anesthetizing location.*
(2) Every patient receiving anesthesia shall have arterial blood pressure and heart rate determined and evaluated at least every five minutes.*
(3) Every patient receiving general anesthesia shall have, in addition to the above, circulatory function continually evaluated by at least one of the following: palpa-

tition of a pulse, auscultation of heart sounds, monitoring of a tracing of intra-arterial pressure, ultrasound peripheral pulse monitoring, or pulse plethysmography or oximetry.

BODY TEMPERATURE
Objective

To aid in the maintenance of appropriate body temperature during all anesthetics.

Methods

There shall be readily available a means to continuously measure the patient's temperature. When changes in body temperature are intended, anticipated or suspected, the temperature shall be measured.

The ASA has adopted the Standards for Basic Intraoperative Monitoring (Box 6-2) as guidelines for patient care. The perioperative nurse should be familiar with these standards and understand their significance in patient safety. If routine or frequent deviation from such standards occur, then a QA alert (notification through the hospital's quality assessment or total quality management program) should be considered.

Monitors considered appropriate include: (1) inspired oxygen analyzer (F_IO_2), which is calibrated to room air on a daily basis; (2) low-pressure disconnect alarm, which senses pressure in the expiratory limb of the patient circuit; (3) inspiratory pressure; (4) respirometer (these four devices are an integral part of most modern anesthesia machines); (5) electrocardioscope; (6) blood pressure (frequently measured with a noninvasive automated unit); (7) heart rate; (8) precordial or esophageal stethoscope; (9) temperature; (10) peripheral nerve stimulator if muscle relaxants are used; (11) pulse oximeter; and (12) $ETCO_2$ monitor. Many facilities also incorporate the analysis of respiratory and anesthetic gases in addition to the other parameters. This is done with an infrared analyzer, a mass spectrometer, or a Raman spectrometer, which uses an argon ultraviolet laser.

The latest models of anesthesia machines have most of the basic monitors (excluding ECG) integrated into a computerized system. This system generally includes: F_IO_2; inspired and expired CO_2; inspired and expired volatile agents; airway pressure and disconnect alarms; tidal volume, respiratory rate, and minute ventilation; noninvasive blood pressure (systolic, diastolic, and mean); SpO_2; pulse rate; temperature; and an event marker. A sophisticated, prioritized system displays the caution/alarm condition(s) in one location, making it unnecessary to scan numerous individual monitors with a variety of displays when an alarm

sounds. The internal computer system stores the digital data for more than 8 continuous hours. These data can be transferred to a computer disk (CD) for later analysis, or it can be reviewed on the display screen. The above features are usually denoted by "CD" in the model number.

Based on the cardiovascular and pulmonary status of the patient, the surgical procedure, and the chance of significant physiologic changes, additional invasive monitors may be used. These include direct arterial and venous pressure measurements, a pulmonary artery (PA) catheter, and continuous mixed-venous O_2 saturation ($S\bar{v}O_2$) measured with a special PA catheter. A newly developed PA catheter can provide a continuous measurement of cardiac output. This new technology employs "pulsed thermodilution" to provide intermittent heat along a distal segment of the catheter. The small changes in the temperature of the blood are proportional to the blood flow (cardiac output). These changes are sensed by a thermistor on the tip of the catheter.

For certain conditions, other equipment such as transcutaneous O_2 and CO_2, transesophageal echocardiography, evoked potentials, electroencephalogram, and cerebral or neurologic function monitors may be used. For procedures at risk of venous air embolism, special monitors (such as a doppler probe over the right atrium) may be used. An indwelling urinary catheter also provides a useful indication of renal function and hemodynamic status.

Despite some controversy, most anesthesiologists believe that the monitoring employed depends upon the physiologic status and stability of the patient; the surgical procedure planned and its potential for sudden changes in cardiopulmonary functions, the extent of blood loss and major fluid shifts; and the anticipated monitoring needs for postoperative management as opposed to whether a general or regional anesthetic technique will be used. However, monitoring of some parameters may be negated by the anesthetic technique selected. For example, a low-pressure disconnect alarm is unnecessary with regional anesthesia when a patient is breathing spontaneously. A peripheral nerve stimulator is not needed if muscle relaxants are not used.

The perioperative utilization of pulse oximetry and end tidal capnography has grown exponentially. A brief review will help the reader understand their use.

PULSE OXIMETRY

Pulse oximetry is based on the principles of spectrometric oximetry, plethysmography, and the Lambert-Beer law, which relates the concentration of solute in suspension to the intensity of light transmitted through the solution. It gives a continuous noninvasive indication of the arterial O_2 saturation of functional hemoglobin and the pulse rate, and thus provides an early warning of hypoxemia.

The O_2-dissociation curve relates the percent of totally saturated hemoglobin with O_2 on the Y axis to the PaO_2 on the X axis. The curve is sigmoid shaped, and therefore the relationship of the pulse oximeter (SpO_2) to PaO_2 is nonlinear. The following values are approximations with SpO_2 in % (PaO_2 in torr): 98-100% (95 torr or greater); 90% (60 torr); 75% (39 torr); 50% (26 torr); and 25% (16 torr). Most pulse oximeters are accurate within ± 2% above 70% and ± 3% from 50-70%, but correlate poorly below 50%. On room air, the SpO_2 for a young, healthy person should be 98-100%; an elderly patient may be in the low 90s, whereas a heavy smoker or someone with severe lung disease may even be in the 80s. It is wise to note the resting SpO_2 of a patient before any O_2, medications or stimulation is introduced. Maintenance of a SpO_2 above 90% corresponds to a PaO_2 of 60 torr or greater.

The sensor combines two low-intensity light-emitting diodes (LED) as light sources and a photodiode as a receiver or light detector. One LED emits red light (approximately 660 nanometers [nm]), and the other LED emits infrared light (approximately 940 nm). These light sources alternate about 480 times a second. When the two frequencies of light are transmitted through blood and tissue, they are absorbed differently by the tissue components and by the reduced hemoglobin and the oxyhemoglobin. Because absorption by the other tissue components is essentially constant, the major variable is the saturation of the hemoglobin with O_2. The internal microprocessor analyzes the variations in the absorption of light emitted from both LEDs and provides a readout of the percent saturation of hemoglobin with O_2. The pulse rate is also provided. Many units also display a waveform that correlates with the arterial pulsations.

The response of the pulse oximeter can be adversely affected by any event that significantly reduces vascular pulsations such as hypoperfusion, hypotension, hypovolemia, vasoconstriction, or hypothermia. Electrosurgery, motion,

or ambient light may also artifactually decrease the readout. Carboxyhemoglobin (carbon monoxide bound to hemoglobin) falsely elevates the saturation, and methemoglobin (hemoglobin that has an oxidized iron molecule and cannot reversibly combine with O_2) falsely lowers the saturation. Intravenous dyes affect the pulse oximeter. Methylene blue may cause a drop to 65% for 1 to 2 minutes, indigo carmine a very slight decrease, and indocyanine green a slightly greater decrease. Nail polish can also decrease the SpO_2. Blue, black, or green polish significantly decreases the SpO_2 reading whereas red polish has only a slight effect. Opaque, acrylic nail coverings may block the light beam. If nail polish or coverings seem to cause problems, the sensor can be turned sideways so that the fingernail is not in the light path.

The sensor is usually placed on the third or fourth finger or on a toe. Some manufacturers have sensors for the ear lobe and the bridge of the nose as well as smaller ones for infants and children. The pulse oximeter does not require user calibration. Care must be taken to prevent localized neurovascular or ischemic damage. For example, a hard-cased sensor placed on a finger may cause ischemia when the arms are tightly secured at the patient's side during a long procedure.

If trouble with the pulse oximeter is encountered during a local anesthetic, the perioperative nurse should evaluate the patient's ventilatory status, verify proper placement of the sensor, and rule out the items listed above, which adversely affect operation of the unit. Pulsatile blood flow in the extremity may be inadequate due to hypovolemia, decreased cardiac output, malpositioning, constriction by the blood pressure cuff, or hypothermia from rapid fluid administration. As a final step, the pulse oximeter unit, cable, and sensor can be checked by placing the sensor on the nurse's finger to verify satisfactory function.

Capnography

A capnometer measures CO_2, and a capnograph displays the CO_2 waveform. In patients with normal circulation and pulmonary function, it provides an excellent method to evaluate alveolar ventilation since there is only a small gradient between the arterial and the alveolar CO_2. With forced expiration the $ETCO_2$ provides a close approximation of the arterial CO_2 ($PaCO_2$). In an anesthetized patient, expiration is passive and the point of measurement is near the connection between the patient circuit and the endotracheal tube. Therefore, the $ETCO_2$ is 5 to 8 torr lower than the $PaCO_2$ measured in arterial blood.

The $ETCO_2$ can be measured by a mass spectrometer, a Raman spectrometer, or an infrared analyzer. Recent advances in the technology of infrared analyzers and microprocessors have resulted in compact units that provide a continuous indication of the $ETCO_2$ and have made these the most widely used units for perioperative monitoring. These units measure the amount of infrared light absorbed by the CO_2 in the sample of gas. Two types of monitors are in use. In the *mainstream* unit, all respired gas passes through the detector, whereas with the *sidestream* unit, a portion of the gas is aspirated at a constant rate (50 to 250 ml/min) through a small-bore tubing into the unit. Each design has advantages. Most units display a waveform of the expiratory CO_2 partial pressure versus time after a short sampling and processing delay. The waveform is important for correctly interpreting the output data. Digital readouts usually give the $ETCO_2$ and respiratory rate. Daily user calibration is rarely required with the newer units. Clinically, the units confirm proper endotracheal intubation and are useful to detect anesthesia circuit disconnection, alveolar ventilation, early return of muscle function after muscle relaxants are used, and acute alterations in metabolic functions such as malignant hyperthermia or thyrotoxicosis.

For emergency use or in remote locations where capnography is not available, disposable colorimetric CO_2 detectors are available that can be connected directly to the endotracheal tube. An indicator in the unit changes color corresponding to the CO_2 present. These units are not for routine use.

GENERAL ANESTHESIA

MECHANISM OF ACTION

Numerous theories have been proposed to explain the action of general anesthetics. Many of the recent investigations have involved inhalation anesthetics. (The terms *volatile anesthetic, potent agent,* and *inhaled anesthetic* are synonymous with *inhalation anesthetic.*) Most evidence indicates that the synaptic transmission of nerve impulses is reversibly inhibited in several areas of the central nervous system. The extent of inhibition and consequently the progressive depression of function are correlated with the partial pressure of the inhaled anesthetic at various sites. The inhibition is believed to occur at a lipophilic site on the biologic membrane of synapses and possibly on small, unmyelinated nerve fibers. Suppression of spinal reflex activity is thought to produce some relaxation of skeletal muscles. Although no single concept explains all the phenomena, a few theories explain many of the actions that have been observed. The following are some of the more widely accepted theories:

1. The *protein receptor theory* proposes that hydrophobic areas of specific proteins in the central nervous system act as receptor sites. The steep dose-response curve of inhaled anesthetics seems to support this theory by indicating that a critical number of receptor sites must be occupied before patient movement in response to noxious stimuli is obtunded.
2. The *Meyer-Overton theory* is also called the *critical volume hypothesis* to explain the correlation between the lipid solubility (oil/gas partition coefficient) and the anesthetic potency. This theory proposes that when enough anesthetic molecules dissolve (that is, a critical volume is reached) at a crucial hydrophobic site such as the lipid cellular membrane, anesthe-

sia is achieved. As the cell membrane expands in response to the dissolved anesthetic molecules, changes in the ionic channels occur and alter the sodium flux involved in cellular depolarization. Because some lipid-soluble compounds are not anesthetics, this theory does not give a complete explanation of anesthetic action.
3. *Endogenous endorphins* or opiate-like substances suppress various pain pathways. Several classes of endorphins have been identified. The action of beta-endorphins is antagonized by naloxone (a specific narcotic antagonist), but the relative potency of inhaled anesthetics is not altered. Although some degree of analgesia may be explained by this mechanism, it does not correlate well with the level of anesthesia achieved by inhaled anesthetics.

Intravenous anesthetics may also function by some of the mechanisms proposed for the inhaled anesthetics. Factors involved in the pharmacokinetics of IV drugs include the volume of distribution, biotransformation, and clearance of the drug by metabolism, excretion, or elimination of the drug and its metabolites.

In summary, no single theory for the mechanism of action can explain all the effects observed with anesthetic agents. The spectrum of anesthetic activity varies with the different anesthetics; the effects on the central nervous system and skeletal muscles are similar but not identical; structural and spatial differences exist among agents; changes at both the membrane and cellular levels occur; and optical isomers produce different responses. Although similar in many respects, anesthetic agents are individually unique and probably work through numerous mechanisms and at multiple sites to produce their effects.

LEVELS OF GENERAL ANESTHESIA

Guedel integrated the signs and stages of ether anesthesia into a system (Fig. 6-1) that was used clinically for more than 60 years. This system applied only to unpremedicated patients breathing spontaneously during ether anesthesia, a technique that is rarely used in modern practice. By evaluating the physiologic changes and reflex responses listed in Fig. 6-1, one can estimate the depth of anesthesia. Stage 1 is from the initial administration of anesthetic agents to loss of consciousness. Stage 2 is from the loss of consciousness to the onset of regular breathing and loss of the eyelid reflex. Stage 2 is also called the *delirium* or *excitement* stage, and thrashing movements may occur. No auditory or physical stimulation should take place during this stage. Stage 3, which begins with the onset of a regular breathing pattern and lasts until cessation of respiration, is divided into four planes and is the stage of surgical anesthesia. Stage 4 is from cessation of respiration to circulatory failure that leads to death.

Although Guedel's system gives us an appreciation for the interrelationships of numerous signs during anesthesia, the variety of drugs and anesthetic techniques used today do not provide such uniform responses suitable for estimat-

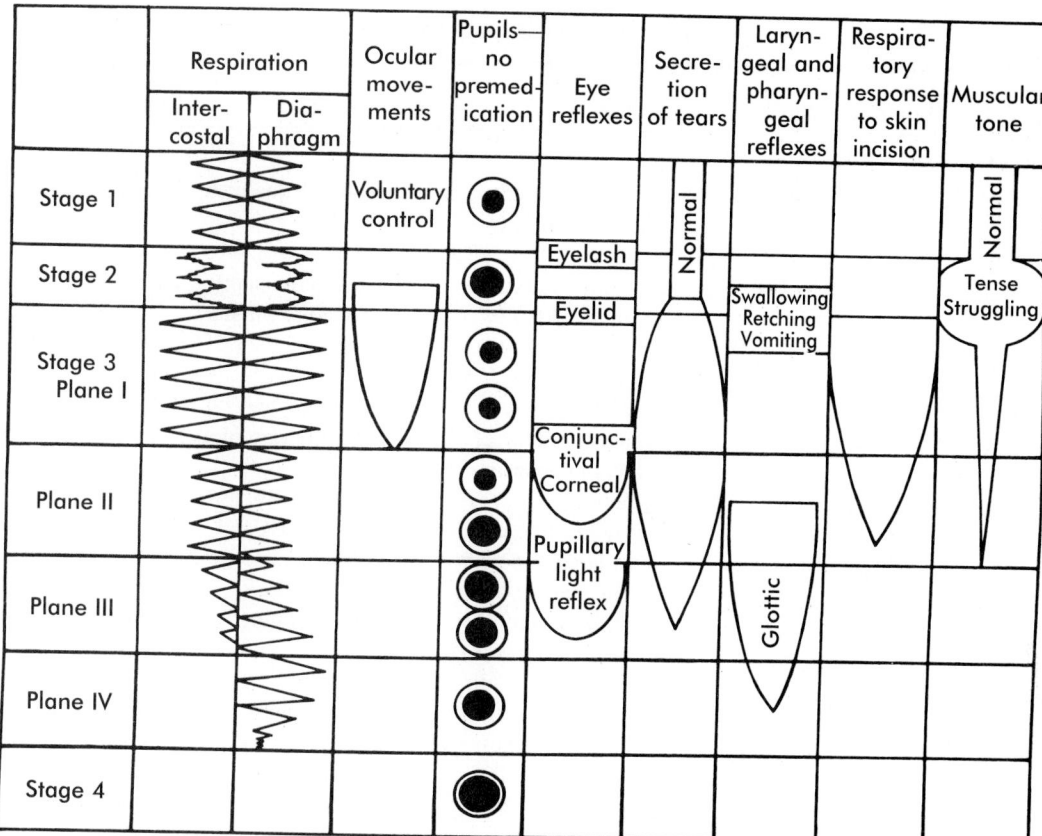

FIG. 6-1 Changes occurring during ether anesthesia. The actions of different anesthetics vary slightly from this.

After Guedel; from Atkinson, R.S., Rushman, G.B., and Lee, J.A.: *A synopsis of anaesthesia,* London, 1982, John Wright & Sons, Ltd., Medical Publishers.

ing the exact depth of anesthesia. Narcotics and anticholinergic drugs given as premedicants alter the pupillary responses. Evaluation of respiratory responses and muscle tone is not valid when controlled ventilation and muscle relaxants are used. Today, general anesthesia is usually induced with the IV injection of a rapid-acting drug such as thiopental or propofol (Diprivan) that takes the patient rapidly to stage 3 and eliminates the untoward responses often seen during stage 2.

For optimal anesthesia and good surgical conditions, several different but interrelated factors are involved. These include hypnosis (sleep), analgesia (freedom from pain), amnesia (lack of recall), appropriate surgical conditions including muscle relaxation and positioning of the patient, and continued homeostasis of the patient's vital functions. Different drugs and anesthetic agents possess various properties that facilitate the above conditions. Combinations of drugs are therefore used to obtain the desired effect. For example, diazepam and midazolam are hypnotics and amnestics, thiopental and etomidate are hypnotics, morphine and fentanyl are analgesics, and pancuronium and succinylcholine are muscle relaxants. Muscle relaxants primarily affect only skeletal muscles and not cardiac or smooth muscles; however, some relaxants may cause side effects such as tachycardia via the autonomic nervous system or hypo-

tension secondary to the release of histamine. The potent inhalational anesthetics (halothane, enflurane, isoflurane, and desflurane) provide sleep, amnesia, analgesia, and muscle relaxation in varying degrees. Hypotensive or hypertensive drugs and cardioactive agents may also be included to achieve the optimum depth of anesthesia while affecting physiologic homeostasis as little as possible. Some of the drugs commonly used in anesthesia are briefly described in Table 6-2.

PHASES OF GENERAL ANESTHESIA

General anesthesia may be divided into three phases: induction, maintenance, and emergence. Induction begins with administration of anesthetic agents and continues until the patient is ready for surgical manipulation or incision. This exact endpoint may vary with the surgical procedure. The maintenance phase continues from this point until near completion of the procedure and may be accomplished with inhalation agents and/or with IV drugs given in titrated doses or by continuous infusions. Emergence varies in length and depends on the depth and duration of anesthesia. Emergence starts as the patient begins to "emerge" from anesthesia and usually ends when the patient is ready to leave the operating room (OR). Intubation occurs during the induction phase, and extubation is usually performed dur-

TABLE 6-2

Commonly Used Anesthetic Drugs

	Common usage	Advantages	Disadvantages	Comments
INHALATIONAL GASES				
Air	Maintenance with O_2; laser surgery near airway	Less support of combustion than N_2O	No anesthetic qualities	Possibly less nausea than N_2O
Oxygen (O_2)	Essential for life	Can slightly increase O_2 available to tissues in low cardiac output states	Can cause retinopathy in premature infants	High concentrations hazardous with lasers in surgery of head/neck & pulmonary areas
Nitrous oxide (N_2O)	Maintenance; frequently for induction	Rapid induction and recovery; additive effects to other anesthetics	No relaxation; can depress myocardium	Hypoxia if overdose given; increases uptake of other volatile agents
Enflurane (Ethrane)	Maintenance; occasionally for induction	Good relaxation; allows larger amounts of epinephrine to be used than with halothane; 2.4% metabolized	Can cause ↑ HR and ↓ BP; lowers seizure threshold; slightly irritating odor	Abnormal EEG at high concentrations
Desflurane (Suprane)	Maintenance in shorter cases	Very rapid emergence & change of anesthetic depth; 0.02% metabolized; good relaxation	May cause transient ↑ HR & BP; some airway irritation; requires heated vaporizer	Rapid recovery phase; can use for emergence after maintenance with another volatile agent
Halothane (Fluothane)	Maintenance; frequently for induction in pediatrics	Rapid induction & recovery; pleasant, nonirritating odor; fair relaxation	Narrow margin of safety—sensitizes myocardium to epinephrine; rare cause of liver damage; 15-20% metabolized	May cause bradycardia & hypotension; PVCs & ventricular fibrillation may occur with epinephrine
Isoflurane (Forane)	Maintenance; occasionally for induction	Good relaxation; allows larger amounts of epinephrine to be used than with halothane; maintains cardiac output; 0.2% metabolized	↑ HR; slightly irritating odor	Isomer of enflurane
OPIOID ANALGESICS				
Morphine sulfate (MS)	Perioperative pain; premedication	Inexpensive; duration of action 4-5 hr; euphoria; good cardiovascular stability	Nausea and vomiting; histamine release; postural ↓ BP (↓ SVR); high first pass effect PO	Used intrathecally & epidurally for post-op pain; elimination half-life 3 hr
Alfentanil (Alfenta)	Surgical analgesia in ambulatory patients	Duration of action 0.5 hr; used as bolus or infusion		Potency: 750 μg = 10 mg MS; elimination half-life 1.6 hr
Fentanyl (Sublimaze)	Surgical analgesia: epidural infusion for post-op analgesia	Good cardiovascular stability; duration of action 0.5 hr		Most commonly used opioid; potency: 100 μg = 10 mg MS; elimination half-life 3.6 hr
Sufentanil (Sufenta)	Surgical analgesia	Good cardiovascular stability; duration of action 0.5 hr; prolonged analgesia	Prolonged respiratory depression	Potency: 15 μg = 10 mg MS; elimination half-life 2.7 hr

TABLE 6-2

Commonly Used Anesthetic Drugs—cont'd

	Common usage	Advantages	Disadvantages	Comments
DEPOLARIZING MUSCLE RELAXANTS				
Succinylcholine (Anectine, Quelicin)	Intubation; short cases	Rapid onset; short duration	Requires refrigeration; may cause fasciculations, post-op myalgias & arrhythmias; ↑ serum K^+ with burns, tissue trauma, paralysis, & muscle diseases; slight histamine release	Prolonged muscle relaxation with serum cholinesterase deficiency & certain antibiotics; trigger agent for malignant hyperthermia
NONDEPOLARIZING MUSCLE RELAXANTS—Intermediate onset & duration				
Atracurium (Tracrium)	Intubation; maintenance of relaxation	No significant cardiovascular or cumulative effects; good with renal failure	Requires refrigeration; slight histamine release	Breakdown by Hofmann elimination & ester hydrolysis
Mivacurium (Mivacron)	Intubation; maintenance of relaxation	Short acting; rapid metabolism by serum cholinesterase; used as bolus or infusion	Expensive in longer cases	New; rarely need to reverse; prolonged effect with serum cholinesterase deficiency
Rocuronium (Zemuron)	Intubation; maintenance of relaxation	Rapid onset; elimination via kidney & liver	Vagolutic; may ↑ HR	Duration similar to Atracurium & Vecuronium
Vecuronium (Norcuron)	Intubation; maintenance of relaxation	No significant cardiovascular or cumulative effects; no histamine release	Requires mixing	Mostly eliminated in bile, some in urine
NONDEPOLARIZING MUSCLE RELAXANTS—Longer onset & duration				
d-Tubocurine (Curare, tubocurine)	Maintenance of relaxation		May cause histamine release & transient ganglionic blockade	
Metocurine (Metubine)	Maintenance of relaxation	Good cardiovascular stability	Slight histamine release	Large bolus may cause ↓ BP
Pancuronium (Pavulon)	Maintenance of relaxation		May cause ↑ HR & ↑ BP	Mostly renal elimination
INTRAVENOUS ANESTHETICS				
Etomidate (Amidate)	Induction	Good cardiovascular stability; fast, smooth induction & recovery	May cause pain with injection and myotonic movements	
Diazepam (Valium)	Amnesia; hypnotic; pre-op medication	Good sedation	Prolonged duration	Residual effects for 20-90 hr; ↑ effect with alcohol
Ketamine (Ketalar)	Induction, occasional maintenance (IV or IM)	Short acting; patient maintains airway; good in small children & burn patients	Large doses may cause hallucinations and respiratory depression	Need darkened, quiet room for recovery; often used in trauma cases
Midazolam (Versed)	Hypnotic; anxiolytic; sedation; often used as adjunct to induction	Excellent amnesia; water soluble (no pain with IV injection); short acting	Slower induction than thiopental	Often used for amnesia with insertion of invasive monitors or regional anesthesia

Continued.

TABLE 6-2

Commonly Used Anesthetic Drugs—cont'd

	Common usage	Advantages	Disadvantages	Comments
Propofol (Diprivan)	Induction & maintenance; sedation with regional anesthesia or MAC	Rapid onset; awakening in 4-8 min	May cause pain if injected in small veins	Short elimination half-life (34-64 min)
Sodium methohexital (Brevital)	Induction	Ultrashort-acting barbiturate	May cause hiccups	Can be given rectally
Thiopental sodium (Pentothal)	Induction	Smooth induction & recovery	Large doses may cause apnea & cardiovascular depression	May cause laryngospasm; can be given rectally
LOCAL ANESTHETICS				
Bupivacaine (Marcaine, Sensorcaine)	Epidural, spinal, or local infiltration	Good relaxation; long acting	Overdose can cause cardiac collapse	Max dose: 200 & 150 mg/70 kg with & without epinephrine, respectively
Chloroprocaine (Nesacaine)	Epidural anesthesia	Ultrashort acting; good relaxation	May cause neurotoxicity if injected into CSF	Maximum dose: 1000 & 800 mg/70 kg with & without epinephrine, respectively
Lidocaine (Xylocaine)	Epidural, spinal, peripheral, IV anesthesia & local infiltration	Short acting; good relaxation; low toxicity	Overdose can cause convulsions	Also used for ventricular dysrhythmias; maximum dose: 7 & 5 mg/kg with & without epinephrine, respectively
Tetracaine (Pontocaine)	Spinal anesthesia	Long acting; good relaxation		Max dose: 1-1.5 mg/kg (epinephrine rarely used)
ANTICHOLINERGICS				
Atropine	Block effects of acetylcholine; decrease vagal tone; reverse muscle relaxants; treat sinus bradycardia	↑HR; suppresses salivation, bronchial & gastric secretions	Depresses sweating; may cause dry mouth, flushing, dizziness, CNS symptoms	Quite selective at muscarinic receptor in smooth & cardiac muscle & exocrine glands
Glycopyrrolate (Robinul)	Similar to atropine	Small ↑HR ; does not cross blood-brain barrier; can raise gastric pH more than atropine	Prolonged duration of effects	Lower incidence of dysrhythmias than atropine

---

ing emergence. Recovery from anesthesia can be considered a fourth phase of general anesthesia.

TYPES OF GENERAL ANESTHESIA

The type of general anesthesia employed for maintenance is often described as IV, inhalation (with a volatile anesthetic agent), or a combination of both IV and inhalation anesthetics. For example, an IV technique traditionally included an induction agent such as thiopental, combined with 30% to 40% O_2 with N_2O, an amnestic drug such as diazepam, an analgesic such as fentanyl or morphine sulfate, and a muscle relaxant.

In contrast, an inhalation technique may utilize thiopental or propofol to facilitate a rapid induction, or patients may "breathe themselves down" with increasing concentrations of a potent agent such as halothane plus N_2O and O_2. An inhalation induction is often used with children to avoid inserting an IV catheter before induction. Depending upon the kind of surgical procedure, maintenance of anesthesia may be accomplished with only inhalation agents and spontaneous, assisted, or controlled ventilation. Effects of the volatile agents are dose-related and provide differing levels of sleep, amnesia, analgesia, muscle relaxation, and cardiovascular system responses. If supplemental muscle relaxation is needed, the dose required is significantly less than the dose necessary during IV anesthesia.

In the past, the term *balanced anesthesia* was used when various combinations of IV drugs were "balanced" to provide complete anesthesia. Today, the term is often used to describe a combination of both IV drugs and inhalation agents employed to obtain specific effects in each patient and procedure.

Recently, many anesthesia providers have been using *total IV anesthesia*. With this anesthetic technique, a short-acting drug such as propofol may be employed for induction. The level of anesthesia is then maintained with intermittent doses or infusions of propofol, alfentanil, fentanyl, or sufentanil and an intermediate muscle relaxant (atracurium or vecuronium) plus O_2 alone or with N_2O. As surgery nears completion, the maintenance drugs are decreased and discontinued, and emergence from anesthesia occurs.

MUSCLE RELAXANTS

Muscle relaxants are primarily used by anesthesia providers to facilitate intubation and provide good operating conditions at lighter planes of general anesthesia. These drugs may be used elsewhere for emergency intubation or less frequently when a patient is being mechanically ventilated. Muscle relaxants primarily affect skeletal muscle and have little effect on cardiac or smooth muscle. Although not always dose dependent, many of these drugs have adverse side effects. The route of metabolism and elimination varies, and this may be important in patients with hepatic or renal disease. Muscle relaxants are classified as *depolarizing* or *nondepolarizing*.

Succinylcholine is the only *depolarizing* muscle relaxant in clinical use. Its action is similar to acetylcholine, and at the neuromuscular junction it causes depolarization of the postjunctional membrane. Generalized skeletal muscle contractions known as fasciculations result from this sustained depolarization. These fasciculations and associated postoperative myalgias may be attenuated by giving a *pretreatment* dose of a nondepolarizing relaxant (such as d-Tubocurine 0.04 mg/kg) 3-5 minutes before administering the intubating dose of succinylcholine. Onset of paralysis (30-90 seconds) is faster and the duration of action (5-10 minutes) is shorter than with other relaxants. The speed of onset makes it the preferred drug for rapid sequence inductions. Adverse side effects associated with the use of succinylcholine include cardiac dysrhythmias, hyperkalemia, myalgias (particularly in young ambulatory patients), and increases in intraocular, intracranial, and intragastric pressures. It can also trigger malignant hyperthermia in susceptible patients. Succinylcholine is hydrolyzed by plasma cholinesterase, and the rare patient with an abnormal or absent enzyme (plasma cholinesterase) will have prolonged muscle paralysis.

Nondepolarizing muscle relaxants competitively block the depolarizing action of acetylcholine at the neuromuscular junction, which results in skeletal muscle paralysis. Fasciculations do not occur. These drugs can be subdivided by the duration of action into intermediate (mivacurium, atracurium, and vecuronium) and long-acting (d-Tubocurine, metocurine, gallamine, pancuronium, pipecuronium, and doxacurium). The potency, duration (metabolism and elimination), and side effects of these drugs vary and may be individually altered in patients with hepatic or renal dysfunction, electrolyte imbalance, hypothermia, or by other drugs administered perioperatively (inhalation and local anesthetics, amino-glycoside antibiotics, calcium entry blockers, magnesium, and cardiac antiarrhythmics). Generally, nondepolarizing relaxants can be used in patients with malignant hyperthermia or plasma cholinesterase deficiencies (except for mivacurium). Side effects vary with the individual drugs and usually are dose dependent and include alterations in blood pressure and heart rate. The effect of the muscle relaxants (neuromuscular blockade) can be monitored with a peripheral nerve stimulator. Paralysis caused by the nondepolarizing relaxants may be antagonized by IV anticholinesterases such as edrophonium, neostigmine, or pyridostigmine. These antagonists compete for receptor sites at the neuromuscular junction and may be associated with bradycardia (which can be treated with atropine or glycopyrrolate).

TYPICAL SEQUENCE OF GENERAL ANESTHESIA

After arriving in the OR suite, the patient is identified, the chart is checked for signed consents and/or an operative permit, and the latest results of laboratory tests and diagnostic studies are reviewed. Although the patient may have been evaluated several days earlier in a pre-anesthesia clinic, certain information must be verified by the perioperative nurse immediately before surgery. The anesthesia provider also reviews the pertinent medical history and data, and confirms that there have been no interval changes in the patient's status. Depending on the practice of the anesthesia department, an IV infusion may be started in a preoperative area or after the patient is transferred to the OR. After arrival in the OR, the appropriate intraoperative monitors are connected to the patient before induction of anesthesia. In the perioperative period, nearly all anesthesia-related drugs are given IV, except, of course, the inhalation agents.

Before induction, the patient is usually preoxygenated (actually denitrogenated) using a mask with 100% O_2 for 3-5 minutes. This practice permits washout of most of the gaseous nitrogen from the body and provides a large reserve supply of O_2 in the lungs. A test dose of the induction agent (e.g., 50 mg of thiopental) is often given to check for any unusual or exaggerated response. If succinylcholine is to be used for intubation, a small pretreatment dose of a nondepolarizing muscle relaxant (such as 3 mg of d-Tubocurarine, 0.5 to 1 mg of pancuronium or vecuronium, or 3 mg of atracurium) is usually given. If the patient can be safely ventilated with a mask, many anesthesia providers now avoid the adverse effects of succinylcholine and use one of the intermediate-acting nondepolarizing muscle relaxants for intubation.

To induce anesthesia, a short-acting barbiturate such as thiopental (2 to 6 mg/kg) or propofol (1.5 to 2.5 mg/kg) is given. When the patient becomes apneic and the eyelash reflex is gone, the airway is checked for patency by ventilating the patient with a mask. Depending on several factors such as the airway and the type and duration of surgery, O$_2$ and anesthetic gases may be delivered to a spontaneously breathing patient via a mask that is held in place with a head strap. Positioning of the head and/or insertion of an oral or nasal airway may be used to maintain a patent airway.

If mask anesthesia is not suitable, then an endotracheal tube may be used to facilitate ventilation or to prevent aspiration. (Typical equipment used for intubation as well as airway control and monitoring is shown in Fig. 6-2.) An intubating dose of a muscle relaxant is administered, which results in temporary paralysis.

To facilitate intubation, a laryngoscope held in the left hand is inserted into the right side of the mouth and then moved to the midline, "sweeping" the tongue to the left.

The endotracheal tube is introduced on the right side of the mouth and gently inserted into the trachea so that the cuff is approximately 1 cm below the vocal cords. The cuff is inflated just enough to occlude any air passage with the peak pressures used for ventilation. Location of the endotracheal tube in the trachea is verified by an appropriate level and waveform of ETCO$_2$, by listening for bilaterally equal breath sounds with a stethoscope, by absence of sounds over the stomach, by symmetrical movement of the thorax with positive pressure ventilation, and by condensation of moisture from expired air in the endotracheal tube and breathing circuit. Proper placement of the endotracheal tube is shown in Fig. 6-3. The vocal cords are the narrowest portion of an adult trachea; however, the smallest portion of a child's airway is below the vocal cords. Therefore, uncuffed endotracheal tubes are usually selected for children because the internal diameter of cuffed tubes in these small sizes would have too much resistance to ventilation and could easily become obstructed. After the initial paralysis from the muscle relaxant has worn off, the patient may be allowed to breathe spontaneously with intermittent assistance, or additional muscle relaxant may be given and the ventilation controlled mechanically.

If the procedure is an emergency or the patient is at risk for aspiration (e.g., in cases of intestinal obstruction, a full stomach, hiatal hernia), the anesthesia provider may elect a rapid sequence induction or an awake fiberoptic intubation. If a rapid sequence induction is performed, the perioperative nurse must be ready to assist by applying down-

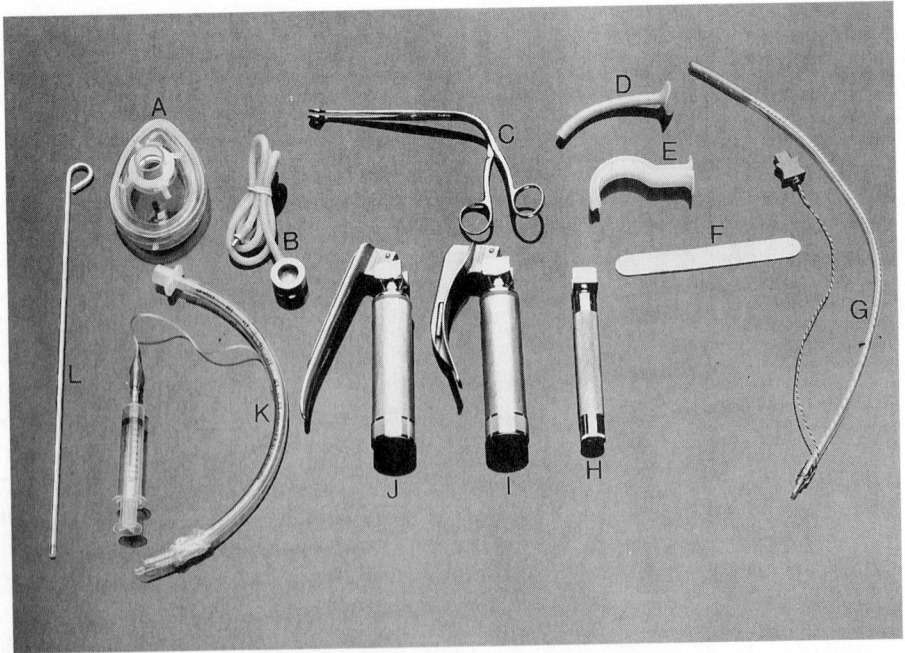

FIG. 6-2   Commonly used anesthesia equipment. **A,** Mask. **B,** Precordial stethoscope. **C,** McGill forceps. **D,** Nasal airway. **E,** Oral airway. **F,** Tongue blade. **G,** Esophageal stethoscope with esophageal temperature monitor. **H,** Pediatric laryngoscope handle. Fiberoptic laryngoscope blades and handles: **I,** MacIntosh; **J,** Miller. **K,** Endotracheal tube. **L,** Intubating stylet for endotracheal tube.

Courtesy Scott & White Memorial Hospital, Temple, Tex.

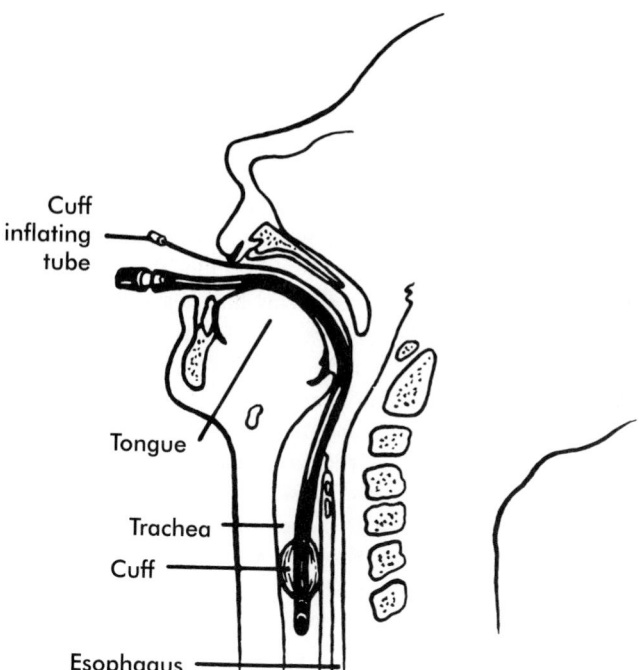

FIG. 6-3 Endotracheal tube in position.

ward pressure on the cricoid cartilage with the thumb and index finger of one hand (Sellick maneuver) while the other hand is placed under the patient's neck for stability. The cricoid cartilage is the only complete ring in the trachea, and downward pressure occludes the esophagus which lies immediately posterior to the trachea.

Additional assistance may be provided by the perioperative nurse if an unexpected difficult intubation occurs and/or the patient cannot be adequately ventilated with a mask. Emergency airway equipment should be brought into the room immediately. The nurse should be familiar with the location of the various pieces of equipment and how to assemble them for use, and should also assist the anesthesia provider in securing the patient's airway. Contents of a typical emergency or difficult airway cart are listed in Box 6-3. If invasive monitors will be placed after induction, the nurse may assist by properly positioning the patient or extremity and prepping the area(s); and may assist with placement, connection, and calibration of the monitors. If the procedure is emergent, the nurse may also assist by obtaining additional IV access, connecting fluid or patient warming units, double-checking blood products, and "pumping" IV fluids as needed. In situations where the anesthesia provider is involved with a critical procedure, the nurse can perform a valuable service by watching the monitors, recording the data, and communicating significant changes to the anesthesia provider.

The laryngeal mask airway (LMA) as shown in Fig. 6-4 is a major advancement in airway management. Before insertion, the LMA must be carefully deflated so that there are no wrinkles in the cuff as shown in Fig. 6-5. The tech-

---

BOX 6-3

Typical Contents of a Difficult (or Emergency) Airway Cart

FIBEROPTIC EQUIPMENT
- Flexible fiberoptic (FO) bronchoscope
- Fiberoptic light source
- Bullard scope (FO)
- Siliconized spray

LARYNGOSCOPE EQUIPMENT
- Assorted pediatric & adult laryngoscope handles & blades
- Extra alkaline batteries

ENDOTRACHEAL TUBES (ETT)
- Regular ETT: uncuffed, 2.5-6.0 mm
- Regular ETT: cuffed, 5.0-9.0 mm
- Oral RAE ETT: uncuffed, 3.0-7.0 mm
- Oral RAE ETT: cuffed, 6.0-8.0 mm
- Nasal RAE ETT: uncuffed, 3.0-7.0 mm
- Nasal RAE ETT: cuffed, 6.0-8.0 mm
- Reinforced ETT: cuffed, 7.0-8.0 mm
- Controllable tip ETT (Endotrol)

AIRWAYS
- Regular oral: assorted pediatric & adult
- Regular nasal: assorted adult
- Intubating airways: assorted (e.g., Ovassapin, Williams)
- Nasopharyngeal airway with inflatable introducer
- Laryngeal mask airways (LMA): assorted sizes
- Tongue blades
- Water-soluble lubricant (K–Y)

INTUBATING EQUIPMENT
- Intubating stylets
- Magill forceps: pediatric & adult
- Esophageal (gastric tube) airway (EGTA)
- Hollow ETT changers

SUCTION EQUIPMENT
- Assorted flexible suction catheters
- Stiff suction catheters (Yankauer)

TOPICAL ANESTHESIA EQUIPMENT
- Atomizers
- Pressurized topical anesthetic spray
- Long Q-Tips
- Lidocaine 4%
- Lidocaine 4% with phenylepiphrine
- Lidocaine 2%-viscous
- Lidocaine 5%-ointment
- Lidocaine 10%

Continued.

BOX 6-3

Typical Contents of a Difficult (or Emergency) Airway Cart—cont'd

---

TRANSTRACHEAL AIRWAY EQUIPMENT
- Transtracheal O_2 jet ventilator with pressure regulator, manual control valve & luer-lock male connector
- Assorted large IV catheters
- Assorted long guide wires, epidural needles & epidural catheters (for retrograde intubation)

MISCELLANEOUS
- Safety glasses
- Heat-moisture exchanger (Humidivent)
- Assorted face masks with port for FO scope
- Right angle connector with port for FO scope
- $ETCO_2$ chemical indicators (Easy Cap)
- Twill tape (to secure ETT)
- Skin adhesive (Mastisol)
- Adhesive tape

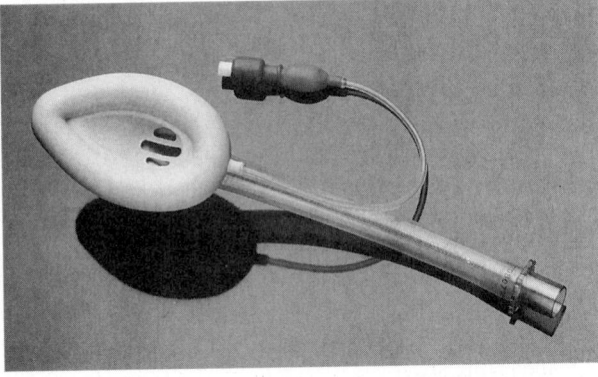

FIG. FIG. 6-4 The Laryngeal Mask Airway inflated.

Courte Courtesy Scott & White Memorial Hospital, Temple, Tex.

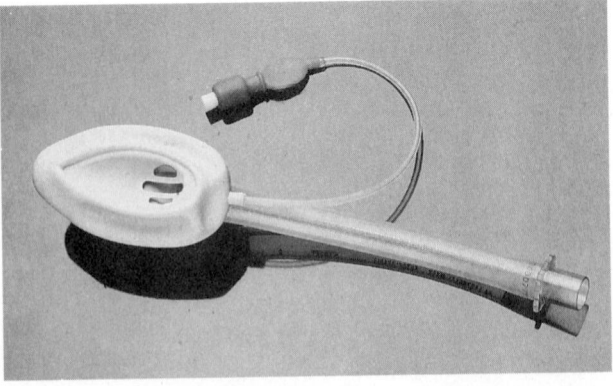

FIG. 6-5 The Laryngeal Mask Airway—deflated and ready for insertion.

Courtesy Scott & White Memorial Hospital, Temple, Tex.

nique for proper insertion of the LMA is shown in Fig. 6-6, and correct placement is shown in Fig. 6-7. It was approved by the Food and Drug Administration for use in the United States in 1991 but was not available for sale in the United States until December 1992, even though it has been used elsewhere in the world in more than 3 million patients. It is available in five sizes, is autoclavable, and is reusable. Placement of the LMA is relatively simple and does not require laryngoscopy or muscle relaxation. For adults, it is recommended that a 2.5-3.0 cm diameter roll of gauze sponges be used as a "bite block" and inserted beside the LMA tube. The LMA and gauze roll can be secured with adhesive tape to the chin to maintain some tension on the inflated cuff of the LMA and maintain the seal. When comparing ease of use, invasiveness, and airway protection, the LMA lies between the face mask and an endotracheal tube. It is ideal for a supine patient under general anesthesia with spontaneous ventilation. The LMA may also be useful in a difficult airway situation where tracheal intubation cannot be achieved easily (Research Highlight 6-2).

Maintenance of anesthesia can be accomplished with either IV or inhalational anesthetic techniques or a combination of both, with or without additional muscle relaxant. A variety of factors are considered by the anesthesiologist in selecting the anesthesia technique for each situation.

Many factors influence emergence. The objective is to be able to move the patient from the OR bed to the postanesthesia care unit (PACU) bed as soon as the dressing is applied. During emergence, the anesthesia provider suctions the oropharynx to decrease the risk of aspiration and laryngospasm following extubation, reverses any residual neuromuscular blockade, and allows the washout of N_2O and volatile anesthetic agents by giving 100% O_2 for several minutes before extubation. Following extubation, the patient is then transported to the PACU to awaken from the anesthetic experience. In some situations the patient may be transferred to the PACU before extubation, and the endotracheal tube is removed when the patient is fully awakened.

Untoward events that can occur with general anesthesia include hypoxia; respiratory, cardiovascular, or renal dysfunction; hypotension; hypertension; fluid or electrolyte imbalance; residual muscle paralysis; dental damage; neurologic problems; hypothermia; and malignant hyperthermia. The anesthesiologist usually directs the treatment and management of such events.

ANESTHESIA MACHINES

The first apparatus resembling an anesthesia machine was used in 1905. Since then, innumerable changes and improvements have been incorporated. The anesthesia machines used for general anesthesia look complicated, but the basic functions are similar and simple to understand. Perioperative nurses should be familiar with the basic function of anesthesia machines as they may need to administer O_2 during local procedures. Many anesthesia machines are still

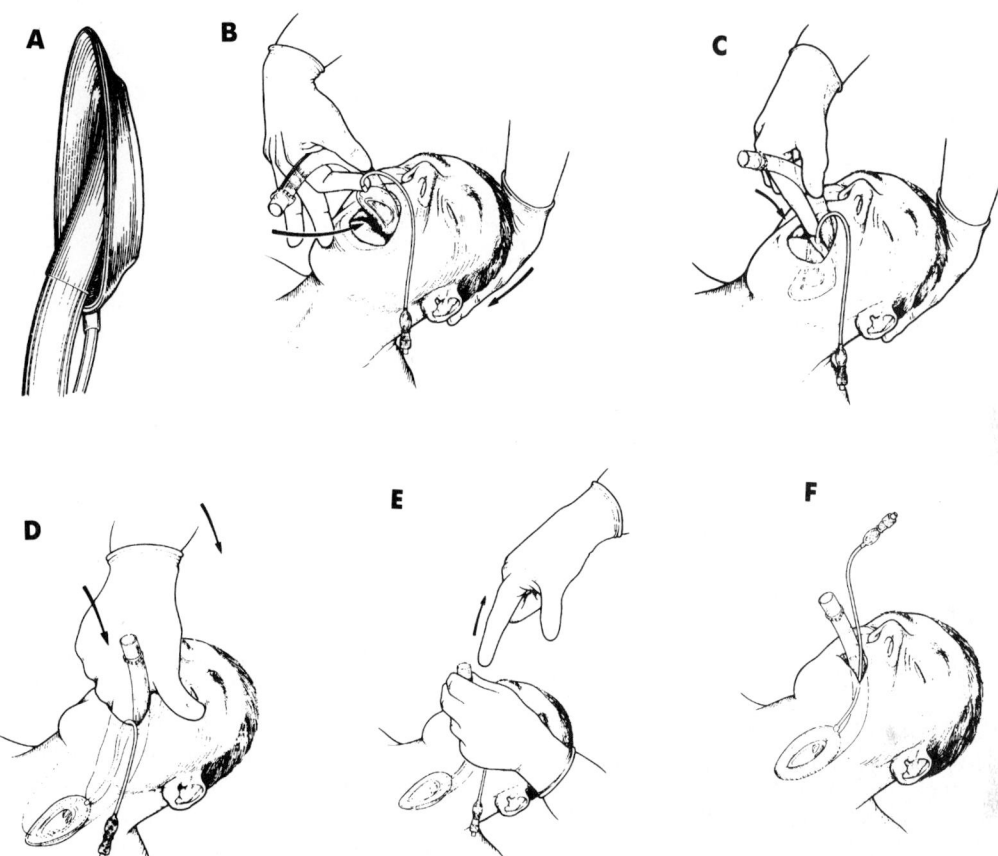

FIG. 6-6   Insertion of the Laryngeal Mask Airway (LMA). **A,** Carefully deflate the LMA as tightly as possible, so that the rim faces away from the mask aperture as shown. There should be no folds near the tip. **B,** Under direct vision, press the tip of the LMA cephalad against the hard palate to flatten it out. Using the index finger, continue pressing the LMA against the palate as the LMA is advanced into the pharynx to ensure that the tip remains flattened and avoids the tongue. **C,** Keeping the neck flexed and the head extended, use the index finger to press the LMA into the posterior wall. **D,** Continue pushing with the ball of the index finger guiding the LMA posteriorly into position. By withdrawing the other fingers and slightly pronating the forearm, it is usually possible to push the LMA fully into position in one fluid movement. **E,** Firmly grasp the tube with the other hand and then withdraw the index finger from the pharynx. Gently press the LMA posteriorly to ensure that it is fully inserted. **F,** Carefully inflate the LMA with the recommended volume of air (size 1: 2-4 ml; size 2: ≤ 10 ml; size 2½: ≤ 15 ml; size 3: ≤ 20 ml; size 4: ≤ 30 ml). Do not overinflate. Do not touch the LMA tube while inflating unless it is obviously unstable (e.g., elderly edentulous patients with loose oropharyngeal tissues). Usually the LMA will move slightly forward out of the hypopharynx as it is inflated. Insert a bite-block (roll of gauze) along side the LMA tube to minimize occlusion of the tube as the patient is awakening.

Courtesy Brain Medical, Ltd.

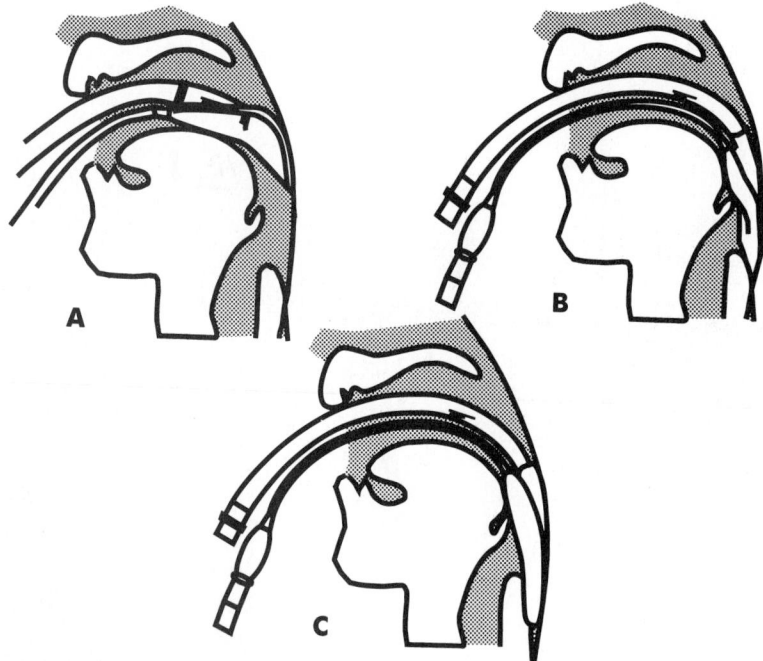

FIG. 6-7   Sagittal views of insertion and proper placement of the Laryngeal Mask Airway. **A,** Insertion of LMA. **B,** proper location of LMA (deflated). **C,** Properly placed and inflated LMA.

Courtesy Scott & White Memorial Hospital, Temple, Tex.

RESEARCH HIGHLIGHT 6-2

Pennant and White presented an extensive review of the laryngeal mask airway (LMA) and its uses in anesthesiology. A total of 202 references were cited. The design, development, and technical aspects of utilization of the LMA are covered in detail. It has been employed extensively in both pediatric and adult patients. Case reports comprise much of the literature with few well-controlled clinical studies. The LMA became commercially available in the United Kingdom in 1988 and is now used in more than 50% of the general anesthetics in some hospitals.

The overall incidence of aspiration with the LMA is unknown, but its protection against aspiration lies between the use of a face mask and an endotracheal tube. It may also be considered as an option in patients with a difficult airway.

Pennant and White concluded that the LMA is easy and atraumatic to insert with little somatic and autonomic responses from the patient. It is a suitable alternative to the face mask or tracheal intubation in many clinical situations. It also facilitates blind and fiber optic assisted intubation. Based on experience elsewhere in the world, the LMA may extensively change the practice of anesthesia in the United States.

Pennant, J.H., & White, P.F. (1993). The laryngeal mask airway. Its uses in anesthesiology. *Anesthesiology* 79:144-163.

in service after 10 to 25 years. An older model is shown in Fig. 6-8 and a newer one in Fig. 6-9. A typical generic schematic is shown in Fig. 6-10. Anesthesia machines sold in the United States after January 1, 1984, are required to meet the criteria set forth in the American National Standards Institute (ANSI) Standard Z79.8. This standard incorporates many safety features that were not required on earlier machines. Because diagrams of anesthesia machines are difficult to find in reference books, the pneumatic circuit for the Ohmeda Modulus II Plus and later machines is shown in Fig. 6-11; the piping diagram for the North American Drager Narkomed models 2B, 2C, 3 and 4 is shown in Fig. 6-12. These references will enable perioperative nurses to become familiar with the anesthesia machines used in their hospital.

Oxygen, N_2O, and air are usually supplied from the hospital pipelines to the anesthesia machine at pressures of 50 to 55 psi. The gas hoses going to the machine are color-coded: O_2 (green); N_2O (blue); and air (yellow). The connectors are specific for each gas so that they cannot be inadvertently cross-connected. If a central gas supply is not available or the hospital piping system fails, the machines are equipped with E-size cylinders of both gases. One or two cylinders of each gas are connected to yokes on the machine. These yokes are pin-indexed so that only the correct gas can be connected in that position. In the pin-indexing safety system, two steel pins are in a unique location on the yoke assembly. The mating gas cylinder (for example, the O_2 tank) has two matching holes in the same

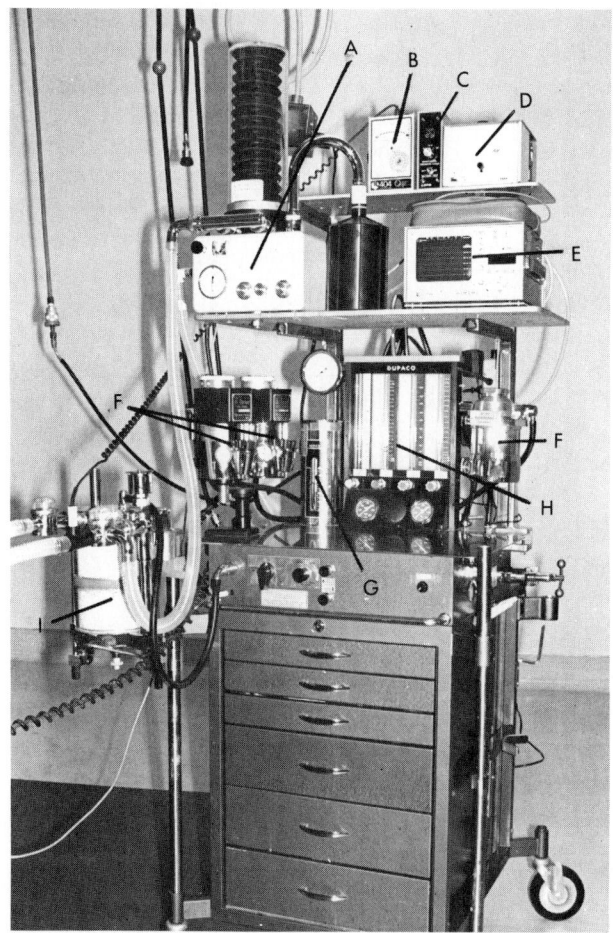

FIG. 6-8 Older anesthesia machine. **A**, Ventilator. **B**, Oxygen analyzer. **C**, Disconnect alarm. **D**, Temperature monitor. **E**, ECG monitor. **F**, Flow-through vaporizers. **G**, Copper Kettle vaporizer. **H**, Flowmeters. **I**, CO_2 absorber and circle system.

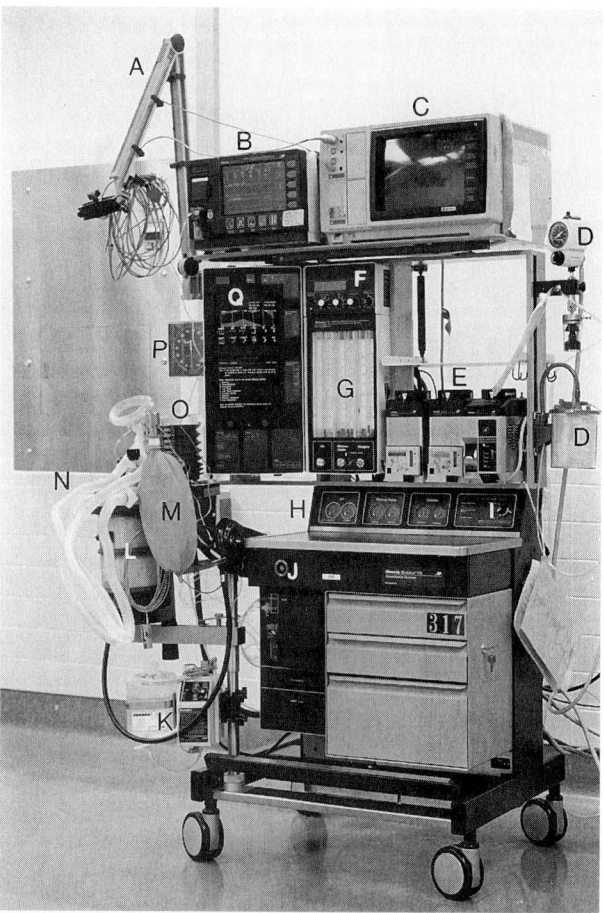

FIG. 6-9 Modern Anesthesia Machine (Ohmeda-Modulus "CD") **A**, Adjustable arm for cables going to patient. **B**, Rascal II (Raman) anesthetic and respiratory gas monitor. **C**, Multichannel physiologic monitor. Channels include ECG (2), pressure (2), temperature (1), and heart rate. **D**, Suction regulator and canister. **E**, Flow-through vaporizers (Isoflurane, Halothane, Desflurane). **F**, Controls for ventilator. **G**, Flowmeters for air, N_2O and O_2. **H**, Gauges for pipeline and E-tank pressures (air, N_2O, O_2). **I**, On/off switch. **J**, Oxygen flush valve. **K**, Heater/humidifier for patient breathing circuit. **L**, CO_2 absorber. **M**, Reservoir "breathing" bag. **N**, Patient circuit. **O**, Ventilator. **P**, Sphygmomanometer for manual blood pressure. **Q**, Integrated monitor/display (noninvasive blood pressure, F_1O_2, tidal volume, respiratory rate, heart rate, % expired anesthetic agent, caution and alarm displays, record of time and vital signs, trends, and output to computer disk).

Courtesy of Scott & White Memorial Hospital, Temple Tex.

locations so that the cylinders cannot be mounted in the wrong place.

In cylinders, O_2 is stored as a compressed gas. A full E-size cylinder contains about 660 L of O_2 at 2000 psi. As the O_2 is used, the pressure falls in direct proportion to the remaining volume. Because the E-size cylinder is used to provide O_2 while transporting patients, knowing how much O_2 is left in a partially used tank is important. Thus 1000 psi would indicate 330 L remaining, and 500 psi would indicate 165 L remaining or sufficient O_2 at 5 L/min flow for more than 25 minutes. When the pressure has dropped to about 250 psi, the cylinder should not be used because it no longer has an adequate reserve.

Nitrous oxide is stored as a liquid in cylinders, and the pressure above the liquid is 750 psi. A full, E-size cylinder contains about 1600 L of N_2O. As the N_2O is used, the pressure above the liquid remains constant. Only when the liquid has been completely vaporized does the pressure begin to fall. Therefore, the N_2O can be almost gone but will

still show the same pressure. In contrast to O_2, the amount remaining in the tank cannot be readily determined.

The gases in the cylinders flow through regulators that reduce the pressure to about 50 psi. The hoses from the hospital gas sources are connected to the machine at the outlet of these regulators. In machines sold after January 1, 1984, a pressure interlock device shuts off the N_2O flow if O_2 pressure is not present. The gases then flow through individual *flowmeters* (or rotameters) on the front of the ma-

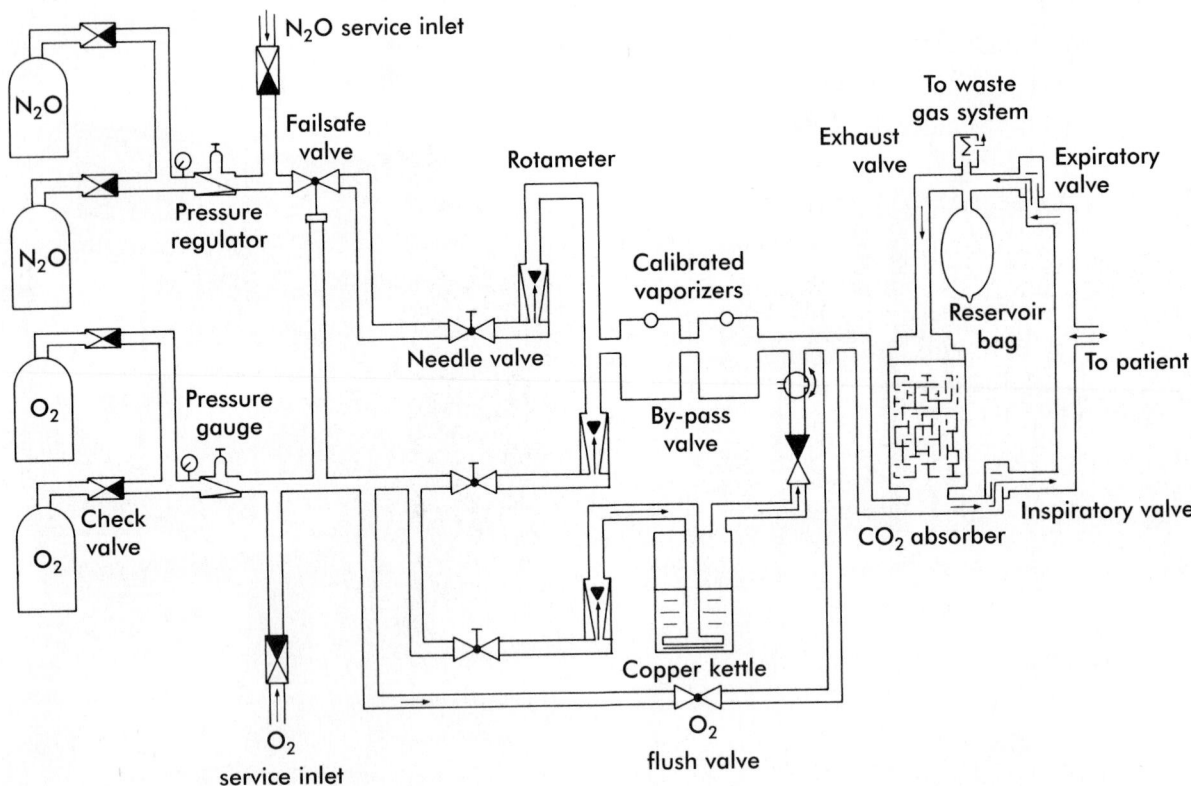

FIG. 6-10 Generic anesthesia machine circuit. Oxygen and nitrous oxide enter the machine from cylinders or from the hospital service supply. Pressure regulators reduce cylinder pressure to about 50 psi. Check valves prevent transfilling of cylinders or gas flow from cylinders to service line. The fail-safe valve prevents flow of nitrous oxide if the oxygen supply fails. Needle valves control flows to rotameters. Calibrated vaporizers provide a preselected concentration of volatile anesthetics. An interlock allows only one vaporizer to be on at a time. The Copper Kettle (no longer manufactured) is a "bypass vaporizer" that delivers saturated anesthetic vapor; thus, the effluent must be diluted. The bypass valve vents vapor from the Kettle when it is not in service. Gases are delivered to the circle absorber, where unidirectional valves assure flow from patient through carbon dioxide absorber. Excess gas is vented through the exhaust valve into a waste gas scavenger system. The reservoir bag compensates for variations in respiratory demand.

Modified from Dripps, R.D., Eckenhoff, J.E., & Vandam, L.D. (1982). *Introduction to anesthesia: the principles of safe practice*, ed. 6. Philadelphia: W.B. Saunders.

chine so that the gas flows and the ratio of O_2 to N_2O or air can be selected by the anesthesia provider. From the top of the flowmeters, the gases are mixed and then flow through a vaporizer in which the inhalational anesthetic of choice is vaporized and added to the gas mixture. The total gas flow is then delivered from the machine to the patient. With a *flow-through vaporizer,* by definition, all of the fresh gas going from the anesthesia machine to the patient flows through the vaporizer. The control dials are usually located on top of these vaporizers and are calibrated in percentages. Most recently manufactured vaporizers are flow and temperature compensated, meaning that they are reasonably accurate at all flows and temperatures used clinically. The filling ports on the vaporizers are usually key indexed so that only the appropriate volatile agent can be used.

Desflurane (Suprane) is a new inhalational anesthetic approved for use in September of 1992. It is unique because it is a liquid below 22.8° C and must be heated slightly to ensure vaporization. Therefore, the vaporizer for desflurane

contains an electric heater. Desflurane also has several other unique characteristics: (1) the solubility in blood (Blood/Gas Partition Coefficient) is lower (0.42) than N_2O (0.47), isoflurane (1.41), or halothane (2.30), which means that it has a faster "wash-in" (induction) and "wash-out" (emergence) than the other agents; (2) there is far less metabolism (0.02%) as a percentage of the anesthetic taken up than isoflurane (0.2%), enflurane (2.4%), or halothane (15 to 20%); (3) emergence and recovery from general anesthesia and discharge from PACU is significantly faster than with thiopental; (4) the cardiovascular effects are to be similar to those of isoflurane; and (5) the muscle relaxant qualities appear similar to the other inhalational agents. The pungency of desflurane precludes its use as an inhalational induction agent. Its clinical use will rapidly increase over the next few years as more experience is gained. Sevoflurane is another new volatile agent currently used in Asia that is not yet approved for use in the United States.

Although no longer approved (by the ANSI Z79.8 stan-

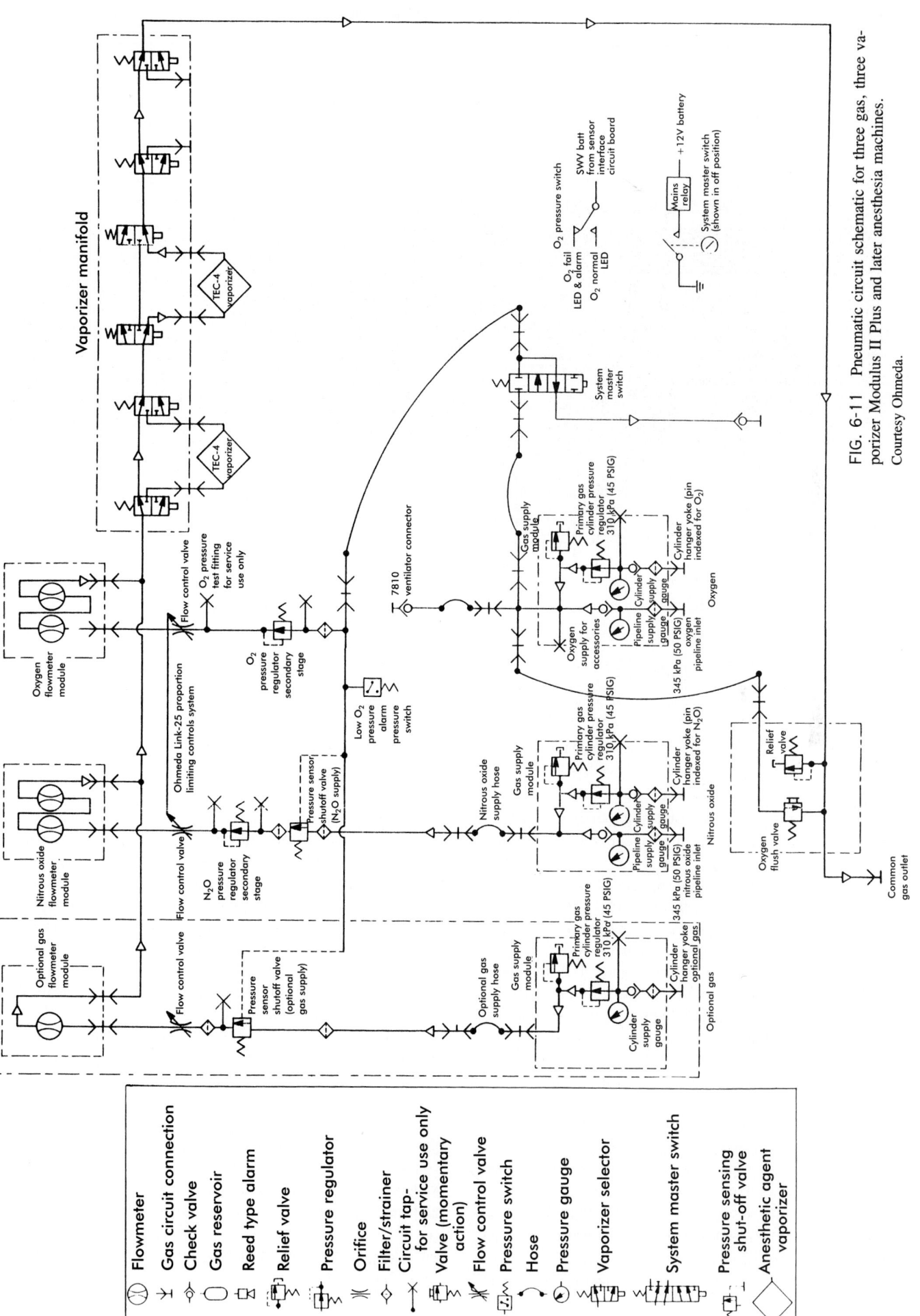

FIG. 6-11 Pneumatic circuit schematic for three gas, three vaporizer Modulus II Plus and later anesthesia machines. Courtesy Ohmeda.

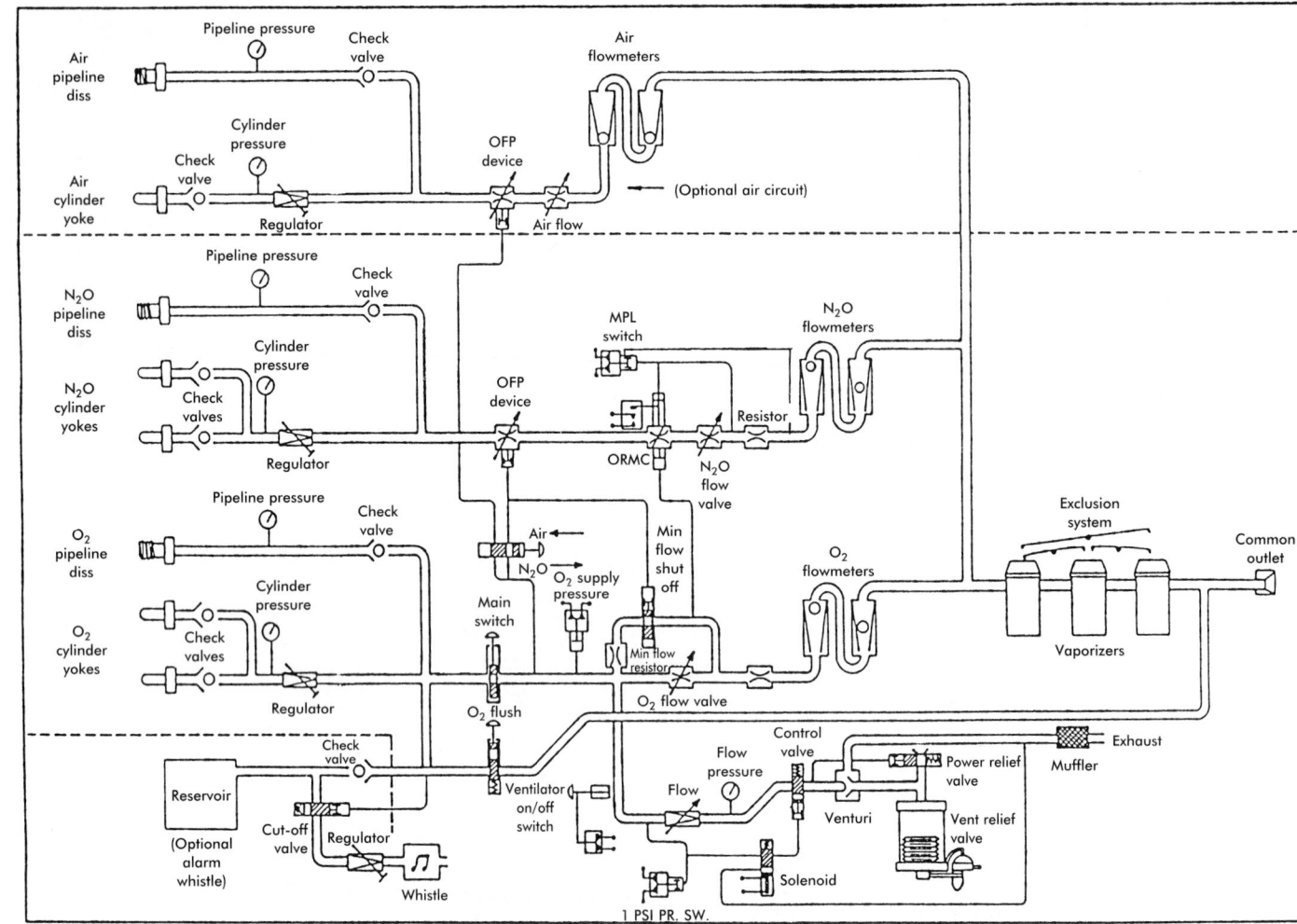

FIG. 6-12 Piping diagram for Narkomed models 2B, 2C, 3, and 4 anesthesia machines.
Courtesy North American Drager.

dard) for sale in the United States, another type of vaporizer, the *bypass vaporizer,* functions in a different manner. The Copper Kettle is one type of bypass vaporizer that may still be found on many older machines. The location in the anesthesia circuit is shown in Fig. 6-10. A low flow of O_2 (usually less than 1 L/min) goes through a separate flowmeter and then through the bypass vaporizer, where this O_2 is totally saturated with the anesthetic vapor. The saturated O_2 is then combined with the gas mixture from the other flowmeters, and the total mixture flows from the machine to the patient. To calculate the concentration of anesthetic going to the patient, the anesthesia provider must know the barometric pressure, the vapor pressure of the anesthetic agent being used, the O_2 flow through the bypass vaporizer, the temperature of the anesthetic liquid in the vaporizer, and the total combined flow of the gas mixture. The major advantage of bypass vaporizers is that any volatile anesthetic agent except desflurane can be used in them. However, serious accidents have occurred when the "wrong" anesthetic was in the vaporizer and the concentration was incorrectly calculated.

Another important feature of the anesthesia machine is the O_2 *flush valve.* With all new machines and on most earlier models, pushing the O_2 flush valve allows 100% O_2 from the 50 psi line to flow directly to the *fresh gas outlet* on the machine and to the patient. This O_2 flow completely bypasses the flowmeters and vaporizers. Caution must be exercised because the pressure is 50 psi and the flow rate is 35-75 L/minute.

In most hospitals in the United States, a semiclosed circle system is used to deliver the fresh gas flow (including anesthetic gases) to patients. The circle system is composed of a container filled with a CO_2-absorbing material (such as soda lime or baralyme), two *one-way (unidirectional) valves,* an *adjustable pressure limiting (APL) valve,* a *reservoir bag,* an inlet connection for fresh gas flow, and two connections to the patient through corrugated breathing (or anesthesia circuit) tubing. As the patient inspires, gases are drawn through the CO_2 absorber and from the fresh gas supply through the inspiratory limb of the corrugated tubing. As the patient exhales, the one-way valve on the inspiratory limb prevents backflow, and the exhaled gases flow into the expiratory limb and through the expiratory one-way valve. The expiratory limb and valve are easily identified by the condensation of water vapor along this portion of the circuit. The reservoir bag absorbs the peak flow of expired gases and allows the anesthesia provider to force gas through the CO_2 absorber, along the inspiratory limb of the circuit, and ventilate the patient. The expired gases flow through the CO_2 absorber where CO_2 is removed. Substances used in the CO_2 absorbent include an indicator that changes color as the soda lime is exhausted. For example, the soda lime may turn from white to blue, indicating that the absorbent material must be changed to prevent a buildup of CO_2 in the patient. Any excess gas is vented through the APL valve into the gas scavenger system. The APL valve is usually mounted just ahead of the CO_2 absorber. A typical circle system is shown in Fig. 6-13.

The *F_IO_2 sensor* is usually mounted in the inspiratory limb just after the one-way valve. It measures the fraction of inspired O_2 (F_IO_2) and can be set to alarm if a low concentration is detected. A low pressure sensor is usually mounted in the expiratory limb near the other one-way valve to detect a ventilator malfunction or a circuit disconnection.

The advantage of the circle system is that much lower flows of O_2, N_2O, and anesthetic gases can be used. This conserves the patient's body heat and respiratory moisture and reduces the cost of volatile agents. A semiclosed circuit (or circle system) is typically used when the fresh gas flows into the system range from 1 to 6 L/min. During exhalation, some of the expired gases are recycled through the CO_2 absorber, and the excess gas is scavenged or eliminated (hence *semiclosed*). With a *closed-circle system,* all of the CO_2 is absorbed. No gas is vented from the system, and only enough O_2 is added to the system to meet the basal requirements of the patient (approximately 3.5 ml/kg/min). In an *open circuit* (such as the Ayres T-piece, Magill, or Bain circuits), a relatively high flow of fresh gas is used, and most of the exhaled gas is vented from the circuit. The fresh gas flowrates/minute vary from approximately two thirds of the patient's minute volume with the Magill circuit to at least 100 ml/kg for the Bain or T-piece circuits. The open-circuit system is commonly used for neonates, infants, and small children.

With all these circuits, the final connection to the patient is via a mask or endotracheal tube. A mask or LMA may be used for a patient with a good airway who is at minimal risk of aspiration, undergoing a relatively short procedure, and when the surgical site is not located in the head or neck area. Endotracheal intubation ensures a patent airway during surgery. When the patient is paralyzed, the ventilation is controlled during the procedure.

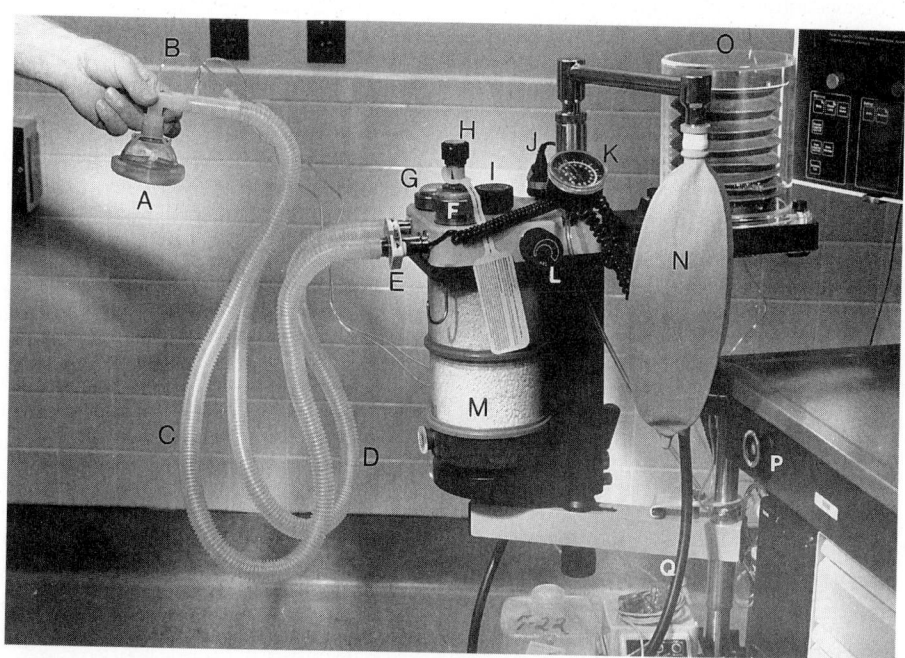

FIG. 6-13 A typical circle system. **A,** Patient mask. **B,** Sensing lines for respiratory and anesthetic gases monitor. **C,** Expiratory limb of patient circuit. **D,** Inspiratory limb of patient circuit. **E,** Flowmeter sensor for expired gases. **F,** One-way expiratory valve. **G,** One-way inspiratory valve. **H,** Adjustable Positive End Expiratory Pressure (PEEP) valve. **I,** Reservoir bag/ventilator selector valve. **J,** F_IO_2 sensor. **K,** Airway pressure gauge. **L,** Adjustable Pressure Limiting (APL) or "pop-off" valve. **M,** CO_2 absorber. **N,** Reservoir ("breathing") bag. **O,** Ventilator. **P,** O_2 flush valve. **Q,** Fresh gas supply hose. Courtesy Scott & White Memorial Hospital, Temple, Tex.

REGIONAL ANESTHESIA

Preoperative preparation for regional anesthesia is essentially the same as for general anesthesia. Preoperative medication is ordered frequently before regional anesthesia to blunt any discomfort that may be experienced during placement of the block. The criteria for monitoring during regional anesthesia is also similar to general anesthesia. Whenever regional anesthesia is performed, resuscitative equipment and drugs must be immediately available. Regional anesthesia (also called conduction anesthesia) can be accomplished by injecting a local anesthetic anywhere along the pathway of a nerve from the spinal cord (spinal anesthesia), epidurally, peripherally, or topically.

During preparation and placement of the regional anesthetic, the perioperative nurse usually provides valuable assistance. This may include: placing the appropriate monitors such as pulse oximetry, ECG, and blood pressure; providing supplemental O₂ if indicated; reassuring the patient; administering sedation such as midazolam as directed; and properly positioning the patient which is crucial for a successful block. Peripheral blocks on the lower or upper extremities or on the head are frequently done in a holding area to allow adequate time for the local anesthetic to penetrate the peripheral nerve before the patient is transferred to the OR. For peripheral blocks, the perioperative nurse may aspirate during needle placement (to detect vascular puncture) and inject the local anesthetic while the anesthesiologist is stabilizing the needle in the precise location. After an initial period of evaluation by the anesthesiologist, the nurse may monitor the patient for any substantial change in vital signs or untoward reactions until the patient is transferred to the OR. For regional anesthesia as well as general anesthesia, an anesthesia provider continuously monitors the patient during the surgical procedure.

SPINAL ANESTHESIA

A local anesthetic (usually lidocaine, tetracaine, or bupivacaine) injected into the cerebral spinal fluid (CSF) in the subarachnoid space is termed a spinal anesthetic. A spinal needle is usually inserted into a lower lumbar interspace with the patient either lying on one side or in a sitting position. The local anesthetic is generally mixed with a dextrose solution for a total of 1 to 4 ml to make a *hyperbaric* (heavier than the CSF) solution. These hyperbaric mixtures settle in a gravity-dependent manner following injection into the CSF. By changing the patient's position, the block can be directed up, down, or to one side of the spinal cord. For example, with prostate surgery the patient may remain in the sitting position for a minute or so after the local anesthetic is injected. A bilateral block of the S1-5 dermatomes results.

For surgery in the upper abdomen, the patient may be placed in a slightly (5 to 10°) head-down position to allow the anesthetic to move cephalad while the anesthesia provider carefully checks the level of sensory block. When an adequate level is obtained, the bed is leveled to minimize further spread. After 10 to 15 minutes, the block is usually

"set" and will not extend farther. The sympathetic nervous system is usually blocked two dermatomes higher and the neuromuscular system two dermatomes lower than the sensory block. The patient may then be positioned as necessary for surgery.

If the local anesthetic is mixed with a larger volume of sterile water, the solution will be *hypobaric* and the drug will move to the nondependent area. Hypobaric spinal anesthesia is usually done after the surgical site is positioned above the site of injection. By mixing the local anesthetic with some CSF withdrawn from the subarachnoid space, the solution becomes *isobaric*. Distribution of this solution is minimally affected by gravity.

Spinal anesthesia may evoke several physiologic responses that can result in major problems if not properly managed:

1. *Hypotension* may occur rapidly following injection of a local anesthetic solution into the subarachnoid space. It is caused by vasodilation as the sympathetic nerves that control vasomotor tone are blocked. This causes peripheral pooling of blood resulting in a reduced venous return to the heart and a decrease in cardiac output. The hypotensive response can usually be avoided by infusing 750-1500 ml of balanced salt solution immediately before the block and placing the patient in a 5° head-down position to improve venous return to the heart. A vasopressor such as ephedrine may also be administered.
2. *Total spinal* anesthesia (or an inadvertently high block) may cause paralysis of the respiratory muscles and necessitate immediate intubation and ventilation. Any symptom of respiratory distress occurring shortly after instituting spinal anesthesia should alert the anesthesia provider to the possibility of a high spinal.
3. *Positioning problems* can occur because pain and sensory inputs to a portion of the patient's body are blocked. Care must be taken in positioning the patient intraoperatively to avoid neurologic damage, burns, or other trauma.
4. *Post spinal cephalgia* or "postspinal or postdural puncture headache" is one of the most frequent postoperative complaints following spinal anesthesia. It occurs more commonly in young parturients or other individuals less than 40 years of age. The incidence is about 1% when a 25- or 26-gauge blunt-bevel needle is used. It is unrelated to how soon the patient is ambulated. The headache is thought to result from leakage of CSF through the hole in the dura, and typically occurs when the patient assumes an upright position. The incidence, severity, and duration of the headache appears to correlate with the size of the hole left in the dura. The headache is usually in the occipital area and generally resolves over 1 to 3 days but may last as long as 2 weeks. A variety of treatment modalities have been advocated to relieve the

headache including strict bedrest for 24 to 48 hours; vigorous hydration; abdominal binders; epidural infusion of saline; PO or IV caffeine; and injection of 5 to 20 ml of autologous blood into the epidural space at the puncture site (that is, a "blood patch").

Recently, many anesthesiologists have begun using different spinal needles, which have a tip shaped like a sharpened wood pencil with the hole on the side of the needle. These 24- or 25-gauge Sprotte or Whitacre spinal needles presumably separate or go between the dural fibers as opposed to cutting the fibers, which may occur when a blunt-bevel spinal needle is used. With these "pencil point" needles, the incidence and severity of postdural puncture headaches is extremely low.

EPIDURAL AND CAUDAL ANESTHESIA

The epidural space is located between the ligamentum flavum and the dura and extends from the foramen magnum to the sacrococcygeal membrane. This potential space is filled with epidural veins, fat, and loose areolar tissue. For epidural anesthesia the local anesthetic is usually injected through the intervertebral spaces in the lumbar region, although it can also be injected in the cervical or thoracic regions. The anesthetic spreads both cephalad and caudad from the site of injection. A comparative location of the needle points and injected anesthetic is shown in Fig. 6-14.

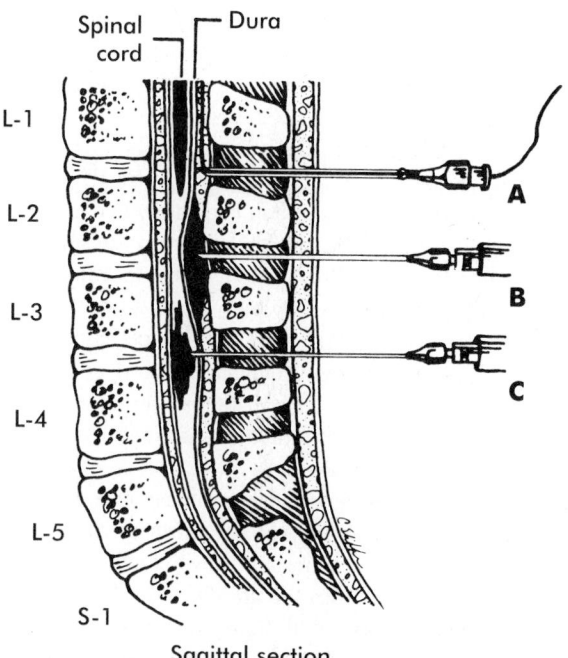

Sagittal section

FIG. 6-14 Location of needle point and injected anesthetic relative to dura. **A,** Epidural catheter. **B,** Single injection epidural. **C,** Spinal anesthesia. (Interspaces most commonly used are L4-5, L3-4, and L2-3.)

For caudal anesthesia the local anesthetic is also injected into the epidural space, but the approach is through the caudal canal in the sacrum. Compared to a lumbar epidural, this approach requires a greater volume of anesthetic to fill the epidural space. Caudal anesthesia has a 5 to 10% technical failure rate. However, due to the ease of administration, it is often employed for pediatric surgical procedures on the lower extremities or the perineal area.

Several techniques may be used for epidural or caudal anesthesia. A "single-shot epidural" involves administration of the local anesthesia through the needle before its removal. For intermittent injections or continuous infusions, a small catheter is inserted into the epidural space for administration of the local anesthetic.

Techniques used to identify the epidural space include the "hanging drop" and the "loss of resistance" to injection of either air or fluid as the needle is slowly advanced through the ligamentum flavum. With the hanging drop technique, the needle is filled with sterile saline or local anesthetic with a meniscus at the needle hub. As the needle is slowly advanced into the epidural space, the negative (less than atmospheric) pressure draws the fluid inward toward the epidural space. Location of the needle tip within the epidural space is verified by injection of an additional 1 to 2 ml of air or saline.

When local anesthetics are injected into the epidural space, the major sites of action are probably the nerve roots as they leave the spinal cord and proceed out the intervertebral foramina beyond the meningeal sheath. However, some of the anesthetic diffuses into the subarachnoid space to the spinal cord. Because local anesthetics diffuse away from the site of injection, segmental anesthesia may be possible in specific areas. In contrast to spinal anesthesia, much larger volumes of local anesthetic are needed with epidural anesthesia; the head-up, head-down, or lateral position of the patient does not have as much effect on the level of the epidural anesthetic; and the onset of anesthesia is much slower with epidural anesthesia. As with spinal anesthesia, hypotension can occur with epidural anesthesia, but the onset is much slower and usually can be managed with the rapid IV infusion of a balanced salt solution or repositioning of the patient.

The local anesthetics most frequently used for epidural anesthesia are lidocaine, bupivacaine, and chloroprocaine. Depending on the concentration of the anesthetic agent, the effect can range from loss of sensory input to complete motor blockade. To help verify that the anesthetic is not being injected into the subarachnoid space or into an epidural vein, a test dose of 3 to 5 ml of lidocaine with a 1:200,000 concentration of epinephrine is frequently used. Injected intravascularly, this test dose causes a transient tachycardia. If injected into the subarachnoid space, it produces a low level of spinal anesthesia. Complications associated with the use of local anesthetics in the epidural and subarachnoid spaces are unique to the agent used. Permanent neurologic sequelae have been reported when chloroprocaine was injected into the subarachnoid space. Bupivacaine is associated with marked cardiac toxicity if injected intravascularly.

With epidural anesthesia, several problems can occur:

1. *Inadvertent dural puncture* with the epidural needle (i.e., a *wet tap*) can cause a postdural puncture headache. This headache is significant in about 50% of patients, and the intensity can be incapacitating. Treatment is essentially the same as discussed previously for postspinal headache.
2. *Subarachnoid injection* occurs if the needle or catheter is unintentionally inserted into the subarachnoid space. If a large volume of local anesthetic is injected as a bolus, it causes "total spinal" anesthesia. This is associated with a rapid onset of hypotension caused by vasodilation, profound bradycardia as the sympathetic nerves to the heart are blocked, and a totally paralyzed and anesthetized patient. Treatment includes intubation, control of ventilation, support of blood pressure and the cardiovascular system, and administration of amnestic drugs until the block has resolved. If properly managed, this problem is not life-threatening, but use of the test dose described previously usually averts it.

   With patient movement over time, the epidural catheter may migrate through the dura. Therefore, a small test dose should be given each time additional local anesthetic is injected through the catheter. In addition, each subsequent dose should be injected in increments of 3 to 5 ml each.
3. *Vascular injection* of the local anesthetic into an epidural vein may inadvertently occur with the initial dose or with subsequent injections. As previously stated, intravenously injected bupivacaine is associated with cardiac arrest. Toxicity from other local anesthetics can cause sudden and profound hypotension, convulsions from the effects on the central nervous system, and tachycardia if the solution contains epinephrine. The convulsions usually dissipate rapidly as the local anesthetic is redistributed throughout the body. Intravenous thiopental or a benzodiazepine may be given to reduce these effects. A vasopressor (such as ephedrine or phenylephrine) can be used to restore blood pressure. If the patient becomes paralyzed, this may require intubation and ventilation until the toxic effects are gone. Use of the test dose with each injection usually prevents these problems.

PERIPHERAL NERVE BLOCKS

A wide variety of peripheral nerves can be effectively blocked by injecting local anesthetic around them to provide adequate surgical anesthesia. Onset and duration of the block are related to the drug used, its concentration and volume, and the addition of epinephrine. Complications are usually caused by an inadvertent intravascular injection or an overdose of the local anesthetic. Rarely, nerve damage may occur from trauma caused by the needle or compression from the volume of local anesthetic injected.

INTRAVENOUS REGIONAL ANESTHESIA

Intravenous regional anesthesia was first described by August Bier in 1908 and is frequently referred to as a *Bier block*. Although it can be used on a lower extremity, it is more often used on the upper extremities. It is highly reliable and easy to accomplish.

A small IV catheter is inserted as distally as feasible, and a single- or double-cuffed pneumatic tourniquet is placed around the limb proximal to the surgical site. The limb is raised upward, and the blood is then exsanguinated from the limb by wrapping it with an Esmarch bandage. The tourniquet is then inflated to approximately 100 mm Hg above the patient's systolic blood pressure, and the Esmarch bandage is removed. Approximately 50 ml of 0.5% lidocaine is injected through the catheter. Onset of anesthesia is rapid and lasts until the tourniquet is deflated.

When a double-cuffed pneumatic tourniquet is used, the proximal cuff is initially inflated. When the patient experiences discomfort from the cuff pressure (usually about 35 to 40 minutes after inflation of the cuff), the distal cuff, which is located over an anesthetized area, is inflated. Then the proximal cuff is deflated. The proximal cuff must remain inflated until the distal cuff has been inflated to prevent loss of the IV anesthetic from the limb. If the patient experiences pain from the tourniquet, an IV analgesic or sedative can be used to supplement the block.

Although problems can occur from an overdose or toxic reaction to the lidocaine, these are rare if the tourniquet has been inflated more than 20 minutes. The risk is also minimized by intermittently deflating the cuff for a few seconds at a time for several cycles when the surgical procedure is over. This reduces the transient peak blood level of the local anesthetic in the central nervous system and the heart. Obviously, loss of pneumatic pressure in the tourniquet can cause both a toxic reaction and a loss of anesthesia.

MONITORED ANESTHESIA CARE

A gentle and patient surgeon can safely accomplish minor and even some major procedures when the surgical site is infiltrated with a local anesthetic. This technique can be employed for normal, healthy individuals as well as sicker, unstable patients who may require extensive invasive monitoring and pharmacological management if general anesthesia is employed. For these patients, the issue is the relative risks and benefits of monitored anesthesia care (MAC) versus general anesthesia.

During MAC, the anesthesia provider may supplement the local anesthetic with an IV analgesic such as fentanyl and with sedative and amnestic drugs (such as midazolam or propofol). In addition, the anesthesia provider carefully monitors the patient's vital signs, respiratory and cardiovascular status, as well as positioning, and may give supplemental low-flow O_2. Depending on the clinical situation, the anesthesia provider may have to induce general anesthesia or utilize one of the regional techniques described previously if a greater degree of anesthesia is necessary.

LOCAL ANESTHESIA

For selected patients, a regional nerve block, "field" block, or infiltration with a local anesthetic is done by the surgeon. Other physicians such as cardiologists, pulmonologists, proctologists, or gastroenterologists may also schedule local procedures in the OR suite. No anesthesia provider is involved in the care of the patient in these circumstances.

For these patients, the physician may order a premedication. The physician is responsible for monitoring the patient and for administration of all perioperative drugs. The terms *local anesthesia, local,* and *straight local* are used interchangeably to describe these procedures. Hospitals and ambulatory facilities should have established guidelines for monitoring, perioperative drugs, and the types of procedures that can be done under local anesthesia. A perioperative nurse is usually responsible for monitoring the patient and administering medications as directed by the attending physician.

Patients receiving local anesthesia may have an IV infusion started before the procedure as adequate venous access can be critical in life-threatening situations when resuscitative drugs must be given immediately. Whenever feasible, intraoperative drugs are given intravenously, carefully titrated, and their effects are closely monitored.

The perioperative nurse should have a basic knowledge of the monitoring equipment that will be used, including the function, patient connections, and interpretation of the data. As a minimum, this monitoring should include an ECG, heart rate, blood pressure, and pulse oximetry.

The nurse should be familiar with the drugs to be administered during the procedure. This knowledge should include the usual dosages, limits on both the rate of injection and maximum dosage (usually stated on a per kilogram basis), the duration of action, the physiologic and psychologic changes to be expected, normal and abnormal reactions to the drugs used, and the appropriate action to take should an untoward reaction occur (Chapter 2). In addition to continuous or very frequent assessment of the patient's status, the vital signs should be recorded at least every 15 minutes. The drug dosage, route and time of administration, and the patient monitoring utilized should also be properly documented. Should any significant change occur in the patient's physiologic or psychologic status, the nurse should immediately notify the physician. Good communication is essential for optimal patient care. Because the patient is awake during the procedure, extraneous or irrelevant conversation and noise pollution should be kept to a minimum.

Following completion of the procedure, the patient's postoperative status must be carefully assessed. The patient may be transferred to the Day Surgery area, to the PACU for recovery and observation, or returned directly to the hospital room. This evaluation and decision should be properly documented on the chart, and a report called to the receiving unit before the patient's transfer. The report should include the type and amount of drugs given as well as any adverse reaction noted, the site and condition of the IV infusion (if applicable), the type and amount of solution infused in the OR, the range of intraoperative vital signs, the surgical procedure performed, and the condition of the dressing. Any special postoperative orders, allergies, and a general statement of the patient's tolerance of the procedure should also be included.

PAIN MANAGEMENT

Because of their experience in analgesia and regional anesthesia, many anesthesiologists have applied this expertise to the management of both acute and chronic pain. Chronic pain is often a multifactorial entity that may occur following a discrete injury or trauma, an amputation, laminectomy, or other surgical procedure. It may also result from prolonged repetitive stress such as "low back pain." Chronic pain frequently has a complex psychologic component that is unrecognized by patients or those closely associated with them. Diagnosis and treatment of such chronic pain problems usually involves multiple medical disciplines and prolonged management.

Management of acute perioperative pain is a different problem. Traditionally, postoperative pain has been treated with IM narcotics every 3 to 6 hours as needed. This is often associated with undesirable side effects including oversedation, respiratory depression, deep venous thrombosis secondary to decreased mobility, and variable degrees of pain relief. Recently, other modalities have been used successfully. Patient controlled analgesia (PCA) is a technique that utilizes a programmable electronic pump, which can continuously infuse a small amount of IV narcotic (basal rate) and, in addition, allows the patient to administer a predetermined bolus "on demand." Safety interlocks limit the frequency of the boluses and the total dose per hour.

When spinal or epidural anesthesia is employed for a surgical procedure, small amounts of a preservative-free narcotic such as fentanyl, sufentanil, or morphine may be added to the local anesthetic mixture. The narcotics act via central receptors and provide analgesia for 24 to 36 hours.

More recently, continuous epidural analgesia is used for prolonged postoperative pain management. This technique is employed for extensive procedures including total hip or knee replacements, knee reconstruction, and major abdominal or thoracic operations. It can also be used for acute trauma such as multiple rib fractures.

Typically, a lumbar or thoracic epidural catheter is inserted before surgery, covered with a transparent occlusive dressing, and injected with local anesthetic. Because of the duration, manipulation, or positioning required for the operative procedure, general anesthesia is often induced for patient comfort. The epidural markedly reduces the analgesic requirements of general anesthesia. For pain control postoperatively, the epidural infusion of local anesthetic is usually ⅛ to ⅟₁₆ the concentration used for surgical anesthesia. A small dose of preservative-free narcotic such as fentanyl, sufentanil, or morphine is often added to enhance analgesia. After the surgical procedure, the infusion rate is adjusted to provide analgesia during the early recovery phase. As the level of pain decreases over time, the infusion rate is reduced. The catheter is removed after 2 to 5 days to minimize the risk of infection. Benefits of epidural analgesia for acute postoperative pain include good analgesia with minimal sedation, early ambulation and physical therapy, and excellent patient satisfaction. Side effects that may occur include nausea, pruritus, and areas of slight numbness. These are controlled with drugs such as diphenhydramine (Benadryl) or Naloxone (Narcan), and by adjusting the infusion rate. A nonsteroidal antiinflammatory drug (NSAID) such as ketorolac (Toradol) is frequently given for any "breakthrough pain" instead of increasing the epidural infusion.

A single caudal injection is often used in pediatric patients having surgery of the lower abdomen, pelvis, or lower extremities. It is usually administered after the induction of general anesthesia, and a long-acting local anesthetic such as bupivacaine with epinephrine is typically used. This provides good analgesia for 8 to 24 hours postoperatively as well as markedly decreasing the intraoperative requirements for general anesthesia.

Epidural infusions have also been used for patients suffering from the intense pain of terminal malignancies. These patients may experience pain that is often so severe that parental analgesics provide inadequate pain relief and produce marked respiratory depression. Epidural infusions for prolonged periods of time have been used in these patients. Transdermal fentanyl patches may also be used in these patients as well as for chronic pain.

TEMPERATURE CONTROL

Increased attention has been directed toward maintaining a normal temperature perioperatively for both pediatric and adult patients. The room temperature can be raised and infrared warming lights used for pediatric patients. Lower fresh-gas flowrates of cool, dry, anesthetic gases can be used. A heat and moisture exchanger (such as HumidiVent) or a heated nebulizer helps to maintain the heat and moisture of inspired gases. Thermia blankets with circulating warm or cool liquid can be placed under or over the patient. A variety of IV fluid warmers are available to warm refrigerated blood products or crystalloid solutions. Some of these units originally designed for major trauma procedures will warm fluids at flowrates up to 500 ml per minute. Blanket-type units that blow heated air onto the upper or lower body surface are also available. These units are usually effective in maintaining body temperature even during a large abdominal procedure and can also be used in the PACU (Chapter 8).

MALIGNANT HYPERTHERMIA

First identified in the late 1960s, malignant hyperthermia (MH) is a rare, life-threatening complication that may be triggered by drugs commonly used in anesthesia. Inhalational anesthetics and succinylcholine are the most frequently implicated triggering agents. Malignant hyperthermia perhaps may also be induced by trauma, strenuous exercise, or emotional stress. It is a multifactorial disease and is genetically transmitted as an autosomal dominant trait with variable expression in affected individuals. Recent studies in a specific breed of MH-susceptible swine have shown a defect in the ryanodine receptor in the calcium release channel from the sarcoplasmic reticulum. However, the genetic identification is far more complex in humans, although a point mutation on chromosome 19 (ryanodine receptor) does occur in some MH-susceptible humans. There is an increased incidence of MH in patients with central core disease (a congenital myopathy) and a number of muscular dystrophies.

The syndrome begins with a hypermetabolic condition in skeletal muscle cells that involves altered mechanisms of calcium function at the cellular level. Characteristics of the syndrome include cellular hypermetabolism resulting in hypercarbia, tachypnea, tachycardia, hypoxia, metabolic and respiratory acidosis, cardiac dysrhythmias, and elevation of body temperature at a rate of 1 to 2° C every 5 minutes. It must be emphasized that the rise in body temperature is one of the late manifestations of MH. These signs may occur during induction or maintenance of anesthesia, although the syndrome can occur postoperatively or even after repeated exposures to anesthesia. It is most frequently seen in children and adolescents. The signs and symptoms associated with MH are listed in Box 6-4.

It is important to remember that: (1) MH is a rare, multifaceted syndrome and it can have variable clinical presentations; (2) many of the signs and symptoms associated with

---

BOX 6-4

Signs and Symptoms Often Seen with Malignant Hyperthermia

1. Hypercarbia
2. Tachycardia
3. Tachypnea (may not be seen in a paralyzed patient)
4. Muscle stiffness or rigidity
5. Hypoxia and dark (desaturated) blood in operative field
6. Unstable or elevated blood pressure
7. Cardiac dysrhythmias
8. Changes in CO_2 absorbant (↑ temperature, color)
9. Metabolic and respiratory acidosis
10. Peripheral mottling, cyanosis, or sweating
11. Rising body temperature (1-2° C every 5 min)
12. Myoglobinuria
13. Hyperkalemia, hypercalcemia, lacticemia
14. Marked elevation in creatinine phosphokinase (may exceed 20,000 units in initial 12-24 hours)

MH can have other causes; and (3) other disorders, such as neuroleptic malignant syndrome (NMS), may also have similar presentations. The NMS occurs after use of neuroleptic drugs (such as haloperidol) and is characterized by muscular rigidity, akinesia, hyperthermia, and autonomic dysfunction. Because MH is such a life-threatening disorder, many anesthesia providers will initiate treatment protocol when some of these early signs and symptoms occur that cannot otherwise be readily explained.

Time is crucial when MH is diagnosed. All OR and anesthesia personnel should be familiar with the protocol for its management. In the past, mortality ranged up to 80%, but the immediate infusion of dantrolene and proper treatment have reduced the incidence of fatalities to about 7%. Dantrolene (Dantrium) is a hydantoin skeletal muscle relaxant that also has effects on vascular and heart muscle. It is postulated that dantrolene alters the calcium transfer into the sarcoplasmic reticulum. In addition to dantrolene, the major modalities of treatment include cooling the patient with ice packs and cold IV solutions, administering diuretics, treating cardiac dysrhythmias, correcting the acid-base and electrolyte imbalances, and monitoring fluid intake and output and the body temperature. Many hospitals maintain an emergency MH kit or cart that contains the drugs, laboratory tubes, other supplies, and instructions to treat MH in the OR area. Location of the iced or cold saline and other equipment should also be listed with the emergency kit. Chilled saline is often kept in the refrigeration unit for blood products. An outline for emergency treatment of MH is given in Box 6-5. The Malignant Hyperthermia Association of the United States (MHAUS) has names of on-call physicians available for consultation in MH emergencies at (209) 634-4917: INDEX ZERO. For patient referral or nonemergency calls, (203) 847-0407 should be used.

BOX 6-5

Emergency Management of Malignant Hyperthermia

1. Immediately discontinue all triggering agents (inhalational anesthetics and succinylcholine).
2. Terminate surgery if possible or continue with safe anesthetic drugs.
3. Hyperventilate with 100% O_2 at highest flowrate.
4. Immediately give dantrolene sodium (Dantrium) 2.5 mg/kg IV. Give additional incremental doses up to 10-20 mg/kg total until the signs of MH are controlled.
5. Give sodium bicarbonate IV to correct the metabolic acidosis. Use arterial blood gases (ABG). If ABG are not available, consider 1-2 mEq/kg.
6. If the patient is hyperthermic, begin active cooling.
   a. Inject iced saline (not Lactated Ringers) IV 15 ml/kg over 15 min × 3.
   b. Use iced saline to lavage stomach, bladder, rectum and open body cavities as feasible.
   c. Cool the body surface with a thermia blanket. Rub with cold, wet towels or ice.
   d. Monitor the temperature to avoid hypothermia.
7. Cardiac dysrhythmias usually resolve with correction of acidosis and hyperkalemia. If not, anti-dysrhythmic agents such as procainamide 3 mg/kg (max of 15 mg/kg) may be used. Avoid calcium entry blockers because they may cause hyperkalemia and cardiovascular collapse.
8. Closely monitor temperature, $ETCO_2$, arterial and central venous blood gases, urine output and myoglobin, K^+, Ca^{++}, lactate, CK, and coagulation studies. Insert a urinary catheter. Consider arterial line and a central venous or PA catheter.
9. Hyperkalemia is common. Treat with hyperventilation, sodium bicarbonate, or 10 units of regular insulin in 50 ml of D_{50} IV titrated to K^+ level or regular insulin 0.15 units/kg and glucose 0.5 g/kg. Life-threatening hyperkalemia may also be treated with calcium (e.g., 2.5 mg/kg of $CaCL_2$).
10. Maintain urine output above 2 mg/kg/hr. Consider volume, mannitol, and furosemide.
11. Males less than 9 years old who have a sudden cardiac arrest after succinylcholine without hypoxia may have subclinical muscular dystrophy. Treat for acute hyperkalemia first. Give $CaCL_2$ with other treatments in #9 above.
12. Transfer patient to ICU when stable. Monitor at least 24 hours for recurrence of MH and for late complications.
13. Administer dantrolene 1 mg/kg IV every 6 hours for 24-48 hours. Then oral dantrolene 1 mg/kg every 6 hours for 24 hours may be given as necessary.
14. Monitor core body temperature (continuously), ABG, K^+, Ca^{++}, CK, serum and urine myoglobin, and coagulation studies until they return to normal.
15. Counsel the patient and family about MH and further precautions. Refer the patient to MHAUS and complete an Adverse Metabolic Reaction to Anesthesia (AMRA) report to the North American Malignant Hyperthermia Registry at (717) 531-6936.
16. MHAUS 24 hour hotline: (209) 634-4917: INDEX ZERO.

After Emergency Therapy for Malignant Hyperthermia, revised 1993. Malignant Hyperthermia Association of the United States (MHAUS).

Patients known or suspected to have this syndrome can be anesthetized with minimal risk if appropriate precautions are taken. If the syndrome is suspected, a muscle biopsy should be done to make a diagnosis before the patient is anesthetized. For their own safety, relatives of persons with MH should be evaluated and tested for presence of the syndrome.

SAFETY OF HEALTH CARE WORKERS

The transmission of diseases including hepatitis B and the human immunodeficiency virus (HIV) from body fluids is a major concern for health care workers in the perioperative setting. All health care workers should therefore observe universal precautions for all body fluids. It has been shown that blood, serum, and cerebrospinal fluid have higher concentrations of HIV than do saliva, tears, urine, breast milk, amniotic fluid, or vaginal secretions. Precautions include use of protective eye wear; face mask; latex gloves; and use of a needleless system, stopcocks, or one-way injection devices for all IV medications given to the patient.

OPERATING ROOM POLLUTION

Contamination and pollution of the OR environment can come from many sources. Every chemical should be considered potentially harmful until proven otherwise. Reaction to chemicals and irritants may vary with age, sex, race, season of the year, and concurrent exposure to other substances. Disinfectants, antiseptics, soaps, aerosol or pressurized sprays, and other compounds contribute to the potential for pollution. Recent attention is also being placed on noise pollution. Of particular interest in the present context is the pollution of the OR with anesthetic gases such as N_2O and the halogenated agents halothane, enflurane, isoflurane, and desflurane. Various surveys taken among personnel exposed to these anesthetic gases (anesthesia providers, other anesthesia personnel, perioperative nurses, dentists, and dental assistants who work with anesthetic gases) and their spouses have implicated such pollution as a possible contributing factor to an increased abortion rate and incidence of lymphoma and other conditions. However, the interpretation of these surveys is controversial.

To minimize the hazards of bacteria and other airborne pollutants, as well as waste anesthetic gases, many OR suites receive 100% fresh "conditioned" air with up to 25 air exchanges each hour. To reduce pollution from trace anesthetic gases and contain costs, many anesthesia providers use "low-flow" anesthetic techniques that greatly reduce the volume of waste gases. However, air pollution with waste anesthetic gases is still a major concern, and all anesthesia machines should have a waste gas scavenging system. In modern OR suites, a dedicated vacuum line is used to scavenge such gases. One such scavenging system is shown in Fig. 6-15. It includes: (1) a reservoir bag so that

less instantaneous vacuum is needed; (2) a positive-pressure relief valve that prevents excessive back pressure in the patient's lungs and that vents excess gas into the room air should the vacuum be occluded or inadequate; (3) a negative-pressure relief valve that prevents excessive vacuum from damaging the patient's lungs; and (4) a needle valve to adjust the vacuum. Evacuation hoses are connected to the ventilator and the adjustable pressure limiting (APL) valve. When the patient is not intubated, however, air pollution may occur from a loose mask fit on the patient's face. According to the National Institute for Occupational Safety and Health (NIOSH), pollution levels should be less than

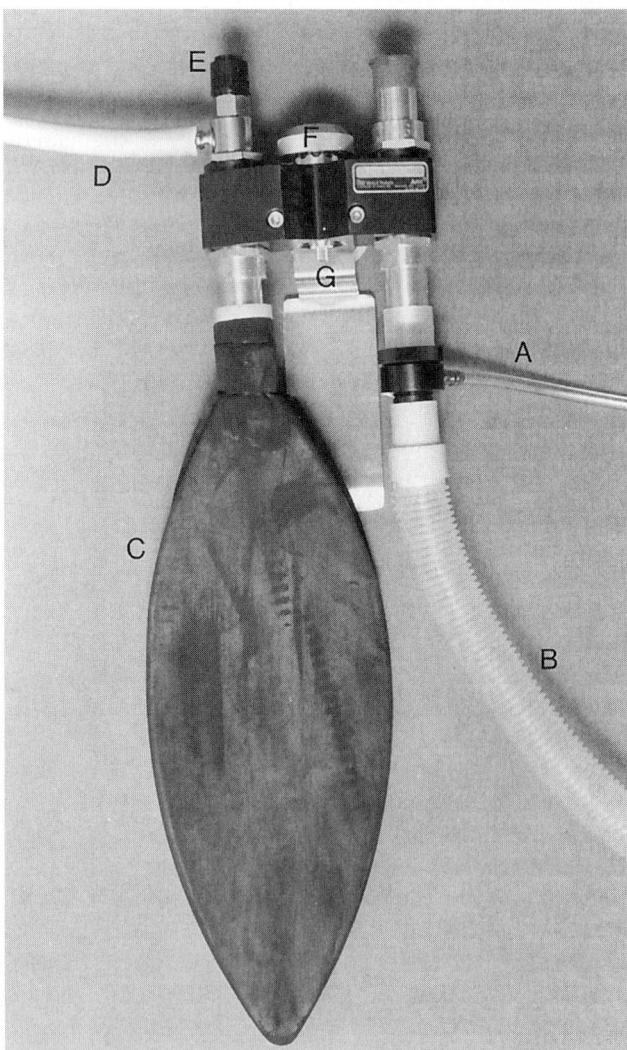

FIG. 6-15 A typical scavenging system for waste anesthetic gases. **A,** Scavenging line from respiratory and anesthetic gases monitor. **B,** Scavenging hose from ventilator and APL valve. **C,** Reservoir bag. **D,** Vacuum line to hospital scavenging exhaust system. **E,** Vacuum adjustment valve. **F,** Positive-pressure relief valve. **G,** Negative-pressure relief valve.

Courtesy Scott & White Memorial Hospital, Temple, Tex.

25 ppm (time-weighted average) for N_2O and 2 ppm for halogenated agents. These levels are difficult to achieve during induction and emergence.

Chronic occupational exposure to trace concentrations of anesthetic gases is of particular concern to pregnant women. A safe exposure level below which one can be assured that no adverse effects will occur has not been established. Individuals with questions about exposure levels should consult a knowledgeable member of the anesthesia department for the latest information.

PERIOPERATIVE NURSING CONSIDERATIONS RELATED TO ANESTHESIA

Care of the surgical patient is a cooperative effort, and personnel involved in the perioperative period should function as a smooth, well-coordinated team. The nurse who checks the chart must verify the patient's identity and the scheduled procedure, confirm that the operative permit is properly signed, identify any patient allergies, and ensure that current reports of laboratory tests and diagnostic studies are complete and on the chart.

In many OR suites a preoperative preparation or *holding area* is utilized for procedures such as the insertion of arterial, central venous, or pulmonary artery catheters and placement of epidural catheters or peripheral nerve blocks. This area may be staffed by nursing personnel from the OR, PACU, or the Department of Anesthesiology. The purpose of this area is to optimize the flow of patients through the OR and to provide support services for the above procedures. The minimum requirement for available monitoring should be an ECG, noninvasive blood pressure, and pulse oximetry. Equipment for emergency airway management should be readily available. It is important that the nursing staff be familiar with such equipment and be readily available to assist in its utilization.

A patient should never be left alone in the OR suite. For example, when there is an anesthetized patient in the OR, a perioperative nurse should always be immediately available to provide assistance if needed. During the insertion of IV, arterial, central venous, or pulmonary artery catheters, the nurse should assist as appropriate.

During induction of anesthesia, particularly with a traumatized patient or for an emergency procedure, the nurse should be ready to apply cricoid pressure to prevent regurgitation of stomach contents and assist the anesthesia provider in visualizing the vocal cords. When cricoid pressure is used to prevent aspiration, it should not be released until the intubation is accomplished, the cuff on the endotracheal tube inflated, and proper placement of the endotracheal tube has been verified. However, when two anesthesia providers are present, one of them will usually provide this support.

Operating room personnel should never move an unconscious patient without first coordinating the positioning or move with the anesthesia provider. When the patient is positioned for surgery, the nurse should always check the arms and legs to ensure that no pressure points exist and that the extremities are appropriately positioned and padded (Chapter 4).

Before transporting the patient from the OR to the PACU, the circulating nurse should call the PACU and give a preliminary status report of the patient's condition. This report includes the surgical procedure performed, type of anesthesia care provided, information specific to the patient's preoperative diagnosis and subsequent outcome related to intraoperative intervention, and any special equipment required (such as a ventilator, T-piece, or arterial pressure monitors).

POSTANESTHESIA RECOVERY

Recovery from anesthesia usually takes place in the *recovery room,* which is now designated the Postanesthesia Care Unit (PACU). Critically ill patients are usually transferred directly to the Surgical Intensive Care Unit (SICU) for recovery and postoperative management. The PACU should be immediately adjacent to the OR suite for rapid access by the anesthesiologist in case any untoward event occurs. The PACU is staffed (ideally one nurse per patient) by nurses specially trained in the prompt recognition and management of postoperative complications. Equipment, support, and drugs available for routine postoperative care should include supplemental O_2, suction, monitors, expertise in treatment of common problems, as well as for full resuscitation if necessary.

When the patient arrives in the PACU, the anesthesia provider gives the receiving PACU nurse pertinent information including the name, age, surgical procedure and complications, type of anesthesia, preoperative medications and anesthetic drugs, preoperative and intraoperative vital signs, estimated blood loss, intraoperative fluid intake and output, allergies, orders for analgesia during recovery, and any special instructions. Any analgesics, sedatives, or other drugs given in the PACU are usually ordered by the anesthesia staff.

The initial vital signs and patient status in the PACU are usually recorded on the anesthesia record. Supplemental O_2 (2-5 L/min) is usually given via nasal cannulae. Vital signs are recorded every 15 minutes or less and charted with other pertinent information on a separate PACU record. To facilitate recovery from general anesthesia, the PACU nurse encourages the patient to wake up, cough, breathe deeply, and change positions. For a summary of the patient's recovery, many institutions use some variation of the postanesthesia recovery score (PARS) originally proposed by Aldrete. The PARS is recorded every 15 to 30 minutes until discharge. A score of 9 or 10 usually indicates that the patient is ready for transfer to the postoperative nursing unit. The parameters typically evaluated are shown in Fig. 6-16. The patient is evaluated and discharged from the PACU by an anesthesiologist. In some hospitals, the patient may be

Criteria for Postanesthesia Recovery Score		Time										
		Arrival										
ACTIVITY												
Able to move 4 extremities voluntarily or on command	= 2											
Able to move 2 extremities voluntarily or on command	= 1											
Able to move 0 extremities voluntarily or on command	= 0											
RESPIRATION												
Able to deep breathe and cough freely	= 2											
Dyspnea or limited breathing	= 1											
Apneic	= 0											
CIRCULATION												
BP ≤ 20% of preanesthetic level	= 2											
BP ± 20 to 50% of preanesthetic level	= 1											
BP ≥ 50% of preanesthetic level	= 0											
CONSCIOUSNESS												
Fully awake	= 2											
Arousable on calling	= 1											
Not responding	= 0											
SKIN COLOR												
Pink	= 2											
Pale, dusky, blotchy, jaundiced, other	= 1											
Cyanotic	= 0											
TOTALS												

TIME														
PACU Score	Activity									**ACTIVITY**		**RESPIRATION**		
	Respiration									Moves 4 extremities		Deep breath & cough		2
	Circulation									Moves 2 extremities		Dyspnea/Limited breathing		1
	Conscious									Moves 0 extremities		Apneic		0
	Skin Color									**CIRCULATION**		**SKIN COLOR**		
	TOTALS									BP ≤ 20% preanesth		Pink, warm to touch		2
REMARKS										BP ± 20-50% preanesth		Pale, cool to touch		1
										BP ≥ 50% preanesth		Cyanotic, clammy to touch		0
										CONSCIOUSNESS				
										Awake, converses, appr. falls asleep at intervals				2
										Arouses on calling, obeys simple commands				1
										Not responding, non-reactive				0

FIG. 6-16   Postanesthetic recovery score factors and a condensed format.

Modified from Aldrete, J.A., and Kroulik, D. (1970). *Anesthesia and Analgesia,* 49:924.

transferred from the PACU by meeting written discharge criteria established by the Department of Anesthesiology.

COMMON PROBLEMS

A number of problems can occur during recovery from anesthesia. The PACU nurse must be aware of the potential problems and frequently assess the patient's status so that early interventional therapy can be initiated.

Nausea and vomiting

Nausea is believed to be caused by stimulation of the vomiting center in the medulla by impulses from the gastrointestinal tract, other cerebral centers, or by drugs. It occurs more frequently in females than males. Contributing factors include a history of motion sickness, phase of menstrual cycle, pain, perioperative medications, anesthetic technique, gastric distention, duration of surgery, surgical site (upper abdomen or thorax more than lower abdomen or extremities), perioperative hypotension, respiratory insufficiency, obesity, patient positioning, and rapid patient movement.

Prophylactic perioperative measures that decrease the incidence of nausea and the risk of aspiration include nonparticulate antacids (0.3 M sodium citrate), H_2 antagonists (cimetidine or ranitidine) to reduce gastric acid secretion, gastrokinetic agents (metoclopramide) to improve gastric emptying, scopolamine patches, droperidol, and ondansetron (Zofran—a new serotonin receptor blocking drug). The choice of anesthetic agents and drugs will also significantly affect the incidence of nausea and vomiting.

Postoperative management for nausea is directed toward minimizing rapid patient movements, prompt and satisfactory relief of pain, ensuring adequate respiratory function and stable vital signs, use of antiemetics, and prevention of aspiration.

Pain

Unsatisfactory pain relief is a common complaint from patients. An adequate amount of promptly administered analgesics is necessary for satisfactory pain control. Generally, all medications in the PACU should be given IV because the absorption and onset of IM drugs are delayed and highly variable. Newer methods of pain relief, including the intraspinal and epidural administration of narcotics and patient-controlled analgesia (PCA), are discussed in the section on Pain Management. Studies have shown that these newer modalities result in shorter ICU and hospital stays and a decrease in the total amount of drug required.

Alteration in mental status

Abnormal neurologic function is common in the first hour. Agitation, shivering, hyperreflexia, hypertonicity, and clonus are frequently observed. Common causes include pain, respiratory dysfunction, gastric or urinary distention, perioperative medications, anesthetic technique, electrolyte imbalance (e.g., dilutional hyponatremia after

prostatic resection), drug abuse, and preexisting psychologic factors. These changes usually resolve with additional recovery time and treatment of the contributing factors. However, sedation and restraint of the patient may be necessary on an interim basis.

Hypoxemia

Hypoxemia is defined as inadequate oxygenation of the blood or a decrease in the arterial O_2 content. Hyperoxia is rarely a problem in the PACU except with premature infants or adults with prolonged (greater than 24 hours) exposure to F_1O_2 above 0.5 (O_2 concentration greater than 50%). Increasing age, obesity, preexisting pulmonary disease, and smoking increase the risk of hypoxemia. The use of pulse oximetry has greatly diminished the incidence of hypoxemia in the PACU. The causes of hypoxemia can be organized as problems with (1) O_2 delivery to the lungs; (2) the pulmonary system; or (3) delivery of O_2 from the lungs to the tissues.

Inadequate F_1O_2 can reduce the amount of O_2 delivered to the lungs. Hypercarbia can displace O_2 in the alveoli. Obstruction of the airway is a common cause of hypoxemia. Pharyngeal obstruction is usually caused by the tongue, surgery on the head or neck with resultant edema, or abnormal anatomy. Management includes supplemental O_2, anterior displacement of the mandible, positioning the patient on the side, or use of an oral or nasal airway. Laryngeal obstruction can be caused by spasm, edema, secretions triggering glottic response, or surgery on the airway. Management includes supplemental O_2 or a mixture of helium and O_2, suctioning of secretions, positive airway pressure with a mask or assisted ventilation, racemic epinephrine, or reintubation. Hemorrhage after neck surgery or carotid endarterectomy can also cause acute obstruction of the airway. The anesthesia provider and surgeon should be notified immediately. Emergency intubation may be required.

Pulmonary causes of hypoxemia are numerous. Hypoventilation secondary to drugs, splinting from surgical pain (particularly of the upper abdomen or thorax), obesity, or positioning can reduce oxygenation. Intrapulmonary shunting of blood past obstructed or poorly oxygenated alveoli reduces the O_2 content of arterial blood. Difficulties in the diffusion of O_2 from the alveoli to arterial blood can be caused by atelectasis, aspiration, adult respiratory distress syndrome, bronchospasm caused by allergies or asthma, pulmonary edema, pneumonia, pneumothorax, or pulmonary embolism.

Changes in the delivery of O_2 from the lungs to the tissues usually result from inadequate cardiac output, bleeding, hypovolemia, or anemia. Increased O_2 consumption from fever, or disease processes such as malignant hyperthermia, thyrotoxicosis, or sepsis can occur.

If the simple maneuvers discussed previously do not improve the oxygenation, the anesthesia provider should be called immediately.

Carbon dioxide elimination

Hypoventilation is one of the most common problems that results in an increase in $PaCO_2$. Changes in $PaCO_2$ can be confirmed by arterial blood gases or recognized by $ETCO_2$ monitoring which is not routine in the PACU unless the patient is intubated. Causes of hypoventilation include the operative procedure and surgical site, preexisting pulmonary disease, depression of the respiratory center (by narcotics, sedatives, or residual anesthetics), obesity, disease states, and muscle weakness secondary to residual muscle relaxant. Increased CO_2 production may occur with shivering, hyperthermia, or excitement on emergence. Treatment should begin with determination of the cause, and then appropriate management should be initiated. Tachypnea causing a decrease in $PaCO_2$ is rarely a problem in the PACU but can be caused by splinting with pain or anxiety.

Hypotension

Verification of the blood pressure (e.g., properly sized BP cuff, transducer calibration) and an assessment of the rapidity of the change are essential in the initial diagnosis and management of hypotension. Hemodynamic stabilization of the patient may be necessary before the precipitating factors can be determined. Possible causes can be organized as problems with preload to the heart, intracardiac difficulties, cardiac afterload, and miscellaneous factors.

A decreased preload secondary to hypovolemia is probably the most common cause of hypotension in the PACU. Hemorrhage or inadequate fluid replacement should be considered first, but decreased venous return (position, compression of major vessels, pulmonary embolism, or pneumothorax) and response to drugs such as venodilators or diuretics must also be considered.

Intracardiac causes of hypotension include ischemia, hypoxia, myocardial infarction, dysrhythmias, congestive heart failure, cardiac tamponade, cardiomyopathy, valvular dysfunction, and the effects of myocardial depressants.

Decreased afterload can be caused by vasodilation from regional anesthetic techniques (such as spinal or epidural), drugs, allergic reactions, or transfusion reactions. Miscellaneous factors include septic shock and Addison's disease.

Treatment depends upon the diagnosis, but the ECG, peripheral pulses, jugular venous engorgement, changes or alterations in the cardiac or pulmonary auscultatory findings, and urinary output should be quickly evaluated.

Hypertension

As with hypotension, verification of the blood pressure and the rapidity of the change must be noted. Pain, hypoxia, hypercarbia, and preexisting hypertension are common causes. Other causes include anxiety, hypervolemia, bladder distention, drug effects, hypoglycemia (reflex sympathetic response), reflex vasoconstriction from hypothermia, autonomic hyperreflexia, and elevated intracranial pressure. Diseases such as malignant hyperthermia, thyrotoxicosis, or pheochromocytoma can also cause acute hypertension.

Treatment of hypertension depends upon the etiology and the rapidity of onset. Unless the cause can be readily identified (for example, pain, hypoxia, hypercarbia, or bladder distention), the anesthesia provider should be notified immediately.

Cardiac dysrhythmias

Multiple cardiac dysrhythmias can occur postoperatively. Common predisposing factors include (1) preexisting cardiac disease; (2) pain; (3) hypothermia; (4) respiratory dysfunction resulting in hypoxia, hypercarbia, or acidosis; and (5) imbalance of fluids, electrolytes, or acid-base status. If the dysrhythmias produce patient symptoms, the anesthesia provider should be notified immediately. Additional information related to postoperative patient care can be found in Chapter 8.

ANESTHESIA FOR AMBULATORY SURGERY

In recent years increasing numbers of surgical procedures have been performed on an ambulatory basis. Many health professionals believe that ambulatory surgery will soon comprise 60 to 80% of all elective surgery. Reasons for this change include evolving concepts for delivery of health care, a significant reduction in the overall cost for such surgical procedures, new surgical techniques such as endoscopic procedures, shorter acting anesthetic agents, an increased emphasis on personal attention to patients' needs, and the overwhelming satisfaction of patients who have ambulatory surgery. Depending on many factors, ambulatory surgery may be performed in a regular OR, elsewhere in the same facility, in a separate building adjacent to the hospital, or at a freestanding facility not directly associated with a hospital.

In addition, for an increasing number of major procedures, the patients are processed through the day surgery area, but postoperatively are admitted for observation of less than 24 hours or transferred to regular hospital units or ICUs. This practice not only reduces health care costs, but also provides the patient with a more restful night preoperatively. As postoperative hospitalization is scheduled in advance, these patients are not true ambulatory patients. To distinguish them from inpatients, however, these patients and procedures are frequently called *ambulatory-observation, ambulatory-admit, ambulatory-inpatient, A.M. admit,* or *admission day surgery.*

Although the anesthetic technique may be similar for inpatient and ambulatory surgery, the concepts of anesthesia care are very different. Because ambulatory surgery is usually reserved for relatively healthy individuals, the preoperative evaluation may be done several days before the surgery, on the day of surgery, or by telephone. Many laboratory tests and diagnostic studies, such as electrocardiograms and chest x-rays, are no longer done routinely before ambulatory surgery because they have not been shown to be cost-effective for healthy asymptomatic individuals. In most instances, the commonly used preoperative medications are omitted because they tend to prolong the postoperative recovery period and may have residual effects for 1 to 3 days after surgery. The goal is to provide high-quality health care in a pleasant, personal, safe, and expeditious manner with minimal disruption of the patient's usual level of activity.

One typical scenario illustrates the general concepts of ambulatory surgery. After an examination in the physician's office, the patient and physician agree that the surgery is needed. A specialized history and physical examination form is completed by the surgeon and the consent for the operation is signed and witnessed. The patient is given a brochure about ambulatory surgery and then scheduled for the elective procedure. Two to five days before the scheduled surgery date, the patient visits the ambulatory surgery center for a preoperative interview, appropriate laboratory tests, and diagnostic studies. An evaluation by the anesthesiologist may take place on that day or on the day of surgery. The patient is instructed regarding NPO status. On the day of surgery, the patient arrives 1 hour before the procedure and changes into a surgical gown plus a robe. In the preoperative area a nursing assessment is done, an IV infusion is started and the patient reads magazines, listens to music, or visits with family or friends until going to the OR. In the OR, the induction of anesthesia using short-acting anesthetic drugs commences. After surgery, the patient is transferred to a stretcher and taken to the phase I PACU. When recovered sufficiently, the patient is assisted to the phase II recovery area and sits in a reclining chair. A family member or responsible adult joins the patient, and the patient may be offered water, ginger ale, cola, tea, or coffee. (Typically, in phase I PACU the patient remains on a stretcher or PACU bed until initially recovered from the effects of anesthesia and able to sit on the side of the bed. Phase II PACU provides a transitional period to ensure that the patient can sit up in a chair, ambulate, and is stable and sufficiently alert to leave the facility.) When ready to go home, the patient is evaluated by a physician or meets the established discharge criteria, and receives discharge instructions from the PACU nurse. A mail-in questionnaire is also given to the patient for comments about the ambulatory surgery experience. The patient may not drive and must be taken home by a responsible adult. Typical times from completion of surgery to discharge are 1½ to 2½ hours. Two to five days after surgery, a follow-up telephone call is made to the patient by one of the nursing staff.

FURTHER READING

The information presented in this chapter is intended to provide an overview of anesthesia concepts and practice.

This should give the perioperative nurse a general understanding of anesthesia care for the surgical patient. To provide additional information relating to anesthesia, some selected resources are listed in the bibliography under Anesthesiology. Some of these books may be available in your hospital library or may be borrowed from the Department of Anesthesiology. Other pertinent references to the topics discussed in this chapter are included in the General section of the bibliography.

BIBLIOGRAPHY

Anesthesiology

American Society of Anesthesiologists. (1992). *Recommendations for infection control for the practice of anesthesiology*. Park Ridge, Ill: A.S.A.

Anderton, J.M., Keen, R.I., & Neave, R. (1988). *Positioning the surgical patient*. Boston: Butterworths.

Atkinson, R.S. (1993). *Lee's synopsis of anaesthesia*, ed. 11. Bristol, England: Butterworths.

Atlee, J.L. (1989). *Perioperative cardiac dysrhythmias: mechanisms, recognition, management*. ed. 2. Chicago: Year Book Medical Publishers.

Barash, P.G., Cullen, B.F., & Stoelting, R.K. (1992). *Clinical anesthesia*, ed. 2. Philadelphia: J.B. Lippincott.

Benumof, J.L. (1992). *Anesthesia and perioperative complications*. St. Louis: Mosby.

Benumof, J.L. (1987). *Anesthesia for thoracic surgery*. Philadelphia: W.B. Saunders.

Berry, F.A. (1990). *Anesthetic management of difficult and routine pediatric patients*, ed. 2. New York: Churchill Livingstone.

Blitt, C.B. (1990). *Monitoring in anesthesia and critical care medicine*, ed. 2. New York: Churchill Livingstone.

Brown, D.L. (1992). *Atlas of regional anesthesia*. Philadelphia: W.B. Saunders.

Brown, D.L., editor (1992). *Risk and outcome in anesthesia*, ed. 2. Philadelphia: J.B. Lippincott.

Bruner, J.M.R., & Leonard, P.S. (1989). *Electricity, safety, and the patient*. Chicago: Year Book Medical Publishers.

Coté, C.J., Ryan, J.F., Todres, I.D., & Goudsouzian, N. (1993). *A practice of anesthesia for infants and children*, ed. 2. New York: Grune & Stratton.

Cousins, M.J., & Bridenbaugh, P.O. (1988). *Neural blockade in clinical anesthesia and management of pain*, ed. 2. Philadelphia: J.B. Lippincott.

Cucchiara, R.F, & Michenfelder, J.D., editors (1990). *Clinical neuroanesthesia*. New York: Churchill Livingstone.

Dornette, W.H.L. (1991). *Legal issues in anesthesia practice*. Philadelphia: F.A. Davis.

Dorsch, J.A., & Dorsch, S.E. (1993). *Understanding anesthesia equipment: construction, care and complications*, ed. 3. Baltimore: Williams & Wilkins.

Eger, E.I., II (1985). *Nitrous oxide/N_2O*. New York: Elsevier.

Ehrenwerth, J. & Eisenkraft, J.B. (1993). *Anesthesia equipment: Principles and applications*. St. Louis: Mosby.

Davison, J.K., Eckhardt, W.F. 3d, & Perese, D.A. (1993). *Clinical anesthesia procedures of the Massachusetts General Hospital*, ed. 4. Boston: Little, Brown & Co.

Gilman, A.G., & others (1990). *Goodman and Gilman's the pharmacological basis of therapeutics*, ed. 8. New York: McGraw-Hill.

Gravenstein, J.S. (1990). *Gas monitoring and pulse oximetry*. Boston: Butterworth-Heinemann.

Gravenstein, J.S. (1991). *Manual of complications during anesthesia*. Philadelphia: J.B. Lippincott.

Gravenstein, J.S. & Holzer, J.F., editors (1988). *Safety and cost containment in anesthesia*. Boston: Butterworths.

Gravenstein, J.S., Paulus, D.A., & Hayes, T.J. (1989). *Capnography in clinical practice*. Boston: Butterworths.

Greene, N. (1993). *Physiology of spinal anesthesia*, ed. 4, Baltimore: Williams & Wilkins.

Gregory, G.A. (1989). *Pediatric anesthesia*, ed. 2, New York: Churchill Livingstone.

Kaplan, J.A., editor (1993). *Cardiac anesthesia*, ed. 3, Philadelphia: W.B. Saunders.

Katz, J. & Steward, D.J. (1993). *Anesthesia and uncommon pediatric diseases*, ed. 2, Philadelphia: W.B. Saunders.

Keys, T.E. (1978). *The history of surgical anesthesia.* Huntington, N.Y.: Robert E. Krieger Publishing.

Longnecker, D.E., & Murphy, F.L. (1992). *Dripps/Eckenhoff/Vandam Introduction to anesthesia*, ed. 8, Philadelphia: W.B. Saunders.

Martin, J.T. (1987). *Positioning in anesthesia and surgery*, ed. 2, Philadelphia: W.B. Saunders.

Miller, R.D., editor (1990). *Anesthesia*, ed. 3, New York: Churchill Livingstone.

Mueller, R.A., & Lundberg, D.B.A. (1992). *Manual of drug interactions for anesthesiology*, ed. 2, New York: Churchill Livingstone.

Newfield, P., & Cottrell, J.E. (1991). *Handbook of neuroanesthesia: clinical and physiologic essentials*, ed. 2, Boston: Little Brown & Co.

Nimmo, W.S., editor (1994). *Anaesthesia*, ed. 2, London: Blackwell Scientific Publications.

Nunn, J.F., Utting, J.E., & Brown, B.R., Jr., editors (1989). *General anaesthesia*, ed. 5, Boston: Butterworths.

Raj, P.P. (1992). *Practical management of pain*, ed. 2, Chicago, Year Book Medical Publishers.

Rogers, M.C. (1992). *Current practice in anesthesia*, ed. 2, St. Louis: Mosby.

Rogers, M.C., Tinker, J.H., Covino, B.G., Longnecker, D.E., editors (1993). *Principles and practice of anesthesiology.* St. Louis: Mosby.

Saidman, L.J. & Smith, N.T., editors (1993). *Monitoring in anesthesia*, ed. 3. Boston: Butterworth-Heineman.

Shapiro, B.A., & others (1993). *Clinical application of blood gases*, ed. 5. Chicago: Year Book Medical Publishers.

Shnider, S.N., & Levinson, G. (1993). *Anesthesia for obstetrics*, ed. 3, Baltimore: Williams & Wilkins.

Stoelting, R.K. (1991). *Pharmacology and physiology in anesthetic practice*, ed. 2. Philadelphia: J.B. Lippincott.

Stoelting, R.K., Dierdorf, S.F., & McCammon, R.L. (1993). *Anesthesia and co-existing disease*, ed. 3. New York: Churchill Livingstone.

Stoelting, R.K., & Miller, R.D. (1989). *Basics of anesthesia*, ed. 2. New York: Churchill Livingstone.

Taylor, T.H. & Major, E. (1993). *Hazards and complications of anesthesia*, ed. 2. New York: Churchill Livingstone.

Wetchler, B.V., editor (1991). *Anesthesia for ambulatory surgery*, ed. 2. Philadelphia: J.B. Lippincott.

White, P.F., editor (1990). *Outpatient anesthesia.* New York: Churchill Livingstone.

Wood, M. & Wood A.J.J. (1990). *Drugs and anesthesia*, ed. 2. Baltimore: Williams & Wilkins.

General

Aldrete, J.A., & Kroulik, D. (1970). A postanesthetic recovery score, *Anesthesia and Analgesia*, 49:924.

Association of Operating Room Nurses, Inc. (1994). Recommended practices for cleaning and processing anesthesia equipment. In *AORN standards and recommended practices for perioperative nursing.* Denver: The Association.

Association of Operating Room Nurses, Inc. (1994). Recommended practices for monitoring the patient receiving intravenous conscious sedation. In *AORN standards and recommended practices for perioperative nursing.* Denver: The Association.

Association of Operating Room Nurses, Inc. (1994). Recommended practices for universal precautions in the perioperative practice setting. In *AORN standards and recommended practices for perioperative nursing.* Denver: The Association.

Association of Operating Room Nurses, Inc. (1994). Recommended practices for monitoring the patient receiving local anesthesia. In *AORN Standards and recommended practices for perioperative nursing.* Denver: The Association.

Brimacombe, J. (1993). The laryngeal mask airway: tool for airway management. *Journal of Post Anesthesia Nursing*, 8(2):88-95.

Christensen, B. (1992). Hemodynamic monitoring: What it tells you and what it doesn't? Part I. *Journal of Post Anesthesia Nursing*, 7(5):330-337.

Christensen, B. (1992). Hemodynamic monitoring: What it tells you and what it doesn't? Part II. *Journal of Post Anesthesia Nursing*, 7(5):338-345.

Derrick, S.J., Waters, H., Kang, S.W., Cwalina, T.F., & Simmons, W. (1993). Evaluation of a nasal/oral discriminant sampling system for capnographic respiratory monitoring. *Journal of American Association of Nurse Anesthetists*, 61:509-523.

Dershwitz, M., Rosow, C.E., Di Biase, P.M., Joslyn, A.F., & Sanderson, P.E. (1992). Ondansetron is effective in decreasing postoperative nausea and vomiting. *Clinical Pharmacology and Therapeutics*, 52:96-101.

Fetzer-Fowler, S. (1992). State of the Art: Regional anesthesia using anesthetic admixtures. *Journal of Post Anesthesia Nursing*, 7(4):229-237.

Fezer, S.J. (1987). Cricoid pressure: how, when and why. *AORN Journal*, 45:1374.

Ghouri, A.F., Bodner, M., & White, P.F. (1991). Recovery profile after desflurane—nitrous oxide versus isoflurane—nitrous oxide in outpatients. *Anesthesiology*, 74:419-424.

Hinojosa, R.J. (1992). Nursing interventions to prevent or relieve postoperative nausea and vomiting. *Journal of Post Anesthesia Nursing*, 7(1):3-14.

Hogenson, K.D. (1992). Acute postoperative hypertension in the hypertensive patient. *Journal of Post Anesthesia Nursing*, 7(1):38-44.

Kenny, G.N.C., Oates, D.L., Leeser, J., Rowbotham, J., Lip, H., Rust, M., Saur, P., Onsrud, M., & Haigh, C.G. (1992). Efficacy of orally administered ondansetron in the prevention of postoperative nausea and vomiting: A dose ranging study. *British Journal of Anaesthesiology*, 68:466-477.

Krasner, P.R. (1991). Avulsed teeth: Management during anesthesia induction, surgery. *AORN Journal*, 53(4):998-1004.

Larijani, G.E., Gratz, I., Afshar, M., & Minassian, S. (1991). Treatment of postoperative nausea and vomiting with ondansetron: A randomized, double-blind comparison with placebo. *Anesthesia and Analgesia*, 73:246-249.

Leeser, J., & Lip, H. (1991). Prevention of postoperative nausea and vomiting using ondansetron, a new, selective, $5-HT_3$ receptor antagonist. *Anesthesia and Analgesia*, 72:751-755.

Longinow, L.T., & Rzeszewski L.B. (1993). The holding room. *AORN Journal*, 57(4):914-924.

Maltby, J.R., Lewis, P., Martin, A., & Sutherland, L.R. (1991). Gastric fluid volume and pH in elective patients following unrestricted oral fluid until three hours before surgery. *Canadian Journal of Anaesthesia*, 38(4):425-529.

McEwan, A.I., & Mason, D.G. (1992). The laryngeal mask airway. *Journal of Clinical Anesthesia*, 4:252-257.

McKenzie, R., Kovac, A., O'Conner, T., Dunclaf, D., Angel, J., Gratz, I., Tolpin, E., McLesky, C., & Joslyn, A. (1993). Comparison of ondansetron versus placebo to prevent postoperative nausea and vomiting in women undergoing ambulatory gynecologic surgery. *Anesthesiology*, 78:21-28.

Moak, E. (1991). Electrosurgical unit safety. The role of the perioperative nurse. *AORN Journal*, 53:744-752.

Pennant, J.H., Pace, N.A., & Gajraj, N.M. (1993). Role of the laryngeal mask airway in the immobile cervical spine. *Journal of Clinical Anesthesia*, 5:226-230.

Pennant, J.H., & White, P.F. (1993). The laryngeal mask airway. Its uses in anesthesiology. *Anesthesiology*, 79:144-163.

Saleh, K.L. (1992). Practical points in the management of malignant hyperthermia. *Journal of Post Anesthesia Nursing*, 7(5):327-329.

Saleh, K.L. (1992). Practical points in understanding local anesthetics. *Journal of Post Anesthesia Nursing*, 7(1):45-47.

Saleh, K.L. (1991). Practical points in understanding spinal anesthesia. *Journal of Post Anesthesia Nursing,* 6(6):407-409.

Scuderi, P., Wetchler, B., Sung, Y.F., Mingus, M., DuPen, S., Claybon, L., Leslie, J., Talke, P., Apfelbaum, J.L., Sharifi-Azad, S., & Williams, M.F. (1993). Treatment of postoperative nausea and vomiting after outpatient surgery with the 5-HT$_3$ antagonist ondansetron. *Anesthesiology,* 78:15-20.

Shevde, K., & Trivedi, N. (1991). Effects of clear liquids on gastric volume and pH in healthy volunteers. *Anesthesia and Analgesia,* 72:528-531.

Summers, S. (1991). Axillary, tympanic and esophageal temperature measurement: Descriptive comparisons in postanesthesia patients. *Journal of Post Anesthesia Nursing,* 6(6):420-425.

Sung, Y.F., Wetchler, B.V., Duncalf, D., & Joslyn, A.F. (1993). A double-blind, placebo-controlled pilot study examining the effectiveness of intravenous ondansetron in the prevention of postoperative nausea and emesis. *Journal of Clinical Anesthesia,* 5:22-29.

Watcha, M.F., White, P.F. (1992). Postoperative nausea and vomiting. Its etiology, treatment, and prevention. *Anesthesiology,* 77:162-184.

Watson, D.S., & Kaempf, G. (1991). *Monitoring the patient receiving local anesthesia,* ed. 2. Denver: The Association of Operating Room Nurses, Inc.

Wenrich, J. (1991). Acute pain service in a community hospital. *Journal of Post Anesthesia Nursing,* 6(5):324-330.

Yelderman, M. (1990). Continuous measurement of cardiac output with the use of stochastic system identification techniques. *Journal of Clinical Monitoring,* 6:322-332.

7

WOUND HEALING, DRESSING, AND DRAINS

NANCYE RUE FEISTRITZER

WOUND HEALING

A primary goal of perioperative intervention is the prevention of surgical wound infections. Actions taken by perioperative personnel can mean the difference between a postoperative wound infection with associated sequelae and the normal healing process. A clear understanding of wound healing and the factors that adversely affect healing is therefore important for the appropriate management of patients undergoing surgery.

Wound healing is a complex and highly organized response by an organism to tissue disruption caused by injury. The ability to heal wounds is one of the most powerful defensive properties human beings possess. This process is infallible in the absence of endogenous and exoge-

nous infections, mechanical interferences, or certain disease processes. Apposition and maintenance of the edges of a cleanly incised wound almost always result in prompt healing.

The etiology of wounds can be described in three categories:

Surgical: caused by an incision or excision
Traumatic: caused by an injury (mechanical, thermal, or chemical)
Chronic: caused by an underlying pathophysiology, such as pressure ulcers or venous leg ulcers, over time.

Fig. 7-1 illustrates the layers of the skin corresponding to different wound depths.

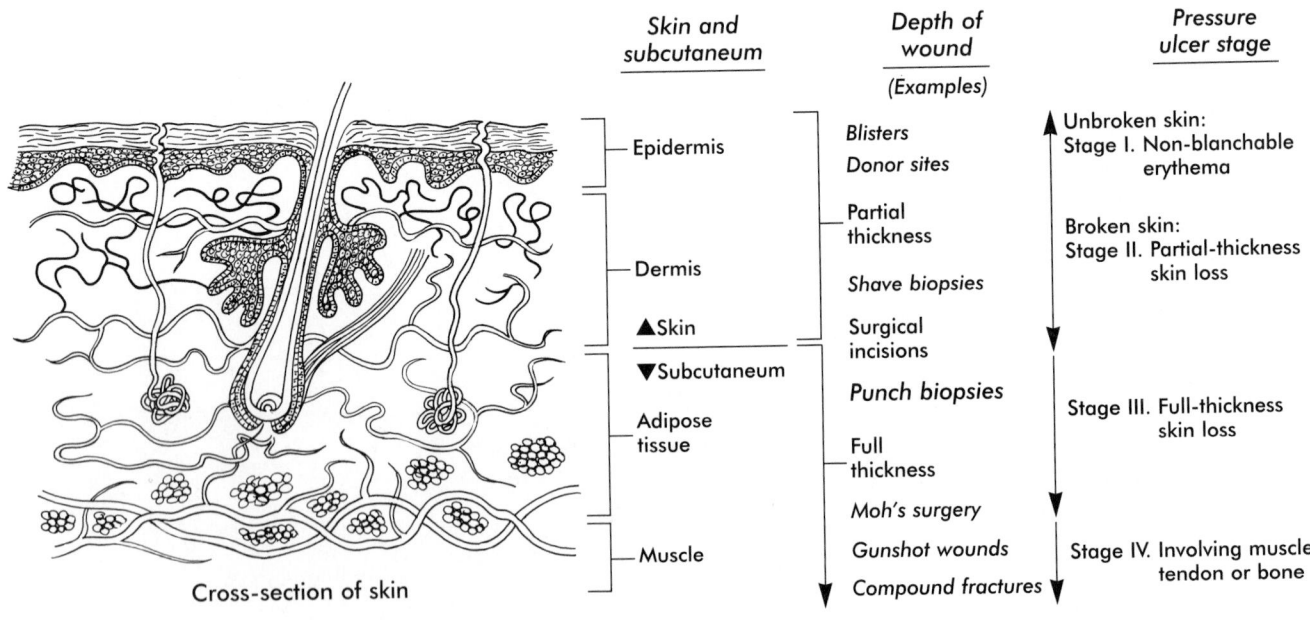

FIG. 7-1 Layers of the skin corresponding to different wound depths.
From Bolton, L., & von Rijswijk, L. (1991). Wound dressings: meeting clinical and biological needs. *Dermatology Nursing. 3*(3), 147.

Clean, full-thickness wound healing is an intricate, exact biologic process that takes place in three phases: (1) inflammatory (also known as the defensive stage), (2) fibroplastic (also known as the proliferative stage), and (3) remodelling (also known as the maturation stage) (Fig. 7-2). These phases do not take place in isolation; overlap between phases occurs. In the *inflammatory phase* an exudate containing blood, lymph, and fibrin begins clotting and loosely binds the cut edges together. Blood supply to the area is increased, and the basic process of inflammation is set in motion. Inflammation is a prerequisite to wound healing and is a vascular and cellular response to dispose of bacteria, foreign material, and dead tissue (Gogia, 1992). Leukocytes increase in number to fight bacteria in the wound area and by phagocytosis help to remove damaged tissues. The severed tissue is quickly glued together by strands of fibrin and a thin layer of clotted blood, forming a scab. Plasma seeps to the surface to form a dry, protective crust. This seal helps to prevent fluid loss and bacterial invasion. During the first few days of wound healing, however, the seal has little tensile strength.

The *fibroplastic phase* allows for new epithelium to cover the wound, beginning the process within hours of the occurrence of injury (Daly, 1990). Epithelial cells migrate and proliferate to the wound area covering the surface of the wound to close the epithelial defect. Epithelialization also provides a protective barrier to prevent fluid and electrolyte loss and to reduce the incidence of infection. While the re-epithelialization takes place, wound contraction and collagen synthesis are occurring. Contraction begins approximately 5 days after the wound onset and peaks at 2 weeks, gradually pulling the entire wound into a smaller area. Epidermal migration is limited to approximately 3 cm from the point of origin. Larger wounds may require skin grafting due to the limited epidermal migration. Collagen synthesis produces fiber molecules that cross-link to provide strength to the wound.

The *remodelling phase* begins after approximately 2 to 4 weeks, depending on the size and nature of the wound. It may last up to a year or longer. During the remodelling phase, the scar tissue formed during fibroplasia changes in bulk, form, and strength. Throughout normal wound healing, new collagen is produced, while old collagen breaks down in a balanced fashion (Gogia, 1992). This collagen turnover allows randomly deposited scar tissue to be arranged in both linear and lateral orientation. As the scar ages, fibers and fiber bundles become more closely packed and ultimately create the final shape and function of the wound. At best, the tensile strength of scar tissue is never more than 80% of the tensile strength in nonwounded tissue.

The amount of tissue loss, the existence of contamination or infection, and damage to tissue are all factors that determine the type of wound healing that will occur. This process of healing takes place in one of three ways.

PRIMARY INTENTION

Healing through primary intention occurs when wounds are created aseptically, with a minimum of tissue destruction and postoperative tissue reaction. This includes wounds closed with sutures, staples, or tape applied as soon after

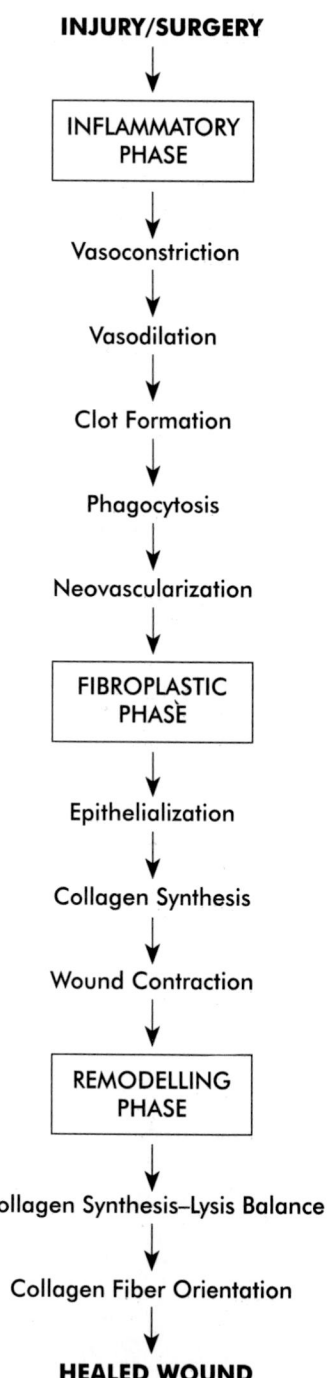

FIG. 7-2 Flow diagram of normal wound healing.

From Gogia, P. (1992). The biology of wound healing. *Ostomy/Wound Management.* 38(9), Nov./Dec., 13.

the time of injury as possible. Healing by primary intention takes place under the following conditions:

1. Edges of an incised wound in a healthy person are promptly and accurately approximated.
2. Contamination is held to a minimum by rigid adherence to aseptic technique.
3. Trauma to the wound is minimal.
4. After closure, no dead space is left to become a potential site of infection.
5. Drainage is minimal.

SECONDARY INTENTION (GRANULATION)

When surgical wounds are characterized by tissue loss with inability to approximate wound edges, healing occurs through secondary intention (Fig. 7-3). This type of wound is usually left open and allowed to heal from the inside toward the outer surface. In infected wounds, this process allows the proper cleansing and dressing of the wound as healthy tissue builds up from the inside. The area of tissue loss gradually fills with granulation tissue comprising fibroblasts and capillaries. Scar tissue is extensive because of the size of the tissue gap that must be closed. Contraction of surrounding tissue also takes place. Consequently, this healing process takes longer than primary intention healing.

DELAYED PRIMARY CLOSURE OR TERTIARY INTENTION

As the name implies, this healing process takes place when approximation of wound edges is delayed by 3 to 5 days or more after injury or surgery. The conditions that contribute to a decision for a delayed closure are:

1. Removal of an inflamed organ
2. Heavy contamination of the wound

FACTORS AFFECTING WOUND HEALING

Patients who have experienced any sort of wound should be assessed for healing status. The patient's nutritional status, oxygenation, and overall recuperative power are of utmost importance in tissue repair and healing. Nutritional status, the inflammatory response, and oxygen tension all depend on microcirculation to deliver components to the wound. It is important to maintain body temperature in the operating room to promote healing. If the patient becomes hypothermic, vasoconstriction will occur, leading to compromised wound healing.

Wound healing depends on adequate oxygenation. Decreased oxygen tension to the wound area inhibits fibroblast migration as well as collagen synthesis, resulting in decreased tensile strength of the wound (Gogia, 1992). Nutritional status also has a profound effect on healing due to the need for an adequate supply of protein necessary for the growth of new tissues. Protein is also required for the regulation of the osmotic pressure of blood and other body

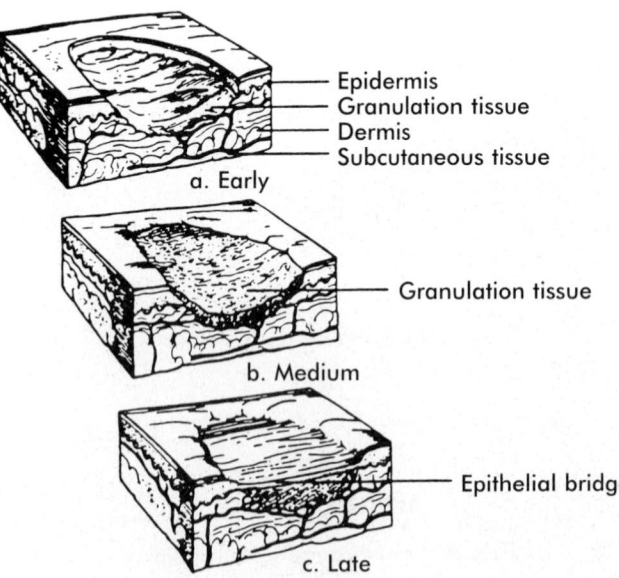

FIG. 7-3 Three stages in secondary intention healing.
Courtesy Johnson and Johnson Patient Care, Inc., New Brunswick, N.J.

BOX 7-1

Definitions of Surgical Site Infection

INCISIONAL SURGICAL SITE INFECTION (SSI)
Superficial incisional SSI
   Within 30 days of surgery
   Skin and subcutaneous tissue
   One of the following: pus, culture, physician's diagnosis, or one symptom (pain, redness, wound separation)
Deep incisional SSI; one of the following:
   Pus from drain into deep tissue not in incision
   Spontaneous dehiscence or is opened by the physician
   Abscess in deep tissues
   Diagnosis of SSI by a physician
Operative field SSI (area contiguous with organ or space of the operating site). Infection within 30 days of surgery and one of the following:
   Pus from drain through stab wound
   Positive culture
   Diagnosis by a physician
Culture obtained by aseptically preparing the site before collection or aspiration of cutaneous tissue or fluid.
If an implant is placed, an infection may be linked to the operation for up to 1 year.

From Barrett, T. (1992). Recognition and treatment of surgical wound infections. *Today's OR Nurse. 14*(10), 12.

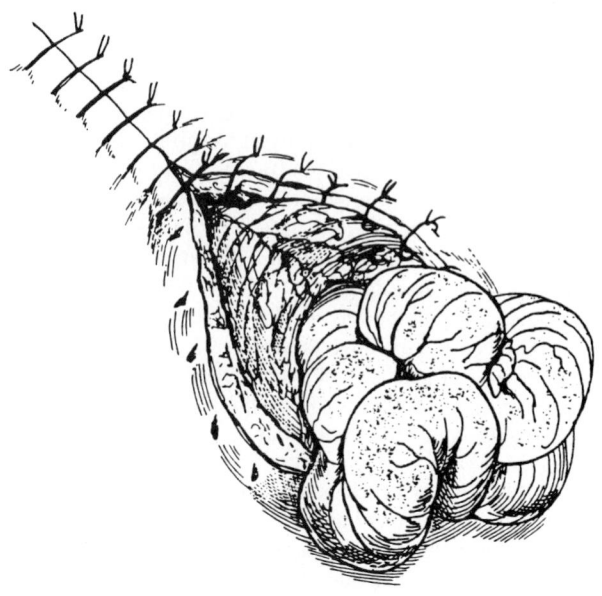

FIG. 7-4 Wound dehiscence and evisceration.
Courtesy Johnson and Johnson Patient Care, Inc., New Brunswick, N.J.

fluids, and the formation of prothrombin, enzymes, hormones, and antibodies. Other nutritional essentials are water; vitamins A, C, B_6, and B_{12}; iron; calcium; zinc; and adequate calories.

The most common cause of delayed wound healing in the operative patient is wound infection. Box 7-1 summarizes the types and definitions of surgical site infections.

BOX 7-2

Additional Terms Used in Connection with Wound Healing

The following are additional terms used in connection with wound healing:

keloid Dense, unsightly connective tissue or excessive scar formation that is often removed surgically

"proud flesh" Overgrowth of granulation tissue

gangrene Anaerobic infection process that may occur instead of healing; implies necrosis (death of tissue) and putrefaction (decomposition); usually caused by failure of nutriment or blood to reach a part

adhesions Adherence of serous membranes to one another, causing fibrous tissue to form; sometimes occurring in healing and inflammatory processes; commonly occurring in or about gastrointestinal tract, where adhesions may form bands and cause obstructions and subsequent surgical emergencies

dehiscence Separation of layers of surgical wound (Fig. 7-4)

evisceration Extrusion of internal organs, or viscera, through gaping wound (Fig. 7-4)

There are a number of possible causes of postoperative wound infections including patient susceptibility and severity of illness; microbial contamination by the patient's microflora; and exogenous wound contamination from the OR environment and personnel. The presence of a foreign body left in place after closure is another factor in wound infections because the body has a diminished capacity to inhibit infection on implanted material. Adherence to strict aseptic principles, careful observation of sterile technique, and thorough antimicrobial preparation of the patient and operative site are essential to minimize the risk of postoperative wound infection.

Wound healing can also be impaired by poor surgical technique. Rough handling of tissue causes trauma that can lead to bleeding and other conditions conducive to infection. Examples of meticulous surgical technique that promotes wound healing are adequate hemostasis, precise cutting and suturing techniques, elimination of dead spaces, and minimal pressure from retractors and other instruments.

Additional factors affecting wound healing are the patient's age, stress level, immunologic status, and smoking history. Preexisting conditions such as diabetes, anemia, malnutrition, cancer, obesity, and cardiovascular or respiratory impairments also contribute to poor wound healing.

Additional terms used in connection with wound healing are shown in Box 7-2.

WOUND CLASSIFICATION

The Centers for Disease Control (CDC) recommends four surgical wound classifications: clean wounds, clean contaminated wounds, contaminated wounds, and dirty or infected wounds (Garner, 1985). This classification scheme reflects the probability of infection and thus enables appropriate preventive measures to be taken. "AORN Recommended Practices for Documentation of Perioperative Nursing Care" states that the patient record should reflect the surgical wound classification (AORN, 1994). Following are descriptions of each classification.

CLEAN WOUNDS

These wounds are uninfected operative wounds in which no inflammation is encountered and the respiratory, alimentary, and genitourinary tracts are not entered. They are primarily closed and can be drained with a closed wound drainage system. They show no sign of infection. Examples are breast biopsy, total hip replacement, or open heart surgery.

CLEAN CONTAMINATED WOUNDS

These wounds are operative wounds in which the respiratory, alimentary, or genitourinary tract is entered under controlled conditions. There is no sign of infection and no break in surgical aseptic technique. Examples of clean contaminated wounds are nonperforated appendectomy, hysterectomy, or thoracotomy.

CONTAMINATED WOUNDS

These wounds are open, fresh, accidental wounds or operations with major breaks in aseptic technique. Incisions with signs of infection or gross spillage from the gastrointestinal tract are also included. Some examples are an appendectomy for ruptured appendix, a penetrating abdominal trauma involving bowel, or a gunshot wound to the abdomen.

DIRTY OR INFECTED WOUNDS

These wounds include old traumatic wounds with retained devitalized tissue and wounds that involve an existing clinical infection or perforated viscera. Examples of dirty or infected wounds are excision and drainage of abscess or delayed primary closure of wound following appendectomy for ruptured appendix.

An alternative system for classification of surgical wounds exists in the National Nosocomial Infections Surveillance System (NNIS). This risk index utilizes a broader and simpler division of wound class into two categories: clean and clean-contaminated (Cardo, 1993) (Research Highlight 7-1).

NURSING DIAGNOSES

The nursing diagnoses—high risk for infection (wound); high risk for impaired skin integrity; altered nutrition; altered tissue perfusion and hypothermia—all point the nurse toward strategies that can be used to prevent wound infections and promote healing.

Box 7-3 provides a guide to nursing actions for preventing wound infection during the perioperative period. Attention should also be given to maintaining skin integrity through proper positioning, the use of therapeutic mattresses as needed, and the safe use of electrosurgery. The nurse plays a vital role in the prevention of wound infections, pressure ulcers as well as burns due to improper grounding.

DRESSINGS

After surgery a dressing may be applied to the wound. Following are the purposes of a dressing:

1. To cushion and protect the wound from trauma and gross contamination
2. To absorb drainage
3. To debride the wound
4. To support, splint, or immobilize the body part and incisional area
5. To aid in hemostasis and minimize edema, as in a pressure dressing
6. To enhance the patient's physical comfort and aesthetic appearance

---

RESEARCH HIGHLIGHT 7-1

Cardo et al (1993) prospectively studied the accuracy of circulating nurses in classifying surgical wounds according to the Centers for Disease Control (CDC) classification system of clean, clean-contaminated, contaminated, and dirty or infected wounds. One hundred surgical procedures (50 general and 50 trauma) were classified by circulating nurses while a physician simultaneously observed and independently classified each surgical procedure.

The overall accuracy of classification by the circulating nurses was 88% compared with the classification of the physician observer. Accuracy increased when surgical wounds were classified into only two categories: clean or clean-contaminated vs. contaminated or dirty/infected.

The researchers concluded that circulating nurses can classify surgical wounds with a high degree of accuracy utilizing the CDC system, and that accuracy increases further when a simplified two-tiered system is utilized.

Cardo, D.M., Falk, P.S., & Mayhall, C.G. (1993, May). Validation of surgical wound classification in the operating room. *Infection Control Hospital Epidemiology*, 14:255-259.

---

7. To maintain a moist environment and prevent cell dehydration
8. To apply medications

Beyond these clinical needs, dressings should be chosen based on each wound's unique characteristics of site, depth, and area as well as the patient's overall condition. Table 7-1 compares various wound dressings and the nursing considerations for each.

Dressings can be grouped into two main categories: *primary* and *secondary* dressings. Primary dressings are placed directly over or in the wound. A variety of dressing materials are available on the market today. The function of these dressings is to absorb drainage and allow it to wick away from the wound edge. Cotton gauze or synthetic dressings may be used for this purpose. Cotton gauze dressings are increasingly passé, as newer, more effective dressing materials have been developed. The layer of dressing directly contacting the wound should be nonadherent unless debridement is desired.

Secondary dressings are placed directly over the primary dressing. These function to absorb excessive drainage, provide hemostasis by compression, and protect the wound from further trauma. These functions are usually accomplished with a bulky dressing such as an abdominal pad. These pads have a cotton filling that provides extra absorbency. Several varieties of transparent "biologic" synthetic

---

BOX 7-3

Guide to Nursing Actions for Preventing Wound Infection

1. Preoperatively assess the patient for pre-existing disposition to wound infection. Note patient's age, weight, nutritional status, history of chronic systemic or metabolic disease, electrolyte values, skin condition at proposed operative site, presence of remote infection (i.e., respiratory, urinary), status of immune system, laboratory values.
2. Report deviations in laboratory values, especially WBC.
3. Check the patient's baseline preoperative vital signs.
4. Establish and maintain a sterile field according to principles of basic aseptic technique.
5. Adhere to institutional policy and protocol for OR attire.
6. Follow institutional policy and protocol for surgical hand scrubs.
7. Create effective barriers to transmission of microorganisms through proper gowning, gloving, and draping procedures.
8. Visually inspect room for total cleanliness before opening the case cart/supplies and instrument sets.
9. Inspect sterile items for contamination before opening. Check package integrity, expiration date, chemical process indicator.
10. Maintain sterility while opening sterile items to preserve the sterility of the item and the integrity of sterile field.
11. Constantly monitor the sterile field.
12. Initiate corrective action when break in technique occurs.
13. Communicate maintenance of a sterile field.
14. Classify surgical wound based on the degree of contamination of the wound and surrounding tissues during the operative procedure (clean, clean contaminated, contaminated, dirty).
15. Control movement of the patient, personnel, and materials in and out of the OR by adhering to established traffic patterns.
16. Minimize risk of cross infection by cleaning and processing anesthesia equipment and all items that have come into contact with the patient and/or sterile field properly.
17. Select materials for inhospital packaging that are: compatible with the sterilization process, effective barriers, easily presented, and non-toxic.
18. Adhere to OR sanitation policies and protocols.
19. Cleanse skin at the operative site through skin preparation procedures.
20. Utilize methods of sterilization and disinfection to decontaminate needed supplies and equipment.
21. Meticulously wash hands following contact with the patient or any object likely to be contaminated with blood or body fluids.
22. Maintain the OR temperature between 20° C and 24° C (68°-75° F) except where contraindicated for patient care.
23. Maintain relative humidity at 50 percent ±10.
24. Keep OR doors closed to maintain pressure gradients.
25. Requisition, or administer, antibiotics as ordered. Check the patient record for drug allergy/sensitivity. Note drug, dosage, route and time of administration.
26. Remove soiled linen from around patient before transfer to postanesthesia care unit.
27. Document additional nursing actions related to prevention of wound infection.
28. The following AORN Recommended Practices may be consulted to modify/expand this care plan:
    - Aseptic technique
    - Traffic patterns in the surgical suite
    - Cleaning and processing anesthesia equipment
    - Protective barrier materials for gowns and drapes
    - Selection and use of packaging systems
    - Sanitation in the surgical practice setting
    - Skin preparation of patients
    - Surgical attire
    - Surgical hand scrubs
    - Steam and ethylene oxide sterilization
    - Disinfection

From Rothrock, J.C. (1990). Generic care planning: AORN patient outcome standards. In Rothrock, J.C. (editor), *Perioperative nursing care planning* (pp 87-88). St. Louis: Mosby.

---

dressings are available and are quite popular. Most are vapor and oxygen permeable, conform to irregular body surfaces, prevent gross outside contamination, and allow visibility of the wound itself. These transparent semiocclusive films keep the wound moist and thereby enable epidermal cells to move more quickly across the wound and bridge the incision. The "scab" stage of wound healing is avoided.

Although these film types of dressings cannot be used on heavily draining wounds, their skinlike qualities seem to aid wound healing and protect delicate healing skin edges.

Dressings may be secured with tape. Tape is available with a variety of backing materials (cloth, paper, taffeta, plastic) and with regular or nonallergenic adhesive. The amount of strength and elasticity required, patient allergies,

TABLE 7-1

Comparing Wound Dressings

Products	Advantages	Disadvantages	Nursing considerations
COTTON MESH GAUZE	• Moderately absorbent	• Bulky	• Can be used dry to cover surgical wounds, wet-to-dry to nonselectively debride some wounds, and moist to pack undermining and tunneling • Combine with normal saline solution for granulation or antibiotic solutions for infection • Use transparent films or occlusive tape to retain moisture, p.r.n. • Cover with nonwoven gauzes to increase absorption
NONADHERENT DRESSING • *Nonimpregnated:* ETE Sterile Protective Dressing, EXU-DRY, Metalline, Release, Telfa • *Impregnated:* Adaptic, Scarlet Red, Vaseline Gauze, Xeroflo, Xeroform	• Occlusive • Nontraumatic	• Minimally absorbent • Some impregnated dressings contain antimicrobial agents that harm fibroblasts	• Nonadhesive • Doesn't require secondary dressing • Useful for skin tears and other friable wounds, wounds near body hair, donor sites, and skin grafts
TRANSPARENT FILM • ACU-Derm, Bioclusive, BlisterFilm, Ensure-It, Hi/moist, Omiderm, OpraFlex, OpSite, Polyderm Picture Frame Film, Polyskin II, Tegaderm, Tegaderm Pouch, Transite Exudate Transfer Film, UniFlex, Vari/Moist, Visi Derm II	• Moisture retentive • Semipermeable • Very comfortable for patient • Not bulky • Allows for easy wound inspection • Water resistant	• Minimally absorbent • Channeling (wrinkling) occurs	• Adhesive • Doesn't require secondary dressing • Useful for autolytic debridement, as well as superficial wounds, donor sites, abrasions, and burns
HYDROCOLLOID • Comfeel, DuoDERM, Hydrapad, Intact, IntraSite, Johnson & Johnson Ulcer Dressing, Restore, Sween-A-Peel, Tegasorb, ULTEC	• Moisture retentive • Occlusive or semipermeable • Very comfortable for patient • Not bulky • Excellent bacterial barriers, high tack • Water resistant • Moderately absorbent	• Melt out occurs, resulting in residue in the wound bed and particles on the wound margins	• Adhesive • Doesn't require secondary dressing • Useful for autolytic debridement, as well as for covering a variety of acute and chronic wounds • Available in powder, wafer, and paste form

TABLE 7-1

Comparing Wound Dressings—cont'd

Products	Advantages	Disadvantages	Nursing considerations
HYDROGEL • Biolex Wound Gel, Carrington Dermal Wound Gel, ClearSite, Elasto-Gel, Geliperm Wet/Granulate, Hydron Wound Dressing, IntraSite Gel, Nu-Gel, Second Skin, Spand-Gel, Vigilon	• Moisture retentive • Moderately absorbent • Cooling, soothing effects • Can be used on infected wounds • Water resistant (if used with secondary transparent film) • Allows for easy wound inspection		• Adhesive or nonadhesive • May or may not require secondary dressing • Useful for autolytic debridement, as well as for covering a variety of acute and chronic wounds • Available in sheet or gel forms • Sheets don't leave a residue; gel easily rinsed off
EXUDATE ABSORBER • Algosteril, Allevyn Cavity Wound Dressings, Bard Absorption Dressing, Debrisan, Envisan, Hydragan, Kaltostat, Mesalt, Sorbsan	• Moisture retentive • Highly absorbent		• Nonadhesive • Requires secondary dressing • Useful for autolytic debridement and for heavily exudating wounds • Available as starches, pastes, beads, hypertonic saline gauzes, and calcium alginate dressings
FOAM • Allevyn, EPIGARD, Epi-Lock, LYOfoam, Mitraflex	• Moisture retentive • Very comfortable for patient • Moderately absorbent • Insulating		• Nonadherent • May or may not require secondary dressing • Useful for friable wounds or wounds near body hair

Note: The products included here are representative of what's available; the lists under each category aren't meant to be inclusive.
From "Selecting Wound Dressings by Category," *NARD Journal* © 1991 National Association of Retail Druggists, Alexandria, Va., May 1991. Adapted with permission of the publisher.
Source: Krasner, D. (1992). The 12 Commandments of wound care. *Nursing 92,* 22(12),38.

and anticipated frequency of dressing change influence which type is selected. When frequent dressing changes are anticipated, Montgomery straps can be selected to secure the dressing (Fig. 7-5). When compression of the wound for hemostasis or reduction of edema is desired, a polyurethane dressing, elastic tape, or elastic bandage may be used to secure the secondary dressing. Immobilization is accomplished with the addition of soft padding, splints, elastic bandages, and casting materials. These immobilizing dressings are discussed in greater detail in Chapter 21.

In some situations the wound is not dressed at all. The air-exposed wound will heal, and having no dressing: (1) allows for optimum observation of the incisional area, (2) aids bathing, (3) prevents possible adhesive tape reactions, (4) increases comfort and maneuverability for many patients, and (5) seems to minimize adverse responses by the patient to the operation.

DRAINS

Drains provide exits through which air and fluids such as serum, blood, lymph, intestinal secretions, bile, and pus can be evacuated from the operative site. Drains may also be used to prevent the development of deep wound infections. They are usually inserted at the time of surgery, directly from the incision or through a separate small incision, known as a *stab wound,* close to the operative site.

In some instances (chest, common bile duct, bladder), drainage is directly through the lumen of the tube (as with a Foley retention catheter) into a closed drainage system.

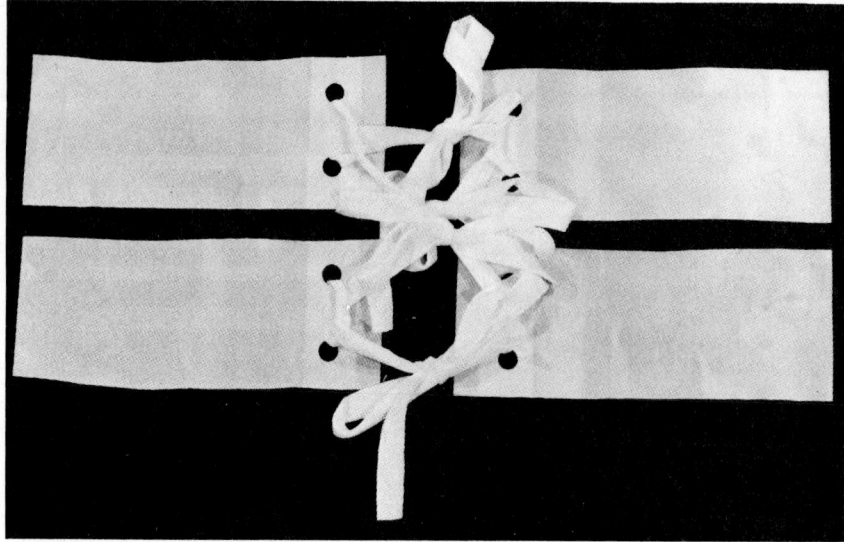

FIG. 7-5   Montgomery straps.

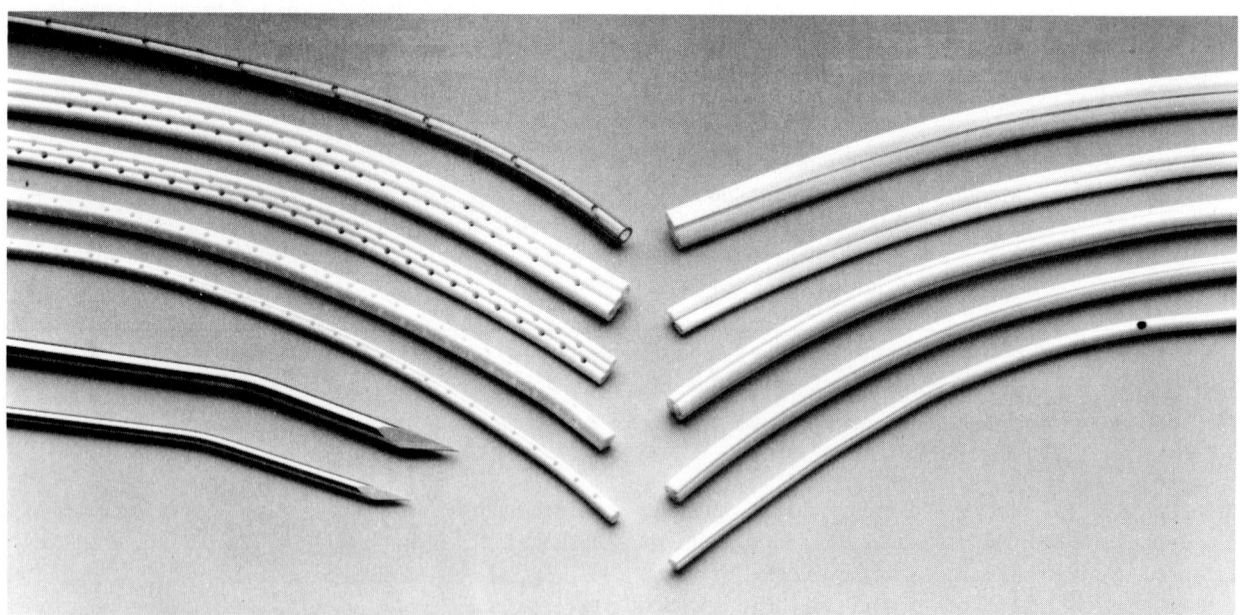

FIG. 7-6   Drains are available in a variety of styles. Pictures are round PVC, flat and round silicone, trocars, and a variety of fluted silicone drains.

Courtesy Johnson and Johnson Patient Care, Inc., New Brunswick, N.J.

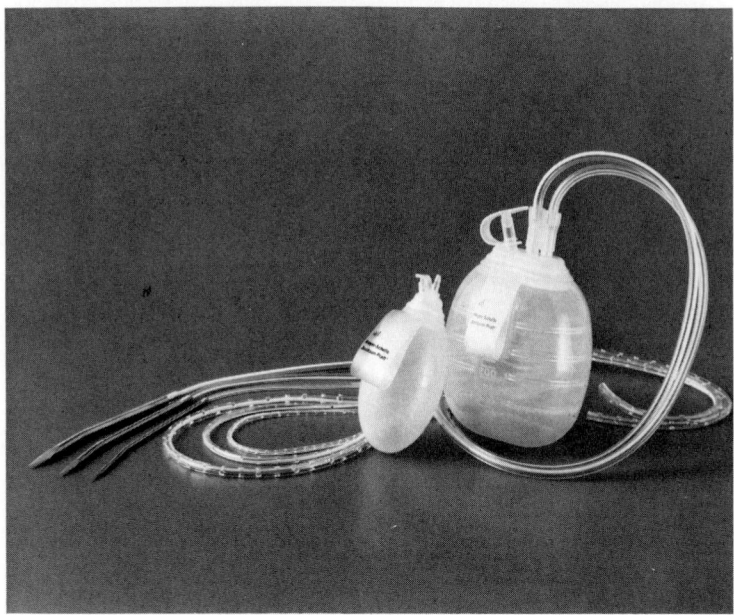

FIG. 7-7   Portable self-contained wound drainage system.
Courtesy Zimmer, Inc., Warsaw, Ind.

In other instances (peritoneal cavity or skin wound), drainage of pus or blood is primarily along the outside surface of the drain by capillary action and gravity (as with the simple Penrose drain).

The selection of a simple versus a closed drainage system depends on the needs of the site to be drained, patient activity, and overall healing capability. Many types of drains are available. The most common are made of latex, PVC (polyvinyl chloride), or silicone (Fig. 7-6). Particular care should be taken to ensure that the patient is not allergic to latex when selecting any latex drain. For many wounds, a portable, self-contained, closed wound suction unit is selected. These units create a negative pressure in a reservoir attached to the drain. Fluid is then gently drawn out of the wound and collected in the reservoir (Fig. 7-7).

The perioperative nurse must clearly document the location and type of drains on the operative record. This information is important to nurses caring for the patient in the postanesthesia and postoperative nursing units. Some wounds yield significant amounts of drainage and as such must be monitored closely during the postoperative course.

SUMMARY

Wound healing is an essential part of the surgical experience. Perioperative nurses should vigilantly guard and enhance their patients' ability to heal with an eye toward prevention of problems before they occur.

REFERENCES

Association of Operating Room Nurses (1994). Recommended practices for documentation of perioperative nursing care. In *AORN standards and recommended practices for perioperative nursing*. pp.III: 4-1-III:4-4. Denver: The Association.

Cardo, D., Falk, P., & Mayhill, C. (1993). Validation of surgical wound classification in the operating room, *Infection Control Hospital Epidemiology, 14* (4), 255-259.

Daly, T. (1990). The repair phase of wound healing: re-epithelialization and contraction, In Kloth, L., McCulloch, J., & Feeder, J. (editors): *Wound healing: alternatives in management*. Philadelphia: FA Davis.

Garner, Julia S. (1985). *Guidelines for prevention of surgical wound infections*. Atlanta: Centers for Disease Control.

Gogia, P. (1992). The biology of wound healing. *Ostomy/Wound Management, 38*(9), Nov./Dec., 12-20.

BIBLIOGRAPHY

Association of Operating Room Nurses. (1994). *AORN standards and recommended practices for perioperative nursing*. Denver: The Association.

Barrett, T. (1992). Recognition and treatment of surgical wound infections. *Today's OR Nurse, 14* (10), 11-14.

Bolton, L., & van Rijswijk, L. (1991). Wound dressings: meeting clinical and biological needs. *Dermatology Nursing, 3*(3), 146-161.

Bryant, R.A. (1992). *Acute and chronic wounds and nursing management*. St. Louis: Mosby.

Krasner, D. (1992). The 12 commandments of wound care. *Nursing 92, 22*(12), 34-41.

Rothrock, J. (1990). *Perioperative nursing care planning*. St. Louis: Mosby.

Wysocki, A. (1989). Surgical wound healing: a review for perioperative nurses. *AORN Journal, 49*, 502-504.

Wysocki, A. (1992). Fibronectin in acute and chronic wounds. *Journal of ET Nursing, 19*(5), 166-170.

8

POSTOPERATIVE CARE AND COMPLICATIONS

JAN ODOM

The postoperative phase of care begins as soon as the surgical procedure is concluded and the patient is transferred to the postanesthesia care unit (PACU). The PACU has been known in the past as the recovery room or postanesthesia room.

An assigned area for the care of the postoperative patient is a fairly recent addition to surgical patient care. Even though surgical procedures have been performed for thousands of years and general anesthesia has been available for almost 150 years, PACUs have become common only in the last 30 to 40 years. A postanesthesia area was first described by Florence Nightingale (1863): "It is not uncommon, in small country hospitals, to have a recess or small room leading from the operating theater in which the patients remain until they have recovered, or at least recovered from the immediate effects of the operation."

There were a few recovery rooms opened in the 1920s and 1930s. In the 1940s a large number of PACUs opened due to the shortage of nurses during the war years and the need to centralize patients, equipment, and personnel for postoperative care. It was soon discovered that use of the PACU decreased patient morbidity and mortality and shortened the period of hospitalization of some patients (Ruth et al., 1947). Many hospitals opened PACUs after this discovery was reported.

PACUs have flourished since that time. Technologic innovation has had an impact there, as in other critical care areas. The complexity of today's anesthesia management demands specially trained nurses. Most patients who receive general anesthesia, major regional anesthesia, or monitored anesthesia care are transferred to a PACU.

The PACU should be adjacent to the surgical suite with easy access provided. The patient's status should be assessed for needs during transfer (such as oxygen, manual positive pressure device, a bed instead of a stretcher).

The perioperative nurse in some cases may actually provide care for the patient in the PACU. It is more common, however, for the perioperative nurse to accompany the patient to the PACU with an anesthesia provider and then give a report on the status of the patient to a postanesthesia nurse. The nurse in PACU assumes the care of the patient after an initial assessment of the patient and a report from the transferring team.

PERIOPERATIVE NURSING CONSIDERATIONS

ASSESSMENT
Admission to PACU

The initial assessment of the postoperative patient begins with an immediate determination of airway and circulatory adequacy. The airway is assessed for patency, humidified oxygen is applied, and respirations are counted. Pulse oximetry is initiated on all patients, and the quality of breath sounds is determined. The patient is then connected to the cardiac monitor, and cardiac rate and rhythm are evaluated. Blood pressure measurement is then obtained by means of a manual cuff or a noninvasive cuff (such as Dinamap). An arterial line can be connected to the monitor at this time.

After the PACU nurse has assessed the ABCs (airway, breathing, circulation), the perioperative nurse and anesthesia provider can then prepare a comprehensive report on the patient. Even though the report is usually given by the anesthesia provider, the perioperative nurse should collaborate and then add and verify important information about the patient (Rothrock, 1990).

The American Society of Post Anesthesia Nurses (ASPAN, 1992) recommends that the report contain (1) relevant preoperative status, such as vital signs, radiology findings, laboratory values, oxygen saturation, allergies, and disabilities, (2) anesthesia technique, (3) anesthetic agents including muscle relaxants, narcotics and reversal agents, (4) length of time anesthesia was administered and time reversal agents were given, (5) type of surgical procedure, (6) estimated fluid/blood loss and replacement, and (7) complications occurring during anesthesia course.

Other useful information that the perioperative nurse can provide includes the status of the airway, presence of tubes, drains and catheters, and intravascular lines. Any postoperative orders to be initiated in PACU can be discussed at this time.

The anesthesia provider should not leave the patient until the PACU nurse accepts responsibility for the patient's care. Standard III-3 of the American Society of Anesthesiologists' Standards for Postanesthesia Care (1991) states, "The member of the anesthesia care team shall remain in the PACU until the PACU nurse accepts responsibility for the nursing care of the patient."

Initial assessment

After the immediate assessment of ABCs and completion of the report, the PACU nurse begins a more thorough postanesthesia assessment. The assessment is performed

quickly and is specific to the type of operative procedure. ASPAN has recommended elements of an initial assessment in the PACU (Box 8-1).

Some PACUs use a head-to-toe assessment to organize the data obtained (Fig. 8-1). Other PACUs have adopted a major body systems approach to assessment (Fig. 8-2). In any case, the PACU nurse assesses the admitting vital signs and the ABCs beginning with the respiratory system. Respiratory assessment consists of rate, rhythm, auscultation of breath sounds, and an oxygen saturation level. Presence of an artificial airway and type of oxygen delivery system are noted.

The cardiovascular system is assessed by monitoring heart rate and rhythm. The patient's initial blood pressure is compared to one or more preoperative readings. Body temperature is obtained and skin condition is examined,

---

BOX 8-1

Initial Assessment in the PACU

Initial assessment to include documentation of:
1. Vital signs
   a. Airway patent, respiratory rate and competency, breath sounds, type of artificial airway, mechanical ventilator settings and oxygen saturations
   b. Blood pressure: cuff or arterial line
   c. Pulse: apical, peripheral
   d. Temperature: oral, rectal, axillary, digital through dermal sensor, tympanic
2. Level of consciousness
3. Pressure readings: central venous, arterial blood, pulmonary artery wedge, and intracranial pressure if indicated
4. Position of patient
5. Condition and color of skin
6. Patient safety needs
7. Neurovascular: peripheral pulses and sensation of extremity (ies) as applicable
8. Condition of dressings
9. Condition of suture line, if dressing absent
10. Type, patency, and securement of drainage tubes, catheters, and receptacle
11. Amount and type of drainage
12. Muscular response and strength
13. Pupillary response as indicated
14. Fluid therapy, location of lines, condition of IV site, and securement and amount of solution infusing (including blood)
15. Level of physical and emotional support
16. Numerical score if used

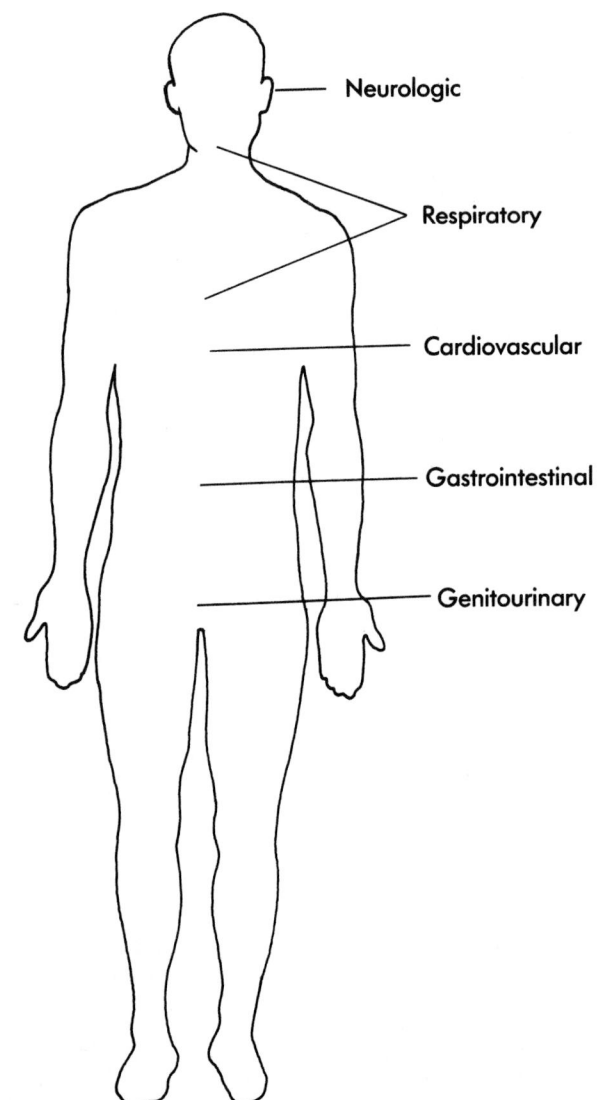

FIG. 8-1   Head-to-toe assessment.

From Litwack, K. (1991). *Post anesthesia care nursing.* St. Louis: Mosby.

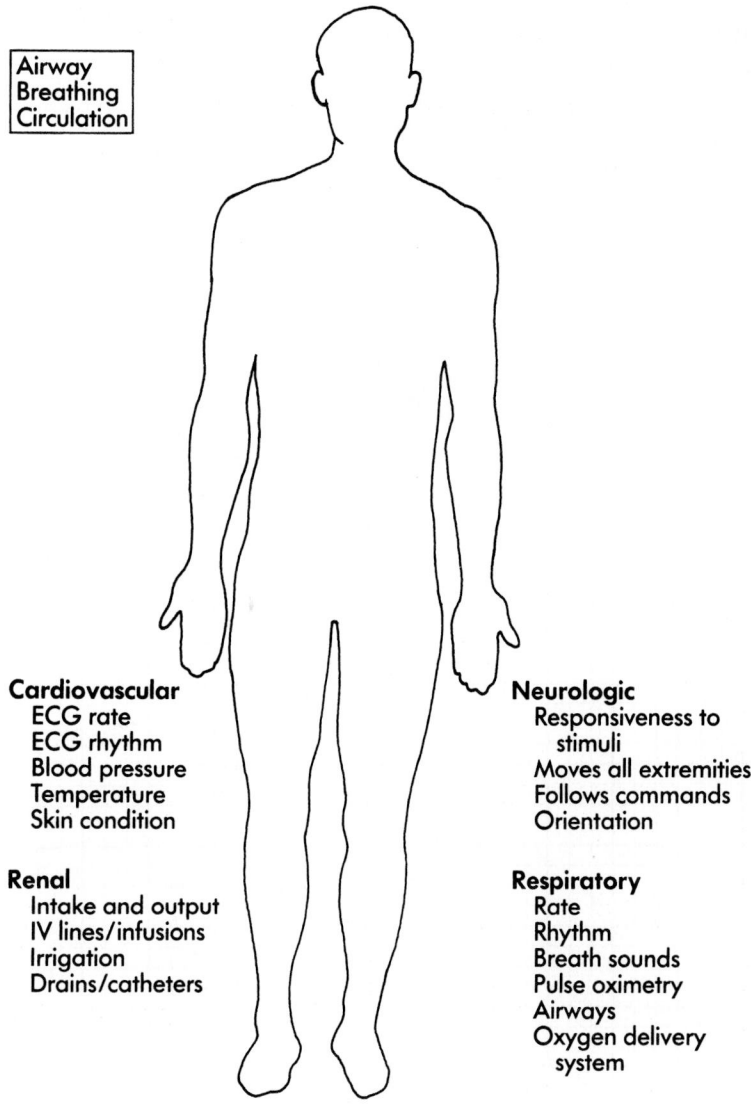

Airway
Breathing
Circulation

Cardiovascular
  ECG rate
  ECG rhythm
  Blood pressure
  Temperature
  Skin condition

Renal
  Intake and output
  IV lines/infusions
  Irrigation
  Drains/catheters

Neurologic
  Responsiveness to
    stimuli
  Moves all extremities
  Follows commands
  Orientation

Respiratory
  Rate
  Rhythm
  Breath sounds
  Pulse oximetry
  Airways
  Oxygen delivery
    system

FIG. 8-2   PACU major body systems assessment.

From Litwack, K. (1991). *Post anesthesia care nursing*. St. Louis: Mosby.

including peripheral pulses, if indicated. The patient is then assessed for neurologic functioning. Has the patient reacted (awakened from anesthesia)? Can the patient follow commands? Is the patient oriented—at least to name and hospital? Can the patient move all extremities? Are there deviations from preoperative neurologic functioning? Some operative procedures require a more detailed assessment.

To assess renal function, the intake and output are examined. The intraoperative fluid total and estimated blood loss are assessed. The intravenous lines, infusions, and irrigation solutions are recorded. Presence of all lines, drains, and catheters is noted; output is noted for color, amount, and consistency.

All of the information obtained from the admission assessment is documented in the PACU record. One example of a PACU record is shown in Fig. 8-3.

NURSING DIAGNOSIS

Common nursing diagnoses related to the care of postanesthesia patients might include the following:

· Ineffective breathing pattern
· Decreased cardiac output
· High risk for altered body temperature
· Altered thought processes
· Pain

OUTCOME IDENTIFICATION

Outcomes identified for the selected nursing diagnoses could be stated as:

· Patient will maintain ventilation, perfusion, and adequate expansion of lungs on discharge from PACU.
· Patient will maintain adequate cardiac output on discharge from PACU.

FORREST GENERAL HOSPITAL
POST ANESTHESIA CARE UNIT RECORD

POST ANESTHESIA RECOVERY SCORE	MINUTES				
	in	30	60	90	out

Activity
Able to move 4 extremities voluntarily or on command = 2
Able to move 2 extremities voluntarily or on command = 1
Able to move 0 extremities voluntarily or on command = 0

Respiration
Able to deep breath and cough freely = 2
Dyspnea or limited breathing = 1
Apneic = 0

Circulation
BP ± 20 of Preanesthetic level = 2
BP ± 20-50 of Preanesthetic level = 1
BP ± 50 of Preanesthetic level = 0

Consciousness
Fully Awake = 2
Arousable on calling = 1
Not Responding = 0

Color
Pink Normal = 2
Pale Dusky Blotchy Jaundiced Other = 1
Cyanosis = 0

TOTAL

Pre-op B.P. _____
Allergies:

Airway: On Adm.
Jawthrust _____
Chin Hold _____
Endotracheal _____
Oral Airway _____
Mask Oxygen _____
Nasal Oxygen _____
Trach _____
T-Tube _____
Nasal Airway _____
Ventilator Settings _____

Addressograph

Time In _____ Time Out _____
Accompanied by _____
Type of anesthesia _____
Surgical Procedure:

PULSE - RESPIRATION - BLOOD PRESSURE graph: 240 220 200 180 160 140 120 100 80 60 40 20; time 15 30 45 (×4)

O₂ Sat.
CVP

CODES: ⊥ A-line T B.P.   V Manual or ∧ NBP   Pulse • Resp. o   Siderails: Yes No   Restraints: Yes No

A-LINE _____

INTAKE
I.V. Running _____
Total
I.V. in Surgery _____
BLood in Surgery _____
BLood in PACU _____
TOTAL IV FLUIDS Given in PACU _____
RN Signature

Foley Cath. _____
Supra pubic _____
Ureteral _____

OUTPUT
Urinary In OR _____
Urinary In PACU _____
Voided _____
Total _____
Levine _____
Hemovac:
Drains:

MEDICATIONS AND TREATMENTS

	AMT.	ROUTE	TIME
Demerol			
Morphine			
Phenergan			
Droperidol			

FIG. 8-3 PACU nursing record.
Courtesy Forrest General Hospital, Hattiesburg, Miss.

DATE	TIME	DESCRIPTIVE NOTES (Sign Each Entry)	DATE	TIME	DESCRIPTIVE NOTES (Sign Each Entry)

DIAGNOSIS (Circle number of any diagnosis made)	GOAL	Goal Achieved	
		YES	NO
1 Alteration in neurological status			
2 Alteration in comfort level			
3 Alteration in emotional status			
4 Alteration in circulation			
5 Alteration in fluid volume			
6 Alteration in mobility			
7 Alteration in respiratory function			
8 Alteration in skin integrity			
9 Alteration in temperature			
10 Alteration in elimination			
11 Alteration in gastrointestinal function			
12 Potential for injury			
13 Potential for bleeding			
14 Other			

30-2-092-4

STANDARD OFFICE SUPPLY - HATTIESBURG

FIG. 8-3, CONT'D. PACU nursing record.

SAMPLE CARE PLAN

NURSING DIAGNOSIS: Ineffective breathing pattern related to medications associated with anesthesia, type of surgical procedure, pain, tracheobronchial obstruction

OUTCOME: Patient will maintain ventilation, perfusion, and adequate expansion of lungs on discharge from PACU: regular respiratory rate and pattern; bilateral breath sounds clear and equal; BP and pulse within preoperative range; oxygen saturation >92% or equal to preoperative status; patent airway; pain controlled.

INTERVENTIONS:

Assess respiratory status on admission to PACU and at intervals until discharge.

Determine level of consciousness (to assess for need to reverse narcotic, benzodiazepine, or muscle relaxant).

Administer humidified oxygen; assess need for continued oxygen after discharge.

Elevate head of bed (if not contraindicated).

Encourage patient to take deep breaths or sustained maximal inspiration (SMI).

Determine need for chin tilt or jaw thrust if patient nonreactive without patent airway. Insert artificial airway if needed. Call physician for further assistance.

Assess patient for level of comfort. Administer pain medication as needed, per order or protocol.

NURSING DIAGNOSIS: Decreased cardiac output related to anesthetic agents and other medications, fluid or blood loss or replacement, peripheral pooling of blood, alteration in preload or afterload, alterations in rate or rhythm

OUTCOME: Patient will maintain adequate cardiac output on discharge from PACU: BP within preoperative range, skin warm and dry, oriented to person and place, pulse strong and regular.

INTERVENTIONS:

Monitor vital signs, ECG, CVP, and/or pulmonary artery catheter.

Assess level of consciousness to determine effect of medication still in circulation.

Monitor drainage from surgical site.

Monitor intake and output.

Administer fluid/blood products if indicated.

If hypotensive, use Trendelenburg position unless contraindicated, increase fluid administration.

Maintain patency of intravenous lines.

Administer medication if needed to improve depressed myocardial contractility, increase cardiac output, and promote diuresis.

Administer vasodilators or antidysrhythmics as ordered.

Warm patient to temperature >96°F.

Administer humidified oxygen.

NURSING DIAGNOSIS: High risk for altered body temperature related to surgical procedure: anesthetic agents, length of surgery, age of patient, environment, irrigation, type of surgery, or genetic predisposition to malignant hyperthermia

OUTCOME: The patient will maintain a normal body temperature (oral or tympanic) of 96° to 99.5°F on discharge from PACU.

INTERVENTIONS:

Measure body temperature (oral or tympanic) on admission.

Assess peripheral circulation.

Monitor vital signs and oxygen saturation.

Observe for shivering.

Initiate measures to warm the patient if hypothermic:
 Place warmed blankets on patient's body and head.
 Utilize forced warm air device to rewarm patient (such as Bair Hugger).

Initiate appropriate measures for malignant hyperthermia, if indicated (see Chapter 6).

Initiate ongoing temperature monitoring until discharge.

· Patient will maintain normal body temperature (96° to 99.5° F) on discharge from PACU.

· Patient will demonstrate appropriate cognitive functioning on discharge from PACU.

· Patient will exhibit a decreased level of pain or pain will have improved and be at tolerable level on discharge from PACU.

PLANNING

Once the nursing diagnoses and desired outcomes are identified for the postoperative patient, the plan of care is designed for the specific patient. Some nursing diagnoses are appropriate for all postanesthesia patients. A Sample Care Plan for the postanesthesia patient is included on pp. 198 and 199.

SAMPLE CARE PLAN—CONT'D

NURSING DIAGNOSIS: Altered thought processes related to the surgical process: anesthetic agents, hypoxia, pain, bladder distention
OUTCOME: The patient will demonstrate appropriate cognitive functioning on discharge from PACU: oriented to person and place, responds to commands, calm appearance.
INTERVENTIONS:
Assess level of consciousness.
Determine type of anesthetic agents used.
Monitor oxygen saturation level.
Evaluate level of anxiety and pain.
Determine if bladder distention is present; catheterize if appropriate.
Reorient patient to person and place.
Administer humidified oxygen.
Administer sedation for anxiety or appropriate pain medication.

NURSING DIAGNOSIS: Pain related to invasive diagnostic tests and/or tissue trauma (surgery)
OUTCOME: The patient will exhibit a decreased level of pain or pain at a tolerable level on discharge from PACU.

INTERVENTIONS:
Assess for subjective signs of pain:
  The patient reports to the nurse that he or she is in pain:
  The patient is given a visual analog or numerical scale to determine perception of the level of pain.
Assess for objective signs of pain:
  Protective guarding behavior
  Moaning, crying, whimpering
  Restlessness
  Irritability
  Diaphoresis
  Dilated pupils
  Facial expression of pain
  Change in vital signs: BP, respiratory rate, or pulse.
Administer pain medication as prescribed: titrate intravenous doses or initiate patient-controlled analgesia (PCA).
Initiate alternate methods of pain relief: transcutaneous electrical nerve stimulation (TENS), music, massage.
Reposition patient if not contraindicated.
Assess causes of pain (such as surgical site versus chest pain).
Evaluate effectiveness of pain relief.

IMPLEMENTATION

Dramatic and life-threatening changes can occur rapidly in the postanesthesia setting. Some studies in the PACU have revealed an incidence of complications from 10% to 18% (Frost, 1992). The following complications are pertinent to the care of all patients during the postoperative period. Prompt recognition and immediate intervention are imperative for the well-being of the patient.

Postoperative complications
Respiratory

The first priority in the care of the postanesthesia patient is to establish a patent airway. A very common cause of airway obstruction is the tongue, which is relaxed due to the anesthetic agents and muscle relaxants used during surgery (Fig. 8-4). The patient may present with snoring, retraction of intercostal muscles, asynchronous movements of the chest and abdomen, and a decreased oxygen saturation level. The nursing action taken may be as simple as stimulating the patient to take deep breaths. If the patient is still unresponsive, the nurse may need to open the airway with a chin tilt or jaw thrust. A chin tilt is

accomplished by lifting the chin with one hand while tilting the forehead back with the other. A jaw thrust is accomplished by displacing the temporomandibular joint forward bilaterally.

If these actions do not open the airway, an artificial airway may need to be inserted (Fig. 8-5). Either an oral or nasal airway may be used. An oral airway is indicated for use with an unresponsive patient; a nasal airway is indicated for patients who are arousable because it is better tolerated by an awake patient.

In certain situations, such as apnea, intubation with ventilation may be required. If intubation is impossible, the patient may require a tracheostomy, although this is rare.

A very serious complication that can occur in the PACU is laryngospasm. The muscles of the larynx contract and either partially or completely obstruct the airway. Laryngospasm is usually due to an irritable airway. Nursing actions include removing the irritating stimulus, hyperextending the patient's head, oxygenating the patient, and possibly administering an aerosol with racemic epinephrine. In most cases positive pressure ventilation must be delivered per mask and bag. If the symptoms last longer than 1 minute

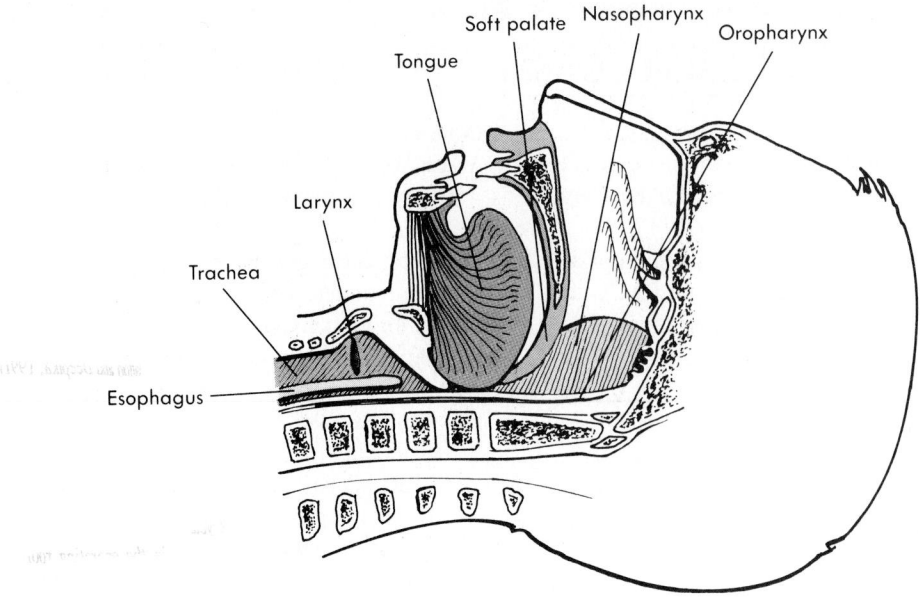

FIG. 8-4   Obstruction of airway by tongue.

From Long, B.C., Phipps, W.J., & Cassmeyer, V.L. (Eds.). (1993). *Medical-surgical nursing: A nursing process approach*. St. Louis: Mosby.

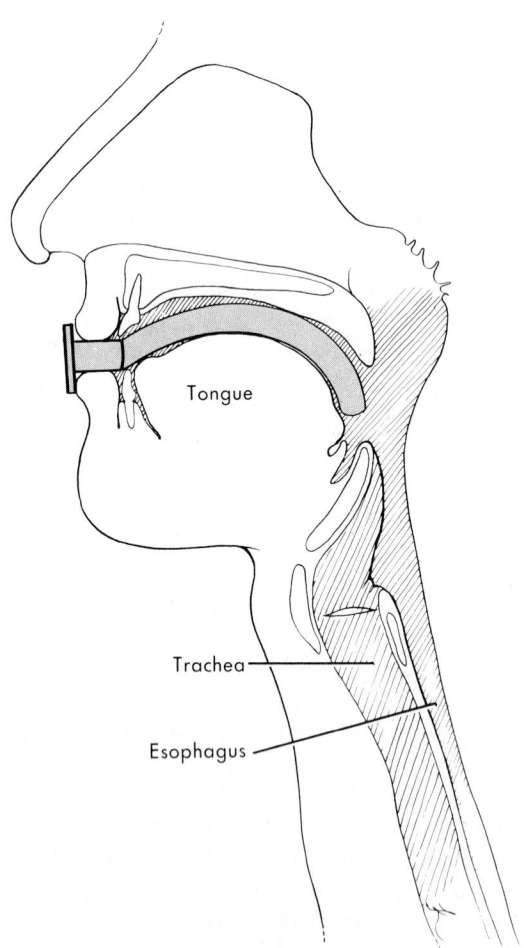

FIG. 8-5   Oropharyngeal airway in place.

From Long, B.C., Phipps, W.J., & Cassmeyer, V.L. (Eds.). (1993). *Medical-surgical nursing: A nursing process approach*, St. Louis: Mosby.

and are unrelieved by positive pressure, administration of a muscle relaxant is required. Reintubation is undesirable and used only as a last resort.

Bronchospasm is a lower airway obstruction caused by spasms of the bronchial tubes. Inhaled bronchodilators are the first choice of therapy for these patients, followed by IV aminophylline. Epinephrine and methylprednisolone may also be administered in some cases.

Cardiovascular

Instability of the cardiovascular system is a frequent finding following surgery (Frost, 1992). Common problems include hypotension, hypertension, and dysrhythmias.

Hypotension is experienced by about 3% of postoperative patients (Frost, 1992). Hypotension has been defined as a blood pressure of less than 20% of baseline or preoperative blood pressure. Many times the clinical signs of hypotension are more reliable as an indicator, especially in the patient with only one recorded preoperative pressure. Clinical signs may include a rapid, thready pulse, disorientation, restlessness, oliguria, or cold pale skin.

Cardiac output and vascular resistance determine blood pressure. Hypotension may be due to a cardiac dysfunction such as myocardial infarction, tamponade, embolism, or medications, including anesthetic agents. In this case the heart is no longer pumping effectively. Oxygen and cardiac stimulants will be used as needed as well as hemodynamic monitoring.

Hypovolemia reduces cardiac output and may be caused by hemorrhage, dehydration, or increased positive end-expiratory pressure (PEEP). Fluid and/or blood replacement is used to treat hypovolemia. If the patient is hemorrhaging at the surgical site, a return to the operating room is indicated.

Decreased vascular resistance can be related to medications, general and regional anesthesia, or anaphylaxis. Vasodilatation can be treated with fluids, vasopressors, or elevation of the patient's legs. Anaphylactic reactions are treated with epinephrine, antihistamines, and additional fluids.

Systemic arterial *hypertension* is usually defined as a blood pressure 20% higher than the patient's baseline or preoperative level. Again, clinical signs are the most important indicator of the severity of the hypertension. Headache, mental status changes, and substernal pain are all indicators of end-organ damage.

Asymptomatic hypertension is a common occurrence in the PACU and is usually considered to be harmless. The solution is usually determined by the cause. Elevated blood pressure does cause increased ventricular wall tension, afterload, and myocardial work. The patient with a history of cardiac disease is more at risk for adverse results.

Hypertension may be due to volume overload or pulmonary edema, which causes an increase in the cardiac output. In this case the patient is given diuretics, fluids are restricted, and the patient is hemodynamically monitored.

Other causes of hypertension are pain and anxiety, hypothermia, hypoxemia, hypercarbia, and viscus distention, all of which cause increased vascular resistance. Patients in pain are medicated and patients with hypothermia are warmed. Patients are oxygenated well and ventilated if necessary to improve hypoxemia or hypercarbia. Patients are encouraged to void or are catheterized to empty a full bladder.

Antihypertensive drugs are used as necessary to control blood pressure. Patients should resume taking prescribed preoperative antihypertensives as soon as possible after surgery. Ambulatory surgical patients, as well as inpatients, should be allowed to take their prescribed antihypertensives the day of surgery.

A common *dysrhythmia* following surgery is sinus tachycardia (a rate greater than 100 in the adult). Frequent causes include pain, hypoxemia, hypovolemia, increased temperature, and anxiety. The underlying cause is treated. Propranolol, metroprolol, or esmolol may be given.

Sinus bradycardia (heart rate less than 60 in the adult) is also a common dysrhythmia in the PACU. Causes include hypoxemia, hypothermia, high spinal anesthesia, vagal stimulation, and some medications that are commonly given during or after surgery. The underlying cause is treated. Atropine is the drug of choice to increase the heart rate, and usually no other treatment is required. Temporary or permanent pacemakers may sometimes be required.

Premature ventricular contractions (PVCs) are repre-

sented by wide, bizarre looking QRS complexes. The most common causes in the postoperative period are hypoxemia and hypokalemia. Those underlying conditions are treated. Many times if cardiac disease or hypotension is not present, the PVCs do not require medication. If intervention is required, lidocaine remains the drug of choice.

Temperature abnormalities

Postoperative *hypothermia,* defined as a temperature less than 36° C or 96.8° F, continues to be a widespread problem in the PACU. As many as 60% of patients in the PACU are believed to be hypothermic (Patton and Deepika, 1991). Often hypothermia is not life threatening; however, it does cause physiologic stress. Hypothermia can prolong recovery time and contributes to postoperative morbidity. Especially vulnerable to the effects of hypothermia are the elderly and children up to 2 years of age.

Prevention of heat loss begins in the operating room. Under general anesthesia the patient does not produce heat and is dependent on ambient temperature. Prevention can include increasing the ambient temperature in the operating room and draping the patient on arrival to minimize exposure. Heated humidifiers and fluid warmers add heat. A recent technique of preventing hypothermia in the operating room is the forced warm air device (Fig. 8-6).

In the PACU tremendous demands are made on the body if the patient begins to shiver. Shivering can increase the need for oxygen by 300% to 400%. Hypothermic patients should have oxygen therapy initiated immediately upon admission. For a patient with a healthy heart, there may be no untoward effects. However, for the patient with coronary artery disease or cardiomyopathy, decompensation can occur.

There are other problems associated with hypothermia. Intravascular volume loss, due to a fluid shift from the extracellular space, is probably related to vasoconstriction. As the patient begins to rewarm, vasodilatation ensues, and the patient can require large amounts of intravenous fluids to avoid hypovolemia.

The central nervous system is depressed by hypothermia. The postanesthesia patient will remain more anesthetized than a warm patient while recovering. Nitrogen loss and hypokalemia can cause a predisposition to wound infection and cardiac problems. Hypothermia delays metabolism and alters effects of some anesthetic drugs. Of special interest is the prolonged elimination of muscle relaxants in hypothermic patients. Clotting abnormalities can occur. Platelet activity declines and fibrinolysis increases with hypothermia. Both of these conditions enhance the tendency to bleed (Feroe and Augustine, 1991).

Rewarming is a priority in the immediate care of the postoperative patient because normothermia reverses all effects of hypothermia. Wet and cold gowns and blankets should be removed and warm, dry gowns and blankets applied to head and body. There are several external

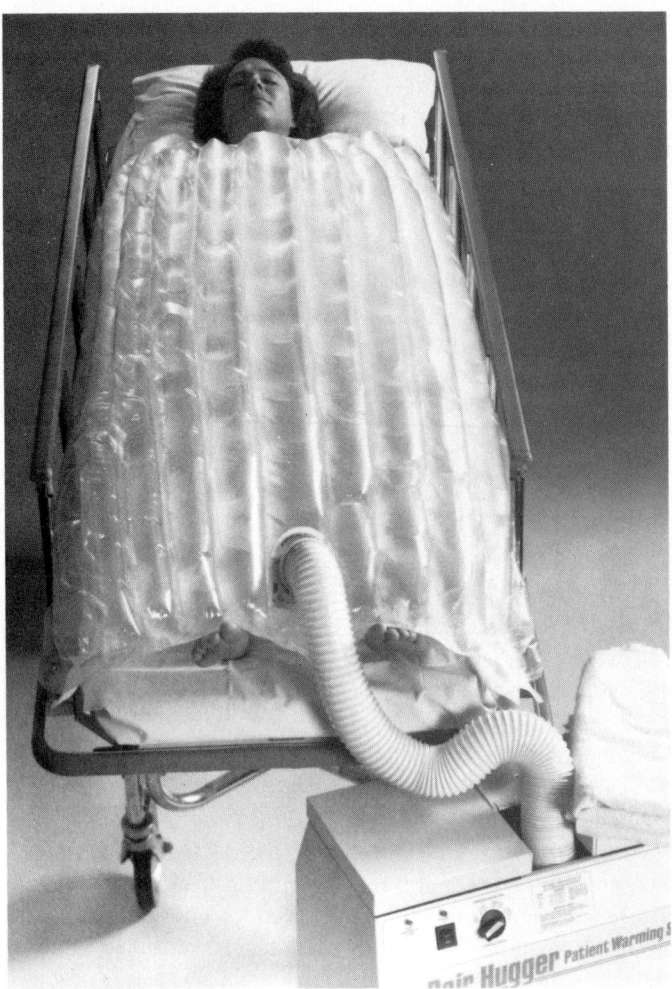

FIG. 8-6 Bair Hugger; focused thermal environment.
From Litwack, K. (1991). *Post anesthesia care nursing*. St. Louis: Mosby.

rewarming techniques available. Application of warm cotton blankets has been the tradition in the PACU. The warm blankets are applied every 5 to 10 minutes until the patient is normothermic. Cotton blankets do gradually increase the patient's temperature. However, they do not actively heat patients and can be a slow process. Continuous fluid-circulating blankets or warm water mattresses have been shown to have little value in rewarming patients due to the size of surface area in contact with the heat source. Radiant heat lamps depend on exposure of large areas of body surface, which is of limited use to adult patients. Fluid and blood warmers are useful for large volumes of cool fluids, but not to reverse hypothermia. Forced warm air devices, a new technology, have been proven effective in rewarming patients (see Research Highlight 8-1). This device produces a thermal focused environment that transfers heat to a patient by blowing warm air through a plastic and tissue paper blanket that covers the patient. These forced warm air devices are now a standard hypothermia treatment in the PACU setting.

Hyperthermia may be an indication of an infectious process or sepsis, or it may indicate a hypermetabolic process—malignant hyperthermia. This is a very serious emergency that is genetic in origin and is triggered by volatile anesthetic agents and the depolarizing muscle relaxant succinylcholine. Death ensues unless malignant hyperthermia is immediately recognized and treated (see Chapter 6).

Altered thought processes

The PACU patient may be disoriented, drowsy, confused, or delirious. The cause may range from residual effects of anesthesia to pain and anxiety. Hypoxemia should always be ruled out first; it remains the most common cause of postoperative agitation. Patients who are chemically dependent or substance abusers many times awaken in an agitated state. Viscus distention can also contribute to agitation in a drowsy, confused patient. The PACU nurse should identify and eliminate the cause of the agitation or confusion, if possible. The patient can be engaged in short conversations and reoriented to place and person. Baseline pre-

RESEARCH HIGHLIGHT 8-1

Lennon and colleagues studied the effectiveness of a forced warm air system versus warmed cotton blankets for treatment of hypothermic postoperative patients. Thirty adult PACU patients whose temperatures were <35° C were randomized into two groups. Group 1 patients were covered with cotton blankets warmed to 37° C; group 2 patients were treated with the Bair Hugger system.

Patients in group 2 were warmer at all time intervals measured. Mean oral temperature was 34.3° C for both groups on admission. Mean oral temperature in the forced-air warming group had risen to 34.8° C 15 minutes after admission to PACU; patients in the cotton blanket group remained at 34.3° C. At 90 minutes the forced-air group was 36° C, the cotton blanket group 35° C. Patients in group 2 spent significantly less time in the PACU than did patients in group 1: 99.7 versus 156 minutes.

The forced warm air system produced a more rapid rate of warming, a decreased incidence of shivering, and earlier discharge from the PACU than patients who were warmed with cotton blankets.

Lennon, R.L., Hosking, M.P., Conover, M.A., & Perkins, W.J. (1990). Evaluation of a forced-air system for warming hypothermic postoperative patients. *Anesthesia and Analgesia, 70*, 424-427.

operative data are important to determine cause. Persistent changes from preoperative status require thorough assessment and possible intervention from the physician.

Pain

Pain is a subjective experience and may or may not be verbalized. Many times health care providers require objective signs of discomfort in addition to subjective reports of pain from the patient. As a result, it is believed that up to 75% of postsurgical patients are undertreated for pain (Frost, 1992.) The Agency for Health Care Policy and Research (AHCPR, 1992) has developed clinical practice guidelines on acute pain management and contends that all patients should be assessed for severity of pain using either a verbal rating scale or visual analog scale (Fig. 8-7). Copies of the guidelines may be obtained free of charge by writing to Center for Research Dissemination and Liaison, AHCPR Publications Clearinghouse, P.O. Box 8547, Silver Spring, MD 20907; or by calling 1-800-358-9295.

Nonpharmacologic interventions that may be used include positioning, verbal reassurance, touch, applications of heat or cold, massage, and transcutaneous electrical nerve stimulation (TENS). If the patient was taught preoperatively, other techniques that can be used are relaxation, imagery, music distraction, and biofeedback.

Evidence has indicated that early analgesia reduces postoperative problems (Frost, 1992). Nonsteroidal antiinflam-

matory drugs (NSAIDs) and opiates are the analgesics of choice. An intramuscular dose of 30 mg of ketorolac is equivalent to 100 mg of meperidine. NSAIDs and opiates are usually used in combination in the PACU. The patient may receive a dose of ketorolac in the operating room or immediately after arrival in the PACU. Pain is then treated intravenously with an opiate such as morphine, meperidine, or fentanyl.

Patient-controlled analgesia (PCA) allows a patient to control the analgesic administration. Dosage, time between doses, and the maximum dosage that can be administered is prescribed by the physician. The PCA can be started in the PACU or immediately upon arrival in the patient's room. Other methods of postoperative pain relief include spinal and epidural opiate placement and direct placement of local anesthetics by the surgeon.

Nausea and vomiting

Nausea and vomiting are postoperative problems that affect a large number of patients in the PACU. The management of nausea and vomiting actually begins preoperatively and continues into the intraoperative period. Preventive therapy has been effective in reducing the incidence. There is no single method of prevention or treatment of nausea and vomiting. Many causative factors are related to anesthesia and surgery.

The PACU nurse must protect the airway of an unconscious or semiconscious patient to prevent the possibility of aspiration of gastric contents. Precipitating factors should be eliminated, such as avoiding conversations that could elicit nausea and vomiting and preventing rapid movement and head elevation of the patient.

Antiemetic therapy is planned to reduce GI symptoms without oversedating the patient. A frequently used drug, especially in the ambulatory surgical setting, is droperidol. Other drugs commonly used are metoclopramide (Reglan), prochlorperazine (Compazine), and promethazine (Phenergan). The antiemetic agent odansetron (Zofran) has recently been approved for prevention of postoperative nausea and vomiting. This drug may become popular due to its lack of side effects such as sedation, hypotension, and tremors. Other useful medications include dimenhydrinate (Dramamine), hydroxyzine (Vistaril, Atarax), and scopolamine (Transderm-Scop).

EVALUATION

The patient is evaluated based on the outcomes identified as significant after the initial assessment.

- The patient maintained an adequate oxygen saturation on room air.
- The blood pressure and heart rate are within normal range for the patient.
- The patient is normothermic.
- The patient is oriented to time and person.
- The patient's pain decreased to a tolerable level. The patient is relaxed and sleeping at intervals. The patient verbalized pain relief.

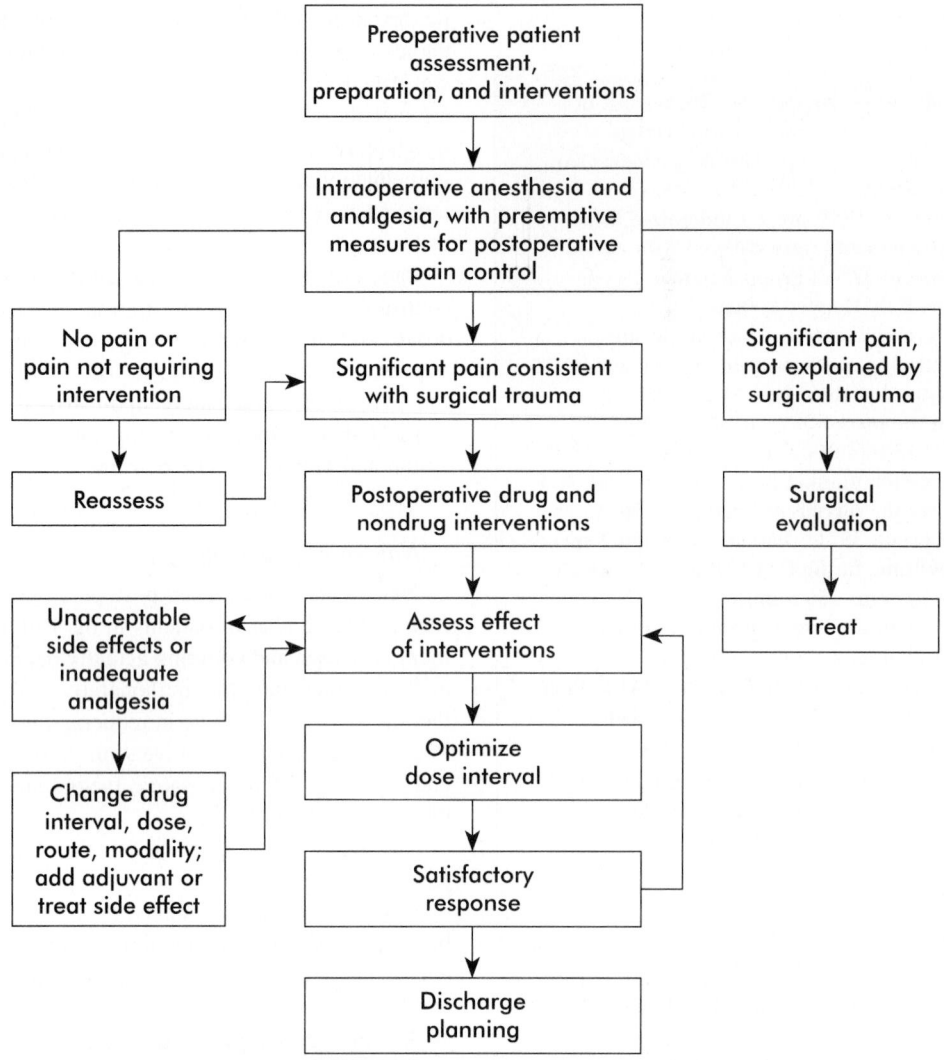

FIG. 8-7   Acute pain management in adults.

From Acute Pain Management Guideline Panel. (1992). *Acute pain management in adults: Operative procedures. Quick reference guide for clinicians.* AHCPR Pub. No. 92-0019. Rockville, Md: Agency for Health Care Policy and Research.

DISCHARGE FROM THE PACU

The PACU nurse completes a thorough assessment immediately before the patient's discharge and transfer to the surgical unit. The nurse assesses the patient's vital signs, level of consciousness, condition of the operative site, comfort level, and other parameters, such as those suggested in Box 8-2.

The patient is usually discharged from the PACU by an anesthesiologist, who may be present and actually write a discharge order. Alternatively, a numeric scoring system approved by the Department of Anesthesia may be used to determine if the patient is ready for discharge. The most common scoring system in use is the Aldrete Score. Activity, respiration, circulation, consciousness, and color are scored from 0-2 (see Fig. 8-3). A total score of 9 or 10 is generally acceptable for PACU discharge with exceptions made by physician's order.

A report on the patient's condition is given to the nurse who will assume care for the patient on the surgical unit. This report may be given by telephone prior to the patient leaving PACU or person-to-person after the patient reaches the surgical unit. The report should include a preoperative history, pertinent information regarding the patient's surgery and recovery, medications the patient was given, physician's orders, and any other appropriate information.

ADMISSION TO THE SURGICAL UNIT

The patient's room is prepared for admission, and any necessary equipment is provided. The patient is placed in the bed with adequate help. The bed siderails should be kept raised until the patient is fully awake to prevent patient falls. The patient is informed to notify the nurse for assistance to ambulate. The family is also instructed and enlisted

---

BOX 8-2

Pain Assessment and Reassessment

PRINCIPLES

- Patients who may have difficulty communicating their pain require particular attention. This includes patients who are cognitively impaired, psychotic or severely emotionally disturbed, children and the elderly, patients who do not speak English, and patients whose level of education or cultural background differs significantly from that of their health care team.
- Unexpected intense pain, particularly if sudden or associated with altered vital signs such as hypotension, tachycardia, or fever, should be immediately evaluated, and new diagnoses such as wound dehiscence, infection, or deep venous thrombosis considered.
- Family members should be involved when appropriate.

PAIN ASSESSMENT TOOLS

- The single most reliable indicator of the existence and intensity of pain—and any resultant distress—is the patient's self report.
- Self-report measurement scales include numerical or adjective ratings and visual analog scales.
- Tools should be reliable, valid, and easy for the patient and the nurse or doctor to use. These tools may be used by showing a diagram to the patient to indicate the appropriate rating. The tools may also be used by simply asking the patient for a verbal response (e.g., "On a scale of 0 to 10 with 0 as no pain and 10 as the worst pain possible, how would you rate your pain?").
- Tools must be appropriate for the patient's developmental, physical, emotional, and cognitive status.

PREOPERATIVE PREPARATION

- Discuss the patient's previous experiences with pain and beliefs about and preferences for pain assessment and management.
- Give the patient information about pain management therapies that are available and the rationale underlying their use.

- Develop with the patient a plan for pain assessment and management.
- Select a pain assessment tool, and teach the patient to use it. Determine the level of pain above with adjustment of analgesia or other interventions will be considered.
- Provide the patient with education and information about pain control, including training in inonpharmacologic options such as relaxation.
- Inform patients that it is easier to prevent pain than to chase and reduce it once it has become established and that communication of unrelieved pain is essential to its relief. Emphasize the importance of a factual report of pain, avoiding stoicism or exaggeration.

POSTOPERATIVE ASSESSMENT

- Assess the patient's perceptions, along with behavioral and psychologic responses. Remember that observations of behavior and vital signs should not be used instead of a self-report unless the patient is unable to communicate.
- Assess and reassess pain frequently during the immediate postoperative period. Determine the frequency of assessment based on the operation performed and the severity of the pain. For example, pain should be assessed every 2 hours during the first postoperative day after major surgery.
- Increase the frequency of assessment and reassessment if the pain is poorly controlled or if interventions are changing.
- Record the pain intensity and response to intervention in an easily visible and accessible place, such as a bedside flow sheet.
- Revise the management plan in the pain is poorly controlled.
- Review with the patient before discharge the interventions used and their efficacy and provide specific discharge instructions regarding pain and its management.

Acute Pain Management Guideline Panel. *Acute Pain Management in Adults: Operative Procedures. Quick Reference Guide for Clinicians.* AHCPR Pub. No. 92-0019. Rockville, MD: Agency for Health Care Policy and Research, Public Health Service, U.S. Department of Health and Human Services.

---

to maintain safety for the patient. The equipment and condition of the patient should be explained to the family members who are present. A special concern is the use of the PCA. Family members should be instructed that the PCA is for the patient's use only; that pushing the PCA button for the patient can have a detrimental effect on the patient's well-being.

POSTOPERATIVE NURSING CONSIDERATIONS

ASSESSMENT

The nurse makes an immediate assessment as soon as the patient is transferred to the bed. The nurse may choose a head-to-toe or systems assessment. Parameters include respiratory, cardiovascular, and neurologic status. The condition of the dressing and surgical site and patient comfort and safety are also assessed (Box 8-3).

NURSING DIAGNOSIS

Nursing diagnoses related to the care of the postoperative patient might include the following:

- High risk for infection
- Ineffective breathing pattern
- Pain
- Altered nutrition, less than body requirements
- Impaired physical mobility

OUTCOME IDENTIFICATION

Outcomes identified for the selected nursing diagnoses could be stated as:

- The patient will be free from infection as indicated by normal vital signs; temperature within normal range;

normal white blood count; clear breath sounds; clear, yellow urine; warm, dry skin.
- The patient's respirations will be easy, unlabored, and adequate.
- The patient will state subjective assertions of comfort ("I am in no pain") and will have no objective signs of discomfort (grimaces, tachycardia).
- The patient eats well from prescribed diet; weight loss is minimal.
- The patient ambulates at appropriate levels and carries out activities of daily living appropriate for condition.

PLANNING

Planning for the postoperative patient requires not only a knowledge of surgical techniques, but also knowledge regarding underlying medical conditions. Throughout the patient's stay, planning must always involve the family or significant other with measurable goals determined by discharge. A Sample Care Plan for the postoperative patient is included on pp. 207-208.

IMPLEMENTATION
Wound healing

The basis for much of the postoperative nursing care is to promote wound healing. Wound care, nutritional requirements, and need for mobility are all related to the promotion of wound healing. For a detailed discussion of the pathophysiology of wound healing, see Chapter 7.

Adequate respirations

The postoperative patient is at very high risk for pulmonary complications due to increased respiratory secretions, decreased lung expansion, depression of the respiratory center, and the possibility of aspiration of gastric contents. The occurrence of these complications can be minimized by appropriate nursing management.

Circulation

Venous stasis in the postoperative patient can lead to thrombophlebitis, which is usually a preventable complication. Platelets adhere to the venous wall and form a thrombus, with a resultant potential for pulmonary embolus.

Prevention may include administration of prophylactic heparin, aspirin, dextran, or warfarin. Application of an intermittent external pneumatic compression device may be ordered or application of antiembolism (AE) hosiery may be required.

Nursing measures that can prevent formation of a thrombus include using the AE hosiery whether the patient is in or out of bed, teaching the patient not to cross the legs, isometric leg exercises, and encouraging early ambulation.

If thrombophlebitis is suspected, the patient should return to bed, and the physician should be notified. Treatment will consist of rest, heat, elastic bandages, and anticoagulant therapy.

BOX 8-3

Patient Assessment on Return from PACU

RESPIRATORY STATUS
Patency of airway
Respirations: depth, rate, character
Breath sounds: presence, character

CIRCULATORY STATUS
Pulse, blood pressure, temperature
Skin color, temperature
Capillary filling

NEUROLOGIC STATUS
Level of consciousness, ability to move extremities

DRESSING
Presence of drainage
Presence of tubes to be connected to drainage systems

COMFORT
Presence of pain, nausea, vomiting
Patient positioned for comfort and to facilitate ventilation

SAFETY
Necessity for side rails
Call cord within reach

EQUIPMENT
Monitors connected and functioning
Intravenous fluids: rate, amount in bag, patency of tubing
Drainage systems (for example, nasogastric, chest, urinary): type, patency of tubing, connection of appropriate container, character and amount of drainage

SAMPLE CARE PLAN

NURSING DIAGNOSIS: High risk for infection related to altered skin integrity, compromised aseptic technique, or malnutrition

OUTCOME: Patient will be free from infection, as indicated by normal vital signs, temperature within normal range, normal white blood count, clear breath sounds, clear, yellow urine, and warm, dry skin.

INTERVENTIONS:

Monitor vital signs every 4 hours or as prescribed.

Monitor temperature every 4 hours or as needed.

Monitor laboratory values for evidence of infection.

Encourage patient to take deep breaths or sustained maximal inspiration (SMI) and/or use respiratory aids.

Preserve closed urinary system and provide catheter care. Remove catheter as soon as possible.

Encourage the patient to eat foods high in protein and vitamin C.

Avoid antiinflammatory drugs to facilitate healing.

Use aseptic technique when changing dressings and change soiled dressings immediately.

Monitor suction of wound catheters to provide drainage from wound.

NURSING DIAGNOSIS: Ineffective breathing pattern related to postoperative pain, decreased energy or fatigue, decreased lung expansion, surgery

OUTCOME: Patient's respirations will be easy, unlabored, and adequate.

INTERVENTIONS:

Monitor respirations and chest expansion frequently for 24 to 48 hours.

Place the bed in high Fowler's position if possible.

Auscultate lungs and evaluate the productiveness of the cough.

Have the patient cough and deep breathe at regular intervals.

Encourage use of respiratory aids if appropriate.

Treat underlying conditions, such as pain.

Splint incisional area with pillow before cough.

Encourage the patient to turn and change positions at least every 2 to 3 hours.

Ambulate as soon as possible.

NURSING DIAGNOSIS: Pain related to invasive diagnostic tests and/or tissue trauma (surgery)

OUTCOME: The patient will state subjective assertions of comfort and have no objective signs of discomfort.

INTERVENTIONS:

Assess for subjective signs of pain:

The patient reports to the nurse that he or she is in pain.

The patient is given a visual analog or numerical scale to determine perception of the level of pain.

Assess for objective signs of pain:

Protective guarding behavior

Moaning, crying, whimpering

Restlessness

Irritability

Diaphoresis

Dilated pupils

Facial expression of pain

Change in vital signs: BP, respiratory rate, or pulse

Administer pain medication as prescribed. Initiate patient-controlled analgesia (PCA) if prescribed.

Initiate alternate methods of pain relief: nerve stimulation (TENS), music, massage, relaxation.

Reposition patient if not contraindicated.

Assess causes of pain (surgical site versus chest pain).

Evaluate effectiveness of pain relief.

NURSING DIAGNOSIS: Altered nutrition, less than body requirements, related to surgery

OUTCOME: Patient will eat well from prescribed diet; weight loss will be minimal.

INTERVENTIONS:

Encourage the patient to eat foods high in protein and vitamin C.

Offer frequent small amounts of food or high-protein liquids to patients who have little or no appetite.

Continued.

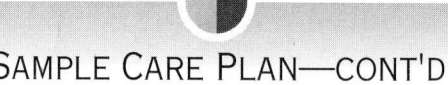

SAMPLE CARE PLAN—CONT'D

Encourage ambulation (improves appetite).
Schedule procedures not to conflict with mealtime.
Administer medication for pain and nausea as needed.
Refer to nutritional support team if appropriate.

NURSING DIAGNOSIS: Impaired physical mobility related to surgical procedures and/or pain
OUTCOME: Patient will ambulate at appropriate levels and carry out activities of daily living (ADL) appropriate for condition.
INTERVENTIONS:
Encourage muscle-strengthening exercises before ambulation.

Encourage ambulation and/or position changes and extremity exercises at least every shift.
Have patient dangle legs over side of bed until pulse has stabilized and patient is not dizzy before attempting to ambulate.
Use two people to help ambulate if the patient is weak and/or obese.
Provide for patient to walk further with each ambulation.
Teach proper use of appropriate devices (such as crutches, slings, Ace bandages) and observe return demonstration.

Urinary function

One of the priorities during surgery and immediately afterward is to keep the patient well hydrated so that voiding will take place 6 to 8 hours after surgery. Usually intake is greater than output for 48 hours, when the fluid and electrolyte balance returns to normal.

Every effort is made to refrain from use of a catheter because of the risk of urinary tract infection. Measures to aid the patient in voiding include a warm bedpan, letting water run, applying warm water to the perineum, and allowing the patient up to the bathroom whenever possible. If discomfort is present and the bladder is palpable, catheterization becomes necessary. In the event several catheterizations are required, an indwelling catheter is inserted. Hydration of the patient becomes a priority. Intake and output are recorded accurately. A urine output of less than 30 ml in 2 hours is reported to the physician.

Bowel elimination

The postoperative patient who has had abdominal or pelvic surgery may have decreased peristalsis for at least 24 hours; this may persist for several days for the patient who has had gastrointestinal surgery. Increased fluid intake and early ambulation can promote the return of peristalsis. Bowel sounds can be heard with a stethoscope to ensure that peristalsis has returned.

Constipation occurs frequently after surgery due to the effects of the anesthetic agents, narcotics, immobility, and decreased gastrointestinal motility. Fluids, roughage, and bulk laxatives can be given to aid in the relief of constipation. Occasionally an enema may be needed to empty the lower bowel.

EVALUATION

Evaluation of the postoperative patient on the surgical unit involves evaluating the outcomes identified as the patient was assessed:

· The patient's vital signs were within normal limits.
· The patient was normothermic.
· The patient's lab values were within normal range.
· The patient's wound is healing properly.
· The patient's breath sounds were clear bilaterally.
· The patient verbalized freedom from pain and was free from facial grimaces, moaning, and other evidence of pain or discomfort.
· The patient was eating well; there were no complaints of nausea or vomiting.
· The patient ambulated as appropriate.
· The patient is capable of performing the appropriate activities of daily living.

DISCHARGE PLANNING

Discharge planning should begin on admission of the patient to the surgical unit. The patient and family should be prepared to assume any care that may be needed after discharge. If needed, community resources may be used. A community health nurse is a valuable resource for the patient with treatment needs after discharge.

The patient and family should be instructed in proper care of the wound or incision. They should be knowledgeable about every medication that the patient will be using at home. A doctor's appointment for the return visit should be scheduled as ordered and the patient taught the importance of the return visit. Normal activities are gradually resumed according to the physician's protocols. Chapter 9 describes patient education and discharge planning in further detail.

REFERENCES

Acute Pain Management Guideline Panel. (1992). *Acute pain management: Operative or medical procedures and trauma. Clinical practice guideline.* AHCPR Pub. No. 92-0032. Rockville, Md: Agency for Health Care Policy and Research, Public Health Service, U.S. Department of Health and Human Services.

ASA. (1991). *Standards for postanesthesia care* (approved by House of Delegates on October 12, 1988 and last amended on October 23, 1990). Park Ridge, Ill: ASA.

ASPAN. (1992). *Standards of postanesthesia nursing practice.* Richmond, Va: ASPAN.

Feroe, D.D., & Augustine, S.D. (1991). Hypothermia in the PACU. *Critical Care Clinics of North America, 3* (1), 135-144.

Frost, E.A.M. (1992). Complications in the post-anesthesia care unit. Part I. *Current Reviews for Post Anesthesia Care Nurses, 14* (14), 113-120.

Nightingale, F. (1863). *Notes on hospitals* (3rd ed.). London: Longman, Green, Longman, Roberts, & Green.

Patton, C., & Deepika, K. (1991). Selected problems in the recovery room: A commentary. *Current Reviews for Post Anesthesia Care Nurses, 13* (7), 49-56.

Rothrock, J.C. (1990). The perioperative nurse in the postanesthesia care unit. In J.C. Rothrock (Ed.), *Perioperative nursing care planning.* St. Louis: Mosby.

Ruth, H.S., Haugen, F.P., & Grove, A.P. (1947). Anesthesia study commission. *The Journal of the American Medical Association, 35,* 881-884.

BIBLIOGRAPHY

Allen, A. (Ed.). (1991). *Core curriculum for post anesthesia nursing practice* (2nd ed.). Philadelphia: W.B. Saunders.

ASPAN. (1990). *Fifty years of progress in post anesthesia nursing: 1940-1990.* Richmond, Va: ASPAN.

Atlee III, J.L. (1990). Diagnosis and management of common dysrhythmias. *Current Reviews for Post Anesthesia Care Nurses, 11* (1), 108.

Baxter, K., Nolan, K., Winyard, J., Roulson, C.J., & Goldhill, D.R. (1993). Are they getting enough? Meeting the oxygen therapy needs of postoperative patients. *Professional Nurse, 8* (5), 310-312.

Benumof, J.L., & Saidman, L.J. (Eds.). (1992). *Anesthesia and perioperative complications.* St. Louis: Mosby.

Breslow, M.J., Miller, C.F., & Rogers, M. (1990). *Perioperative management.* St. Louis: Mosby.

Burden, N. (1993). *Ambulatory surgical nursing.* Philadelphia: W.B. Saunders.

Daleiden, A. (1993). Physiology and treatment of hemorrhagic shock during the early postoperative period. *Critical Care Nursing Quarterly, 16* (1), 45-59.

Drain, C.B., & Christoph, S.S. (1987). *The recovery room: A critical care approach to post anesthesia nursing* (3rd ed.). Philadelphia: W.B. Saunders.

Erickson, R.S., & Yount, S.T. (1991). Comparison of tympanic and oral temperatures in surgical patients. *Nursing Research, 40* (2), 90-93.

Fraulini, K. (1987). *After anesthesia: A guide for PACU, ICU, and medical-surgical nurses.* Norwalk, CT: Appleton & Lange.

Frost, E.A.M. (1992). Complications in the post-anesthesia care unit. Part II. *Current Reviews for Post Anesthesia Care Nurses, 14* (15), 121-128.

Frost, E A.M. (1990). *Post anesthesia care unit: Current practices* (2nd ed.). St. Louis: Mosby.

Giuffre, M., Finnie, J., Lynam, D., & Smith, D. (1991). Rewarming postoperative patients: Lights, blankets, or forced warm air. *Journal of Post Anesthesia Nursing, 6,* 387-393.

Hamlin, W., Schnobel, L., & Smith, B. (1991). The patient with noncardiogenic pulmonary edema. *Journal of Post Anesthesia Nursing, 6,* 43-49.

Hardy, E.B., Cirillo, B.L., & Gutzeit, M.N. (1988). Rewarming patients in the PACU: Can we make a difference? *Journal of Post Anesthesia Nursing, 3,* 313-316.

Hayden, R.A. (1992). What keeps oxygenation on track? *American Journal of Nursing, 92* (12), 32-42.

Hines, R., Barash, P.G., Watrous, G., & O'Connor, T. (1992). Complications occurring in the postanesthesia care unit. *Anesthesia and Analgesia, 74,* 503-509.

Hinojosa, R.J. (1992). Nursing interventions to prevent or relieve postoperative nausea and vomiting. *Journal of Post Anesthesia Nursing, 7,* 3-14.

Hogenson, K.D. (1992). Acute postoperative hypertension in the hypertensive patient. *Journal of Post Anesthesia Nursing, 7,* 38-44.

Jacobsen, W.K. (1992). *Manual of post anesthesia care.* Philadelphia: W.B. Saunders.

Jurf, J.B., & Nirschl, A.L. (1993). Acute postoperative pain management: A comprehensive review and update. *Critical Care Nursing Quarterly, 16* (1), 8-25.

Litwack, K. (Ed.). (1991). Pain and post anesthesia management. *Critical Care Clinics of North America, 3* (1), 1-164.

Litwack, K. (1991). *Post anesthesia care nursing.* St. Louis: Mosby.

Long, B.C., Phipps, W.J., & Cassmeyer, V.L. (Eds.). (1993). *Medical-surgical nursing: A nursing process approach* (4th ed.). St. Louis: Mosby.

Marshall, M. (1993). Postoperative confusion: Helping your patient emerge from the shadows. *Nursing, 23* (1), 44-47.

McConnell, E.A. (1991). Preventing postop complications: Respiratory problems. *Nursing, 21* (11), 35-39.

McFarland, G.K., & McFarlane, E.A. (1993). *Nursing diagnosis and intervention: Planning for patient care.* St. Louis: Mosby.

Metzler, D.J., & Fromm, C.G. (1993). Laying out a care plan for the elderly postoperative patient. *Nursing, 23* (4), 66-74.

Odom, J L. (1993). Airway emergencies in the post anesthesia unit. *Nursing Clinics of North America, 28,* 483-491.

Phoenix, J. (1990). Low blood pressure: How to investigate this ominous sign. *Nursing, 20* (11), 34-40.

Redmond, M.C. (1993). The importance of good communication in effective patient-family teaching. *Journal of Post Anesthesia Nursing, 8,* 109-112.

Rowland, M.A. (1990). Myths—and facts—about postop discomfort. *Nursing, 90* (5), 60-64.

Saleh, K.L. (1992). Practical points in the management of malignant hyperthermia. *Journal of Post Anesthesia Nursing, 7,* 327-329.

Shapiro, G. (1990). Postanesthesia care unit problems. *Anesthesiology Clinics of North America, 8* (2), 223-439.

Smeltzer, S.C., & Bare, B.G. (Eds.). (1992). *Brunner and Suddarth's textbook of medical-surgical nursing* (7th ed.). Philadelphia: J.B. Lippincott.

Stein, R.H. (1991). The importance of communication between the anesthesiologist and the postanesthesia care unit nurse. *Journal of Post Anesthesia Nursing, 6,* 279-281.

Strong, A.G. (1991). Nursing management of postoperative dysrhythmias. *Critical Care Nursing Clinics of North America, 3* (4), 709-715.

Strong, N.S. (1993). Assessing the postanesthesia patient. *Critical Care Quarterly, 16* (1), 1-9.

Thompson, J.M., McFarland, G.K., Hirsch, J.E., & Tucker, S.M. (1993). *Mosby's clinical nursing* (3rd ed.). St. Louis: Mosby.

Tirk, J. (1992). Defining discharge priorities. *Nursing, 22* (7), 55.

Vendor, J.S., & Spiess, B.D. (1992). *Post anesthesia care.* Philadelphia: W.B. Saunders.

Welter, E.R., & Reiff, P.A. (1989). Transferring patients from the OR: What the postanesthesia room nurse needs to know. *AORN Journal, 50,* 1248-1252.

Whitman, G.R. (1991). Hypertension and hypothermia in the acute postoperative period. *Critical Care Clinics of North America, 3* (4), 661-673.

9

PATIENT EDUCATION AND DISCHARGE PLANNING

VICKI J. FOX

IMPORTANCE OF PATIENT EDUCATION

Patient education and discharge planning create a vital, emerging role for the perioperative nurse because of the growing emphasis on home care and shortened hospital stays, the increasing number of ambulatory surgery procedures, and managed competition. Cross-training between nursing units, such as the operating room, postsurgical units, and postanesthesia care units may become commonplace. The perioperative nurse has the unique opportunity and knowledge base to coordinate efforts to meet the education needs of surgical patients. This chapter examines four questions about patient education: (1) Why teach? (2) When should patient education occur? (3) What is the appropriate content for patient teaching? and (4) How should nurses teach?

HISTORICAL DEVELOPMENT

One answer to the question "Why teach?" is that patient education is a long-standing nursing tradition. Nursing has used patient education as a tool for providing safe, cost-effective, and quality health care since the middle of the nineteenth century. Nurses themselves highly value patient education and consider it an important part of their job (Kruger, 1991; Johnson, 1989) (Research Highlight 9-1). Patient education began in an era when the sick were cared for in the home. Operative procedures also were often done at home. Nurses taught families about sanitation and cleanliness when caring for the sick, as well as how to care for those convalescing from home surgery (Redman, 1993). The National League of Nursing Education, in its 1918 *Standard Curriculum Guide for School of Nursing,* considered "preventive and educational factors" an essential element of routine nurse training, especially in new specialties such as public health, school nursing, infant welfare, and industrial welfare. In 1937 the curriculum guide described the nurse as a teacher and an agent for health. In 1950 the guide identified teaching and contributing subject

---

RESEARCH HIGHLIGHT 9-1

Kruger surveyed staff nurses, nurse administrators, and nurse educators for answers to two questions: (1) How do nurses perceive their role as patient educators? and (2) How well do nurses believe they meet patients' education needs? A 16-item, five-point Likert-type scale questionnaire was used. The subjects were a stratified random sample of nurses who belonged to the American Nurses' Association (ANA). Of the 1230 nurses surveyed, 756 responded (61.4% return rate). The data analysis showed that nurses in all three roles believed that nurses have a high level of responsibility for patient education with a mean above 4. The majority (74%, n = 549) selected the nurse providing patient care as the one to assume primary responsibility for patient education, over the patient educator and physician. The respondents were asked to rate how well they were able to achieve three areas of patient education: (1) preparing patients to receive care, (2) preparing patients for discharge, and (3) documenting patient education activities.

Achievement of preparing a patient to receive care was rated highest (M = 2.99); achievement of preparing patients for discharge was rated next (M = 2.80); achievement of documentation of patient education activities was rated next (M = 2.65). All nurse groups rated the overall achievement of patient education activities below 3 (the "good" rating) on the Likert-type scale. Kruger attributed this below-satisfactory rating to the shorter hospital stays and lack of administrative support for patient education activities. Of all respondents 97% (n = 733) believed nurses' responsibility for patient education would increase in the future.

Kruger, S. (1992). The patient educator role in nursing. *Applied Nursing Research, (4),* 19-24.

matter, such as psychology, knowledge of principles of teaching and learning, and teaching skills as areas common to all nursing curricula.

ACCREDITATION MANDATES

In answering the question "Why teach?" one could argue that, as health care providers, nurses are ethically and legally bound to teach. Illness prevention and patient education have long been nursing priorities. Traditionally, however, physicians' first priority was protecting the patients from harm. Complete disclosure about the disease and treatment was a secondary concern. More recently, in medical care the emphasis has changed from simply treating the disease to health maintenance and wellness. In the 1970s and 1980s, organized medicine recognized patient education as an ethical obligation. The American Hospital Association's "A Patient's Bill of Rights" (Box 9-1) affirms the patient's right to information about their illness and to give informed consent for treatment. If the hospital adopts the "Bill of Rights" as policy, then it becomes as legally binding as the hospital's medical bylaws and standards of nursing practice. Several nurse practice acts have made patient education an explicit legal responsibility for the individual nurse (Redman, 1993; Sundeen et al., 1994). Failure to teach or to document that teaching was done is considered below reasonable and prudent nursing practice and has been the basis of malpractice litigation involving nurses (Smith, 1987). Courts have repeatedly maintained that the right of self-determination in a democratic society is fundamental. To limit it in health care decision-making is an injustice. Nowhere is this better demonstrated than in the perioperative setting when obtaining informed consent. The Joint Commission for the Accreditation of Healthcare Organizations (JCAHO) *1993 Accreditation Manual for Hospitals* (AMH) consolidated functions of patient and family education from eight chapters in the previous AMH into one new chapter, "Patient and Family Education" (Box 9-2).

DEFINITIONS AND GOALS

A third answer to the question "Why teach?" comes from the ultimate goal of patient education, which is to enable patients to be responsible for their own health care (Sundeen, et al., 1994). Patient education is a planned experience designed to change behavior. The goal of patient education is for the patient to improve health behaviors and health status. Patient education may use a combination of methods to accomplish this: behavior modification, counseling, and teaching.

Patient teaching is an activity that may increase the patient's knowledge. The goals of patient teaching are to give information and to improve knowledge. Changes in knowledge may be needed before the patient is motivated to change behaviors. Teaching is a systematic way of introducing new information, events, skills, or objects into the patient's environment. When viewed as an interpersonal interaction between the patient and nurse, teaching is a distinctive form of communication that is uniquely structured and sequenced to produce learning. Theoretically, teaching should meet the patient's need for new information and skills. Neither the definition of patient education nor patient teaching contains assurance that the patient will actually learn or that behavior will change (Redman, 1993; Lorig, 1992).

Learning, on the patient's part, is demonstrated in changed behavior (Smith, 1989). Nurses can assess educational needs, provide information, instruction, and resources, and communicate with family and colleagues to enable learning. Nurses cannot, however, force patients to learn. Ultimately patients are responsible for changing their own behaviors (Ruzicki, 1989).

BENEFITS OF PREOPERATIVE PATIENT EDUCATION

A fourth answer to the question, "Why teach?" are the benefits for the patient, for the patient's family, support system and significant others, for nurses, and for institutions. Lindeman and other nurse researchers have confirmed the value of preoperative patient teaching (Research Highlight 9-2) when based on scientific content and structured either for a group or the individual (Lindeman and Van Aernam, 1971; Lindeman, 1972, 1973; Devine and Cook, 1983; Hathaway, 1986; Good-Reis and Pieper, 1990). The benefits of patient education for the patient undergoing a surgical intervention include the following: (1) speeds recovery (Midgley and Osterhage, 1973), (2) relieves anxiety (Wolfer and Davis, 1970), (3) increases self-esteem by increasing self-efficacy (Oetker-Black et al. 1992), (4) reduces cost of hospitalization, (5) prevents complaints about care, and (6) decreases the amount of perceived immediate and residual pain.

The benefits for the patient's family and support system (Research Highlight 9-3) are as follows: (1) alleviates anxiety and fear, (2) reduces cost, (3) hastens family's return to normal functioning, (4) increases self-esteem, and (5) develops support for caregiver's efforts (Raleigh et al. 1990; Lindeman, 1972). A primary benefit of patient education for nurses is increased job satisfaction. Patient education makes the nurse's job easier in the long run by saving time. It reduces the nurse's stress level and increases self-esteem. The institution benefits from patient education by reduced litigation potential, decreased length of hospital stay, and compliance with JCAHO requirements.

TRENDS IN PATIENT EDUCATION

The focus of health care moved from the home to institutions between 1925 and 1975. Ironically, since 1975 the focus has returned to the home setting. Patient education has come full circle. Ambulatory surgery and shortened hospital stays with early ambulation require preparation for convalescence at home. Homes have also become the site of preventive care, such as reducing the risk of highly communicable diseases (for example, HIV), appropriate nutri-

---

BOX 9-1

A Patient's Bill of Rights

1. The patient has the right to considerate and respectful care.
2. The patient has the right to and is encouraged to obtain from physicians and other direct caregivers relevant, current, and understandable information concerning diagnosis, treatment, and prognosis.

   Except in emergencies when the patient lacks decision-making capacity and the need for treatment is urgent, the patient is entitled to the opportunity to discuss and request information related to the specific procedures and/or treatments, the risks involved, the possible length of recuperation, and the medically reasonable alternatives and their accompanying risks and benefits.

   Patients have the right to know the identity of physicians, nurses, and others involved in their care, as well as when those involved are students, residents, or other trainees. The patient also has the right to know the long-term financial implications of treatment choices, insofar as they are known.
3. The patient has the right to make decisions about the plan of care prior to and during the course of treatment and to refuse a recommended treatment or plan of care to the extent permitted by law and hospital policy and to be informed of the medical consequences of this action. In case of such refusal, the patient is entitled to other appropriate care and services that the hospital provides or transfer to another hospital. The hospital should notify patients of any policy choice that might affect patient choice within the institution.
4. The patient has the right to have an advance directive (such as a living will, health care proxy, or durable power of attorney of health care) concerning treatment or designating a surrogate decision maker with the expectation that the hospital will honor the intent of that directive to the extent permitted by law and hospital policy.

   Health care institutions must advise patients of their rights under state law and hospital policy to make informed medical choices, ask if the patient has an advance directive, and include that information in patient records. The patient has the right to timely information about hospital policy that may limit its ability to implement fully a legally valid advance directive.
5. The patient has the right to every consideration of privacy. Case discussion, consultation, examination, and treatment should be conducted so as to protect each patient's privacy.
6. The patient has the right to expect that all communications and records pertaining to his/her care will be treated as confidential by the hospital, except in cases such as suspected abuse and public health hazards when reporting is permitted or required by law. The patient has the right to expect that the hospital will emphasize the confidentiality of this information when it releases it to any other parties entitled to review information in these records.
7. The patient has the right to review the records pertaining to his/her medical care and to have the information explained or interpreted as necessary, except when restricted by law.
8. The patient has the right to expect that, within its capacity and policies, a hospital will make reasonable response to the request of a patient for appropriate and medically indicated care and services. The hospital must provide evaluation, service and/or referral as indicated by the urgency of the case. When medically appropriate and legally permissible, or when a patient has so requested, a patient may be transferred to another facility. The institution to which the patient is to be transferred must have accepted the patient for transfer. The patient must also have the benefit of complete information and explanation concerning the need for, risks, benefits, and alternatives to such a transfer.
9. The patient has the right to ask about and be informed of the existence of business relationships among the hospital, educational institutions, other health care providers, or payers that may influence the patient's treatment and care.
10. The patient has the right to consent or decline to participate in proposed research studies or human experimentation affecting care and treatment or requiring direct patient involvement, and to have those studies fully explained prior to consent. A patient who declines to participate in research or experimentation is entitled to the most effective care that the hospital can otherwise provide.
11. The patient has the right to expect reasonable continuity of care when appropriate and to be informed by physicians and caregivers of available and realistic patient care options when hospital care is no longer appropriate.
12. The patient has the right to be informed of hospital policies and practices that relate to patient care, treatment, and responsibilities. The patient has the right to be informed of available resources for resolving disputes, grievances, and other conflicts, such as ethics committees, patient representatives, or other mechanisms available in the institution. The patient has the right to be informed of the hospital's charges for services and available payment methods.

From The American Hospital Association. (1992). A patient's bill of rights. Chicago: The Association.

RESEARCH HIGHLIGHT 9-2

In a landmark study, Lindeman demonstrated the value of preoperative instruction. The study design was a static pretest-posttest. The subjects were a convenience sample of 261 adult patients (135 subjects in the control group and 126 subjects in the experimental group) scheduled for surgical procedures other than eye, ear, nose and throat procedures under nonemergency conditions. All were to have a general anesthetic, were able to cooperate for pulmonary function tests, and were not on intermittent positive pressure breathing treatments. The purpose of the study was to determine what the effect of structured and unstructured teaching was on (1) the ability of a surgical patient to cough and deep breathe 24 hours postoperatively, (2) length of hospital stay, and (3) the need for postoperative analgesics. Unstructured teaching was of the type nurses did when and how each nurse thought to be appropriate. The control group received only unstructured teaching preoperatively. The experimental group received structured teaching. Structured teaching defined and described the postoperative stir-up routine, which required the patient to adequately inflate his lungs, cough, and turn or be moved. Structured teaching also included a formal teaching plan with content and process for instruction and teaching aids developed for nurse use when teaching. The nursing staff on the surgical units were retrained to the structured teaching plan. Patients' forced vital capacity (VC), forced expiratory volume (FEV_1), and expiratory flow rate were checked preoperatively and 24 hours postoperatively in both groups.

The experimental group scored higher postoperatively in all three ventilatory function tests than the control group. These findings supported that structured preoperative teaching significantly increased the adult surgical patient's ability to cough and deep breathe. When the length of stay of the two groups was compared, the experimental group's average stay was 1.9 days shorter than the control group, also statistically significant. The use of postoperative analgesics was shown to be lower in the experimental group, but not at a statistically significant level.

Lindeman, C. A., & Aernam, B. V. (1971). Nursing intervention with the presurgical patient: The effects of structured and unstructured preoperative teaching. *Nursing Research, 20,* 319-332.

tion for specific health states (such as diabetes), and early screening for diseases (breast self-exam). The home is the site of follow-up care, such as exercise programs for cardiac patients. Long-term care of the frail elderly in the home is also an educational need. Home care can even involve the use of high-technology equipment. Home care is based on a self-care philosophy aimed at moving the patient from the dependent role limited to compliance with instruction into a more contractual arrangement with the health care provider (Redman, 1993). Self-care philosophy is based on self-reliance, personal responsibility, and individual initiative. Educational support is an integral part of the self-care philosophy. The perioperative nurse has a unique opportunity to manage the educational partnership among health care professionals, patients, and their families (Smith, 1989).

ASSESSMENT

This section examines what content is appropriate for patient teaching and when a patient is ready to learn. This section also introduces the interrelatedness of the nursing process and the process of teaching. The first step in the nursing process and the teaching process is assessment. Table 9-1 illustrates the relationship of these two processes.

⚜
RESEARCH HIGHLIGHT 9-3

Raleigh and co-workers studied the amount of knowledge and anxiety level of spouses and significant others of patients preparing for coronary artery bypass surgery. The convenience sample subjects were selected from volunteers who attended a preoperative class for cardiac bypass surgery with a friend or family member at two large metropolitan hospitals. The classes were held from 1 day to 1 week prior to planned hospital admission. Two questionnaires were administered to the subjects before the class. One questionnaire rated each subject's state of anxiety, a transitory emotional state that varies in intensity and over time. The second questionnaire rated each subject's knowledge of the surgical experience. Alternate forms of the questionnaires were administered after the class. Data analysis revealed that significant others were statistically more anxious than patients before the preoperative class. The researcher postulated this could be because of a sense of helplessness on the part of the significant other, denial on the part of the patient, or that patients may actually get more social support than the family. The anxiety level of the significant other after the class decreased and knowledge increased. Neither were at the .05 level of significance set by the researchers.

Raleigh, E. H., Lepczyk, M., & Rowley, C. (1990b). Significant others benefit from preoperative information. *Journal of Advanced Nursing, 15*, 941-945.

ASSESSMENT OF INDIVIDUAL PATIENT EDUCATION NEEDS

The most important activity the perioperative nurse can carry out is assessment because it is the foundation for the entire patient education process. Collecting accurate assessment data about what a patient needs to know and the level of readiness to learn assists the perioperative nurse in setting realistic priorities. Not all patient needs are the same, nor do all patients need to know everything. The key question the nurse must ask when assessing the patient's educational needs is "What does this patient need to know?" The question is not "What would it be nice for this patient to know?" The dramatic increase in ambulatory surgery procedures, drastically shortened hospital stays, and the proliferation of high-tech treatments do not allow the nurse the luxury of teaching everything it would be nice for the patient to know (Ruzicki, 1989). The patient needs to know enough to (1) grant informed consent to an invasive procedure, (2) facilitate intraoperative cooperation, (3) provide self-care at home, and (4) survive until more teaching can be provided. A patient's hospitalization may involve enough discomfort and anxiety to prevent retention of any information on complicated subjects, such as pathophysiology. Highly technical content may actually confuse the patient. Patient compliance has more to with an understanding of what the patient needs to do and an ability to carry it out than on knowledge. Patients learn information about events directly related to their hospitalization (Ruzicki, 1989). The need-to-know assessment should be based on critical activities that the patient will be expected to accom-

---

TABLE 9-1

Relationship of the Teaching Process to the Nursing Process

Assessment	Diagnosis/planning	Implementation	Evaluation
NURSING PROCESS			
General nursing assessment to determine patient's need to learn; if positive, use teaching process	Nursing diagnosis and planning of nursing interventions	Nursing activities may include teaching/learning interactions	Evaluation against outcome criteria
TEACHING PROCESS			
Assessment of need to learn Assessment of readiness and motivation	Learning diagnosis; specific content areas to include in other nursing interventions	Teaching/learning interactions	Evaluation of learning

Adapted from Redman, B. K. (1993). *The process of patient education* (7th ed.). St. Louis: Mosby.

plish right away. Naturally, the plan is different if the patient actively seeks highly technical information. Assessment should also include determining what the patient already knows.

Even though discharge planning is often considered a postoperative activity, assessment of the patient's needs upon discharge should begin in the preoperative phase, especially in the ambulatory surgery setting. A preliminary assessment of the patient's and family's understanding of the knowledge and skills required to care for the patient will often make educational needs apparent.

NEEDS ASSESSMENT OF GROUPS

Informal assessment of the individual patient is the best way to gather preliminary data for the learning needs of groups of patients. Patients who will be going home with a new or changed medication regimen need to be taught how and why to take the medicine. Other informal methods of data collection may include talking to patients and staff, reviewing patient charts, or determining what type of patient teaching is currently being done. For a group of individuals with similar needs, a more formal method of assessment is appropriate. Assessing the needs of patients undergoing a surgical intervention can be accomplished in a variety of ways, including (1) interested party analysis, (2) checklist surveys, (3) focus groups discussion, and (4) structured interviews (Lorig, 1992).

Interested party analysis

For interested party analysis, select a general topic such as cardiac surgery. Make a list of all parties interested in the cardiac surgery. The patients may wish to have information about the procedure, length of stay, and rehabilitation; however, the spouses may be interested in dietary changes and how to prepare "heart healthy" meals. The needs of patients and families are often different. The next step is to find out what all of these interested parties want from an educational program and how it will affect other programs. For example, cardiac surgery patients want to know about postoperative rehabilitation. Teaching them about rehabilitation may require involving the cardiac rehabilitation department. Teaching spouses about dietary changes may involve the dietitian. This assessment can be done either by written questionnaire or personal interview. When and where to conduct interested party interviews and questionnaires may require targeting specific populations creatively. For example, if your general topic is ambulatory surgery, the interviews could be done or questionnaires administered in the discharge lounge of the ambulatory surgery unit.

Checklists

One of the most common and easiest forms of needs assessment is a checklist. List a variety of topics and let the potential participants check off topics of interest. Advan-

tages are that checklists are quick and easy to administer. Patients and families rarely object, and the results are easy to tally. One problem with a checklist is that it may reflect what the nurse wants to teach, not necessarily what the patient wants to know. A checklist may include changes in diet after a gastrectomy for stomach cancer, but may not include living with the possibility of the cancer recurring. Using the checklist in combination with another needs assessment method is wise.

Focus groups

Another way of conducting a needs assessment is to assemble eight to 12 potential participants. Focus groups work best if members are similar, such as mothers with small children. Start by asking for their input using statements such as "If my child was having surgery, I would want. . . ." The leader of a focus group discussion should be as nondirective as possible. The discussion can be tape recorded for analysis later. Focus groups are especially useful in program redesign by identifying weaknesses and strengths and suggesting new content or formats.

Structured interviews

A structured interview is another method of assessing the needs of a group. Opinion polls are good examples of structured interviews. Structured interviews have a specific format similar to that used in the interested party interview. Each participant is interviewed using the same format in person or by telephone. This type of assessment is easy to administer and tally, but the interviewer will not get information the format does not cover. The addition of open-ended questions can overcome this disadvantage.

ASSESSMENT OF INDIVIDUAL READINESS TO LEARN

The timing of preoperative teaching is critical. When to teach has more to do with the patient's readiness to learn than the actual number of weeks, days, or hours before a surgical procedure (Lepczyk et al., 1990) (Research Highlight 9-4). The literature is replete with articles on the importance of assessing the learner's readiness to learn, but little on how to go about it. Assessment of readiness to learn is similar to other kinds of nursing assessments. A continuous process, it requires expertise in observation, communication skills, especially listening, collaboration with nurse and physician colleagues, and assimilation of chart data (Ruzicki, 1989). Much of the literature on readiness to learn refers to healthy students in the classroom setting. Although there are some similarities between readiness to learn in an academic setting and readiness to learn in the context of health care, there are notable differences. The differences are time and health (Narrow, 1979). Health affects readiness to learn because the patient and family may be profoundly concerned, rationally or irrationally, about basic issues such as pain, disability, self-esteem, and dying. Time

RESEARCH HIGHLIGHT 9-4

Lepczyk and co-workers (1990) studied the hypothesis that cardiac patients who received a preoperative teaching program prior to admission would have less anxiety and greater knowledge preoperatively than patients who received preoperative teaching after admission. The convenience sample was selected from patients who came to preoperative classes before coronary artery bypass surgery at two large metropolitan hospitals. Group 1 (n = 32), chosen from one hospital, received teaching 2 to 7 days prior to admission. Group 2 (n = 42), chosen from the other hospital, received teaching on the afternoon of hospital admission. The subjects were asked to complete two questionnaires before and after the teaching intervention took place. The heart surgery questionnaire, developed by the researchers, measured the subjects' knowledge of the procedure. It included questions about anatomy, physiology, procedures, policies, activities, and sensations.

The researchers' hypothesis that patients who received preoperative teaching 2 to 7 days prior to admission would have greater knowledge than patients who received preoperative teaching after admission was supported. However, Lepczyk's team noted that one group had significantly higher knowledge scores in the pretest than the other group, which probably affected the posttest scores. The researchers also noted that the 58 patients who reported knowing someone who had had cardiac surgery had higher knowledge scores overall than those who did not. In addition, 50 patients (81%) reported seeking knowledge, a primary indicator of being ready to learn, when told of the need for surgery. The State-Trait Anxiety Inventory (STAI) measured the subjects' level of anxiety. The researchers' hypothesis that patients receiving the teaching intervention 2 to 7 days prior to admission would score lower on the STAI was not supported by repeated data analysis. There was no significant relationship between the amount of anxiety and the length of time between learning the need for surgery and the actual surgical procedure.

Lepczyk, M., Raleigh, E. H., & Rowley, C. (1990). Timing of preoperative patient teaching. *Journal of Advanced Nursing, 15,* 300-306.

Factors that influence readiness to learn

Nurses do not have time to teach patients who are not physically and emotionally ready. Assessing the patient's readiness to learn should occur before each teaching/learning interaction as a distinct activity, even though it may occur as the nurse is assessing other needs or providing other kinds of nursing care. The assessment may be done quickly. The instruction that follows will be influenced by the patient's readiness to learn. The quality, nature, method, and scope of instruction may well affect the patient's future levels of readiness to learn. Readiness to learn is being both willing and able to make use of instruction (Johnson & Jackson, 1989). Readiness establishes evidence of motivation (Narrow, 1979). The degree of readiness to learn depends on the degree of willingness and ability. The difference between teaching and instruction is important to note. Teaching includes, among other things, both the assessment of readiness and the activities of instruction. Instruction is only a part of teaching.

Several factors influence readiness to learn (Narrow, 1979). The first is comfort, both physical and psychologic. The six most common sources for physical discomfort are pain, nausea or dizziness, itching, fatigue or weakness, hunger or thirst, and the need to urinate or defecate. Since these conditions are not always directly observable, the perioperative nurse may be able to get the information from the chart. Asking the patient directly is usually the best way to get the information. One cannot assume that absence of complaints indicates comfort. Psychologic comfort implies the patient is not currently having uncomfortable emotions to a degree that would impair abilities.

The six most common uncomfortable emotions are fear, anxiety, worry, grief, anger, and guilt. The perioperative nurse may be able to observe behaviors or body language that indicate the present of psychologic discomfort. Any intense emotion, including pleasant ones, will preclude the possibility of effective involvement in learning. One attribute of a skillful perioperative nurse is to be able to modify planned intervention to accommodate the patient's comfort. If the patient is either physically or psychologically uncomfortable, the appropriate intervention is to relieve the discomfort before proceeding. Patients faced with the prospect of a thoracotomy for a suspected malignant lesion may be so overwhelmed with the fear of cancer that they are unable to listen to procedural information. The wise intervention is to be supportive and wait for patients to advance to a higher level of adaptation to the illness when their level of readiness will be greater.

The amount of energy currently available to the learner is a critical factor. The patient's energy is limited. If large amounts of energy, physical or psychic, are being expended, there may be none available for learning. The amount of energy patients have is closely related to their physical condition, their reaction to the stage of illness, the current number of stressors in their lives, and the degree of the situational or maturational crisis. For example, a pa-

constraints are very different. In the academic setting the teacher and learner have agreed on a time period: 6 weeks, a semester, or a year. In the health care setting the nurse is most often concerned with the patient's readiness to learn at this moment in time. The moment may be the brief span of time the nurse sees the patient preoperatively and postoperatively. The nurse's assessment must be brief, basic, concrete, specific, and useful.

tient who is fighting for every breath has no energy for anything else; a person actively denying the illness has little energy to learn about it.

A third factor influencing readiness to learn is motivation. Behaviors that indicate a person is motivated may include leaning forward, asking questions, taking notes, asking for a more complete explanation, seeking out the perioperative nurse for help or information, and requesting books or pamphlets. The perioperative nurse's goal is to help the patient and family learn whatever it is they wish to learn. The goal is to assess the level, not the basis, of motivation. If the behaviors that reflect motivation to learn were placed on a continuum, they would range from an overall posture of eagerness through lack of eagerness and apathy to rejection of any effort to teach. Motivation is discussed in greater depth later in this chapter.

The patient's capability to learn affects readiness to learn. The first three factors that influence readiness to learn can be assessed primarily by subjective data. The patient's capabilities can be assessed on more or less objective data. Prerequisite capabilities include physical ability, intellectual ability, knowledge, attitudes, and skill. Capability is influenced or determined by age, maturation, stage of development, past learning, physical and mental health, and environment. Both physical and intellectual capability should be assessed. When assessing physical ability, the perioperative nurse should ask these questions:

1. Are the patient's height and weight adequate to accomplish the task involved? For example, can this child reach the light switch?
2. Is the patient strong enough? For instance, can this frail elderly woman lift a long leg cast?
3. Does this patient have the coordination and dexterity to accomplish the task? For example, can the patient whose hands are crippled with arthritis manage to change a colostomy bag?
4. Can the patient see, hear, smell, taste, and feel well enough to accomplish the task? Can this patient see well enough to adequately compare the color chart on a reagent strip for urinalysis?

Assessment of intellectual ability includes the following:

1. Basic math skills (Can this patient read a thermometer?)
2. Reading skills (Can this patient read the directions on a prescription bottle?)
3. Verbal skills (Can this patient communicate with others who are involved in care and express himself?)
4. Problem-solving skills (Can this patient recognize situations in which she should seek help and would she know how to seek help? For instance, will the patient know what to do if she becomes febrile at home?)
5. Comprehension and ability to follow instructions (Is there some factor, such as recently administered pain

medication, that may impair this patient's ability to receive the instruction the perioperative nurse has to offer?)

Knowledge influences readiness to learn. Does the patient have the basic concepts and facts to understand the new material? For instance, does the patient know where the organ to be operated on is located? A related factor influencing the patient's readiness to learn is the patient's acquired skills. Has this patient already acquired skills from past experiences? Will past experiences attract or detract the patient from the goal? Discrepancies between expectations and capabilities should be discovered early as a result of careful assessment rather than later as a result of the patient's failure to reach the goals. The patient's attitude and value system are powerful influences on readiness to learn. These are influenced by factors such as ethnicity, religious beliefs, values about health care, and socioeconomic status. What is important to the patient? In teaching a new mother about immunizations for her child, does the mother share the belief that immunizations are safe? The discussion on the Health Belief Model in this chapter helps illustrate this.

Motivation

Motivation is the force that "initiates, directs, and maintains behavior" (Redman, 1993). This section looks at general theories of motivation in a teaching-learning context. No single motivation theory, but rather a combination of two or more of these theories, is likely to account for a patient's behavior. The six theories are reinforcement, needs, cognitive dissonance, attribution, personality, and expectancy (Redman, 1993). Behaviors that have been positively reinforced, rather than punished or ignored, are far more likely to be repeated. The positive social reinforcement a cardiac rehabilitation patient gets from exercising in groups, rather than alone, provides motivation to continue the behavior. Another reinforcer is the verbal encouragement from other patients and the cardiac rehabilitation nurse.

According to Maslow, people are motivated by a hierarchy of needs, in which higher level needs emerge as lower level needs are met. In other words, unmet needs create motivation. A satisfied need has no power to motivate, but it permits a higher level need to emerge, which in turn motivates the individual. For example, if the patient perceives a surgical procedure is life threatening, his safety needs motivate him to learn more about it than to interact in meaningful ways with friends, which serves to meet a higher level social need.

Cognitive dissonance theory maintains that people become uncomfortable when a deeply held value or belief is challenged. To resolve the discomfort, a person may rationalize to justify the belief or behavior: "Well, everybody has to die of something. I'll really enjoy smoking while I'm alive, and just die a little sooner." The person may also be motivated to change the behavior or belief:

"Smoking is less socially acceptable than it used to be. It does contribute to heart disease and lung cancer. I will quit smoking."

Attribution is identifying a cause for what is happening. Patients frequently do this after the diagnosis, an accident, or a cure of a disease. Attribution answers the "Why did this happen to me?" question. A concept essential to understanding attribution is locus of control. People with an internal locus of control believe their own efforts contribute to the success or failure of a situation. A postoperative patient with an internal locus of control may be highly motivated to cough, deep breathe, and ambulate. She believes these activities are in her control and will positively affect her health. On the other hand, people with an external locus of control attribute success or failure to causes external to themselves such as luck, the difficulty of the task, or other people's behavior. A postoperative patient with an ex-

ternal locus of control may be poorly motivated to cough, deep breathe, and ambulate. He may see these activities as something the nurse requires of him rather than being in control of them himself. He may not connect participation in those activities to a shorter hospital stay.

In personality theory, motivation is a relatively stable characteristic that exhibits a tendency toward a desire for one of the following: (1) affiliation, having positive relationships with others, (2) achievement, being productive and reaching goals, or (3) power, influencing and controlling others. Patients with strong affiliation desires may be motivated to learn if they believe it will improve their relationships with their family or health care provider. A patient with strong achievement desires may be motivated to learn because of a sense of accomplishment. This is especially true of learning specific tasks. Coping styles can be a stable personality characteristic. Table 9-2 describes var-

---

TABLE 9-2

Coping Styles when Faced with Illness

Coping style	Description	Strategy
Confronting	Making an observation about one's behavior	Not useful in dealing with the illness itself; useful in dealing with another's positive or negative response to illness
Distancing	Separating oneself from the problem	Convincing themselves that their problem is unique, therefore, they believe they cannot learn from someone else's experience
Self-control	Taking an active interest in by taking control	Practicing self-care and participating in decision making; must learn the difference between what can be controlled and what cannot
Seeking social support	Through supportive interaction with friends, family, church groups, etc.	The perception of having support is more important than the actual support received
Accepting responsibility	Buying into the treatment plan	Useful when encouraging life-style changes; harmful when used for blaming
Escape/avoidance	Failure to deal with or address the problem	May be useful as a short-term strategy, but harmful in the long run
Problem solving	Critical thinking skills	One of the more useful strategies; most educational programs teach solutions, not the problem-solving process
Positive reappraisal	Reinterpreting or reframing a negative to a positive	Instead of dwelling on what one cannot do, emphasize what one is successful at doing; looking at the illness as a challenge
Activity/distraction	Physical activity such as walking, jogging, swimming, or less active activity, such as painting or reading; humor, laughter, and relaxation are other forms	The idea that doing something is better than doing nothing; especially helpful in dealing with pain, depression, and changing habits such as eating or smoking; keeps the mind occupied
Self-talk	A variation of positive thinking	Can be either positive or negative; goal is to change negative self-talk to positive self-talk
Prayer	Private conversations with a higher power; meditation	Useful for segments of the population who find it a source of inner strength

Data in Lorig, K. (1992). *Patient education: A practical approach.* St. Louis: Mosby.

ious coping styles people use in the face of illness. Dysfunctional coping occurs when coping styles do not change as one matures or adapts in new situations, such as illness.

Expectancy theory maintains that a person's motivation is based on an expectation of success or failure. If the patient expects to go home the morning after a laparoscopic cholecystectomy, she is more likely to do so than a patient who expects to stay in the hospital 2 or 3 days. Learners try to live up to the expectations set both by themselves and by others. Learned helplessness is the idea that one is doomed to failure, no matter what. Depression is a common result.

Learned helplessness has three causes (Lorig, 1992). The first separates helplessness caused by the patient himself and helplessness caused by other factors. For example, a smoker may believe he has a personality flaw—lack of will power—that will defeat his efforts to quit smoking. He believes his inability to quit smoking is caused by his own personal failure. He may, however, blame his inability to quit smoking on peer pressure. His inability to quit is caused by factors out of his control or external to himself. Notice how similar these concepts are to locus of control discussed earlier.

The second cause of learned helplessness differentiates between global and specific causes. Global helplessness means that the patient lacks confidence in his ability to do a wide range of things, from losing weight to graduating from school to quitting smoking. Specific helplessness focuses on one activity. The patient may be certain he can quit smoking but does not believe he can graduate from school.

The third cause of learned helplessness distinguishes between what occurs occasionally and what occurs consistently, or a trait-state distinction. A trait is a stable personality characteristic. A state is temporary or transitory. Occasional or transient helplessness accounts for the patient's inability to lose weight during the Christmas holidays, even though he may be able to at other times during the year.

Self-efficacy is a concept closely related to learned helplessness and locus of control. Perceived self-efficacy is a person's judgment of her capabilities to organize and follow through a course of action required to achieve a designated level of performance (Lorig, 1992). Perceived self-efficacy has more to do with the person's belief that she is capable of accomplishing the goal than with her actual skill. Judgments about self-efficacy are based on skill mastery, modeling other's behaviors, verbal persuasion from others, and physiologic states. Self-efficacy has been positively related to activities such as coughing, deep breathing, and ambulation to prevent postoperative complications (Oetker-Black et al., 1992). Self-efficacy theory is the connection between what we believe about ourselves and how we behave. Oetker-Black and colleagues (1992) suggest self-efficacy is the vehicle by which preoperative teaching effects behavior change (Research Highlight 9-5).

☼

RESEARCH HIGHLIGHT 9-5

The purpose of this study was to determine if there was a relationship between perceived self-efficacy—what a person believes he is capable of accomplishing—and postoperative deep breathing and ambulation. The convenience sample was selected from patients who were scheduled for a cholecystectomy under general anesthesia in a private hospital in the Midwest. The 68 subjects met these criteria: (1) female, (2) over 18 years of age, (3) oriented to person, time, and place, and (4) able to walk unassisted for at least 10 minutes preoperatively. The Preoperative Self-Efficacy Scale (PSES), a tool the researcher had developed and validated in a previous study, was used to collect data preoperatively. The researcher or an assistant observed and used a stopwatch to time ambulation preoperatively and on the second postoperative day. Deep breathing was assessed by a mechanical device that measures vital capacity in liters of air both preoperatively and postoperatively. When analyzed, the data supported the idea that high PSES scores positively influenced postoperative ambulation and deep breathing.

Oetker-Black, S. L., Hart, F., Hoffman, J., & Geary, S. (1992). Preoperative self-efficacy and postoperative behaviors. *Applied Nursing Research, 5*, 134-139.

Stages of psychosocial adaptation to illness

Stages in emotional adjustment occur in all patients; however, the duration of each stage varies depending on the patient, the support system, and coping patterns. Transitions between stages are usually gradual and not clearly defined. The perioperative nurse will be able to assess the correct stage by listening to the patient. Several authors have proposed stages of psychosocial adjustment to illness (Table 9-3). All have similar components. Lee (1970) describes these four stages as (1) impact, (2) regression, (3) acknowledgment, and (4) reconstruction. Fig. 9-1 compares Lee's four stages to Maslow's hierarchy of needs (McHatton, 1985; Fox, 1986).

Impact corresponds with the foundation of Maslow's pyramid—physiologic and safety needs. Patients experience fear, anxiety, and loss of control. They may feel threatened. This may be a patient's first encounter with mortality. Patients may be very discouraged and become present oriented, seeing only the here-and-now. They focus all their energy inward because they perceive survival as their primary goal. Those with an external locus of control wonder if they can influence the outcome of the situation. Those with an internal locus of control may begin to operate from a learned helplessness mode.

Regression corresponds to Maslow's third level—social needs. Regression occurs when patients are forced to deal with the reality and attempt to return to a time when they felt more emotionally comfortable. After regressing for a short time, they will be able to handle this crisis and mourn the loss of body image or self-esteem. In this stage, the sense of belonging is threatened. Patients may lash out in anger at the family or staff. If they succeed in driving people away, their fears of not being able to give or receive love will be reinforced. Accept the patient, but do not support the behavior. To help the patient through this stage, use realistic terms and specific time frames. "It will be 3 or 4 days before your intestines start to work again." They may joke about their illness or reveal unrealistic plans upon discharge. "I plan to play golf with my buddies on Wednesday." Again, respond in realistic terms, but try not to overwhelm them. Having been provided with a measure of psychologic safety, they will move on to the next stage.

Many perioperative nurses do not recognize teaching as such during the impact and regression stages. Though little response is produced, therapeutic instruction helps the patient when moving into subsequent stages. At this point, families may benefit more from teaching than the patient because families may be ahead of patients in terms of adjusting to the crisis. In turn, they will be able to reinforce information when the patient is ready.

Acknowledgment parallels Maslow's fourth level—esteem needs. Patients have little self-confidence and self-respect and may express loss and fear of abandonment: "I'm such a burden to my family like this." As unlikely as it seems, this is the time when effective teaching, in the traditional sense, may begin. Patients realize they have survived their crisis and are reviewing the events in an attempt to prevent them from recurring. Patients give subtle signs that they have accepted changes in body image: "I thought the colostomy would be bigger." This indicates the patient has actually looked at it. They also begin to make provisions for the future: "Can I get this incision wet? I'd like to take a shower." Soon they will perceive their own need for information, leading them to the last stage.

Reconstruction parallels Maslow's fifth level—self-actualization. This is the most creative and positive stage because patients perceive hope for the future. Even though many patients cannot resume their lives exactly where they left off, they experience a renewed sense of self-worth. Patients start to plan new approaches for old behaviors. They will be very concerned about the future; therefore, instruction should be positive.

NURSING DIAGNOSIS

The nursing care plan provides a structured framework through which the nurse delivers nursing care. In the planning phase of the nursing/teaching process, the perioperative nurse diagnoses the patient's educational needs, identifies desired outcomes, and plans nursing interventions. Only one of the nursing diagnoses that follow deals directly with an educational need. The other nursing diagnoses indirectly reflect the need for patient teaching. Many nursing diagnoses have an inherent educational component. The perioperative nurse cannot isolate planning interventions to meet educational needs from the continuous reassessment and planning that occurs when providing other nursing care.

Nursing diagnoses related to the educational needs of the preoperative patient may include:

- Decisional conflict regarding the treatment options
- Anxiety
- Knowledge deficit regarding planned surgical intervention

A nursing diagnosis related to the educational needs of the postoperative patient may include:

- Pain

Decisional conflicts arise when the decision maker must consider one or more options. A classic example is the surgical treatment options for breast cancer with a tumor mass less than 2 cm in size and no skin involvement. Different options afford the patient an excellent 10-year survival rate. The options have advantages and disadvantages. The decision maker may take or avoid opportunities to seek further information. Decisional conflict and the accompanying emotional distress occur when one of three conditions is present (Pierce, 1993). First, a conflict can arise when the patient has a treatment preference, such as nutritional or faith healing, but was not offered this option or was discouraged from using it. Second, a conflict can arise when neither treatment option seems to have any advantages from the patient's perspective, and yet the patient must choose one. Third, conflict can occur when the patient prefers one of the offered treatment options, but a significant person prefers the other alternative. For example, when the surgeon strongly recommends mastectomy and the patient prefers lumpectomy and radiation, the situation can be particularly stressful because the patient depends on the physician for medical care. Families can also contribute to the conflict by adding their views for what the patient should do. A patient's decision-making ability may be so impaired by anxiety, fear, and interpersonal conflict that she is unable to make the choice and definitive treatment is delayed significantly (Kim et al., 1992).

Anxiety is present in most surgical patients to a certain degree. Anxiety is the uneasiness and apprehension the patient feels without being able to identify the precise cause. Anxiety interferes with the patient's ability to concentrate, recall information, and process new information. In the preoperative patient, anxiety may be due to threats to the patient's self-concept, socioeconomic status, role functioning, patterns of interacting, or fear of dying. The surgical patient may be anxious about the way the surgical intervention will alter essential values and life goals. Clues that the patient is experiencing high levels of anxiety are increased heart and respiratory rates, elevated blood pressure, voice and hand tremors, insomnia, and poor eye contact. He may be able to say he is "uptight" or "nervous" or express concern about changes in his life (Kim et al., 1992; Rothrock, 1990).

TABLE 9-3

Stages of Psychosocial Adaptation to Illness

Disbelief	Development of awareness	Reorganization	Resolution and identity change
CRATE*			
This begins when person learns by diagnosis or change in function (symptoms) that he or she has a particular condition. He or she may express denial by "I don't have it," a claim to have something else, avoidance by forgetting or refusing to do things required of him or her, attempts to control treatment, or diverting attention to other issues. Nurse should allow patient to deny but does not join him or her in the denial.	Patient becomes less able to maintain denial, more aware of what has happened to him or her and the implications of it. Dependence on others causes conflict yielding anger, at first diffuse and later more specifically focused on being sick. Anger may be expressed openly, projected, or directed inward in depression. Nurse should avoid joining patient in his or her anger. Nurse assumes responsibility for care so that patient is free to deny.	Patient accepts increased dependence. There is reorganization of feelings between family members. Nurse is safety valve when family cannot accept patient.	Patient resolves his or her loss; he or she begins to acknowledge changes in how he or she sees himself or herself. He or she begins to identify with others who have same problem. Nurse encourages patient to express his or her views of himself or herself. Goal of this process is for patient to be better able to live with his or her illness, rather than repressing it. If he or she has chronic illness, he or she is likely to undergo this process again and again.

Transition from health to illness	Accepted illness	Convalescence	
LEDERER†			
Apprehension and anxiety are present. Many patients ignore symptoms and use denial to allay anxieties, reinforced by plunge into health. Denial may be expressed by minimizing importance of symptoms by identifying them with common, benign, or trivial indispositions. Some patients meet anxiety aggressively and are irascible and ill humored. Others allay anxiety by passivity and are compliant. Patient is driven by his or her symptoms to seek diagnosis and therapy but is anxious and so displays vacillating behavior, reflecting indecision. Urgent requests for diagnostic examinations are rapidly alternated with failure to appear for examination.	Patient has accepted diagnosis and initial therapeutic procedures. He or she views himself as ill and abandons pretenses of health. He or she is preoccupied with symptoms and illness, is greatly concerned with functioning of his or her body, and is dependent. He or she assumes that physician and nurse share these preoccupations and is highly subjective in judging things. In people who have elaborate defenses against regression and expression of dependency, there is little or no phase of "accepted illness." These people continue to deny and do not follow medical advice; rather, they challenge it. This phase ends gradually after pathologic process has been reversed or arrested.	There is return of physical strength and reintegration of personality. This stage may be prolonged if previous life pattern was not satisfying or if person believes he or she cannot return to a life that will be satisfying. Some patients wrench themselves quickly from dependency and overdo. This stage has been likened to adolescence. Nurse must not encourage dependency with protection.	

Symptom experience	Assumption of sick role	Medical care contact	Dependent patient role	Recovery or rehabilitation
SUCHMAN[‡]				
Decision that something is wrong is made in these ways: 1. Physical experience (pain, discomfort, change of appearance) 2. Cognitive aspect (interpretation of physical experience) 3. Emotional response of fear or anxiety There is often denial of illness or "flight of health."	Person decides that he or she is sick and needs professional care. He or she seeks symptom alleviation, information and advice, and temporary acceptance of his or her condition by family and friends. How they react has much to do with his or her ability to enter sick role. Patient wants confirmation of his or her feelings and permission to suspend normal obligations.	Patient seeks professional medical diagnosis and course of treatment. He or she seeks authoritative sanction to become "legitimately" ill or return to normal activities. If he or she refuses to accept diagnosis or treatment, this stage is prolonged as he or she searches for another diagnosis. Patients who perceive their symptoms as less serious use self-treatment rather than going to the physician.	There is decision to transfer control to physician and to accept and follow prescribed treatment—to be a "patient"; 74% of people studied felt this task to be difficult for them.	Person relinquishes patient role. For many with chronic illnesses or physical impairments, this is a long and demanding stage with recurring episodes of illness. Person reestablishes relationships changed by illness.
Stage I: Denial	**Stage II: Resistance**	**Stage III: Affirmation**	**Stage IV: Integration**	
MATSON AND BROOKS[§]				
"It's not true; it can't be happening to me." Concealing symptoms. Seeking an authority who will deny the diagnosis. Refusing help. Holding to past life and values.	"It won't get me down." Searching for a cure or treatment. Active in programs seeking other patients. Reluctant to accept help. Initial recognition of change in life orientation.	"I guess I have to face it." Grieving for loss of former self. Publicly explaining diagnosis (e.g., multiple sclerosis). Learning to accept help. Subjectively rearranging priorities in life.	"I know it's there, but I don't think much about it." Living with it. Spending time and energy on other matters. Accepting help when necessary. Integration of life style with new values.	

From Redman; B. K. (1993). *The process of patient education* (7th ed.). St. Louis: Mosby.
*Crate, M. A. (1965, October). *American Journal of Nursing, 65,* 72-76.
†Lederer, H. E. (1952). *Journal of Social Issues, 84*(4), 4-15.
‡Suchman, E. A. (1965). *Health and Human Behavior, 6,* 114-128.
§Matson, R. R., & Brooks, N. A. (1977). *Social Science and Medicine, 11,* 245-250.

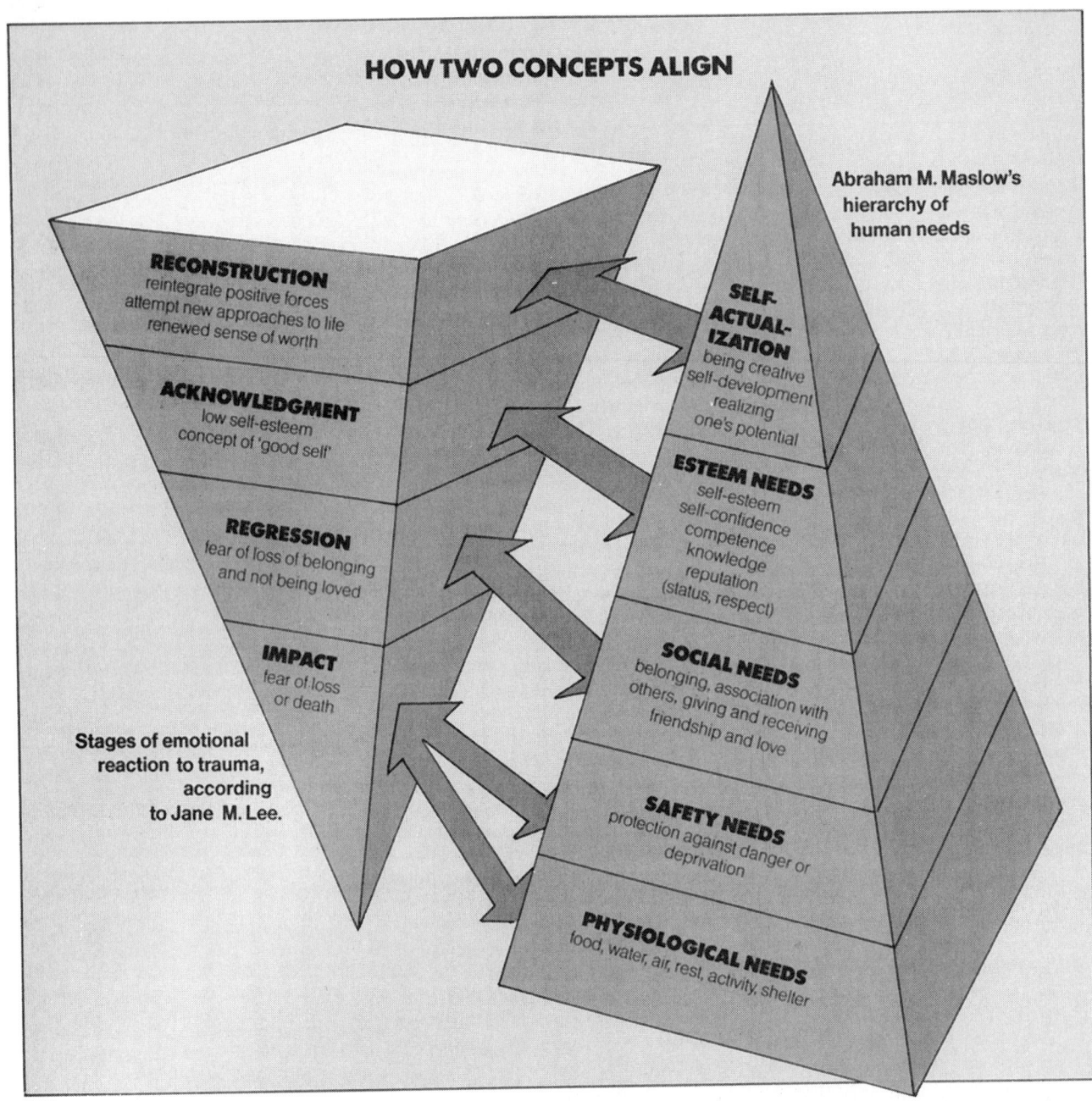

FIG. 9-1   How two concepts align.

From McHatton, M. (1985). A theory for timely teaching. *American Journal of Nursing, 85,* 799.

Knowledge deficit occurs when the patient lacks specific information. The unknown is often the cause of anxiety in preoperative patients. Signs of knowledge deficit are inappropriate or exaggerated behaviors such as hysteria, overt hostility, agitation, or apathy, inaccurate follow-through of instruction, inadequate return demonstration, a request for more information, or verbalization of the problem (Kim et al., 1992). When the knowledge deficit relates directly to the surgical procedure, the surgeon is responsible for informing patients of the nature, risks, and benefits of the pro-

cedure. The perioperative nurse's role is to enhance and reinforce this information. The perioperative nurse may be responsible for ensuring that an informed consent has been obtained and documented in the health record according to institutional policy (Rothrock, 1990).

Pain for the postoperative patient is most often inadequately controlled incisional pain. Signs of pain include guarding or protecting the incision, facial expression such as grimace or rigid affect, increased respiratory and pulse rates, diaphoresis, and elevated blood pressure. The patient

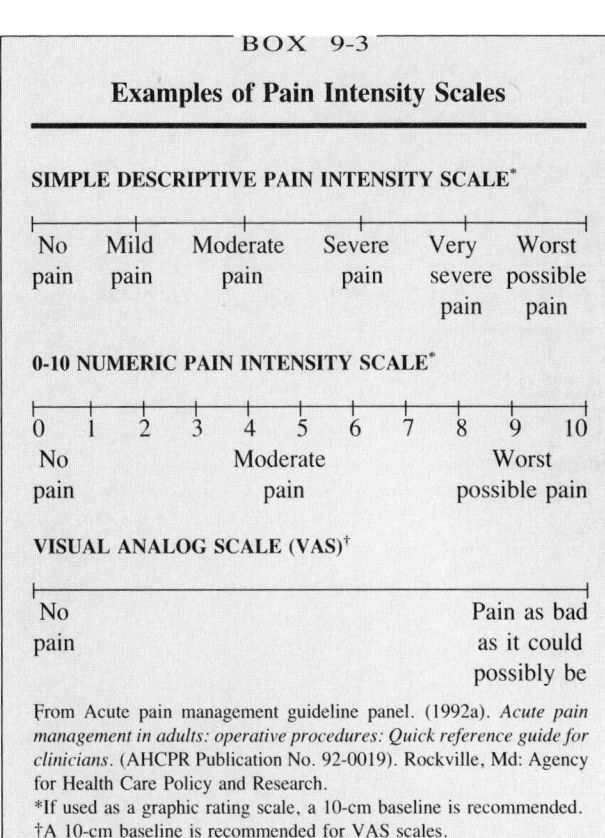

BOX 9-3

Examples of Pain Intensity Scales

SIMPLE DESCRIPTIVE PAIN INTENSITY SCALE*

| No pain | Mild pain | Moderate pain | Severe pain | Very severe pain | Worst possible pain |

0-10 NUMERIC PAIN INTENSITY SCALE*

| 0 | 1 | 2 | 3 | 4 | 5 | 6 | 7 | 8 | 9 | 10 |
| No pain | | | | Moderate pain | | | | | Worst possible pain | |

VISUAL ANALOG SCALE (VAS)†

| No pain | | Pain as bad as it could possibly be |

From Acute pain management guideline panel. (1992a). *Acute pain management in adults: operative procedures: Quick reference guide for clinicians.* (AHCPR Publication No. 92-0019). Rockville, Md: Agency for Health Care Policy and Research.
*If used as a graphic rating scale, a 10-cm baseline is recommended.
†A 10-cm baseline is recommended for VAS scales.

may withdraw from contact with friends and family and focus energy inward in an attempt to deal with the pain. Pain interferes with the patient's perception of time and critical thinking skills (Kim et al., 1992). The simplest and most reliable method to diagnose pain is to ask the patient (Acute pain management, 1992b). Behavior or vital signs cannot substitute for self-report because patients may hide pain from the nurse and family as a coping mechanism. Pain assessment tools are extremely useful in diagnosing the intensity and affective distress of pain. Samples of commonly used pain intensity scales appear in Box 9-3.

OUTCOME IDENTIFICATION

As was true with diagnosis, outcomes may not explicitly state that an educational need was met. A behavior in the outcome may indicate the educational need was met. Many outcomes imply that learning occurred and motivated the patient to change a behavior. Outcomes identified for the selected nursing diagnoses could be stated as:

· The patient will consent to a specific treatment option.
· The patient will verbalize feeling a lower level of anxiety.
· The patient will demonstrate knowledge of the physiologic and psychologic responses to surgery (Rothrock, 1990).
· The patient will identify a lower level of pain on a pain intensity scale.

PLANNING

MODELS FOR PLANNING PATIENT EDUCATION

Two models widely used to plan and organize patient education programs are the PRECEDE model and the Health Belief Model (Lorig, 1992). A model is a structure or conceptual framework for organizing things. Models can also help us understand why people behave the way they do and what works when changing behaviors. The PRECEDE model suggests looking at predisposing, enabling, and reinforcing factors when planning an educational program (Fig. 9-2).

Predisposing factors can be either beliefs or benefits. The nurse's goal is to determine what the predisposing factors are and in which category they fall. People generally have rational reasons for doing what they do. We may not agree with the reason, but that doesn't matter. For example, if a patient believes spinal anesthesia always causes headaches, it's not surprising when she chooses general anesthesia instead. To change beliefs, the nurse must first find out what they are. An excellent way to do this is to ask, "What do you think will happen if . . ." then add the desired behavior ". . . you have a spinal anesthetic?" Once you know the belief, the plan can include information to change it: "Headaches after a spinal happen only rarely." Be prepared for those times when you cannot change a belief, particularly if it is a dearly held cultural or religious belief. In these cases, helping a person broaden an interpretation of the belief may accomplish behavior change and improve self-efficacy. "I know you have prayed to God to cure you. Perhaps He has answered your prayers by letting you know there is a surgical procedure that can help you. The health care team could be instruments of God's love in your life." The second category of predisposing factors is benefits—the secondary gain from having this illness. Is this illness being used to get out of work or get attention from family and friends? Behavior change is unlikely to occur until the benefits for maintaining cease. For example, the number of smokers has decreased with the decline in the social acceptability of smoking.

Enabling factors help people do what they should do and want to do, but are unable to do. Two ways to enable people are by finding resources and by skills mastery. Putting resources where the person is can enable learning; skills mastery enables perpetual problem solving rather than simply fixing the situation at hand. Being too helpful too often can encourage dependence.

Reinforcing factors support the person's decision to change. Nurses can provide reinforcement through modeling, persuasion, and including families and friends and other health care providers in educational efforts. (More examples of reinforcement are discussed in the Facilitating Learning section of this chapter.) One final reinforcing factor is that, if behavior changes, people feel better. If a person consents to a cholecystectomy, the acute attacks of cholecystitis may stop.

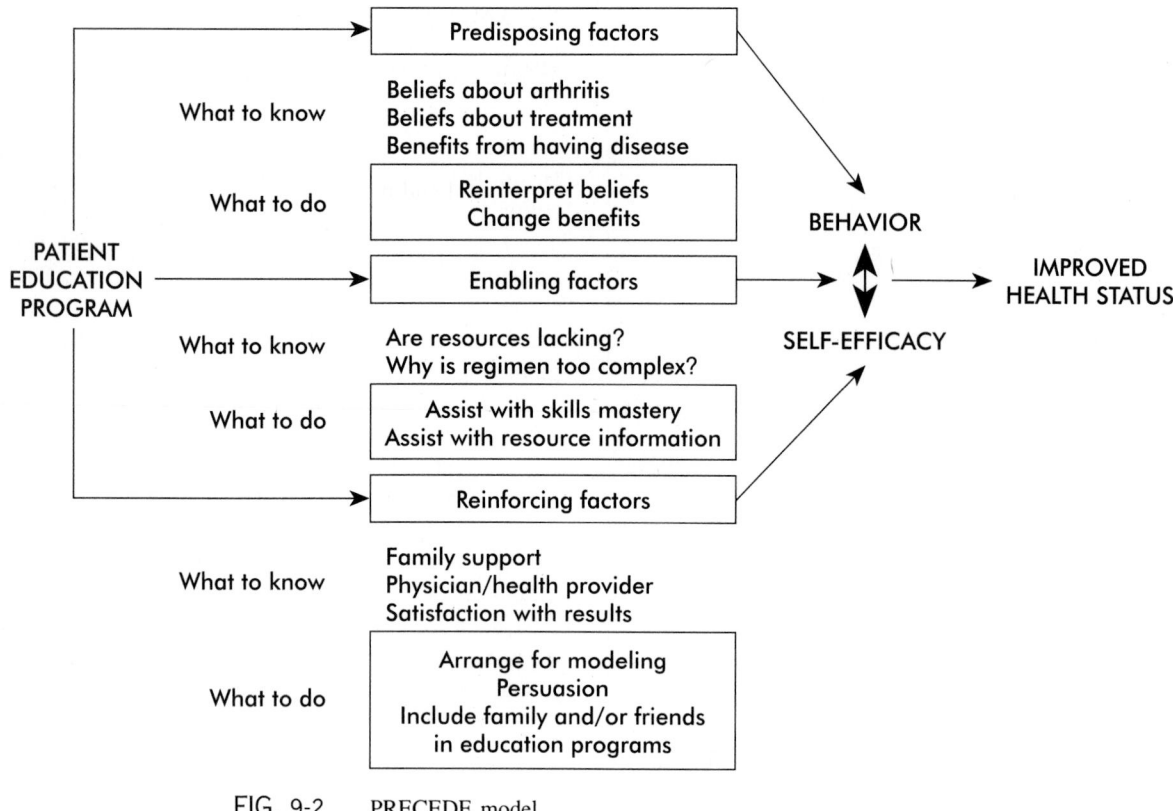

FIG. 9-2   PRECEDE model.

From Lorig, K. (1992). *Patient education: A practical approach.* St. Louis: Mosby.

The Health Belief Model is one of the oldest and best known educational models (Fig. 9-3). It is based on the concept that people act based on perceived threats or expectations. Perceived threat has two components: perceived susceptibility and perceived severity. For example, although most health care providers believe that AIDS is a severe and deadly disease (high perceived severity), many demonstrate low perceived susceptibility by failing to wear gloves when they should. To change behaviors, people must have expectations that the new behavior will reduce their susceptibility or the severity of the condition, that the benefits to changing are greater than the barriers, and that the behavior change can be accomplished. People engage in a subconscious or conscious cost/benefit analysis (Pierce, 1993): "If I have my uterus removed, it will hurt for several days and I will miss several weeks of work. But on the other hand, if I have my uterus out, I will stop bleeding so much. I will feel better and do a better job at work." Difficulty arises when the barriers to behavior change are obvious and the benefits are unpredictable. A good example is exercising and eating properly now to avoid vascular disease later in life.

CARE PLANS SPECIFIC TO EACH DIAGNOSIS

After diagnosing the educational needs and specifying outcomes, the perioperative nurse must plan interventions to help the patient achieve those outcomes. The University of Iowa's Nursing Intervention Classification (NIC) re-

search project defines nursing interventions, nursing activities, nurse-initiated treatments, and physician-initiated treatments as follows (McCloskey & Bulechek, 1992, p. xvii):

Nursing Interventions

Any direct care treatment that a nurse performs on behalf of the client. Nursing interventions include nurse-initiated treatments and physician-initiated treatments. Nursing intervention labels are at the conceptual level and require a series of actions or activities to carry them out.

Nursing Activities

Those behaviors or actions that nurses do to assist clients to move toward a desired outcome. Nursing activities are at the concrete level of action.

Nurse-Initiated Treatment

Interventions initiated by the nurse in response to a nursing diagnosis: "an autonomous action based on scientific rationale that is executed to benefit the client in a predicted way related to the nursing diagnosis and stated goals."

Physician-Initiated Treatments

Interventions that are initiated by the physician in response to a medical diagnosis and carried out by the nurse in response to a "doctor's order."

A care plan for the preoperative patient that incorporates the selected diagnoses and outcomes follows. Interventions in these care plans suggest how the nurse may directly or indirectly meet the patient's educational needs for each diagnosis. Again, planning to meet the educational needs of the patient is impossible to separate from planning other in-

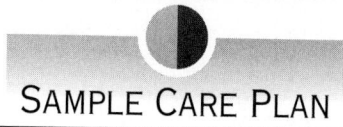

SAMPLE CARE PLAN

NURSING DIAGNOSIS: Decisional conflict regarding the treatment options

OUTCOME: The patient will consent to a specific treatment option.

INTERVENTIONS:

Active Listening—Attending closely to and attaching significance to a patient's verbal and nonverbal messages

Cognitive Restructuring—Challenging a patient to alter distorted thought patterns and view self and the world more realistically

Decision-Making Support—Providing information and support for a patient who is making a decision regarding health care

Family Involvement—Facilitating family participation in the emotional and physical care of the patient

Referral—Arrangement for services by another care provider or agency

Self-Esteem Enhancement—Assisting a patient to increase his or her judgment of self-worth

Teaching: Disease Process—Assisting the patient to understand information related to a specific process

NURSING DIAGNOSIS: Anxiety

OUTCOME: The patient will verbalize feeling a lower level of anxiety.

INTERVENTIONS:

Admission Care—Facilitating entry of a patient into a health care facility

Anxiety Reduction—Minimizing apprehension, dread, foreboding, or uneasiness related to the unidentified source of anticipated danger

Learning Readiness Enhancement—Improving the ability and willingness to receive information

Surgical Preparation—Providing care to a patient immediately prior to surgery and verifying required procedures, tests, and documentation in the clinical record

Teaching: Preoperative—Assisting the patient to understand and mentally prepare for surgery and the postoperative recovery period

Touch—Providing comfort and communication through purposeful tactile contact

NURSING DIAGNOSIS: Knowledge deficit regarding planned surgical intervention

OUTCOME: The patient will demonstrate knowledge of the physiologic and psychologic responses to surgery (Rothrock, 1990).

INTERVENTIONS:

Learning Facilitation—Promoting the ability to process and comprehend information

Teaching: Disease Process—Assisting the patient to understand information related to a specific process

Teaching: Preoperative—Assisting a patient to understand and mentally prepare for surgery and postoperative recovery period

NURSING DIAGNOSIS: Pain

OUTCOME: The patient will identify a lower level of pain on a pain intensity scale.

INTERVENTIONS:

Pain Management—Alleviation of pain or a reduction in pain to a level of comfort that is acceptable to the patient

Patient Controlled Analgesia (PCA)—Facilitating patient control of analgesic administration and regulation

Touch—Providing comfort and communication through purposeful tactile contact

Simple Relaxation Therapy—Use of techniques to encourage and elicit relaxation for the purpose of decreasing undesirable signs and symptoms such as pain, muscle tension, or anxiety

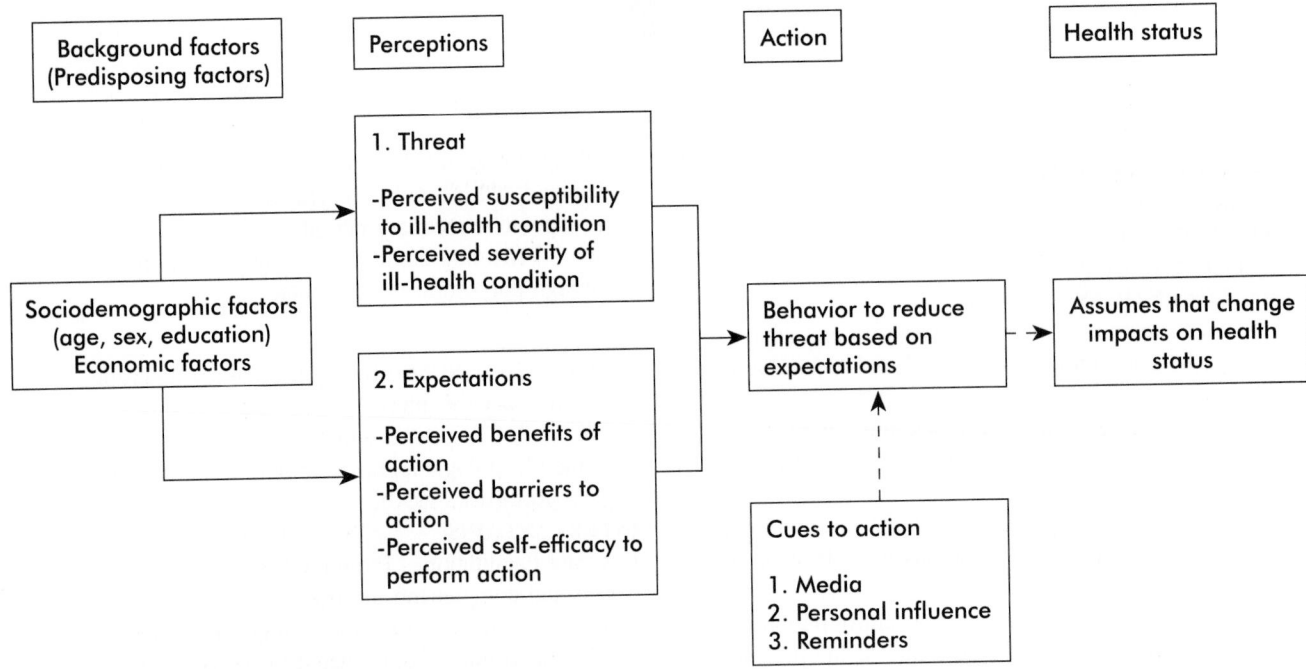

FIG. 9-3   Health belief model.

From Lorig, K. (1992). *Patient education: A practical approach*. St. Louis: Mosby.

terventions. Each intervention is defined according to the NIC (McCloskey & Bulechek, 1992).

IMPLEMENTATION

NURSING ACTIVITIES—CASE STUDIES

This section discusses the "how to" of patient education. Nursing interventions are conceptual labels that require activities to carry them out. Nursing activities are how nurses help patients reach a specified outcome. They are the concrete behaviors. Nursing activities can be either nurse initiated or physician-initiated (McCloskey & Bulechek, 1992). This section analyzes the implementation of nursing activities for selected nursing interventions in the planning section. In the case studies to follow, there may not be a separate nursing intervention that deals with meeting education needs. However, there are nursing activities within every intervention that deal directly or indirectly with meeting educational needs. These nursing activities involve more than merely instructing or informing the patient. Teaching is an interpersonal interaction that includes assessing readiness and current knowledge, facilitating learning, establishing rapport, trust, and mutual respect, reducing anxiety, and evaluating learning and the activities of instruction. The perioperative nurse adjusts nursing activities to meet the educational needs of the individual patient in the following case studies. Many nursing activities specific to one diagnosis will overlap nursing activities specific to another diagnosis.

Decisional conflict regarding treatment options

Mrs. Adams is a 44-year-old bookkeeper who underwent a left breast biopsy 1 week ago. The pathologic diagnosis is invasive intraductal carcinoma. The surgeon discussed treatment options with both Mr. and Mrs. Adams. Mrs. Adams has been scheduled for a quadrantectomy and left axillary lymphadenectomy at a free-standing ambulatory surgery center. The perioperative nurse visits Mr. and Mrs. Adams in the preoperative admitting area. As soon as Mr. Adams leaves the room, Mrs. Adams confides to the nurse she is not all that sure about having this procedure. She then berates herself for being "wishy-washy" about making a decision. She confesses that she and her mother have had considerable conflict over her original decision to have lumpectomy and radiation rather than mastectomy. Mrs. Adams asks the nurse if she has heard anything about radiation causing cancer rather than curing it.

Nursing diagnosis. Decisional conflict regarding the treatment options.

Outcome. The patient will consent to a specific treatment option.

Intervention. Active listening—attending closely to and attaching significance to a patient's verbal and nonverbal messages.

Nursing activities. Active listening requires undivided attention. Fiddling with IV lines and doing paperwork while listening will send the message that the perioperative nurse is too busy or uninterested. Display an interest by maintaining eye contact and leaning toward the patient. Acknowledge understanding by saying "I see" or "I hear you." Encourage the patient to say more by saying "I'm listening" or "Go on." Clarify ambiguous messages from the patient. "You said 'they' don't think lumpectomy is a good choice. Who are 'they'?" Reflecting or repeating the patient's own words back to her can produce more detail.

Patient: "The idea of radiation really scares me."
Nurse: "Having radiation scares you?"
Patient: "Yes, my mother says radiation can cause this problem."

Interpreting what the patient means can also facilitate the active listening process. Notice what words the patient may be avoiding. These are nonverbal clues to underlying fears.

Patient: "Yes, my mother says radiation caused this problem."
Nurse: "Are you fearful of getting cancer somewhere else if you choose radiation over mastectomy?"

Reactions that betray disgust, disapproval, embarrassment, impatience, or boredom will block communication. Although the perioperative nurse may be inwardly horrified that the patient may be considering no treatment at all, responses should be unbiased and empathetic. "What you're feeling is understandable. This decision must be very difficult for you." If a series of interactions with the patient is possible, you may identify predominant themes.

Intervention. Cognitive restructuring—challenging a patient to alter distorted thought patterns and view self and the world more realistically.

Nursing activities. Help the patient accept that self-statements elicit emotional arousal and that the inability to make this decision may be due to irrational self-statements. The self-statement "I'll never be able to make such an awful decision, I'm so wishy-washy" is self-defeating. The self-statement "I'm having difficulty making a decision right now" presents a challenge. Help the patient recognize that some of her beliefs are inaccurate. Overgeneralization, polarized thinking, and magnification of the problem can lead to dysfunctional thinking. "What evidence supports your mother's belief that radiation to the breast will cause you to have cancer somewhere else?" Replace faulty interpretations with accurate information and reality-based interpretations of the situation. Help the patient to label the uncomfortable emotions and identify perceived stressors (such as interactions with family, the diagnosis). "Are you feeling hopeless (angry, fearful, etc.) since you've been diagnosed with breast cancer?"

Intervention. Decision-making support—providing information and support for a patient who is making a decision regarding health care.

Nursing activities. These nursing activities build on those used in cognitive restructuring. Establishing a relationship with the patient early in admission may give the perioperative nurse more time. Determine if there is a difference between the patient's view and your view of the patient's condition. The patient may believe the diagnosis of any kind of cancer is an automatic death sentence. The nurse knows that, since the tumor was smaller than 2 cm and there are no palpable axillary nodes, the patient's chances for cure are very high. Determine if the patient understands the difference in the two alternative treatment options for breast cancer. Help the patient identify the advantages and disadvantages of each option. Assist the patient in articulating what she believes the goals of treatment should be. The nurse can serve as a liaison between Mrs. Adams and her husband as well as the surgeon. You should be familiar with the policies of the institution regarding informed consent.

Intervention. Family involvement—facilitating family participation in the emotional and physical care of the patient.

Nursing activities. When involving the family in Mrs. Adams's care, you must first determine which family members she prefers, how much information she will allow to be given to the family, and which family members are capable of and desire to be involved in her care. You must also identify what the family expects of Mrs. Adams in this situation and how informed they are about Mrs. Adams's situation and care. In doing so, you will be able to assess the learning needs of the family members to be involved and initiate nursing activities to meet those needs.

Intervention. Referral—arrangement for services by another care provider or agency.

Nursing activities. In Mrs. Adams's case, you should refer her to the surgeon. Relate your observations and professional opinion of the causes of the decisional conflict to the surgeon. Decisional conflicts are frequently caused by lack of understanding or misconceptions. The solutions to decisional conflict are often found in patient teaching. Assist the surgeon in knowing what information Mrs. Adams needs. Furthermore, you can clarify misconceptions and reinforce accurate information after the surgeon leaves. You may be asked to begin physician-initiated interventions, such as teaching about the disease process, after the surgeon and Mr. and Mrs. Adams have talked.

Anxiety

Mr. Caldwell is a 66-year-old retired football coach scheduled for an inguinal herniorrhaphy through the ambulatory surgery department of a small community hospital with two operating rooms. Ambulatory surgery patients are admitted directly to the holding area for admission procedures. Mr. Caldwell is to have local anesthesia and IV sedation monitored by a CRNA. He is accompanied by his wife and adult son. When the perioperative nurse enters the holding area, Mr. Caldwell is pacing beside the stretcher and has refused to change into a hospital gown.

Nursing diagnosis. Anxiety.

Outcome. The patient will verbalize feeling a lower level of anxiety.

Intervention. Admission care—facilitating entry of a patient into a health care facility.

Nursing activities. Begin by introducing yourself and

briefly describing the role you will play in Mr. Caldwell's procedure. Pull the drapes around the bed to provide privacy for the patient and family. In the initial interview, document the admission history, nursing assessment (physical exam, psychosocial history, educational needs), and informed consent as required by institutional policy. Ensure the patient is properly identified. Begin planning for Mr. Caldwell's needs upon discharge. Carry out the admitting physician's orders.

Intervention. Anxiety reduction—minimizing apprehension, dread, foreboding, or uneasiness related to the unidentified source of anticipated danger.

Nursing activities. Establish and cement the patient/nurse relationship through active listening while providing admission care. Create an atmosphere of trust by displaying respect. Allow Mr. Caldwell to remain in his street clothes as long as possible. He may feel safer, less vulnerable, and more in control in his own clothes. Begin by making an observation about his behavior and stating what your expectations for his behavior are: "You seem a little jittery. I'd like to help you feel calmer." Explain all procedures, including the sensations likely to be experienced during the procedure. "You will feel a burning sensation while the numbing medicine is being injected. After that, you may feel pressure and pulling. You should not feel anything sharp." Seek to understand Mr. Caldwell's perspective of this stressful situation. Reinforce his behavior when his anxiety level decreases. "You seem calmer. You are sitting down instead of pacing." Judicious use of humor can also lower anxiety levels. "I'm here to take you to the room. That means it's about 5 minutes to kick-off." Stay with the patient as long as possible. Allow time for addressing his concerns.

Intervention. Surgical preparation—providing care to a patient immediately prior to surgery and verification of required procedures/tests and documentation in the clinical record.

Nursing activities. Verify Mr. Caldwell's identity verbally and by checking his arm band. Determine his level of anxiety. Reinforce preoperative teaching information. Complete preoperative documentation as required by the institution, such as checklists, consent forms, and nursing assessment. Administer, explain, and document the use of preoperative medications as appropriate. Ensure that required preoperative lab work, ECG, and history and physical are on the chart. Start IV therapy, explaining the procedure, tubing, and equipment as needed. Support the family's needs with reassurance and information. Use supportive touch as appropriate. Solicit family assistance in keeping Mr. Caldwell's personal valuables.

Intervention. Teaching: preoperative—assisting the patient to understand and mentally prepare for surgery and the postoperative recovery period.

Nursing activities. Involve both Mr. Caldwell and his family in this intervention. Inform them of the scheduled time of surgery, keeping them updated if delays occur. Ensure that they know the approximate length of the procedure and stay in PACU. Familiarize the family with the locations of the waiting room and cafeteria. Discuss postoperative routines (medication, surgical dressings, ambulation, diet, activity). Discuss how Mr. Caldwell can assist in his own recovery (early ambulation, techniques for incision splinting and getting out of bed, coughing and deep breathing, limits on activity). Determine Mr. Caldwell's expectations of surgery and correct unrealistic expectations. Discuss possible pain control measures. Provide information on what Mr. Caldwell will hear, see, taste, and feel during the procedure and immediately after.

Knowledge deficit regarding treatment options

Mrs. Rhines is a 77-year-old retired English literature professor. She is a widow and has no children. She is accompanied by Mrs. Campbell, a friend who lives across the street. Mrs. Rhines still enjoys an occasional round of golf. She experienced a transient ischemic attack (TIA) that caused her to faint in her kitchen last week. She was admitted through the ambulatory surgery department for carotid arteriograms this morning. She is scheduled for a right carotid endarterectomy this afternoon. During the preoperative assessment Mrs. Rhines says, "I wish I understood more about this block in the vein in my neck. My surgeon explained some of it, but I didn't get it all."

Nursing diagnosis. Knowledge deficit regarding planned surgical intervention.

Outcome. The patient will demonstrate knowledge of the physiologic and psychologic responses to surgery.

Intervention. Teaching: disease process—assisting the patient to understand information related to a specific process.

Nursing activities. Begin by determining what Mrs. Rhines knows about carotid artery disease. Reinforce and elaborate on information provided by other health care team members. Show her a drawing of the vessel. Point out on her neck where it is located. Draw in the distribution of plaque around the bifurcation. After the arteriogram, show her the exact location of the lesion. Explain the cause of the TIA. Discuss factors in the etiology of vascular disease (genetic, life-style, aging, dietary, and physiologic responses to stress). Provide information about the diagnostic tests, carotid Doppler studies, and digital subtraction arteriography. Determine what she understands about the surgical procedure. Preoperative teaching may be necessary and can be included in this intervention.

Pain

Elliot Chambers is a 54-year-old man who owns his own construction company. He has undergone a sigmoid colon resection for severe diverticular disease. On the first postoperative day the perioperative nurse visits him in the surgical unit. He is pale and tense. When asked, he reports pain relief to be inadequate. He has a PCA pump set to give 3 mg of morphine every 15 minutes. When shown a 0-10 Numeric Pain Intensity Scale (see Box 9-3), he chooses the number 8.

Nursing diagnosis. Pain.

Outcome. The patient will identify a lower level of pain on a pain intensity scale.

Intervention. Patient-controlled analgesia (PCA)—facilitating patient control of analgesic administration and regulation.

Nursing activities. Determine if Mr. Chambers received preoperative teaching on the use of the PCA pump. Preoperative teaching in its use enhances the patient's ability to manage postoperative pain (Timmons & Bower, 1993; Shade, 1992) (Research Highlight 9-6). Validate that Mr. Chambers and his family understand the use of the PCA pump, how to deliver the medication, the lockout interval, the effect of the medication, and the maximum dose feature. Teach him how to monitor the intensity and duration of pain. Collaborate with the surgical unit nurses in documenting inadequate pain relief at the current dosage. Rec-

ommend to the physician a loading dosage of 3 to 5 mg every 5 minutes until current pain is diminished, then 2 to 3 mg every 10 minutes prn with a 10-mg hourly maximum dose (Acute Pain Management Guideline Panel, 1992a). Use the pain intensity scale to evaluate pain after loading dose. Collaborate with unit nurses for ongoing reassessment of pain relief using the pain intensity scale.

Intervention. Simple relaxation therapy—use of techniques to encourage and elicit relaxation for the purpose of decreasing undesirable signs and symptoms such as pain, muscle tension, or anxiety.

Nursing activities. Describe the reason for and benefits of relaxation therapy. Determine if Mr. Chambers has any previous experiences with relaxation therapy. Consider his willingness and ability to participate. Create a quiet, soothing atmosphere by dimming lights and closing the door. Use a slow, rhythmic tone of voice. Use one of the relaxation exercises in Box 9-4.

SELECTING CONTENT IN PREOPERATIVE AND POSTOPERATIVE TEACHING

Nursing research has recommended that selection of content for preoperative teaching be based on what the patient wants to know and needs to know (Research Highlight 9-7). The perioperative nurse can select content for an individual patient based on input from not only the patient and the nurse's own observations, but also from other health care team members. Preoperative information falls into four broad categories (Wallace, 1985): (1) procedural, (2) sensory/temporal, (3) coping, and (4) reassurance. Not every patient needs or wants to know everything. Content should be selected on a need-to-know basis. The perioperative nurse selects the content appropriate for each patient, the institution, the amount of time allotted, and resources available.

Procedural information is a concrete description of which procedures are to be carried out and why. Box 9-5 lists the possible procedural information that could be included in preoperative and postoperative content. Sensory and temporal information includes how the procedures will feel and how long they will take (Box 9-6). Table 9-4 has procedural, sensory, and temporal content for specific surgical procedures. Coping suggestions inform the patient of ways to control the emotional responses. These can include any of those listed in Table 9-4. Perioperative nurses frequently give global reassurances rather than specific information they believe the patient will find alarming or when time is extremely limited, as in emergency situations like trauma. "Your surgical team is highly skilled at this procedure. This hospital has the latest equipment." A combination of the salient points of all categories is the appropriate content. Booklets that provide simple procedural information, sensory and temporal experiences, suggestions on how to cope, as well as practical information about hospital admission procedures are welcomed by patients (Wallace, 1985).

RESEARCH HIGHLIGHT 9-6

Timmons and Bower (1993) studied the effect of structured teaching on postoperative patients' understanding of PCA use and their ability to manage their pain. The study design was a control group posttest only. The subjects (n=89) were chosen from a private community on the West Coast who had undergone an orthopedic procedure. Selection criteria included the 16 to 86 age bracket and the ability to read English, understand the teaching program, and complete the posttest. The subjects were randomly assigned to two groups, nearly identical in makeup. Although both the control group and the experimental groups received preoperative instruction from their physicians, only the experimental group was given a structured teaching program 2 hours before surgery. The researchers developed an educational booklet for use in the teaching program. The posttest was designed to determine if subjects understood how PCA worked and how well they used the information to manage their pain. The posttest was given on the third postoperative day.

When the data were analyzed, the experimental group scored higher on every score. There was a statistically significant difference, at the .03 level, between the groups on the management of pain scores. When the data were analyzed by each question on the posttest, the experimental group subjects had better understanding of how to use the PCA to relieve pain before coughing and deep breathing, how to avoid drowsiness, and what to do if the pain control was inadequate.

Timmons, M. E, & Bower, F. L. (1993). The effect of structured preoperative teaching on patients' use of patient-controlled analgesia (PCA) and their management of pain. *Orthopaedic Nursing, 12,* 23-31.

BOX 9-4

Relaxation Exercises

EXAMPLE 1: DEEP BREATHE/TENSE, EXHALE/RELAX, YAWN FOR QUICK RELAXATION

1. Clench your fists; breathe in deeply and hold it a moment.
2. Breathe out slowly and go limp as a rag doll.
3. Start yawning.

Additional points: Yawning becomes spontaneous. It is also contagious, so others may begin yawning and relaxing too.

EXAMPLE 2: SLOW RHYTHMIC BREATHING FOR RELAXATION

1. Breathe in slowly and deeply.
2. As you breathe out slowly, feel yourself beginning to relax; feel the tension leaving your body.
3. Now breathe in and out slowly and regularly, at whatever rate is comfortable for you. You may wish to try abdominal breathing. If you do not know how to do abdominal breathing, ask your nurse for help.
4. To help you focus on your breathing and breathing slowly and rhythmically: Breathe in as you say silently to yourself, "in, two, three." Breathe out as you say silently to yourself, "out, two, three," *or* each time you breathe out, say silently to yourself a word such as peace or relax.
5. You may imagine that you are doing this in a place you have found very calming and relaxing for you, such as lying in the sun at the beach.
6. Do steps 1 through 4 only once or repeat steps 3 and 4 for up to 20 minutes.
7. End with a slow deep breath. As you breathe out say to yourself "I feel alert and relaxed."

Additional points: If you intend to do this for more than a few seconds, try to get in a comfortable position in a quiet environment; you may close your eyes or focus on an object. This technique has the advantage of being very adaptable in that it may be used for only a few seconds or for up to 20 minutes.

EXAMPLE 3: PEACEFUL PAST

Something may have happened to you a while ago that brought you peace and comfort. You may be able to draw on that past experience to bring you peace or comfort now. Think about these questions:

1. Can you remember any situation, even when you were a child, when you felt calm, peaceful, secure, hopeful, comfortable?
2. Have you ever daydreamed about something peaceful? What were you thinking of?
3. Do you get a dreamy feeling when you listen to music? Do you have any favorite music?
4. Do you have any favorite poetry that you find uplifting or reassuring?
5. Have you ever been religiously active? Do you have favorite readings, hymns, or prayers? Even if you haven't heard or thought of them for many years, childhood religious experiences may still be very soothing.

Additional points: Very likely some of the things you think of in answer to these questions can be recorded for you, such as your favorite music or a prayer. Then you can listen to the tape whenever you wish. Or, if your memory is strong, you may simply close your eyes and recall the events or words.

Modified with permission from McCaffery, M., & Beebe, A. (1989). *Pain: Clinical manual for nursing practice*. St. Louis, Mosby.

Selecting educational content specifically for families and significant others is also important. In addition to the procedural, sensory, temporal, coping, and reassurance content that the patient receives, families and significant others need information about what they can do as helping caregivers (Silva, 1987).

FACILITATING LEARNING

Facilitating learning can take a variety of forms. Since readiness to learn is an essential factor, nurses can enhance readiness to learn by addressing the patient's specific concerns first, minimizing sensory overload in the environment, providing time for the patient to ask questions, assisting the patient to realize what ability he has to control the illness, and helping him to have confidence in his judgment (Rakel, 1992).

The perioperative nurse can use basic principles of motivation to enhance teaching/learning interactions (Redman, 1993). Use the environment to focus the patient's attention on what he needs to know. A warm yet businesslike atmosphere is a successful strategy. Visual and tactile aids, such as a drawing of the biliary system or a sample of a vascular prosthesis, capture and hold the learner's interest.

Incentives stimulate the motivation to learn. For some individuals the pay-off for learning is approval and praise from their family or health care providers. For others the enjoyment of reaching a goal is motivation enough. Others need more concrete incentives such as having special food as a treat.

Internal, self-directed motivation to learn will last longer than external motivation. External motivation requires frequent positive reinforcement. Assessment data can give the

---

Two concurrent studies examined the extent to which patients welcomed additional preparation about surgery and their preferences for the type of information, the timing, and the format of the preparation given. The patients in both studies were women undergoing laparoscopy for sterilization or infertility investigation. Data were collected in structured interviews in the outpatient clinic immediately after the physician had explained they were to undergo a laparoscopy in 6 to 8 weeks. Each patient was again interviewed the morning of the procedure just prior to being taken to the surgical suite or the evening before surgery.

Ninety percent of the patients welcomed additional preparation. Patients in all categories consistently preferred procedural information and preferred to receive it in the outpatient clinic regardless of when or where the data were collected. In the outpatient clinic patients were asked to state their preferences for the format of preparation. Most preferred to talk to the physician (46.6%) or receive a booklet (29.8%). Other preferences were a film presentation (7.6%), talking to a nurse (5.3%), talking to a psychologist (2.3%), and audiocassette presentation (0.8%). This study revealed that 10% wanted no preparation in any format.

The second study examined what preferences patients had for preparatory materials. The researcher constructed six booklets to provide information about hospitalization and the surgical procedure. Patients were interviewed as in the first study in the outpatient clinic. Then each subject was given each booklet in a predetermined random order and asked to rate each booklet on the booklet rating form before reading the next booklet. Finally, they were asked to express an overall preference among all six booklets or no booklet. The six booklets provided the following types of information: (1) procedural information (information about which procedures are carried out and why); (2) procedural plus sensory and temporal information (the addition of information about how procedures feel to the patient, how long they will take); (3) procedural and coping suggestions (addition of information about how to control emotional responses through means such as cognitive restructuring, relaxation, and affiliation); (4) global reassurances (reassurances only rather than specific procedural information); (5) directions about hospital admission procedures (explanation of admission and dismissal procedures); and (6) a composite of the information illustrated in booklets 1 through 5.

This study's results replicated the same preferences for additional preparation and timing of the first study. The introduction of the booklets revealed different results in the format preferences. Most (62.5%) chose the composite booklet. Of the other booklets, 12.5% chose either the procedural information or procedural plus sensory and temporal information booklets. Only 6% chose the booklets on coping and directions. Although the first study indicated procedural information to be the information of choice, the second study revealed procedural information alone was insufficient. Patients in both studies preferred information to be presented by the surgeon. However, making well-designed booklets available was welcomed by the patient as well. This format is far more cost-effective.

Wallace, L. M. (1985). Surgical patients' preferences for preoperative information. *Patient Education and Counseling, 7,* 377-387.

---

nurse a place to start, but unless the patient buys into the plan, behavior change will be short-lived or not occur at all.

An individual will learn most effectively when she is ready to learn. Factors affecting readiness to learn and ways to enhance readiness have been discussed. If the need for change is urgent, the perioperative nurse is in a good position to encourage the development of readiness and supervise the patient's progress.

Motivation is enhanced by structured educational materials. Better organized material is more meaningful and more effective.

Success motivates better than failure. Design a learning experience that allows the learner to succeed. Learning takes place in small increments. The patient can easily be overwhelmed by too much, too soon. Practice and return demonstrations done in sequence allow the patient to succeed one step at a time.

Learning is likely to create anxiety because it may require changes in beliefs and behavior. During high anxiety or stress periods, keep teaching/learning interactions to a minimum.

The perioperative nurse must help the learner set personal goals and provide feedback about progress toward those goals. Goals are more likely to be met if the patient's behavior is reinforced and praised, if the content is tailored to the individual, if the perioperative nurse helps the patient take action, if the content is relevant, and if the teaching methods are meaningful and appealing to the patient.

As discussed earlier, there are three ways to enhance self-efficacy that, when used properly, can enhance learning (Lorig, 1992). First, skills mastery is based on the principle that success motivates better than failure. Skills mastery is accomplished by breaking the task into small manageable subtasks and ensuring that each subtask is completed successfully. Modeling is another way to enhance self-efficacy. Ideally, the model should be an ordinary person who has the same problem as the patient and has to

---

BOX 9-5

Procedural Information in Preoperative Teaching

Location of surgery suite
Location of holding area
Location of surgery waiting area
Location of PACU
Location and tour of postsurgical unit and waiting area
Incision site
Planned alterations to anatomy and physiology by surgical intervention
Use of PCA pump
Splinting of the incision
Technique for getting out of bed postoperatively
Coughing and deep breathing
Use of incentive spirometer
Leg exercises
Description of preoperative routines
   Bowel preparation
   Diet/NPO
   Preoperative lab tests/diagnostic procedures
   Voiding
   Skin preparation
   ECG
   Preoperative sedation
Anesthesia
Description of postoperative routines
   Support hose
   Surgical dressings
   Diet
   Medications
   Respiratory treatments
   Machines
   Drains
   Nature of postoperative nursing assessments

BOX 9-6

Sensory and Temporal Information in Preoperative Teaching

Date and time of surgery
Time patient will leave room
Amount of time spent in the preoperative holding area
Length of surgical procedure
Length of stay in PACU
Length of hospital stay
Estimated time to full recovery
When diet can resume
When drains, cast, dressings, etc. will be removed
Hours of family visitation
Sights, sounds, and smells of preoperative holding area, OR, and PACU
Sensations during administration of local anesthesia
Sensations produced by preoperative medications
Taste of certain drugs used in anesthesia induction
Postoperative pain sensations
Sensations of the stretcher transport to and from surgery
Postoperative sensations specific to certain procedures (sore throat from endotracheal intubation)

---

cope with it daily. An excellent example of learning enhancement through modeling is the American Cancer Society's Reach for Recovery program. Women who have had mastectomies teach new mastectomy patients how to do arm and shoulder exercises. A third way of facilitating learning by enhancing self-efficacy is through persuasion. This is probably the most used and least effective. It can be used to urge patients to do more than they are currently doing.

Teaching materials are divided into two major categories: printed and nonprint materials. Printed materials include booklets, brochures, and pamphlets. Although printed material can limit feedback, it is useful for relaxing time requirements. Printed material is always available to the learner and can be referred to as often as needed. The following are considerations in selecting printed material (Ruzicki, 1989):

1. Is the content written at the appropriate skill level of the target audience? The mean literacy level in the United States is the eighth grade level or below; 20% of adult learners are functionally illiterate; 34% have marginal reading skills. Materials should be written for a sixth grade level. Simplify printed material by eliminating medical jargon and pathophysiology. In addition, illness or stress can lower one's ability to comprehend even more. For patients with higher levels of literacy and the desire to know, additional information can be provided.

2. Are sentences clear, short, and concise? Material presented should be the very least needed to convey the message. The content should be essential material. Focusing on required behaviors, such as "Do not eat or drink anything after midnight the day of your surgery," increases the chances the patient will follow through.

3. Is the material logically organized? The most important points should be presented first and highlighted. Headings and graphics can draw attention to important content. The purpose and summary should be clearly stated.

4. Are the visuals and graphics pleasing and do they help convey the message? Visuals should relate to the topic and not detract from the message.

5. Is the content accurate?

6. Is the type large and easy to read?

7. Does the material foster interaction between the nurse and patient? This helps develop the nurse/patient relationship and assists the patient to individualize and personalize the instructions.

Text continued on p. 243.

TABLE 9-4
Selecting Content for Teaching

	Inguinal herniorrhaphy	Sigmoid colectomy	Thoracotomy	Cholecystectomy (open or laparoscopic)	Carotid endarterectomy
PREOP POINTERS					
Medical diagnosis	Inguinal hernia	CA of sigmoid colon; diverticulitis	CA, primary or metastatic; for diagnosis; drain abscesses	Cholecystitis; cholelithiasis	Carotid stenosis
Diagnostic tests	History and physical exam	Barium enema, colonoscopy	CT of chest; bronchoscopy; needle biopsy; CME; thoracoscopy	Sonogram; HIDA scan; oral cholecystogram; blood work for amylase and bilirubin	Dopscan; arteriogram; CT of head
Routine proper tests	CBC, ECG	SMA 6/20, T&C if H&H low, bowel prep, ECG	Pulmonary functions, SMA 20, T&C, ECG	SMA 20, ECG	SMA 6/20, ECG
Incision site	Right or left lower quadrant	MD preference; lower midline or transverse	Lateral chest, fourth or fifth interspace	Open: right subcostal; lap: umbilicus, rt subcostal, RLQ, upper midline	Neck
Resume eating	ASAP	4-5 days when ileus resolves	2-3 days	Open: 2-3 days; lap: 8-12 hr	ASAP
Pain control	PO or IM	IM or PCA	PCA or epidural	IM, PCA, or PO	IM or PO
Estimated length of procedure	1-1½ hr	2½-3 hr	3-4 hr	1-1½ hr	1-1½ hr
Estimated length of hospital stay	Day surgery or overnight	7-10 days	7-8 days	Open: 3-5 days; lap: 12-24 hr	2-4 days
Long-term effects of surgery	Return to normal activities	Potential for temporary colostomy	Potential for reduced pulmonary functions	Potential for rare bile salt imbalance	Potential for permanent or temporary neurologic deficit
Drains or tubes	None	Potential for colostomy bag; Foley catheter	2 chest tubes and suction; needed 2-4 days	Open: potential for T-tube/Penrose drain; lap: none	Potential for Penrose drain; needed 1-2 days

From Fox, V. J. (1993, June). Preop and postop pointers. In *Getting ready for RNFA certification*. Association of Operating room Nurses, Inc. Symposium, Lake Tahoe, NV. *CA*, Cancer; *CT*, computed tomography; *CME*, Cervical Mediastinal Exploration; *HIDA*, Hepatobiliary imaging (HIDA is actually an acronym for the radioisotope used in a hepatobiliary scan); *CBC*, complete blood count; *ECG*, electrocardiogram; *RLQ*, right lower quadrant; *PCA*, patient-controlled analgesia; *T&C*, Type and Crossmatch; *CEA*, carcinoembryonic antigen; *PSA*, Prostate-specific antigen; *PT*, prothrombin time; *PTT*, partial thromboplastin time; *lap*, laparoscopic; *ERCP*, endoscopic retrograde cholangiopancreatography; *H&H*, hematocrit and hemoglobin; *IOL*, intraocular lens; *IVP*, intravenous pyelogram; *MRI*, magnetic resonance imaging; *PTCA*, Percutaneous Translumenal Coronary Angioplasty.

Continued.

TABLE 9-4

Selecting Content for Teaching—cont'd

POSTOP POINTERS—HOME INSTRUCTIONS

	Inguinal herniorrhaphy	Sigmoid colectomy	Thoracotomy	Cholecystectomy (open or laparoscopic)	Carotid endarterectomy
Food	ASAP	Regular or low-residue diet	Regular diet	Regular diet	Regular or cardiac diet
Wound care	Change dressing PRN × 1-2 days, then none required except for comfort; ice pack is OK	Bathe or shower daily	Bathe or shower daily	Bathe or shower daily	Bathe or shower daily
Bathing	12-24 hr	Daily	Daily	Daily	Daily
Driving	4 days to 4 weeks; MD preference	In 5-7 days when soreness less	10-14 days when soreness less	Open: 5-7 days when soreness less; lap: 2-4 days	In 5-7 days when soreness less
Sex	Restricted only by limits of pain	Restricted only by limits of pain	Restricted only by limits of pain	Restricted only by limits of pain	Restricted only by limits of pain
Return to work	2-6 weeks, depending on nature of work	4-6 weeks	4-6 weeks	Open: 2-4 weeks; lap: 5 days to 2 weeks	2 weeks
Medications	As prescribed	As prescribed	As prescribed	As prescribed	As prescribed
Follow-up	MD preference; 7-10 days	MD preference; 7-10 days	MD preference; 10-14 days	MD preference; 7-10 days	MD preference; 7-10 days
Special restrictions	Heavy lifting 4-6 weeks	Within limits of pain and energy	Within limits of pain and energy	Within limits of pain and energy	Within limits of pain and energy
Worrisome but normal	Swelling and bruising of penis and scrotum	Temporary colostomy closure 6-8 weeks	Noticeable incision pain 3-4 months		Temporary or permanent numbness of earlobe

TABLE 9-4

Selecting Content for Teaching—cont'd

	Mastectomy	Ventral herniorrhaphy	Small bowel resection	Abdominal perineal resection	Common duct exploration
PREOP POINTERS					
Medical diagnosis	CA of breast	Incisional hernia	Small bowel obstruction; small bowel strangulation	CA of rectum	Common duct stone; common duct stricture
Diagnostic tests	History and physical exam; mammogram; breast biopsy	History and physical exam	History and physical exam; abdominal x-ray	Digital rectal exam; colonoscopy; rigid sigmoidoscopy	History and physical exam; ERCP
Routine preop tests	CBC, ECG	CBC, ECG	CBC, ECG	CEA, SMA 6/20, CBC, ECG, T&C, bowel prep	SMA 6/20, ECG, CBC, amylase, bilirubin
Incision site	Right or left upper chest	Previous incision site	Midline or transverse	Midline or transverse	Right subcostal
Resume eating	ASAP	ASAP	May be 4-5 days before ileus resolves	May be 4-5 days before ileus resolves	1-3 days
Pain control	PO or IM	PO, IM, or PCA	IM or PCA	IM, PCA or epidural	IM or PCA
Estimated length of procedure	1-1½ hr	1½-2 hr	1-2 hr	3-4 hr	1-1½ hr
Estimated length of hospital stay	2-4 days	3-5 days	5-7 days	7-10 days	3-5 days
Long-term effects of surgery	Potential for restricted movement in arm, lymphedema	Possibility of recurrence	Possibility of recurrence	Permanent colostomy	Potential for common duct stricture
Drains or tubes	1-2 Jackson-Pratt drain to stay 2-5 days	Jackson-Pratt drain to stay 2-5 days		Colostomy bag; Jackson-Pratt to stay 2-4 days	T-tube to stay 10 days; potential for Penrose drain to stay 2-3 days

Continued.

TABLE 9-4

Selecting Content for Teaching—cont'd

	Mastectomy	Ventral herniorrhaphy	Small bowel resection	Abdominal perineal resection	Common duct exploration
POSTOP POINTERS—HOME INSTRUCTIONS					
Food	Regular diet	Regular diet	Regular diet	Regular diet	Regular diet
Wound care	Shower daily; empty drain and redress daily for comfort; ice pack is OK	Bathe or shower daily	Bathe or shower daily	Bathe daily; change peripad to posterior wound PRN	Shower daily; redress T-tube daily
Bathing	Daily	Daily	Daily	Daily	Daily
Driving	7-10 days when soreness less	7-10 days when soreness less	7-10 days when soreness less	10-14 days when soreness less	7-10 days when soreness less
Sex	Restricted only by limits of pain	Restricted only by limits of pain	Restricted only by limits of pain	Restricted only by limits of pain	Restricted only by limits of pain
Return to work	4-6 weeks	4-6 weeks	4-6 weeks	6-8 weeks	2-4 weeks
Medications	As prescribed	As prescribed	As prescribed	As prescribed	
Follow-up	MD preference; 7-10 days; 2-4 days if going home with drain	MD preference; 7-10 days	MD preference; 10-14 days	MD preference; 10-14 days	MD preference; 10-14 days
Special restrictions	Begin arm and shoulder exercises within prescribed limits	Heavy lifting 4-6 weeks	Within limits of pain and energy	Within limits of pain and energy	Within limits of pain and energy
Worrisome but normal	Numbness and tingling from elbow to axilla			Drainage from posterior wound particularly if left open	Leaking of bile around T-tube

TABLE 9-4

Selecting Content for Teaching—cont'd

	Cesarean delivery	Vaginal hysterectomy	Total hip replacement	Cataract extraction	Craniotomy
PREOP POINTERS					
Medical diagnosis	Cephalopelvic disproportion; cord prolapse; fetal distress; abruptio placentae; placenta previa; breech presentation; previous cesarean section	Uterine prolapse; dysfunctional uterine bleeding; benign or malignant lesions	Degenerative joint disease	Cataracts	Subdural hematoma; malignant or benign lesions
Diagnostic tests	History and vaginal exam; fetal monitor	History and pelvic exam; biopsy of lesions; transvaginal sonogram	History; physical exam; x-ray	History and slit-lamp eye exam; keratometer, A scan	CT of head; neurologic assessment
Routine preop tests	CBC, ECG, T&C blood	SMA 6/20, T&C if H&H low	SMA 20, T&C, ECG	SMA 6, ECG if warranted	SMA 20, ECG
Incision site	Vertical or transverse	Through the vaginal opening; abdominal punctures if lap-assisted	In line with vertical axis of joint	Conjunctival flap	Head, depending on location of lesion
Resume eating	ASAP	1 day postop	ASAP	ASAP	ASAP
Pain control	PO or IM	IM or PO	PCA; epidural; IM; PO	PO, nonnarcotic	IM, PO, PCA
Estimated length of procedure	1 hr	1-1½ hr	2-3 hr	½-1 hr	1-1½ hr
Estimated length of hospital stay	3 to 4 days	2-4 days	7-8 days	4-6 hr	Variable depending on diagnosis and neurologic status
Long-term effects of surgery	May require subsequent cesarean delivery	Permanent sterilization	Reduced pain; potential for dislocation of prosthesis	Improved or restored vision; rarely change IOL	Potential for permanent or temporary neurologic deficit
Drains or tubes	Foley catheter	Foley catheter	Hemovac for 2 days	None	None
Food	Regular diet	Regular diet	Regular diet	Regular diet	Regular diet
Wound care	Change dressing PRN × 1-2 days, then none required	Bathe or shower daily	Shower may be easier than bathing	Eye patch and shield for 24 hr; then shield at night	Bathe or shower daily

Continued.

TABLE 9-4

Selecting Content for Teaching—cont'd

	Cesarean delivery	Vaginal hysterectomy	Total hip replacement	Cataract extraction	Craniotomy
PREOP POINTERS—cont'd					
Bathing	12-24 hr	Daily	Daily	May bathe or shower after 24 hr	Daily
Driving	7 days to 4 weeks; MD preference	In 7-14 days when soreness lessens	Varies with MD preference; may be 2-6 weeks	2-7 days due to impaired depth perception	Depends on existence and extent of neurologic deficit
Sex	Restricted only by limits of pain	MD preference; may be as long as 6 weeks	MD preference limited by restrictions on internal and external rotation of joint	Limited only by restrictions on rigorous activity	Restricted only by limits of pain
Return to work	6 weeks, depending on nature of work	2-4 weeks	6-12 weeks	3-7 days if work does not require rigorous activity	6-12 weeks
Medications	As prescribed	As prescribed	As prescribed	Antibiotic and antiinflammatory drops; artificial tears	As prescribed
Follow-up	MD preference; 7-10 days	MD preference; 7-10 days	MD preference; 7-10 days	First day postop, then 7 days; in 3-4 weeks	MD preference; 7-10 days
Special restrictions	Within limits pain and energy	Within limits of pain and energy	Must keep knees lower than hips; may recline but may not sit in low chair or commode seat if lower than knees	Heavy lifting, bending, or rigorous activities for 7 days	Within limits of pain and energy
Worrisome but normal	Vaginal drainage	Vaginal drainage	Prolonged discomfort	Foreign body sensation; dry eye; may see floaters	Lingering neurologic deficit

TABLE 9-4

Selecting Content for Teaching—cont'd

PREOP POINTERS	Retropubic prostatectomy	Nephrectomy	Radical neck dissection	Arthroscopy of knee	Coronary artery bypass graft
Medical diagnosis	Malignant lesions	Malignant lesions; infectious or inflammatory processes that destroy kidney function	Malignant lesions of the mouth and neck	Torn meniscus; diagnostic purposes	Coronary artery occlusive disease
Diagnostic tests	Rectal sonogram control for needle biopsy	Arteriogram; sonogram; CT; IVP with retrograde pyelogram; radionucleotide renogram	Physical exam; CT; nasopharyngoscopy	Physical exam; MRI	ECG; stress test; chest x-ray; thallium scan; cardiac catheterization; interventions: PTCA, arthrectomy, laser
Routine preop tests	CBC, ECG, T&C blood, PSA and acid phosphatase	Renal functions (creatinine and electrolytes)	SMA 20, ECG	SMA 6, ECG if indicated	SMA 20, ECG, T&C, pulmonary function, PT, PTT
Incision site	Pfannenstiel or midline	Lateral for inflammatory disease; anterior for malignant lesions	T shape; horizontal extends along underside of mandible; vertical from jaw to sternal notch	3-4 stab incisions around patella	Midsternal, multiple leg incisions for vein harvest
Resume eating	ASAP	Lateral: ASAP; anterior: 2-3 days	ASAP	ASAP	2-3 days after removal of endotracheal and nasogastric tubes
Pain control	PO or IM	IM or PCA	IM or PO	PO	IM, PO, PCA
Estimated length of procedure	2-2½ hr	2 hr	2-2½ hr	1-2 hr	4-6 hr
Estimated length of hospital stay	4-6 days	5-7 days	3-5 days	4-6 hr	6-8 days
Long-term effects of surgery	Probably impotence; possibly incontinence	Remaining kidney hypertrophies up to ⅓ in size	Poor cosmetic effect; possible loss of trapezius muscle	Possibility of arthritic changes	Loss of saphenous vein, possible intermittent lower leg edema

Continued.

TABLE 9-4

Selecting Content for Teaching—cont'd

	Retropubic prostatectomy	Nephrectomy	Radical neck dissection	Arthroscopy of knee	Coronary artery bypass graft
PREOP POINTERS—cont'd					
Drains or tubes	Jackson-Pratt for 2-4 days; Foley catheter	Jackson-Pratt or Penrose drain for 2-4 days	Jackson-Pratt for 2-4 days	None	2 days: mediastinal chest tube; 2-3 days: pleural chest tube; 2-3 days: Hemovac in leg wounds
POSTOP POINTERS—HOME INSTRUCTIONS					
Food	Regular diet	Regular diet	Regular diet	Regular diet	Cardiac diet
Wound care	Bathe or shower daily	Bathe or shower daily	Bathe or shower daily	Bathe or shower daily	Wounds covered if draining; redress after shower or bathe
Bathing	Daily	Daily	Daily	Daily	Daily
Driving	10 days to 2 weeks when soreness less	10 days to 2 weeks when soreness lessens	5-10 days when soreness lessens	2-4 days when soreness lessens	Not before 2 weeks and not recommended before 6 weeks (automatic shift only)
Sex	Restricted by limits of pain and ability	Restricted by limits of pain	Restricted by limits of pain	Restricted by limits of pain	Restricted by limits of ability to bear weight on upper arms and chest
Return to work	6-8 weeks	4-6 weeks	3-4 weeks	2-4 days, depending on nature of work	8-12 weeks
Medications	As prescribed	As prescribed	As prescribed	As prescribed	As prescribed
Follow-up	MD preference; 7-10 days	MD preference; 7-10 days	MD preference; 7-10 days	MD preference; 7-10 days	MD preference; 7-14 days
Special restrictions	Within limits of pain and energy	Within limits of pain and energy; should always avoid dangerous contact sports	Within limits of pain and energy	Limited weight bearing as tolerated	Upper body movement restricted for 6 weeks for sternal healing
Worrisome but normal	Impotence; incontinence		Inability to raise shoulder		Fatigue, swelling in leg, leg discomfort 4-6 weeks

Nonprint materials include audio and visual programs, such as videotapes, television, flip charts, pictures and slides, cassette tapes, and models (Ruzicki, 1992). Videotapes and television are very effective tools for instructing hospitalized patients (Redman, 1993). These may be rented or purchased. Some hospitals are part of a nationwide satellite network that televises patient education programs, and some produce their own videotapes and live broadcasts. Audiotapes and phone teaching are available in some hospitals via a toll-free dial access system. Another technique is to tape an educational session and give it to the patient when the session is completed. Cassette tapes or videotapes of the teaching session can be replayed at the patient's convenience. Select audio or video programs that are appropriate to the subject matter, accurate in content, simple, and appealing to the target audience (Ruzicki, 1992).

DOCUMENTATION

Unfortunately, patient education is often not thoroughly documented. Perioperative nurses may not recognize the value of teaching/learning interactions or not consider the interaction patient education because it was not a formal process with written objectives (Ruzicki, 1989). As the JCAHO focuses on quality of care and outcomes, standardized documentation of all kinds of patient education is becoming very important. A simple narrative in the nursing notes is adequate for informal teaching/learning interactions. Be sure to include the outcomes of the interaction as well as assessment data and content. Effective forms for documentation combine teaching protocols, objectives, and outcomes on a single page. Equally as important to document are those times when the patient was not ready to learn. It should include the assessment data that indicated lack of readiness and what the nurse did to enhance readiness. Be sure to document when portions of the content are referred to another provider. Referral is an important nursing intervention for perioperative nurses to utilize given the limited amount of time available to spend with patients. Box 9-7 is a good example of how to document the nursing diagnosis, activities, and outcomes in a quick, concise form.

DISCHARGE PLANNING

Discharge planning is "preparing for moving the patient from one level of care to another within or outside the current health care agency" (McCloskey and Bulechek, 1992). Discharge *planning* is a misnomer. A more accurate label is *implementing* discharge activities. Perioperative nurses are becoming more responsible for discharge planning because of the tremendous increase in same-day surgical procedures. Having assessed the patient's needs upon discharge during the preoperative and postoperative phases, the perioperative nurse helps the patient and family prepare for discharge. This requires collaboration with and coordinating the efforts of the other members of the health care team. The perioperative nurse may be the individual that determines if the patient meets the criteria for discharge as well as communicates and documents discharge plans. These plans may include: (1) arranging for maintenance or follow-up care with the physician or nurse practitioner, (2) helping the family create a supportive environment at home, (3) encouraging self-care philosophy, (4) coordinating referrals to financial or social services, home care agencies, or outreach programs, (5) evaluating and arranging the need for caregiver support, and (6) arranging for discharge.

EVALUATION

Evaluation of patient education activities should be considered early in the teaching process. Evaluation measures if and how well a patient learned the desired behavior. Does the patient willingly change behavior? Evaluation criteria (outcome criteria) are set during the planning phase. Evaluation can serve many purposes (Redman, 1993). It can motivate continued learning or behavior change because it provides concrete evidence that the patient accomplished or failed to accomplish the goal. It reinforces desired behavior on the part of the patient and helps the perioperative nurse determine the adequacy of the instruction and teaching materials.

In evaluation the evidence of learning is compared to the outcome criteria. Although there are a variety of methods to measure outcomes (Table 9-5), the most frequent method used by the perioperative nurse is some form of observation. Direct observation is more effective in evaluating learning in health care than in other areas. Whereas it may be difficult to evaluate cognitive skills and thinking processes by direct observation, we know that motor skills rely on and reflect cognitive processes. For example, for the outcome criteria "The patient will consent to a specific treatment option" the nurse can directly observe whether the patient signed the operative permit. Recording observations or documenting outcomes is essential when using observation as the evaluation method. Narrative form is the best method to document critical incidents or anecdotal events that do not lend themselves to a simpler, quicker method of documentation. Checklists and rating scales save time and produce uniform documentation. Box 9-7 is a good example of a checklist format. Rating scales are another useful way to document outcomes. Box 9-3 illustrates three types of pain rating scales. Rarely will the perioperative nurse be able to evaluate using more extensive self-reports and self-monitoring methods. Although these are excellent methods of evaluation, they are time consuming. Time is a resource in critically short supply. These methods are best used for group educational programs.

Although evaluation is the final step in the teaching/nursing process, it rarely means the end of the process. Evaluation frequently points the perioperative nurse back to other steps in the process.

TABLE 9-5

Methods of Evaluating Learning

Technique	Advantages	Disadvantages
Direct observation	Performance under real or simulated conditions can be assessed.	Awareness of the observer may affect performance.
	Task is credible to patient.	Training, supervising, using observers is costly.
	Measure has good content validity.	Number of patients who may be studied and their locale may be restricted because of the high per-patient cost of observing.
Observational checklist	Simple, objective task to record observations	Checklist may be long if a multifaceted behavior is measured.
	Observer error low	
Anchored rating scale	Simple, objective task to record observations	Difficult to write behavioral descriptions that differ by equal amounts over an ordered scale
	Observer error low	
	More gradations of judgment allowed than typical of an observational checklist	Descriptions may introduce several dimensions into a single rating
Observational record	Permits routine recording of simple, repetitive behaviors	Inferences depend on sample of time and fineness of recording unit
Anecdotal notes	May provide unique insights, illustrations	May be irrelevant to outcomes of interest
Critical incidents	Characterize adaptive and maladaptive behavior	Time consuming to collect and analyze
	May serve as the basis for more structured measurement	Focus on behavioral extremes; ignore typical behavior that is not outstandingly adaptive or maladaptive.
Physiologic measures	Measure is accurate.	Measure may be multiply determined; not affected by teaching outcomes alone.
	Measure is a good indicator of health status.	
	Measure is responsive to compliance with health care regimen.	Measure may depend on patient's willingness and ability to perform routine self-testing and recording.
		Measurement may be costly to obtain and analyze.
		Measurement may be invasive.
Self-report	Provides data and insights not available for other sources	Subject to faking, socially desirable response set
	Measures cognitive, affective, and performance outcomes directly	Requires skill in construction of instrument
Oral self-report	Little reading and no writing required of patient	Recording burden for interviewer.
	Contingent questions, probing, and question clarification possible	Responses may be biased by interviewer.
		Data collection individualized and costly
Written self-report	Cost-effective group administration of instruments is possible.	Reading and recording burdens are placed on patient.
		Questions are fixed; probes and clarifications cannot be introduced.
		Possible reduction in response rate of quality resulting from respondent burden

TABLE 9-5

Methods of Evaluating Learning—cont'd

Technique	Advantages	Disadvantages
Open-ended questions	Respondent free to shape reply	Extent of reply depends on verbal fluency of respondent Heavy recording burden for respondent or interviewer Inconsistent dimensions of response across patients Responses difficult to code and analyze
Closed, fixed-alternative questions	Easy recording, coding, processing of data Limited dimensions for replies Relative insensitivity to verbal fluency	Construction of instrument is time consuming Dimensions on which choices will vary must be anticipated Choices may be forced among nonsalient options
Single questions per topic Scales of questions per topic Self-monitoring	Speed, ease of response Stability of response Recording occurs concurrently with behavior Access to all behaviors, covert and overt, is possible.	Instability of response Increased length of instrument Recording process may be reactive. Quality of record is dependent on patient's cooperation Self-monitored data may differ from externally observed data.
Records	*Noninvasive*—supply data without added demands on patients *Nonreactive*—relatively insensitive to external manipulation to claim desired outcomes Relatively low cost of collection	May not be organized to permit easy access retrieval Incomplete and/or inconsistent records Indirect measures; may not be directly relevant to teaching outcomes
Patient charts, physician records		May require health care professional to record and interpret relevant data Privacy considerations may restrict access to records or require hierarchy of obtained consents.
Agency service records, public records and reports	Data may be collected by relatively unskilled workers.	Data come from a variety of sources with varying degrees of accessibility, reporting standards, and variable conceptualization

From: Redman, B. K. (1993). *The process of patient education* (7th ed.). St. Louis: Mosby.

BOX 9-7

Example of Checklist Documentation

GENERIC CARE PLAN The patient demonstrates knowledge of the physiologic and psychologic responses to surgery

Patient Data:

Nursing Diagnosis:
Risk for knowledge deficit regarding planned surgical intervention.

Patient Outcome:
The patient will demonstrate knowledge of the physiologic and psychologic responses to the planned surgical intervention.

Outcome Criteria:
The patient will demonstrate knowledge by:
1. Remaining oriented to person, place, and time
2. Confirming, in writing or verbally, consent for the operative procedure
3. Describing the sequence of events during the perioperative period
4. Stating outcomes in realistic terms
5. Expressing feelings about the surgical experience

Evaluation of Patient Outcomes

	Outcome met	Outcome met with additional outcome criteria	Outcome met with revised nursing care plan	Outcome not met	Outcome not applicable to this patient
1. The patient remained oriented to person, place, and time.	☐	☐	☐	☐	☐
2. Physical and emotional factors which impacted on the patient's response to the planned surgical intervention were alleviated.	☐	☐	☐	☐	☐
3. The patient was physically and emotionally prepared for the planned surgical intervention.	☐	☐	☐	☐	☐
4. The patient correctly reviewed anticipated perioperative events.	☐	☐	☐	☐	☐
5. The patient signed the operative permit.	☐				

Nursing Actions

	Yes	No	N/A
1. Patient identified?	☐	☐	☐
2. Sensory aids/prosthetic devices removed?	☐	☐	☐
3. Sensory impairments?	☐	☐	☐
4. LOC: Alert?	☐	☐	☐
5. Verbal verification of operative site?	☐	☐	☐
6. Consent signed?	☐	☐	☐
7. Language barrier?	☐	☐	☐
8. Special religious needs?	☐	☐	☐
9. Special cultural beliefs?	☐	☐	☐
10. Perioperative routine explained?	☐	☐	☐
11. Patient expressed understanding?	☐	☐	☐
12. Patient has additional questions?	☐	☐	☐

Nursing Actions (continued)

	Yes	No	N/A

Document additional nursing actions/care plan revisions here:

_____

_____

_____

Signature: _____ Date: _____

From Rothrock, J.C. (1995). Generic care planning: AORN patient outcome standards. In J.C. Rothrock (Ed.), *Perioperative nursing care planning* (2nd ed.). St. Louis: Mosby.

REFERENCES

Acute pain management guideline panel. (1992a). *Acute pain management in adults: operative procedures: Quick reference guide for clinicians* (AHCPR Publication No. 92-0019). Rockville, Md: Agency for Health Care Policy and Research.

Acute pain management guideline panel. (1992b). *Acute pain management: operative or medical procedures and trauma: clinical practice guidelines* (AHCPR Publication No. 92-0032). Rockville, Md: Agency for Health Care Policy and Research.

American Hospital Association. (1992). A patient's bill of rights. Chicago: The Association.

Devine, E. C., & Cook, T. D. (1983). A meta-analytic analysis of effects of psychoeducational interventions on length of hospital stay. *Nursing Research, 32,* 267-274.

Fox, V. J. (1986). Patient teaching: Understanding the needs of the adult learner. *AORN Journal, 44,* 234-242.

Good-Reis D. V., & Pieper, B. A. (1990). Structured vs unstructured teaching: A research study. *AORN Journal, 51*(5), 1334-1339.

Hathaway, D. (1986). Effect of preoperative instruction on postoperative outcomes: A meta-analysis. *Nursing Research, 35,* 269-275.

Johnson, E. A., & Jackson, J. (1989). Teaching the home care client. *Nursing Clinics of North America, 24,* 267.

Johnson, S. (1989). Preoperative teaching: A need for change. *Nursing Management, 20,* 80B-80H.

Joint Commission for the Accreditation of Healthcare Organizations. (1992). *1993 Accreditation Manual for Hospitals.* Chicago: The Commission.

Kim, M. J., McFarland, G. K., & McLane, A. M. (1995). *Pocket guide to nursing diagnosis* (6th ed.). St. Louis: Mosby.

Kruger, S. (1991). The patient educator role in nursing. *Applied Nursing Research, 4,* 19-24.

Lee, J. M. (1970). Emotional reactions to trauma. *Nursing Clinics of North America, 5,* 577-587.

Lepczyk, M., Raleigh, E. H., & Rowley, C. (1990). Timing of preoperative patient teaching. *Journal of Advanced Nursing, 15,* 300-306.

Lindeman, C. A., & Aernam, B. V. (1971). Nursing intervention with the presurgical patient: The effects of structured and unstructured preoperative teaching. *Nursing Research, 20,* 319-332.

Lindeman, C. A. (1972). Nursing intervention with the presurgical patient. *Nursing Research,* 196-209.

Lindeman, C. A. (1973). Influencing recovery through preoperative teaching. *Heart and Lung, 2,* 515-521.

Lorig, K. (1992). Patient education: A practical approach. St. Louis: Mosby.

McCloskey, J. C., & Bulechek, G. M. (Eds.). (1992). *Nursing classification interventions (NIC).* St. Louis: Mosby.

McHatton, M. (1985). A theory for timely teaching. *American Journal of Nursing, 85,* 798-800.

Midgley J. W., & Osterhage, R. A. (1973). Effect of nursing instruction and length of hospitalization on postoperative complications in cholecystectomy patients. *Nursing Research, 22,* 69-72.

Narrow, B. W. (1979). *Patient teaching in nursing practice: A patient and family centered approach.* New York: John Wiley & Sons.

National League for Nursing Education. (1918). *Standard curriculum for schools of nursing.* Baltimore: The Waverly Press.

National League for Nursing Education. (1937). *A curriculum guide for schools of nursing.* New York: The League.

National League for Nursing Education. (1950). *Nursing organization curriculum conference.* Glen Gardener, NJ: Libertarian Press.

Oetker-Black, S. L., Hart, F., Hoffman, J., & Geary, S. (1992). Preoperative self-efficacy and postoperative behaviors. *Applied Nursing Research, 5,* 134-139.

Pierce, P. F. (1993). Deciding on breast cancer treatment: A description of decisional behaviors. *Nursing Research, 42,* 22-28.

Rakel B. A. (1992). Interventions related to patient teaching. *Nursing Clinics of North America, 24,* 397-423.

Raleigh, E. H., Lepczyk, M., & Rowley, C. (1990). Significant others benefit from preoperative information. *Journal of Advanced Nursing, 15,* 941-945.

Redman, B. K. (1993). *The process of patient education* (7th ed.). St. Louis: Mosby.

Rothrock, J. C. (1990). Generic care planning: AORN patient outcome standards. In J. C. Rothrock (Ed.), *Perioperative nursing care planning.* (pp. 72-117). St. Louis: Mosby.

Ruzicki, D. A. (1989). Realistically meeting the educational needs of hospitalized acute and short-stay patients. *Nursing Clinics of North America, 24,* 629-637.

Shade, P. (1992). Patient-controlled analgesia: Can client education improve outcomes? *Journal of Advanced Nursing, 17,* 408-413.

Silva, M. C. (1987). Needs of spouses of surgical patients: A conceptualization within the Roy adaptation model. *Scholarly Inquiry for Nursing Practice: An International Journal, 1,* 29-44.

Smith, C. E. (1987, July). Patient teaching: It's the law. *Nursing 87,* pp. 67-68.

Smith, C. E. (1989). Overview of patient education: Opportunities and challenges for the twenty-first century. *Nursing Clinics of North America, 24,* 583-587.

Sundeen, S. J., Stuart, G. W., Rankin, E. A. D., & Cohen, S. A. (1994). *Nurse-client interaction: Implementing the nursing process* (5th ed.). St. Louis: Mosby.

Timmons, M. E., & Bower, F. L. (1993). The effect of structured preoperative teaching on patients' use of patient-controlled analgesia (PCA) and their management of pain. *Orthopaedic Nursing, 12,* 23-31.

Wallace, L. M. (1985). Surgical patients' preferences for preoperative information. *Patient Education and Counseling, 7,* 377-387.

Wolfer, J. A., & Davis, C. E. (1970). Assessment of surgical patient's preoperative emotional condition and postoperative welfare. *Nursing Research, 19,* 402-414.

PART TWO

SURGICAL INTERVENTIONS

10

GASTROINTESTINAL SURGERY

LYNDA R. PETTY

Many gastrointestinal diseases are treated by surgery, and many surgical procedures of the abdomen begin with an exploratory laparotomy as a means of diagnosis, assessment of extent of disease, and treatment. In several diseases, such as cancer, the planned procedure may be changed due to the laparotomy findings. In other instances a first plan of care is made only after laparotomy findings are ascertained. Many different procedures involving the abdominal viscera are performed using a laparotomy approach; examples include resection of a portion of the bowel due to disease or obstruction, procedures performed on the stomach such as gastrectomy, and procedures performed to diagnose a problem that has resulted in physiologic symptoms.

Surgical procedures involving the gastrointestinal tract are usually performed through an abdominal incision; however, endoscopic possibilities and laparoscopic procedures are rapidly changing the approach to surgical interventions. The surgeon chooses an incision that affords maximum exposure of the involved structures, ensures minimal trauma and postoperative discomfort, and provides for primary wound healing with maximal wound strength. Although surgical interventions have changed drastically over the years, the types of laparotomy incisions used to expose the affected organs of the GI tract have remained relatively constant. In few other types of surgery can attention to detail and technique so profoundly affect the ultimate result as in the opening and closing of abdominal incisions.

The abdominal wall consists of various tissue layers through which dissection is necessary to enter the abdominal cavity (Figs. 10-1 and 10-2). Beneath the skin and subcutaneous fat, the layers include fascia, muscles (external and internal oblique, rectus abdominis, and transversus abdominis), preperitoneal fat, and peritoneum. Fascia, which consists of bands of tough, fibrous connective tissue, surrounds the muscles anteriorly and posteriorly (Fig. 10-3). The peritoneum is a serous membrane lining the abdominal cavity. Incision of this tissue layer exposes abdominal cavity contents.

SURGICAL ANATOMY

The alimentary canal comprises a series of organs joined to form a tubelike structure that extends the entire length of the trunk (Fig. 10-4). The alimentary tract includes the mouth; pharynx; esophagus; stomach; small intestine, consisting of the duodenum, jejunum, and ileum; and large intestine, which comprises the cecum, ascending colon, transverse colon, descending colon, sigmoid colon, rectum, and anus. These organs are responsible for the supply of nourishment to the body and the elimination of solid wastes.

The esophagus extends from the pharynx, at the level of the sixth cervical vertebra, and passes through the neck, posterior to the trachea and heart and anterior to the vertebral column. The lower portion of the esophagus passes in front of the aorta and through the diaphragm, slightly to the left of the midline, to join the cardia of the stomach.

Blood is supplied to the esophagus from branches of the inferior thyroid, thoracic aorta, and celiac arteries. The nerve supply comes from branches of the vagi and sympathetic chain. The esophagus of an adult is about 10 inches in length and is a collapsible musculomembranous tube.

The stomach is situated between the esophagus and the duodenum and lies in the upper left abdominal cavity, slightly to the left of the midline and beneath the diaphragm. The stomach is divided into three parts: the fundus, the body, and the antrum (Fig. 10-5). The fundus lies beneath the left dome of the diaphragm, behind the apex of the heart, and the body and antrum lie in an oblique direction within the abdominal cavity. The stomach is stabilized indirectly by the lower portion of the esophagus and directly by its attachment to the duodenum, which is anchored to the posterior parietal peritoneum. The omentum, the peritoneal ligaments, and branches of the celiac vessel provide additional support to the stomach.

The convex, or lower, margin of the stomach is known as the greater curvature; the concave, or upper, margin is the lesser curvature. Attached to the greater curvature is the greater omentum, which is a double fold of peritoneum containing fat. It covers the intestines loosely and is not to be

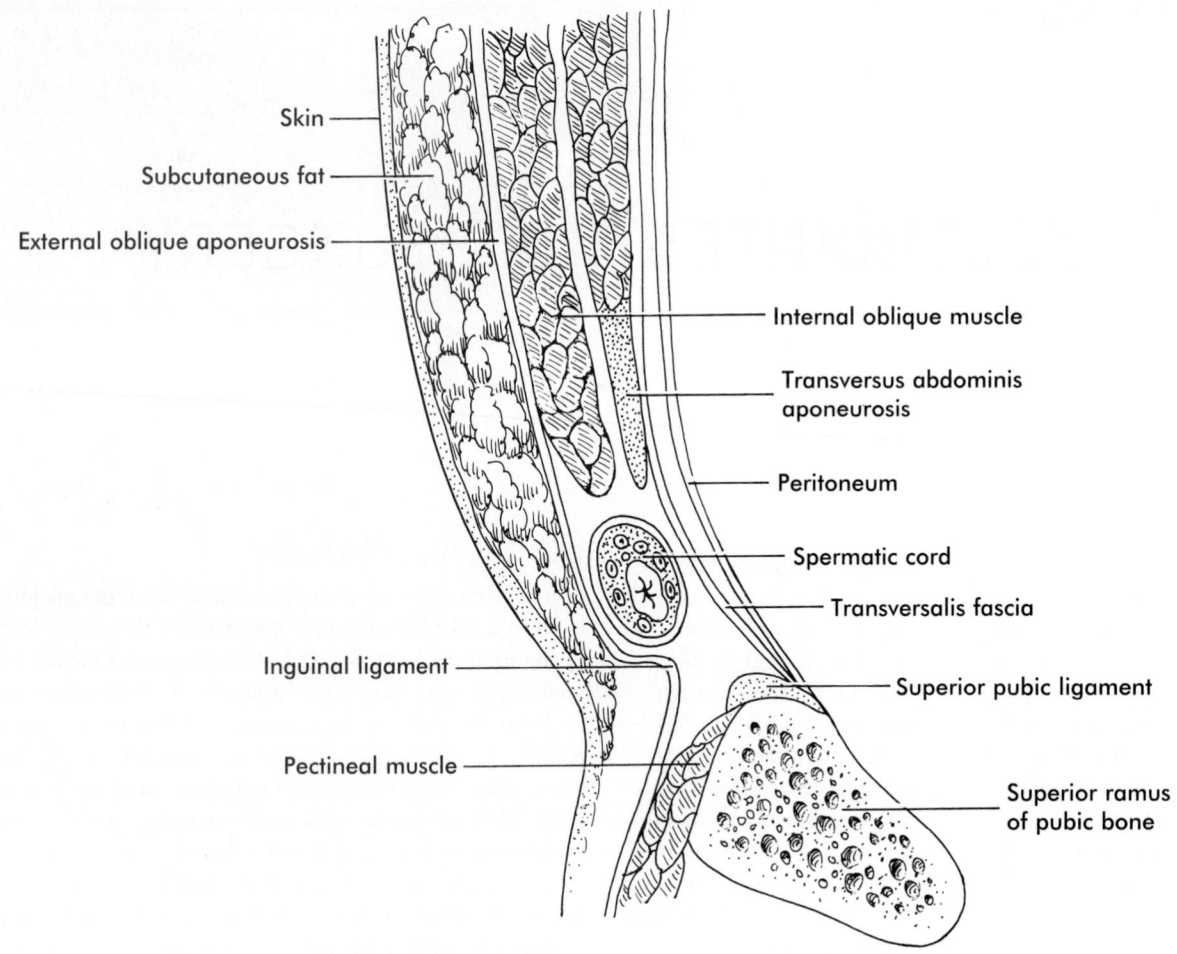

Skin

Subcutaneous fat

External oblique aponeurosis

Internal oblique muscle

Transversus abdominis
aponeurosis

Peritoneum

Spermatic cord

Transversalis fascia

Inguinal ligament

Superior pubic ligament

Pectineal muscle

Superior ramus
of pubic bone

FIG. 10-1   Vertical section of abdominal wall.

confused with the mesentery, which connects the intestines with the posterior abdominal wall. The left gastroepiploic branch of the splenic artery and the right gastroepiploic branch of the hepatic artery run through the greater omentum. The lesser omentum, which is attached to the lesser curvature of the stomach, contains the left gastric artery, a branch of the celiac axis, and the right gastric branch of the hepatic artery (Fig. 10-6). During a gastrectomy, these vessels are clamped and ligated.

The small intestine begins at the pylorus and ends at the ileocecal valve (Fig. 10-7). It is also divided into three parts: the duodenum, which is about 10 inches long; the jejunum, which is about 7½ feet long; and the ileum, which is about 10½ feet long in an adult. The small intestine varies in size with the degree of contraction but is usually about 20 feet in length and 1 inch in diameter (Fig. 10-7). The duodenum, the proximal portion of the small intestine, begins at the pylorus, is continuous with the jejunum, and is stabilized by a fusion between the pancreas and the posterior parietal peritoneum. The duodenum is divided into four portions: superior (I), descending (II), transverse (III), and ascending (IV) (Fig. 10-8). Nearly all of the first portion

mucosa is characterized by the lack of folds; it appears slightly dilated, and is referred to as the duodenal bulb. The characteristic circular folds of the small intestine mucosa begin just proximal to the end of the first portion of the duodenum and extend through the jejunum. They become less prominent in the ileum. The purpose of the circular mucosal folds, called plicae circulares of Kerckring or valvulae conniventes, is to provide greater mucosal surface area (Thompson, 1992).

The common duct enters the pancreas posterior to the duodenal bulb. The common bile duct and the main pancreatic duct enter the medial wall of the middle of the second portion of the duodenum at the ampulla of Vater. The first, second, and third portions of the duodenum curve in a C-loop concavity in which the head of the pancreas lies. The fourth portion of the duodenum ascends to the duodenojejunal flexure. The duodenojejunal flexure is stabilized by the ligament of Treitz, which suspends the duodenum from the posterior body wall. The ligament of Treitz serves as an important landmark during any abdominal exploration because it provides the surgeon with a reliable orientation of the patient's anatomy.

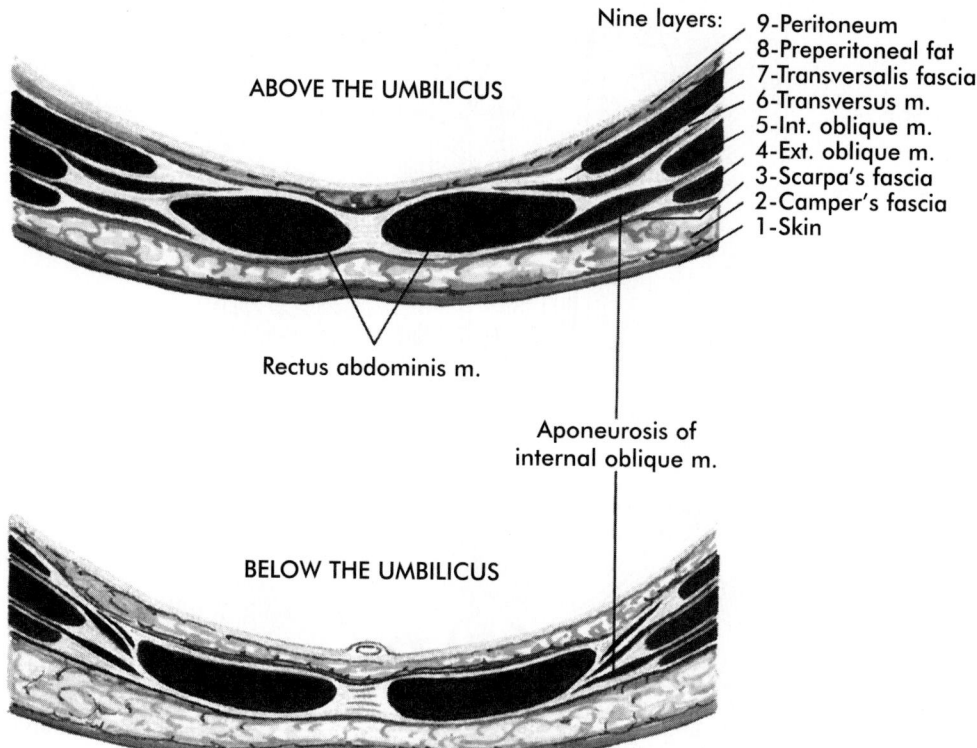

Nine layers:
9-Peritoneum
8-Preperitoneal fat
7-Transversalis fascia
6-Transversus m.
5-Int. oblique m.
4-Ext. oblique m.
3-Scarpa's fascia
2-Camper's fascia
1-Skin

ABOVE THE UMBILICUS

Rectus abdominis m.

Aponeurosis of internal oblique m.

BELOW THE UMBILICUS

FIG. 10-2 Horizontal section of abdominal wall. Aponeurosis of internal oblique muscle splits into two sections, one lying anterior and the other posterior to rectus abdominis muscle, thereby forming encasing sheath around muscle above umbilicus. Below umbilicus, aponeuroses of all muscles pass anterior to rectus.

From Thibodeau, G.A. (1990). *Anthony's textbook of anatomy and physiology*, ed. 13, St. Louis: Mosby.

The blood supply of the duodenum comes from the arterial branches of the celiac axis. The gastroduodenal artery branches off the hepatic artery and is located behind the duodenal bulb. At the inferior margin of the bulb the gastroduodenal artery divides into the right gastroepiploic artery and a superior pancreaticoduodenal branch. The superior pancreaticoduodenal artery supplies blood to the proximal duodenum and head of the pancreas. The inferior pancreaticoduodenal artery branch of the superior mesenteric artery supplies blood to the third and fourth portions of the duodenum as well as to the head and body of the pancreas (Fig. 10-9).

The jejunum, which is situated in the upper portion of the abdomen, joins the ileum, which is situated in the lower portion of the cavity. The ileum empties into the large intestine through the ileocecal valve. The jejunum and ileum are suspended by the mesentery, which is attached to the posterior abdominal wall (Fig. 10-10). The free border of the mesentery, which is about 18 feet long, contains branches of the superior mesenteric artery, many veins, lymph nodes, and nerve fibers. The blood supply to the jejunum and ileum comes entirely from the superior mesenteric artery. The small bowel contains major deposits of lymphatic tissue, known as Peyer's patches in the ileum. The rich lymphatic drainage of the small bowel plays a major role in fat absorption. Lymphatic drainage from the mucosa proceeds through the wall of the small intestine to lymph nodes adjacent to the mesentery. Lymphatic drainage then proceeds to larger lymphatics that communicate to the retroperitoneal cisterna chyli and from there to the thoracic duct. The lymphatics of the intestine play a major role in the body's immune defense as well as in the spread of cells arising from intestinal neoplasms (Thompson, 1992).

The jejunum has a larger circumference and is thicker than the ileum. The mesenteric vessels usually form only one or two arcades, a series of anastomosing arterial arches, in comparison to the multiple vascular arcades of the ileum. The jejunal mucosa is thick and has prominent plicae circulares. The ileum mucosa is thinner with few plicae (Thompson, 1992) (Fig. 10-11).

The large intestine begins at the ileocecal valve and terminates at the anus. It is divided into the cecum, colon and rectum. The cecum is attached to the ileum and extends

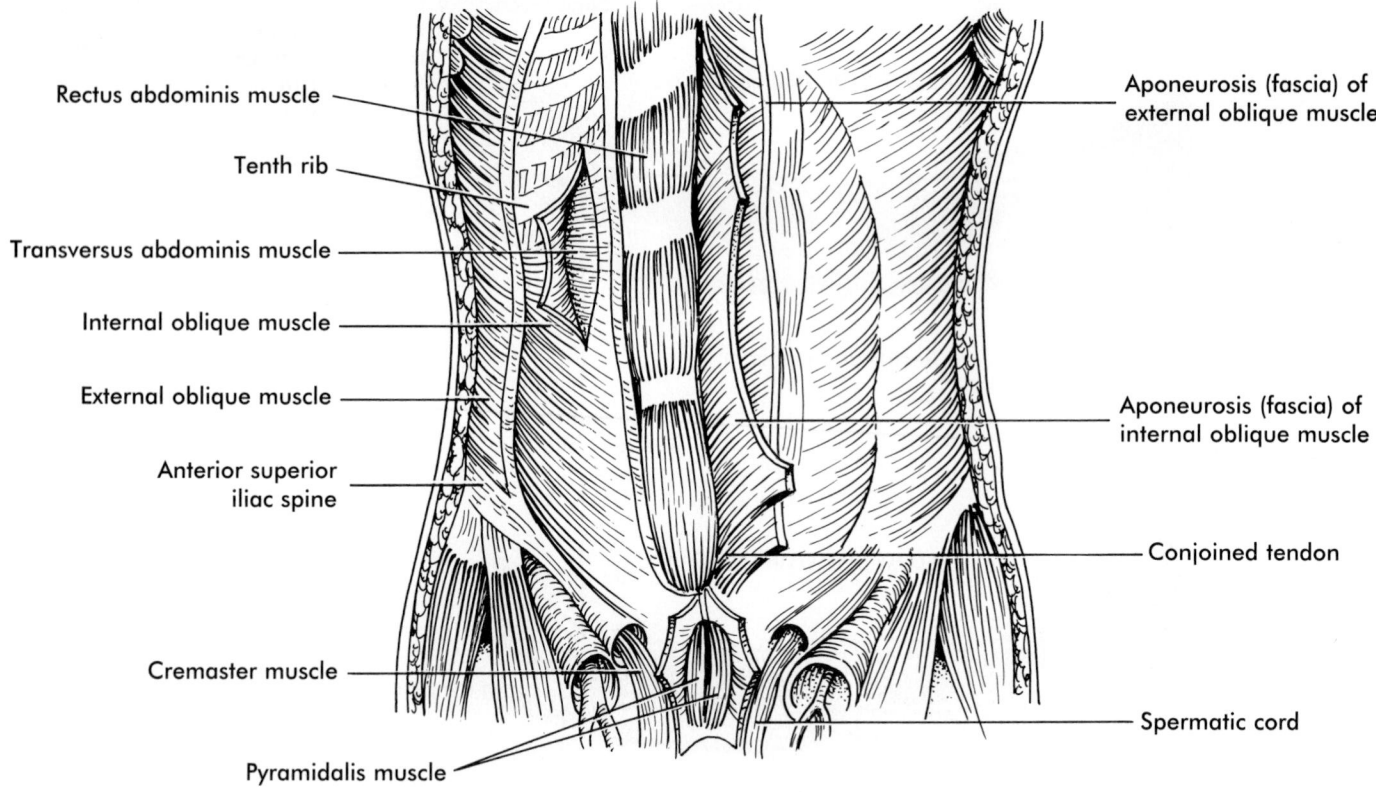

Rectus abdominis muscle

Tenth rib

Transversus abdominis muscle

Internal oblique muscle

External oblique muscle

Anterior superior
iliac spine

Cremaster muscle

Pyramidalis muscle

Aponeurosis (fascia) of
external oblique muscle

Aponeurosis (fascia) of
internal oblique muscle

Conjoined tendon

Spermatic cord

FIG. 10-3   Superior muscles of abdominal wall.

about 2½ inches below it (Fig. 10-12). The cecum in an adult is usually adherent to the posterior wall of the peritoneal cavity and has a serosal covering on its anterior wall only. The cecum forms a blind pouch from which the appendix projects.

The colon is divided into four parts: the ascending colon, the transverse colon, the descending colon, and the sigmoid colon (Fig. 10-12).

The ascending colon is about 6 inches long and extends upward from the ileocecal valve to the hepatic flexure. The upper portion of the ascending colon lies behind the right lobe of the liver and in front of the anterior surface of the right kidney.

The transverse colon, which is about 20 inches long, begins at the hepatic flexure and ends at the splenic flexure. It lies below the stomach and is attached to the transverse mesocolon.

The descending colon extends downward from the splenic flexure to the area just below the iliac crest and is about 7 inches long. The iliac portion of the sigmoid colon, which is about 6 inches long, lies on the inner surface of the left iliac muscle. The remaining portion of the colon passes over the pelvic rim into the pelvic cavity and lies partly in the abdomen and partly in the pelvis. It then forms

an S curve in the pelvis and terminates in the rectum at the level of the third segment of the sacral vertebrae.

The blood supply to the ascending colon, hepatic flexure, and transverse colon comes from the superior mesenteric artery, whereas the blood supply to the descending colon and rectum comes from the inferior mesenteric artery (Fig. 10-13).

The wall of the colon is made up of taeniae coli, epiploic appendices, and haustra. The taeniae coli are three longitudinal, or axial, strips of muscles distributed around the circumference of the colon. They represent the longitudinal muscle layer, which is not complete in the colon. The small intestine and rectum have both circular and complete longitudinal muscle layers. The epiploic appendices are fatty appendages along the bowel that have no particular function; the haustra are sacculations that are the outpouchings of bowel wall between the taeniae coli. The diameter of the colon varies in size from about 3½ inches in the cecum to an average of about ½ inch in the sigmoid colon.

The rectum originates at the sigmoid colon and terminates in the anus. A slightly curved passage about 6 inches long, it is surrounded by the pelvic fascia as it lies on the anterior surface of the sacrum and coccyx. In the male the rectum lies behind the prostate gland, seminal vesicles, and

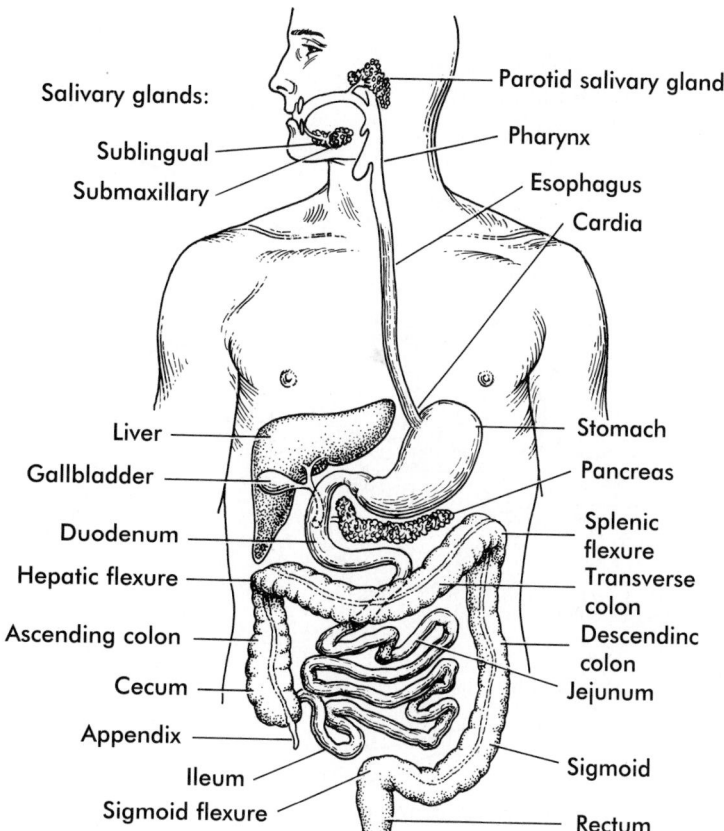

FIG. 10-4 Alimentary canal and its appendages.

the bladder. In the female the rectum lies behind the uterus and the vagina. A rectovesicale septum, also called Denonvilliers' fascia, separates the rectum from the urogenital structures. The rectum is suspended in the pelvis by fascia extending from the right and left pelvic sidewalls. Rectosacral fascia extending from the sacrum to the anorectal junction suspends the rectum posteriorly. The rectum dilates just before it becomes the anal canal, and this dilatation or ampulla presents folds called Houston's valves. The wall of the rectum consists of four layers, similar to those of the small intestine.

The anal canal is a narrow passage about 1 inch long, which passes downward and slightly posterior. It is surrounded and controlled by two circular muscle groups, which form the external and internal anal sphincters. The internal sphincter is a continuation of the longitudinal muscle layer.

The esophagus serves as the route from which food enters the stomach from the mouth. When food enters the stomach, it undergoes chemical and mechanical changes and then enters the duodenum, where it is mixed with bile and pancreatic juices. The stomach is never entirely empty

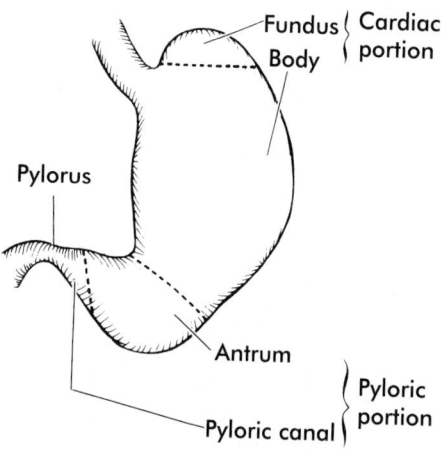

FIG. 10-5 Regional anatomy of stomach.

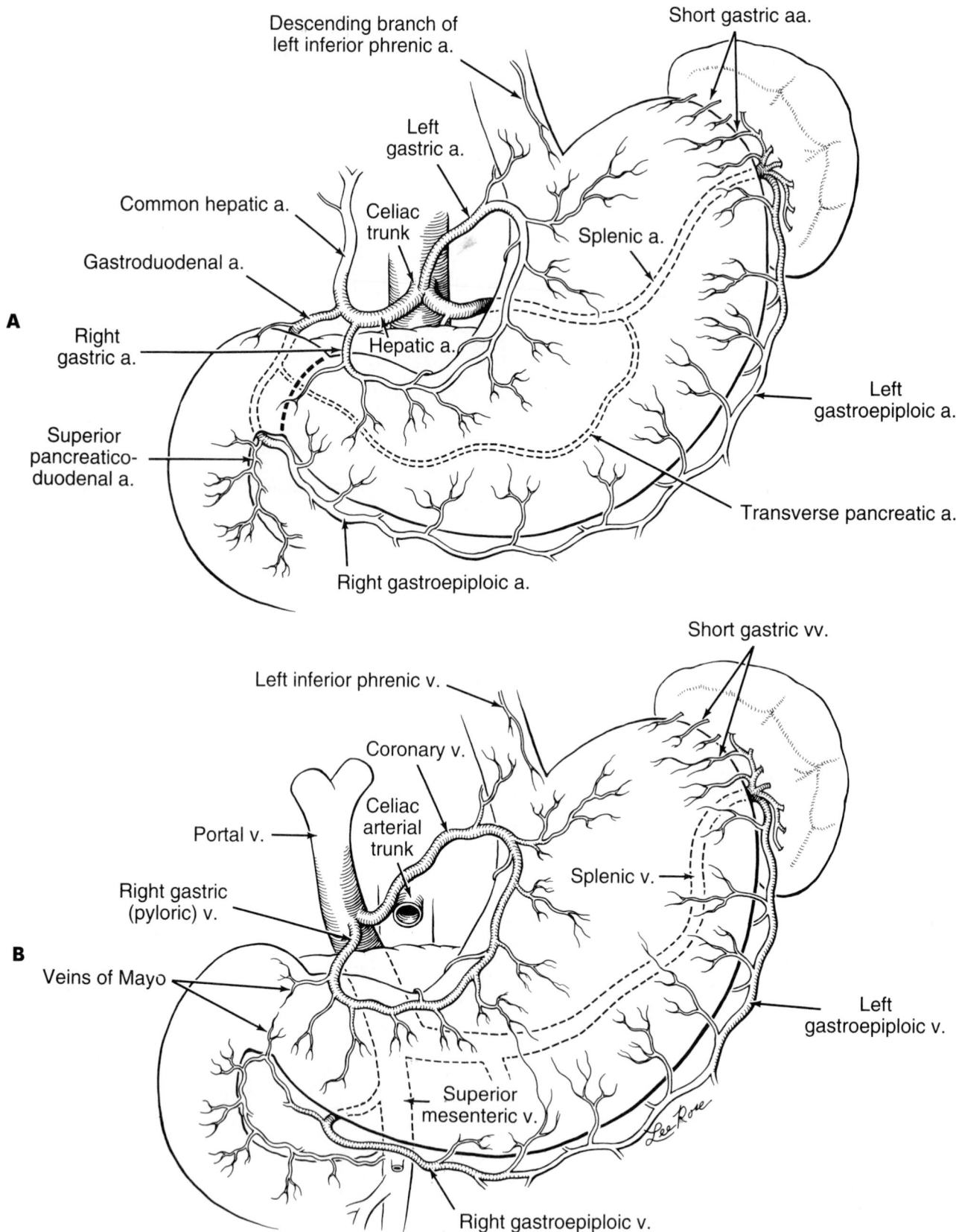

Descending branch of
left inferior phrenic a.

Short gastric aa.

Left
gastric a.

Common hepatic a.

Celiac
trunk

Splenic a.

Gastroduodenal a.

A

Right
gastric a.

Hepatic a.

Left
gastroepiploic a.

Superior
pancreatico-
duodenal a.

Transverse pancreatic a.

Right gastroepiploic a.

Short gastric vv.

Left inferior phrenic v.

Coronary v.

Celiac
arterial
trunk

Portal v.

Splenic v.

Right gastric
(pyloric) v.

B

Veins of Mayo

Left
gastroepiploic v.

Superior
mesenteric v.

Right gastroepiploic v.

FIG. 10-6 For legend see opposite page.

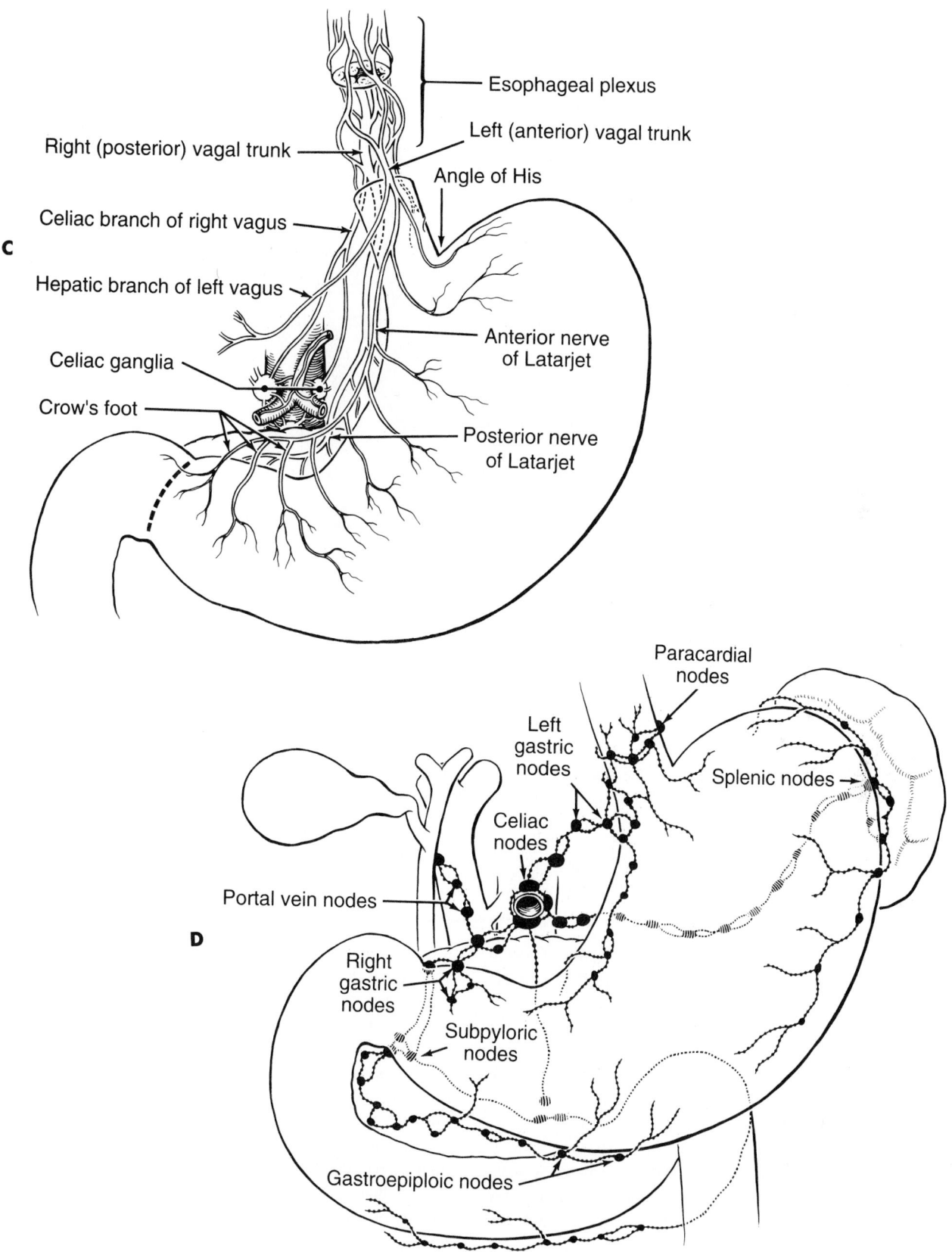

FIG. 10-6 **A,** Arterial supply of stomach. **B,** Venous supply of the stomach. **C,** Innervation of the stomach and distal esophagus. **D,** Lymphatic drainage of the stomach, duodenum, and periportal region.
From Thompson, J.C. (1992). *Atlas of surgery of the stomach, duodenum, and small bowel,* St. Louis: Mosby.

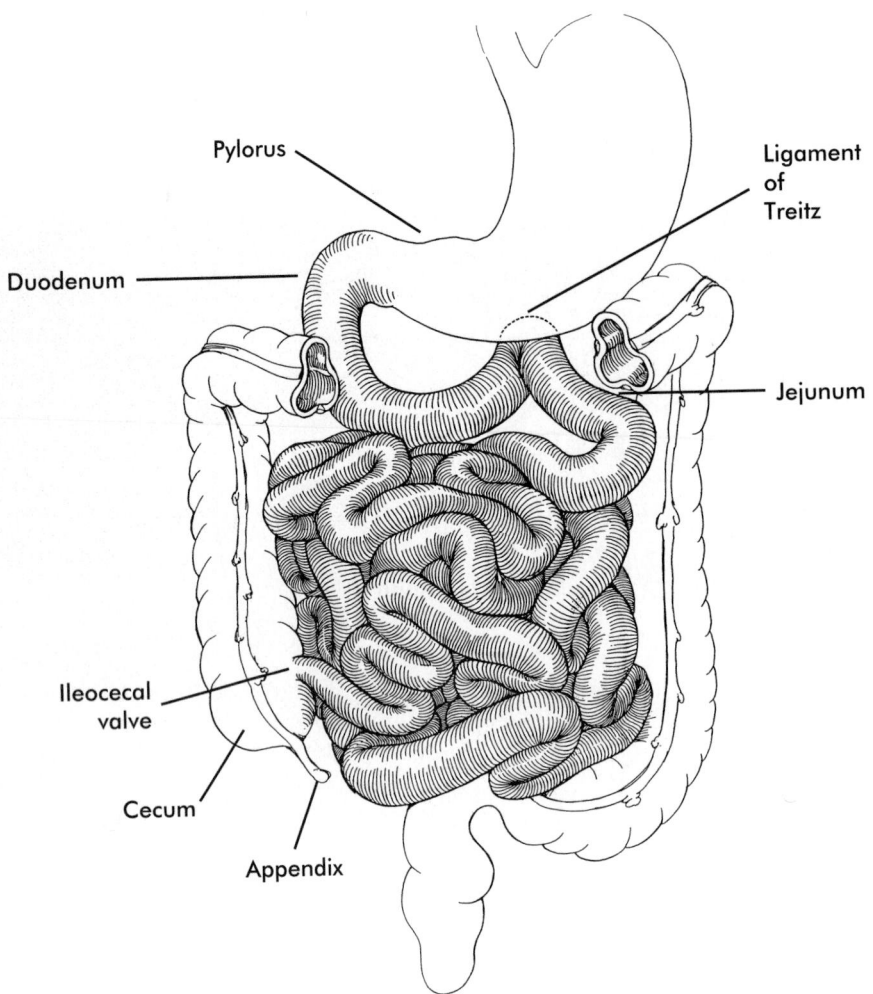

FIG. 10-7   Illustration of the small bowel; the duodenum originates at the pylorus and flexes at the ligament of Treitz where the jejunum begins. The jejunum extends into the ileum which terminates at the ileocecal valve at the cecum.

From Thompson, J.C. (1992). *Atlas of surgery of the stomach, duodenum, and small bowel*, St. Louis: Mosby.

because it always contains some gastric juice, which is acid in nature and produced by numerous tubular glands in the wall of the stomach.

Food enters the stomach by passing through the lower esophageal sphincter and leaves by passing through the pyloric sphincter. When food is in the stomach, the stomach becomes distended and the rugae, or folds, flatten out. Little absorption takes place in the stomach, and liquid enters the duodenum within 30 minutes after ingestion. Food is moved through the stomach and intestines by peristalsis, which consists of waves of motion caused by successive contractions of the muscles in the walls of the stomach and intestines.

Absorption of nutrients is a function of the small intestine. The large intestine absorbs water from the contents and expels the indigestible residue from the body. The res-

idue is composed primarily of cellulose from carbohydrates, connective tissue, and undigested fats. The act of defecation is accomplished by contraction of the rectal and abdominal muscles, the descent of the diaphragm, and the relaxation of the anal sphincter muscles.

The gastrointestinal tract is probably affected by psychologic factors at least as much as are other body systems. In our high-pressured society, people tend to overeat or undereat, and the pressures of everyday living frequently show their effects on the gastrointestinal tract. Although there is no conclusive evidence, some disease entities—for example, pylorospasm, peptic and duodenal ulcers, colitis, and obesity—seem to be exacerbated by psychologic factors. Some of these diseases can be treated medically; others require adjunctive psychotherapy. All of them necessitate diagnostic studies, and many require surgery.

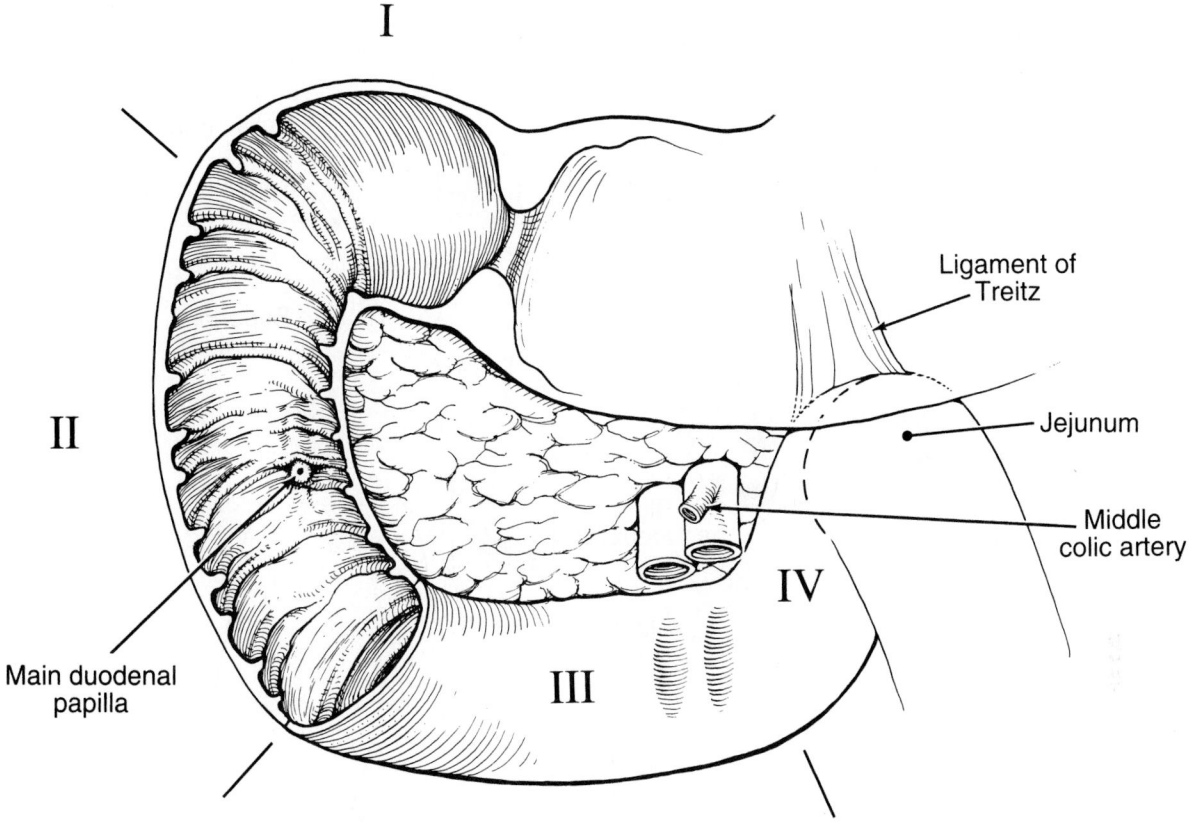

FIG. 10-8 The duodenum consists of four portions as illustrated.
From Thompson, J.C. (1992). *Atlas of surgery of the stomach, duodenum, and small bowel*, St. Louis: Mosby.

TYPES OF ABDOMINAL INCISIONS

VERTICAL MIDLINE INCISION

The vertical midline is the simplest abdominal incision to perform. It is an excellent primary incision and generally preferred because it offers good exposure to any part of the abdominal cavity. With this incision hemostasis is easily achieved, and fewer layers are traversed. The incision can be extended from just below the sternal notch, distally around the umbilicus (which is avascular, tough connective tissue), back to the midline, and down to the symphysis pubis (Fig. 10-14). The peritoneum is incised, and the round ligament of the liver may be divided.

To close the wound, the peritoneum and posterior fascia are usually sutured as a single layer. Sometimes the suture line is supported by using retention sutures, which extend through most or all layers of the wound. Anterior fascia, subcutaneous tissue, and skin are closed as layers. An alternative closure uses figure-of-eight, monofilament, nonabsorbable sutures, for one-layer closure of peritoneum and fascia.

OBLIQUE INCISIONS

McBurney muscle-splitting incision

The McBurney muscle-splitting incision is used for removal of the appendix. It is an 8-cm oblique incision that begins well below the umbilicus, goes through McBurney's point, and extends upward toward the right flank (Fig. 10-14). The external oblique muscle and fascia are split in the direction of their fibers and are retracted. The internal oblique muscle, transversalis muscle, and fascia are split and retracted. The peritoneum is incised transversely. This incision is quick and easy to close and allows a firm wound closure. However, it does not permit good exposure and is difficult to extend. To extend the incision medially, the inferior epigastric vessels are ligated, and the rectus sheath is incised transversely.

Subcostal incision

The subcostal incision is usually made on the right side and may be used for operations on the gallbladder, common duct, or pancreas. When made on the left side, it is

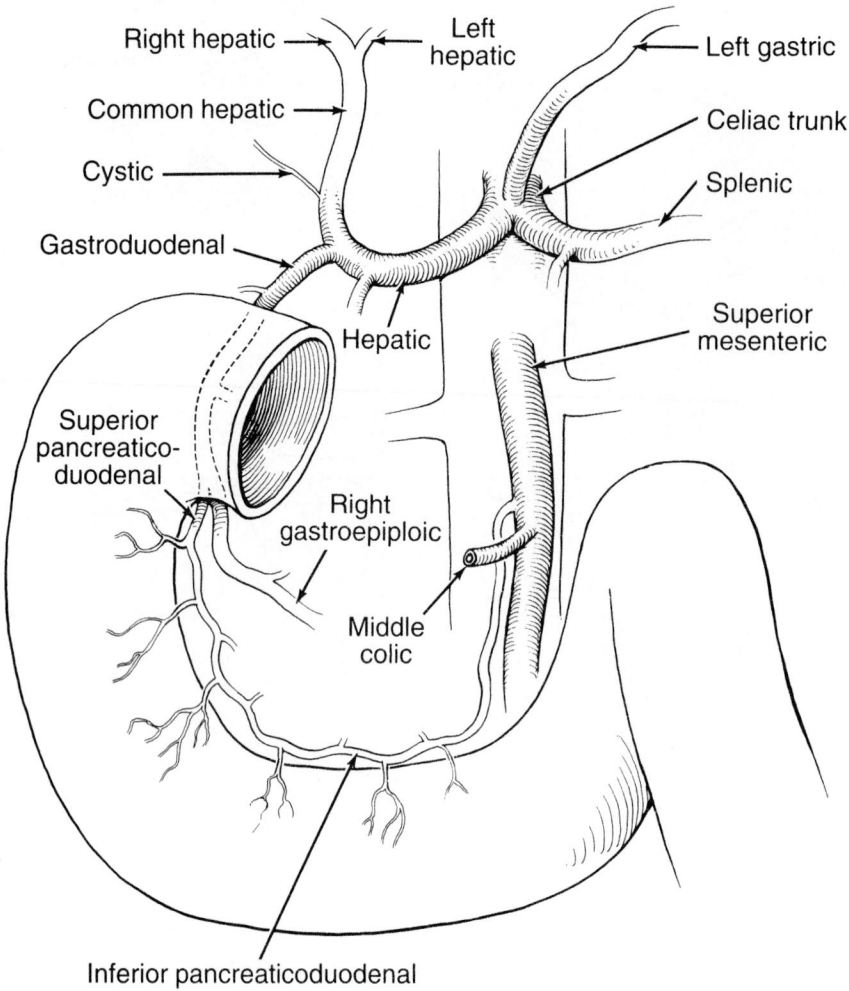

FIG. 10-9 Blood supply of the duodenum.

From Thompson, J.C. (1992). *Atlas of surgery of the stomach, duodenum, and small bowel,* St. Louis: Mosby.

used for splenectomy. This incision usually gives only limited exposure unless the patient is short with a wide abdomen and wide costal margins. The advantages of this type of incision are that it provides good cosmetic results because it follows the skin lines and the nerve damage is limited because only one or two nerves are cut, most commonly the eighth intercostal nerve. Also, tension on the incisional edges is less than in a vertical incision, it can readily be extended for wide exposure, and it causes less respiratory impairment.

This oblique incision begins in the epigastrium, extending laterally and obliquely downward to just below the lower costal margin (Fig. 10-15). Each muscle contains and arteries requiring ligation. If more exposure is needed, the incision is extended across the rectus muscle of the other side. The rectus muscle is either retracted or transversely divided. Vessels in the muscle must be ligated.

The closure of this incision includes approximation and closure of the falciform ligament, peritoneum, posterior rectus sheath, and anterior rectus sheath with interrupted, nonabsorbable sutures. The subcutaneous tissue and skin are closed as described for a vertical midline incision. Absorbable sutures may be used in conjunction with staples.

TRANSVERSE INCISIONS
Pfannestiel incision

The Pfannestiel incision is used frequently for pelvic surgery. It is a curved transverse incision across the lower abdomen through the skin, subcutaneous tissue, and rectus sheaths (Fig. 10-16). This incision is made approximately ½ inch above the symphysis pubis. The rectus muscles are separated in the midline, and the peritoneum is entered through a midline vertical incision. This incision provides

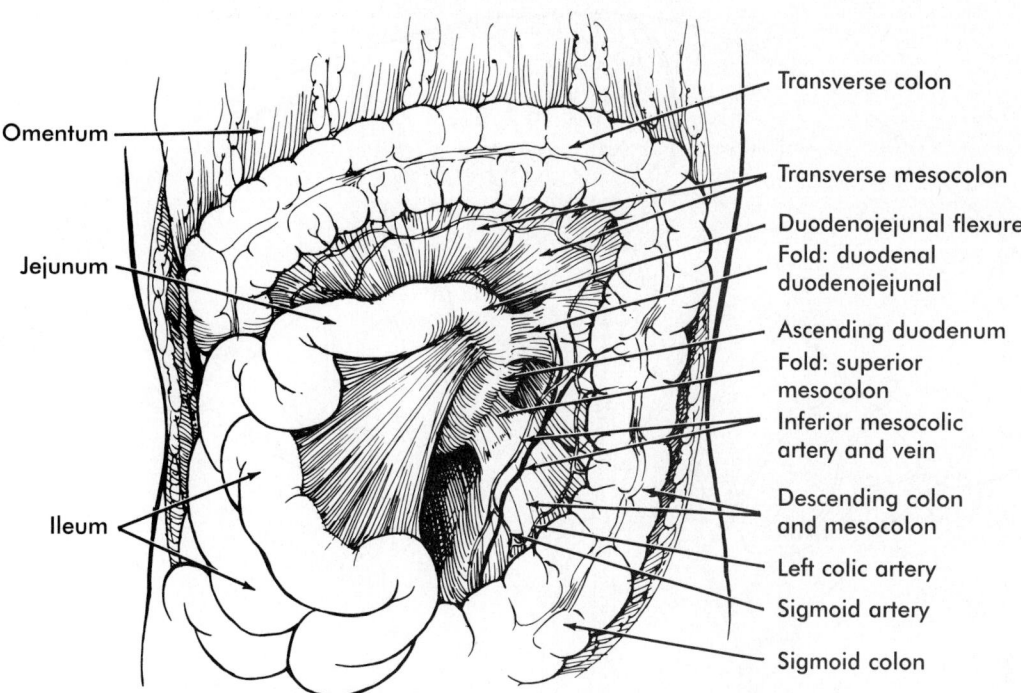

Omentum

Jejunum

Ileum

Transverse colon

Transverse mesocolon

Duodenojejunal flexure
Fold: duodenal
duodenojejunal

Ascending duodenum
Fold: superior
mesocolon

Inferior mesocolic
artery and vein

Descending colon
and mesocolon

Left colic artery

Sigmoid artery

Sigmoid colon

FIG. 10-10   Mesentery, as seen when intestine is pulled aside.

for a strong closure; when the rectus muscles contract, there is less strain on the fascial sutures.

Midabdominal transverse incision

The midabdominal transverse incision is used on the left or right side or for a retroperitoneal approach. The incision begins slightly above or below the umbilicus on either side and is carried laterally to the lumbar region at an angle between the ribs and crest of the ilium. The skin and subcutaneous tissue are incised, the anterior rectus sheath is split, the rectus muscle is divided, and the vessels within the rectus are clamped and ligated. The posterior rectus sheath and peritoneum are cut in the direction of the fibers, preserving the intercostal nerves. The peritoneum is incised near the midline, and the incision is extended laterally to the oblique muscle. The lateral muscles are incised to provide wide exposure. The closure is in layers with interrupted sutures; the subcutaneous tissue and skin are closed as for laparotomy (see pp. 278-279). The rectus muscle usually cannot be closed because its fibers run vertically. Approximation of the rectus sheath brings the edges of the rectus muscle into excellent apposition, thus eliminating the need to suture the muscle itself.

Thoracoabdominal incision

The thoracoabdominal incision is used for operations on the proximal portion of the stomach and the distal section of the esophagus. Often the abdominal part of the incision is made first for exploration and then if necessary is extended across the costal margin into the chest.

The incision begins at a point midway between the xiphoid process and the umbilicus and extends across to the seventh or eighth interspace and to the midscapular line. The rectus and oblique abdominal muscles are divided in the line of the incision down to the peritoneum and pleura. The costal cartilage and the diaphragm are then divided (Fig. 10-17).

The wound is closed in layers with interrupted sutures. Absorbable sutures may be used for the peritoneum and intercostal muscles. Nonabsorbable suture may be used for the muscle and fascial layers. Skin edges are approximated with staples or a nonabsorbable suture.

Upper inverted U abdominal incision

An upper inverted U abdominal incision is seldom used today; however, it can be used for gastrectomy, transverse colon resection, transverse colostomy, and biliary and pancreatic procedures. The incision extends from a point below the costal margin on one side in the anterior axillary line to the same point on the opposite side. It is curved, with the midpoint lying midway between the xiphoid process and the umbilicus. The intercostal nerves are preserved.

An upper abdominal transverse incision is closed by placing interrupted sutures in the peritoneum and anterior and posterior rectus sheaths. The muscle and fat need not

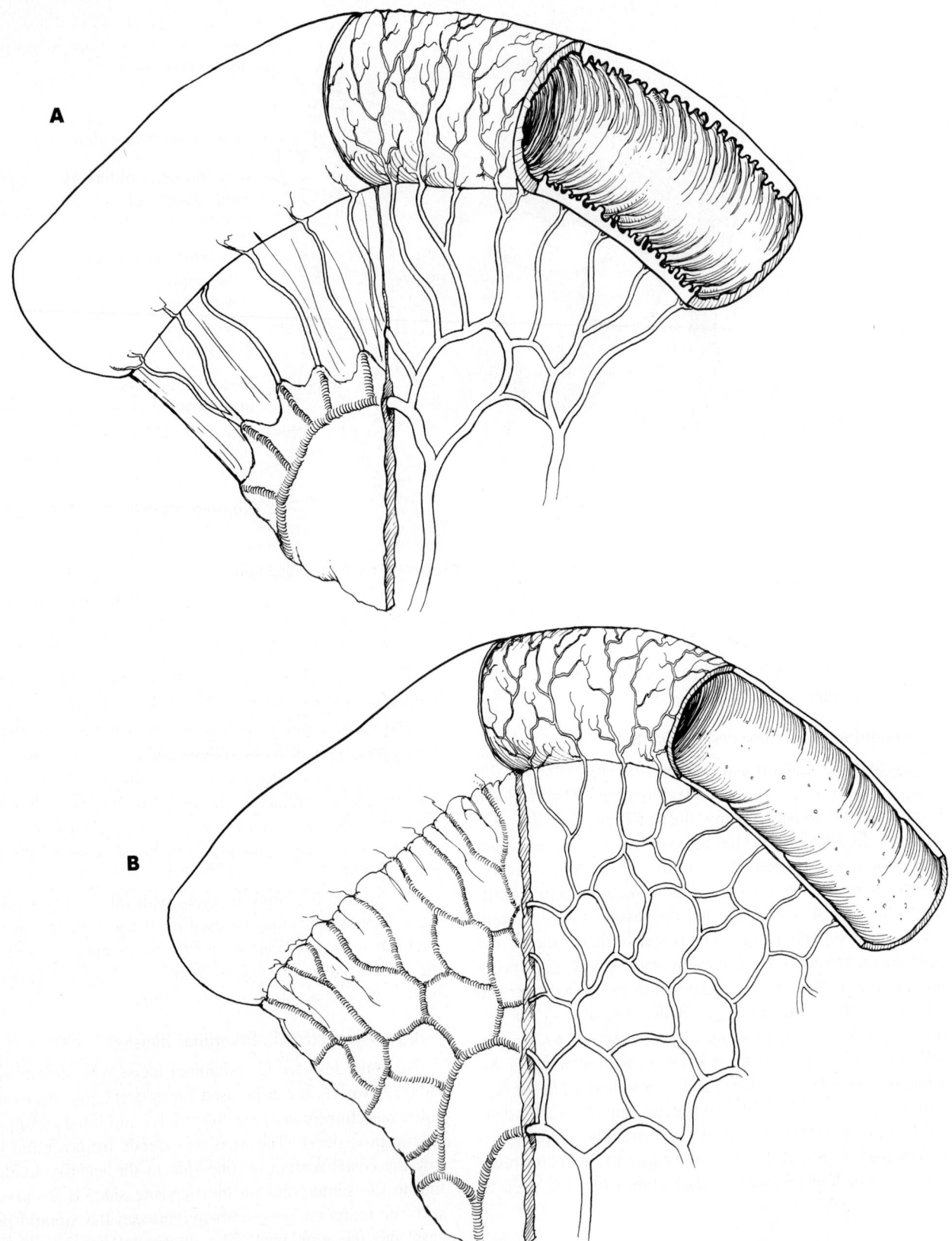

FIG. 10-11   Comparison of jejunum to ileum. **A,** Jejunum has larger circumference, thick mucosa, and one or two vascular arcades. **B,** Ileum has smaller circumference, thin mucosa, and multiple vascular arcades.

From Thompson, J.C. (1992). *Atlas of surgery of the stomach, duodenum, and small bowel,* St. Louis: Mosby.

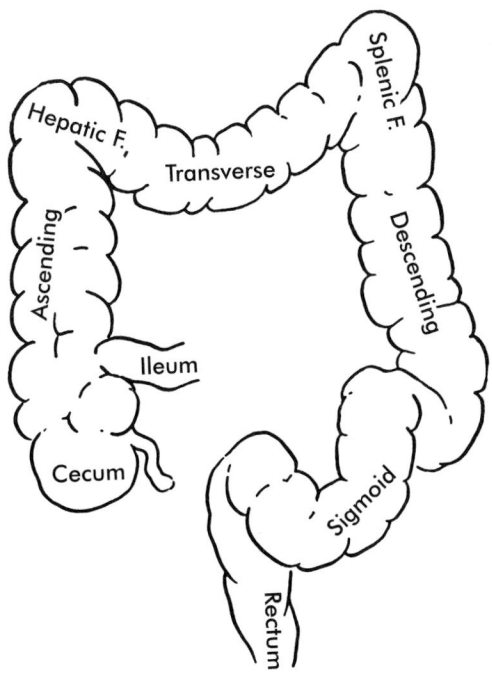

FIG. 10-12 Anatomic division of large intestine, showing placement of ileocecal valve, hepatic flexure, and splenic flexure.

be sutured. The skin edges are approximated and closed using the suture material or mechanical staple applier according to surgeon's preference.

PERIOPERATIVE NURSING CONSIDERATIONS

ASSESSMENT

Nursing care for patients undergoing gastrointestinal surgery begins with assessment. Individualized care, integrating physiologic with psychologic preparation, is afforded each patient. Patients undergoing gastrointestinal surgery should understand why they need preoperative preparation, what the intended surgical intervention will be, and how it will affect them postoperatively. A preoperative nursing assessment of the patient is essential for appropriate planning and implementation of intraoperative nursing care and evaluation of patient outcomes. The nurse should ensure that the patient understands the nature of the surgery and the site of the incision. Turning, coughing, and deep breathing are taught preoperatively and reinforced after surgery. If an ostomy is anticipated, an enterostomal nurse specialist should be consulted to prepare the patient for the realization of an abdominal stoma. The enterostomal specialist can also assist in allaying fears and anxieties for the patient and the family. The patient's abdomen can be marked preoperatively, indicating the most optimal placement for the abdominal stoma.

The nursing assessment of the patient having gastrointestinal disease should include the following information:

> Demographic data
> Present problems/chief
>   complaint/symptoms
>   which lead the patient
>   to seek medical atten-
>   tion (Box 10-1)
> Medical history
> Family history
>   Personal and social history

Examination of the patient's abdomen should include inspection, palpation, and auscultation of bowel sounds.

Pertinent serum studies related to the patient with gastrointestinal disease might include complete blood count (CBC) with differential, serum electrolytes, platelet count, serum osmolality, cholesterol level, vitamin and mineral levels, serum enzymes, bilirubin metabolism, serum proteins, and pancreatic function studies (Table 10-1). Laboratory indices of nutritional status may also be relevant for patients with gastrointestinal disease (Table 10-2).

Carcinoembryonic antigen (CEA) is a serum tumor marker that has been found to be a valuable monitoring tool for patients having a history of colon or rectal cancer. CEA is a glycoprotein found in the cell membranes of many tissues, including tumors of the gastrointestinal tract. It is not used as a screening tool because patients with primary colon or rectal cancer may have normal CEA levels. The normal range is 0 to 5 ng/ml. A baseline CEA is usually obtained on patients diagnosed with cancer of the colon or rectum so that their levels can be closely followed after surgery. Any rise in the patient's CEA level following resection of the primary tumor is cause for concern and will be closely monitored. When a definite pattern of elevation is established, the patient will be advised to undergo an aggressive regimen of diagnostics to detect possible metastasis. CEA-directed second-look laparotomy may be indicated even if scans are negative. This procedure is reviewed later in this chapter (pp. 314, 317).

NURSING DIAGNOSIS

The value of nursing care plans has been well documented in the literature. Perioperative nurses are challenged to diagnose, plan, implement, and evaluate care in a very short time. They must have the ability to prioritize patient needs and act accordingly. The first step in this process, patient assessment, leads to the formulation of nursing diagnoses and identification of desired outcomes and is essential to all other steps. Nursing diagnoses related to the care of patients undergoing gastrointestinal surgery might include the following:

- Anxiety related to fear of the unknown
- Body image disturbance related to potential postoperative ostomy

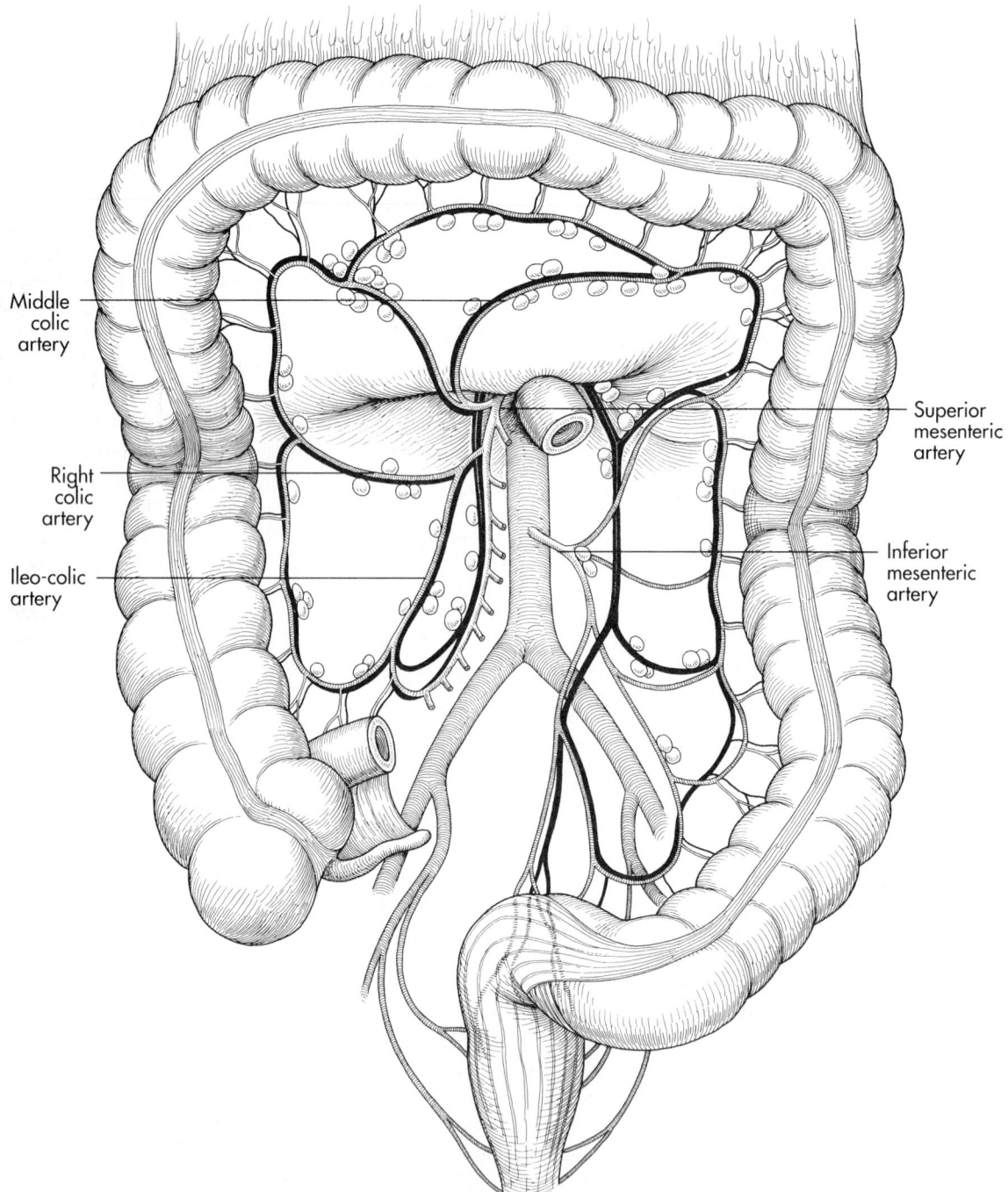

Middle
colic
artery

Right
colic
artery

Ileo-colic
artery

Superior
mesenteric
artery

Inferior
mesenteric
artery

FIG. 10-13   Blood supply of the colon.

From Bauer, J.J. (1993). *Colorectal surgery illustrated*, St. Louis: Mosby.

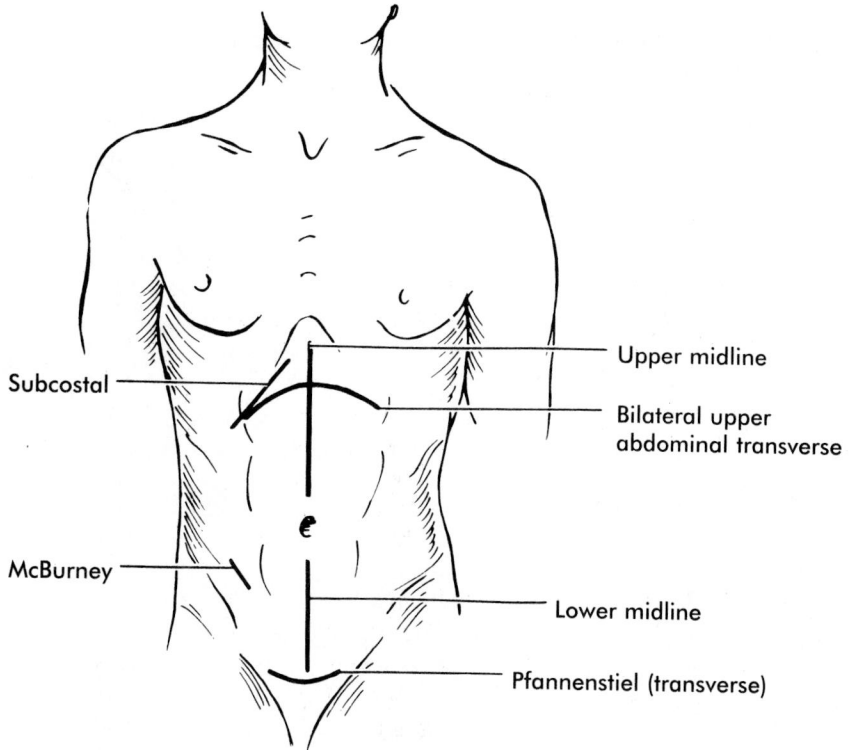

Subcostal

Upper midline

Bilateral upper
abdominal transverse

McBurney

Lower midline

Pfannenstiel (transverse)

FIG. 10-14   Incisions made through the abdominal wall.

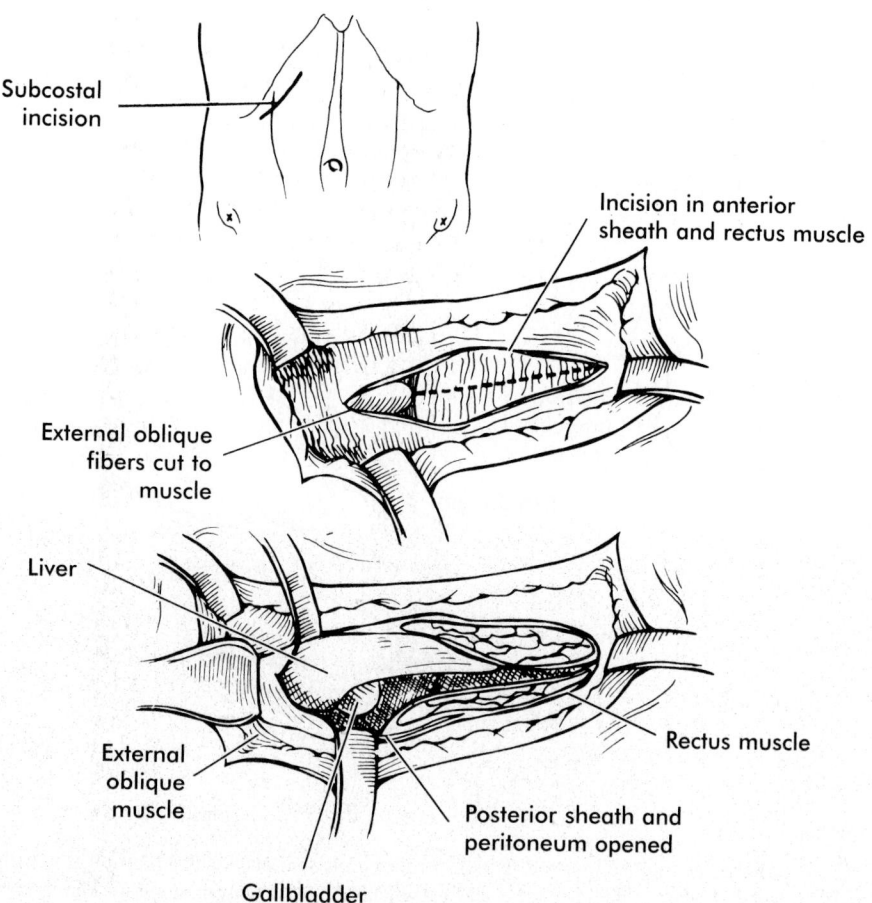

Subcostal
incision

Incision in anterior
sheath and rectus muscle

External oblique
fibers cut to
muscle

Liver

Rectus muscle

External
oblique
muscle

Posterior sheath and
peritoneum opened

Gallbladder

FIG. 10-15   Subcostal incision in upper right quadrant. Anterior sheath has been divided transversely, and muscle is exposed. Posterior sheath and peritoneum have been opened transversely.

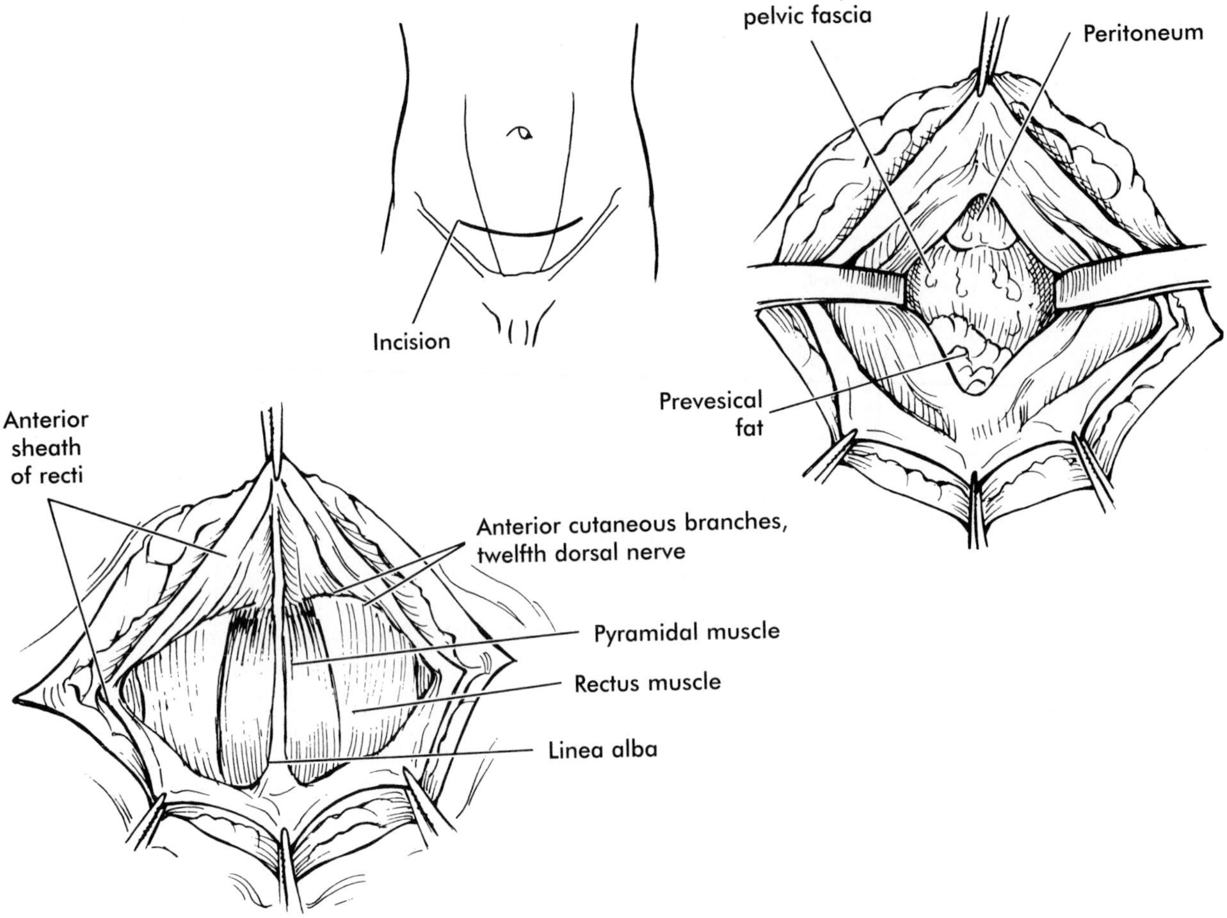

Incision

Vesical layer,
pelvic fascia

Peritoneum

Prevesical
fat

Anterior
sheath
of recti

Anterior cutaneous branches,
twelfth dorsal nerve

Pyramidal muscle

Rectus muscle

Linea alba

FIG. 10-16   Pfannenstiel incision (transverse).

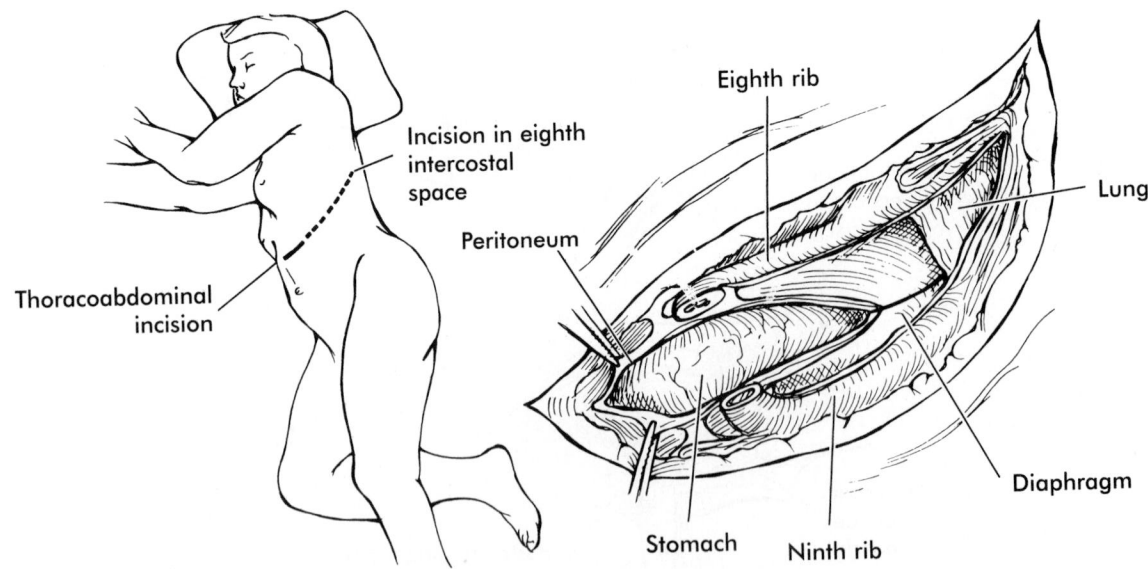

Eighth rib

Incision in eighth
intercostal
space

Peritoneum

Lung

Thoracoabdominal
incision

Stomach

Ninth rib

Diaphragm

FIG. 10-17   Thoracoabdominal incision. Patient is placed on unaffected side. Incision is usually made from point midway between xiphoid process and umbilicus to costal margin at site of eighth costal cartilage. Dissection is carried down to peritoneum and pleura. Costal cartilage and diaphragm are divided, and stomach is exposed.

BOX 10-1

Assessment Data

GENERAL DATA

Usual height and weight

Nutrient intake:

    Types of food usually eaten at each meal or snack

    Food likes and dislikes

    Religious or medical food restrictions

    Food intolerances

    Patient's perception and concerns pertaining to diet and weight

    Effects of life-style on diet, weight gain or loss

    Vitamins and nutritional supplements used

Oral hygiene

Bowel elimination patterns

Use of medications/laxatives

    Stool softeners

    Antiemetics

    Antidiarrheals

    Antacids

    Frequent or high doses of aspirin, acetaminophen, or ibuprofen

SPECIFIC DATA

Oral lesions

Appetite

Digestion or indigestion

Dysphagia

Nausea

Vomiting

Hematemesis

Change in stool

    Color (clay color, black)

    Contents (undigested food, blood, mucus)

Constipation

Diarrhea

Flatulence

Hemorrhoids

Abdominal pain

Hepatitis

Jaundice

Ulcers

Gallstones

Polys

Tumors

Anal discomfort

Fecal incontinence

Exposure to infectious disease

- High risk for fluid volume deficit related to loss of blood and electrolyte-rich gastric and intestinal juices
- High risk for infection related to invasive gastrointestinal procedures
- Hypothermia related to room temperature, skin exposure, and an open wound

OUTCOME IDENTIFICATION

Outcomes identified for the selected nursing diagnoses could be stated as the following:

- The patient will verbalize knowledge of the perioperative experience.
- The patient demonstrates knowledge of the ostomy and a desire to perform self-care.
- The patient's fluid and electrolyte balance is maintained.
- The patient will demonstrate no clinical signs of wound infection.
- The patient will be free from injury related to heat loss.

PLANNING

Preoperative assessment enables the perioperative nurse to plan for the specific needs of the individual patient. For example, the size of the patient influences positioning during surgery and may necessitate additional instruments, such as deeper retractors and longer forceps and scissors. The perioperative nurse has to provide the patient with reassurance and emotional support for effective management of anxiety. The perioperative nurse must also understand the potential for altered body image with some gastrointestinal procedures.

Once the nursing diagnosis is made, desired outcomes are identified and the care plan is developed to assist the patient to meet the outcomes. The care plan is an essential component in ensuring high-quality perioperative nursing care. A typical care plan for a patient undergoing gastrointestinal surgery follows.

TABLE 10-1

Common Nonspecific Serum Studies

Test name	Normal values
COMPLETE BLOOD COUNT WITH DIFFERENTIAL COUNT (CBC AND DIFF)	
Red blood cell count (RBC)	Men: 4.7-6.1 million/mm^3 Women: 4.2-5.4 million/mm^3 Low values indicate anemia resulting from blood loss, hemolysis, dietary deficiency, drug ingestion, bone marrow failure, or chronic illness; high values may indicate compensation for high altitudes, chronic anoxia, or polycythemia vera
Hemoglobin (Hb) concentration	Men: 14-18 g/dl Women: 12-16 g/dl Low and high values tend to be caused by the same processes that cause low or high values for RBC; dehydration causes an artificially high value
Hematocrit (Hct)	Men: 42%-52% Women: 37%-47% Low and high values tend to be caused by the same processes that cause low or high RBC and Hb values
Mean corpuscular volume (MCV)	Adults: 80-95/μm^3 High values may be seen in megaloblastic anemias (e.g., vitamin B$_{12}$ deficiency); low values may be seen with iron-deficiency anemia or thalassemia
Mean corpuscular hemoglobin (MCH)	Adults: 27-31 pg Low and high values tend to be caused by the same processes that cause low or high values for MCV
Mean corpuscular hemoglobin concentration (MCHC)	Adults: 32-36 g/dl Low values indicate hemoglobin deficiency and are seen in iron-deficiency anemia and thalassemia
White blood cell count (WBC)	Adults: 5000-10,000/mm^3
Differential	Neutrophils: 55%-70% Lymphocytes: 20%-40% Monocytes: 2%-8% Eosinophils: 1%-4% Basophils: 0.5%-1% Elevated WBC commonly indicates infection or leukemia; decreased WBC may indicate bone marrow failure, overwhelming infection, dietary deficiency, or autoimmune disease; elevated neutrophil count may be seen in acute suppurative infection; decreased neutrophil count may be seen with overwhelming bacterial infection (especially in the elderly) or dietary deficiency; elevated lymphocyte count may be seen with chronic bacterial infection or viral infection; decreased lymphocyte count may be seen with sepsis; elevated eosinophil count may be seen with parasitic infestation, allergic reactions, or autoimmune diseases; a "shift to the left" means there is an increased percentage of neutrophils and immature leukocytes, which occurs with infection
Platelet count	150,000-400,000/mm^3 Reduced levels of platelets may result from decreased platelet production, increased sequestration (as is seen in hypersplenism), increased platelet destruction or consumption (e.g., disseminated intravascular coagulation), or loss of platelets through hemorrhage Elevated levels may be seen with severe hemorrhage, polycythemia vera, postsplenectomy syndromes, and some malignant disorders

TABLE 10-1

Common Nonspecific Serum Studies—cont'd

Test name	Normal values
SERUM ELECTROLYTES	
Sodium (Na)	136-145 mEq/L
	Elevated levels may be seen with excessive sweating, extensive burns, osmotic diuresis, and excessive sodium intake or reduced sodium excretion; reduced levels may be seen with inadequate sodium intake, increased sodium losses (e.g., vomiting, nasogastric suction, diarrhea), renal disease, or third-space losses of sodium)
Potassium (K)	3.5-5 mEq/L
	Elevated levels may be seen with excessive intake or reduced excretion of potassium (e.g., renal failure), crushing injuries causing release of intracellular potassium, or with metabolic acidosis; reduced levels may be seen with inadequate intake or excessive losses (e.g., diarrhea, vomiting, use of diuretics, hyperaldosteronism) or as a result of metabolic alkalosis or administration of glucose, insulin, or calcium (which causes a shift of potassium from the bloodstream into cells)
Chloride (Cl)	90-110 mEq/L
	Changes in chloride concentration usually parallel changes in sodium concentration
Carbon dioxide (CO_2)	23-30 mEq/L
	Elevated levels are seen with acidosis; reduced levels are seen with alkalosis
BLOOD GAS STUDIES (ARTERIAL)	
pH	7.35-7.45
	High levels indicate alkalosis; low levels reflect acidosis
Partial pressure of carbon dioxide (P_{CO_2})	34-45 mm Hg
	High levels indicate carbon dioxide retention due to respiratory depression or pulmonary disease (respiratory acidosis); low levels reflect excessive loss of carbon dioxide through hyperventilation (e.g., respiratory alkalosis due to overventilation or emotional trauma; may also be seen as compensatory response in metabolic acidosis)
Bicarbonate (HCO_3^-)	22-26 mEq/L
	Low levels indicate metabolic acidosis due to excessive acid production, resulting in depletion of HCO_3^- (e.g., diabetic acidosis); failure to eliminate H^+ ions, resulting in depletion of HCO_3^- (e.g., renal failure); or excessive loss of HCO_3^- (e.g., intestinal losses through diarrhea or fistula drainage); low levels may also be seen with insulin overdose, insulinoma, hypothyroidism, hypopituitarism, Addison's disease, and extensive liver disease
	High levels indicate metabolic alkalosis resulting from bicarbonate overdose or excessive gastric losses; may also be seen as a compensatory response in a patient with prolonged respiratory acidosis; pancreatic disorders (e.g., adenoma, pancreatitis), corticosteroid therapy, diuretics, Cushing's disease, and hyperthryoidism

From Doughty, D.B., & Jackson, D.B.: *Gastrointestinal disorders.* 1993, St. Louis: Mosby, pp. 65-66.

TABLE 10-2

Laboratory Indices of Nutritional Status

Test name	Normal values
Albumin (serum)	3.5-5.5 mg/dl Decreased levels are seen in protein malnutrition and with hepatocellular injury.
Transferring (serum)	250-300 mg/dl Decreased levels are seen in protein malnutrition; transferring levels may be used to monitor a patient's response to nutritional support therapy, because transferrin's half-life is 8 to 10 days, whereas albumin's half-life is 19 to 20 days (this means that transferrin levels reflect changes in the patient's visceral protein status much faster than do albumin levels).
Prealbumin (serum)	15-32 mg/dl Decreased levels are seen in protein malnutrition; because the half-life of prealbumin is 2 to 3 days, these values reflect changes in the patient's visceral protein status even faster than transferrin levels.
Total lymphocyte count (serum)	$>150,000/mm^3$ Decreased levels may be seen in protein malnutrition; however, many other conditions affect the total lymphocyte count (e.g., infection or conditions affecting WBC production).
24-hour urine for urea nitrogen (UUN)	Reflects renal excretion of nitrogen; used to determine nitrogen balance, which should be positive Formula: $$\frac{\text{24-hour nitrogen intake (g of protein)}}{6.25} - (\text{24 hours UUN} + 4) = \text{Balance}$$

From Doughty, D.B., & Jackson, D.B.: *Gastrointestinal disorders.* 1993, St. Louis: Mosby, p. 70.

IMPLEMENTATION

Preoperative mechanical preparation of the gastrointestinal tract is often employed for elective surgery, and often bactericidal and bacteriostatic agents are used in an attempt to eliminate pathogenic microorganisms, especially in the lower gastrointestinal tract. Many patients require nasogastric tubes. Fluid and electrolyte balance must be maintained before, during, and after surgery. Often an indwelling urinary catheter is inserted preoperatively or immediately after induction to monitor output and renal function during surgery and to keep the bladder empty, thereby allowing more space in the lower abdomen for the surgeon to perform the operation.

If required, hair removal from the proposed incisional site should be accomplished as close to the time of incision as possible, especially if removal is by shaving so there is no time for bacteria to grow in the disturbed hair follicle. A wet shave is performed to reduce the abrasion to the skin surface and prevent hair from becoming airborne and possibly contaminating the sterile fields. Hair should be removed according to the protocol for the type of surgery the patient is to have, as well as the surgeon's preference.

If the surgeon anticipates the need to replace blood, the patient's blood is typed and cross-matched before the operation. Preadmission arrangements may have been made for the availability of autotransfused blood or donor-directed units.

The circulating nurse should be well informed of what the procedure will entail and should ensure that all necessary supplies and equipment are on hand and that the integrity of the equipment is uncompromised. An electrosurgical unit and accessories may be used for the cutting and coagulation of tissue.

As in all surgery, careful consideration should be given to positioning the patient so that the surgeon can gain optimum exposure without compromising the respiratory, circulatory, and nervous systems and without producing undue pressure on any body part (see Chapter 4).

Suture materials used on gastrointestinal tissue have traditionally been chromic and silk. With the increased number of synthetic absorbable and nonabsorbable suture materials available, surgeons have a variety of materials from which to choose. Polyester fiber sutures and polyglycolic acid sutures are frequently employed on gastrointestinal tissue. Generally, 3-0 and 4-0 sutures are used on intestinal tissues. Checking the surgeon's preference card for appropriate suture materials not only ensures the availability of necessary supplies but also is a cost-effective measure.

Surgical stapling instruments have had a great impact on the technical aspects of gastrointestinal surgery. For some

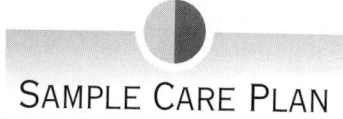

SAMPLE CARE PLAN

NURSING DIAGNOSIS: Anxiety related to fear of the unknown

OUTCOME: Patient will verbalize knowledge of the perioperative experience.

INTERVENTIONS:

Explain preoperative procedures that will facilitate the surgery, such as intravenous lines, skin preparation, bowel preparation.

Explain all procedures done in the OR prior to induction.

Explain postoperative drains, catheters, dressings.

Minimize stimuli in the OR.

Remain with the patient during induction.

Allow time for the patient to verbalize feelings and fears.

NURSING DIAGNOSIS: Body image disturbance related to potential postoperative ostomy

OUTCOME: Patient demonstrates knowledge of the ostomy and a desire to perform self-care.

INTERVENTIONS:

Participate in therapeutic communication during the preoperative visit; include family members if appropriate.

Be aware of nonverbal cues.

Refer patient to ostomy nurse.

Encourage patient participation in all aspects of care.

NURSING DIAGNOSIS: High risk for fluid volume deficit related to loss of blood and electrolyte-rich gastric and intestinal juices

OUTCOME: The patient's fluid and electrolyte balance is maintained.

INTERVENTIONS:

Obtain baseline data from the chart relating to fluid and electrolyte balance.

Assess nutritional status, skin turgor, or medications affecting fluid and electrolyte balance.

Periodically inform the surgical team of estimated blood loss.

Record all solutions being administered from the surgical field.

NURSING DIAGNOSIS: High risk for infection related to invasive gastrointestinal procedure

OUTCOME: Patient will demonstrate no clinical signs of wound infection.

INTERVENTIONS:

Check the integrity and expiration date of all sterile packages and containers.

Ensure aseptic technique is maintained; communicate and correct breaks in asepsis.

Contain contaminants appropriately.

NURSING DIAGNOSIS: Hypothermia related to room temperature, skin exposure, and an open wound

OUTCOME: Patient will be free from injury related to heat loss.

INTERVENTIONS:

Provide the patient with a warm blanket prior to induction.

Ensure that irrigating solutions are warm.

Keep room temperature at a level that provides for maintenance of body temperature.

Cover patient with a warm blanket prior to transport to postanesthesia care unit (PACU).

surgeons the use of these devices has to an extent replaced conventional suturing techniques. The stapling instruments can be employed to divide and ligate, resect and anastomose. The **B** design of the implanted staple does not compromise the vascularity of the resected tissue edges. These devices are available in reusable and disposable models. Personnel must be familiar with the types of available stapling equipment, applications, assembly if indicated, and proper loading (see Chapter 5).

Irrigating solution is frequently used during gastrointestinal procedures. The surgeon specifies the solution of choice, which frequently contains a broad-spectrum antibiotic. Normal saline, an isotonic solution, may be used to moisten laparotomy sponges and for irrigation. Moist packs are used to isolate open and diseased portions of the stomach and bowel from the abdominal cavity and to protect other viscera. Solutions should be warm when used for these purposes.

As in all operations, the excised specimen is handled carefully and prepared for examination by the pathologist. The surgeon usually determines how the specimen will be handled before examination. It may be sent to the pathology department fresh, in saline, or in a preservative solution. Tissue also may be sent for frozen-section examination to verify the pathologic condition and determine whether tissue margins are free from malignant cells.

To reduce tissue trauma, the jaws of heavy intestinal forceps may be protected by pieces of soft rubber tubing or other smooth material. These guards (shods) should fit the jaws firmly but not tightly and should extend slightly beyond the tips of forceps. Before sterilization the rubber shods must be separated from the forceps to facilitate and ensure steam penetration.

Whenever a portion of the gastrointestinal tract is entered, bowel technique must be performed. *Bowel technique* means that any instrument coming in contact with the gastrointestinal mucosa is used only on that mucosa, not any other tissue. These instruments are discarded in a separate basin and do not come in contact with other instruments.

For closure, some surgeons may desire a new set of instruments, additional draping materials, and a change of gown and gloves.

Instruments used during gastrointestinal surgery should include a basic laparotomy set combined with instruments specifically designed for use with gastrointestinal tissue. The basic laparotomy set may include the following instruments.

Cutting instruments
(Fig. 10-18)

3 Knife handles: two no. 3 handles with blade no. 10; one no. 7 with blade no. 15
1 Mayo scissors, straight, 6¼ inches
1 Mayo scissors, curved, 6¼ inches
1 Metzenbaum scissors, 7 inches
1 Suture scissors

Holding instruments
(Fig. 10-19)

2 Debakey forceps, 8 inches
2 Tissue forceps without teeth, 5½ inches
2 Tissue forceps with teeth, 5½ inches
2 Tissue forceps without teeth, 7 and 10 inches
2 Tissue forceps with teeth, 7 and 10 inches
2 Russian tissue forceps, 7 and 10 inches
2 Adson forceps with teeth
4 Sponge-holding forceps, 10 inches
6 Towel clamps, 3½ or 5½ inches
4 Allis forceps, 6 and 9 inches
4 Babcock intestinal forceps, 6 inches

Clamping instruments
(Fig. 10-20)

10 Crile forceps, straight or curved, 5½ inches
10 Rochester-Pean forceps, curved, 6¼ inches
8 Rochester-Pean forceps, curved, 10 inches
4 Ochsner or Kocher forceps, straight, 6¼ inches
4 Ochsner or Kocher forceps, straight, 9 inches

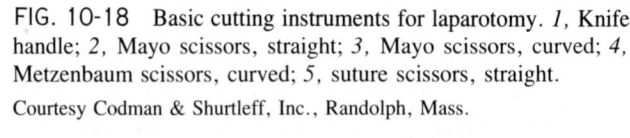

FIG. 10-18 Basic cutting instruments for laparotomy. *1,* Knife handle; *2,* Mayo scissors, straight; *3,* Mayo scissors, curved; *4,* Metzenbaum scissors, curved; *5,* suture scissors, straight.

Courtesy Codman & Shurtleff, Inc., Randolph, Mass.

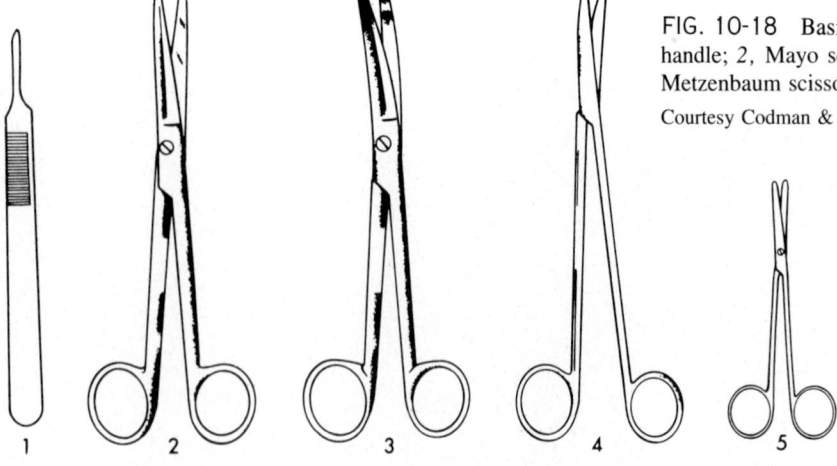

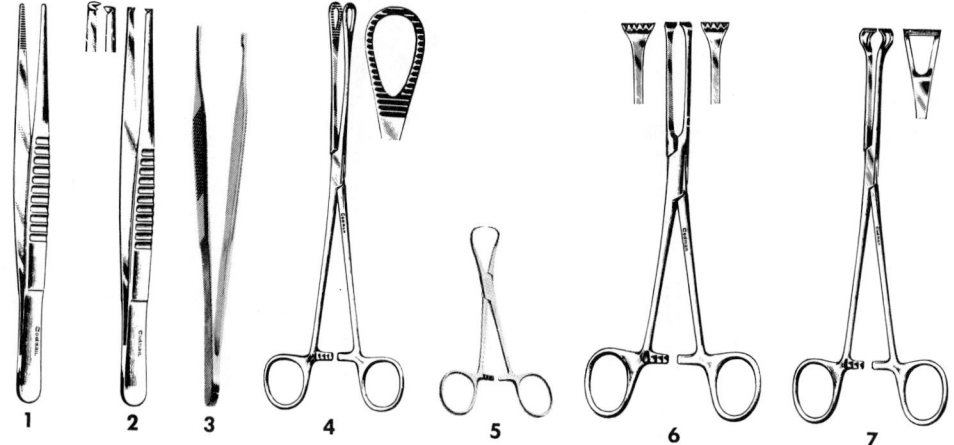

FIG. 10-19 Basic holding instruments for laparotomy. *1,* Tissue forceps, smooth; *2,* tissue forceps with teeth; *3,* Adson tissue forceps; *4,* sponge-holding forceps; *5,* towel clamps; *6,* Allis forceps; *7,* Babcock intestinal forceps.

Courtesy Codman & Shurtleff, Inc., Randolph, Mass.

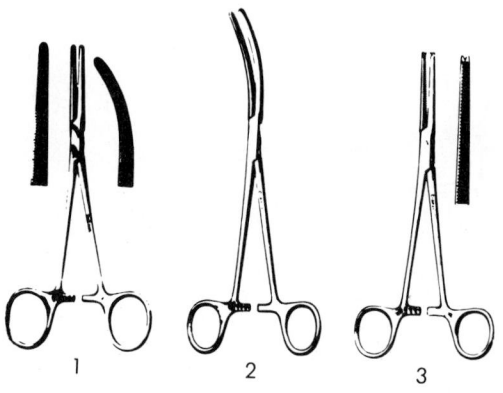

FIG. 10-20 Basic clamping instruments for laparotomy. *1,* Crile hemostatic forceps; *2,* Rochester-Pean hemostatic forceps; *3,* Ochsner or Kocher hemostatic forceps.

Courtesy Codman & Shurtleff, Inc., Randolph, Mass.

Exposing instruments
(Fig. 10-21)

2 Malleable retractors,
   1- to ½-inch width
2 Vein retractors, small
2 Parker, Roux,
   Greene, or Army-
   Navy retractors
6 Richardson or Kelly
   retractors, small, me-
   dium, and large
4 Rake retractors, four-
   and six-pronged
   pairs, dull

3 Deaver retractors,
   small, medium, and
   large
1 Weitlaner retractor
1 Balfour self-retaining
   retractor with blades
1 Bookwalter or Omni-
   tract retractor system
   (see Fig. 11-7).

Suturing instruments

6 Needle holders, 6 and
   8 inches
2 Skin hooks (optional)

Accessory items
(Fig. 10-22)

1 Frazier suction tip
1 Poole (sump) suction
   tube and tubing

2 Yankauer suction
   tubes and tubing
1 Silver probe
1 Grooved director

The gastrointestinal set may include the following instruments.

Cutting instruments

1 Metzenbaum scissors,
   9 inches
2 Metzenbaum scissors,
   5¾ inches, 1 straight
   and 1 curved

2 Mayo scissors, 9
   inches, 1 straight and
   1 curved

Clamping instruments
(Fig. 10-23)

1 Best colon clamp
4 Allen intestinal anas-
   tomosis clamps
4 Rochester-Carmalt
   forceps, straight, 8
   inches
4 Doyen intestinal for-
   ceps, longitudinal
   serrations, 9 inches, 2
   straight and 2 curved
2 Mayo vessel clamps,
   angled, 9 inches

2 Mayo-Robson intesti-
   nal forceps, straight
2 Dennis intestinal
   clamps
6 Ochsner forceps, 6¼
   inches
6 Ochsner forceps, 9
   inches
1 Pace-Potts clamp
4 Gallbladder forceps,
   right-angled, assorted
   sizes

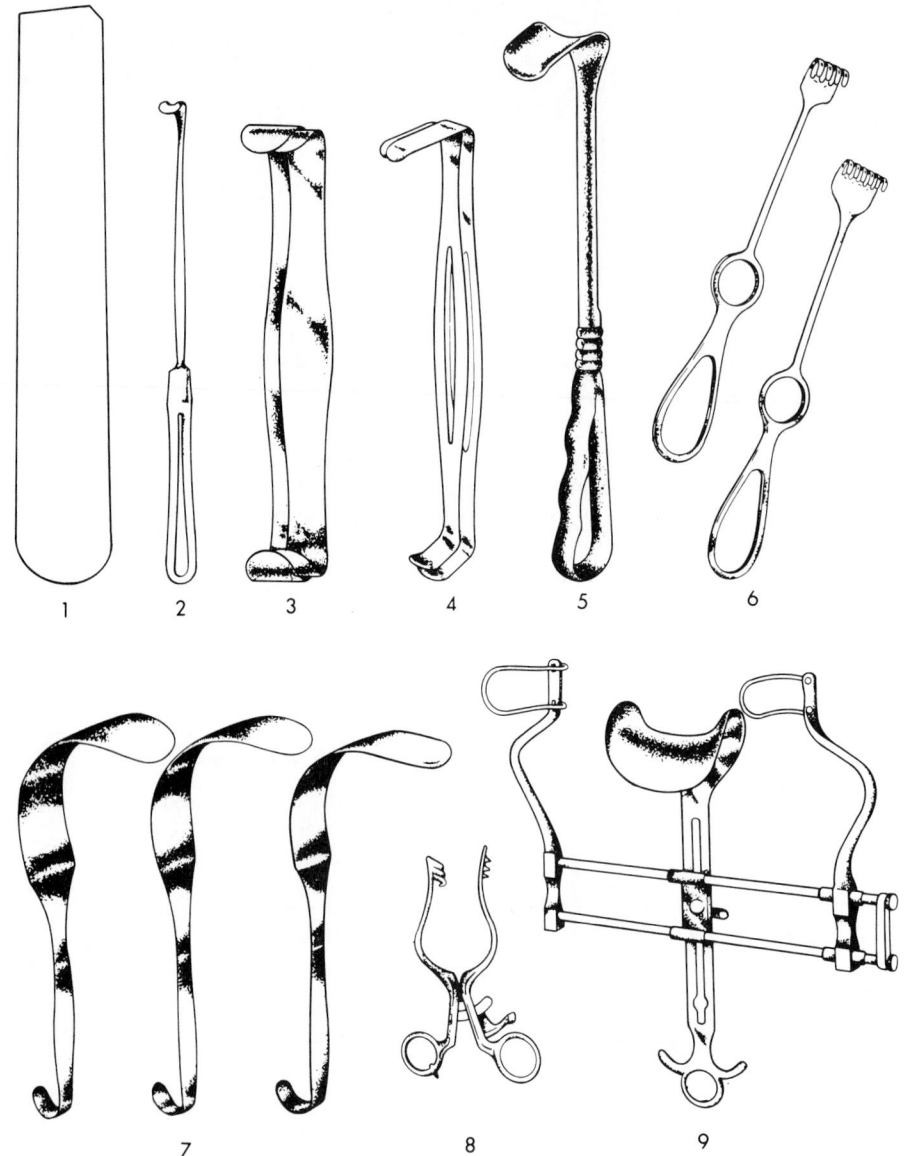

FIG. 10-21   Basic exposing instruments for laparotomy. *1*, Malleable copper retractor; *2*, vein retractor; *3*, Parker retractors; *4*, Army-Navy retractors; *5*, Richardson retractor; *6*, Volkmann rake retractors; *7*, Deaver retractors; *8*, Weitlaner retractor; *9*, Balfour self-retaining retractor with blades.

Courtesy Codman & Shurtleff, Inc., Randolph, Mass.

Clamping
instruments—cont'd

4 Rochester-Pean forceps, curved, 8 inches

10 Rochester-Pean forceps, curved, 6¼ inches

10 Crile hemostats, curved, 5½ inches

36 Halsted mosquito hemostats, 5 inches, 24 curved and 12 straight

Holding instruments

2 Debakey forceps, 8 inches

2 Tissue forceps without teeth, 5½ inches

2 Fixation or Adson forceps, 5 inches

2 Potts-Smith dressing forceps, 8 inches

6 Babcock intestinal forceps, 6¼ inches

6 Allis forceps, 6¼ inches

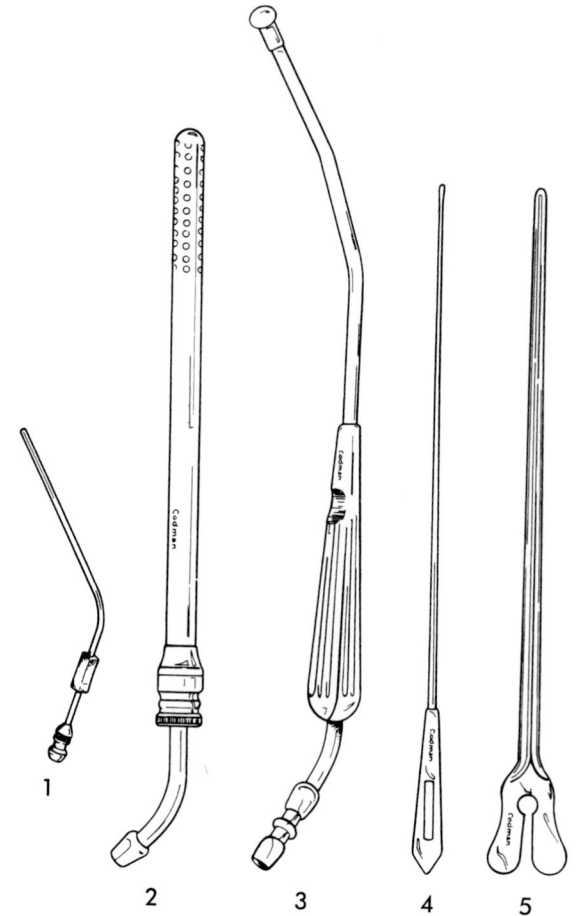

Exposing instruments

1 Doyen retractor, large blade, 2¼ inches wide × 3½ inches deep
2 Kelly retractors, large blade, 2½ inches wide × 3 inches deep

Suturing items

2 Mayo-Hegar needle holders or Crile-Wood needle holders, 8 inches
2 Fine needle holders, 6 inches
2 Medium ligating clip appliers with clips
2 Long ligating clip appliers with clips
Suture materials
  Ligatures for small blood vessels: synthetic absorbable and nonabsorbable suture, 3-0 and 4-0
  Ligatures for larger blood vessels: synthetic absorbable no. 0 or nonabsorbable no. 2-0 or 0

Self-retaining retractor and blades; this may include a Balfour retractor or more extensive retracting systems such as the Bookwalter or Omnitract retractor systems

Closure of gastrointestinal layers
  Mucosal—synthetic absorbable suture no. 4-0 or 3-0 with curved atraumatic intestinal needle; usually continuous
  Seromuscular—synthetic absorbable suture 3-0 or 2-0 and nonabsorbable suture no. 4-0 or 3-0 with curved or straight atraumatic intestinal needles; interrupted silk sutures on intestinal needles may be used
GI stapling devices
Abdominal closure and retention sutures (if indicated), as previously described

FIG. 10-22   Accessory items. *1*, Frazier suction tip; *2*, Poole suction tube; *3*, Yankauer suction tube; *4*, silver probe; *5*, grooved director.

Courtesy Codman & Shurtleff, Inc., Randolph, Mass.

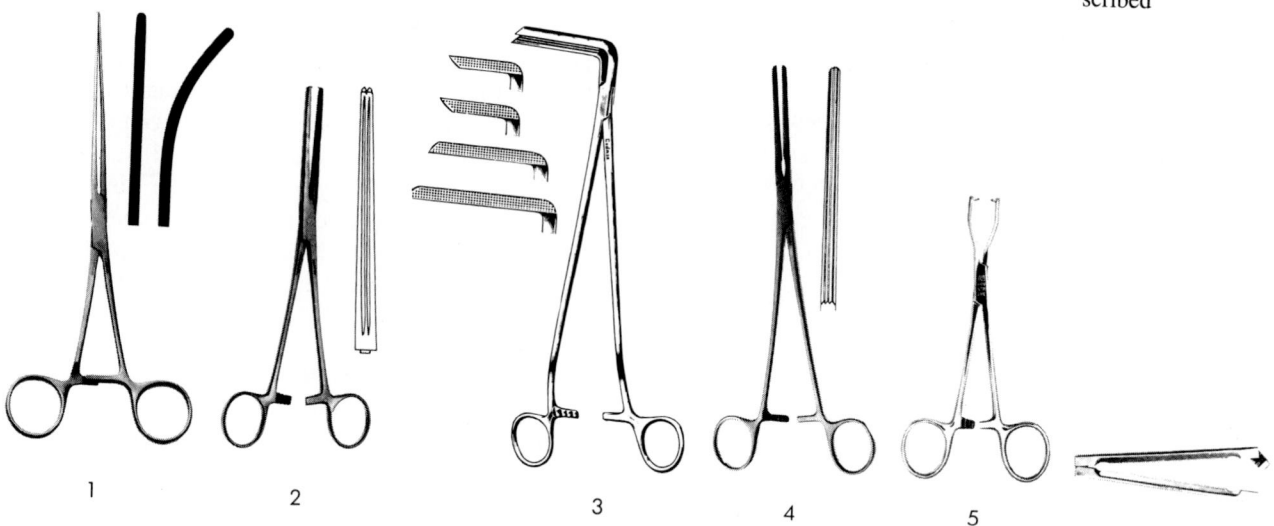

FIG. 10-23   Instruments for stomach and intestinal operations. *1*, Doyen intestinal forceps, straight and curved; *2*, Allen intestinal anastomosis clamp; *3*, Best colon clamps; *4*, Dennis intestinal clamp, *5*, Pace-Potts clamp.

1, 2, and *4. Courtesy Codman & Shurtleff, Inc., Randolph, Mass; 3,* Courtesy American V. Mueller, Deerfield, Ill; *5,* Courtesy Edward Weck & Co., Research Triangle Park, N.C.

Accessory items

2 Malecot, Pezzer, or
  Foley catheters in
  desired size for gas-
  trostomy tube
1 Robinson catheter,
  desired size
1 Baker jejunostomy
  tube
1 Closed wound drain-
  age system

Sump drain
Suction drain
2 Poole suction tubes
  with tubing
1 Yankauer suction tube
  with tubing
Electrosurgical unit with
  accessories, if desired

EVALUATION

As with any surgical procedure, evaluation of nursing care must be done throughout the surgery and before the patient is transported to the postanesthesia care unit (PACU) or a surgical intensive care unit (SICU) if indicated. The dressing and drains are securely placed to avoid damage during transfer to the PACU stretcher or SICU bed. Skin is assessed for reddened or bruised areas; if such areas are present, treatment is initiated immediately. The electrosurgical dispersive pad is removed, the site is inspected, and the condition of the skin is documented. The circulating nurse ensures that the patient is covered with a clean, warm blanket before being transported to PACU or SICU. Any variances postoperatively are reported to the surgeon, documented in the nursing notes, and included in the report given to the nurse in PACU or SICU. Patient outcomes, based on the perioperative nursing diagnoses, should be reviewed. Based on the nursing diagnoses selected for the patient undergoing gastrointestinal surgery, documenting and reporting perioperative patient care might include the following statements:

- The patient verbalized knowledge and expressed feelings about the perioperative experience.
- The patient verbalized feelings about body image disturbance.
- The patient's fluid volume status was maintained.
- The patient will demonstrate no clinical signs of wound infection postoperatively. Contamination related to the invasion of the GI tract was confined.
- Normothermia was maintained.

SURGICAL INTERVENTIONS

ENDOSCOPIC PROCEDURES

Endoscopic procedures that permit direct visual inspection of the contents and walls of the esophagus, stomach, and colon may be pertinent to establishing a diagnosis or determining preferred treatment of a disease process. A neodymium:uttrium-aluminum-garnet (Nd:YAG) laser may also be used in conjunction with endoscopic procedures as a treatment modality for ulcers, esophageal varices, malignancies, and gastrointestinal bleeding (see Chapter 31).

Care must be taken in handling fiberoptic equipment. Flexible scopes can be easily damaged if handled improp-

erly. The endoscopic equipment is terminally cleaned according to the manufacturer's instructions and stored so that drainage of liquid from the lumens can occur.

Endoscopic procedures may be performed with local anesthesia, with sedation only, or during the course of a procedure being performed with general anesthesia. Although medications may be used for sedation, the nurse must be immediately available to provide emotional support and appropriately monitor the patient's physiologic and psychologic status.

Gastroscopy

Gastroscopy is visual inspection of the stomach, with aspiration of contents and biopsy, if necessary, by an instrument known as a gastroscope (Fig. 10-24). When gastroscopy is performed with local anesthesia or sedation, the patient is usually not allowed to eat solid food 4 to 6 hours before the procedure but may take liquids up to 2 hours before it.

Procedural considerations

The patient's position for gastroscopy depends on the areas of the stomach to be visualized. For inspection of lesions in the gastric fundus and cardia, an upright sitting position may be used. Instrumentation is as follows:

Local anesthesia set
Gastroscope and video
  camera (optional)
Light source with air
  infusion capability
  and water bottle for
  irrigation

Biopsy forceps
Suction set
Lubricating jelly
Aspiration tubes
Electrosurgical unit
Protective bite block

Operative procedure

1. The gastroscope is thinly but completely covered with water-soluble lubricating jelly.
2. During introduction of the gastroscope, the patient's head and neck must remain in the sagittal plane of the spine so the axis of the mouth is in line with the esophagus.
3. The gastroscope is slowly passed into the stomach.
4. The stomach is inspected, and stomach contents may be aspirated for cytologic analysis. A biopsy can be performed. Laser treatment may be carried out as indicated.

Colonoscopy/sigmoidoscopy

Colonoscopy is visual inspection of the entire large intestine by means of a colonoscope. Sigmoidoscopy is the direct visualization of the sigmoid colon and rectum. The colonoscope is an important diagnostic tool and may be used for biopsy, removal of polyps, or laser treatment of tumors or bleeders. The patient must receive a liquid diet for 2 days before the colonoscopy/sigmoidoscopy and may receive bowel cleansing agents such as citrate of magnesium or GoLytely. Enemas may be necessary before the procedure.

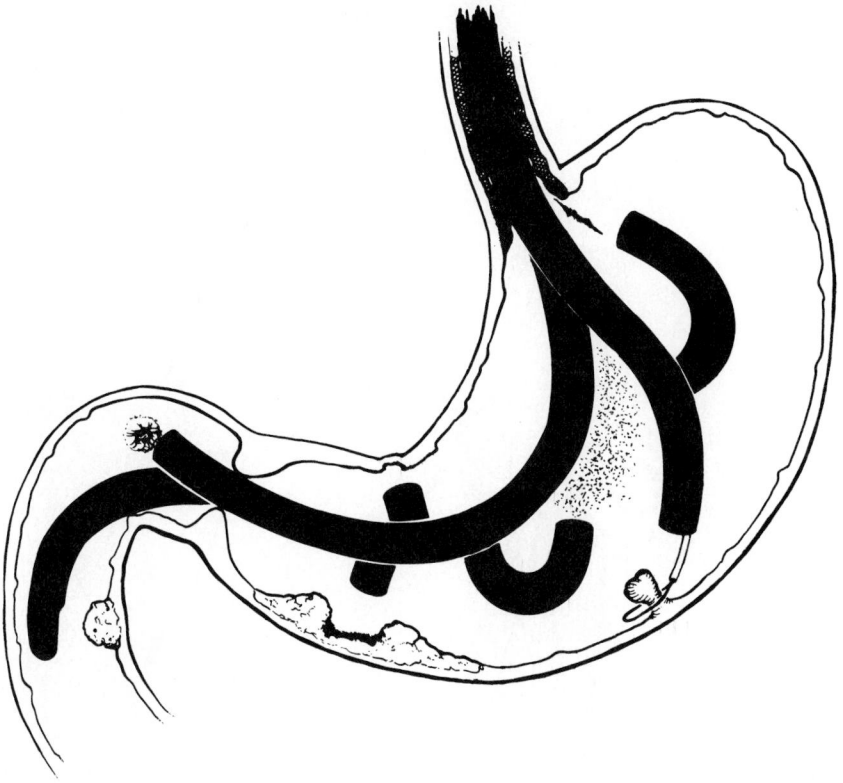

FIG. 10-24 Gastroscope in lumen of stomach illustrating the visualization capabilities and potential uses gastroscopy affords.

From Thompson, J.C. (1992). *Atlas of surgery of the stomach, duodenum, and small bowel*, St. Louis: Mosby.

Procedural considerations

The following instruments must be available:

Colonscope or flexible sigmoidoscope	Biopsy forceps
Video camera and monitors (optional)	Snares
	Brush
Light source	Electrosurgical unit and accessories
Air insufflation capability with water bottle for irrigation	Lubricating jelly
	Suction

Operative procedure

1. Analgesia is induced intramuscularly or intravenously.
2. The well-lubricated colonoscope is passed slowly into the anal canal and advanced continuously until it reaches the cecum for colonoscopy. With sigmoidoscopy, only the left colon is examined.
3. Following the endoscopic examination, the patient should be observed carefully to ensure that neither postprocedural bleeding nor signs of perforation occur.

Laparoscopy

A small incision is made in the fold of the umbilicus through which a percutaneous needle or trocar and sheath are placed. The peritoneal cavity is insufflated with CO_2 and a rigid wide-angle laparoscope is placed into the operative sheath for direct visualization of the abdominal viscera. This can be for diagnostic purposes or to assist or accomplish surgical interventions when additional operative ports are established. Specific laparoscopic procedures are described later in this chapter.

LAPAROTOMY

An opening made through the abdominal wall into the peritoneal cavity is called a laparotomy. Surgical intervention may be necessary to repair or remove traumatized tissue, to cure disease processes by organ removal, and to examine by biopsy or otherwise visualize internal organs for diagnosis. Surgery may be indicated for diagnostic, therapeutic, palliative, or prophylactic reasons. Most procedures requiring a laparotomy involve the organs of the alimentary canal.

Operative procedure
Laparotomy opening

1. The suction tube and tubing are connected, tested, and secured to the field.
2. The skin incision is made and carried to fascia (Fig. 10-25, *A*).

A   **B**   **C**

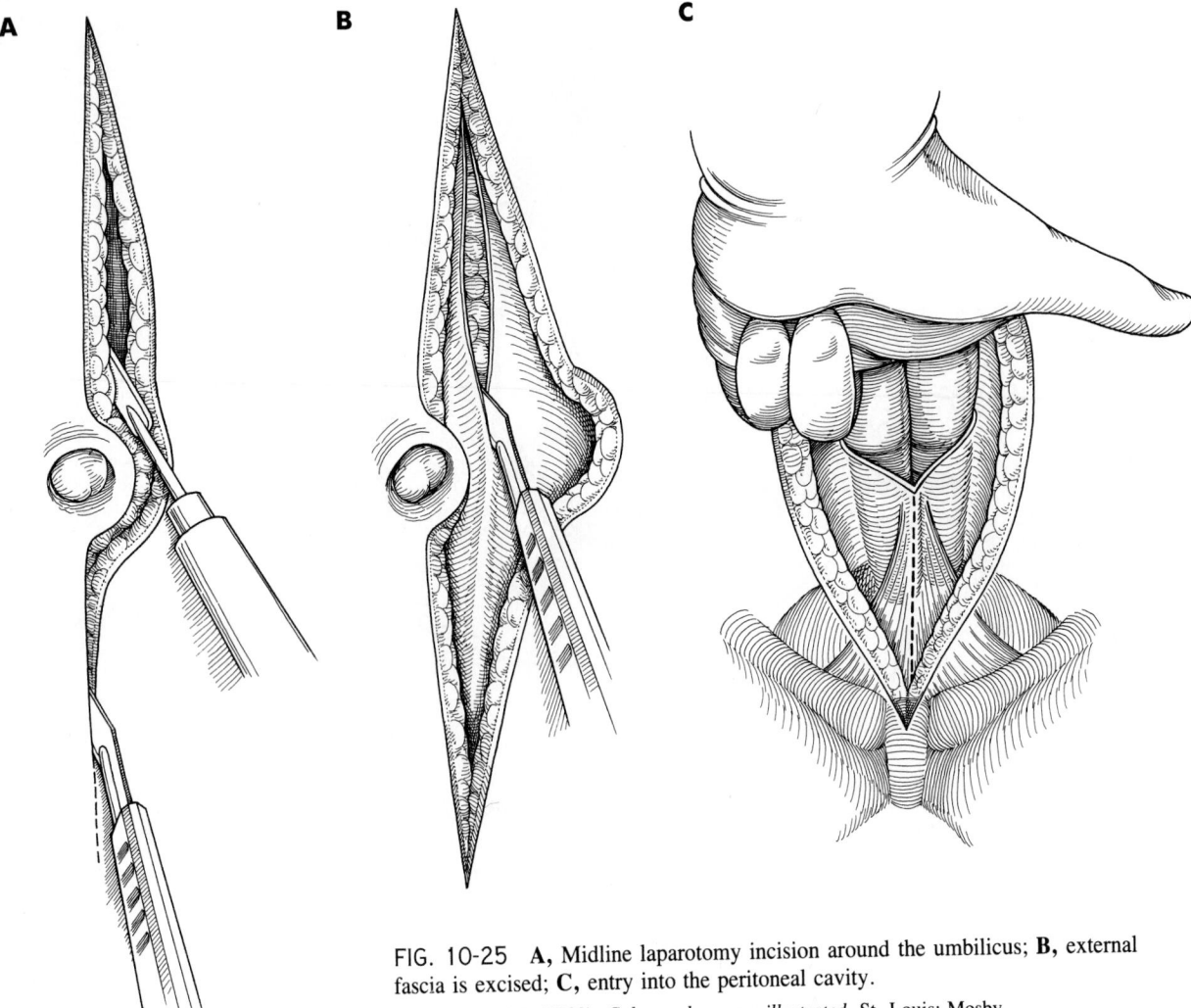

FIG. 10-25   **A,** Midline laparotomy incision around the umbilicus; **B,** external fascia is excised; **C,** entry into the peritoneal cavity.

From Bauer, J.J. (1993). *Colorectal surgery illustrated,* St. Louis: Mosby.

3. Hemostats or ligating clips are used to control bleeding vessels. Clamped vessels are ligated with fine absorbable ligatures or nonabsorbable suture, or they are electrocoagulated.
4. The wound edges are retracted with small retractors.
5. With tissue forceps and scalpel, the external fascia is incised (Fig. 10-25, *B*).
6. With Metzenbaum or curved Mayo scissors, electrocautery, or knife, the external oblique muscle is split the length of the incision. Bleeding vessels are controlled with hemostats, ligating clips, or medium or fine ligatures.
7. The external oblique muscle is retracted.
8. The internal oblique and transverse muscles are split, parallel to the fibers, up to the rectus sheath with a scalpel or scissors. These muscles are then retracted.
9. The peritoneum is exposed, grasped with smooth tissue forceps, and nicked with a no. 10 blade (Fig. 10-25, *C*).
10. Sponges, laparotomy pads, and suction are used as needed. Culture samples may be taken at this time.

11. The peritoneal incision is extended the length of the wound with Metzenbaum or Mayo scissors.
12. The peritoneum is retracted with large Richardson retractors for initial exploration.
13. Once the affected organs are identified, a self-retaining retractor, such as the Bookwalter retractor system, may be used to ensure adequate exposure.

Laparotomy closure

1. Two tissue forceps or clamps are used to approximate the peritoneal edges, and the peritoneum is closed with a continuous synthetic absorbable suture or interrupted nonabsorbable sutures. The internal oblique fascia is usually closed with the peritoneum. Muscle tissue is approximated and may or may not be sutured.
2. The external oblique fascia is closed with interrupted sutures, staples, or both. Retraction is necessary as the various layers are closed and Richardson retractors are utilized.
3. Fine, interrupted, absorbable sutures are usually employed to close the subcutaneous tissue. Retraction is

provided with laparotomy pads or small retractors.

4. Skin edges are held with Adson forceps and approximated with interrupted fine silk, nylon, or other nonabsorbable sutures on a cutting needle. Skin staples or clips are often used to approximate skin edges. Retention sutures of heavy nonabsorbable material may be used. Usually prepackaged retention bridges or rubber tubing bolsters are used to protect the incision site.

SURGERY OF THE ESOPHAGUS

Esophagectomy and intrathoracic esophagogastrostomy

Esophagectomy and intrathoracic esophagogastrostomy involve the removal of diseased portions of the stomach and esophagus through a thoracoabdominal incision in the left side of the chest—including a resection of the seventh, eighth, or ninth rib or separation of the two appropriate ribs—and establishment of an anastomosis between the esophagus and the stomach. These procedures are performed to remove strictures in the lower esophagus that may develop after trauma, infection, or corrosion or to remove tumors in the cardia of the stomach or in the distal esophagus.

Procedural considerations

The basic thoracotomy set (Chapter 24), basic laparotomy set, and gastrointestinal set are required.

Operative procedure

1. The skin incision is carried downward midway between the vertebral border of the scapula and the spinous processes to the eighth rib and then forward along this rib to the costochondral junction. The extent of the vertical portion of the incision depends on the location of the tumor. The wound is retracted, and bleeding vessels are ligated or coagulated.
2. The chest cavity is opened, and the rib spreader is placed. Moist packs are placed, and the lung is retracted with a Deaver or Harrington retractor.
3. The mediastinal pleura is incised with long Metzenbaum scissors and long plain forceps in line with the esophagus and the lesion. The esophagus is dissected free from the aorta with dry dissectors. Suture ligatures of nonabsorbable material nos. 2-0 and 3-0 are used for controlling bleeding vessels.
4. The diaphragm is opened, and a series of traction sutures is attached. The stomach is mobilized by dissection of its ligamental attachment with long scissors and curved thoracic clamps.
5. The left gastric artery is clamped, cut, and doubly ligated with nonabsorbable suture no. 2-0 and a suture ligature of nonabsorbable material no. 3-0.
6. The sterile field is prepared for the open method of anastomosis. The stomach is transsected well below the lesion with the selected resection instruments. Closure of the stomach is completed with two rows of intesti-

nal sutures of synthetic absorbable suture no. 2-0 and sometimes with an additional row of nonabsorbable no. 3-0 sutures for reinforcement. A separate circular opening is usually made in the upper portion of the stomach for anastomosis to the esophagus.

7. Two Allen clamps or a stapler type of clamp is applied above the stricture, and the freed esophagus is divided.
8. The circular opening in the stomach and the transsected end of the esophagus are anastomosed. The mucosal layers are approximated. The muscular layers of the esophagus and stomach are closed by two rows of interrupted sutures.
9. A mechanical end-to-end anastomosing surgical stapling device may also be used to accomplish the gastroesophageal anastomosis.
10. The stomach is anchored to the pleura, and the edges of the diaphragm are sutured to the wall of the stomach with interrupted sutures of nonabsorbable material, no. 3-0 or 2-0.
11. The pleura is cleansed with warm, normal, saline irrigation that is suctioned off. A thoracic catheter is inserted for closed drainage. The chest wall is closed as described for thoracotomy (see Chapter 24).

Excision of esophageal diverticulum

Excision of an esophageal diverticulum, sometimes referred to as Zenker's diverticulum, is removal of a weakening in the wall of the esophagus that collects small amounts of food and causes a sensation of fullness in the neck. Because diverticula usually occur in the cervical portion of the esophagus, excision gives complete relief of symptoms.

Procedural considerations

A thyroid set (see Chapter 15) or equivalent set of instrumentation, two Pennington clamps, six Halsted curved mosquito hemostats, two 5-inch Adson forceps, and two lateral retractors are required.

Operative procedure

An incision is made over the inner border of the sternocleidomastoid muscle and is extended from the level of the hyoid bone to a point 2 cm above the clavicle. The sac of the diverticulum is freed and ligated, and the pharyngeal muscle and surrounding tissues are closed. In conjunction with this procedure, an esophageal myotomy is often performed distal to the diverticulum. A myotomy seems to lessen the likelihood of recurrence.

Esophageal hiatal hernia repair/antireflux procedure

Hiatal herniorrhaphy is performed to restore the cardioesophageal junction in its correct anatomic position in the abdomen, to secure it firmly in place, and to correct gastroesophageal reflux. A hiatal hernia is a special type of hernia in which a defect, either congenital or accidental, in

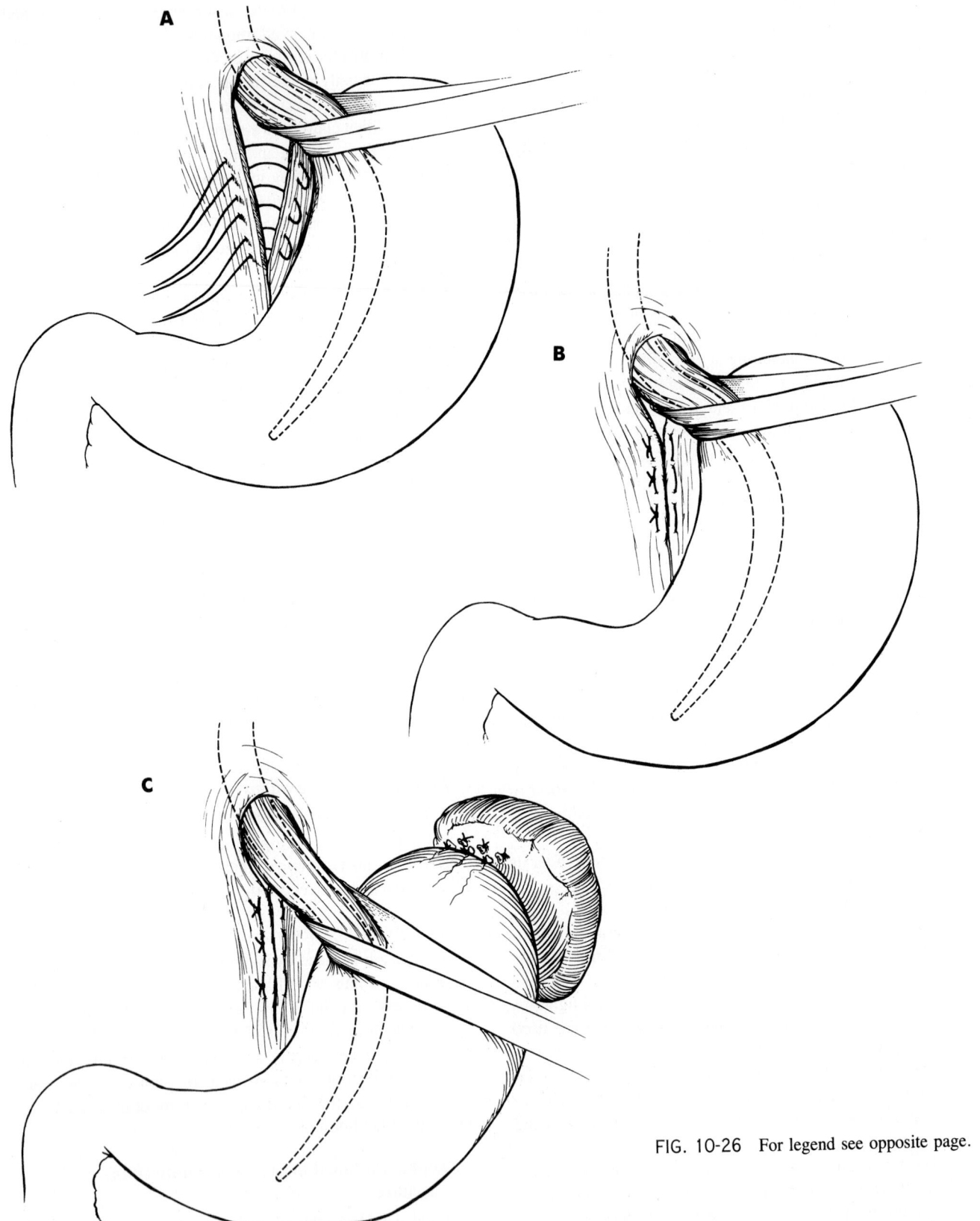

FIG. 10-26 For legend see opposite page.

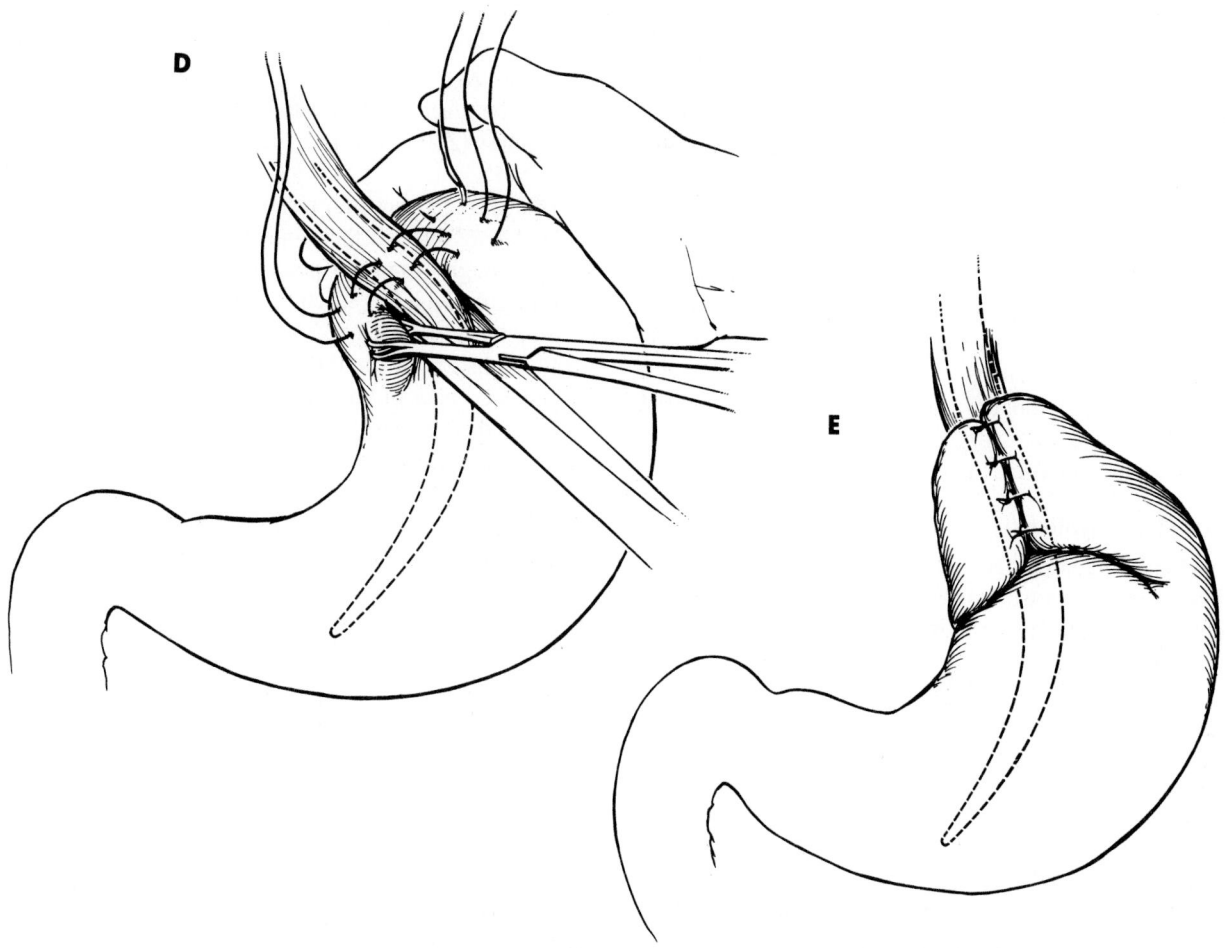

FIG. 10-26 The Nissen Fundoplication procedure begins with: **A,** mobilization of the esophagus and placement of a penrose drain around the gastroesophageal junction to allow for traction to pull the esophagus downward and out of the hernia after a Maloney dilator (40 to 48Fr.) has been passed into the lumen of the stomach from the patient's oral cavity in the same manner as passing an NG tube. **B,** Shown are three heavy sutures (#0 braided absorbable) placed to narrow the hiatal aperture but not so tight as to constrict the esophagus, thus the purpose of stenting the esophagus with the Maloney dilator. **C,** Further traction is applied to the distal esophagus while the proximal stomach and fundus are freed from all peritoneal attachments. **D,** The posterior wall of the stomach is brought up around the distal esophagus. **E,** The stomach walls are wrapped and sutured around the intraabdominal esophagus, with the Maloney stent in place.

From Thompson, J.C. (1992). *Atlas of surgery of the stomach, duodenum, and small bowel,* St. Louis: Mosby.

the diaphragm permits a portion of the stomach to enter the thoracic cavity.

Hiatal hernias are usually of two distinct types—paraesophageal and sliding. Symptoms vary from none to severe heartburn, reflux (backward flow), regurgitation, and dysphagia. When symptoms are severe, a repair of the hernia is done, usually through a transabdominal approach.

An antireflux procedure, which prevents reflux of gastric juices into the esophagus, is also done when the hernia is repaired. The three most frequently performed antireflux procedures are the Nissen (Fig. 10-26), Hill, and Belsey Mark IV procedures.

Procedural considerations

A transthoracic approach is used in patients who previously had left upper quadrant surgery or are extremely obese, or if a Belsey Mark IV procedure is selected.

Instrumentation is as follows:

Laparotomy set	2 Crile nerve hooks
Thoracotomy set (Chapter 24), if requested	2 Schnidt thoracic forceps, long
2 Forceps, smooth, extra long	2 Vessel clip appliers, long, with clips
1 Semb ligature carrier	

Operative procedure

1. Through a transabdominal incision, the hernia is located, and a crural repair is done.
2. The fundus of the stomach is wrapped around the lower 4 to 6 cm of the esophagus and is sutured in place (Nissen fundoplication); the upper part of the lesser curvature of the stomach and the cardioesophageal junction are sutured to the median arcuate ligament (Hill procedure); or the stomach is plicated around approximately 270 degrees of esophageal circumference (Belsey Mark IV procedure). The Nissen fundoplication procedure is illustrated in Fig. 10-26.
3. Vagotomy, pyloroplasty, or both may be performed at the same time.
4. The wound is closed.

Esophagomyotomy

Esophagomyotomy (Heller cardiomyotomy) is myotomy of the esophagogastric junction and is done to correct esophageal obstruction resulting from cardiospasm.

Procedural considerations

Selection of a transthoracic or transabdominal incision depends on the patient's general condition and other existing pathologic factors. The surgeon may elect to perform a pyloroplasty to prevent reflux.

Operative procedure

1. After exposure of the esophagogastric junction, a Maloney dilator is inserted to distend the esophagus.
2. A scalpel with a no. 15 blade is used to make a longitudinal incision through the muscular wall of the distal esophagus and proximal stomach, leaving the mucosa intact.
3. A small portion of the fundus of the stomach may be plicated to the lateral wall of the esophagus.
4. The wound is closed.

Esophageal dilatation

Esophageal dilatation may be indicated in patients having esophageal stricture related to past surgery, chemical or thermal injury, or anatomic anomalies. An upper gastrointestinal series is required prior to the procedure to determine the location of the stricture.

Procedural considerations

The following equipment and supplies are needed:

Flexible gastroscope
  and light source
Bougie dilators in grad-
  uated sizes: Hurst or
  Maloney
Water-soluble lubricant
Gauze sponges

Operative procedure

1. The patient is positioned supine under general anesthesia or IV sedation. The perioperative nurse has the bougies arranged in graduated order beginning with the smallest (24 Fr) and progressing to the largest size (60 Fr).
2. The surgeon may first perform gastroscopy and pass a guidewire through the esophageal stricture.
3. The bougies are then passed one at a time gently but firmly through the strictures in an attempt to dilate the esophageal lumen.
4. Continuation of the dilatation to the largest bougie depends on ease of passage and patient tolerance.
5. Laser therapy may be indicated for palliation if tumor mass is causing the stricture. The Nd:YAG laser energy may be delivered to the mass/stricture via a flexible quartz fiber passed through the operative channel of the gastroscope.

SURGERY OF THE STOMACH
VAGOTOMY

Truncal vagotomy

Truncal vagotomy is the identification of the two vagal trunks on the distal esophagus and resection of a segment of each, including any additional nerve fibers running separately from the trunks. By interrupting the parasympathetic innervation, this procedure reduces the gastric acid secretion in patients with duodenal ulcers. When truncal vagotomy was initially performed alone, a high incidence of gastric stasis resulted from the loss of cholinergic innervation to the smooth muscle of the stomach; thus pyloroplasty or another gastric drainage procedure almost always accompanies truncal vagotomy. Truncal vagotomy deprives not only the stomach but also the liver, gallbladder, bile duct, pancreas, small intestine, and half of the large intestine of the parasympathetic nerve supply (Fig. 10-27). Truncal vagotomy with antrectomy or drainage procedure is the most common operation for duodenal ulcers.

Selective vagotomy

Selective vagotomy is the transsection of each abdominal vagus at a point just beyond its bifurcation into the gastric and extragastric divisions. Thus the hepatic branch of the anterior vagus and the celiac branch of the posterior vagus are preserved. Selective vagotomy possesses theoretical advantages over truncal vagotomy because vagal innervation of the viscera other than the stomach is preserved. However, selective vagotomy also denervates the entire stomach, so the addition of a drainage procedure is still necessary. Selective vagotomy may cause less postvagotomy diarrhea than truncal vagotomy, but the incidence of dumping syndrome is probably the same or even higher. Both procedures are about equally effective in controlling duodenal ulcers.

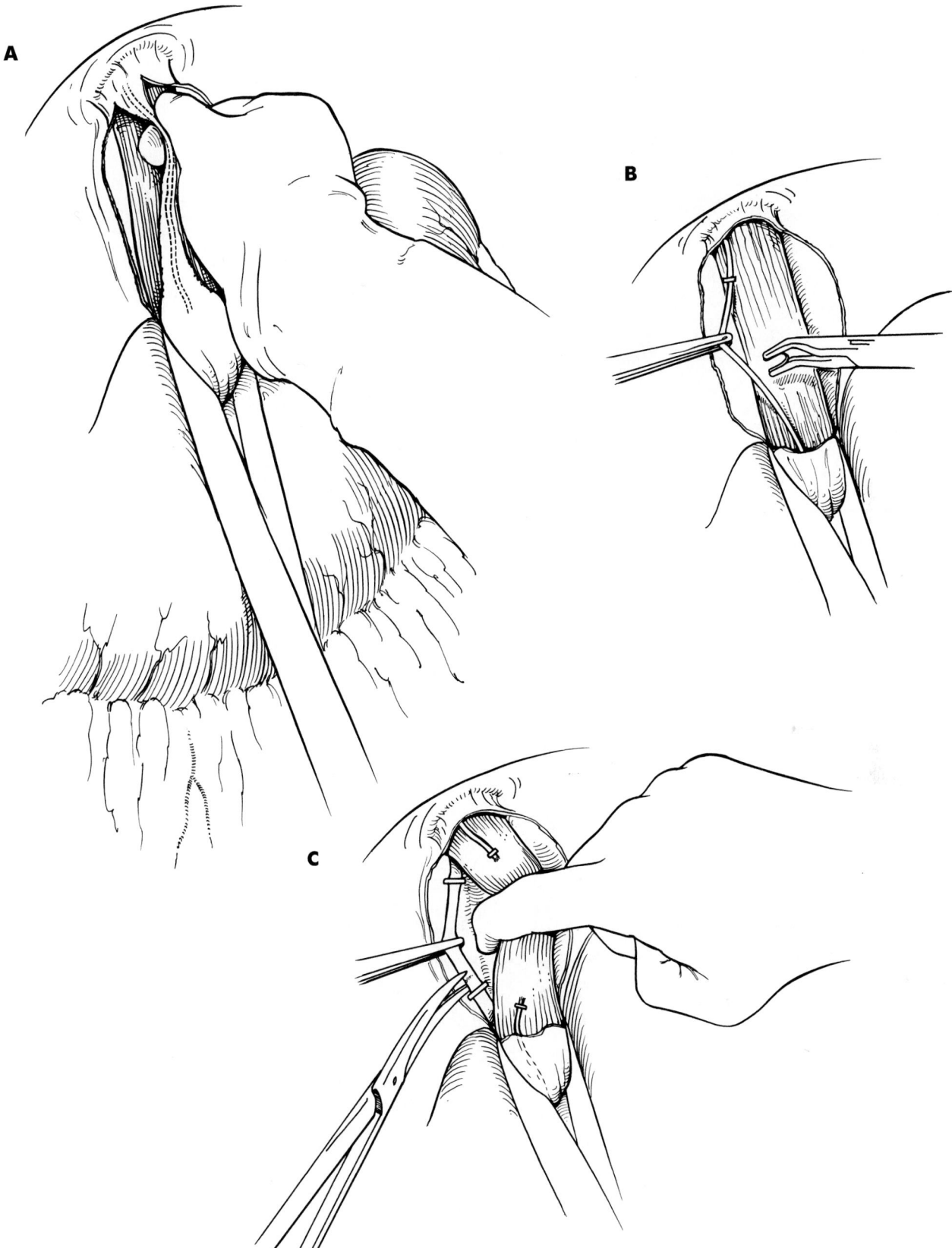

FIG. 10-27   Truncal vagotomy. **A,** The phrenoesophageal ligament is lifted from the surface of the esophagus and the vagal trunks are identified. **B,** Ligating clips are applied to the vagus nerve. **C,** Ligating clips have been applied to the larger posterior nerve in preparation for resecting a 2 cm segment between the clips.

From Thompson, J.C. (1992). *Atlas of surgery of the stomach, duodenum, and small bowel*, St. Louis: Mosby.

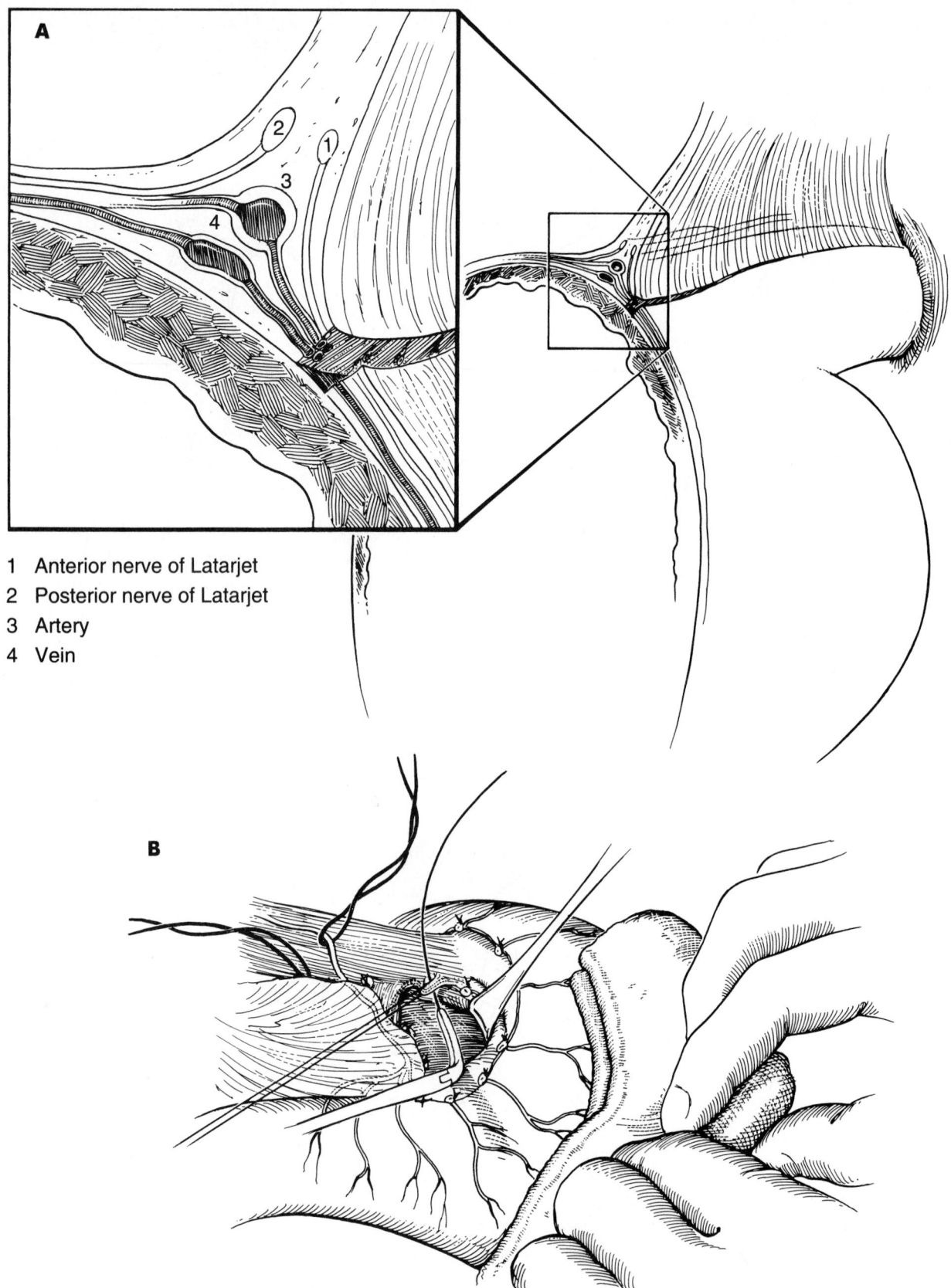

1 Anterior nerve of Latarjet
2 Posterior nerve of Latarjet
3 Artery
4 Vein

FIG. 10-28 Selective Proximal Vagotomy. **A,** Illustrates the junction of the gastrohepatic ligament with the lesser curve of the stomach and demonstrates the (1) anterior and (2) posterior nerves of Laterjet, along with the (3) artery and (4) vein. **B,** The lesser curve is lifted with a vein retractor to facilitate serial ligation of the intermediate and posterior neurovascular attachments.

From Thompson, J.C. (1992). *Atlas of surgery of the stomach, duodenum, and small bowel,* St. Louis: Mosby.

Parietal cell vagotomy

Parietal cell vagotomy is the vagal denervation of only the parietal cell area of the stomach. The technique spares the main nerves of Latarjet but divides all vagal branches that terminate on the proximal two thirds of the stomach. The operation has also been called proximal gastric vagotomy (Fig. 10-28) and highly selective vagotomy. Because antral innervation is preserved, gastric emptying is unimpaired and a drainage procedure is unnecessary. The incidence of dumping and diarrhea following parietal cell vagotomy is much lower than after truncal or selective vagotomy.

Procedural considerations

Instrumentation is as follows:

Basic thoracotomy set (if a thoracoabdominal incision is to be used)	2 Vessel clip appliers, 10 inches, with clips
Laparotomy set	1 Metzenbaum dissecting scissors, 10 inches
Gastrointestinal set	
2 Blunt nerve hooks (Smithwick)	

Operative procedure

1. A midline incision is made, and the esophagus is identified and retracted with Penrose drains.
2. The vagus nerves or their branches, depending on which type of vagotomy is being done, are identified, clamped with either a ligature or a hemostatic clip, and resected.
3. The wound is closed in layers.

PYLOROPLASTY

Pyloroplasty is the formation of a larger passageway between the prepyloric region of the stomach and the first or second portion of the duodenum with excision of peptic ulcer, if present. A pyloroplasty may be performed for the treatment of a peptic ulcer under selected conditions but is more frequently employed to remove cicatricial bands in the pyloric ring, thus relieving spasm and permitting rapid emptying of the stomach. In adults a vagotomy is usually performed in conjunction with a pyloroplasty.

Procedural considerations

A laparotomy set and a gastrointestinal instrument set are required.

Operative procedure

1. The abdominal cavity is opened through a midline incision.
2. An incision is made through the stomach and the duodenum.
3. The pyloroplasty is closed with nonabsorbable or synthetic, absorbable intestinal sutures.
4. The abdominal wound is closed in layers, and a dressing is applied.

GASTROSTOMY

In a gastrostomy, through a high left rectus abdominal or midline incision, a temporary or permanent channel is established from the gastric lumen to the skin. This lumen permits liquid feeding or retrograde dilatation of an esophageal stricture. Gastrostomy is a palliative procedure performed to prevent malnutrition and starvation, which may be caused by a lesion or stricture situated in the esophagus or in the cardia of the stomach. A temporary procedure is done when the obstruction is capable of being corrected.

Procedural considerations

For an extensive lesion of the esophagus, some surgeons advise a permanent gastrostomy in which a stomach flap is formed around the catheter. The catheter is brought out of the abdomen through a separate stab wound. When the incisional area is avoided, tissue healing is improved, and the incidence of postoperative wound healing problems decreases.

Operative procedure

1. The abdominal cavity is opened through an upper midline or transverse incision.
2. The stomach is held with Allis or Babcock forceps, and a pursestring suture is placed at the proposed site for the catheter.
3. A scalpel with a no. 15 blade is used to make an incision within the pursestring suture, and the contents of the stomach are suctioned.
4. Bleeding points are controlled. The catheter is inserted, and the pursestring suture is tied around it.
5. The catheter is brought through a stab wound in the area of the left rectus muscle.
6. The stomach may be sutured to the peritoneal layer, and the abdominal wound is closed in layers.

PERCUTANEOUS ENDOSCOPIC GASTROSTOMY (PEG)

Percutaneous endoscopic gastrostomy utilizes a flexible gastroscope and a uniquely designed gastrostomy tube for placement through the abdominal wall. The patient may remain awake with sedation while the procedure is performed in the operating room or endoscopy suite. There are push and pull techniques to insert a PEG tube. The pull technique is reviewed here.

Procedural considerations

A PEG tube kit containing the following is required:

Percutaneous needle
Long silk suture with end strengthened
Percutaneous gastrostomy tube and bolster
A flexible gastroscopy system is required as well as snare forceps

Operative procedure

1. With the patient in supine position, the gastroscope is passed into the stomach through the oral cavity and down the esophagus: the end of the scope is angled anteriorly to the left anterolateral wall of the stomach's fundus. The light from the gastroscope can be seen through the abdominal wall. The stomach is insufflated with air.

2. Local anesthesia is injected at the site if the patient is awake. A small stab wound is made with a no. 10 blade. The percutaneous needle is inserted into the abdominal wall and into the stomach lumen under direct visualization of the gastroscope.

3. The long silk suture is threaded into the lumen of the needle and passed into the stomach where it is snared with the forcep. A clamp is applied to the exterior distal end of the suture after the needle is removed.

4. The gastroscope is removed and the suture extends out of the patient's oral cavity. The suture is then attached to the tapered end of the gastrostomy tube.

5. The gastrostomy tube is gently guided into the patient's oral cavity, down the esophagus, and into the lumen of the stomach and pulled through the abdominal wall. The tube is secured with an internal bolster by reinserting the gastroscope and snugging it up to the gastric wall under direct visualization. An external bolster is applied over the tube and snugged to the abdominal wall. Care is taken to ensure the bolsters are not compressing the tissues.

6. The distal end of the tube is cut and a connector is applied.

7. The patient's stomach is deflated and the procedure is complete.

GASTROTOMY

Gastrotomy is the opening of the anterior stomach wall through a left paramedian abdominal incision and exploration of the interior. This procedure is usually done to explore for upper gastrointestinal tract bleeding, perform a tissue biopsy, or remove a gastric lesion or foreign body.

Procedural considerations

A laparotomy set and gastrointestinal instrument set are required.

Operative procedure

1. A longitudinal incision is made through the anterior wall of the stomach, halfway between the curvatures.

2. The stomach wall is grasped and elevated by Allis or Babcock forceps.

3. An incision is made, and a suction tube is inserted into the stomach to remove gastric contents.

4. The lesion or foreign body is removed, and the stomach wall and abdominal wall are closed.

CLOSURE OF PERFORATED GASTRIC OR DUODENAL ULCER

Closure of a perforation in the stomach or duodenum is performed through a high right rectus or midline abdominal incision.

Procedural considerations

A perforated gastric or duodenal ulcer is treated as a surgical emergency, and the operation is performed as soon as the diagnosis is made. The patient's blood should be typed and cross-matched so an adequate supply will be available for emergency replacement. A gastric lavage is not performed, but continuous suction is used. A laparotomy set and gastrointestinal set are required. Linear stapling instruments are available.

Operative procedure

1. Through a right rectus or midline abdominal incision the perforation is located.

2. Suction is used to remove exudate in the peritoneal cavity.

3. The perforation is closed with a pursestring suture by inverting the raw edges and suturing a piece of omentum over the closure.

4. The abdomen is irrigated with warm saline, which may contain a broad-spectrum antibiotic.

5. The abdominal wound is closed in layers, and a dressing is applied.

GASTROJEJUNOSTOMY

Gastrojejunostomy is the establishment of a permanent communication, either between the proximal jejunum and the anterior wall of the stomach or between the proximal jejunum and the posterior wall of the stomach, without removing a segment of the gastrointestinal tract (Fig. 10-29). It is accomplished through a midline or a paramedian abdominal incision. Gastrojejunostomy may be performed to treat a benign obstruction at the pyloric end of the stomach or an inoperable lesion of the pylorus when a partial gastrectomy would not be feasible. It also provides a large opening without sphincter obstruction.

Procedural considerations

A laparotomy and gastrointestinal instrument set are required. Linear stapling instruments should be available. An indwelling catheter is placed into the urinary bladder prior to abdominal prep.

Operative procedure

1. Through an upper midline or paramedian abdominal incision exploration of the peritoneal cavity is completed, as described for routine laparotomy. The pathologic condition is confirmed.

2. Warm, moist packs are placed, and a loop of proximal jejunum is grasped with Babcock forceps and freed from the mesentery. It is approximated to either the anterior

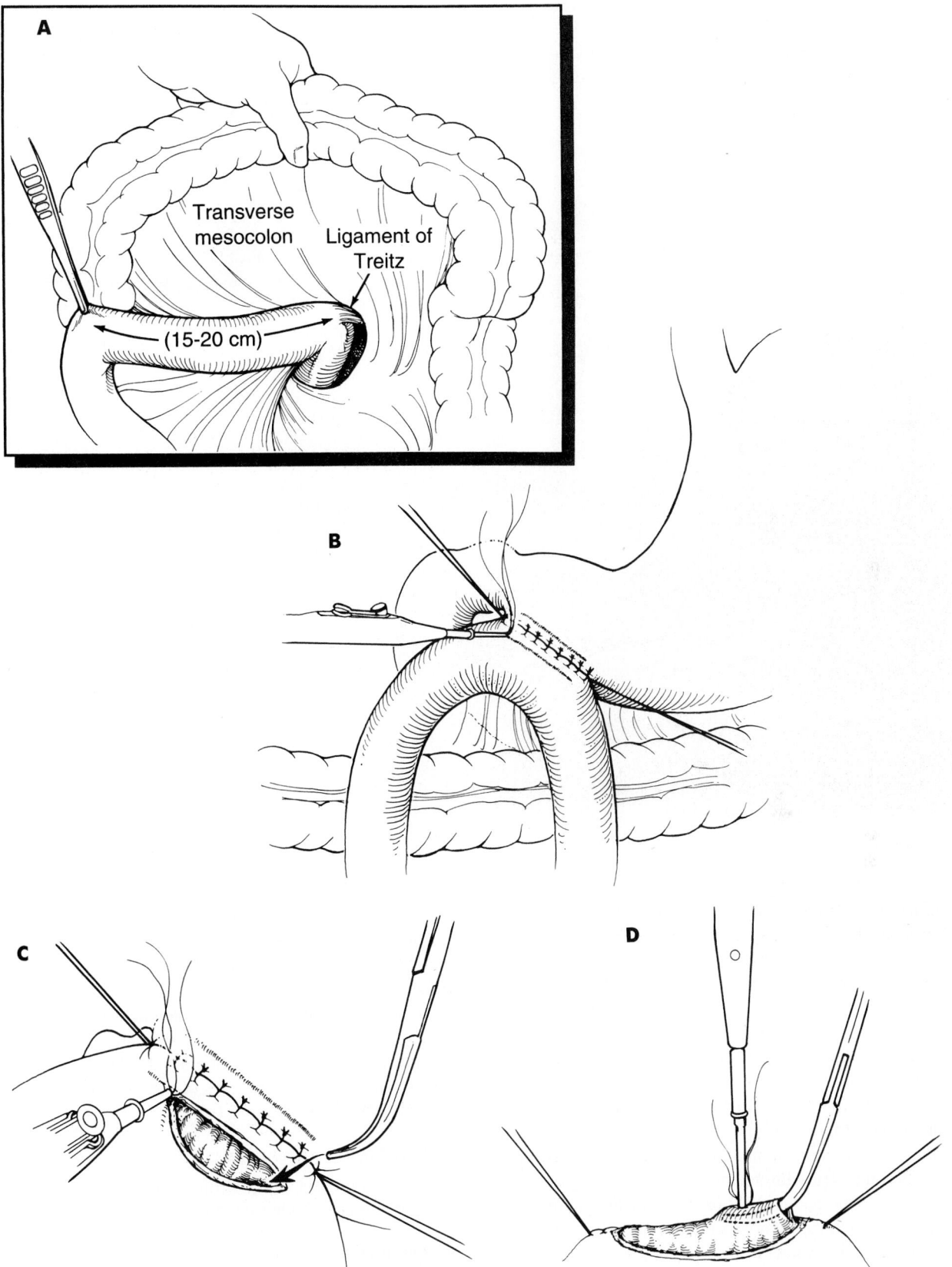

FIG. 10-29 Gastrojejunostomy. **A,** Illustrates the selection of a segment of jejunum that will be anastomosed to the stomach; the distance between the ligament of Treitz and the anastomosis should not be excessively long or under any tension. **B,** A posterior row of interrupted suture is placed between the gastric and jejunal serosae and the sites of the gastric and jejunal stomas are scored with the electrosurgical pencil. **C,** The jejunal stoma is created by dissecting through the serosa and muscularis with the electrosurgical pencil. An opening is made in the mucosa and a right-angled clamp is inserted into the lumen. **D,** The clamp is opened and elevated.   *Continued.*

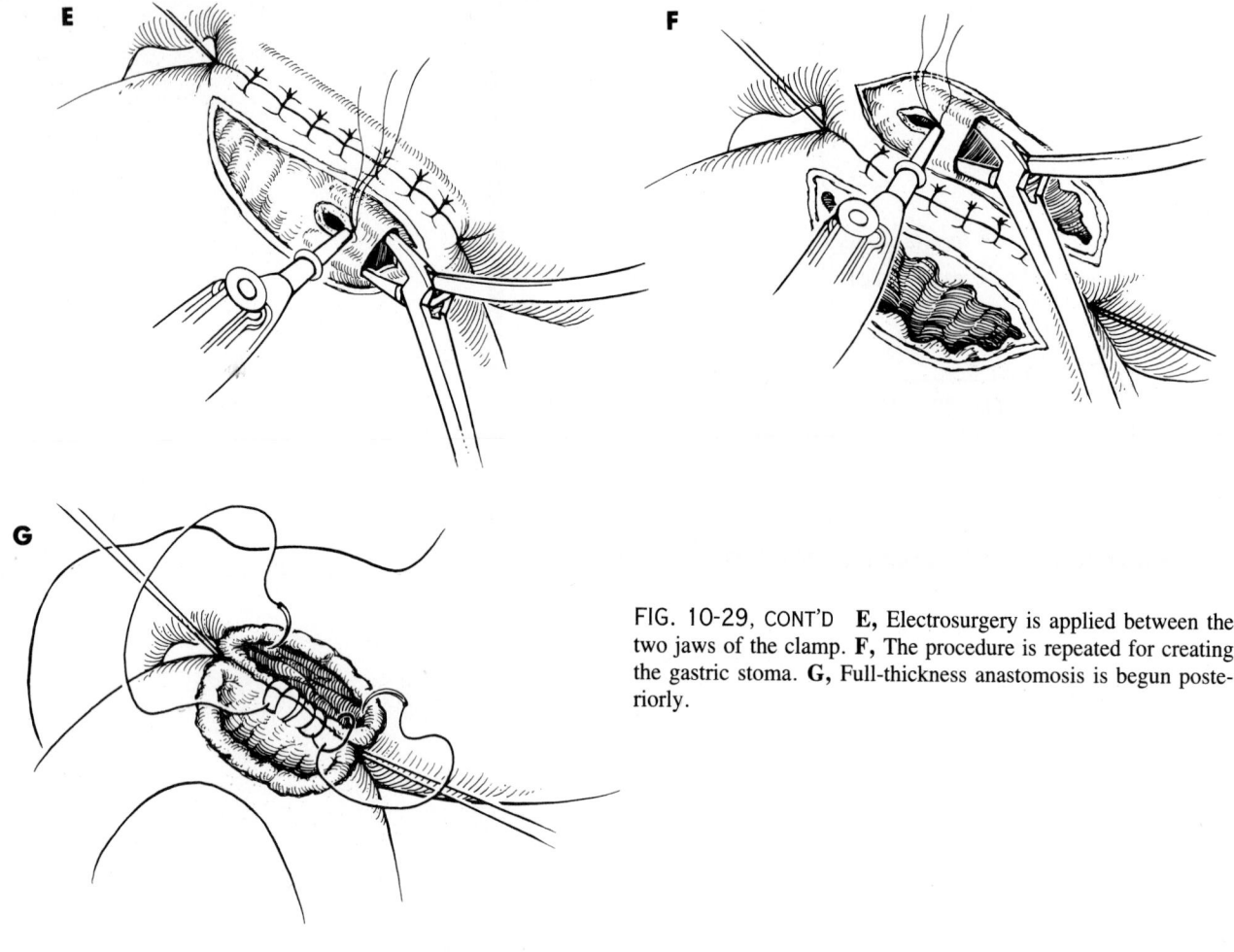

FIG. 10-29, CONT'D **E,** Electrosurgery is applied between the two jaws of the clamp. **F,** The procedure is repeated for creating the gastric stoma. **G,** Full-thickness anastomosis is begun posteriorly.

or posterior stomach wall several centimeters from the greater curvature. Nonabsorbable no. 2-0 traction sutures are placed through the serosal layers at each end of the selected portion of the jejunum and stomach. Gastroenterostomy clamps may be placed before insertion of the posterior interrupted nonabsorbable no. 3-0 or 2-0 serosal sutures.

3. The field is draped for open anastomosis. The jejunum and stomach are opened. Bleeding points are clamped with mosquito hemostats and ligated with no. 3-0 synthetic absorbable sutures. The inner posterior row of sutures is placed, using continuous synthetic absorbable suture no. 2-0 or 3-0 with atraumatic intestinal needles, and continued for the first anterior row. The anastomosis is completed with anterior serosal sutures of nonabsorbable material, no. 3-0 or 2-0. Traction sutures are removed. Interrupted nonabsorbable no. 4-0 sutures may be used for reinforcement.

4. The contaminated instruments are discarded. The abdominal wound is closed in layers and a dressing applied.

PARTIAL GASTRECTOMY
Billroth I

A Billroth I gastrectomy is the resection of the diseased portion of the stomach through a right paramedian or midline abdominal incision and the establishment of an anastomosis between the stomach and duodenum. It is performed to remove a benign or malignant lesion located in the pyloric, or upper half of the stomach. One of several techniques may be followed to establish gastrointestinal continuity, including the Schoemaker, the von Haberer-Finney, and other modifications of the Billroth I procedure (Fig. 10-30).

Procedural considerations

A laparotomy set and gastrointestinal instrument set are required. Linear stapling instruments should be available.

Operative procedure

1. The abdominal wall is incised, and the peritoneal cavity opened and explored. Bleeding vessels are clamped and ligated or coagulated.
2. The abdominal wound is retracted, and the surrounding organs are protected with warm, moist packs.

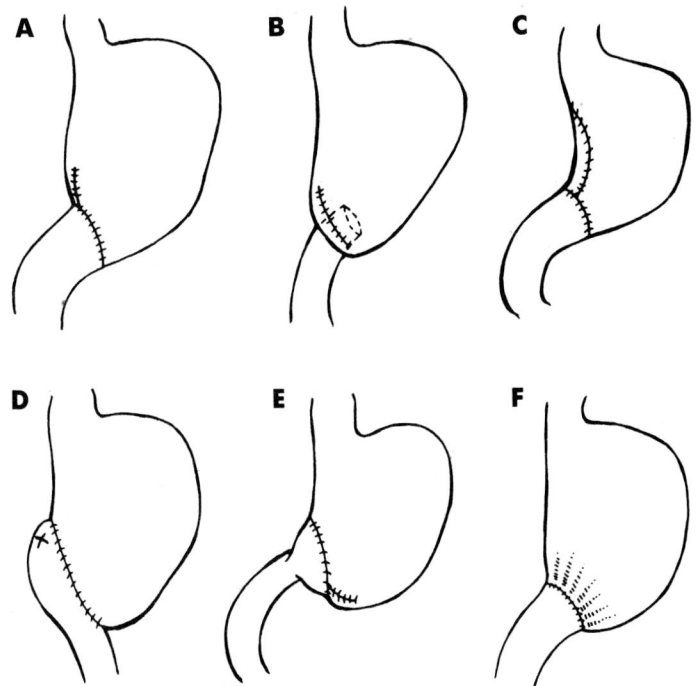

FIG. 10-30 Diagrams illustrating resections of stomach with anastomosis of stomach and duodenum (gastroduodenal anastomosis). All are modifications of Billroth I technique, in which stomach is brought to duodenum. **A,** Billroth I: after pylorus is removed, lesser curvature is partially closed, and duodenum is sutured to open end of stomach at its lower margin. **B,** Kocher: distal end of stomach is closed, and duodenum is brought up to posterior margin of closed stomach. **C,** Schoemaker: lesser curvature of stomach is sutured and brought down to same size as duodenum, and end-to-end anastomosis is done. **D,** von Haberer-Finney: side of duodenum is brought up to end of stomach so that entire end of stomach is open for direct anastomosis. **E,** Horsley: lesser curvature end of stomach is used to suture to duodenum and closes greater curvature end. **F,** von Haberer: modification of operation shown in **D.** Stomach is, so to speak, narrowed or puckered so that it fits end of duodenum. Modification of this is done by some as follows: duodenum is split longitudinally, and its ends are flared open so that opening is large enough to fit open end of stomach.

3. The gastrocolic omentum is freed from the colon mesentery to prevent injury to the middle colic artery. With hemostats and Metzenbaum scissors, the right and left gastroepiploic arteries and veins are clamped, divided, and ligated with nonabsorbable no. 2-0 and suture ligatures of nos. 2-0 and 3-0, thereby freeing the greater curvature of the stomach. The gastrohepatic vessels are also clamped, divided, and ligated to free completely the diseased portion of the stomach.

4. The operative field is prepared for open anastomosis. Two Allen intestinal anastomosis clamps or other suitable clamps are placed on the upper portion of the duodenum just distal to the pylorus. Division is accomplished by scalpel or electrosurgery, as preferred. Additional moist packs are placed for protection, and two sets of anastomosis clamps are placed across the stomach. Division is completed by the surgeon's preferred method.

5. At the lower margin the opened stomach is approximated to the duodenum by a series of interrupted sutures placed in the serosa layers. No. 3-0 nonabsorbable suture on an atraumatic intestinal needle is used. Suture ends are held with hemostats, and the intestinal clamps are removed. Stumps of the stomach and duodenum are cleansed with moist sponges, and bleeding vessels are ligated with fine suture or coagulated. During the anastomosis the involved segments may be held with rubbershod clamps.

6. The excess of the lesser curvature in the stomach is closed on completion of the anastomosis. Soiled instruments are discarded into a separate basin.

7. Routine laparotomy closure is completed.

Billroth II

A Billroth II gastrectomy is a resection of the distal portion of the stomach through an abdominal incision and the establishment of an anastomosis between the stomach and jejunum. It is performed to remove a benign or malignant lesion in the stomach or duodenum. This technique and modifications may be selected because the volume of acidic gastric juice will be reduced, and the anastomosis can be made along the greater curvature or at any point along the stump of the stomach. Modifications of the Billroth II procedure include the Polya and Hofmeister operations, which also establish gastrointestinal continuity through bypassing the duodenum.

After surgery, duodenal and jejunal secretions empty into the remaining gastric pouch. The stomach empties more rapidly because of the larger opening, and a limited amount of gastric juice remains.

Procedural considerations

A laparotomy set and gastrointestinal instrument set are required. Linear stapling instruments should be available.

Operative procedure

1. Through an abdominal incision the distal portion of the stomach is resected, and an anastomosis is established between the stomach and jejunum (Fig. 10-31).

2. The abdomen is closed.

TOTAL GASTRECTOMY

Total gastrectomy is the complete removal of the stomach and establishment of an anastomosis between the jejunum and the esophagus (Fig. 10-32). It may include an en-

Text continued on p. 294.

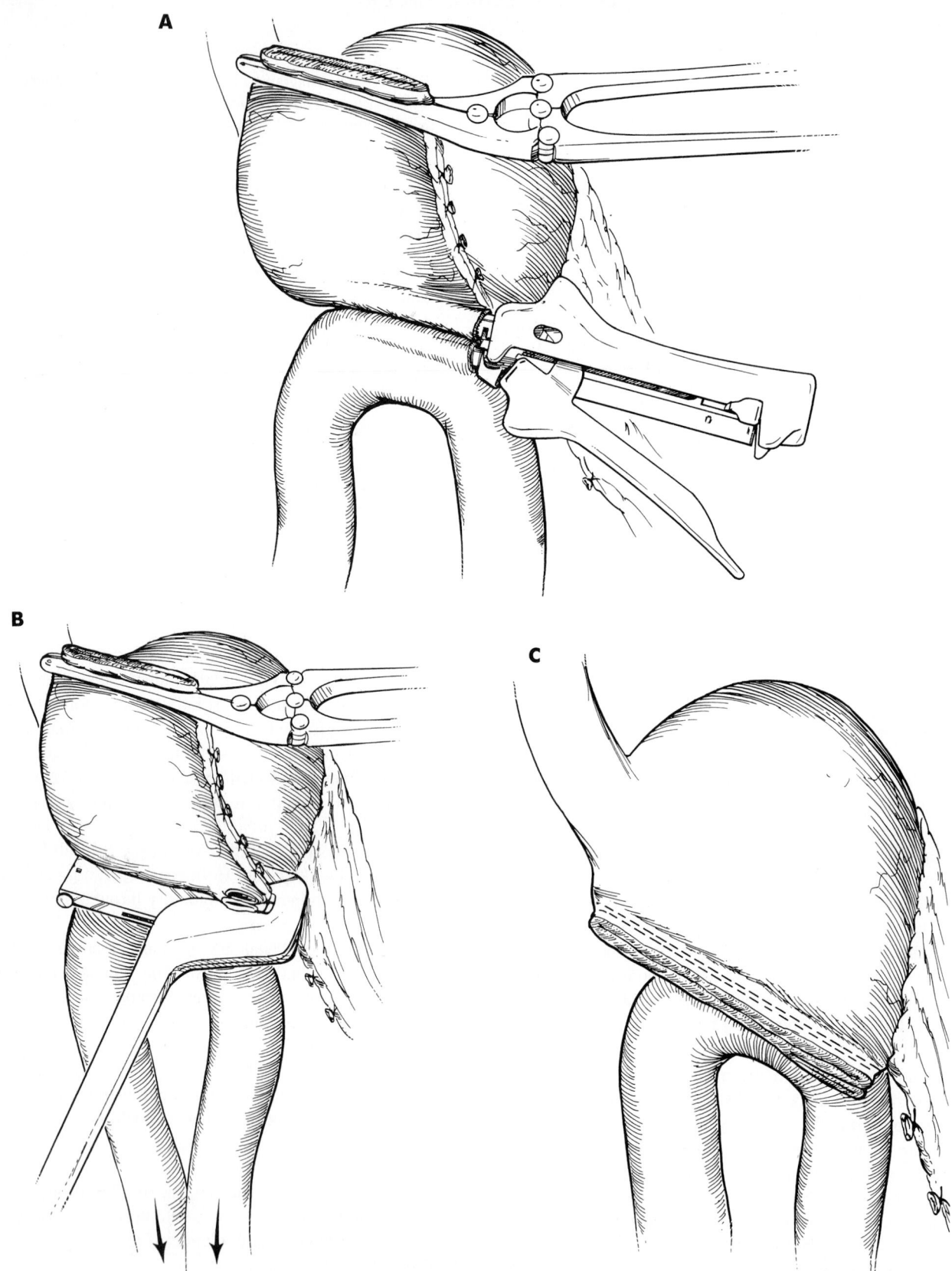

FIG. 10-31 Subtotal gastrectomy with stapled Billroth II anastomosis. **A,** The distal stomach has been dissected free and resected just distal to the pylorus. A proximal limb of jejunum is brought up to anastomose to the posterior wall of the stomach with a linear stapling instrument that transects between two parallel staple lines. **B,** The stomach is elevated and a 90 staple mechanical stapling device is placed across the distal stomach. **C,** Illustration of the completed subtotal gastrectomy with stapled antecolic gastrojejunostomy.

From Thompson, J.C. (1992). *Atlas of surgery of the stomach, duodenum, and small bowel*, St. Louis: Mosby.

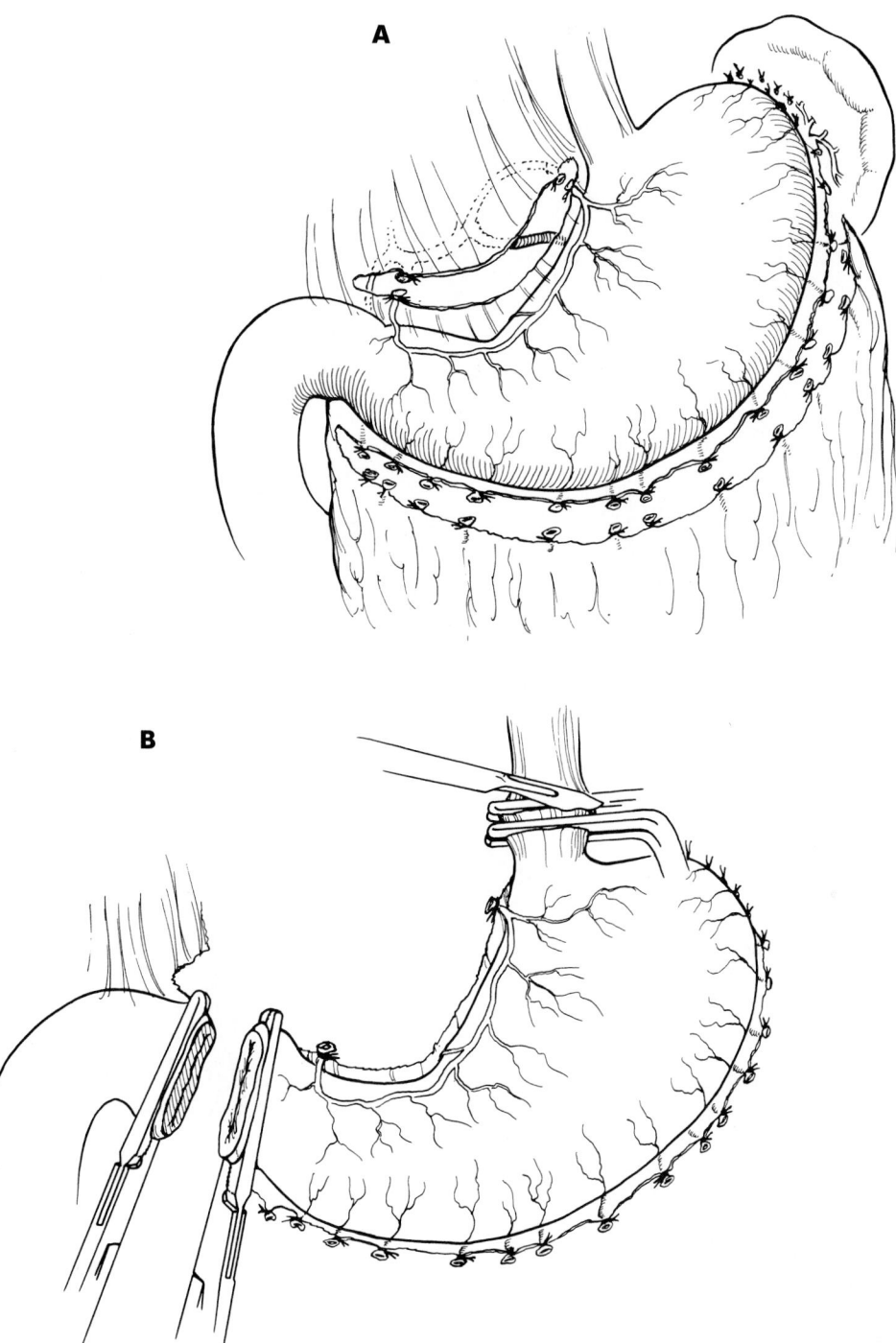

FIG. 10-32   Total gastrectomy may be performed for benign or malignant disease. **A** demonstrates the mobilization of the stomach for benign disease. Serial division of the vessels in the gastrocolic ligament and gastrohepatic ligament are performed to free the greater and lesser omentum. The short gastric vessels connecting the stomach to the spleen are divided and the spleen is preserved. **B,** The duodenum is divided distal to the pylorus and the proximal line of division is at the distal intraabdominal esophagus.

Continued.

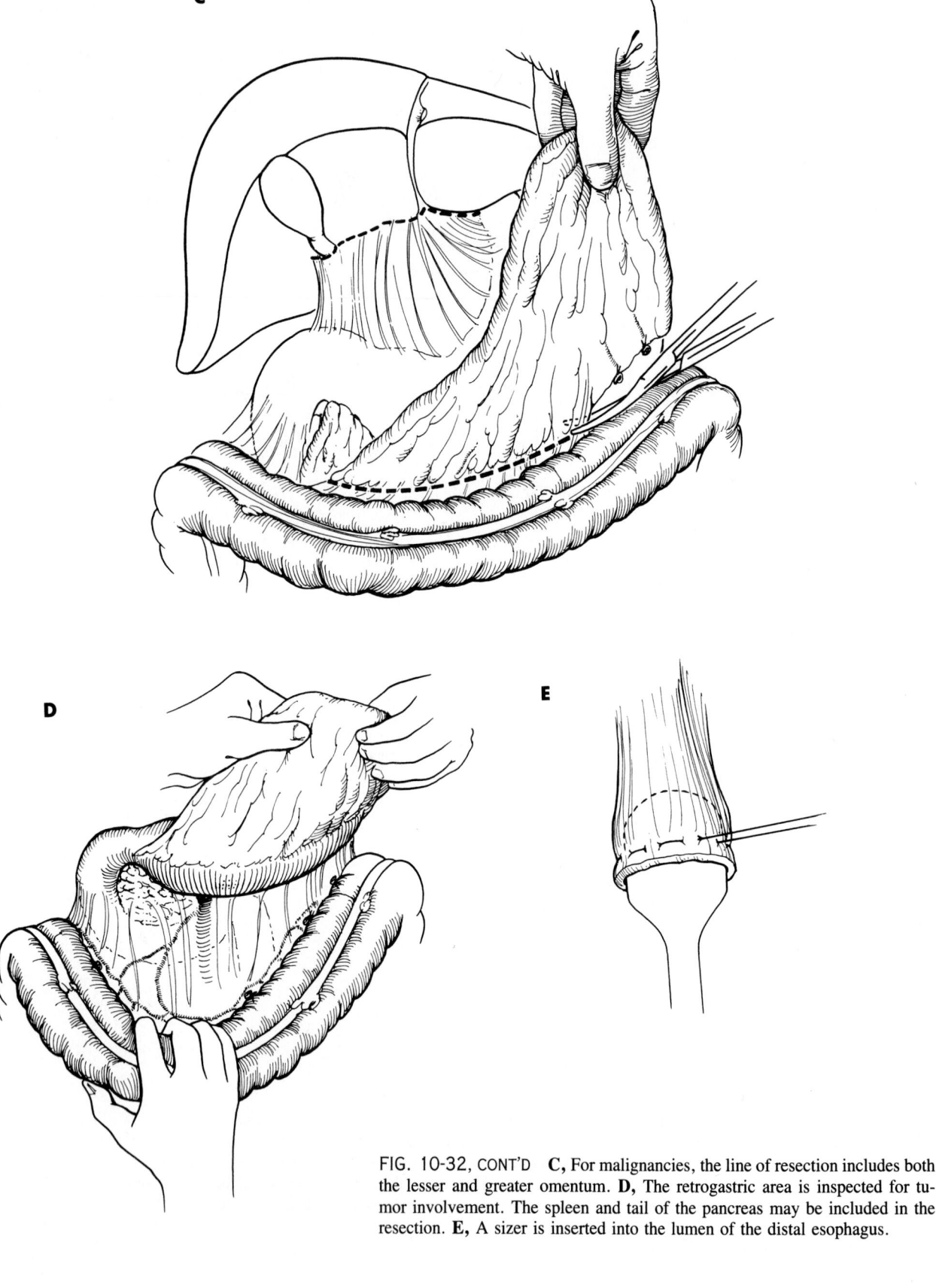

FIG. 10-32, CONT'D   **C,** For malignancies, the line of resection includes both the lesser and greater omentum. **D,** The retrogastric area is inspected for tumor involvement. The spleen and tail of the pancreas may be included in the resection. **E,** A sizer is inserted into the lumen of the distal esophagus.

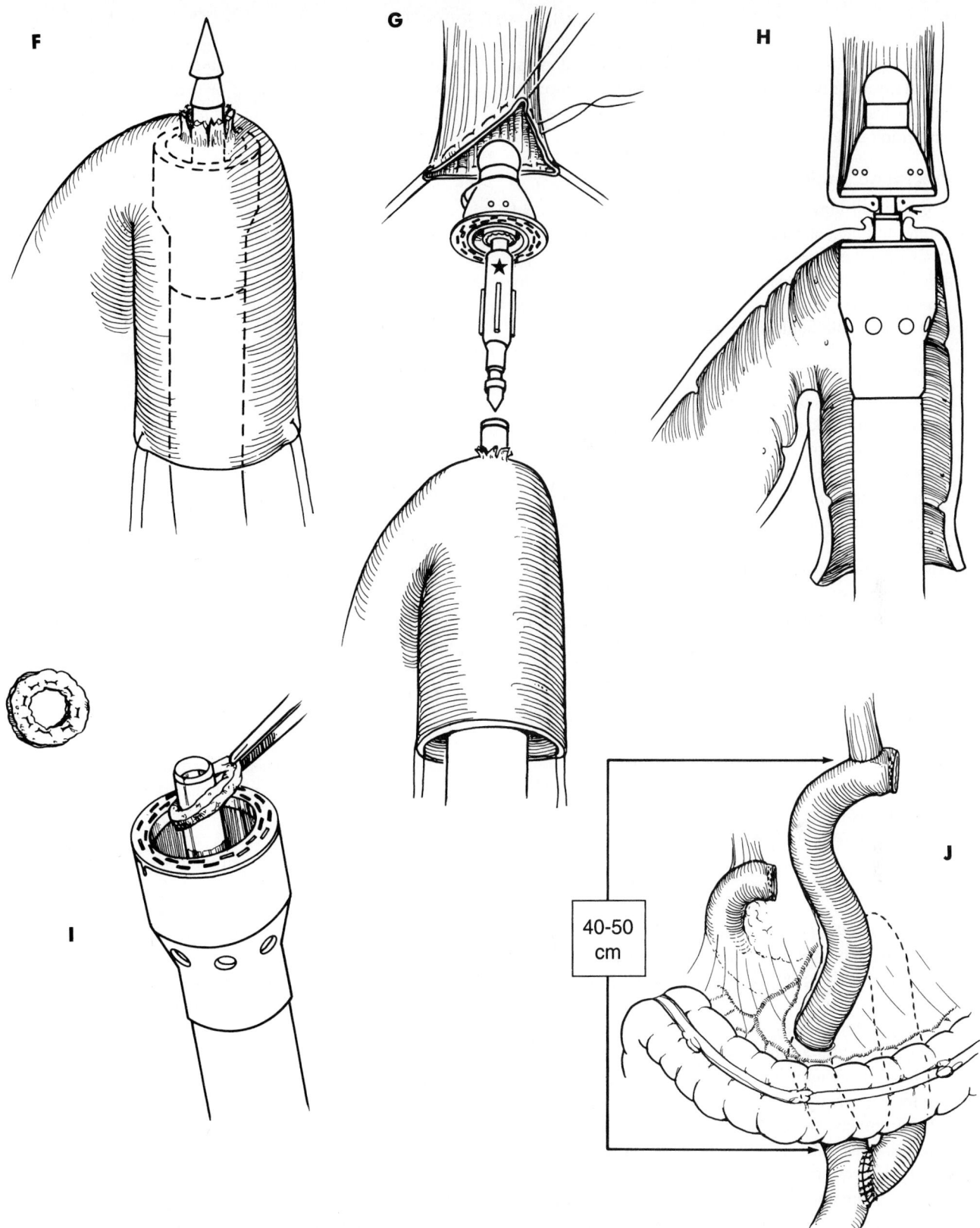

FIG. 10-32, CONT'D **F,** The EEA or ILA is inserted into the lumen of the jejunum to facilitate esophagojejunostomy. **G,** The anvil is inserted into the distal esophagus where purse-string sutures will be
snugged around the protruding arm of the anvil. **H,** The distal esophagus and the jejunum are brought
together by the mechanism of the stapling device, and the interluminal anastomosis will be performed. **I,**
The "donuts," distal esophagus and jejunal tissues, are examined for integrity and completeness. **J,** Illustration of the esophagojejunostomy completed.

From Thompson, J.C. (1992). *Atlas of surgery of the stomach, duodenum, and small bowel,* St. Louis: Mosby.

teroenterostomy, if indicated. Total gastrectomy is done as a potentially curative or palliative procedure to remove a malignant lesion of the stomach and metastases in the adjacent lymph nodes.

Procedural considerations

The incision may be bilateral subcostal, long transrectus, long midline, or thoracoabdominal. A basic throacotomy set (if a thoracoabdominal incision is to be used; see Chapter 24), a gastrointestinal set, as well as a laparotomy set are necessary. Also, two long, blunt, nerve hooks and two 10-inch needle holders are used.

Operative procedure

1. The abdomen is opened, and the wound edges are protected and retracted, as previously described.
2. Careful and complete exploration for the extent of metastasis is carried out.
3. The omentum is freed from the colon, using sharp dissection; vessels are ligated with nonabsorbable no. 2-0 suture.
4. The splenic vessels are ligated and transfixed with nonabsorbable suture, nos. 2-0 and 3-0, at the tail of the pancreas; the spleen is left attached to the omentum.
5. The duodenum is mobilized, intestinal clamps are applied, and the operative field is protected for transsection and closure of the distal duodenum.
6. The right gastric artery is ligated and transfixed with nonabsorbable suture nos. 2-0 and 3-0, and the gastrohepatic omentum is separated from the liver. Following ligation of the left gastric artery, the mobilized stomach, spleen, omentum, and lesser and greater curvature ligamentous attachments are delivered into the wound.
7. Division of the coronary ligament of the left lobe of the liver permits exposure of the diaphragmatic peritoneum over the esophagogastric junction. The liver is protected by moist packs, and gentle retraction is maintained with a Harrington, Deaver, or malleable retractor.
8. A flap of peritoneum is freed from the diaphragm, and branches of the vagus nerves are divided.
9. A loop of jejunum is selected and delivered antecolic to the esophagogastric junction for anastomosis. With the specimen for traction, the posterior layer of interrupted nonabsorbable no. 3-0 sutures is inserted or stapling devices are utilized.
10. As the jejunum and the esophagus are incised, bleeding is controlled by mosquito hemostats and ligatures of synthetic absorbable suture no. 3-0. The posterior layer is reinforced with synthetic absorbable suture no. 3-0, intestinal, interrupted sutures, or a linear staple line.
11. Division of the esophagus is completed, and the entire specimen is removed. Interrupted, synthetic absorbable no. 4-0 sutures also are used to approximate the mu-

cosal anterior wall of the anastomosis. A second layer of sutures, nonabsorbable or synthetic absorbable no. 3-0, is placed anterior in the seromuscular and muscular coat of the intestine. A flap of the peritoneum is attached to the jejunum with interrupted no. 3-0 nonabsorbable sutures to relieve traction on the anastomosis. A lateral jejunojejunal anastomosis is completed to permit irritating bile and pancreatic fluids to bypass the anastomosis line, thereby preventing esophageal regurgitation. The alternative to using suture materials is the use of mechanical stapling devices. Another method of establishing continuity is a combination of a Roux-en-Y jejunojejunstomy and a jejunoesophagostomy.

12. The abdominal wound is closed in layers. If retention sutures are used, they must be placed extraperitoneally because of the absence of omentum to protect the small bowel.

SURGERY OF THE SMALL BOWEL
OPERATION FOR MECKEL'S DIVERTICULUM

Meckel's diverticulum is removed to prevent inflammation and obstruction from intussusception of the diverticulum. Meckel's diverticulum consists of an unobliterated congenital duct at the umbilicus that is attached to the distal ileum (Fig. 10-33). The diverticulum may contain gastric mucosa, which may ulcerate, perforate, or bleed.

Procedural considerations

A laparotomy set and gastrointestinal instrument set are required. A linear stapling instrument should be available.

Operative procedure

1. The abdomen is opened, and the diverticulum is identified.
2. If the diverticulum is long and narrow with a narrow base, the procedure is similar to that of an appendectomy.
3. If the base is broad, the loop of bowel containing the diverticulum is isolated from the mesentery, and a limited small bowel resection is performed.
4. An anastomosis of the divided ends is completed with an inner continuous layer of synthetic absorbable suture no. 3-0 and an interrupted outer layer of nonabsorbable no. 4-0 sutures.
5. The wound is closed as in a laparotomy.

APPENDECTOMY

Appendectomy is the severance and removal of the appendix from its attachment to the cecum through a right lower quadrant muscle-splitting (McBurney) incision. This procedure is performed to remove an acutely inflamed appendix, thereby controlling the spread of infection and reducing the danger of peritonitis. A normal appendix is sometimes removed when the abdomen is opened for another procedure.

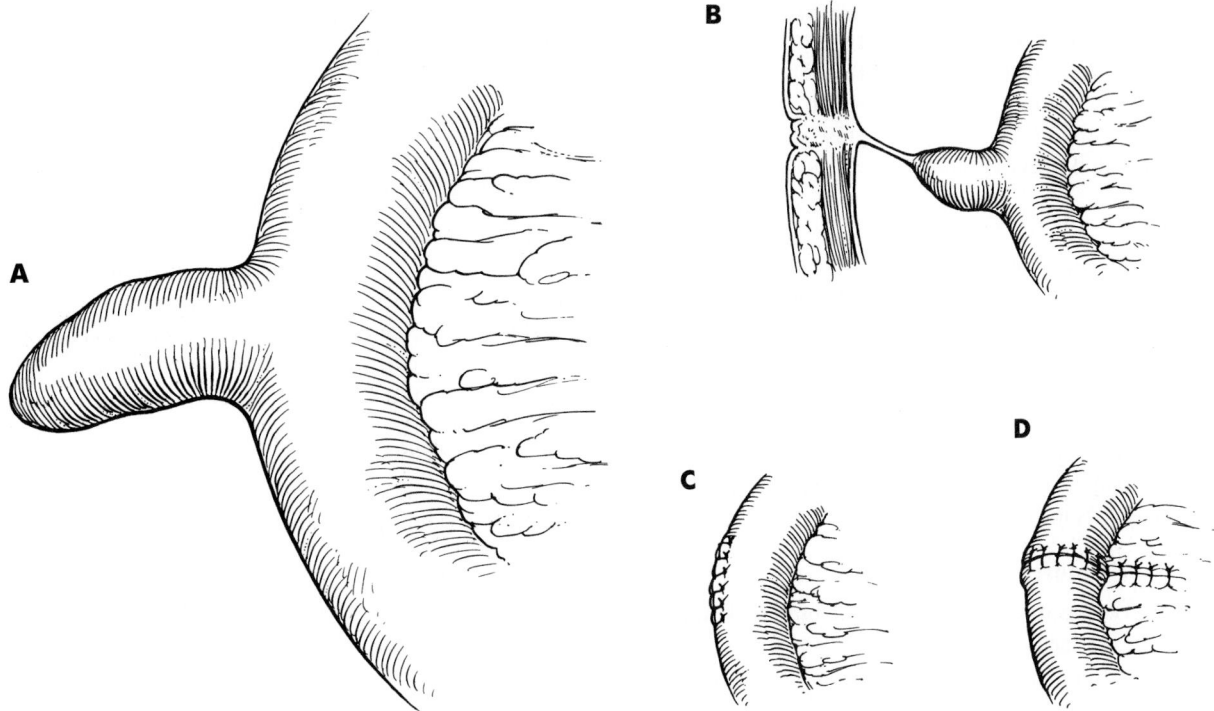

FIG. 10-33 **A,** The most common nonpathologic appearance of Meckel's diverticulum arises from the antimesenteric border of the distal ileum. **B,** A persistent fibrous band of tissue connects the apex of the diverticulum to the anterior abdominal wall at the umbilicus. **C,** Demonstrates the suture line of a local Meckel's diverticulectomy. **D,** Illustration of completed ileoileal anastomosis after excision of 1 to 2 cm of ileum on each side of a Meckel's diverticulum.

From Thompson, J.C. (1992). *Atlas of surgery of the stomach, duodenum, and small bowel,* St. Louis: Mosby.

Procedural considerations

Instrumentation is the same as for a laparotomy.

Operative procedure

1. A right lower quadrant muscle-splitting incision usually is made.
2. Muscles are retracted with Richardson or Parker retractors to expose the peritoneum.
3. The peritoneum is grasped with tissue forceps or Allis forceps, and a small incision is made with a scalpel using a no. 15 blade. A culture sample may be taken. The incision is completed with Metzenbaum scissors.
4. The mesoappendix is grasped near the tip with a Babcock forceps or a hemostat for gentle traction. The mesoappendix is dissected from the appendiceal wall by hemostats and ligated with nonabsorbable no. 3-0. If a suture ligature is required, synthetic absorbable suture no. 2-0 on an atraumatic gastrointestinal needle is preferred.
5. The appendix is elevated as a pursestring suture of synthetic absorbable suture no. 2-0 is placed in the cecal wall at the appendiceal base.
   a. The base of the appendix is crushed with a straight hemostat, a synthetic absorbable suture no. 3-0 tie is placed over the crushed area, and a hemostat is placed above the ligature.
   b. A basin is provided for the specimen and discarded instruments that have come in contact with gastrointestinal mucosa.
   c. Protective gauze sponges are placed over the cecum around the base of the appendix. The appendix is amputated between the clamp and synthetic absorbable suture with a scalpel. Sometimes the stump is swabbed with alcohol or betadine solution to reduce bacterial flora.
   d. The appendiceal stump may be inverted into the lumen of the cecum as the pursestring suture is tightened and tied by means of a fine straight hemostat and a small sponge on a holder. Soiled instruments are discarded in the basin.
   e. The abdomen is closed in the usual manner.
6. If the appendix has ruptured, copious amounts of liquid are used to irrigate the peritoneal cavity. A drain may be inserted down to the appendiceal bed to allow continuous drainage. Deeper layers are closed, leaving the

subcutaneous tissue and skin open. The wound may then be packed open with moist, fine-mesh gauze, and healing by secondary intention is permitted. This packing method may be used in any case in which bowel contamination or abscess formation is present. It allows clean healing and prevents pocketing of pus.

LAPAROSCOPIC APPENDECTOMY

A laparoscopic approach to appendectomy is gaining popularity and may be the surgeon's preferred technique at many institutions.

Procedural considerations

The procedure involves the placement of three trocars with the standard laparoscopic equipment and supplies available. The patient is positioned supine, and the pneumoperitoneum is obtained in the usual manner.

Operative procedure

1. An 11- or 12-mm trocar is placed in the umbilicus for insertion of the laparoscope.
2. An 11- or 12-mm trocar is placed in the right upper quadrant (RUQ) to serve as the working port.
3. The 5-mm trocar placed in the midline suprapubic site serves as the traction trocar.
4. A laparoscopic Babcock instrument is inserted into the RUQ trocar to grasp the cecum and retract it toward the liver.
5. The appendix is grasped at its tip by a grasping forcep that has been inserted through the suprapubic trocar and is held in an upward position.
6. The Babcock forceps are removed and a dissecting instrument is inserted through the RUQ trocar to create a mesenteric window in the mesoappendix. Dissection is performed in close proximity to the appendix beginning directly under the base and progressing to a 1- to 2-cm length.
7. Depending on the surgeon's preferred technique, the appendix may be transsected in several different ways:
   a. By an endoscopic linear stapling instrument
   b. By a ligating loop instrument
   c. By a suturing instrument
8. If an endoscopic linear stapling instrument is used, the lower jaw of the stapling device is passed through the mesenteric window previously created via the RUQ trocar.
9. The grasping forceps are used to rotate the tip of the appendix so that the stapling device can be snugged to the base of the appendix and closed.
10. The stapling instrument is fired and withdrawn, and the staple line is inspected.
11. The remainder of the mesoappendix is dissected, hemostasis is achieved, and the appendix is removed via the RUQ port. If the appendix is too thick, a specimen pouch may be necessary to facilitate its extraction.

12. The abdomen is irrigated, the irrigation fluid is aspirated with a suction/irrigation device, and then the abdomen is desufflated.
13. Trocar sites are closed and dressed in the usual fashion.

RESECTION OF THE SMALL INTESTINE

Resection of the small intestine involves excision of the diseased intestine through an abdominal incision and frequently includes some type of bowel reanastomosis. It is performed to remove certain tumors, a gangrenous portion of the intestine caused by strangulation from bands of adhesions, a herniation of the intestine, or a volvulus.

Procedural considerations

A laparotomy set and gastrointestinal instrument set are required. Linear stapling instruments should be available.

Operative procedure

1. The abdominal wall is incised and retracted; the peritoneal cavity is explored and protected with moist, warm packs.
2. The clamps are placed above and below the diseased segment of the bowel and mesentery. The involved area is removed with a linear stapling instrument such as a GIA, electrosurgical blade, or a scalpel.
3. The continuity of the gastrointestinal tract is established by an end-to-end, and end-to-side, or a side-to-side anastomosis.
4. The wound is closed and dressed.

An alternative approach to a traditional suture anastomosis is the use of a mechanical stapling device (Fig. 10-34). The device allows the surgeon to perform an end-to-end, end-to-side, or side-to-side anastomosis. An enterotomy is made close to the anatomosis site. The stapler is inserted, and the distal bowel is secured between the anvil and the head of the stapler (Fig. 10-35). The anvil is then inserted into the proximal loop of bowel and secured to the center rod. The gap is closed, and the stapler fired. The stapler is extracted through the enterotomy. The integrity of the anastomosis is verified, and the enterotomy is closed with sutures.

ILEOSTOMY

Ileostomy is the formation of a temporary or permanent opening into the ileum. This procedure is generally done when an extensive lesion is present either to reduce activity in the colon by means of diversions or when all the large bowel has been resected.

Procedural considerations

A laparotomy set and gastrointestinal instrument set are required. Linear stapling instruments will be used. An ostomy appliance for the stoma should be available.

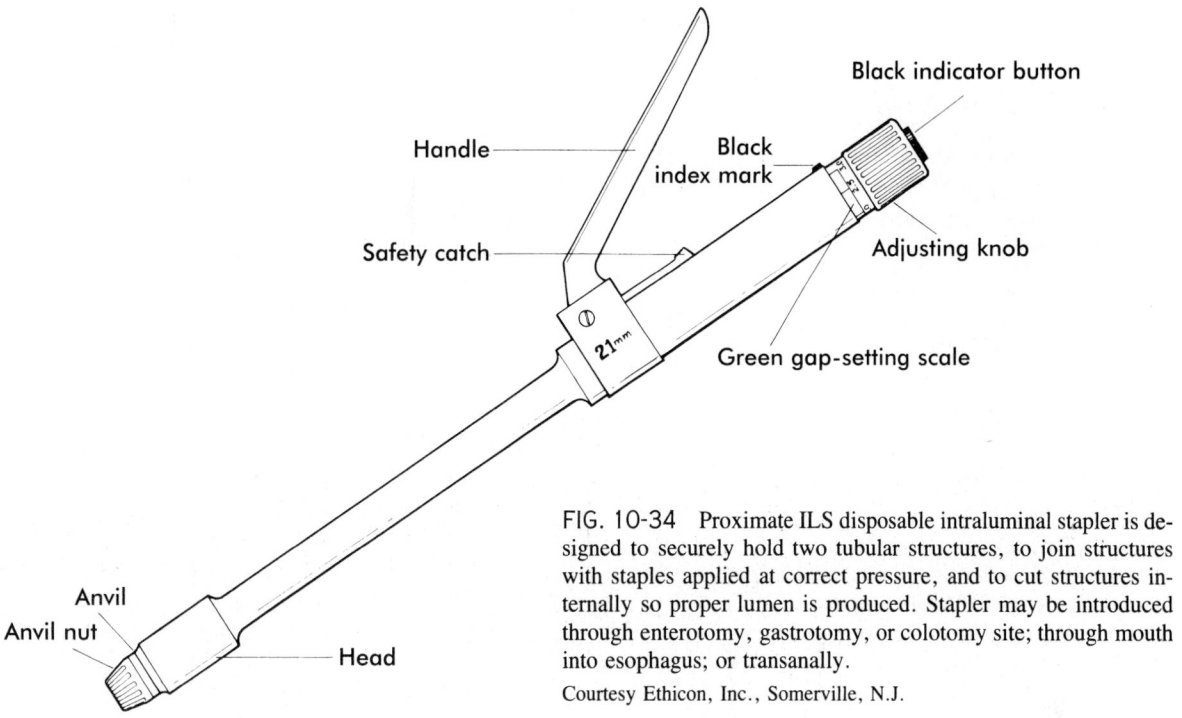

Handle

Safety catch

Black index mark

Black indicator button

Adjusting knob

Green gap-setting scale

21mm

Anvil
Anvil nut
Head

FIG. 10-34 Proximate ILS disposable intraluminal stapler is designed to securely hold two tubular structures, to join structures with staples applied at correct pressure, and to cut structures internally so proper lumen is produced. Stapler may be introduced through enterotomy, gastrotomy, or colotomy site; through mouth into esophagus; or transanally.

Courtesy Ethicon, Inc., Somerville, N.J.

Operative procedure

1. Through a midline incision the peritoneal cavity is explored and the pathologic condition determined.
2. The ileum is mobilized with Metzenbaum scissors and hemostatic clamps. The mesentery is clamped, divided, and ligated with nonabsorbable no. 3-0 sutures at the proposed site, usually about 15 cm from the ileocecal junction.
3. Two intestinal clamps are placed on the bowel, and the ileum is divided with a scalpel or linear stapling instrument (GIA) between the two clamps.
4. The distal end of the ileum is closed with synthetic absorbable suture no. 2-0 on a general closure needle if a stapling device has not been used.
5. The proximal end is brought out to the skin through an opening on the right side and is held in place by clamps, making sure that the ileum is not overstretched or its blood supply compromised. The mesentery of the ileum is sutured to the parietal wall to eliminate a potential internal hernia. The abdomen is then closed.
6. The stoma is sutured to the skin after the ileum is everted to form a protective cover over the exposed ileal serosa.
7. A disposable ostomy appliance is placed over the stoma to collect small bowel contents.

An alternative to a conventional ileostomy for selected patients is the Kock pouch, or continent ileostomy. The internal pouch is constructed of small intestine with an outlet to the skin. When it is functioning properly, no stool spontaneously exits from the stoma. A catheter is inserted into the stoma three or four times daily to evacuate the contents. This procedure eliminates the need for an external appliance.

SURGERY OF THE COLON

LAPAROSCOPIC COLECTOMY

Resection of a segment of bowel and an anastomosis can be accomplished using laparoscopic techniques (Quilici, 1992). The advantages of laparoscopic colectomy are the reduction of postoperative ileus and a potential shortening of the recovery period.

Procedural considerations

Depending on the intended segment of bowel to be resected, the patient may be positioned supine or in a modified lithotomy for access to the rectum for end-to-end anastomosis. Laparotomy instrumentation should be available.

To assist the surgeon in accurately identifying the segment of bowel to be resected, a colonoscope may be used preoperatively or during the laparoscopic procedure to tattoo the lesion with methylene blue.

Operative procedure

1. Pneumoperitoneum is created and the 10-mm umbilical trocar is placed for insertion of the laparoscope.
2. Usually two 12-mm trocars are placed in locations dependent on the anatomic segment of colon that will be resected.

TA® PRODUCTS

MULTIFIRE TA™ Reloadable Disposable Surgical Staplers with TITANIUM Staples

- MULTIFIRE TA™ 30-3.5
- MULTIFIRE TA™ 30-4.8
- MULTIFIRE TA™ 55-3.5
- MULTIFIRE TA™ 55-4.8

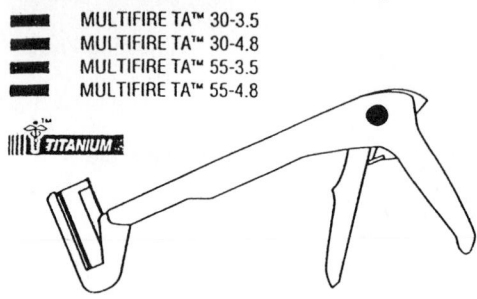

MULTIFIRE TA™ Disposable Loading Units with TITANIUM Staples

- MULTIFIRE TA™ 30-3.5
- MULTIFIRE TA™ 30-4.8
- MULTIFIRE TA™ 55-3.5
- MULTIFIRE TA™ 55-4.8

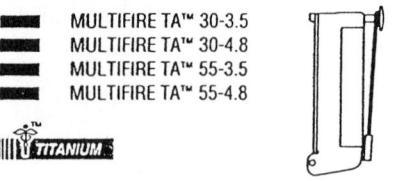

Disposable TA® Long Staplers

- Disposable TA® 30 V-3 Long
- Disposable TA® 90 Long-3.5
- Disposable TA® 90 Long-4.8

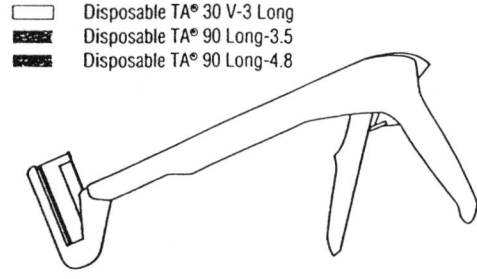

ROTICULATOR® PRODUCTS

ROTICULATOR® Disposable Surgical Staplers with TITANIUM Staples

- ROTICULATOR® 30-3.5
- ROTICULATOR® 30-4.8
- ROTICULATOR® 30-V3
- ROTICULATOR® 55-3.5
- ROTICULATOR® 55-4.8

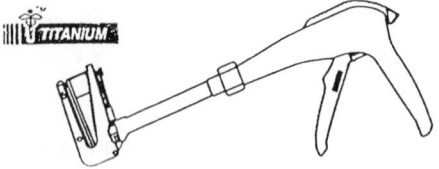

TA PRODUCTS ARE USED TO DELIVER A LINEAR LINE OF STAPLES THAT PROVIDE FOR CLOSURE AND HEMOSTASIS OF TISSUE WHILE PERMITTING TISSUE PERFUSION AND OXYGENATION.

THE STAPLES ARE PROVIDED IN VARIOUS MATERIALS, ABSORBABLE AND NONABSORBABLE.

THE LENGTH OF THE STAPLE USED IS DEPENDENT UPON THE TYPE AND THICKNESS OF TISSUE APPLICATION.

MANUFACTURER'S RECOMMENDATIONS FOR USE OF THE MECHANICAL STAPLING DEVICES ARE FOLLOWED FOR PATIENT SAFETY.

TA PRODUCTS ARE COMMONLY USED ON SUCH TISSUES AS STOMACH, BOWEL, AND THE RECTUM IN GASTROINTESTINAL PROCEDURES. TA PRODUCTS MAY ALSO BE USED ON VASCULAR STRUCTURES AND THE BRONCHUS.

THE ROTICULATOR TA PRODUCTS ASSIST THE SURGEON IN THE RESECTION OF STRUCTURES SUCH AS THE RECTUM, IN WHICH MANIPULATION OF THE STAPLING DEVICE COMPROMISED BY THE SURROUNDING ANATOMICAL STRUCTURES.

FIG. 10-35   Various linear stapling instruments that are both disposable and reloadable.

GIA™ PRODUCTS

GIA 50 PREMIUM™
GIA 90 PREMIUM™
MULTIFIRE GIA™ 60
MULTIFIRE GIA™ 80

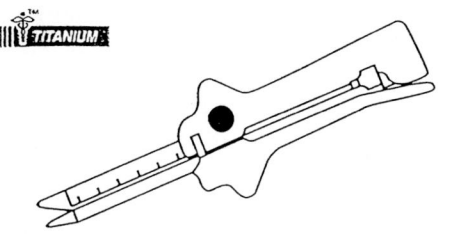

GIA PRODUCTS DELIVER A
PARALLEL LINE OF STAPLES
THEN TRANSECT THE TISSUES.
THE GIA PRODUCTS PROVIDE THE
SURGEON WITH A CHOICE OF
STAPLE LENGTHS AND MATERIALS.
THE LENGTH OF THE STAPLE
LINE IS DEPENDENT ON THE
WIDTH OF THE STRUCTURE
BEING TRANSECTED.

GIA™ Disposable Loading Units

MULTIFIRE GIA™ 60
MULTIFIRE GIA™ 80
GIA 50 PREMIUM™
SGIA 50 PREMIUM™
GIA 90 PREMIUM™
SGIA 90 PREMIUM™

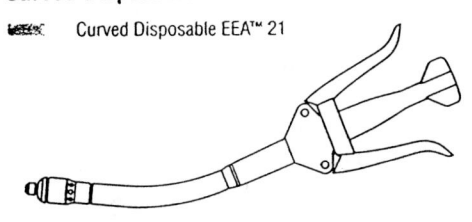

GIA PRODUCTS ARE COMMONLY USED
ON THE STOMACH, SMALL BOWEL,
PANCREAS, COLON, AND RECTUM
IN GASTROINTESTINAL SURGERY.
GIA PRODUCTS MAY ALSO BE
USED FOR THORACIC SURGERY.

EEA™ PRODUCTS

Curved Disposable EEA™ 21

    Curved Disposable EEA™ 21

EEA PRODUCTS ARE INTENDED FOR
INTRALUMINAL AND END-TO-END
ANASTOMOSIS OF TISSUES. THE EEA
PRODUCTS PROVIDE A CIRCULAR
STAPLE LINE TO THE PROXIMAL
AND DISTAL TISSUES AND TRANSECT
THE TISSUE CIRCULARLY. THE TISSUE
TRANSECTED IS REMOVED WITH THE
INSTRUMENT. RESEMBLING "DONUTS",
THE RESECTED TISSUE IS EXAMINED
FOR CONTINUITY TO ENSURE AN
OPTIMAL ANASTOMOSIS.

PREMIUM CEEA™ Disposable Surgical Staplers

    PREMIUM CEEA™ 25
    PREMIUM CEEA™ 28
    PREMIUM CEEA™ 31

THE EEA PRODUCTS ARE COMMONLY
USED FOR SUCH PROCEDURES AS
LOW ANTERIOR RESECTION,
ESOPHAGOGASTRECTOMY, AND
ESOPHAGECTOMY.

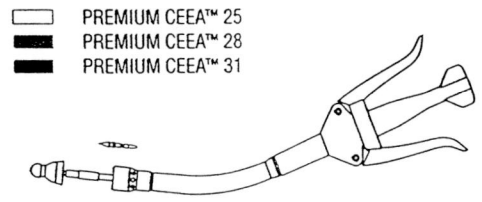

FIG. 10-35, CONT'D   Various linear stapling instruments that are both disposable and reloadable.

Continued.

LDS™ PRODUCTS

Powered Disposable LDS™ Stapler with TITANIUM staples

Powered Disposable LDS™ -15W

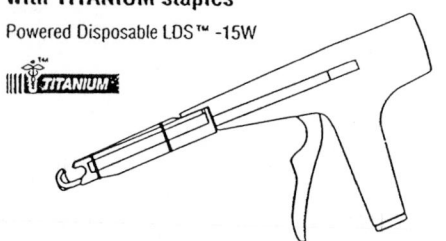

LDS PRODUCTS ARE USED TO LIGATE AND DIVIDE VASCULAR TISSUE SUCH AS IN THE OMENTUM. THE POWERED LDS DELIVERS THE LIGATING CLIPS AND TISSUE DISSECTION IN A QUICK AND EFFICIENT MANNER, REDUCING GRASPING FATIGUE FOR THE SURGEON.

LDS™ Disposable Loading Units for use with LDS™-2 Instrument

LDS™-6
LDS™-6W
LDS™-15
LDS™-15W

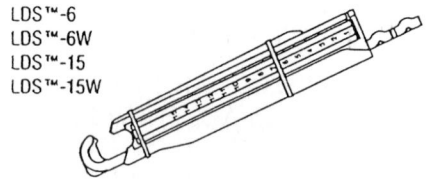

THIS LDS CARTRIDGE FITS THE NONDISPOSABLE LDS DEVICE.

OCCLUDING CLIPS

PREMIUM SURGICLIP™ Clip Appliers with TITANIUM Clips

PREMIUM SURGICLIP™ S-9.0˚
PREMIUM SURGICLIP™ M-9.75˚
PREMIUM SURGICLIP™ M-11.5˚
PREMIUM SURGICLIP™ L-13.0˚

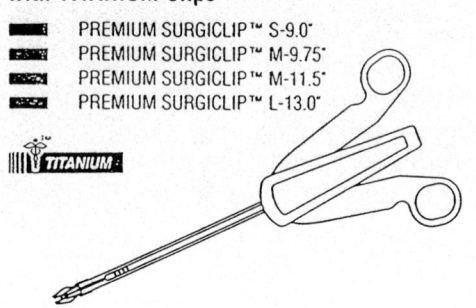

OCCLUDING CLIPS ENABLE THE SURGEON THE CONVENIENCE AND EFFICIENCY OF A LOADED APPLIER, THUS PROVIDING CONTINUITY IN APPLICATION TO VASCULAR STRUCTURES.

THE LENGTH OF THE APPLIER AND SIZE OF OCCLUDING CLIP USED IS DEPENDENT UPON THE DEPTH AND VOLUME OF TISSUE BEING ADDRESSED.

SURGICLIP® Clip Appliers with TITANIUM Clips

SURGICLIP® M-9.5˚
SURGICLIP® M-11.0˚

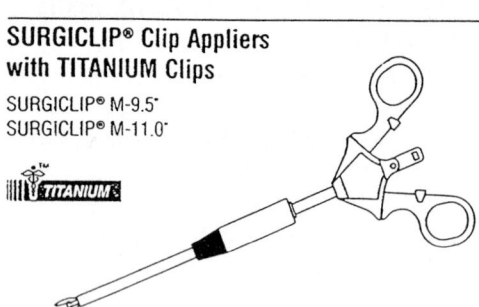

FIG. 10-35, CONT'D   Various linear stapling instruments that are both disposable and reloadable.

3. Dissecting forceps are used to establish a mesenteric window as the bowel segment is held with Babcock forceps.
4. A multifire endoscopic linear stapling device (GIA) is positioned appropriately over the segment of bowel and fired to both transsect and staple the segment.
5. Unless an end-to-end anastomosis can be performed, as in a low sigmoid or rectal resection, a small incision is made over the area of the abdomen, which will provide the best access to the segments for anastomosis.
6. The segment of bowel to be resected is brought through the small laparotomy incision and transsected, and anastomosis is performed by the surgeon's preferred manner.
7. The anastomosed bowel is then dropped back into the peritoneal cavity, the cavity is well irrigated and suctioned, and closure commences after hemostasis is ensured.

COLOSTOMY

Colostomy is mobilization of a loop of colon through a right rectus incision to expose the transverse colon. A left rectus incision can also be made to expose the descending sigmoid colon. The layers of the wound beneath or around the colostomy are subsequently closed. A colostomy is performed to treat an obstruction in the sigmoid colon resulting from a malignant lesion. Another possible indication for this procedure is advanced inflammation or trauma that has caused distention or obstruction of the proximal portion of the colon. A temporary colostomy is often done to decompress the bowel or to give the bowel a rest (Fig. 10-36).

Procedural considerations

A laparotomy set and gastrointestinal instrument set are required. Linear stapling instruments may be used. Stoma appliances as determined by the surgeon are required. These items may include a glass rod, rubber tubing, or a loop ostomy bridge.

Operative procedure
First-stage loop colostomy

1. The abdomen is opened, and the wound edges are protected and retracted. The peritoneal cavity is opened and walled off with moist laparotomy packs, and appropriate retractors are inserted.
2. A small opening is made in the mesentery near the bowel with curved hemostats and Metzenbaum scissors. A piece of tubing is passed around the colon, and the two ends are held with a hemostat to maintain gentle traction.
3. The loop of colon is brought out through an incision made on the left side of the midline.
4. The abdomen is closed.
5. A loop ostomy bridge is used to keep the loop of colon in proper position.
6. The loop of intestine is dressed with petrolatum gauze.

Second-stage loop colostomy

After 48 hours the loop of colon is completely severed by an electrosurgical blade. By this time, if there is no tension, healing has advanced sufficiently to allow protection from feces contamination onto the wound. This procedure is simple and painless and is usually performed in the patient's room or in a treatment room.

Transverse colostomy

1. A short incision, vertical or preferably transverse, is made to reach the transverse colon.
2. A loop of transverse colon, freed of omentum, is withdrawn (Fig. 10-37). A loop ostomy bridge is passed through an avascular area of the mesocolon, preventing the loop from returning to the peritoneal cavity. A mushroom catheter, which is held in place with a pursestring suture, brings about immediate decompression.
3. The bowel is opened 24 to 36 hours later.
4. The bridge may be removed in about 7 to 10 days.

Closure of a colostomy

Closure of a colostomy involves the reestablishment of internal intestinal continuity and repair of the abdominal wall.

Procedural considerations

When the loop has been completely divided, a closed or open anastomosis may be performed. A laparotomy set and gastrointestinal instrument set are required. Linear stapling instruments may be used.

Operative procedure

1. A circumferential incision is made around the colostomy to free the skin margin. Moist packs, a scalpel with a no. 10 blade, Metzenbaum scissors, and Crile hemostats are used as the layers of the abdominal wall are identified and dissected free.
2. An end-to-end anastomosis is completed in two layers, the inner with synthetic absorbable suture no. 3-0 and the outer with nonabsorbable no. 3-0 on an intestinal needle, using interrupted sutures. This anastomosis may be completed with a surgical stapling device.
3. The abdominal wound is closed in layers. A dressing is applied. The surgeon may elect to leave the subcutaneous tissue and skin open. In this instance the wound is packed and permitted to heal by secondary intention.

Right hemicolectomy and ileocolostomy

Right hemicolectomy and ileocolostomy involve the resection of the right half of the colon—including a portion of the transverse colon, the ascending colon, and the cecum—and a segment of the terminal ileum and mesentery (Fig. 10-38, *A*). An end-to-end, side-to-side, or end-to-side anastomosis is done between the transverse colon and the ileum. A right hemicolectomy and ileocolostomy are per-

Text continued on p. 306.

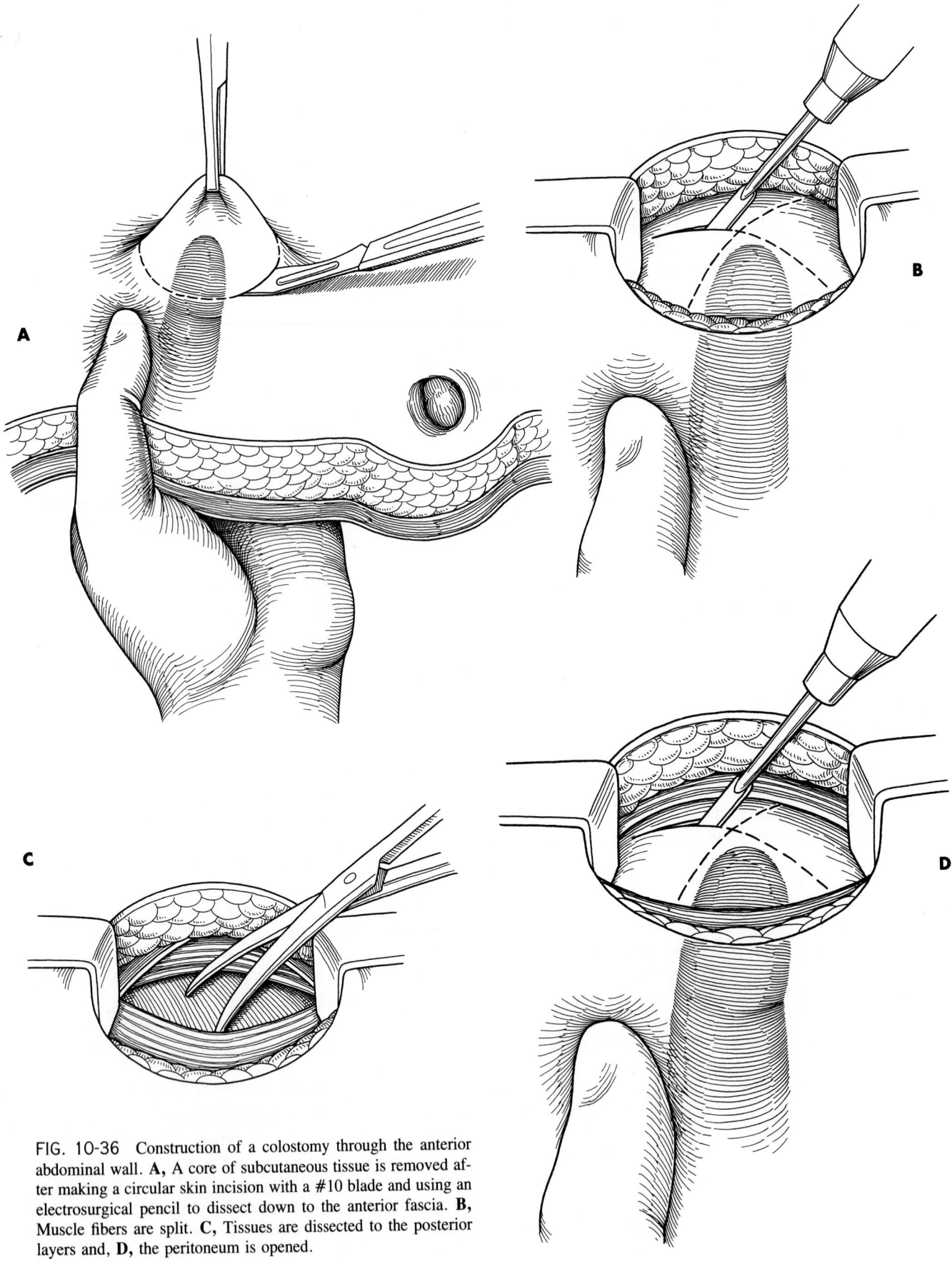

FIG. 10-36 Construction of a colostomy through the anterior abdominal wall. **A,** A core of subcutaneous tissue is removed after making a circular skin incision with a #10 blade and using an electrosurgical pencil to dissect down to the anterior fascia. **B,** Muscle fibers are split. **C,** Tissues are dissected to the posterior layers and, **D,** the peritoneum is opened.

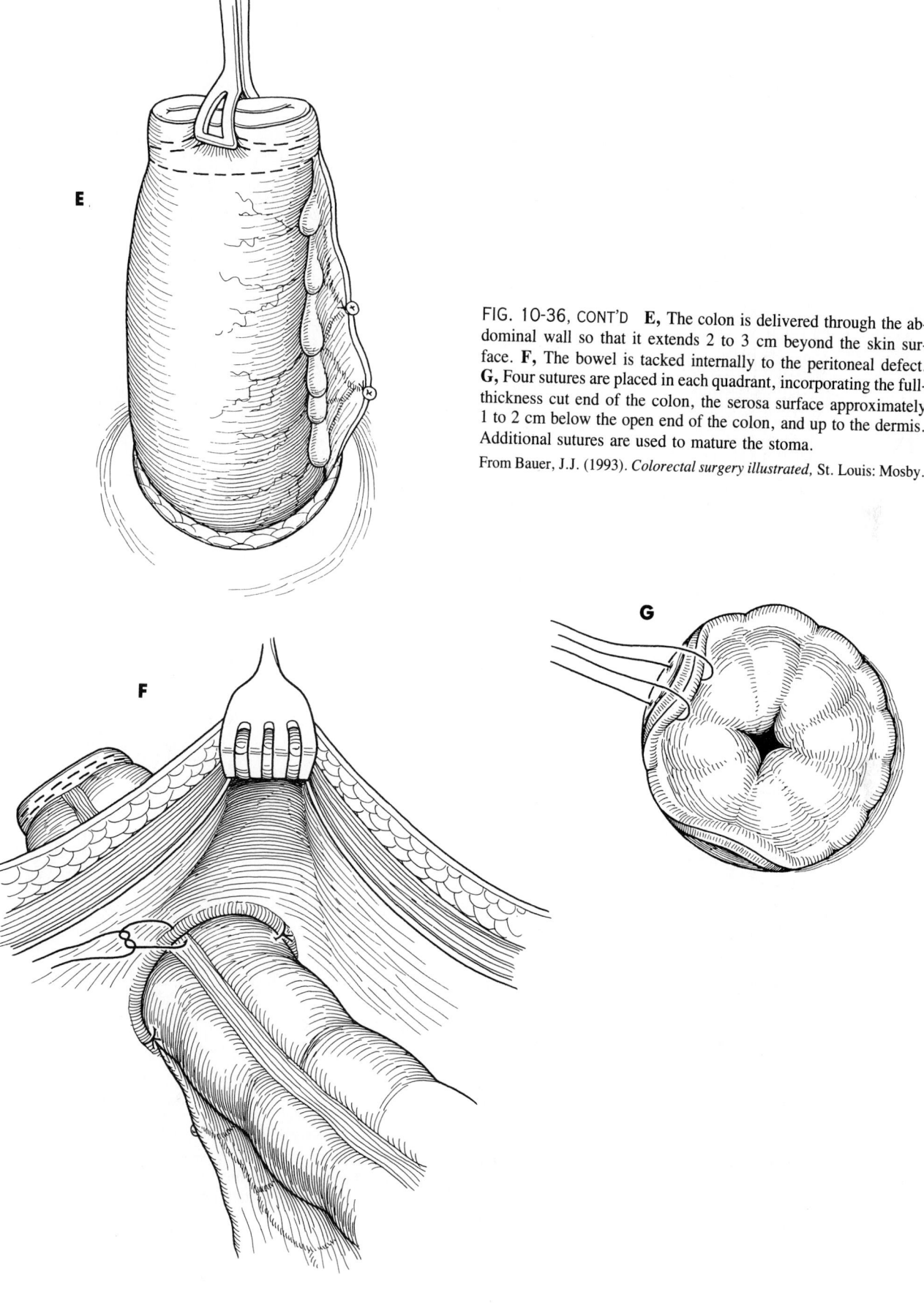

FIG. 10-36, CONT'D **E,** The colon is delivered through the abdominal wall so that it extends 2 to 3 cm beyond the skin surface. **F,** The bowel is tacked internally to the peritoneal defect. **G,** Four sutures are placed in each quadrant, incorporating the full-thickness cut end of the colon, the serosa surface approximately 1 to 2 cm below the open end of the colon, and up to the dermis. Additional sutures are used to mature the stoma.

From Bauer, J.J. (1993). *Colorectal surgery illustrated,* St. Louis: Mosby.

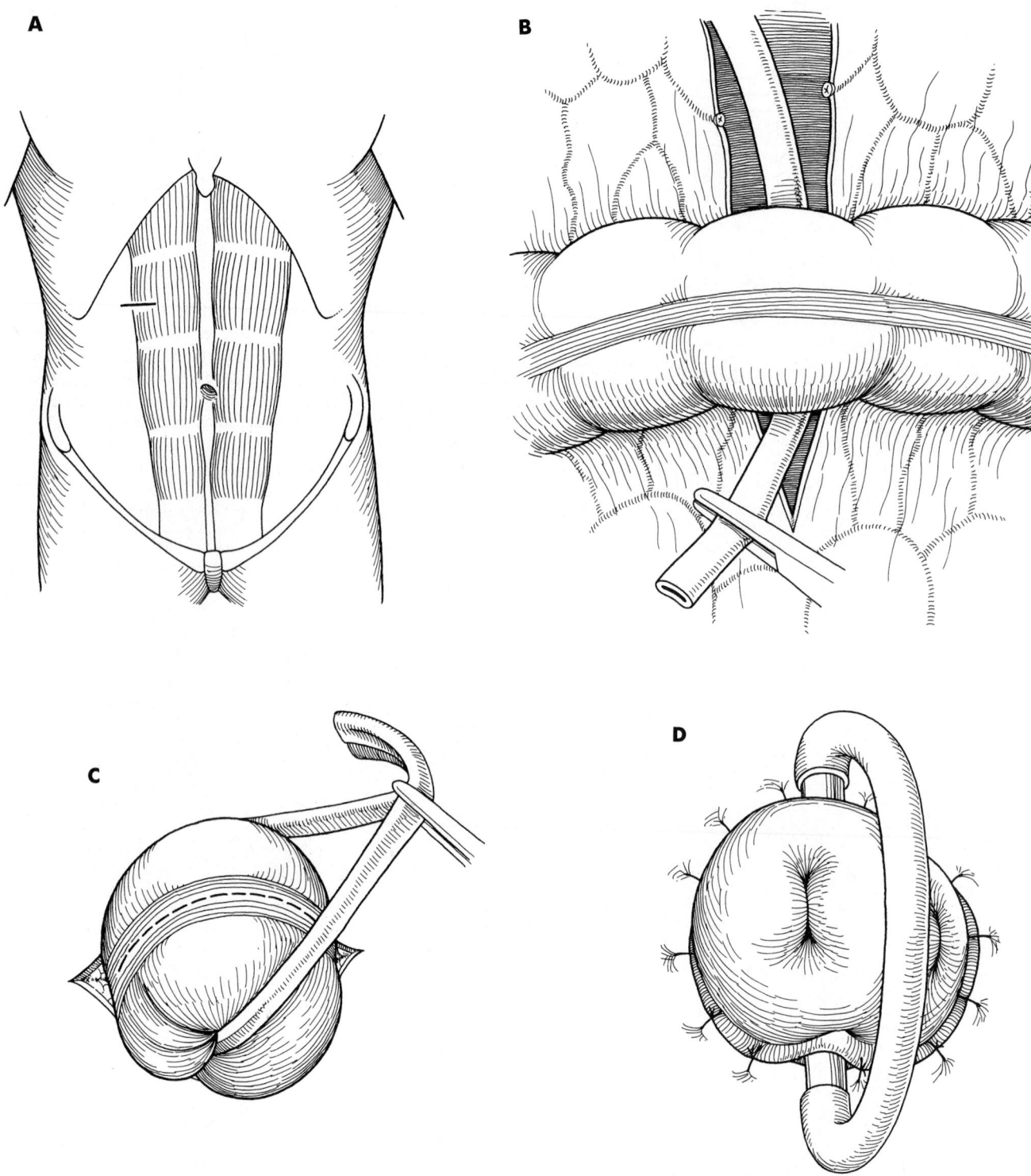

FIG. 10-37 Transverse loop colostomy. **A,** Illustrates a small transverse incision into the abdomen. **B,** The mesentery adjacent to the colon is taken down so that a Penrose drain may be passed beneath the colon. **C,** The colon is pulled through the transverse incision and opened longitudinally along the teniae. **D,** An apparatus or rod is placed underneath the stoma, sutures are used to mature the colostomy. The rod can be removed after the 7th postoperative day.

From Bauer, J.J. (1993). *Colorectal surgery illustrated,* St. Louis: Mosby.

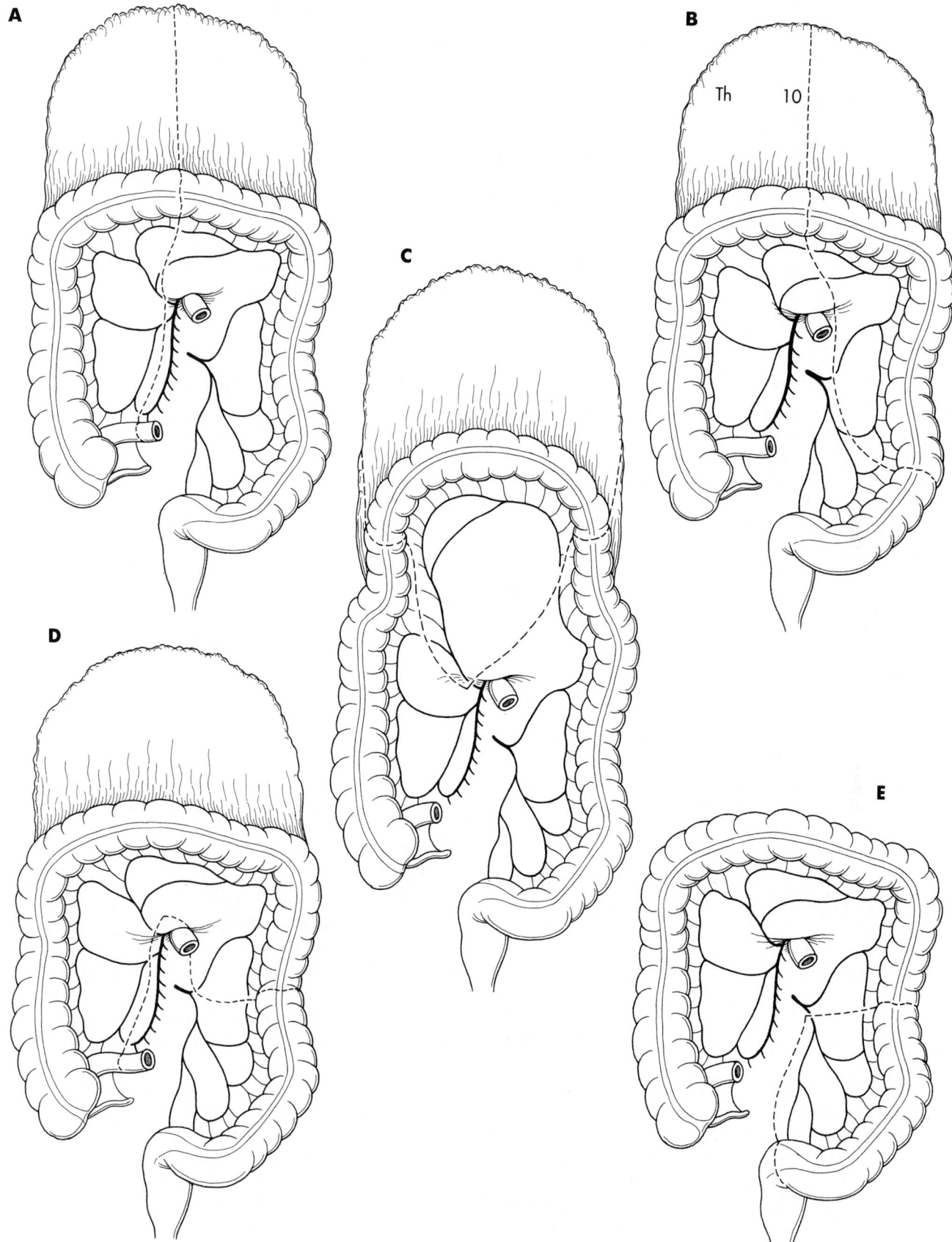

FIG. 10-38 The resection lines for various types of colon resection. **A,** Right hemicolectomy and ileocolostomy; **B,** left hemicolectomy; **C** and **D,** transverse colectomy; and **E,** anterior resection of sigmoid colon and rectosigmoidostomy.

From Bauer, J.J. (1993). *Colorectal surgery illustrated*, St. Louis: Mosby.

formed to remove a malignant lesion of the right colon and in some cases to remove inflammatory lesions involving the ileum, cecum, or ascending colon.

Procedural considerations

When a side-to-side anastomosis is carried out, the transsected stumps of the ileum and the transverse colon are closed before the anastomosis is done. It is completed between the side portions of the ileum and the transverse colon. When an end-to-end anastomosis is performed, the layers of the transsected stumps of the ileum and the transverse colon are sutured together. Linear stapling devices may be used for anastomosis.

A laparotomy set and gastrointestinal instrument set are required.

Operative procedure

1. The abdomen is opened, and the peritoneal cavity is retracted and packed with warm, moist sponges.
2. The mesentery of the transverse colon and the terminal ileum is incised at the points where the resection is to be done. Moist packs, Metzenbaum scissors, hemostats, and nonabsorbable no. 3-0 ligatures are used.
3. The lateral peritoneal fold along the lateral side of the right colon is incised, and the right colon is mobilized medially. Metzenbaum scissors, hemostats, and sponges on holders are used. The ureter and duodenum are carefully identified.
4. The same procedure is carried out on the terminal ileum.
5. The mesenteric vessels are clamped and ligated with nonabsorbable no. 2-0 ligatures.
6. The operative field is prepared for anastomosis. Resection clamps are placed on the transverse colon and ileum. Division is completed with a scalpel, and the specimen is removed.
7. An end-to-end anastomosis is completed between the severed ends of the terminal ileum and the transverse colon.
8. Instruments and supplies that have come in contact with bowel mucosa are discarded.
9. The mesentery and posterior peritoneum are closed with interrupted sutures of nonabsorbable no. 3-0.
10. The abdominal wound is closed. A dressing is applied.

TRANSVERSE COLECTOMY

Transverse colectomy is excision of the transverse colon through an upper midline or transverse incision (Fig. 10-38, *C* and *D*). Bowel integrity is reestablished by an end-to-end anastomosis. A transverse colectomy is performed for malignant lesions of the transverse colon. A more radical procedure may be required when the lesion has perforated the greater curvature of the stomach. If the entire lesion is resectable, a partial gastrectomy may also have to be performed.

Procedural considerations

A laparotomy set and gastrointestinal instrument set are required. Linear stapling instruments should be available. A self-retaining retractor system is an asset.

Operative procedure

1. The abdomen is opened, and the peritoneal cavity is explored to determine the extent of the pathologic area.
2. Moist packs are used to wall off surrounding structures to expose the hepatic and splenic flexures.
3. The colon is mobilized by incising the lateral peritoneum on either side and transsecting the transverse mesocolon. Hemostats, Metzenbaum scissors, and nonabsorbable no. 3-0 ligatures are used.
4. The operative field is prepared for resection. Two Allen intestinal resection clamps are applied. Transsection is completed with a scalpel, and an end-to-end or side-to-side stapled anastomosis is completed.
5. Contaminated articles are discarded. Approximation of mesentery and lateral peritoneum is completed with nonabsorbable no. 3-0 sutures.
6. The abdominal wound is closed. Retention sutures may be used. The wound is dressed.

ANTERIOR RESECTION OF THE SIGMOID COLON AND RECTOSIGMOIDOSTOMY

Anterior resection of the sigmoid colon and rectosigmoidostomy involve the removal of the lower sigmoid and rectosigmoid portions of the rectum (Fig. 10-38, *E*). This is usually done through a laparotomy incision, and an end-to-end anastomosis is completed. This operation is selected to treat lesions in the lower portion of the sigmoid and rectum that permit excision with a wide margin of safety and still retain sufficient tissues with adequate blood supply for a viable rectosigmoid end-to-end anastomosis.

Procedural considerations

A laparotomy set and gastrointestinal instrument set are required. Linear stapling instruments as well as the end-to-end curved mechanical stapling instruments (EEA) are used. Long instruments for dissecting into the pelvis may be necessary. A rigid sigmoidoscope is utilized prior to patient prep and after the anastomosis. A self-retaining retractor set is required. The patient is placed in a modified lithotomy position with legs extended into Allen universal stirrups.

An indwelling catheter is inserted into the patient's urinary bladder prior to the abdominal and peritoneal prep.

If there is an assisting surgeon, a table with a basic minor set and rectal instruments should be available to facilitate the end-to-end stapling of the anastomosis. Cross-contamination from the table of instruments utilized on the patient's rectum to the table of laparotomy instruments is prevented. A table with closure instruments may be the surgeon's preference. This should require only a laparotomy set of instruments.

Operative procedure

1. The abdomen is entered through a laparotomy incision. The peritoneal cavity is explored for metastasis and resectability of the lesion.
2. Before the colon is mobilized, the tumor-bearing segment is isolated by ligatures to the lymphovenous drainage (that is, provided these structures are accessible).
3. A loop of sigmoid colon is elevated as the small intestines are walled off with moist packs; retractors are placed.
4. The peritoneum on the left side of the colon is incised with a long scalpel, scissors, hemostats, and sponge forceps. Traction sutures of nonabsorbable no. 2-0 may be used as the peritoneum is reflected. Bleeding vessels are ligated with nonabsorbable no. 2-0 or 3-0 ligatures.
5. The pelvic peritoneum is exposed and dissected free to form the left side of the reconstructed pelvic floor. Long dissecting instruments are used. Vessels are ligated with 30-inch nonabsorbable ligatures. Extreme care must be exercised throughout to protect the ureters from injury. Identification of the ureters during extensive deep abdominal procedures is best achieved by the preoperative placement of ureteral catheters via transurethral approach. Often the surgeon will have consulted a urologist to perform the ureteral catheter placement at the start of the patient's scheduled procedure. Preparation and assembly of transurethral endoscopes, supplies, and equipment are necessary.
6. The sigmoid colon is turned toward the left, and the procedure that was described in step 4 is carried out on the right side of the pelvis. The two incisions are then curved and joined in front of the rectum.
7. The rectum is freed anteriorly and posteriorly from the adjacent structures.
8. The sigmoid colon is clamped with resection clamps after mobilization of the proximal portion. As the sigmoid colon is divided distally to the clamp, the transsected rectal edges are grasped with Allis or Ochsner forceps, and the rectal opening is exposed. The diseased portion is removed, and, the soiled instruments discarded into a separate basin.
9. Continuity is established by an end-to-end anastomosis of the proximal colon and the rectum using a curved mechanical stapling instrument (EEA) (Fig. 10-39). "Donuts" of tissue removed during EEA stapling (Fig. 10-32, *I*) are examined closely for thickness and continuity, then sent as specimens to the pathology lab.
10. The assisting surgeon passes a rigid sigmoidoscope into the lumen of the bowel transanally. Warm irrigating solution is poured into the peritoneal cavity and the lumen of the bowel is insufflated. The surgeon observes for air leak from the anastomosis and oversews the site if indicated.
11. The pelvic floor is reperitonealized, and drains may be placed.
12. The abdominal wound is closed in the routine manner, and a dressing is applied.

ABDOMINOPERINEAL RESECTION

Abdominoperineal resection is the mobilization and division of a diseased segment of the lower bowel through a midline incision. The proximal end of bowel is exteriorized through a separate stab wound as a colostomy. The distal end is pushed into the hollow of the sacrum and removed through the perineal route (Fig. 10-40).

An abdominoperineal resection is performed for malignant lesions and inflammatory diseases of the lower sigmoid colon, rectum, and anus that are too low for the use of EEA stapling devices.

Procedural considerations

The choice of patient position depends on the surgeon. Some surgeons prefer to start with the patient in the supine position and move the patient to the lithotomy position for the perineal portion of the operation. Others initially place the patient in a modified lithotomy position; thus surgery may be performed simultaneously by two teams, which may require two scrub nurses with two different setups. An indwelling urinary catheter is inserted after induction.

A gastrointestinal set and an ostomy appliance are required for the abdominal portion of the procedure. A perineal set is used for the perineal portion of the procedure; it consists of basic laparotomy instruments plus the following:

2 Volkmann rake retractors, four-pronged, sharp	1 Anal retractor
	1 Rectal speculum
2 Hill retractors	4 Pennington forceps, 6 inches

Operative procedure

1. A midline incision is made.
2. After thorough exploration of the abdominal cavity, the surgeon determines the extent and operability of the lesion.
3. If a resection is to be done, the surgeon retracts the sigmoid colon to the right side. The peritoneum on the left of the mesocolon is divided.
4. The incision into the peritoneum is made opposite the main branches of the inferior mesenteric vessels and extended into the pelvis and around anterior to the rectum.
5. The pelvic peritoneum is mobilized by blunt dissection to form the left side of the new pelvic floor and permit early visualization of the left ureter.
6. The peritoneum is incised on the right side until the incision connects with that made on the left. The right ureter is identified and protected.
7. The blood supply of the portion of intestine to be removed is isolated and ligated.

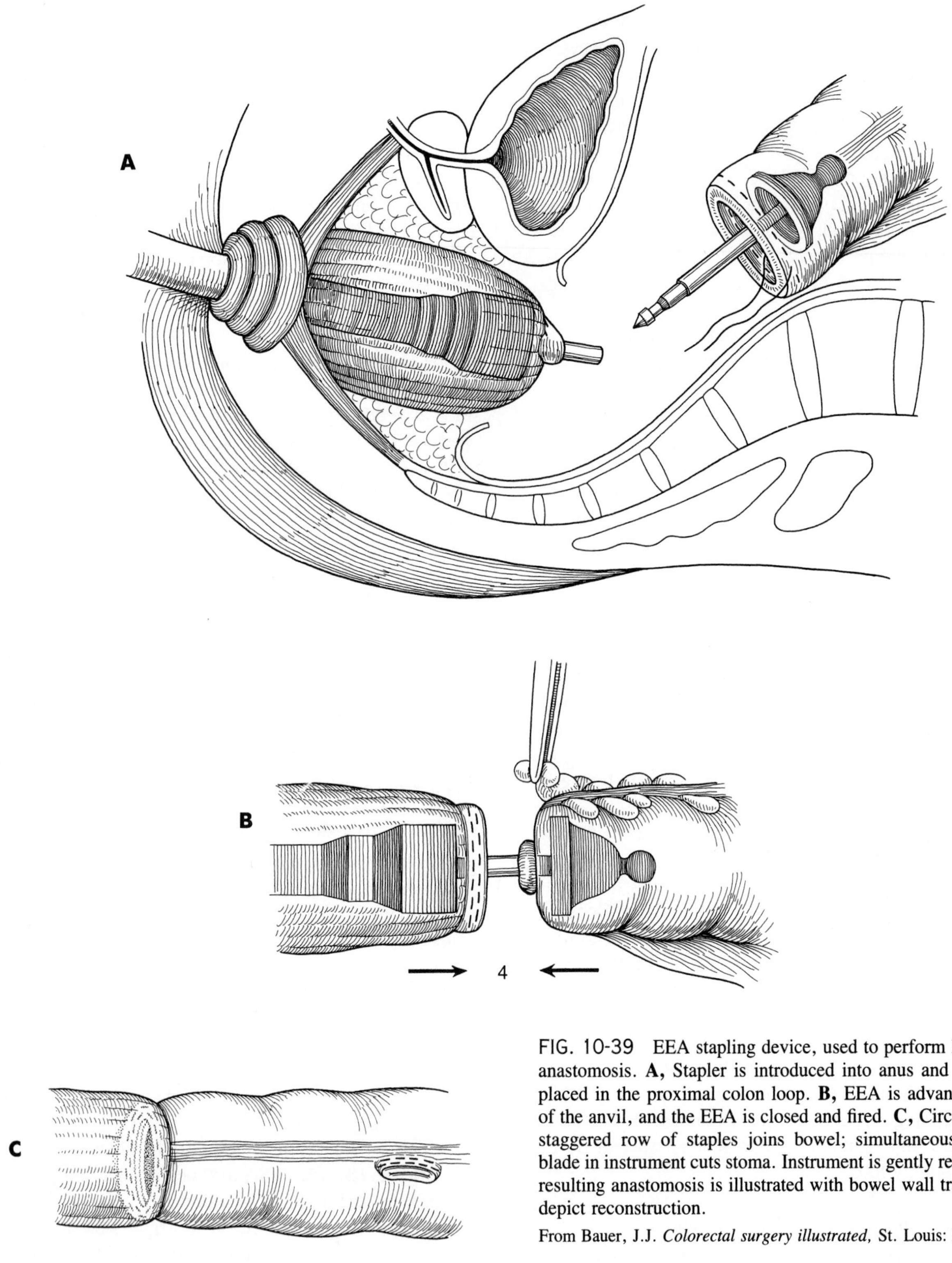

A

B

4

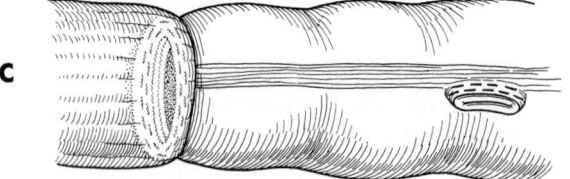

C

FIG. 10-39 EEA stapling device, used to perform low anterior anastomosis. **A,** Stapler is introduced into anus and the anvil is placed in the proximal colon loop. **B,** EEA is advanced to level of the anvil, and the EEA is closed and fired. **C,** Circular double-staggered row of staples joins bowel; simultaneously, circular blade in instrument cuts stoma. Instrument is gently removed. The resulting anastomosis is illustrated with bowel wall transparent to depict reconstruction.

From Bauer, J.J. *Colorectal surgery illustrated,* St. Louis: Mosby.

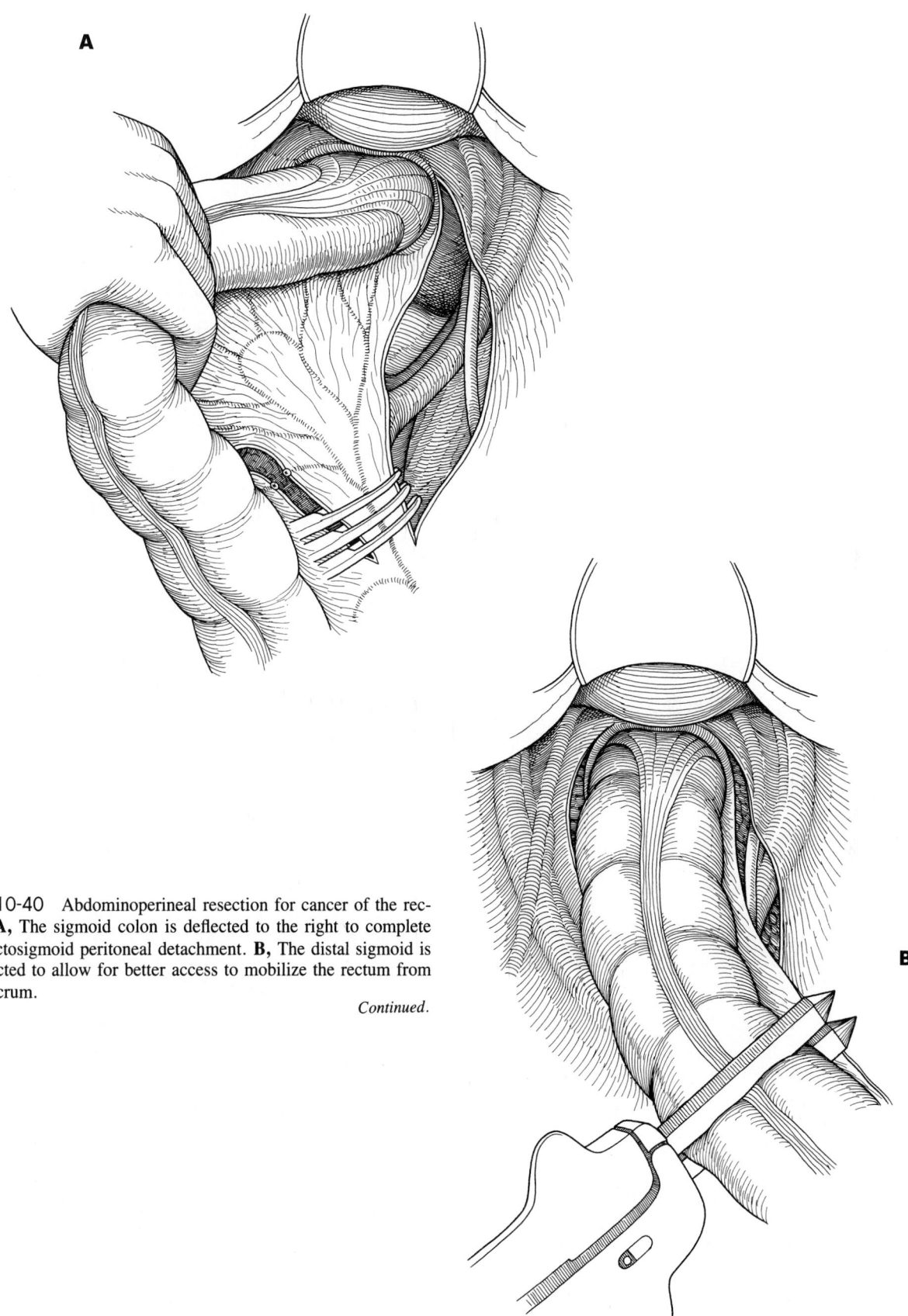

FIG. 10-40   Abdominoperineal resection for cancer of the rectum. **A,** The sigmoid colon is deflected to the right to complete the rectosigmoid peritoneal detachment. **B,** The distal sigmoid is transected to allow for better access to mobilize the rectum from the sacrum.

Continued.

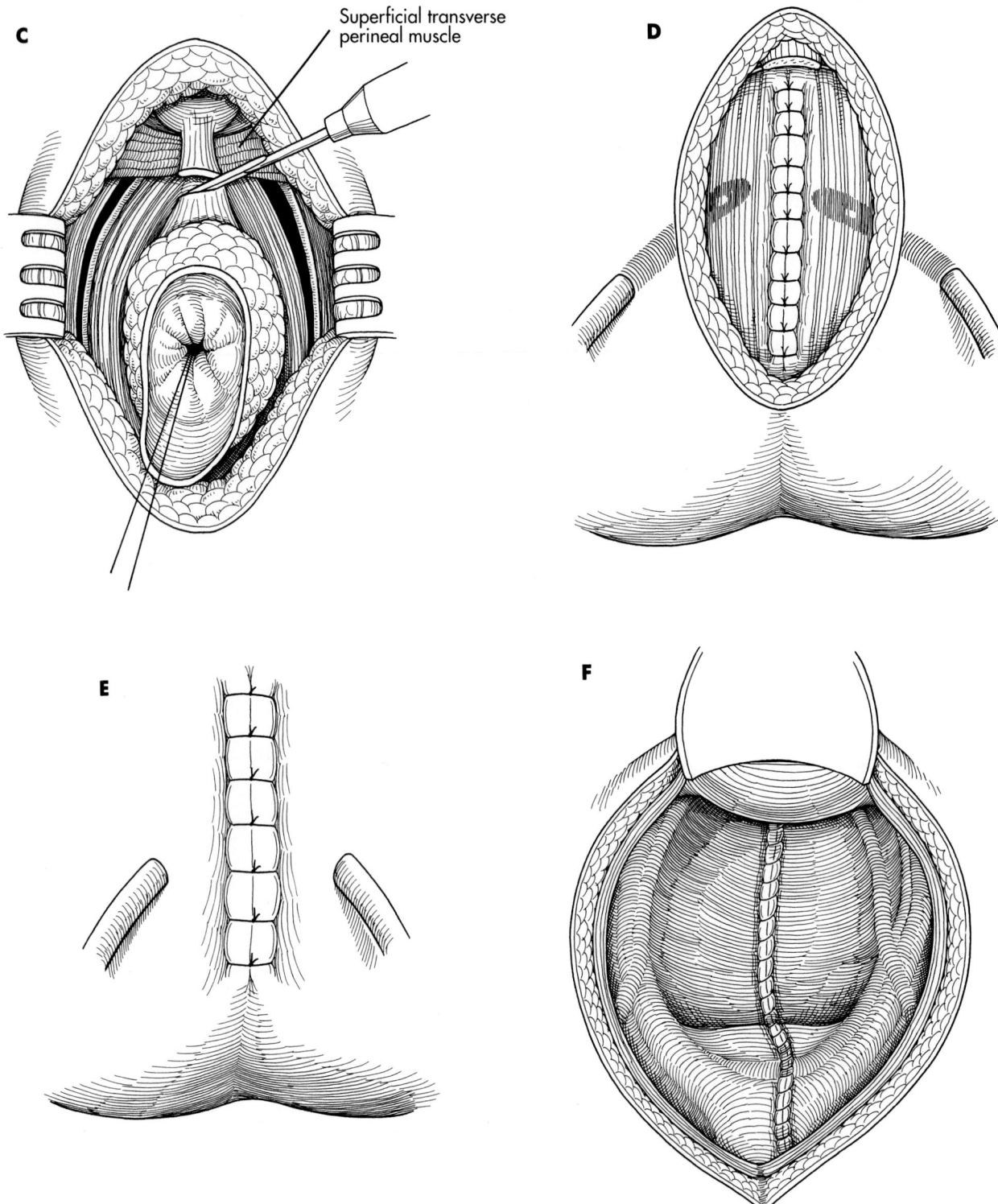

C

Superficial transverse
perineal muscle

D

E

F

FIG. 10-40, CONT'D **C,** The rectal stump is excised from the perineal approach. **D,** Drains are placed and brought through stab wounds; the levator tissues are reapproximated with 2-0 synthetic absorbable sutures. **E,** The perineal skin is closed. **F,** The pelvic peritoneal floor is closed from the abdominal approach.

From Bauer, J.J. (1993). *Colorectal surgery illustrated,* St. Louis: Mosby.

8. Care must be taken not to damage the left colic artery, which will supply the blood to the colostomy.

9. The mesentery is tied to permit greater exposure in the operative field.

10. The surgeon frees the rectum, usually as low as the sacrococcygeal junction. Care is taken to avoid injury to the presacral nerves, which could result in sexual and bladder dysfunction.

11. After the bowel is freed, the distal segment is transsected with a linear stapling instrument (Fig. 10-40, *B*). The proximal margin of resection is examined and transsected. The bowel and mesentery are removed from the abdominal cavity. The surgeon prepares the permanent colostomy by extending the stump through the abdominal wall. The colostomy will be "matured" following abdominal closure.

12. The combined excision and perineal dissection is initiated when the lesion is determined to be resectable. If two teams are not available for synchronous excision of the perineum, the perineal portion of the operation is performed after the abdominal resection is complete. In this case the abdomen is closed and the remaining rectosigmoid stump is excised perineally. To prevent contamination, the anus is often closed with a pursestring suture. An incision is made around the anus in an elliptical manner outside of the sphincter muscles with a generous margin of perianal skin.

13. The anus is grasped with Allis or Ochsner forceps and tipped upward to enable its attachment to the coccyx to be severed more readily. Electrodissection is used.

14. The levator ani muscle is exposed; while the finger of the surgeon is held beneath it, it is divided as far from the rectum as possible.

15. All bleeding points are clamped and tied.

16. The Foley catheter allows the surgeon to get as close to the bladder as possible without damaging it.

17. After the anococcygeal raphe is divided, the surgeon's hand is thrust up into the hollow sacrum to free the rectum by blunt dissection, grasp the upper end of the distal fragment, and deliver the stump through the perineum.

18. Drains may be placed in the pelvic cavity and exteriorized through stab wounds in the buttocks (Fig. 10-40, *D*).

19. The surgeon is regloved before returning to the abdominal wound.

20. When all bleeding is controlled, the incision is closed.

ILEOANAL ENDORECTAL PULL-THROUGH

Ileoanal endorectal pull-through is the removal of the entire colon and the proximal two thirds of the rectum. It includes a mucosectomy of the remaining distal rectum, creation of a pouch from the distal small bowel, and anastomosis of the pouch to the anus. The operation is performed to relieve the symptoms of ulcerative colitis and familial polyposis (diarrhea, pain, cramping, bleeding, and others)

RESEARCH HIGHLIGHT 10-1

An estimated 43,000 new rectal cancers will be diagnosed in 1993 in the United States. A large percentage of these patients will have low rectal cancers, which will probably be treated by abdominal perineal resection and permanent colostomy.

Colostomy-sparing treatment options can be performed for smaller lesions of the lower rectum; however, the potential of residual pelvic disease remains problematic. The use of rectal ultrasound in evaluating tumor invasion into the layers of the rectal mucosa muscularis and subsequent lymph node involvement has afforded better patient selection.

Radioimmunoguided surgery (RIGS), using a radiolabeled monoclonal antibody (MAb) and a hand-held gamma-detecting probe (GDP), the Neoprobe 1000, has proven useful in detecting tumor metastasis not found on inspection or palpation.

A pilot study at a large midwestern academic medical center was completed on eight primary rectal cancer patients who were evaluated preoperatively by three different methods:

1. Transanal GDP probing following administration of the MAb CC49
2. Rectal ultrasound
3. CT scan of the abdomen and pelvis

The objective of the study was to determine if the use of the GDP and rectal ultrasound would provide better evaluation of the patient's tumor and therefore support a more appropriate preoperative decision for resection in comparison to the standard CT scan findings.

Five of the eight patients were considered candidates for transanal excision (TAE) alone to remove their rectal tumor. In 3 of the 5 patients TAE was abandoned due to the additional pelvic tumor demonstrated by rectal ultrasound and transanal GDP probing. At least 2 of the patients had significant metastatic disease in the pelvis, which would have gone undetected without the use of RIGS. This was pathologically confirmed.

This pilot study represents very early results and requires further study. The data indicate rectal ultrasound and RIGS GDP transanal probing are complementary tests that can be used preoperatively for better selection of the appropriate surgical management in rectal cancer patients.

Arnold M.W. (1993). Unpublished manuscript, The Ohio State University College of Medicine, Columbus, OH.

A

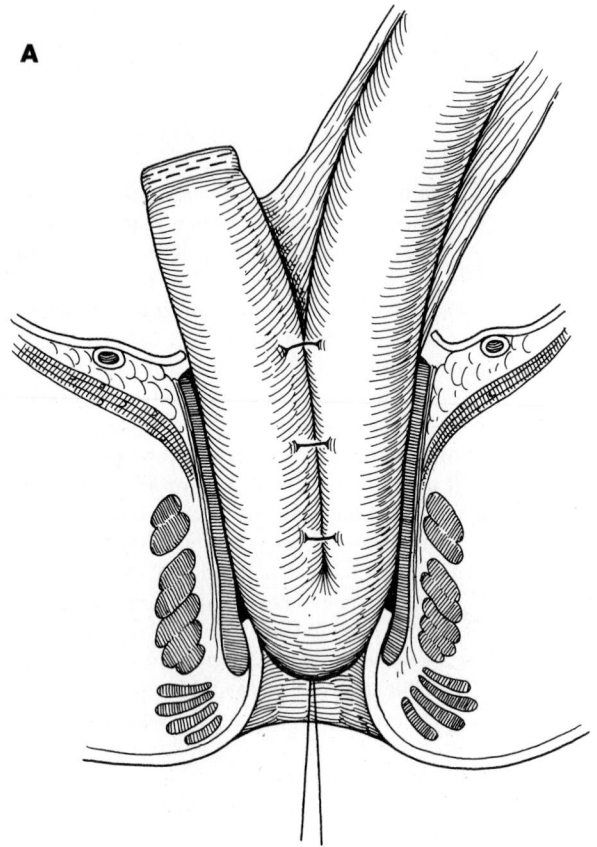

B

Mesentery vascular
division alternative

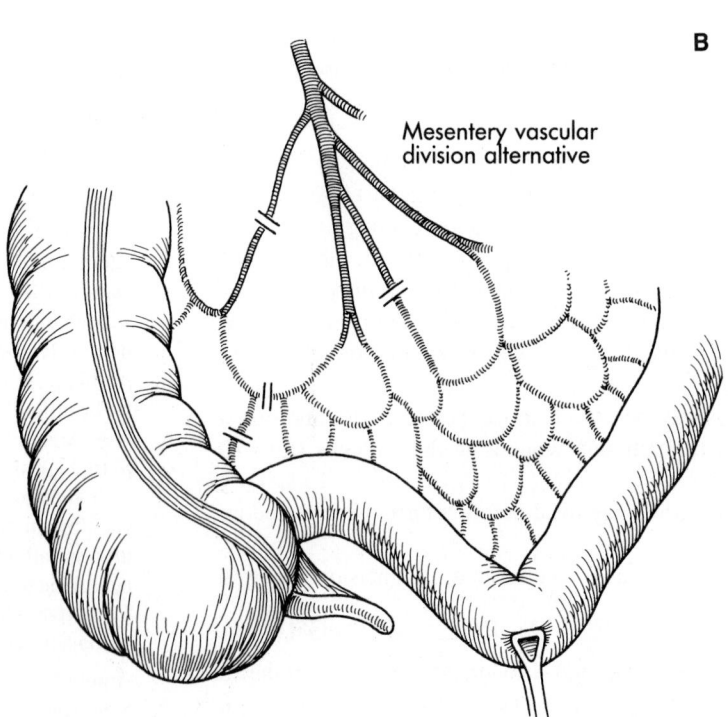

FIG. 10-41   J pouch for ileoanal endorectal pull-through. **A,** The J pouch is created at terminal ileum by folding two adjacent loops of small bowel, approximately 10 to 15 cm each, parallel with each other. **B,** Mesenteric vascular arcades may need to be divided to provide adequate length for anal anastomosis.

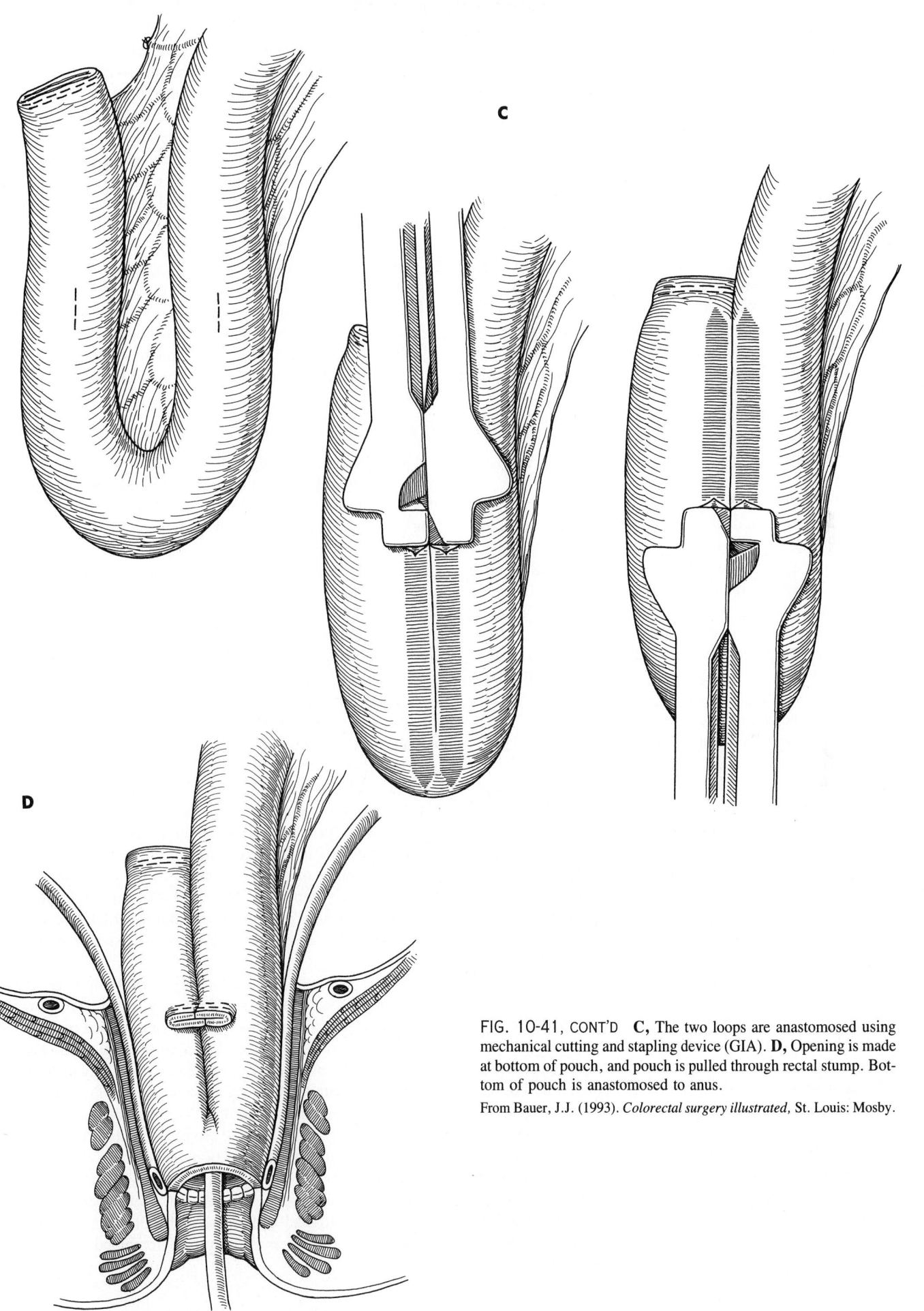

C

D

FIG. 10-41, CONT'D **C,** The two loops are anastomosed using mechanical cutting and stapling device (GIA). **D,** Opening is made at bottom of pouch, and pouch is pulled through rectal stump. Bottom of pouch is anastomosed to anus.

From Bauer, J.J. (1993). *Colorectal surgery illustrated*, St. Louis: Mosby.

and to prevent colon malignancies. This procedure is an anal sphincter-saving operation that is done to avoid the need for a traditional ileostomy.

Procedural considerations

The patient is usually placed in a modified lithotomy position. Some surgeons prefer to perform the mucosectomy with the patient in a jackknife position and then place the patient in a modified lithotomy position for the remainder of the procedure.

A gastrointestinal set, a perineal set, and rectal instrumentation are required. Separate instrument sets are used for the rectal and abdominal approaches. Additional draping and gowning supplies should be available because redraping and regowning occur after the mucosectomy and after the ileoanal anastomosis. An epinephrine solution should be available for injection into the submucosal tissue, proximal to the anus, to separate the mucosa from the muscularis layer. An ileostomy appliance is applied immediately postoperatively.

Operative procedure

1. The anal canal is dilated and inspected through an anoscope. Starting at the dentate line, the anal-rectal junction, the epinephrine solution is injected circumferentially, separating the mucosa from the muscularis layer. The mucosectomy is then performed by making a circular incision at the dentate line, cutting only through mucosa. The mucosa is peeled off the muscularis tissue for a distance of 2 to 8 cm and resected. When all bleeding is controlled, the patient is repositioned, if necessary, for the abdominal approach.

2. A midline incision is made, and the abdomen explored. The entire large intestine from the ileocecal junction through the upper two thirds of the rectum is freed and immobilized. All vessels are ligated. The terminal ileum is separated from the cecum using a mechanical cutting and stapling device (GIA). The mesocolon is ligated using suture ligatures or a ligating, dividing, and stapling instrument. The rectum is resected down to the level of the mucosectomy. The colon and resected portion of the rectum are removed en bloc.

3. The pouch is created. Most surgeons use either the J pouch or the S pouch. The J pouch is created at the terminal ileum by folding two adjacent loops of small bowel, approximately 10 to 15 cm each, parallel with each other and anastomosing them using a GIA. An opening is made at the bottom of the pouch, and the pouch is pulled through the rectal stump. The bottom of the pouch is anastomosed to the anus with interrupted absorbable sutures (Fig. 10-41). An S pouch is created by aligning the distal ileum in an S configuration with each of the three limbs approximately 10 cm in length. The most distal 2 cm of the ileum is not incorporated into the pouch but is preserved for the anastomosis to the anus. The three limbs are manually incised and anastomosed to create a pouch. Mucosal tissue is approxi-

mated with absorbable suture, and nonabsorbable suture is used for the serosal layer. The preserved distal end of the ileum and the pouch are pulled through the rectal stump and anastomosed to the anus (Fig. 10-42). This completes the anal portion of the procedure.

4. The scrubbed team changes gowns and gloves, redrapes, and completes the abdominal procedure by creating a loop ileostomy on a previously designated site through the abdominal wall. The abdominal incision is closed in the usual manner.

5. Approximately 2 to 6 months are required after the initial operation for adequate healing of the ileoanal anastomosis to occur and to ensure the absence of postsurgical complications. When the patient's status is determined to be satisfactory, a second procedure is performed to restore bowel continuity and close the loop ileostomy.

CEA-DIRECTED SECOND-LOOK LAPAROTOMY

Carcinoembryonic antigen (CEA) serum levels are followed closely in patients with a history of adenocarcinoma of the colon or rectum. When a persistent rise in the patient's CEA level is demonstrated, noninvasive diagnostics such as CT scan or MRI scans are obtained. Colonoscopy may be performed to directly visualize the anastomotic site for recurrence or a secondary primary tumor. CT scans and MRI scans may not detect tumor metastasis less than 0.5 cm in size. Lymph nodes in the periportal area may, however, be identified as enlarged or suspicious. Negative diagnostic workup does not negate the justification for exploratory laparotomy when the patient's CEA level rises persistently two standard deviations above the individual's baseline level. Normal CEA levels vary according to the type of assay conducted to measure CEA serum levels. Generally, CEA levels are normal in the 0 to 5 ng/ml range. A patient's baseline may be 0.2 ng/ml, but a rise to 4.2 ng/ml is cause for alarm. Thus obtaining baseline CEA levels in all patients undergoing surgical intervention for the primary resection of adenocarcinoma of the colon or rectum is extremely important. These patients can be educated as to the importance of periodic monitoring of CEA serum levels and readily accept this as justification to undergo laparotomy.

Potential findings upon exploratory laparotomy vary. If carcinomatosis is found, a simple biopsy may be taken to confirm diagnosis. The patient signing an informed consent for CEA-directed second-look laparotomy understands the potential for extensive radical resection, which may include hysterectomy with bilateral salpingo-oophorectomy, partial or total cystectomy, retroperitoneal lymph node dissection, hepatic resection, gastrohepatic lymph node dissection, colon resection, small bowel resection, omentectomy, and abdominal wall resection. For patients with a history of rectal adenocarcinoma, pelvic exenteration may be performed. The informed surgical consent should reflect the possible interventions, as well as the potential for blood loss and complications.

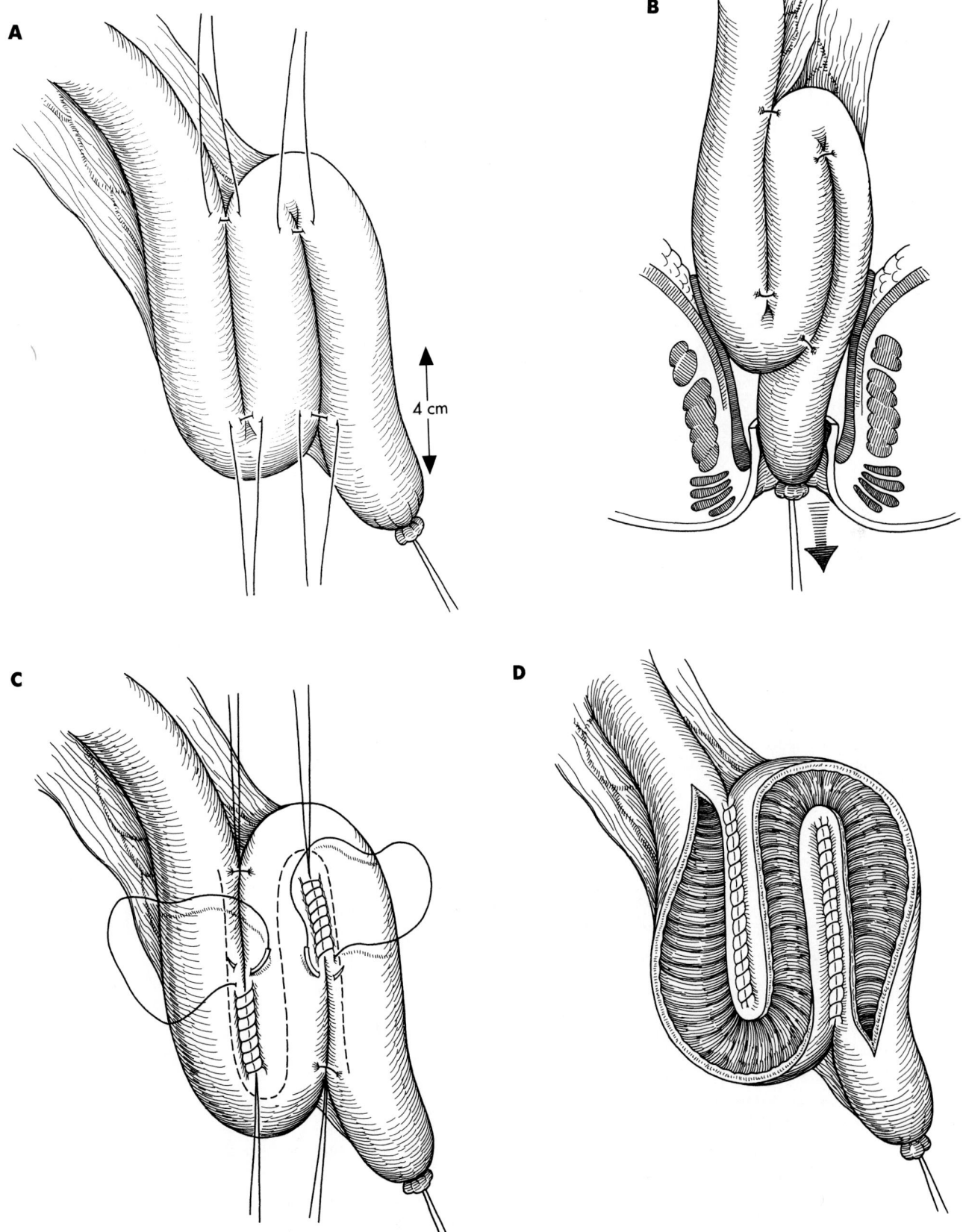

FIG. 10-42 S pouch for ileoanal endorectal pull-through. **A,** Pouch is created by aligning distal ileum in S configuration with each limb (three in total) approximately 12 cm in length. **B,** The length is measured before anastomosis begins. **C,** Three limbs are incised and anastomosed to create pouch. **D,** Incision is made as illustrated.

Continued.

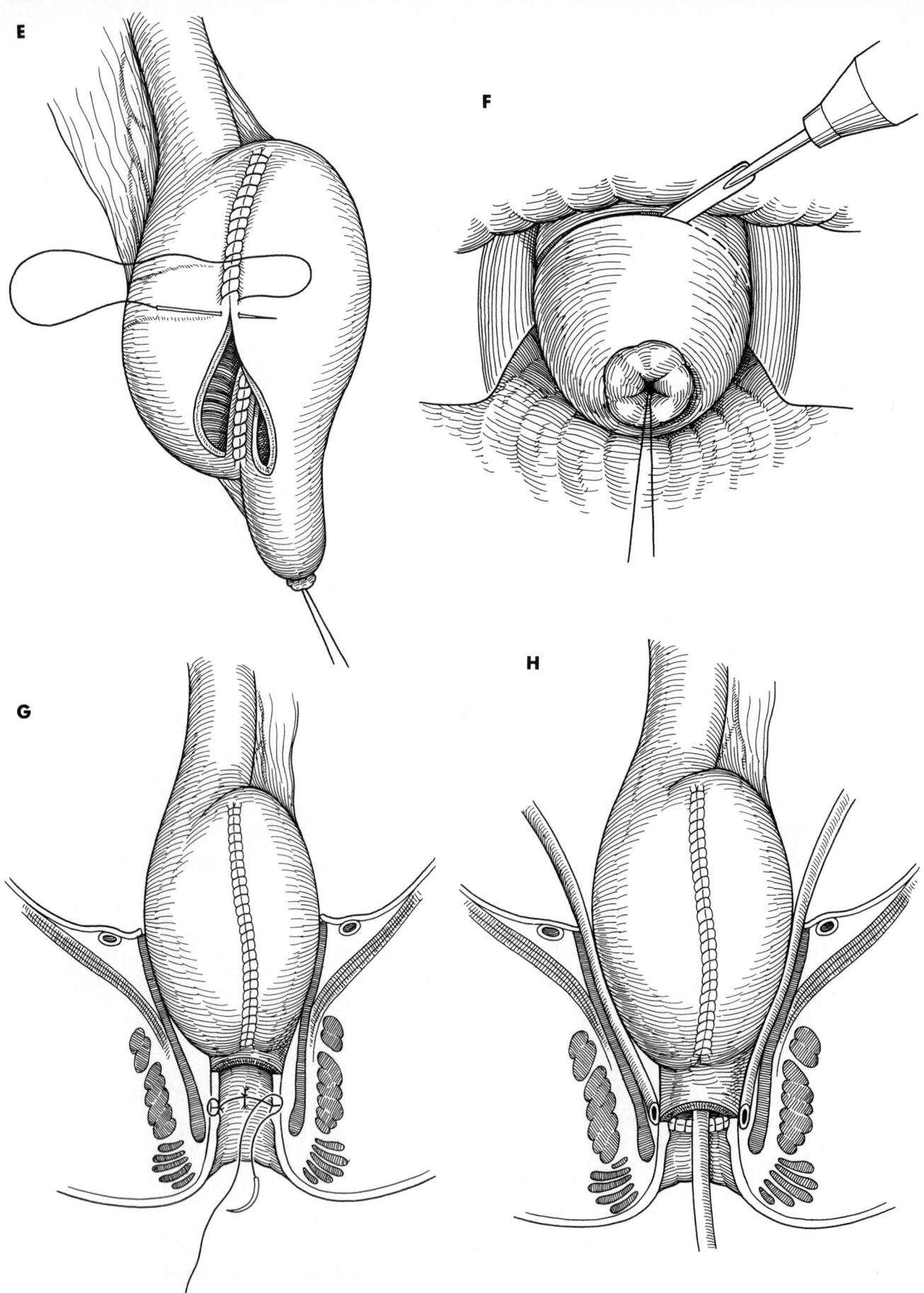

FIG. 10-42, CONT'D **E,** The pouch is closed using suture for the formation of the reservoir. **F,** The distal ends of ileum and pouch are pulled through the rectal stump and the lower outflow tract is trimmed. **G,** With 3-0 absorbable sutures, the outflow tract is anastomosed to the anus at the dentate line. **H,** Demonstrates a drain in place in the lumen of the newly created ileoanal-rectal canal.

From Bauer, J.J. (1993). *Colorectal surgery illustrated*, St. Louis: Mosby.

Procedural considerations

A basic laparotomy instrument set is required as well as Richardson retractors and a Bookwalter retractor system. Gastrointestinal instruments, vascular instruments and linear stapling instruments should be readily available. Intraoperative ultrasound and the Cavitron Ultrasonic Surgical Aspirator (CUSA) should also be available.

Operative procedure

1. The patient is placed in supine position. A Foley catheter is inserted into the urinary bladder and the patient's abdomen is prepped from nipple line to midthigh. A nasogastric tube is inserted for stomach decompression.
2. A midline incision is made from the xiphoid, around the umbilicus, to the pubis.
3. The peritoneum is entered after removal of any sutures from earlier surgical procedures.
4. Abdominal adhesions may be extensive and require hours of tedious dissection using Metzenbaum scissors, Debakey forceps, gauze dissectors, and electrodissection.
5. An extensive inspection and palpation of all the abdominal viscera is required in a systematic approach.
6. Samples of suspicious tissues are collected for biopsy. Frequent specimens may be sent for frozen section to confirm diagnosis.
7. The liver is examined by palpation, inspection, and intraoperative ultrasound.
8. If the patient has been prepared for RIGS by receiving a radiolabeled MAb prior to surgery, abdominal exploration using the Neoprobe is performed. The Neoprobe is a hand-held gamma-detecting probe used to detect the minute amount of radioactive ^{105}I bonded to an MAb that is injected intravenously 2 to 3 weeks prior to the patient's scheduled surgery. The MAb is a glycoprotein that will bind to the antigen on cancer cell membranes. Remaining circulating MAb is excreted from the body via the kidneys during the weeks before surgery. During exploration with the Neoprobe, an audible tone sounds when the instrument is in proximity with tissues in which the MAb-antigen bonding has occurred. The surgeon can then detect an occult tumor that might otherwise remain concealed. The radioimmunoguided surgery concept is currently being tried with a number of carrier substances such as the MAb. Future applications may apply to malignancies other than adenocarcinoma.
9. Necessary resection of organs and tissues is performed.
10. The abdomen is closed according to surgeon preference. Retention sutures may be used.
11. The abdomen is cleaned and dried and dressings are applied.

SURGERY OF THE RECTUM
HEMORRHOIDECTOMY

Hemorrhoidectomy is the excision and ligation of dilated veins in the anal region to relieve discomfort and control bleeding. The frequency of hemorrhoidectomies performed in the operating room has decreased due to banding procedures now being done on an ambulatory surgery basis.

Procedural considerations

Preoperative anal dilatation aids in exposing the vessels and contributes to the patient's comfort in the immediate postoperative period. Many surgeons prefer to precede the operation with a sigmoidoscopy. Spinal, caudal, or local anesthesia may be used. A minor set plus two 8-inch tissue forceps without teeth or 8-inch Debakey forceps, and rectal instruments similar to the following are required:

2 Hill retractors	1 Set of rectal dilators
1 Anoscope	Buie pile forceps
1 Rectal speculum	1 Crypt hook

The CO_2 laser may also be used for vaporization and coagulation of hemorrhoidal tissue.

Operative procedure

1. The patient is usually placed in the lithotomy or jackknife position.
2. The anal canal is dilated and inspected through an anoscope.
3. Four Allis forceps are applied several centimeters from the anal margin to expose the anus.
4. The base of the hemorrhoid and tissue are grasped with Allis forceps and held.
5. An intestinal suture of synthetic absorbable suture no. 2-0 is placed and tied at the proximal end of the hemorrhoid, and a Buie pile forceps is applied across the base and above the proposed incision line. Excision is completed with a scalpel. Suturing is completed by loosely placed continuous sutures over the Buie forceps. The suture is tightened as the forceps are removed, and the suture ends are tied.
6. Traction may be maintained as hemostatic forceps are applied and dissection is completed segmentally. Suture ligatures of synthetic absorbable suture no. 2-0 are used as each hemostat is removed.
7. Remaining hemorrhoids are excised in a similar manner.
8. Petrolatum gauze packing may be placed in the anal canal. A dressing is applied.

EXCISION OF ANAL FISSURE/LATERAL SPHINCTEROTOMY

Excision of an anal fissure involves the dilatation of the anal sphincter and removal of the lesion. Anal fissures are benign lesions of the anal wall.

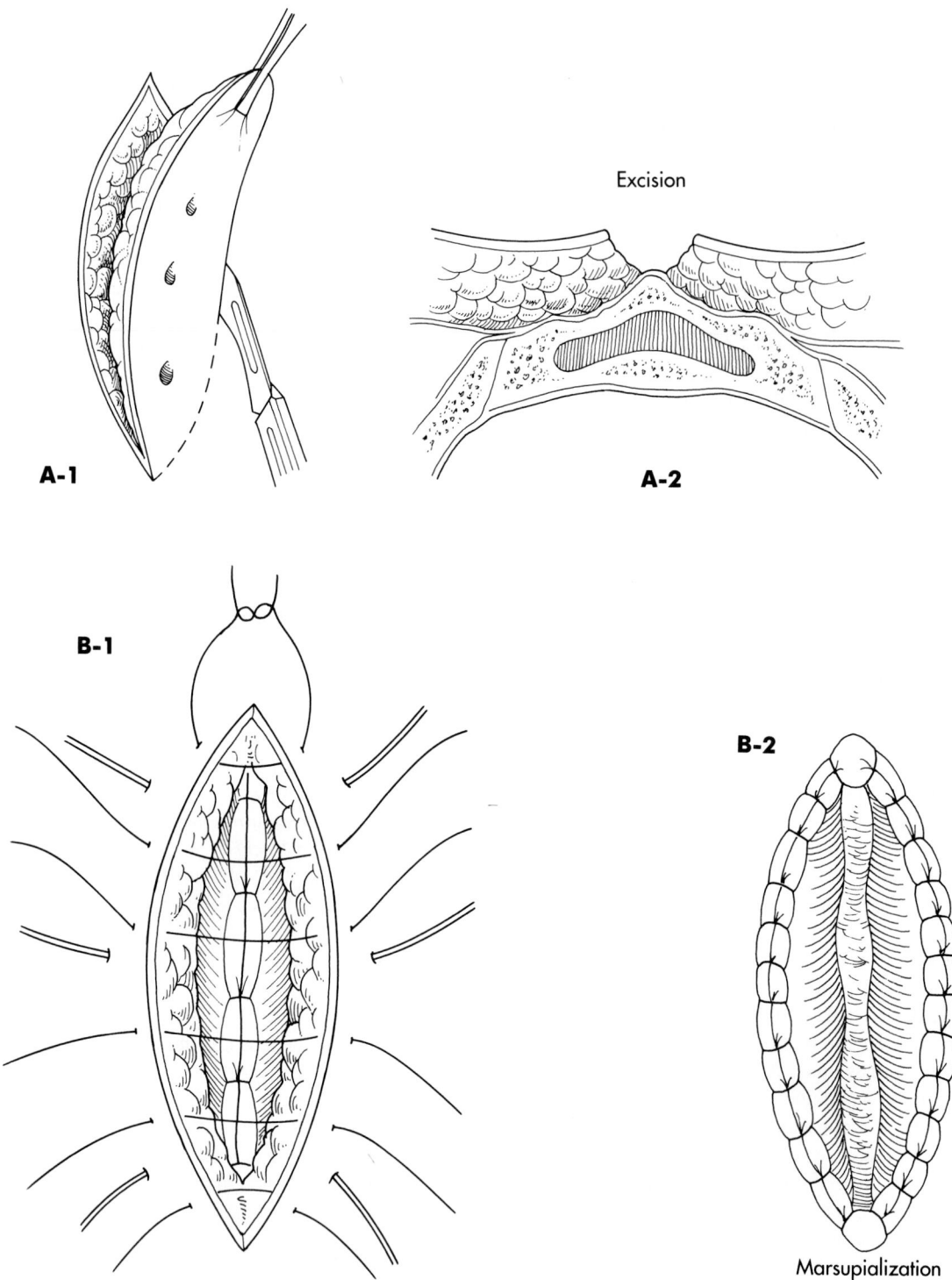

FIG. 10-43   Pilonidal cyst. The pilonidal sinus tract is identified with injection of methylene blue into the tract. **A,** A wide elliptical incision (A-1) is made to include all the subcutaneous tracts and tissue to the fascia overlying the sacrum and coccyx (A-2). **B,** Closure of the wound can be primary (B-1) or secondary (B-2).

From Bauer, J.J. (1993). *Colorectal surgery illustrated,* St. Louis: Mosby.

Procedural considerations

A minor set and rectal instruments, as listed previously, are required.

Operative procedure

1. The patient is placed in the lithotomy or jackknife position.
2. Dilatation of the anal sphincter is completed.
3. The fissure is excised, and bleeders are ligated or electrocoagulated.
4. A lateral incision is made, and the internal sphincter is incised. The mucosa is approximated over the incision.
5. A drain or packing is inserted.
6. A dressing is applied.

EXCISION OF PILONIDAL CYST AND SINUS

Excision of a pilonidal cyst and sinus is removal of the cyst with sinus tracts from the intergluteal fold on the posterior surface of the lower sacrum (Fig. 10-43). A pilonidal cyst and sinus, which may have a congenital origin, rarely become symptomatic until the individual reaches adulthood. Inflammatory reaction varies from a mild, irritating, draining sinus tract to an acute abscess with secondary recurrences. Treatment consists of drainage in the acute stage and total surgical excision during remission.

The excision of the cyst and sinus tracts must be complete to prevent recurrence. The defect resulting from recurrences may become too large for primary closure. In this case the wound is left open to heal by granulation.

Procedural considerations

A minor set and rectal instruments, as listed previously, are required, as well as methylene blue, a 10- or 20-ml syringe, and a blunt-tip needle.

Operative procedure

1. The patient is placed in the jackknife position.
2. The sinus tracts are identified with probes.
3. The tract is marked by injecting methylene blue with a blunted needle into the tract.
4. An elliptical incision is made down to the fascia. A curette is used to remove gelatinous tissue. Excision of cyst and sinus tracts is completed.
5. Bleeding is controlled.
6. If the wound is to be left open, it is packed, and a pressure dressing is applied. If the wound is closed, 2-0 nonabsorbable sutures are used for stay sutures on the deeper tissue, and fine nonabsorbable suture is used on the skin.

REFERENCES

Bauer, J.J. (1993). *Colorectal surgery illustrated.* St Louis: Mosby.

Daly, J.M., & Cady, B. (1993). *Atlas of surgical oncology.* St. Louis: Mosby.

Doughty, D.B., & Jackson, D.B. (1993). *Gastrointestinal disorders.* St. Louis: Mosby.

Thompson, J.C. (1992). *Atlas on surgery of the stomach, duodenum, and small bowel.* St. Louis: Mosby.

Quilici, J.P. (1992). *New developments in laparoscopy.* Norwalk, Conn: The U.S. Surgical Corp.

BIBLIOGRAPHY

Brunner, L.S., & Suddarth, D.S. (1988). *Textbook of medical-surgical nursing* (6th ed.). Philadelphia: J.B. Lippincott.

Thibodeau, G.A., & Patton, K.T. (1993). *Anatomy and physiology* (2nd

11

Surgery of the Liver, Biliary Tract, Pancreas, and Spleen

Lynda R. Petty

Diseases of the liver, biliary tract, pancreas, and spleen have a great influence on the wellness of the patient. Because these organs are highly vascular and control many of the metabolic and immune functions of the body, pathology in one or more of them requires urgent intervention. Surgical interventions relating to the liver, biliary tract, pancreas, or spleen may be indicated for tumor, infection, cystic anomalies, congenital anomalies, metabolic diseases, or trauma.

In the past decade, surgeries of the liver and biliary tract have become more advanced as research and new technology have permitted more complete diagnosis of pathology involving this complex organ and portal system. Resection of the liver for carcinomas has achieved a recognized role for cure or substantial palliation with safety and low morbidity.

Cholecystectomy is an operation commonly performed in most hospital operating rooms. Approximately 20 million people in the United States have gallstones, and nearly 300,000 operations are performed each year for this disease and its complications (Way & Pellegrini, 1987).

Laparoscopic cholecystectomy has become the most common mode of surgical intervention for the treatment of cholecystitis. It offers the advantages of reduced trauma to tissues as well as a significant reduction in the length of postoperative recovery. The introduction and success of laparoscopic cholecystectomy have evolved into a number of abdominal procedures now being performed or assisted through the laparoscope.

New diagnostic technology and the intraoperative use of ultrasound, biliary endoscopy, and radiography have enabled surgeons to better treat diseases of the biliary tract. Solid organ transplantation, as with the liver, pancreas, and kidneys, has achieved commonality as a means of treatment for primary hepatic tumors, end-stage liver disease, and insulin-deficient diabetes. Liver transplant now offers the patient the option of living-related organ donation. The pioneers in transplantation are now attempting animal-to-human organ transplants as a possible means of providing more organs for the ever-growing list of waiting recipients.

This chapter contains information pertaining to the most common and innovative procedures and technology related to surgery of the liver, biliary tract, pancreas, and spleen.

SURGICAL ANATOMY

The liver is in the right upper quadrant of the abdominal cavity, beneath the dome of the diaphragm and directly above the stomach, duodenum, and hepatic flexure of the colon. The external covering, known as Glisson's capsule, is composed of dense connective tissue. The visceral peritoneum extends over the entire surface of the liver, except at the point of posterior attachment to the diaphragm. This connective tissue branches at the porta hepatis into a network of septa that extends into an intrahepatic network of support for the more than 1 million hepatic lobules. The porta hepatis is located on the inferior surface of the liver and is the location of entry and exit for the major vessels, ducts, and nerves. The arterial blood supply is maintained by the hepatic artery, and venous blood from the stomach, intestines, spleen, and pancreas is carried to the liver by the portal vein and its branches (Fig. 11-1). The hepatic venous system returns blood to the heart by way of the inferior vena cava.

The lobules are the functional units of the liver. Each lobule contains a portal triad that consists of a hepatic duct, hepatic portal vein branch, a branch of the hepatic artery, nerves, and lymphatics. A central vein is located in the center of each lobule and provides for venous drainage into the hepatic veins.

The lobules also contain hepatic cords, hepatic sinusoids, and bile canaliculi. The hepatic cords comprise numerous columns of hepatocytes, the functional cells of the liver. The hepatic sinusoids are the blood channels that communicate between the columns of hepatocytes. The sinusoids have a thin epithelial lining composed primarily of

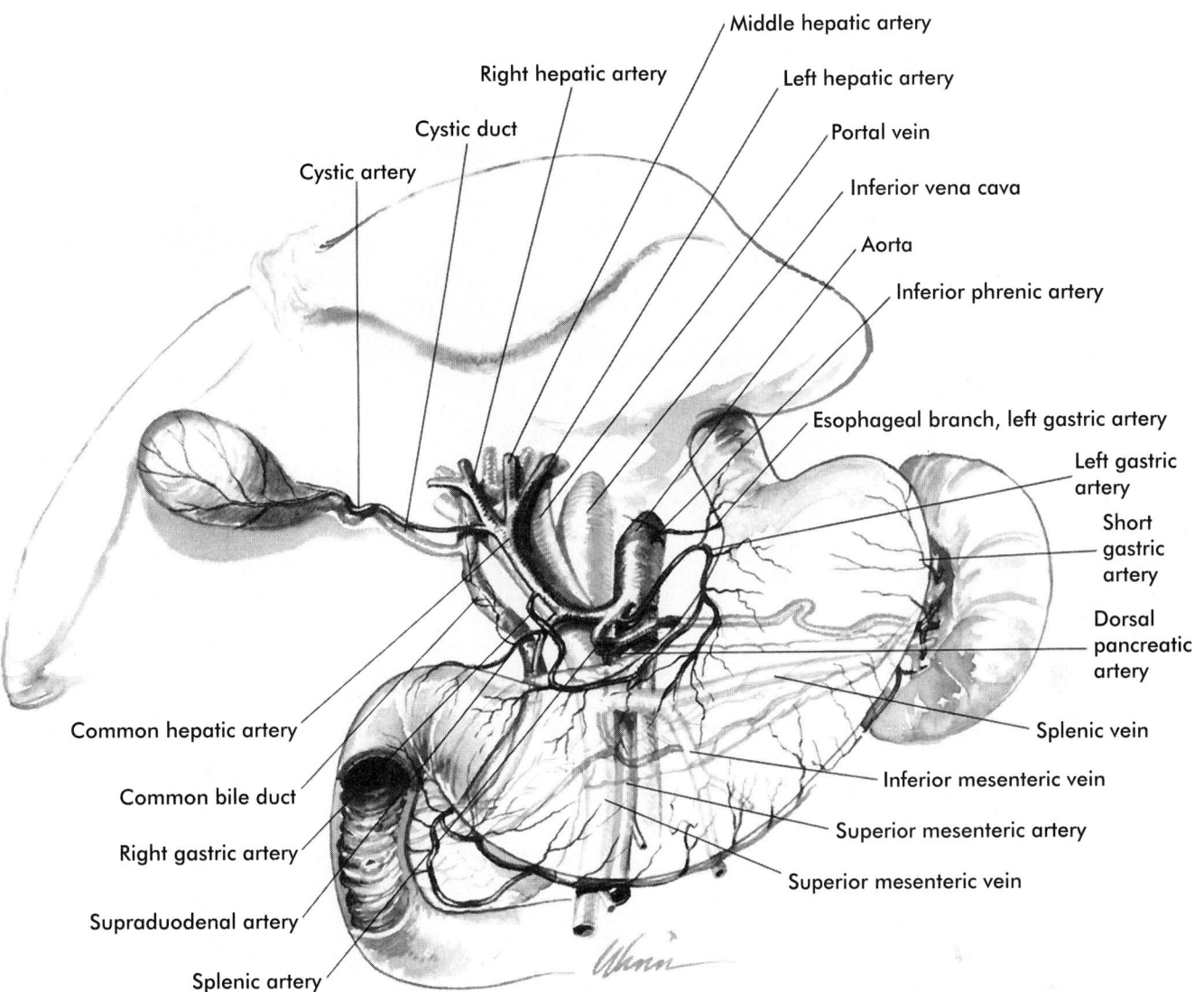

FIG. 11-1 Intricate relationships of the arterial and venous blood supply of the liver, gallbladder, pancreas, spleen, and the biliary ductal system.

From Davis, J.H., et al. (1987). *Clinical surgery* (Vol. 2). St Louis: Mosby.

Kupffer's cells, phagocytic cells that engulf bacteria and toxins. The sinusoids drain into the central vein.

Bile is manufactured by the hepatocytes. The bile canaliculi are tiny bile capillary vessels that communicate between the columns of hepatocytes. The bile canaliculi collect bile and transport it to the bile ducts in the portal triad of each lobule, and subsequently it flows into the hepatic ducts at the porta hepatis. These ducts join immediately to form one common hepatic duct that merges with the cystic duct from the gallbladder to form the common bile duct (Fig. 11-2). The common bile duct opens into the duodenum in an area called the ampulla or papilla of Vater, located about 7.5 cm below the pyloric opening from the stomach.

Bile contains bile salts, which facilitate digestion and ab-

sorption, and various waste products. The liver is essential in the metabolism of carbohydrates, proteins, and fats. It metabolizes nutrients into glycogen stores for regulation of blood glucose levels and energy sources for the brain and body functions.

The liver plays several important roles in the blood-clotting mechanism. It is the organ that synthesizes plasma proteins, excluding gamma globulins but including prothrombin and fibrinogen. Vitamin K, a cofactor to the synthesis of prothrombin, is absorbed by the metabolism of fats in the intestinal tract as a result of bile formation by the liver. Patients with liver disease may have alterations in their blood coagulation abilities.

The liver also synthesizes lipoproteins and cholesterol. Cholesterol is an essential component of the blood plasma.

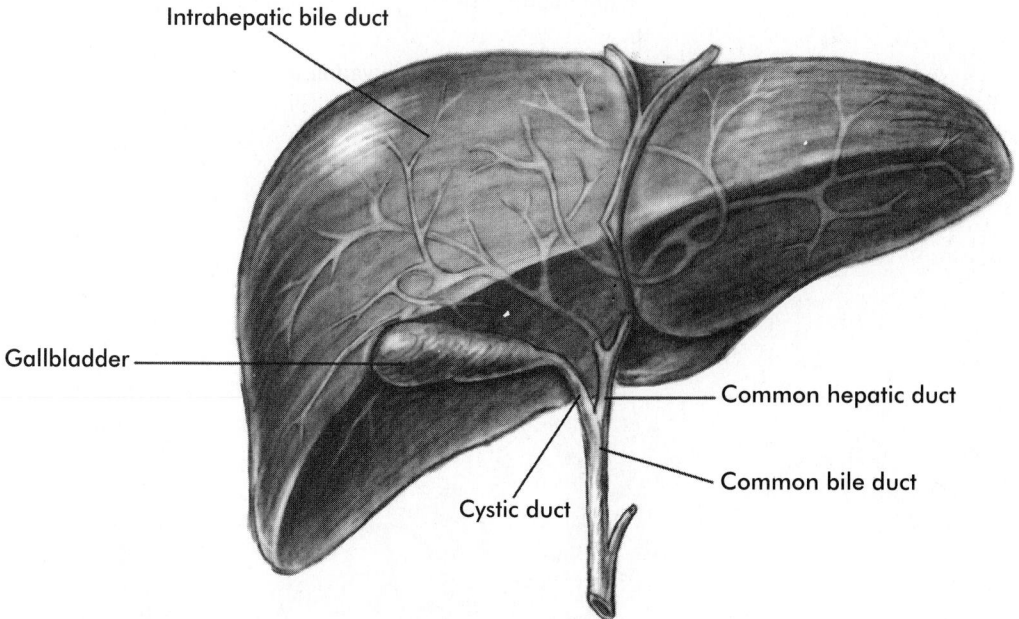

FIG. 11-2   Biliary system can be divided into three anatomic areas: the intrahepatic bile duct, the extrahepatic bile duct (common hepatic and common bile ducts), and the gallbladder and cystic duct.

From Davis, J.H., et al. (1987). *Clinical surgery* (Vol. 2). St. Louis: Mosby.

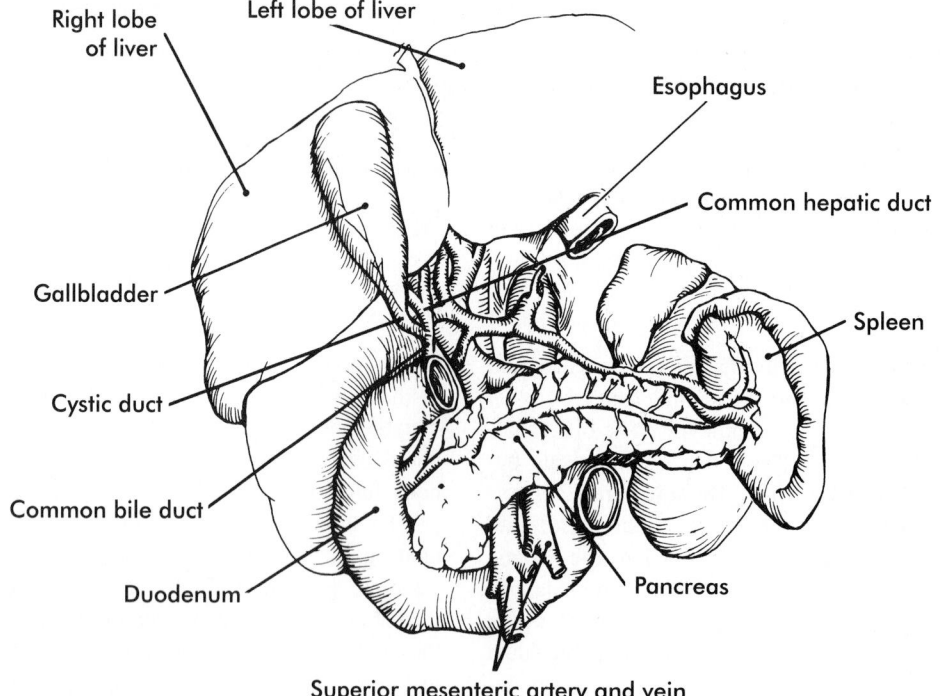

FIG. 11-3   Gallbladder and surrounding anatomy.

It serves as a precursor for bile salts, steroid hormones, plasma membranes, and other specialized molecules. A diet high in cholesterol reduces the amount that must be synthesized by the liver. When diet is deficient in cholesterol, the liver increases synthesis to maintain the levels necessary for the production of the vital chemical molecules.

The liver also serves in the metabolic alteration of foreign molecules or biotransformation of chemicals. The microsomal enzyme system (MES) plays a major role in the body's response to foreign chemicals such as pollutants, drugs, and alcohol. Patients with liver disease may have alterations in their response to chemical substances. This consideration is most important in the induction and management of general anesthesia for patients with liver disorders.

The gallbladder, which lies in a sulcus on the undersurface of the right lobe of the liver, terminates in the cystic duct (Fig. 11-3). This ductal system provides a channel for the flow of bile to the gallbladder, where it becomes highly concentrated during the storage period. Approximately 600 to 1000 ml of bile are produced by the liver daily. The gallbladder's average storage capacity is 40 to 70 ml. As food, especially fats, is ingested, cholecystokinin is released by the duodenal cells when food enters the small intestine. The musculature of the gallbladder contracts, forcing bile into the cystic duct and through the common duct. As the sphincter of Oddi in the ampulla of Vater relaxes, bile pours forth, flowing into the duodenum to aid in digestion by emulsification of fats. The gallbladder receives its blood supply from the cystic artery, a branch of the hepatic artery. Innervation for the gallbladder and biliary tree is controlled by the autonomic nervous system. The parasympathetic innervation stimulates contraction, whereas sympathetic innervation inhibits contraction.

The pancreas (Fig. 11-3) is a fixed structure lying transversely behind the stomach in the upper abdomen. The head of the pancreas is fixed to the curve of the duodenum. Blood is supplied to the pancreas and the duodenum via the celiac axis and the superior mesenteric artery (Figs. 11-4 and 11-5). The body of the pancreas lies across the vertebrae and over the superior mesenteric artery and vein. The tail of the pancreas extends to the hilum of the spleen. In total, the pancreas extends approximately 25 cm. The pancreatic secretions, containing digestive enzymes, are collected in the pancreatic duct, or duct of Wirsung, which unites with the common bile duct to enter the duodenum about 7.5 cm below the pylorus. The ampulla of Vater is formed by the dilated junction of the two ducts at the point of entry.

The pancreas also contains groups of cells, called islets or islands of Langerhans, that secrete hormones into the blood capillaries instead of into the duct. These hormones are insulin and glucagon, and both are involved in carbohydrate metabolism.

The spleen (Fig. 11-6) is in the upper left abdominal cavity, with full protection provided by the tenth, eleventh, and twelfth ribs; the lateral surface is directly beneath the dome of the diaphragm. The anterior medial surface is in proximity to the cardiac end of the stomach and the splenic flex-

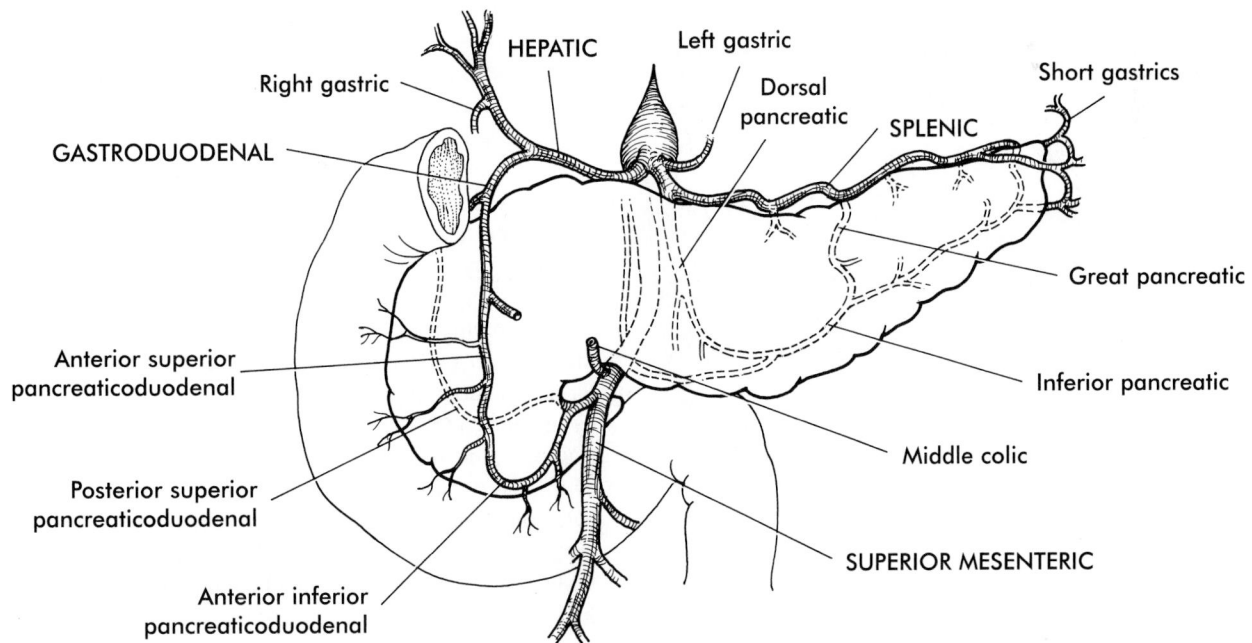

FIG. 11-4 Arterial supply to the pancreas arises from the celiac axis (hepatic and splenic arteries) and the superior mesenteric artery. The blood supply to the head of the gland is via the pancreaticoduodenal (anterior and posterior) arcades, which arise from the gastroduodenal artery (superior) and superior mesenteric arteries (inferior).

From Cooperman, A.M., & Hoerr, S.O. (Eds.). (1978). *Surgery of the pancreas: A text and atlas.* St. Louis: Mosby.

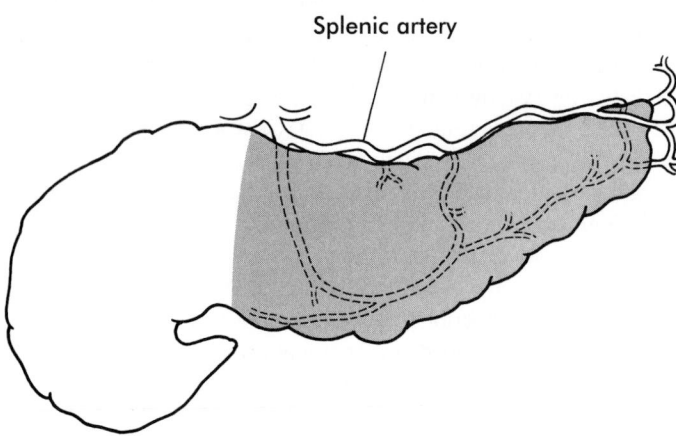

FIG. 11-5 Major arterial supply to the body and tail of the pancreas is derived from branches of the splenic artery.

From Cooperman, A.M., & Hoerr, S.O. (editors.). (1978). *Surgery of the pancreas: A text and atlas.* St. Louis: Mosby.

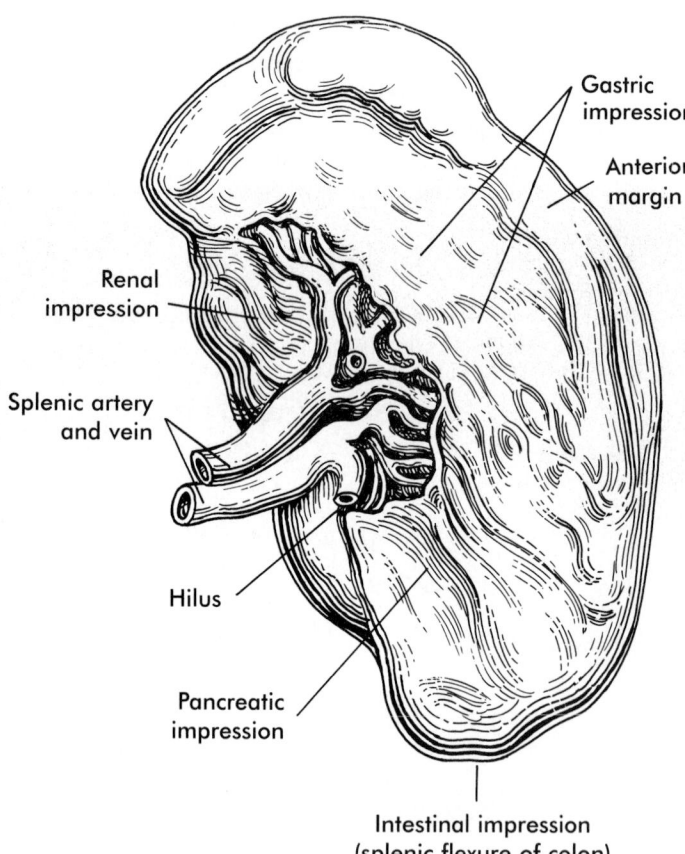

FIG. 11-6 Spleen, medial aspect. Arrangement of vessels at hilum is highly variable.

From Anthony, C.P., & Thibodeau, G.A. (1983). *Textbook of anatomy and physiology* (11th ed.). St. Louis: Mosby.

ure of the colon. The spleen is covered with peritoneum that forms supporting ligaments. The arterial blood supply is furnished by the splenic artery, a branch of the celiac axis. The splenic vein drains into the portal system.

The spleen has many functions. Among them are the defense of the body by phagocytosis of microorganisms, formation of nongranular leukocytes and plasma cells, and phagocytosis of damaged red blood cells. It also acts as a blood reservoir.

PERIOPERATIVE NURSING CONSIDERATIONS

ASSESSMENT

The patient with hepatobiliary disease may have extreme jaundice, urticaria, petechiae, lethargy, and irritability. Depending on the extent of the disease, the patient may have increased bleeding and coagulation times and a decreased platelet count, thus predisposing to bruising easily. A thorough nursing history is necessary to properly assess the health status of patients with dysfunctions of the hepatobiliary system, the pancreas, or the spleen. Assessment should include data pertaining to the patient's perception of his or her disease, comfort status, nutritional status, fluid and electrolyte balance, bowel and elimination patterns, energy level and independence, and exposure to toxins.

Establishing the objective database for a person with hepatobiliary or pancreatic dysfunction requires comprehensive assessment. Particular attention should be directed toward observing for characteristic signs of dysfunction. Increased abdominal girth and distention, palmar erythema, distended periumbilical veins, hemorrhagic areas, spider nevi, muscle wasting, and dry mucous membranes are a few of the characteristic signs and symptoms of dysfunction. Vascular volume can be assessed by monitoring vital signs, including orthostatic changes, assessment of skin turgor, temperature, appearance, and weight gain or loss.

Physical examination of the patient's abdomen should include palpation and percussion to evaluate tenderness, ascites, and organ enlargement.

The common laboratory tests to assess liver function are those which evaluate fat metabolism, protein metabolism, blood coagulation properties, bilirubin metabolism, and antigens and antibodies of hepatitis (Tables 11-1 and 11-2). Radiographic studies commonly used to evaluate function of the liver, pancreas, and spleen include ultrasound studies, computed tomography (CT scan), radioisotope scanning, nuclear magnetic reasonance imaging (MRI), angiography, cholecystography, and cholangiography. An abdominal flatplate radiograph and upper gastrointestinal series may also aid in diagnosing gross anomalies of the liver, pancreas, and spleen.

Endoscopy and biopsy are more invasive diagnostic procedures that may be used in evaluation of the liver, pancreas, and spleen. Endoscopic retrograde cholangiopancreatography (ERCP) is a procedure that allows for direct vi-

TABLE 11-1

Liver Function Studies

Test name	Normal values
SERUM ENZYMES	
Alkaline phosphatase	13-39 U/ml
	Elevated levels are seen with biliary obstruction and cholestatic hepatitis.
Aspartate aminotransferase (AST; previously SGOT)	5-40 U/ml
	Elevated levels are seen with hepatocellular injury.
Alanine aminotransferase (ALT; previously SGPT)	5-35 U/ml
	Elevated levels are seen with liver dysfunction; the ratio of AST/ALT usually is more than 1 in alcoholic cirrhosis and liver congestion and less than 1 in acute hepatitis, viral hepatitis, and infectious mononucleosis.
Lactic dehydrogenase (LDH)	200-500 U/ml
	Elevated levels are seen with hepatitis and untreated pernicious anemia, as well as in a number of other conditions (e.g., acute myocardial infarction, renal disease, muscle disease, or malignant tumors).
5'-Nucleotidase	2-11 U/ml
	Elevated levels may be an early indication of metastasis to the liver.
Leucine aminopeptidase (LAP)	Men: 80-200 U/ml
	Women: 75-185 U/ml
	Elevated levels may be seen with liver metastasis and choledocholithiasis.
Gamma-glutamyltranspeptidase (GGTP)	Men: 8-38 U/L
	Women <45 yr: 5-27 U/L
	Elevated levels are seen in 75% of chronic alcoholics.
BILIRUBIN METABOLISM	
Serum bilirubin	
Indirect (unconjugated)	<0.8 mg/dl
	Elevated levels are seen with hemolysis (lysis of RBCs).
Direct (conjugated)	0.2-0.4 mg/dl
	Elevated levels are seen with hepatocellular injury or obstruction.
Total	<1 mg/dl
	Elevated levels may be seen with biliary obstruction.
Urine bilirubin	0
	Bilirubin in the urine may be seen with hepatic disease or biliary obstruction; only conjugated bilirubin spills into the urine, because unconjugated bilirubin is bound to albumin in the serum and thus cannot pass the glomerular membrane.
Urine urobilinogen	0-4 mg/24 h
	Increased levels are seen with hemolytic processes, shunting of portal blood flow, or increased intestinal bacteria.
Fecal urobilinogen	40-280 mg/24 h
	Reduced levels cause clay-colored stools and are seen in biliary obstruction.
AMMONIA	Adult: 15-110 μg/dl
	Elevated levels may be seen with liver dysfunction, hepatic failure, or congestive heart failure.

Continued.

TABLE 11-1

Liver Function Studies—cont'd

Test name	Normal values
SERUM PROTEINS	
Albumin	3.5-5.5 g/dl
	Reduced levels are seen with hepatocellular injury.
Globulin	2.5-3.5 g/dl
	Increased levels are seen with hepatitis.
Total	6-7 g/dl
	Decreased levels may be seen with hepatocellular injury.
Albumin/globulin (A/G) ratio	1.5/1-2.5/1
	Ratio may be reversed with chronic hepatitis or other chronic liver disease.
Transferrin	250-300 μg/dl
	Reduced levels may be seen with liver damage; increased levels may be seen with iron deficiency.
BLOOD CLOTTING FUNCTIONS	
Prothrombin time (PT)	11.5-14 sec *or* 90%-100% of control
	Increased levels may be seen with chronic liver disease (e.g., cirrhosis) or vitamin K deficiency.
Partial thromboplastin time (PTT)	25-40 sec
	Increased levels may be seen with severe liver disease or heparin therapy.

From Doughty, D.B., Jackson D.B.: *Gastrointestinal disorders.* 1993, St. Louis, Mosby, p. 68.

TABLE 11-2

Tests of Pancreatic Function

Test name	Normal values
Serum amylase	60-180 Somogyi units/ml
	Elevated levels are seen with pancreative inflammation.
Serum lipase	1.5 Somogyi units/ml
	Elevated levels may indicate pancreatic inflammation.
Urine amylase	35-260 Somogyi units/h
	Elevated levels are seen with pancreatic inflammation.
Secretin test	Volume 1.8 ml/kg/h
	HCO_3^- concentration >80 mEq/L
	HCO_3^- output >10 mEq/L/30 sec
	Reduced volumes are seen with pancreatic disease.

sualization of the biliary tract, the injection of radiographic dye into the ductal system, and biopsy when indicated. Percutaneous transhepatic cholangiography (PTC) involves percutaneous insertion of a long flexible needle into a bile duct of the liver. Contrast medium is injected and serial x-rays are taken. Arteriography of the liver, biliary tree, pancreas, and spleen is accomplished by femoral arteriotomy and the placement of a catheter into the celiac branch of the abdominal aorta under fluoroscopic visualization.

Contrast medium is then injected and serial x-rays are taken as the vessels are visualized during the perfusion and drainage phases.

NURSING DIAGNOSIS

Following a thorough nursing assessment of all subjective and objective data related to the patient with dysfunction of the liver, biliary tract, pancreas, or spleen, nursing diagnoses are formulated. Nursing diagnoses related to the care of patients undergoing surgery of the liver, biliary tract, pancreas, or spleen might include the following:

- Anxiety related to impending surgical procedure and knowledge deficit
- High risk for fluid volume deficit related to hemorrhage or large volume blood loss
- High risk for alteration in body temperature
- High risk for infection related to invasive gastrointestinal procedure
- High risk for injury related to positioning and length of surgical procedure

OUTCOME IDENTIFICATION

Outcomes identified for the selected nursing diagnoses could be stated as:

- The patient will maintain a manageable level of anxiety as evidenced by the ability to communicate appropriately and to verbalize knowledge and understanding of the perioperative events.
- The patient will maintain fluid volume equilibrium throughout the operative procedure.
- The patient will demonstrate a consistent core body temperature of 96° to 99° F.
- The patient will demonstrate no clinical symptoms of wound infection.
- The patient will maintain neuromuscular function and tissue integrity normal for him or her.

PLANNING

Planning for the care of the patient having surgery of the liver, biliary tract, pancreas, or spleen requires assimilation of knowledge of the anatomy and subsequent physiologic complications that may occur with surgical interruption of tissues. Principles of proper positioning of the patient, maintenance of asepsis, prevention of biologic and electrical hazards, and providing proper instrumentation and equipment are a few constituents of the plan of care.

Assessment and patient interview will give insight as to the specific needs of the individual patient. The patient's past medical and surgical history, as well as age, size, and nutritional status will assist the perioperative nurse in developing an effective plan of care. A typical care plan for a patient undergoing surgery of the liver, biliary tract, pancreas, or spleen follows.

IMPLEMENTATION

Patients having surgery of the liver, biliary tract, pancreas, or spleen are usually given general anesthesia. The following pertinent factors are to be considered in caring for the patient undergoing biliary surgery.

Positioning the patient

The patient is placed in a supine position. A small positioning aid placed under the lower right thorax may be requested by the surgeon. This elevates the lower rib cage to provide better exposure and access to the viscera in the right upper quadrant of the abdomen.

Positioning the patient for laparoscopic procedures requires the nurse to exercise caution when applying the safety strap(s). Because of the potential for the patient to be placed in a severe side tilt and/or reverse Trendelenburg's position, the nurse must ensure the security of the safety strap placement. Close monitoring of the patient is essential during positional changes due to the decrease lighting in the room.

When an operative cholangiogram is anticipated, the operating room bed is prepared with an x-ray cassette holder before the patient is positioned. A preliminary x-ray film may be taken to ensure correct placement of the cassette. The holder must be directly beneath the patient's right upper quadrant because correct positioning is imperative to ensure accurate visualization of the biliary tract. The use of fluoroscopy for operative cholangiogram is becoming more prevalent. If it is the technology of choice for the operative cholangiogram, the nurse must ensure that the patient's OR table has been equipped and positioned so that C-arm image intensification can be efficiently accomplished.

Attention is given to proper alignment of the patient's body and extremities. Areas of pressure and bony prominences are padded well to prevent interruption of circulation and pressure injury to tissues. This precaution is especially important with diabetic, circulatory impaired, and elderly patients.

Draping the patient

Following the abdominal prep, sterile towels are arranged to accommodate the intended incision. A sterile drape sheet is applied over the patient's lower torso and a laparotomy sheet is then placed to provide a wide sterile field and cover all exposed body surfaces except the incisional site.

Instrumentation

Instrumentation includes a basic laparotomy set (see Chapter 10) with instruments available for dilating and exploring the ducts adjacent to the pancreas and biliary tract. Vascular clamps, gastrointestinal clamps, ligating clips of all sizes with appliers, and linear stapling instruments should be available. A self-retaining retractor system such as the Bookwalter or the Omni-tract allows optimal safe retraction of tissues and excellent exposure of the abdominal viscera (Fig. 11-7). Specific biliary tract instruments should be included as follows:

Cutting instruments

1 Metzenbaum or Nelson scissors, 9¼ inches
1 Potts-Smith scissors

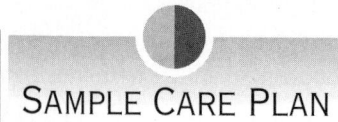

SAMPLE CARE PLAN

NURSING DIAGNOSIS: Anxiety related to impending surgical procedure and knowledge deficit
OUTCOME: Patient will maintain a manageable level of anxiety as evidenced by the ability to communicate appropriately and to verbalize knowledge and understanding of the perioperative events.
INTERVENTIONS:
Complete as much of the setup as possible before the patient's arrival to the OR suite, especially those activities that create noise.
Greet the patient positively and professionally.
Introduce the patient to the OR team.
Avoid hasty movements or gestures of indecision.
Speak slowly and clearly when addressing the patient, and use terminology the patient can understand.
Offer emotional reassurance through touch, facial expression, and allowing the patient to talk about feelings.

NURSING DIAGNOSIS: High risk for fluid volume deficit related to hemorrhage or large volume blood loss
OUTCOME: Patient will maintain fluid volume equilibrium throughout surgical procedure.
INTERVENTIONS:
Have available blood products in close, refrigerated storage for timely access.
Measure and record accurate fluid volume loss throughout surgical procedure.
Anticipate and communicate potential for fluid volume deficit to blood bank personnel.
Check lab values intraoperatively.

NURSING DIAGNOSIS: High risk for alteration in body temperature
OUTCOME: Patient will demonstrate a consistent core body temperature of 96° to 99° F.

INTERVENTIONS:
Adjust room temperature and humidity to accommodate preservation of body temperature.
Cover all possible body surfaces to maintain body heat.
Use only warm irrigation solutions.
Warm IV fluids and blood products prior to infusion.

NURSING DIAGNOSIS: High risk for infection related to invasive gastrointestinal procedure
OUTCOME: Patient will demonstrate no clinical symptoms of wound infection.
INTERVENTIONS:
Ensure aseptic technique is maintained; communicate and correct breaks in asepsis.
Contain contaminants appropriately.
Ensure that all sterilization procedures and expiration dates have been properly observed.

NURSING DIAGNOSIS: High risk for injury related to positioning and length of surgical procedure
OUTCOME: Patient will maintain neuromuscular function and tissue integrity normal to the individual.
INTERVENTIONS:
Ensure patient is in optimal anatomic alignment following induction of anesthesia.
Adequately pad all bony prominences.
Secure limbs with nonflexible safety strap to ensure position is maintained and to prevent limb from falling from positioning device.
Ensure safe and proper placement of electrosurgical dispersive pad.
Ensure that no fluid pooling occurs beneath patient during surgical procedure.
Ensure that no weight or stress is placed on body parts and structures.
Ensure padding is in place beneath all self-retaining retractors.

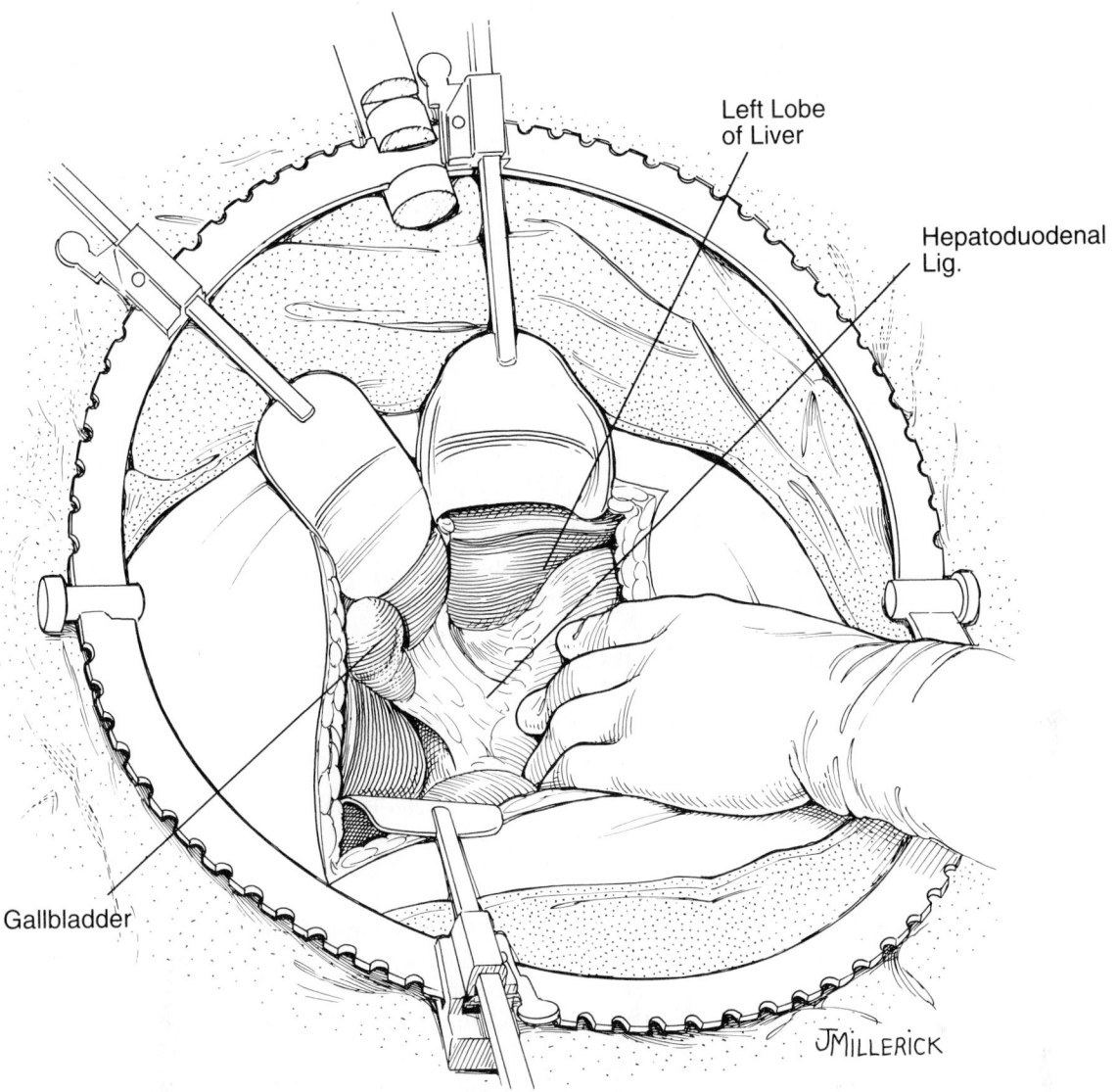

FIG. 11-7 Bookwalter self-retaining retractor in place to provide optimal exposure to the abdominal viscera.

From Daly, J.M., & Cady, B. (1993). *Atlas of surgical oncology.* St. Louis: Mosby.

Clamping and exposing instruments (Fig. 11-8)

2 Harrington retractors
2 Mixter gallbladder forceps, 7¼ inches
2 Johns Hopkins gallbladder forceps, 8 inches, or

Duct instruments (Fig. 11-9)

1 Mayo common duct scoop, malleable shaft, 10½ inches
1 Set gall duct spoons, malleable, sizes 1 to 5

2 Lahey gall duct forceps, 7¼ inches
6 Schnidt gall duct forceps

1 Ochsner gallbladder aspirating trocar
2 Potts-Smith tissue forceps

Stone instruments (Fig. 11-10)

1 Set Randall kidney stone forceps (may be used instead of Blake and Desjardin gallstone forceps)
2 Blake gallstone forceps, 1 straight and 1 curved, 8¼ inches

Accessory items

Drainage catheters, as desired
Sutures, surgeon's preference
Fogarty biliary catheters

1 Desjardin gallstone forceps, 9 ¼ inches
1 Set Bakes common duct dilators
1 Moynihan bile duct probe and scoop

Contrast medium (Hypaque, Conray, or Reno-M)
Culture tubes

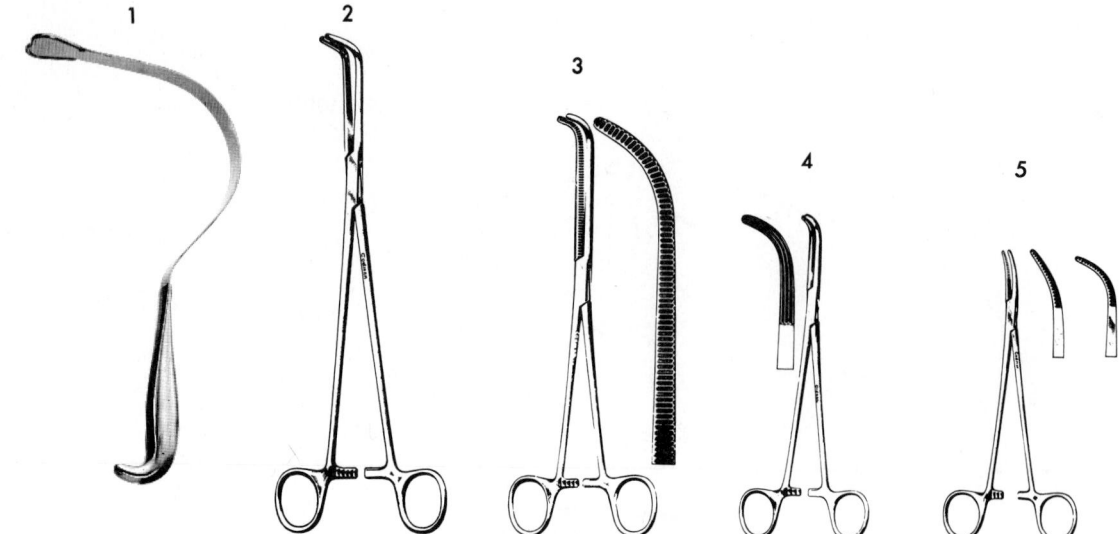

FIG. 11-8   Clamping and exposing instruments for gallbladder surgery. *1,* Harrington retractor; *2,* Mixter (right-angle) gallbladder forceps; *3,* Johns Hopkins gallbladder forceps; *4,* Lahey gall duct forceps, *5,* Schnidt gall duct forceps.

Courtesy Codman & Shurtleff, Inc., Randolph, Mass.

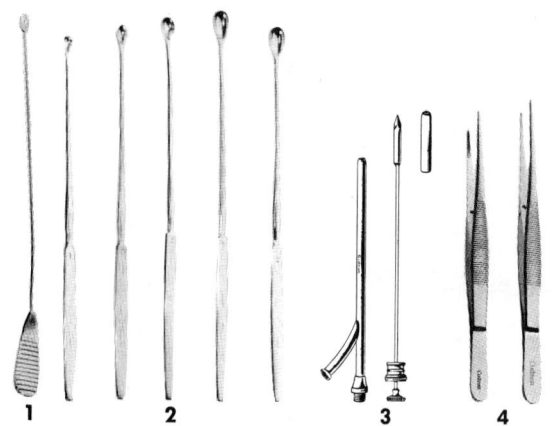

FIG. 11-9   Duct instruments. *1,* Mayo common duct scoop; *2,* gall duct spoons; *3,* Ochsner gallbladder trocar; *4,* Potts-Smith tissue forceps.

Courtesy Codman & Shurtleff, Inc., Randolph, Mass.

Equipment and supplies

An electrosurgical unit, laser, argon beam coagulator, surgical headlight, intraoperative ultrasound handpiece and unit, Cavitron Ultrasonic Suction Aspirator (CUSA) unit (Fig. 11-11), and cell saver system may be required for the operative procedure, according to the surgeon's preference.

Thrombin, Gelfoam, Surgicel, Avitene, and other hemostatic agents should be available in the operating room suite. Radiographic dye and supplies for intraoperative radiography or angiography may also be required.

Drainage materials

Tubes and catheters must be in optimal condition and suitable for the areas to be drained. If a defective drain is used, a free fragment may remain in the wound on removal of the tube.

The scrub nurse should note the condition of all drainage materials and should test them for patency before they are placed in the patient.

Soft rubber or latex tissue drains may be used after a cholecystectomy or a choledochotomy. A latex rubber T tube drain of suitable size is prepared by the surgeon after the duct has been explored. The center of the crossbar is notched opposite the junction of the vertical limb so that its ends will bend more readily during removal. The ends are beveled and tailored to fit the duct.

Drains are usually exteriorized through separate stab wounds and anchored to skin edges to prevent their retraction. The perioperative nurse should document the types of drains and reservoirs inserted during the operative procedure and identify them with an applied label. All drains and their locations should be included in the perioperative nurse's report to the nursing unit to which the patient is transferred postoperatively.

Aseptic considerations

When the common duct is opened or an anastomosis is established between a duct and other parts of the tract, care should be exercised to isolate contaminated instruments and materials from the remainder of the operative field, as described for gastrointestinal surgery (see Chapter 10). Instruments and materials used for the exteriorization of a drain should be treated as contaminated.

FIG. 11-10   Stone instruments. *1* to *4,* Randall kidney stone forceps (four shapes); *5,* Blake gallstone forceps; *6,* Desjardin gallstone forceps; *7,* Bakes common duct dilators; *8,* Moynihan gall duct probe and scoop.

Courtesy Codman & Shurtleff, Inc., Randolph, Mass.

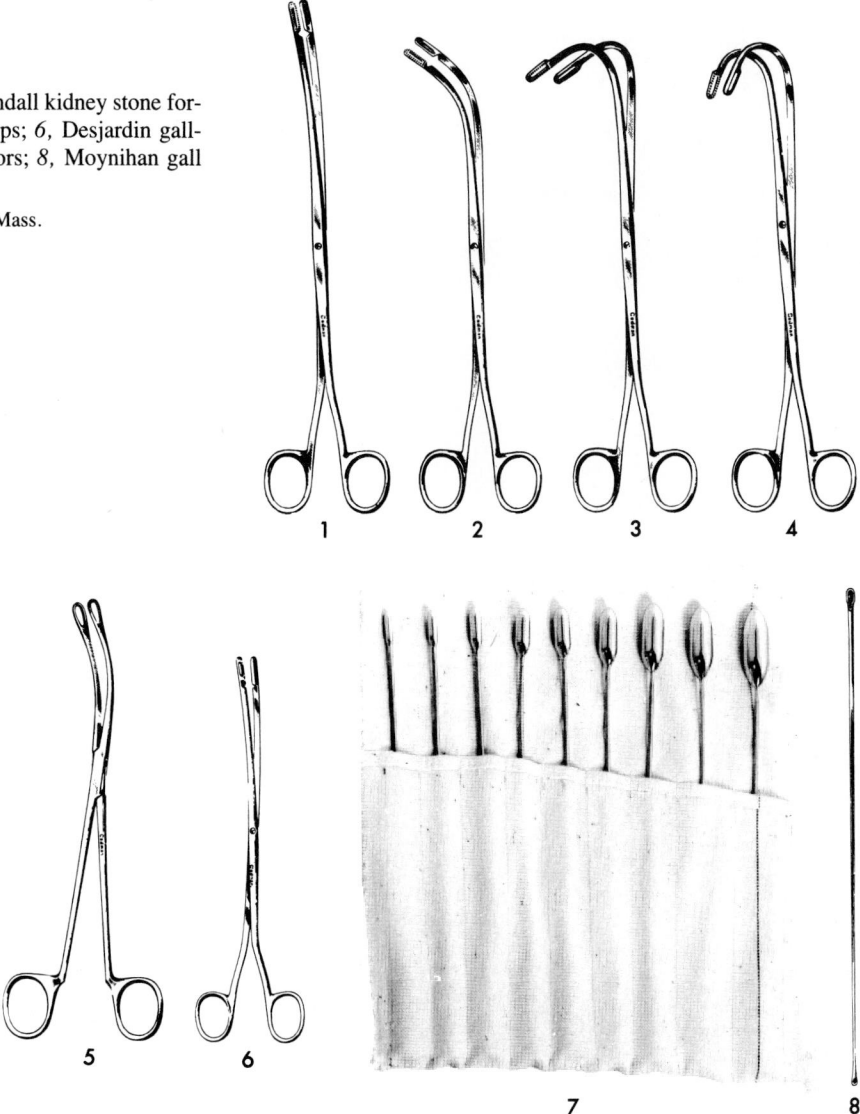

Blood products

The perioperative nurse should be aware of the type and amount of blood products available for the patient having surgery of the liver, biliary tract, pancreas, or spleen. Constant evaluation of blood loss is communicated to the anesthesia and surgical team as well as to the blood bank personnel so that blood products are readily available.

EVALUATION

Evaluation of the patient following surgery includes examination of all skin surfaces and comparison to the preoperative assessment data. Abdominal drains, chest drainage systems, urinary drainage systems, and peripheral infusion lines are assessed for patency and labeled appropriately. Fluid volume use and loss are documented and communicated appropriately. A thorough report of the patient's history, preoperative assessment, intraoperative events, and postoperative evaluation is communicated to the PACU or SICU nurse.

The evaluation of patient status can be phrased as outcome statements such as the following:

- The patient expressed a positive recollection of perioperative events upon postoperative visit.
- The patient's hematocrit is in the 30% to 35% range; vital signs are stable.
- The patient's core body temperature remained consistently in the 96° to 99° F range.
- The patient's surgical incision is dry and intact. There are no clinical signs of infection.
- All skin surfaces are clear, intact, and free from stress markings; capillary filling is noted following blanching of tissues. The patient demonstrates normal range of motion in extremities. Pulses are palpable in all distal extremities.

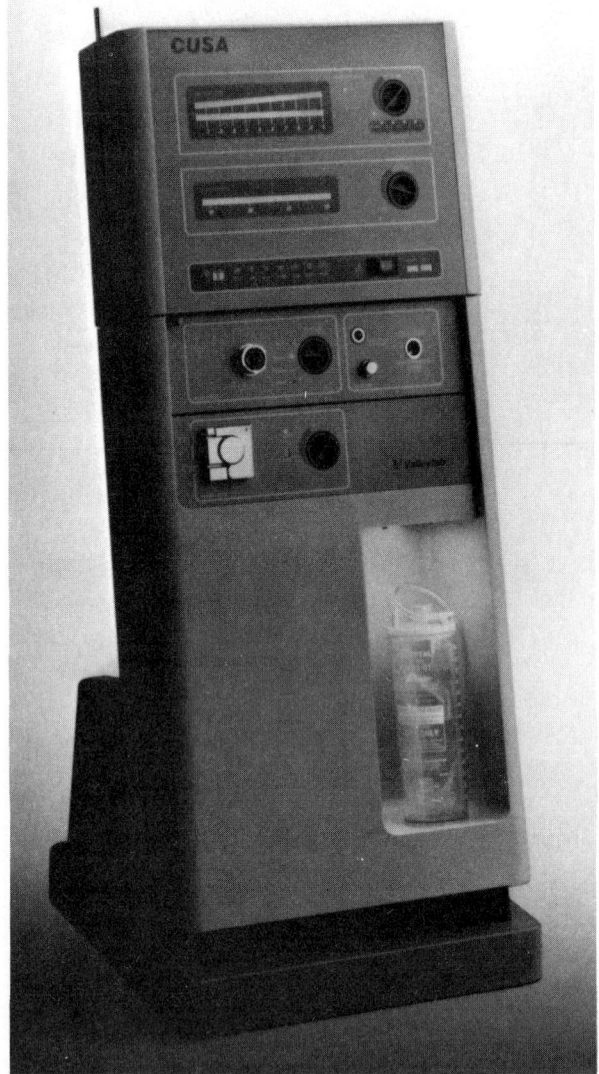

FIG. 11-11   Valleylab CUSA System 200 ultrasonic surgical aspirator manufactured by Valleylab, Inc., Boulder, Colo.

SURGICAL INTERVENTIONS

SURGERY OF THE BILIARY TRACT

Cholecystectomy

Cholecystectomy is removal of the gallbladder. It is performed for the treatment of diseases such as acute or chronic inflammation (cholecystitis), stones (cholelithiasis), or the presence of polyps or carcinoma.

Procedural considerations

A basic laparotomy set and biliary instruments are utilized when cholecystectomy is performed through an open abdominal incision.

Operative procedure (Fig. 11-12)

1. Through a right subcostal, right paramedian, or midline incision the abdominal cavity is opened. Hemostasis of capillary vessels is achieved with electrocoagulation. Larger vessels are clamped with hemostats and tied with suture material. Retractors and laparotomy packs are employed as the abdominal cavity is carefully examined.
2. The common duct is palpated for evidence of stones, and the pathologic conditions determined. Harrington or Deaver retractors, moist laparotomy packs, long tissue forceps, and suction are used.
3. The surrounding organs are walled off from the gallbladder region by laparotomy packs and deep retractors.
4. To facilitate gentle traction, Pean forceps are usually placed on the body of the gallbladder (Fig. 11-12, *A*).
5. The peritoneal fold overlying the junction of the cystic and common duct is incised with a no. 7 knife handle and a no. 15 blade, long Metzenbaum scissors, and forceps. Suction is available, and bleeding points are clamped and ligated or electrocoagulated.
6. Adhesions are separated by blunt dissection with small, round, dry dissector sponges, sponges on holders, and blunt right-angled clamps. Dissection is continued to expose the neck of the gallbladder, the cystic artery, and the cystic duct (Fig. 11-12, *B* and *C*).
7. Dissection is continued to expose the cystic artery as it enters the wall of the gallbladder. On complete exposure and visualization of the branches, the cystic artery is doubly ligated with silk or clamped with ligating clips and divided (Fig. 11-12, *B*). Occasionally a third ligature or clip may be used. If the cystic artery has more than one branch, each is ligated and divided separately. Abnormalities of the arterial and ductal anatomy are common (Fig. 11-13), and the surgeon works with meticulous care to identify these structures.
8. The true junction of the cystic duct with the common bile duct is visualized. The cystic duct is identified and carefully dissected down to its junction with the hepatic duct. Any stones in the cystic duct are milked back into the gallbladder, and a tie is placed around the proximal cystic duct. If necessary, a cholangiogram is performed at this time (see procedure for intraoperative cholangiogram).
9. If a cholangiogram is not done, the cystic duct is doubly ligated and divided (Fig. 11-12, *C*). A transfixion suture of fine absorbable suture may be used on the stump of the cystic duct near the common bile duct. The gallbladder is freed from the liver, working upward to the fundus, and it is removed (Fig. 11-12, *D*). In some cases working from the fundus downward to the neck of the gallbladder may be necessary.
10. All bleeding is controlled; reperitonealization of the liver bed, if indicated, is accomplished with interrupted or continuous fine, absorbable intestinal sutures.

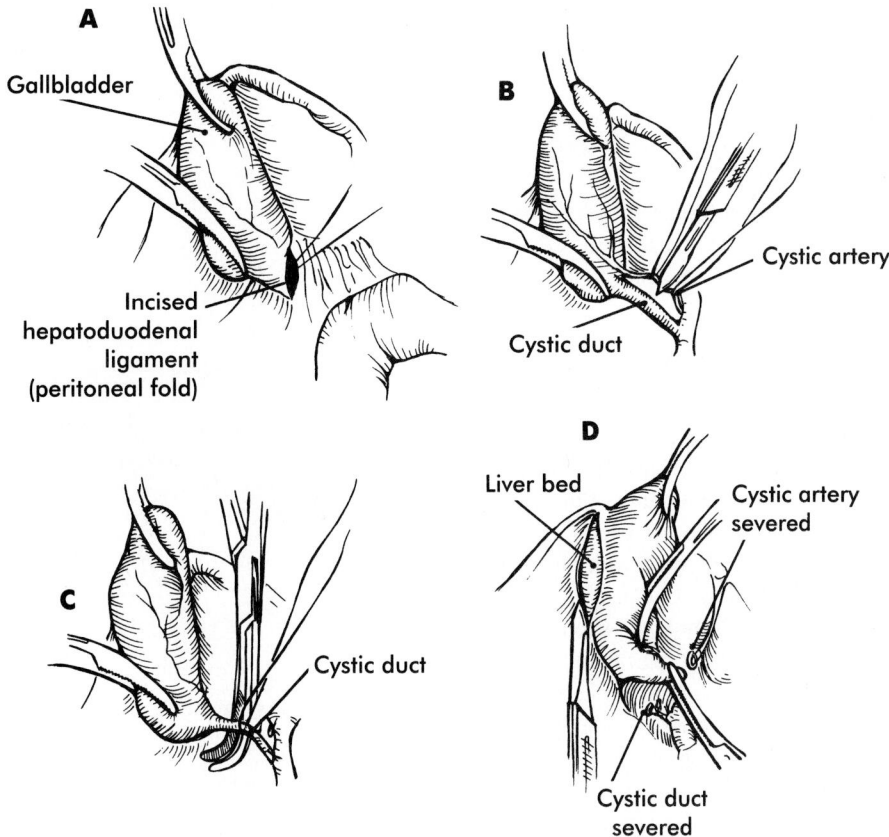

FIG. 11-12 Cholecystectomy. **A,** With Pean forceps in place, gentle traction is maintained as peritoneum over Calot's triangle is incised. **B,** Cystic artery is clearly visualized, doubly ligated, and divided. **C,** Cystic duct is carefully dissected and identified before forceps and ligatures are applied. **D,** Dissection of gallbladder from liver bed is completed.

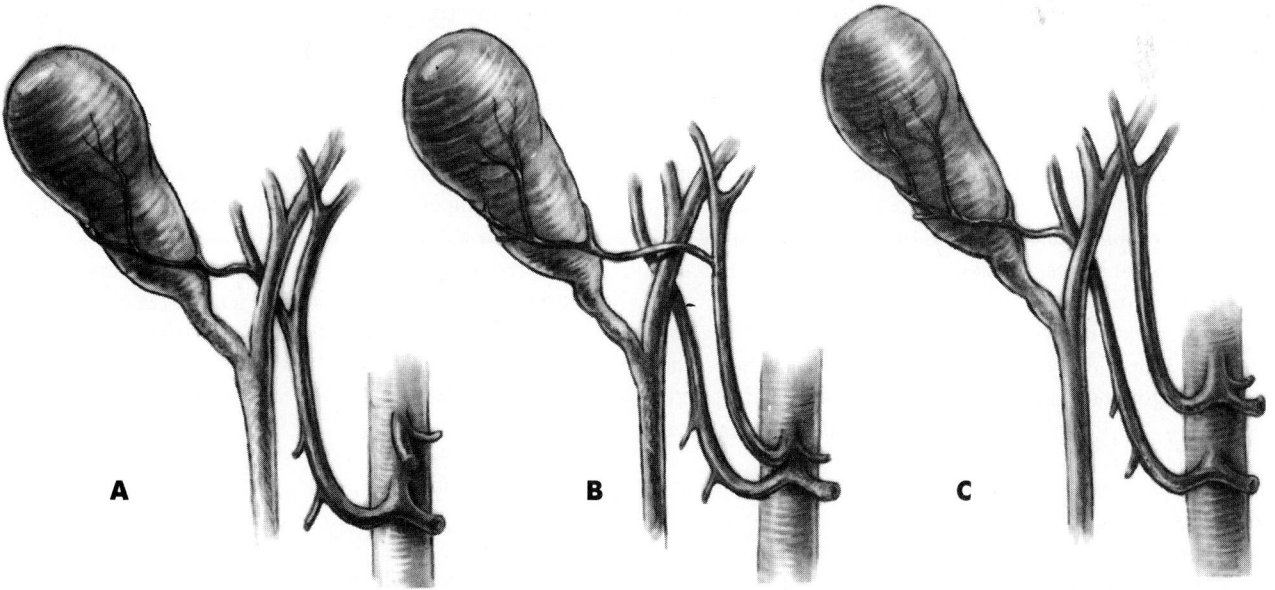

FIG. 11-13 Arterial blood supply of the liver and biliary system is quite variable. **A,** The most common anatomic arrangement is a cystic artery arising from the right hepatic artery. **B,** A dual hepatic blood supply is found in 15% to 20% of patients, with the right hepatic artery arising from the superior mesenteric artery in a significant number, as in **C.**

From Davis, J.H., et al. (1987). *Clinical surgery* (Vol. 2). St Louis: Mosby.

11. A drain may be inserted near the cystic duct stump. The free end of the drain is exteriorized through a stab wound in the lateral abdominal wall.
12. The wound is closed in layers and a dressing applied.

Intraoperative cholangiogram

An intraoperative cholangiogram is usually performed in conjunction with cholecystectomy to visualize the common bile duct and the hepatic ductal branches and to assess patency of the common bile duct.

Procedural considerations

An intraoperative cholangiogram requires the use of x-ray. The OR bed should be prepared with radiographic attachments that permit easy insertion of the x-ray film cassette beneath the patient. If the surgeon prefers fluoroscopy to visualize the filling of the ducts, the OR bed is prepared before the patient's arrival in the OR suite with an image-intensification attachment.

The perioperative nurse should ensure the patient has not had previous allergic reactions to the x-ray medium before dispensing the pharmaceutical agent to the sterile field.

Protection such as x-ray aprons or leaded shields should be readily available for all members of the surgical team. Because the patient's abdomen remains open while the x-ray equipment is positioned directly over the operative site, appropriate draping to maintain asepsis is necessary. Radiopaque sponges and any unnecessary instrumentation are removed from the abdominal site to avoid obscuring the view of the contrast medium filling the ducts.

The scrub nurse prepares a cholangiocath by attaching a stopcock with a 20-ml syringe of saline and a 20-ml syringe of contrast medium to the Luer-Lok ports. All air bubbles are removed because they might be misinterpreted as gall duct stones on the x-ray.

Operative procedure

1. The cholangiocath is irrigated with saline before and during the insertion of the catheter into the cystic and common bile ducts (Fig. 11-14). Irrigation during insertion facilitates dilatation and reduces trauma to the ductal lumen.
2. The cholangiocath is anchored in the lumen of the common bile duct by the surgeon's preferred method. The more common methods are applying a ligaclip proximal to the insertion site, tying or suturing the catheter in place, or using a ring-jawed holding clamp, such as a Swenson clamp, that has been designed specifically for this purpose.
3. With placement of the cholangiocath confirmed and anchored, the surgeon informs the surgical team that x-ray is now required.
4. All radiopaque sponges, instruments, and obstructing equipment are removed from the field.
5. The surgical field is draped with a sterile drape sheet to maintain asepsis of the wound and field.

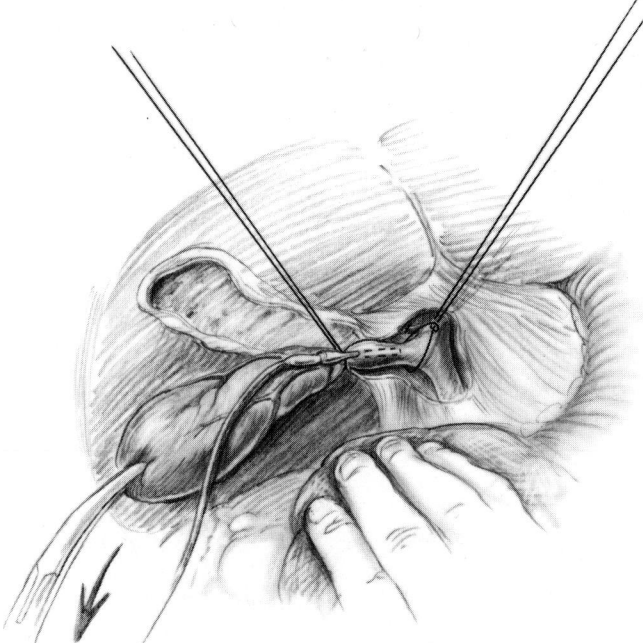

FIG. 11-14   Cholangiocath inserted into the cystic duct through a small opening proximal to a silk tie placed at the cystic duct–gallbladder junction. The gallbladder has been dissected from the liver bed, and the cystic duct is dissected down to its junction with the hepatic duct.

From Davis, J.H., et al. (1987). *Clinical surgery* (Vol 2). St. Louis: Mosby.

6. The x-ray equipment is positioned, as the surgeon redirects the stopcock to allow for injection of the contrast medium.
7. The surgeon directs the radiology technician as to the precise time to take the radiograph.
8. The x-ray equipment is removed from the operative site and the drapes covering the incisional site are carefully removed and discarded.
9. The x-ray is developed immediately to ensure that appropriate visualization of the ductal structures has been achieved. (Fig. 11-15 illustrates a stone in the distal bile duct.)
10. Once the surgeon studies the radiograph hung on the x-ray view box in the OR, the decision is made to repeat the intraoperative cholangiogram, to explore the common bile duct, or to proceed with the conclusion of the patient's surgery.

Laparoscopic cholecystectomy

Laparoscopic-guided cholecystectomy using electrodissection for detachment of the gallbladder from the liver bed has gained popularity as the surgical treatment of choice in patients with gallbladder disease who meet the appropriate criteria for safe laparoscopic intervention. The preoperative

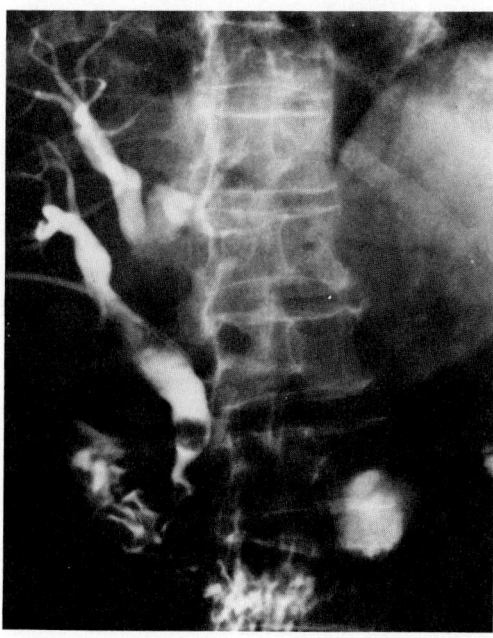

FIG. 11-15   Cholangiogram shows a retained stone in the distal bile duct.

From Davis, J.H., et al. (1987). *Clinical surgery* (Vol. 2). St. Louis: Mosby.

evaluation of patients having laparoscopic cholecystectomy differs little from that for patients scheduled for laparotomy. An abdominal ultrasound may be performed to document the presence or absence of gallstones as well as intrahepatic or extrahepatic bile duct dilatation, which may suggest intraductal stones. If stones are not present and the patient does not have a history of pancreatitis or jaundice, the patient becomes a candidate for the laparoscopic-guided procedure. For patients with a history of peptic ulcer disease, a flexible esophagogastroduodenoscopy may be performed to rule out existing disease. In patients with suspected ductal stones, a preliminary ERCP is advised. A laparoscopic procedure always has the potential to convert to a laparotomy, an option the patient should be informed about.

Procedural considerations

Patients are generally admitted to the hospital on the morning of surgery. General anesthesia is commonly utilized; however, a combination of regional and local anesthetics with IV sedation may be requested.

The following instrumentation, supplies, and equipment are required:

Laparoscope
3 trocars and sheaths, 5 mm, or 2 trocars and sheaths, 5 mm, and 1 trocar and sheath, 7 mm
2 trocars and sheaths, 10 or 11 mm
Converters to adapt sheath size to instrument size
No. 7 knife handle with no. 11 blade
Multiple clip appliers

Blunt grasping forceps (an assortment of alligator, Babcock, and spatula)
Laparoscopic scissors
Laparscopic video unit and secondary "slave" monitor
Laparoscopic camera and control unit
Light source
CO_2 tank and insufflation unit
Electrosurgical unit
Filtered insufflation tubing (disposable)
Electrocautery or electrocautery suction-irrigator (disposable)
Pressure bag for IV saline 0.9%
Laparotomy instrumentation and supplies should be readily available in the operating room if needed

Operative procedure

1. The patient is positioned supine with the usual comfort and safety measures observed. A Foley catheter is inserted into the urinary bladder via the urethra, and a nasogastric tube is inserted for decompression of the stomach. The patient is then placed in a reverse Trendelenburg position of 10 to 20 degrees.

2. A small skin incision is made in the folds of the umbilicus with a no. 11 blade on a no. 7 knife handle. Pneumoperitoneum is accomplished by two options:
   a. A Veress needle is placed percutaneously through the umbilicus into the peritoneal cavity and insufflation with CO_2 gas prior to the introduction of the trocar and sleeve.
   b. Open laparoscopy, sometimes termed the Hasson technique, which is the surgical opening into the peritoneum and placement of the operative sleeve to which the insufflation tubing is then attached and pneumoperitoneum is achieved. This technique is suggested in patients who have had a prior abdominal incision near the umbilicus or those having potential for intraperitoneal adhesions. CO_2 is the gas of choice for pneumoperitoneum because it does not support combustion and is relatively innocuous to the patient. Should air emboli occur, CO_2 is safer in preventing intracardiac foaming and subsequent complications.

3. Gas flow is initiated at 1 to 2 L/minute. The intraabdominal pressure is normally in the 8 to 10 mm Hg range and is commonly used as an indicator for proper Veress needle placement by the surgeon. If the pressure gauge indicates a higher pressure, the needle may be in a closed space such as fat, buried in the omentum, or in the lumen of the intestine.

4. The perioperative nurse should set the insufflation unit to a maximum pressure of 15 mm Hg. When intraabdominal pressure reaches 15 mm Hg, the flow will stop. Pressure higher than 15 mm Hg may result in bradycardia or a change in blood pressure, or may force a gas emboli into an exposed blood vessel during the operative procedure. Most insufflation units are equipped with an alarm mechanism to alert the operative team if

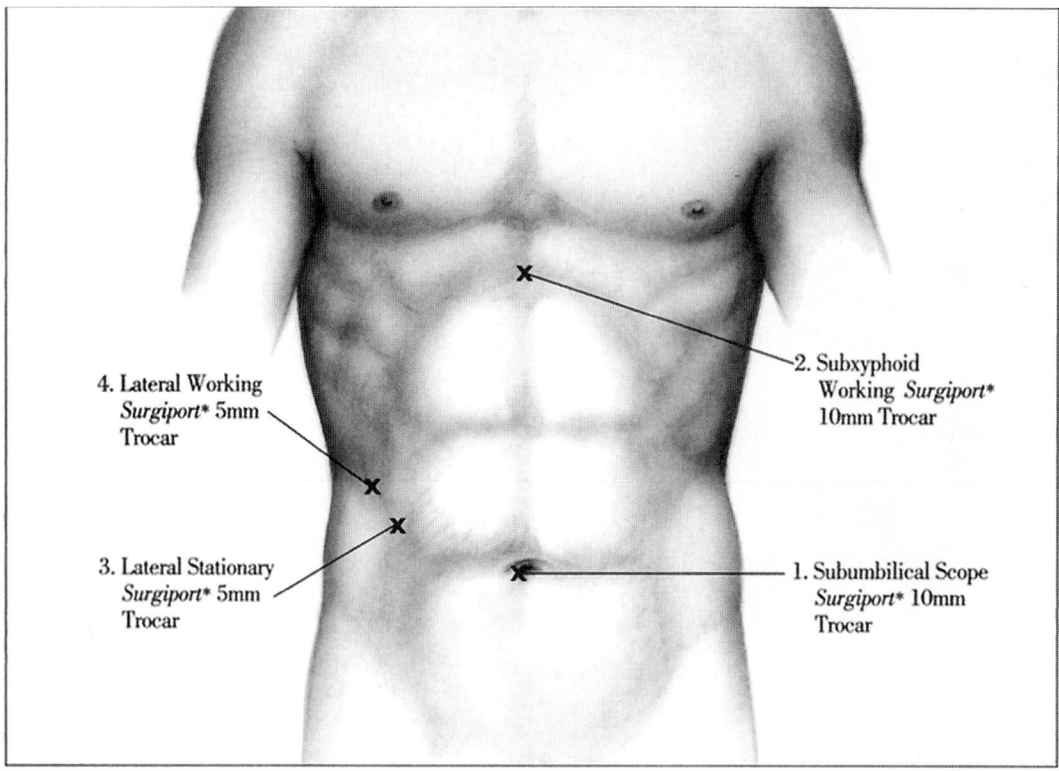

4. Lateral Working *Surgiport* 5mm Trocar

3. Lateral Stationary *Surgiport* 5mm Trocar

2. Subxyphoid Working *Surgiport* 10mm Trocar

1. Subumbilical Scope *Surgiport* 10mm Trocar

FIG. 11-16   Trocar placement for laparoscopic cholecystectomy demonstrating anatomic placement and the usual size of trocar used at each site.

the intraabdominal pressure is exceeded. The surgeon may frequently ask what the pressure reading is, as might the anesthesiologist.

5. When 3 to 4 L of gas have been used and the abdomen is rounded, the insufflation needle is removed. The skin incision is extended using the no. 11 blade so that a 10- or 11-mm trocar and sheath can be inserted. The surgeon grasps the abdominal skin cephalad to the trocar and sheath and in a firm motion inserts the sharp trocar point slightly angled toward the pelvis.

6. The trocar is removed, leaving the sheath in place. The laparoscope is then placed through the sheath, and the camera is attached to view and explore the peritoneal cavity on the video screen. The surgeon usually stands on the left side of the patient while the first assistant stands on the right. Video monitors are positioned at eye level at both the right and left sides of the operative field.

7. The patient is then placed in a 30-degree, reverse Trendelenburg's position and tilted slightly to the left.

8. Three additional skin incisions are made for the insertion and placement of the operative sheaths (Fig. 11-16). The trocars and sheaths are inserted into the peritoneal cavity under the direct visualization of the laparoscopic view. Two sheaths are usually 5 mm and one

is 10 mm to accommodate the accessory instrumentation. A fifth trocar and sheath may be needed to accomplish grasping or retracting during the procedure.

9. Blunt grasping forceps are inserted through the 5-mm sheaths. Convertor pieces are placed atop the sheath ports to prevent gas from escaping. The gallbladder is manipulated with one pair of forceps while the porta hepatis is exposed with the other.

10. Using the midline sheath the surgeon dissects the cystic duct and artery with blunt forceps beginning at the gallbladder and proceeding toward the cystic and common bile duct junction. (Fig. 11-17, A).

11. The cystic artery and the cystic duct are dissected free from the surrounding tissues (Fig. 11-17, B). Two clips are applied proximally and distally to the intended line of division on both the duct and artery (Fig. 11-17, C). The use of a disposable, preloaded multiple clip applier assists in the placement of ligating clips in a more efficient manner than a singly loaded reusable applier. A pretied suture loop may be used if the surgeon desires.

12. The cystic duct and artery are divided.

13. Attention is then given to dissection of the gallbladder from the liver. This is accomplished using electrosurgery set at 25 to 35 W. The electrosurgical instrument may have a channel through which suction can be ap-

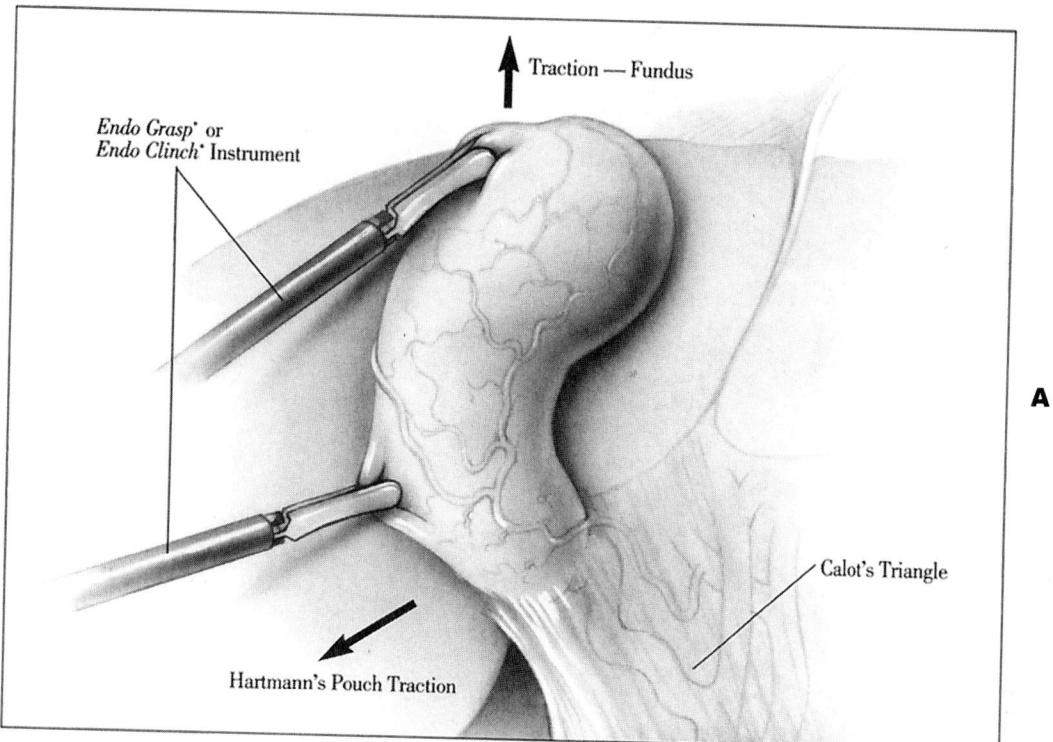

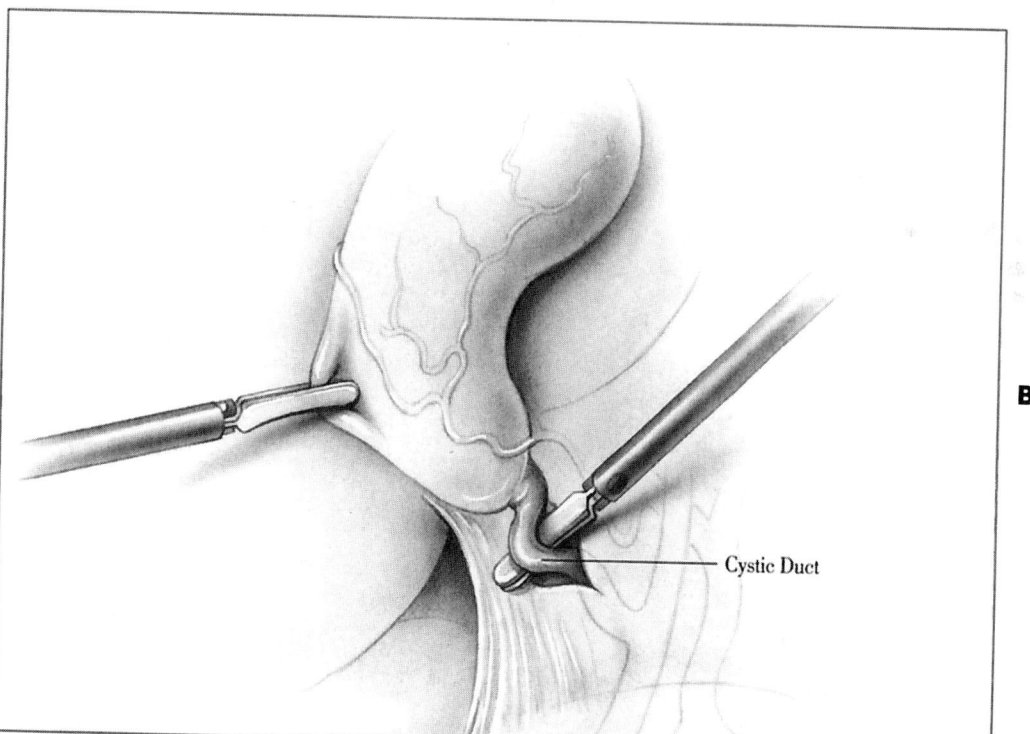

FIG. 11-17 Laparoscopic cholecystectomy. **A,** The gallbladder is grasped with blunt grasping forceps and the cystic duct and artery are identified by gentle retraction anteriorly. **B,** The cystic duct and artery are isolated from the surrounding tissue.

From Quilici, P.J. (1992). *New developments in laparoscopy.* Norwalk, Conn.: U.S. Surgical Corporation.

Continued.

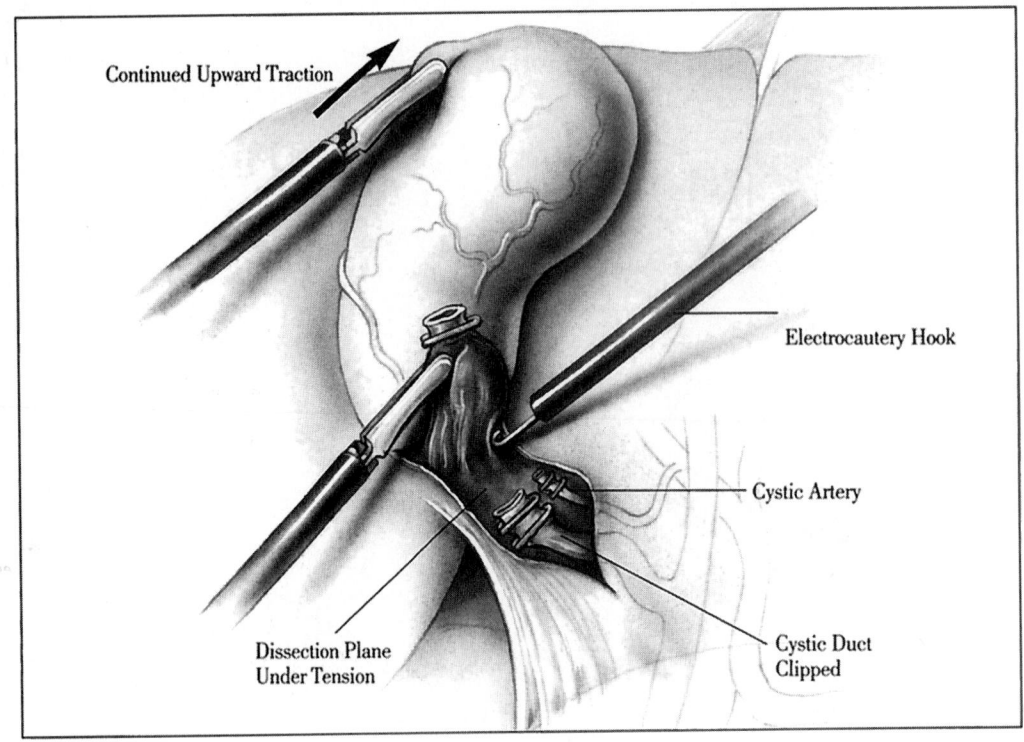

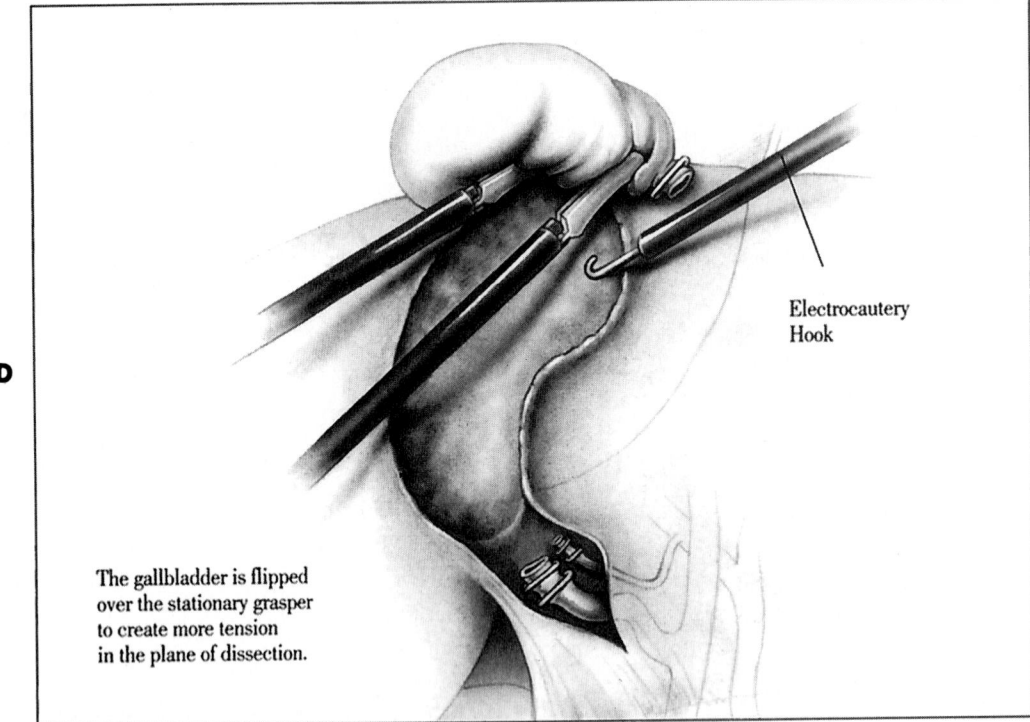

FIG. 11-17, CONT'D   **C,** Ligating clips are applied via an endoscopic multiple clip applier. **D,** The gallbladder is dissected from the liver bed.

From Davis, J.H., et al. (1987). *Clinical surgery* (Vol. 2). St. Louis: Mosby.

plied. This is particularly useful in evacuating the smoke plume during the procedure. Some disposable instruments employ suction, electrocoagulation, and irrigation through the same instrument.

14. The gallbladder is retracted using the forceps inserted through the 5-mm sheaths. It is manipulated to allow the medial and lateral attachments to be dissected with the electrosurgical instrument (Fig. 11-17, *D*).

15. Irrigation of the liver bed is performed prior to the detachment of the gallbladder. Once it is determined to have no visible bile leak or bleeding in the liver bed, the laparoscope and camera are moved to the upper midline sheath. Large grasping forceps are inserted through the umbilical sheath and are placed on the neck of the gallbladder. An endobag or similar specimen-containing accessory may be used to secure the gallbladder for extraction, or the gallbladder may be brought out through the umbilical incision. If the gallbladder is too large to be extracted, the neck is brought above the surface of the incision, Kelly clamps are applied, and bile is suctioned out of the gallbladder for decompression.

16. The stab wounds are closed following decompression of the peritoneal cavity.

17. The patient's hospital stay is usually overnight with discharge the following morning.

Cholecystostomy

Cholecystostomy is establishment of an opening into the gallbladder to permit drainage of the organ and removal of stones. This procedure is usually selected for patients with acute gallbladder disease and a general physical condition that does not permit more extensive surgery.

Procedural considerations

A large Toomey syringe (50 ml) or an Asepto syringe may be needed for irrigation purposes. If a local anesthetic is used, the anesthetic drug and syringes and needles are necessary. Specified drainage tubes or catheters should be available.

Operative procedure

1. Although many surgeons prefer the right subcostal incision, cholecystostomy procedures are often performed as emergencies, and so a quicker midline or transverse incision may be used.

2. The fundus of the gallbladder is grasped with Allis or Babcock forceps, and the proposed opening is encircled by means of an absorbable pursestring suture, leaving the ends long.

3. To protect the abdominal cavity from contamination, the gallbladder is isolated with laparotomy packs, and suction is available.

4. Within the pursestring suture, the gallbladder contents are aspirated by means of a suction tubing attached to a trocar sheath.

5. As the contents are aspirated, culture specimens should

be taken. The contaminated trocar and sheath are removed and discarded.

6. The opening can be enlarged with Metzenbaum scissors; gallstones are removed with malleable scoops and stone forceps. Irrigating the gallbladder with isotonic saline solution is necessary to remove small stones, grit, or pastelike material. A syringe with a catheter or an Asepto syringe may be used for irrigation. Contaminated instruments are placed in a basin on the operative field.

7. A drainage tube is inserted in the gallbladder opening. The pursestring suture is tightened around the catheter, care being taken not to occlude it. A second pursestring suture or separate mattress sutures may be used to secure the gallbladder to the peritoneum and the posterior rectus fascia.

8. The free end of the catheter or tube is exteriorized through a stab wound and then anchored to the skin edges, as described for cholecystectomy.

9. Drainage of the abdominal cavity is established. The exterior end of each drain is secured.

10. The wound is closed in layers, as described for laparotomy, and dressings are applied without disturbing the drains.

Choledochotomy and choledochostomy

Choledochotomy is an incision made into the common bile duct (Fig. 11-18). Choledochostomy is the establishment of an opening into the common bile duct with placement of a drainage T tube. Choledochotomy with subsequent choledochostomy are performed to treat choledocholithiasis or to relieve an obstruction in the common bile duct.

Procedural considerations

Before exploration is begun, operative cholangiography may be performed to locate all stones within the ductal system. X-ray films are repeated after the T tube drain is in place to confirm the successful evacuation and patency of the ducts. A subcostal or upper right rectus incision is made. Instrumentation is the same as that described for biliary surgery, with the addition of the following instruments and supplies:

1 Set Bakes common duct dilators, malleable shafts, sizes 3 to 11 mm (see Fig. 11-10)

1 Ochsner flexible spiral gallstone probe, 14 inches

1 Malleable silver probe, 8 inches

1 Asepto syringe, 60 ml

4 Syringes, 2, 20, 30, and 50 ml

Fogarty biliary catheters

3 Aspirating needles: 24 gauge, ¾ inch; 19 gauge, 3½ inches; and 16 gauge, 2 inches

1 Catheter adapter for saline solution irrigation

2 Ampules contrast media

3 Robinson catheters, 8, 11, and 16 Fr

3 T tubes, 8 to 26 Fr, as desired

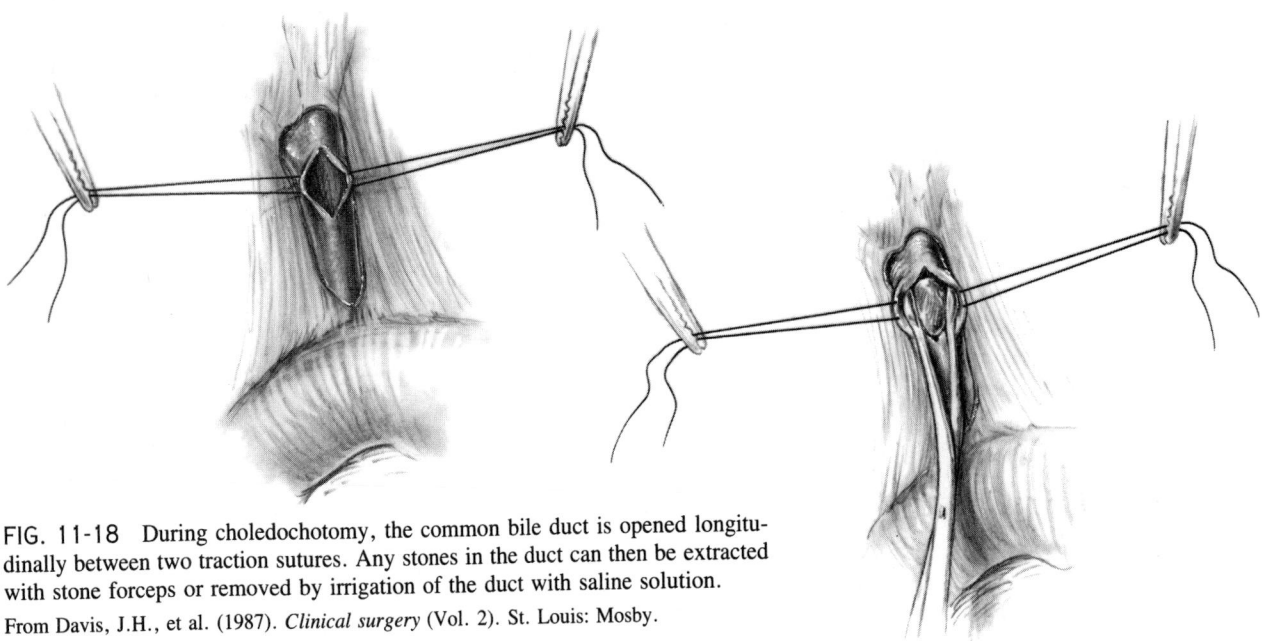

FIG. 11-18   During choledochotomy, the common bile duct is opened longitudinally between two traction sutures. Any stones in the duct can then be extracted with stone forceps or removed by irrigation of the duct with saline solution.

From Davis, J.H., et al. (1987). *Clinical surgery* (Vol. 2). St. Louis: Mosby.

Operative procedure

1. The abdomen is opened as for cholecystectomy. If the gallbladder has not been previously removed, it is exposed and removed or retracted by means of laparotomy packs and retractors.
2. The common duct may be identified by means of an aspirating syringe and fine-gauge needle to make certain that the suspected duct is not a blood vessel. Culture specimens may be obtained.
3. Two fine traction sutures are placed in the wall of the duct, below the entrance of the cystic duct.
4. The common duct region is walled off with laparotomy packs and narrow blade retractors. A discard basin for contaminated instruments is placed at the lower end of the operative field; a suction apparatus is made ready for immediate use.
5. A longitudinal incision is made in the common duct (Fig. 11-19, *A*), between the traction sutures, with a long no. 3 knife handle and a no. 15 or no. 11 blade. Constant suction is maintained with a Yankauer suction tube to keep the field free from oozing bile as the incision is enlarged with Potts angled or Metzenbaum scissors. Additional stay sutures may be applied to the ductal opening.
6. Visible stones are removed with gallstone forceps, after which exploration of the duct is begun with small malleable scoops proximal and then distal to the opening. Probing is continued as stones are removed from both the common and hepatic ducts. Isotonic saline solution in an Asepto syringe and a small-lumen catheter or a Fogarty-type, balloon-tipped catheter are used to facilitate the removal of small stones and debris, as

well as to demonstrate patency of the common bile duct through to the duodenum (Fig. 11-19, *B* to *D*).
7. A duodenotomy may be performed if patency of the sphincter of Oddi and ampulla of Vater cannot be demonstrated.
   a. An area of the duodenum is walled off with laparotomy packs. The incision is made longitudinally, using a scalpel with a no. 15 blade and Metzenbaum scissors.
   b. Bleeding vessels are clamped with mosquito hemostats and ligated with fine silk or absorbable sutures or electrocoagulated.
   c. Fine silk traction sutures are inserted, and exploration is continued.
   d. The duodenal opening is usually closed transversely in two layers with fine absorbable and silk intestinal sutures.
8. The T tube is prepared by the surgeon (Fig. 11-19, *E*), irrigated for patency, and introduced into the common duct with fine vascular forceps.
9. The common duct incision is closed with fine absorbable intestinal sutures. Contaminated instruments are placed in the discard basin.
10. The T tube is irrigated to demonstrate patency (Fig. 11-19, *E*), and a cholangiogram is done.
11. The gallbladder may be removed as described for cholecystectomy.
12. A drain is introduced into the foramen of Winslow. Both drain and T tube are exteriorized through a stab wound.
13. The wound is closed in layers; the T tube and drain are carefully anchored to the skin, and each wound is

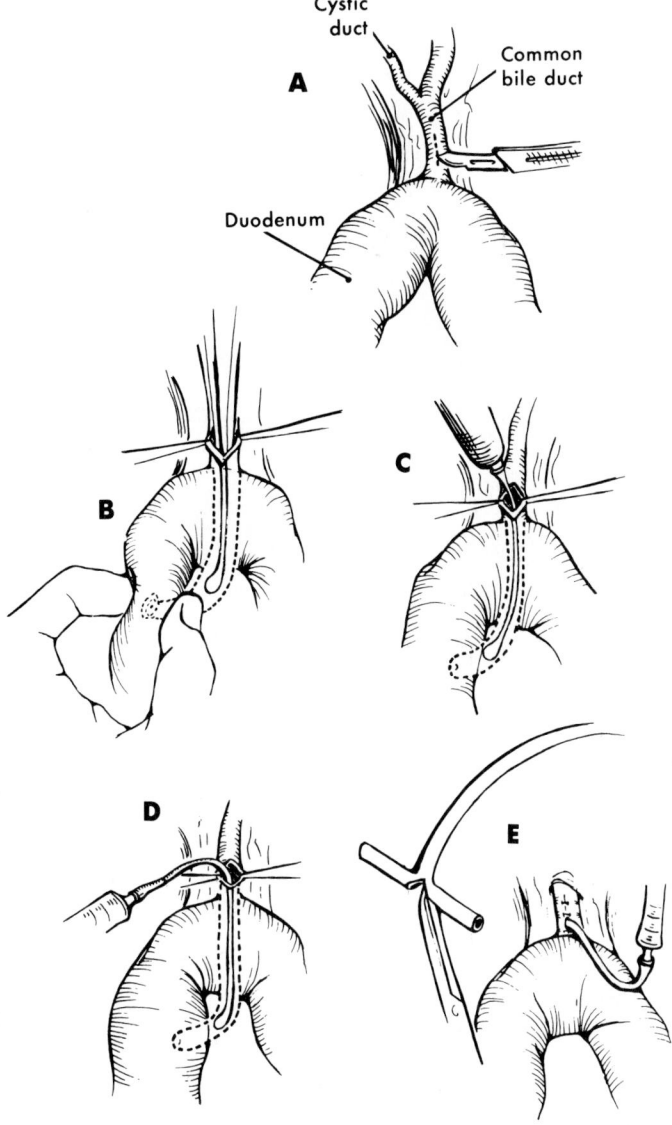

FIG. 11-19   Choledochotomy with choledochostomy. **A,** Opening common duct. **B,** Introducing stone forceps. **C,** Probing common duct. **D,** Irrigating duct. **E,** Preparing and irrigating T tube.

copious amounts of sterile saline. A pressure bag is placed around an IV bag of 0.9% saline, and pressure is applied to 300 mm Hg. Sterile tubing is then passed from the sterile field and attached to the saline bag. The scrub nurse attaches the distal end of the sterile IV tubing directly to the irrigating stopcock on the scope.

Instrumentation is as described for biliary surgery, with the addition of the following instruments:

Choledochoscope with accessories: biopsy forceps, stone-grasping forceps, and a sheath that can be used to direct other instruments into various portions of the biliary tract	Video camera and viewing screen Light cord Normal saline, 1000-ml bag Sterile IV tubing IV pole Pressure bag Light source

Operative procedure

1 to 5. As described for choledochotomy.
6. The choledochoscope is inserted into the common duct, which is then flushed with saline. Stones are grasped with the stone forceps and removed. The choledochoscope allows visualization of the entire duct to ensure no stones remain. After all stones are removed, the common duct is again thoroughly flushed with saline. Closure of the duct and wound is completed.

Cholecystoduodenostomy and cholecystojejunostomy

Cholecystoduodenostomy and cholecystojejunostomy are the establishment of continuity by creating an anastomosis between the gallbladder and duodenum or the gallbladder and jejunum to relieve an obstruction in the distal end of the common duct.

An obstruction in the biliary system may be caused by a tumor of the ducts involving the head of the pancreas or the ampulla of Vater, the presence of an inflammatory lesion, a stricture of the common duct, or the presence of stones.

Procedural considerations

Instrumentation is as described for cholecystostomy, plus two Doyen intestinal forceps, curved with guards, or similar nontraumatic holding forceps.

Operative procedure

1. The abdomen is opened, the gallbladder is exposed and contents aspirated, and the pathologic condition is confirmed, as described for cholecystostomy.
2. The anastomosis site is prepared, posterior serosal silk sutures are placed, and open anastomosis is performed. The surgical technique for anastomosis of the gallbladder to the duodenum or loop of jejunum is usually performed as a two-layer anastomosis. The serosa of the duodenum or loop of jejunum is sutured to the full thick-

dressed individually to prevent undue tension that could result in displacement of the tube and drain.
14. Sterile tubing is used to connect the T tube to a small drainage container or bag.

Choledochoscopy

Choledochoscopy is direct visualization of the common bile duct by introduction of a choledochoscope. Surgeon's preference may require a rigid or flexible scope. Choledochoscopy may take the place of operative cholangiography. It provides a means for extraction of stones that are difficult to remove.

Procedural considerations

Distending the common duct is necessary for better visualization and is accomplished by irrigating the duct with

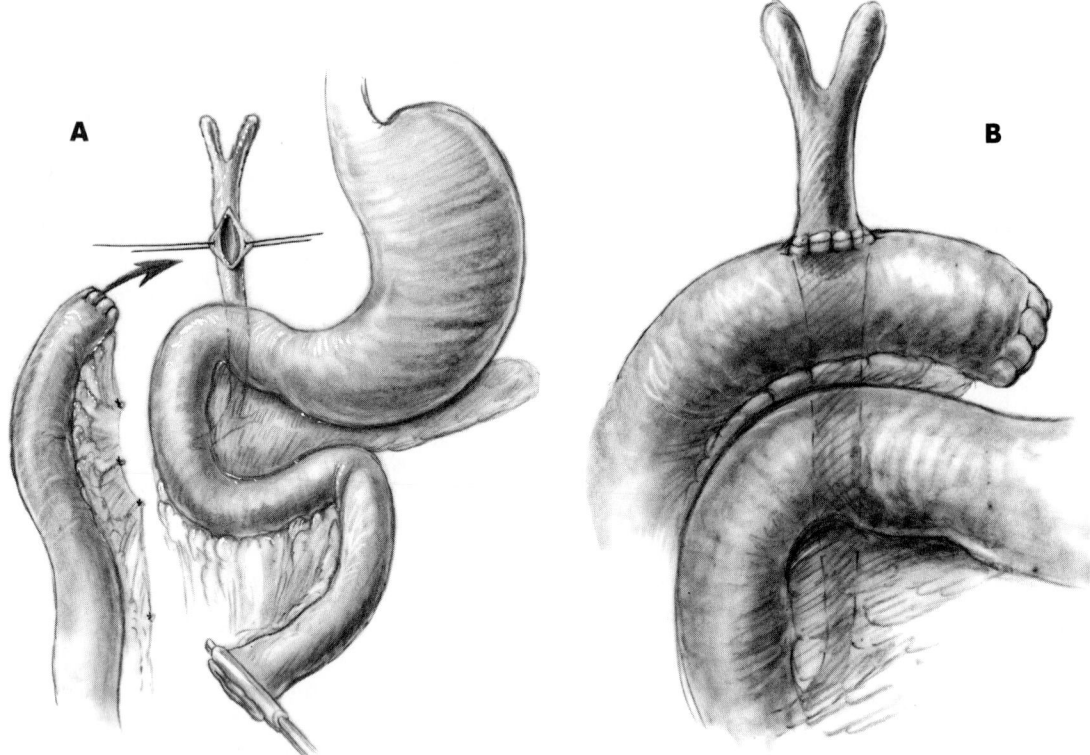

FIG. 11-20   Choledochojejunostomy. **A,** The divided end of the jejunum is closed, and an end-to-side choledochojejunostomy is made in two layers to the jejunum. **B,** A jejunal-jejunostomy completes the operative procedure.

From Davis, J.H., et al. (1987). *Clinical surgery* (Vol. 2). St. Louis: Mosby.

ness of the fundus of the gallbladder. A 1- to 1.5-cm opening is made into the small bowel and gallbladder in corresponding positions. Interrupted 4-0 sutures of surgeon's preference are then placed around the entire circumference.

3. Contaminated instruments are placed in the discard basin, and the operative field is prepared for closure.
4. A drain may be introduced; the wound is closed in layers, and dressings are applied.

Choledochoduodenostomy and choledochojejunostomy

Choledochoduodenostomy is anastomosis between the common duct and duodenum, and choledochojejunostomy is anastomosis between the duct and the jejunum. These procedures are usually necessary in postcholecystectomy patients to circumvent an obstructive lesion and reestablish the flow of bile into the intestinal tract.

Procedural considerations

Surgical approaches are similar to those for choledochostomy and cholecystojejunostomy.

Operative procedures
Choledochoduodenostomy

1. The abdomen is opened, and the common duct and duodenum are exposed.
2. The common duct is identified and dissected free.
3. The common duct and duodenum are approximated, either side-to-side or the end of the common duct to the side of the duodenum, and an anastomosis is established.
4. An intraluminal catheter is inserted, the wound is closed in layers, and dressings are applied.

Choledochojejunostomy

1. The abdomen is opened, the jejunum is mobilized, and the common duct is identified and opened (Fig. 11-20, *A*).
2. Anastomosis is established between the common duct and the transected jejunum. A catheter is introduced, as described for cholecystoduodenostomy.
3. Jejunal continuity is reestablished by jejunojejunostomy (Fig. 11-20, *B*).
4. As an alternative, anastomosis may be fashioned from the end of the severed duct to the side of a loop of jejunum, with a side-to-side jejunal anastomosis.

5. Contaminated instruments are removed from the operative field.
6. A drain is exteriorized, the wound is closed in layers, and dressing are applied.

Repair of strictures of the common and hepatic ducts

Repair of strictures of the common and hepatic ducts relieves biliary obstruction either by resection or a stricture of the duct and an end-to-end anastomosis over a T tube splint or by means of an anastomosis between the duct or ducts and the intestinal tract. These operations are usually difficult because they follow previous unsuccessful operations on the biliary tract with resultant scarring, stricture, and fistulas.

Operative procedure

1. The abdomen is opened, and the anastomosis to be performed is selected after careful exploration and evaluation of the existing pathologic condition.
2. After anastomosis, the selected T tube is inserted. Extreme caution is exercised to prevent displacement of the vital drainage tubes.
3. The wound is closed.

Transduodenal sphincteroplasty

Transduodenal sphincteroplasty is a method of producing a choledochoduodenostomy between the distal end of the common duct and the side of the duodenum. The sphincters normally affecting the distal common and pancreatic ducts are rendered functionless because the stoma is noncontractile and remains permanently open. Indications for transduodenal sphincteroplasty include a history of recurrent bile stones, impacted distal common duct stones, papillary stenosis, distal common bile duct strictures, recurrent idiopathic pancreatitis, and postcholecystectomy pain.

Procedural considerations

Instrumentation is as described for choledochotomy, with the addition of a gastrointestinal set, since the duodenum is entered through a longitudinal incision. The patient is positioned supine on the operating room bed.

Operative procedure

1. The abdomen is prepped from nipple line to pubis.
2. A right subcostal or midline incision is made, and exposure of the biliary tract is achieved.
3. All structures are inspected, and the normal configuration is established before any structure is tied, clamped, or divided during biliary tract dissection (Way & Pellegrini, 1987).
4. Operative cholangiography is then performed by placing a cholangiocath through a small incision made with a no. 11 blade into the cystic duct.
5. The surgeon examines the films and makes the final

decision to proceed with the sphincteroplasty.
6. If the gallbladder is present, cholecystectomy is performed.
7. The duodenum is mobilized by dividing the peritoneal reflection that covers the lateral portion of the second part of the duodenum and holds it in place (Way & Pellegrini, 1987).
8. The common duct is incised longitudinally between two stay sutures and explored. Any residual stones are removed.
9. Duodenotomy is performed with a longitudinal incision, and the location of the papilla of Vater is identified (Fig. 11-21, *A*).
10. The sphincter of Oddi is divided at the 11 o'clock position with angled Potts scissors, and the ductal mucosa is sutured to the duodenal mucosa with a fine absorbable suture on a small urologic needle (Fig. 11-21, *B*).
11. The duodenum is then closed in two layers.
12. The common bile duct is joined to the apex of the mobilized duodenum in a two-layer anastomosis.
13. A T tube is inserted to splint the anastomosis (Fig. 11-21, *C*).
14. The abdominal cavity is drained, and the wound is closed.

SURGERY OF THE PANCREAS
Drainage or excision of pancreatic cysts

Pancreatic cysts may be drained internally into the small intestine or stomach or may require excision or external drainage (marsupialization).

Cysts of the pancreas have been classified according to the following etiologic factors: developmental or congenital, inflammatory, traumatic, neoplastic, and parasitic. Their etiology, size, location, and anatomic relationships are important factors in selection of the surgical procedure. Pancreatic pseudocysts result from pancreatic fluid exudate in the lesser sac region.

Procedural considerations

Internal or external drainage of the cyst is the preferred procedure. Appropriate drains must be available.

Operative procedure

1. Simple external drainage is established by direct introduction of a retention catheter into the cyst, following decompression and inspection.
2. Internal drainage may be accomplished by an incision into the anterior wall of the stomach, directly opposite the cyst as it adheres to the posterior wall. A fistula is established between the anterior wall of the cyst and the posterior wall of the stomach, thereby providing drainage through the gastrointestinal tract (Fig. 11-22). Many surgeons prefer an anastomosis between the cyst and a Roux-en-Y loop of jejunum or into the duodenum directly, depending on the location of the cyst.

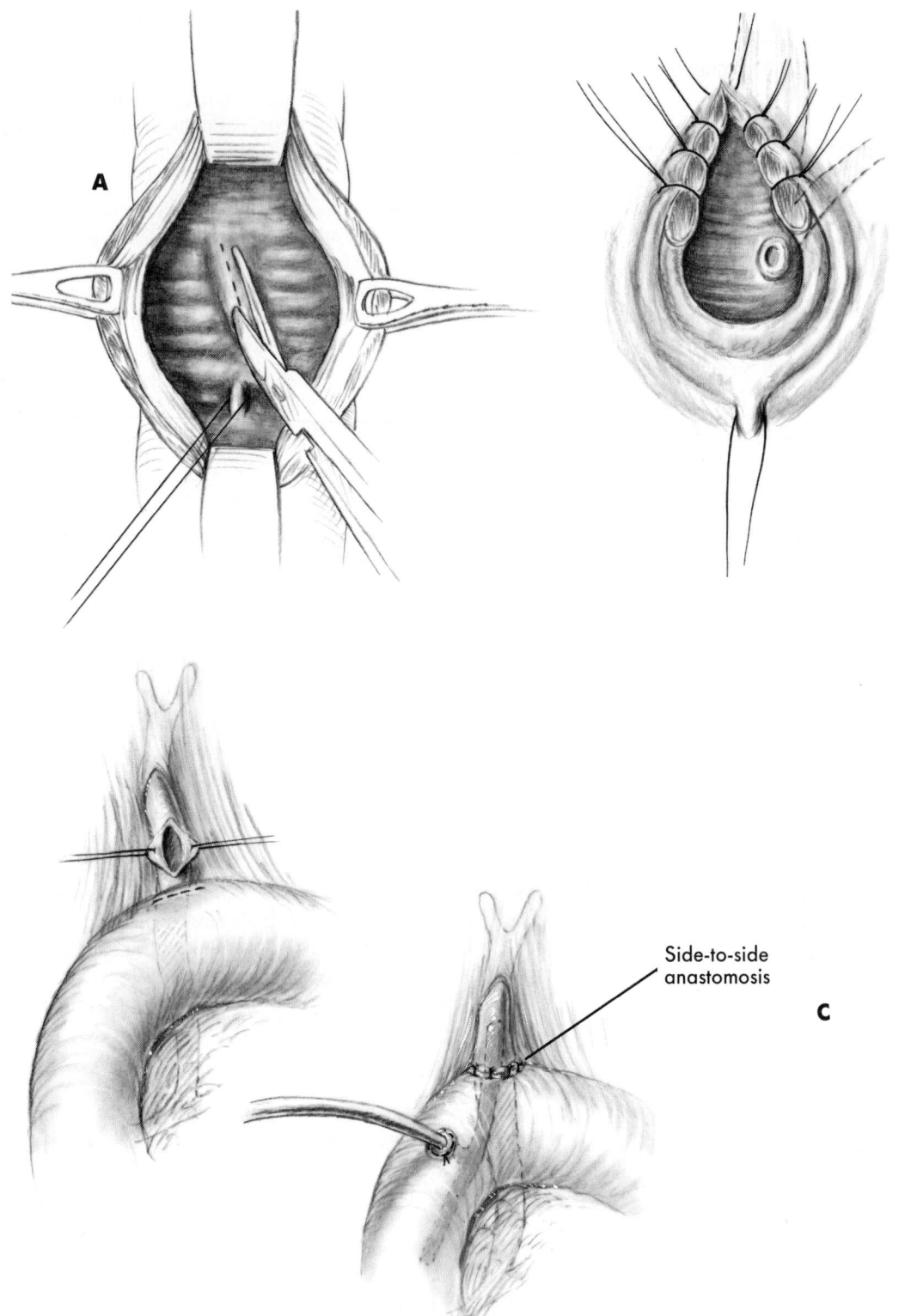

FIG. 11-21   Tranduodenal sphincteroplasty. **A,** The duodenum is opened longitudinally. **B,** The sphincter of Oddi is divided at 11 o'clock with angled Potts scissors, and the ductal mucosa is then sutured to
the duodenal mucosa with 4-0 absorbable suture. The duodenum is then closed longitudinally in two
layers. **C,** Choledochoduodenostomy. The common bile duct is joined to the apex of the mobilized duodenum in a two-layer anastomosis. A T tube is placed to stent the anastomosis with the external stem of
the tube brought out through the bile duct or through the wall of the duodenum.

From Davis, J.H., et al. (1987). *Clinical surgery* (Vol. 2). St. Louis: Mosby.

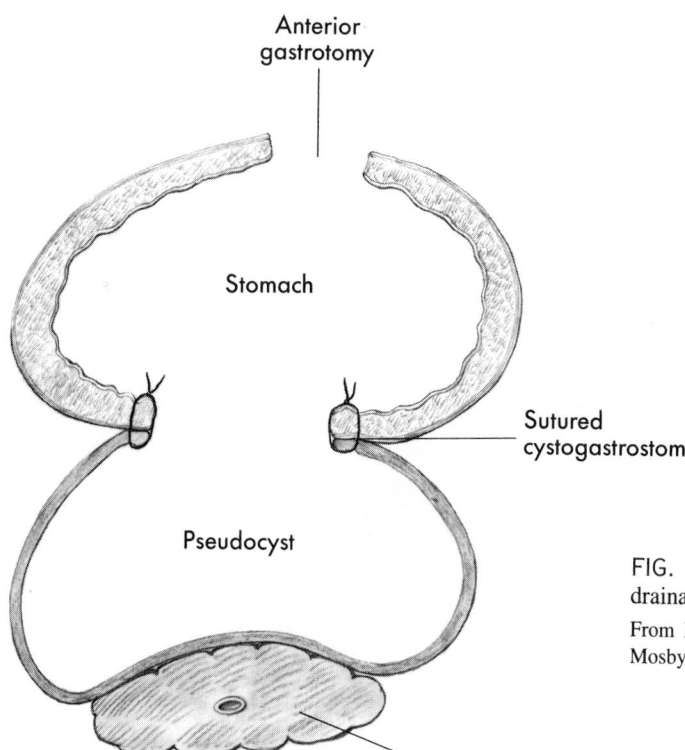

Anterior gastrotomy

Stomach

Sutured cystogastrostomy

Pseudocyst

Pancreas

FIG. 11-22 Cross-section diagram of cystogastrostomy for drainage of pseudocyst of the lesser sac.
From Davis, J.H., et al. (1987). *Clinical surgery* (Vol. 2). St. Louis: Mosby.

3. The anterior gastrotomy is closed, and the wound closure is completed.

Pancreatoduodenectomy (Whipple's operation)

Pancreatoduodenectomy is the removal of the head of the pancreas, the entire duodenum, a portion of the jejunum, the distal third of the stomach, and the lower half of the common bile duct, with the reestablishment of continuity of the biliary, pancreatic, and gastrointestinal tract systems.

Radical excision of the head of the pancreas for carcinoma is a technically hazardous procedure because it involves many vital structures and organs. Resectability of the tumor in the presence or absence of metastasis and the general overall condition of the patient are evaluated carefully before resection.

Procedural considerations

General laparotomy and gastrointestinal instruments, plus appropriate drains and catheters, are used for this procedure. After the surgeon opens and explores the abdomen, including the liver, pancreas, and biliary tree, the blood bank should be advised if the patient will require extensive surgery. Pancreatoduodenectomy may require 5 to 6 hours and the transfusion of many units of blood or blood products.

The patient is commonly sent to the SICU immediately from the OR suite. After surgery the surgeon must reevaluate the patient's insulin requirements and supplementary pancreatin.

Operative procedure

1. The abdomen is entered through an upper transverse, bilateral subcostal, or long paramedian incision. Laparotomy packs and retractors are used to expose the operative site and protect vital structures.
2. Mobilization of the duodenum is achieved with an adequate Kocher maneuver, which consists of incision of peritoneal reflection, lateral to the second portion of the duodenum, with Metzenbaum scissors and subsequent blunt dissection of loose areolar tissue.
3. Mobilization of the duodenum continues, and bleeding vessels are ligated with silk.
4. The gastrocolic ligament and the gastrohepatic omentum are divided between curved forceps and are ligated or transfixed.
5. The gastroduodenal and right gastric arteries are clamped, divided, and ligated.
6. The prepyloric area of the stomach is mobilized. The operative field is prepared for open anastomosis. By placing two long Allen or Payr clamps near the midportion of the stomach, the transsection is completed.
7. The duodenum is reflected, the common duct is divided, and the hepatic end is marked or tagged for later anastomosis.
8. The jejunum is clamped with two Allen forceps, and the duodenojejunal flexure is divided.
9. The pancreas is divided, and the duct is carefully identified.
10. Further mobilization of the duodenum and division of

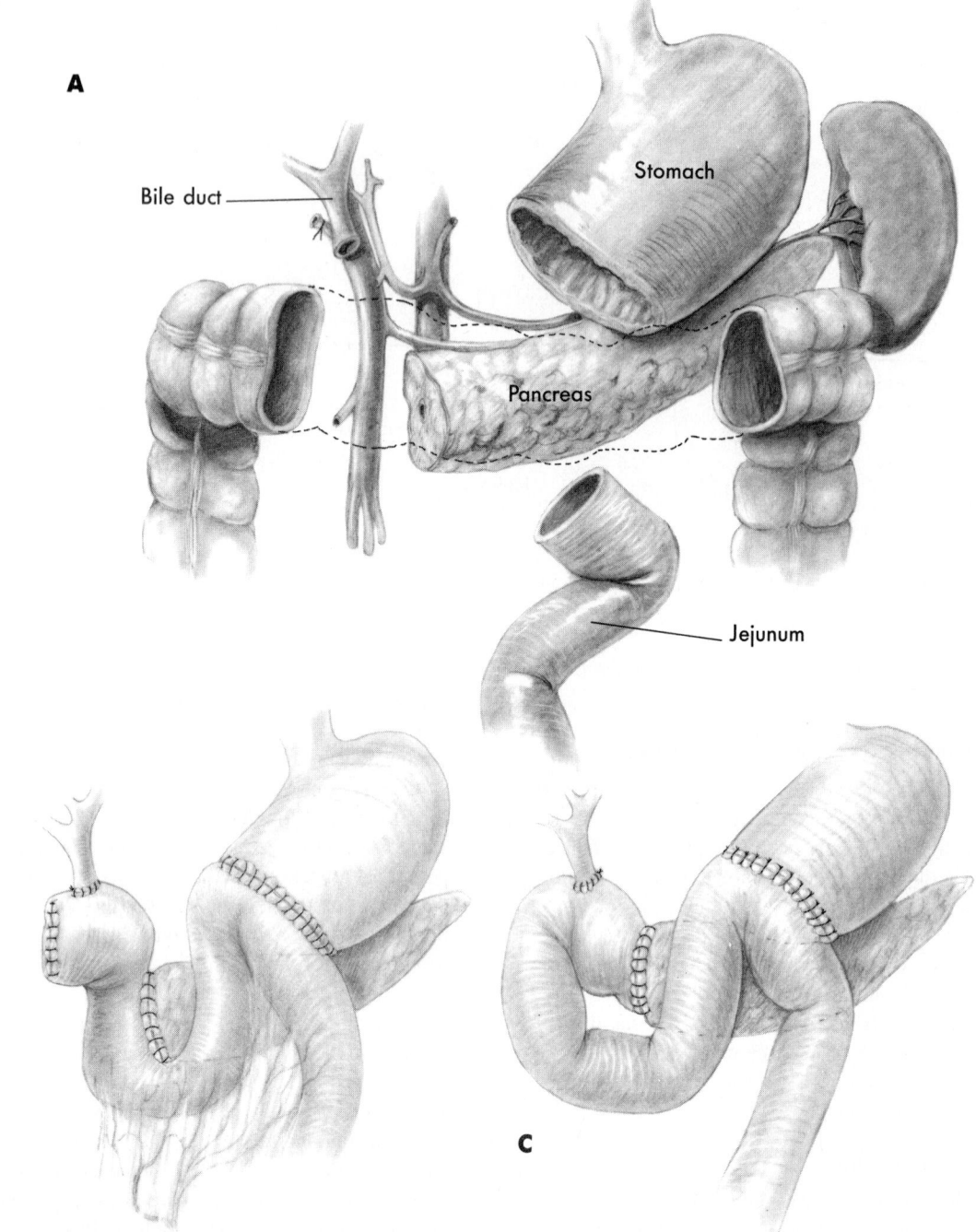

FIG. 11-23   **A,** Resection margins of bile duct, pancreas, stomach, and jejunum following a Whipple procedure. **B,** Reconstruction following a Whipple procedure showing biliary anastomosis preceding pancreas and stomach. **C,** Reconstruction showing pancreatic anastomosis preceding bile duct and stomach.

From Davis, J.H., et al. (1987). *Clinical surgery* (Vol. 2). St. Louis: Mosby.

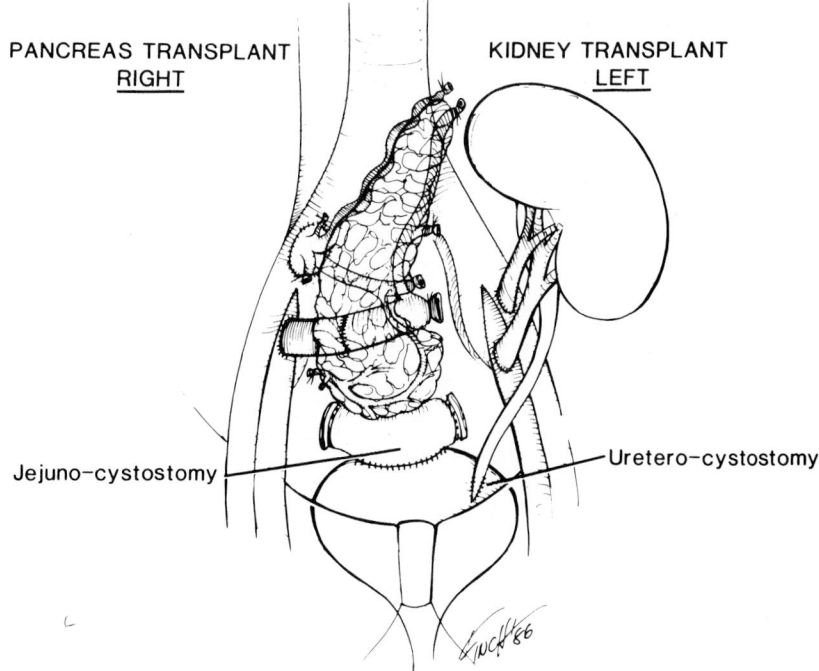

FIG. 11-24   Whole pancreas transplantation with simultaneous or serial kidney transplantation illustrating the position of the two donor grafts in the recipient.

From Cerilli, G.J. (1988). *Organ transplantation and replacement*. Philadelphia: J.B. Lippincott.

the inferior pancreatoduodenal artery are done to permit complete removal of the specimen.

11. Reconstruction of the gastrointestinal tract is completed by the following anastomoses: retrocolic end-to-end pancreatojejunostomy, retrocolic end-to-side choledochojejunostomy, and an antecolic long-loop isoperistaltic gastrojejunostomy (Fig. 11-23).

12. Drains are introduced, as for cholecystostomy. Some surgeons prefer to place a sump drain near the pancreatic anastomosis.

13. The wound is closed in layers, usually including wire sutures.

Pancreatic transplantation

Pancreatic transplantation is the implantation of a pancreas from a donor into a recipient. This procedure is considered a possible means of treatment for type I diabetes. Pancreatic transplantation differs from other organ transplants in that it does not have immediate life-saving results. Insulin therapy is a more common alternative medical treatment. Pancreatic transplantation is indicated for long-established, totally insulin-deficient diabetics with end-stage renal disease. Since nephropathy, retinopathy, and neuropathy are secondary complications to long-established, insulin-deficient diabetes, pancreatic transplantation may interrupt their progression.

Pancreatic transplantation can be combined with the re-

nal transplant procedure (Fig. 11-24). Serial transplantation is an alternative for patients who have already received a transplanted kidney.

The surgical technique for pancreatic transplantation varies between segmental pancreatic grafting and whole-organ transplantation. With either procedure, vascular anastomosis and management of the pancreatic duct are performed. Managing pancreatic ductal exocrine secretions remains one of the major technical problems with the transplantation procedure. The segmental pancreatic graft can be placed in a paratopic position just superior to the native pancreas of the recipient or in a heterotopic position in the retroperitoneum or in a intraperitoneum. The pancreatic duct is then routed into the stomach, intestine (Fig. 11-25, *A*), or urinary bladder (Fig. 11-25, *B*). A pancreaticocutaneous fistula, with external drainage via a catheter (Fig. 11-25, *C*), may also be an alternative for managing the exocrine secretions from the pancreatic duct. Occlusion of the pancreatic duct with polymer injection (Fig. 11-25, *D*) prior to transplantation or 3 to 6 weeks following the transplant is another means of managing the exocrine secretions. Whole-organ pancreatic transplantation has achieved popularity over segmental pancreatic transplantation. Better blood supply of the whole-organ graft and an increased number of islet cells for insulin production are the advantages that have changed the trend to whole-organ pancreatic transplantation in recent years.

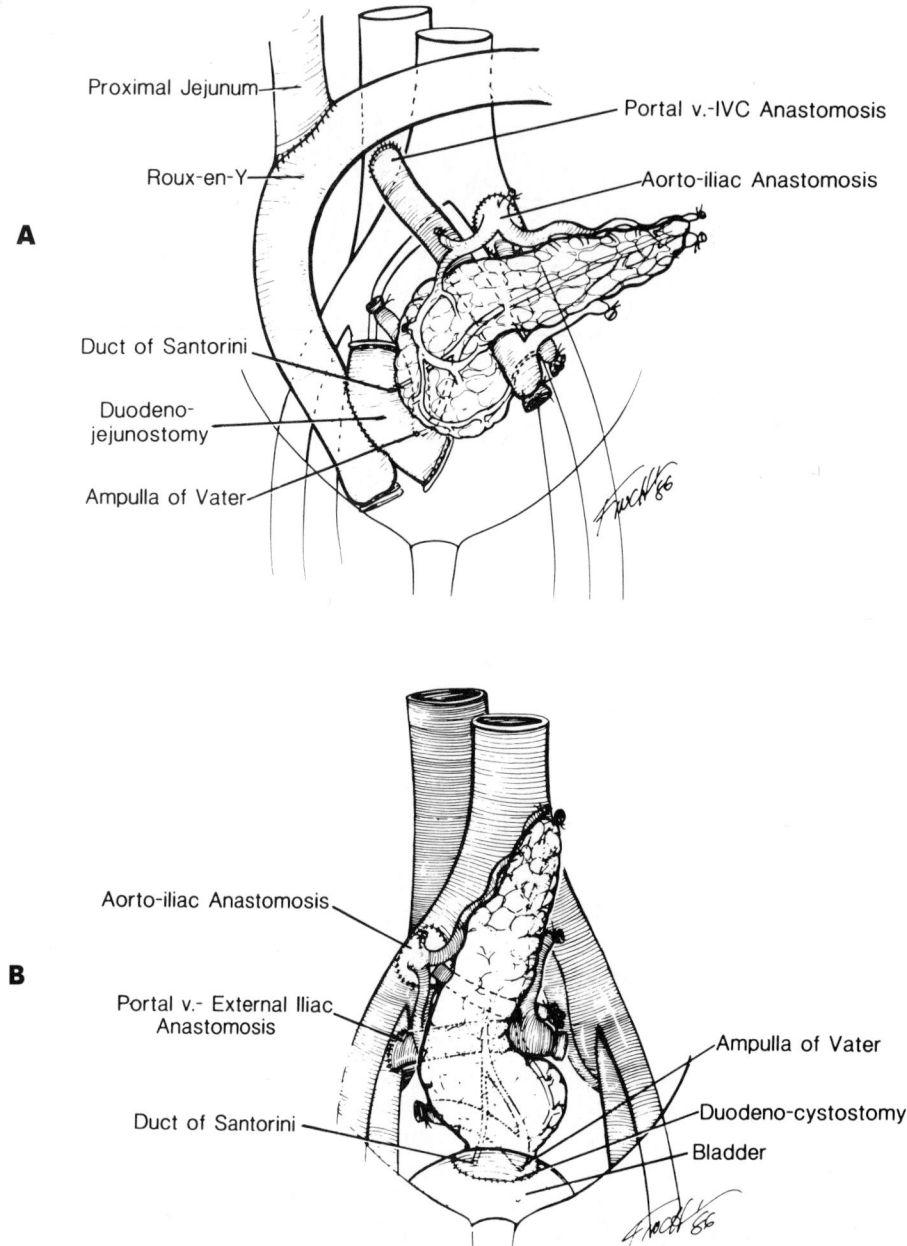

Proximal Jejunum

Roux-en-Y

A

Duct of Santorini

Duodeno-
jejunostomy

Ampulla of Vater

Portal v.-IVC Anastomosis

Aorto-iliac Anastomosis

B

Aorto-iliac Anastomosis

Portal v.- External Iliac
Anastomosis

Duct of Santorini

Ampulla of Vater

Duodeno-cystostomy

Bladder

FIG. 11-25 **A,** Enteric drainage of a whole-pancreas graft showing a side-to-side anastomosis of the donor duodenal patch and the recipient's jeunal segment of a Roux-en-Y. **B,** Whole-pancreas transplantation showing donor duodenal patch anastomosed to dome of urinary bladder. **C,** Enteric drainage of a segmental pancreas graft to a Roux-en-Y limb of the recipient jejunum, showing an external drain exteriorized through the abdominal wall. **D,** Segmental pancreas transplantation showing polymer injection into pancreatic duct of graft.

From Cerilli, G.J. (1988). *Organ transplantation and replacement.* Philadelphia: J.B. Lippincott.

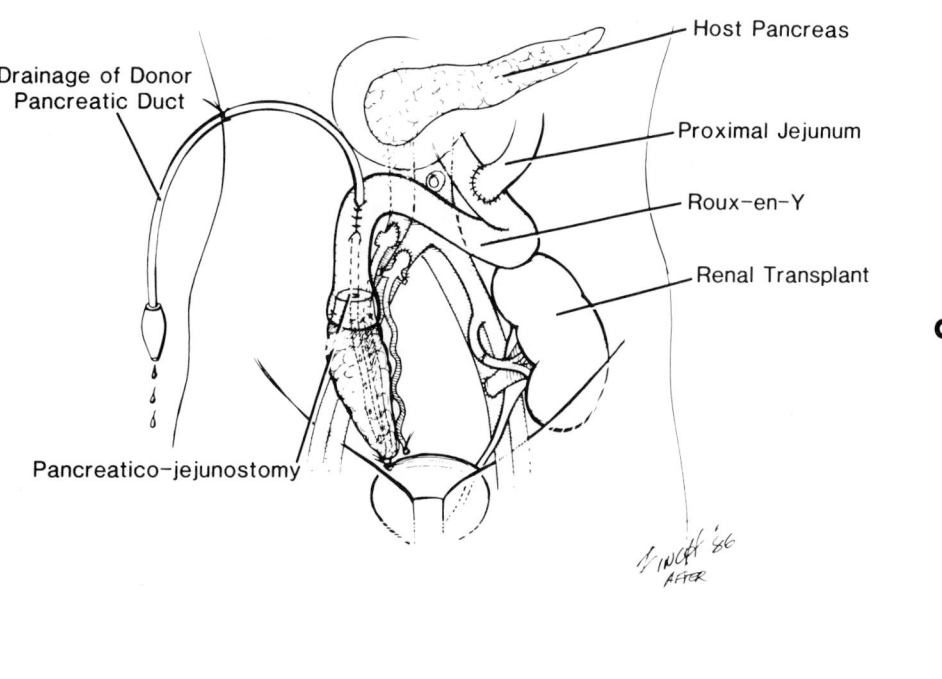

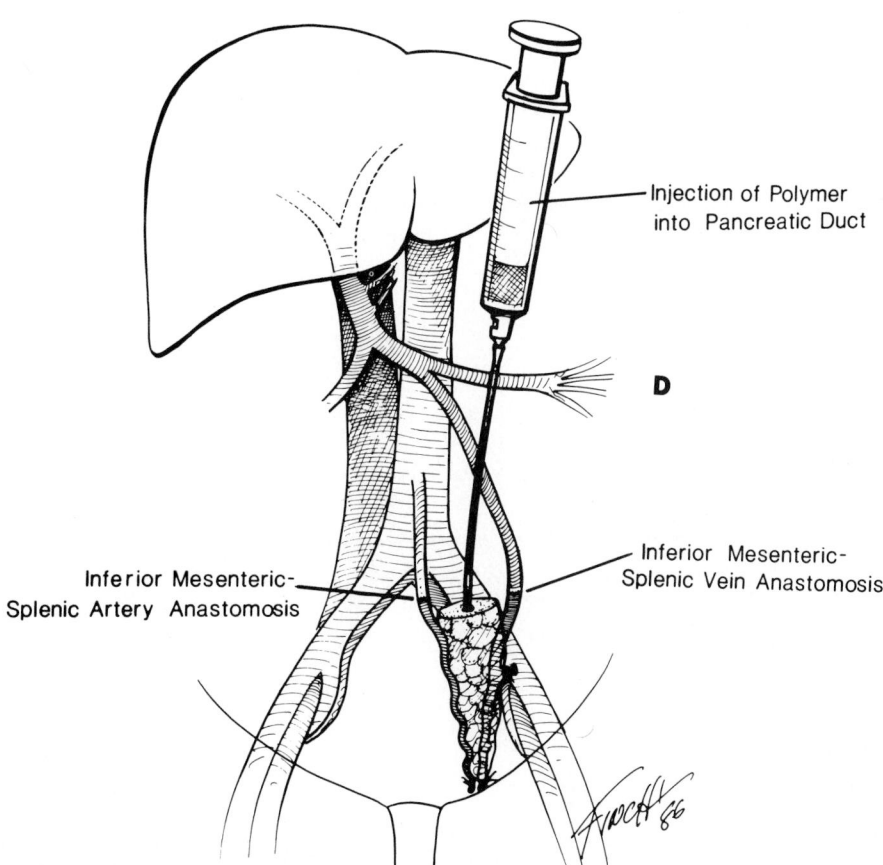

FIG. 11-25, CONT'D   For legend see opposite page.

Procedural considerations

Instrumentation for pancreatic transplantation includes a transplant set as described for kidney transplantation in Chapter 14. In addition to the transplant set, consideration must be given to the resection of the duodenal segment and the management of the pancreatic duct. A gastrointestinal instrument set and linear stapling devices with two loads are required for grafting the duodenal segment that contains the pancreatic duct into an enteric route of drainage.

Operative procedure

1. The whole-organ pancreatic transplantation procedure is performed through an oblique incision opposite the side of the renal transplant in the lower abdominal quadrant. A midline incision may also be used for pancreatic transplant.
2. The external iliac artery and vein are skeletalized, and lymphatics are tied off with 4-0 silk strands.
3. The external iliac vein is clamped with noncrushing vascular clamps, and venotomy is achieved with a no. 11 blade. The venotomy incision is extended with Potts scissors.
4. An end-to-side anastomosis of the donor portal vein to the recipient's external iliac vein is achieved with four double-armed 5-0 polypropylene sutures.
5. The external iliac artery is then clamped, and arteriotomy is achieved with an aortic punch.
6. An end-to-side anastomosis of the recipient's external iliac artery with the donor aortic patch containing the origin of the superior mesenteric artery and the celiac axis is performed with four double-armed 6-0 polypropylene sutures.
7. Management of the pancreatic duct is then performed. The whole-organ pancreatic transplantation may also be performed as a pancreaticoduodenal transplantation or a pancreaticoduodenal-splenic transplantation.

Management of the pancreatic duct depends on the type of an bloc procedure performed. Various enteric procedures for drainage of pancreatic duct secretions have been performed with whole-organ transplants en bloc with a segment of duodenum and the spleen. They include cutaneous jejunostomy, drainage into an ileal loop, and duodenojejunostomy with an end-to-end or side-to-side anastomosis.

Direct grafting of the pancreatic duct into the enteric or urinary system is also performed for management of exocrine secretions. Surgical procedures would include pancreaticojejunostomy with an established Roux-en-Y loop of jejunum, pancreaticoductoureterostomy, and pancreaticocystostomy.

SURGERY OF THE LIVER
Drainage of intrahepatic, subhepatic, or subphrenic abscess

Abscesses of the liver may require incision and drainage. Hepatic abscesses may be pyogenic or parasitic and single or multiple.

Extreme care is used in removal of an *Echinococcus* (hydatid) cyst because the fluid is under high tension, and any spillage into the peritoneal cavity may result in anaphylactic reaction. Even more important is the possible escape of daughter cysts that can spread through the abdomen and produce multiple cysts, an extremely difficult condition to treat. Hydatid cysts of the liver are rare in the United States.

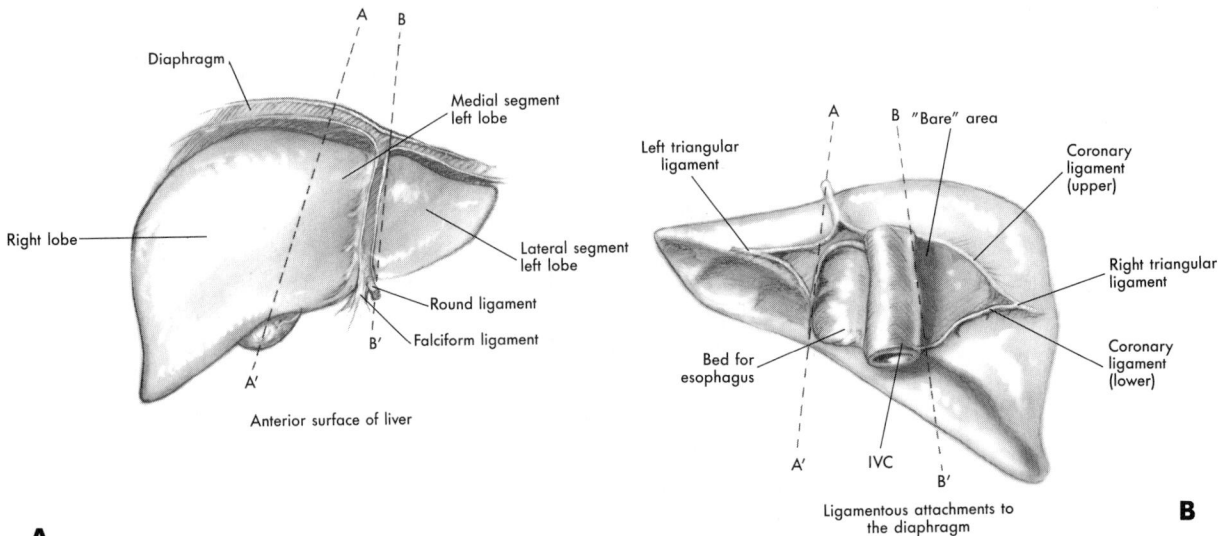

A

B

FIG. 11-26   **A,** Anterior surface of the liver. Plane *A-A'* divides the liver into the right and left lobes. Plane *B-B'* divides the left lobe into the medial and lateral segments. **B,** The ligamentous attachments to the diaphragm.

From Davis, J.H., et al. (1987). *Clinical surgery* (Vol. 2). St. Louis: Mosby.

Procedural considerations

A basic laparotomy set is used. Biliary instrumentation, drainage materials, and aerobic and anaerobic culture tubes should be available.

Operative procedure

1. The incision and type of procedure selected depend on the cause and location of the abscess. For the anterior approach, a right transperitoneal incision is made. For the posterior approach, the patient is prepped and the incision selected as described for a posterior thoracotomy.
2. Drainage of an abscess may be treated in one or two stages. In the one-stage procedure, the approach is through the outer third of the right twelfth rib to reach the liver abscess retroperitoneally and extrapleurally. A two-stage operation, which is rarely done, obliterates the right pleural cavity. The objective of the first stage is to seal off the pleural cavity by stimulating adhesions with the insertion of iodoform packing. When the second stage is performed at a higher level, the chest cavity does not become contaminated.

Hepatic resection

The liver is divided into the left lobe and the right lobe, with the caudate lobe lying in the dorsal segment. Resection of the liver is according to the lobe and segment involved (Figs. 11-26 to 11-28); a small wedge biopsy, excision of simple tumors, or a major lobectomy may be per-

formed. Increased knowledge of liver function and circulatory physiology as well as improved methods of hemostasis now permit the surgeon to offer safe, definitive treatment to the patient with liver disease or trauma.

Procedural considerations

Supplies and equipment should be available for hypothermia, electrosurgery, measurement of portal pressure, thoracotomy drainage, and replacement of blood loss. Special blunt needles for suturing liver tissue are also necessary.

The patient is placed in the supine position. The abdomen is prepped from nipple line to midthigh. A midline abdominal incision, occasionally with division of the lower sternum, provides access to the liver. Vertical abdominal incisions are advantageous because they can be made and closed more rapidly and permit better exposure of all abdominal organs.

Instrumentation includes a basic laparotomy set, biliary instruments, vascular instruments, and additional items as follows:

Long clamps	Vessel loops and umbilical tapes
Self-retaining retractor system such as the Bookwalter retractor	Hemostatic material, such as Gelfoam, Surgicel, or Avitene, absorbable collagen sheets
Liver sutures, absorbable or nonabsorbable, according to surgeon's preference	

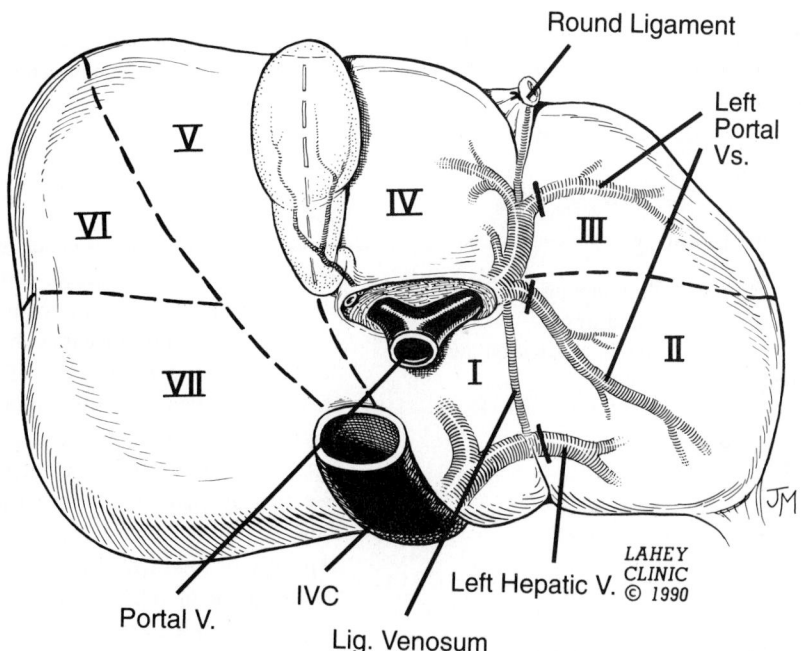

FIG. 11-27 Eight segments of the liver.

From Daly, J.M., & Cady, B. (1993). *Atlas of surgical oncology*. St. Louis: Mosby.

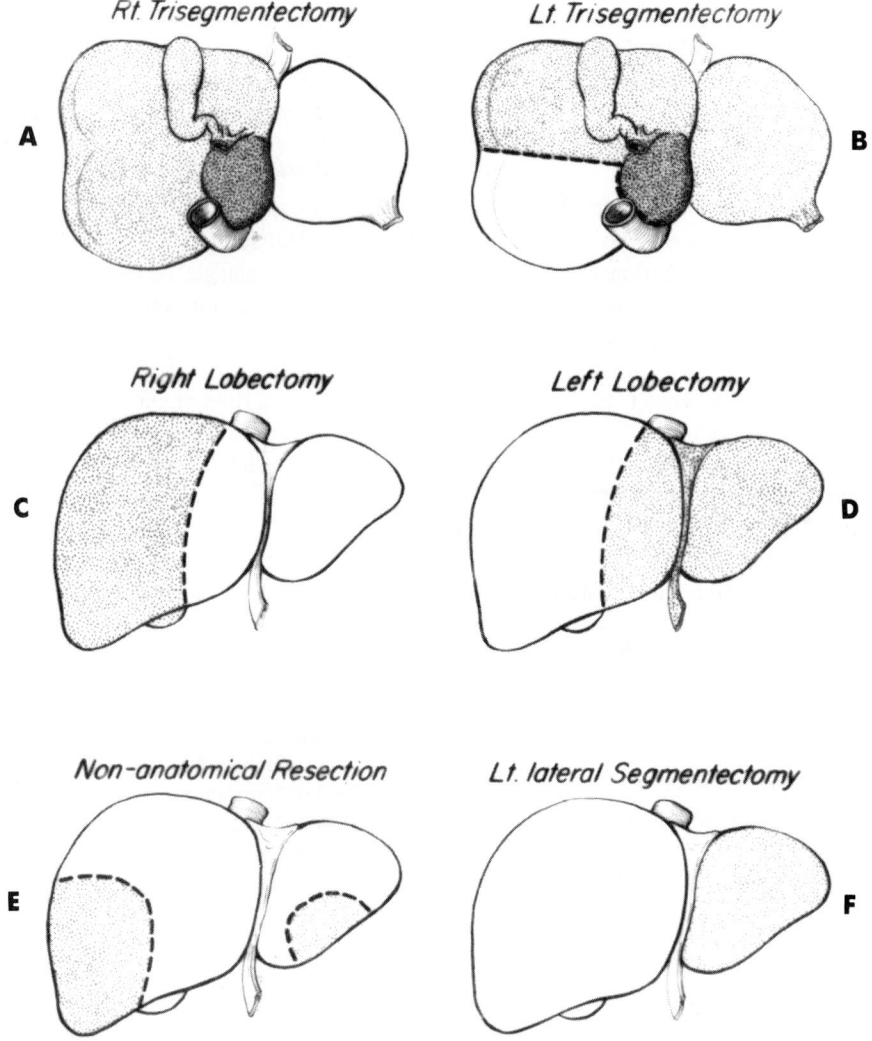

FIG. 11-28 Techniques for hepatic resection. **A,** Right trisegmentectomy. **B,** Left trisegmentectomy. **C,** Right lobectomy. **D,** Left lobectomy. **E,** Nonanatomic resection such as a wedge resection. **F,** Left lateral segmentectomy.

From Daly, J.M., & Cady, B. (1993). *Atlas of surgical oncology.* St. Louis: Mosby.

Equipment should include the following:

Intraoperative ultrasound 7-mHz probe and unit	Two suction tubings and tips
Cavitron Ultrasonic Surgical Aspirator (CUSA)	Smoke evacuation system
Electrosurgical unit (set on blend 3 and coagulation at 100 to 110 during resection)	Surgeon's headlight

Operative procedure

1. Through an upper midline or chevron type incision, the abdominal cavity is opened and examined. Pathologic condition is determined, and resectability evaluated.

2. Moist laparotomy packs are inserted, and a self-retaining retractor is placed. Intraoperative ultrasound is performed to assess all segments of the liver (Fig. 11-29). If the tumor appears to be confined to one lobe, the procedure will proceed. If the tumor is diffuse or unresectable, a simple biopsy is performed for diagnostic confirmation. Lymph nodes in the porta hepatis and along the gastrohepatic ligament are then assessed by palpation to determine extrahepatic metastasis.

3. Exposure of the hilar structures is obtained by upward displacement of the right lobe toward the right chest cavity. The falciform ligament is disconnected using electrodissection until it approaches division into the triangular ligament. Displacement of intestines is accomplished with moist packs and retractors.

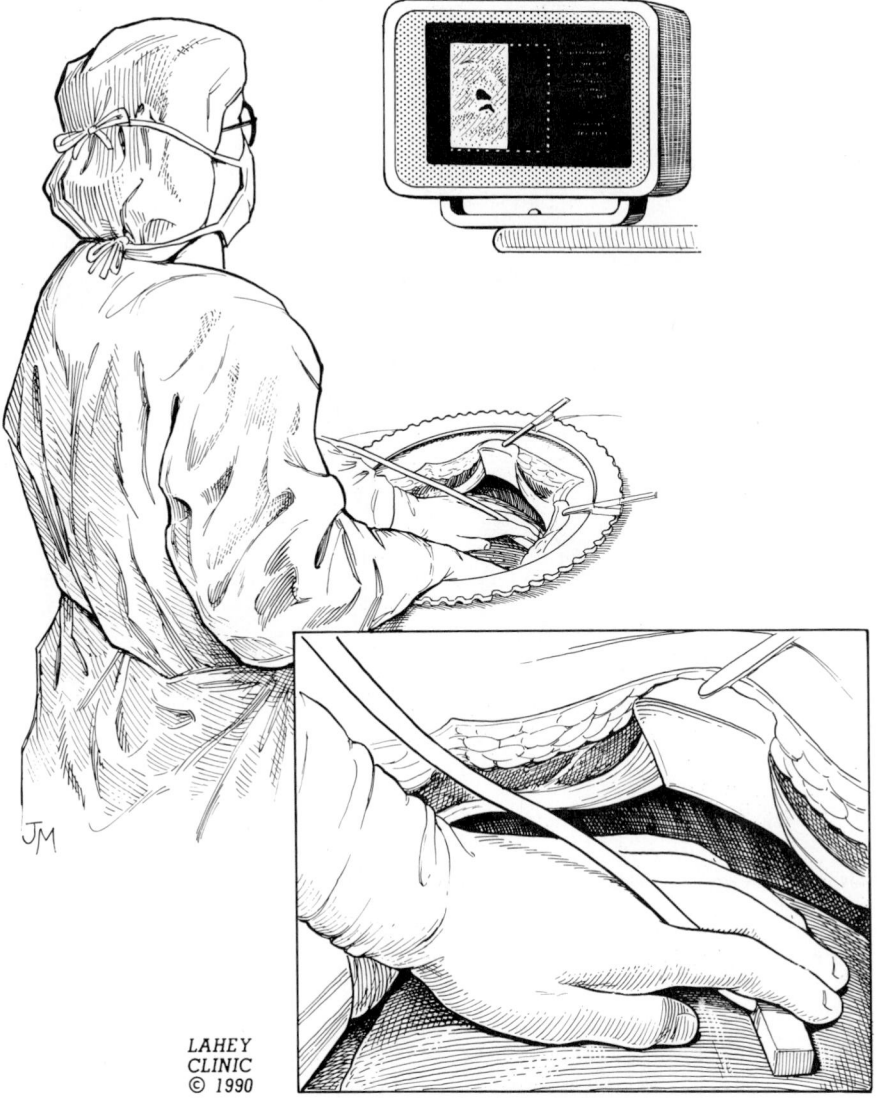

FIG. 11-29   Demonstrating the use of intraoperative ultrasound using a 7-mHz T probe to assess the liver.

From Daly, J.M., & Cady, B. (1993). *Atlas of surgical oncology*. St. Louis: Mosby.

4. The cystic duct is carefully exposed, using Metzenbaum scissors, vascular forceps, small dry dissectors on curved clamps, and fine right-angled forceps. It is clamped, transsected, and double ligated with chromic or silk ligatures and transfixion sutures.

5. The involved hepatic duct, branch of hepatic artery, and branch of the portal vein are also transected and doubly ligated with silk ligatures and transfixion sutures.

6. The liver is rotated forward, and the multiple hepatic veins are assessed and isolated.

7. The intended resection line is scored using an electrosurgical pencil with blade tip and coagulation set at 100 (Fig. 11-30).

8. The liver parenchyma is then delicately resected using the CUSA handpiece set at 5 (Fig. 11-31).

9. Large vascular structures are identified and clamped, ligaclips are applied, and the structures are ligated (Fig. 11-32). The surgeon may choose suture material for vessel occlusion.

10. Use of the CUSA handpiece continues for dissection through the parenchyma. Electrosurgical charring of surfaces or use of the argon beam coagulator is intermittent.

11. Once the portion of the liver is resected, the remaining liver resection margins are assessed for bleeding and bile leakage. A laparotomy sponge is placed against the transsected surface for several minutes. The

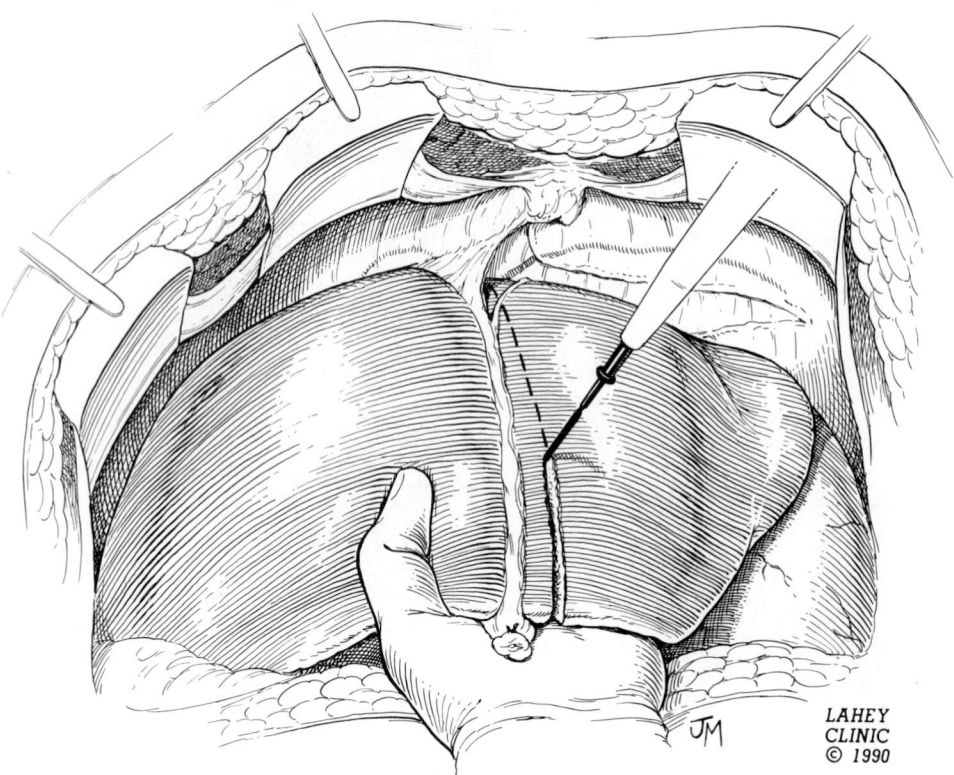

FIG. 11-30   Use of electrosurgical pencil with blade tip to score the line of resection on the surface of the liver.

From Daly, J.M., & Cady, B. (1993). *Atlas of surgical oncology*. St. Louis: Mosby.

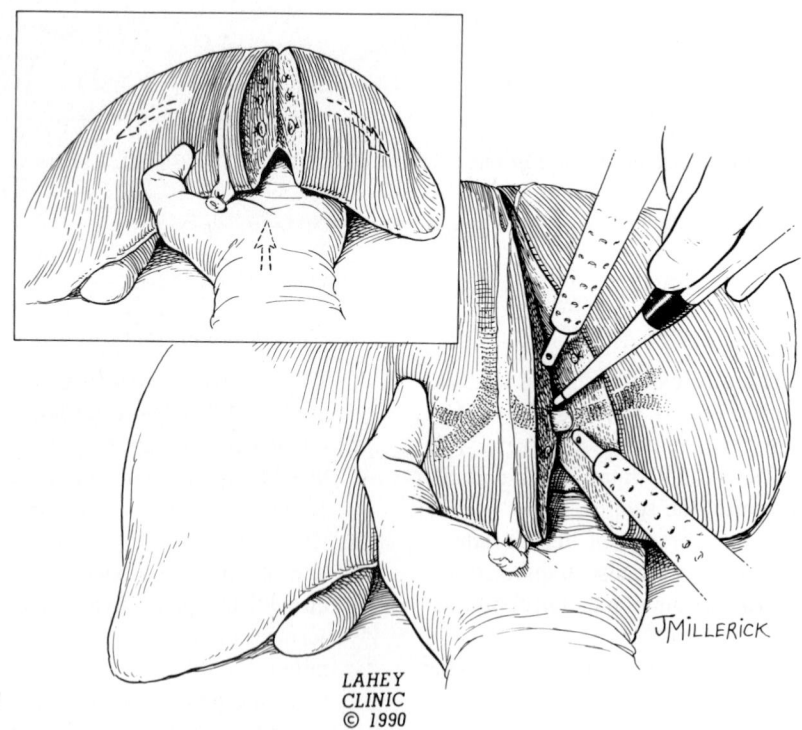

FIG. 11-31   Use of the Cavitron Ultrasonic Surgical Aspirator (CUSA) handpiece to dissect through the hepatic parenchyma.

From Daly, J.M., & Cady, B. (1993). *Atlas of surgical oncology*. St. Louis: Mosby.

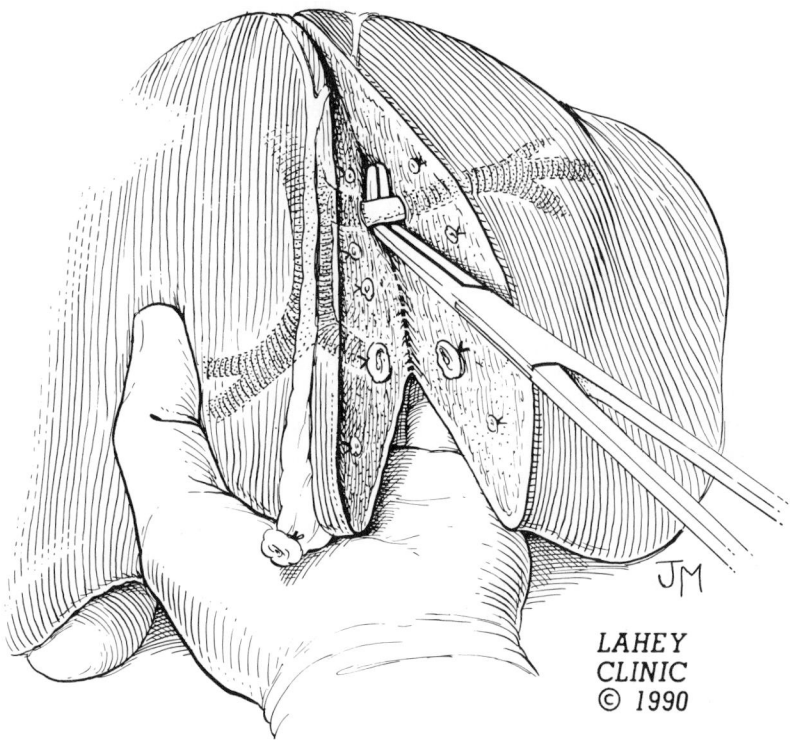

FIG. 11-32 Large intrahepatic vascular structures are isolated with blunt dissection, clamped, and ligated before division. Ligating clips or suture may be used to ensure hemostasis.

From Daly, J.M., & Cady, B. (1993). *Atlas of surgical oncology.* St. Louis: Mosby.

laparotomy sponge is gently rolled from the surface and examined for bile leakage. Areas may then be oversewn with 2-0 or 3-0 absorbable suture or an intended layer of eschar applied using electrocoagulation or the argon beam coagulator.

12. Abdominal drains may be placed along the liver bed and brought out through the abdominal wall through separate stab wounds. The abdominal wound is then closed.

Wedge resection of metastatic hepatic tumors

Patients with primary colon or rectal cancer can have metastasis to the liver occur within 5 years of primary resection of the colon or rectal lesion. These patients are followed closely by monitoring CEA levels in their blood at scheduled intervals that depend on the findings. When a rise in CEA levels is noted, x-rays, MRI, and CT scans are often used for diagnosis.

Wedge resection of metastatic hepatic lesions is an abbreviated procedure for isolated lesions in which lobectomy or segmentectomy is not indicated. The criteria for candidacy except those who have metastases outside the abdominal cavity, in lungs, or in bones.

Procedural considerations

Intraoperatively, the surgeon can confirm suspicion of liver metastasis by bimanual examination of each lobe, intraoperative ultrasonography, biopsy, or Neoprobe scanning of the liver. This is sometimes scheduled as a CEA-directed second-look procedure, and equipment and supplies for bowel or liver resection should always be available. This procedure and considerations are discussed in depth in Chapter 10.

An elongated electrosurgical blade with the unit set on a high blend 2 setting is used to initiate the resection of the metastatic tumor. The CO_2 laser with smoke evacuator and/or the CUSA aspirator, and the argon beam coagulator provide valuable technologic assistance for resection of metastatic lesions of the liver.

The surgeon's intent is to achieve a 1-cm margin of normal liver tissue dissection around each lesion.

Metastatic lesions may range from 0.5 to 20 cm in diameter. Following resection or excision of the metastatic lesions from the liver, localized chemotherapy lines may be indicated for postoperative, self-administered chemotherapy. A boviac catheter is inserted into the hepatic artery, and a Hickman catheter is inserted into the portal vein via a gastroepiploic artery and vein. The catheters exit the skin in the right upper quadrant of the abdomen and are labeled accordingly.

Procedure for wedge resection of metastatic carcinoma lesions follows the hepatic resection technique.

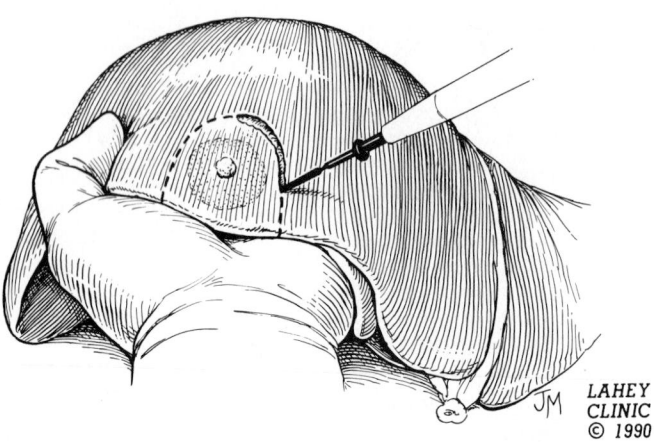

FIG. 11-33 Hepatic wedge resection demonstrating the use of electrocautery to score a reasonable clear margin around the liver lesion.

From Daly, J.M., & Cady, B. (1993). *Atlas of surgical oncology*. St. Louis: Mosby.

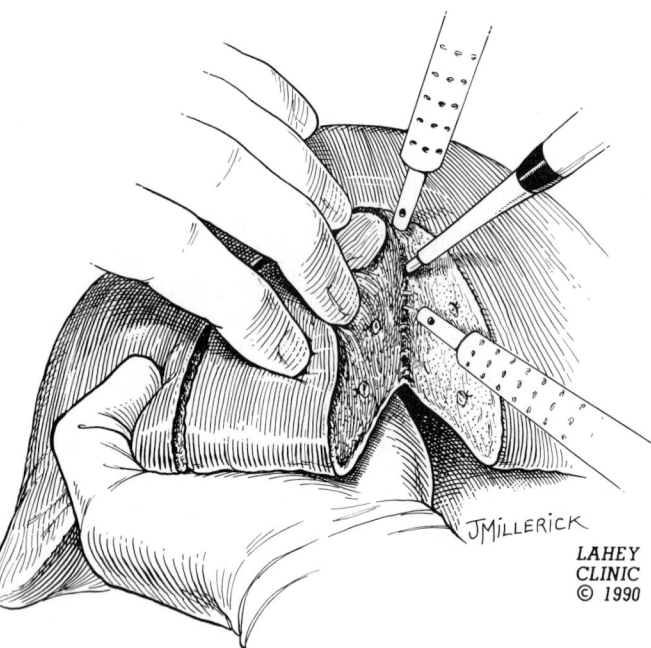

FIG. 11-34 The surgeon places a hand beneath the liver lobe while using the CUSA handpiece to dissect through the parenchyma. The assistant affords gentle manual retraction and suction to the site.

From Daly, J.M., & Cady, B. (1993). *Atlas of surgical oncology*. St. Louis: Mosby.

Operative procedure

1. The liver is examined by palpation and visualization. Intraoperative ultrasound is used to assess all eight segments of the liver.
2. Procedures are taken to mobilize the intended lobes of the liver from which the wedge resection will be performed.
3. Electrosurgery is used to score the surface of the resection line (Fig. 11-33).
4. The CUSA is then used for dissection of the parenchyma (Fig. 11-34).
5. Hemostasis is achieved by electrocoagulation, application of ligaclips, and the use of Surgical or Avitene sheets.
6. Once the wedge resection is accomplished, the margins are assessed for remaining tumor, hemostasis, and bile leakage. If no further resection is indicated, a layer of eschar may be applied to the parenchymal margin.
7. The abdominal wound is then closed.

Hepatic trisegmentectomy

As the field of extensive surgical procedures for treatment of liver diseases evolves, an aggressive approach to the resection of hepatic metastases has also become more common. Trisegmentectomy refers to an extensive resection of the liver. With right trisegmentectomy, the right lobe of the liver and the medial segment of the left lobe are removed. The caudate lobe may be included in the right trisegmentectomy if indicated by tumor involvement. In left trisegmentectomy the left lobe of liver and the anterior segment of the right lobe are resected. Again, the caudate lobe may or may not be included in the resection.

Operative procedure

1. Various types of incisions may be performed according to surgeon's preference:
   a. A basic bilateral subcostal with an upper midline extension; the right subcostal incision is longer
   b. A J-shaped incision, beginning at the xiphoid process and extending down and across the abdominus rectus muscle then anterior and lateral
   c. A midline incision extending from the xiphoid to the pubis
   Variations in these incisions may be applied.
2. Once the patient's abdomen is opened, the liver is assessed for resectability. Intraoperative ultrasound must confirm an absence of tumor in the segment of liver that is to remain. The vascular structures supporting the remaining segment must also have margins free from tumor involvement.
3. The surgeon then assesses the porta hepatis and foramen of Winslow by palpation for extrahepatic disease. Should enlarged or suspicious lymph nodes be found along the gastrohepatic ligament or in the area of the celiac axis, a decision to abandon resection of the liver may be made. It is critical for the surgeon to carefully

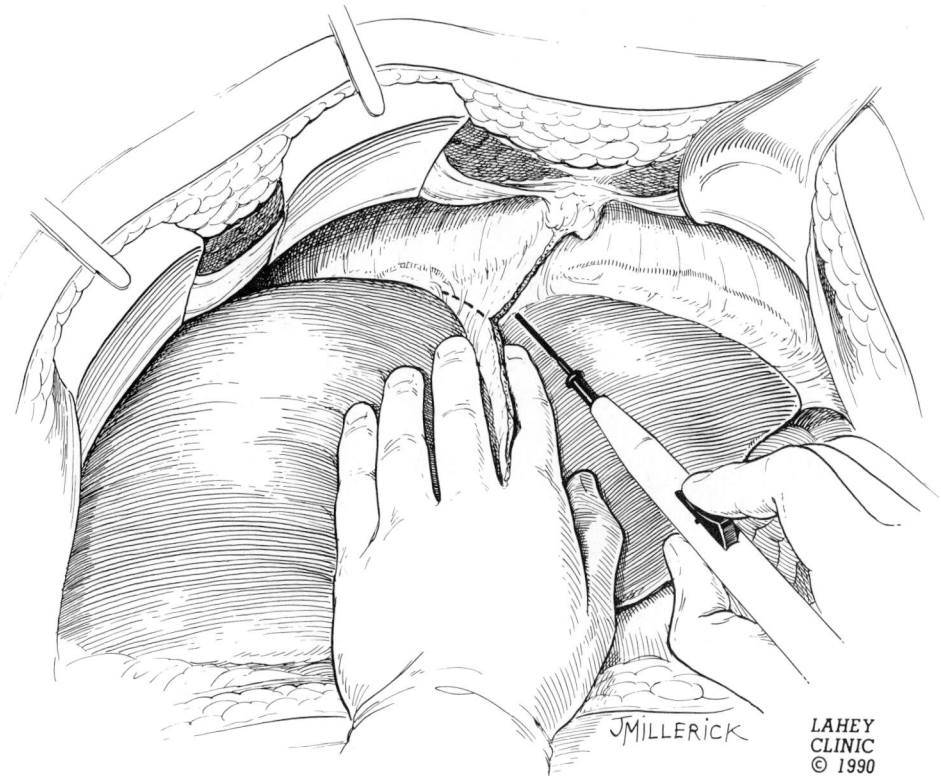

FIG. 11-35   With the Bookwalter self-retaining retractor in place the liver is mobilized by separating the falciform ligament using electrocautery. Curved Metzenbaum scissors may also be used.

From Daly, J.M., & Cady, B. (1993). *Atlas of surgical oncology.* St. Louis: Mosby.

weight this decision. Lymph node dissection may be performed in an attempt to remove all extrahepatic disease or for pathologic confirmation of lymph node metastasis. Surgeons' philosophies differ in regard to extrahepatic disease–defining resectability. Radioimmunoguided surgery (RIGS) is an innovative intraoperative technology that has been developed to better assist the surgeon in assessing lymph node metastasis. This technique is discussed later in this chapter.

4. When a decision to resect is made, the surgeon begins with mobilization of the liver (Fig. 11-35). The falciform ligament is disconnected, and the attachment of the hepatocolic ligament and the renohepatic ligament is separated from the inferior surface of the right lobe of the liver. The right lobe of the liver is then manipulated so that the triangular ligament can be dissected using long Metzenbaum scissors.

5. For right trisegmentectomy, the hilar dissection is the same as for right lobectomy. The cystic duct and artery are dissected, ligated, and divided. The peritoneum and lymphatics are then dissected clear for access to the right branch of the portal vein. If applicable, clamps are applied for ligation and division of the vessel. Suture may be required to close the proximal end of the vessel, depending on the length.

6. Care is taken to identify the biliary ducts that are to be included in resection and especially to identify the duct that passes into the segment that will be retained.

7. The exact location of the umbilical fissure is then identified. It is the landmark to identify vascular structures and hepatic ducts that will be ligated and divided and those which must remain intact for viability of the remaining segment.

8. The right lobe of the liver is retracted anteriorly and to the left to expose the vena cava. A vessel loop is placed to encircle the right hepatic vein. Small branches are ligated and divided, and the right hepatic vein is then clamped, ligated, and divided with care.

9. The resection line is scored with the electrosurgical pencil. For right trisegmentectomy the falciform ligament on the anterior surface and the umbilical fissure or round ligament on the inferior surface mark the transsection line.

10. The CUSA is used to dissect through the parenchyma.

11. Devascularization of the three segments is achieved and those become cyanotic.

12. Upon removal of the liver segments, the remaining segment is assessed for vascularization and hemostasis. Appearance of the remaining left segment is almost alarming, considering 75% to 80% of the patient's liver has been removed.

13. The abdominal wound is closed.

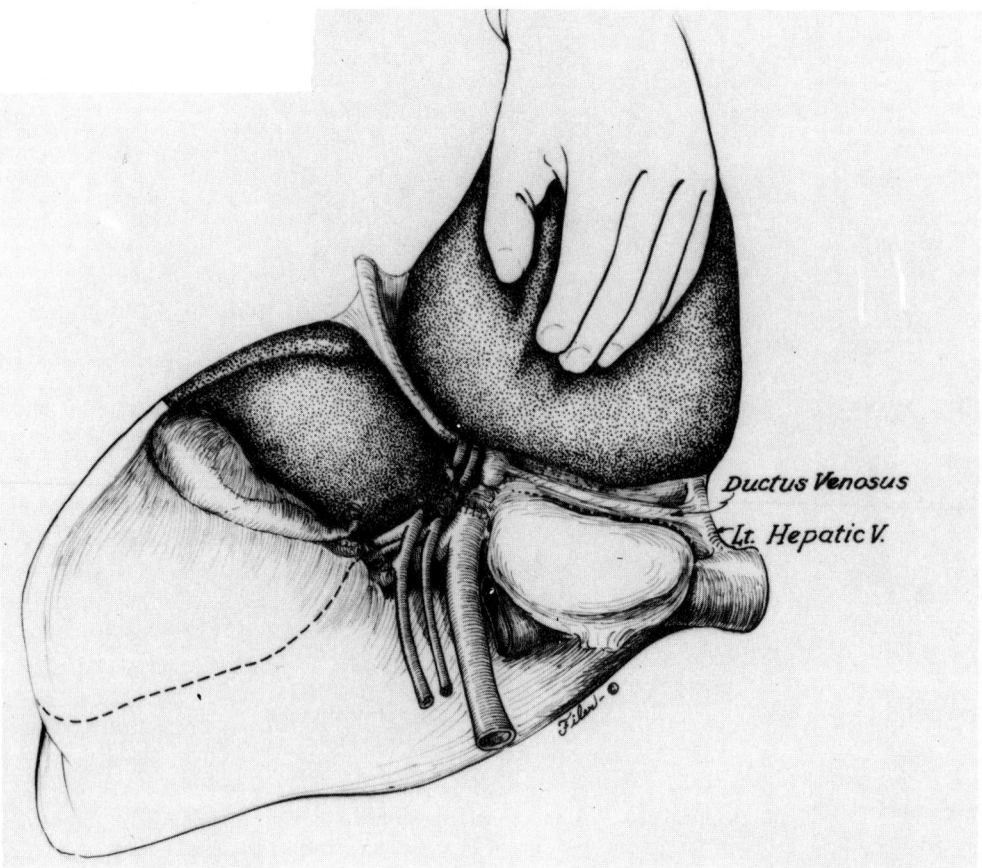

FIG. 11-36 Left trisegmentectomy. The lobe of the liver is retracted anteriorly to demonstrate the ductus venosus and the intended resection line through the right lobe.

From Daly, J.M., & Cady, B. (1993). *Atlas of surgical oncology.* St. Louis: Mosby.

Left trisegmentectomy

Left trisegmentectomy refers to the resection of the left lobe and right anterior lobe of the liver. As with right trisegmentectomy, decision is contemplated only after inspection, palpation, and ultrasonic examination of the liver indicate the remaining right inferior segment is free from tumor. Extrahepatic disease is also assessed.

Operative procedure

1. The ligament teres hepatis is divided and the falciform ligament is disconnected. The left triangular and coronary ligaments are divided.
2. The left lobe of the liver can be lifted anteriorly and retracted to the right to expose the vena cava and left hepatic vein (Fig. 11-36).
3. The left branch of the portal vein, left hepatic artery, and the left hepatic duct are identified, ligated, and divided.
4. Parenchymal transsection begins in front of the vena cava at the ductus venosus. Using the CUSA, an intersegmental plane is transsected from the hilum of the liver toward the diaphragm (Fig. 11-37, A to D).
5. Complete hemostasis and attention to bile leaks is achieved.

6. Abdominal drains may be placed.
7. The abdomen is closed.

Radioimmunoguided surgery (RIGS)

Radioimmunoguided surgery (RIGS) is an innovative technique used intraoperatively to detect cancer that may not be readily detected by inspection or palpation. This technique has been found to be very useful in determining safe margins of resection for metastatic colon cancer lesions in the liver. Current studies have also identified RIGS to be efficacious in assessing extrahepatic disease and occult tumor in patients with rising serum CEA levels.

Two to 3 weeks before surgery, patients receive an intravenous injection of radiolabeled monoclonal antibody, which binds reactive antigen on or near the surface of tumors cells. The antigen-antibody bond keeps minute amounts of radioactivity, or gamma emissions, localized in tumor tissue. An intraoperatively used, hand-held, gamma-detecting probe connected to a microcomputer emits an audible signal when the radioactive waves hit the crystal in the distal end of the probe (Martin et al., 1988). The Neoprobe instrument (Fig. 11-38) gives a digital reading as well as an audible pitch that rises or falls when placed on the gamma-emitting tissue. This advance in the intraop-

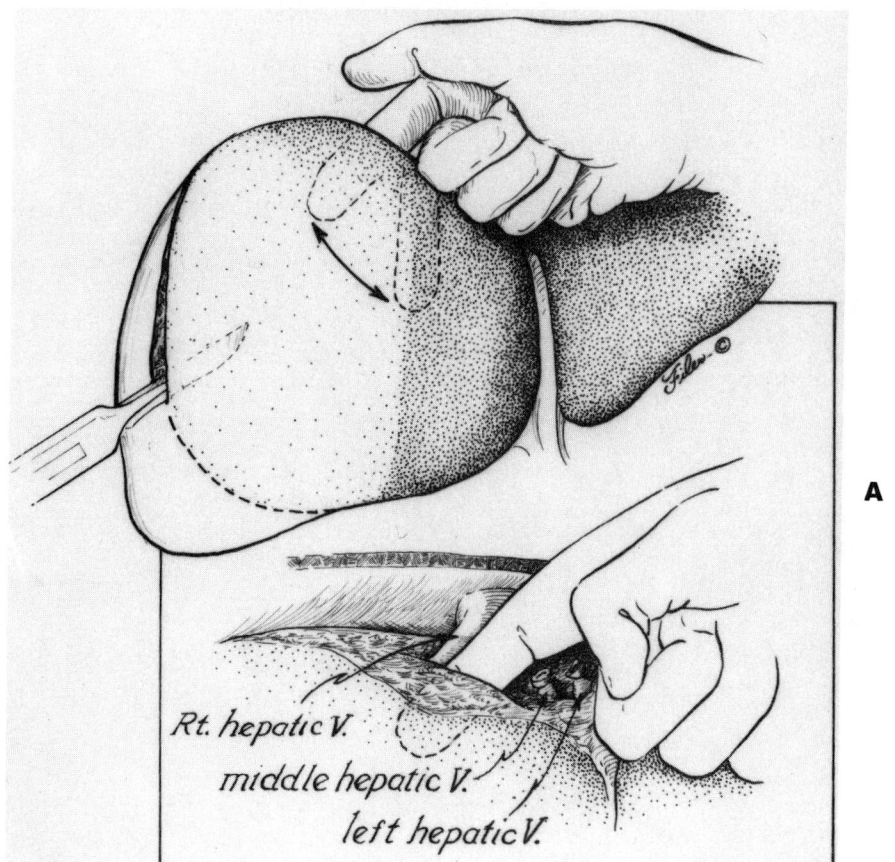

Rt. hepatic V.
middle hepatic V.
left hepatic V.

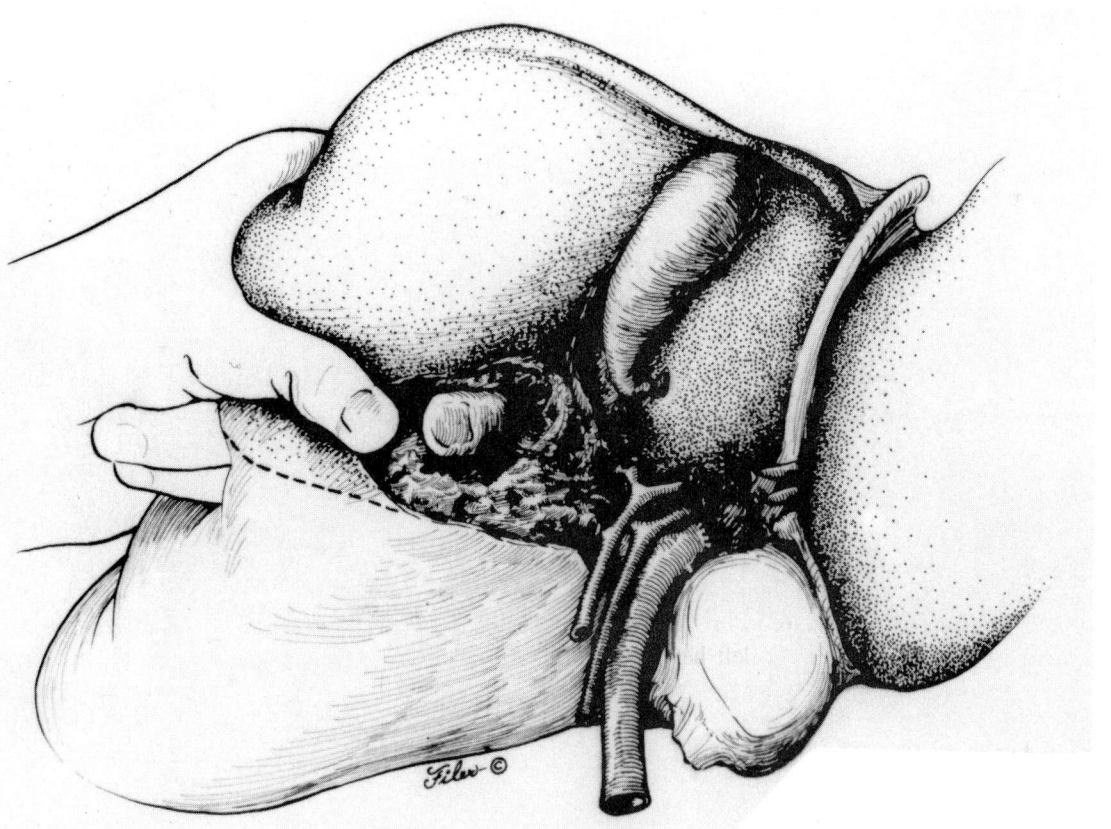

FIG. 11-37 Left hepatic trisegmentectomy. **A,** Demonstrates the intended resection from the anterior viewpoint. **B,** Manual retraction of the segments included in left trisegmentectomy and finger-fracture through the parenchyma.

From Daly, J.M., & Cady, B. (1993). *Atlas of surgical oncology.* St. Louis: Mosby.   *Continued.*

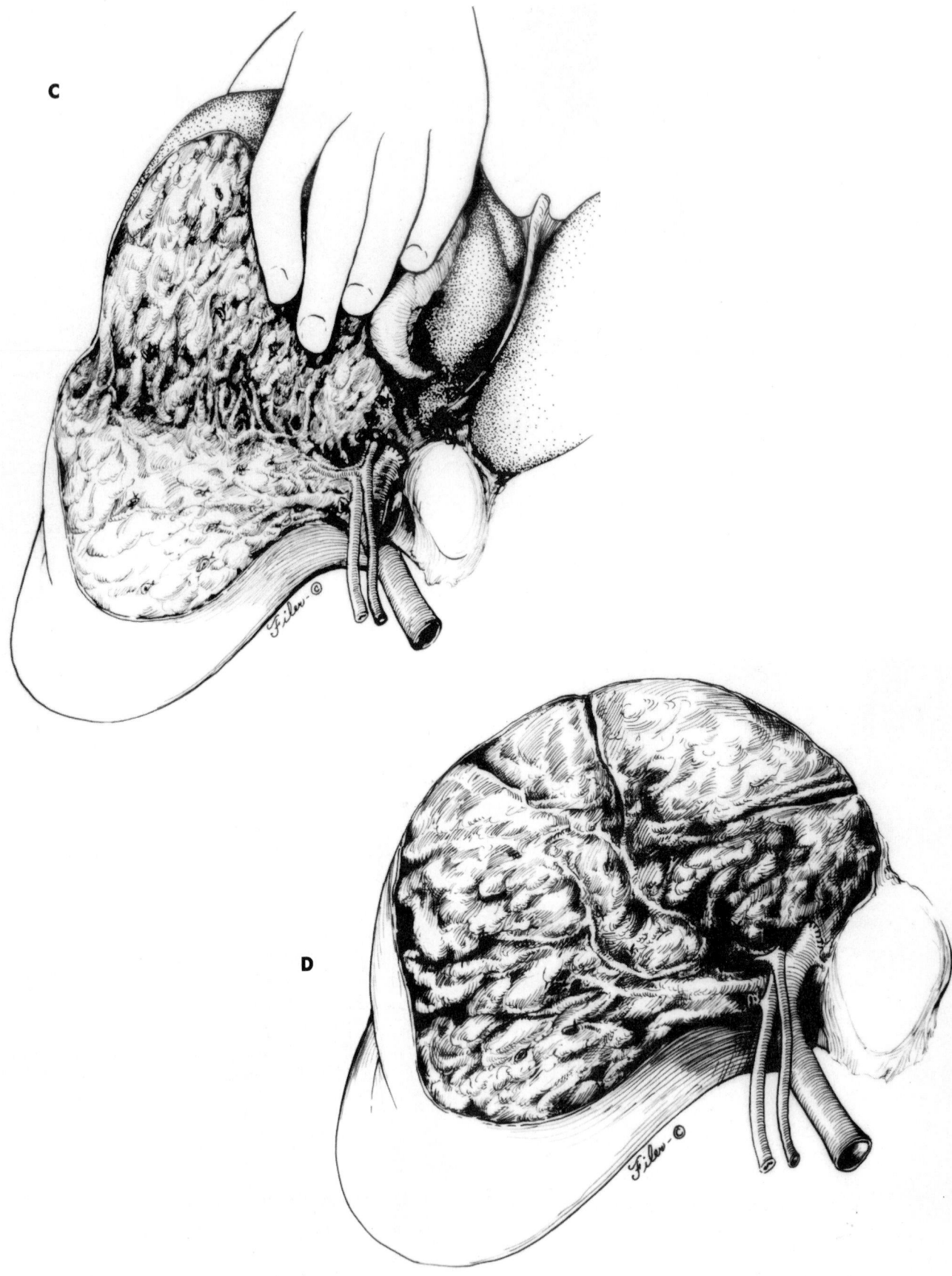

FIG. 11-37, CONT'D   **C,** The liver parenchyma is transsected in the right lobe. **D,** Illustration of the remaining liver following left trisegmentectomy.

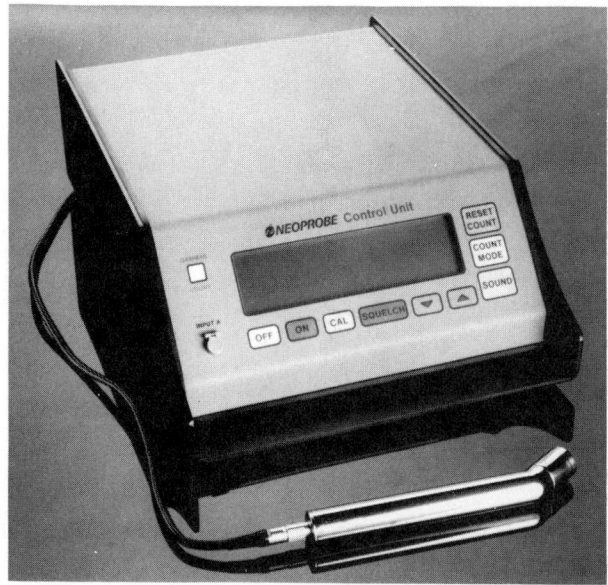

FIG. 11-38   Neoprobe instrument.
Courtesy Neoprobe Corp., Columbus, Ohio.

erative detection of adenocarcinoma and metastases can greatly assist in decision making and resection of diseased tissue (Research Highlight 11-1).

Procedural considerations

A basic laparotomy set of instruments is used. A gastrointestinal instrument set should be available.

Operative procedure

1. The operative procedure is identical to the second-look laparotomy procedure as described previously.
2. A midline abdominal incision is made from the xiphoid process to the pubis.
3. Intraoperative scanning of the liver and abdominal viscera is performed using the probe. The digital readings as well as the anatomic structures being scanned are recorded. Great care is taken to scan mesenteric, pelvic, and periaortic lymph nodes individually.
4. The liver is scanned, and areas emitting strong-pitched tones are marked with a sterile marking pen. A very distinct change in pitch may be noted on liver tissue within a 2- to 3-cm radius of the tumor site.
5. Intraoperative ultrasound and a review of the CT and MRI scans of the patient's liver are used to further confirm the liver lesions.
6. Margins for resection are drawn using an electrosurgical knife on a blend 2 setting at 40. Resection of the lesion may be segmental, circumferential, or lobar.
7. Following each resection the margins of healthy liver tissue adjacent to the resection site are scanned, and readings are recorded.
8. This procedure continues until all tissue emitting high gamma waves has been resected.

RESEARCH HIGHLIGHT 11-1

At a large midwestern academic medical center, a phase I/II study was completed on 60 patients with primary or recurrent colrectal cancer. The patients received the monoclonal antibody (MAb) CC-49 in preparation for the RIGs procedure applicable to each patient's specific preoperative diagnostic findings. Eighteen of 21 (86%) of the primary tumors were localized by the CC-49 MAb and the gamma-detecting probe. Twenty-nine of 30 (97%) recurrent tumors demonstrated localization. Antibody dose did not affect primary tumor localization.

Specimens located by the RIGS system were grouped into those tissues found by traditional methods (inspection and palpation) and those found only by RIGS (occult). There were 79 separate specimens removed from 30 patients with recurrent cancer. Nine specimens removed were histologically confirmed occult tumor sites found by the RIGS system. Sixteen specimens removed were RIGS positive but histologically negative. Forty-five specimens found by traditional means were histologically confirmed RIGS-positive tissues. For the 30 patients receiving second-look surgery for recurrent disease, RIGS findings changed 17 operative procedures in 14 patients (47%).

This study has lead to a more in-depth investigation to ascertain the ability of the RIGS system to identify adenocarcinoma at an early state than present pathologic examinations provide. A phase III study of the CC 49 Mab and the RIGS system is currently underway in at least 25 centers across the United States.

Arnold, M.W., Schneebaum, S., Petty, L.R., & Martin, E.W. (1993). Carcinoembrionic antigen-directed second-look surgery. In Wanebo, H.J. (editor). *Colorectal cancer*. St Louis: Mosby.

9. Specimens are sent to the pathology lab for further pathologic and histologic analysis. The perioperative nurse greatly enhances the correlation of pathologic diagnosis with the intraoperative RIGS findings by specifically and accurately identifying the tissue specimens.

Liver transplantation

Liver transplantation is the implantation of a liver from a donor into a recipient. The total procedure involves retrieving, or procuring, the liver from a donor, transporting the donor liver to the recipient's hospital, performing a hepatectomy on the recipient, and implanting the donor liver, including reanastomosis of suprahepatic vena cava, infrahepatic vena cava, portal vein and hepatic artery, biliary reconstruction with end-to-end anastomosis of donor and recipient common bile ducts, or Roux-en-Y anastomosis if the recipient bile duct is absent as a result of biliary atresia.

Liver transplantation is indicated for patients with end-stage liver disease resulting from postnecrotic cirrhosis, primary biliary cirrhosis, sclerosing cholangitis, Budd-Chiari syndrome, biliary atresia, metabolic disorders, and sometimes alcoholic cirrhosis. Patients with primary hepatic malignancies and metastatic malignancies confined to the liver are also candidates for liver transplant. When malignancies are the cause of the end-stage liver disease, intraoperative radiation of the right upper quadrant following hepatectomy and before the transplant may be performed in institutions employing this advanced technology.

Procedural considerations

Successful transplantation requires the cooperative efforts of the organ procurement agency and the staffs of the donor and recipient hospitals. Usually two members of the surgical team from the recipient's hospital travel to the donor's hospital to procure the donated liver. Multiple transplant teams may arrive at the donor hospital to procure the various organs available and viable for transplant.

The donor operating room is set up for a major laparotomy procedure. Basic instrumentation and equipment include the following:

Major abdominal instrument set	Nephrectomy instruments
Cardiovascular instruments	Intravenous volumetric pumps on stands
Power sternal saw	Extra suction bottles

The procurement team provides special Collins solution for flushing the organs, sterile plastic containers and ice chest for organs, and in situ flush tubing. The liver is generally placed in two Lahey bags immediately after procurement. Common practice is to procure the kidneys as well as the liver; other organs, tissues, and bone may also be procured.

Each transplant surgeon has preferred instruments, supplies, and sutures. In general, the following are needed in the recipient operating room:

Major abdominal instrument set	Overhead table and drape
Cardiovascular instrument set	Ring stand with basin
Set of T tubes	Large sterile draped instrument table for scrub nurse
Slush unit or means of providing iced lactated Ringer's solution	Medium sterile draped instrument table for preparation of liver
2 Electrosurgical units	Prep table and set
Thermia unit	Gram scale for measuring blood loss in sponges and laparotomy pads
Temperature probe	
Intravenous volumetric pumps on stands	
2 Blood warmers or water baths	4 Calibrated suction reservoirs for measuring blood loss through suction unit
Foley catheter and urinometer	
1 Sterile gown and glove table	

Large-bore cannulas for intravenous monitoring and fluid or blood replacement lines	Syringes, 50, 10, and 20 ml, 6 each
2 Headlights and light sources	Cold intravenous Ringer's solution
Venovenous bypass system	1 Sterile intravenous administration set for flushing the new liver
Extra drape sheets, table covers, gowns, towels, gloves, sponges, and laparotomy pads	Umbilical tape, booties, and vessel loops
50 Tuberculin syringes or 1-ml blood tubes (for blood specimens)	Sutures, as designated by surgeon
	Loupes, as desired by surgeon

A cart containing sutures and the numerous other small items should be set up and placed in the room for each procedure. This practice eliminates the circulating nurse running for extra supplies.

The procedure requires a bilateral subcostal incision with possible midline extension and removal of the xiphoid. The right side of the chest may be entered to provide more exposure when needed.

In addition to previously noted nursing diagnoses, patient goals, and nursing interventions, the following aspects of implementing the perioperative care plan deserve special attention.

Patient positioning. The patient is placed in the supine position with knees slightly flexed and padded. Accurate body alignment is essential. Foam padding should be used under all potential pressure areas. Heel protectors are applied and an eggcrate pad is placed over both legs and secured with the safety strap. As much body surface as possible should be in contact with the heating blanket to assist in maintaining the patient's temperature. A stocking cap may be helpful in preventing heat loss from the patient's head.

Blood loss and replacement. Blood loss may be extensive, and replacement must be timely. Blood products normally available at the beginning of the procedure include 10 units each of packed cells, fresh-frozen plasma, and platelets. Sufficient clot should be available in the blood bank to process additional blood products if needed. As in all surgical procedures, care must be exercised by all members of the surgical team in handling bloody sponges and instruments. Universal precautions should be strictly enforced. Nursing and medical team members should have previously been tested for immunity to hepatitis B and should have received Heptavax or another appropriate vaccine if indicated. Needle sticks must be reported and treated according to hospital policy.

Intraoperative laboratory testing. Thirty to 50 blood specimens can be drawn for analysis during the procedure. This blood must be recorded on the blood loss record and calculated into replacement needs. The specimens are delivered to the laboratory immediately. A telephone in the operating room is most useful for receiving reports directly from the laboratory.

Length of procedure. Procedures may last from 6 to 20 hours but normally last 8 to 10 hours. Special attention must be directed toward maintaining the integrity of the sterile environment from the standpoint of time and the numbers of people moving in and out of the room.

Communication with family. Frequent reports to the family are important. Family members usually are knowledgeable about liver function tests and laboratory values and want this information, in addition to reports on the condition of their loved one. One person should be assigned in advance to make regular contacts with family and support persons.

Operative procedure

1. Bilateral subcostal incisions are made with a midline incision extended toward the umbilicus.
2. Initial dissection of the underlying tissues is achieved with electrosurgery and suture ligatures.
3. Isolation of all hilar structures and dissection to mobilize the lobes of the native liver are performed.
4. The retrohepatic vena cava is skeletalized, as are the hepatic artery, portal vein, common bile duct, and inferior vena cava.
5. Nothing irreparable is done to the native liver before the arrival and examination of the donor liver.
6. Following the arrival of the donor organ, the patient is prepared for venovenous bypass, if indicated, by incision into the left external iliac vein and the left axillary vein. Cannulation into both the femoral and axillary sites allows for bypass of the portal system and inferior vena cava.
7. The infrahepatic vena cava and the suprahepatic vena cava are clamped, as are the portal vein, the hepatic artery, and the common bile duct. Native hepatectomy is then performed.
8. Revascularization of the donor organ begins with an end-to-end anastomosis of the suprahepatic vena cava with double-armed 3-0 vascular suture. The infrahepatic vena cava anastomosis is performed, followed by the end-to-end anastomosis of the portal vein. At this point, all venous clamps are removed, and blood flow through the vena cava and portal vein is restored. Hemostasis of the anastomosis sites is then achieved. Venovenous bypass is discontinued, and the cannulation sites are closed.
9. In situations in which the portal vein anastomosis may obstruct the ability to anastomose the hepatic artery, the hepatic artery anastomosis may be performed before that of the portal vein. Clamps are removed from the vena cava sites, the portal vein, and the hepatic artery simultaneously.
10. Modifications in the method of arterial reconstruction may be necessary, depending on the anatomic structure of the donor organ and the recipient's remaining hepatic arterial stump.
11. The postrevascularization phase focuses on achieving hemostasis. Complete hemostasis may require extensive time at this point. Bleeding may be exacerbated by a fibrinolytic episode associated with the reperfusion of the donor organ.
12. Biliary reconstruction varies with the status of the recipient's biliary tract. If biliary atresia is the cause of the patient's end-stage liver disease, choledochoenterostomy into a Roux-en-Y loop of jejunum is performed (Fig. 11-39, *A*). Sclerosing cholangitis also necessitates this biliary reconstruction procedure. An end-to-end reconstruction of the common bile duct may be possible if the recipient's biliary tract is free from disease and a T tube can be placed in the native duct (Fig. 11-39, *B*).
13. Drains are inserted and exit through the right abdominal wall.
14. The abdomen is then closed.

Donor hepatectomy

Donor hepatectomy is performed for procurement of a healthy liver for transplant into a patient suffering from end-stage liver failure. This procedure occurs only after the donor patient has been determined to be brain dead and family consent for organ donation has been obtained.

Donor hepatectomy can be performed at any hospital. Organ procurement agencies arrange contact with transplant centers when a viable organ donor has been identified. Candidates for liver transplants are placed on a national network waiting list and are matched according to urgency of need, blood type, and body size.

Procedural considerations

Once the liver transplant candidate has been identified, the procurement team from that transplant center travels to the institution where the organ donor is hospitalized. If multiple organs are being donated, surgeons from several transplant centers may arrive to procure the organs they will be transplanting at their respective centers.

The procedure for procurement of multiple organs may differ according to the transplant centers represented. Most commonly the systemic cooling of the donor's body temperature is started prior to the procurement of the heart. Cannulation sites may also vary according to which organs are procured.

The perioperative nurses at the donor hospital are responsible for supplying a basic laparotomy setup with instrumentation to open the sternum. Basic vascular clamps are also required for clamping the major vascular structures. Cold lactated Ringer's solution for parenteral infusion and cold Ringer's solution for irrigation are usually used in large amounts.

Perioperative nurses involved in organ procurement procedures must first consider their ethical and moral beliefs. Often the organ donor is a young and otherwise healthy individual who does not exhibit outward signs of death. The donor is brought to the surgical suite on life-support sys-

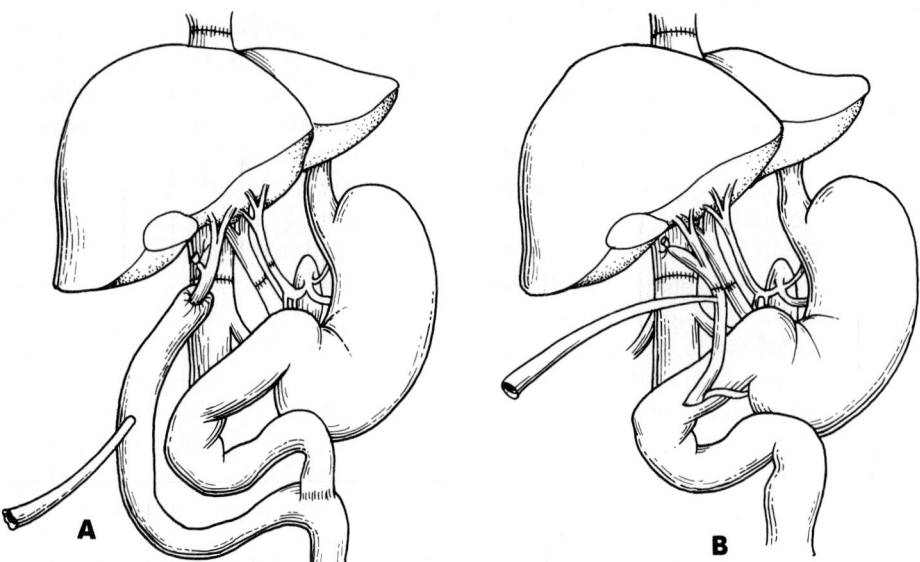

FIG. 11-39   Completed orthotopic liver transplant with Roux-en-Y biliary reconstruction **(A)**, and **(B)** end-to-end anastomosis of the donor-to-recipient common bile ducts.

From Anscher, N.L., et al. (1984). In Simmons, R.L., et al. (editors). *Manual of vascular access, organ donation, and transplantation.* New York: Springer-Verlag.

tems. The donor may appear as any patient would under general anesthesia. Strong feelings of uncertainty, denial, and internalization of fear for one's own loved ones must be dealt with appropriately. Perioperative nurses involved with organ procurement procedures must support and respect each person's feelings, since that individual may be grieving for the donor and his or her family during and long after the procedure is completed.

Operative procedure

1. The donor is positioned supine on the OR bed. The skin area from neck to midthigh is prepped and draped.
2. A midline incision is made from the suprasternal notch to the pubis. A subcostal incision is performed bilaterally on the abdomen for better exposure of the abdominal viscera.
3. Retractors are placed to provide optimal exposure of the organs that will be procured. The aorta and vena cava, superior and inferior to the liver and kidneys, are skeletalized by dissection and ligation of the lymphatics and smaller vasculatures. The porta hepatis is dissected; the superior mesenteric artery and celiac trunk are dissected and delicately exposed as close to the aorta as is convenient.
4. The superior mesenteric vein is dissected and prepared for cannulation. The donor is heparinized and systemically cooled.
5. If the heart is to be procured, at this point in the procedure the patient is pronounced dead, and the procurement of the heart is achieved.
6. Further cooling and flushing of the pancreas, liver, and kidneys are achieved by cannulation and infusion of

cold Ringer's lactate via the inferior vena cava just superior to the bifurcation. One to 2 L of lactated Ringer's solution are infused before the organs have been properly cooled.

7. The liver, pancreas, spleen, and a segment of the duodenum harboring the pancreatic duct are procured en bloc by placing clamps on the suprahepatic and infrahepatic venae cavae. The superhepatic vena cava is transsected with a surrounding cuff of diaphragm intact. The infrahepatic vena cava is transsected above the level of the renal veins. The celiac axis is detached from the aorta with an aortic patch or taken with a full aortic circumference. The duodenal segment is procured, using a linear stapling device at opposite ends of the segment.
8. The en bloc organs are taken to a back table for further dissection and ligation to separate the liver from the en bloc pancreas, spleen, and duodenal segment graft. Meanwhile, other members of the procurement team continue working to free the kidneys and ureters if they are to be taken.
9. The liver is placed in a basin of very cold Ringer's solution, double-bagged in sterile Lahey bags, and placed in an ice chest for transport to the recipient's hospital.
10. The kidneys are placed in sterile cassettes and mechanically perfused.
11. The pancreatic en bloc graft is also placed in a basin of cold Ringer's solution, bagged, and transported in a thermal chest of ice.
12. The abdomen is closed with a single layer of nonabsorbable no. 1 or 0 suture.
13. Drapes are removed, and the body is cleaned and

washed. Tubes and infusion lines are tied off or clamped.

14. Sometimes the family of the donor requests to view the body following organ donation. This factor may be important in helping them face the loss of their loved one. The perioperative nurse can assist them in their grieving process by providing them with a quiet and private environment in which to say good-bye to their family member. Removing the donor's body from the OR where the surgical procedure took place is best. The nurse should make sure that the donor is clothed and covered with a warm blanket and then stay with the family to support them through this most painful realization.

15. Morgue care is performed, and the donor is transported via stretcher to the morgue.

Living related liver transplantation

Just as kidney transplantation has evolved into cadaveric donor and living related donor possibilities, so too has liver transplantation. On November 27, 1989, a 21-month-old girl received the left lobe of her mother's liver at the University of Chicago Medical Center. The capacity of the liver to regenerate provided the scientific basis for development of the living related donor transplantation procedure. Surgeons in Australia, Brazil, and Japan had attempted such operations before in an attempt to save desperately ill children in end-stage liver failure (Fox & Swazey, 1992).

Where the field of transplantation will go is an ethical question. As technique and technology increase the possibilities, the only limiting factor in transplantation may be our social paradigms.

SPLENECTOMY

Splenectomy is removal of the spleen. It is usually performed for trauma to the spleen, for specific conditions of the blood such as hemolytic jaundice or splenic anemia, or for tumors, cysts, or splenomegaly. Another common indication for splenectomy is accidental injury to the spleen during vagotomy or other gastric procedures or operations involving mobilization of the splenic flexure of the colon. If accessory spleens are present, they are also removed, since they are capable of perpetuating hypersplenic function.

Procedural considerations

Massive splenomegaly may occasionally require a thoracoabdominal approach. Abdominal suction apparatus should be available throughout all splenectomies.

Instrumentation is as described for a basic laparotomy, plus two large, right-angled pedicle clamps, long instruments, and hemostatic materials or devices.

Operative procedure

1. The abdomen is opened through an upper midline or left subcostal incision. Retractors are placed over laparot-

omy packs, and gentle retraction is employed as exploration is carried out. The costal margin is retracted upward.

2. The splenorenal, splenocolic, and gastrosplenic ligaments are clamped and divided with long dressing forceps, long hemostats, sponges on holders, and long Metzenbaum or Nelson scissors. Adhesions posterior to the spleen are freed.

3. The spleen is delivered into the wound after these attachments are freed. The short gastric vessels are now easily identified, clamped, divided, and ligated.

4. The cavity formerly occupied by the spleen is packed with moist laparotomy pads, if necessary.

5. The splenic artery and vein are dissected free with fine dissecting scissors and forceps.

6. The artery is clamped and double ligated with silk. The artery is ligated first, and then the vein, thus permitting disengorgement of blood from the spleen and facilitating the return of venous blood to the circulatory system.

7. The splenic vein is clamped, divided, and ligated.

8. The specimen is removed; all bleeding vessels are controlled.

9. The wound is closed in layers, as described for laparotomy, and dressings are applied. Drainage is usually required only if many adhesions to the diaphragm were divided or if significant clotting abnormalities exist.

REFERENCES

Arnold, M.W., Schneebaum, S., Petty, L.R., & Martin, E.W. (1993). Carcinoembrionic antigen-directed second-look surgery. In H.J. Wanebo (Ed.), *Colorectal cancer*. St. Louis: Mosby.

Fox, R.C., & Swazey, J.P. (1992). *Spare parts*. New York: Oxford University Press.

McDermott, W.V. (1989). *Surgery of the liver*. Boston: Blackwell Scientific Publications.

Martin, E.W., et al. (1988). Radioimmunoguided surgery using monoclonal antibody. *American Journal of Surgery, 156*, 386-392.

Quilici, P.J. (1992). *New developments in laparoscopy*. Norwalk, Conn: Auto Suture Company, Division of United States Surgical Corporation.

Way, L.W., & Pellegrini, C.A. (1987). *Surgery of the gallbladder and bile ducts*. Philadelphia: W.B. Saunders.

Zucker, K.A. (1991). *Surgical laparoscopy*. St. Louis: Quality Medical Publishing.

BIBLIOGRAPHY

Davis, J.H., et al. (1987). *Clinical surgery* (Vol. 2). St. Louis: Mosby.

Daly, J.M., & Cady, B. (1993). *Atlas of surgical oncology*. St. Louis: Mosby.

Doughty, D.B., & Broadwell Jackson, D. (1993). *Gastrointestinal disorders*. St Louis: Mosby.

Maddrey, W.C. (1988). *Transplantation of the liver*. New York: Elsevier Science Publishing Co.

Minton, J.P., et al. (1989). Results of surgical excision of one to 13 hepatic metastases in 98 consecutive patients. *Archives of Surgery, 114-*124.

Moody, F.G., Carey, L.C., et al. (1990). *Surgical treatment of digestive disease*. Chicago: Year Book Medical Publishers, Inc.

Ricker, L.E., et al. (1989). Colorectal carcinoma: Using a gamma counter to find recurrent tumors. *AORN Journal, 50*, 5.

Toledo-Pereyra, L.H. (1988). *Pancreas transplantation*. Boston: Kluwer Academic Publishers.

12

REPAIR OF HERNIAS

AMY B. SHANNON

A hernia is a protrusion or the displacement of intraabdominal tissue or viscus through a congenital or acquired opening or fascial defect in the abdominal wall. In general, hernias of the abdominal wall occur far less frequently in women than in men, with the greatest disparity in the incidence of indirect and direct inguinal hernias.

Groin hernias were originally documented 3500 years ago, with surgical intervention starting approximately 1500 years after that (Cameron, 1992). Before the intervention of surgical repair of the hernia, external supports called trusses were used to contain hernias that protruded from the body. In the late nineteenth century, Edoardo Bassini introduced a surgical technique that is still the foundation for modern hernia repair (Long & Sandler, 1990).

The incidence of abdominal wall hernias is 15 per 1000 population (Sabiston, 1991). Femoral hernias are more common in females (84%) than males and account for 6% of all hernias (Davis et al., 1991). About 75% of hernias occur in the groin, with the remaining 25% distributed among ventral, umbilical, femoral, and other types. As the frequency and magnitude of abdominal surgeries have increased in recent years, so has the incidence of incisional hernia.

Herniorrhaphy is one of the most common operative procedures performed and is the preferred treatment for all population groups when a defect is detected.

Hernias have a tremendous economic significance in the United States. The amount of work days lost is substantial, and the trend toward ambulatory surgery for hernia repair can save $3000 per procedure, or $1.5 billion per year (Lichtenstein et al., 1990).

A hernia can occur in several places in the abdominal wall, with protrusion of a portion of the parietal peritoneum and often a part of the intestine. The weak places or intervals in the abdominal aponeurosis are (1) the inguinal canals, (2) the femoral rings, and (3) the umbilicus. Any number of conditions causing increased pressure within the abdomen can contribute to the formation of a hernia. Contributing factors to hernia formation include age, sex, previous surgery, obesity, nutritional state, and pulmonary and cardiac disease. Loss of tissue turgor occurs with aging and in chronic debilitating diseases.

SURGICAL ANATOMY

A hernia is a sac lined by peritoneum that protrudes through a defect in the layers of the abdominal wall. Generally, a hernial mass is composed of covering tissues, a peritoneal sac, and any contained viscera. Hernias may be acquired or congenital.

Depending on their location, hernias are classified as direct inguinal, indirect inguinal, femoral, umbilical, or epigastric. Hernias in any of these groups are either reducible or irreducible; that is, the contents of the hernia sac either can be returned to the normal intraabdominal position or are trapped in the extraabdominal sac (incarcerated). The conditions preventing the return of the hernial contents to the abdomen can result from (1) adhesions between the contents of the sac and the inner lining of the sac, (2) adhesions among the contents of the sac, or (3) narrowing of the neck of the sac. Patients with incarcerated hernias may have signs of intestinal obstruction, such as vomiting and distention. The great danger of an incarcerated hernia is that it may become strangulated. In a strangulated hernia the blood supply of the trapped sac contents becomes compromised, and eventually the sac contents necrose. When bowel is trapped in such a hernia, resection of necrosed bowel, in addition to the repair of the hernia defect, becomes mandatory.

INGUINAL HERNIAS

The anterolateral abdominal wall consists of an arrangement of muscles, fascial layers, and muscular aponeuroses lined interiorly by peritoneum and exteriorly by skin (Figs. 12-1 and 12-2). The abdominal wall in the groin area is composed of two groups of these structures: a superficial group—Scarpa's fascia, external and internal oblique muscles, and their aponeuroses, and a deep group—the internal oblique muscle, transversalis fascia, and peritoneum.

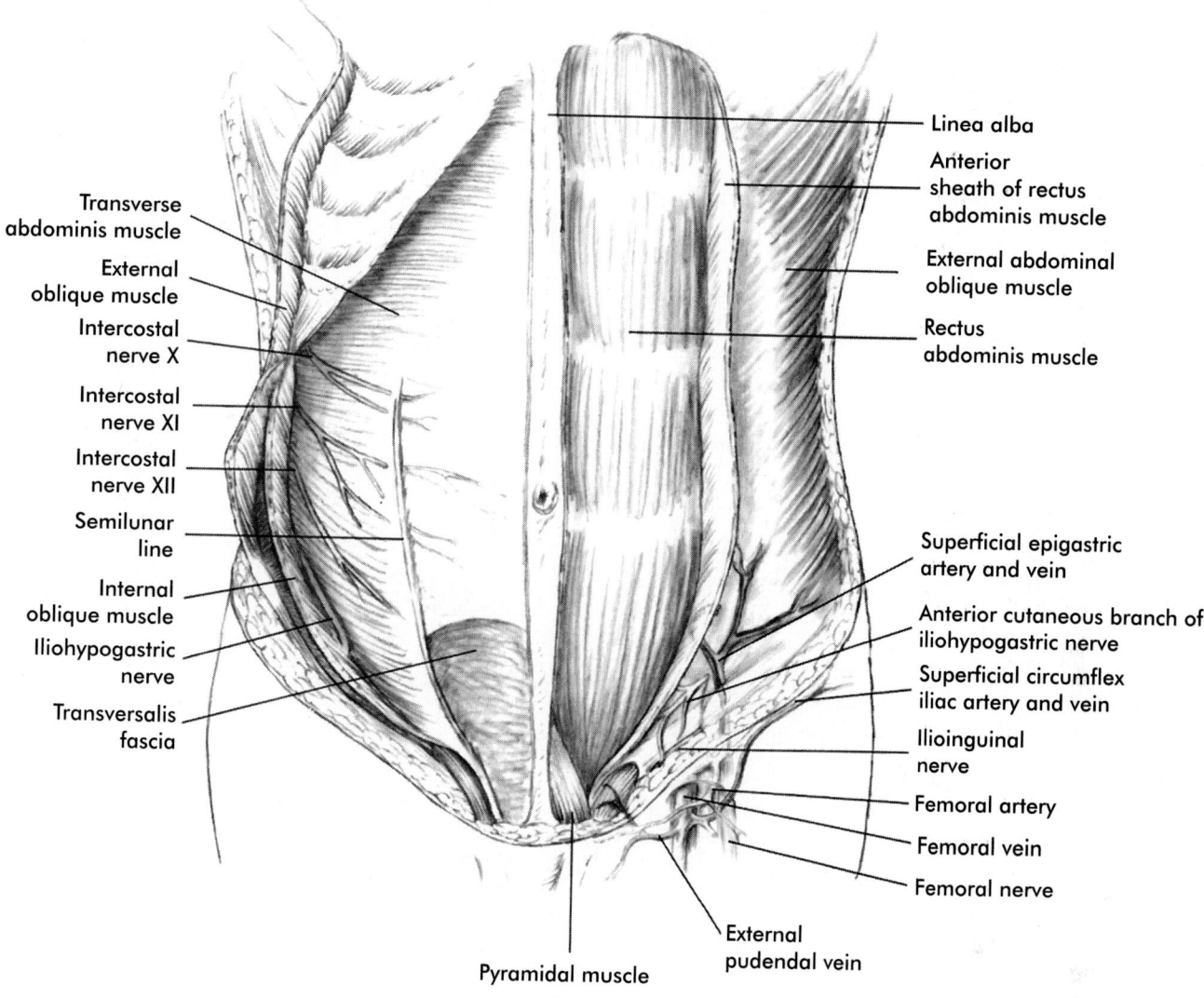

FIG. 12-1   Perspective of the anterior abdominal wall illustrating the layers of musculature, aponeurotic extensions, vasculature, and innervation.

From Davis, J.H., et al. (1987). *Clinical surgery* (Vol. 2). St. Louis: Mosby.

Essential to an understanding of inguinal hernia repair is an appreciation of the central role of the transversalis fascia as the major supporting structure of the posterior inguinal floor. The inguinal canal, which contains the spermatic cord and associated structures in males and the round ligament in females, is approximately 4 cm long and takes an oblique course parallel to the groin crease. The inguinal canal is covered by the aponeurosis of the external abdominal oblique muscle, which forms a roof (Fig. 12-3). A thickened lower border of the external oblique aponeurosis forms the inguinal (Poupart's) ligament. This ligament stretches from the anterior superior iliac spine to the pubic tubercle. Structures that traverse the inguinal canal enter it from the abdomen by the internal ring, a natural opening in the transversalis fascia, and exit by the external ring, an opening in the external oblique aponeurosis, to go to either

the testis or the labium. If the external oblique aponeurosis, is opened and the cord or round ligament mobilized, the floor of the inguinal canal is exposed. The posterior inguinal floor is the structure that becomes defective and is susceptible to indirect, direct, or femoral hernias (Figs. 12-4 and 12-5).

The key component of the important posterior inguinal floor is the transversalis muscle of the abdomen and its associated aponeurosis and fascia. The posterior inguinal floor can be divided into two areas. The superior lateral area represents the internal ring, whereas the inferior medial area represents the attachment of the transversalis aponeurosis and fascia to Cooper's ligament (iliopectineal line). Cooper's ligament is the site of the insertion of the transversalis aponeurosis along the superior ramus from the symphysis pubis laterally to the femoral sheath. Note that the in-

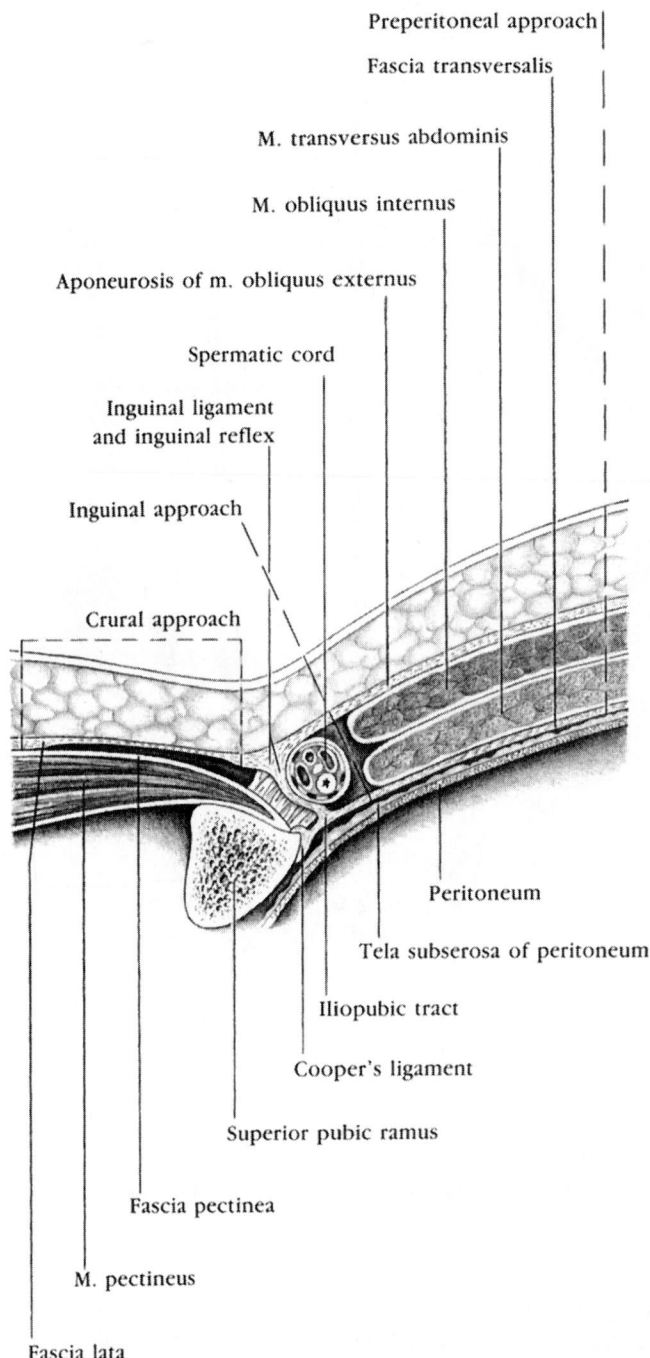

FIG. 12-2 Anatomy and approach routes *(broken lines)* to the inguinal and femoral region in cross section.

From Schumpelick, V. (1990). *Atlas of hernia surgery*. Toronto: B.C. Decker.

guinal portion of the transversalis fascia arises from the iliopsoas fascia and not from the inguinal ligament.

Medially and superiorly, the transversalis muscle becomes aponeurotic and fuses with the aponeurosis of the internal oblique muscle to form anterior and posterior rectus sheaths. As the symphysis pubis is approached, the contributions from the internal oblique muscle become fewer and fewer. At the pubic tubercle and behind the spermatic cord or round ligament, the internal oblique muscle makes no contribution, and the posterior inguinal wall (floor of the inguinal canal) is composed solely of aponeurosis and fascia of the transversalis muscle.

None of the three groin hernias develops in the presence of a strong transversus abdominis layer and in the absence of persistent stress on the connective tissue layers (Nyhus & Condon, 1989). When a weakening or a tear in the apo-

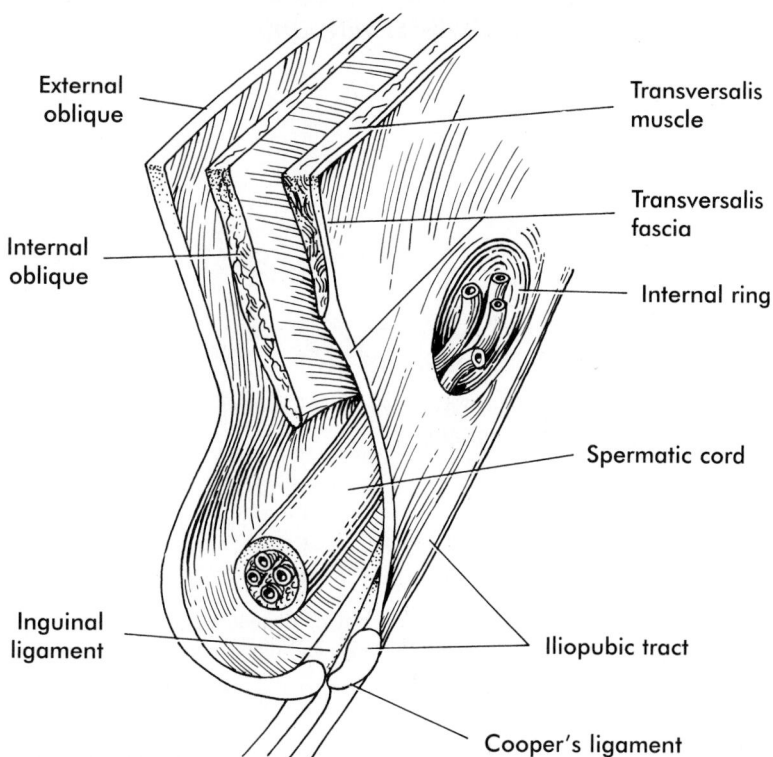

FIG. 12-3 Right inguinal region, parasagittal section. Roof of inguinal canal is formed by external oblique aponeurosis, and floor is formed by transversalis aponeurosis and fascia.

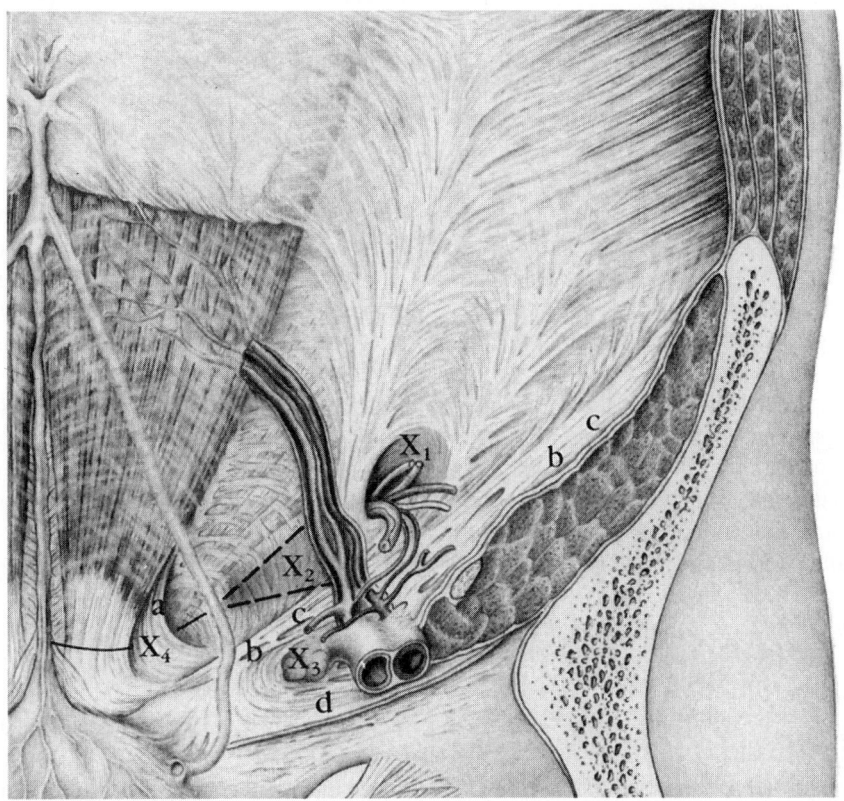

FIG. 12-4 Anatomic representation of the abdominal wall. Internal view in the area of the hernia orifices, showing the hernial orifice of the indirect and direct inguinal hernia, the femoral hernia, and the supravesical hernia $(X_1$ to $X_4)$. *a*, Falx inguinalis; *b*, inguinal ligament; *c*, iliopubic tract; *d*, pectineal ligament; X_1, indirect hernia; X_2, direct hernia; X_3, femoral hernia; X_4, supravesical hernia.

From Schumpelick, V. (1990). *Atlas of hernia surgery*. Toronto: B.C. Decker.

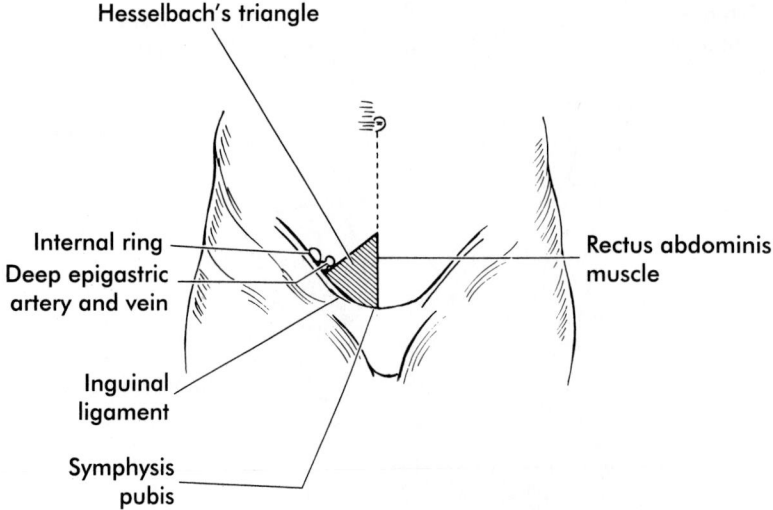

FIG. 12-5   Schematic representation of Hesselbach's triangle. Boundaries of Hesselbach's triangle are deep epigastric vessels laterally, inguinal ligament inferiorly, and rectus abdominis muscle medially.

neurosis of the transversus abdominis and the transversalis fascia occurs, the potential for development of a direct inguinal hernia is established.

FEMORAL HERNIAS

When the transversus abdominis aponeurosis and its fascia are only narrowly attached to the Cooper's ligament, a femoral hernia may develop. Dilation of the femoral ring and canal, which allows for the prominence of the iliofemoral vessels, can also result in femoral herniation.

The walls of the femoral sheath are formed anteriorly and medially from the transversalis fascia, posteriorly from pectineus and psoas fascia, and laterally from iliaca fascia. The pelvis ostium consists of a relatively fixed rim of bone and connective tissue: anterior and medial, the iliopubic tract; posterior, the superior ramus; and lateral, the iliopectineal arch.

The femoral sheath is subdivided into three compartments. The lateral compartment contains the femoral artery, and the intermediate compartment the femoral vein. The medial compartment is the smallest and constitutes the femoral canal, which is formed anteriorly and medially by the iliopubic tract. Laterally this opening is bound by the iliofemoral vessels and posteriorly by the superior pubic ramus and pectineus fascia. Superiorly, laterally, and inferiorly the fossa is formed by the falciform margin of the fascia lata.

ABDOMINAL HERNIAS

The anterior abdominal wall is composed of external abdominal oblique muscles attached to a thick sheath of connective tissue called the rectus sheath. The linea alba extends superior and inferior from above the xiphoid process to the pubis. Beneath the rectus sheath lies the rectus abdominis muscles, lateral to the right and left of the linea

alba. Lateral to the rectus abdominis is the linea semilunaris. The transversus abdominis muscles originate from the seventh to the twelfth costal cartilages, lumbar fascia, iliac crest, and the inguinal ligament and insert on the xiphoid process, the linea alba, and the pubic tubercle. The third layer of abdominal wall includes the internal abdominal oblique muscles originating from the iliac crest, inguinal ligament, and lumbar fascia and inserting on the tenth to twelfth ribs and rectus sheath.

DIRECT AND INDIRECT HERNIAS

The deep epigastric vessels (inferior epigastric) arise from the external iliac vessels and enter the inguinal canal just proximal to the internal ring. The triangle formed by the deep epigastric vessels laterally, the inguinal ligament inferiorly, and the rectus abdominis muscles medially is referred to as Hesselbach's triangle (Fig. 12-5).

Hernias that occur within Hesselbach's triangle are called direct inguinal hernias. Indirect inguinal hernias occur lateral to the deep epigastric vessels. Therefore both direct and indirect hernias represent attenuations or tears in the transversalis fascia (Fig. 12-6).

Direct hernias protrude into the inguinal canal but not into the cord and therefore rarely into the scrotum. Direct inguinal hernias usually result from heavy lifting or other strenuous activities. Indirect hernias leave the abdominal cavity at the internal inguinal ring and pass with the cord structures down the inguinal canal. Consequently the indirect hernia sac may be found in the scrotum. Indirect hernias may be either congenital, representing a persistence of the processus vaginalis, or acquired. In a congenital hernia, the hernia sac has a small neck, is thin walled, and is closely bound to the cord structures. In an acquired indirect hernia the neck is wide, and the sac is both short and thick walled. When both direct and indirect hernias are

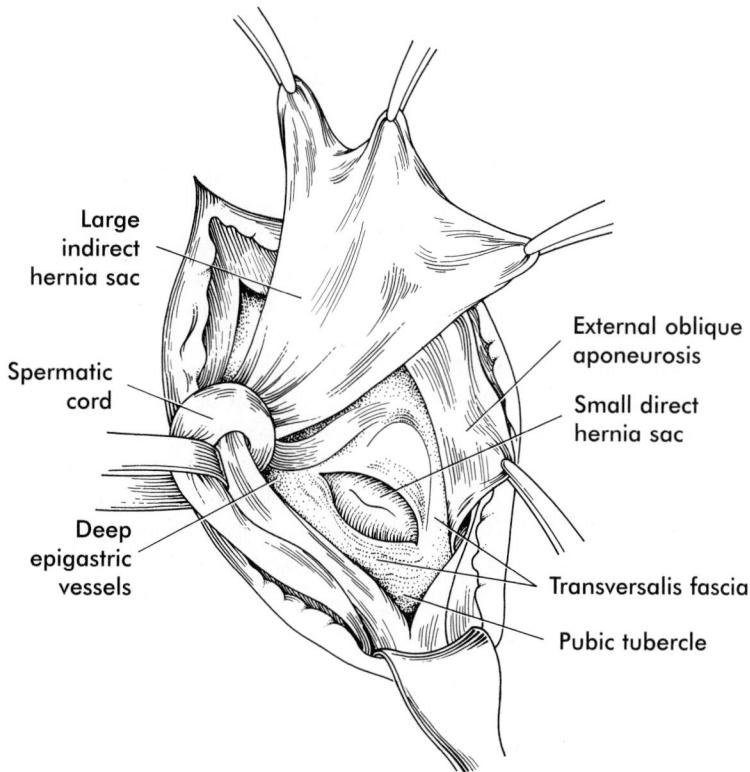

FIG. 12-6   Defect in transversalis fascia, medial to deep epigastric vessels, gives rise to direct hernia. Defect lateral to deep epigastric vessels results in indirect hernia.

present, the defect is called a pantaloon hernia after the French word for pants, which this situation suggests.

PERIOPERATIVE NURSING CONSIDERATIONS

ASSESSMENT

Assessment of the patient with a hernia begins with a nursing history of past surgeries related to the herniated area. The patient's occupation and physical activities may be contributing factors to the development of the hernia. A thorough nursing history includes information relating to a familial history of hernias, the patient's nutritional status, when the symptoms occurred, a history of obesity, increased intraabdominal pressure, chronic cough, constipation, a history of benign prostatic hypertrophy, intestinal obstruction, colon malignancy, and for females pregnancy (Nyhus et al., 1990).

Pain is often a notable symptom for the patient. An accurate description of the type and degree of pain is included in the assessment. Patients often describe the feeling of a foreign body at the hernia site.

Physical examination is the most common means for diagnosis. Palpation of the herniated area reveals the contents of the hernia sac. Fingertip palpation allows the nurse to feel the edges of the ring or abdominal wall. Having the patient stand and cough during the examination also assists in the evaluation of the herniated area.

The diagnosis of hernias is almost always accomplished by a clinical physical examination and a thorough health history. If a definitive diagnosis is not confirmed, ultrasonic scanning and imaging techniques (such as computed tomography, herniography, and standard x-ray) may be employed.

A hernia may cause no symptoms; its only sign may be a swelling or protrusion in a restricted area of the abdominal wall. If the hernia is unilateral, the patient notes the lack of a protrusion on the other side in comparison. The area may be visible when the patient stands or coughs and may disappear on reclining. Femoral hernias can be difficult to diagnose and may resemble an enlarged lymph node.

Preoperative testing for a hernia repair facilitates safe and efficient perioperative care. Baseline data are obtained by a complete blood count. Prior to surgery, patients over 40 years of age may need an ECG and chest x-ray. Patients with a history of more complex medical problems must be fully evaluated with appropriate laboratory tests.

NURSING DIAGNOSIS

Nursing diagnoses related to the care of the patient undergoing hernia surgery might include the following:

• Activity intolerance related to pain
• High risk for urinary retention
• Altered tissue perfusion of the scrotal area causing scrotal edema and ecchymosis

OUTCOME IDENTIFICATION

Outcomes identified for the selected nursing diagnoses could be stated as the following:

• The patient will return to previous level of activity.
• The patient will not experience urinary retention.
• The patient will preoperatively verbalize an understanding of potential scrotal edema and ecchymosis. The patient will not experience scrotal edema.

PLANNING

The perioperative nurse formulates a plan of care for the patient having hernia repair surgery by assimilating knowledge pertaining to the anatomy involved and principles of asepsis. Instrumentation, draping, and positioning for the patient's surgery depend on the type of hernia.

A typical care plan for a patient having surgery for repair of a hernia is shown in the Sample Care Plan.

IMPLEMENTATION

The patient may undergo general anesthesia, spinal or epidural block, regional anesthesia with sedation, or local anesthesia. Routine monitoring equipment such as a three-lead ECG, oxygen saturation monitor, and blood pressure cuff are utilized for a hernia repair. An IV line is inserted for fluid replacement and medication administration. During inguinal herniorrhaphy the surgeon may want the patient to cough or bear down.

The patient is usually positioned supine with basic prepping and draping procedures followed (see Chapter 3). Instruments used for herniorrhaphies are those found in standard laparotomy sets (see Chapter 10) or minor sets. A typical minor instrument set contains the following:

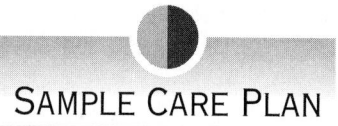

SAMPLE CARE PLAN

NURSING DIAGNOSIS: Activity intolerance related to pain
OUTCOME: The patient will return to his previous level of activity.
INTERVENTIONS:
Determine the patient's baseline activity level.
Encourage early postoperative ambulation.
Instruct the patient to use prescribed pain medications before physical activity and as needed.
Advise the patient to gradually increase activity as tolerated.
Explain the anticipated postoperative activity recommendations.

NURSING DIAGNOSIS: High risk for urinary retention
OUTCOME: The patient will not experience urinary retention.
INTERVENTIONS:
Encourage patient to void before surgery.
Monitor and record intake and output status.

Postoperatively assess bladder for signs of urinary retention (palpable bladder or patient discomfort).
Encourage and assist patient with early ambulation as soon as choice of anesthesia permits.
Catheterize the patient if urinary retention occurs.

NURSING DIAGNOSIS: Altered tissue perfusion of the scrotal area causing scrotal edema and ecchymosis
OUTCOME: The patient will preoperatively verbalize an understanding of the potential for scrotal edema and ecchymosis. The patient will not experience any scrotal edema or ecchymosis.
INTERVENTIONS:
Preoperatively discuss the possibility of swelling and ecchymosis.
Apply scrotal support intraoperatively.
Assess scrotum for evidence of swelling, ecchymosis, and redness.
Apply ice packs as ordered.
Reassure the patient and instruct him on the importance of wearing the scrotal support.
Reassure the patient that the swelling and ecchymosis will subside.

8 Towel clamps, non-
perforating
6 Halsted mosquito for-
ceps, straight
6 Halsted mosquito for-
ceps, curved
10 Crile artery forceps,
5½ inches, curved
4 Allis forceps
2 Ochsner forceps,
straight
2 Babcock forceps
2 Mayo-Hegar needle
holders, 6 inches
2 Webster needle hold-
ers, 4½ inches
Metzenbaum dissecting
scissors, 5½ inches,
curved
Mayo dissecting scis-
sors, 6¾ inches,
straight
Metzenbaum dissecting
scissors, 7 inches,
straight
Forester sponge forceps,
7 inches, straight
2 Adson tissue forceps,
4¾ inches

2 Tissue forceps, 5½
inches
Dressing forceps, 5
inches
2 Brophy tissue forceps,
8 inches
2 USA retractors
2 Volkmann rake retrac-
tors, 4-prong, blunt
2 Volkmann rake retrac-
tors, 4-prong, sharp
2 Richardson retractors,
¾ inch × 1 inch
2 Richardson retractors,
1⅛ × 1⅛ inches
2 Senn retractors
2 Weitlaner retractors,
6½ inches
2 Cushing vein retrac-
tors
2 Single skin hooks
2 Double skin hooks
2 Knife handles, no. 3
Knife handle, no. 7
Knife handle, no. 4
2 Frazier suction tips, 8
Fr and 12 Fr
Yankauer suction tip

1 Laparoscope, 25 de-
grees
1 Panoview laparo-
scope, 10 mm
1 Endoscopic hernia
stapler
1 Endoscopic clip ap-
plier
2 Trocars and sleeves,
no. 11
3 Trocars and sleeves,
no. 5
2 Trocar reducers, 11
mm to 5 mm
1 Applicator for endo-
ligature, 2 mm
1 Aspiration needle
1 Two-way suction irri-
gator with stylet
1 Microdissecting scis-
sors
1 Cabot claw forceps

1 Double-action scis-
sors
1 Randall stone for-
ceps
1 Hasson set
1 Dissecting hook can-
nula
1 Dissecting spatula
1 Hook scissors
2 Dissecting graspers
1 Grasping forceps
1 Light cord
1 2-way stopcock
1 Veress needle
2 Sealing caps, 10
mm
2 Sealing caps, 12
mm
3 Rubber seals, 11
mm
3 Rubber seals, 5.5
mm

A self-retaining retractor, such as a Weitlaner, facilitates the separation of tissue layers. A Penrose drain is used to retract the spermatic cord structures for better exposure. Because the peritoneal cavity may be entered in this procedure, accurate sponge, sharp, and instrument counts must be performed.

With a sliding hernia or an incarcerated hernia, the possibility of having to enter the peritoneal cavity must be considered. If the hernia is strangulated, necrotic bowel must be resected, and instruments for doing a bowel anastomosis must be ready. Antibiotics may be added to the irrigation to prevent an infection.

Repair of the inguinal hernia includes approximation of the transversalis fascia with a heavy, nonabsorbable type of suture. With some indirect hernias, only two or three sutures may be necessary. In other cases, however, up to 10 sutures in succession may be needed. Numerous types of needles are used for hernia repair. Scarpa's fascia is approximated with absorbable sutures, and the skin is closed by one of several methods.

Implementation of a laparoscopic hernia repair is technically similar to the open laparotomy, but the instrumentation includes laparoscopic equipment. A typical laparoscopic hernia set includes basic laparoscopic instrumentation, such as the following:

There is always a possibility that a laparoscopy may become a laparotomy, and instrumentation for this change in procedure must always be available.

EVALUATION

Evaluation of the patient having repair of a hernia should include examination of all skin surfaces to assess variances with the preoperative assessment data. The patient should awaken from general anesthesia in a reasonable amount of time without exhibiting signs of anxiety or extreme disorientation. Extubation should be timely to avoid stress on the repaired hernia site. The evaluation of the patient's status can be phrased in outcome statements such as:

- The patient will return to his previous level of activity.
- The patient does not experience urinary retention.
- The patient has minimal edema and ecchymosis of the scrotum. The patient will verbalize an understanding of the importance of utilizing the scrotal support.

The perioperative nurse gives a detailed report to the PACU nurse pertaining to the relative events and patient status during the operative procedure.

Urinary retention may occur after a herniorrhaphy, and measures must be taken to prevent overdistention of the bladder. Early ambulation is permitted to encourage the resumption of bladder and bowel functions. If the bowel has been resected because of strangulation, a nasogastric tube and suction may be required to reduce the incidence of postoperative vomiting and distention with subsequent strain on the suture line (Research Highlight 12-1).

Postoperative inflammation or swelling of the scrotum from manipulation is reduced with the application of either

a scrotal support (suspensory), ice packs, or both. The patient is reassured that ecchymosis and discomfort will diminish within a few days and that sexual functioning should
not be affected.

Hospital stays for hernia patients are usually only a day
or two. An uncomplicated herniorrhaphy may also be performed as an ambulatory surgery procedure with the patient
going home a few hours after surgery. More patients and
their physicians are electing to have herniorrhaphies performed as ambulatory surgery procedures due to decreased
cost and earlier return to normal activities. Consequently,
the perioperative nurse is responsible for discharge and
home care planning for the patient. A patient who has had
elective surgery for a hernia should be restricted from strenuous activity for at least a week and should be informed
that good body alignment is necessary. If the patient's occupation involves heavy lifting or straining, some modifications may be necessary.

SURGICAL INTERVENTIONS

SURGERY FOR REPAIR OF GROIN HERNIAS

Repair of inguinal hernias

Several operative procedures for repair of inguinal hernias are currently used. Approaches that reestablish the integrity of the transversalis fascia and simultaneously reestablish and strengthen the posterior inguinal floor are favored. A surgical repair in which transversalis fascia is
sewn to transversalis fascia accomplishes this goal.

Procedural considerations

The patient is in the supine position for abdominal wall
and inguinal and/or femoral hernia repairs. The patient's
skin surface area from above the umbilicus to midthigh is
exposed, prepped with antimicrobial solutions, and draped
with sterile drapes. A sterile drape should be placed under
the scrotum in the event it becomes necessary to enter the
scrotum.

Operative procedures

McVay or Cooper's ligament repair. A McVay or
Cooper's ligament repair approximates transversalis fascia
superior to the inferior insertion of the transversalis fascia
along Cooper's ligament.

1. An oblique incision is made parallel to the inguinal ligament, ending two fingerbreadths lateral to the pubic
   tubercle. Frequently the skin is lightly crosshatched to
   facilitate later closure (Fig. 12-7).
2. The incision is carried through the superficial and deep
   (Scarpa's) fascia to the external oblique aponeurosis.
   Hemostasis is maintained with fine ties or electrocoagulation.
3. The external oblique aponeurosis is opened in the direction of its fibers to the external ring, and the aponeurotic flaps are reflected back along the iliohypogas-
   tric and ilioinguinal nerves, which are usually identified and preserved at this point (Fig. 12-7).
4. The cremaster muscles that form an envelope around
   the spermatic cord and represent the continuation of the
   internal oblique muscles are opened and the cord exposed.
5. By gentle dissection the spermatic vessels and the vas
   deferens are separated. While this is being done, the
   cord is examined for an indirect hernia, which arises
   from the internal ring and is initially adherent to the
   cord.
6. If an indirect sac is identified, it is carefully dissected
   away from the cord until the neck of the hernia is
   clearly delineated (Fig. 12-8).
7. The sac is opened, and any abdominal contents are returned to the abdominal cavity.
8. A suture ligature or purse-string suture is placed high
   in the neck of the sac, and the excess peritoneum of
   the hernia is excised. The ligated stump quickly retracts
   into the peritoneal cavity. If only a direct sac is present,
   usually no resection of the hernia is done because the
   sac easily returns to the abdominal cavity.
9. If transversalis fascia is present on both sides of the
   hernia defect, it is sutured together (Fig. 12-9). Suturing begins at the symphysis pubis and continues laterally to the internal ring. If the inferior transversalis fascia is weak or not present, the superior portion is sutured to Cooper's ligament, the site of insertion of the
   transversalis fascia. In this case, suturing again begins
   at the pubic tubercle and is continued laterally along
   Cooper's ligament to the medial border of the femoral
   sheath, where a transition stitch is place. The repair is
   then carried laterally, approximating transversalis fascia to inguinal ligament (Fig. 12-10).
10. When the transveralis fascia is pulled down to Coo-
    per's ligament, a relaxing incision in the rectus sheath
    is sometimes necessary to relieve excess tension. Es-
    sentially this incision is 5 to 7 cm long in the anterior
    rectus sheath. The incision begins immediately above

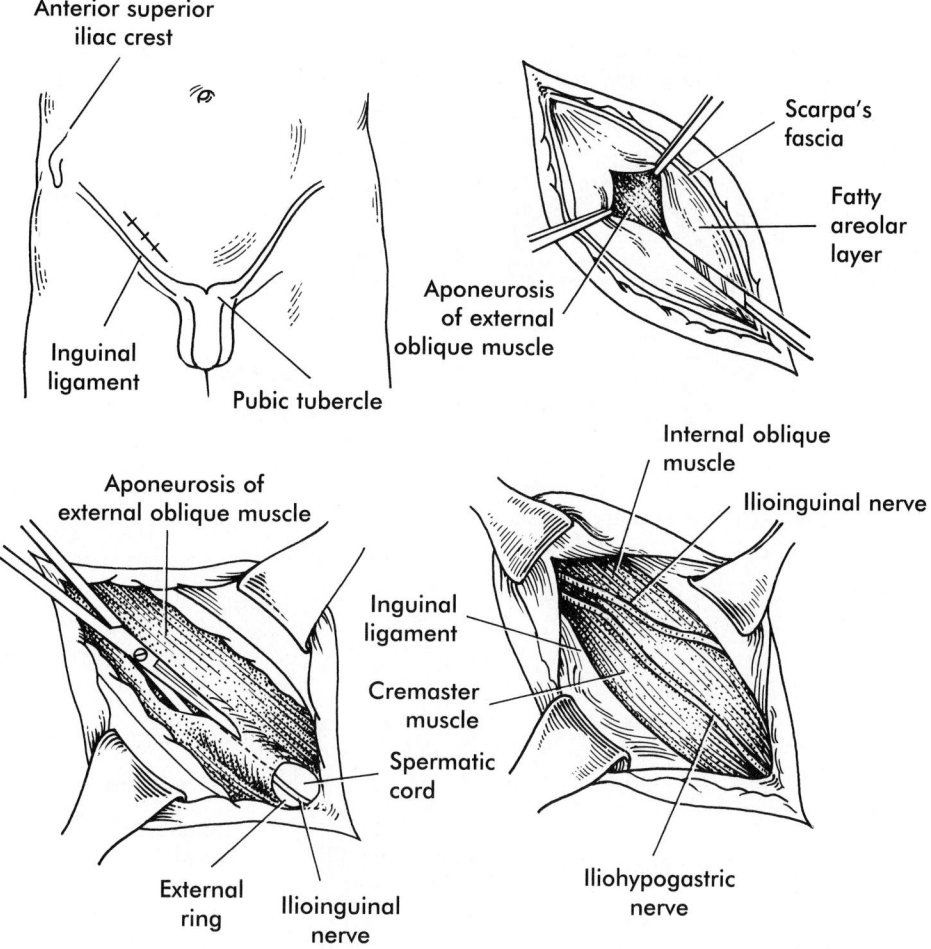

FIG. 12-7 Skin incision with division of superficial muscle and fascial layers.

the pubic crest, approximately 1 cm from the midline, and extends cephalad, following the line of fusion of the external oblique aponeurosis with the rectus sheath. The posterior rectus sheath and the rectus muscle itself guard against later herniation at the point where the relaxing incision is made. In some situations a prosthetic material, such as Marlex mesh, may be used to cover the hernia defect to allow repair and healing without undue stress.

11. After the integrity of the posterior inguinal floor has been reestablished, the cremaster muscles are reapproximated around the cord. Repair is completed with the approximation of the external oblique aponeurosis, Scarpa's fascia, and the skin.

Bassini repair. The Bassini repair approach to the hernia and the treatment of the sac is identical to that previously described. The major difference with this repair is that the superior transversalis fascia is sutured to the inguinal ligament with no attempt made to approximate it to the inferior portion of the transversalis fascia or Cooper's ligament. Critics of this procedure claim that it is not anatomic because layers that originally are not one (transversalis fas-

cia and inguinal ligament) now are approximated. Nonetheless, this repair is extremely popular and is used successfully by many surgeons.

Shouldice repair. Again the approach to the hernia is the same as previously described, but in the Shouldice repair a double layer of transversalis fascia is sutured to the inguinal ligament. It is reinforced by a layer of internal oblique muscle and conjoined tendon approximated to the undersurface of the fascia of the external oblique. At the Shouldice Clinic in Toronto, where this procedure was developed and now is used exclusively, the hernia recurrence rate is about 0.6% (Nyhus and Condon, 1989).

Although the Shouldice repair is controversial, it remains a practiced alternative for those surgeons who have studied the technique.

Laparoscopic hernia repairs. Ger was the first surgeon to perform a laparoscopic herniorrhaphy. In 1982 he described a laparoscopic transabdominal hernia approach for patients who were undergoing laparotomies for other conditions. Variations in techniques for laparoscopic hernia repair continue to develop as surgeons gain experience with these procedures (Filipi et al., 1992).

Three types of laparoscopic hernia approaches are out-

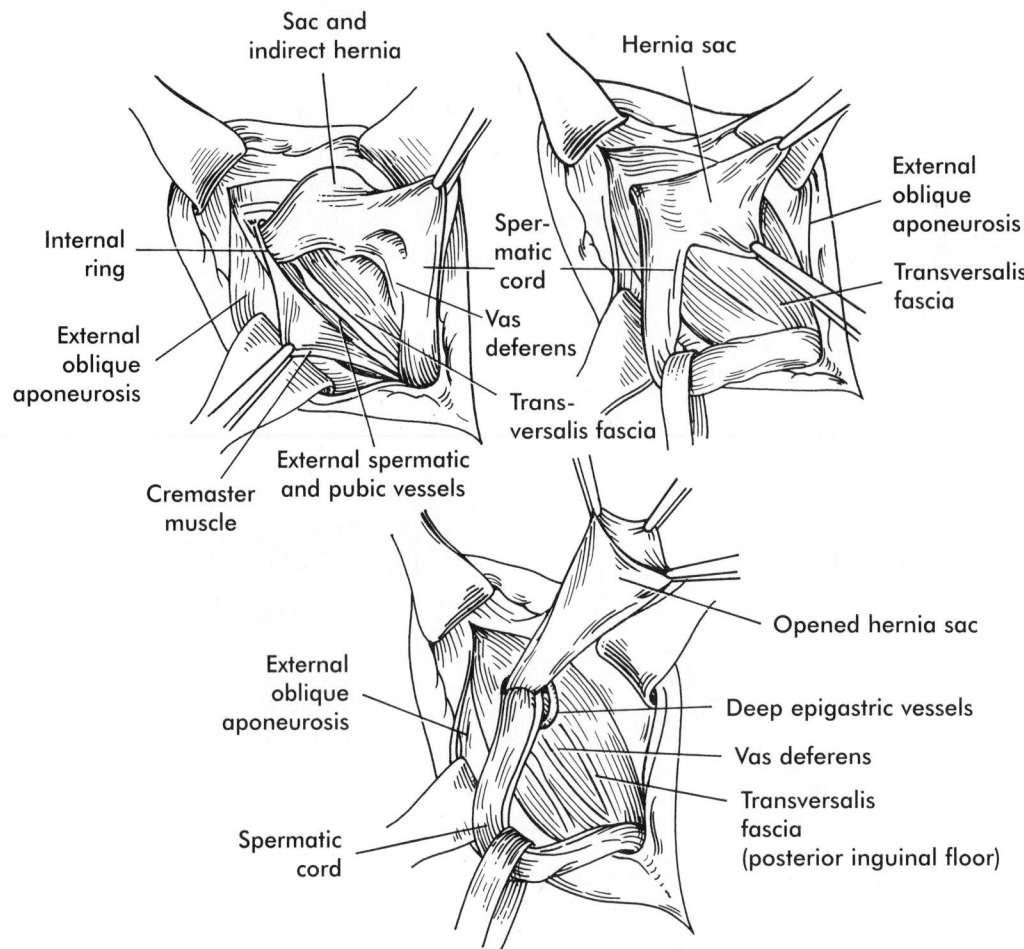

Sac and
indirect hernia

Hernia sac

External
oblique
aponeurosis

Transversalis
fascia

Internal
ring

External
oblique
aponeurosis

Sper-
matic
cord

Vas
deferens

Trans-
versalis fascia

Cremaster
muscle

External spermatic
and pubic vessels

Opened hernia sac

Deep epigastric vessels

Vas deferens

Transversalis
fascia
(posterior inguinal floor)

External
oblique
aponeurosis

Spermatic
cord

FIG. 12-8   Indirect hernia sac is identified along with cord structures and dissected away from cord.
Neck of hernia sac is clearly delineated, and sac is opened to check for abdominal contents.

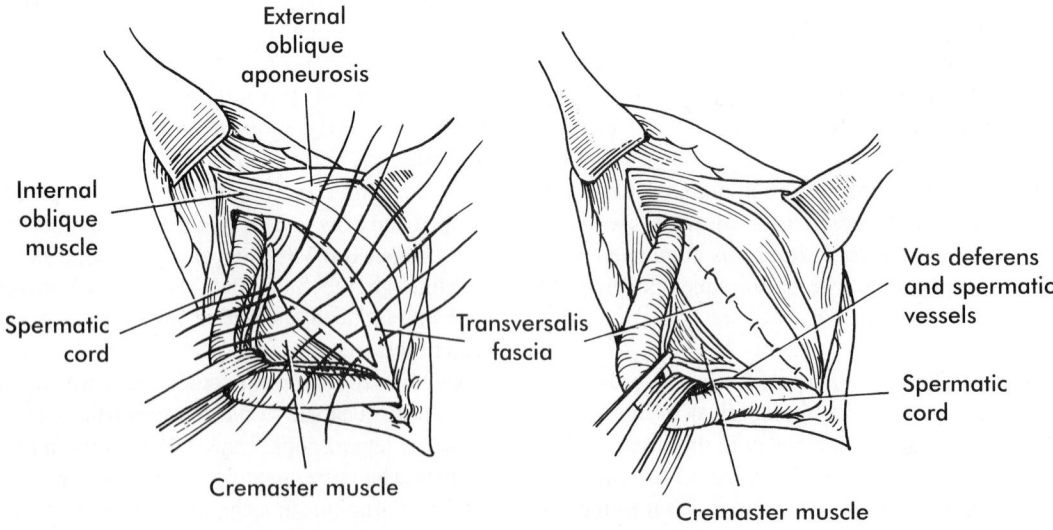

External
oblique
aponeurosis

Internal
oblique
muscle

Spermatic
cord

Transversalis
fascia

Vas deferens
and spermatic
vessels

Spermatic
cord

Cremaster muscle

Cremaster muscle

FIG. 12-9   Transversalis fascia on either side of large hernia defect is approximated.

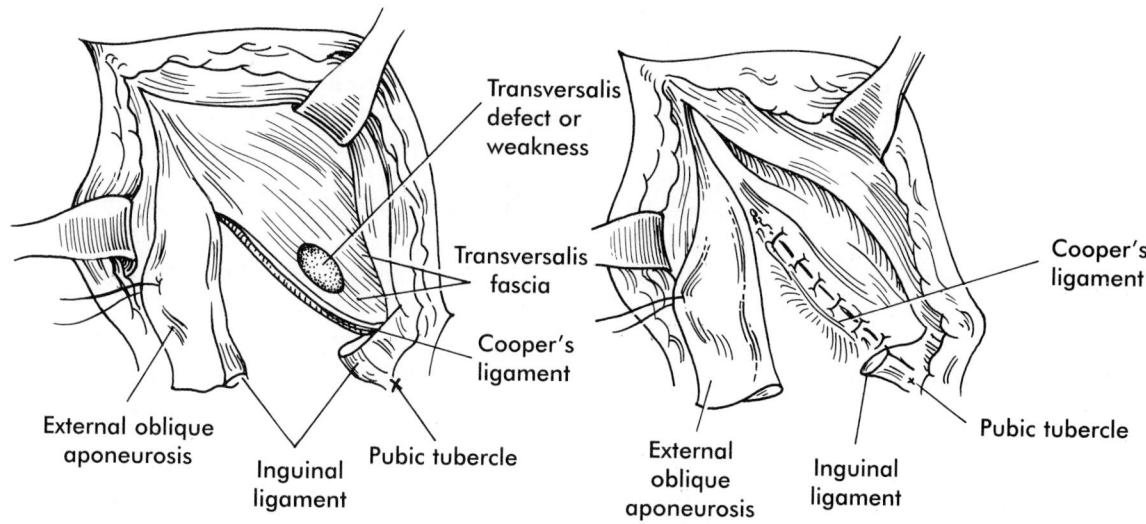

FIG. 12-10 Defect in transversalis fascia repaired by approximation of fascia to Cooper's ligament.

lined by Filipi and co-workers (1992). In a transabdominal preperitoneal repair (TAPP), a laparoscopy is performed and a second incision in the peritoneum provides entry into the preperitoneal space. The second technique is the intraperitoneal onlay mesh repair (IPOM). Synthetic mesh is placed intraperitoneally over the defect. The laparoscopic extraperitoneal herniorrhaphy (LEP) involves an extraperitoneal approach utilizing a laparoscope. These repairs are facilitated by a laparoscopic rotating stapler or with sutures.

Long-term studies indicating postoperative hernia recurrence and complication rates are not yet available. A laparoscopic hernia repair has the advantages of a quicker return to normal activity and some reduction of postoperative adhesions. The disadvantages of a laparoscopic repair include longer operating times, the potential for nerve injury, and the need for a general anesthetic. The open hernia repair will remain the gold standard for technique until the medical community has evaluated long-term studies of laparoscopic hernia repair.

Repair of inguinal hernias in females. Regardless of the specific technique used, the initial approach to the repair of a hernia in the female is the same as that used in the male. After the cremaster muscles are opened to expose the round ligament, variations that may be encountered include the following: (1) with the sac exposed and cleared from the round ligament, the round ligament and accompanying vessels are dissected free from the inguinal floor to the labium; (2) at the labium the round ligament is clamped, ligated, and divided; (3) the sac at the internal ring is opened, checked to be sure that no abdominal contents are present, and ligated at its neck, together with the round ligament and associated vessels; or (4) the sac distal to the ligature is removed with the distal round ligament, while the ligated stump retracts promptly into the abdomen. The remainder of the repair is the same as that previously described.

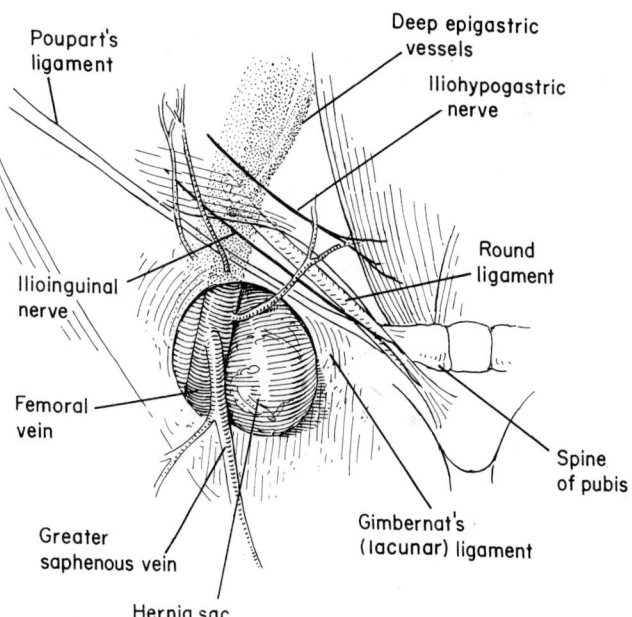

FIG. 12-11 Bulge from femoral hernia occurring below inguinal ligament.

From Zollinger, R.M., & Zollinger, R.M., Jr. (1993). *Atlas of surgical operations* (7th ed.) New York: McGraw-Hill.

Repair of femoral hernias

A femoral hernia protrudes from the groin below the inguinal ligament into the thigh (Fig. 12-11). In its most obvious form, a femoral hernia is an inflamed, tender mass with bowel sounds below the inguinal ligament. Unfortunately, the presentation is frequently more subtle, and the diagnosis is completely missed or confused with enlarged inguinal lymph nodes, a psoas muscle abscess, a saphenous varix, or a lipoma. The defect is usually small and frequently irreducible. Femoral hernias are highly likely to incarcerate and strangulate; elective repair is clearly indicated unless serious contraindications to surgery exist (Davis et al., 1987).

Operative procedure

The general approach is surgical treatment to free the tightly bound hernia, closely examine the contents of the hernia for ischemic change, and repair the hernia defect. The principles for repair of this type of hernia are the same as those described for inguinal herniorrhaphies. Ultimately, repair of the transversalis fascia must be accomplished. Repair of femoral hernia requires approximating the aponeurotic margins of the femoral canal. The sutures are placed through the iliopubic tract superiorly and through the Cooper's ligament and pectineus fascia inferiorly. Care should be taken to not compromise the femoral artery and vein.

Preperitoneal (properitoneal) repair

Preperitoneal (properitoneal) repair also is based on the essential role of the transversalis fascia in the cause and sub-sequent correction of a hernia. This repair is suitable for direct, indirect, and femoral hernias. It is particularly applicable in dealing with recurrent hernias because exposure is obtained by operating through virgin surgical fields rather than through previous scars.

Operative procedure

1. A transverse incision is made 2 cm above the symphysis pubis, through the rectus abdominis muscle on the affected side (Fig. 12-12, A).
2. The wound is deepened by cutting the external oblique, internal oblique, and transversalis muscles.
3. The transversalis fascia is then cut, and the preperitoneal space is entered. This is the proper plane of dissection for the remainder of the operation.
4. Retraction on the lower side of the incision reveals the posterior inguinal wall and the hernia defect.

Variations in the procedure are performed for different types of hernias.

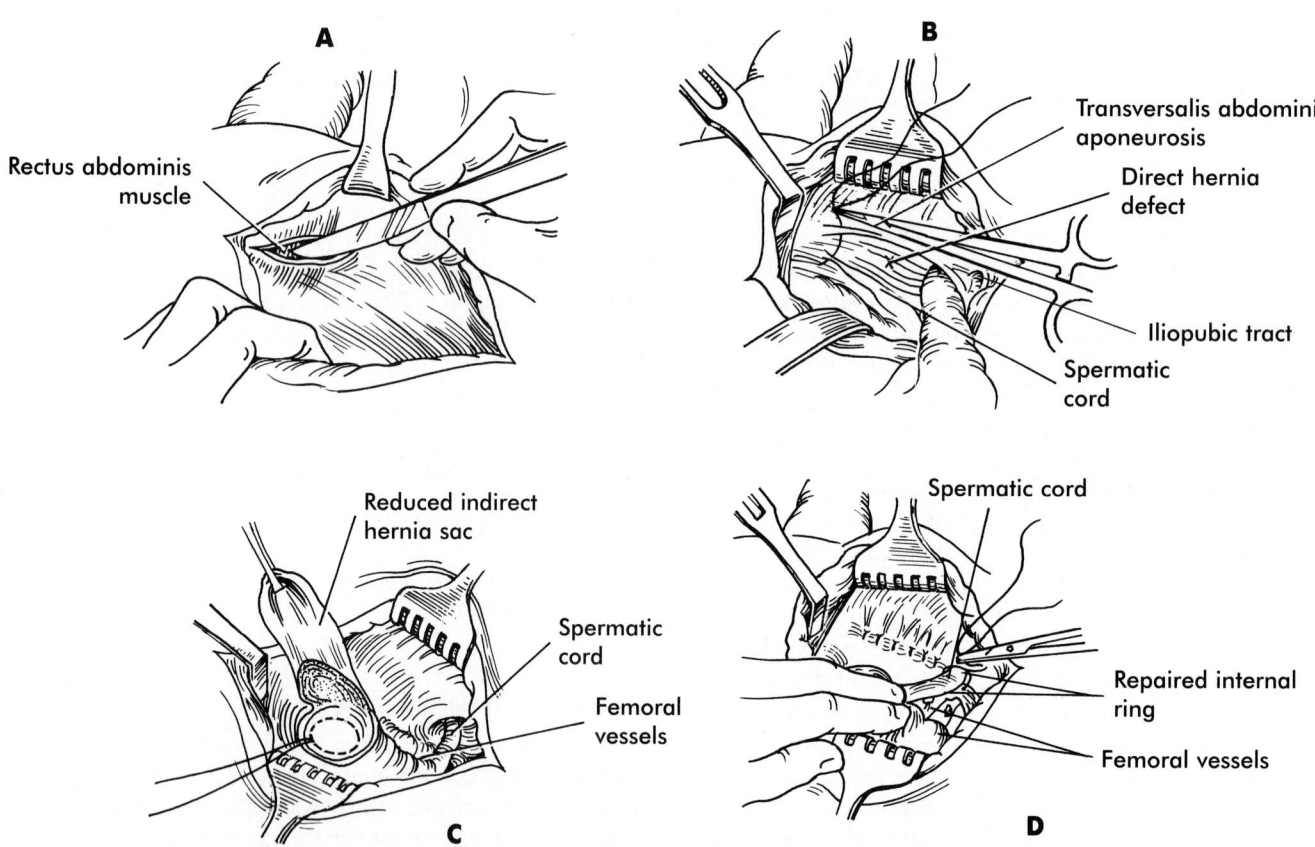

FIG. 12-12 Preperitoneal repair. **A,** Skin incision starts 2 cm above symphysis pubis and is extended through external oblique, internal oblique, and transversalis muscles. **B,** With finger in direct hernia defect, surgeon sutures transversalis abdominis aponeurosis to iliopubic tract. **C,** In case of indirect defect, sac is reduced and then excised, with high ligation being achieved by use of a purse-string suture. **D,** Internal ring is tightened after transversus abdominis aponeurosis has been approximated to iliopubic tract.

1. If the hernia is direct, it can be reduced easily, and the superior edge of the hernia defect (the transversalis fascia) is sutured to the iliopubic tract (origin of the transversalis fascia) (Fig. 12-12, *B*).
2. In an indirect hernia, the sac is gently retracted from the inguinal canal. A pursestring suture is placed around the peritoneal defect as the sac is excised (Fig. 12-12, *C*). The lateral aspect of the internal abdominal ring is closed, and the posterior wall is reinforced as with the direct hernia.
3. In repair of a femoral hernia, the sac is again reduced by traction. After the sac is inspected for contents, a high ligation is performed. As it approaches Cooper's ligament, the defect in the posterior inguinal floor, the transversalis fascia is clearly identified and is repaired by direct approximation (Fig. 12-12, *D*). After repair of any of the aforementioned hernias the preperitoneal space is irrigated with saline solution, and the appropriate layers are approximated.

Repair of sliding hernias

Direct or indirect hernias may occur as sliding hernias. A sliding inguinal hernia occurs when the wall of a viscus forms a portion of the wall of the hernia. The most common sliding hernias involve the bladder in direct hernias,

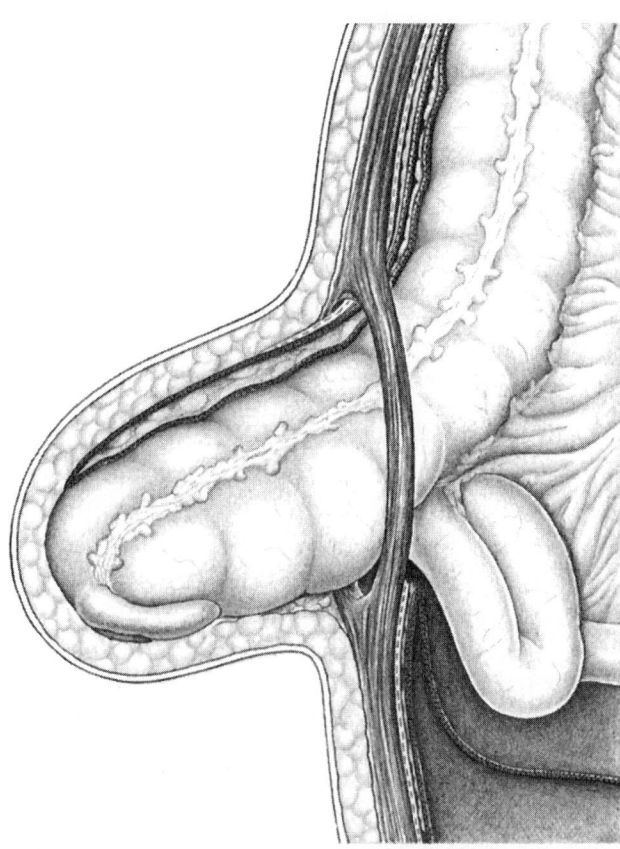

FIG. 12-13   Sliding hernia.
From Schumpelick, V. (1990). *Atlas of hernia surgery*. Toronto: B.C. Decker.

the sigmoid colon in left indirect hernias, and the cecum in right indirect inguinal hernias (Fig. 12-13). This hernia must be recognized early in the repair because attempts at surgical removal of the entire sac will injure the sliding viscus.

Operative procedure

All operations designed to repair sliding hernias adhere to the basic principle of repairing the defect in the transversalis fascia. To free the bowel from the sac, the following steps must be taken:

1. The sac is opened in an area where no bowel is present and is excised medially and laterally to a point at which the bowel can be mobilized (Fig. 12-14).
2. The lateral and medial peritoneal margins are approximated.
3. The bowel is reduced to the peritoneal cavity, and high ligation of the sac is performed.
4. Repair of the transversalis fascia is done by one of the methods previously described.

Littre's hernia, Maydl's hernia, and Richter's hernia

An inguinal hernia containing a Meckel's diverticulum is called Littre's hernia, and one containing two loops of bowel is called Maydl's hernia. A special type of strangulated hernia is Richter's hernia (Fig. 12-15). In this case only a part of the circumference of the bowel is incarcerated or strangulated in the hernia. Frequently it is described as a knuckle of bowel that becomes trapped and ischemic. Because initially a very small area is necrotic, diagnosis may be delayed and the probability of mortality becomes significant. Richter's hernia most frequently occurs in femoral hernias because of the small size and sharp, relatively inflexible nature of the fascial ring in this area. A strangulated Richter's hernia may be reduced spontaneously, and the gangrenous piece of intestine may be overlooked at the time of operation. Most commonly, the distal ileum is involved in Richter's hernia; however, omentum is frequently encountered in the sac. The favored approach for repair is through the preperitoneal space.

SURGERY FOR REPAIR OF HERNIAS OF THE ANTERIOR ABDOMINAL WALL
Ventral or incisional hernias

Ventral hernias can appear either spontaneously or after previous operations. Spontaneously occurring ventral hernias include epigastric and umbilical hernias. Postoperative ventral hernias, called incisional hernias, appear more frequently when the original incision was T shaped or a vertical midline. Operations that involve a potential for contamination, such as for acute perforated ulcer or other perforated abdominal viscera, are more prone to developing subsequent ventral hernias. A poor nutritional state with re-

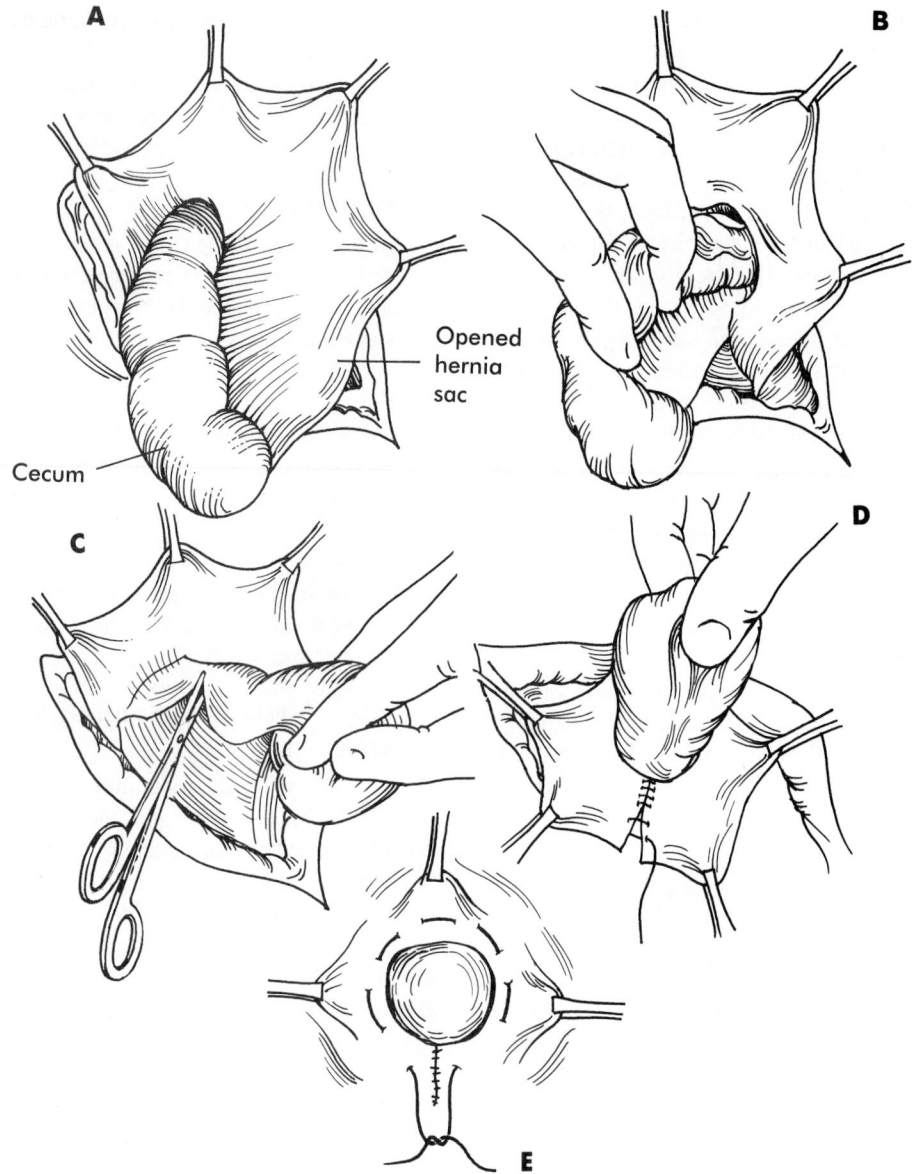

FIG. 12-14   Right sliding hernia. **A,** Cecum forms posterior wall of hernia sac. **B,** Peritoneum is excised medially **(C),** and laterally **(D),** allowing mobilization of cecum for subsequent reduction to peritoneal cavity. Lateral and medial margins are approximated. **E,** After reduction, high ligation is accomplished by using purse-string suture.

sulting hypoproteinemia predisposes some individuals to ventral hernia formation. Finally, faulty surgical technique, such as the choice of inappropriate suture materials, may result in the ultimate appearance of a ventral hernia.

Several methods have been developed for repairing ventral hernias. If all layers of the abdominal wall are easily identified, anatomic layer-by-layer repair may be done. Frequently a type of overlap method for repair is employed. Vertical and transverse overlap procedures are referred to as vest-over-pants repairs. For large defects, in which approximation of tissue would result in closure with exces-

sive tension or would cause either circulatory or respiratory compromise, synthetic materials such as Marlex mesh or Gore-tex patch are employed.

When a very large fascial defect is present, a recent technique that extrapolates on the principles of tissue expansion may be used. A Tenckhoff catheter is placed percutaneously into the peritoneal cavity. Gradual expansion of the abdominal fascia is accomplished by insufflation of the abdomen with 1 to 2 L nitrous oxide gas, similar to the procedure for laparoscopy. The patient's vital signs are monitored during and after the insufflation procedure, which may

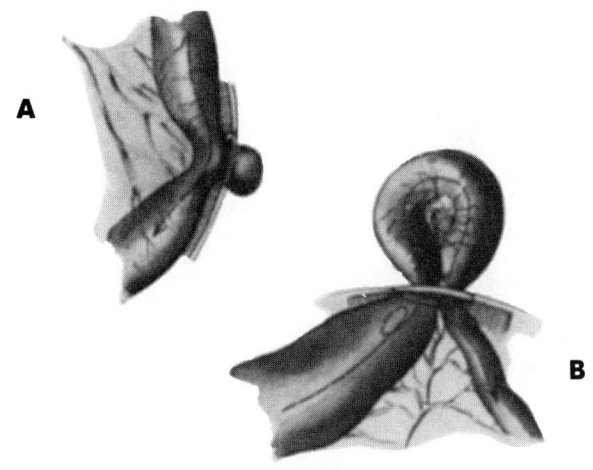

FIG. 12-15 **A,** Richter's hernia. Only a portion of bowel passes through hernial ring; *arrow* indicates that bowel need not be obstructed mechanically even with strangulation. **B,** Incarcerated hernia. Distended bowel in hernia cannot return to abdomen through narrow fascial defect.

From Liechty, R.D., & Soper, R.T. (1985). *Synopsis of surgery* (5th ed.). St. Louis: Mosby.

be performed on a nursing unit or possibly in an outpatient clinical setting. The graduated expansion of the tissues sometimes allows for primary closure of the defect without the use of synthetic mesh or Gore-tex patch.

Umbilical hernias

Umbilical hernias are extraperitoneal and occur as small fascial defects under the umbilicus. They are common in children and frequently disappear spontaneously by age 2. If the defect is persistent, a simple approximation of the overlying fascia is all that is necessary for repair. In adults, umbilical hernias represent a defect in the linea alba just above the umbilicus. These hernias tend to occur more frequently in obese people, making diagnosis more difficult. Umbilical hernias are potentially dangerous because they have small necks and frequently incarcerate. Surgical repair is indicated for all adults with asymptomatic umbilical hernias.

Epigastric hernias

Epigastric hernias are protrusions of fat through defects in the abdominal wall between the xiphoid process and the umbilicus. Patients with epigastric hernias can have nausea, vague abdominal pain, or epigastric pain similar to that observed with cholecystitis or duodenal ulcers. Surgical repair of epigastric hernias is simple and very successful.

Spigelian hernias

The linea semilunaris, often referred to as Spigelius's line, marks the transition from muscle to aponeurosis in the transversus abdominis muscle. The area of aponeurosis that lies between the linea semilunaris and the lateral edge of

the rectus muscle is referred to as the spigelian zone. Protrusion of a peritoneal sac, preperitoneal fat, or other abdominal viscera through a congenital or acquired defect in this area is called a spigelian hernia. It is usually located between the different muscle layers of the abdominal wall. For this reason the spigelian hernia may be referred to as an interparietal, interstitial, or intramuscular hernia.

Spigelian hernias are uncommon and are generally difficult to diagnose. Ultrasonic scanning has improved the diagnosis of such intramural hernias. When ultrasonic scanning is not conclusive, CT can better visualize the hernia orifice.

Interparietal hernias

An interparietal hernia lies between the layers of the abdominal wall. These hernias may be classified by dividing them into those which present with ventral swelling and those without ventral swelling (Nyhus and Condon, 1989). Diagnosis is often made during an exploratory laparotomy for symptoms of intestinal obstruction.

Repair follows the same procedure as that done for a strangulated hernia. The sac contents are closely examined for ischemia, the sac is resected, and the defect is repaired.

Synthetic mesh and patch repairs

Synthetic meshes, such as Mersilene, Marlex, Prolene, and Dacron, have been particularly helpful in repairing recurrent or large ventral hernias. Closure of the defect is obtained with minimal or no tension on the suture line. These synthetic materials are strong and durable, promoting fibrovascular growth within their pores, which lends extra strength to the repair. A major criticism of synthetic meshes is that, as with any foreign body implant, the risk of infection is increased.

Another synthetic material, Gore-tex patch, has become popular for the reconstruction of abdominal wall defects and repair of soft tissue. Gore-tex soft-tissue patch comes in both 1-cm and 2-cm thicknesses. It has been associated with reduced incidence of infection. Gore-tex is very expensive, and the same results can often be achieved with a less expensive mesh.

Essential to the use of mesh or patch in a hernia repair are the identification and cleaning of tissue planes to which the mesh or patch will be attached (Fig. 12-16, *A*). In a ventral hernia the peritoneum is dissected from the undersurface of the rectus abdominis muscle, and the mesh or patch is placed between the peritoneum and the rectus (Fig. 12-16, *B*). After the mesh or patch is positioned, it is sutured in place on one side, using the synthetic suture material compatible with the type of mesh or patch employed (Fig. 12-16, *C*). After the mesh is in place, the surgeon often sprinkles an antibiotic powder over the mesh.

At this point the peritoneum can be closed, if possible. If the peritoneum cannot be closed, mesh or patch can be placed directly over the omentum. The mesh or patch is then placed and sutured to the other side of the defect, with

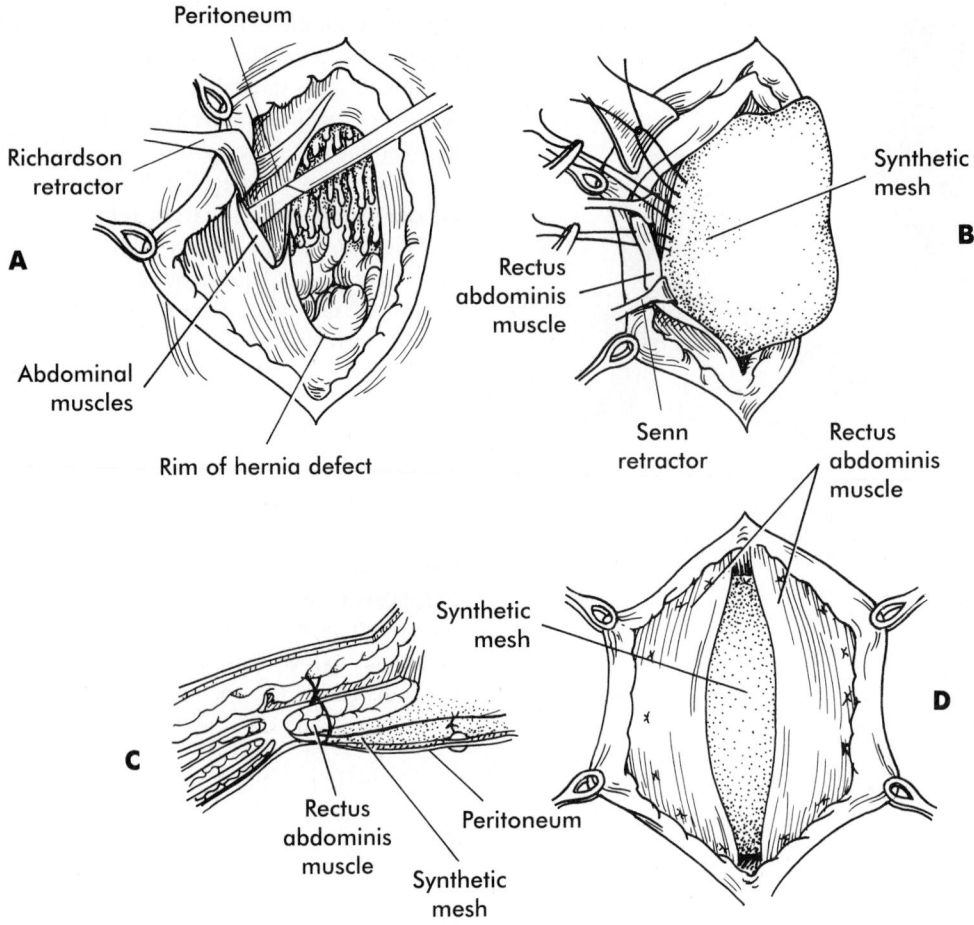

FIG. 12-16   Use of mesh in hernia repair. After layers of abdominal wall surrounding ventral hernia are identified (**A**), mesh is inserted between rectus and peritoneum (**B**). **C**, Mesh is sutured into place on one side. **D**, With moderate tension, mesh is inserted between appropriate layers on opposite side and is sutured into place.

moderate tension maintained (Fig. 12-16, *D*). If possible, the mesh or patch is then covered with a fascial or muscular layer before the subcutaneous fat and skin are closed. Closed-wound drainage catheters are usually placed in the wound, and antibiotics are frequently used prophylactically. Using mesh or patch to repair inguinal hernias is based on the same principles used for closing ventral hernias. With inguinal hernias the mesh or patch is sutured to transversalis fascia on both sides of the defect.

REFERENCES

Davis, J.H., Foster, R.S., & Gamelli R.C., Jr. (1991). *Essentials of clinical surgery,* St. Louis: Mosby.

Fogel, S. (1992). Groin hernia. In Cameron, J.S. (editor). *Current surgical therapy* (4th ed.). St. Louis: Mosby.

Filipi, C.J., Fitzgibbons, R.J., Salerno, G.M., & Hart, R.O. (1992, October). Laparoscopic hernia. *Surgical Clinics of North America, 72*(5), 1109-1125.

Lichtenstein, I.L., Shulman, A.G., Amid, P.K., & Willis, P.A. (1990, September). Hernia repair with polypropylene mesh. *AORN Journal, 52*(3), 559-565.

Long, J.D., & Sandler, J. (1990, October). Outpatient hernia repair: The Shouldice technique. *AORN Journal, 52*(4), 801-816.

Nyhus, L.M., & Condon, R.E. (1989) *Hernia*. Philadelphia: J.B. Lippincott.

Nyhus, L.M., Klein, M.S., Robers, F.B., & Kowalczyk, S. (1990, August). Inguinal hernia repairs. *AORN Journal, 52*(2), 292-304.

Petros, J.G., Rimm, E.B., Robillard, R.J. & Argy, O. (1991, April). Factors influencing postoperative urinary retention in patients undergoing elective inguinal herniorrhaphy. *The American Journal of Surgery, 161,* 431.

Sabiston, D.C. (1991). *Textbook of surgery: The biological basis of modern surgical practice* (14th ed.). Philadelphia: W.B. Saunders.

Schumpelick, V. (1990). *Atlas of hernia surgery.* Toronto: B.C. Decker.

BIBLIOGRAPHY

Zollinger, R.M., & Zollinger, R.M. Jr. (1993). *Atlas of surgical operations* (7th ed.). New York: McGraw-Hill.

13

GYNECOLOGIC SURGERY AND CESAREAN BIRTH

GWEN LYNN NELSON

Historical advancements in gynecology have been based on increasing the quality of health care provided for women. Descriptions of gynecologic examinations have been traced back to the time of Hippocrates. For years the midwife performed the roles of gynecologist and obstetrician in society. As knowledge increased regarding female anatomy and its abnormalities, surgeons began to develop techniques in abdominal and pelvic surgery. In 1794 Jesse Bennett is recorded as having performed one of the earliest pelvic surgeries. Effective surgical corrections of gynecologic disorders continued into the nineteenth century. Through the years, the efficiency of laparoscopy, along with improvements in diagnostic techniques and surgical interventions have evolved to promote the health care of women.

Today's gynecologic surgery has built on this foundation. Some of the gynecologic specialties that have evolved are oncology, endocrinology, and infertility. The numerous developments and techniques within each of these specialty areas represent challenges for today's perioperative nurse.

Operations on the structures of the female reproductive system are performed for diagnostic or therapeutic purposes, for conditions such as abnormal bleeding from the reproductive organs, for suspected malignant or benign neoplasms, and for infertility. Procedures are also done to remove or repair weakened anatomic structures.

SURGICAL ANATOMY

The female reproductive organs and their relationships are shown in Fig. 13-1. The adult female structures associated with the process of reproduction are the bony pelvis, the associated ligaments and muscles, the soft tissues and contents of the pelvic cavity, the external organs (vulva) (Fig. 13-2), and the breasts (mammary glands).

BONY PELVIS

The Latin word *pelvis* means basin. The pelvis is that portion of the trunk below and behind the abdomen. The bony pelvis is composed of the ilium, symphysis pubis, ischium, sacrum, and coccyx. The so-called pelvic brim divides the abdominal false portion, located above the arcuate line, from the true portion of the pelvis, located below this line. It forms the passageway through which the fetus passes during parturition.

The true pelvis may be considered as having three parts: inlet, cavity, and outlet. The muscles lining the pelvis facilitate movement of the thighs, give form to the pelvic cavity, and provide firm elastic lining to the bony pelvic framework. All organs located in the pelvis are covered by pelvic fascia (Fig. 13-3), which is extremely important in the maintenance of normal strength in the pelvic floor.

The fascia covering the muscles is usually dense and firm, whereas that covering organs is often thin and elastic. The nerves, blood vessels, and ureters coursing through the anatomic structures are closely associated with muscular and fascial structures.

The pelvic fascia may be divided into three general groups: parietal, diaphragmatic, and visceral. The parietal pelvic fascia covers the muscles of the true pelvic wall and perineum. The diaphragmatic fascia covers both sides of the pelvic diaphragm, which is made up of the levator ani and coccygeal muscles (Fig. 13-4). The visceral fascia is thin and flexible and covers the pelvic organs. The floor of the pelvis, known as the pelvic diaphragm, gives support to the abdominal pelvic viscera in this region. It consists of the levator ani and coccygeal muscles with their respective fascial coverings and separates the pelvic cavity from the perineum (Fig. 13-4).

The levator ani muscles, varying in thickness and strength, may be divided into three parts: the iliococcygeal,

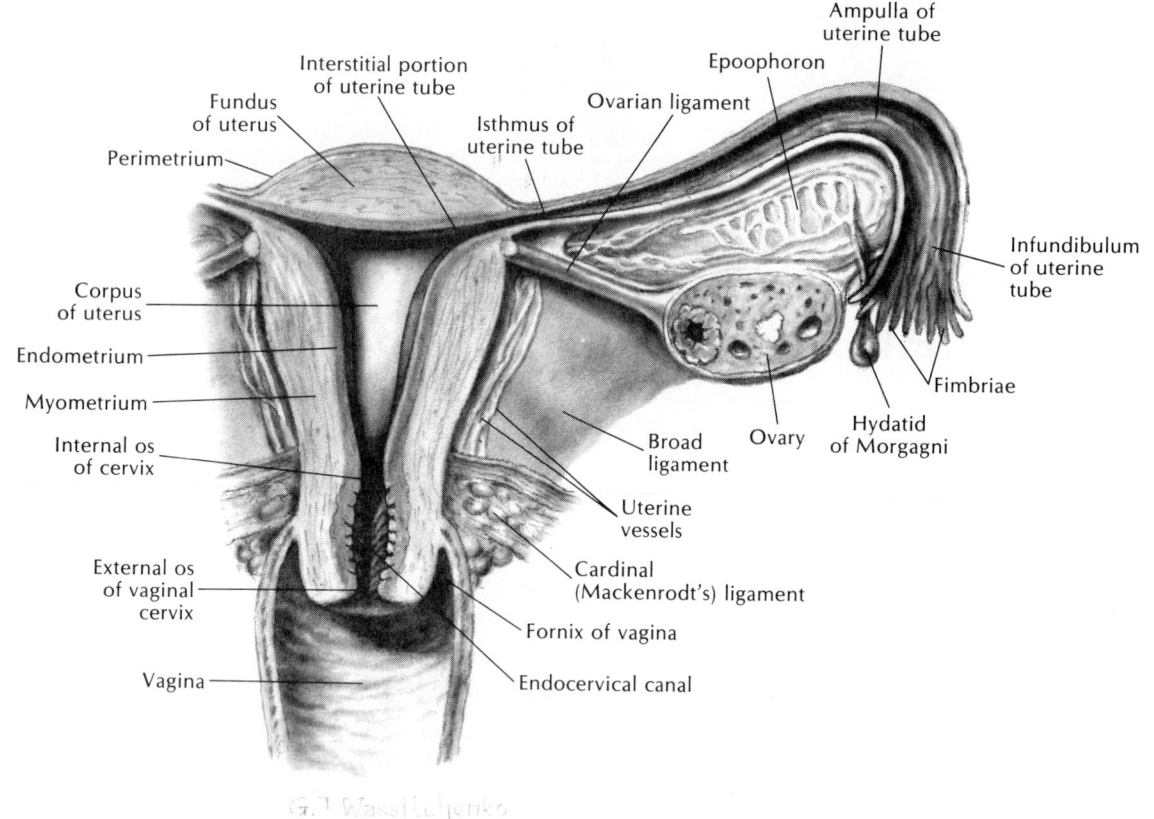

FIG. 13-1   Female reproductive organs.

From Bobak, I.M., & Jensen, M.D. (1993). *Maternity and gynecologic care* (5th Ed.). St. Louis: Mosby.

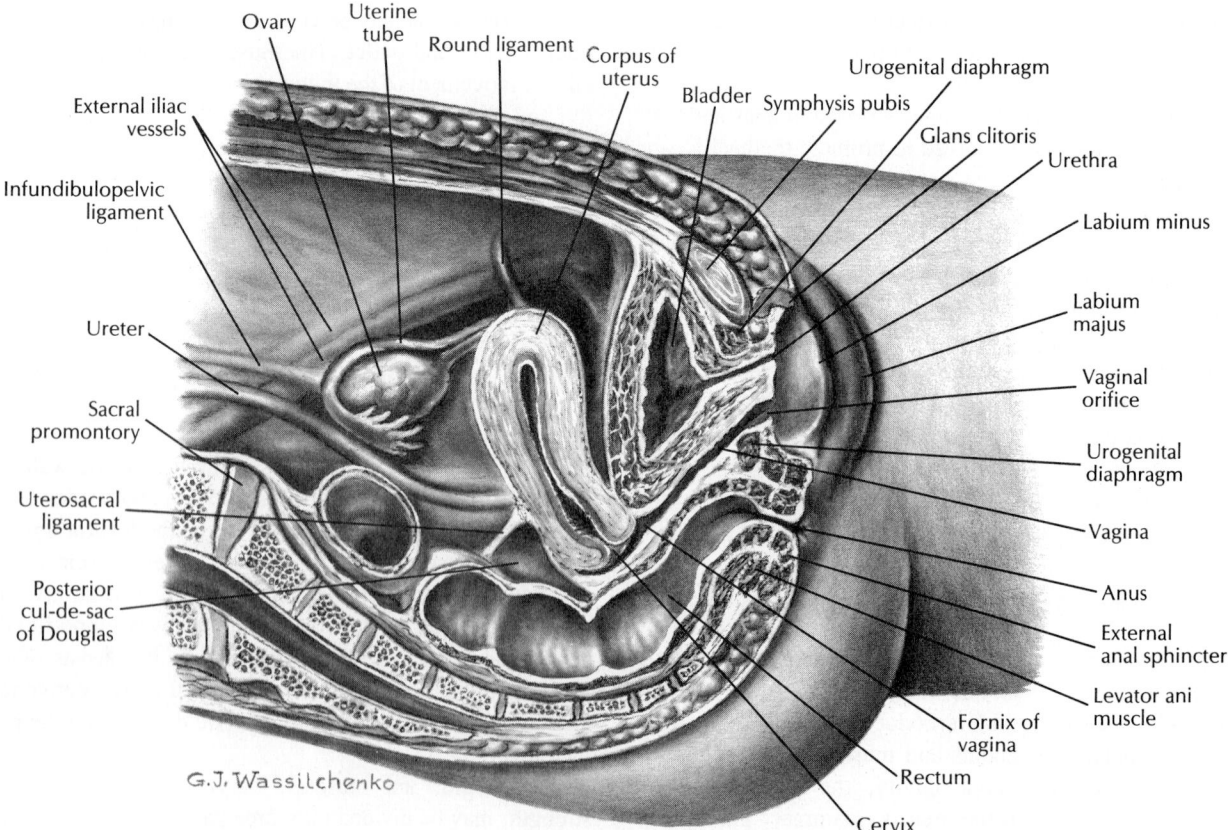

FIG. 13-2   Female pelvic organs as viewed in midsagittal section.

From Bobak, I.M., & Jensen, M.D. (1993). *Maternity and gynecologic care* (5th Ed.). St. Louis: Mosby.

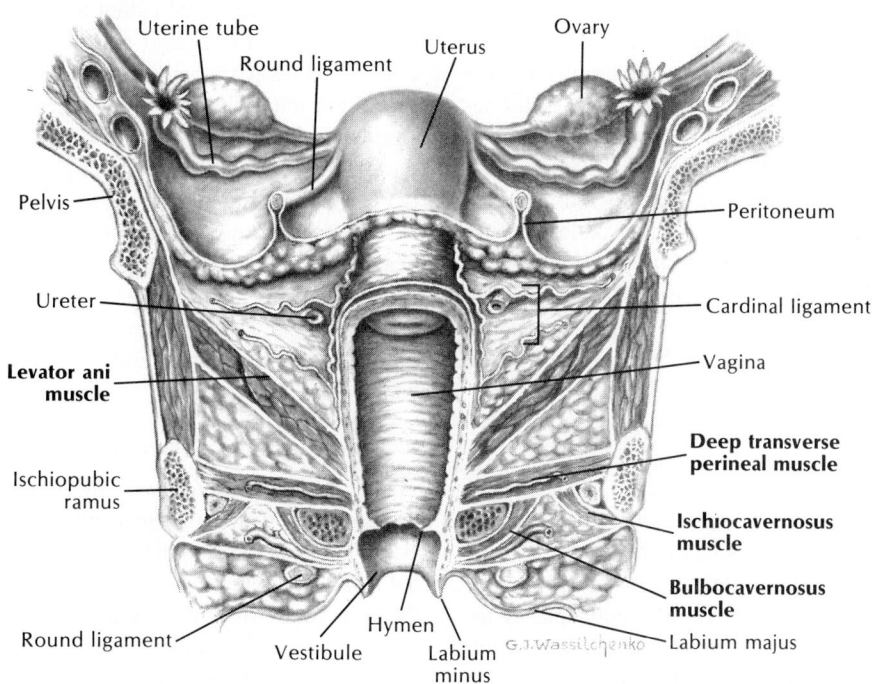

FIG. 13-3 Relationship of female sexual organs to anterior abdominal wall.

From Bobak, I.M., & Jensen, M.D. (1993). *Maternity and gynecologic care* (5th Ed.). St. Louis: Mosby.

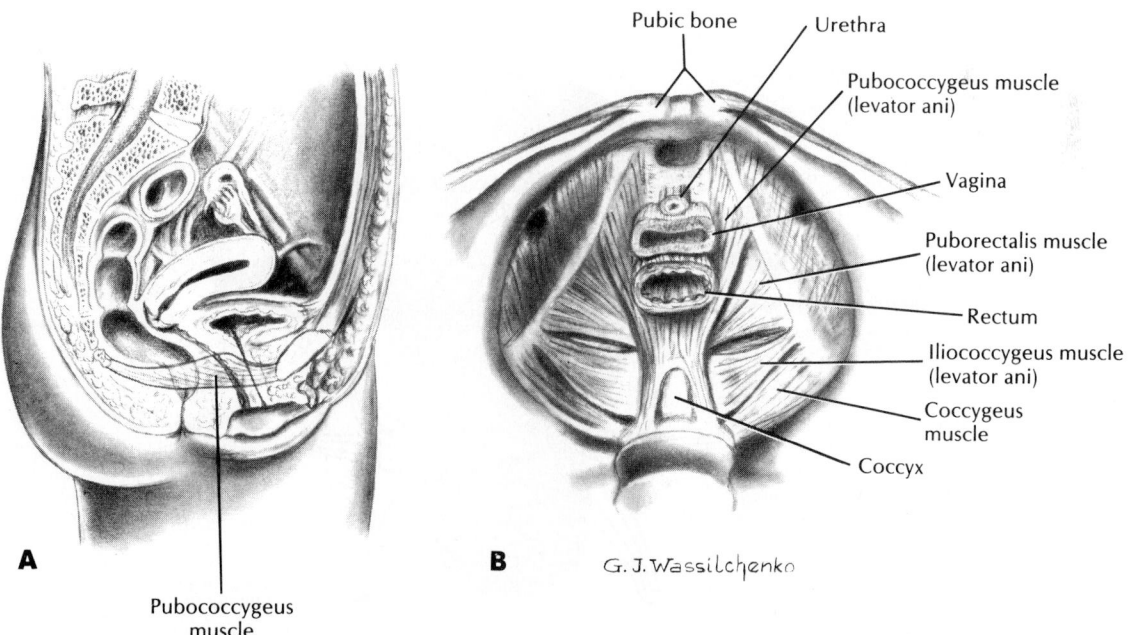

FIG. 13-4 Perineal musculature.

From Bobak, I.M., & Jensen, M.D. (1993). *Maternity and gynecologic care* (5th Ed.). St. Louis: Mosby.

the pubococcygeal, and the puborectal muscles (Fig. 13-4). The fibers of the levator ani muscles blend with the muscle fibers of the rectum and vagina. The pubovaginal fibers of the pubococcygeal portion of the levator ani muscles, lying directly below the urinary bladder, are involved in the control of micturition. The pubococcygeal fibers of the levator ani muscles control and pull the coccyx forward and assist in the closure of the pelvic outlet. The fibers pull the rectum, vagina, and bladder neck upward toward the symphysis pubis in an effort to close the pelvic outlet and are responsible for the flexure at the anorectal junction. Relaxation of the fibers during defecation permits a straightening at this junction. During parturition the action of the levator ani muscles directs the fetal head into the lower part of the passageway.

PELVIC CAVITY
Uterus

The uterus (from the Greek word *hystera*) is a pear-shaped organ situated in the pelvic cavity between the bladder anteriorly and the rectum posteriorly. It gains much of its support by its direct attachment to the vagina and by indirect attachments to nearby structures such as the rectum and pelvic diaphragm. The uterus is supported on each side by the broad, round, cardinal, and uterosacral ligaments and levator ani muscles (Figs. 13-4 and 13-5). The upper lateral points, the uterine cornua, receive the fallopian tubes (see Fig. 13-1). The fundus of the uterus is the upper rounded portion situated above the level of the tubal open-

ings and just below the pelvic brim. Below, the body of the uterus joins the cervix, from which it is separated by a slight constriction canal called the isthmus. The cervix lies at the level of the ischial spines. The body of the uterus communicates with the cervical canal at the internal orifice, called the internal os. The constriction (canal) ends at the vaginal portion of the cervix at the external orifice, called the external os. This is a small oval aperture situated between two lips.

The uterine body has three layers: (1) the outer peritoneal, or serous, layer, which is a reflection of the pelvic peritoneum; (2) the myometrium, or muscular layer, which houses involuntary muscles, nerves, blood vessels, and lymphatics; and (3) the endometrium, or mucosal layer, which lines the cavity of the uterus.

Fallopian tubes or oviducts

The Greek word *salpinx,* meaning trumpet or tube, is used to refer to the fallopian tubes (see Fig. 13-1). Bilateral tubes, each consisting of a musculomembranous channel about 4 to 5 inches long, form the canals through which the ova from either ovary are conveyed to the uterus. The outer surfaces of the tubes are covered by peritoneum. Each tube receives its blood supply from the branches of the uterine and ovarian arteries. Each fallopian tube leaves the upper portion of the uterus, passes outward toward the sides of the pelvis, and ends in fringelike projections called fimbriae. These fimbriae are situated just below the ovaries.

How the ova are transported from the ruptured follicles

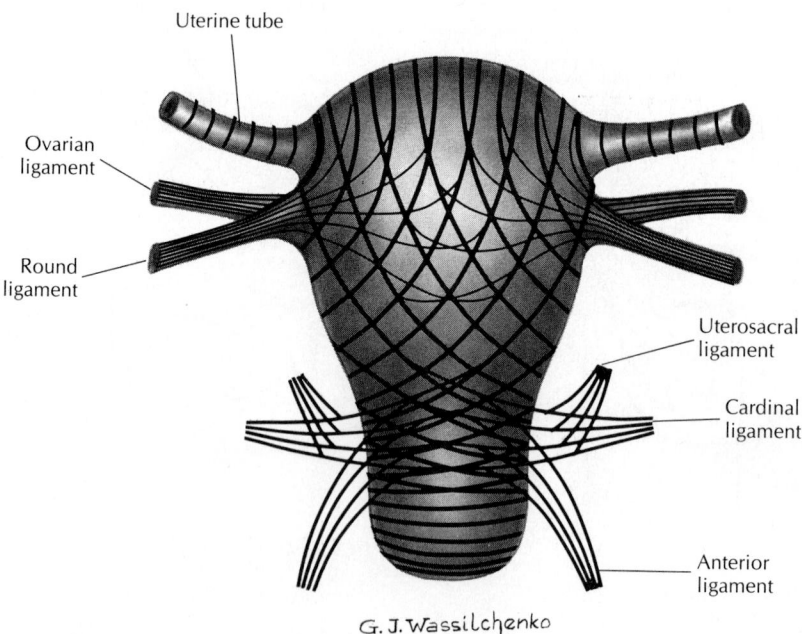

G. J. Wassilchenko

FIG. 13-5 Scheme to show relative positions of eight uterine ligaments formed by folds of peritoneum: two broad ligaments, double folds extending from uterus to side walls of pelvic cavity; two uterosacral ligaments, foldlike extensions of peritoneum from uterus to sacrum; posterior ligament, fold between uterus and rectum; and two round ligaments, folds from uterus to deep inguinal ring.

From Bobak, I.M., & Jensen, M.D. (1993). *Maternity and gynecologic care* (5th Ed.). St. Louis: Mosby.

into the uterus is unknown. One theory is that transfer is accomplished through vascular changes, which occur with contraction of the smooth muscle fibers of the tube, and the peristaltic movements of the tube push the ova toward the uterus.

The right tube and ovary are in close relationship to the cecum and appendix; the left tube and ovary are situated near the sigmoid flexure. The close proximity of the fallopian tubes to the ureters should be noted.

Ovaries

The ovaries are situated on each side of the uterus. Each ovary lies within a depression (ovarian fossa) on the lateral wall of the pelvic cavity and above the broad ligament (see Fig. 13-1). The anterior border of each ovary is attached to the posterior layer of the broad ligament by a peritoneal fold (mesovarium) and is suspended by the ovarian ligament.

The ovaries, small, almond-shaped organs, are composed of an outer layer, known as the cortex, and an inner vascular layer, known as the medulla. The medulla consists of connective tissue containing nerves, blood, and lymph vessels. The ovary is covered by epithelium, not peritoneum. The cortex contains ovarian (graafian) follicles in different stages of maturity. After ovulation the corpus luteum arises from the graafian follicle that expelled the ovum.

The ovaries are homologous with the testes of the male. They produce ova after puberty and also function as endocrine glands, producing hormones, such as estrogen, secreted by the ovarian follicles. Estrogen controls the development of the secondary sexual characteristics and initiates growth of the lining of the uterus during the menstrual cycle. Progesterone, which is secreted by the corpus luteum, is essential for the implantation of the fertilized ovum and for the development of the embryo.

Ligaments of the uterus

The uterine ligaments are the broad, round, cardinal, and uterosacral ligaments (see Figs. 13-3 and 13-5).

From each side of the uterus the pelvic peritoneum extends lateral, downward, and posterior. A double fold of pelvic peritoneum forms the layers of the broad ligament, enclosing the uterus (see Fig. 13-3). These layers separate to cover the floor and sides of the pelvis. The fallopian tube is situated within the free border of the broad ligament. The free margin of the upper division of the broad ligament, lying immediately below the fallopian tube, is termed the mesosalpinx. The ovary lies behind the broad ligament.

Round ligaments are fibromuscular bands attached to the uterus (see Figs. 13-2 and 13-3). Each round ligament passes forward and lateral between the layers of the broad ligament to enter the deep inguinal ring.

Cardinal ligaments are composed of connective tissue with smooth muscle fibers and provide strong support for the uterus.

Uterosacral ligaments are a posterior continuation of the peritoneal tissue. The ligaments pass posterior to the sacrum on either side of the rectum (see Fig. 13-5).

Vagina

The vagina is like a collapsed tube and is lined with mucous membrane. It functions as the organ for copulation, the excretory duct for products of menstruation, and the birth canal. The anterior wall measures 6 to 8 cm in length and the posterior wall 7 to 10 cm (see Figs. 13-1 and 13-2). The anterior wall of the vagina is in close proximity to the bladder and urethra. The lower posterior wall is anteriorly adjacent to the rectum. The upper portion of the vagina lies above the pelvic floor and is surrounded by visceral pelvic fascia. The lower half is surrounded by the levator ani muscles.

The cervix consists of a supravaginal portion, which is closely associated with the bladder and the ureters, and a vaginal portion, which projects downward and backward into the vaginal vault. The projection of the cervix into the vaginal vault divides the vault into four regions, called fornices: anterior and posterior and right and left lateral.

The posterior fornix is in close contact with the peritoneum of the pouch of Douglas or cul-de-sac. The rectovaginal septum lies between the vagina and rectum. The dense connective tissue separating the anterior wall of the vagina from the distal urethra is termed the urethrovaginal septum.

FEMALE EXTERNAL GENITAL ORGANS (VULVA)

The external organs, referred to collectively as the vulva, include the mons pubis, the labia majora and minora, the clitoris, the vestibule, the urethral orifice, the hymen, and various glandular structures (Fig. 13-6).

The mons pubis is a rounded elevation of tissue covered by skin and, after puberty, by hair. It is situated over the anterior surface of the symphysis pubis.

The labia majora are two folds of skin that extend downward and backward from the mons pubis. They unite below and behind to form the posterior commissure and in front to form the anterior commissure. The labia minora comprise the two delicate folds of skin that lie within the labia majora (see Fig. 13-6). Each labium splits into lateral and medial parts. The lateral part forms the prepuce of clitoris, and the medial part forms the frenulum. The posterior folds of the labia are united by a delicate fold extending between them. This forms the fossa navicularis.

The clitoris is the homologue of the penis in the male. It hangs free and terminates in a rounded glans (small, sensitive vascular body). Unlike the penis, the clitoris does not contain the urethra.

The vestibule is a smooth area surrounded by the labia minora, with the clitoris at its apex and the fossa navicularis at its base. It contains openings for the urethra and the vagina.

The urethra, which is about 4 cm long, is close to the anterior vaginal wall and connects the bladder with the ure-

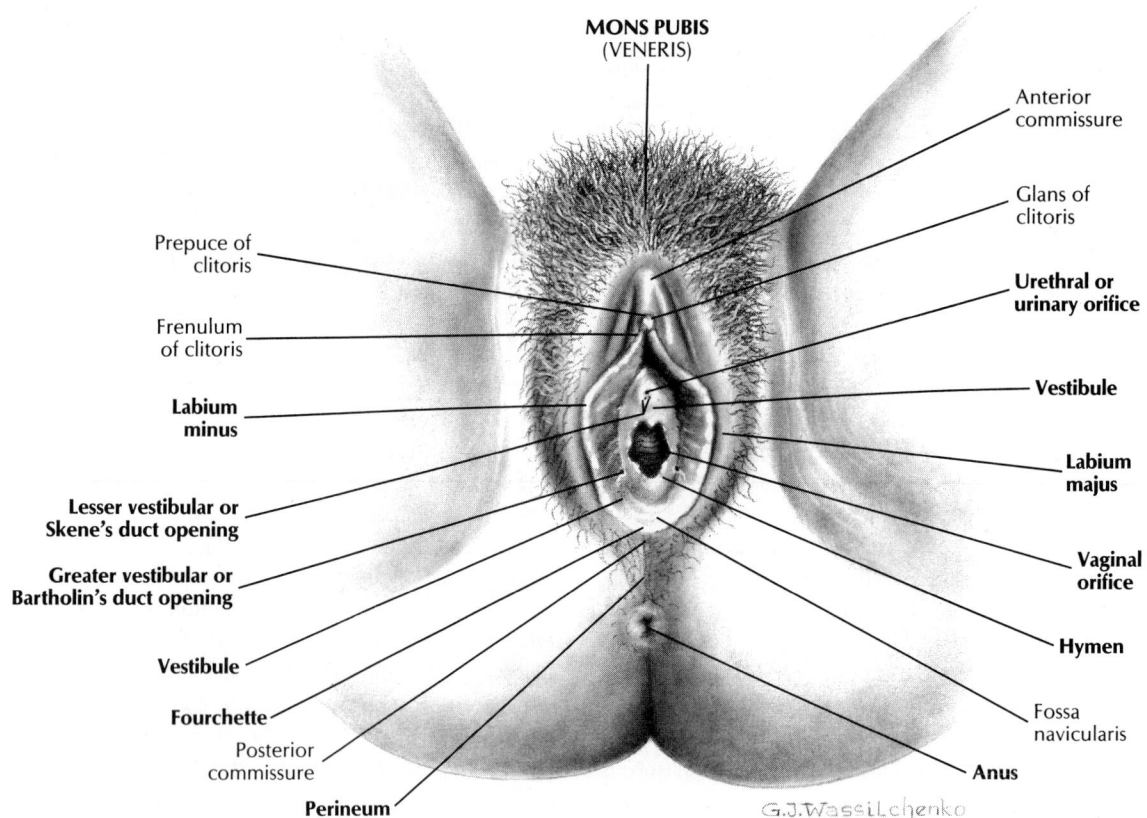

MONS PUBIS
(VENERIS)

Anterior commissure

Glans of clitoris

Prepuce of clitoris

Urethral or urinary orifice

Frenulum of clitoris

Vestibule

Labium minus

Labium majus

Lesser vestibular or Skene's duct opening

Vaginal orifice

Greater vestibular or Bartholin's duct opening

Hymen

Vestibule

Fossa navicularis

Fourchette

Posterior commissure

Anus

Perineum

G.J.Wassilchenko

FIG. 13-6   External female reproductive organs.
From Bobak, I.M., & Jensen, M.D. (1993). *Maternity and gynecologic care* (5th Ed.). St. Louis: Mosby.

thral meatus. On either side of the urethral meatus lie two small paraurethral ducts, which are commonly known as Skene's ducts (see Fig. 13-6).

The vaginal orifice lies below the urethral meatus. This opening extends through the hymen, which was originally a septum. The configuration and size of the opening vary and cannot be used as a determinant of a virginal state.

Bartholin's glands and ducts lie one on each side of the lower end of the vagina. They are homologues of the bulbourethral glands in the male. These narrow ducts open into the vaginal orifice on the inner aspects of the labia minora.

VASCULAR, NERVE, AND LYMPHATIC SUPPLY OF THE REPRODUCTIVE SYSTEM

The blood supply of the female pelvis is derived from the internal iliac branches of the common iliac artery and is supplemented by the ovarian, superior rectal, and median sacral arteries—branches of the aorta.

The nerve supply of the female pelvis comes from the autonomic nerves, which enter the pelvis in the superior hypogastric plexus (presacral nerve). The lymphatics of the female pelvis either follow the course of the vessels to the iliac and preaortic nodes or empty into the inguinal glands (Fig. 13-7).

PERIOPERATIVE NURSING CONSIDERATIONS
ASSESSMENT

The provision of quality perioperative nursing care depends on thorough perioperative assessment and care planning. Data are gathered on the gynecologic patient through the review of systems, physical examination, nursing/medical histories, and diagnostic test results located in the patient record.

Initial review of the patient record permits the perioperative nurse to prioritize and validate information on which the care plan is formulated. Through review of the history and physical exam the perioperative nurse interprets and applies information to the plan of care for the individual patient and the surgical interventions to be performed.

Application of interpersonal communication techniques is vital during nursing assessment. The interview may be conducted on the patient care unit or in the holding area of the surgical suite. Open-ended questions, progressing from general to specific, are incorporated throughout this process. For example, the perioperative nurse may initially inquire about the patient's understanding of the surgical intervention to be performed, and then proceed to questions

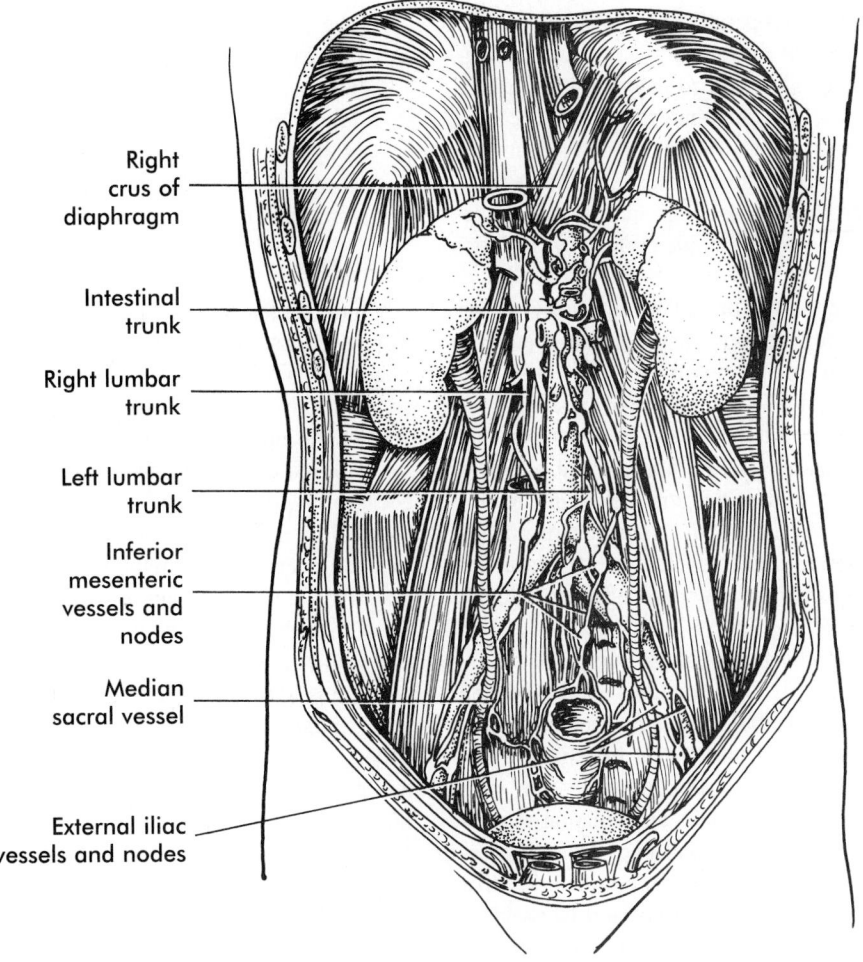

Right crus of diaphragm

Intestinal trunk

Right lumbar trunk

Left lumbar trunk

Inferior mesenteric vessels and nodes

Median sacral vessel

External iliac vessels and nodes

FIG. 13-7 Lymphatic system of abdomen and pelvis.

pertaining to intraoperative positioning, which would include the presence of back pain and limitations in joint mobility.

The assessment includes identification of the gynecologic patient's chief complaint, present problem, social history, and relevant medical and surgical histories. A family history includes such information as maternal use of diethylstilbestrol and deaths related to gynecologic disorders, cancer, hypertension, diabetes, and heart disease. Cultural, psychologic, and religious beliefs are identified and incorporated into the care plan. Throughout this process the perioperative nurse must remain open and supportive to assist in establishing a trusting therapeutic relationship. These factors can greatly affect the patient's perception of her intended surgery and play a major role in the patient outcomes.

The gynecologic patient's history includes a chronologic listing of each pregnancy with length of gestation, type of delivery, complications during pregnancy, duration of labor, and fetal weight. The menstrual cycle is discussed to include age at onset, length of each cycle, amount of flow,

duration of bleeding, and pain or discomfort associated with menses. The amount of flow is described in relation to the number of sanitary napkins and tampons used. The perioperative nurse should inquire about a history of vaginal infections or discharge. If bleeding is present, the duration, color, and consistency of blood are noted. Questions about use of vaginal douches, creams, and contraceptives are included in the assessment.

A medication history is taken, including use of analgesics, oral contraceptives, estrogen therapy, diuretics, antihypertensives, and cardiac medications. Medication frequency, dosage, and duration of use are noted.

Gynecologic disorders may be associated with urinary problems. Stress incontinence or loss of urine while coughing, sneezing, or laughing should be identified. Pain or burning sensations upon urination are noted. The gynecologic patient may have urologic studies ordered preoperatively, especially in the presence of uterine prolapse.

Results of the physical examination are reviewed by the perioperative nurse. Baseline vital signs, height, weight, and findings from assessment of the thyroid, chest, heart, lungs, breasts, abdomen, pelvis, and rectum are analyzed for their relationship to intraoperative care planning.

The gynecologic patient may undergo numerous diagnostic studies. The studies performed depend on the gynecologic problem or disorder. A laparoscopy may be performed for diagnostic or therapeutic reasons, for example, infertility, pelvic pain, pelvic inflammatory disease, ova retrieval for in vitro fertilization, lysis of adhesions, evaluation of pelvic mass, removal of ectopic pregnancy, or tubal sterilization.

Gynecologic surgery is performed in proximity to the kidneys, ureters, and bladder and may warrant preoperative studies such as an intravenous pyelogram (IVP) and barium enema (BE) to establish an anatomic baseline.

Pelvic ultrasound helps diagnose ectopic pregnancy and adnexal and uterine disease. Uterine fibroids and blood or fluid in the pelvis may be identified via ultrasound. Computed tomography (CT scanning) and magnetic resonance imaging (MRI) may be utilized in evaluation of the patient with suspected malignancy in the retroperitoneal lymph nodes or bone.

Preoperatively the gynecologic patient may have a hysterosalpingogram to identify abnormalities in the uterine cavity and occlusions in the tubal folds. This diagnostic tool is useful in detecting potential reasons for infertility.

A colposcopy, with colpomicroscopy, is often performed in the physician's office. This examination is indicated for the patient with an abnormal Pap smear suggestive of dysplasia. It identifies cellular abnormalities that may involve the vulva, vagina, or cervix and helps identify areas of dysplasia and carcinoma in situ. Endocervical curettage may be obtained during the colposcopic procedure to rule out invasive carcinoma or to detect early adenocarcinoma.

NURSING DIAGNOSIS

Comprehensive perioperative nursing care is a planned process that is implemented to ensure high-quality patient care. Nursing diagnoses are formulated after reviewing the patient record and conducting a complete patient assessment. All significant data collected are reviewed and prioritized, then incorporated into the perioperative care plan. The gynecologic patient may have multiple nursing diagnoses that warrant perioperative nursing intervention. Nursing diagnoses for the gynecologic patient may include the following:

- Anxiety related to surgery and surgical outcome
- High risk for urinary retention
- High risk for impaired skin integrity
- Body image disturbance
- High risk for injury related to surgical position

OUTCOME IDENTIFICATION

Outcomes identified for the selected nursing diagnoses could be stated as the following:

- The patient will experience reduced anxiety.
- The patient will maintain or regain normal patterns of urinary elimination.
- The patient's skin will remain intact.
- The patient will effectively cope with disturbance in body image.
- The patient will be free from injury related to the surgical position.

PLANNING

Planning determines the ability of the perioperative nurse to provide patient care in an organized and individualized manner. Planning involves preparation for both the psychosocial and physiologic needs of the gynecologic patient. Part of the nursing care plan is therefore the gathering of the required equipment and supplies and the positioning of accessories, devices, and adjuncts requisite to gynecologic surgical interventions. For example, if the gynecologic patient is undergoing a lengthy surgical intervention, the perioperative nurse will plan to have a warming blanket, gel-filled mattress, and antiembolic stockings available. These will aid in maintaining the patient's body temperature, in promoting skin integrity, and in preventing venous stasis. Once nursing diagnoses and desired outcomes are established, nursing interventions are identified that will assist the gynecologic patient to reach the desired outcomes. Some examples of interventions for the gynecologic patient are shown in the Sample Care Plan.

IMPLEMENTATION

During implementation of the plan of care, the perioperative nurse performs the identified nursing interventions. Part of perioperative care plan implementation includes selecting the appropriate instruments and patient care supplies, patient positioning on the OR bed, antimicrobial skin preparation, insertion of urinary catheters, draping, creation and maintenance of a sterile field, initiation of safety measures, and patient monitoring. Data continue to be collected, the care plan is documented, and reports are given to relief personnel, ensuring continuity of the patient's plan of care.

Principles and methods of patient positioning for different types of surgical procedures are described in Chapter 4. Patient positions may be modified based on the surgical procedure and surgeon preference. The patient is placed in the lithotomy position for most vaginal and vulvar surgery. For abdominal gynecologic surgery, the Trendelenburg's position may be used. Some surgeons use low lithotomy with Trendelenburg's positions for abdominal oncology procedures to facilitate access to pelvic and paraaortic nodes. Patients placed in Trendelenburg's position for prolonged gynecologic procedures are at increased cardiovascular risk, due to decreased tidal volume. Care should be taken to protect the patient from nerve injury and ensure adequate circulatory, renal, and respiratory functions.

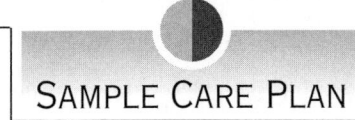

SAMPLE CARE PLAN

NURSING DIAGNOSIS Anxiety related to surgery and surgical outcome
OUTCOME: The patient will experience reduced anxiety.
INTERVENTIONS:
Introduce self and establish rapport.
Determine signs and symptoms indicating presence of anxiety:
    Diaphoresis
    Restlessness
    Hyperventilation
    Tachycardia
    Urinary frequency
    Nausea
Identify maladaptive and adaptive responses to anxiety.
Encourage use of adaptive coping mechanisms.
Evaluate strengths and resources available to assist patient in coping with anxiety.
Encourage use of relaxation techniques, guided imagery, or music when appropriate for patient.
Identify patient's readiness to learn and provide individualized teaching based on these findings.
Describe sequence of perioperative events to patient in a brief, clear manner.
Use short, simple sentences.
Use calm, firm tone of voice.
Minimize environmental stimuli.
Encourage patient to ventilate feelings and concerns.
Develop therapeutic relationship with patient.
Use active listening skills.
Offer, clarify, and further validate information as needed.

NURSING DIAGNOSIS: High risk for urinary retention
OUTCOME: The patient will maintain or regain normal patterns of urinary elimination.
INTERVENTIONS:
Instruct patient on importance of adequate postoperative fluid intake and early ambulation.

Before surgery, explain that indwelling urinary catheter will be inserted (as applicable). Review important elements of catheter care, management of drainage system, catheter removal, and signs and symptoms of urinary tract infection.
Encourage patient to verbalize feelings and concerns regarding ability to void postoperatively, presence of indwelling catheter, and catheter removal.
Clarify any misperceptions the patient may have.
Insert indwelling urinary catheter using aseptic technique.
Obtain urine specimen as required. Connect catheter to closed drainage system.
Document size of catheter inserted and specimens obtained.
Secure tubing to patient to prevent inadvertent stretching or stress on catheter.
Place urinary drainage bag where it is readily observable.
Keep drainage bag below level of bladder.
Check patency of catheter and drainage system whenever patient is repositioned.
Observe color and amount of urine; report abnormalities.
Record urinary output; report amount of urine to anesthesia provider.

NURSING DIAGNOSIS: High risk for impaired skin integrity
OUTCOME: The patient's skin will remain intact.
INTERVENTIONS:
Note the presence of any skin rashes, bruises, lacerations, ecchymoses, petechiae, or other alterations, and record them.
Select an appropriate site of placement for electrosurgical dispersive pad (close to the operative site, on area with good muscle mass, free of excessive hair or skin oil).
Verify that patient has no known allergies to antimicrobial skin preparation agents.
Prepare operative site according to institutional procedure.

Continued.

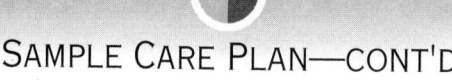

INTERVENTIONS—*cont'd*

Keep dependent skin areas around preparation site and electrosurgical pad dry; do not allow solutions to pool.

Keep OR bed surface free from wrinkles.

Pad bony prominences, which may include the heels, ankles, and buttocks, depending on patient position.

Place safety and restraining straps so that they are snug but not tight.

Apply dressings to surgical incision line and drain exit sites before surgical drapes are removed to prevent contamination of the incision; use aseptic technique.

After dressing has been applied, cleanse area surrounding incision and drain sites of blood and exudate.

Apply tape gently but firmly to secure dressing in place; allow room for postoperative swelling to prevent tape burns.

Document location of electrosurgical dispersive pad site and ECG leads, antimicrobial skin preparation solution, placement of safety and restraining straps, and presence of drains.

NURSING DIAGNOSIS: Body image disturbance

OUTCOME: The patient will effectively cope with disturbance in body image.

INTERVENTIONS:

Encourage patient to express feelings about her diagnosis and surgery and how she believes it will affect her body image.

Clarify any misconceptions.

Maintain the patient's privacy.

Express understanding and assurance to the patient that her feelings and concerns are normal.

Determine patient's readiness to learn, and teach patient information relevant to her body image alteration.

Be nonjudgmental.

Demonstrate empathy and positive regard.

Identify effective coping skills previously used by patient and encourage use of these if appropriate in current situation.

Assist patient to value her present self realistically.

Encourage patient to identify her strengths.

Encourage attendance at self-help groups when appropriate.

NURSING DIAGNOSIS: High risk for injury related to surgical position.

OUTCOME: The patient will be free from injury related to the surgical position.

INTERVENTIONS:

Note the presence of any preexisting patient conditions (nutritional status, weight, preoperative chemotherapy, limitations in mobility or range of motion, neurovascular impairments) that place the patient at risk for positional injury. Document them.

Preoperatively, assess and document condition of dependent skin areas.

If possible, have the patient assume the planned surgical position prior to induction of anesthesia. Modify plan for patient positioning in presence of pain or discomfort.

Gather positioning accessories appropriate to the planned position.

Pad OR bed (foam, water or gel-filled mattress) as appropriate to identified patient risk factors.

Pad dependent pressure sites.

Protect vulnerable neurovascular bundles from injury.

Reassess padding and protection on any positional changes.

Maintain body alignment.

Secure patient in position with safety and body straps.

Accomplish all positioning and positional changes slowly, gently, and gradually.

Document position (and positional changes), safety measures, and accessories used.

Because pelvic and vaginal procedures involve manipulation of the ureters, bladder, and urethra, indwelling urinary drainage systems are frequently established before or during surgery. Either an indwelling urethral Foley catheter or a suprapubic cystostomy (Silastic) catheter may be used, depending on the surgeon's preference and the type of procedure. The size of sutures, needles, and drains also varies, depending on surgeon's preference.

Skin preparation and routine draping procedures are described in Chapter 3. A basic vaginal instrument set is required for vaginal and vulvar surgery. A basic abdominal gynecologic instrument set is required for abdominal gynecologic surgery. Surgeons' instrument preferences may vary, and the following instrument sets are not meant to be all-inclusive.

INSTRUMENTATION
Vaginal prep set

Disposable prep sets may be used for the vagina. If they are not available, the perioperative nurse may prepare a basic vaginal prep set that includes the following:

1 Graves vaginal speculum
1 Urethral catheter, 16 or 18 Fr
1 Bozeman dressing forceps
3 Foerster sponge-holding forceps

Gauze sponges
2 Towels
Stainless steel cups
Antimicrobial solutions, as desired

Basic vaginal instrument set

The basic vaginal instrument set includes the following:

Cutting instruments

1 Bard-Parker knife handle no. 4 with blade no. 20
2 Bard-Parker knife handles no. 3 with blade no. 10
2 Mayo dissecting scissors, 1 curved and 1 straight, 6¾ inches
1 Metzenbaum scissors, curved, 7 inches
1 Suture scissors

1 Set Sims uterine curettes, sharp (Fig. 13-8)
1 Set Thomas uterine curettes, blunt (Fig. 13-8)
1 Endometrial biopsy suction curette (Fig. 13-8)
1 Gaylor biopsy forceps (Fig. 13-8)

Holding instruments

4 Foerster sponge-holding forceps, 9½ inches
6 Backhaus towel clamps, 5¼ inches
2 Dressing forceps, 5½ inches
2 Tissue forceps with 1 × 2 teeth, 5½ inches
1 Dressing forceps, 10 inches
1 Tissue forceps with 1 × 2 teeth, 10 inches
2 Russian tissue forceps, 8 inches
8 Allis-Adair tissue forceps, 6¼ inches

6 Allis intestinal forceps, 6 inches
2 Babcock intestinal forceps, 6¼ inches
2 Babcock intestinal forceps, 9½ inches
2 Lahey vulsellum forceps, 6 inches
1 Jacobs vulsellum forceps (Fig. 13-9)
1 Uterine tenaculum (Fig. 13-9)
1 Staude uterine tenaculum (Fig. 13-9)
1 Bozeman dressing forceps (Fig. 13-9)

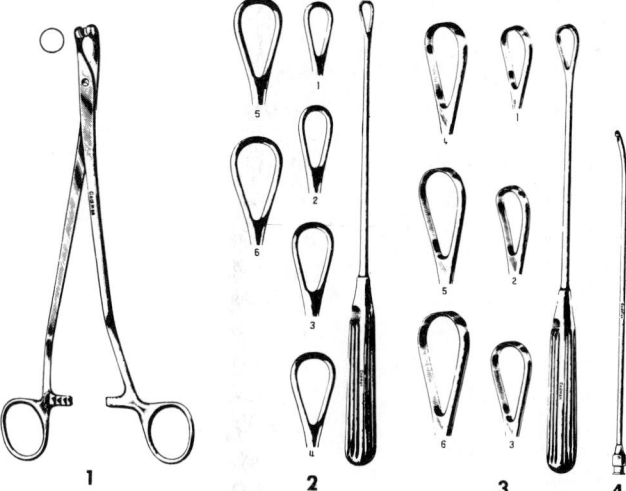

FIG. 13-8 Vaginal instruments: cutting. *1,* Gaylor biopsy forceps; *2,* Thomas uterine curettes (blunt); *3,* Sims uterine curettes (sharp); *4,* endometrial biopsy suction curette.

Courtesy Codman & Shurtleff, Inc., Randolph, Mass.

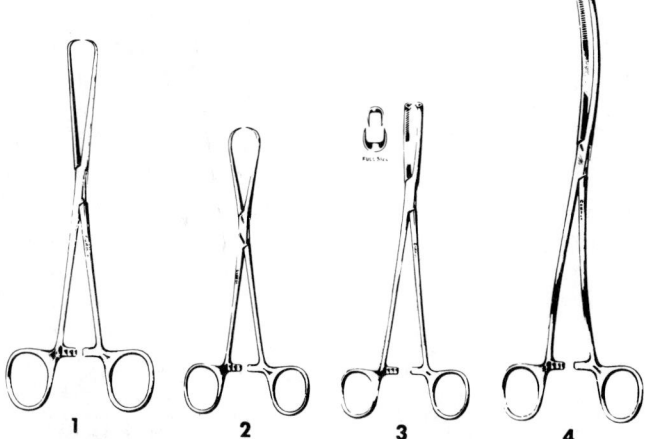

FIG. 13-9 Vaginal instruments: holding. *1,* Uterine tenaculum; *2,* Staude uterine tenaculum; *3,* Jacobs vulsellum forceps; *4,* Bozeman dressing forceps.

Courtesy Codman & Shurtleff, Inc., Randolph, Mass.

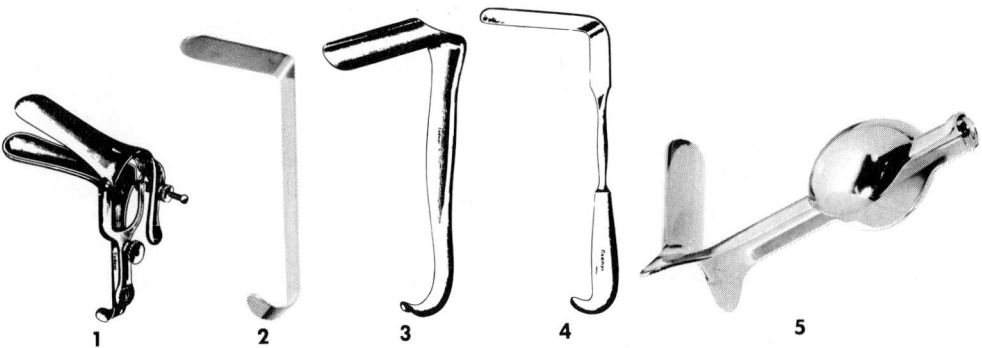

FIG. 13-10 Vaginal instruments: exposing. *1*, Graves self-retaining vaginal speculum; *2*, Heaney hysterectomy retractor; *3*, Doyen vaginal retractor; *4*, Glenner vaginal retractor; *5*, Auvard vaginal speculum (weighted).

Courtesy Codman & Shurtleff, Inc., Randolph, Mass.

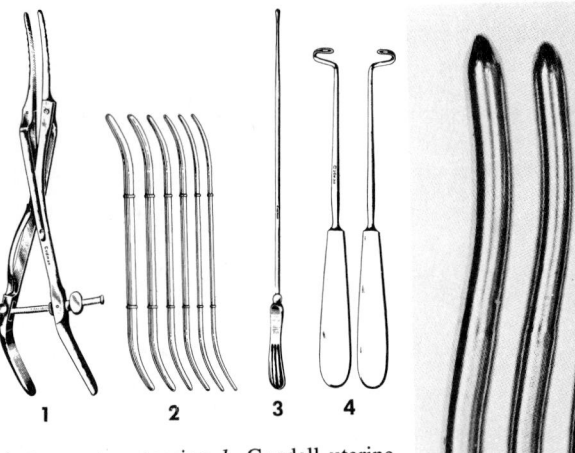

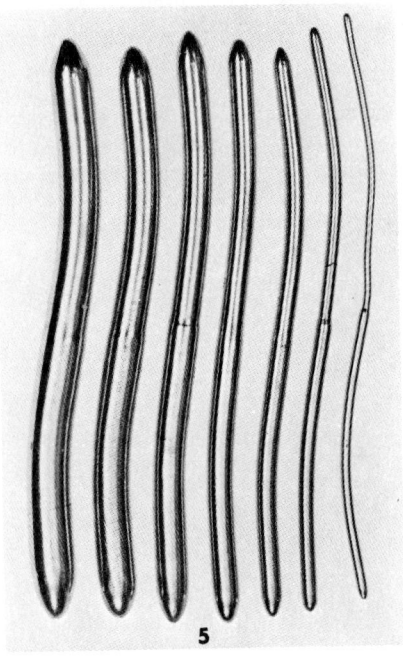

FIG. 13-11 Vaginal instruments: exposing *1*, Goodell uterine dilator; *2*, Hank uterine dilators; *3*, uterine sound (graduated); *4*, Deschamp ligature carriers (right and left); *5*, Hegar dilators.

1, 3, 4, 5 Courtesy Codman & Shurtleff, Inc., Randolph, Mass., *2* Courtesy DISC Co., Inc., Malvern, Pa.

FIG. 13-12 Abdominal gynecologic instruments: cutting and suturing. *1*, Heaney needle holder; *2*, Mayo dissecting scissors (straight, 6¾ inches); *3*, Mayo dissecting scissors (curved, 6¾ inches).

Courtesy Codman & Shurtleff, Inc., Randolph, Mass.

Clamping instruments

6 Crile hemostats, straight, 6¼ inches
12 Kelly hemostats, curved, 5½ inches
2 Pean forceps, curved, 6¼ inches
2 Ochsner forceps, straight, 6¼ inches

4 Ochsner forceps, straight, 8 inches
4 Heaney hysterectomy forceps, 8¼ inches
6 Rochester-Pean hysterectomy forceps, curved, 9 inches

Exposing instruments

1 Self-retaining vaginal speculum (Fig. 13-10)
1 Jackson vaginal retractor
2 Heaney retractors (Fig. 13-10)
2 Deaver retractors
1 Auvard vaginal speculum, weighted (Fig. 13-10)

1 Doyen vaginal retractor (Fig. 13-10)
1 Uterine sound, graduated (Fig. 13-11)
1 Set Hegar or Hank uterine dilators (Fig. 13-11)
1 Goodell uterine dilator (Fig. 13-11)

Suturing instruments

2 Mayo-Hegar needle holders, 8 inches
2 Heaney needle holders (Fig. 13-12)

2 Crile-Wood needle holders, 6 inches

Accessory items

Suction tubing
Suction tip
Asepto syringe (optional)

Metal tray for surgeon's lap (optional)

Indwelling urinary drainage items: Foley catheter or suprapubic cystostomy (Silastic) catheter

Drain (optional)
Lubricant, water-soluble
Electrosurgical unit, if desired

A basic vaginal prep set is required for abdominal gynecologic surgery. The basic abdominal gynecologic instrument set consists of the basic laparotomy set (Chapter 10), plus the following:

Cutting instrument

1 Jorgenson scissors

Holding instruments

1 Somer uterine elevating forceps (Fig. 13-13)

2 Barrett tenaculum forceps, 7 inches
1 Lahey goiter vulsellum forceps, 6 inches

Clamping instruments

4 Heaney hysterectomy forceps, 8 inches (Fig. 13-13)

Exposing instruments

1 Martin or O'Sullivan-O'Connor abdominal retractor with blades (Fig. 13-14)

1 Balfour self-retaining retractor with blades (Fig. 13-14)

Suturing instruments

2 Heaney needle holders, 8½ inches

2 Masson needle holders, 10¼ inches

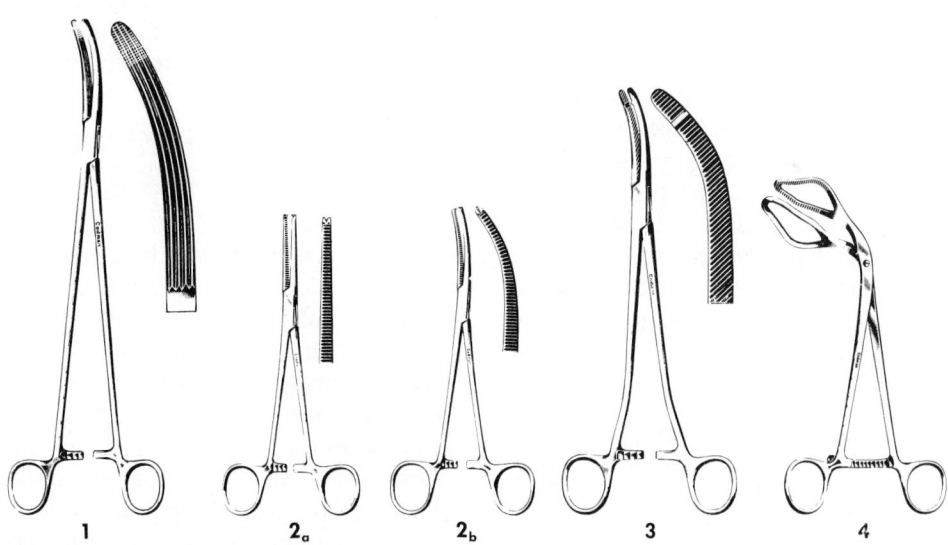

FIG. 13-13 Abdominal gynecologic instruments: clamping. *1,* Rochester-Pean forceps; *2a,* Rochester-Ochsner (straight) forceps; *2b,* Rochester-Ochsner (curved) forceps; *3,* Heaney hysterectomy forceps; *4,* Somer uterine elevating forceps.

Courtesy Codman & Shurtleff, Inc., Randolph, Mass.

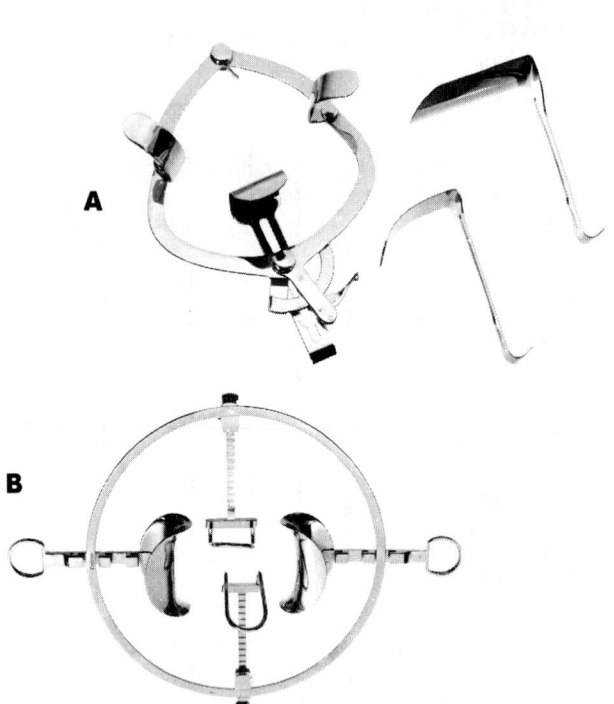

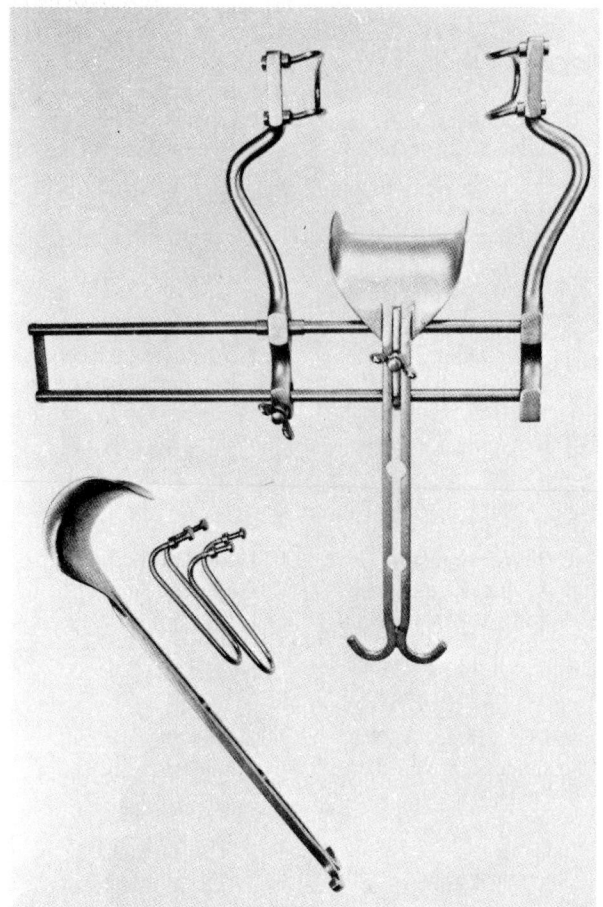

FIG. 13-14 Abdominal gynecologic instruments: exposing. **A,** O'Sullivan-O'Connor self-retaining abdominal retractor; **B,** Martin self-retaining abdominal ring retractor, **C,** Balfour self-retaining retractor with blades.

Courtesy Codman & Shurtleff, Inc., Randolph, Mass.

For most abdominal gynecologic procedures, a dilatation and curettage set should be available.

EVALUATION

During evaluation the perioperative nurse determines whether the patient met the established goals. Some goals can be reached during the preoperative and intraoperative phases of care; they are evaluated prior to the patient's discharge from the operating room. Others require ongoing monitoring and measurement in the postoperative phase; these are denoted by the word "will" to indicate their ongoing nature. Part of the perioperative nursing report to the recovery area (PACU, ambulatory recovery) should include the goals of the nursing care plan. They can be phrased as outcome statements, as follows:

- The patient's anxiety was reduced; she verbalized concerns and used personally effective coping strategies.
- Urinary elimination patterns were maintained; urinary output was adequate, and catheter patency was maintained.
- Skin integrity was maintained; there were no reddened areas at dependent pressure sites or at the placement site of the dispersive pad; the incision was aseptically dressed.

- The patient will effectively cope with her disturbance in body image; questions will continue to be answered and misconceptions clarified.
- There was no evidence of injury related to surgical positioning; range of motion and neurovascular status were consistent with preoperative levels.

LASERS IN GYNECOLOGIC SURGERY

The carbon dioxide (CO_2) laser, neodymium:yttrium-aluminum-garnet (Nd:YAG) laser, and argon laser have been used in gynecology to treat extrauterine disease such as pelvic endometriosis, cervical dysplasia, condylomata acuminata, pelvic adhesive disease, and premalignant diseases of the vulva and vagina. They are usually used in conjunction with the colposcope and operating microscope, or the laparoscope. A laser plume evacuator or suction system is necessary to remove smoke and fumes from the operative field. All accessories and instrumentation used should be laser safe, secure, and tested or examined for working order prior to use. Safety precautions must be implemented by the OR team when the laser is used (see Chapter 31).

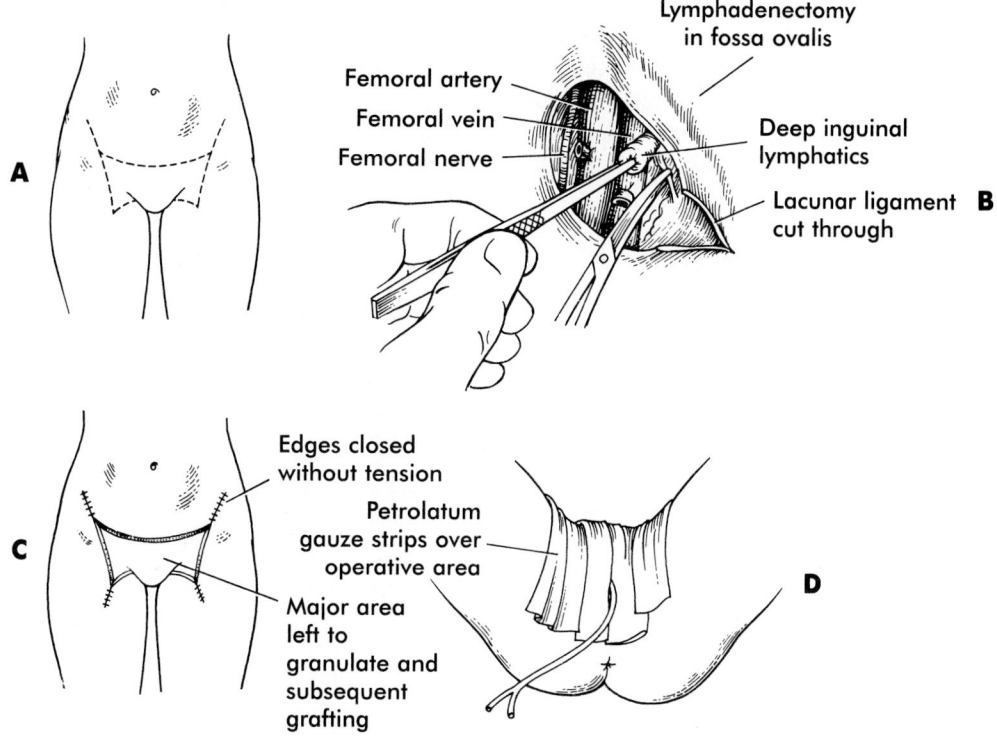

FIG. 13-15 **A,** Outline of incisional lines for simple or radical operations for vulvar cover. **B,** Dissection is completed, involving nerves, saphenous veins, and muscles, when dissection of distal half of femoral canal has been completed. **C,** Upper edges of abdominal incisions may be partially closed. **D,** With indwelling catheter in bladder, wound is dressed with layers of gauze and held in place with light pressure dressing.

SURGICAL INTERVENTIONS

VULVAR SURGERY

The treatment of early malignant disease of the vulva is accomplished by a skinning technique, local wide excision, or, for more multicentric or extensive lesions, simple vulvectomy. These procedures may also be accomplished by use of a laser.

Simple vulvectomy

Simple vulvectomy is removal of the labia majora and labia minora, possibly but not preferably the glans clitoris, and occasionally tissue from the perianal area, with a plastic closure. A simple vulvectomy is usually done for the treatment of carcinoma in situ of the vulva when it is multicentric or for the treatment of Bowen's or Paget's disease. Occasionally a vulvectomy is necessary for the treatment of either leukoplakia or intractable pruritus, especially when a skinning procedure is impractical or has failed.

Procedural considerations

The basic vaginal instrument set is required, plus an electrosurgical unit, if desired. The patient is positioned in lithotomy.

Operative procedure

1. The affected skin is incised, usually starting anteriorly above the clitoris. The incision is continued laterally to the labia majora, to the midline of the perineum, and around the anus, if it is involved (Fig. 13-15, *A*). A knife, hemostats, gauze sponges on sponge-holding forceps, tissue forceps, and Allis forceps are needed. Bleeding vessels are clamped. Bleeding is also controlled by electrocoagulation or sutures.

2. Periurethral and perivaginal incisions are made. Bleeding of this vascular area can be controlled by means of Kelly or Crile hemostats and electrocoagulation. Ligation of blood vessels should be minimal. Allis-Adair forceps are used for holding diseased tissues.

3. All skin and subcutaneous tissues are undermined and mobilized with curved dissecting scissors, tissue forceps, Allis forceps, and sponges on holding forceps.

4. The wound is closed, usually by simple bilateral Z-plasty or other plastic closure. In some cases skin is excised around the anus to accomplish a sliding skin flap.

5. Closed wound drainage catheters may be placed in the dependent areas, an indwelling urinary catheter is inserted, and vaginal gauze packing may be placed in the vagina. Dressings are applied.

Skinning vulvectomy

Skinning vulvectomy is the simple removal of the external skin from the affected area, which has been previously identified with a stain such as toluidine blue. The purpose of this procedure is to preserve the underlying structures of the external genitalia. A skinning procedure may be done to treat leukoplakia, intractable pruritus, or other types of skin lesions, such as kraurosis, vitiligo, and chronic venereal granulomas.

Procedural considerations

The instrumentation required and patient position are as described for simple vulvectomy.

Operative procedure

The external skin is simply excised from the affected area.

Groin lymphadenectomy and radical vulvectomy

Groin lymphadenectomy and radical vulvectomy are the en bloc dissection of the following structures: a large segment of skin from the abdomen and groin, the labia majora, labia minora, clitoris, mons veneris, and terminal portions of the urethra, vagina, and other vulvar organs, as well as the superficial and deep inguinal nodes, portions of the round ligaments, portions of the saphenous veins, and the lesion itself. It also involves reconstruction of the vaginal walls and pelvic floor and closure of the abdominal wounds (Fig. 13-15). Placement of full-thickness pinch or split-thickness grafts may be done if the denuded area of the vulva appears too large for normal granulation. A plastic surgeon may immediately complete skin grafts or rotation flaps to cover defects (see Chapter 23).

Groin lymphadenectomy and radical vulvectomy involve abdominoperineal dissection and groin dissection, which may be performed as a one- or two-stage operation. When performed as a one-stage operation, it is optimally done by a four-person team. The skin prep is usually extensive, including the abdomen and thighs; if a skin graft will be done, the donor site will also need to be prepped.

Procedural considerations

The patient lies supine and may be placed in Trendelenburg's and low lithotomy positions, as required for the various stages. The skin prep includes both the abdomen and vulva, and the skin of the thighs is usually prepped down to the knees. An indwelling urinary catheter may be placed to act as a urethral marker and to prevent postoperative urethral trauma. As in other radical surgery, the nursing team should be prepared to measure blood loss and anticipate procedures to combat shock.

For groin lymphadenectomy the basic abdominal gynecologic instrument set is required, plus the following:

Clamping instruments

8 Schnidt tonsil forceps, 7¼ inches	Ligating clips and appliers
4 Kantrowitz thoracic clamps, 7½ inches	

Assessory items (optional)

2 Closed-wound drainage systems

For radical vulvectomy the basic vaginal instrument set is required, plus the following:

Exposing instruments

Richardson retractors, assorted sizes	2 Volkmann rake retractors, three-pronged, dull
2 Richardson appendectomy retractors, long blade	2 Skin hooks

Accessory items (optional)

2 Closed-wound drainage systems

Operative procedures
Groin lymphadenectomy

1. The first skin incision is made on the side opposite the primary lesion. The end of the incised skin is grasped with Allis forceps. The incision is carried down to the aponeuroses of the external oblique muscle.

2. The fascia over the inguinal ligament and the fascia lata of the upper thigh are exposed, separated, and freed with retractors, knife, scissors, hemostats, and sponges.

3. Bleeding vessels, including the superficial iliac artery and vein, the epigastric artery and vein, and the superficial external pudendal artery and vein, are clamped and ligated. Smaller bleeding vessels are controlled by electrocoagulation.

4. The fibers of the inguinal, hypogastric, and femoral nerves are resected using Metzenbaum scissors, tissue forceps without teeth, and long-bladed retractors.

5. The lymphatic node beds may be identified with silk sutures or metal clips. Fine, long, sharp dissection scissors are needed.

6. The large tissue surfaces are exposed for complete dis-

section by means of retractors and are protected by warm, moist laparotomy packs. High saphenous vein ligation is performed with scissors, forceps, and hemostats and should be doubly tied with nonreactive suture.

7. The femoral canal is cleaned of its lymphatics; the round ligament is clamped, cut, and ligated.
8. The peritoneum is freed from the muscles; the fascia is dissected free; deep lymphatic nodes and areolar tissue are removed; and vessels and their attachments are clamped, cut, and ligated, using long curved scissors, long tissue forceps, hemostats, and ligatures (Fig. 13-15, *B*).
9. The lesion is removed. In deep pelvic lymphadenectomy, the ureter may be exposed and the area drained.
10. The inguinal canal is reconstructed, and the wound is partially closed with a nonabsorbable suture (Fig. 13-15, *C*). An indwelling urethral catheter is inserted and the wound is dressed.

Radical vulvectomy

1. The skin incisions of the abdomen and thigh join with those for vulvectomy. The incisions in the vulva encircle the urethra.
2. In the vulvar dissection, terminal portions of the urethra and vagina, the mons veneris, the clitoris, the frenulum, the prepuce of the clitoris, Bartholin's and Skene's glands, and fascial coverings of the vulva are removed with the specimen.
3. Reconstruction of the vaginal walls and the pelvic floor is completed. An indwelling urinary catheter is inserted, closed wound drainage catheters are placed in the denuded area, and the wound is dressed with a pressure dressing (Fig. 13-15, *D*).

VAGINAL SURGERY
Plastic reconstructive repair of the vagina (anterior and posterior repair: colporrhaphy)

A vaginal repair is done to correct a cystocele or a rectocele and to reestablish the support of the anterior and posterior vaginal walls, which will restore the bladder and rectum to their normal positions.

A cystocele is a herniation of the bladder that causes the anterior vaginal wall to bulge downward (Fig. 13-16). A defect in the anterior vaginal wall is usually caused by obstetric or surgical trauma, age, or an inherent weakness. A large protrusion may cause a sensation of pressure in the vagina or present a mass at or through the introitus; it may also cause voiding difficulties.

A rectocele is formed by a protrusion of the anterior rectal wall (posterior vaginal wall) into the vagina. In general, the anterior rectal wall forms a bulging mass beneath the posterior vaginal mucosa (Fig. 13-16). As the mass pushes downward into the lower vaginal canal, the rectum may be torn from the fascial and muscular attachments of the urogenital diaphragm and the pelvic wall. The levator ani mus-

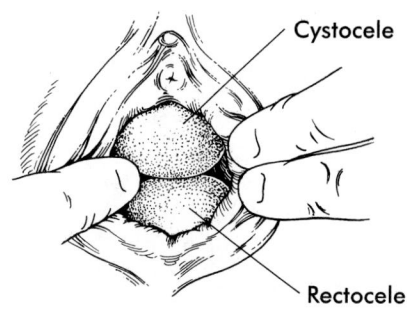

FIG. 13-16 Cystocele and rectocele resulting from unrepaired tears of muscles of pelvic floor and those under bladder, usually resulting from childbirth, surgical trauma, age, or inherent weakness.

cles (see Fig. 13-4) become stretched or torn. The symptomatic signs are a mass protruding into the vagina, difficulty in evacuating the lower bowel, hemorrhoids, and a feeling of pressure.

An enterocele is a herniation of Douglas's cul-de-sac and almost always contains loops of the small intestine. An enterocele herniates into a weakened area between the anterior and posterior vaginal walls.

Procedural considerations
The basic vaginal instrument set is required.

Operative procedures
1. Dilatation and curettage may be done in conjunction with the repair.
2. Vaginal retractors are used for exposure. The labia may be sewn back if the exposure is inadequate.

Anterior wall repair
1. The bladder may be drained, or an indwelling urinary catheter or suprapubic cystostomy catheter may be inserted (surgeon's preference). Areolar tissue between the bladder and vagina at the bladder reflection is exposed. The full thickness of the vaginal wall is separated up to the bladder neck by a knife, curved scissors, tissue forceps, Allis-Adair or Allis forceps, and gauze sponges. Bleeding vessels are clamped and tied with ligatures or electrocoagulated.
2. The urethra and bladder neck are mobilized with a knife, gauze sponges, and curved scissors.
3. Sutures are placed adjacent to the urethra and bladder neck in such a manner that, after they have been tied, a narrowing of the bladder neck and a delineating of the posterior urethrovesical angle occur (Fig. 13-17, *A*).
4. The connective tissue on the lateral aspects of the cervix is sutured into the cervix to shorten the cardinal ligaments.
5. Allis-Adair forceps are applied to the edges of the inci-

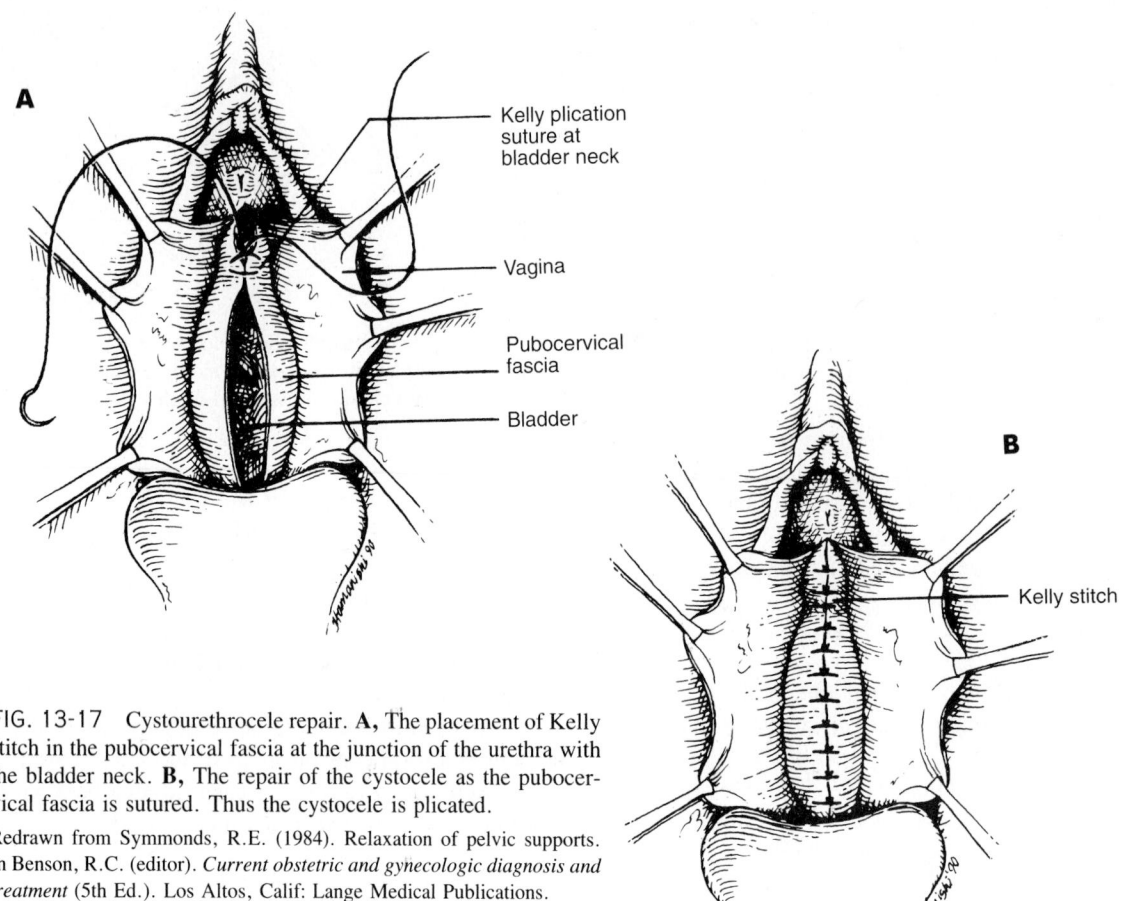

FIG. 13-17 Cystourethrocele repair. **A,** The placement of Kelly stitch in the pubocervical fascia at the junction of the urethra with the bladder neck. **B,** The repair of the cystocele as the pubocervical fascia is sutured. Thus the cystocele is plicated.

Redrawn from Symmonds, R.E. (1984). Relaxation of pelvic supports. In Benson, R.C. (editor). *Current obstetric and gynecologic diagnosis and treatment* (5th Ed.). Los Altos, Calif: Lange Medical Publications.

sion, and the left flap of the vaginal wall is drawn across the midline. Edges are trimmed according to the size of the cystocele. This process is repeated on the right flap of the vaginal incision.

6. The anterior vaginal wall is closed in a manner resulting in reconstruction of an anterior vaginal fornix (Fig. 13-17, *B*).

Posterior wall repair

1. Allis forceps are placed posterior at the mucocutaneous junction on each side, at the hymenal ring, and just above the anus (Fig. 13-18, *A*).
2. Skin and mucosa are incised and dissected from the muscles beneath with a knife, tissue forceps, curved scissors, and gauze sponges.
3. Allis-Adair forceps are placed on the posterior vaginal wall, scar tissue (from obstetric trauma) is removed, and dissection is continued to the posterior vaginal fornix and laterally, depending on the size of the rectocele (Fig. 13-18, *A* and *B*).
4. The perineum is denuded by sharp dissection, and the trimming of the posterior vaginal wall is carried out with Allis forceps, curved scissors, and gauze sponges (Fig. 13-18, *C*).

5. The rectal wall proximal to the puborectal muscle is strengthened by placement of sutures.
6. Bleeding is controlled, and the vaginal wall is closed from above, downward to the anterior edge of the puborectal muscle. The rectocele is repaired from the posterior fornix to the perineal body. Remains of the transverse perineal and bulbocavernosus muscles are used to build up the perineum. The anterior edge of the levator ani muscle may be approximated (Fig. 13-18, *D*).
7. The mucosa and skin are trimmed, and the remaining closure is effected by interrupted sutures.
8. The vagina may be packed with 2-inch vaginal gauze packing to which sulfa cream may be added. An indwelling urinary catheter or suprapubic cystostomy catheter is inserted, according to the surgeon's preference.

Enterocele repair. The procedure is illustrated in Fig. 13-19. The peritoneal sac must be carefully dissected from the underlying rectum, the overlying bladder, or both, so that the peritoneal tissues are completely freed from the surrounding structures. The sac is opened to establish true identification and is then closed as high as possible by permanent purse-string sutures. The portion of peritoneal tis-

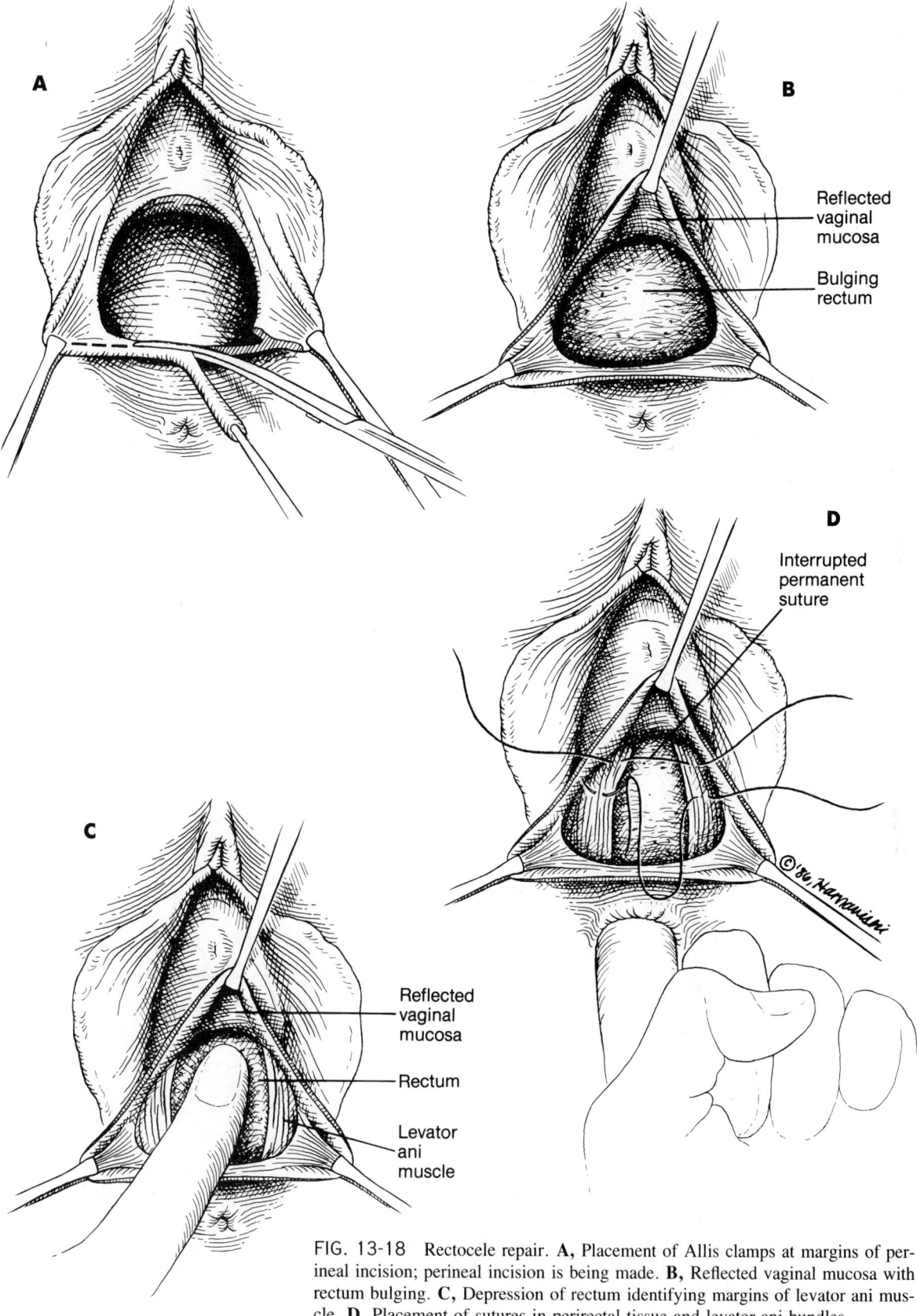

FIG. 13-18 Rectocele repair. **A,** Placement of Allis clamps at margins of perineal incision; perineal incision is being made. **B,** Reflected vaginal mucosa with rectum bulging. **C,** Depression of rectum identifying margins of levator ani muscle. **D,** Placement of sutures in perirectal tissue and levator ani bundles.

From Herbst, A.L., et al. (1992). *Comprehensive gynecology* (2nd Ed.). St. Louis: Mosby.

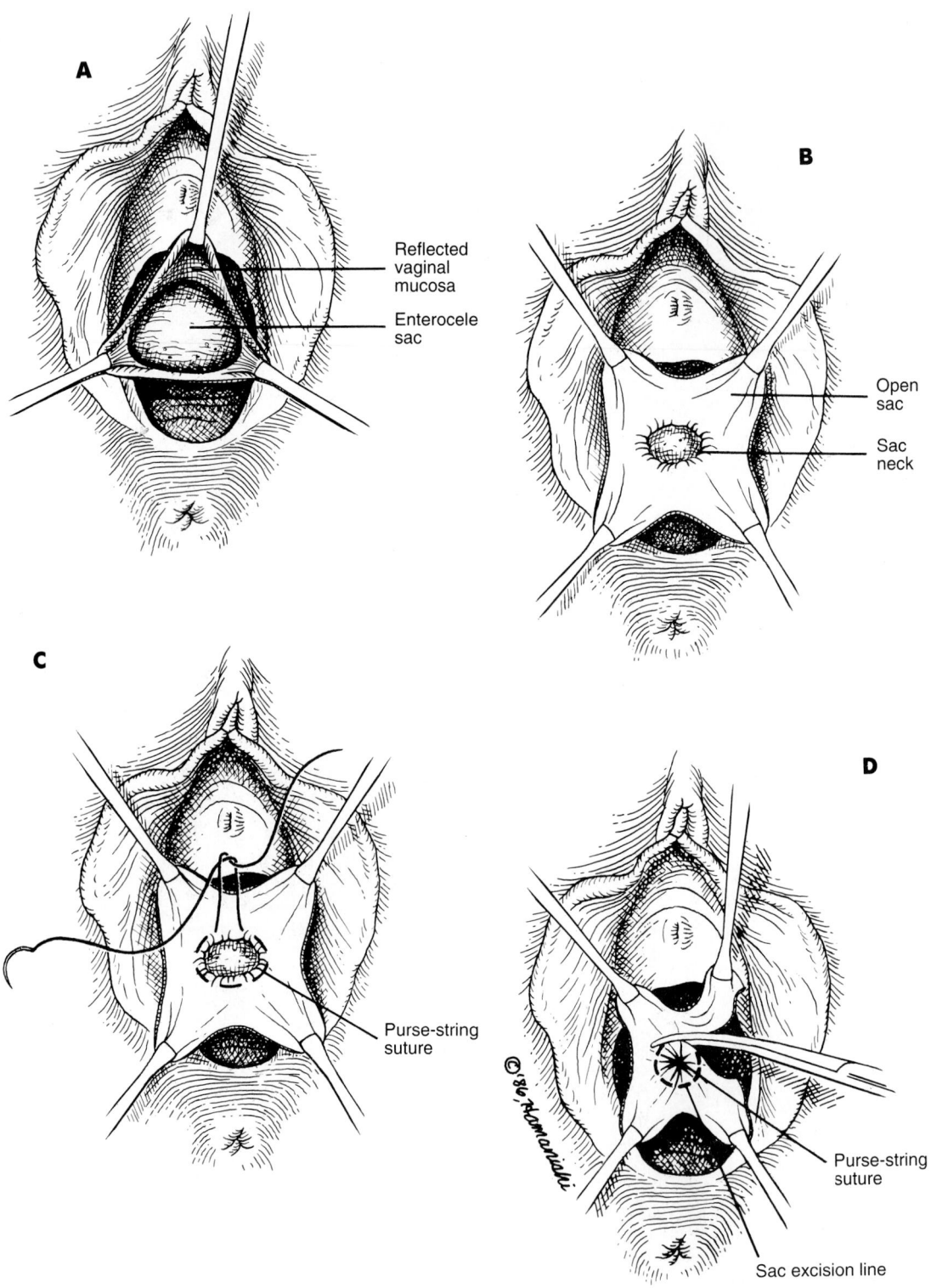

FIG. 13-19 Enterocele repair. **A,** Appearance of enterocele sac with vaginal wall reflected. **B,** Appearance of open enterocele sac with sac neck identified. **C,** Placing of purse-string suture at neck of enterocele sac. **D,** Excision of enterocele sac.

From Herbst, A.L., et al. (1992). *Comprehensive gynecology* (2nd Ed.). St. Louis: Mosby.

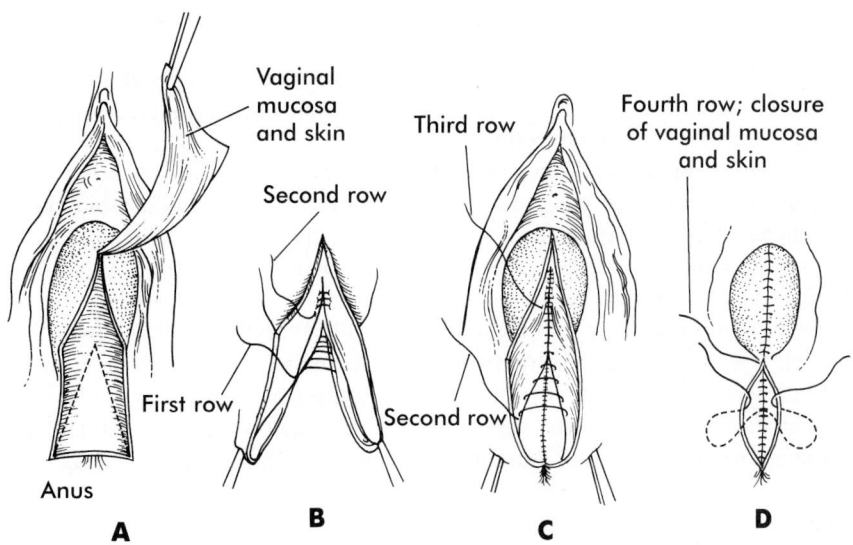

FIG. 13-20 Repair of complete lacerations of the perineum. **A,** Lower margins of incision. **B,** Placement of first and second rows of sutures. **C,** Second and third rows of sutures. **D,** Fourth row of sutures.

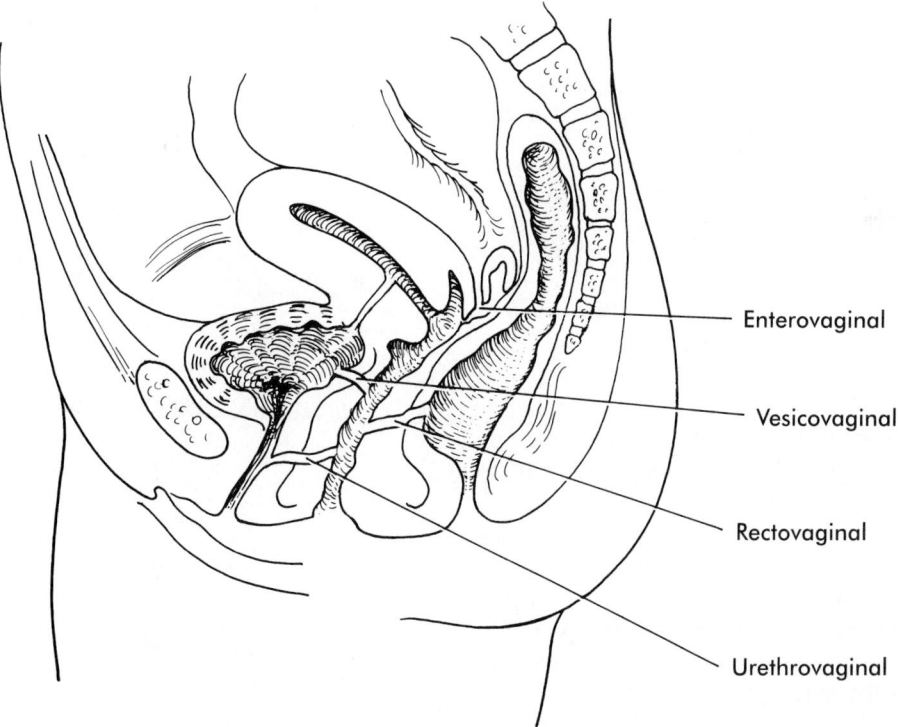

FIG. 13-21 Types of genital fistula. Urogenital fistula is communication between urethra, bladder, or one of ureters and some part of genital tract. Urethrovaginal, vesicovaginal, and ureterovaginal fistulas, most common types, empty into vaginal canal.

sue distal to the purse-string ties is then excised, and the area is reinforced locally by transverse suture closures of whatever supportive tissues may be available. This technique is used to prevent recurrence.

Perineal repair. The procedure is illustrated in Fig. 13-20.

Vesicovaginal fistula repair

A vesicovaginal fistula is repaired by free dissection of the mucosal tissue of the anterior vaginal wall, closing of the fistula tract, and repair of the fascial attachments between the bladder and vagina, with establishment of urinary drainage. Fistulas vary in size from a small opening that permits only slight leakage of urine into the vagina to a large opening that permits all urine to pass into the vagina (Fig. 13-21). They may result from radical surgery in the management of pelvic cancer, from radiation therapy without surgery, from chronic ulceration of the vaginal structures, from penetrating wounds, or from obstetric trauma.

A urethrovaginal fistula usually causes constant incontinence or difficulty in retaining urine. This condition occurs after damage to the anterior wall and bladder or following radiation therapy or parturition. A ureterovaginal fistula develops as a result of injury to the ureter. In some cases reimplantation of the ureter in the bladder or ureterostomy may be done.

Urethrovaginal fistula repair (vaginal approach)
Procedural considerations. The basic vaginal instrument set is required, plus the following:

1 Kelly fistula scissors	Frazier suction tips,
1 Dressing forceps, 7	desired sizes
inches	2 Ureteral catheters,
2 Probes	desired size
2 Skin hooks	Sterile water for irrigation

Operative procedure

1. Traction sutures are placed about the fistulous tract; tissues are grasped with Allis-Adair forceps and plain tissue forceps.
2. The scar tissue around the fistula is excised, cleavage between the bladder and vagina is located, and flaps are mobilized with scissors, forceps, and gauze sponges.
3. The bladder mucosa is inverted toward the interior of the bladder with interrupted sutures. The sutures are passed through the muscularis of the bladder down to the mucosa.
4. A second layer of inverting sutures is placed in the bladder and tied, thereby completely inverting the bladder mucosa toward the interior.
5. The vaginal wall is closed with interrupted sutures in a direction opposite the closure of the bladder wall.
6. The bladder is distended with sterile water to determine any leaks. An indwelling urinary catheter is left in place.

Vesicovaginal fistula repair (transperitoneal approach)

In the presence of a high vesicovaginal fistula, a suprapubic incision is used. The opening from the bladder into the vagina is closed, and the fascial attachments are repaired.

Procedural considerations. The patient is placed in slight Trendelenburg's position. Ureteral catheters may be inserted just before surgery (see Chapter 14). The vagina is cleansed and packed with moist gauze saturated with an antibiotic or antimicrobial solution. The abdominal operative site is prepped, and the patient is draped.

An abdominal gynecologic instrument set is required.

Operative procedure

1. A midline abdominal incision is usually made, as described for laparotomy.
2. The fistulous tract is identified; the vaginal vault and the adjacent adherent bladder are separated with scissors, forceps, and sponges.
3. The vesicovaginal septum is dissected down to the healthy tissue beyond the site of the fistula.
4. The fistulous tract is mobilized. The bladder site of the fistula is inverted into the interior of the bladder with two rows of inverting sutures. The muscularis and mucosa layers of the vagina are inverted into the vaginal vault by means of two rows of sutures.

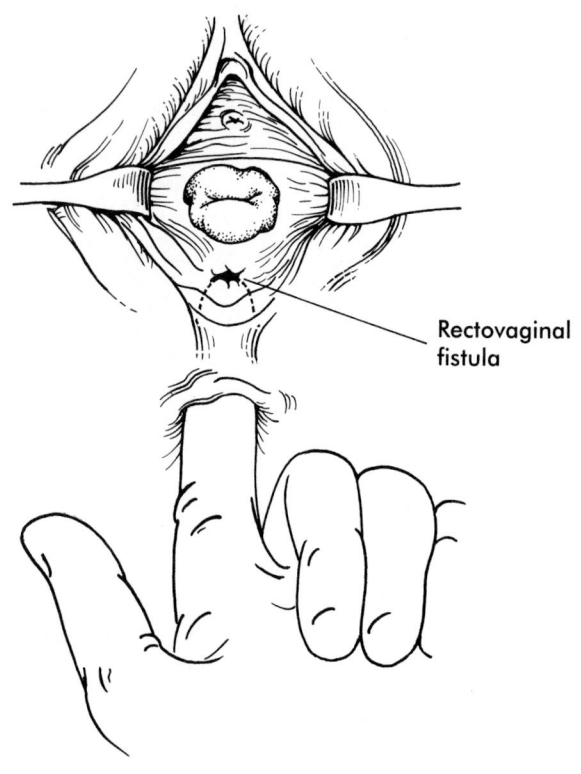

Rectovaginal fistula

FIG. 13-22   Rectovaginal fistula. Examiner's finger puts tension on rectovaginal septum.

5. The flaps of peritoneum are mobilized, both from the bladder and from the adjacent vaginal vault, and are closed to form a new vesicovaginal reflection of peritoneum below the site of the old fistulous tract.
6. The wound is closed in layers, as for laparotomy. Abdominal dressings are applied. An indwelling urinary catheter is left in the bladder.

Rectovaginal fistula repair (vaginal approach)

Rectovaginal fistula repair by the vaginal approach includes repair of the perineum, fascia, and muscle-supporting structures between the rectum and vagina, thereby closing the fistula formed between the rectum and the vagina (Fig. 13-22). In the presence of a large rectovaginal fistula, as in patients who have incurable cancer, a colostomy may be done (see Chapter 10).

Procedural considerations

The basic vaginal instrument set is required for a rectovaginal fistula repair.

Operative procedure

1. The scar tissue and tract between the rectum and vagina are excised (Fig. 13-23); edges of fresh tissue are approximated with absorbable sutures.
2. The rectum and vaginal walls are mobilized; the rectum is closed with inversion of the mucosa into the rectal canal.
3. The vagina is closed transversely or in a sagittal plane different from that of the rectal canal. The vaginal mucosal layer is inverted into the vaginal wall; an indwelling urinary catheter is inserted.

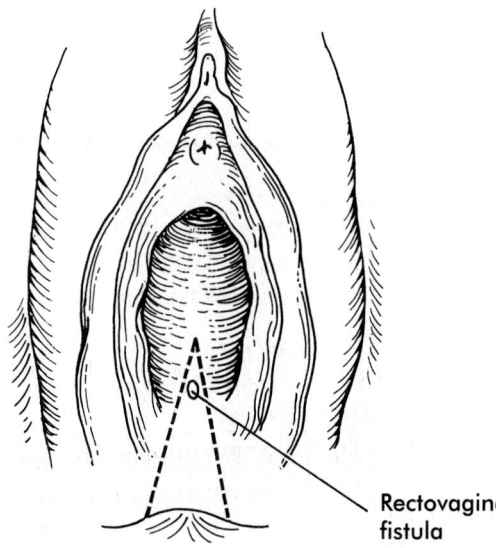

Rectovaginal
fistula

FIG. 13-23 Repair of rectovaginal fistulas of all types essentially same as shown here. Portion of scar tissue to be excised is included within *dotted lines;* repair is as described for complete lacerations of perineum (see Fig. 13-20).

Operations for urinary stress incontinence

Surgery for urinary stress incontinence entails repair of the fascial supports and the pubococcygeal muscle (see Fig. 13-4) surrounding the urethra and the bladder neck through a vaginal or abdominal approach.

The proper operative approach for the treatment of stress incontinence must be selected specifically for each patient. Normal micturition depends on a finely coordinated group of voluntary and involuntary movements. As a result of volitional impulses, voiding may be inhibited or stopped by the intrinsic muscles of the bladder neck and proximal urethra and the puborectalis division of the levator ani muscle (see Chapter 14).

The type of operation selected depends on the severity of stress incontinence, the extent of the condition causing it, the patient's ability to use the anatomic mechanism for voluntary inhibition of urination, and the operations that have previously been performed. States of stress incontinence are classified in relation to frequency and degree of incontinence, the presence of other diseases, and the function of the pubococcygeus muscle (levator ani) (see Fig. 13-4).

Previous pelvic operations may have resulted in scarring and distortion, with displacement of the bladder neck to an unfavorable position for proper functioning. Conditions such as uterine prolapse, cystocele, urethrocele, cystourethrocele, or urogenital fistulas following radiation therapy may be associated with stress incontinence.

The outcome of any operation for urinary stress incontinence is to improve the performance of a dislodged or dysfunctional vesical neck, to restore normal urethral length, and to tighten and restore the anterior urethral vesical angle. The Agency for Health Care Policy and Research developed clinical practice guidelines for the treatment of female stress incontinence in 1992. These are presented in Box 13-1.

Operative procedures
Vaginal approach

1. An indwelling urinary catheter or suprapubic cystostomy catheter is inserted, according to the surgeon's preference. The posterior vaginal wall is retracted, and an incision is made through the anterior vaginal wall down to the urethra and bladder.
2. The vaginal wall is dissected from the bladder and urethra; the neck of the bladder is sutured together. The wound is closed, as described for anterior vaginal wall repair (p. 399).

Vesicourethral suspension. See the Marshall-Marchetti procedure (Chapter 14). Basic steps of the procedure follow.

1. Through a suprapubic abdominal incision the space of Retzius is entered, and the bladder and urethra are freed from the underlying structures.
2. Mattress sutures are inserted through the perivaginal fas-

BOX 13-1

Algorithm Recommendations for Treatment of Female Stress Incontinence

In a broad-based review of the literature, the Agency for Health Care Policy and Research (AHCPR) concluded that the following steps be implemented in making decisions regarding treatment of female stress incontinence:

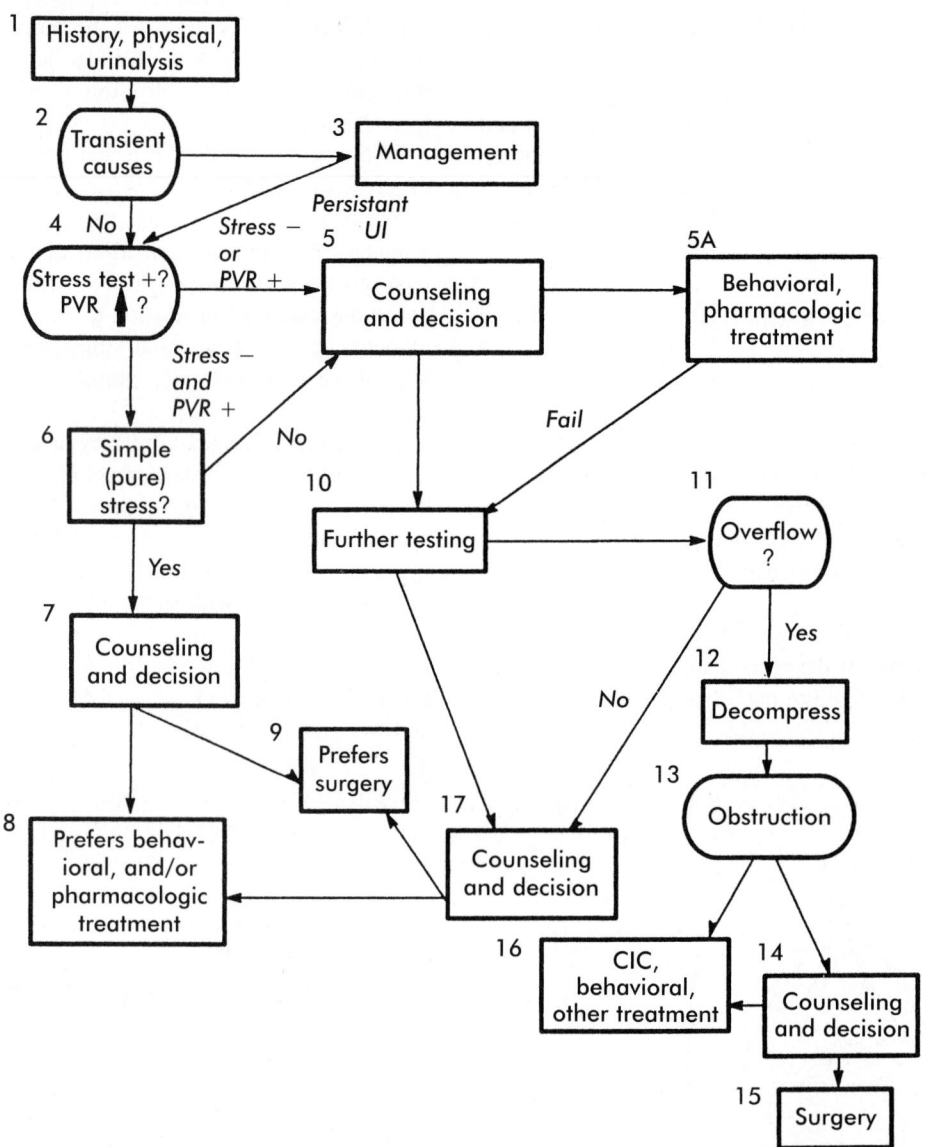

1. History, physical, and urinalysis.
2 and 3. Transient causes are identified and managed. If UI persists, go to node 4.
4. Provocative stress testing and measurement or estimation of postvoid residual (PVR) volume should be performed at this point.

Possibilities include:
• Stress test positive for leakage and PVR normal— simple stress (pure), go to node 6.
• Abnormal PVR regardless of stress test result—not simple stress, mixed stress and urge symptoms, go to node 5.
• Stress test negative and PVR normal, go to node 5.

Urinary Incontinence Guideline Panel. (1992). *Urinary incontinence in adults: Clinical practice guideline.* AHCPR Pub. No. 92-0038. Rockville, Md: Agency for Health Care Policy and Research, Public Health Service, U.S. Department of Health and Human Services.

BOX 13-1

Algorithm Recommendations for Treatment of Female Stress Incontinence—cont'd

STRESS URINARY INCONTINENCE OTHER THAN SIMPLE

5. After stress testing and PVR estimation/measurement, all patients except those with simple stress UI will need further counseling and evaluation of disposition. The types of patients that will be encountered include:
   - Stress test negative and PVR normal
   - Stress test positive and PVR normal and symptoms are mixed/other/not simple stress UI
   - PVR elevated regardless of stress test result or symptom
   - Anatomically reversible condition including prolapsing cystocele, rectocele, enterocele, or uterus

5A. Stress test negative and PVR normal

If the symptom of stress UI is simple and the PVR volume is low but incontinence cannot be documented with the stress test, the patient can be counseled either for a trial of behavioral therapy and/or pharmacologic treatment. Perform further testing if the initial therapy is not preferred or has failed.

Stress test positive and PVR normal and symptoms are mixed/other/not simple stress

If the patient has mixed symptoms (stress/urge) or other symptoms and the stress test is positive and the PVR is low, the patient can be counseled for either trial of behavioral or pharmacologic therapy or surgical therapy. Further testing is recommended for patients who already failed initial therapeutic trial or have other comorbid conditions complicating the UI symptom.

PVR abnormal

If the PVR is elevated regardless of the symptoms (simple stress UI, complex or mixed), further testing is recommended.

SIMPLE (PURE) STRESS URINARY INCONTINENCE

6. Simple stress urinary incontinence is defined as follows:
   - Urine loss only with physical exertion (history and stress test)
   - Normal voiding habits (less than or equal to 8×/d and no more than 2× at night)
   - No neurologic history or neurologic findings
   - No prior antiincontinence or radical pelvic surgery
   - Pelvic examination documenting hypermobility of the urethra and bladder neck, pliable and compliant vaginal wall, and adequate vaginal capacity
   - PVR normal
   - Not pregnant

Any patient with stress incontinence who fails any of these criteria will be considered not to have simple or pure stress UI; go to node 5.

7. Patients with simple stress UI may be counseled regarding behavioral, pharmacologic, and surgical treatment options.
8. Treatment. If the patient prefers behavioral therapy, the recommended techniques are pelvic muscle exercises or bladder training with or without biofeedback and/or vaginal cones.

   If the patient prefers pharmacologic therapy, the recommended agent is an alpha-adrenergic agent. For women with vaginal atrophy, a trial of estrogen therapy may be initiated alone or in combination with an alpha agonist.
9. In patients with simple stress incontinence who prefer surgery, preoperative evaluation should include a comprehensive history, physical examination, urinalysis, urine culture, and PVR volume measurement. Document incontinence directly (positive stress test). For further corroboration, cystoscopy, cystogram with straining, Valsalva leak point pressure, and/or dynamic urethral profilometry may be used. The goal of surgical intervention in this case is to correct urethral hypermobility.

Anatomically reversible conditions such as prolapsing cystocele, uterine prolapse, etc.

If an anatomically reversible condition is present, see the algorithm for urge UI (node 8).
10. Numerous specialized diagnostic tests are available, and the choice of tests must be tailored to the question to be answered.

    Tests for bladder and urethral function include filling cystometry, stress cystourethrogram, dynamic profilometry or Valsalva leak-point pressure, pressure flow, and/or cystoscopy. Tests should be performed according to the need of the patient as described below.

Suspected condition	Recommended test
Unstable bladder	Filling cystometry
Stress UI	Dynamic profilometry or Valsalva leak-point pressure and/or stress cystourethrogram or videourodynamics
Overflow UI	Voiding cystometrogram (pressure flow study), cystoscopy, and/or stress cystourethrogram; videourodynamics is another option

11. If overflow incontinence is found, the patient will need counseling regarding initial decompression of the bladder.
12. Decompression of the bladder may be accomplished with either intermittent self-catheterization or indwelling Foley catheter.

Continued.

Algorithm Recommendations for Treatment of Female Stress Incontinence—cont'd

13. Obstruction in women, as diagnosed in node 10, is usually due either to an anatomically reversible condition or to postsurgical obstruction of the urethra.
14. If the patient is a good surgical risk and is willing to undergo surgery, relief of obstruction is an option with the risk of recurrent stress UI. If the patient is a poor risk or prefers nonsurgical therapy, then clean intermittent catheterization (CIC) and other nonsurgical treatments should be instituted.
15. The patient should be counseled regarding the procedure for repair of the prolapse or relief of postsurgical urethral obstruction and told whether suspension of the bladder neck will be performed.
16. If there is no obstruction, as determined in node 10, and the patient has an acontractile or underactive detrusor, or if obstructed and the patient is either not a

surgical candidate or prefers nonsurgical treatment, counseling regarding the use of CIC, behavioral voiding techniques, use of pessary, etc., is necessary. If bladder neck suspension is a consideration in the face of persistent abnormal residual volume, the patient must be counseled that persistent retention may result after the suspension procedure.

17. If the patient is found to have no overflow incontinence in node 10, the specific condition identified after testing and the patient preference will determine treatment option. Options include behavioral, pharmacologic, and surgical treatment. For surgical treatment of intrinsic sphincter deficiency (ISD), recommend bulking technique, sling, or artificial urinary sphincter. If hypermobility is found, see node 7.

cia on either side of the vesicourethral angle area and preferably at a right angle to the long axis of the urethra and bladder. These are then passed through the central portion of the undersurface of the symphysis pubis under direct vision. The application of the sutures to the perivaginal connective tissue is done with the surgeon's hand in the vagina to ensure that the suture material is not passed through the vaginal mucosa (see Figs. 13-2 and 13-4).

3. The wound is closed and may be drained if the vascularity of the area warrants. An abdominal dressing is applied.

Excision of fibroma of the vagina

Excision of fibroma of the vagina involves the removal of the lesion through a transverse or longitudinal incision of the vaginal wall. Small cysts or small benign tumors that distort the vagina or those that are ulcerated and infected are treated surgically.

Procedural considerations

A dilatation and curettage set is required, plus six Halsted mosquito hemostats.

Operative procedure

1. The vaginal vault is retracted with lateral retractors. Sutures may be placed on each side of the tumor. The posterior lip of the cervix is grasped with a tenaculum and is drawn anterior to expose the operative site.
2. The vaginal wall is incised, and the edges are grasped with traction sutures on curved, taper-point needles or with Allis forceps.
3. The base and its capsule are excised with a knife and curved scissors; bleeding vessels are clamped with Hal-

sted mosquito hemostats and ligated with fine sutures.
4. The vaginal incision is closed with interrupted sutures.

Construction of a vagina

Two basic approaches are used for repairing or overcoming a congenital or surgical defect of the vagina: obtaining a skin graft, which is applied to a mold and placed in the area of vaginal reconstruction, and a simple opening of the area of vaginal reconstruction and the placing of a mold to permit the spontaneous epithelialization of the area.

Procedural considerations

For a skin graft the plastic local instrument set (see Chapter 23) is required, plus the following:

Dermatome of choice
Marking pen
Nonadherent gauze
　dressing

For vaginal construction the basic vaginal instrument set is required, plus the following:

2 Iris scissors, 1 straight and 1 curved, 4½ inches	12 Halsted mosquito hemostats, 6 straight and 6 curved, 5 inches
2 Skin hooks	
Vaginal mold	Ruler

Operative procedure

1. The skin graft is taken from the abdomen or anterior thigh. The donor site is dressed in the routine manner with nonadherent gauze and a pressure dressing.
2. The skin graft is kept in a moist gauze sponge until it is ready to be used.
3. A vaginal orifice is created by sharp dissection. Great

care must be taken to prevent damage to the rectum and bladder. A mold is used to apply the donor skin or simply to hold the dissected area open to permit spontaneous epithelialization.

Trachelorrhaphy

Trachelorrhaphy is removal of torn surfaces of the anterior and posterior cervical lips and reconstruction of the cervical canal. It is performed to treat deep lacerations of a cervix that is relatively free from infection.

Procedural considerations

The basic vaginal instrument set is required, plus a conization loop electrode, if desired. An indwelling urinary catheter may be inserted in the bladder, depending on the surgeon's preference.

Operative procedure

1. The labia may be retracted with Allis-Adair tissue forceps or sutures. The cervix is grasped with a tenaculum.
2. The infected tissue of the exocervix is denuded with a knife. The flaps are undermined by means of a knife and curved scissors. Bleeding vessels are clamped and ligated. The mucosa is dissected from the cervix.
3. A small distal portion of the cervical canal is coned with a knife or a loop electrode to remove infected tissue. Bleeding vessels are clamped and ligated.
4. The denuded and coned areas are covered by transversely suturing the mucosal flaps of the exocervix, using interrupted sutures. Tissue forceps, hemostats, and gauze sponges are needed. The sutures are placed in such a manner that the fibromuscular tissue of the cervix is included, thereby eliminating dead space where a hematoma may form and providing a complete reconstructed cervical canal.
5. A vaginal pack may be inserted.

Dilatation of the cervix and curettage

In this procedure instruments are introduced through the vagina for the purpose of dilating the cervix to permit evacuation of uterine contents or scraping of the endometrium. Dilatation of the cervix can also take place by inserting laminaria tents into the cervical os before surgery; these tents are removed immediately before the procedure.

Dilatation and curettage are done either for diagnostic purposes or as a form of therapy for a variety of pelvic conditions such as incomplete abortion, therapeutic abortion, abnormal uterine bleeding, or primary dysmenorrhea. Dilatation and curettage may also be performed when carcinoma of the endometrium is suspected, in the study of infertility, or before amputation of the cervix or an operation for prolapse of the uterus.

Procedural considerations

The dilatation and curettage set includes the following:

Exposing instruments

2 Jackson vaginal retractors
1 Sims vaginal retractor
1 Auvard vaginal speculum, weighted (see Fig. 13-10)
2 Deaver retractors

1 Uterine sound, graduated (see Fig. 13-11)
1 Set Hegar or Hank uterine dilators (see Fig. 13-11)
1 Goodell uterine dilator (see Fig. 13-11)

Holding instruments

2 Barrett tenaculum forceps (see Fig. 13-9)
1 Jacobs vulsellum forceps (see Fig. 13-9)
2 Foerster sponge-holding forceps
1 Bozeman dressing forceps (see Fig. 13-9)
1 Fletcher-Van Doren polyp forceps

2 Backhaus towel clamps, 5¼ inches
1 Tissue forceps with 1 × 2 teeth, 5½ inches
1 Russian tissue forceps, 8 inches
1 Dressing forceps, 7¼ inches
2 Allis forceps, 6 inches

Cutting instruments

1 Bard-Parker knife handle no. 3 with blade no. 10
2 Mayo dissecting scissors, 1 curved and 1 straight, 6¾ inches
1 Set Sims uterine curettes, sharp (see Fig. 13-8)

1 Set Thomas uterine curettes, blunt (see Fig. 13-8)
1 Heaney uterine curette
1 Gaylor biopsy forceps (see Fig. 13-8)

Clamping instruments

2 Crile hemostats, 5½ inches

2 Pean forceps, 6¼ inches

Suturing instruments

1 Mayo-Hegar needle holder, 8 inches

Suture of surgeon's preference, if desired

Accessory items

1 Urethral catheter, 16 or 18 Fr
1 Telfa dressing
1 Ampule oxytocic drug, if desired

Iodoform or plain gauze packing, as desired
Vaginal gauze packing, as desired

Operative procedure

1. A Jackson or Auvard retractor is placed posterior in the vagina. A Sims or Deaver retractor is placed anterior to expose the cervix. The anterior lip of the cervix is grasped with a tenaculum (Fig. 13-24).
2. The direction of the cervical canal and the depth of the uterine cavity are determined by means of a blunt probe or graduated uterine sound.
3. The cervix is gradually dilated by means of graduated

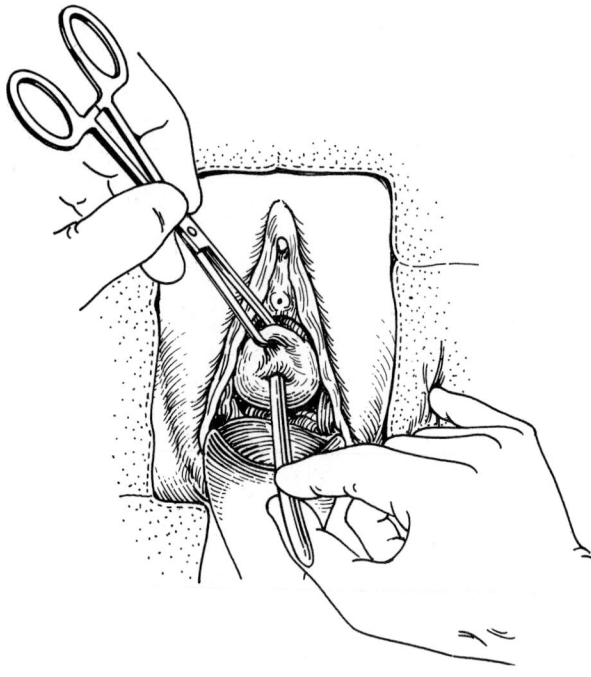

FIG. 13-24   Dilatation of cervix and curettage. Vaginal wall retracted; cervix held by tenaculum; cervix dilated with dilator. Uterine cavity curetted with sharp curettes.

From Ball, T.L. (1963). *Gynecologic surgery and urology* (2nd Ed.). St. Louis: Mosby.

Hegar or Hank dilators and possibly a Goodell uterine dilator.

4. Exploration for pedunculated polyps or myomas may be done with a polyp forceps.
5. The interior of the cervical canal and the cavity of the uterus are curetted to obtain either a fractional or a routine specimen. For specific identification of the site of specimens, the endocervix is scraped with the curette first, and the specimen is separated from the curettings of the uterine endometrium. In a routine curettage, all curettings are sent together for identification of tissue cells.
6. Fragments of endometrium or other dislodged tissues may be removed with warm, moist gauze sponges on sponge-holding forceps or with a teaspoon, and are then collected on Telfa.
7. Multiple-punch biopsies of the cervical circumference (at the 3, 6, 9, and 12 o'clock positions) may be taken with the Gaylor biopsy forceps to supplement the diagnostic studies.
8. Retractors are withdrawn; iodoform or plain gauze packing may be inserted into the uterus, using dressing forceps. The tenaculum is removed from the cervix. A vaginal pack may be inserted.

Suction curettage

Suction curettage is vacuum aspiration of the uterine contents. Aspiration has proved to be a safe and effective method for early termination of pregnancy and for use in missed and incomplete spontaneous abortions. Advantages are smaller dilatation of the cervix, less damage to the uterus, less blood loss, less chance of uterine perforation, and reduced danger of infection. Laminaria tents may be inserted approximately 4 to 24 hours before suction curettage to dilate the cervix.

Procedural considerations

The instrumentation required includes the dilatation and curettage set, plus the following:

1 Set of Pratt or Hawkin or Hank uterine dilators	Sterile cannulas, desired sizes
1 Placenta forceps, if desired	Aspirator tubing
	Vacuum aspirator unit
1 Urethral catheter, 16 or 18 Fr	Oxytocic drugs

Operative procedure

1. The cervix is exposed with an Auvard weighted speculum and an anterior retractor; then the cervix is grasped with a sharp tenaculum and is drawn toward the introitus.
2. The laminaria tents are removed, and the cervix can be further dilated in the routine manner, allowing 1 mm of cannula diameter for each week of pregnancy.
3. The appropriate size cannula is inserted into the uterus until the sac is encountered. The suction is turned on with immediate disruption and aspiration of the contents. Continued gentle motion of the cannula removes the uterine contents (Fig. 13-25). Use of uterine curettes may supplement suction in removing the entire uterine contents.
4. Retractors and tenaculum are removed.
5. The specimen, contained in the suction bottle, is removed for pathologic examination.

Removal of pedunculated cervical myoma

Cervical polyps (small pedunculated lesions) stem from the endocervical canal and consist almost entirely of columnar epithelium with or without squamous metaplasia. They may vary in size and are soft, red, and friable. Bleeding may result from the slightest trauma. Pedunculated lesions may be removed by the snare method or by dissection from the cervical canal with a knife, cold-knife conization, or resectoscope. Usually the surgeon performs an endometrial and endocervical curettage, and a cytologic smear is taken.

Procedural considerations

A dilatation and curettage set, a tonsil snare with medium snare wire, glass slides, an electrosurgical unit and a blade electrode or resectoscope are required.

Operative procedure

1. The anterior lip of the cervix is grasped with a Jacobs

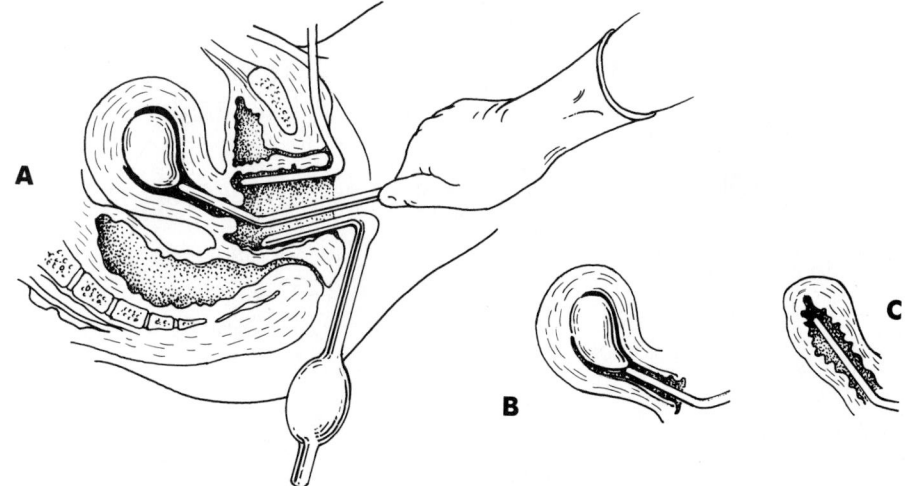

FIG. 13-25   Suction curettage. **A,** Insertion of cannula. **B,** Gentle suction motion to aspirate contents. **C,** Uterine contents evacuated.

vulsellum forceps or a tenaculum. The canal is sounded and dilated either to visualize or palpate the base of the pedicle.

2. If the pedicle of the tumor is thin, a tonsil snare may be placed over the body of the tumor, permitting the snare to crush the base of the tumor and to control bleeding. If the tumor is large, its base is dissected out with a knife. Bleeding may be controlled by the use of warm, moist gauze sponges and/or electrocoagulation. A resectoscope with the use of electrosurgery may be used to dissect the tumor.

3. Iodoform or plain gauze packing may be introduced into the cervical os. The tenaculum is removed from the cervix, and the retractors are withdrawn. A vaginal pack may be inserted for hemostasis.

Shirodkar operation (postconceptional)

Incompetence of the cervix is a condition characterized by habitual midtrimester spontaneous abortions. Surgical intervention is designed to prevent cervical dilatation that results in release of uterine contents. The postconceptional Shirodkar operation is placement of a collar-type ligature of Mersilene, Dacron tape, heavy nylon suture, or plastic-covered braided-steel suture at the level of the internal os to close it (Fig. 13-26).

Procedural considerations

Gentle vaginal preparation is carried out. The instrumentation includes the basic vaginal instrument set, plus the following:

2 Deschamps ligature carriers, right and left	Sutures as noted plus the surgeon's preference for closure of mucosa
2 Trocar needles	

Operative procedure

1. Anterior and posterior vaginal retractors are placed, and the cervix is pulled down with smooth ovum or sponge-holding forceps. With smooth tissue forceps and dissecting scissors, the mucosa over the anterior cervix is opened to permit the bladder to be pushed back (see Fig. 13-26).

2. The cervix is lifted, and the posterior vaginal mucosa is similarly incised at the level of the peritoneal reflection. The corners of the anterior and posterior incisions are bilaterally approximated in the area of the lateral mucosa with curved tonsil or Allis forceps.

3. The prepared ligature is placed at the desired level by passage of the material through the approximated tissue and is drawn tight posteriorly to close the cervix. The suture material for the ligature is then tied. It is not necessary to suture the ligature to the underlying tissues. The suture material used for this ligation is 5-mm Dacron or Mersilene tape. The anterior and posterior mucosal incisions are usually closed with absorbable no. 2-0 suture to complete the procedure.

Conization and biopsy of the cervix

Diseased cervical tissue is removed to treat strictures of the cervix, chronic cervicitis, epithelial dysplasia, and carcinoma in situ. The conization may be performed by scalpel, electrosurgery, or laser. The laser may be used to treat severe dysplasia and carcinoma in situ.

Endometrial biopsy is done to determine the menstrual phase and carry out histologic study of the endometrium. Conizations are done for diagnostic purposes, such as when a patient has a positive Papanicolaou (Pap) smear. Conization of the cervix, instead of hysterectomy, may be done in some cases to preserve reproductive function. It may also

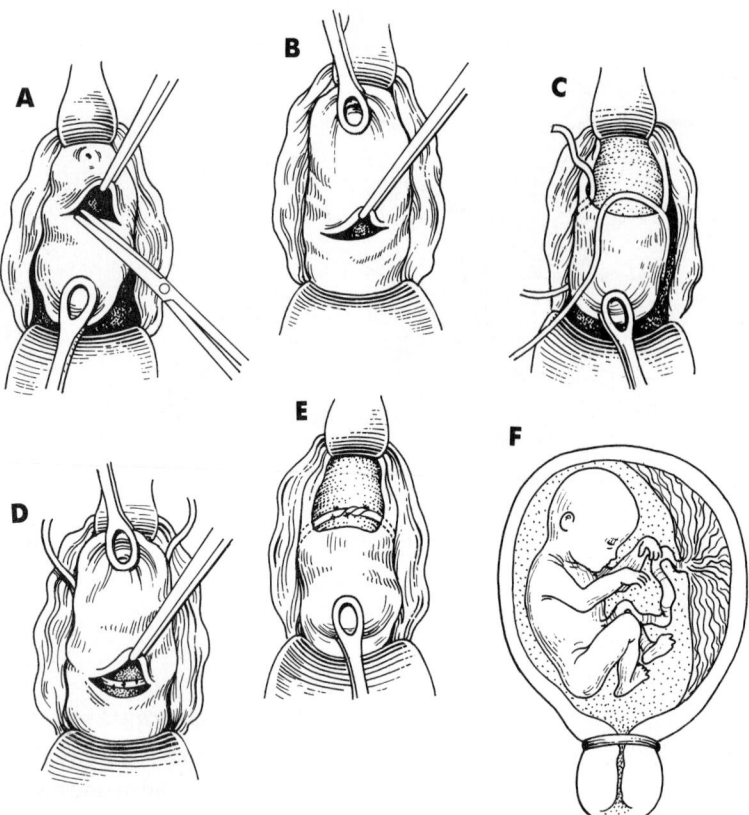

FIG. 13-26   Principles of Shirodkar operation for treatment of incompetent internal cervical os during pregnancy.

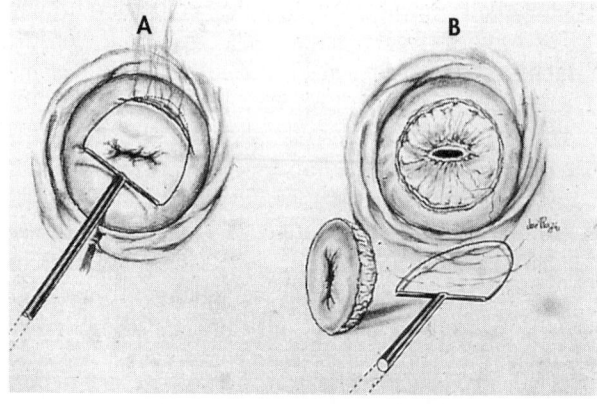

FIG. 13-27   The electrical loop (0.2 mm) vaporizes across at 1.5- to 2-cm front; therefore it cuts more rapidly than a laser.

From Nichols, D.H. (editor). (1993). *Gynecologic and obstetric surgery.* St. Louis: Mosby.

be done for benign or malignant diseases of the cervix and in cases in which total hysterectomy is not feasible. The loop electrical excision cone (LEEC) (Fig. 13-27) and the laser excisional cone (Fig. 13-28) appear to provide an adequate histologic specimen while promoting hemostasis and possibly eradicating the disease process.

Procedural considerations

The instruments required include a dilatation and curettage set. An electrosurgical unit or laser, conization electrical loop, and ball-tip electrodes may be indicated.

Operative procedure

1. The posterior vaginal wall is retracted by a speculum and the anterior vaginal wall by lateral retractors. The outer portions of the cervix are grasped with a tenaculum, and the cervix is drawn toward the introitus. Cystic areas of the cervix may be treated with a needle electrode or laser. Endometrial biopsy may be done (Fig. 13-29, *A*). Bleeding points are coagulated or lasered.
2. For cauterization the electrode is passed into the cervical canal, and the diseased tissue is treated. Ferrous subsulfate (Monsel's solution) may be used for hemostasis.
3. The electrical loop (Fig. 13-29, *B* and *C*) or the laser may be used to remove the diseased tissue and provide a histologic specimen, which is sent to the pathology lab for examination.
4. If a wide conization is performed, the cervix may be sutured and vaginal packing may be used. An indwelling urinary catheter may be inserted.

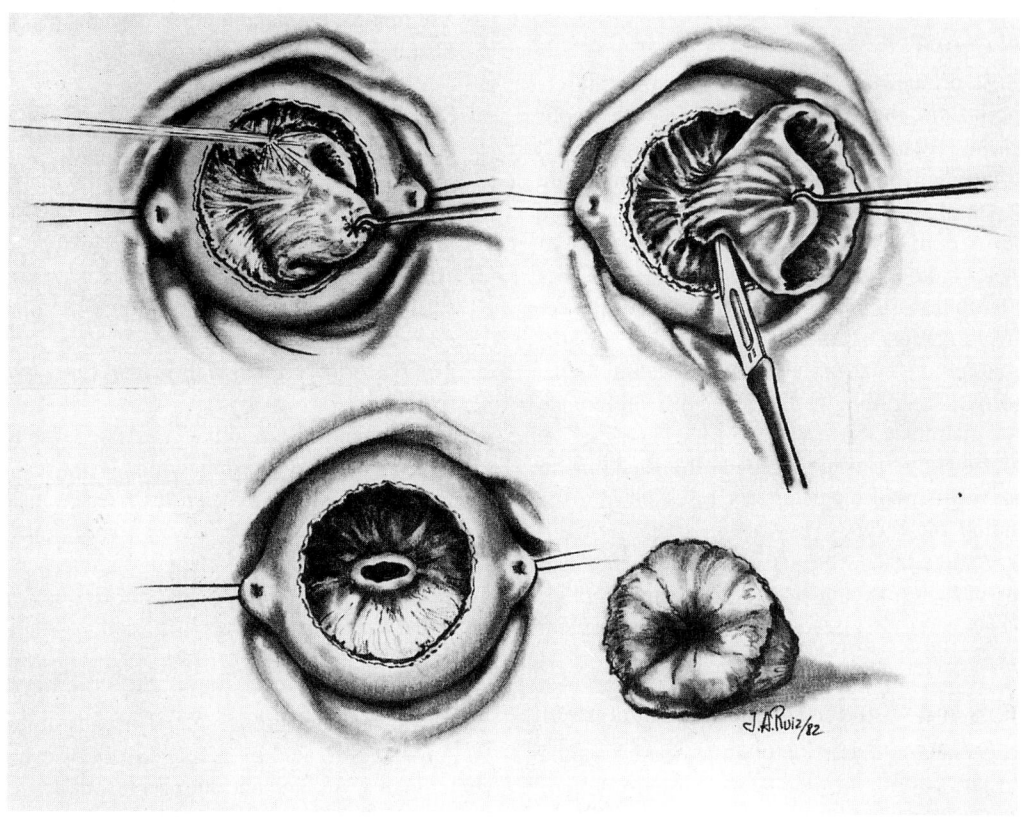

FIG. 13-28 The laser creates a 0.3- to 0.5-mm spot, which cuts as it is swept across the tissue plane. A hook provides traction as the laser cuts and permits shaping of the cone.

From Nichols, D.H. (editor). (1993). *Gynecologic and obstetric surgery*. St. Louis: Mosby.

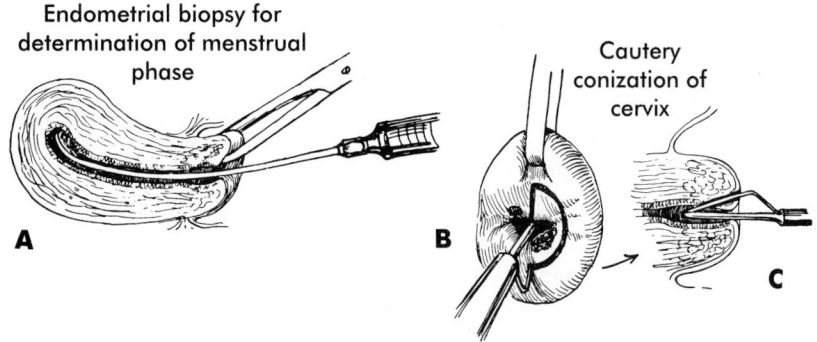

Endometrial biopsy for determination of menstrual phase

Cautery conization of cervix

A

B

C

FIG. 13-29 **A,** Endometrial biopsy technique. **B** and **C,** Methods of treating cervical conditions or obtaining specimens for diagnostic tests.

Modified from Ball, T.L. (1963). *Gynecologic surgery and urology* (2nd Ed.). St. Louis: Mosby.

Cesium insertion for cervical and endometrial malignancy

Cesium has generally replaced radium insertions for treatment of malignancy of the cervix and endometrium.

Procedural considerations

The patient is brought to the operating room for insertion of the applicators; the cesium is loaded into the applicators later in the radiation department, or in the patient's room under controlled conditions in which all personnel are monitored by use of a dosimeter.

The bladder is drained with an indwelling urinary catheter. The catheter balloon is inflated with a radiopaque medium for radiographic visualization after insertion of the cesium. An indwelling rectal marker is also placed by the surgeon for radiographic visualization. Various cesium applicators may be used according to the surgeon's preference and the area of malignancy.

Interstitial therapy. Cesium needles are available in various lengths with small diameters for insertion into the tissue surrounding the cervix. They are inserted vaginally with a needle applicator and are used as a supplement to intravaginal or intrauterine sources. To facilitate removal, the needles have wires or threads attached to their distal ends.

Culdocentesis and posterior colpotomy (culdotomy)

Needle culdocentesis is insertion of an aspirating needle through the posterior fornix of the vagina. Posterior colpotomy (culdotomy) is incision through the vagina and peritoneum into the cul-de-sac.

Diagnostic needle culdocentesis is done to diagnose ectopic pregnancy and to detect intraperitoneal bleeding or cul-de-sac hematoma. This procedure is rarely done today as a result of advancements in diagnostic laparoscopy. Posterior colpotomy can be done to carry out definitive operative procedures: various kinds of tubal ligations, aspiration or the removal of ovarian cysts, the occasional management of an ectopic pregnancy, and exploratory diagnostic operative procedures.

Procedural considerations

The basic vaginal instrument set is required, plus the following:

1 Needle, 15 gauge, 3½ inches	2 Culture tubes
1 Syringe	2 Drains, if desired

An abdominal gynecologic instrument set should be available in case laparotomy is indicated.

Operative procedures
Needle culdocentesis

1. A 15-gauge needle attached to a syringe is inserted through the posterior fornix of the vagina. Suspected intraperitoneal bleeding is confirmed if dark or red blood flows freely into the syringe. Failure to obtain blood does not rule out the possibility of intraperitoneal bleeding.
2. Bleeding of the vaginal wall is controlled by sutures. Vaginal packing and an indwelling urinary catheter may also be used.

Posterior colpotomy

1. A transverse incision is made through the posterior vaginal wall with curved scissors. This incision is carried into the peritoneum, behind the cervix at the superior point of the posterior fornix.
2. Allis forceps are used to facilitate exposure, and hemostasis is obtained by placing a number of sutures in the corners or angles of the wound.
3. The posterior vaginal wall is held open with a weighted retractor.
4. In case of infection in the cul-de-sac, the opening is enlarged enough to permit drainage from the cul-de-sac. The cavity is explored; drains may be inserted.
5. Bleeding of the vaginal wall is controlled by sutures. The peritoneum and the vaginal mucosa are closed with a continuous suture. Vaginal packing and an indwelling urinary catheter may also be used.

Marsupialization of Bartholin's duct cyst or abscess

A cyst in a Bartholin's gland usually follows acute infection and is treated by marsupialization when it is quiescent. Such cysts are not neoplastic but result from retention of glandular secretions caused by blockage somewhere in the duct system. Marsupialization of Bartholin's duct cyst or abscess entails removal or incision of the cyst through the vaginal outlet and drainage of the area. In true marsupialization the cyst is surgically exteriorized by resecting the anterior wall and suturing the cut edges of the remaining cyst to the adjacent edges of the skin.

Procedural considerations

The basic vaginal instrument set is required, plus the following:

1 Needle, 15 gauge, 3½ inches	Iodoform or plain gauze packing
1 Syringe	1 Drain, if desired
2 Culture tubes (aerobic and anaerobic)	

Operative procedure

1. The labia minora may be sutured to the perineal skin on each side to expose the vaginal introitus.
2. An elliptic incision is made in the mucosa, which is distended over the cyst.
3. The cyst wall is dissected, and, if indicated, removal of the gland is completed with blunt-pointed scissors. The tissue may be everted with sutures and left open. A drain or packing may be inserted, and a dressing is applied.

Hysteroscopy

Hysteroscopy is endoscopic visualization of the uterine cavity and tubal orifices. A fiberoptic hysteroscope is introduced vaginally and aids in the diagnosis and treatment of intrauterine disease. The common indications for hysteroscopy include evaluation of abnormal uterine bleeding, with possible endometrial ablation, location and removal of "lost" intrauterine devices (IUDs), evaluation of infertility, diagnosis and surgical treatment of intrauterine adhesions, verification of submucous leiomyomas or endometrial polyps, resection of uterine septa or submucous leiomyomas, and tubal sterilization. Laparoscopy may be done in association with hysteroscopy to assess the external contour of the uterus. Contraindications to either diagnostic or operative hysteroscopy include pelvic infection, cervical malignancy, and in some instances heavy bleeding.

Procedural considerations

The instrumentation required includes a dilatation and curettage set, plus the following:

1 Hysteroscopy set
(Fig. 13-30)
2 Syringes, 50 ml
Polyethylene tubing
Fiberoptic light source
Electrosurgical unit, if
desired

Laser, if desired
Hysteroscopic insufflator, if desired
Hysteroscopic pump, if
desired
Video camera and monitor, if desired

Operative procedure

1. The cervix is exposed with an Auvard weighted speculum and an anterior retractor; the anterior lip of the cervix is grasped with a tenaculum and is drawn toward the introitus.
2. The direction of the cervical canal and the depth of the uterine cavity are determined by means of a graduated uterine sound.
3. The endocervical canal is dilated by means of graduated Hegar or Hank uterine dilators to 6, 7, or 8 mm, depending on the size of the hysteroscope.
4. A self-retaining vacuum cannula with obturator may be

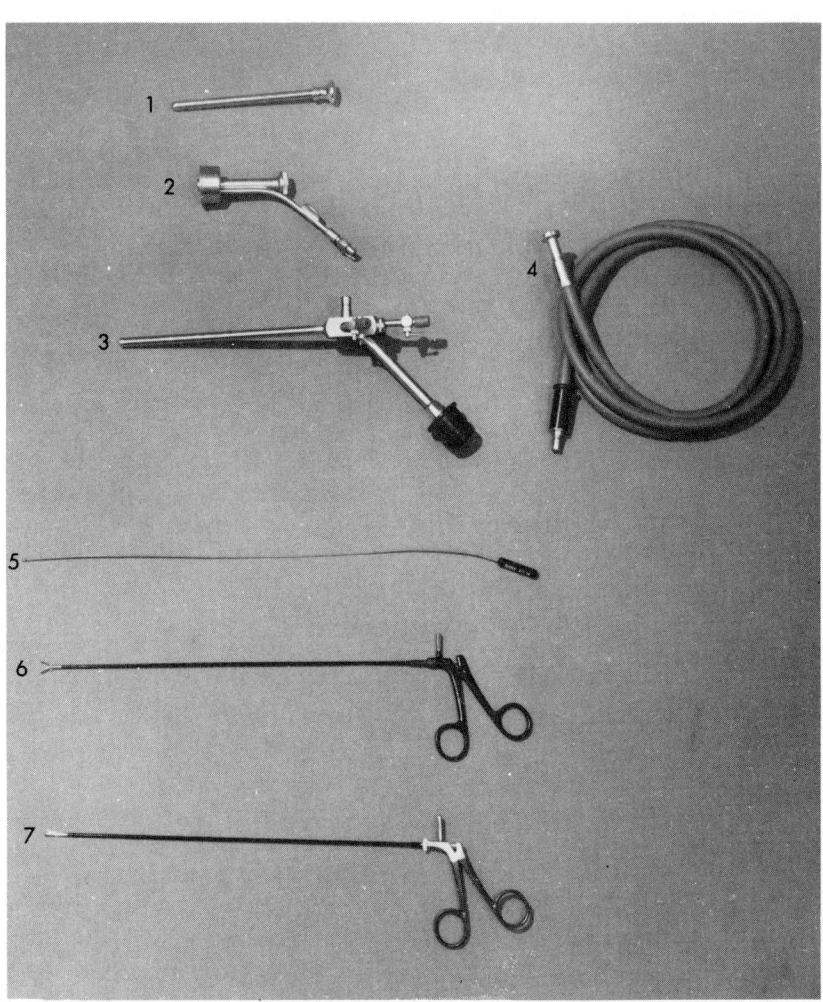

FIG. 13-30   Instruments for hysteroscopy. *1*, Obturator for cannula; *2*, self-retaining vacuum cannula, small; *3*, hysteroscope; *4*, fiberoptic light cord; *5*, coagulation electrode; *6*, grasping forceps; *7*, scissors.

placed in contact with the cervix. The cannula is firmly applied to the cervix by vacuum created with a negative pressure.

5. The obturator is withdrawn and the hysteroscope is introduced to the level of the internal cervical os.

6. To achieve satisfactory visualization and sustained intrauterine pressure, the uterine cavity must be distended with one of the following media: 32% Dextran 70 in dextrose (Hyskon), dextrose 5% in water (D5W), or carbon dioxide gas insufflation. Air or gas used for uterine insufflation may result in gas or air embolism. Therefore CO_2 pressures must be monitored closely. Injection of 32% Dextran 70 in dextrose (Hyskon) may be under continuous pressure from a 50-ml syringe or delivered via the hysteroscopic pump into the irrigating channel of the hysteroscope. When the syringe is used, care must be taken to prevent air bubbles, which distort the view or could lead to air embolism. Uterine distention with D5W may be achieved by inserting a 500-ml plastic bag containing the medium into an intravenous pressure infusor or the hysteroscopic pump. The fluid runs freely via polyethylene tubing through the channel of the hysteroscope. However, a satisfactory hysteroscopy may not be done if bleeding occurs because D5W is miscible with blood. Distention with CO_2 is achieved by a controlled pressure system.

7. Exploration of the uterine cavity is begun. A video camera monitor may be used to enhance visibility for the OR team, and the procedure may be videotaped for record keeping and reevaluation.

8. Ancillary instruments such as rigid and flexible biopsy forceps, scissors, grasping forceps, insulated coagulation electrodes, resectoscope/"rollerball" electrode, laser fiber/tips, and tubal occlusive devices may be introduced for intrauterine manipulation or surgical intervention through the operating channel of the hysteroscope.

9. Upon completion of the procedure, the hysteroscope is withdrawn and the self-retaining vacuum cannula is removed.

10. If 32% Dextran 70 in dextrose (Hyskon) is used for uterine distention, the instruments must be rinsed immediately and cleaned in hot water because Dextran has a tendency to harden and is difficult to remove if permitted to dry.

Endometrial ablation

Endometrial ablation is performed to treat abnormal uterine bleeding. The overall goal of endometrial ablation is to create amenorrhea or to reduce menstrual bleeding to a normal, tolerable flow for the patient (Research Highlight 13-1). It may be an alternative to hysterectomy in some patients with chronic menorraghia. Endometrial ablation may be performed after unsuccessful dilatation and curettage, or in conjunction with it. This procedure is performed through

---

⚛ RESEARCH HIGHLIGHT 13-1

In this study operative hysteroscopy was employed in over 1000 women (15% postmenopausal). Ninety percent of the premenopausal patients received some type of preoperative endometrial suppression. All patients had a laminaria tent placed prior to surgery. All surgery was performed under general anesthesia. Follow-up occurred from 6 months to 4 years. Success was based on patients' satisfaction with the overall results. In women with normal to slightly enlarged uteri (that is, in under 10 weeks), over 95% reported being satisfied. Complications in less than 0.05% were reported in this study. Success rates, however, cannot be determined until 2 years after the surgical intervention, since patients experience bleeding sometimes as late as 3 years after the procedure. As a result, operative hysteroscopy, when properly performed, is a safe, effective option for managing women with abnormal uterine bleeding.

Townsend, D.E., Fields, G.A., & McCausland, A.M. (1992). Operative hysteroscopy: Results in 1,000 patients. *American Association of Gynecologic Laparoscopists Annual Meeting Proceedings.*

the hysteroscope with the use of energy from either the laser or electrosurgical unit.

The Nd:YAG laser destroys the endometrium and results in scarring of the uterine lining. It is often the laser of choice for this procedure because of its ability to penetrate deep in the tissue, which results in greater tissue destruction. The Nd:YAG, argon, and KTP 532 lasers may be used hysteroscopically.

There are two endometrial ablation techniques when the Nd:YAG laser is used: blanching and dragging. In the blanching technique the tip of the laser fiber is held away from tissue. In the dragging technique the laser fiber tip is in direct contact with the endometrium. The endometrial lining is treated from the fundus to approximately 4 cm above the external cervical os. Air or gas is not used in cooling the laser fiber due to the risk of air or gas embolism. Because of the systemic effects of fluid absorption through open capillaries, 32% Dextran 70 in dextrose (Hyskon) is not generally used as an irrigant for endometrial laser ablation.

Electrical energy delivered through an adapted urologic resectoscope, using continuous flow irrigation, either coagulates or resects the endometrium. Endometrial ablation with the use of a resectoscope, with a rollerball electrode attached, is not an option for a patient who desires to remain fertile. When using the resectoscope, often 32% Dextran 70 in dextrose is chosen as the distending media, since it is electrolyte free and compatible with electrosurgery.

Reported complications associated with endometrial ablation using the Nd:YAG laser and electrosurgery have included hemorrhage, fluid overload, uterine perforation, recurrent bleeding, injury to bowel and bladder, cervical lacerations, and rupture of a fallopian tube.

The patient usually has general anesthesia, yet endometrial ablation can be performed using a local anesthetic. The patient is placed in the lithotomy position and all potential pressure points are padded. If the Nd:YAG laser is to be used, all laser safety precautions for the patient and the OR team are followed (see Chapter 31). If electrosurgery is being used for the procedure, an electrosurgical dispersive pad is applied. The length of the procedure is typically less than that for a hysterectomy. Therefore the patient requires less anesthesia and may be discharged the same day, provided her condition remains stable.

Vaginal hysterectomy

Vaginal hysterectomy is removal of the uterus through an incision made in the vaginal wall and the pelvic cavity. Contraindications to a vaginal approach are (1) when a large uterine tumor is present, (2) in pelvic malignancy because of an associated inflammatory process involving the fallopian tubes and ovaries, and (3) the possibility of missing metastatic disease that might be present.

Procedural considerations

The instrumentation includes the basic vaginal instrument set; two needles, 22 gauge, 1½ or 3 inches; and two syringes, 10 ml. An abdominal gynecologic instrument set should be available in case laparotomy is indicated. To facilitate dissection and decrease bleeding, the vaginal walls may be infiltrated with normal saline or a local anesthetic (vasoconstrictors are optional).

Operative procedure

1. The labia may be retracted with sutures. A vaginal retractor is inserted to retract the vaginal wall.
2. Dilatation and curettage may be performed, as previously described (see Fig. 13-24).
3. A Jacobs vulsellum forceps, tenaculum, or suture ligature is placed through the cervical lips to permit traction on the cervix (Fig. 13-31).
4. The vaginal wall is incised with a knife anteriorly through the full thickness of the wall. The bladder is freed from the anterior surface of the cervix by sharp and blunt dissection. The bladder is then elevated to expose the peritoneum of the anterior cul-de-sac, which is entered by sharp dissection (Fig. 13-31, *B*).
5. The peritoneum of the posterior cul-de-sac is identified and incised.
6. The uterosacral ligaments containing blood vessels are clamped, cut, and ligated (Fig. 13-31, *C* and *D*). The ends of the ligatures are left long and are tagged with a clamp.

7. The uterus is drawn downward and the bladder held aside with retractors and moist, small laparotomy packs.
8. The cardinal ligament on each side is clamped, cut, and ligated. The uterine arteries are doubly clamped, cut, and ligated.
9. The fundus is delivered with the aid of a uterine tenaculum.
10. When the ovaries are to be left, the round ligament, the uterovarian ligament, and the fallopian tube on each side are clamped together (Fig. 13-31, *E*) and cut, and the uterus is removed. These pedicles are then ligated.
11. The peritoneum between the rectum and vagina is approximated with a continuous suture. The retroperitoneal obliteration of the cul-de-sac is done by sutures that pass from the vaginal wall through the infundibulopelvic ligament and round ligament, through the cardinal ligament, and out the vaginal wall. The sutures are tied on the vaginal aspect of the new vault (Fig. 13-31, *F* and *G*). The round, cardinal, and ureterosacral ligaments may be individually approximated for additional support.
12. Any existing cystocele and rectocele and the perineum are repaired, as described for vaginal plastic repair (see Figs. 13-18 and 13-20). In the presence of prolapse, reconstruction of the pelvic floor may be required.
13. An indwelling urethral or suprapubic catheter is usually inserted. The vagina may be packed, and a drain may be inserted.

ABDOMINAL GYNECOLOGIC SURGERY
Laparoscopy

Laparoscopy is endoscopic visualization of the peritoneal cavity through the anterior abdominal wall after the establishment of a pneumoperitoneum. It is used in investigating and diagnosing the causes of abdominal and pelvic pain, determining causes of infertility, and evaluating pelvic masses. Ancillary procedures such as adhesiolysis, fulguration of endometriotic implants, aspiration of cysts, biopsy of tissue, aspiration of peritoneal fluid for cytologic study, and tubal sterilization may be performed. Laparoscopy also can be used for oocyte retrieval in in-vitro fertilization procedures. Lasers and electrosurgery may be used with the laparoscope.

Procedural considerations

A general or local anesthetic is administered. The patient is placed in lithotomy position. The abdomen, perineum, and vagina are prepped. The abdomen and perineum are then draped for a combined procedure. Specially designed drapes with openings for the umbilical and perineal areas may be used. The bladder should be emptied.

Dilatation and curettage may be done with laparoscopic procedures when indicated. After the cervix is exposed and the position and depth of the uterus are confirmed, Hulka

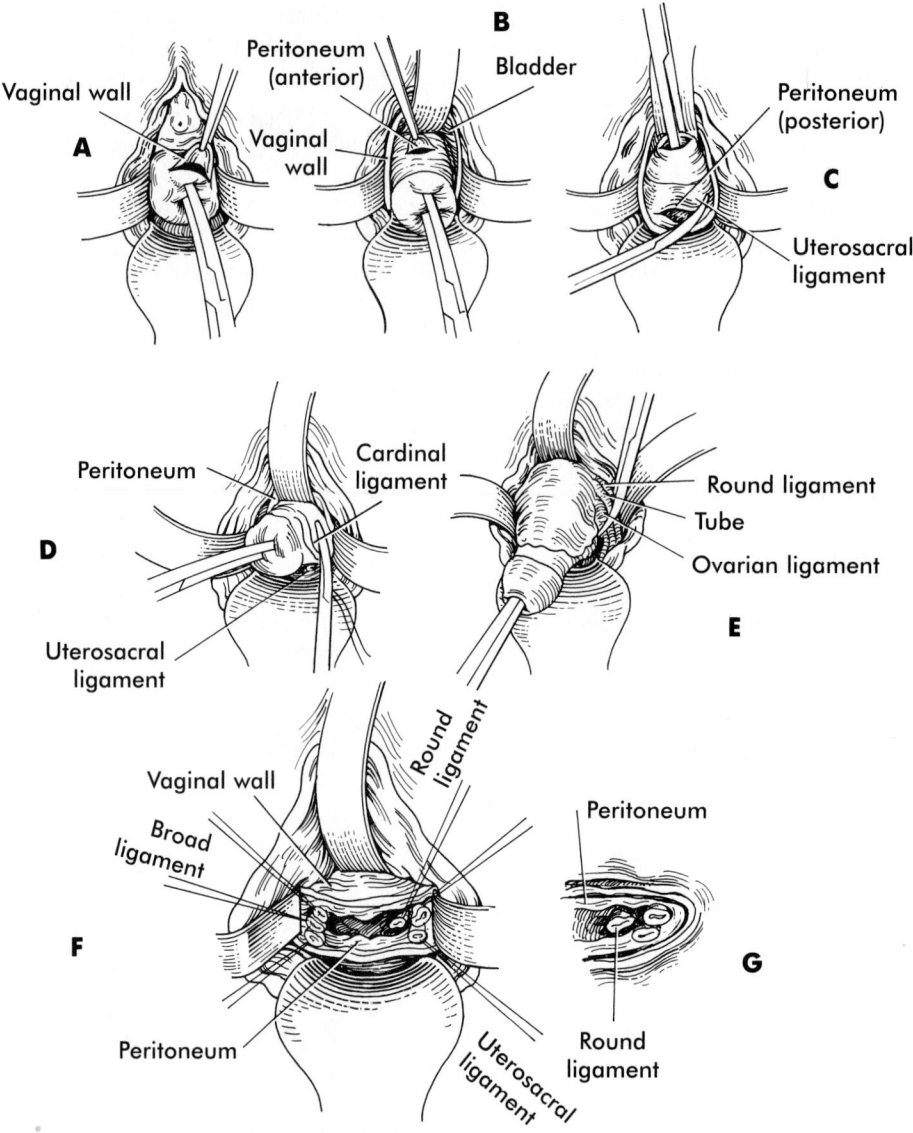

FIG. 13-31   Vaginal hysterectomy. **A,** Incision of vaginal wall around cervix. Anterior vaginal wall slightly elevated. **B,** Deaver retractor on each side; one Deaver retractor under bladder. Peritoneum opened. **C,** Posterior cul-de-sac opened. Heaney clamp applied to left uterosacral ligament. **D,** Left uterosacral ligament cut and tied. Clamp applied to left cardinal ligament. **E,** Clamp applied to ovarian ligament, round ligament, and fallopian tube. **F,** Uterosacral ligament, broad ligament, and round ligament shown in their respective normal positions. **G,** Peritoneum closed and cardinal broad ligament and uterosacral ligaments reattached to angle of vagina. Left uterosacral and broad ligaments anchored.

forceps or a uterine dilator may be introduced into the cervix to manipulate the uterus during the laparoscopy so that the surgeon has better visibility. If chromotubation to evaluate the patency of the fallopian tubes will be performed during the laparoscopy, an intrauterine cannula is placed in the cervical canal at the time of dilatation and curettage.

The usual instrumentation for the vaginal portion of the procedure includes a dilatation and curettage set, and the following may be indicated:

1 Hulka forceps
1 Intrauterine cannula
1 Syringe, 20 ml, if desired

Diluted methylene blue or indigo carmine solution, if desired

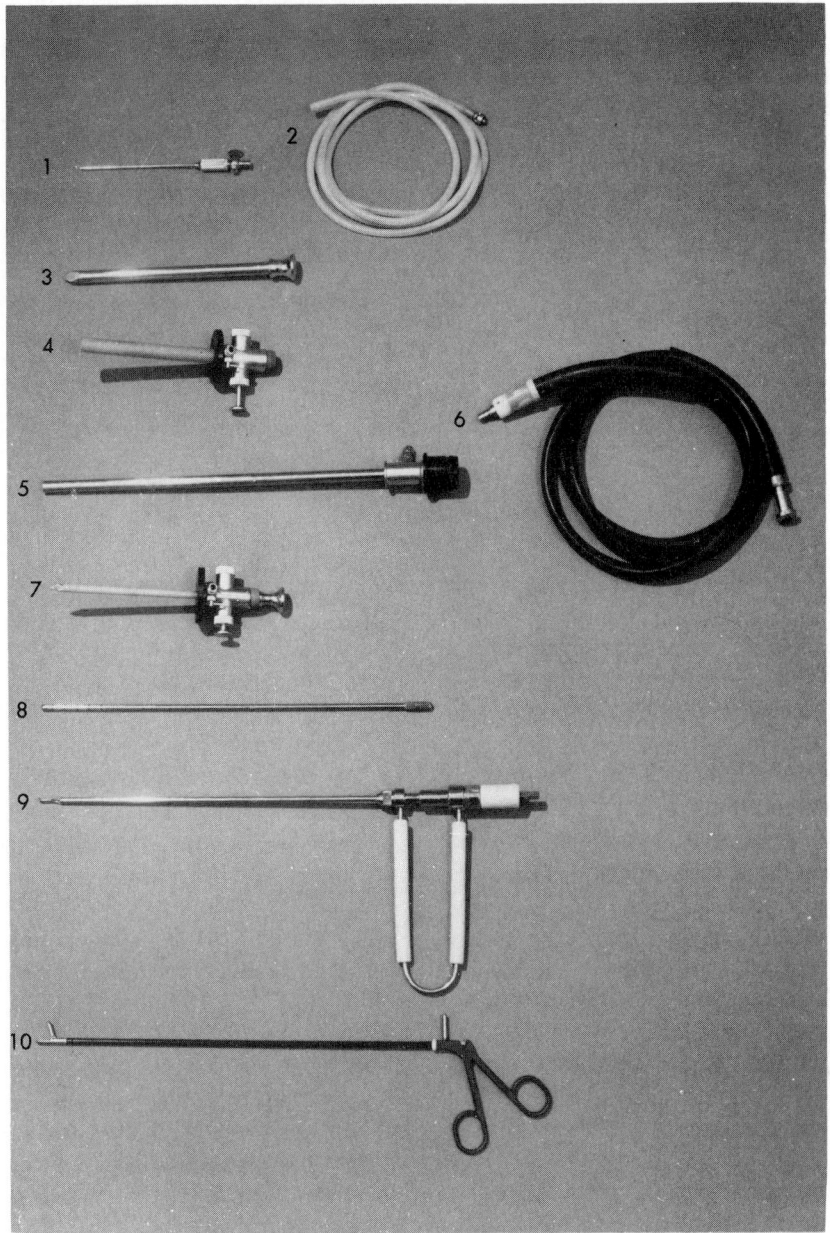

FIG. 13-32   Instruments for laparoscopy. *1,* Verres needle; *2,* Silastic tubing with connector; *3,* trocar with pyramidal tip; *4,* trocar sleeve with trumpet valve; *5,* laparoscope; *6,* fiberoptic light cord; *7,* secondary trocar sleeve and trocar; *8,* calibrated probe; *9,* bipolar forceps; *10,* biopsy forceps.

The setup for laparoscopy may include:

1 Laparoscopy set (Fig. 13-32)
1 Syringe, 10 ml
1 Bard-Parker no. 3 knife handle with blade no. 15 or 11
6 Backhaus towel clamps, 5¼ inches
2 Allis forceps, 6 inches

2 Crile hemostats, 5½ inches
1 Mayo-Hegar needle holder, 6 inches
1 Suture scissors
2 Adson forceps with teeth
2 Skin hooks, if desired
1 Suture for skin closure

Band-Aids, if desired
Steri-Strips, if desired
Electrosurgical unit
Fiberoptic light source
Gas insufflator for achieving pneumoperitoneum
Video camera/monitor system, if desired

Laser, if desired
Electrosurgical unit, if desired
Suction-irrigation-dissection system, if desired

An abdominal gynecologic instrument set should be readily available in the event that a laparotomy is indicated.

Common complications that may led to laparotomy are (1) perforation of hollow viscus, such as the intestine, (2) hemorrhage from a punctured vessel or biopsy site, (3) gas embolism from intravascular injection, and (4) burns of the bowel and abdominal wall.

Operative procedure

1. A small incision (0.7 to 1.2 cm) is made at the inferior margin of the umbilicus.
2. Elevating the skin with a towel clamp on either side of the umbilicus or grasping below the umbilicus with a gauze sponge for traction, the surgeon inserts a Verres needle through the layers of the abdominal wall into the peritoneal cavity.
3. Once the Verres needle is inserted into the peritoneal cavity, a 10-ml syringe partially filled with sterile saline is attached to the needle for aspiration. If the needle has entered a blood vessel, blood is aspirated. If a loop of intestine or the stomach has been entered, aspiration of bowel contents or malodorous gas occurs. If the needle is free in the peritoneal cavity, nothing is aspirated.
4. A plastic or Silastic tubing is attached to the Verres needle and the gas insufflator. Approximately 2 to 3 L of carbon dioxide or nitrous oxide gas are then delivered into the peritoneal cavity to achieve pneumoperitoneum. Carbon dioxide is commonly used as the insufflation medium because it is nontoxic, highly soluble in blood, and rapidly absorbed from the peritoneal cavity. The intraabdominal pressure must be closely monitored to prevent overdistention of the abdomen and to ensure free passage of gas into the peritoneal cavity.
5. After insufflation is completed, the Verres needle is withdrawn.
6. The trocar covered by the trocar sleeve is inserted boldly through the abdominal wall into the peritoneal cavity. The angle taken by the trocar is approximately 45 degrees toward the concavity of the pelvis. The plastic or Silastic tubing is attached to the trocar sleeve and insufflation is resumed. Some surgeons prefer a direct trocar insertion technique or open laparoscopy technique of Hassan to establish the pneumoperitoneum through the valve of the trocar sleeve rather than through a Verres needle.
7. With the trocar sleeve in place, the trocar is withdrawn and the laparoscope is introduced (Fig. 13-33). Visualization of the pelvis and lower abdomen and the visceral contents is begun. If the lens of the laparoscope becomes foggy, touching the lens to a loop of intestine is one method of clearing it. Before use, warming the tip of the scope in warm saline or towels may prevent fogging of the distal lens.
8. The patient is placed in Trendelenburg's position.
9. The video camera may be attached to the scope to aid in the OR team's visualization, and the procedure may

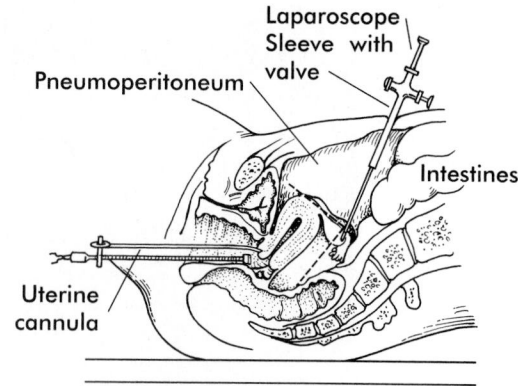

FIG. 13-33   Technique of laparoscopy.

be recorded for future reference. If an ancillary instrument such as biopsy forceps or bipolar forceps is needed, a second trocar with sleeve is inserted under direct laparoscopic visualization through an incision made suprapubically.

10. To test for tubal patency, diluted methylene blue or indigo carmine solution is injected through the intrauterine cannula in the cervical canal. If the fallopian tubes are patent, dye can be seen at the fimbriated ends.
11. On completion of the intraabdominal procedure, the laparoscope is withdrawn and the insufflated gas is allowed to escape from the trocar sleeve. The trocar sleeve is removed.
12. Application of skin clips or subcuticular closure of the primary skin incision is followed by placement of a Band-Aid or Steri-Strip.

PELVISCOPY

Pelviscopy is a fast-growing alternative to abdominal surgery for many procedures (Levine, 1990). Pelviscopic surgery has historically been utilized in treating infertility in younger women, yet now it is being used to benefit older women as well. Some benefits associated with pelviscopic surgery have been shown to be shorter hospital stay, decreased total cost, lower morbidity, and quicker return to full activity (Research Highlight 13-2).

Pelviscopy is an endoscopic approach to pelvic and intraabdominal examination or surgery. It differs from operative laparoscopy in two ways: (1) a 10-mm pelviscope with a 30-degree angle replaces the standard 7-mm laparoscope with a 0-degree angle; (2) the instrumentation utilized is capable of intraabdominal hemostasis and suturing. A 30-degree angle telescope is used to visualize the intrapelvic and intraabdominal structures. There is a wide field of vision, and the size, depth, and mobility of the organs can be assessed throughout the procedure.

Procedural considerations

Many of the procedural considerations for pelviscopy are similar to those associated with laparoscopy. The patient

☀
RESEARCH HIGHLIGHT 13-2

One hundred seventy women who underwent operative pelviscopy over a 67-month period were evaluated in this study. Each participant followed a preoperative screening, involving CA-125 and ultrasound, to decrease the risk of affecting the prognosis of potentially malignant ovarian tumors. CA-125 is a tumor marker which has a high degree of sensitivity and specificity for ovarian cancer. Forty-four women were over 40 years of age. Participants' ages ranged up to 68 years. The mean age was 45 years. The operations performed ranged from pelviscopic lysis of adhesions to bilateral oophorectomy. Eighty-six percent of the patients were hospitalized for 2 days or less; 45% were outpatients and 36.4% were 23-hour admission patients. Many postmenopausal women undergo laparotomy with its high financial cost and increased morbidity. Women of this age group may now have a choice, provided they have adequate preoperative screening, and may be spared the long recovery time and increased cost with little, if any, increased risk.

Levine, R.L. (1990, June) Pelviscopic surgery in women over 40. *Journal of Reproductive Medicine, 35,* 597.

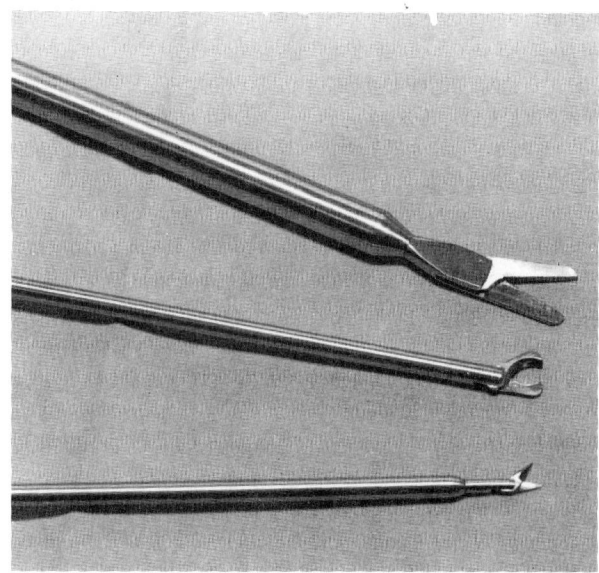

FIG. 13-34   Graspers have been designed for work on various pelvic organs.

From Nichols, D.H. (editor). (1993). *Gynecologic and obstetric surgery.* St. Louis: Mosby.

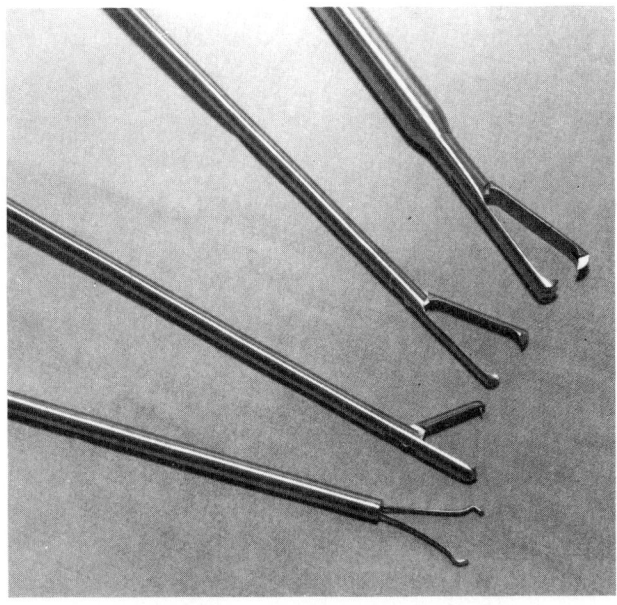

FIG. 13-35   Scissors range from microscissors with delicate tips to heavy scissors designed to go through an 11-mm trocar.

From Nichols, D.H. (editor). (1993). *Gynecologic and obstetric surgery.* St. Louis: Mosby.

may be typed and crossmatched for blood preoperatively, as in the instance of ectopic pregnancy. If the pelviscopic surgery is elective, autologous blood donation may be an alternative. The patient may be placed in the supine position, with a warming blanket in place. An indwelling urinary catheter is inserted and antiembolic stockings are applied. Bony prominences are padded and a dispersive electrosurgical pad is applied. In the instance of possible ectopic pregnancy, dilatation and curettage may be performed to rule out an intrauterine pregnancy. There are usually two or three puncture sites established for the necessary accessory instrumentation.

The surgeon and assistants manipulate instruments through trocar sheaths, as described with laparoscopy. The OR team utilizes the video screens placed on opposite sides of the operating room bed for visualization. Accessory instruments used with the pelviscope include dissecting forceps, grasping forceps, scissors, sponge holders, needle holders, suture forceps, knot tiers, appendix extractors, suction manipulators, fulgurating electrodes, laser probes, and applicators for loop ligature (Figs. 13-34 to 13-36). A tissue morcellator may be used to slowly fragment the tissue using jaws; the tissue is then loaded into the barrel of the morcellator for removal. Endocoagulation and endoligation may be accomplished (Fig. 13-37). Intraabdominal ligation is accomplished using loops of synthetic and natural suture materials.

Procedures performed through the pelviscope include adhesiolysis, ovarian biopsy, ovarian cystectomy, oophorec-tomy, adnexectomy, enucleation of intramural myomas, appendectomy, fimbrioplasty, removal of ectopic tubal pregnancy, tuboplasty, uterosacral neurectomy, and lymphadenectomy. The complications associated with pelviscopy are similar to those described with laparoscopy. An abdominal gynecologic instrument set should be readily available in case laparotomy is indicated.

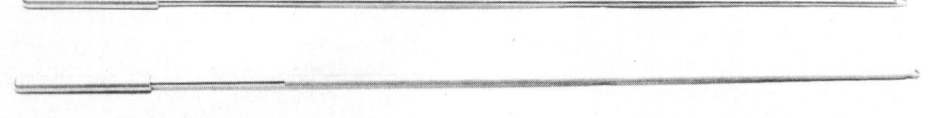

FIG. 13-36 Suturing technique can be aided by extracorporeal ties with the knot pushed by ligating devices such as the Clarke-Reich ligators.

Marlow Surgical Technologies, Inc.

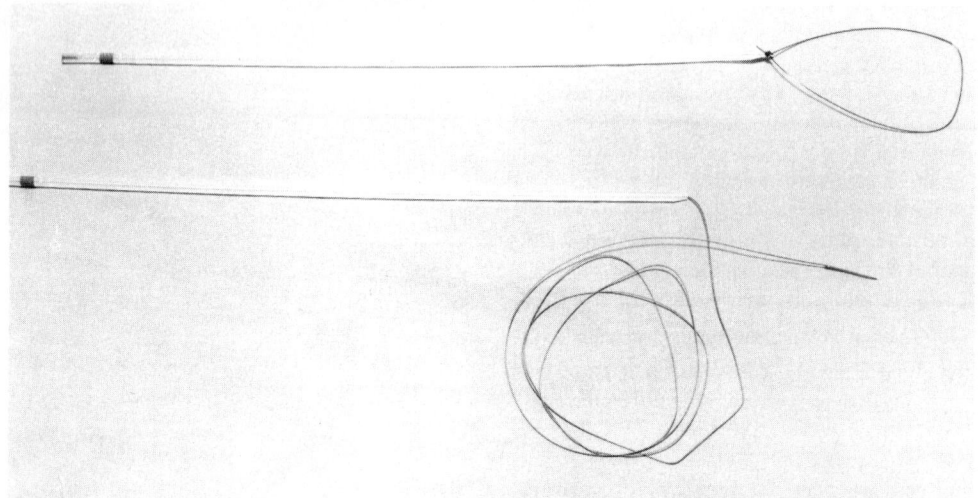

FIG. 13-37 Endoloops and Endoknots (Ethicon, Inc.) have been easy to place and use at laparoscopy.

From Nichols, D.H. (editor). (1993). *Gynecologic and obstetric surgery*. St. Louis: Mosby.

The setup for pelviscopy may include:

Pelviscopy set
1 Syringe, 10 ml
1 Bard-Parker no. 3
   knife handle with
   blade no. 15 or 11
6 Backhaus towel
   clamps, 5¼ inches
2 Allis forceps, 6
   inches
2 Crile hemostats, 5½
   inches
1 Mayo-Hegar needle
   holder, 6 inches
1 Suture scissors
2 Adson forceps with
   teeth

2 Skin hooks, if desired
Suture/clips for skin
   closure
Steri-Strips or Band-
   Aids, if desired
Electrosurgical unit/
   argon beam
   coagulator/laser, if
   desired
Fiberoptic light source
Gas insufflator
Suction-irrigation-
   dissection system, if
   desired
2 Video camera/monitor
   systems

Ectopic tubal pregnancy

A majority of tubal pregnancies occur in the ampullary region of the fallopian tube, and nearly 67% are within the lumen of the fallopian tube (Leach & Ory, 1989). The selection of an operation is determined by (1) location of the pregnancy within the fallopian tube, (2) the capabilities of the surgeon, and (3) the availability of special instrumentation (Leach & Ory, 1989). The overall goal is tubal preservation. Adhesion formation and tubal damage may be minimized by ensuring hemostasis, atraumatic tissue handling, prevention of serosal drying, and the use of fine nonreactive sutures throughout the pelviscopic surgery.

Pelviscopic salpingostomy

Pelviscopic salpingostomy may be used in the treatment of unruptured ampullary gestations.

Operative procedure

1. After successful pelviscopic entry, the distal fallopian tube is mobilized and the adhesiolysis is completed. Grasping forceps are placed on either side of the fallopian tube and gentle traction is applied.
2. Prior to making an incision, cauterization of the serosal vessels on both sides of the anticipated incision may be

performed. A dilute solution of vasopressin may also be injected into the mesenteric margin to avoid excessive bleeding.

3. A single incision is made with scissors from the mesenteric to the antimesenteric side of the fallopian tube, where the products of conception are exposed.

4. The tissue is removed gently with forceps while constant irrigation is maintained with an isotonic solution. Care needs to be taken to avoid vigorous evacuation, so that the highly vascular underlying interstitium is not disturbed.

5. Small bleeding vessels can be ligated with a fine, nonreactive suture, or simple atraumatic compression of bleeding margins will promote hemostasis. Mesosalpingeal vessel ligation may be performed.

6. The tubal incision may be closed by second intention or, as in the instance of salpingotomy, the incision may be closed in one or two layers, with 6-0, interrupted, nonreactive sutures.

7. Upon completion, the pelviscope and instrumentation are removed. The insufflated gas is permitted to escape from the trocar sleeves. Trocar sleeves are then removed.

8. Application of skin clips, or subcuticular closure of the primary skin incisions, is followed by placement of Band-Aids, Steri-Strips, or dressings.

Other methods to pelviscopically treat ectopic pregnancy include salpingotomy, segmental resection, fimbrial expression, and salpingectomy.

Ovarian cystectomy

Ovarian cystectomy is frequently performed via pelviscopic surgery.

Operative procedure

1. After successful pelviscopic entry, adhesiolysis is achieved.

2. Upon entry, peritoneal washings for cell block are obtained, if indicated.

3. The ovarian cyst is mobilized, and the cortex is grasped with a biopsy instrument.

4. The cortex is then incised by scissors or laser, exposing the cyst wall.

5. The incision is then enlarged with scissors, and aquadissection is used to separate the cyst from the ovarian stroma.

6. The cyst is dissected and may be removed intact via a culdotomy incision, or the cyst may be opened, evacuated, thoroughly lavaged with the aquadissector, and removed.

7. If the cyst is opened intraperitoneally, the patient should be taken out of Trendelenburg's position while the fluid is removed, and the pelvis lavaged.

8. Arterial bleeders are identified and desiccated.

9. The ovary usually does not require suturing; however, if the edges gape widely, they may be loosely approximated with interrupted, 4-0, synthetic absorbable suture.

10. Upon completion, the pelviscope and accessory instrumentation are removed. The insufflated gas is permitted to escape from the trocar sleeves. Trocar sleeves are then removed.

11. Application of skin clips or a subcuticular closure of the primary skin incisions is followed by placement of Band-Aids, Steri-Strips, or dressings.

Laparoscopic-assisted vaginal hysterectomy

Laparoscopic-assisted vaginal hysterectomy (LAVH) or pelviscopic-assisted vaginal hysterectomy (PAVH) offers an alternative to total abdominal hysterectomy (TAH) and vaginal hysterectomy (VH). The patient does not have the large abdominal incision, long hospital stay, and long recovery period that would be necessary with a total abdominal hysterectomy. Patients who are not candidates for traditional vaginal hysterectomy may be candidates for laparoscopic-assisted vaginal hysterectomy.

The surgeon uses laparoscopy to visualize the pelvis and thereby determine whether disease is present. This is not possible with traditional vaginal hysterectomy. Conditions leading to LAVH include postmenopausal bleeding, pelvic pain, uterine leiomyomata, and adnexal masses. Indications for LAVH may be absence of genital prolapse, required adnexectomy, history of abdominopelvic surgery, salpingitis or endometriosis, lymphadenectomy, and endometrial cancer.

Procedural considerations

Procedural considerations and accessory instrumentation and approach are similar to that used in other pelviscopic surgical procedures. The patient may be placed in lithotomy position or with legs spread, and padding is applied to bony prominences and all potential pressure areas to prevent nerve damage.

Operative procedure

Operative procedure may include the following steps:

1. Aquadissection of the broad ligament
2. Dessication of round and infundibulopelvic ligaments with bipolar coagulation
3. Dissection of the broad ligaments
4. Freeing the urinary bladder from the lower uterine segment
5. Opening the vaginal vault with endoscopic scissors or monopolar electrode, and removing the uterus vaginally.

Future advancements in endoscopic technology will promote the advancement and safety of pelviscopic surgical intervention.

TOTAL ABDOMINAL HYSTERECTOMY

Total abdominal hysterectomy (TAH) is removal of the entire uterus, including the corpus and the cervix. When TAH is combined with bilateral salpingo-oophorectomy, the procedure is commonly termed panhysterectomy or complete hysterectomy. TAH may be performed for symptomatic pelvic relaxation or prolapse, pain associated with pelvic congestion, pelvic inflammatory disease, endometriosis, recurrent ovarian cysts, fibroids (myomas), bleeding with no apparent cause in postmenopausal women, adenomyosis, or dysfunctional uterine bleeding. TAH, usually with bilateral salpingo-oophorectomy, is also indicated in anatomic disease, malignancy, premalignant states, and conditions of high risk for development or recurrence of malignancy. The procedure can also be used to accomplish sterilization.

Procedural considerations

Diagnostic dilatation and curettage usually have already been performed. However, an instrument set should be readily available. Before the abdominal skin prep, an internal vaginal prep is done. An indwelling urinary drainage catheter is inserted to provide constant bladder drainage during the operation. Supine and Trendelenburg positions are used. Instrumentation includes the abdominal gynecologic set. Provisions are made to remove from the abdomen and field those instruments used in separating the cervix from the vagina, thereby avoiding vaginal contamination of the pelvis.

Operative procedure

1. In an obese patient or for exploration of the upper abdominal cavity, a left rectus or midline incision may be made. For simple hysterectomy a Pfannenstiel incision may be used. The abdominal layers and the peritoneum are opened as described for laparotomy.
2. As the peritoneal cavity is opened, the patient is usually placed in Trendelenburg's position to provide better visualization of the pelvic organs.
3. The round ligament is grasped with forceps, clamped, and ligated with sutures on long needle holders. Pedicles are cut with a knife or Metzenbaum scissors; sutures are tagged with a hemostat to be used as traction later. This procedure is done on both sides (Fig. 13-38, A).
4. By use of the surgeon's fingers, the layer of the broad ligament close to the uterus is separated on each side, bleeding vessels are clamped and ligated, and a moist laparotomy pack is inserted behind the flap. The fallopian tube and the uteroovarian ligaments are double-clamped together, incised, and double-tied with suture ligatures (Fig. 13-38, B).
5. The uterus is pulled forward to expose the posterior sheath of the broad ligament, which is incised with a knife or Metzenbaum scissors. Ureters are identified. The uterine vessels and uterosacral ligaments are

double-clamped, divided by sharp dissection at the level of the internal os, and ligated with suture ligatures (Fig. 13-38, C).
6. The severed uterine vessels are bluntly dissected away from the cervix on each side with the aid of sponges on sponge-holding forceps, scissors, and tissue forceps.
7. The bladder is separated from the cervix and upper vagina with sharp and blunt dissection assisted by sponges on sponge-holding forceps.
8. The bladder may be retracted with a moist laparotomy pack and a retractor with an angular blade. The vaginal vault is incised close to the cervix with a knife or scissors (Fig. 13-38, D).
9. The anterior lip of the cervix is grasped with an Allis, Kocher, or tenaculum forceps. With scissors, the cervix is dissected and amputated from the vagina. The uterus is removed. Potentially contaminated instruments used on the cervix and vagina are placed in a discard basin and removed from the field (including sponge-holding forceps and suction). Bleeding is controlled with hemostats and sutures.
10. The vaginal vault is reconstructed with interrupted sutures. Angle sutures anchor all three connective tissue ligaments to the vaginal vault. The pedicles, fallopian tubes, and ovarian ligaments are left free of the vault.
11. Vaginal mucosa is approximated with a continuous suture on a long needle holder. The muscular coat of the vagina may be closed with figure-of-eight sutures to make the vault of the vagina firm and provide resistance against prolapse. A drain may be placed in the vagina.
12. The peritoneum is closed over the bladder, vaginal vault, and rectum (Fig. 13-38, E). The laparotomy packs are removed, and the omentum is drawn over the bowel.
13. The abdominal wound is closed as described for laparotomy closure (see Chapter 10).

Abdominal myomectomy

Uterine fibroids are benign tumors that arise from the muscular wall of the uterus. Abdominal myomectomy is removal of fibromyomas, or fibroid tumors, by carefully separating each fibroid from the uterine wall and its blood supply. Myomectomy is usually done in young women who have symptoms that indicate the presence of tumors and who wish to preserve their potential fertility. Also, tumors may be removed because of infertility, habitual abortion, excessive bleeding during menses, pain, or pressure on the bladder or bowel. Myomectomy may be performed as a prophylactic measure in conjunction with other abdominopelvic surgery.

Procedural considerations

The basic abdominal gynecologic instrument set is required.

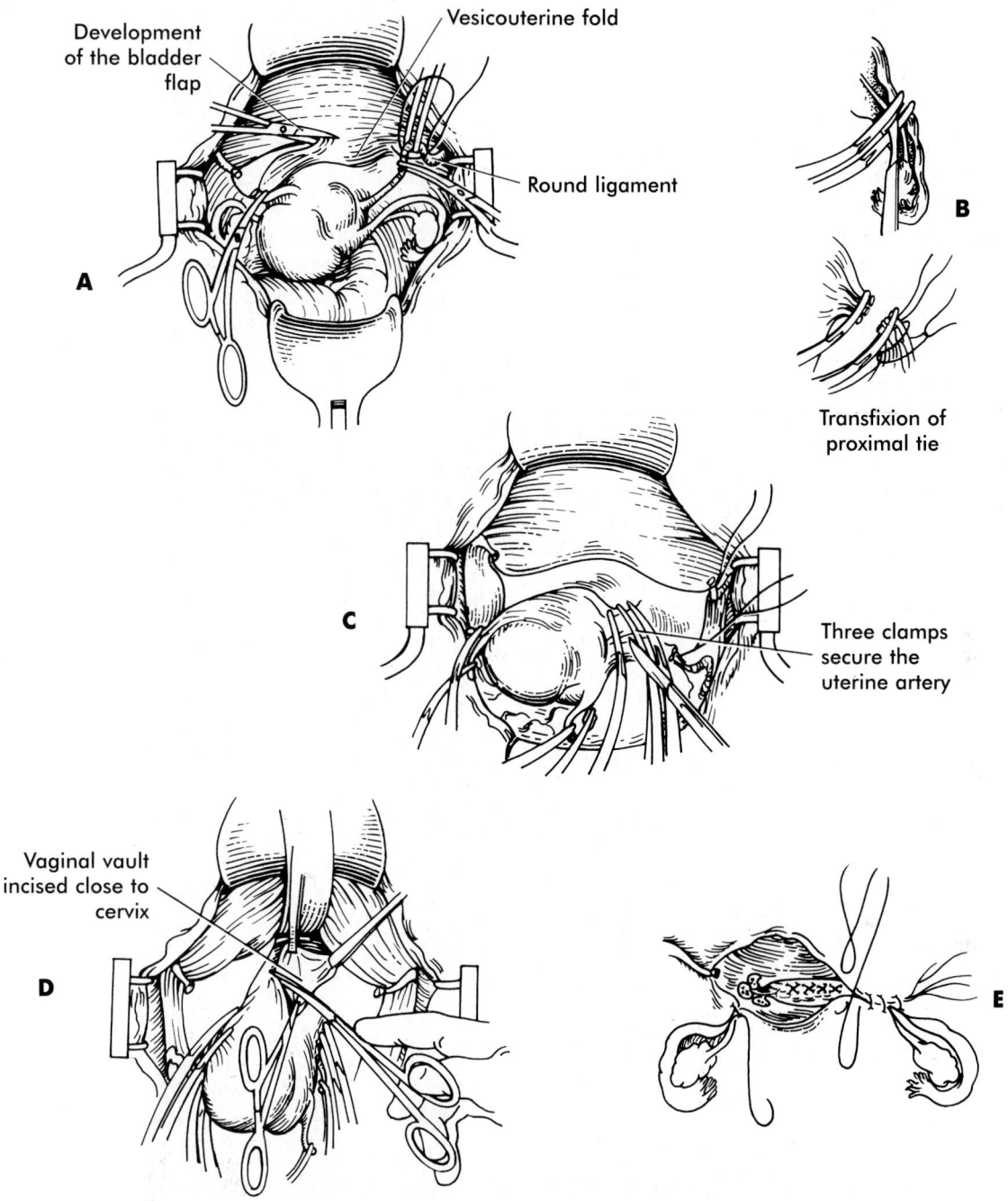

FIG. 13-38 Abdominal hysterectomy for single fibroid uterus. **A,** Peritoneum retracted with self-retaining retractors, and organs protected with laparotomy packs saturated in warm normal saline solution. Transverse incision made through uterine peritoneum and carried to each side of uterine attachments of round ligaments. Bleeding vessels clamped and ligated. Round ligament grasped, ligated, and cut. **B,** Tube and ovarian ligaments clamped, cut, and sutured. **C,** Uterus pulled forward, posterior sheath of broad ligaments divided, and uterine artery and veins secured by three heavy curved clamps. Pedicle divided, leaving two hemostats on proximal pedicle. **D,** Bladder separated from cervix and upper vagina. Vaginal vault opened and grasped with Allis forceps. Allis forceps placed on anterior lip of cervix, and dissection of cervix carried out to complete its amputation from vagina. **E,** Three connective tissue thickenings anchored to vaginal vault, vaginal mucosa approximated, and vault closed. As shown, peritoneum closed with continuous suture.

From Ball, T.L. (1963). *Operative gynecology and urology* (2nd Ed.). St. Louis: Mosby.

Operative procedure

1. The patient is prepared as described for abdominal hysterectomy. A midline or Pfannenstiel incision is used, and the uterus is exposed.
2. To contract the musculature of the uterine wall, a suitable drug may be injected into the fundus.
3. The fibroid tumor is grasped with a tenaculum. The broad ligament may be opened with curved hemostats and Metzenbaum scissors to determine the course of the ureter or to free the bladder.
4. Each tumor is shelled out of its bed, using blunt and sharp instruments, or lasered. Bleeding vessels are clamped and ligated or electrocoagulated.
5. The uterus is reconstructed with interrupted or continuous sutures.
6. The perimetrium is closed over the operative site. The abdominal wound is closed.

Radical hysterectomy (Wertheim)

Radical hysterectomy is en bloc dissection with careful removal of all recognizable lymph nodes in the pelvis, together with wide removal of the uterus, tubes, ovaries, supporting ligaments, and upper vagina (Fig. 13-39). Extensive dissection of the ureters and of the bladder is also involved.

Radical abdominal hysterectomy is performed in the presence of cervical carcinoma, with or without attendant radiation therapy. Abdominal exploration determines lymph node involvement. With no lymph node involvement, a wide-cuff hysterectomy is performed. The uterus, tubes, and ovaries, together with most of the parametrial tissues and the upper portion of the vagina, are dissected en bloc. Dissection of the ureters from the paracervical structures takes place so that the ligaments supporting the uterus and vagina can be removed. Radical abdominal hysterectomy can also be used in certain cases of endometrial carcinoma.

Procedural considerations

Careful estimation of blood loss and calculation of urinary output are needed throughout the operative procedure. The patient is prepped as described for total abdominal hysterectomy. An indwelling urinary catheter is inserted. The basic abdominal gynecologic instrument set is required, plus the following long/deep instrumentation may be used:

8 Schnidt tonsil forceps, 7¼ inches
6 Mixter forceps, 9 inches
1 Bard-Parker no. 4 long knife handle with blade no. 20
2 Long Cushing vein retractors (Fig. 13-40)
2 DeBakey tissue forceps, 12 inches (Fig. 13-40)
Ligating clips and appliers
Kitner sponges
2 Closed wound drainage systems
4 Lemon retractors (Fig. 13-40)

2 Deaver retractors (Fig. 13-40)
Russian tissue forceps, 12 inches (Fig. 13-40)
Long ring forceps (Fig. 13-40)
Long right angles (Fig. 13-40)
Long regular/Heaney needle holders (Fig. 13-40)
Long straight and curved Allis clamps (Fig. 13-40)
Long scissors (Fig. 13-40)

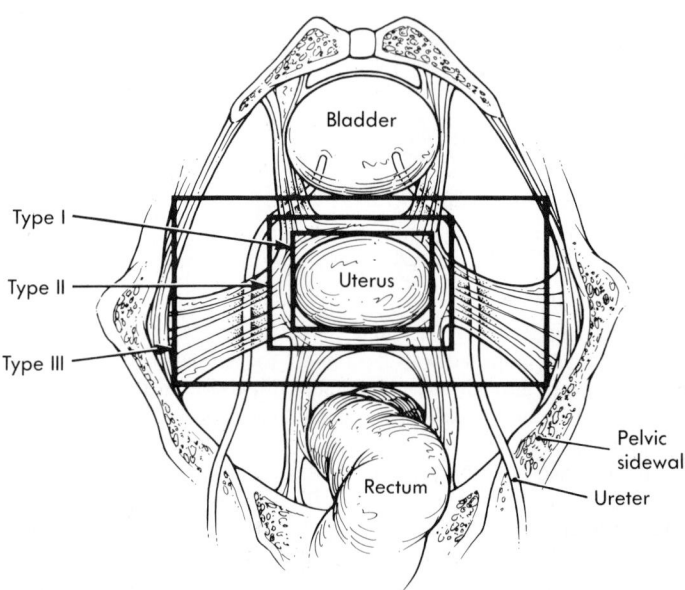

FIG. 13-39 Different types of hysterectomy: type I simple hysterectomy, type II modified radical hysterectomy, type III radical hysterectomy.
From Nichols, D.H. (editor). (1993). *Gynecologic and obstetric surgery*. St. Louis: Mosby.

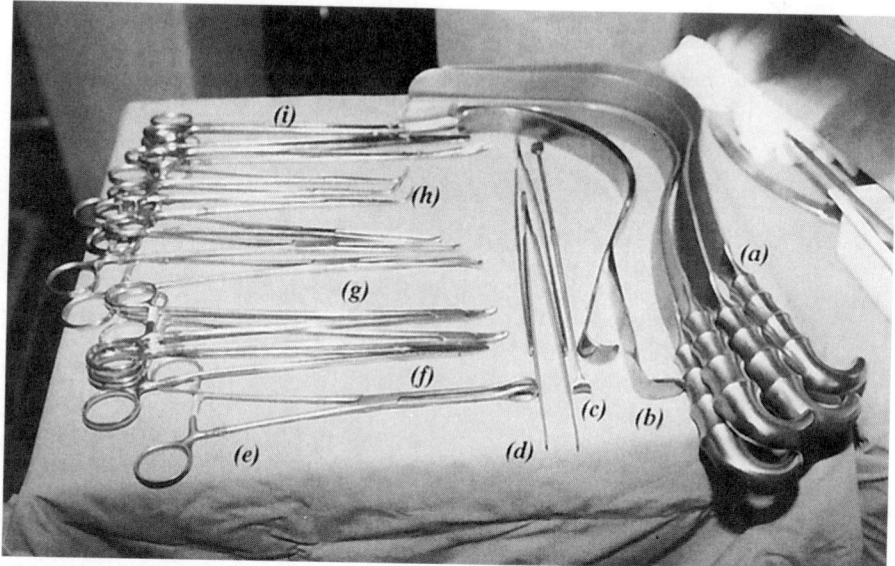

FIG. 13-40 Deep instruments used for radical hysterectomy include four Lemon retractors *(a)*, two Deaver retractors *(b)*, long vein retractor *(c)*, long Russian and DeBakey forceps *(d)*, ring forceps *(e)*, long regular and Heaney needle holders *(f)*, long straight and curved Allis clamps *(g)*, long right angles *(h)*, and long scissors *(i)*.

From Berger, P.H., & Saul, H.M. (1990, December). Radical hysterectomy: Treatment for advanced cervical carcinoma. *AORN Journal, 52,* 1212. Reprinted with permission. Copyright © AORN Inc., 2170 South Parker Road, Suite 300, Denver, CO 80231-5711.

Operative procedure

1. The skin is incised, and the abdominal layers are opened, as described for laparotomy.
2. The peritoneum is cut at its reflection on the anterior surface of the uterus between the round ligaments (Fig. 13-41, *A*). By blunt dissection, the bladder surface is freed from the cervix and vagina.
3. The right round and infundibulopelvic ligaments are clamped, cut with a knife or Metzenbaum scissors, and ligated with sutures to expose the external iliac artery. The ureter is identified and retracted with a vein retractor (Fig. 13-41, *B*).
4. The lymph and areolar tissues are dissected from the iliac artery, obturator fossa, and ureter with Lahey forceps, Kitner sponges, and Metzenbaum scissors. A complete lymph gland dissection removes the tissue from Cloquet's node to the bifurcation of the iliac arteries bilaterally. The uterine artery and vein are clamped, cut, and doubly ligated.
5. The uterus is elevated, the cul-de-sac is opened (Fig. 13-41, *C*), and the uterosacral and cardinal ligaments are clamped, cut with scissors, and doubly ligated with suture ligatures. The pararectal and paravesical areolar tissues are dissected free to skeletonize the upper vagina, and the paraurethral tissues are removed as near to the pelvic walls as possible.
6. The upper third of the vagina is cross-clamped with Heaney forceps (Fig. 13-41, *D*) and divided with a long

no. 4 knife handle and no. 20 blade. The uterus and surrounding tissues are removed. Electrocoagulation is useful in minimizing venous oozing from small venules and capillaries. Lowering the head of the operating bed 15 degrees is also helpful in reducing the oozing of blood and serum. Careful apposition of the skin edges with interrupted mattress sutures must take place to prevent overlapping of the skin edges and a resulting delay in healing.

7. The vagina is sutured open with a running locked stitch, and closed wound drainage is provided from above (Fig. 13-41, *E*). The pelvis is peritonealized with a continuous suture.
8. The abdominal wound is closed (retention sutures may be used) and dressed in the usual manner. Vaginal packing and drains may be used. A suprapubic indwelling catheter may be placed. The catheter helps prevent postoperative bladder spasm and allows for bladder drainage if the patient is unable to void after removal of the urinary catheter.

Pelvic exenteration

Pelvic exenteration is en bloc removal of the rectum, distal sigmoid colon, the urinary bladder and the distal ureters, the internal iliac vessels and their lateral branches, all pelvic reproductive organs and lymph nodes, and the entire pelvic floor with the accompanying pelvic peritoneum, levator muscles, and perineum. A partial exenteration, ei-

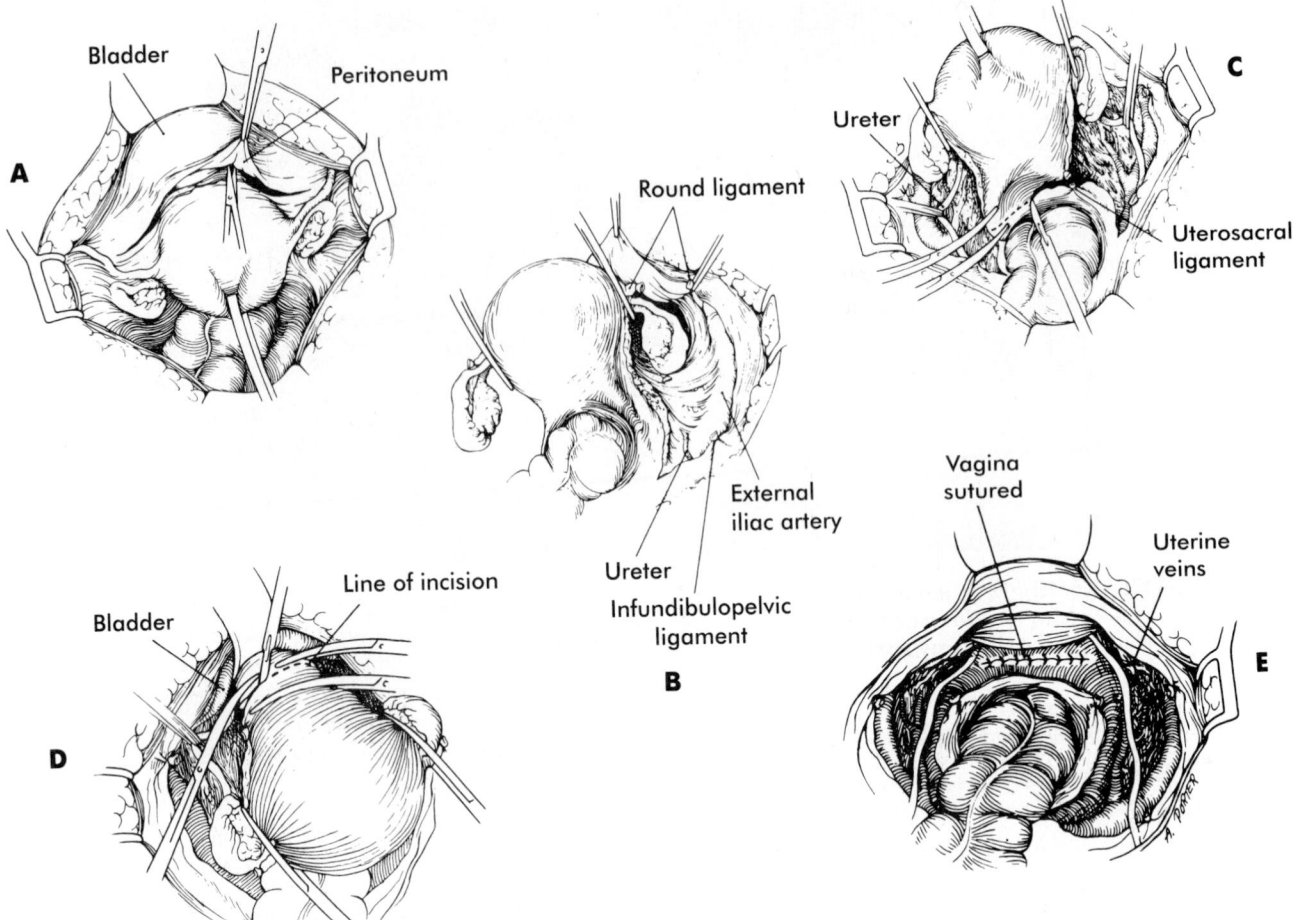

FIG. 13-41   Wertheim radical hysterectomy. **A,** With upward traction applied on uterus, peritoneum is incised from round ligament to round ligament. **B,** Right round and infundibulopelvic ligaments are ligated and cut, thus exposing right external iliac artery. **C,** Uterus is held upward and forward, exposing cul-de-sac, which is incised as shown by *dotted line*. **D,** After dissection is completed, vagina is doubly clamped preparatory to transsection, after which entire specimen is lifted out en masse. **E,** Vagina is closed. Peritoneum remains to be reperitonealized.

ther anterior or posterior, may be performed, depending on the origin of the carcinoma and the extent of local tissue invasion.

The success of modern deep pelvic surgery for malignant abdominoperineal lesions is attributable to increased knowledge regarding aseptic and surgical techniques, anesthesia, transfusions, intravenous antibiotic therapy, and the pathophysiology of involved organs. Current therapeutic techniques evolved after determination of the modes of metastasis, resective possibilities, and means of reestablishing modified physiologic function.

Pelvic exenteration is the preferred treatment for recurrent or persistent carcinoma of the cervix after radiation therapy; it is also applicable to carcinomas of the endometrium or rectum. Exenteration is considered only after a thorough investigation of the patient and disease status to determine if there is a reasonable chance of cure and of return to a productive life. The surgeon can determine with

finality the chance of resectability with cure at the time of abdominal exploration.

The need for creation of urinary and bowel diversions must also be considered, together with the patient's ability to cope with these diversions postoperatively. Plastic surgery may be required for creation of a neovagina. Total pelvic exenteration has been advocated as the definitive procedure of choice in a critical clinical situation.

Psychologic preparation of the patient and family by the perioperative nurse and physician is a prime requisite. Perioperative nursing care should be directed toward supporting the patient during therapy and helping the patient maintain personal dignity.

Procedural considerations

The bowel is cleansed preoperatively with antibiotics and enemas. A nasogastric tube, indwelling urinary catheter, and rectal tube are inserted before or during surgery.

Antiembolic stockings are placed on both legs. A hyperthermia blanket and radiant hat, leg, and arm covers are applied to maintain body temperature. Cardiac and central venous pressure monitoring is maintained throughout the procedure.

Utmost care must be taken in positioning the patient, due to duration of surgery. Strict attention should be paid to the knees, hips, and lower back to prevent vascular and nerve damage. The patient is placed in the supine position with legs abducted in the ski position or elevated in a modified lithotomy position to allow access to the perineum without disruptive position changes; antiembolic devices are applied. Skin prepping includes the abdomen, thighs, perineum, and the internal vaginal vault.

The circulating and scrub nurses must be alert to fluid and blood loss, irrigation solutions must be accurately measured, laparotomy packs must be weighed to assess blood volume loss, and the anesthesiologist and surgical team must be apprised of the measurements.

When the colon is transsected or ureteral drainage is diverted into an ileosegment, the gastrointestinal technique as described in Chapter 10 should be followed.

Separate instrument setups are required for the abdominal and perineal approaches. Extra drapes, gowns, and gloves should be available. For the abdominal approach, the basic abdominal gynecologic instrument set and instrumentation described previously for abdominoperineal resection (see Chapter 10) are required, plus the following:

1 Bard-Parker no. 4 long knife handle with blade no. 20
1 Nelson dissecting scissors, 11 inches
8 Schnidt tonsil forceps, 7¼ inches
6 Mixter forceps, 9 inches
6 Allis forceps, 9¼ inches
8 Rochester-Pean hysterectomy forceps, 9 inches
4 Right-angled clamps, 12 inches

2 Stille kidney clamps, 9 inches
2 Cushing vein retractors
2 DeBakey tissue forceps, 12 inches
2 Mayo-Hegar needle holders, 12 inches
Ligating clips and appliers
Red rubber catheters, assorted sizes
Colostomy bag
Ileostomy bag

For the perineal approach, the basic vaginal instrument set is required. To prevent contamination, the anus may be closed with a purse-string suture.

Operative procedure

1. A long midline incision from the symphysis pubis to the umbilicus is made, and the abdomen is opened in the usual manner. A second incision within the perineum encircling the vestibule and anus is also made.
2. The peritoneal cavity is explored for metastasis to the liver, the nodes of the celiac axis, the superior mesenteric artery, and the paraaortic tissues.
3. The pelvis is explored, and the peritoneum along the brim of the pelvis examined for lymph node involvement. Frozen sections may be indicated. The obturator fossa and the region of the uterosacral ligaments are explored. When findings at exploration are negative, retractors are placed and the small bowel is packed off with moist laparotomy packs (Fig. 13-42).
4. The sigmoid mesocolon is freed and sectioned by means of intestinal clamps and a scalpel or a stapling device. The proximal end is exteriorized through an opening in the left side of the abdomen; an intestinal clamp is left across the lumen until later, when the permanent colostomy will be secured to the skin.
5. The remaining sigmoid mesentery is clamped with Rochester-Pean forceps, cut, and ligated down to and including the superior hemorrhoidal vessels. Long instruments and sutures are used to facilitate reaching the deep pelvic structures.
6. The distal sigmoid colon is closed with an inverting suture. The sigmoid colon and rectum are freed from the sacrococcygeal area by blunt and sharp dissection.
7. The lateral pelvic peritoneum is cut along the iliac vessels; the ovarian vessels and round ligaments on each side are clamped with Rochester-Pean forceps, cut, and doubly ligated.
8. The peritoneum is incised over the dome of the bladder with a long knife and Metzenbaum scissors, and the bladder is separated from the symphysis pubis down to the urethra.
9. The ureters are identified and divided 2 to 3 cm below the brim of the pelvis. The proximal end is left open to allow urinary drainage while the distal end is ligated.
10. The hypogastric artery, the internal iliac vein, and the superior and inferior gluteal vessels are exposed, clamped with hemostats, doubly ligated, and cut. The external iliac vein is retracted to allow evacuation of the contents of the obturator fossa, leaving the obturator nerve intact. Care must be taken in dissection not to damage the sacral plexus and sciatic nerve.
11. The internal pudendal vessels are isolated, ligated with transfixion sutures, and cut. The remaining soft tissue attachments of the pelvis are clamped and cut. Steps 10 and 11 are then performed on the opposite side.
12. The perineum is incised by an elliptic incision that includes the clitoris and anus. The ischiorectal fat is incised up to the area of the levator muscle.
13. The coccygeal attachment of the rectum is severed. The levator muscles are severed at their lateral attachments by means of a long no. 4 knife handle with no. 20 blade; hemostasis is maintained by pressure and traction.
14. The paravesical and paravaginal tissues are resected from the periosteum of the symphysis pubis and superior pubic rami by means of a knife. The specimen is completely freed and removed from the pelvis (Fig. 13-43).

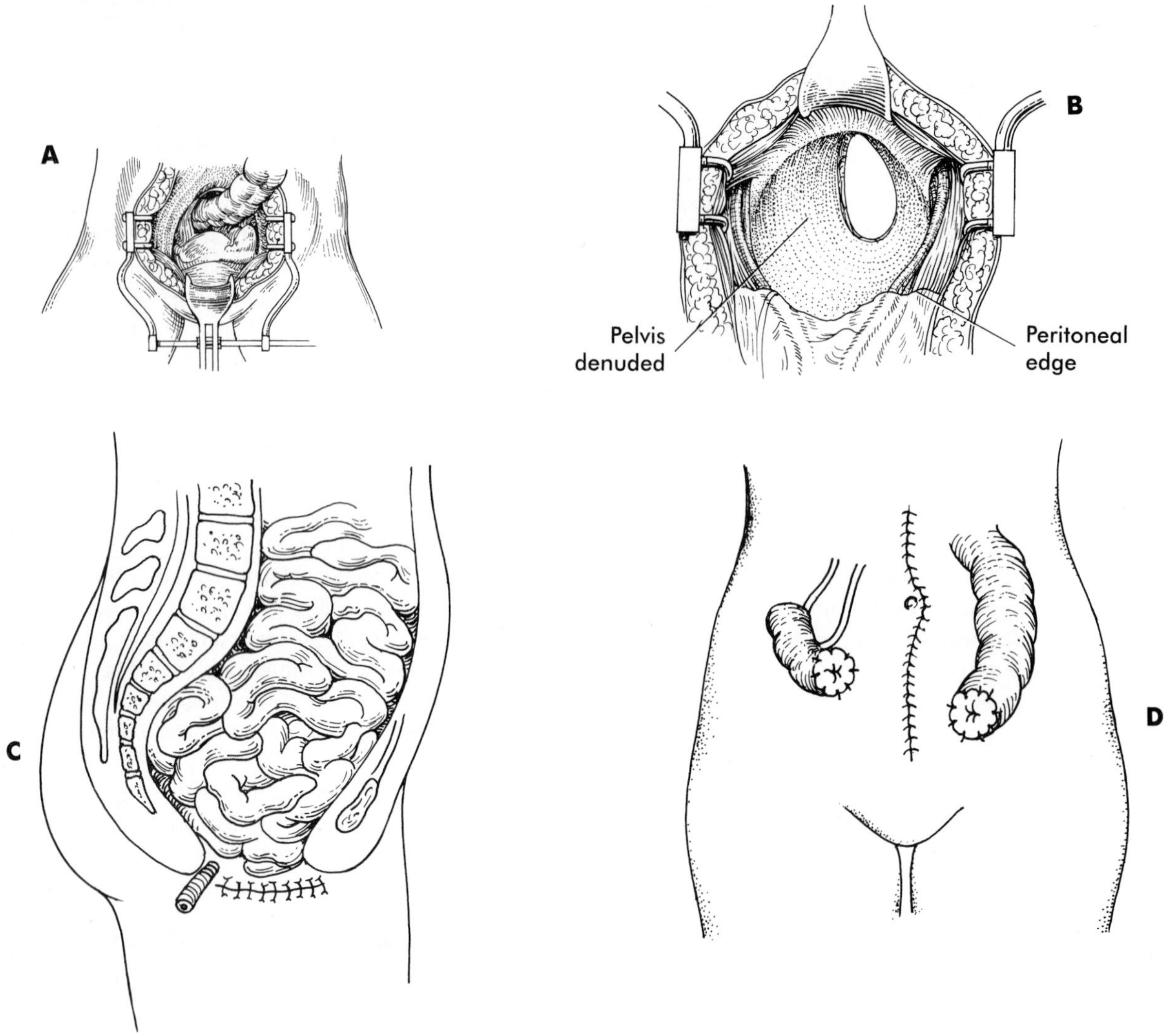

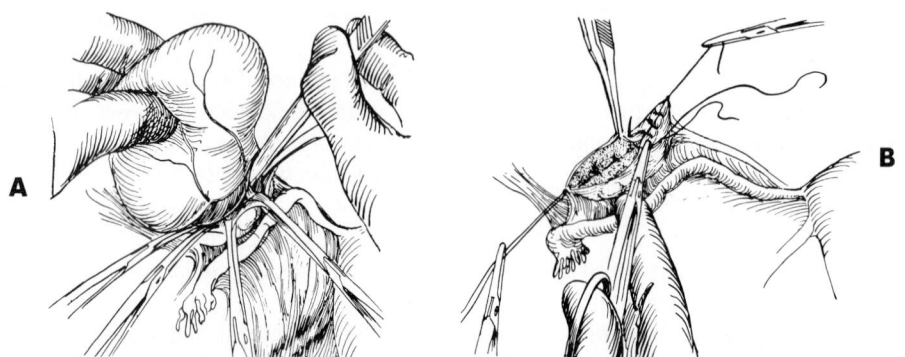

FIG. 13-42   Pelvic exenteration. **A,** Pelvic viscera in situ as viewed from operating surgeon's vantage point after retractors are placed and small bowel is packed off. **B,** Empty pelvis after dissection of paravesical and paravaginal tissues and removal of specimen en bloc. **C,** Sagittal view of small bowel above pelvic defect. Perineal packing and/or drain may be used. **D,** After closure of abdominal wall, colostomy and ileostomy stomas are sutured to skin edges.

FIG. 13-43   Resection of small cyst from ovary. **A,** Incision made around ovary near junction of cyst wall and normal ovarian tissue. Knife handle is convenient instrument for shelling out cyst. **B,** Wound in ovary closed.

From Ball, T.L. (1963). *Operative gynecology and urology* (2nd Ed.). St. Louis: Mosby.

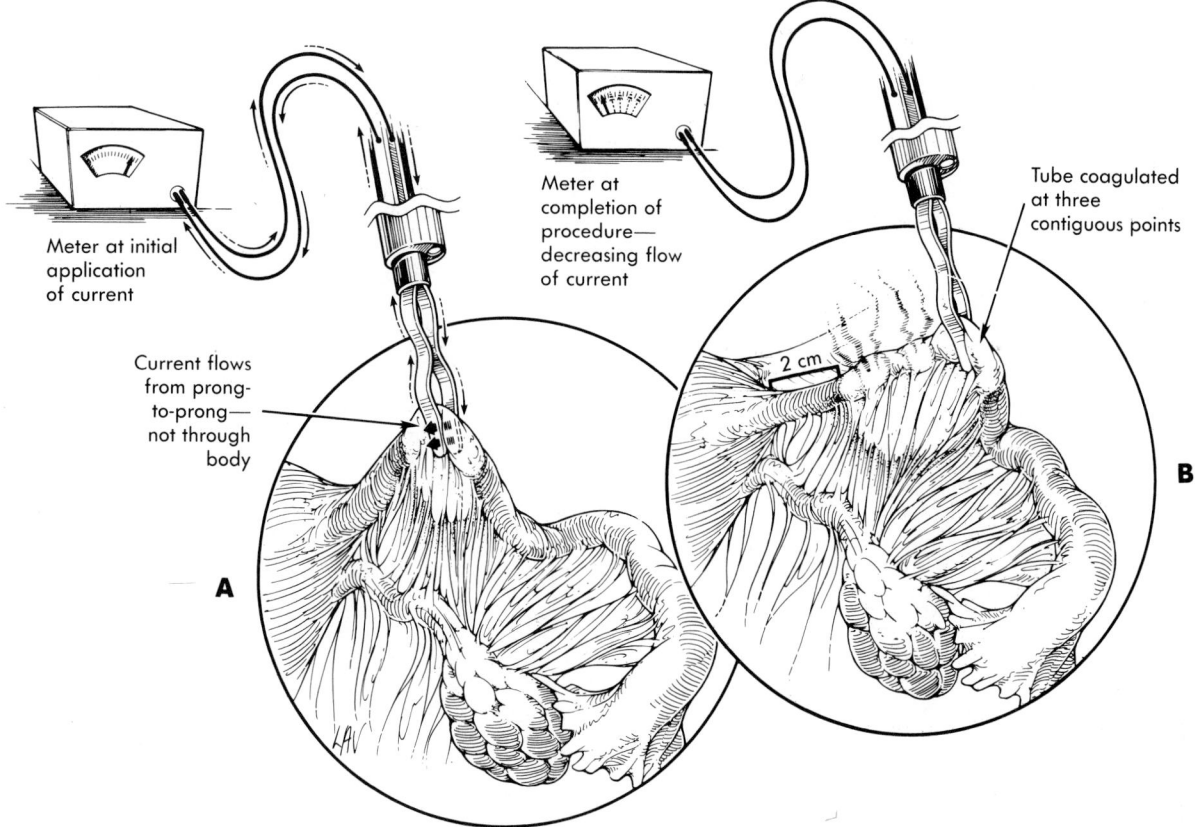

Meter at initial application of current

Meter at completion of procedure—decreasing flow of current

Tube coagulated at three contiguous points

Current flows from prong-to-prong—not through body

2 cm

A

B

FIG. 13-44   Bipolar coagulation. **A,** Current passes only through the tube from prong to prong of the forceps. **B,** Three contiguous burns are needed to prevent spontaneous recanalization. The end point for coagulation is tissue desiccation, at which point current ceases to flow through the dry, nonconducting tube. A meter on the generator to monitor current flow is therefore necessary.

From Nichols, D.H. (editor). (1993). *Gynecologic and obstetric surgery.* St. Louis: Mosby.

15. After residual bleeding vessels are identified and controlled by transfixing ligatures, the subcutaneous tissue is closed by interrupted sutures. A drain is placed in the wound, and the skin is closed.
16. In the abdomen, further residual bleeding vessels are controlled. Packs may be left in the pelvis to be removed through the perineum after 48 hours.
17. The ileosegment is then fashioned and the ureters anastomosed to it. The external stoma of the ileosegment is placed on the right side of the abdomen.
18. A red, rubber, multieyed tube, size 16 Fr, is inserted into the proximal jejunum for the length of the jejunum and the ileum to aid in postoperative bowel decompression. It is connected to the bowel with a purse-string suture and brought out to the skin, where it is sutured in place.
19. A gastrostomy tube is placed in the stomach in the same manner.
20. Hemostasis is checked. The small intestines are carefully repositioned into the pelvis. Packs and retractors are removed (Fig. 13-44).
21. The peritoneum, rectus muscles, and fascial sheaths are closed with interrupted figure-of-eight sutures. The skin is closed with interrupted sutures.

22. The colostomy stoma is prepared by removing the intestinal clamp from the sigmoid colon, opening the colon, and suturing the stoma to the skin edges (Fig. 13-45).
23. The abdominal wound and tube sites are dressed in the usual manner. Drainage bags are applied to the colostomy and ileostomy stomas. A perineal dressing may be secured by means of a T binder.

SURGERY FOR CONDITIONS THAT AFFECT FERTILITY

UTERINE SUSPENSION

Uterine suspension is shortening of the ligaments of the uterus and positioning them retroperitoneally. The ligaments are then sutured bilaterally to the undersurface of the abdominal fascia in the corners of the transverse incision to ensure the maintenance of an anterior position of the uterus. This prevents the fallopian tubes and ovaries from entrapment in the cul-de-sac. Uterine suspension is done as part of a conservative surgical treatment of pelvic inflammatory disease or endometriosis. It is also indicated in patients who require lysis of extensive pelvic adhesions, for

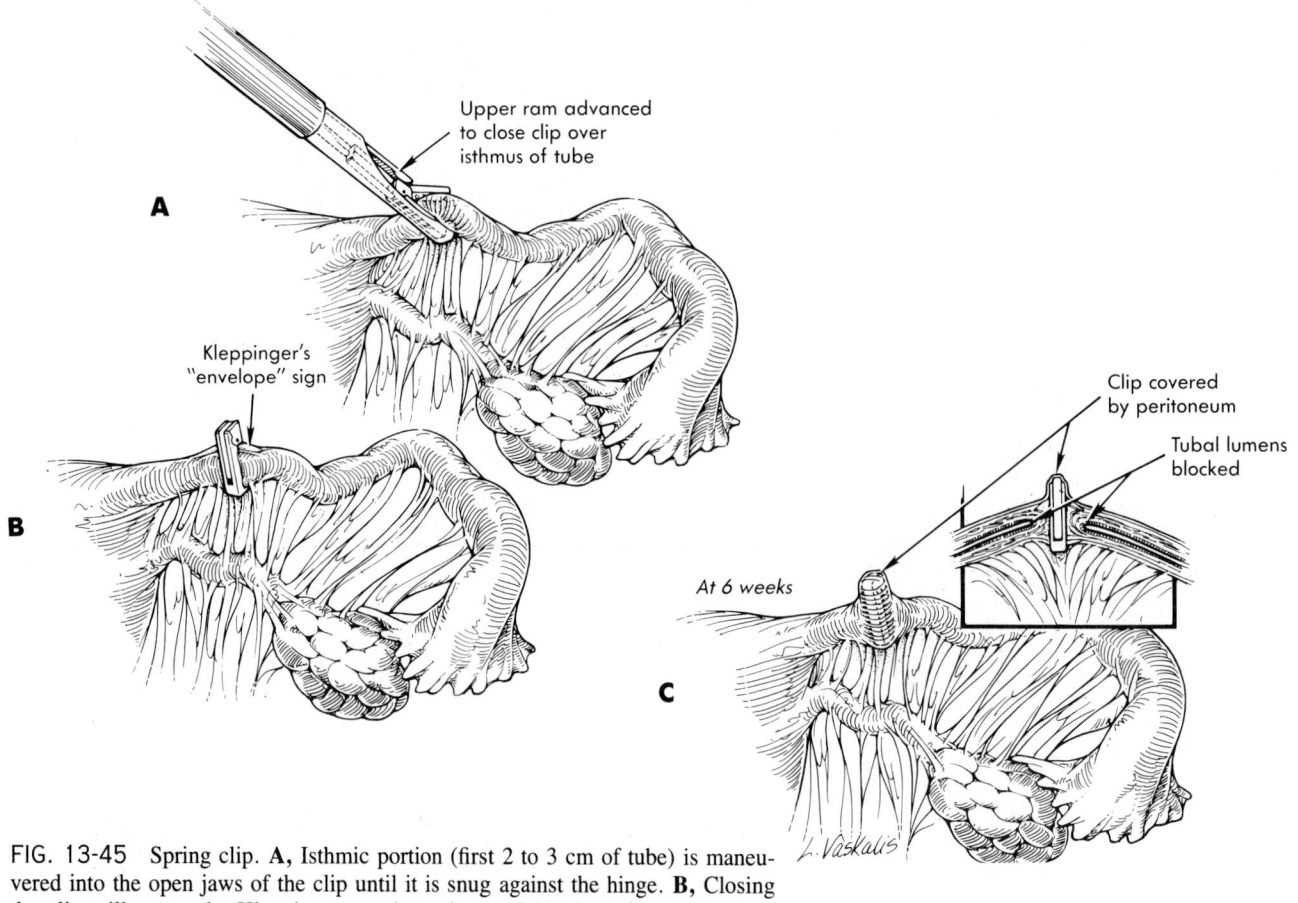

FIG. 13-45   Spring clip. **A,** Isthmic portion (first 2 to 3 cm of tube) is maneuvered into the open jaws of the clip until it is snug against the hinge. **B,** Closing the clip will create the Kleppinger envelope sign, a fold of tubal peritoneum in the hinge of the clip **(C).** Failure to get the clip completely across the isthmus results in pregnancy. Some routinely use two clips close together on each tube.

From Nichols, D.H. (editor). (1993). *Gynecologic and obstetric surgery.* St. Louis: Mosby.

the correction of the symptoms of uterine retroversion, and for uterine prolapse in young women.

Procedural considerations

The basic abdominal gynecologic instrument set is required.

Operative procedure

1. The abdomen is opened as described for myomectomy.
2. The suspension is accomplished. If it is being done to correct uterine prolapse, a strip of Mersilene material is placed retroperitoneally to elevate the uterus at the level of the internal os posteriorly and to correct the prolapse into the vagina.
3. The wound is closed in layers, as described for laparotomy.

OOPHORECTOMY AND OOPHOROCYSTECTOMY

Oophorectomy is removal of an ovary. Oophorocystectomy is removal of an ovarian cyst (Fig. 13-46). Functional cysts comprise the majority of ovarian enlargements; fol-

licular cysts are the most common. Functional cysts develop in the corpus luteum; these cysts are usually larger than other functional cysts. The true ovarian epithelial tumors, serous cystadenomas and pseudomucinous cystadenomas, are prone to malignant change.

The choice of operation depends on the patient's age and symptoms, findings during physical examination, and direct examination of the adnexa during exploration. If the ovarian tumor is recognized as benign, only the visibly diseased portions of the adnexa are removed. In the presence of dermoid, follicular, and corpus luteum cysts, the cyst is usually enucleated, and most of the ovarian parenchyma is preserved. In tubal pregnancy the ectopic pregnancy may be removed from the tube or the pregnant fallopian tube may be removed and, in some instances, the ovary.

Procedural considerations

The basic abdominal gynecologic instrument set is required, plus the following:

1 Trocar and cannula
Suction tubing
1 Syringe, 10 ml

1 Needle, 21 gauge, 1½ inches

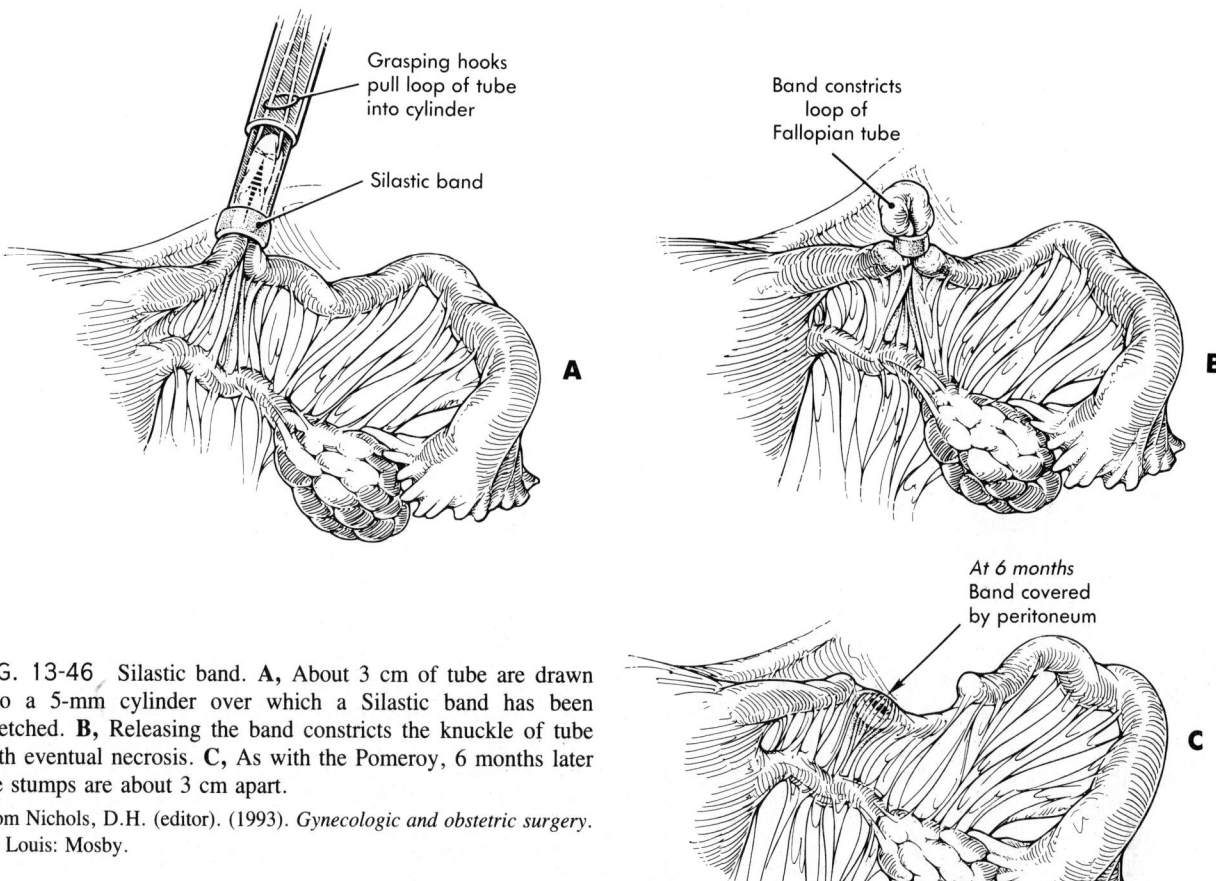

Grasping hooks
pull loop of tube
into cylinder

Silastic band

A

Band constricts
loop of
Fallopian tube

B

At 6 months
Band covered
by peritoneum

C

L. Vaskalis

FIG. 13-46 Silastic band. **A,** About 3 cm of tube are drawn into a 5-mm cylinder over which a Silastic band has been stretched. **B,** Releasing the band constricts the knuckle of tube with eventual necrosis. **C,** As with the Pomeroy, 6 months later the stumps are about 3 cm apart.

From Nichols, D.H. (editor). (1993). *Gynecologic and obstetric surgery.* St. Louis: Mosby.

Operative procedure

1. The abdominal cavity is opened, as described for laparotomy.
2a. For removal of a large ovarian cyst, a purse-string suture may be placed in the cyst wall, and a trocar is introduced in its center; the suture is tightened around the trocar as the fluid is aspirated. The trocar is removed, and the purse-string suture is tied. All normal ovarian tissue is preserved.
   b. *For removal of a dermoid cyst,* the field is protected with laparotomy packs because the contents of such cysts produce irritation if they are spilled into the peritoneal cavity. An incision is made along the base of the cyst between the wall and normal ovarian tissue. The cystic wall is dissected away. The ovary is closed with interrupted or continuous sutures.
   c. *For decortication of the enlarged ovary and wedge resection,* a large segment of the ovarian cortex opposite the hilum is removed. The cysts are punctured with a needlepoint and collapsed. A wedge of ovarian stroma, extending deep in the hilum, is resected with a small knife; the cortex of the ovary is closed with interrupted or continuous sutures.
3. To prevent prolapse of the tube into the cul-de-sac, it

may be sutured to the posterior sheath of the broad ligament.
4. The abdominal wound is closed as described for laparotomy.

SALPINGO-OOPHORECTOMY

Salpingo-oophorectomy is removal of a fallopian tube and all or part of the associated ovary. Unilateral salpingo-oophorectomy may be done in some young women who are anxious to have children after all other methods of treatment have failed to cure chronic salpingo-oophoritis, in patients with ectopic tubal gestation, or in those with certain disease conditions of the adnexa or large adnexal cysts. If both tubes and ovaries are diseased, they are removed with total hysterectomy.

Procedural considerations

The basic abdominal gynecologic instrument set is required.

Operative procedure

1. The abdominal cavity is opened, as described for laparotomy.
2. The affected tube is grasped with Allis or Babcock for-

ceps. The infundibulopelvic ligament is clamped with hemostats, cut, and ligated.

3. The mesosalpinx is grasped with hemostats and divided with the suspensory ligament of the ovary.

4. The cornual attachment of the tube is excised with a knife or curved scissors. Bleeding vessels are clamped and ligated.

5. The edges of the broad ligament are peritonealized from the uterine horn to the infundibulopelvic ligament, as described for total hysterectomy.

6. The wound is closed, as described for laparotomy; dressings are applied.

MICROSCOPIC RECONSTRUCTIVE SURGERY OF THE FALLOPIAN TUBE

The obstructed portion of a fallopian tube may be removed and the tube reconstructed to create patency of the remaining portion of the tube to promote the possibility of fertilization. Reconstructive surgery of the tube, categorically called tuboplasty, includes reanastomosis, salpingoneostomy, fimbrioplasty, and lysis of adhesions.

Microsurgical correction of tubal pathology is the most successful way to perform tuboplasties and may be employed in all previously mentioned methods. The laser may be adapted to the operating microscope or the free-hand approach may be utilized in tubal reconstructive surgery (see Chapter 31).

Procedural considerations

The patient is placed in the supine position. The vagina is prepped as described previously. An indwelling urinary catheter is inserted into the bladder. A Kahn, Calvin, Rubin, Hui, or Humi cannula or a pediatric Foley catheter may be placed in the uterine cavity for intraoperative chromotubation with diluted methylene blue or indigo carmine solution. Intraoperative chromotubation can also be achieved by applying a Buxton uterine clamp around the lower segment of the uterus and inserting an Angiocath catheter through the fundus into the cavity. A vaginal pack may be inserted to help elevate the uterus.

The basic abdominal gynecologic instrument set is required, plus the following:

2 Iris scissors, 1 curved and 1 straight

2 Adson forceps without teeth

8 Halsted mosquito hemostats, 4 curved and 4 straight

1 Set Bowman lacrimal probes

2 Webster needle holders

1 Frazier suction tip, no. 2

1 Kirschner retractor, if desired

1 Buxton uterine clamp, if desired

Basic microsurgical instruments

2 Microscissors, 1 curved and 1 straight

1 Bayonet microscissors, curved

2 Jeweler's forceps, no. 5

2 Jeweler's forceps, no. 7

1 Microforceps with platform

1 Microforceps with platform and very fine teeth

1 Fallopian tube forceps

1 Petit-point mosquito hemostat

2 Microneedle holders, 1 curved and 1 straight

1 Ball tipped nerve hook

2 Serrefines

3 Glass or Teflon rods

Accessory items

2 Microneedle electrodes

1 Electrosurgical pencil with fingertip control

1 Swolin electrosurgical handpiece, if desired

1 Bipolar forceps with cord

1 Irrigator for microsurgery with 2 irrigator cannulas, if desired

Syringes and blunted needles for irrigation of the tissues

Plastic or Silastic tubing and connectors

Diluted methylene blue or indigo carmine solution

Diluted heparinized, lactated Ringer's solution

Microscope drape

Microscope or operative loupes

Electrosurgical unit with monopolar and bipolar capabilities

Video monitoring system, if desired

Operative procedure

Operative procedures for correction of postsurgical tubal occlusion are usually performed under the operating microscope. Other reconstructive procedures vary according to the nature of the pathologic condition of the tube and may be done under the operating microscope or by use of operative loupes.

In microsurgery the surgeon must make sure that virtually no instruments are used in contact with the fallopian tube except those necessary to carry out the surgical technique. Microsurgery for infertility requires the use of specialized and delicate instruments. Each of these instruments is designed to permit gentle, atraumatic handling of tissues and prevent abrasions, lacerations, and vascular damage.

The tissues must be continually irrigated to prevent drying of the serosal surfaces. Ringer's lactate solution alone or with heparin added may be used as the irrigating solution. Meticulous hemostasis is required in microsurgery. Irrigation is used to identify the bleeders. Hemostasis can be achieved by electrocoagulation with a microneedle electrode or very fine bipolar forceps. When a CO_2 laser beam is used, the smoke from laser vaporization should be evacuated through suction to prevent carbon deposits on the tissue.

Tubal ligation

Tubal ligation is interruption of fallopian tube continuity, resulting in sterilization of the patient. In general, the indication for sterilization depends entirely on the desire of the patient. Certain medical indications and concern for the psychosocial needs of the patient are factors, and occasionally an obstetric indication exists, such as inherited fetal deformity. However, at least in the United States, sterilization is entirely a voluntary procedure. In many states a sterilization permit does not have to be signed by the husband. Good presurgical counseling is needed for the patient and her husband or significant other because this procedure is not predictably reversible. Approximately 1% of sterilized women seek reversals as a result of sterilization performed at an early age, death of a child, or remarriage. Patients may elect to have the procedure performed on an ambulatory surgery basis at a time that is convenient for them.

The optimal time for sterilization is approximately 24 hours after vaginal delivery. This method may not delay the normal discharge time for the patient. An objection to this practice is that the danger of hemorrhage still exists soon after delivery. With a normal delivery, tubal ligation is done on the first or second postpartum day. If a cesarean section is done, the tubes may be ligated at that time.

Operative procedures

Many surgical methods and techniques are available for tubal ligation. The objective of each method is to achieve complete closure of the fallopian tube so that conception is prevented. When a segment of each fallopian tube is excised, it is preserved for pathologic examination. General surgical considerations are directed to excising a section of each fallopian tube, ligating the severed ends, achieving hemostasis, and incorporating the proximal stump within layers of the mesosalpinx.

Laparoscopic tubal occlusion

1. Operative procedure is the same as for laparoscopy.
2. An accessory suprapubic incision may be made for the occluding instrument.
3. Sterilization may take place by electrocoagulation/thermal coagulation, or by the placement of a spring clip or silastic band after the tube has been identified and isolated in the grasping forceps.
   a. *Bipolar coagulation* occurs when electrical current passes only through the tube from prong to prong (Fig. 13-47, *A*). At least 3 cm of the tube is destroyed, which therefore prevents spontaneous recanalization. It has been recommended that the tube be grasped at least 2 to 3 cm away from the uterocornual junction at the time of this procedure so that a stump of isthmus remains to absorb the intrauterine fluid under pressure and minimize fistula formation, which could result in an ectopic pregnancy for the patient in the future.
   b. *Spring clip* offers a mechanical alternative to elec-

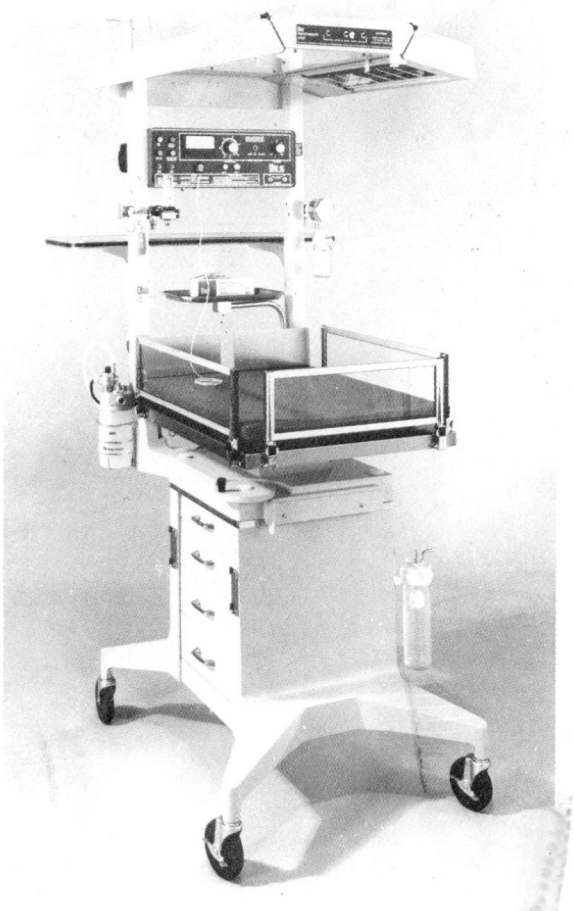

FIG. 13-47 Neonatal intensive care unit.
Courtesy Ohio Medical Products, Madison, Wis.

trocoagulation. The spring clip occludes the isthmus of the tube by two plastic jaws (Fig. 13-48, *A* and *B*). The tube is compressed by a stainless steel spring that presses the jaws together. Spring clip application requires careful surgical technique to assure that the clip is completely across the isthmus of the tube (Fig. 13-48, *C*). Some surgeons may prefer to apply two spring clips positioned close together on each tube when utilizing this approach.
   c. *Silastic band* offers another mechanical alternative to electrocoagulation. The tube is drawn 1.5 cm into a 0.5 cm diameter metal cylinder, which destroys approximately 3 cm of the tube (Fig. 13-49, *A*). A Silastic ring stretched on the outside of the cylinder is released to form an occlusion (Fig. 13-49, *B*). In time about 3 cm of the constricted tube undergoes necrosis and the tubes separate (Fig. 13-49, *C*).

Vaginal approach (posterior colpotomy)

1. Operative procedure is the same as for posterior colpotomy.
2. Sterilization can take place by the placement of a spring clip or Silastic band, by fimbriectomy, or by ligation of

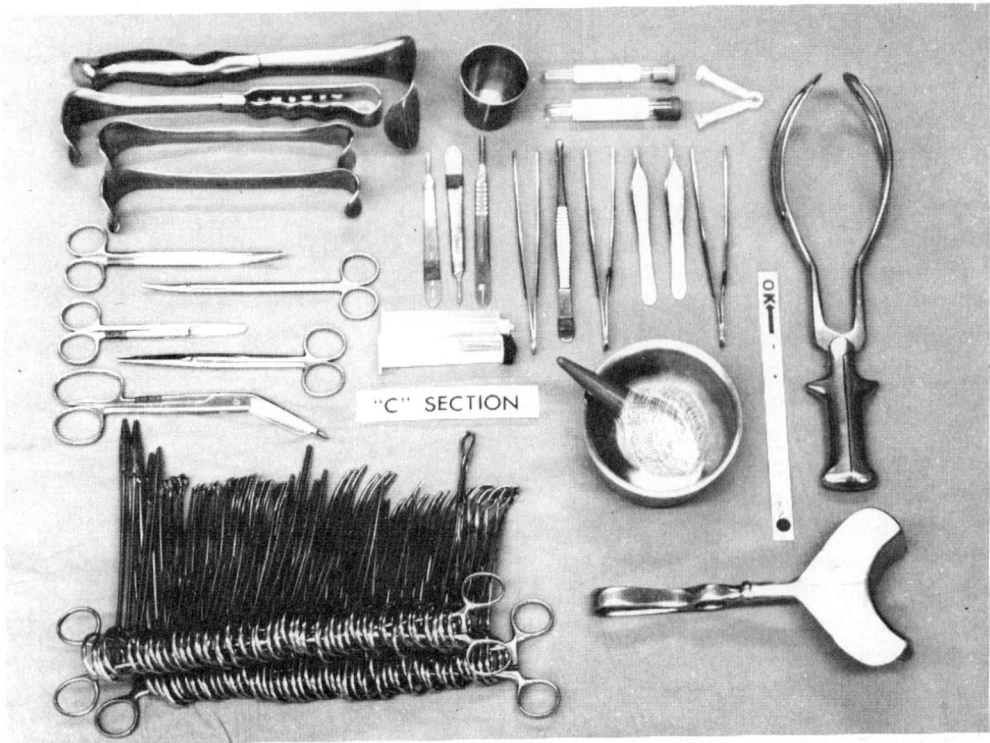

FIG. 13-48   Instrument setup for cesarean birth.
Courtesy Edward Weck & Co., Research Triangle Park, N.C.

the proximal portion of the fallopian tubes with a permanent suture.

Minilaparotomy approach

1. A 2-cm transverse incision is made above the pubic hairline.
2. A large bivalved speculum may be placed through the incision and into the peritoneal cavity. The large Graves bivalve speculum serves as a small abdominal retractor and permits easy access to the tubes.
3. Spring clips or Silastic bands can be applied, or the original Pomeroy method of ligation can be carried out. The Pomeroy technique provides a tissue specimen of each tube. Suture material is tied around each tube and a section of tube is removed. Over time the tubes pull apart, destroying the passage between the ovary and the uterus.

IN VITRO FERTILIZATION AND EMBRYO TRANSFER

Infertility may be described as the inability of a couple to conceive a biologic child after a year or more of repeated attempts. This is an emotionally stressful process for both partners. There are various coping strategies utilized by individuals with infertility, and the perioperative nurse needs to be aware of these in providing effective care (Research Highlight 13-3).

RESEARCH HIGHLIGHT 13-3

A study was conducted to examine the coping patterns of women who were infertile. The sample consisted of 30 infertile women who were clients of a physician specializing in infertility. Each participant had a private interview in which she was asked what she had done to cope with feelings and experiences associated with her infertility. The researchers identified six common coping strategies used by the women: (1) increasing space between themselves and reminders of infertility; (2) regaining control; (3) being the best; (4) looking for hidden meaning: (5) giving in to feelings; and (6) sharing the burden.

These findings may be utilized in providing nursing care in a sensitive, yet informed, manner. Nurses can promote an atmosphere in which the woman can give in to her feelings and share her burden. The nurse can assure the woman that her feelings are normal and might direct the couple to an organized support group for couples experiencing common concerns. Further research to examine the coping strategies of males and couples experiencing infertility will aid the nurse in caring for these individuals.

Davis, D.C., & Dearman, C.N. (1991). Coping strategies of infertile women. *Journal of Obstetric, Gynecologic, and Neonatal Nursing, 20*(3), 221.

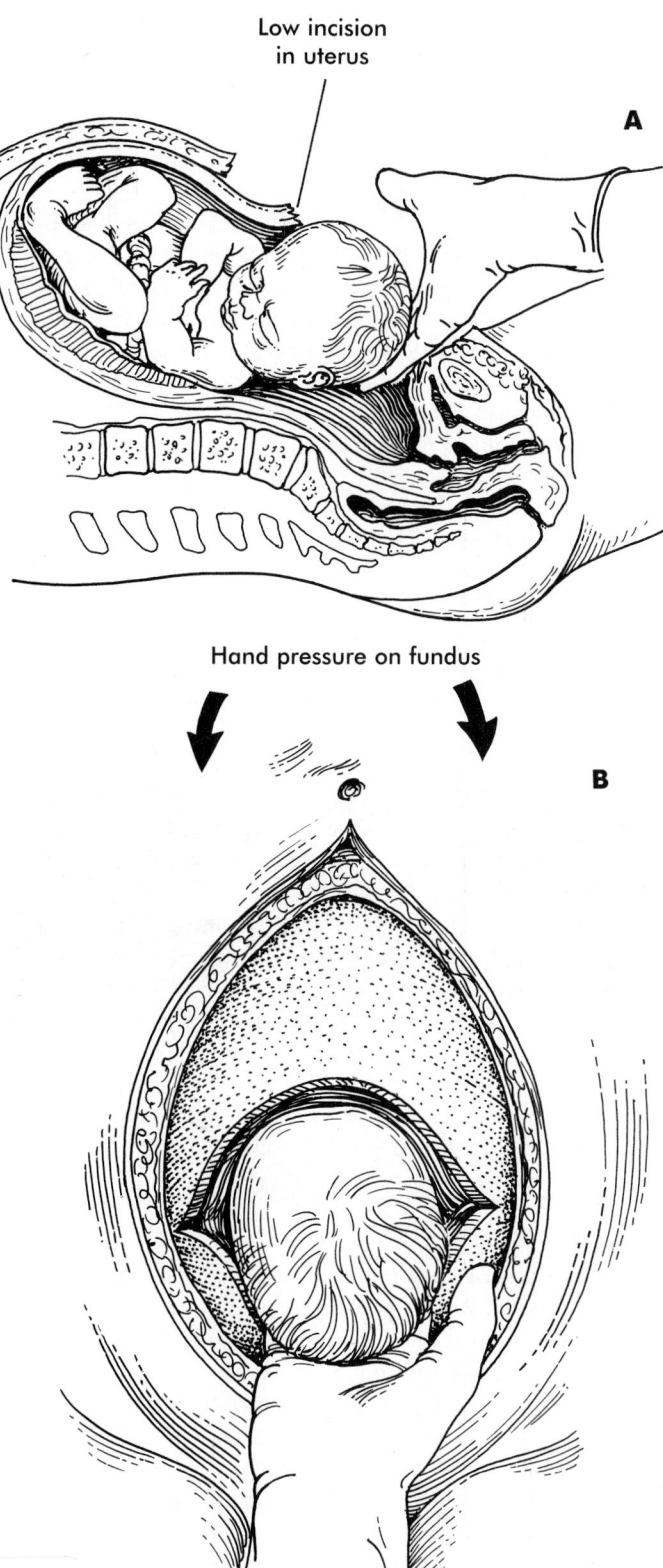

Low incision
in uterus

A

Hand pressure on fundus

B

FIG. 13-49   Manual delivery of fetal head at low uterine segment cesarean section. **A,** Lateral view. **B,** Anterior view.

Both individuals undergo extensive testing to identify possible organic or functional causes for their infertility. For example, there may be a structural defect in either partner, past or present infections, genetic or immunologic abnormalities, or endocrine imbalance or deficit.

Today there are options couples may select to assist them in the reproduction process. Fertilization may be achieved by retrieval of oocytes from the ovary, followed by in vitro fertilization with sperm and implantation of the fertilized oocytes (embryos) into the uterine cavity (IVF).

In vitro fertilization and embryo transfer are indicated for women who have had bilateral absence or irreparable obstruction of the fallopian tubes, for women who have undergone tubal reconstructive surgery and have not conceived within 1 year after surgery, for women who have cervical or immunologic factors and have not conceived following treatment or for whom no treatment is available, for women who have failed to conceive following conservative surgery and hormonal suppressive therapy for endometriosis, for couples who have unexplained infertility, and for oligospermia as a cause of infertility. This procedure has raised many legal and ethical issues in its early stage of development. For example, with IVF the fertilization process takes place in a culture dish or test tube in a laboratory environment. Some individuals might view this as being unnatural and therefore ethically unacceptable.

To be a candidate for in vitro fertilization and embryo transfer, a woman must have at least one functioning ovary. The ovaries must be physically accessible for laparoscopic follicular aspiration unless aspiration is done under ultrasound-guided transabdominal or transvaginal puncture. The uterus must be normal and have functioning endometrium. The partner's semen must have sufficient motile sperm for insemination.

The treatment cycle for in vitro fertilization and embryo transfer can be divided into five stages: follicular development, aspiration of the mature preovulatory follicles, sperm preparation, in vitro fertilization, and embryo transfer. Laparoscopic aspiration of the follicles is the only stage that may occur in the operating room. Embryo transfer may or may not take place in the operating room. The treatment cycle is extremely stressful, and both partners need emotional support from all members of the in vitro fertilization team. It is important that the perioperative nurse be knowledgeable about the treatment cycle to promote a feeling of empathy and participate effectively in patient teaching.

Follicular development

Although a spontaneous ovulatory cycle was used for recovery of the oocyte in the early development of in vitro fertilization, all programs at present use a stimulated cycle to obtain multiple oocytes.

With a stimulated cycle, induction of ovulation is achieved by one of three regimens. The first is clomiphene citrate (Clomid) and human chorionic gonadotropin (HCG).

The patient receives 50 to 150 mg/day of Clomid for 5 days starting at a specified point in her menstrual cycle. On the day following the last dose of Clomid, the patient begins daily ultrasonic scanning and determination of serum level of estrogen to monitor follicular growth. The timing for HCG administration is based on the size and rate of growth of the follicles and the level of serum estradiol. To ensure follicular maturation, 4000 to 10,000 units of HCG are then administered to the patient.

The second regimen is human menopausal gonadotropin (HMG) and HCG. The patient receives 1 to 3 ampules of HMG daily starting on day 3 or day 5 of her menstrual cycle, depending on the protocol. Monitoring methods and timing of the HCG are similar to the Clomid regimen.

The third regimen is a combination of Clomid, HMG, and HCG. The patient receives Clomid for 5 days, followed by daily administration of HMG. In all three regimens, oocyte retrieval is performed 34 to 36 hours after the administration of HCG.

Aspiration of the mature preovulatory follicles

Follicular aspiration may be performed via an ultrasound-guided transabdominal or transvaginal puncture or via laparoscopic technique. When the laparoscopic follicular aspiration technique is used, a regular laparoscopic instrument setup is utilized. In addition, grasping forceps, an aspirating needle with needle sleeve, a trap to collect the follicular fluid and ovum, a suctioning device, and a warming unit for the traps may be needed. A closed-circuit television monitoring system may be used, and the procedure videotaped or portions photographed.

In preparation for the procedure the operating room temperature may be increased. Perioperative considerations when opening sterile supplies and setting up the sterile field include the elimination of talc power and antimicrobial solutions from the instrument setup. These substances may be toxic if they are permitted to contact the follicular fluid or ovum.

The laparoscopy is performed with the patient in the supine or modified lithotomy position. Routinely, instruments are not placed in the cervix or vagina. The pneumoperitoneum may be achieved with 100% carbon dioxide or a gas mixture of 90% nitrogen, 5% oxygen, and 5% carbon dioxide.

1. Follicular aspiration may be performed using a double-puncture or a triple-puncture technique.
2. The ovary is stabilized against the pelvic side wall by grasping the uteroovarian ligament with grasping forceps.
3. The aspirating needle is placed in contact with the surface of the follicle.
4. Suction is applied as the follicle is punctured. The needle tip is moved within the follicle in an attempt to dislodge the cumulus mass from the follicle wall.

5. After the follicle has collapsed, suction is disconnected before the needle is removed from the follicle; this disconnection prevents aspiration of carbon dioxide.
6. After the needle is outside the peritoneal cavity, suction is reapplied to empty the fluid contained within the tubing into the ovum trap.
7. The ovum trap is changed, and culture medium is aspirated into another ovum trap to rinse the needle and ensure that the oocyte is not retained within the tubing.
8. The follicular aspirate is transferred immediately to the embryo laboratory where it is inspected microscopically for the presence of an oocyte. If an oocyte is not identified, the aspirating needle is reintroduced into the follicle. The follicle is redistended with culture media and is reaspirated.
9. The laparoscopic procedure is completed after all available follicles are aspirated.

Sperm preparation

A semen sample is obtained from the partner. After liquefaction, the semen is washed of seminal plasma by centrifugation twice in culture medium and incubated at 37° C until the time of insemination.

In vitro fertilization

The oocytes and surrounding cumulus are transferred to culture medium to complete maturation. The oocytes are incubated for different periods of time, depending on the degree of maturation of the oocytes before insemination. Oocytes may be inseminated with 50,000 to 200,000 motile sperm to each oocyte.

Evaluation of fertilization in the tissue culture dish requires visualization of the oocyte approximately 18 hours after insemination. The presence of two pronuclei is taken as presumptive evidence of fertilization, and the oocyte is transferred to growth medium. The embryo should be at the four-cell stage by 32 to 40 hours after insemination.

Embryo transfer

No anesthesia is required. The patient may be placed in the knee-chest or lithotomy position. A Graves vaginal speculum is inserted into the vagina. A single-tooth tenaculum may be used to grasp the cervix.

As soon as the patient is ready, the embryos are loaded into the transfer catheter with a minute amount of transfer medium and two small air bubbles. The catheter is carefully introduced into the uterine cavity, and the embryos are expelled. The catheter is withdrawn and returned to the laboratory, where it is examined for retained embryos. If the embryos have not been retained in the catheter, the speculum is removed.

Following embryo transfer, the patient is placed in the supine or modified jackknife position, depending on the position of the uterus, for 4 to 24 hours.

Another approach to in vitro fertilization is the gamete

intrafallopian transfer (GIFT). It has been proven successful for women with long-standing infertility who have at least one patent fallopian tube. Oocyte retrieval for the GIFT approach may be accomplished by laparoscope, minilaparotomy, or vaginal aspiration using ultrasound guidance. Egg fertilization occurs within the fallopian tube. Ovulation is stimulated and the ova are aspirated via laparoscopy and are loaded into a catheter with prepared sperm. The material loaded in the catheter are then expelled in the fallopian tube, where fertilization normally occurs.

In vitro fertilization program development now includes cryopreservation of embryos, donor eggs, donor sperm, and embryo sitters (implantation of embryos into surrogate mothers). Technical problems have been overcome and moral and ethical issues are being resolved. Established use of these advances is becoming a reality.

CESAREAN BIRTH

Cesarean birth, also referred to as cesarean section or C-section, is delivery of the fetus or fetuses through abdominal (laparotomy) and uterine (hysterotomy) incisions. In general, cesarean birth is employed whenever further delay in delivery may seriously compromise the fetus, the mother, or both, and vaginal delivery cannot be safely accomplished. In recent years the use of cesarean birth has increased as a result of fetal monitoring, fetal scalp blood sampling for pH determination, and the widespread emphasis on recognition of actual or suspected impairment of fetal well-being if delivery were delayed or vaginal delivery attempted. Reasons for cesarean birth include malposition and malpresentation, cephalopelvic disproportion, abruptio placentae, toxemia, fetal distress, uterine dysfunction, placenta previa, prolapsed cord, previous pelvic surgery, cervical dystocia, active herpes progenitalis, and diabetes. Multiple pregnancy may also be indications for cesarean delivery.

Cesarean delivery is the most frequently performed major surgical operation in the United States. Approximately 25% of all births are cesarean deliveries. From the mid-1960s to the late 1980s, the cesarean delivery rate has increased from less than 5% to approximately 25%. Reasons include increased use of electronic fetal monitoring, an increase in the number of first-time pregnancies, pregnancy at an older age, and a high incidence of repeat cesarean deliveries (Bobak & Jensen, 1993). There are institutional differences in primary cesarean delivery rates.

Cesarean delivery may take place in the obstetric labor delivery suite or in the OR suite. Patients about to undergo cesarean birth need careful assessment and emotional support. Because cesarean birth frequently involves emergency situations, the patient may express grave concern for the infant's well-being. If the patient has participated in childbirth classes, she may feel that she has failed in some way. The nurse must be aware of the psycho-logic, as well as physiologic, needs of this patient population. Mothers may choose to remain awake under regional anesthesia; her significant other may be permitted to accompany and support her in the OR and witness the birth (based upon hospital policy). The significant other may need the perioperative nurse's assistance in preparing for the delivery by washing hands and donning scrub attire or a protective gown. The perioperative nurse may need to reassure and encourage the significant other to coach and lend support to the mother during this intensely stressful time. The significant other can be included in the bonding process that is initiated at birth. The mother, if awake and stable, is shown and encouraged to hold the infant. The perioperative nurse promotes a positive family-oriented experience.

If the cesarean delivery is performed as an emergency, the family-oriented approach may not be feasible. In this emergency situation the mother's support people need to be directed to the surgical waiting area. The nurse and physician need to communicate the condition of the mother and infant. Support people may then be able to accompany the infant as he or she is transferred to the nursery.

PROCEDURAL CONSIDERATIONS

The patient should be in a supine position with elevation of the right side to ensure adequate venous return during preparation and surgery. Bony prominences are padded and the patient positioned in good body alignment with a safety strap above the knees. It may be necessary to assist the anesthesia team with the administration of regional anesthesia prior to placing the patient in the supine position. Throughout this process the maternal vital signs are monitored and recorded according to the institutional protocol. Fetal heart tones are also monitored and recorded per institutional protocol. The perioperative nurse is caring for two patients.

If a general anesthetic is to be employed *all* preparations, including skin prep, bladder drainage, draping, suction connection, counts, and gowning and gloving of all scrubbed personnel, must be done before induction. In many hospitals, health care providers qualified to deliver newborn care and resuscitation are in attendance for the delivery. A radiant warmer (Fig. 13-50) and resuscitative equipment for immediate postdelivery care of the infant are available in the operating rooms, since these infants are considered to be at risk until there is evidence of physiologic stability.

In preparation for delivery, if indicated, the mother's hair is clipped or shaved from the abdomen above the umbilicus to the level of the mons pubis and laterally to above the level of the iliac crests. The skin is prepped for abdominal surgery. The vagina is not prepared. An indwelling urinary catheter is inserted. Instrumentation includes the basic abdominal gynecologic set, plus the following may be indicated:

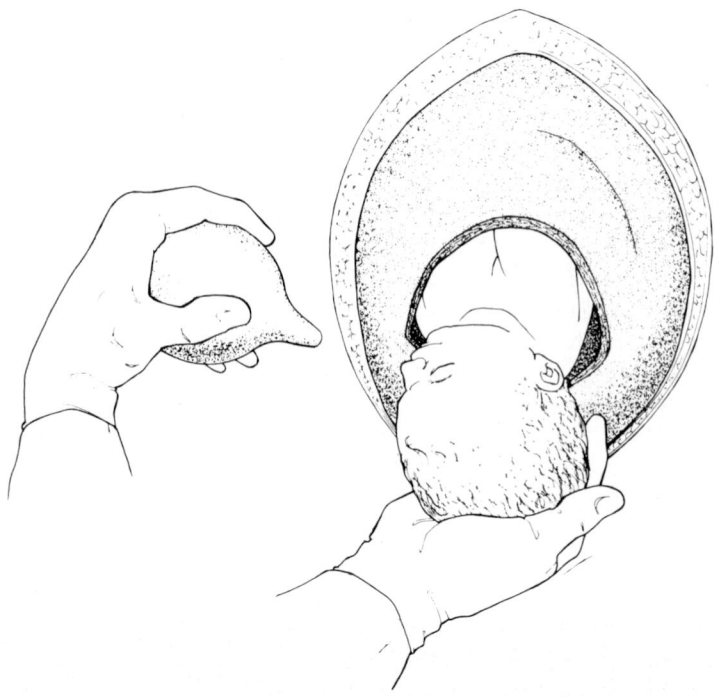

FIG. 13-50   Cesarean birth. Delivery of head; bulb syringe used to clear nares and mouth of amniotic fluid.

Cutting instrument

1 Lister bandage scissors

Holding instruments

4 Foerster sponge-
  holding (ring) for-
  ceps, 7 inches   6 Pennington forceps

Clamping instruments

2 Cord clamps

Exposing instrument

1 DeLee retractor

Obstetric instruments

1 Pair delivery forceps,   1 Head extractor, if de-
  if desired   sired

Accessory items

2 Laboratory tubes for   1 Drain (optional)
  cord blood   1 Bulb syringe

OPERATIVE PROCEDURE

1. An infraumbilical vertical incision or lower transverse Pfannenstiel incision is made. The incision should be long enough to allow the infant to be delivered without difficulty, but no longer. Therefore the length of the incision varies with the estimated size of the fetus.

2. The abdominal wall is opened in layers. The rectus and pyramidalis muscles are separated in the midline by sharp and blunt dissection to expose the underlying transversalis fascia and peritoneum.

3. The peritoneum is elevated with two Crile hemostats about 2 cm apart. The peritoneum between the two clamps is palpated to rule out the inclusion of bowel, omentum, or bladder. The peritoneum is opened and the abdominal cavity entered.

4. Bleeding sites anywhere in the abdominal incision may be clamped but not ligated until later, unless the clamps obstruct exposure. When the patient is under general anesthesia, speed is important to prevent an anesthetized infant. Electrosurgery may be used at this point to stop bleeding, especially if the patient is awake and under regional anesthesia.

5. The uterus is quickly but carefully palpated to determine the size and presenting part of the fetus as well as the direction and degree of rotation of the uterus.

6. The reflection of peritoneum (serosa) above the upper margin of the bladder and overlying the anterior lower uterine segment is gently separated by sharp and blunt dissection.

7. The developed bladder flap is held downward beneath the symphysis with a bladder retractor such as the DeLee.

8. The uterus is opened with a knife through the lower uterine segment about 2 cm above the detached bladder. Once the uterus is opened, the incision can be ex-

tended by cutting laterally with a large bandage scissors or by simply spreading the incision by means of lateral pressure applied with each index finger when the lower uterine segment is thin.

9. The presenting membranes are incised. Suction is imperative here, and many surgeons prefer no suction tip (only the large open end of the suction tubing) during the expulsion and suctioning of amniotic fluid.

10. All retractors are removed. The fetal head is gently elevated, either manually or by use of obstetric forceps, through the incision, aided by transabdominal fundal pressure. The pressure helps expel the fetus.

11. As soon as the head is delivered, a bulb syringe or aspirator tip is used to aspirate the exposed nares and mouth to minimize aspiration of amniotic fluid and its contents.

12. About 20 units of oxytocin per liter of fluid may be administered intravenously as soon as the shoulders are delivered (or after delivery of the infant), so that the uterus contracts; this minimizes blood loss.

13. On delivery of the entire infant, the cord is clamped and cut and the infant given to the member of the team who is responsible for resuscitation efforts as needed. A sterile gown and/or sheet should be provided to the individual receiving the infant to avoid any break in aseptic technique and to maintain universal precautions during transfer of the infant.

14. The edges of the uterine incision are promptly clamped with Pean forceps, ring forceps, or Pennington clamps.

15. The placenta is delivered and placed in a large receptacle provided from the back table. Fundal massage or manual removal may be employed to hasten delivery of the placenta and reduce bleeding.

16. One or two separate layers of suture may be used to close the uterine incision.

17. Following determination that there is no further bleeding after closure of the uterine incision, the cut edges of the serosa overlying the uterus and bladder are approximated with a continuous suture.

18. Any blood, blood clots, vernix, and amniotic fluid in the pelvis and peritoneal cavity are removed. The fallopian tubes and ovaries are also inspected. Tubal ligation may be carried out at this point.

19. The peritoneum and each abdominal layer are closed.

REFERENCES

Bobak, I.M., Jensen, M.D. (1993). *Maternity and gynecologic care: The nurse and the family* (5th Ed.). St. Louis: Mosby.
Leach, R.E., & Ory, S.J. (1989). Modern management of ectopic pregnancy. *Journal of Reproductive Medicine, 34*(5), 324-335.
Levine, R.L. (1990). Pelviscopic surgery in women over 40. *Journal of Reproductive Medicine, 35,* 597.

BIBLIOGRAPHY

Atkinson, L.J. (1992). *Berry & Kohn's operating room technique* (7th Ed.). St. Louis: Mosby.
Baggish, M.S., Barbot, J., & Valle, R.F. (1989). *Diagnostic and operative hysteroscopy, a text and atlas.* St. Louis: Mosby.
Berger, P.H., & Saul, H.M. (1990). Radical hysterectomy treatment for advanced cervical carcinoma. *AORN Journal, 52*(6), 1212-1222.
Garuffi, G., Strobino, D.M., & Paine, L.L. (1990, September/October). Investigation of institutional differences in primary cesarean birth rates. *Journal of Nurse-Midwifery, 35,* 274.
Gray, H. (1989). *Anatomy of the human body* (37th Ed.). Philadelphia: Lea & Febiger.
Hawkins, J.W., & Higgins, L.P. (1989). *Maternity and gynecological nursing: women's health care.* Philadelphia: J.B. Lippincott.
Hunt, R.B. (1992). *Atlas of female infertility surgery* (2nd Ed.). St. Louis: Mosby.
Jackson, K.D. (1991). Endometrial ablation with rollerball electrode: An alternative to hysterectomy. *AORN Journal, 54*(2), 265-282.
Minelli, L., et al. (1991). Laparoscopically-assisted vaginal hysterectomy. *Endoscopy, 23* (2), 64-66.
Mishell, D.R., Kirschbaum, T.H., & Morrow, C.P. (1992). *Yearbook of obstetrics and gynecology.* St. Louis: Mosby.
Nezhat, C., et al. (1989). Endoscopic infertility surgery. *Journal of Reproductive Surgery, 34,* 127.
Nichols, D.H. (1993). *Gynecologic and obstetric surgery.* St. Louis: Mosby.
Peterson, H.B., Hulka, J.F. & Phillips, J.M. (1990). American Association of Gynecologic Laparoscopists' 1988 Membership Survey on Operative Hysteroscopy. *Journal of Reproductive Medicine, 35*(6), 590-591.
Raber, F.G. (1991). Gamete intrafallopian transfer, another approach for the treatment of infertility. *AORN Journal, 53*(6), 1466-1475.
Rothrock, J.C. (1990). *Perioperative care planning.* St. Louis: Mosby.
Thibodeau, G.A., & Patton, K.T. (1992). *Anatomy and physiology* (2nd Ed.). St. Louis: Mosby.
Thompson, J.M., et al. (1993). *Mosby's manual of clinical nursing.* (3rd Ed.). St. Louis: Mosby.
Vasilev, S.A., & Liming, P.R. (1991). Ectopic pregnancy: etiology, diagnosis, treatment. *AORN Journal, 54*(5), 1030-1039.

14

GENITOURINARY SURGERY

GRATIA M. NAGLE

Over the past decade major changes in genitourinary surgery have occurred. The influences of the neodymium:YAG (Nd:YAG), KTP (a variation of the YAG), carbon dioxide (CO_2), and Candela lasers, ultrasonography, electrohydraulic (EHL), ultrasonic, and electrocorporeal shock wave lithotriptors (ESWL), as well as other innovative diagnostic measures and minimally invasive surgical approaches have expanded treatment options. Urologic surgery is now more complex and far more precise.

The perioperative urology nurse has new challenges to face with these advancements. For the perioperative urology nurse to function optimally, up-to-date knowledge and peak technical skills are priorities. Pressures to contain the rising cost of health care are resulting in more procedures being done on an ambulatory or short-stay basis, and in limited time being available for preoperative teaching and discharge planning. Frequently this important task falls to the perioperative nursing team. The success of surgical intervention depends greatly on the perioperative nurse's ability and knowledge in developing a perioperative plan of care.

SURGICAL ANATOMY

A comprehensive understanding of the anatomic structures involved in genitourinary surgery is required to facilitate safe patient positioning and proper selection of instrumentation and equipment. Collaboration with the urologist's plan of care is necessary in preparing the patient for surgery.

The normal urinary tract comprises a pair of kidneys, two ureters, the urinary bladder, and the urethra. Urine is excreted by the kidneys and conveyed to the bladder through the ureters, muscular tubes 25 to 30 cm long. Urine is stored in the bladder, which serves as a reservoir, until its full capacity (350 to 700 ml) is reached, and is eliminated from the body by way of the urethra. Normal urinary output ranges from 0.5 to 1 ml per kilogram of body weight per hour for the average adult. Normal range in the child is generally considered 1 to 1.5 ml/kg/hour.

KIDNEYS

The kidneys are located in the retroperitoneal space along the lateral borders of the psoas muscle, one on each side of the vertebral column at the level of the twelfth thoracic to the third lumbar vertebra. Usually the right kidney is several centimeters lower than the left because the liver rests above and anterior to the right kidney (Fig. 14-1).

Each kidney is surrounded by a mass of fatty and loose areolar tissue known as perirenal fat. A capsule enclosing the renal space is known as fascia renalis, or Gerota's fascia. These structures help keep the kidneys in their normal anatomic position. The anterior and posterior relationships of the kidneys are shown in Fig. 14-2.

On the medial side of each kidney is a concave area known as the hilum through which the renal artery and vein enter and leave. The renal pelvis, a funnel-shaped structure that lies posterior to the renal vascular pedicle, divides into several branches within the kidney called calyces (Fig. 14-3). When surgery is indicated in these structures, a posterior flank approach is preferred. When surgery for removal of a mass is anticipated, a transabdominal or thoracoabdominal incision is often chosen.

The kidneys are highly vascular organs that process approximately one fifth of the entire volume of blood at any one time. The blood supply to the kidney is conveyed through the renal artery, a large branch of the aorta (Fig. 14-4), and leaves through the renal vein. On entering the kidney, the renal artery divides into anterior and posterior sections. These undergo further division into interlobular arteries from which smaller afferent branches pass to the glomeruli. Efferent arterioles in the glomeruli then pass to the tubules of the nephron. Renal arteriography is commonly performed preoperatively to help identify the patient's renal vascular anatomy when renal hypertension and horseshoe kidney are suspected, and as part of the routine workup prior to renal transplantation.

The renal lymphatic supply originates beneath the capsule of the kidney and empties into the lumbar lymph nodes at the junction of the renal vascular pedicle and aorta. The nerves of the autonomic (involuntary) nervous system come

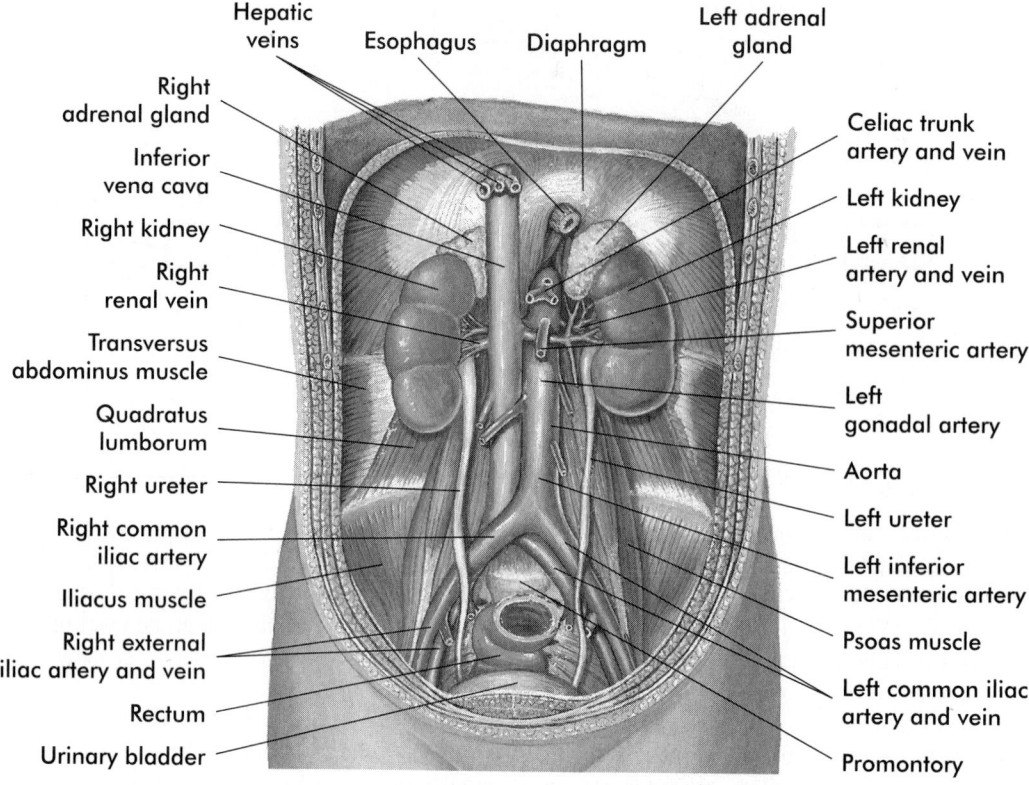

FIG. 14-1 Location of urinary system organs.

Modified from Seidel, H.M., et al. (1995). *Mosby's guide to physical examination* (3rd Ed.) St Louis: Mosby.

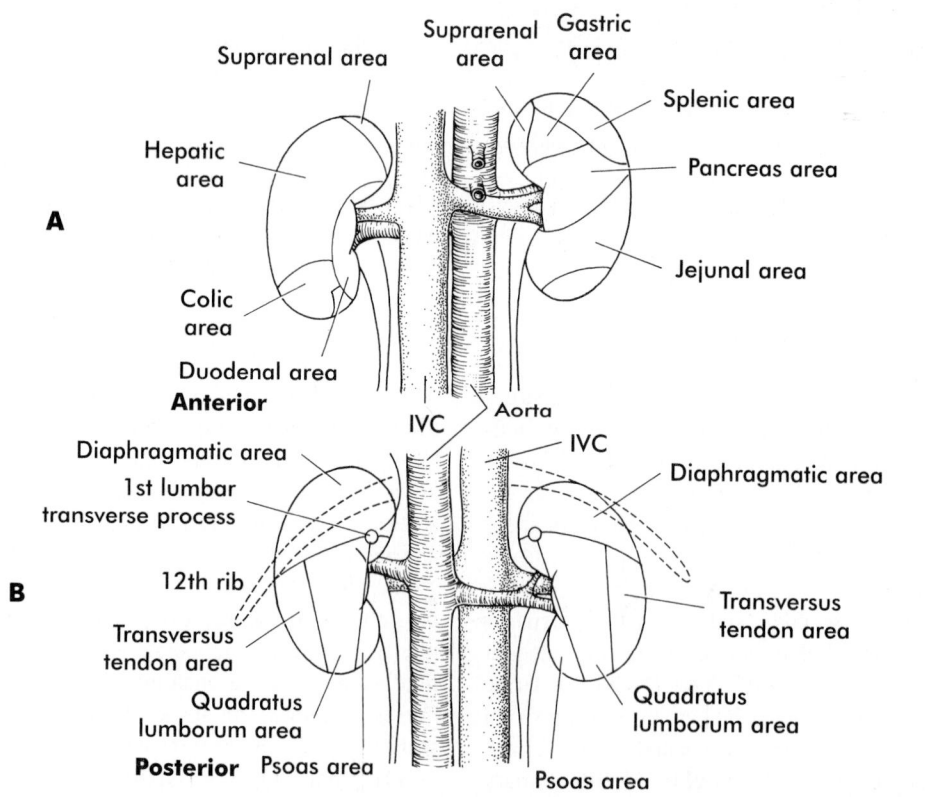

FIG. 14-2 Anterior (**A**) and posterior (**B**) relationship of kidneys and ureters to organs in peritoneal cavity, to vertebral column posteriorly, and to main arteries and veins.

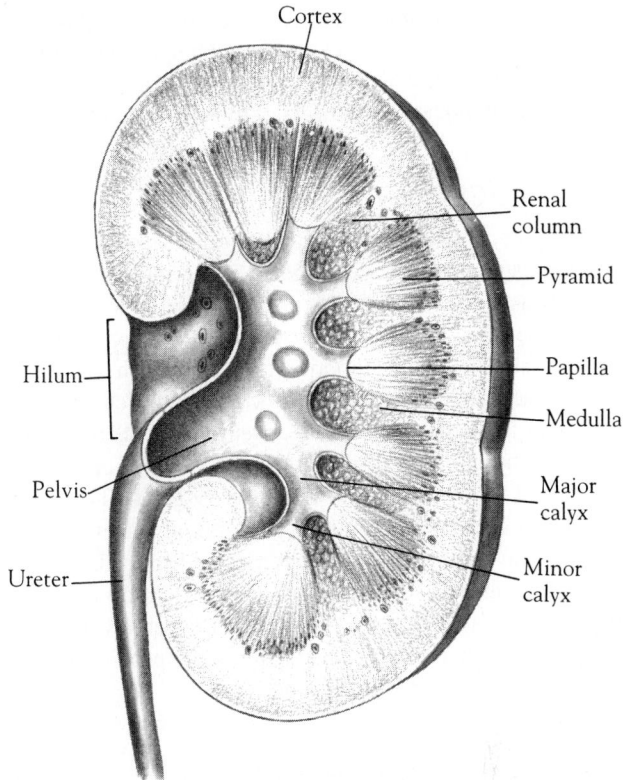

FIG. 14-3 Normal kidney.

From Thompson, J.M., et al. (1993). *Mosby's clinical nursing* (3rd Ed.).
St Louis: Mosby.

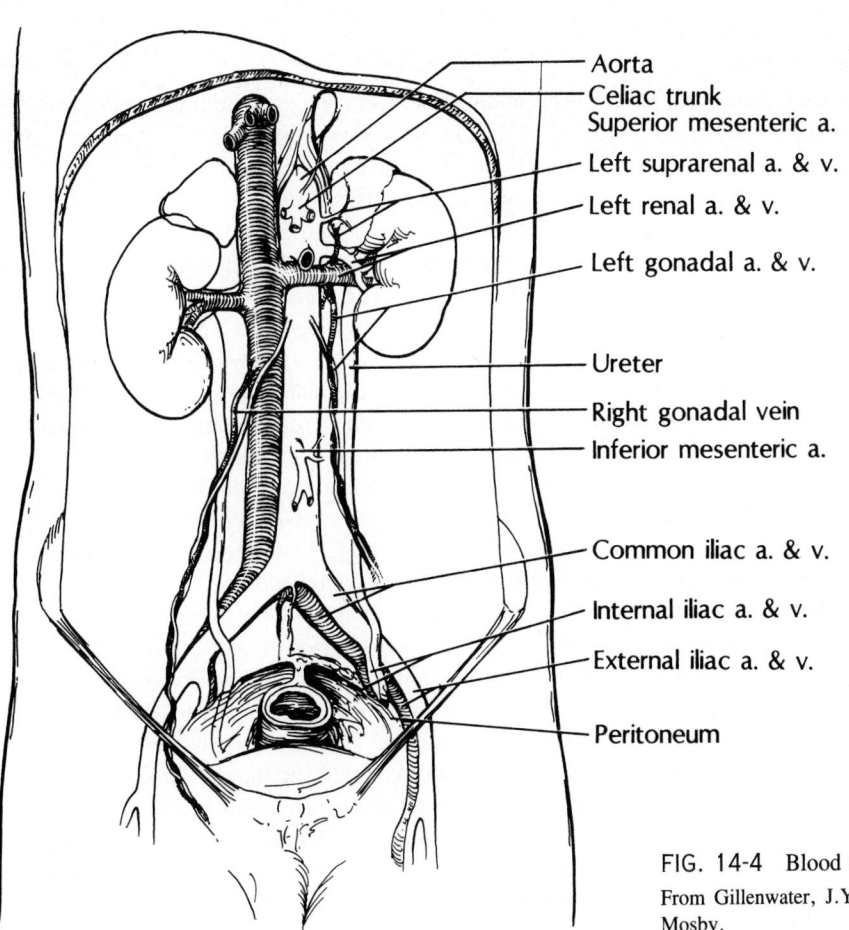

FIG. 14-4 Blood supply of kidneys.

From Gillenwater, J.Y. (1991). *Adult and pediatric urology*. St Louis:
Mosby.

from the lumbar sympathetic trunk and from the vagus. Removal of the nerve pathways does not impair renal function. The renal artery and vein with their accompanying nerves and lymphatics are referred to as the pedicle of the kidney.

ADRENAL GLANDS

The adrenal glands lie retroperitoneally beneath the diaphragm capping the medial aspects of the superior pole of each kidney. On the right side the triangular gland is adjacent to the inferior vena cava; on the left side it is a rounded, crescent-shaped gland posterior to the stomach and pancreas. Each adrenal gland has a medulla, which secretes adrenalin (epinephrine), and a cortex, which secretes steroids and hormones. Secretions from the adrenal cortex are influenced by the activity of the pituitary gland. The adrenal glands are liberally supplied with arterial branches from the inferior phrenic and renal arteries and from the aorta. Venous drainage is accomplished on the right by the inferior vena cava and on the left by the left renal vein. The lymphatic system accompanies the suprarenal vein and drains into the lumbar lymph nodes.

URETERS

Each ureter is a continuation of the renal pelvis. The ureter extends in a smooth S curve from the renal pelvis to the base of the bladder. It is approximately 25 to 30 cm long and 4 to 5 mm in diameter in the adult (see Fig. 14-4). This fibromuscular cylindrical tube is lined by transitional epithelium (urothelium) and lies on the psoas muscle, passing medial to the sacroiliac joints and lateral to the ischial spines. As urine accumulates in the renal pelvis, slight distention initiates a wave of muscular contractions. This peristaltic activity continues down the ureter, propelling urine into the bladder.

The ureter has three areas of narrowing where calculi may become lodged and pose a potential problem with pain and obstruction: (1) the ureteropelvic junction, (2) the crossing of the ureter over the external iliac vessels, and (3) the ureterovesical junction (Fig. 14-5). Urine may sometimes cause calculi to be washed down the ureter to produce severe ureteral colic. Of all renal calculi, 90% are spontaneously passed into the bladder. However, if they become lodged in the ureter, an ESWL, ureteroscopy, stone manipulation, EHL, laser or sonic lithotripsy, or ureterolithotomy may be indicated. During pelvic or intestinal surgery, ureteral catheters or stents are often inserted to facilitate positive identification of the ureters and reduce the potential for severing or ligating them. These stents are generally removed postoperatively, although some surgeons prefer to leave them in place through the early recovery period.

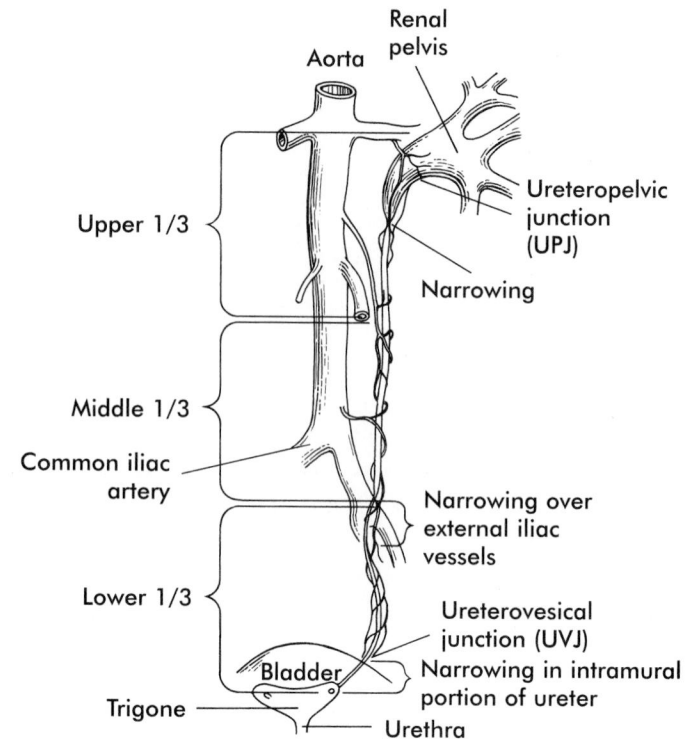

FIG. 14-5   Anatomy of ureter.

URINARY BLADDER

The adult urinary bladder is a hollow muscular viscus that acts as a reservoir for urine until micturition (voiding) occurs. It has an outer adventitial and inner urothelial layer. The trigone, a triangular area, forms the base of the bladder. The three corners of the trigone correspond to the orifices of the ureters and the bladder neck (opening of the urethra) (Fig. 14-6). The ureteral orifices, on the proximal trigone at the interureteric ridge, are 2.5 cm apart. The bladder neck (internal sphincter) is formed from converging detrusor muscle fibers of the bladder wall that pass distally to form the smooth musculature of the urethra. Physiologically the bladder fills with urine and expands into the abdominal cavity. The extraperitoneal location is advantageous because a suprapubic (above pubic arch) incision may be performed without violating the peritoneum and potentially causing intraperitoneal complications.

The main arterial supply of the bladder comprises the superior, middle, and inferior vesical arteries. These vessels are derived from the internal iliac (hypogastric) artery, the obturator and inferior gluteal arteries, and in females the uterine and vaginal arteries. The bladder has a rich venous supply that drains into the internal iliac (hypogastric) vein. The lymphatic system is served by the vesical, external and internal iliac, and common iliac lymph nodes.

The bladder's size, position, and relation to the bowel, rectum, and reproductive organs vary according to the bladder's distention. In a female the vagina lies dorsal to the

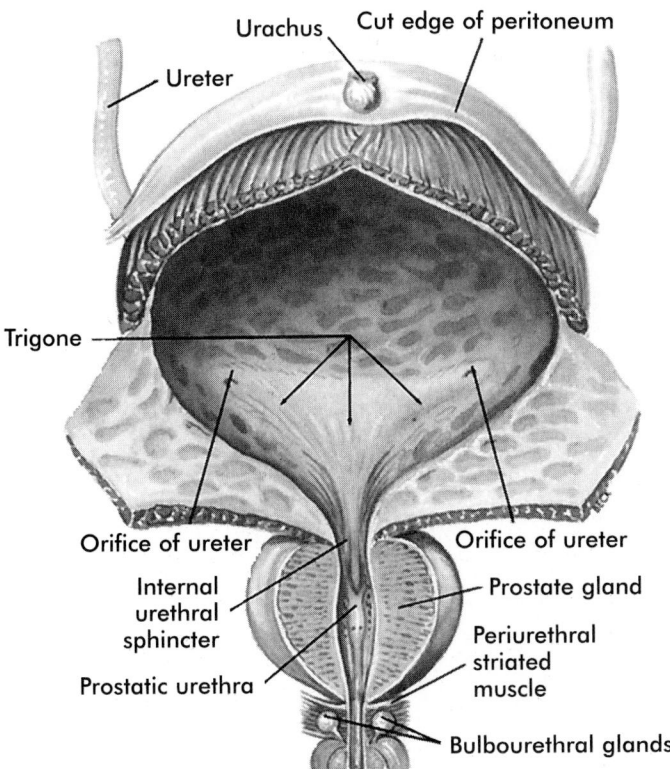

Urachus   Cut edge of peritoneum

Ureter

Trigone

Orifice of ureter

Internal urethral sphincter

Prostatic urethra

Orifice of ureter

Prostate gland

Periurethral striated muscle

Bulbourethral glands

FIG. 14-6 Male urinary bladder cut to show interior.

From Thibodeau, G.A., & Patton, K.T. (1993). *Anatomy and physiology* (2nd Ed.). St Louis: Mosby.

base of the bladder and parallel to the urethra (Fig. 14-7). In a male the prostate gland is interposed between the bladder neck and the urethra (Fig. 14-8). These anatomic relationships influence the symptoms patients experience preoperatively and are important landmarks during pelvic surgery.

The process of bladder evacuation appears to be initiated by nerve cells from the sacral division of the autonomic nervous system. These sacral reflex centers are controlled by higher voluntary centers in the brain. Stimulation of the sacral centers results in contraction of the bladder muscles and relaxation of the bladder outlet sphincters. Muscles inside and adjacent to the urethral wall, and from the pelvic floor, maintain closure of the sphincters of the bladder, thus enabling continence.

URETHRA

The male urethra, normally 20 to 25 cm long, extends from the bladder neck to the tip of the penis and varies in diameter from 7 to 10 mm. It is divided into two portions: the proximal (sphincteric) and the distal (conduit or anterior) urethra, both of which undergo further subdivision. The proximal urethra is commonly referred to as the posterior urethra, where it is elevated by the verumontanum, extending from the bladder neck through the prostate and the membranous portion. Within the posterior urethra lie the prostatic and membranous portions (Fig. 14-9). As the urethra exits the prostate and crosses the pelvic (urogeni-

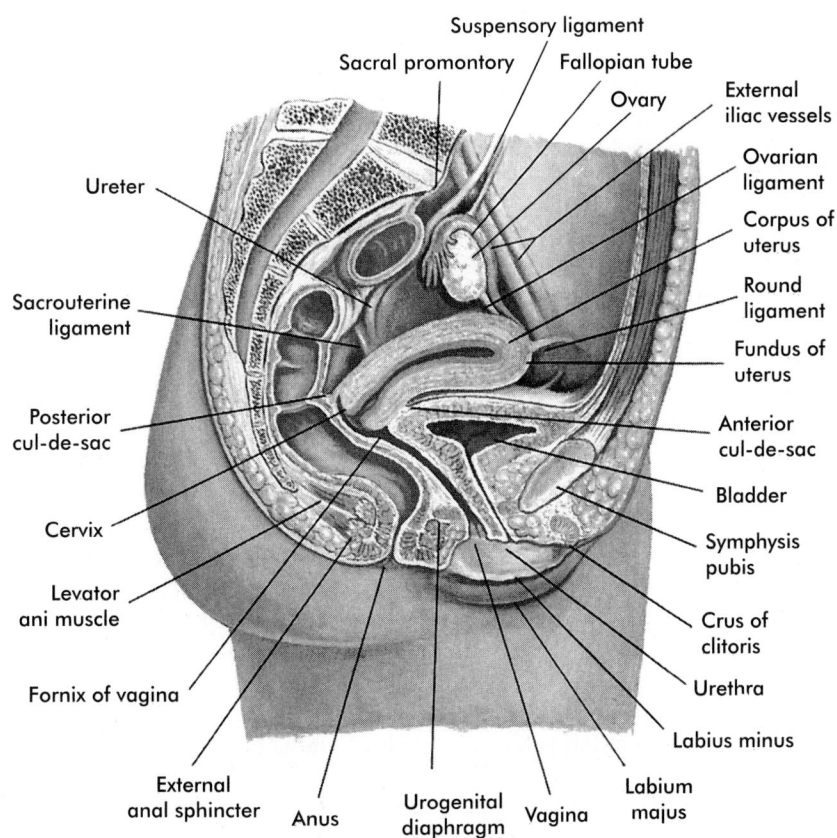

Suspensory ligament

Sacral promontory   Fallopian tube

Ovary

External iliac vessels

Ovarian ligament

Corpus of uterus

Round ligament

Fundus of uterus

Anterior cul-de-sac

Bladder

Symphysis pubis

Crus of clitoris

Urethra

Labius minus

Labium majus

Vagina

Urogenital diaphragm

Anus

External anal sphincter

Fornix of vagina

Levator ani muscle

Cervix

Posterior cul-de-sac

Sacrouterine ligament

Ureter

FIG. 14-7 Female genitourinary and reproductive anatomy.

From Seidel, H.M., et al. (1995). *Mosby's guide to physical examination* (3rd Ed.). St Louis: Mosby.

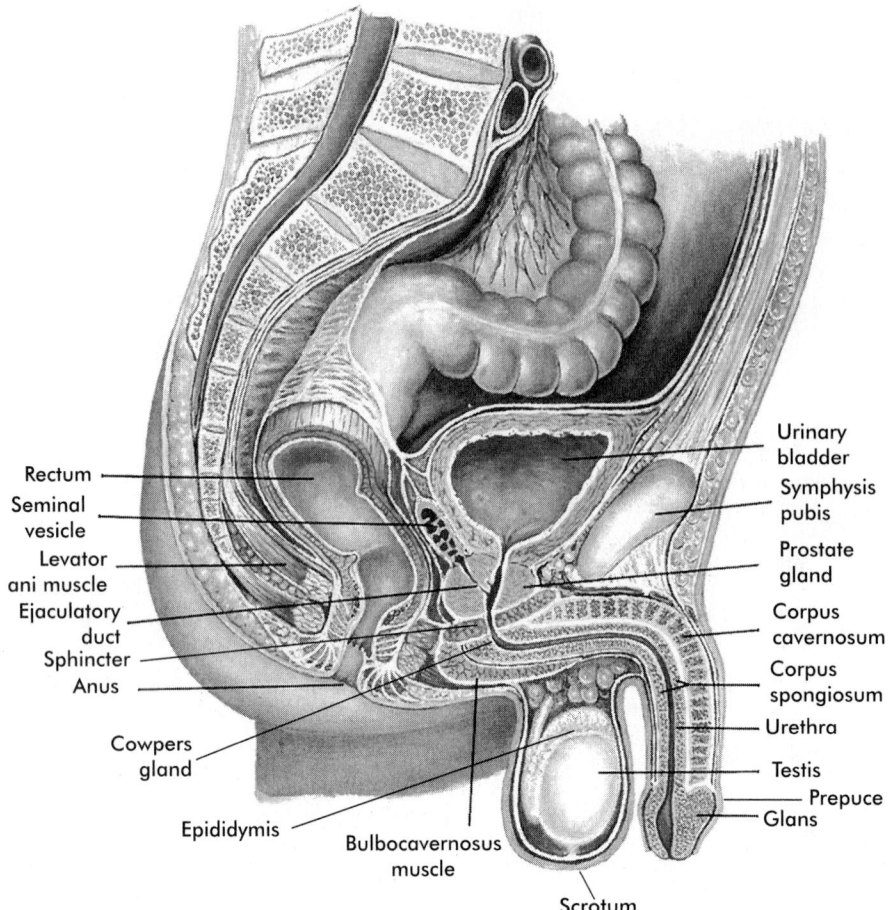

Rectum

Seminal
vesicle

Levator
ani muscle

Ejaculatory
duct

Sphincter

Anus

Cowpers
gland

Epididymis

Bulbocavernosus
muscle

Scrotum

Urinary
bladder

Symphysis
pubis

Prostate
gland

Corpus
cavernosum

Corpus
spongiosum

Urethra

Testis

Prepuce

Glans

FIG. 14-8   Male genitourinary and reproductive anatomy.
From Seidel, H.M., et al. (1995). *Mosby's guide to physical examination* (3rd Ed.). St Louis: Mosby.

tal) diaphragm, it is called the membranous urethra (Fig. 14-9). The distal urethra, commonly called the anterior urethra, is subdivided into the bulbar, pendulous (penile), and glandular urethras (Fig. 14-9). The bulbar urethra is the area most prone to urethral strictures in the male.

The prostatic urethra is approximately 3 cm long and is the widest portion of the urethra. On the floor of the prostatic urethra is the verumontanum, which contains the openings of the ejaculatory ducts.

The membranous urethra is the shortest portion, measuring approximately 2.5 cm and extending from the external sphincter to the apex of the prostate (Fig. 14-9).

The penile, or pendulous, urethra lies within the corpus spongiosum. The urothelium of the urethra is continuous with that of the bladder.

The female urethra is a narrow, membranous tube about 3 to 5 cm in length and 6 to 8 mm in diameter. Slightly curved, it lies behind and beneath the symphysis pubis, anterior to the vagina. It passes through the internal and external sphincter and the urogenital diaphragm. The periurethral glands of Skene open on the floor of the urethra just

inside the meatus. Because the female urethra is so short, microorganisms find easy access to the bladder and can cause urinary tract infections.

MALE REPRODUCTIVE ORGANS

The male reproductive organs include several paired structures: the testes, epididymides, seminal ducts (vas deferens), seminal vesicles, ejaculatory ducts, and bulbourethral glands. Other organs of the reproductive tract are the penis, prostate gland, and urethra.

The scrotum is located behind and below the base of the penis and in front of the anus. Each loose sac contains and supports a testis, an epididymis, and some of the spermatic cord. The two sides of the scrotum are separated from each other by a median raphe (septum). Within the scrotum are two cavities or sacs that are lined with smooth, glistening tissue, the tunica vaginalis. Normally, a small amount of clear fluid is contained in the tunica vaginalis. The condition known as hydrocele is an abnormal accumulation of this fluid.

The testes manufacture the spermatozoa and also con-

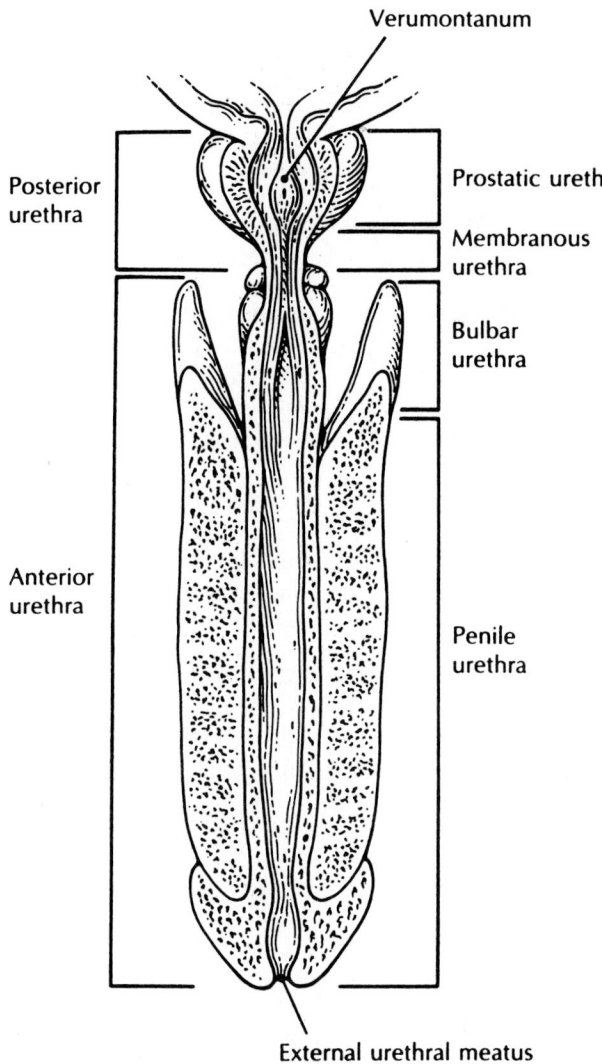

Verumontanum

Posterior
urethra

Prostatic urethra

Membranous
urethra

Bulbar
urethra

Anterior
urethra

Penile
urethra

External urethral meatus

FIG. 14-9   Anatomy of male urethra.

From Glenn, J.F., (editor). (1991). *Urology surgery* (4th Ed.). Philadelphia: JB Lippincott.

tain specialized Leydig cells that produce the male hormone testosterone. Each testis consists of many tubules in which the sperm are formed, surrounded by dense capsules of connective tissue. The tubules coalesce and continue into the adjacent epididymis, where the sperm mature and are stored. At the upper pole of the testis is the appendix testis, a small body that may be pedunculated (stalked) or sessile (flat).

The epididymis is a long, convoluted duct located along the posterolateral surface of the testis. It is closely attached to the testicle by fibrous tissue and secretes seminal fluid, which gives the sperm a liquid medium in which to migrate. The vas deferens (ductus deferens, or seminal duct) is a distal continuation of the epididymis as it enters

the prostate gland and conveys the sperm to the seminal vesicle.

The vas deferens lies within the spermatic cord in the inguinal region. The spermatic cord also contains veins, arteries, lymphatics, nerves, and surrounding connective tissue (cremaster muscle), which give support to the testes. The terminal portion of each vas deferens is called the ejaculatory duct; it passes between the lobes of the prostate gland and opens into the posterior urethra.

The accessory reproductive glands include the seminal vesicles, prostate gland, and bulbourethral gland. The seminal vesicles unite with the vas deferens on either side, are situated behind the bladder, and produce protein and fructose for the nutrition of the sperm cell. Sperm and prostatic fluid are discharged at the time of ejaculation.

The prostate gland is a fibromuscular organ located at the base of the bladder neck and the triangular ligament completely surrounding the urethra. The gland is about 4 cm at its base and about 2 cm in depth and weighs approximately 20 g (see Fig. 14-9).

There are four glandular regions within the prostate: two major regions, the peripheral zone and central zone, and two minor regions, the transitional and periurethral zone. Many clinicians still prefer to divide the prostate into the intraurethral lobe (right and left lateral) and the extraurethral lobe (posterior and median). The posterior lobe is readily palpable during rectal examination and prone to cancerous degeneration. Benign prostatic hypertrophy generally occurs in the transitional zone (intraurethral lobe).

Behind the prostatic capsule is a fibrous sheath known as the true prostatic capsule, which separates the prostate gland and the seminal vesicles from the rectum. This fascia is important when perineal prostatectomy is contemplated.

The lobes of the prostate gland secrete highly alkaline fluid that dilutes the testicular secretion as it is excreted from the ejaculatory ducts. These sections are believed to be essential to the passage of spermatozoa and helpful in keeping them alive. The arterial supply to the prostate is derived from the pudendal, inferior vesical, and hemorrhoidal arteries.

Cowper's glands (bulbourethral glands) are located on each side at the juncture of the membranous and bulbar urethras. Each gland, by way of its duct, empties mucous secretions into the urethra.

The penis is suspended from the pubic symphysis by the suspensory ligaments. The penis contains three distinct vascular spongelike bodies surrounding the urethra: two outer bodies called the right and left corpus cavernosum, and an inner body, the corpus spongiosum urethra. These tissues contain a network of vascular channels that fill with blood during erection (see Fig. 14-9). At the distal end of the penis the skin is doubly folded to form the prepuce, or foreskin, which serves as a covering for the glans penis. The glans penis contains the urethral orifice.

TABLE 14-1

Common Preoperative Laboratory Analyses for Patients with Genitourinary Disorders

Laboratory studies	Normal range (adult values)	Laboratory studies	Normal range (adult values)
COAGULATION PROFILES		**SERUM PROFILES (LOW: FEMALE; HIGH: MALE)— CONT'D**	
Bleeding time	1-9 min	Creatinine	0.5-1.2 mg/dl
Partial thromboplastin time (PTT)	60-70 sec	Glucose (blood sugar)	70-105 mg/dl
Platelet count	150,000-400,000/mm^3	Osmolality	285-295 mOsm/kg H_2O
Prothrombin time (PT)	11-12.5 sec	Potassium (K)	3.5-5 mEq/L
		Phosphorus (P)	3-4.5 mg/dl
FERTILITY PROFILES (MALE)		Prostate specific antigen (PSA)	<4 ng/ml
Follicle-stimulating hormone (FSH)	1-15 mIU/ml	Prostatic acid phosphatase (PAP)	0.11-0.6 U/L
Luteinizing hormone (LH)	7-24 mIU/ml	Protein	6-8 g/dl
Testosterone (total)	300-1000 ng/dl	Sodium (Na)	136-145 mEq/L
Sperm count	50-200 million/ml, 60%-80% motile	Uric acid	2-8.5 mg/dl
		URINE PROFILES (VALUES NOT LISTED SHOULD BE NEGATIVE)	
HEMATOLOGIES (LOW: FEMALE; HIGH: MALE)		Calcium (Ca)	100-300 mg/day
Hematocrit (Hct)	37%-52%	Chloride (Cl)	110-250 mEq/L
Hemoglobin (Hgb)	12-18 g/dl	Creatinine clearance	88-137 ml/min
Red blood cells (RBCs)	4.2-6.1 million/mm^3	Glucose (24 hr)	0.5 g/day
White blood cells (WBCs)	5000-10,000 million/mm^3	Hyaline casts	Occasional
		Osmolality (random)	50-1400 mOsm/kg H_2O
SERUM PROFILES (LOW: FEMALE; HIGH: MALE)		Phosphorus	4.5-8
Bicarbonate	21-28 mEq/L	Potassium (K)	25-120 mEq/L/day
Blood urea nitrogen (BUN)	10-20 mg/dl	Protein	30-150 mg/day
Calcium (Ca)	9-10.5 mg/dl	Red blood cells (RBCs)	0-2
Chloride (Cl)	90-110 mEq/L	Sodium (Na)	40-220 mEq/L/day
Cholesterol	150-200 mg/dl	Uric acid	250-750 ml/day
HDL (High-density lipids)	>45-55 mg/dl	White blood cells (WBCs)	0-4
LDL (Low-density lipids)	60-180 mg/dl	pH	4.6-8 (ave.:6)
VLDL (triglycerides)	25%-50%	Specific gravity	1.005-1.030

From Pagana, K. (1992). *Diagnostic and laboratory test reference*. St. Louis: Mosby; Tanagho, E. (1992). *Smith's general urology*. Norwalk, Conn: Appleton & Lange; and Gray, M. (1992). *Genitourinary disorders*. St. Louis: Mosby.

PERIOPERATIVE NURSING CONSIDERATIONS

ASSESSMENT

Patients entering a hospital or ambulatory surgery unit for genitourinary surgery exhibit many emotions and reactions. These feelings encompass fear, embarrassment, helplessness, hostility, anger, and grief. To most, a successful surgical outcome is of prime importance. The urology patient population varies from infants with congenital anomalies to the elderly with physiologic impairments. Owing to the dramatic increase in ambulatory surgery, the nursing staff must prepare to meet patients' specific needs, from preoperative teaching to postoperative home care. The families of patients need to be involved in this preparation process. Patient education begins in the urologist's office. Communication between the office and perioperative nursing staff allows continuity of care and increases the efficiency and effectiveness of surgical procedures.

In addition to routine admission information, urologic

and cardiac histories are usually obtained. This information includes, but is not limited to, vital signs, allergies, the patient's primary problem, history of the present illness, nature of symptoms, and limitations imposed by the disease condition. All data pertinent to the proposed operative procedure should be reviewed. Nursing observation should include the patient's general physical appearance, as well as nonverbal behaviors such as restlessness, which may indicate discomfort or anxiety. Any limitations in mobility or sensory deficits should be noted. Urologic procedures frequently require positions that create unusual stress for the patient, both anatomic and physiologic. Assessment must provide the perioperative nurse with data adequate to support preoperative planning and postoperative evaluation.

Many urologic surgical interventions require the patient to be in a flank position, causing compression of the vena cava. Additionally, large amounts of irrigating fluids are frequently used intraoperatively. For these reasons a current cardiac and electrolyte status should be available for review. Laboratory studies that have been done preoperatively may include serum and urine electrolytes, blood sugar, BUN, urinalysis and urine cultures, cardiac enzymes, CBC, prothrombin time (PT) and partial thromboplastin time (PTT), blood chemistry profiles (Table 14-1), electrocardiogram (ECG), and chest x-rays. The medical history, including a list of medications and any infectious processes or chronic diseases, should be reviewed. Specific genitourinary studies can also be found in the patient's medical record. They may encompass all or some of the following: computed tomography (CT) scans, magnetic resonance imaging (MRI), intravenous pyelograms (IVPs), KUBs (genitourinary flat plate), urinary flow studies, fluoroscopic exams (angiography, cavernosography), prostatic specific antigen (PSA), and ultrasound. After the medical record is reviewed, assessment information compiled, and perioperative nursing diagnoses identified, the perioperative plan of care is formulated.

NURSING DIAGNOSIS

Nursing diagnoses related to the care of patients undergoing genitourinary surgery might include the following:

- Anxiety
- High risk for injury
- Altered patterns of urinary elimination
- Fluid volume excess or deficit
- Impaired gas exchange

OUTCOME IDENTIFICATION

Outcomes identified for the selected nursing diagnoses could be stated as:

- The patient will verbalize feelings to the perioperative nurse.
- The patient will be free from injury related to surgical position.

- The patient's pattern of urinary elimination will remain patent and within the normal range.
- The patient will exhibit no signs of hypernatremia, hyponatremia, hypervolemia, or hypovolemia.
- The patient will maintain adequate gas exchange.

PLANNING

Care plans are the organizing framework for perioperative nursing activities. Frequently the urology patient presents a complex medical picture. Any alterations in the patient's physical or emotional status may impact both the surgical and postoperative course. A review of the patient record, communication with the patient and/or family, recognition of specific psychosocial needs of the patient and family, and knowledge gained from other members of the patient care team should be used to formulate the nursing data base. A typical care plan for a patient undergoing genitourinary surgery follows.

IMPLEMENTATION

Care plan implementation begins during the patient interview. Patient education that is concise and simply explained enhances the final surgical outcome. Meeting the patient's emotional needs is a nursing priority. A calm patient absorbs more and is more receptive to perioperative teaching. Explanations of what to expect throughout the operative period allay fears and nurture confidence in the nursing care provided. Perioperative nursing care requires not only the collection of pertinent patient data, but also the provision of numerous supplies and equipment to support the smooth implementation of the care plan.

Positioning

Thorough understanding of the urologic OR bed and its functions is essential to provide optimum patient positioning for each operative procedure. The position in which the patient is placed for surgery is determined by the particular operation to be performed. For urologic operative procedures the patient may be placed in the lateral, supine, prone, or lithotomy position, which may be exaggerated to give optimum access to the organ involved, particularly in radical surgery of the prostate and bladder. Considerable care must be taken to ensure that the patient's position does not interfere with respiration or circulation. It is essential to avoid displacement of the joints and undue tension on neurovascular bundles or ligaments, particularly in an aged or debilitated patient.

A patient positioned laterally (flank position) for renal surgery has the spine extended for greater access to the retroperitoneal space. Padding and stabilized support with gel pads, pillows, sandbags, and straps should be available for precise anatomic positioning and safety. If an electrosurgical unit is to be used, care must be taken that the patient does not contact metal equipment.

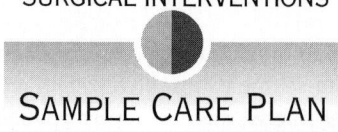

SAMPLE CARE PLAN

NURSING DIAGNOSIS: Anxiety

OUTCOME: Patient will verbalize feelings to the perioperative nurse.

INTERVENTIONS:

Provide an accepting and supportive environment.

Use touch (as appropriate) to convey caring and support.

Encourage expression of feelings.

Promote feelings of self-worth.

Offer suggestions to cope with anxieties.

Facilitate or assist patient in using coping strategies (relaxation, deep breathing, music, imagery).

Maintain patient privacy.

Encourage participation of patient and family in plan of care.

NURSING DIAGNOSIS: High risk for injury

OUTCOME: Patient will be free from injury related to surgical position.

INTERVENTIONS:

Maintain proper body alignment.

Pad all bony prominences.

Avoid compression of vulnerable nerves and neurovascular bundles.

Secure patient to operating room bed without friction or pressure.

Provide support stockings or antiembolism device as indicated.

NURSING DIAGNOSIS: Altered patterns of urinary elimination

OUTCOME: The patient's pattern of urinary elimination will remain patent and within the normal range.

INTERVENTIONS:

Include catheter care and measures to facilitate voiding following catheter removal as part of preoperative teaching to patient and family.

Instruct patient in importance of any postoperative antibiotic or anticholinergic therapy.

Follow aseptic technique during catheter insertion and connection to drainage device.

Maintain closed gravity drainage system.

Note color and character of urine; report abnormalities.

Keep drainage tubing and collection devices below the level of the patient's bladder.

Keep urine draining freely; avoid kinks in tubing.

Check patency of catheter after all positional changes.

Anchor drainage tubing to patient to prevent pulling and retraction of tubing.

Assess bladder for distention.

NURSING DIAGNOSIS: Fluid volume excess or deficit

OUTCOME: Patient will exhibit no signs of fluid or electrolyte imbalance.

INTERVENTIONS:

Provide appropriate intravenous solutions.

Monitor patency of all intravenous lines.

Assess volume of intravenous or irrigating fluids instilled.

Monitor ECG, vital signs, cardiopulmonary status as appropriate.

Monitor blood loss and volume replaced.

Monitor urinary output, note color, report output less than 30 ml/hour and changes in color or clarity.

Maintain accurate intake and output records.

Monitor serum electrolyte status.

NURSING DIAGNOSIS: Impaired gas exchange

OUTCOME: Patient will maintain adequate gas exchange.

INTERVENTIONS:

Review breathing exercises with patient preoperatively.

Position patient to provide maximum lung perfusion.

Monitor and report alterations in ventilation or perfusion from preoperative status.

Administer oxygen as required; assist with intubation and maintenance of airway during positioning.

Assist with collection of arterial blood gases; report results promptly.

Apply cardiac monitor, blood pressure cuff, and pulse oximeter.

In some procedures involving stones of the kidneys or ureters, intraoperative x-ray examinations or fluoroscopy may be required. If x-ray films are to be taken, the patient must be on an operating room bed with an x-ray cassette holder. If the OR bed design does not accommodate x-ray cassettes, an x-ray cassette holder must be placed under the patient who is in the supine, prone, or lithotomy position before the procedure begins. If the patient is in the lateral position with the bed flexed and kidney rest up, the x-ray cassette, encased in a sterile bag, is held lateral to the patient's flank at the time of x-ray exposure. When fluoroscopy (C-arm) is to be employed, the patient must be placed on an OR bed compatible with its use. Whenever possible, the patient should be protected from undue radiation exposure to the thyroid and chest areas by the use of small leaded shields. In urologic procedures it is not generally feasible to shield the reproductive organs.

Aseptic techniques and safety measures

Prevention of infection is an important nursing goal in the care of the genitourinary patient. It is, however, seldom possible to confirm freedom from infection intraoperatively or immediately postoperatively. Aseptic techniques must be carefully maintained and monitored. Skin preparation and draping procedures (see Chapter 3) vary, depending on the surgery to be performed and individual hospital policy. Special care must be taken when cleansing the perineal area to avoid contamination from the rectum to the urethra. Prepping solutions should be applied with downward strokes and the sponge discarded once it has contacted the inner vaginal or anal areas. Transurethral passage of instruments and catheters requires meticulous technique to prevent retrograde infections of the urinary tract.

Visualization of the bladder during transurethral procedures is enhanced by darkening the room. Provision should be made for proper adjustments to lighting. Electrosurgical units and fiberoptic light systems are frequent adjuncts in urologic surgery. The staff must be familiar with the manufacturer's safety precautions and recommendations during their use.

Use of irrigating fluids

When the bladder is to be entered, sterile distilled irrigating fluid is administered to distend the bladder for effective visualization. Commercially prepared sterile irrigation solutions with appropriate closed administration sets are highly recommended. Such closed systems prevent the inherent risks of cross-contamination. Large volumes of irrigating solutions are frequently used, particularly during the more extensive endoscopic procedures. When these solutions are at room temperature, they are a shock to the patient's internal body temperature and can cause hypothermia. Solution warming units are available commercially and are a useful tool to help decrease this risk. The drawback to these units may be that the warmth causes clotting to be delayed, thus increasing blood loss.

For simple observation cystoscopy, retrograde pyelography, and simple bladder tumor fulgurations, sterile distilled water may be used without complication. However, during transurethral resection of the prostate, venous sinuses may be opened, and varying amounts of irrigant are invariably absorbed into the bloodstream. Studies indicate that the use of distilled water for transurethral resection of the prostate may result in hemolysis of erythrocytes and possible renal failure. Other important complications include dilutional hyponatremia and cardiac decompensation.

Ideally, a clear, nonelectrolytic, and isosmotic solution should be used. The most widely used urologic irrigating fluids are 3% sorbitol, an isomer of mannitol, and 1.5% glycine, an aminoacetic solution. Other acceptable solutions include 5% mannitol, 1.8% urea, and 4% glucose. In dilute solutions sorbitol and glycine have many properties that make them particularly useful for irrigation during transurethral prostatectomy. At slightly hypotonic concentrations they do not produce hemolysis. Because the solutions are nonelectrolytic, they do not cause dispersion of high-frequency current with consequent loss of electrosurgical cutting capacity, as occurs with normal saline.

Commercially prepared sterile irrigation solutions are available in collapsible bags and rigid plastic containers, both of which have the same advantage; neither depends on air, and each may be hung in series, thus providing continuous irrigation without interruption. Air bubbles, a problem that distorts visibility during the procedure, are eliminated with these systems.

Thorough knowledge of the potential hazards encountered intraoperatively during transurethral surgery is extremely important. Although complications are more prevalent in the postoperative stage, close observation during the intraoperative period is essential. Symptoms such as sudden restlessness, apprehension, irritability, slow pulse, and rising blood pressure may suggest transurethral resection (TUR) syndrome, a shift of body fluids and electrolytes caused by a decrease of extracellular sodium. Serum electrolyte laboratory studies should be obtained without delay. Minimum amounts of fluids should be given. Irrigation fluid should be under as little pressure as possible, and the bladder emptied before it reaches full capacity to prevent intravesical pressure. Occasionally an operating room has the capacity to perform these crucial laboratory tests intraoperatively, so results are available for interpretation in a short time. If a low serum sodium value is reported, hypertonic sodium chloride is added to the intravenous line, or intravenous diuretics such as furosemide (Lasix) may be used. If the patient's reaction is severe, surgery may have to be terminated.

Endoscopic and ancillary equipment

Cystoscopic and ancillary equipment may vary from one institution to another. Therefore it is valuable to have a reference manual or Kardex system that illustrates and de-

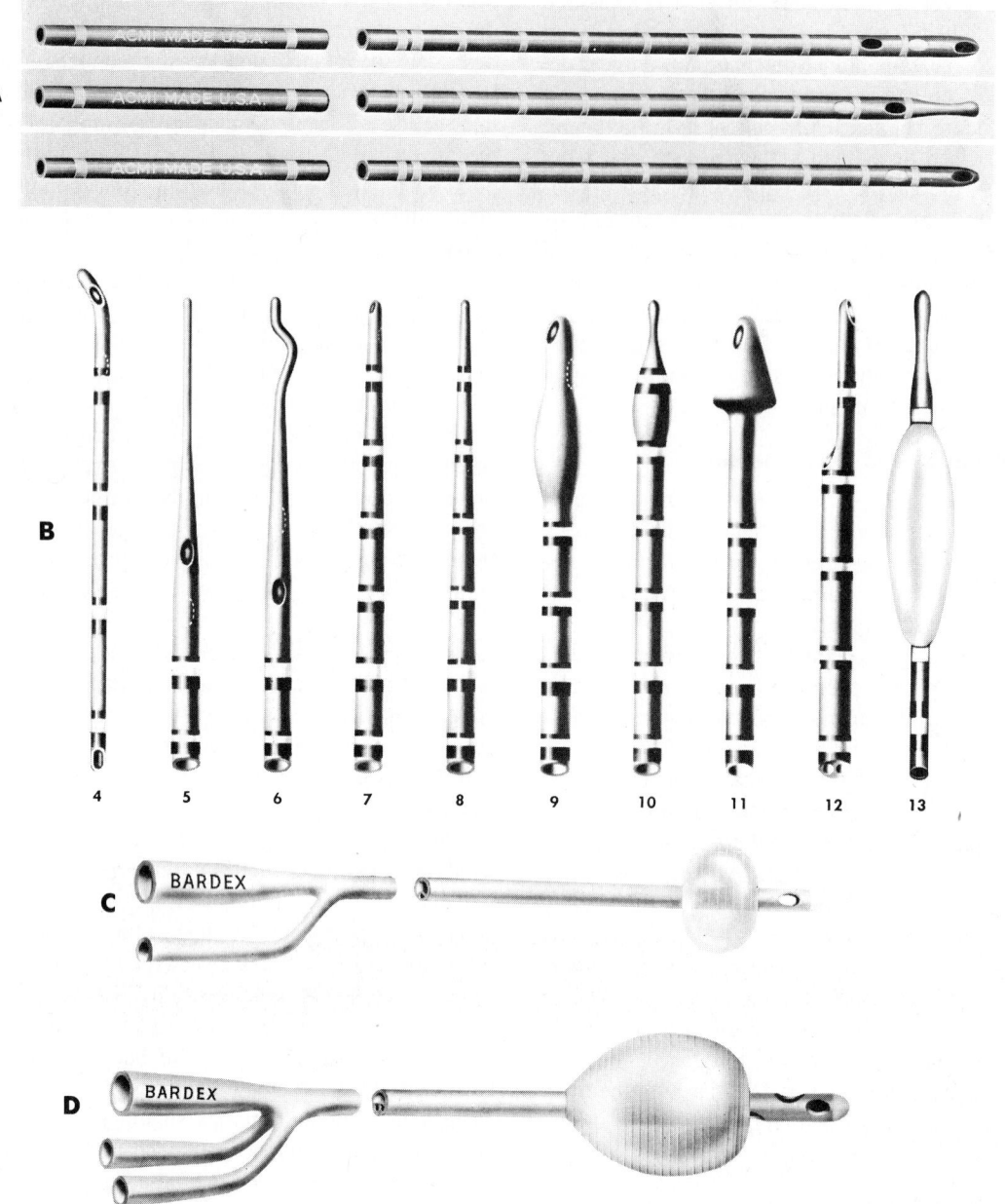

FIG. 14-10 **A,** X-ray graduated woven ureteral catheters of nylon or polyurethane material with outer surfacing to provide flexibility, for easy entry without kinking. Eyes provide adequate high-flow rate. Catheter tips constructed for specific procedures as shown. *1,* Whistle tip; *2,* olive tip; *3,* round tip. **B,** X-ray graduated woven ureteral catheters and bougies. *4,* Wishard catheter with flat, coude tip; *5,* Bla-succi catheter with flexible filiform tip; *6,* Blasucci catheter with flexible spiral filiform tip; *7,* Garceau catheter, tapered for dilatation, with whistle tip; *8,* Garceau bougie, tapered for dilatation, with conical tip; *9,* Braasch bulb catheter with whistle tip; *10,* Braasch bougie with bulb tip; *11,* cone tip catheter (for ureteropyelography); *12,* Hyams double-lumen catheter; *13,* Dourmashkin dilator with inflation balloon and olive tip. **C,** Foley retention catheter. **D,** Bard three-way hemostatic catheter.

Courtesy Circon Corp., Santa Barbara, Calif.

scribes in detail the required instrumentation for each specific procedure.

The basic cystoscopy tray should include instruments and accessory items that are routinely used for all cystoscopy procedures. If ureteral catheterization is planned, catheterizing telescopes or an Albarrán bridge of the appropriate size, which can be packaged and gas sterilized separately, may be easily added to the basic cystoscopy setup. Instruments for transurethral surgery and other special procedures may be wrapped and gas sterilized and placed on separate trays so they are available on request. This concept minimizes handling of the delicate lensed instruments and ultimately reduces costly repairs.

Cystoscopic procedures frequently require additional instrumentation. Instruments of various types and sizes, for example, a visual obturator, biopsy forceps, urethral sounds, Phillips filiforms and followers, and Ellik evacuators, are available as prepackaged, sterile, disposable items. The reusable products may also be packaged separately and sterilized.

Urethral and ureteral catheters

A variety of urethral and ureteral catheters is necessary in the management of urologic disease. Catheters are designed for specific procedures to meet the individualized needs of particular patients. Ureteral catheters are manufactured of polyvinyl or polyurethane material and are graduated so that the urologist may determine the exact distance the catheter has been inserted into the ureter. Most manufacturers provide disposable catheters double-wrapped in peel-open packages to allow aseptic handling during ureteral insertion. Some indications for the use of ureteral catheters are to (1) perform retrograde pyelography, (2) identify the ureters during pelvic or intestinal surgery, and (3) bypass partial or complete obstruction that may be present as a result of ureteral tumors, calculi, or strictures.

Frequently used ureteral catheters include the whistle tip, round, Braasch bulb, spiral, bone, open ended, and olive tip (Fig. 14-10). The spiral Blasucci is useful when difficulty occurs in introducing a ureteral catheter past the ureterovesical junction. When a retrograde ureterogram is indicated, a Braasch bulb or cone-tip ureteral catheter may be helpful in occluding the ureteral orifice to accomplish the x-ray study effectively. When a ureteral catheter is left indwelling, a special adapter (Fig. 14-11) can be connected to the end of the ureteral catheter to facilitate connection to a closed urinary drainage system. A small slit may also be created in the Foley catheter and the distal end of the ureteral catheter slipped into it and taped in place.

Indwelling double-pigtail or double-J stents are now available (Fig. 14-12). These catheters are passed cystoscopically to reside within the ureter. When the guidewire is removed from the core of the stent, a proximal and distal J or pigtail forms in the tubing to retain the stents. Many now have nonabsorbable suture attached to the distal end, which extends through the urethral meatus. A suture may

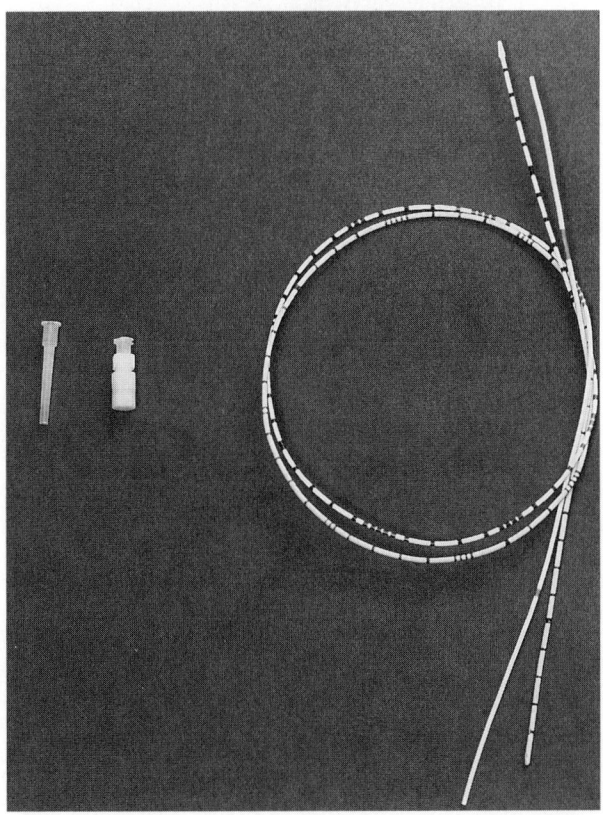

FIG. 14-11 Ureteral catheters and adapters.

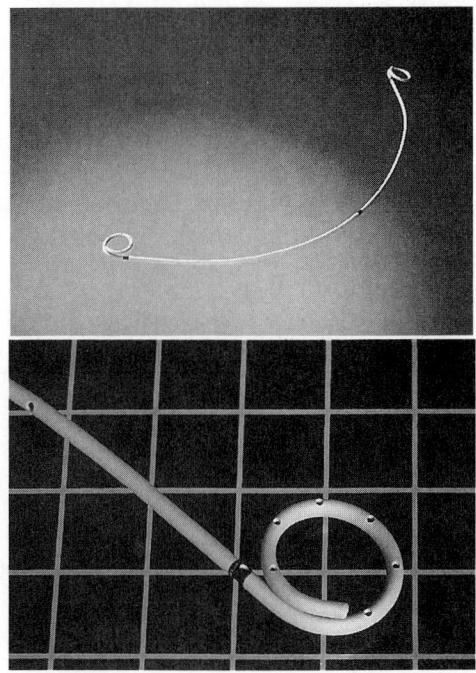

FIG. 14-12 Double-pigtail stent set.
Courtesy Cook Urological, Spencer, Ind.

be easily tied to the distal end of those which do not. The surgeon can then remove the stent in the office setting postoperatively.

Urethral catheters have a multitude of functions as stents, drainage tubes, and in diagnostic studies in the operating room. They are generally divided into two categories, plain and indwelling (retention), and range in different French sizes, most commonly 10 through 30. The Foley catheter is the most frequently used retention catheter and is manufactured with a variety of balloon sizes, tip styles, lengths, and eye arrangements (see Fig. 14-10, C).

After prostatic surgery a three-way Foley catheter with a 30-ml balloon capacity may be left indwelling (see Fig. 14-10, D). This type of catheter is preferred because it facilitates continuous bladder irrigation (CBI), and the large balloon aids in achieving hemostasis in the prostatic bed. The urologist may apply light traction on the Foley catheter, with tape or a leg strap. This causes pressure against the bladder neck and aids in hemostasis (Fig. 14-13). A hematuria catheter, a three-way Foley, specifically for patients with excessive clot formation is also available. This catheter is reinforced with a stretch spiral wire within the catheter lining that permits vigorous aspiration without fear of lumen collapse.

Diagnostic studies are also performed in the cystoscopy suite and require special catheters for specific studies. For example, the Davis double-balloon urethrographic catheter (Fig. 14-14) is used to diagnose lesions of the female urethra, such as urethral strictures, diverticula, and fistulas. To accomplish female urethrography, the catheter is inserted through the urethra into the bladder; the two balloons on the catheter are inflated, one in the bladder and one at the external urethral orifice, effectively isolating the urethra. Contrast medium is injected to visualize the entire urethra.

Another type of self-retaining catheter frequently used in the operating room is a Pezzer, also known as a mushroom catheter. It may be straight or angulated with a large single channel and preformed tip in the shape of a mushroom. The flexible mushroom tip helps keep the catheter

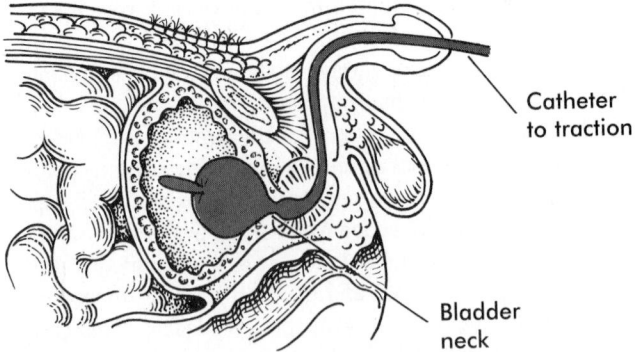

FIG. 14-13 Balloon of Foley catheter inflated to size that prevents catheter from being pulled into prostatic fossa.

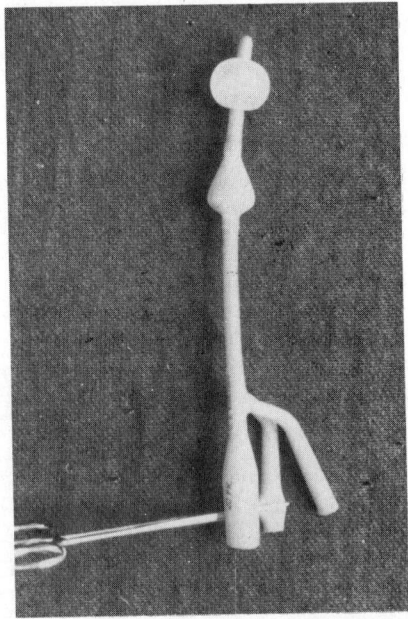

FIG. 14-14 Double-balloon Davis urethrographic catheter.

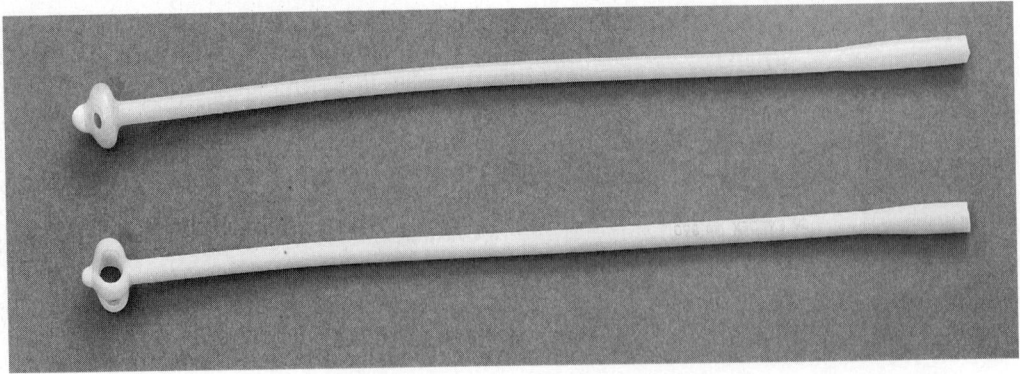

FIG. 14-15 Pezzer (mushroom) catheter and Malecot (bat-wing) four-winged catheter.

in place. This catheter is used primarily for suprapubic bladder drainage, often for poor-risk patients who have uremia, neurogenic bladder syndrome, or possibly long-standing urinary retention. The catheter is inserted in the bladder through a midline or small transverse abdominal wall incision and secured to the abdomen with suture or tape. The Malecot four-winged catheter, often used as a nephrostomy tube to provide temporary or permanent diversion of urine after kidney surgery and when renal tissue needs to be restored, may also be used for suprapubic drainage (Fig. 14-15). A Foley catheter of preferred size is frequently chosen for either purpose. Nephrostomy tube replacement is accomplished by introducing the catheter into the surgical tract with a straight catheter guide and securing it in place with a suture or a nephrostomy retention disk, one size smaller than the nephrostomy tube being used. The flanges of the disk are taped or sutured to the skin. The use of other variations of urethral catheters is described later in the text.

Photography in urology

The use of photographic and video imaging equipment in urologic surgery serves to document the patient's disease, the progress of a disease process, and long-term follow-up. It is also an important teaching resource. Video equipment adapts to endoscopic instrumentation and has the capability of projecting an enhanced image on a television monitor, permitting members of the surgical team to observe and learn during the actual surgical procedure (Figs. 14-16 and 14-17). Other visual aids, such as slides and photographs,

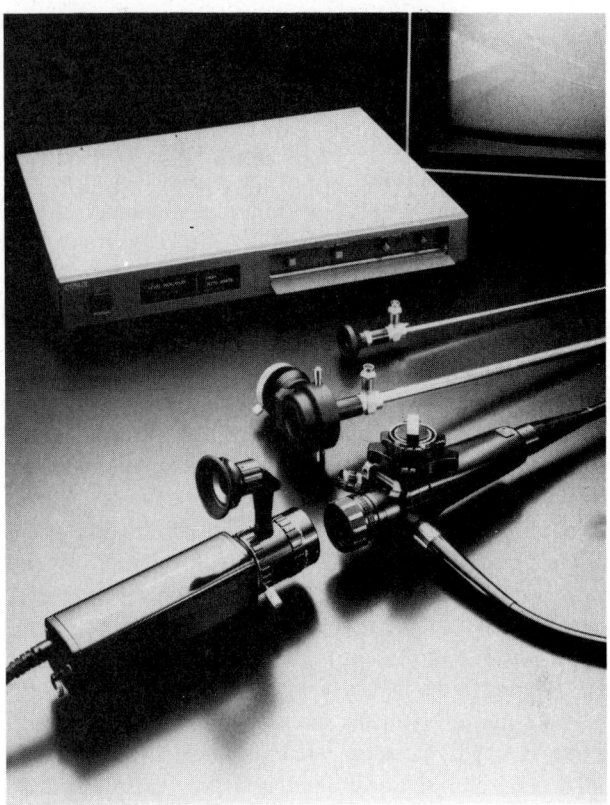

FIG. 14-16 Olympus video system, indicating attachment capabilities of both rigid and flexible instruments.
Courtesy Olympus Corp., Lake Success, N.Y.

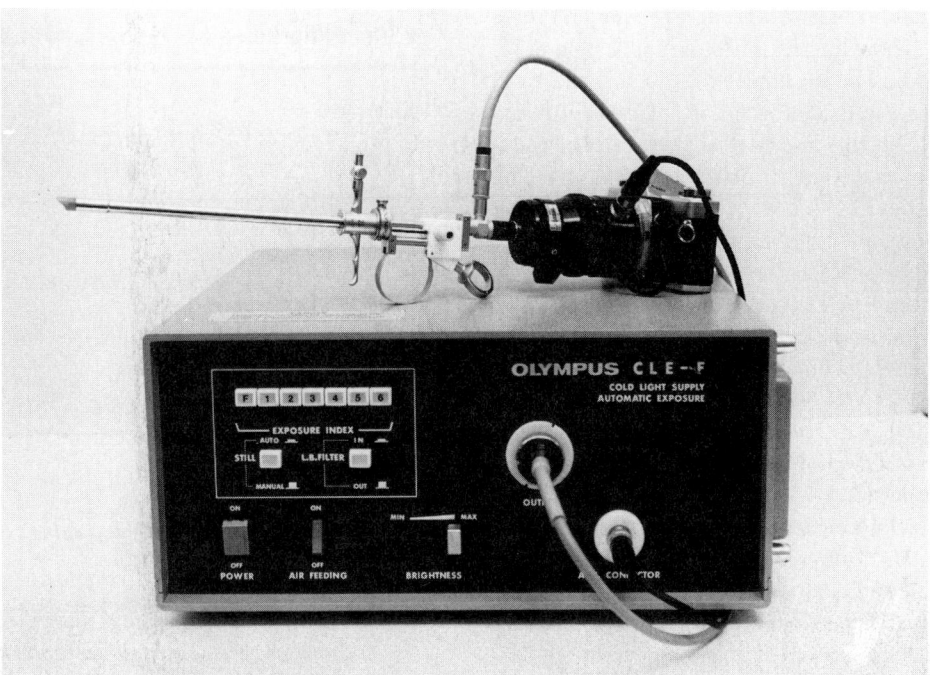

FIG. 14-17 Automatic exposure light source, Olympus camera and adapter, and resectoscope.
Courtesy Olympus Corp., Lake Success, N.Y.

are used in teaching, as visual references in publication, and as documentation in patient records.

When any form of photography or video imaging is used, the patient's privacy must be ensured and an informed consent should be obtained. Special release forms should also be signed preoperatively by the patient for any videotapes or photographs to be used in teaching or publications.

EVALUATION

Before the patient is taken to the postanesthesia care unit (PACU) or observation unit, his or her general condition is evaluated. The general appearance of the skin is assessed. Bony prominences, prepped and draped areas, and areas contacted by the attachment of ancillary equipment are noted for signs of pressure, irritation, or other changes from the preoperative status. Ancillary attachments include, but are not limited to, the electrosurgical dispersive pads or indifferent electrode (ESU) pad and ECG lead pads. Because many urology patients are nutritionally deficient and consequently have friable tissues, the trend has been to minimize the use of tape and to coat the skin with a protective sealant prior to the use of tapes.

Many urology patients are discharged to PACU with drains inserted, including urethral, ureteral, suprapubic, and wound drains. Local anesthesia may have been used for either primary analgesia or postoperative pain management. A complete report to the PACU nurse should include intraoperative position, problems encountered specific to the patient, and the patient's preoperative physical status as well as comprehension and anxiety levels. Documentation of medications administered from the sterile field or by the perioperative nurse intraoperatively should include time of administration, medication, dosage, site and route of administration, and who performed the application or injection. Drains should be documented as to size and type, insertion site, time and date of insertion, type of collection device, who performed the insertion, and character of drainage. When several drains are in place, additional labeling on the collection devices is beneficial. Any postoperative observations prior to or during transport should be recorded. Evaluation should also address whether the patient met the identified outcomes related to specific nursing diagnoses in the perioperative nursing care plan. These outcomes, included in the documentation and report to the PACU, may be phrased as follows:

- Preoperatively, the patient verbalized concerns to the perioperative nurse.
- The patient had no evidence of positional injury; neurovascular status was consistent with preoperative level, and skin integrity was intact.
- The patient maintained patency of the urinary catheter with no signs of infection, blockage, or retention. Urinary output remained within normal limits. The patient should void without difficulty following catheter removal.

- The patient evidenced no signs of fluid or electrolyte imbalance; vital signs were stable, arterial blood gases were within normal limits, and urinary output was maintained at acceptable levels.
- The patient maintained adequate gas exchange; lung expansion and O_2 saturation were satisfactory.

MEDICAL INTERVENTIONS: ALTERNATIVES TO SURGERY

Patients with various types of cancer may be treated in the urology office setting with various therapeutic modalities. These measures may be initiated instead of surgery or as an adjunct to surgery.

SUPERFICIAL BLADDER CANCER

Patients with bladder cancer that has been staged as Ta, Tis, and T1 (Table 14-2) are being treated with intravesical, antineoplastic chemotherapy agents such as thiotepa, mitomycin (Mutamycin), doxorubicin (Adriamycin), Epodyl and BCG. These medications are proving effective in both the eradication of obvious tumor and the prevention of recurrence. BCG has been found, through an unknown mechanism, to strengthen the body's immune reaction to cancer and is considered the most effective therapy for re-

---

TABLE 14-2

Clinical/Pathologic Staging for Bladder Cancer

Finding	AJC-UICC*
No tumor	T0/P0
Carcinoma in situ	Tis/Pis
Noninvasive papillary tumor	TA/PA
Lamina propria invasion	T1/P1
Superficial muscle invasion	T2/P2
Deep muscle invasion	T3a/P3
Invasion of perivesical fat	T3b/P3
Invasion of contiguous organ	T4/P4
Regional lymph node metastases	—/N1-3
Juxtaregional lymph node metastases	—/N3
Distant metastases	M1/M1

From Gillenwater, J. (1991). *Adult and pediatric urology.* St. Louis: Mosby.

*Grading refers to microscopic cell differentiation by the appearance of individual tumor cells and their relationship to each other. The higher the grade the greater the malignancy.

AJC (the American Joint Commission) uses a Grade 1-4 system (well to poorly differentiated tumors).

UICC (Union Internationale Contre Center) uses a Grade 0-3, papillomas.

current and residual bladder cancer. Currently the complete response rate of BCG is 80%. Other therapies show complete response of 60% with a 30% recurrence, compared to 70% recurrence with no treatment.

PROSTATE CANCER

In an attempt to provide cost-effective, curative treatment with a low morbidity, recent trials have initiated a treatment protocol that may provide an alternative to the open surgery approach. Following a thorough workup, including digital rectal exam, serum PSA and acid phosphatase as well as bone scans, CT, or MRI scans of the pelvis, transrectal guided ultrasound biopsies, and histologic grading of the malignancy (Table 14-3), select patients with well or moderately differentiated lesions may be candidates for transperineal ultrasound-guided implantation of radium seeds. The seeds are inserted in the operating room during a short-stay patient admission. The radiation dose is doubled or tripled from that delivered by standard radiation techniques. There is decreased risk to the surrounding tissue because of the limited 1 cm penetration range of the seeds. The radium employed is iodine-125 or palladium-103.

TABLE 14-3

Clinical Staging for Carcinoma of Prostate

Description	AJC (TNM)*
Localized	
Clinically unsuspected	T1
Focal, low grade	T1a
Intragland lump (diffuse/high grade)	T1b
Clinically suspected	T2
<1.5 cm, confined to one lobe	T2a
>1.5 cm, confined to one lobe	T2a
Bilateral lobes	T2b
Disseminated	
Periprostatic	T3, T4
Base seminal vesicle/lateral sulcus	T3
Base seminal vesicle/other structures	T4
Distant	
Pelvic lymph node	T1-4/N1
Bones, lung, etc.	T1-4/N0-3
Elevated PAP only	T1-4/N3

From Gillenwater, J. (1991). *Adult and pediatric urology*. St. Louis: Mosby.
*TNM refers to Tumors, Nodes, Metastases, the counterpart staging system to the Jewett, Marshall, strong system of tumor staging.

PENILE CANCER

Options are now available to limit the extent of the disfiguring surgery previously indicated for penile cancer. Chemotherapy agents, often combined with irradiation, are proving effective in shrinking penile carcinomas that would have previously mandated radical penectomy. Bleomycin, usually combined with irradiation, is showing great success in patients with known metastasis. Methotrexate is another relatively new and effective agent. A third therapy involves the use of cisplatin.

SURGICAL INTERVENTIONS

DIAGNOSTIC AND ENDOSCOPIC PROCEDURES

Cystoscopy

Cystoscopy is an endoscopic examination of the lower urinary tract, including visual inspection of the interior of the urethra, the bladder, and the ureteral orifices using the cystoscope, a versatile optical instrument with a variety of telescopic lenses. In a male patient special attention is given to the examination of the verumontanum (which contains the ejaculatory ducts), the bladder neck, and the median and lateral lobes of the prostate. In a female patient the urethra, bladder neck, and bladder are examined.

Cystoscopy is an important diagnostic tool that provides the urologist with valuable information concerning the patient's urologic condition. Indications for cystoscopy include hematuria, urinary retention, urinary tract infection, tumors, fistulas, vesical calculus disease, and urinary incontinence. Contrary to popular belief, urinary incontinence is not a normal part of the aging process. Although aging contributes to incontinence, it is not the cause (Research Highlight 14-1).

Procedural considerations

Once in the OR, before entering the cystoscopy suite, all patients should be greeted by name and identified by their identification bracelet and number. The perioperative nurse should check the chart for operative consent and pertinent laboratory reports, IVPs, any diagnostic studies, and chest x-ray films ordered preoperatively should also be available for review. Customarily, the patient voids immediately before transport to the OR. The time of urination and the output volume should be documented for ruling out residual urine in the bladder.

After the patient is placed on the cystoscopy bed, correct positioning requires optimum relaxation of muscles of the legs and perineum. Proper positioning of the knee crutches on the cystoscopy bed is a vital consideration for patient safety and comfort. When knee crutches are properly positioned, the curve of the yoke suspension should flow outward from the perineum, as do the patient's legs. Padding the knee crutches is beneficial in reducing pressure on the popliteal areas. If sling stirrups that support only the feet are employed, the post should be padded and po-

Dysfunctions that involve the detrusor muscle, urethra, or alterations in sensation may be associated with involuntary loss of urine. Detrusor instability results from a detrusor muscle that contracts when trying to inhibit voiding or that contracts insufficiently to allow for complete emptying. Diminished sensation of bladder filling often leads to delay in voiding until it is too late. Sphincter incompetence may result from detrusor pressure that overrides it or by detrusor-sphincter dyssynergia. These underlying causes in the elderly are often treatable.

Changes in the lower urinary tract are related to aging and place one at risk for urinary incontinence, but the underlying cause of incontinence is not the aging process. In the elderly, with diminished body defense mechanisms, medical problems associated with incontinence include skin rash, breakdown and infection, urinary tract infection, and psychosocial as well as physical difficulty. Only one in 12 people seeks professional help, while the others continue to believe that incontinence and aging go together.

Education of health care professionals and paraprofessionals is urgently needed. An unpublished study by Ouslander and Morishita raised questions about the attitudes of health care professionals toward incontinence and aging. Professional schools and nurse specialist programs need to consider adding incontinence to the curriculum. This is a treatable problem that is too often neglected by the health care profession. Recognition and assessment must be done to provide diagnosis and treatment for the elderly.

Wozniak-Petrofsky, J. (1993). Urinary incontinence in the elderly: not a normal part of aging. *Urologic Nursing, 13* (1), 12-16.

sitioned to prevent pressure on the peroneal nerve. Currently there are special pads on the market for use with both of these stirrups. Allen stirrups are a boot style that supports the foot and calf. These have thick gel padding within the stirrup and provide optimum patient comfort and protection, relieving pressure on the popliteal space. They are especially beneficial with the patient who has limited hip mobility and altered peripheral circulatory status. Bilateral pedal pulses should be assessed preoperatively and postoperatively when using any stirrups. Care must be taken to adjust the stirrups so that there is no undue pressure on the calf.

After the patient is properly positioned, the bed may be tilted so that the patient's head is slightly higher than the buttocks to allow the prep solution to drain into the collecting pan. The pooling of solutions beneath the patient may cause skin reaction and severe irritation, as well as the potential for burns, if an electrosurgical unit is used. If the cystoscopic procedure requires the use of an electrosurgical unit, the ESU pad is placed on the patient in direct contact with the skin as close to the operative site as practical, and accessible to the circulating nurse, usually on the upper thigh. When placing the ESU pad it is important to avoid hairy areas, bony prominences, and proximity to prosthetic joint implants or pacemakers.

After proper positioning of the patient, the nurse or urologist dons gloves and preps the entire pubic area, including the scrotum and perineum, with an antimicrobial solution. A screen is placed over the drainage pan on the cystoscopy bed (Fig. 14-18). Disposable draping systems with a sterile screen material incorporated into them are available. The patient is then draped according to procedure. Adequate draping is important to ensure that aseptic technique is maintained during the urologic procedure. If a general or spinal anesthetic is required, it is administered before prepping and draping. If a local anesthetic is preferred, it is instilled into the urethra of the male patient after prepping and draping but before instrumentation. For a female patient, a cotton applicator that has been dipped into the anesthetic solution is placed in the urethral meatus. Lidocaine 1% (Xylocaine), or 2% (Anestacon), is usually used. If the patient is allergic to lidocaine, instillation of 50 to 60 ml of lubricant accompanied by anesthesia-monitored sedation is often adequate to afford painless access to the urethra and bladder. The patient should be informed that a sensation of pressure is to be expected.

The cystoscopy setup should include the following:

Prep set and solutions	Medicine glass for dye,
Cystourethroscope (Fig. 14-19)	anesthetic solution, or gel
1 Short bridge	Syringe, disposable 10
1 Fiberoptic light cord	or 20 ml, to instill
1 Lateral telescope	dye
1 Foroblique telescope	Penile clamp (to oc-
1 Luer-Lok stopcock	clude male urethra
and irrigation tubing	after local anesthetic
Lubricant, water-soluble	is instilled)
1 Calibrated container	Urethral syringe for an-
to measure residual	esthetic or Uro-Jet
urine	(sterile, prepackaged
2 Test tubes, screwtop,	prefilled syringe of
for urine specimens	2% lidocaine)
Gauze sponges	Cystoscopy drape pack
1 Albarrán bridge	Irrigation system
2 Rubber catheter nip-	Gown and gloves
ples or adapters	Fiberoptic light source
	Electrosurgical unit

The flexible cystoscope (Fig. 14-20) is used for patients with obstructive symptoms resulting from prostatic hyperplasia and rigid prostatic urethra. In addition, the flexible cystoscope can be used for patients who cannot assume a lithotomy position, such as those with spinal cord injuries or severe arthritis. Flexible cystoscopy may be accomplished with the use of a local anesthetic, although it is not

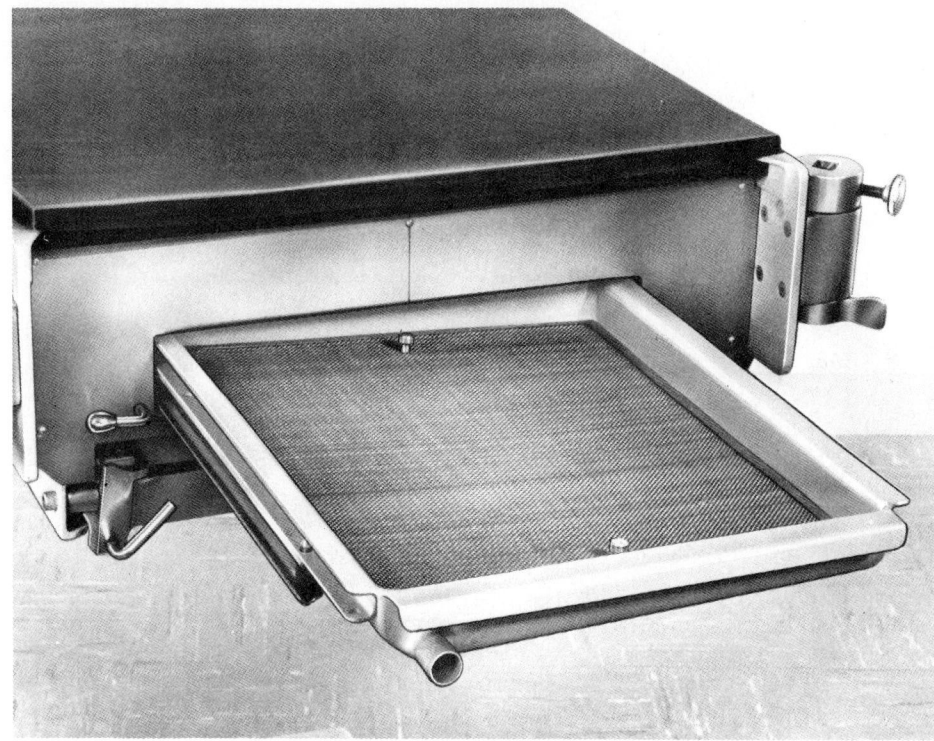

FIG. 14-18   Screen over drainage drawer on cystoscopy bed.

usually necessary. It affords the patient a higher degree of comfort, is less traumatic to the urethra, and can be performed in the patient's bed on the nursing unit.

Cleaning, sterilization, disinfection, and maintenance of endoscopic equipment are important procedures in the care of fiberoptic lensed instruments. Ultimately this process reduces costly repairs and ensures the availability of properly functioning instruments.

Protective padding should be placed on the countertop and on the bottom of the sink in the instrument decontamination area to prevent possible damage to lensed telescopes. After each surgical procedure, components of each cystoscopic set should be disassembled and washed in a solution of warm water and germicidal detergent with endozymatic action (breaks down proteins). All stopcocks and sheaths should be cleaned thoroughly with a soft brush to remove blood, dried lubricant jelly, or other debris. Instruments should then be thoroughly rinsed in warm water, placed on protective padding, and allowed to dry. Although warm water is appropriate for washing the instrumentation, lensed instruments should not be allowed to soak in warm water for too long. Lengthy soaking can cause the seals to loosen, allowing water to leak into the scope, resulting in cloudiness and bubbles. All moving parts must be individually evaluated for mobility. A lubricating instrument milk solution may be applied as required. The patency of all outlets must be maintained to ensure proper sterilization or dis-

infection. Fiberoptic light cords must not be tangled, twisted, or sharply angulated because the fibers inside the cord are easily broken.

Sterilization of instruments provides the greatest assurance of eliminating the risk of infections transmitted by contaminated instruments (see Chapter 3). According to the Centers for Disease Control and Prevention (CDCP), however, sterilization is not essential for items classified as semicritical, for example, cystoscopes. High-level disinfection with an agent such as activated glutaraldehyde or dialdehyde that can destroy vegetative microorganisms, most fungal spores, tubercle bacilli, and small nonlipid viruses is recommended. In most situations meticulous cleaning of endoscopic instruments followed by appropriate high-level disinfection provides reasonable assurance that the items are safe to use. The level of disinfection is based on the contact time, temperature, and concentration of the active ingredients of the disinfectant, as well as the nature of microbial contamination.

For sterilization or disinfection, instruments should be assembled on a covered tray and protected with padding. Because the lens system is delicate and costly, a plastic covering available from some manufacturers may be used to protect the lens. Various instrument manufacturers provide sterilization containers for endoscopy equipment and have written recommendations for the cleaning, sterilization, and disinfection of their equipment.

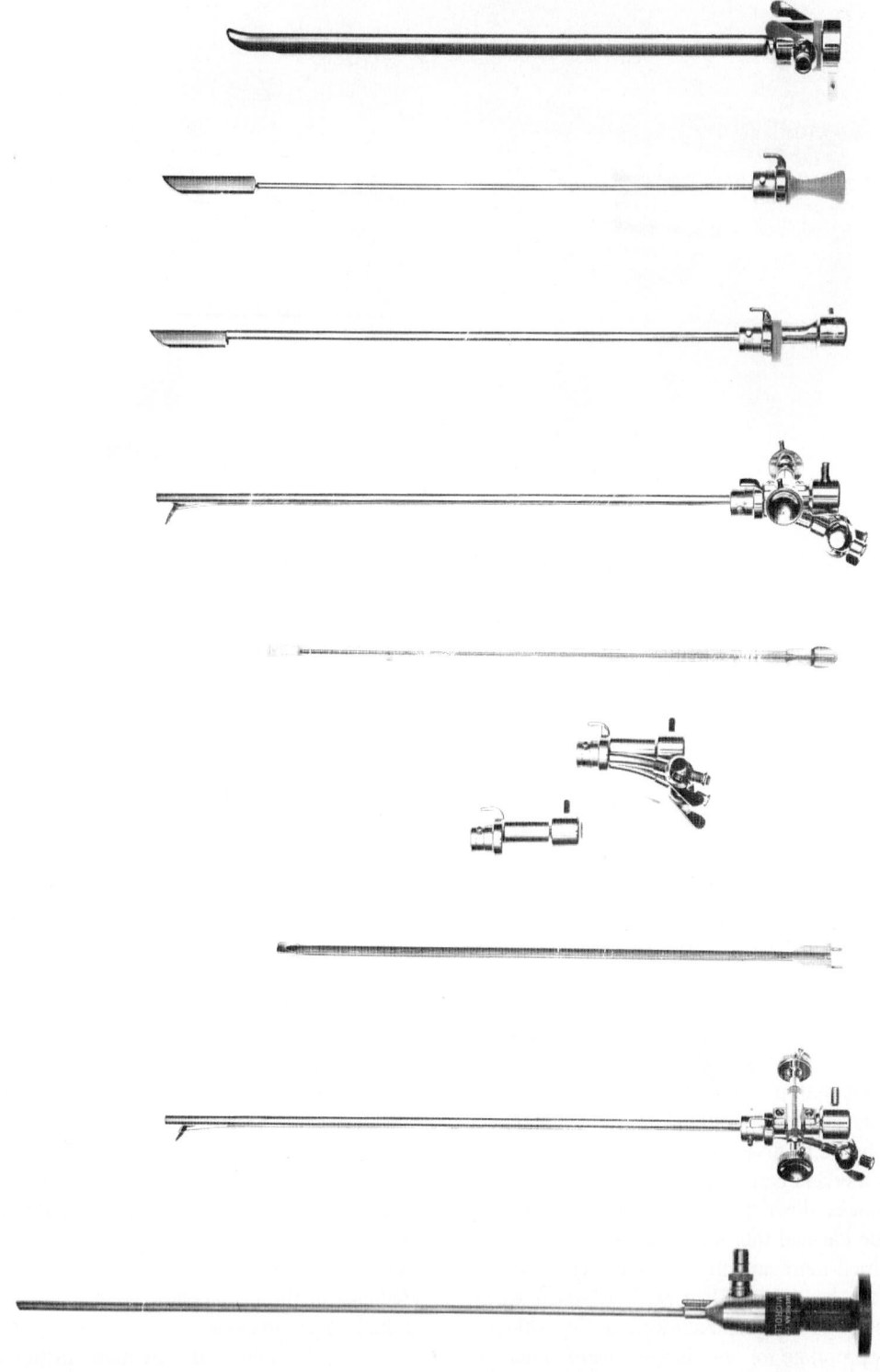

FIG. 14-19   Instruments for cystoscopy, catheterization, and retrograde ureteral pyelography. *Top* to *bottom,* Cystoscope sheath, obturator, visual obturator, double-catheterizing Albarran bridge, double-catheterizing fin, double-catheterizing bridge, examining bridge, stationary deflector, operating Albarran bridge, telescope.

Courtesy Circon Corp., Santa Barbara, Calif.

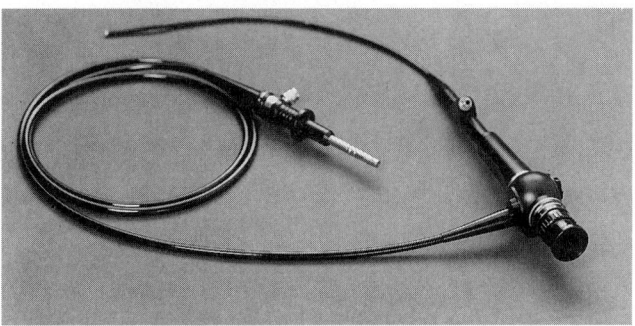

FIG. 14-20 Flexible cystoscope.
Courtesy Circon Corp., Santa Barbara, Calif.

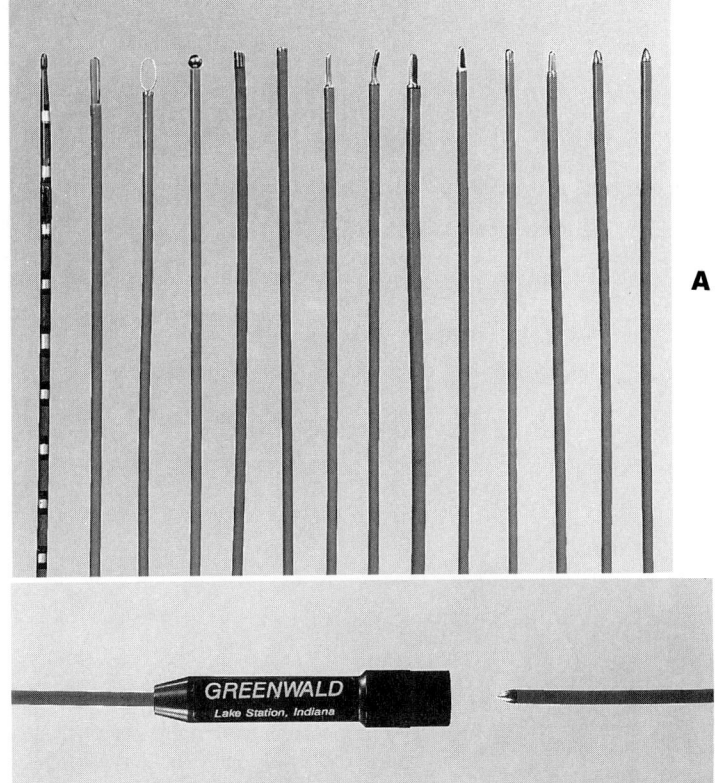

FIG. 14-21 **A,** Flexible fulgurating electrode tips. **B,** Detail of tip and connector end.
Photo courtesy Greenwald Surgical Co., Inc., Lake Station, Ind.

Operative procedure

1. After the urologist has scrubbed, gowned, and gloved, the fiberoptic light cord is connected to the light source and tested for proper intensity. The irrigating system is set up, and, if required, the high-frequency cord is connected to an electrosurgical unit.

2. The cystourethroscope is lubricated and introduced into the urethra, the obturator withdrawn, and residual urine obtained, provided the patient voided before the examination. The specimen may be saved for cultures or cytologic studies. The cystourethroscope is connected to the irrigating system, and the telescope is inserted and locked in place. The urologist controls the flow and volume of fluid by adjusting the stopcock on the scope. If difficulty is encountered during insertion, the visual obturator may be used to introduce the scope under direct vision. This accessory is constructed to smooth the fenestral edges of the cystourethroscope. It requires the use of the telescope for direct vision and permits irrigation during introduction. If the patient is awake, telling him or her to try to urinate also helps facilitate passage of the scope.

3. Stone removal, bladder biopsy, and bladder fulguration may be performed by using special cystoscopic accessories such as the Hendrickson-Bigelow lithotrite, which crushes large bladder calculi. This procedure is called a litholapaxy. Lowsley forceps, Wappler rigid cup forceps, and flexible foreign body forceps may also be employed. Bladder fulguration requires the use of flexible stem electrodes available in various French sizes and tip configurations such as the ball, cone, dome, and bayonet (Fig. 14-21).

4. For retrograde ureteral catheterization and pyelography,

ureteral catheters are passed through the cystoscope sheath and directed by the Albarrán bridge deflector through the ureteral orifice and into the ureter. A radiopaque substance, such as 30% Renografin or 50% Hypaque, is then injected, and an x-ray film is taken to outline the entire upper urinary collecting system.

Pediatric cystoscopy

Pediatric cystoscopy is the endoscopic examination of the lower urinary tract of pediatric patients. The major difference between adult and pediatric cystoscopy is the size of the instruments used and consideration of the small, delicate orifices of the pediatric patient. Indications for pediatric cystoscopy include urinary tract infection, enuresis, urethral valves, vesicoureteral reflux, diverticula, bladder neck contractures, bladder tumors, and urinary tract obstructions.

Procedural considerations

The pediatric patient is not a small adult. It is important to remember this when caring for them; speak to them on their level of understanding, and provide the special emo-

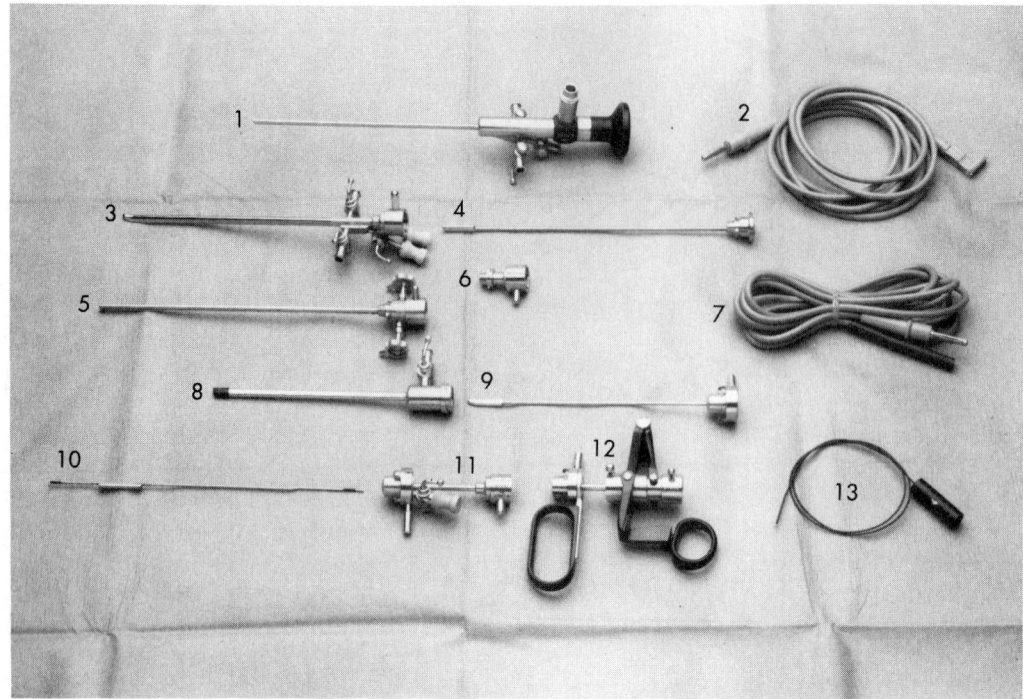

FIG. 14-22   Pediatric cystoscopy instrumentation. *1*, 8 Fr cystoscope; *2*, fiberoptic light cord; *3* and *4*, 13 Fr cystoscope sheath and obturator; *5*, deflector; *6*, bridge; *7*, high-frequency cable; *8* and *9*, 13 Fr resectoscope sheath and obturator; *10*, resectoscope loop; *11*, bridge; *12*, working element; and *13*, ball tip electrode.

Courtesy Karl Storz Endoscopy—America, Inc., Culver City, Calif.

tional support these young patients require (see Chapter 28). The chart will contain essentially the same data as for the adult cystoscopy patient and should be reviewed preoperatively. The cystoscopy setup will have the same type of components as that for the adult cystoscopy patient except that the size of the cystourethroscope system will be specific to the pediatric patient's needs (Fig. 14-22).

Each pediatric cystourethroscope is designed to fit specific component parts and is very delicate. Therefore the perioperative nurse must be familiar with the proper use of the system and handle the components carefully. The resectoscope loop is commonly used to resect urethral valves and occasionally bladder tumors. The cold knife may be used with the resectoscope to cut urethral strictures and occasionally to resect a urethral valve.

The most common anesthesia used for the pediatric patient is general anesthesia. Following induction of anesthesia, the child is placed in a lithotomy or frog-leg position and prepped and draped according to established procedure.

Maintenance of body temperature is of special concern in children. Every effort should be made to limit exposure of the body surface. Chapter 28 provides a thorough discussion of important perioperative nursing considerations for pediatric patients.

Operative procedure

The pediatric cystourethroscope is lubricated and inserted through the urethra into the bladder. The light cord and irrigation tubing are attached to the telescope and cystoscope, and the examination is performed.

Transurethral ureteropyeloscopy

Transurethral ureteropyeloscopy is an endoscopic examination of the ureters and renal pelvis. The use of rigid or flexible ureteroscopes or ureteropyeloscopes provides the opportunity to diagnose filling defects in the ureter and renal pelvis, congenital anomalies, hematuria, ureteral obstruction, and damage from trauma. Manipulation, fragmentation, basketing of ureteral and renal calculi, and retrieval of foreign bodies are possible with transurethral ureteropyeloscopy. Often ESWL, EHL, sonic or laser lithotripsy accompanies the procedure. It may also be used to manage residual sludge and *steinstrasse* (stream of stones) following these treatments. ESWL and EHL are addressed in more detail later in the chapter.

Ureteral strictures may also be treated transurethrally, and biopsies of tumors of the ureter and renal pelvis may be performed under direct visualization. Internal ureteral stents may also be inserted for ureteral patency. These range

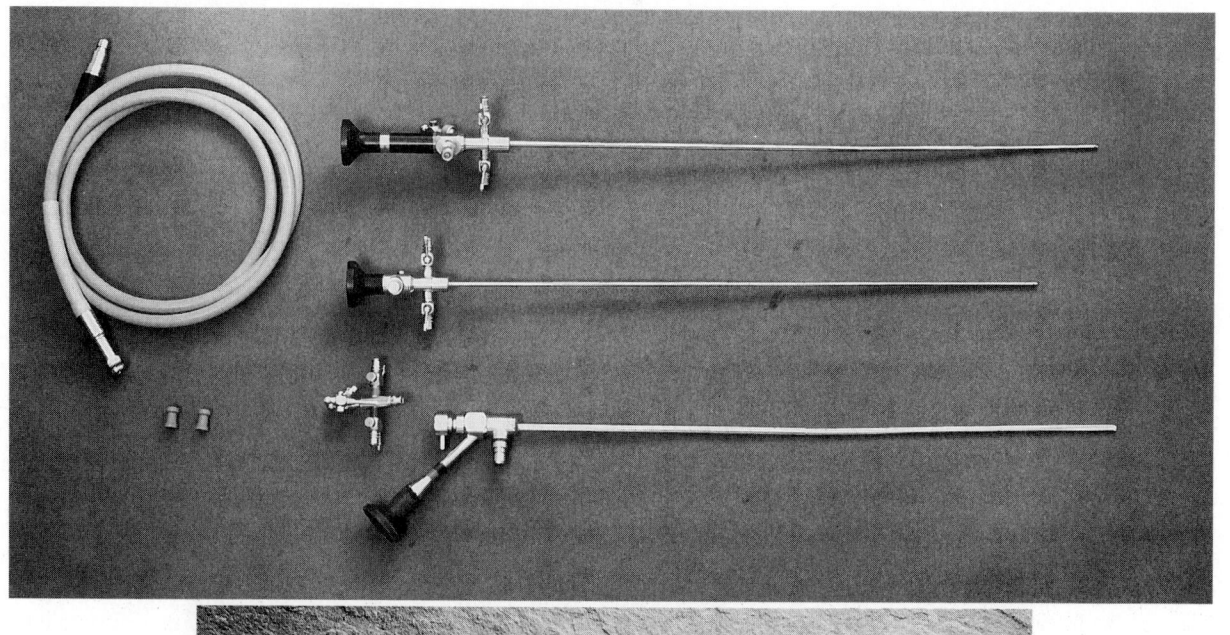

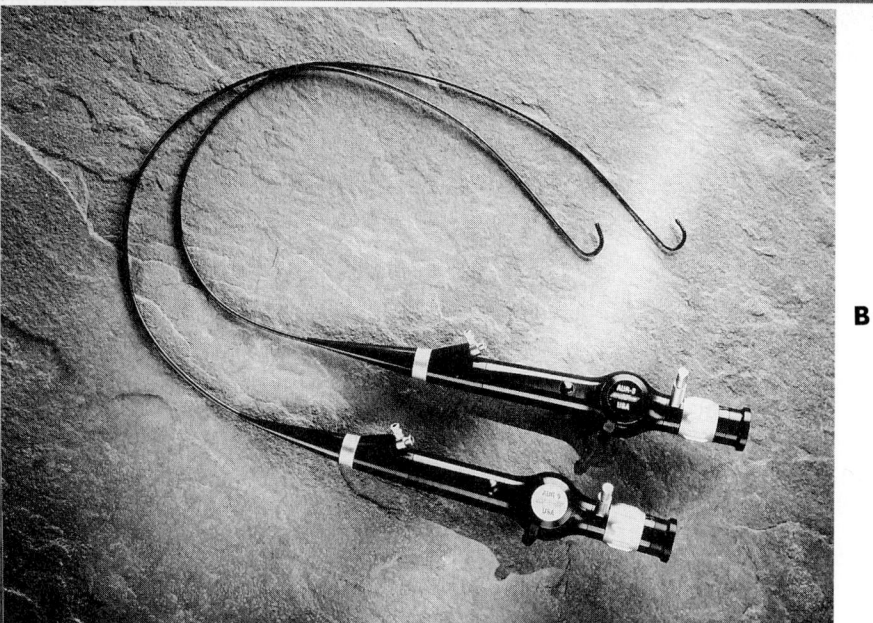

FIG. 14-23 **A,** Rigid ureteroscope system. **B,** AUR8 and AUR9 flexible ureteropyeloscopes.
Courtesy Circon Corp., Santa Barbara, Calif.

in size from 3 to 8.5 Fr and are available in single and double-J and pigtail configurations.

Procedural considerations

The setup is similar to that for a cystoscopy with the addition of a rigid or flexible ureteroscope system (Fig. 14-23). A critical factor in this procedure is allowing enough time for careful dilation of the ureter under C-arm fluoros-

copy. The flexible ureteroscope has gained popularity because of its inherent tip mobility, which provides a more panoramic view of the entire circumference of the ureter. The perioperative nurse must be able to tilt the radiolucent operative bed at head and foot and laterally, as well as raise the bed height.

In addition to the standard cystoscopy setup, the following equipment should be available:

Ureteroscope, rigid
 and/or flexible
Ureteral dilators, gradu-
 ated sizes and styles
Ureteral stone baskets,
 3 to 5 Fr, of various
 styles
1 Ureteral grasping for-
 ceps
1 Ureteral snare

1 Ureteral biopsy for-
 ceps
1 Ureteral scissors
Ureteral catheters, vari-
 ous styles and sizes
Ureteral stents
Ureteral guidewires
Ureteral balloon dilators
Radiographic dye

SURGERY OF THE PENIS AND THE URETHRA

Laser ablation of condylomata and penile carcinoma

Laser ablation of condylomata or penile cancer is the eradication of diseased tissue by means of a laser beam. Laser therapy has been determined, through clinical trials, to be effective therapy for condylomata and penile cancers that are refractive to other treatments. One of the major advantages of the laser is that heat is distributed evenly to the tissue underlying the lesion. The recurrence rate following laser ablation has been extremely low, with cure rates ranging from 88% to 95%. When any laser is being used, precautions appropriate to that system must be initiated (see Chapter 31).

Procedural considerations

Laser treatment may be performed successfully with a local infiltration of anesthetic. A U-shaped craterlike lesion of predetermined depth with a 2-mm radius can be created. A power setting ranging from 2 to 20 W on continuous or superpulse mode is generally used. With laser ablation less edema and necrosis occur, fibrosis is minimized, and rapid healing is facilitated. The argon, CO_2, KTP, and Nd:YAG lasers are all suitable for this therapeutic application.

Operative procedure

The operator moves the beam transversely across the tissue and then in a crosshatch matrix, thereby treating all perimeters of the lesion. Periodically the area should be wiped with a sponge moistened in acetic acid (3% to 5% vinegar). This treatment causes diseased tissue to stand out and allows therapy to deeper layers.

Postoperatively the affected areas may be coated with polymyxin ointment or a similar antibiotic. Wounds are generally left uncovered. A mild oral pain medication is usually adequate for postoperative discomfort.

Circumcision

Circumcision is the excision of the foreskin (prepuce) of the glans penis. Circumcision may be done prophylactically in infancy. The surgery may be performed for religious reasons, as is required in specific faiths. Provision should be made to observe the religious needs and preferences of the parents.

Circumcision is also performed for the relief of phimo-

sis, a condition in which the orifice of the prepuce is stenosed or too narrow to permit easy retraction behind the glans. Another condition, balanoposthitis, results in an inflamed glans and mucous membrane with purulent discharge and may require circumcision. In addition, circumcision may be done to prevent recurrent paraphimosis, a condition in which the prepuce cannot be reduced easily from a retracted position.

Procedural considerations

Newborns are generally positioned on a specially constructed board that facilitates restraint by immobilizing the limbs and exposing the genitals. Generally, only minimal anesthesia is necessary in this age group. Older children require general anesthesia. Adults may be offered the option of regional or general anesthesia.

For infants the setup includes fine plastic instruments. A Gomco clamp of the appropriate size, a Plastibell, or the Hollister disposable circumcision device may be employed. The Hollister device includes sutures that are sealed in a sterile packet ready for use. For older patients there is no need for the circumcision clamp and only a plastic instrument set is used. Petrolatum gauze for dressing should be available.

Operative procedure

1. If the prepuce is adherent, a probe or hemostat may be used to break up adhesions. The prepuce is clamped in the dorsal midline and incised toward the coronal margin (Fig. 14-24, *A*), leaving about 5 cm of coronal mucosa intact. A similar procedure is performed ventrally. The two incisions are then joined circumferentially. Alternatively, a superficial, circumferential incision is made in the skin with a scalpel at the level of the coronal sulcus and the mucosa at the base of the glans. The redundant skin is undermined between the circumferential incisions and removed as a complete cuff (Fig. 14-24, *B*).
2. Bleeding vessels are coagulated or clamped with mosquito hemostats and tied with fine absorbable ligatures. Prior to closure, the area may be cleansed with an appropriate antiseptic solution.

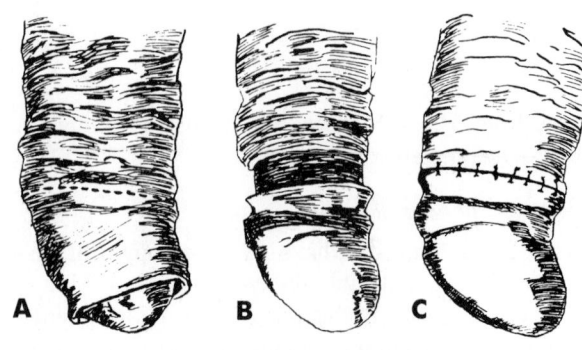

FIG. 14-24 Circumcision.

3. The raw edges of the skin incision are approximated to a coronal cuff of mucosal prepuce, generally with no. 4-0 or 5-0 absorbable sutures on atraumatic, plastic cutting or fine gastrointestinal needles (Fig. 14-24, *C*). The wound is usually dressed with petrolatum gauze.

Excision of urethral caruncle

A urethral caruncle is a benign lesion or inflammatory prolapse of the external urinary meatus in the female. Excision entails the removal of papillary or sessile tumors from the urethra.

Procedural considerations

The patient is placed in the lithotomy position. A minor or plastic set, an electrosurgical unit, and a local anesthetic are used. A urethral catheter of an appropriate size may be required if the distal urethral prolapse is severe.

Operative procedure

With a small, fine-tipped Metzenbaum or plastic scissors the tumor is exposed and excised within a wedge of ventral urethral tissue. Figure-of-eight no. 4-0 absorbable sutures at the edge of the incision are usually sufficient to achieve good hemostasis.

Urethral meatotomy

Urethral meatotomy is an incisional enlargement of the external urethral meatus to relieve stenosis or stricture at the external meatus that is either congenital or acquired.

Procedural considerations

A male patient is placed in the supine position. Prepping and draping are as described for urethral catheterization. For a female patient the lithotomy position is used. Local anesthesia is generally employed. A plastic instrument set is needed. A petrolatum gauze dressing is usually applied.

Operative procedure

A straight hemostat is placed on the ventral surface of the meatus. An incision is made along the frenum to enlarge the opening and overcome the stricture. Bleeding vessels are clamped and ligated with fine absorbable sutures. The mucosal layer is sutured to the skin with fine absorbable sutures. A dressing of petrolatum gauze may be applied.

Urethral dilatation and internal urethrotomy

Urethral dilatation and internal urethrotomy entail the gradual dilatation and lysis of a urethral stricture to provide relief of distal lower urinary tract obstruction. Urethral strictures or narrowing of the urethra may be caused by a congenital malformation that is usually found at the external urinary meatus. Infection or trauma may also contribute to stricture of the membranous and pendulous urethra. One method of treating urethral stricture disease is by pe-

riodic dilatation with Phillips filiforms and followers or Van Buren sounds. Balloon catheters designed for intermittent dilatation are also available.

Procedural considerations

The male patient may be placed in a supine position for routine urethral dilatation and in lithotomy position for other procedures. Prepping and draping are as required for male catheterization. A local anesthetic such as lidocaine (Xylocaine gel or Anestacon) should be used. The female patient is placed in the lithotomy position. A cotton-tipped applicator dipped in the local anesthetic or a urethral syringe filled with anesthetic is placed in the urethral opening. Female urethral dilatation is performed with short, straight metal dilators or with hollow McCarthy dilators, through which a urine specimen can also be obtained.

The setup includes the following:

Urethrotomes (Fig. 14-25)	Van Buren sounds
Direct viewing telescope and bridge for ureteral catheters	Irrigation system
	Prep set and solutions
	Silicone Foley catheter
Resectoscope working element, sheath, obturator, and cold knives	Syringe, 20 ml
	Lubricant, water-soluble
	Fiberoptic light cord
	Luer-Lok water adapter
Urethral dilators	Cystoscopy drape pack
Phillips filiforms and followers	Sterile gown and gloves
	Cystoscopy setup, if required

Operative procedures

Gradual dilatation. In a male patient the urethra is lubricated and anesthetized with a viscous anesthetic that is instilled into the urethra with a urethral or Uro-Jet syringe. A penile clamp occludes the penile urethra at the coronal sulcus and keeps the anesthetic within the urethra. Phillips filiforms of various tips and sizes are introduced first in an attempt to pass an instrument beyond the urethral stricture. Followers of increasing size are connected to the filiforms and passed through the strictured area of the urethra, stretching the scarred area (Fig. 14-26, *A*). Slow dilatation is also achieved with a small catheter or filiform left in the urethra. It leads to softening of the stricture over the course of several days. Before use or sterilization, the filiforms and followers should be carefully inspected for damaged or weak points, particularly around the score thread end. Van Buren sounds (Fig. 14-26, *B*) or a balloon dilatation catheter may also be used for urethral dilatation.

Internal urethrotomy. Under direct vision the assembled visualizing urethrotome is inserted into the urethra. When necessary, a filiform or ureteral catheter is fed into the catheterizing channel to help identify the patent portion of the urethra. The urethrotome is advanced to the desired position, and the blade is used to incise the urethral scar. The normal urethra must be increased 1 cm proximally and distally beyond the stricture to achieve good results. A sil-

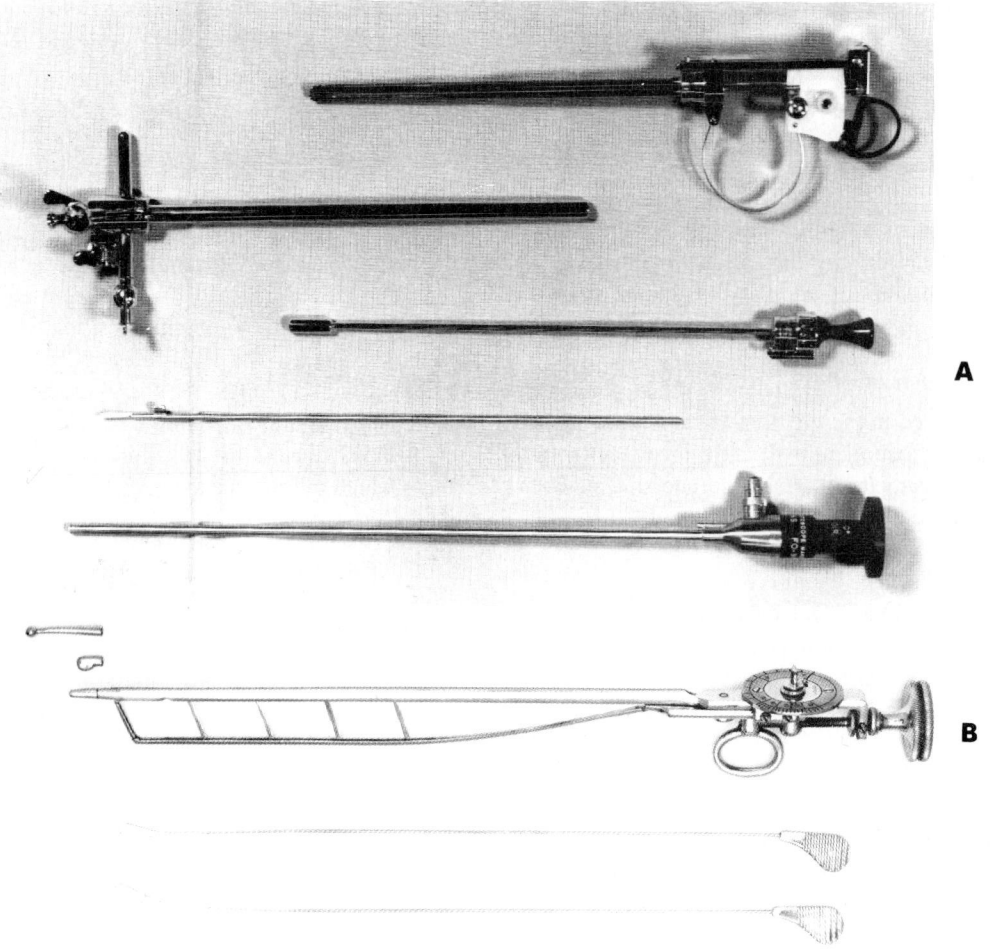

FIG. 14-25 **A,** Circon Corporation internal urethrotome components. **B,** Otis urethrotome components.
Courtesy Circon Corp., Santa Barbara, Calif.

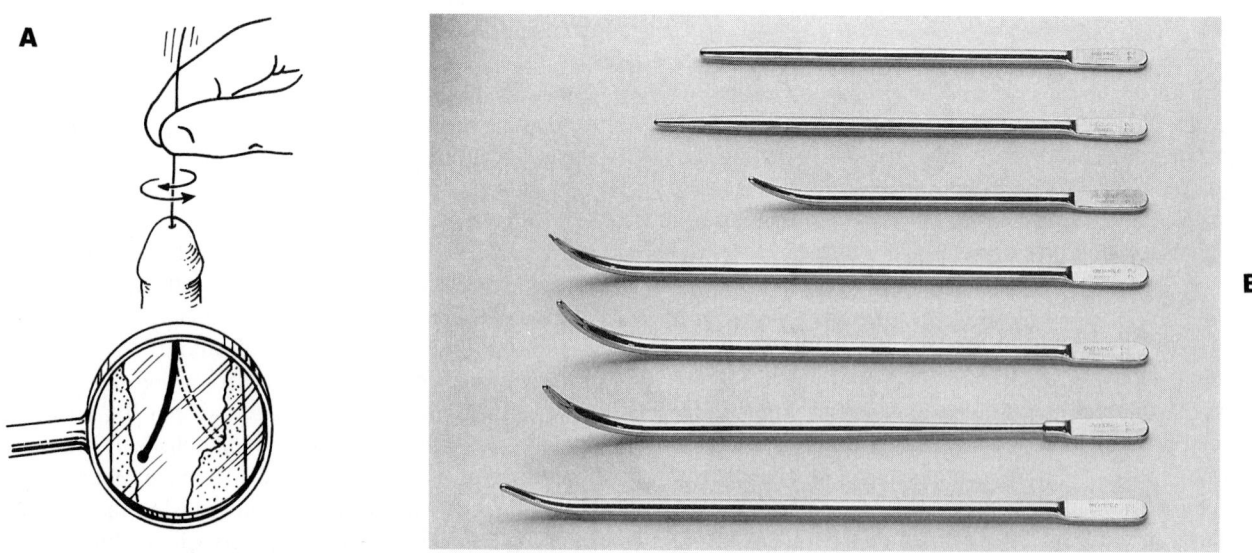

FIG. 14-26 **A,** Method of using coude-tipped bougie for passing stricture. **B,** Variety of urethral sounds
(dilators).
B courtesy Greenwald Surgical Co., Inc., Lake Station, Ind.

icone Foley catheter is usually left in place for 3 to 5 days after surgery.

Hypospadias repair

Hypospadias is a urethral meatus that is proximal to its normal glandular position at the tip of the penis. There are varying degrees of hypospadias. The meatus may be on the ventral surface of the glans, on the corona, anywhere along the shaft, in the scrotum, or even in the perineum. The more proximal the opening, the greater the degree of chordee (ventral curvature of the penis). Chordee are fibrous bands that extend from the hypospadiac urethral meatus to the tip of the glans and represent the abnormally developed urethra and its investing layer of Buck's fascia, dartos, and skin. In some cases of clinical curvature, however, these fibrous bands may not be present. Although these curvatures are still termed chordee, they are not true fibrous chordee.

Principles of hypospadias repair consist of meatoplasty and glanuloplasty, orthoplasty (release of chordee, thereby straightening the penis), urethroplasty (reconstruction of the urethra), skin cover, and scrotoplasty. These may be done in one- or two-stage repairs depending on the extent of the condition. Recently there has been an increase in efforts to relocate the meatus to the apex of the glans, especially in the more extensive one-stage repairs.

One complication of hypospadias repair is urethral fistula formation, which can be repaired without much difficulty. Correction of strictures is more troublesome.

Procedural considerations

The patient (the majority are infants and young children) is placed in the supine position with legs apart. The urine is diverted with a urethral catheter intraoperatively. The instrument setup varies according to the surgeon's preference. However, a minor set with fine plastic instruments is generally required, and sutures, polyethylene infant feeding tubes, silicone tubing or silicone Foley catheters, and drains may be desired. Owens gauze, Elastomull, Coban, and Elastoplast, as well as adhesive tape, are generally required for the dressing, which is an important part of the hypospadias repair.

Operative procedures
Meatoplasty and glanuloplasty (MAGPI procedure)

1. A subcoronal, circumferential incision is made about 8 mm proximal to the meatus and corona. The skin is stripped back from the phallus by subcutaneous dissection (Fig. 14-27, *A* to *C*).
2. A bridge of tissue between the meatus and granular groove is made with a transverse closure of the dorsal meatal edge to the distal granular groove (Fig. 14-27, *D* to *F*).
3. Three traction sutures are placed where the foreskin stops, at the apex of the ventral meatus and lateral glans (Fig. 14-27, *G*).

4. The edges of the glans are sutured together ventrally in a V configuration, and the redundant edges are excised (Fig. 14-27, *H*). Vertical mattress sutures are used to approximate the glans beneath the meatus.
5. If foreskin is excessive at the extremities it may be trimmed, followed by sleeve style reapproximation of the penile skin (Fig. 14-27, *I*). If a ventral skin defect is present, a rotational skin flap closure is used.
6. An indwelling catheter is placed, and the wound is dressed.

Orthoplasty. Orthoplasty is the proper designation for the plastic procedure performed to straighten the penis. Chordee repair is the more common term employed. In true fibrous chordee the penis is curved ventrally with the meatus and glans in close proximity to one another.

Artificial erection is achieved by injecting 0.9% saline solution into the corpus cavernosum. Both corporal bodies fill, making it possible to determine the degree of curvature before and after the resection of the fibrous bands.

1. An incision is made circumferentially around the corona and carried distal to the urethral meatus and well below the glans cap (Fig. 14-28, *A*). Dissection continues to the level of the tunica albuginea of the corpora cavernosa.
2. With proximal dissection the adherent fibrous plaque is freed, working in a side-to-side fashion. The urethra is elevated from the corpora during this process (Fig. 14-28, *B*).
3. The chordee generally surrounds the urethral meatus and often extends for some distance. It is important to free it completely along the entire penile shaft to the penoscrotal junction, or in severe cases into the scrotum or perineum.
4. Following release of the chordee the glans penis is closed with 4-0 absorbable sutures in a circular manner (Fig. 14-28, *C*).
5. If urethroplasty is either delayed or unnecessary, excess dorsal skin is excised (Fig. 14-28, *D*) and the incision closed along the dorsal midline with interrupted, absorbable mattress sutures (Fig. 14-28, *E*). The wound is dressed according to established protocol.

Urethroplasty. Many procedures are described for reconstruction of a urethra. They may be divided into three general groups: adjacent skin flaps, free skin grafts, and mobilized vascular flaps. There are also many combinations of these procedures. In all the procedures some type of temporary urinary diversion, such as a perineal urethrostomy, may be used. The procedural considerations are the same as for chordee repair.

Adjacent skin flap.
It is possible to tubularize skin adjacent to the meatus to create a neourethra in a one-stage repair. Transfer of dorsal skin to the ventrum will also provide graft material close to the meatus. However, this is generally done in two stages, and the vascularity of this thin

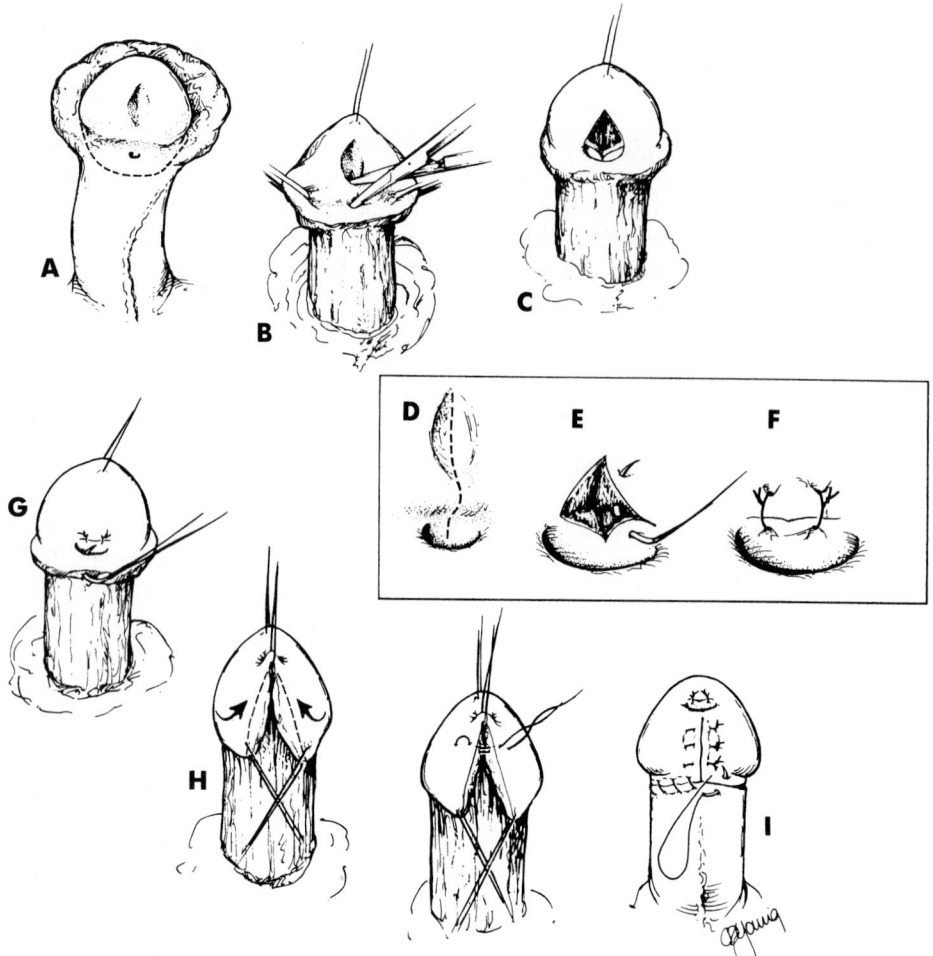

FIG. 14-27   MAGPI chordee procedure in hypospadias repair.
Modified from Gillenwater, J.Y. (1991). *Adult and pediatric urology*. St. Louis: Mosby.

rotational flap is less than optimum with results that are more prone to complication.

1. Traction sutures are placed in the tip of the penis and in the glans wings for stabilization and exposure.
2. The distance between the glans tip and the lower edge of the meatus is measured. An outline of the proposed incision is drawn on the penile shaft (Fig. 14-29, *A*). In a one-stage approach the distal length must be increased to compensate for the added penile length following chordee release.
3. An incision is made around the outlined flap and carried proximally to a point on the shaft that corresponds to the distance required to reach the glans tip (Fig. 14-29, *B*). A flap width of 14 to 16 mm is usually sufficient to ensure good circumference of the neourethra.
4. Once incised, the tube is rolled over a number 8 or 10

Fr catheter (Fig. 14-29, *B*) with an inverted running stitch of 4-0 or 5-0 absorbable suture.
5. The glans penis is incised and the glans wings are undermined and freed. The neourethra is carried to the distal portion of the glans and sutured in place (Fig. 14-29, *C*).
6. The glans wings are sutured around the neourethra with absorbable, interrupted mattress sutures. The redundant foreskin is split down the midline and the flaps are brought around in a Z-plasty manner (Fig. 14-29, *D*).
7. A dry sterile pressure dressing is applied. The patient can often be discharged on the same day, without the need for an indwelling catheter.

Free skin graft. Free skin grafts should be full thickness. Since the free graft must be revascularized, it is important that it have a perfect skin cover of dorsal, prepu-

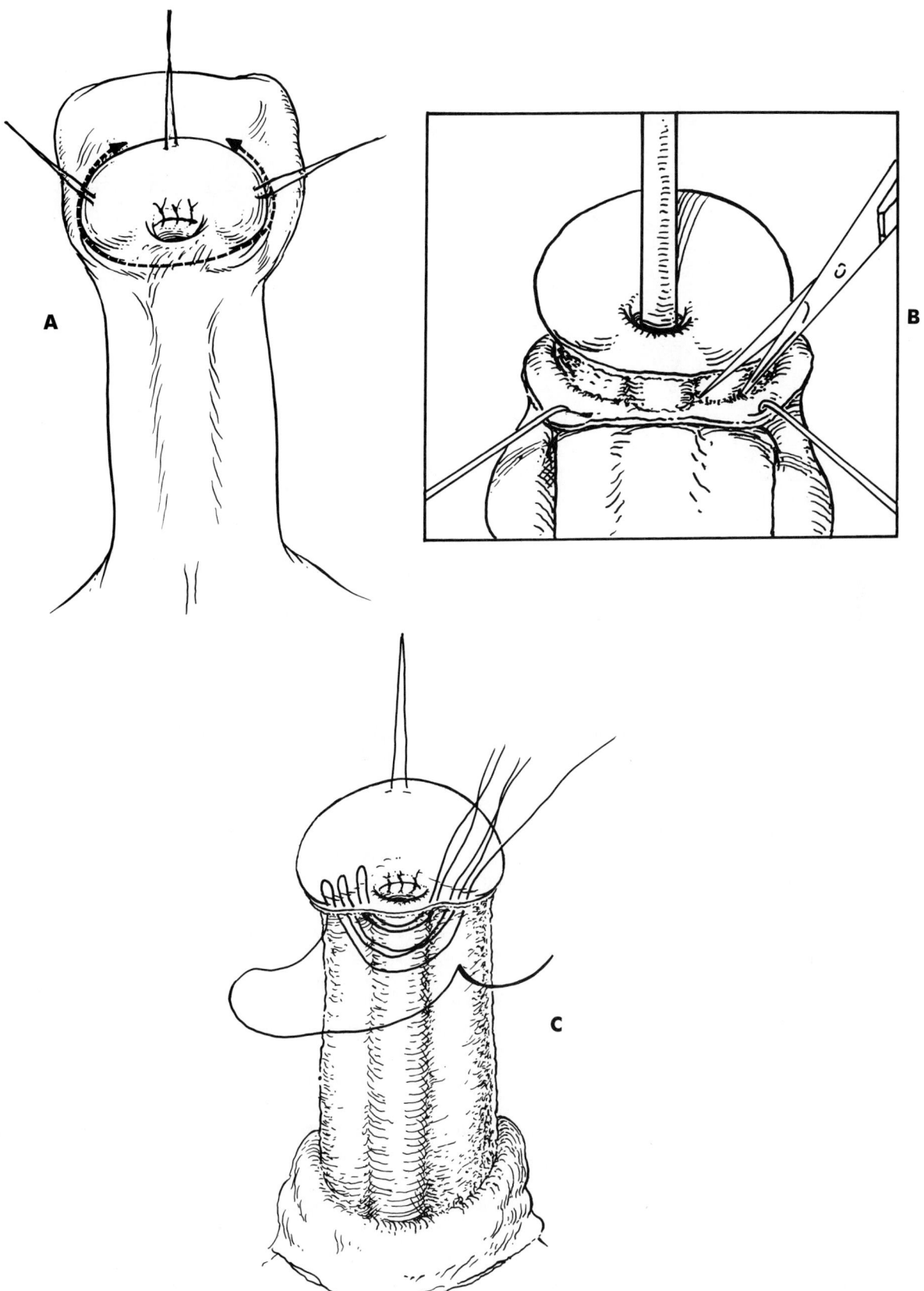

FIG. 14-28 Orthoplasty.

Modified from Droller, M.J. (1992). *Surgical management of urologic disease*. St. Louis: Mosby.

Continued.

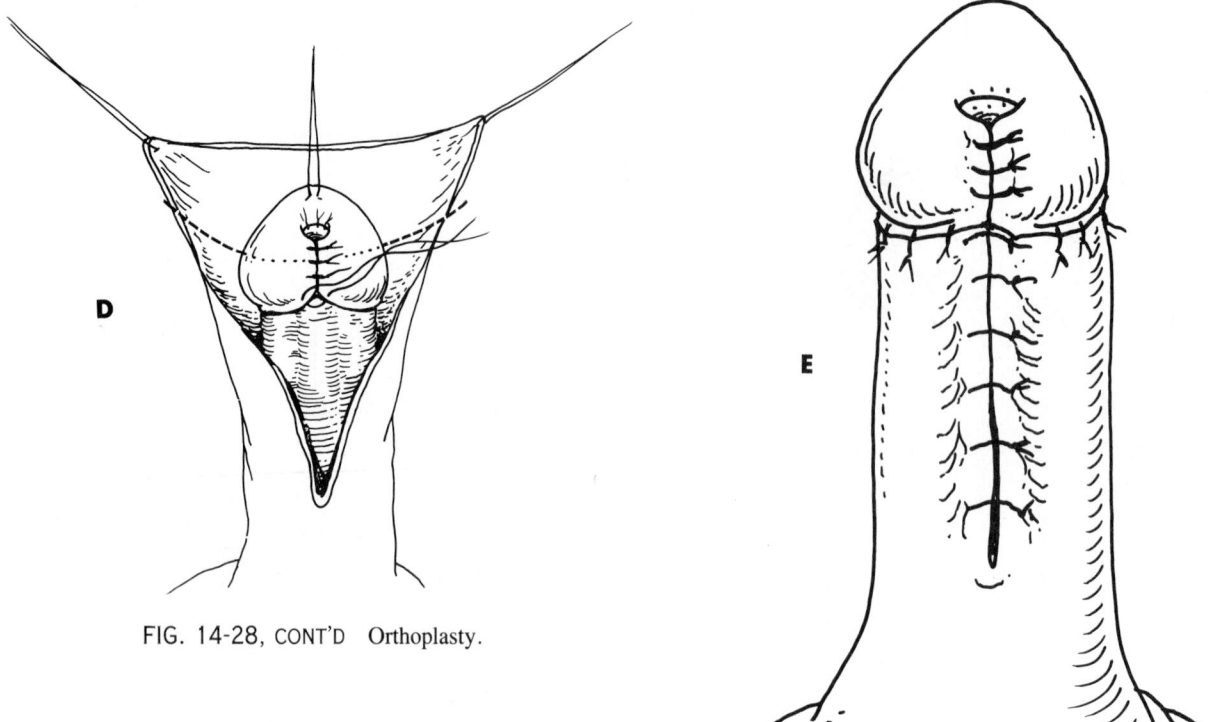

FIG. 14-28, CONT'D   Orthoplasty.

tial, penile skin that is well vascularized. This type of graft is generally used with a one-stage hypospadias repair.

1. A V-shaped incision is made on the glans, and the penile skin is mobilized following the chordee release (Fig. 14-30, *A*).
2. Glans wings are developed in a triangular fashion, and ventral preputial skin is used for the full-thickness free graft (Fig. 14-30, *B*).
3. The graft is formed into a neourethra over a stenting catheter (Fig. 14-30, *C*).
4. The graft is anastomosed proximally to the urethra with the suture line of the graft next to the corpora. The middle glans dart is fixed to the corpora (Fig. 14-30, *D*).
5. A meatoplasty with the dorsal glans dart is accomplished.
6. Fine, absorbable, interrupted sutures are placed around the meatus and glans and along the dorsal penile shaft (Fig. 14-30, *E*).
7. The wound is dressed according to established protocol.

Mobilized vascularized flaps. Vascularized flaps of preputial or penile skin may be mobilized to the ventrum by leaving them attached to the outer surface of the prepuce or as an island flap. One modification is the transverse preputial island flap neourethra with glans channel positioning for the meatus. Preputial skin seems to be preferred due to its rich reliable blood supply.

1. The chordee is released (Fig. 14-31, *A*).
2. Ventral preputial skin is dissected free and fanned out (Fig. 14-31, *B*).
3. The rectangle of skin is rolled into the neourethra and measured (Fig. 14-31, *C*).
4. The island flap is developed by dissection of the subcutaneous tissue from the dorsal penile skin (Fig. 14-31, *D* and *E*).
5. A glans channel is created with plastic scissors in a plane just above the corpora. The glans tissue is removed with the 14 Fr channel, and the island flap urethra is spiraled to the ventrum (Fig. 14-31, *F*).

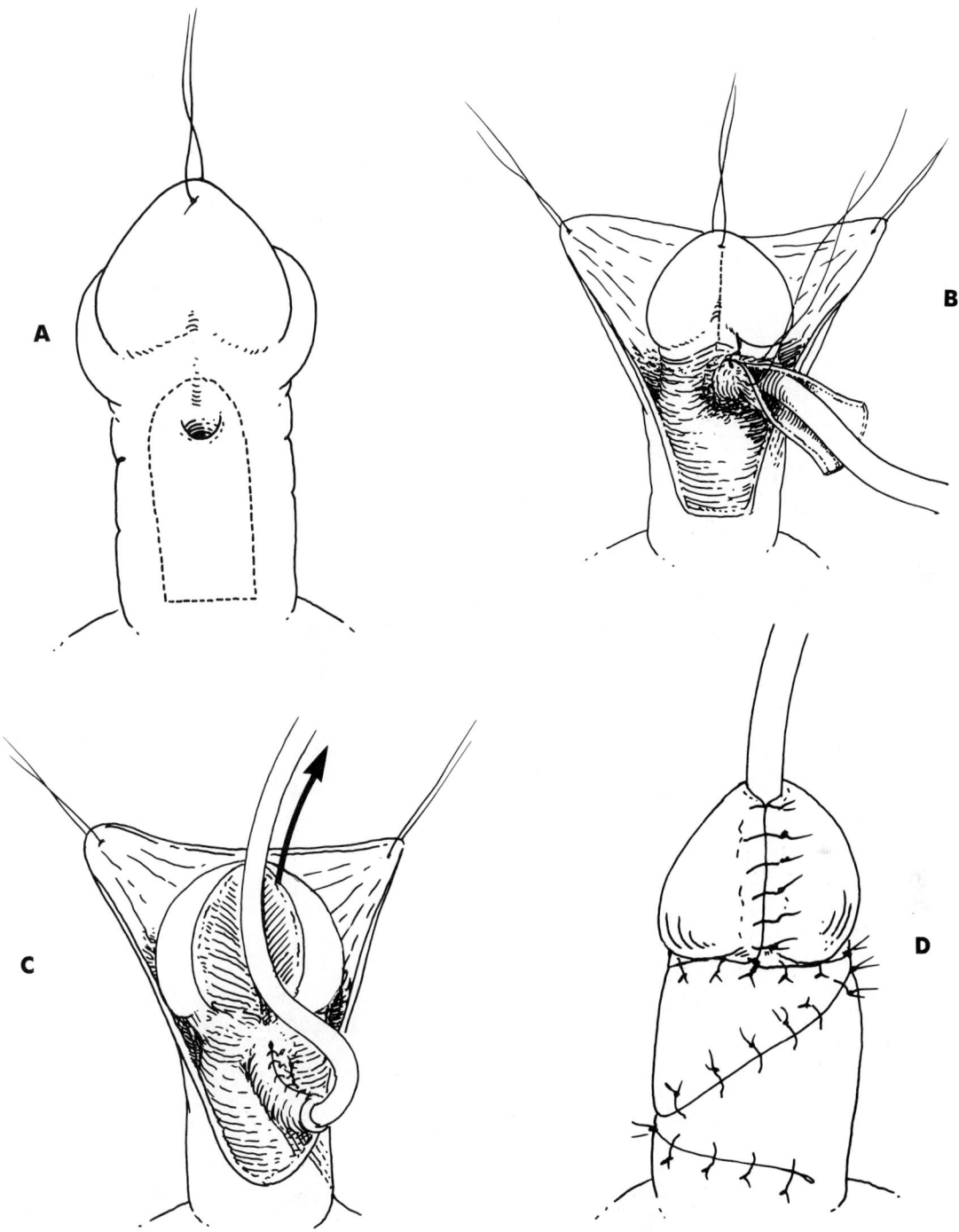

FIG. 14-29   Urethroplasty with adjacent skin flap.

Modified from Droller, M.J. (1992). *Surgical management of urologic disease*. St. Louis: Mosby.

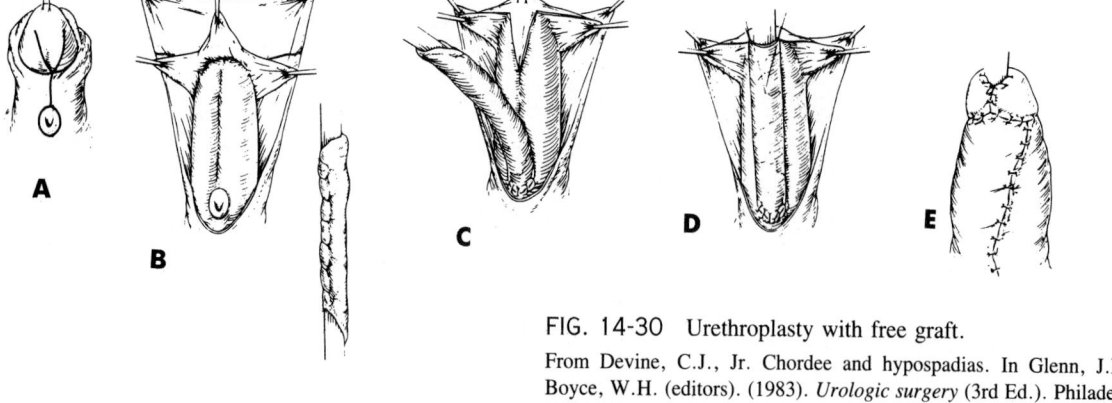

FIG. 14-30 Urethroplasty with free graft.

From Devine, C.J., Jr. Chordee and hypospadias. In Glenn, J.F., &
Boyce, W.H. (editors). (1983). *Urologic surgery* (3rd Ed.). Philadelphia:
JB Lippincott.

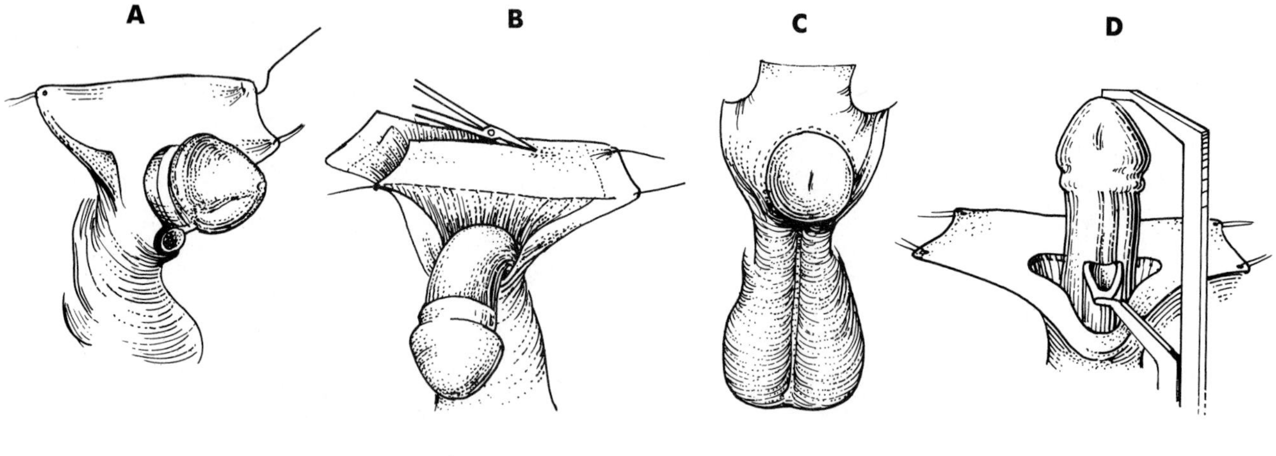

FIG. 14-31 Urethroplasty, island flap.

6. The neourethra is anastomosed proximally to the urethra (Fig. 14-31, *G*).
7. The neourethra is carried to the tip of the glans (Fig. 14-31, *H*).
8. The dorsal penile flaps are transposed laterally to the midline and excess skin is excised. Closure is with fine, absorbable, interrupted mattress sutures around the glans and down the penile shaft (Fig. 14-31, *I*).
9. Dressings are applied according to established protocol.

Skin cover. Following orthoplasty and urethroplasty, the penis must be resurfaced with skin. Abundant, excess dorsal foreskin is usually adequate to achieve the desired results.

1. Preputial tissue is transposed through a small buttonhole opening in the midline (Fig. 14-32, *A*).
2. The vasculature is spread laterally and the glans penis is delivered through the hole (Fig. 14-32, *B*).
3. The skin flap is then sutured with fine, absorbable, interrupted mattress sutures (Fig. 14-32, *C*).

Scrotoplasty. When the penis is caught between two scrotal halves and becomes engulfed, this penoscrotal transposition must be corrected. This condition occurs only in rare instances. The plastic repair of the prepenile scrotal halves is generally accomplished with rotational skin flaps.

Epispadias repair

An epispadias repair is the correction of the absence of the dorsal wall of the urethra and the position of the corpora cavernosa, ventral to the urethra. The surgical procedures employed in the correction of epispadias depend on the extent of the deformity. In mild incomplete defects the repair is the same as a simple hypospadias repair. Complete deformity is always associated with urinary incontinence because of little or no development of the bladder neck; thus the operation is much more involved. The least severe form of the exstrophy epispadias complex is balanitic epispadias, in which the urethra opens on the dorsum of the glans, or penile epispadias, in which the urethra opens on the shaft of the penis. The more severe variety, which occurs when the urethra opens on the proximal shaft or in the penopubic position, is generally associated with severe dorsal chordee and urinary incontinence.

Procedural considerations

The setup for an epispadias repair is as described for hypospadias repair.

Operative procedures

First-stage epispadias repair. A vertical incision is made distal to the epispadiac meatus and carried circumferentially to the dorsal coronal margin. The foreshortened dorsal urethral strip is lifted off the corpora cavernosa, and the ventral prepuce (foreskin) is rotated dorsally to cover the dorsal skin defect created by penile straightening.

Second-stage epispadias repair

1. A vertical suprapubic incision is made, exposing the anterior bladder wall and widened vesical neck. A wedge section of the anterolateral prostatic urethra is removed on either side, so that when it is reconstructed a more normal caliber prostatic urethra is formed.
2. The roof of the membranous urethra is removed.
3. The prostatic urethra is closed, including muscle that is sutured together in the midline, with absorbable sutures. The bladder is closed, leaving an indwelling suprapubic catheter. The abdomen is closed in layers.
4. The anterior urethra is closed after outlining an appropriate size octagonal strip of dorsal penile skin.
5. The remainder of the repair—the creation of the urethra and its coverage with lateral penile skin—is the reverse procedure of a second-stage hypospadias repair.

Urethroplasty

Urethroplasty is reconstructive surgery of the urethra. Strictures, urethral fractures, and narrowing of the urethral lumen are congenital, inflammatory, or traumatic in origin. Various surgical techniques are described in the section on surgical treatment of stricture disease.

Procedural considerations

The patient is placed in the exaggerated lithotomy position. Routine prepping and draping procedures are employed with precautions for protecting the anus (that is, the use of an impervious plastic adherent drape). The setup includes a minor instrument set with fine plastic instruments for dissection and plastic repair. Strictures may be located deep, requiring special instruments such as Turner-Warwick needles and retractors (Fig. 14-33, *A*). A Denis-Browne ring retractor is also helpful (Fig. 14-33, *B*). Fiberoptic lighting is desirable, and an electrosurgical unit may be required.

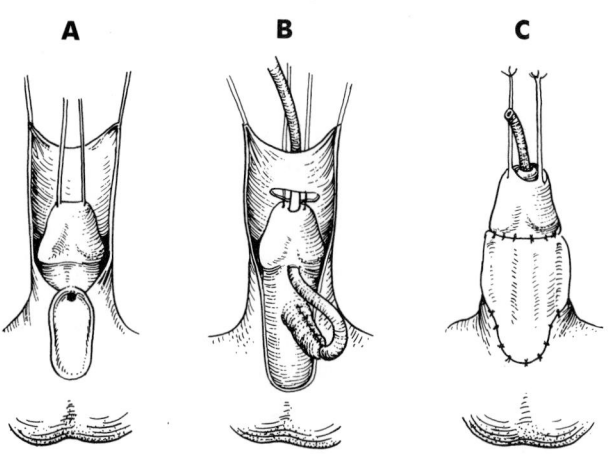

A   B   C

FIG. 14-32   Mustarde procedure skin cover.

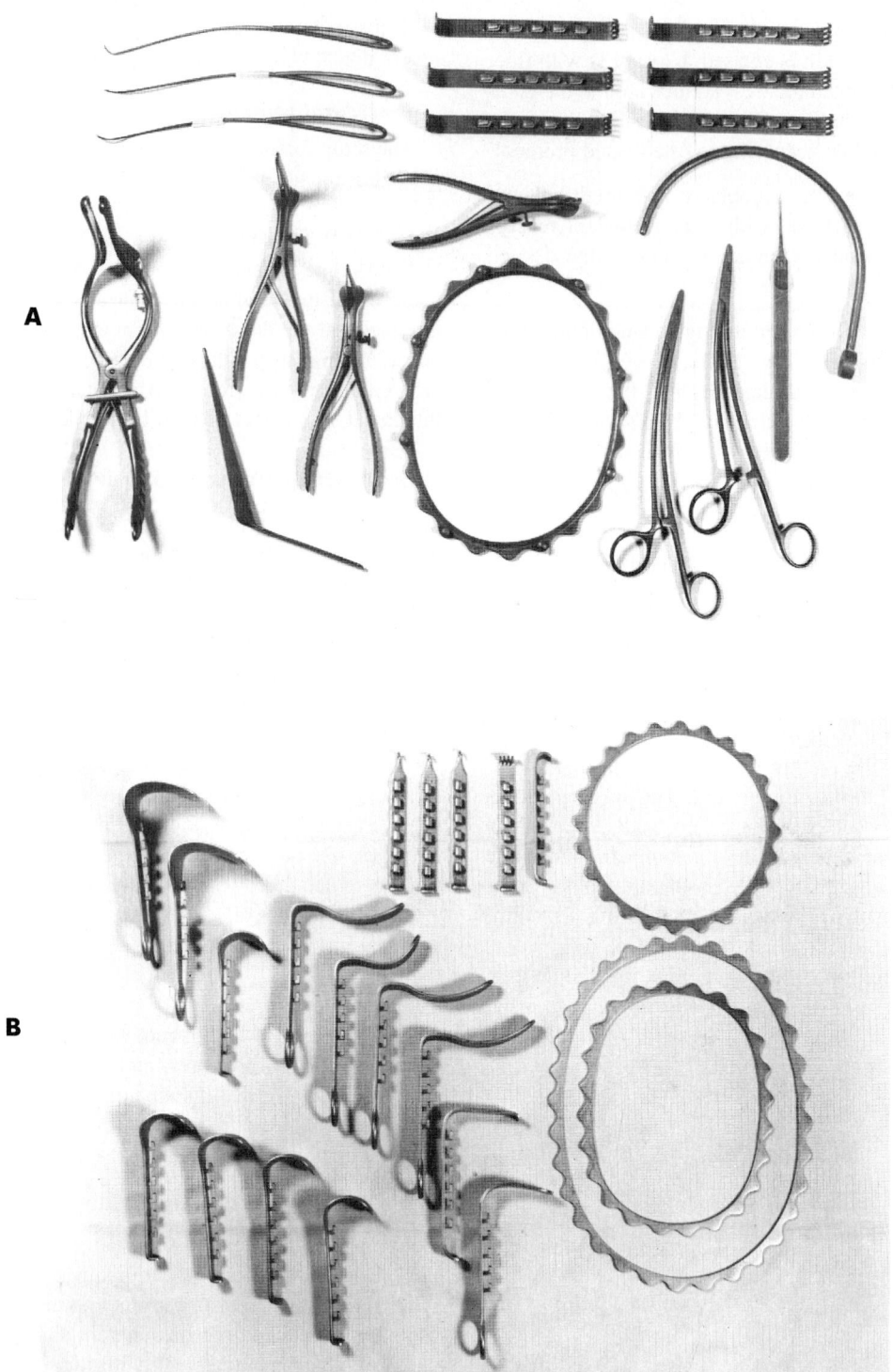

FIG. 14-33   **A,** Turner-Warwick urethroplasty instruments. **B,** Denis-Browne self-retaining ring retractor.

Operative procedures

First-stage Johanson urethroplasty

1. An inverted U incision is made in the perineum from the inner borders of the ischial tuberosities up to and including the base of the scrotum. A Van Buren sound is passed into the urethra up to the stricture. The bulbocavernosus muscle is dissected and retracted laterally.
2. An incision is made in the urethra over the strictured area and is extended at least 1 cm beyond the diseased area of the urethra in each direction.
3. The abnormal scar tissue is excised or simply incised because scrotal skin ultimately increases the lumen. A no. 28 sound is passed through the proximal and the distal urethral lumina to rule out further stricture. The remaining urethral mucosa is sutured with fine absorbable suture to the scrotal skin. A cystotomy tube to divert the urinary stream may be left indwelling and removed in 5 to 7 days.

Approximately 3 months after the first stage, if the operative site is healing and the patient is voiding adequately, a second-stage procedure is performed.

Second-stage Johanson urethroplasty

1. A Robinson catheter is temporarily inserted into the bladder through the proximal urethral stoma. The skin is incised along prolongitudinal lines, and flaps of skin are developed to construct a new urethra.
2. The flaps are brought together in the midline and closed with a continuous or interrupted, fine absorbable suture to a predetermined caliber.
3. Layers of subcutaneous tissue are dissected free, then sutured over the newly constructed urethra with interrupted absorbable sutures.
4. A bulky pressure dressing is applied. Suprapubic cystostomy drainage is an option, but a urethral catheter usually suffices.

Horton-Devine urethroplasty (urethral patch graft).

Urethral patch graft is a one-stage operative procedure for the correction of a urethral stricture, similar to the Johanson urethroplasty.

1. The patient is placed in the lithotomy position.
2. A no. 17 cystoscope is passed into the posterior urethra.
3. A no. 20 urethral dilator is passed into the posterior urethra. A vertical incision in the midline of the perineum is made into the urethral lumen. The cystoscope is reinserted, and whether the incision traversed the stricture is determined.
4. The defect is measured.
5. A circumferential incision on the posterior penile shaft is made to harvest an oval piece of skin the size of the defect.

6. The epidermal side of the graft is defatted, and absorbable sutures of 4-0 are placed at the apex and base.
7. The apex is sutured into position at the verumontanum end of the stricture and then at the distal ends, with the epidermal side toward the urethral lumen.
8. Interrupted absorbable 4-0 sutures are placed to hold the graft in position.
9. The cystoscope is again inserted and the urethra irrigated to check for suture line leaks.
10. A Foley or fenestrated catheter is inserted to serve as a stent.
11. The corpora spongiosa are approximated and closed over the patched area as a separate layer with interrupted 3-0 absorbable sutures.
12. Subcutaneous 4-0 absorbable sutures are placed.
13. The skin and the graft site are closed with interrupted 4-0 sutures.
14. A suprapubic catheter is inserted to divert urine for healing.
15. Petrolatum gauze is wrapped around the penis and covered with gauze sponges and fluffed dressings. A scrotal supporter is applied to provide support and pressure.

PENECTOMY

Penectomy is the partial or total removal of a cancerous penis. The procedure selected depends on the extent of involvement and disease stage. Invasive penile cancer not suited for irradiation owing to its size, depth, or location is best dealt with by penectomy. Excision of a 2-cm gross tumor margin is adequate for local management. Partial penectomy may afford a sufficient length for directable and upright urination. At least 3 cm of viable proximal shaft is necessary for considering a partial penectomy. If the residual stump is inadequate in length, detachment and mobilization of the suspensory ligaments may be an option in selected patients. A total penectomy is generally required when tumor margins are beyond a 2-cm retrievable length from the penoscrotal junction.

Reconstruction is possible following penectomy. Evaluation must take into account sexual, urinary, and cosmetic factors. Extensive or proximally invasive lesions that include the scrotum, perineum, abdominal wall, and pubis necessitate emasculation as well as expanded resection of involved tissues.

Procedural considerations

The setup necessary is similar to that for any inguinal surgery, with the addition of a medium Penrose drain for use as a tourniquet.

Operative procedures
Partial penectomy

1. The lesion is excluded by a towel attached to the planned amputation line. A penile tourniquet is applied at the base (Fig. 14-34, *A*).

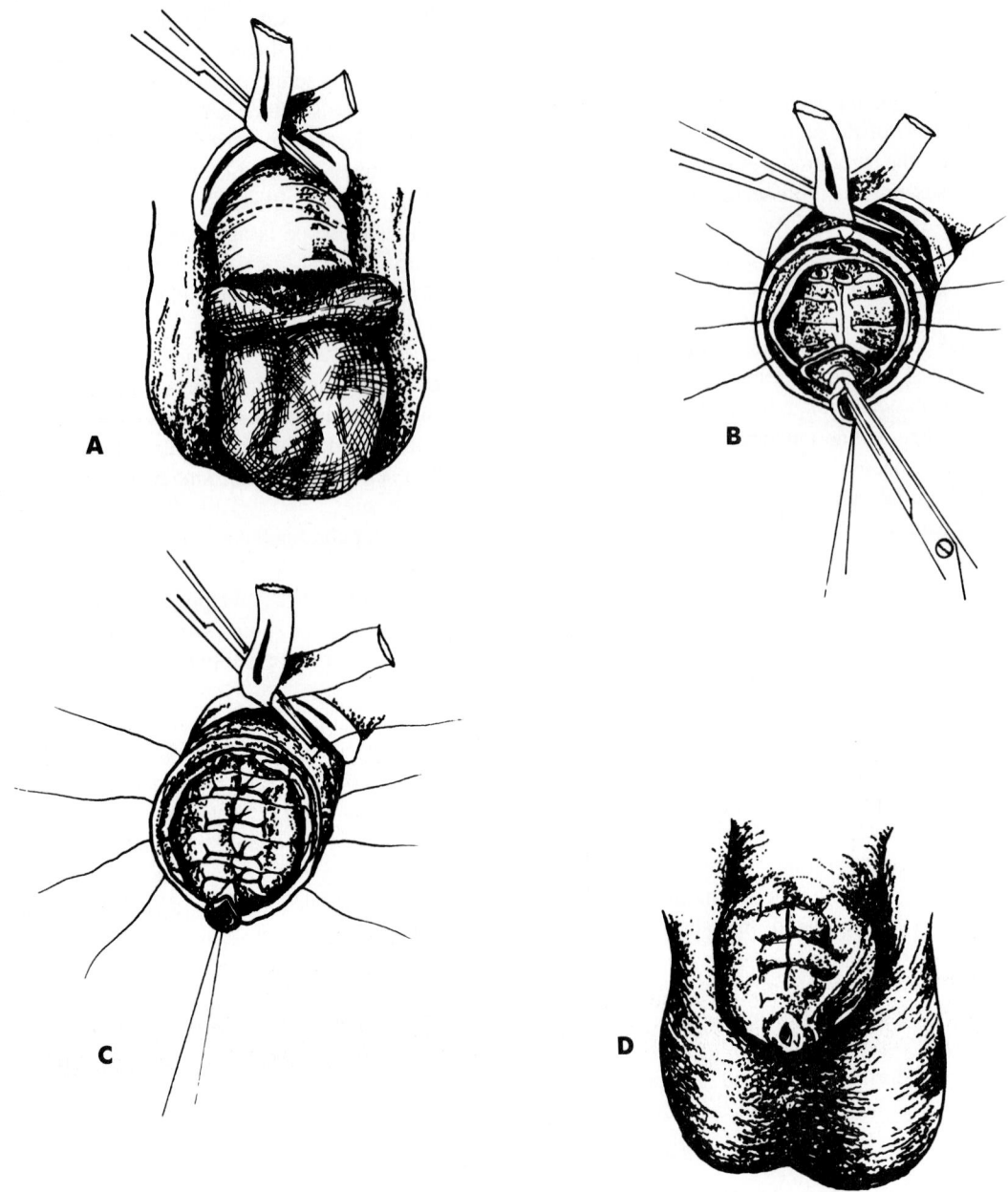

FIG. 14-34   Partial penectomy.

2. Following circumferential skin incision, the cavernous bodies are divided to the urethra with a 2-cm gross margin (Fig. 14-34, *B*).

3. Dorsal vessels are ligated, margins of the tunica albuginea are approximated, and the urethra is dissected proximally and distally (spatulated) to obtain a 1 cm redundant flap (Fig. 14-34, *C*).

4. Without sacrificing the tumor margin, the urethra is then divided. Interrupted sutures are placed on the opposite margins of the tunica albuginea to secure the corpora.

5. The tourniquet is removed, and hemostasis is achieved.

6. Following the dorsal urethrotomy, a skin-to-urethra anastomosis is performed. The redundant skin flap is then dorsally approximated (Fig. 14-34, *D*).

7. A small urinary catheter is inserted, and a nonadherent dressing applied. They are generally removed in 3 or 4 days.

Total penectomy

1. A vertical elliptic incision is made around the penile base (Fig. 14-35, *A*).

2. The distal urethra and its ventral traction are divided through an incision in Buck's fascia, mobilizing the urethra and aiding its dissection, which extends from the

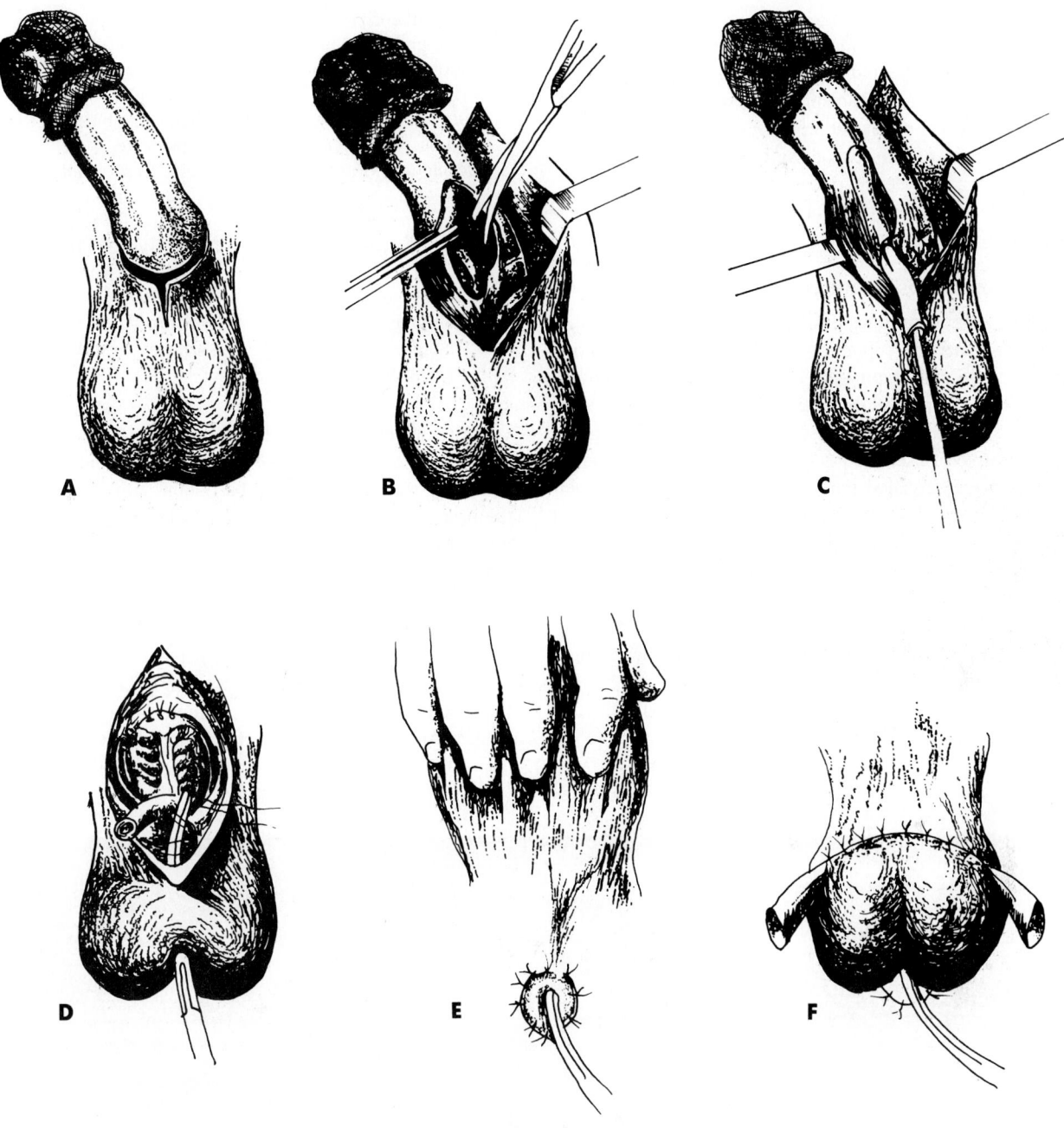

FIG. 14-35 Total penectomy.

corpora to the bulbar region. Then the corpora are separated and ligated (Fig. 14-35, *B*).

3. The suspensory ligaments and dorsal vessels are divided as corporal dissection is carried out. The urethra is transected from the corpora (Fig. 14-35, *C*).

4. An ellipse of skin approximately 1 cm in size is taken from the perineal area. A tunnel is fashioned in the perineal subcutaneous layer of tissue. A traction suture through the tunnel, at the penile base, aids dissection for transposition of the urethra to the perineum (Fig. 14-35, *D*).

5. The urethra is grasped with forceps and transferred to the perineum.

6. The urethra is spatulated and a skin-to-urethra anastomosis is performed through a buttonhole incision in the perineum (Fig. 14-35, *E*).

7. The primary incision is closed horizontally, elevating the scrotum away from the urethral opening (Fig. 14-35, *F*).

8. A urinary catheter is inserted, and the wound covered with a nonadherent dressing.

PENILE IMPLANT

A penile prosthesis is implanted for treatment of organic sexual impotence. Sexual impotence may be caused by (1) diabetes mellitus, (2) priapism, (3) Peyronie's disease, (4) penile trauma, (5) pelvis surgery, (6) neurologic disease (in selected cases), (7) vascular disease, (8) hypertension, and (9) idiopathic impotence (in carefully screened patients). The penile implant serves as a stent to enable vaginal penetration for sexual intercourse.

Procedural considerations

Spinal or general anesthesia is required. The patient is placed in either the supine or lithotomy position. Routine skin prepping and draping are carried out. To prevent urethral injury and potential urinary retention, a no. 14 or 16 Fr Foley catheter may be inserted to identify the urethra intraoperatively. Electrosurgery may be required. Often, a penile block is instilled intraoperatively, prior to the incision, into the corpus cavernosa and the incisional sites. This enables the surgeon to evaluate erectile size and provides some postoperative pain management.

A separate sterile Mayo stand or small table covered with a plastic drape is generally set up for the implants. It is recommended that the implants not be in contact with paper or cloth, which may shed fiber particles.

The instrument setup includes a minor set with fine instruments, plus the following:

Hegar dilators
Penile prosthesis of urologist's choice (Fig. 14-36)
Furlow inserter (Fig. 14-37, A and B)
Closing tool (Fig. 14-37, C)
Denis-Browne or Lone-Star retractor (optional)
Assembly tool for clamping connectors (Fig. 14-38, A)
1% Lidocaine, 50 ml
Connectors of choice (Fig. 14-38, B)
Injectable 0.9% NS, 150 ml
Methylene blue, 1 ml
Papaverine, 2 ml
0.5% Bupivacaine (Marcaine) or 1% etidocaine (Duranest)
25% Hypaque (normal saline if patient allergic to dye)
Bacitracin, 50,000 U
Kanamycin, 80 mg

A serious complication to a penile implant is infection. Meticulous aseptic technique and careful draping are essential. The sterile team should be double gloved throughout the procedure. Some surgeons coat their hands with Betadine just before donning sterile gloves. A 5-minute Betadine scrub of the operative area is critical in reducing skin flora. The anus should be isolated in the perineal approach. Intraoperatively, and before insertion of the implant components, a prophylactic antibiotic irrigant of bacitracin and kanamycin in normal saline is used on the implants and in the insertion sites. Systemic antibiotics may also be required. As with any implant procedure, it is vital to main-

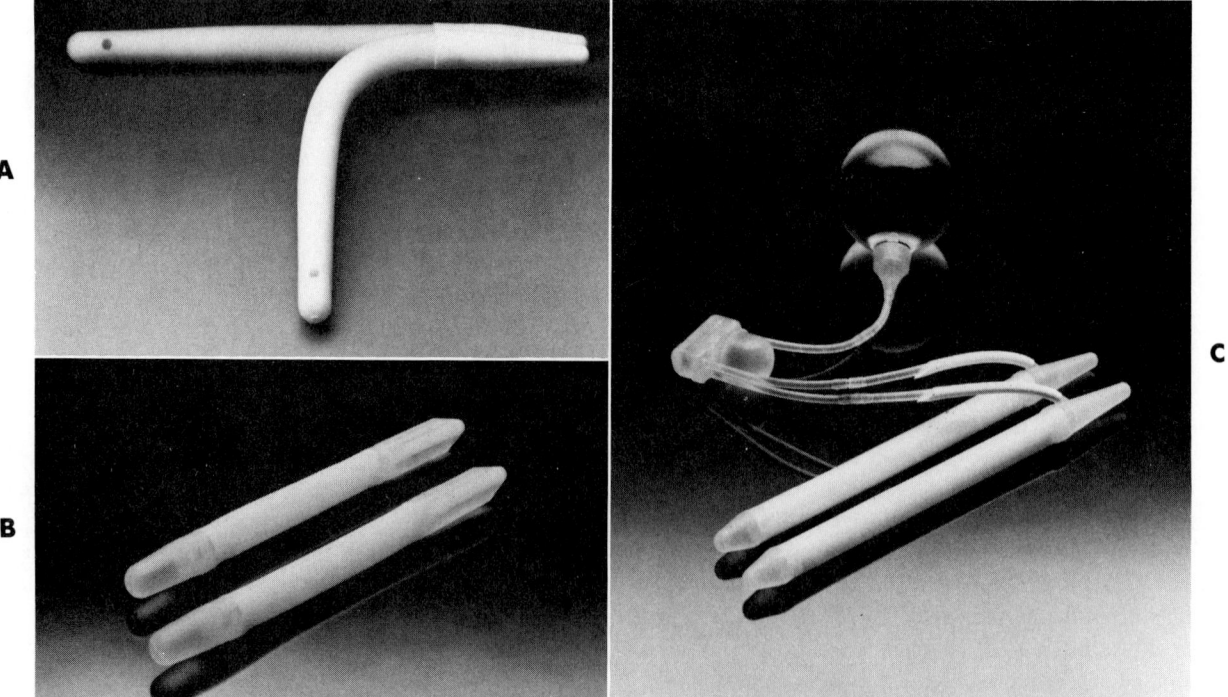

FIG. 14-36   **A,** AMS malleable 600 penile prosthesis. **B,** AMS Hydroflex penile prosthesis. **C,** AMS 700CX inflatable penile prosthesis.

Courtesy American Medical Systems, Minnetonka, Minn.

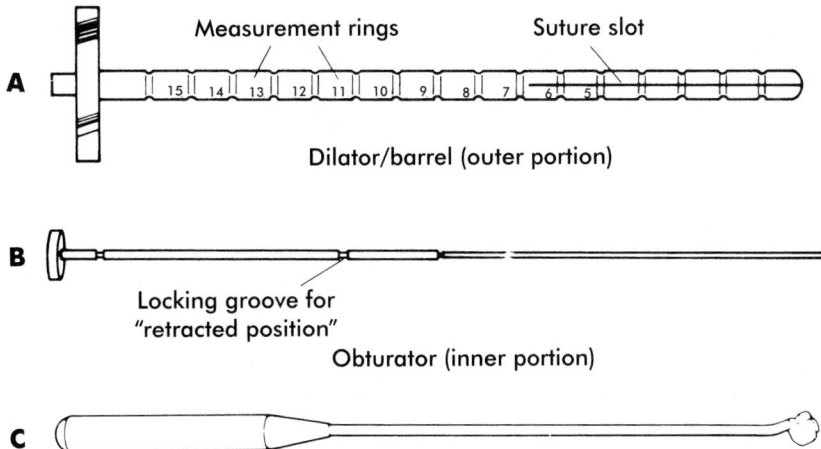

FIG. 14-37 Furlow insertion device. **A,** Dilator/barrel (outer portion). **B,** Obturator (inner portion). **C,** Closing tool.

Courtesy American Medical Systems, Minnetonka, Minn.

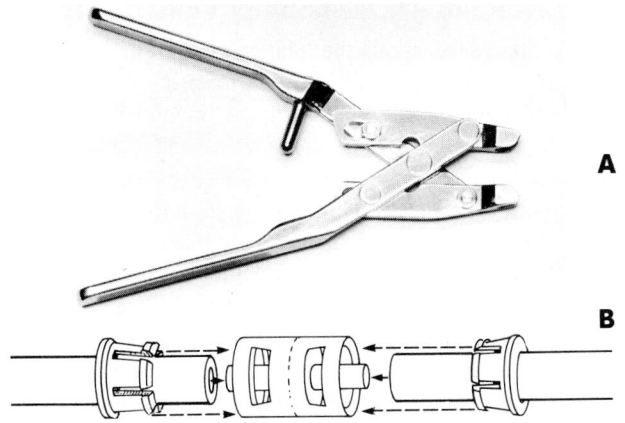

FIG. 14-38 **A,** Assembly tool. **B,** Quik-connectors.

Courtesy American Medical Systems, Minnetonka, MN.

tain an environment conducive to infection prevention. Traffic in and out of the room should be minimized.

Operative procedures
Implantation of non-inflatable (semi-rigid) prosthesis

1. A midline incision is made from the base of the penis into the scrotum for approximately 3 cm. Some surgeons may choose a suprapubic or dorsal penile approach.
2. The tunica albuginea is incised over the most proximal portion of the corpora in a longitudinal manner, and stay sutures are placed. The corpora are dilated proximally and distally with 7- to 11-mm Hegar dilators. Care must be taken not to perforate the urethra. Measurements of the entire corporal length are taken with the Furlow inserter.
3. Following placement of the closure sutures, the prosthe-

ses are inserted in the corpora. Proper placement is evident immediately by change in the configuration of the penis with no buckling of the glans. The tunica albuginea is then closed with the previously placed no. 2-0 absorbable continuous suture; no. 3-0 or 4-0 absorbable interrupted sutures are used for skin closure.

4. Petrolatum gauze or 2-inch Kling tube gauze may be used for the dressing.
5. A Foley catheter is inserted, and the amount and color of urine are noted. Some surgeons divert the urine intraoperatively.

Implantation of inflatable prosthesis

1. A midline incision is made from the base of the penis into the scrotum for approximately 3 cm (Fig. 14-39, *A*). A Foley catheter is inserted to identify and retract the urethra out of the operative field.
2. The tunica albuginea of each corpus is incised in the most proximal portion, and stay sutures are placed. The corpora are dilated distally and proximally with 7- to 11-mm Hegar dilators. The Furlow inserter is used for measuring the entire corporal length.
3. Corporal sutures of no. 2-0 absorbable material are placed along the tunica incision, left uncut with needle attached, and tagged.
4. The cylinders are packaged with attached traction sutures at the distal end. These are placed through the eye of a Keith needle and slid into the groove of the Furlow inserter. The Furlow inserter is slid up the corporal tunnel and the plunger pushed to release the Keith needle, which punctures the glans (Fig. 14-39, *B*). The needle is grasped with a heavy hemostat and pulled through the glans, allowing the cylinders to slide to the channel opening.
5. The Furlow inserter is removed and the cylinder is in-

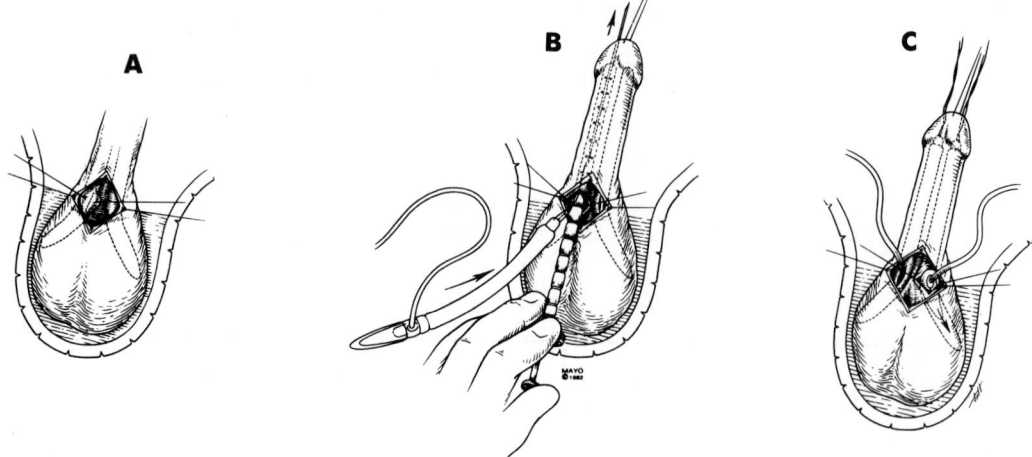

FIG. 14-39   Penoscrotal approach for inflatable penile implant.
From Droller, M.J. (1992). *Surgical management of urologic disease.* St. Louis: Mosby.

serted and guided to the proper position beneath the glans penis (Fig. 14-39, *C*). If necessary, rear tip extenders are added to the proximal cylinder end. The proximal end is positioned in the crus. The procedure is repeated on the other channel.

6. The external inguinal ring is palpated and a path bluntly created (Fig. 14-39, *D*).

7. Dissecting scissors are used to separate the transversalis fascia on the inguinal floor. The perivesical space is enlarged to allow palpation of Cooper's ligament. The reservoir is then positioned into the perivesical space.

8. The reservoir is filled with the appropriate amount of solution for its capacity (different sizes are available) and pulled against the floor of Hesselbach's triangle.

9. The pump is then placed in the most dependent portion of the scrotum. It is generally positioned on the patient's dominant side. The space is created by blunt dissection lateral to the testicle (Fig. 14-39, *E*). The tunica of the scrotum is closed over the pump with a running stitch of no. 3-0 absorbable suture.

10. The rods and reservoir tubings are connected to the pump with the connectors of choice, using the assembly tool to clamp them in place, and tested for inflation and deflation (Fig. 14-39, *F*).

11. The prosthetic device is left in a partially inflated position to reduce bleeding and promote healing (Fig. 14-40). The Foley catheter is left in place during the immediate postoperative period.

12. The incision is closed in a subcuticular fashion with no. 4-0 absorbable suture and a dressing applied (Fig. 14-39, *G*). The penis is positioned flush with the lower abdomen for patient comfort. Mesh pants are useful as a nonadherent support dressing.

DEEP DORSAL AND EMISSARY VEIN LIGATION

This procedure entails the ligation and/or elimination of the penile deep dorsal vein and its tributaries. It is a treatment undertaken for vascular-related impotence. Care is taken to avoid damage to the arteries and nerves lying alongside the deep dorsal vein.

A common cause of erectile dysfunction in patients with organic impotence is vascular compromise. Before surgical intervention is undertaken, a definitive diagnosis of a corporal leak is made through dynamic infusion cavernosometry and cavernosography. Diagnostic results may indicate failure-to-store or failure-to-fill impotence. Patients with vascular compromise in a given anatomic region tend be compromised elsewhere as well. Many are diabetic or hypertensive. Because of this, the perioperative nurse must exercise great care in positioning the patient to prevent further damage to the patient's altered tissue perfusion.

Procedural considerations

In addition to a standard herniorrhaphy setup (see Chapter 12), the perioperative nurse needs to have the following supplies and equipment available for the procedure:

Denis-Browne or Lone Star retractor	Angled vascular scissors, 5 inch
Right-angle retractors	Debakey forceps
Short, narrow Deaver retractors	Bipolar coagulator with microtip
Gemini clamps	Kittner dissectors
Delicate, curved mosquito hemostats	Doppler probe and unit (probe must be sterile)
Schnidt hemostats	
Blunt delicate dissecting scissors	4-0 absorbable suture on a microvascular needle
Sharp delicate dissecting scissors	

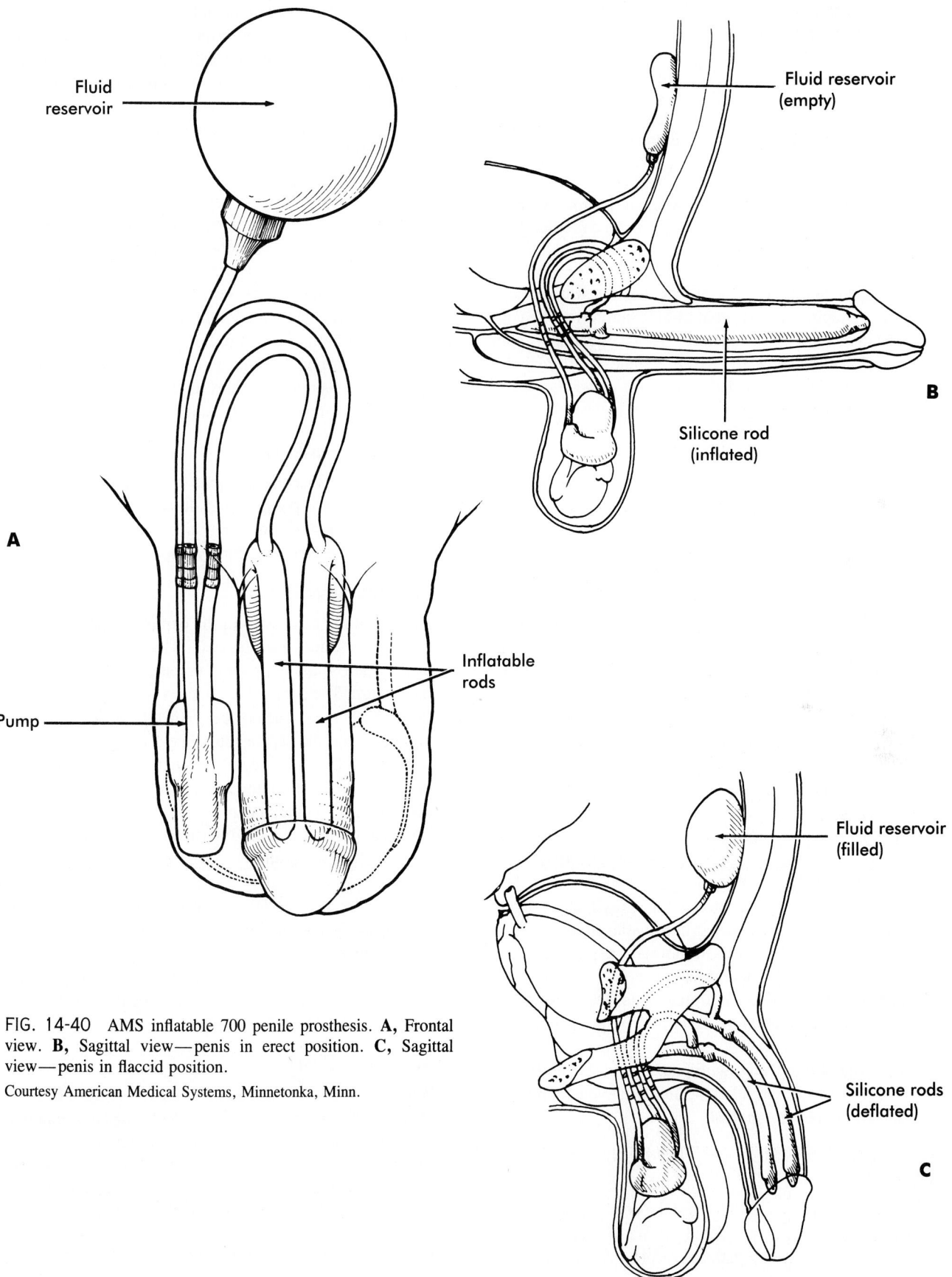

FIG. 14-40 AMS inflatable 700 penile prosthesis. **A,** Frontal view. **B,** Sagittal view—penis in erect position. **C,** Sagittal view—penis in flaccid position.

Courtesy American Medical Systems, Minnetonka, Minn.

3-0 absorbable suture
   on a T-16 or TB-1
   needle
Vascular ties
Papaverine
Prostaglandin
Methylene blue
1% Lidocaine
0.9% Normal saline
0.5% Bupivacaine
   (Marcaine) or 1%
   etidocaine (Duranest)

Thrombin, topical
Doppler gel, sterile
   packet
No. 16, 5-ml balloon
   Foley catheter and
   attached drainage bag
Butterfly needle, 21
   gauge, and 60-ml
   syringe
Medium Penrose drain
Hypodermic needle, 27
   gauge

The patient is placed in the supine position with the legs separated. Draping is carried out as for a herniorrhaphy with the genitalia exposed. The operative area is squared off with five towels, one under the scrotum, and the remainder placed at the iliac crests, umbilicus, and under the penis. The Foley catheter is inserted before the incision is made.

Operative procedure

1. An infrapubic incision is made at the base of the penis and deepened until the neurovascular bundle is identified.
2. The penis is degloved, and dissection is carried out toward the glans penis through Colles' fascia and Buck's fascia to the deep dorsal vein.
3. The deep dorsal vein is separated from the surrounding tissue and ligated at the suspensory level and at the glans penis. It is then excised from the corporal base, extending from the distal to the proximal ligatures.
4. The cavernous and crural veins are suture ligated.
5. All circumflex and emissary branches are ligated or coagulated.
6. The suspensory ligament is detached, and the entire deep and accessory dorsal vein is removed.
7. Hemostasis is established, and the suspensory ligaments are reattached with no. 2-0 nonabsorbable suture in an interrupted figure-of-eight pattern. The fascial layers are approximated and closed in an interrupted fashion with no. 4-0 absorbable suture.
8. The penis is returned to its normal position, and the closure is carried out in three layers.
9. Bupivacaine (Marcaine) or etidocaine (Duranest) is injected during wound closure to afford a more comfortable recovery period.
10. The wound is covered with gauze sponges. Fluffs are placed over the scrotal area, and an athletic supporter or mesh pants are applied.

REVASCULARIZATION OF THE PENILE ARTERIES

The relationship of focal arterial occlusive disease to sexual dysfunction has prompted efforts to rectify the resulting impotence. Investigational reconstructive surgery is taking place in patients who demonstrate correctable vascular disease in the large arteries. The most widely attempted repairs are end-to-end and end-to-side microscopic anastomosis of the distal inferior epigastric artery to the proximal deep dorsal artery near the pubic level, below the rectus muscle and Buck's fascia. Paramedian and infrapubic incisions are made, and the arteries freed and tunneled. This procedure requires both a urologist and a vascular surgeon. Currently the success rate is about 60%.

BLADDER EXSTROPHY REPAIR

Bladder exstrophy repair corrects a more severe form of epispadias, in which the anterior bladder wall as well as the roof of the urethra are absent. Bladder exstrophy is always accompanied by wide separation of the rectus muscles of the lower abdominal wall and by diastasis of the pubic bone with anterior displacement of the anus. Repair of bladder exstrophy requires an adequate size bladder for ultimate continence to be achieved. It is preferable to perform this procedure in the neonatal period.

Procedural considerations

The infant is placed in a supine position, and the abdomen and thighs are prepped and draped. (See Chapter 28 for a full discussion of considerations for pediatric patients.) Instruments are as required for hypospadias repair.

Operative procedure

1. An incision is made around the exposed bladder medial to the paravesical neck mucosa. The incision is carried distally across the epispadiac urethra distal to the verumontanum. The paravesical mucosa is preserved for urethral lengthening. The bladder is then freed from the rectus fascia and the peritoneum. The dorsal chordea is released, and the mobilized paravesical mucosa is apposed in the midline and sutured to the proximal urethra just distal to the verumontanum.
2. The bladder wall is closed vertically in two layers with no. 3-0 absorbable sutures; a suprapubic tube is inserted for drainage.
3. The bladder neck is loosely reconstructed by approximating the interpubic ligament, which extends between the proximal end of the phallus and the pubic bone.
4. The symphysis pubis is approximated with a heavy no. 2 nonabsorbable suture. During this step the assistant rotates the iliac bones anteriorly.

ILIAC OSTEOTOMY

When closure of the bladder exstrophy is delayed beyond the neonatal period, bilateral iliac osteotomies are required to bring the symphysis pubis together in the midline. A vesical neck plasty is performed at a later date with bilateral ureteral reimplantation. The penis may be closed before, during, or some time after the vesical neck plasty.

Procedural considerations

The infant is placed in the prone position with a folded towel under the pelvis.

Operative procedure

A vertical incision is made 0.5 cm lateral to the sacro-iliac joints. The iliac bone is exposed, and osteotomy is performed through both tables to bring the pubic bones together in the midline after reconstruction of the bladder.

SURGERY OF THE SCROTUM AND TESTICLES

HYDROCELECTOMY

A hydrocele is an abnormal accumulation of fluid within the scrotum. The fluid is contained within the tunica vaginalis. Excessive secretion or accumulation of hydrocele fluid may be the result of infection or trauma. A hydrocelectomy is the excision of the tunica vaginalis of the testis to remove the enlarged, fluid-filled sac.

Procedural considerations

The patient is placed in the supine position. Preparation and draping of the patient include routine cleansing of the external genitals and draping of the patient with a fenestrated sheet. A minor instrument set is required, plus a small drain, a 30-ml syringe with a 20-gauge, 2-inch aspirating needle, and a suspensory dressing.

Operative procedure

1. An anterolateral incision is made in the skin of the scrotum over the hydrocele mass by a scalpel with a no. 10 or 15 blade (Fig. 14-41, *A*). Bleeding is controlled with fine-tipped hemostats, and vessels are ligated with no. 3-0 absorbable ligatures.
2. Small retractors may be placed, after which the fascial layers are incised to expose the tunica vaginalis (Fig. 14-41, *B*). With fine scissors, forceps, and blunt dissection the hydrocele is dissected free and delivered (Fig. 14-41, *C*). The sac is opened, and the fluid contents are aspirated.
3. The sac is inverted so that it surrounds the testis, epididymis, and distal cord. Excess tunica vaginalis is excised, and the edges of the remaining tunica are sutured

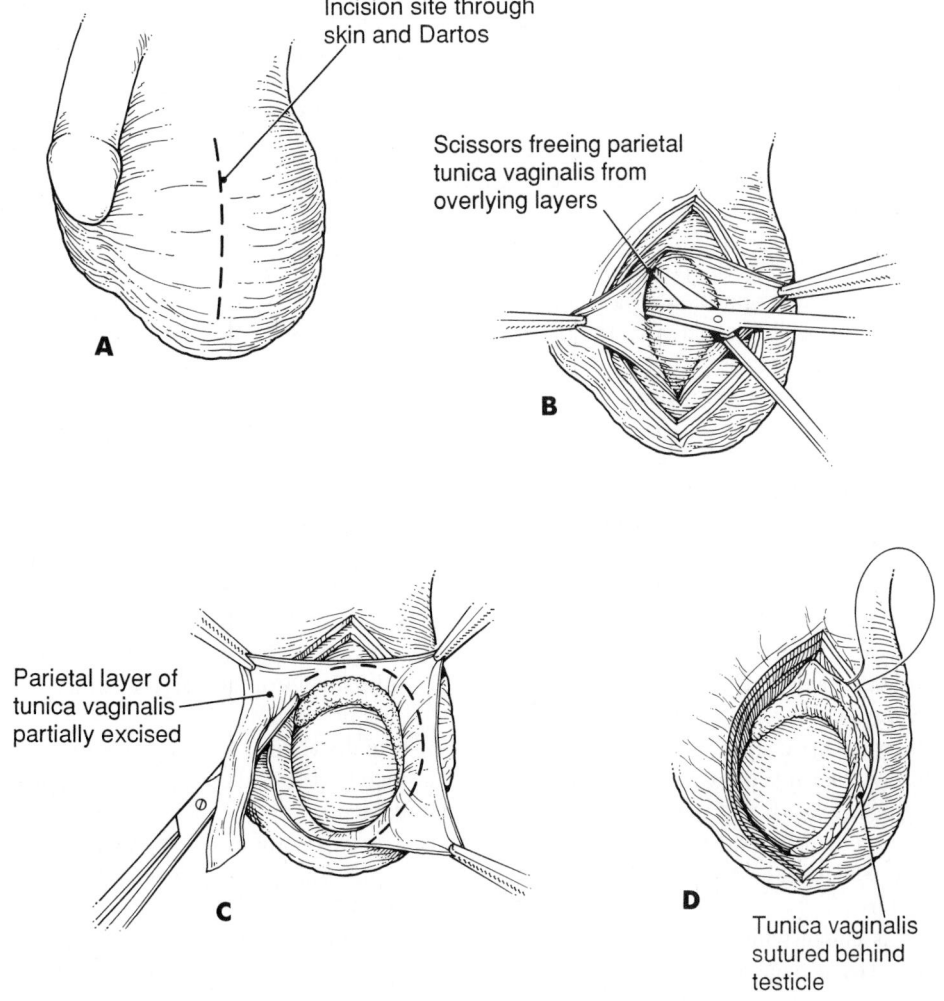

FIG. 14-41 Hydrocelectomy.
Modified from Droller, M.J. (1992). *Surgical management of urologic disease*. St. Louis: Mosby.

with a continuous no. 4-0 absorbable suture behind the testicle (Fig. 14-41, *D*). The testicle is "bottled" by the inverted tunica vaginalis, and the testis may then be returned to the sac.

4. A drain is placed within the scrotum and brought out through a stab wound in the most dependent portion of the scrotum. The scrotal incision is closed in layers with no. 3-0 and no. 4-0 absorbable sutures. A fluff compression dressing contained in a scrotal support (suspensory) aids in reducing postoperative scrotal edema.

VASECTOMY

A vasectomy is the excision of a section of the vas deferens. The operation may be performed selectively as a permanent method of sterilization and also before prostatectomy to prevent possible postoperative epididymitis. Because of the serious implications of permanent sterilization, particular attention must be paid to acquiring informed consent. Recent studies have raised the question of a correlation between prostate cancer and vasectomy; definitive causal relationships have not been established.

The patient having elective sterilization for birth control is encouraged to return to the office setting for sperm count analysis. Generally two successive negative counts are sufficient to indicate sterility has been achieved. Elective vasectomies are seen far less often in the operating room as more surgeons perform the procedure in the office setting.

Procedural considerations

The patient usually lies in the supine position, although the patient can be in the lithotomy position if vasectomy is performed prior to transurethral prostatectomy. The patient is given regional anesthesia for this procedure. A minor instrument set and scrotal suspensory are needed.

Operative procedure

1. The vas is located by digital palpation of the upper part of the scrotum. A small incision is made in the skin over the vas.
2. An Allis forceps, vas clamp, or small towel clamp is inserted into the scrotal incision to grasp the vas and deliver it to the surface of the wound. The vas is denuded of surrounding tissues, and straight hemostats are placed on either side of the Allis forceps to crush the vas.
3. The vas is cut between the clamps, and a section is removed. The cut ends are ligated with no. 2-0 absorbable ties or electrocoagulated, and the severed ends of the vas are allowed to return to the scrotum. Some surgeons bury the vasal ends in the perivasal sheath or seal them with hemoclips.
4. The skin incision is closed with no. 4-0 absorbable interrupted sutures. The patient is instructed to wear a scrotal support of the appropriate size for approximately 3 to 4 days.

VASOVASOSTOMY

Vasovasostomy is the surgical reanastomosis of the vas deferens, utilizing the operative microscope. The number of vasal reanastomosis procedures has increased dramatically. One complication of vasectomy is chronic testicular pain. Reanastomosis may often alleviate this condition. Additionally, a significant number of men who have had a vasectomy want to regain their fertility. A precise reconnection can be performed with the use of a microscope and a modified two-layer anastomosis. Success rates vary from 40% to 70%. When there are not two viable segments of vas deferens, a similar procedure, the epididymovasostomy, may be performed. This involves anastomosis of vas deferens to a segment of the epididymis.

Procedural considerations

A minor instrument set is required, with the addition of selected microsurgical instruments and sutures:

Castroviejo needle holders	10-0 monofilament non-absorbable suture on a microsurgery needle
Westcott scissors, sharp and blunt	Zoom microscope with foot pedals for focus, magnification, and position
2 Straight Bishop-Harmon forceps	
2 Straight tying forceps	
Jeweler's forceps	Bipolar coagulator with micropoint
Lacrimal probes, 000-0	
Vasectomy clamps	Blunt irrigating needle, 27 gauge
Microbulldogs	
8-0 or 9-0 monofilament nonabsorbable suture	Bulb syringe

Operative procedure

1. After the vas deferens has been located by external manipulation, a vertical scrotal incision is made.
2. The testicle, epididymis, and vas are displaced from the scrotum.
3. The vasectomy site is identified and the scarred area excised.
4. The proximal end of the vas deferens is cut back until fluid is expressed.
5. Fluid is collected on a glass slide and examined for the presence of live sperm. Surgery continues even if results for sperm are negative unless an epididymal obstruction exists.
6. The distal end of the vas is resected until a normal lumen is visible. The distal and proximal lumina are then dilated.
7. The two portions of the vas are placed in an approximator clip with background material placed underneath.
8. Six stitches of no. 10-0 nonabsorbable microsuture are placed in the inner layer. The proximal end is sutured through the serosa to the mucosa, and the distal end through the mucosa to the serosa.

9. A second layer of eight to 10 stitches of no. 9-0 nonabsorbable suture is placed without penetrating the lumen of the vas.
10. The incision is closed in two layers with interrupted no. 3-0 and 4-0 absorbable sutures.
11. Gauze sponges and a suspensory support are placed on the patient to provide a pressure dressing.
12. Postoperative precautions include no lifting or ejaculation for a minimum of 2 weeks. The sperm count and viability of sperm are rechecked at 3- and 6-month intervals.

EPIDIDYMECTOMY

An epididymectomy is the excision of the epididymis from the testis. Epididymectomy is rarely performed today but may be indicated to treat degenerative cystic disease or infection of the epididymis.

Procedural considerations

The patient is placed in the supine position with the legs slightly abducted. A general, spinal, or regional anesthetic is required. Setup is as described for hydrocelectomy, plus an electrosurgical unit, if desired.

Operative procedure

1. An anterolateral incision is made over the testis in the scrotum to expose the tunica vaginalis.
2. The tunica is incised to expose the testis and overlying epididymis.
3. An incision is made along the superior head of the epididymis, which is then sharply dissected from the testis. A portion of the vas deferens may also be excised.
4. Bleeding is controlled by electrocoagulation and absorbable ties. The skin wound is closed with no. 4-0 absorbable sutures. A small drain may be left intrascrotally for 24 to 48 hours.

SPERMATOCELECTOMY

Spermatocelectomy is removal of a spermatocele, a lobulated intrascrotal cystic mass attached to the superior head of the epididymis. It is usually caused by an obstruction of the tubular system that conveys the sperm. This is a not infrequent complication following vasectomy that does not exhibit itself immediately.

Procedural considerations

The setup for a spermatocelectomy is as described for a hydrocelectomy, plus a microscope and slides, if desired.

Operative procedure

1. The mass is approached through a scrotal incision as described for hydrocelectomy (see Fig. 14-41).
2. The structures of the testis and spermatic cord are identified, and the cystic structure is dissected free. Bleeding is controlled with electrocoagulation.

3. The wound is closed and dressed as described for hydrocelectomy.

VARICOCELECTOMY

A varicocelectomy is the high ligation of the gonadal veins of the testes. Varicocelectomy is done to reduce venous backflow of blood into the venous plexus around the testes and to improve spermatogenesis. When surgery for this condition was originally devised, the veins of the pampiniform plexus were ligated and divided individually.

This condition occurs more frequently on the left side because the gonadal vein of the left testis units retroperitoneally with the renal vein at a 90-degree angle and is consequently under greater back-pressure. As a result of this unusual back-pressure, the pampiniform plexus of the spermatic cord becomes tortuous and engorged, resembling a bag of worms.

A variation of the standard inguinal or scrotal approaches has recently appeared on the surgical scene—the laparoscopic varicocelectomy. Often this procedure may be combined with a laparoscopic herniorrhaphy.

Procedural considerations

The setup for inguinal varicocelectomy is as described for an inguinal hernia repair (see Chapter 12). The setup for laparoscopic varicocelectomy is as for a laparoscopic hernia repair (see Chapter 12) with the exclusion of the mesh implant.

Operative procedures
Inguinal approach

1. The incision may be through a suprainguinal approach or an oblique inguinal approach over the external inguinal ring. The structures of the spermatic cord are identified, and the vessels are dissected free from the vas deferens (Fig. 14-42, *A* and *B*).
2. The abnormal dilated veins in the inguinal canal are clamped and ligated (Fig. 14-42, *C*). The redundant portions are excised.
3. A drain may be placed. The incision is closed in layers.

Laparoscopic approach

1. Intrabdominal instillation of CO_2 through an umbilical incision and the Veress needle is accomplished.
2. The procedure is performed through primary 10- 11-mm umbilical and suprapubic ports and a 5-mm ipsilateral port.
3. The peritoneum is entered lateral to the spermatic cord and incised in a T configuration across the cord.
4. The spermatic cord is elevated and its major components separated with blunt dissection following identification of the spermatic artery.
   NOTE: Irrigation of the area with papaverine mixed with 0.9% injectable saline will cause the artery to pulsate and make identification easier.

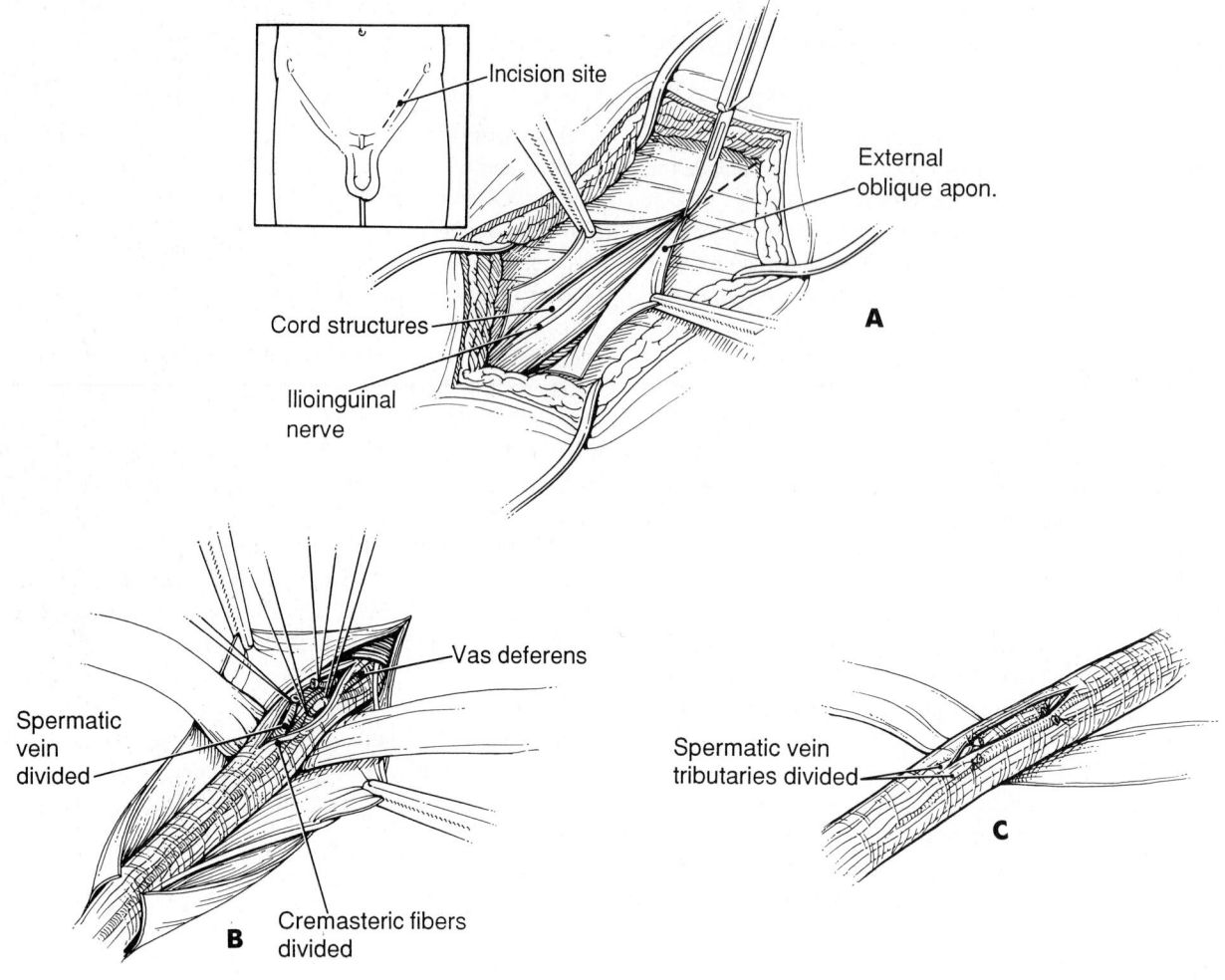

FIG. 14-42   Varicocelectomy.
Modified from Droller, M.J. (1992). *Surgical management of urologic disease*. St. Louis: Mosby.

5. The involved veins are ligated with small and medium vascular endoclips.
6. The incisions are closed and dressed as for other laparoscopic procedures with Steri-Strips, Telfa, and Tegaderm.

TESTICULAR BIOPSY

A biopsy of the testicle involves a wedge excision of suspicious tissue for diagnostic confirmation. There are two primary indications for a testicular biopsy. Men suffering from infertility, who are azospermatic or oligospermatic, with normal or minimally elevated follicle-stimulating hormone, may be evaluated through this means. Children with leukemia may also be evaluated to determine testicular relapse following chemotherapy. Although controversial, if a surgeon is prepared to proceed with an orchiectomy, he or she may choose to first take a biopsy specimen and evaluate a testicular lesion with a frozen section microscopic exam. This occurs in a circumstance where a suspicion of carcinoma is questionable and the patient refuses an orchi-

ectomy without diagnostic confirmation. In some situations a needle biopsy of the testicle has been adequate and appropriate.

Procedural considerations

If required, hair may be removed from the scrotum, which is then aseptically cleansed. General, regional, or spinal anesthesia may be selected. A minor instrument set is used. Special fixatives, such as Bouin's or Zenker's solution, must be available. Formalin destroys the germinal epithelium and should not be used.

Operative procedure

1. The scrotum is held firmly on its posterior aspect. This causes the skin on the anterior aspect to stretch tightly over the incisional site, forcing the epididymis to remain posterior and allowing the scrotal skin to part without retraction.
2. A 1- to 2-cm vertical incision is made, with care taken to avoid injury to the epididymis.

3. The incision is continued to the tunica vaginalis. As the tunica is incised, there should be a normal efflux of clear fluid.

4. Absorbable no. 4-0 stay sutures are placed in the tunica vaginalis. Two more are placed in the tunica albuginea.

5. A small ellipse of tunica with its tubules is resected with a scalpel in a shaving action, with no-touch technique.

6. The specimen is placed in the fixative and the wound closed in three layers with no. 3-0 and no. 4-0 absorbable suture.

7. Gauze sponges and fluffed dressings are placed over and around the scrotum. A suspensory support is applied to provide pressure and support.

ORCHITECTOMY

An orchitectomy is the removal of the testis or testes. Removal of both testes is castration and renders the patient sterile and deficient of the hormone testosterone, which is responsible for development of secondary sexual characteristics and potency. This operation, like vasectomy, has legal implications that require attention to acquiring informed consent for surgery. Bilateral orchiectomy is usually performed to control symptomatic metastatic carcinoma of the prostate gland. A unilateral orchiectomy is indicated because of testicular cancer, trauma, or infection. In many situations a prosthesis may be implanted for cosmetic or psychological reasons. Prostheses are usually made of silicone and molded to approximate normal testicular consistency.

Procedural considerations

The patient is placed in the supine position and draped according to established procedure. A minor instrument setup is required, plus a testicular prosthesis, if specified.

Operative procedure

1a. For *benign conditions* the incision is made over the anterolateral surface of the midportion of the scrotum. The skin incision is carried through the subcutaneous and fascial layers through the tunica vaginalis, exposing the testicle. Retractors are placed, and bleeding vessels are clamped and tied. The spermatic cord is divided into two or three vascular bundles. Each vascular bundle is doubly clamped, cut, and ligated, first with no. 0 absorbable suture ligature and then with a proximal free no. 0 absorbable tie. The vas is separately ligated with a no. 0 absorbable tie. The testis is removed.

This procedure has recently been approached through laparoscopic techniques, usually in conjunction with laparoscopic herniorrhaphy.

1b. For *malignant conditions* the incision is begun just above the internal ring, extending downward and inward over the inguinal canal to the external inguinal ring. The inguinal canal is exposed, and the spermatic cord is dissected free, cross-clamped, and divided into vascular bundles at the internal ring. Gentle forward traction is applied to the cord, which is dissected from its bed. The testis is everted into the wound from the scrotum and excised.

2. Bleeding is controlled with electrocoagulation. A small drain may be placed in the empty hemiscrotum if desired. The external oblique fascia is reapproximated with no. 2-0 absorbable interrupted sutures. Subcutaneous tissue, including Scarpa's fascia, is closed with no. 4-0 absorbable sutures. The skin is reapproximated with surgical staples or no. 4-0 subcuticular suture.

RADICAL LYMPHADENECTOMY (RETROPERITONEAL LYMPH NODE DISSECTION)

Radical lymphadenectomy is a bilateral resection of retroperitoneal lymph nodes. Dissection usually includes lymph nodes, channels, and fat around both renal pedicles, the vena cava, and the aorta, including the bifurcation of the aorta. Lymph node dissection is performed for treatment of nonseminomatous testicular tumors. The procedure is performed after radical inguinal orchiectomy.

Procedural considerations

The patient is placed in the supine position. If the dissection is unilateral, the patient is supine with the operative side tilted upward. Routine skin preparation from nipples to midthigh and draping procedures are carried out. Long fine dissection instruments along with basic laparotomy instruments are required.

Operative procedure

1. A midline abdominal incision is made from the xiphoid process to the symphysis pubis. The abdominal contents are explored to determine the degree of gross nodal involvement. The colon is either packed within the abdominal cavity or mobilized and kept moist outside the abdomen.

2. The posterior peritoneum is opened between the aorta and the vena cava.

3. By blunt and sharp dissection, the lymphatic structures and fat are removed en bloc from around both renal pedicles, the vena cava, and the aorta from above the renal hilum to beyond the bifurcation of the iliac vessels on the side of the original testicular neoplasm.

4. The spermatic vessels of the affected side are removed down to and including the stump of the previous orchiectomy.

5. The inferior mesenteric artery may be sacrificed if technically necessary, but the superior mesenteric artery is not disturbed. The ureter on the affected side is skeletonized to remove any perilymphatic tissue.

6. If reperitonealization is desired, the posterior peritoneum is closed with a no. 2-0 absorbable continuous suture. The viscera are repositioned into the abdominal cavity, and the wound is closed, usually without placement of a drain.

ORCHIOPEXY

An orchiopexy (orchidopexy) is the surgical placement and fixation of the testicle in a normal anatomic position in the scrotal sac. If the testis fails to descend into the scrotum during gestation, then it is considered undescended. An undescended testis becomes arrested somewhere along its normal path of descent. If it is palpable in a position other than its normal path of descent, its position is considered to be ectopic.

A retractile testis has fully descended into the scrotum but retracts out of the scrotum as a result of contraction of the cremaster muscle. Gentle manipulation allows replacement of the testis in the most dependent portion of the scrotum. Retractile testes require no surgical or hormonal treatment.

All testes that are undescended after 1 year, including those which are unresponsive to hormone injections, require surgical placement in the scrotum for optimum maturation.

Procedural considerations

The setup is as described for hydrocelectomy. General anesthesia is required. Preparation and draping include the lower abdomen, genitals, and thighs. Because this operation is usually performed on children, a setup containing small, delicate instruments and sutures is required.

Operative procedure

1. An inguinal incision is generally employed for exploration of undescended testes (Fig. 14-43, *A*). Most undescended testes are located in the superficial inguinal pouch or inguinal canal.

2. The external oblique aponeurosis is opened through the external inguinal ring, exposing the inguinal canal; the gubernacular attachments of the undescended testis are dissected free as high as the internal inguinal ring or into the abdominal cavity (Fig. 14-43, *B* and *C*).

3. All adhesions and the associated inguinal hernial sac are freed to lengthen the cord, allowing the testis to reach the scrotal cavity. The hernia sac is transsected, twisted, and ligated with sutures (Fig. 14-43, *D* and *E*).

4. To draw vessels into the inguinal canal, more proximal to the scrotum, the floor of the inguinal canal may have to be divided at the internal ring (Fig. 14-43, *F* and *G*).

5. The lateral portion of the internal ring is closed to prevent herniation. A scrotal pocket is created, and the testis is anchored in a normal anatomic position within the scrotum with absorbable sutures (Fig. 14-43, *H*).

NOTE: Orchiopexy may be accomplished by several surgical methods. The dependent portion of the undescended testis may be sutured to the base of the scrotum with absorbable or nonabsorbable sutures brought out through the scrotal wall and tied over a peanut dissector or pledget. The most popular method is to anchor the testis into a dissected subdartos pouch. In this procedure a small midtransverse scrotal incision is made, and space between the skin and the dartos muscle is dissected. The testis is then brought through a small hole in the dartos into the subdartos pouch and anchored in position by the traction suture. The overly-

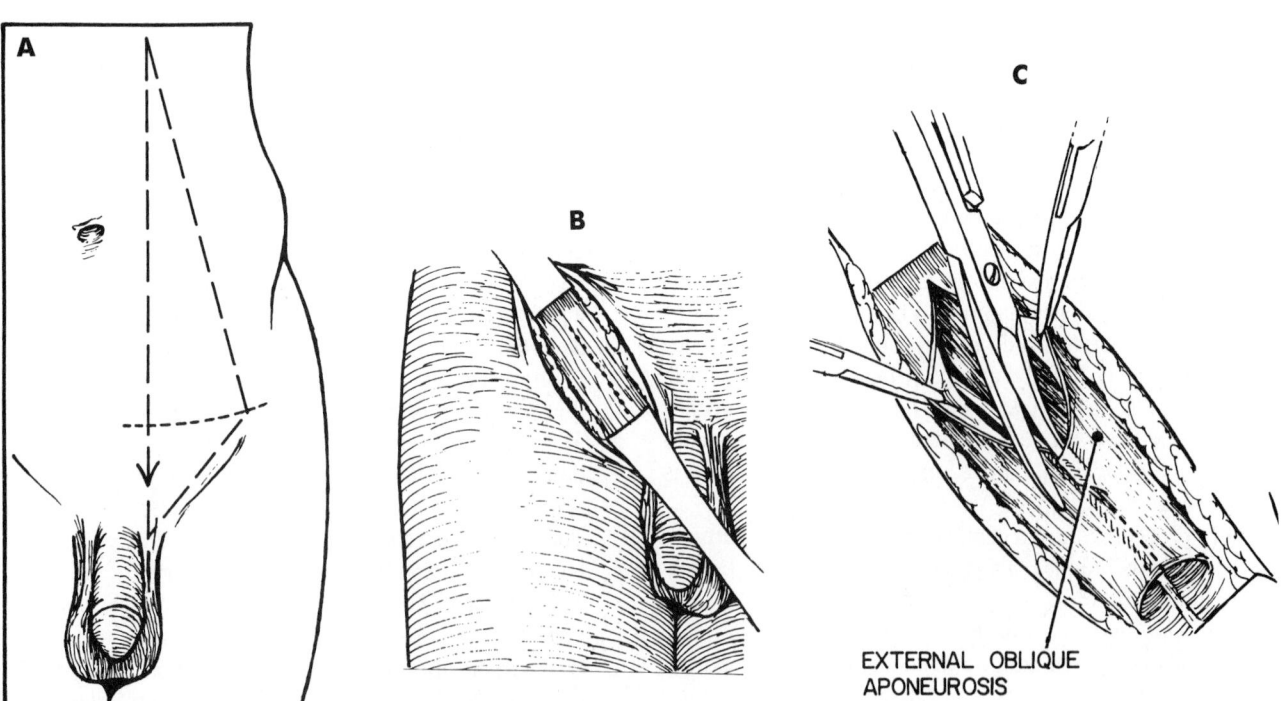

EXTERNAL OBLIQUE
APONEUROSIS

FIG. 14-43   Orchiopexy.
Modified from Culp, D.A., et al. (1985). *Surgical urology* (5th Ed.). Chicago: Year Book Medical Publishers.

ing skin of the subdartos pouch is closed with fine absorbable suture material. The inguinal incision is repaired in layers with no. 3-0 absorbable sutures. The skin is closed with a subcuticular suture; Steri-Strips are used for dressing.

TESTICULAR DETORSION

Torsion of the testicle, spermatic cord, appendix testis, or testis epididymis may be extravaginal or intravaginal in presentation. Intravaginal torsion is generally due to the absence of the usual attachment of the posterior aspect of the testes to the scrotal wall. In this instance the tunica covers the epididymis and testis. Twisting of the vascular pedicle can result, causing extreme pain. It is more commonly found in pubescent boys and young adults.

Procedural considerations

These patients generally present on an emergency basis. Surgery must occur as soon as possible to prevent death of the affected testicle. Emotional support is important, since the patient may fear loss of sexuality and disturbances in body image. Instrumentation required includes a setup as described for hydrocelectomy.

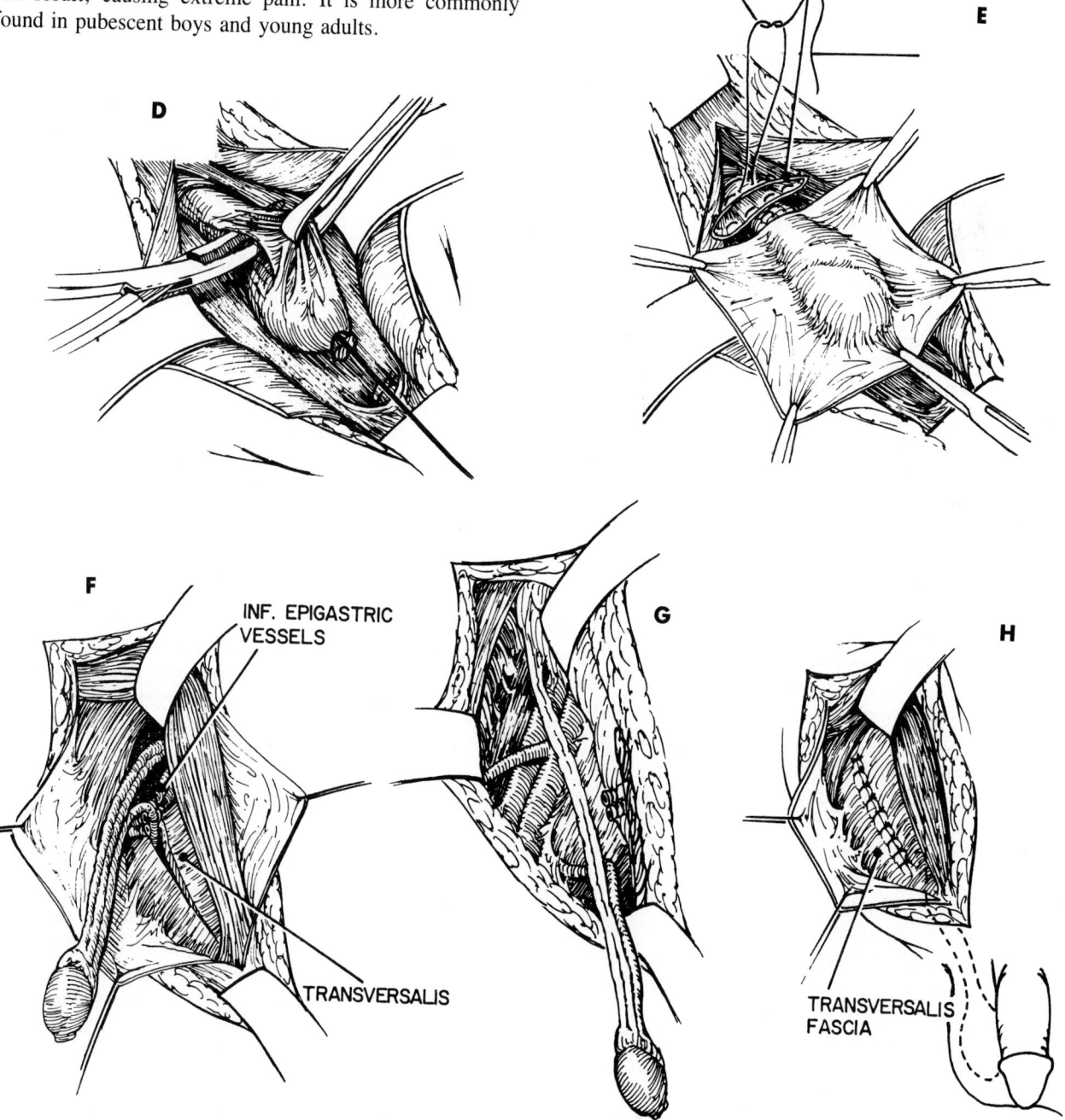

FIG. 14-43, CONT'D   Orchiopexy.

Operative procedure

1. A scrotal incision is made through the tunica vaginalis, and the spermatic cord is untwisted.
2. If normal color returns to the testis, it is anchored with three nonabsorbable sutures through the tunica to the scrotal wall or median septum.
3. The contralateral scrotal compartment is usually opened and the other testicle and spermatic cord examined. To prevent a future torsion on the unaffected side, the testis is often anchored to its surrounding structures.
4. Closure may be done in two or three layers with no. 3-0 and no. 4-0 absorbable interrupted sutures.
5. A support dressing of gauze sponges, fluffs, and a scrotal supporter is applied.

SURGERY OF THE PROSTATE GLAND

Glandular hyperplasia of the prostatic urethra usually manifests itself after the age of 50. Prostatic enlargement may occur in one or more lobes of the prostate but most frequently occurs in the lateral or median lobes. Progressive growth of the hyperplastic gland compresses the remaining normal prostatic tissue, forming what is called a *surgical capsule*. The growth of adenomatous tissue slowly encroaches on the prostatic urethral lumen, causing obstruction of urinary outflow.

Prostatic enlargement may be benign or malignant. In benign prostatic hypertrophy only the periurethral adenomatous portion of the gland is removed. Operable prostatic malignancy requires radical prostatectomy, which includes removal of the entire prostate gland and the seminal vesicles.

A blood sample is drawn to determine the prostatic specific antigen level (PSA), followed by a digital rectal exam. The blood is often drawn first, since manipulation of the gland has been known to alter the efficacy of the PSA test. The PSA test is considered a most valuable tool available for early detection of carcinoma of the prostate. If this test is elevated, the patient is at risk for carcinoma of the prostate. Clinical evaluation and an elevated PSA may indicate the need for a transrectal ultrasound needle biopsy or Franzen transrectal aspiration biopsy to confirm the diagnosis. When the results of the biopsy are positive for malignancy, a bone scan and skeletal survey are necessary to rule out metastasis. An older blood study, which is still being used, is the prostatic acid phosphatase level (PAP). When elevated, it usually indicates that tumor extension beyond the prostatic capsule has occurred. The possibility of hemolytic anemia, Gaucher's disease, or Paget's disease of the bone should be evaluated if diagnostic measures are negative for carcinoma.

Three open surgical approaches are possible in removing the benign hyperplastic obstructive prostate gland: retropubic prostatectomy, suprapubic prostatectomy, and perineal prostatectomy. Of these, the one most commonly employed is the suprapubic prostatectomy. All open prostatectomies hold a risk of loss of sexual potency.

Transurethral prostatectomy (TURP) is an endoscopic (closed) surgical approach that may be performed on some patients. Alternative modalities that have had some success in the treatment of benign prostatic hypertrophy (BPH) are the transurethral incision of the prostate (TUIP), transurethral laser incision of the prostate (TULIP), and the visual laser ablation of the prostate (VLAP). The TULIP and VLAP require the use of the Nd:YAG laser and specially designed fibers. Results seem to indicate a decrease in postoperative blood loss and a low recurrence rate of BPH.

If the prostate gland is cancerous, a radical retropubic or radical perineal prostatectomy, in conjunction with open or laparoscopic retroperitoneal lymph node dissection, is performed. Many patients desire to retain sexual function. The surgeon may attempt to save the neurovascular bundles in what is termed a *nerve sparing* approach. The site and size of the prostatic lesion, however, often determine if this can be achieved successfully and without undue risk to the patient.

Several factors must be taken into account to determine the best route for removal of the prostatic obstruction: the age and medical condition of the patient, the size of the gland and location of the pathologic condition, and the presence of associated medical disease.

PROSTATIC NEEDLE BIOPSY

Needle biopsy of the prostate is indicated for patients in whom prostatic cancer is clinically suspected. It may be accomplished transperineally or transrectally with a needle designed for this purpose.

Procedural considerations

Needle biopsy of the prostate has the risk of both intraoperative and postoperative bleeding. Although seldom needed, an electrosurgery unit should be available. A cystoscopic examination often accompanies a needle biopsy. More and more frequently, needle biopsies are being performed in the office or ultrasound department of the hospital.

Operative procedures
Core needle biopsy

Transrectal approach. The Tru-Cut or Vim-Silverman biopsy needle is inserted into the rectum along the volar aspect of the surgeon's index finger. The needle is advanced to abut the nodule. The obturator is removed, and the cutting blades are inserted or advanced. When the blades are in position, the outer sheath is advanced over them and twisted to receive a slender thread of prostate tissue. This technique is believed to be easier to accomplish than transperineal biopsy.

Transperineal approach. The examining finger is inserted in the rectum and the induration identified. The needle is inserted through the perineal skin and guided ahead until the tip abuts the lesion. The biopsy specimen is taken in the same fashion as described for the transrectal approach. Transperineal biopsy is thought to hold less risk of infection and postoperative bleeding. Some surgeons have incised the site with a no. 11 or 15 scalpel blade and placed a no. 4-0 absorbable closing suture.

Fine needle aspiration biopsy

A finger is inserted in the rectum and the nodule identified. The Franzen biopsy needle is inserted, with the index finger of the free hand guiding it into the rectum. A finger cot may be slipped over both the finger and the needle. A 22-gauge needle is passed into the guide needle and advanced. Suction is applied with an aspiration syringe while the tip is moved back and forth within the lesion. The suction is then released and the needle withdrawn. The aspirate is placed on a glass slide and smeared or expressed into a sterile glass jar.

Prostatic ultrasonography

A transrectal transducer is covered with a sleeve and used to provide linear and radial scans on an imaging screen. The patient is in a lateral position, and the probe is introduced into the rectum to about 10 cm above the anal verge. The needle penetrates the rectal mucosa with spring-loaded biopsy guns or a core biopsy system. This technique is practically painless and is frequently performed in the office setting if ultrasound is available there. Lesions as small as 2 to 3 cm are visible with this procedure. Transurethral ultrasound with biopsy is twice as sensitive as standard techniques in diagnosing carcinoma of the prostate.

TRANSURETHRAL RESECTION OF THE PROSTATE GLAND

By means of a resectoscope passed into the bladder through the urethra, successive pieces of tissue are removed from around the bladder neck and the lobes of the prostate gland are resected, leaving the capsule intact. The resectoscope uses a stabilized cutting loop to resect tissue and coagulate blood vessels by means of electric current. The electric current that powers the electrode is supplied by a high-frequency electrosurgical unit. The current settings are as specified by the urologist, who activates the cutting or coagulating current with a foot pedal during the course of the procedure.

TURP is one of four acceptable surgical methods of treating obstructive enlargement of the prostate gland. Several factors influence the surgical approach: size of the gland and location of the pathologic condition, age and condition of the patient, and presence of associated diseases.

Controversy continues in regard to the efficacy of prophylactic vasectomy to prevent the postoperative complication of epididymoorchitis. If vasectomy is to be done, it should be performed immediately before the transurethral

procedure. The patient must be well informed and have full understanding of the implications of the procedure. Operative consent is mandatory.

Procedural considerations

The instrument setup for transurethral resection of the prostate is as described for cystoscopy with additional necessary instruments. The four principal types of resectoscopes are McCarthy, Nesbit, Iglesias, and Baumrucker (Fig. 14-44). Adult resectoscopes range in size from 24 to 28 Fr and have the following components: Foroblique telescope, operating element, postresectoscope sheaths and obturators, and cutting loops (Fig. 14-45). Supplementary instruments include a resectoscope adapter and a lateral telescope.

A transurethral resection of the prostate requires the following instrument setup:

Resectoscope (multiple working elements)	Toomsy syringe
Foroblique telescope as well as a backup telescope	Syringe, 20 ml
	Ellik or Uro Vac evacuator
Stabilized or unstabilized cutting loops	Van Buren sounds
Postresectoscope sheath with corresponding Timberlake obturator	Strainer and small basin
	Lubricant, water-soluble
	Foley catheter, no. 22 or no. 24, 30 ml, three-way
Cystourethroscope	Disposable urologic drape with rectal sheath
Fiberoptic light cord	
Stopcock water adapter	
High-frequency cord	Cystoscopy drape pack
Resectoscope adapter	Sterile gowns and gloves as required
Short bridge	
Brush (to clean tissue from cutting loops)	Irrigation system
	Fiberoptic light source
Towel clamps (optional)	Electrosurgical unit
Plain forceps	Urinary drainage system
Prep set and solutions	

A continuous flow of isotonic and nonelectrolytic irrigating fluid is necessary to ensure transmission of electrical current and clear visualization throughout surgery. Irrigating solution such as 1.5% glycine or 3% sorbitol, 3 to 6 L, may be connected in tandem to provide a constant flow. Warming units are now available for these solutions. These units help to eliminate the hypothermia often experienced when large amounts of cold irrigants are employed. On the other hand, when solutions are warm, the patient will show a tendency to bleed more intraoperatively. At all times perioperative nursing personnel must be alert to replace the irrigation solution as required.

During transurethral prostatic surgery, return of irrigation fluid must be monitored because extravasation and absorption of fluid into open prostatic venous sinuses or bladder perforation may occur. The perioperative nurse should be aware of the early symptoms and measures employed to

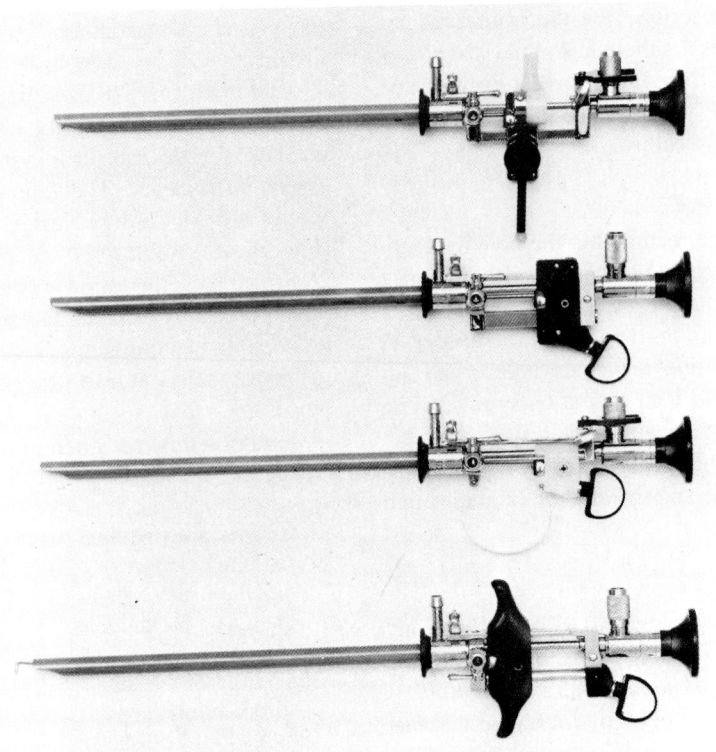

FIG. 14-44   Adult resectoscopes. *Top* to *bottom*, McCarthy, Nesbit, Iglesias, and Baumrucker.
Courtesy Circon Corp., Santa Barbara, Calif.

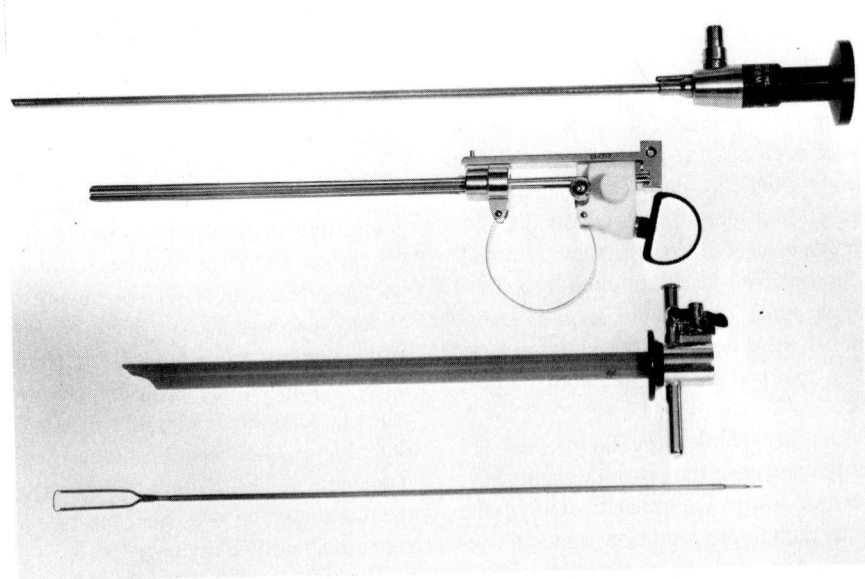

FIG. 14-45   Resectoscope components: Foroblique telescope, Iglesias operating element, postresectoscope sheath, and cutting loop.
Courtesy Circon Corp., Santa Barbara, Calif.

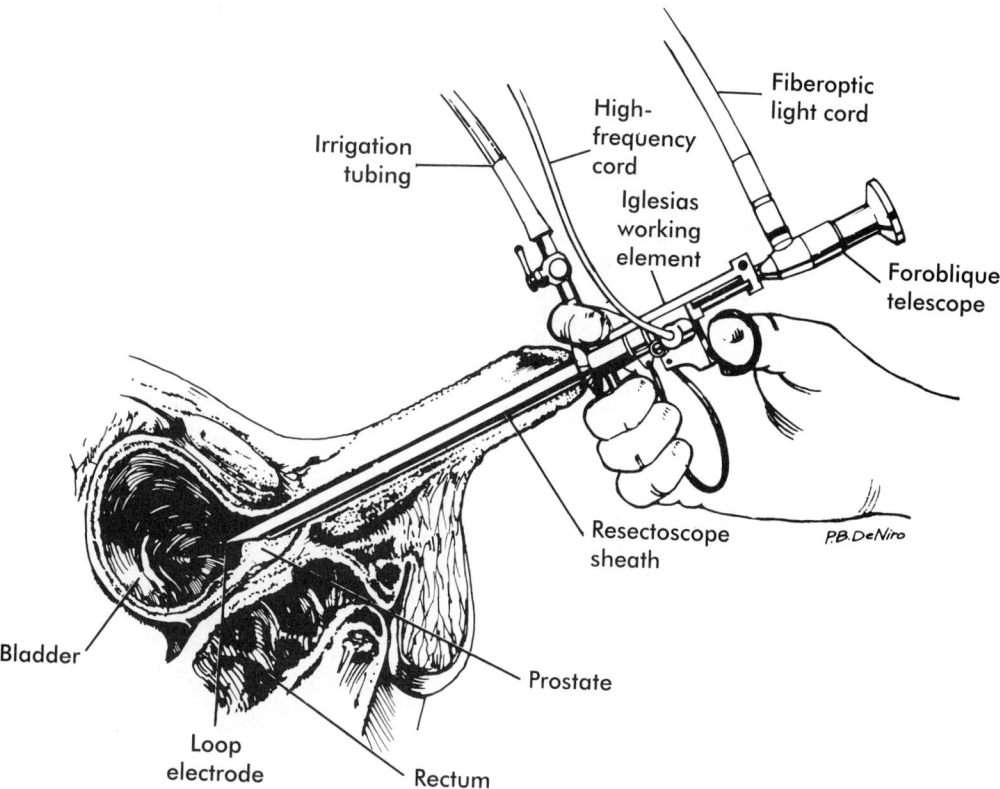

FIG. 14-46   Sectional view illustrating removal of portion of hypertrophied middle lobe of prostate gland with Iglesias resectoscope.

remedy these complications. The patient usually experiences significant respiratory changes and abdominal discomfort. Other important observations are rigidity and swelling of the lower abdomen, coupled with changes in sensorium. If extravasation of irrigating fluid is evident, the surgical procedure is discontinued and a cystogram is obtained immediately to determine if bladder perforation has occurred. Insertion of a Foley catheter is generally all that is necessary to control the situation. In the rare instance of a major perforation, surgical closure may be accomplished through a cystotomy incision.

Operative procedure

1. The urologist checks the endoscopic instruments before performing the transurethral procedure. In transurethral prostatic surgery the urethra is usually first dilated with sounds from 20 to 30 Fr.
2. Cystourethroscopy is performed to assess the degree of prostatic obstruction, as well as to inspect the bladder. Some urologists perform this diagnostic procedure several days before surgery, whereas others perform the examination in the operating room immediately before surgery.
3. A well-lubricated postresectoscope sheath with its fitted Timberlake obturator is passed into the urethra. The Timberlake obturator is removed, and the working element (resectoscope), assembled with the Foroblique

telescope and cutting loop, is inserted through the sheath. The irrigation tubing, light cord, and high-frequency cord are appropriately connected. Irrigation fluid is allowed to fill the bladder. Initial inspection of the prostatic urethra and bladder trigone is carried out. After determining the location of the ureteral orifice, the urologist initiates electrodissection, alternating cutting and coagulating currents as required (Fig. 14-46). At intervals the bladder is drained, washing out prostatic tissue and small blood clots. At times it is necessary to employ the Ellik evacuator to remove resected prostatic tissue. To do this the urologist must remove the working element of the resectoscope. The nozzle of the evacuator is fitted onto the resectoscope sheath, and by manual pulsatile pressure the bladder contents are removed. An Ellik or Uro Vac evacuator or Toomey syringe should be readily available for manual irrigation. Fluid may be drawn from the irrigant directly into the resectoscope sheath through the already attached tubing.
4. When the prostatic resection is completed, the prostatic fossa is inspected to ensure that all bleeding points have been coagulated. The resectoscope is then removed and a Foley catheter (22 or 24 Fr, two- or three-way, 30-ml balloon) is inserted into the bladder for urinary drainage. The balloon is inflated (Fig. 14-47, *A*) and pulled gently in traction against the bladder neck to help control venous bleeding (Fig. 14-47, *B*). The Foley balloon

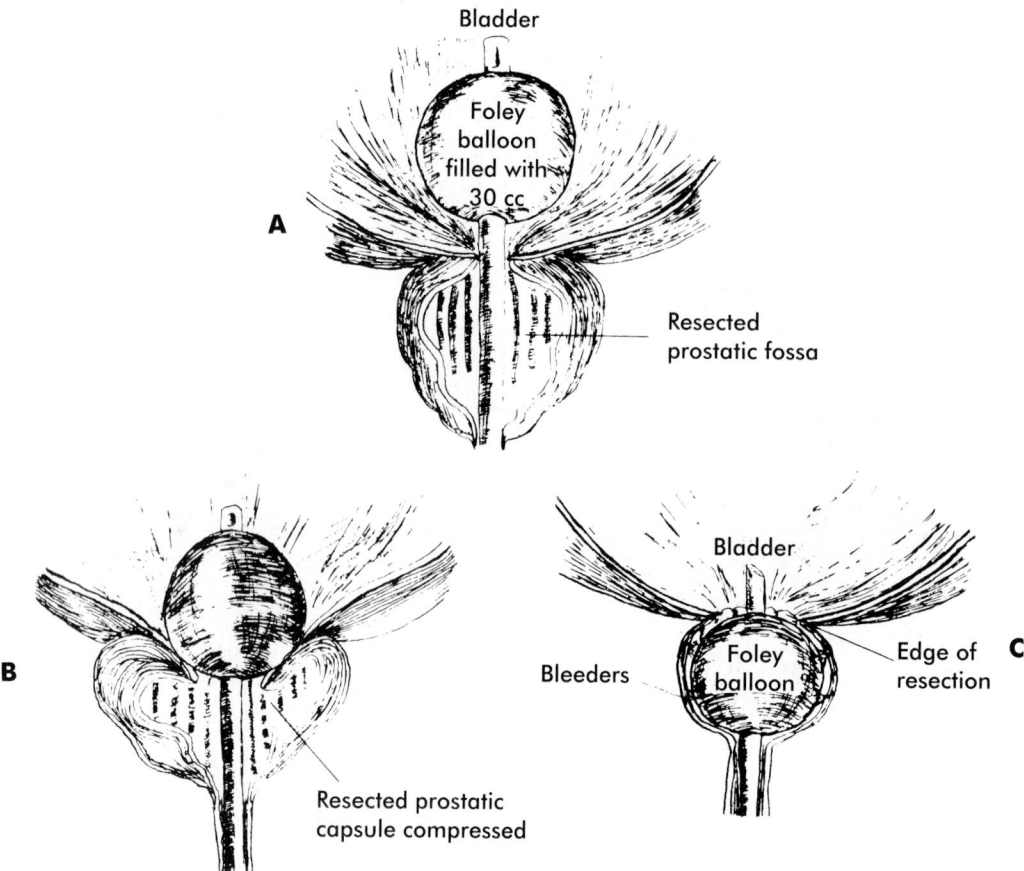

FIG. 14-47   Proper position for Foley catheter with inflated balloon beyond prostatic capsule.

must not be inflated within the prostatic fossa (Fig. 14-47, *C*), where it may cause excessive bleeding from the resected prostatic capsule.

5. If desired, continuous irrigation with gravity drainage is initiated with normal saline as the bladder irrigant, instead of sorbitol or glycine. A 3- to 4-L urinary drainage system is suggested to avoid frequent emptying of the drainage bag.

6. When VLAP or TULIP is performed, the surgeon may choose to place a standard 18 Fr Foley with a 5- or 30-ml balloon connected to straight drainage. If irrigation is required postoperatively, it is then performed manually with sterile solution and a Toomey syringe.

TRANSURETHRAL RESECTION WITH A CONTINUOUS FLOW RESECTOSCOPE

Prostatic tissue or bladder tumors are resected via a transurethral approach, using a continuous flow resectoscope (CFR) (Fig. 14-48). Unique components of the CFR include an outlet stopcock to which a suction tube is attached, an inflow tube on the inner sheath, and outflow holes on the outer sheath. These features enable the urologist to resect

tissue without interruption to empty the bladder, as must be done with the standard resectoscope.

The continuous flow technique decreases intravesical pressure on the bladder during the procedure, provides a clearer field of vision owing to the constant inflow and outflow of irrigant, reduces the operating time because the resection process need not be interrupted to evacuate the bladder, and provides a "still" bladder for the resection of bladder tumors.

Procedural considerations

The setup is as described for the standard transurethral resection of the prostate, with the addition of the CFR, a thick-walled Silastic suction tubing, and possibly a continuous flow pump.

Operative procedure

The procedure for transurethral resection with a CFR is as described previously for transurethral resection of prostate. The manufacturer's recommendations relating to the height of irrigation fluids and placement of the CFR pump should be followed.

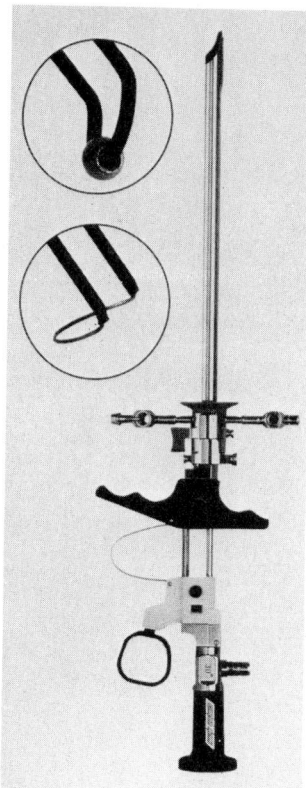

FIG. 14-48 CFR resectoscope.
Courtesy Circon Corp., Santa Barbara, Calif.

BALLOON DILATATION OF THE PROSTATIC URETHRA (TRANSCYSTOSCOPIC URETHROPLASTY)

Balloon dilatation is an alternative approach to surgical TURP, resulting from advances in radiologic techniques and balloon catheter technology. In many patients with urinary outlet obstruction the prostatic urethra can be stretched to promote a more acceptable urinary flow. Patient selection is generally based on age, extent of obstruction, and medical health. Other standard methods of treatment may be employed if the patient does not respond to balloon dilatation. The 5-year success rate is 60%.

Procedural considerations

In addition to a standard cystoscopy setup, the uroplasty TCU dilatation catheter system is needed (Fig. 14-49). It includes the following equipment:

Dilatation catheter (a triple-lumen catheter with a 15-ml capacity)	Calibration catheter Sheath and obturator, 26 Fr Inflation device

Operative procedure

1. A routine cystoscopy is carried out.
2. The length of the prostatic urethra (bladder neck to ex-

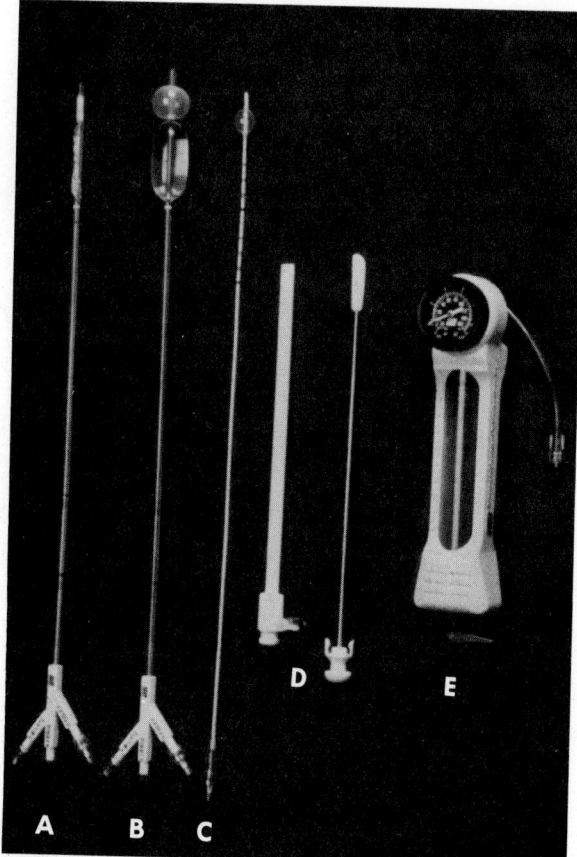

FIG. 14-49 Uroplasty TCU dilatation catheter system. **A,** Urethral dilatation catheter, deflated. **B,** Urethral dilatation catheter, inflated. **C,** Urethral calibration catheter. **D,** Disposable 26 Fr sheath obturator. **E,** Inflation device.
Courtesy Advanced Surgical Intervention, San Clemente, Calif.

ternal sphincter) is calibrated by manual exam, direct vision, and measurements with the calibration catheter (Fig. 14-50, *A*).

3. The urologist selects the balloon catheter of the appropriate size and length.
4. The dilatation catheter is placed through the 26 Fr sheath so that the proximal end of the balloon is beyond the external sphincter (Fig. 14-50, *B*), and the Foley balloon is inflated with sterile water (Fig. 14-50, *C*).
5. The balloon is inflated with the inflation device for 10 minutes at a pressure of 3 to 4 atm while under direct endoscopic control (Fig. 14-50, *D*).
6. A Foley catheter is inserted following the procedure to control bleeding and swelling of the tissue. The catheter remains in place for 48 hours.

SIMPLE RETROPUBIC PROSTATECTOMY

Simple retropubic prostatectomy is the enucleation of hypertrophic prostatic tissue through an incision in the anterior prostatic capsule by an extravesical approach. The

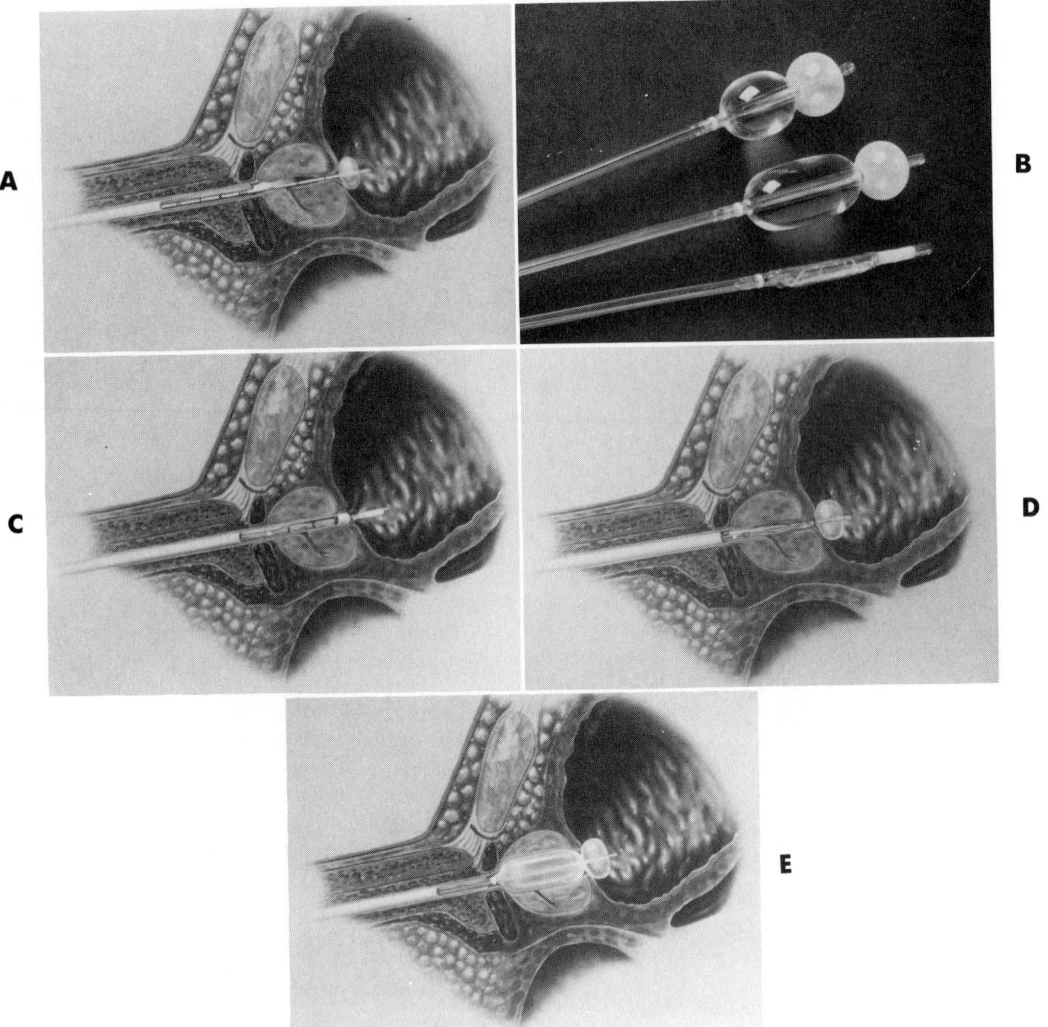

FIG. 14-50 Technique of balloon dilatation of the prostatic urethra.
Courtesy Advanced Surgical Intervention, San Clemente, Calif.

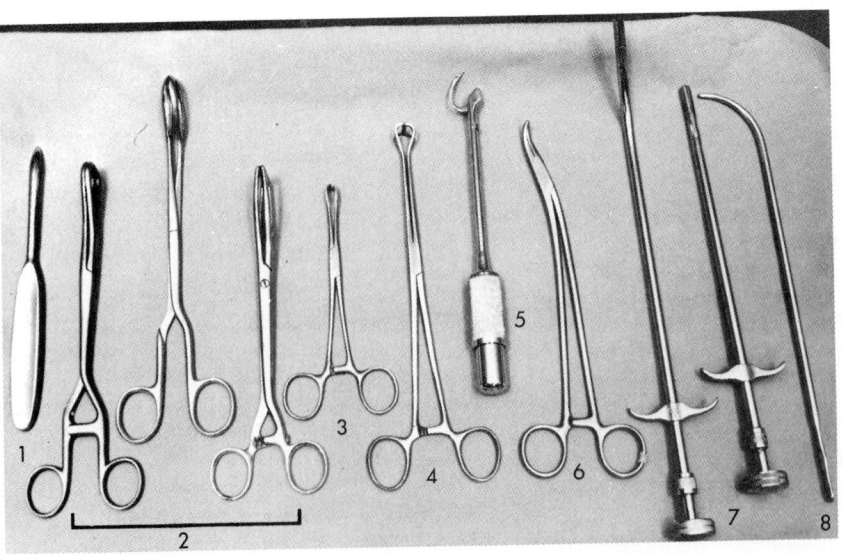

FIG. 14-51 Prostatic instruments. *1*, Prostatic enucleator; *2*, three prostatic lobe forceps; *3*, Lahey forceps; *4*, long Babcock forceps; *5*, boomerang; *6*, Heaney needle holder; *7*, two Lowsley prostatic tractors; *8*, urethral sound.

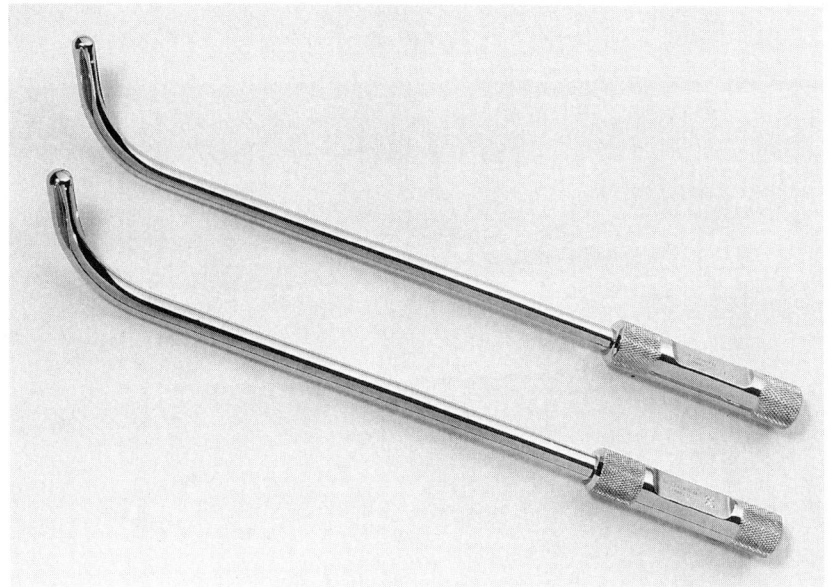

FIG. 14-52   Roth urethral suture guides, 24 Fr and 28 Fr.
Courtesy Greenwald Surgical Co., Inc., Lake Station, Ind.

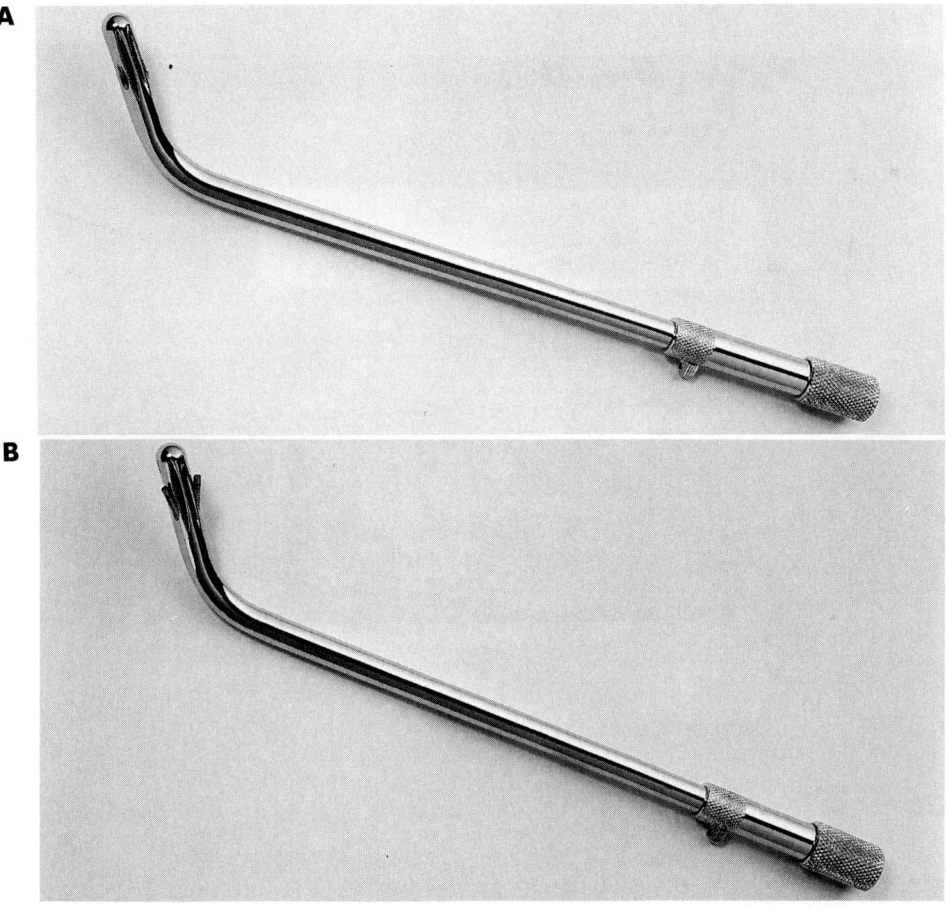

FIG. 14-53   Roth Grip-Tip suture guide, 28 Fr. **A,** Retracted. **B,** Extended.
Courtesy Greenwald Surgical Co., Inc., Lake Station, Ind.

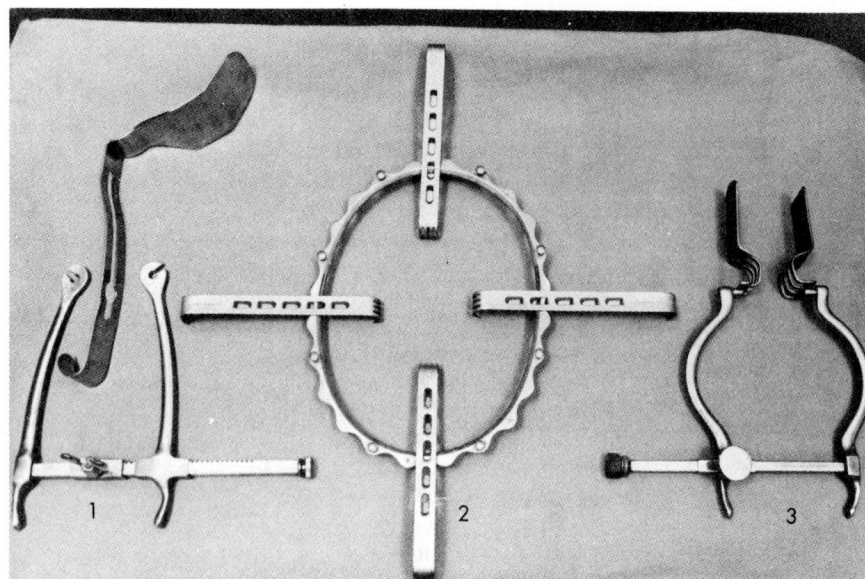

FIG. 14-54   Retractors for prostatectomy. *1,* Millin retropubic bladder retractor; *2,* Denis-Browne ring retractor (perineal); *3,* Masson-Judd bladder retractor (suprapubic).

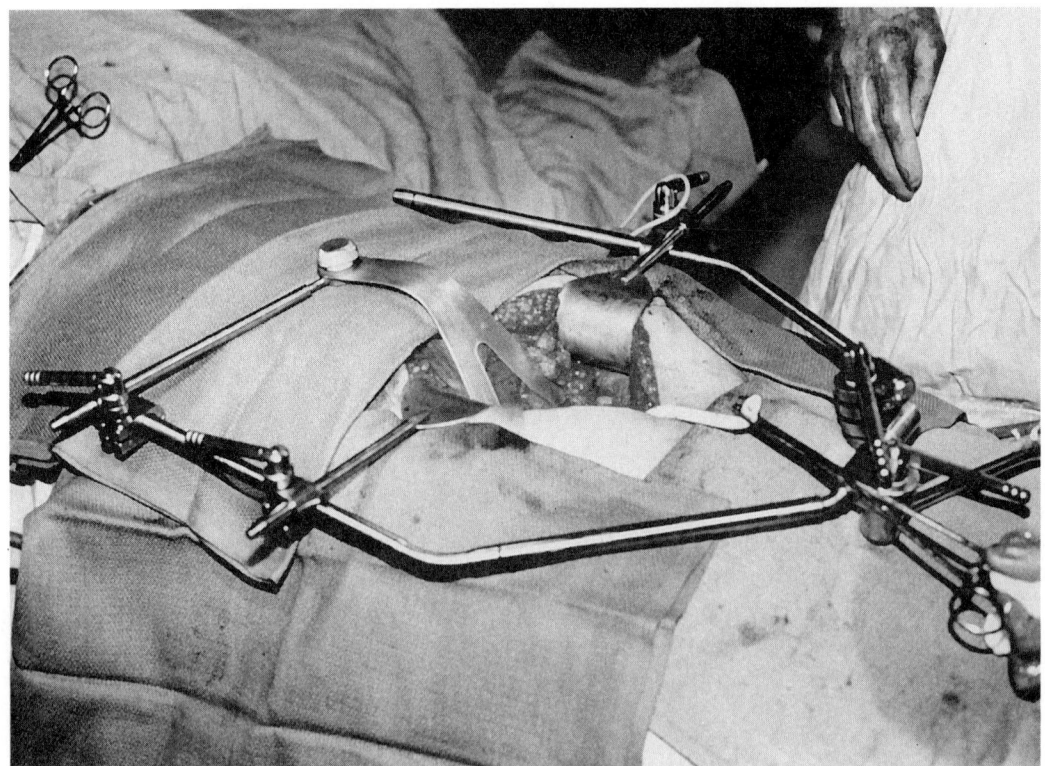

FIG. 14-55   Omni-Tract adjustable US200 urology retractor system.
Courtesy Omni-Tract Surgical, division of MN Scientific, Inc., St. Paul, Minn.

retropubic approach offers ideal exposure of the prostate bed and vesical neck; excellent hemostasis is obtained, and intraoperative and postoperative bleeding is readily controlled.

Procedural considerations

The patient is placed in a slight Trendelenburg position with the pelvis elevated and the legs slightly abducted. Routine skin preparation is carried out. Electrosurgery is usually employed. The draping procedure conforms to individual operating room policy, and the following procedure is suggested for draping the patient.

1. The first towel, with a cuff, is placed under the scrotum.
2. The next three towels are placed around the lower abdominal incision site, followed by a sterile laparotomy sheet.
3. A fifth towel, folded in half, is placed over the penis and scrotum below the retropubic incision site and secured with two towel clamps.

The instrument setup includes a basic laparotomy set and bladder and prostatic instruments (Figs. 14-51 to 14-54). The following supplies should be readily available:

Jackson-Pratt drains	Foley catheter, 22 or 24
Lubricant, water-soluble	Fr, 30-ml balloon
Toomey syringe	Syringes, 10 and 30 ml
Urinary drainage system	Self-retaining retractor
Foley catheter, 20 Fr,	such as the US200
5-ml balloon	adjustable urology
	retractor (Fig. 14-55)

Operative procedure

1. Through a Pfannenstiel or low vertical midline incision the anterior rectus sheath is incised along with portions of the internal and external oblique muscles. The rectus abdominis muscles are retracted laterally to expose the space of Retzius.
2. Following the placement of traction sutures, the anterior portion of the prostatic capsule is incised transversely (Fig. 14-56, A). The prostatic adenoma may be dissected or finger enucleated from the surgical capsule (Fig. 14-56, B).
3. Care is taken to place hemostatic sutures at the 5 and 7 o'clock positions, encompassing the vesical neck and prostatic capsule to ligate the primary blood supply to the prostate. Other bleeding points within the capsule may be suture ligated with no. 2-0 absorbable sutures.
4. A Foley catheter is inserted in the urethra and through the bladder neck and inflated within the bladder. Frequently a three-way catheter is used to afford continuous bladder irrigation.
5. The prostatic capsule incision is closed with either a continuous or an interrupted no. 0 absorbable suture (Fig. 14-56, C). A drain is placed in the space of Retzius and

brought out through the fascia and skin through a separate stab incision. The abdominal incision is then closed in layers, and the wound is dressed.
6. If continuous bladder irrigation is to be used, normal saline solution irrigation is initiated through a 4-L closed irrigation system.

SUPRAPUBIC PROSTATECTOMY

Suprapubic prostatectomy is the removal, through a transvesical approach, of benign periurethral glandular tissue obstructing the outlet of the urinary tract. A low midline or Pfannenstiel incision may be used. One advantage of the suprapubic approach is that it allows access for surgical correction of any existing bladder condition such as vesical calculi or vesical diverticula. Control of bleeding is a major consideration in any prostatectomy and is one disadvantage of the suprapubic approach. Because the prostate is located beneath the symphysis pubis, ligation of bleeding capsular vessels is difficult. However, control of hemorrhage and replacement of blood loss, coupled with skilled perioperative nursing care and early mobilization of the patient, have greatly minimized complications.

Procedural considerations

Spinal, epidural, and general anesthesia may be equally acceptable types of anesthesia for patients having a suprapubic prostatectomy, depending on their medical condition. The patient is placed in a slight Trendelenburg position with the umbilicus elevated and the legs slightly abducted. Skin preparation, draping, and instrumentation are as described for retropubic prostatectomy.

Operative procedure

1. Bilateral vasectomy may be performed to decrease the postoperative incidence of epididymitis and orchitis. A meatotomy may also be required if the penile meatus is too small to accommodate a Foley catheter.
2. A Foley catheter is inserted through the urethra into the bladder, and the bladder is inflated with a preferred irrigating fluid. This maneuver facilitates identification of the bladder.
3. A transverse or midline lower abdominal incision is made through the skin and the two layers of superficial fascia (Fig. 14-57, A). The external and internal oblique muscles are cut along the lines of the original incision. Bleeding vessels are clamped, coagulated, or tied with fine absorbable ties.
4. The rectus muscles are separated in the midline and retracted laterally.
5. Following the placement of traction sutures, the bladder is opened at the dome with a scalpel. Liquid contents are aspirated, and the bladder incision is enlarged. The bladder is visually and manually explored for calculi, a tumor, or diverticula.
6. The tip of the index finger of the operating hand is inserted through the vesical neck into the prostatic ure-

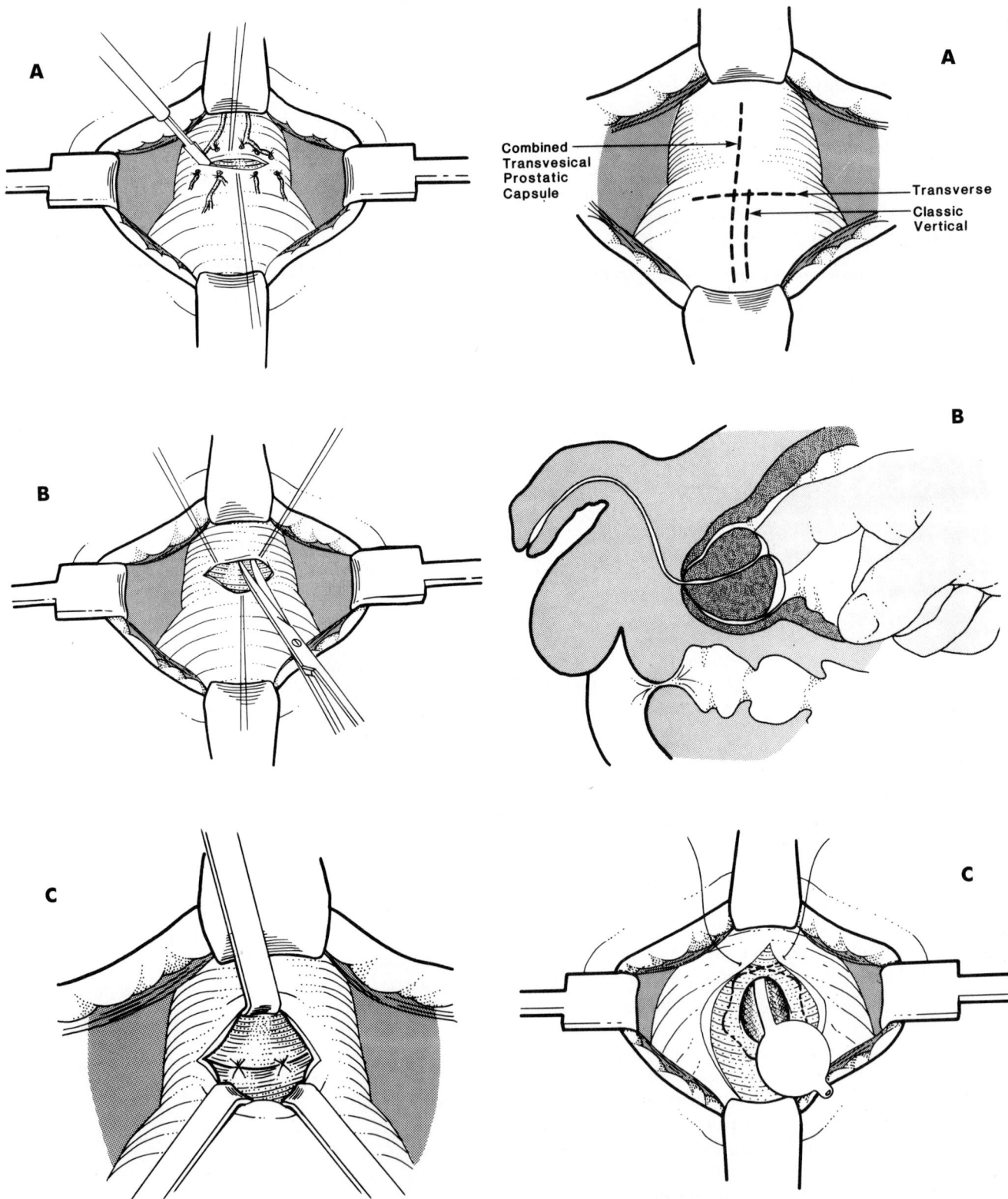

FIG. 14-56 Retropubic prostatectomy.
Modified from Droller, M.J. (1992). *Surgical management of urologic disease*. St. Louis: Mosby.

FIG. 14-57 Suprapubic prostatectomy.
Modified from Droller, M.J. (1992). *Surgical management of urologic disease*. St. Louis: Mosby.

thra, and the adenomatous tissue is enucleated (Fig. 14-57, *B*). If difficulty is experienced with the enucleation, a finger may be placed in the rectum to elevate the prostate gland. Aseptic technique is maintained during enucleation with the use of a sterile second glove on the hand used in the rectum.

7. After enucleation is completed, attention is directed to maintaining good hemostasis by suture ligation of the vesical neck at the 5 and 7 o'clock positions. Other significant bleeding points may also be ligated.

8. A suprapubic catheter of the urologist's choice is placed into the bladder lumen through a small stab incision. A 22 or 24 Fr two- or three-way Foley catheter with a 30-ml balloon is inserted into the urethra, and the balloon is inflated to a size that prevents the catheter from falling or being pulled into the prostatic fossa (Fig. 14-57, *C*). The cystotomy incision is then closed with interrupted no. 2-0 absorbable sutures. A drain is left along the cystotomy incision, brought out through a separate stab wound, and secured to the skin with a silk suture. The muscles, fascia, and subcutaneous tissues are closed in layers, and a dressing is applied.

9. Normal saline irrigation solution may be connected to the Foley catheter to provide continuous irrigation to the bladder to reduce clot formation and maintain catheter patency. Continuous irrigation may be initiated during closure.

SIMPLE PERINEAL PROSTATECTOMY

Simple perineal prostatectomy is the removal of a prostatic adenoma through a perineal approach. A perineal approach to the prostate gland is most suitable when open prostatic biopsy is desired and, after receipt of pathologic confirmation, radical excision is to follow. Other advantages include preservation of the bladder neck, improved urethrovesical anastomosis, and easier control of bleeding. Some surgical disadvantages are (1) inability to perform biopsy of the iliac and obturator nodes for determining extension of disease and (2) urethrorectal fistulas.

Procedural considerations

The patient is placed in an exaggerated lithotomy position with the legs above the level of the pelvis (Fig. 14-58). A bolster beneath the sacrum allows the perineum to be as parallel to the operating room bed as possible, with the buttocks extending several inches over the bed edge. Stirrups should be well padded to protect the popliteal fossa. The Ted sequential alternating compression device is recommended to assist peripheral vascular flow. The patient is often placed in steep Trendelenburg's position. Well-padded shoulder braces, placed over the acromial processes in a manner to prevent stretch or pressure injury, will help prevent the patient from sliding upward on the operating room bed. Routine skin preparation is carried out and includes an interior rectal prep. Special draping is as follows:

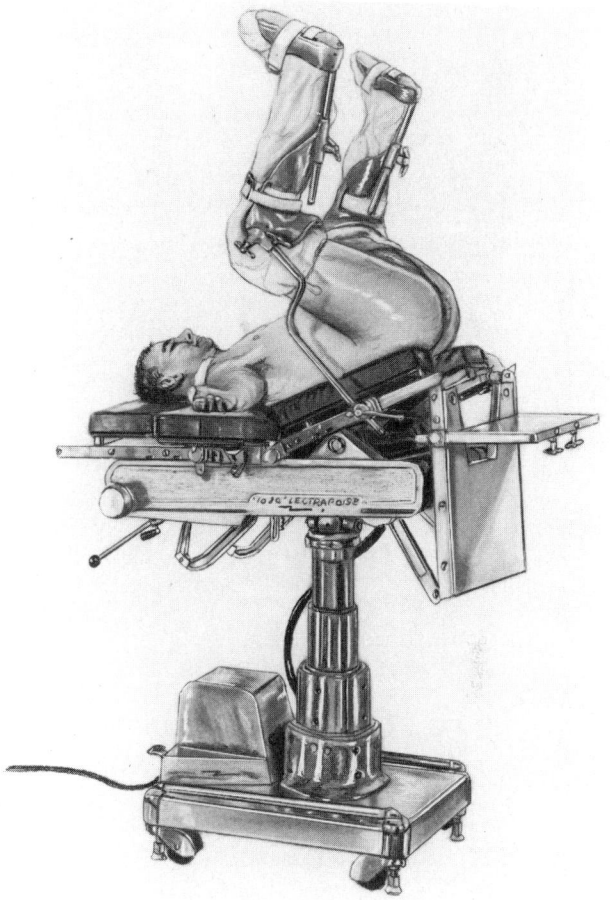

FIG. 14-58   Exaggerated lithotomy position for perineal prostatectomy.

From Droller, M.J. (1992). *Surgical management of urologic disease.* St. Louis: Mosby.

1. A towel folded in half is placed over the pubic area. Two towels with a cuff are placed on either side of the perineum.

2. Two leggings, with points down, are placed over the legs.

3. One impervious drape is placed over the anus.

4. A large sheet fully opened with a large cuff is placed across from one stirrup to the other and secured by towel clamps.

5. A laparotomy sheet follows, with the short end to the floor.

The instrument setup is as described for suprapubic prostatectomy, omitting abdominal self-retaining retractors and adding the following:

Straight and curved
   Lowsley tractors (Fig.
   14-59)
Roux retractors
Jackson retractors, short
   and long blades
Doyen vaginal retractors

Perineal prostatic retractors (Fig. 14-60)
Sauerbruch retractors,
   narrow and wide
Self-retaining perineal
   retractor such as the
   UM150 (Fig. 14-61)

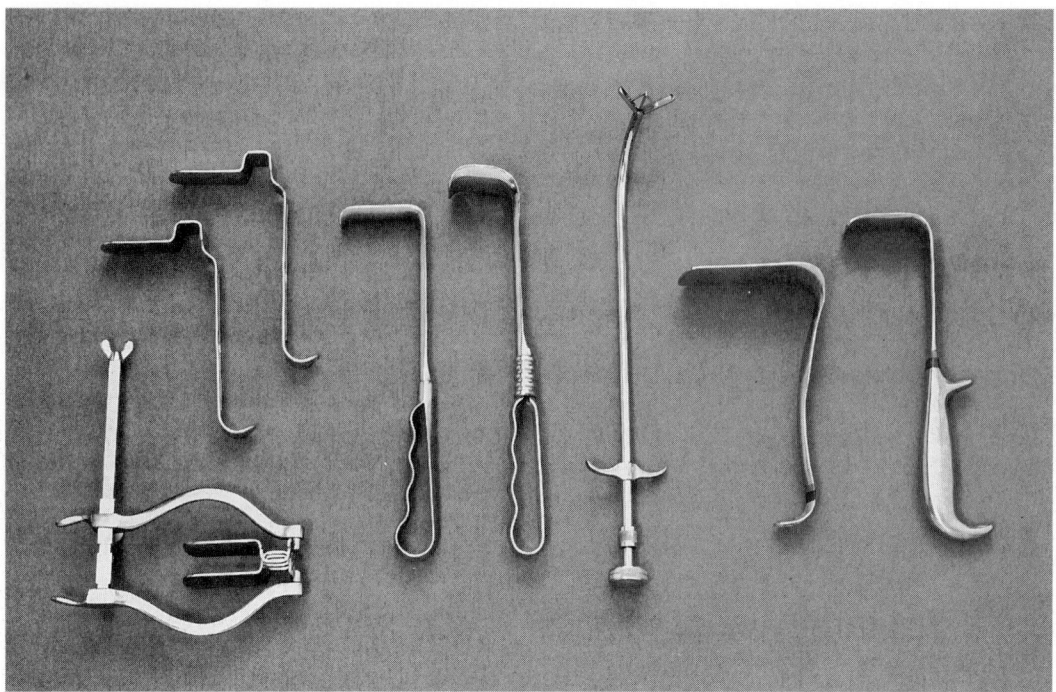

FIG. 14-59   Perineal and suprapubic prostatectomy instruments, including straight and curved Lowsley retractors.

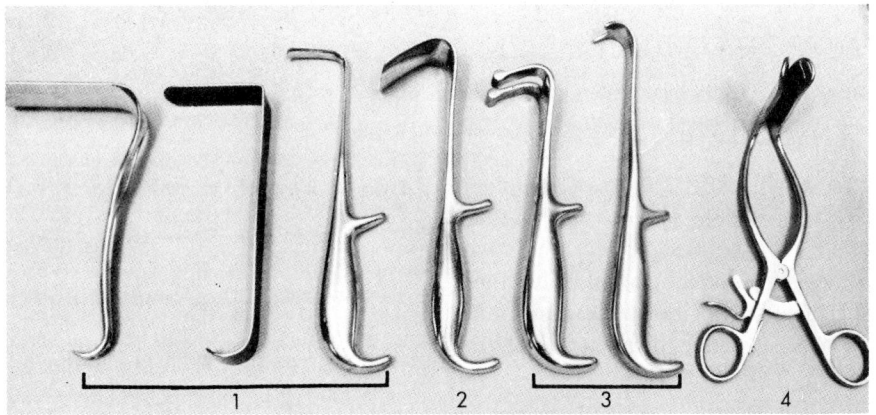

FIG. 14-60   Perineal prostatectomy retractors. *1,* Three prostatic lateral retractors; *2,* prostatic anterior retractor; *3,* two prostatic bifurcated retractors; *4,* self-retaining retractor.

Operative procedure

1. A curved Lowsley tractor is placed through the urethra into the bladder and held back by the surgical assistant, causing the prostate to be pushed down toward the perineum.
2. An inverted U-shaped incision is made from one ischial tuberosity to another, curving just anterior to the anus (Fig. 14-62, *A*).
3. Three Allis clamps are secured to the posterior edge of the incision and retracted downward, over the anal drape.

4. Subcutaneous bleeders are clamped with straight mosquitoes and coagulated or tied with no. 3-0 absorbable ligatures.
5. The central tendon is isolated, clamped, and cut distal to the external anal sphincter (Fig. 14-62, *B*). The rectourethral muscle is incised and pushed downward from the central tendon. The levator ani muscle is exposed and retracted laterally (Fig. 14-62, *C*). The prostate gland is then exposed.
6. Biopsy of the prostate may be performed for pathologic confirmation. If the results are negative, the prostatic

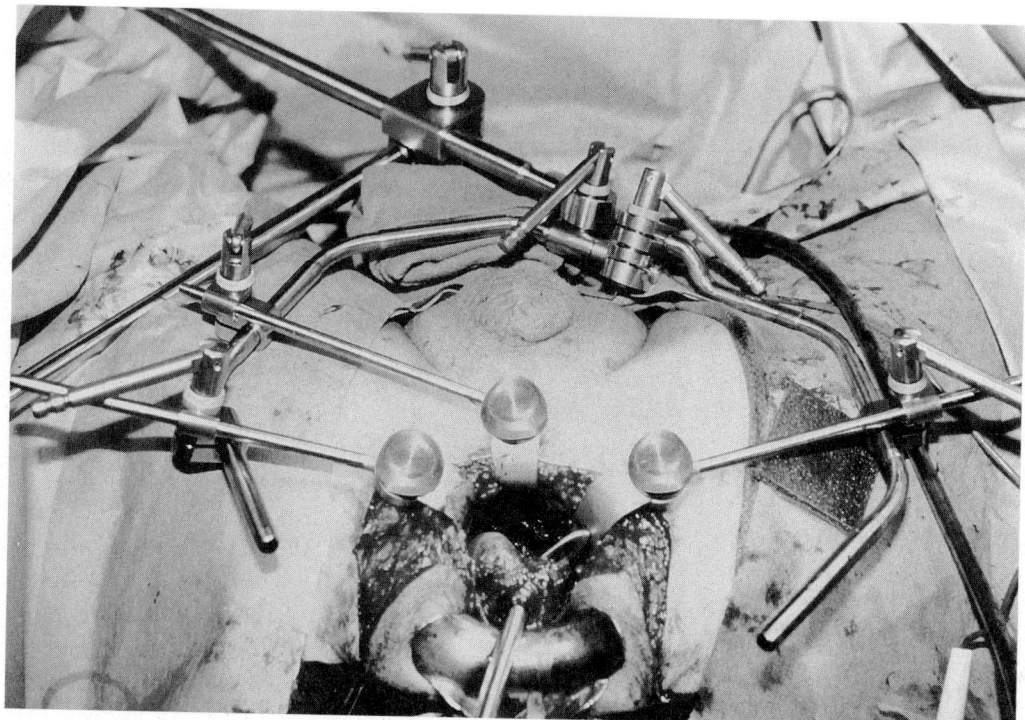

FIG. 14-61 Omni-Tract adjustable urology perineal minitractor.
Courtesy Omni-Tract Surgical, division MN Scientific, Inc., St. Paul, Minn.

adenoma is removed. If the frozen section reveals malignancy, the urologist may choose to do a radical prostatectomy at this time.

7. If simple enucleation is to be performed, the prostatic capsule is incised and the Lowsley tractor is removed (Fig. 14-62, *D*). The urethra is divided and the Young prostatic retractor is inserted into the prostatectomy. The blades are opened, drawing the prostate down, and the adenoma is manually enucleated from the surgical capsule.

8. A 22 Fr Foley catheter with a 30-ml balloon is inserted through the urethra into the bladder.

9. Bleeding is controlled at the 5 and 7 o'clock positions. The capsulotomy incision is repaired with a continuous no. 2-0 absorbable suture (Fig. 14-62, *E*). A drain is left in place at the level of the capsulotomy incision.

10. The subcutaneous tissue is reapproximated with no. 3-0 absorbable suture. The skin incision is reapproximated with no. 4-0 absorbable subcutaneous sutures.

11. The wound is dressed according to the surgeon's preference and taped or held with a supportive device such as mesh pants.

12. A vasectomy may be performed prior to the prostatectomy.

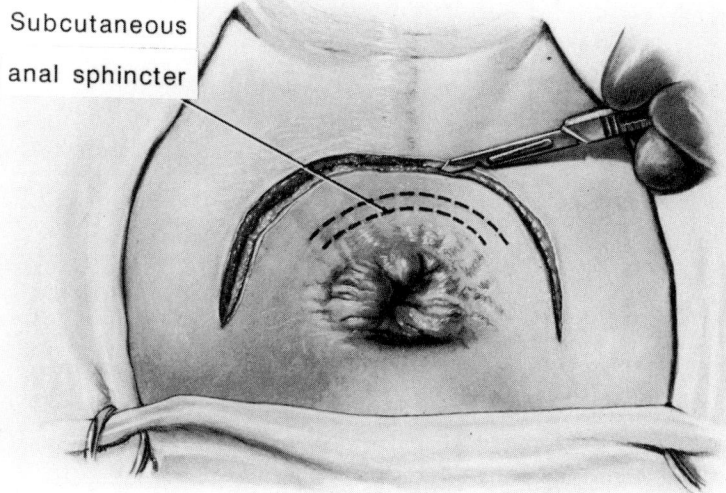

Subcutaneous
anal sphincter

A

FIG. 14-62 Perineal prostatectomy.

Continued.

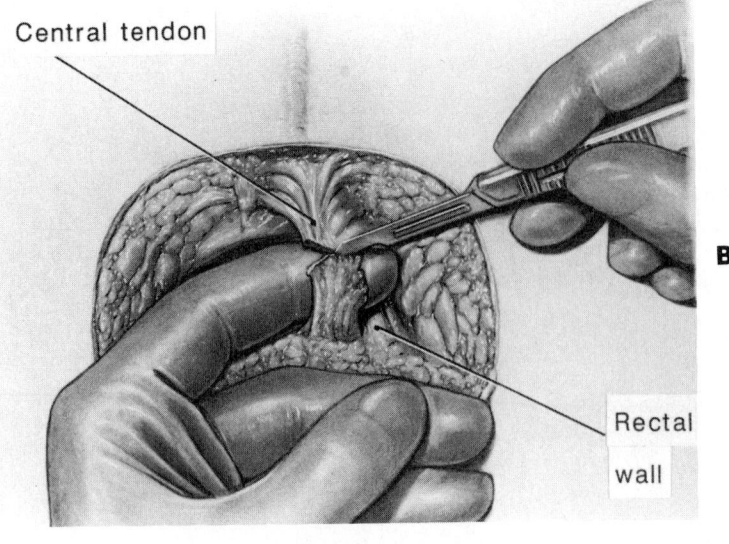

Central tendon

Rectal
wall

B

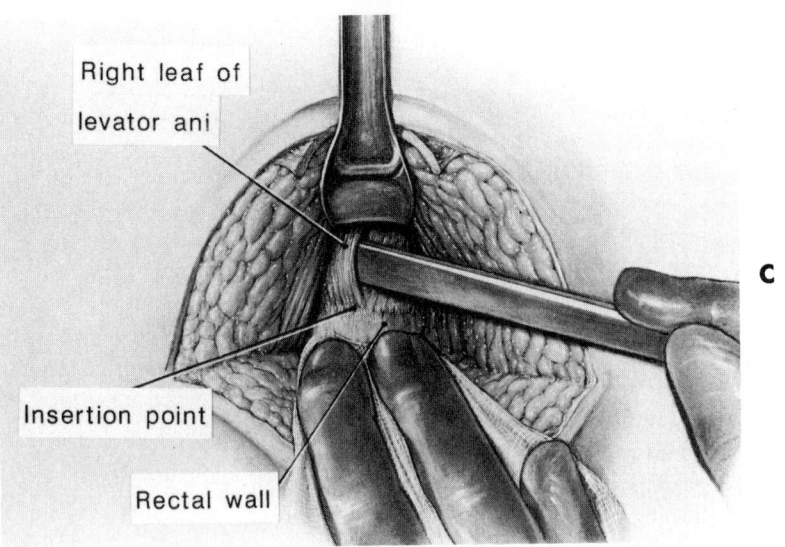

Right leaf of
levator ani

Insertion point

Rectal wall

C

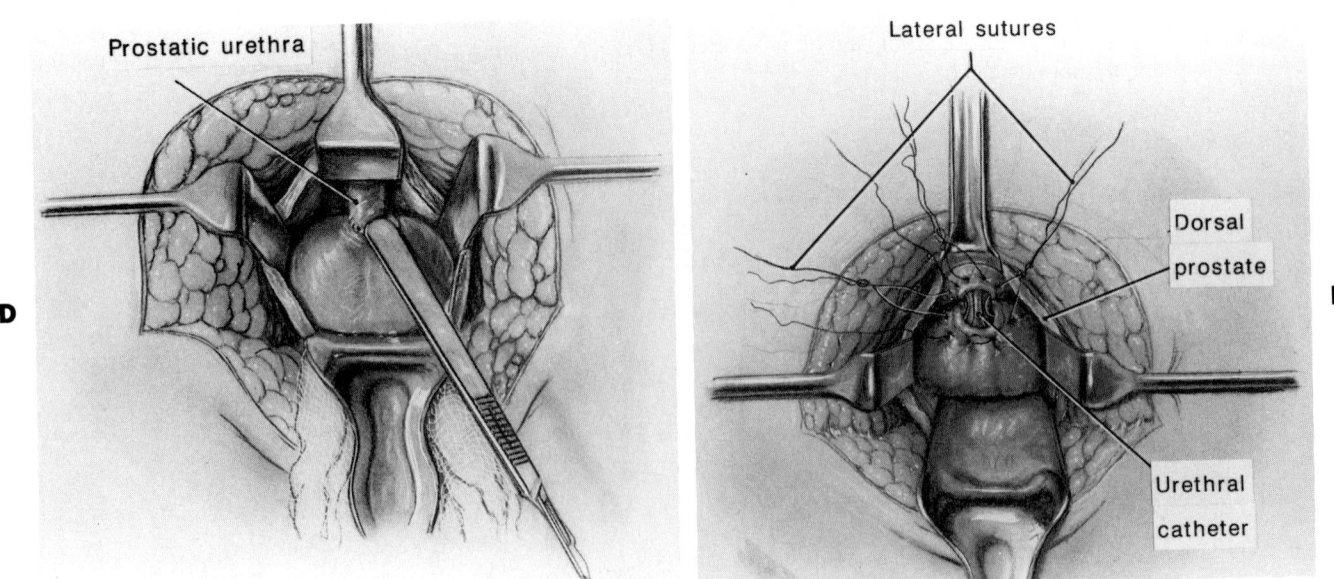

Prostatic urethra

D

Lateral sutures

Dorsal
prostate

Urethral
catheter

E

FIG. 14-62, CONT'D   Perineal prostatectomy.

Modified from Droller, M.J. (1992). *Surgical management of urologic disease*. St. Louis: Mosby.

NERVE SPARING RADICAL RETROPUBIC PROSTATECTOMY

Radical prostatectomy is the treatment preferred for patients with organ-confined carcinoma of the prostate. This procedure involves removal of the entire gland, its capsule, and the seminal vesicles. Until recently the risk of impotence was extremely high following this approach. Now, with careful anatomic consideration, the posterolateral neurovascular bundles, supplying the corpora cavernosa, may be spared for erectile potency in many patients. Urinary incontinence is generally not the threat it used to be. Those with tumors confined in the prostatic capsule (see Table 14-3) are the best candidates. Often, however, in the presence of more advanced tumor extension, one of the bundles may still be spared, allowing potency.

Procedural considerations

Patient preparation and basic surgical instrumentation are as for the simple retropubic approach. Additional supplies include:

Deep, long-tipped right-angle clamps	Bookwalter or Wishbone (UB200) retractor (see Fig. 14-55)
Urethral suture guides (see Figs. 14-52 and 14-53)	Straight and right-angle clip appliers and clips
Long Allis clamps	Right-angle scissors

Operative procedure

1. Following insertion of a 20 or 22 Fr Foley catheter, a vertical midline, lower abdominal, extraperitoneal incision is made.
2. A bilateral pelvic lymphadenectomy is performed, removing the external iliac, obturator, and hypogastric nodes en bloc. This is done primarily for tumor staging. Theories differ on whether to proceed with radical surgery if nodal packets reveal metastatic disease.
3. The puboprostatic ligaments are exposed and the endopelvic fascia is incised on each side of the gland to the puboprostatic ligaments (Fig. 14-63, A).
4. Right-angle scissors are employed to divide the puboprostatic ligaments. The dorsal vein complex is easily subject to injury, and excessive venous bleeding may occur during this phase of the procedure. The perioperative nurse needs to be alert to this potential complication.
5. A plane is developed between the lateral prostatic border and the levator ani muscles with sharp and blunt dissection. Once visualized, the muscle is dissected laterally to the urogenital diaphragm.
6. Collateral veins originating from the levator ani muscle and running lateral to the puboprostatic ligaments are ligated and divided to free the apex of the prostate. The perioperative nurse may hear the surgeon refer to these tributaries as the veins of Kelley. The dor-

sal venous complex, supplying the penis, is carefully retracted medially. Once a plane is developed, the venous complex is separated from the urethra with a long-tipped right-angle clamp. The venous complex is tied off using no. 0 or 2-0 absorbable ligatures. Some surgeons opt to use a stapler designed for this purpose. The complex is then transsected with a no. 15 scalpel.

7. Back bleeding, from the vessels on the anterior surface of the prostate, is suture ligated.
8. The right-angle clamp mobilizes the urethra from the rectourethralis muscle between the two neurovascular bundles, avoiding damage to them. A Penrose drain or vessel loop is passed around the urethra and it is elevated and divided with long-handled scissors or scalpel (Fig. 14-63, B).
9. The catheter is clamped proximally and pulled upward through the urethral incision where it is cut and held cephalad. The posterior urethra is transsected (Fig. 14-63, B).
10. The rectourethralis fibers are dissected free from and medial to the neurovascular bundles (Fig. 14-63, C and D). Enucleation of the prostate, division of the bladder neck, and clip ligation of the seminal vesicles follow (Fig. 14-63, E and F).
11. Once bleeding is controlled, the urethral suture guide is inserted in place of the Foley and six no. 2-0 absorbable sutures on a ⅝ needle are placed inside to outside on the distal urethral segment. These are tagged and left uncut to be anastomosed to the bladder neck (Fig. 14-63, G).
12. The bladder neck is trimmed and everted and a rosebud stoma fashioned. The sutures are placed from the urethra to a corresponding position on the bladder neck. When all are placed, they are brought together in single fashion and tied (Fig. 14-63, G).
13. Closure is as for simple retropubic prostatectomy. Continuous postoperative irrigation is rarely used. A 22 Fr 30-ml Foley is inserted and placed to gentle traction. Dressings follow simple routine.

RADICAL PERINEAL PROSTATECTOMY

Patient preparation and instrumentation are identical to simple perineal prostatectomy. Additionally, however, the radical approach is accompanied by laparoscopic or low abdominal lymph node dissection, if not previously performed as a separate procedure. Currently, laparoscopy outweighs the standard incisional approach. Additional supplies needed for laparoscopy include:

Standard laparoscopic instrumentation	Camera unit
3 10-mm trocars	CO_2 insufflator
1 5-mm trocar	Scissors/coagulator
2 5-mm downsizers	Instruments for open lymph node dissection
Veress needle	

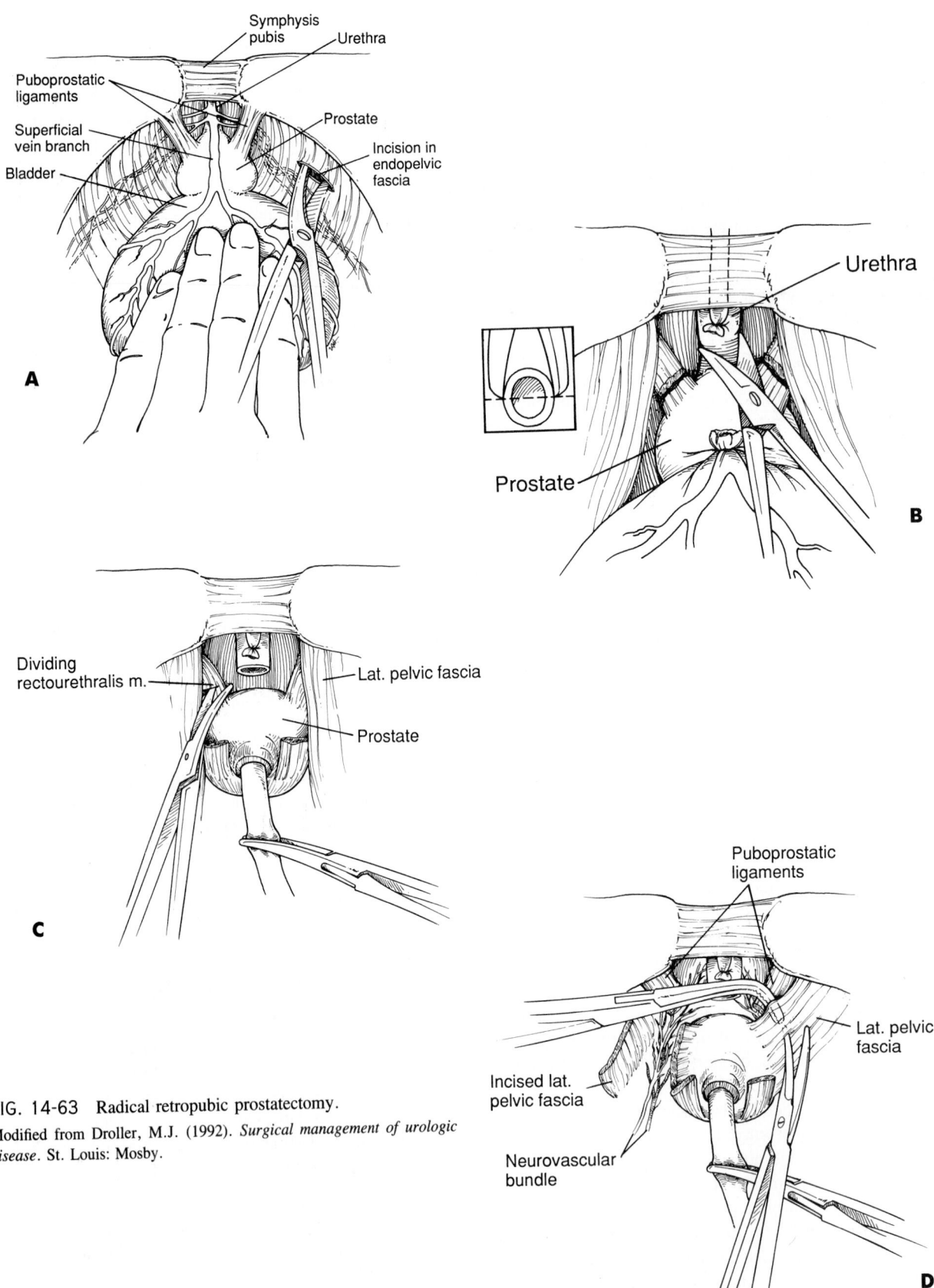

FIG. 14-63   Radical retropubic prostatectomy.

Modified from Droller, M.J. (1992). *Surgical management of urologic disease.* St. Louis: Mosby.

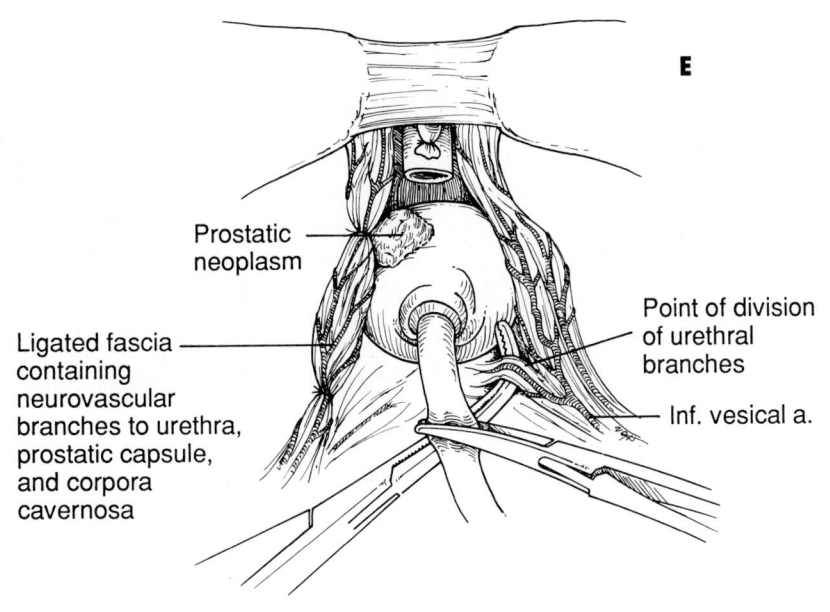

Prostatic
neoplasm

Ligated fascia
containing
neurovascular
branches to urethra,
prostatic capsule,
and corpora
cavernosa

Point of division
of urethral
branches

Inf. vesical a.

E

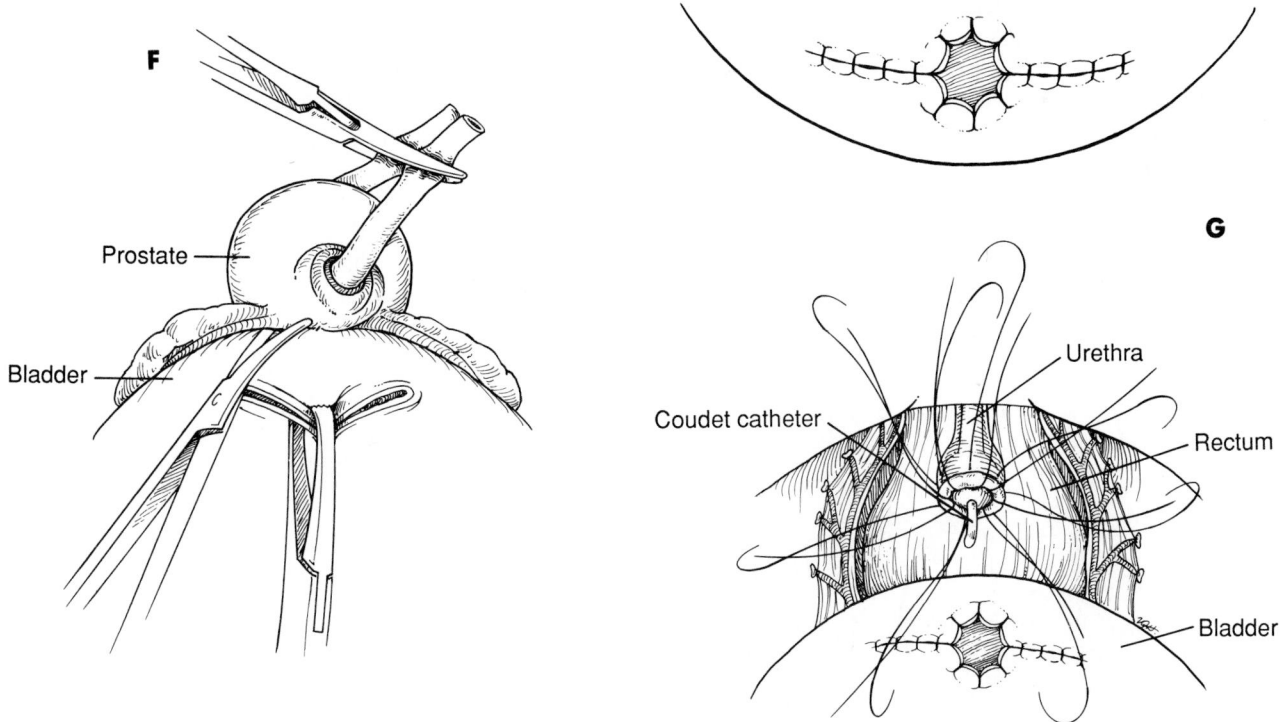

F

Prostate

Bladder

G

Coudet catheter

Urethra

Rectum

Bladder

FIG. 14-63, CONT'D   Radical retropubic prostatectomy.

Procedural considerations

Two operative setups are necessary. Most commonly, laparoscopy precedes prostatectomy. The patient is in the supine position for the laparoscopy with the area of the umbilicus slightly elevated. Sequential compressive stockings and preoperative Foley catheterization are necessary. Instruments should be available in the operating room to do an open procedure if necessary.

Lymph nodes are sent for frozen section, primarily for tumor staging. Theories differ about proceeding if positive nodes are discovered.

Operative procedures
Laparoscopic lymph node dissection

1. Following initial instillation of CO_2 gas through the umbilical Veress needle, 10 mm trocars are placed at the 12 o'clock (umbilicus), 3 o'clock, and 9 o'clock positions. A 5-mm trocar is placed at the 6 o'clock position. The placement of the last three trocars is observed with the laparoscope.
2. The peritoneum is grasped over the vas deferens and an incision is made with scissors.
3. The vas is identified, clipped or coagulated, and divided. The peritoneal dissection is continued lateral and cephalad to the sigmoid colon on the left and the ascending colon on the right.
4. Following identification of the spermatic cord structures, iliac vessels, ureters and psoas muscle, the incision is developed to the pubic ramus.
5. Cloquet's node is identified and freed from under the external iliac vein. Dissection continues until the obturator nerve is isolated. At the level of the bifurcation of the common iliac vein, the large lymph channel is located and removed. Endoclips or scissor-coagulation

may be employed. Clips offer a lower risk of postoperative lymphocele.
6. In a similar fashion the tissue overlying the external iliac artery is removed.
7. The procedure is repeated on the opposite side.
8. Trocars are removed once hemostasis has been achieved. Each trocar is removed under direct observation with the laparoscope, to allow for identification of inner abdominal wall bleeding sites.
9. After evacuation of the gas from the abdomen, the fascia layers are closed at the 12, 3, and 9 o'clock position. The skin is then closed with no. 4-0 absorbable subcuticular sutures.
10. The wounds are dressed with Steri-Strips, Telfa, and Tegaderm. The patient is then repositioned and prepared for radical perineal prostatectomy.

Radical perineal prostatectomy

1. Surgical approach is as for simple perineal prostatectomy (Fig. 14-64, *A* and *B*). A layer of subcutaneous fascia is incised and a space developed within the ischial rectal fossa (Fig. 14-64, *C*).
2. The central tendon is incised, permitting dissection to be carried out beneath the triangle formed by the superficial external anal sphincter (Fig. 14-64, *D*).
3. The sphincter is retracted cephalad and the rectourethralis is visualized (Fig. 14-64, *E*).
4. The true prostatic capsule is exposed by incision of the overlying fascia (Fig. 14-64, *F*).
5. Following dissection of the periprostatic fascia unilaterally, a right-angle clamp is passed around the membranous urethra and it is sharply incised (Fig. 14-64, *G*).
6. The posterior bladder neck is severed and the bladder retracted superiorly (Fig. 14-64, *H*). A plane is then developed between the anterior bladder and the posterior prostate and seminal vesicles (Fig. 14-64, *I*).

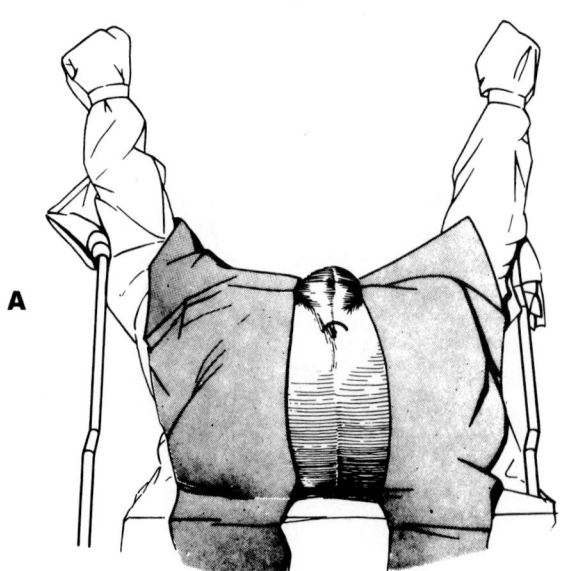
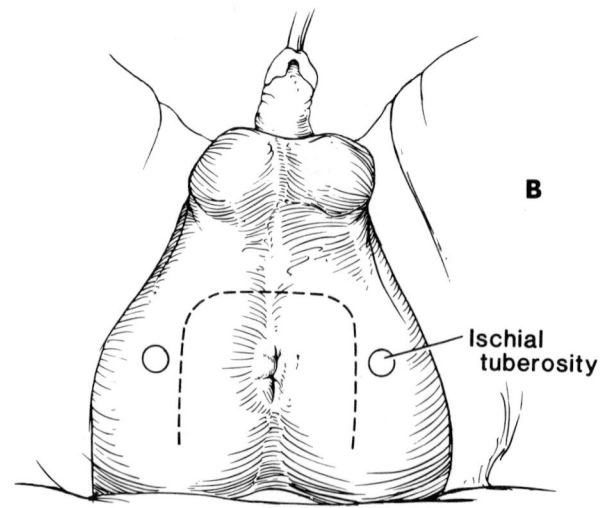

FIG. 14-64 Radical perineal prostatectomy.
Modified from Droller, M.J. (1992). *Surgical management of urologic disease*. St. Louis: Mosby.

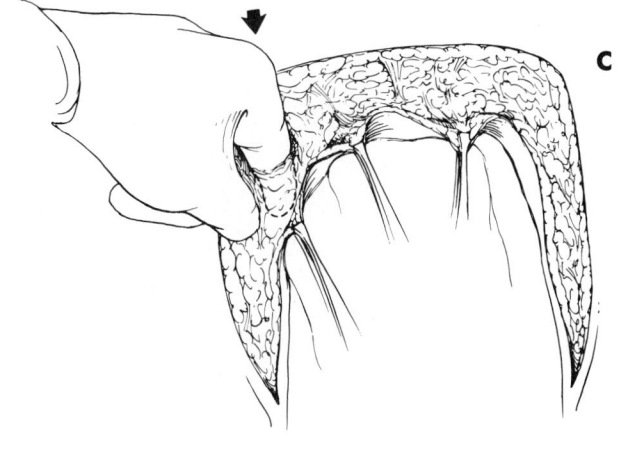

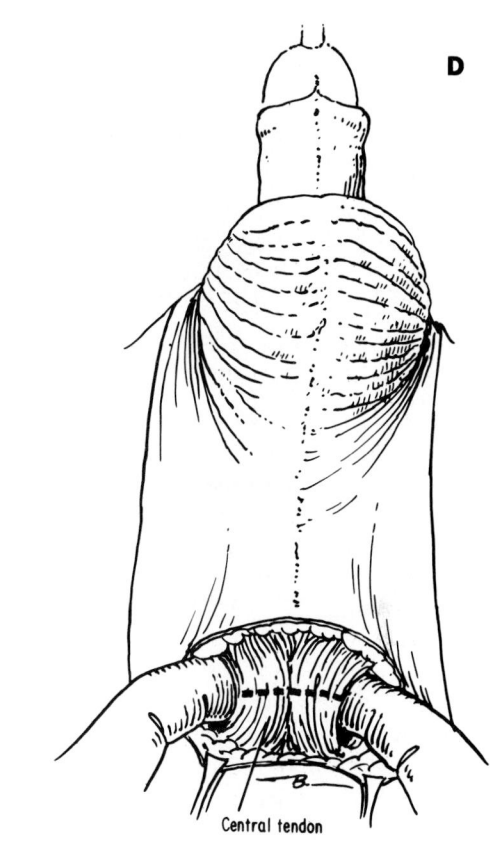

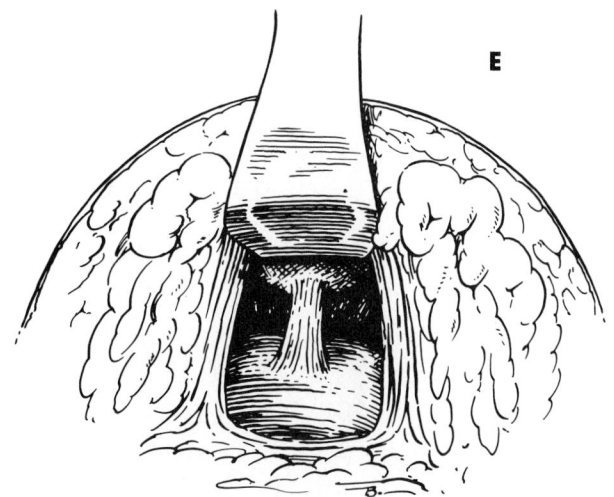

Central tendon

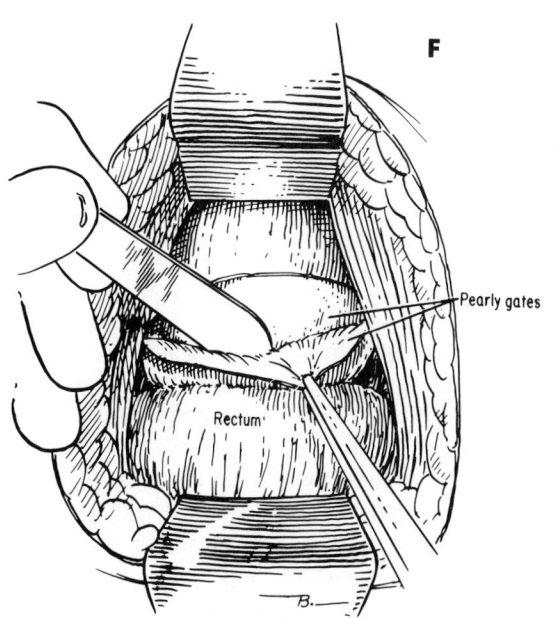

Pearly gates

Rectum

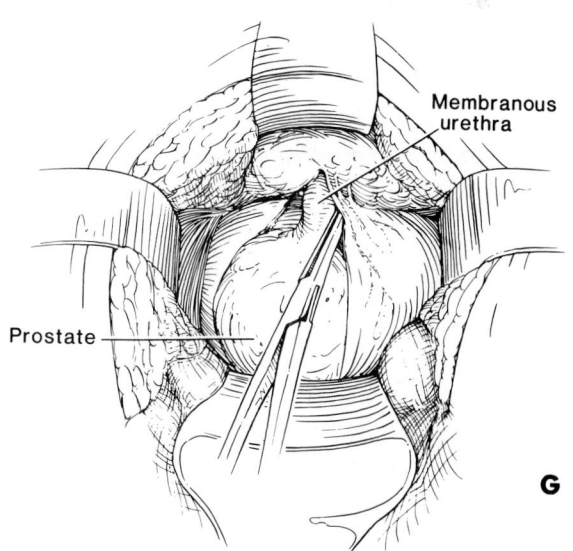

Membranous urethra

Prostate

FIG. 14-64, CONT'D Radical perineal prostatectomy.

Continued.

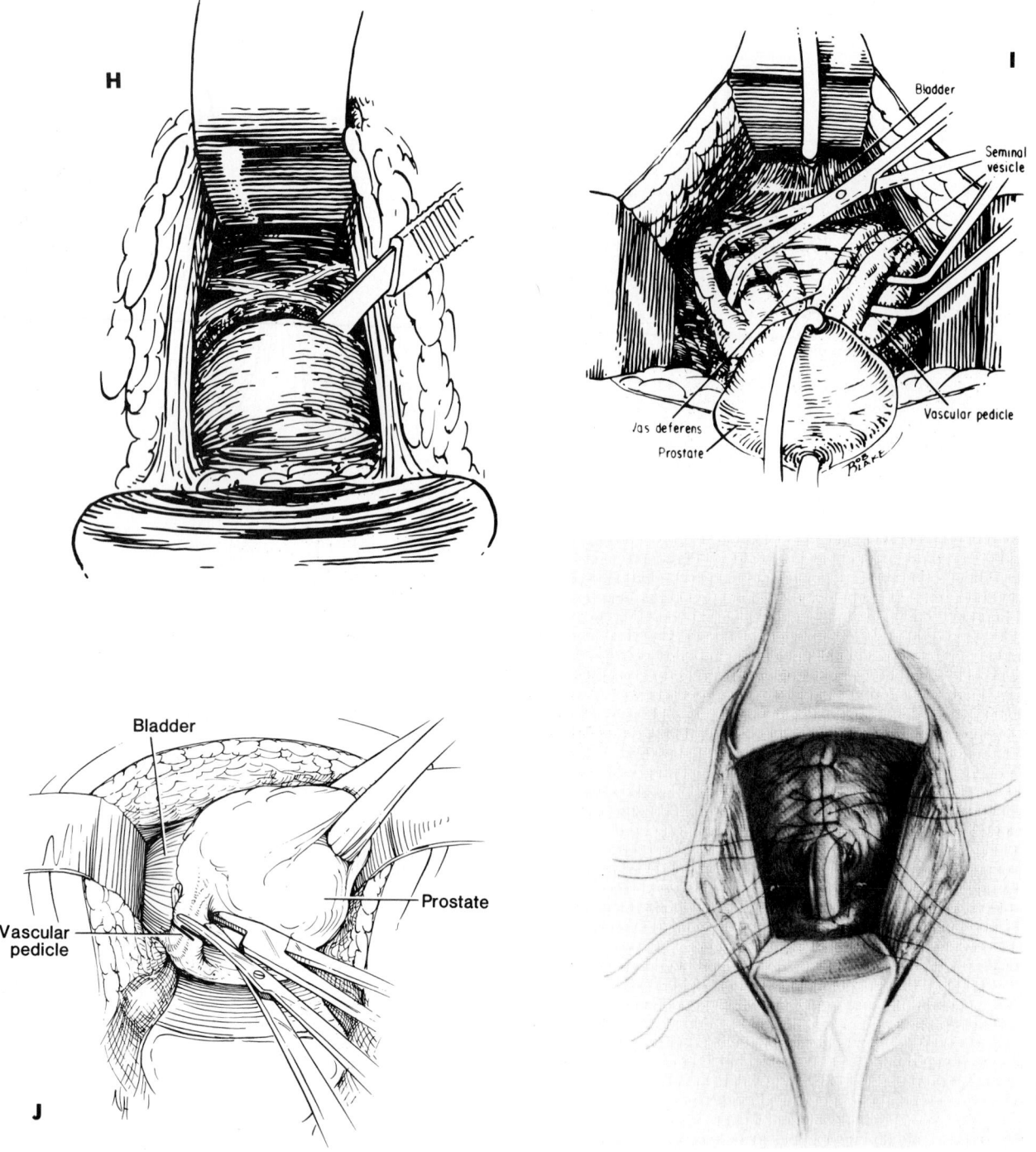

FIG. 14-64, CONT'D   Radical perineal prostatectomy.

7. The vascular pedicles are identified at the 5 and 7 o'clock positions, incised and divided (Fig. 14-64, *J*).

8. Before closure of the bladder neck, vest sutures of no. 0 or 2-0 absorbable sutures are placed in a mattress fashion in the open bladder neck at the 2 o'clock and 10 o'clock positions. These are left long for later lateral perineal placement (Fig. 14-64, *K*).

9. Following placement of the Foley catheter, the urethra is reanastomosed to the bladder neck with four to six

no. 2-0 absorbable sutures, placed at the 2, 4, 8, and 10 o'clock positions. Some surgeons opt to place sutures at the 6 and 12 o'clock positions as well.

10. Once reanastomosis is accomplished, the vest sutures are crossed and brought through the perineal body laterally and parallel to the urethra, anterior to the incision. These are secured just beneath the skin or to the skin with suture buttons.

11. A drain of the surgeon's preference is placed anterior

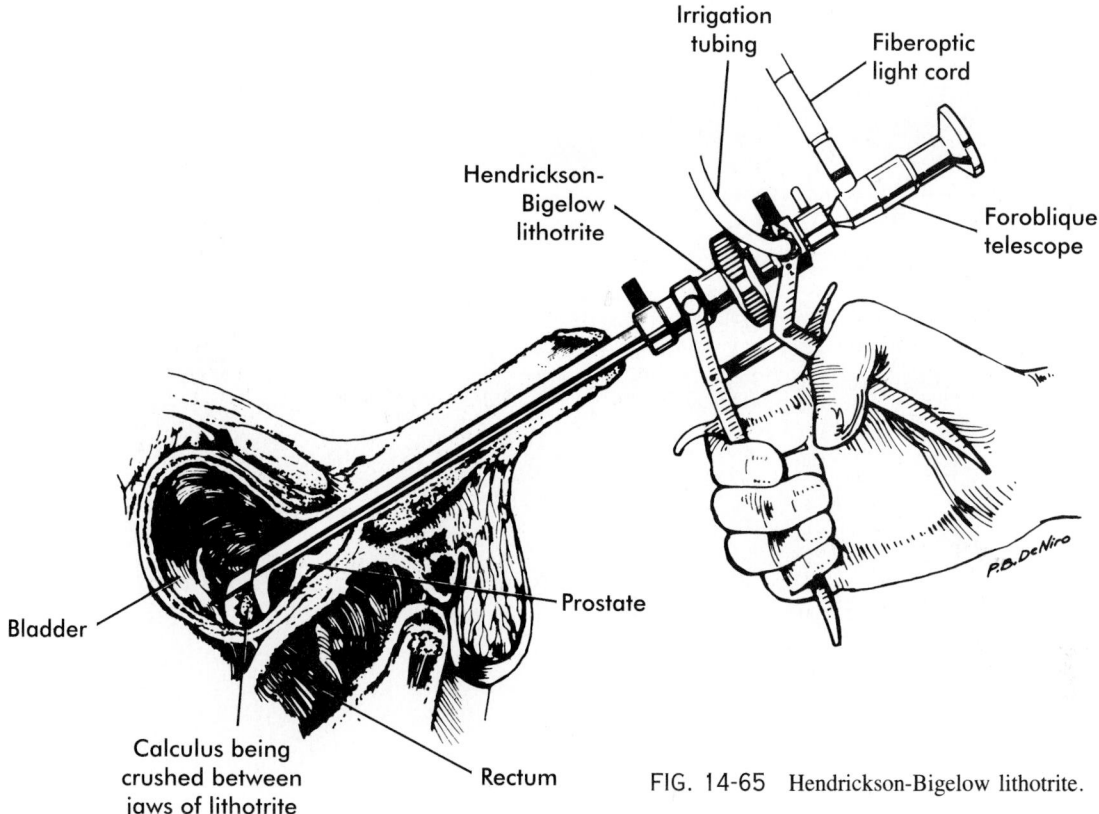

Irrigation tubing

Fiberoptic light cord

Hendrickson-Bigelow lithotrite

Foroblique telescope

Bladder

Prostate

Calculus being crushed between jaws of lithotrite

Rectum

FIG. 14-65   Hendrickson-Bigelow lithotrite.

to the rectal surface and drawn out through a separate stab wound.

12. Final closure and dressings are as described in the simple procedure.

SURGERY OF THE BLADDER

Operations on the urinary bladder may be performed through an open abdominal incision or a transurethral route. Special transurethral instruments such as the lithotrite may be used to crush vesical calculi manually (Fig. 14-65). An electrohydraulic cystolithotriptor may be used to fragment the stone within the bladder by using shock waves initiated by electric current (Fig. 14-66).

Ultrasonic lithotripsy is another procedure used in the management of vesical calculi. Ultrasound waves are transmitted through a hollow metal probe (sonotrode), which creates vibration at the tip. When applied to the surface of a calculus, the vibrating tip drills and fragments the calculus. This mechanical disintegration is continued until the stone is reduced to small fragments that are evacuated by suction through the hollow center of the probe (Fig. 14-67).

Stones may also be removed from the bladder through a suprapubic incision (cystolithotomy). Bladder tumors, diverticula, congenital defects, or trauma may necessitate an open abdominal approach. A thorough diagnostic workup and endoscopic examination can help to determine the ap-

propriate surgical approach to be employed. Radical procedures, such as total cystectomy, are performed for the treatment of invasive carcinoma of the bladder and require permanent urinary diversion.

For most open bladder surgery the patient is placed in the supine position with a bolster under the pelvis. Trendelenburg position may be desired because this position tilts the head down and allows the viscera to fall cephalad. This allows excellent exposure of the pelvic organs, including the bladder. The patient is draped as described for routine suprapubic prostatectomy, using a disposable impermeable drape that is placed immediately below the bladder incision. A catheter of choice may be inserted into the urethra and the bladder distended with sterile saline at the start of surgery for easy identification. Electrosurgery may be desired. The instrument setup for open bladder operations requires a basic laparotomy set, plus the following:

2 Mason-Judd bladder retractors (see Fig. 14-54)	1 Trocar (optional) Closed wound suction drains
3 Thyroid traction forceps, long	Assorted Foley, Pezzer, and Malecot catheters
3 Thyroid traction forceps, short	Vessel loops Catheter stylet
2 Retropubic needle holders or other long needle holders as desired	Electrosurgical unit

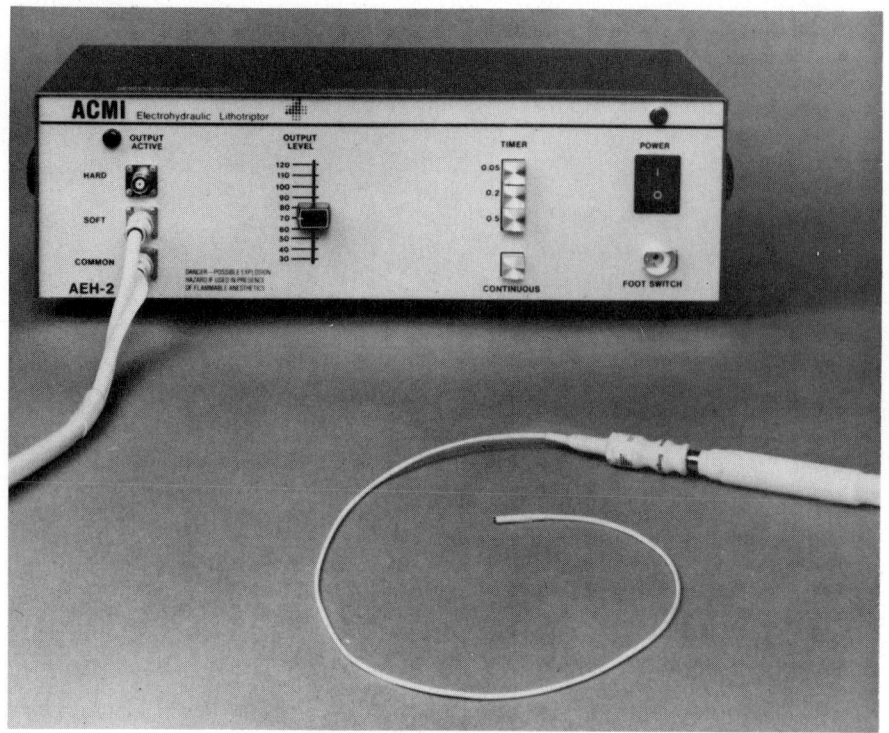

FIG. 14-66   ACMI electrohydraulic lithotriptor and probe.
Courtesy Circon Corp., Santa Barbara, Calif.

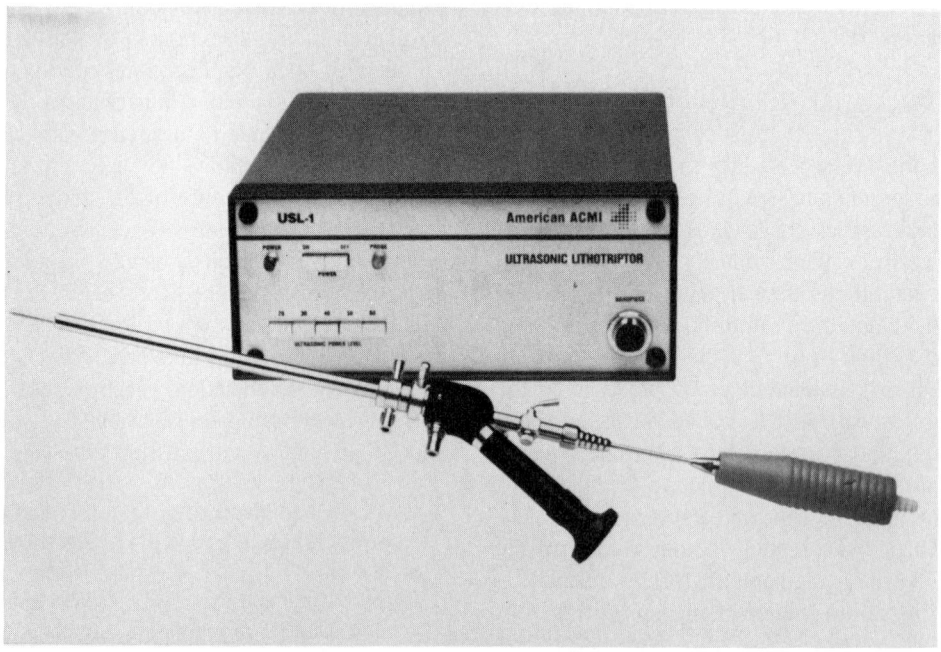

FIG. 14-67   Ultrasonic lithotriptor with rigid nephroscope.
Courtesy Circon Corp., Santa Barbara, Calif.

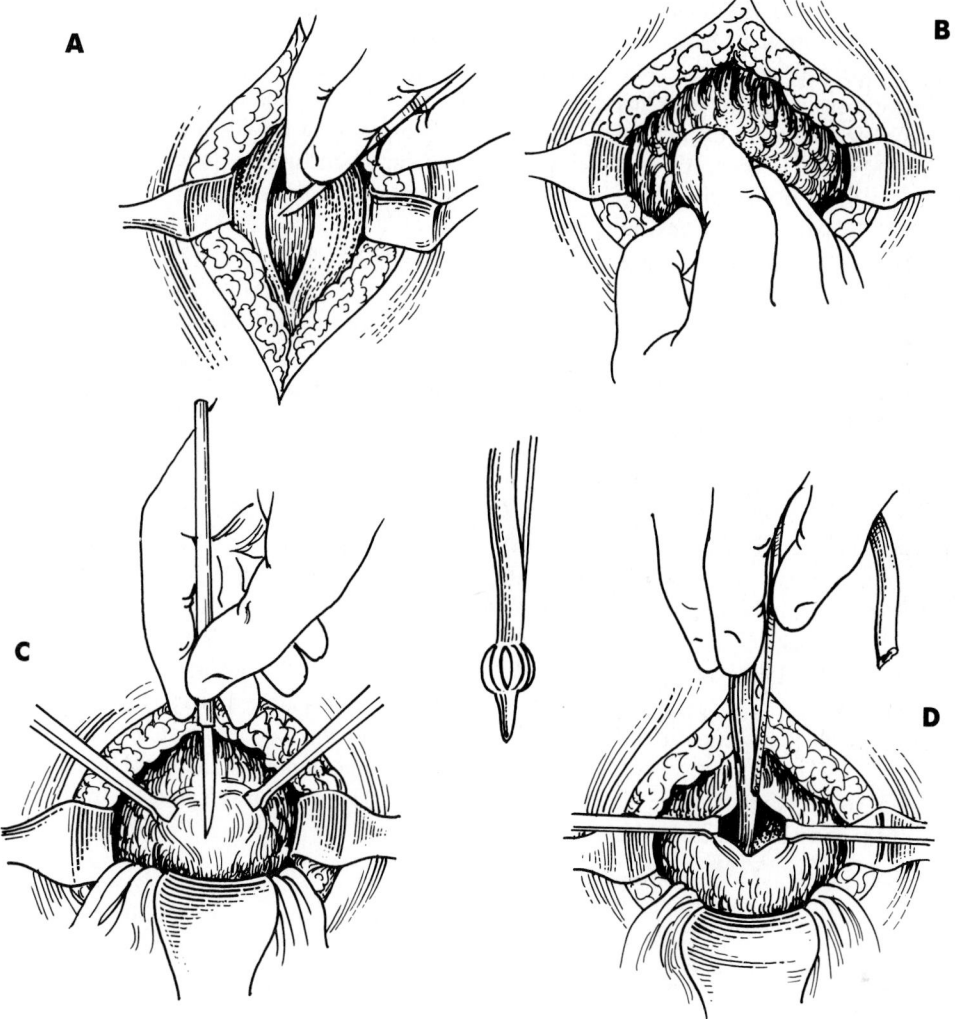

FIG. 14-68   Suprapubic cystostomy.

SUPRAPUBIC CYSTOTOMY (CYSTOSTOMY)

Cystotomy is an opening made into the urinary bladder through a low abdominal incision. When a drainage tube is inserted into the bladder through an abdominal incision, the procedure is a cystostomy.

Procedural considerations

The patient is in the supine position. A basic laparotomy set is generally sufficient for the procedure. Foley catheters ranging from 22 to 30 Fr should be available as well as Malecot suprapubic catheters and a drainage bag. Anesthesia may be general, spinal, or local with sedation. Frequently the urologist will incorporate a flexible cystoscopy into the procedure.

Operative procedure

1. A vertical or Pfannenstiel incision (transverse) is used. The rectus fascia is divided in the midline (Fig. 14-68,

A). The surgical approach is as described for suprapubic prostatectomy.

2. The bladder is distended with saline solution that is instilled with an Asepto syringe through a catheter. The dome of the bladder is then dissected free with Metzenbaum scissors and blunt dissection (Fig. 14-68, B). The wall of the bladder is grasped on either side of the midline with Allis forceps (Fig. 14-68, C). Two traction sutures may be placed through the bladder wall and held with straight hemostats. The bladder is then incised downward with a scalpel. Bleeding vessels in the bladder wall are clamped and ligated. The bladder contents are aspirated with a Poole suction device.

3. The bladder opening may be extended if the bladder is to be explored for diverticula or calculi. A large size Malecot or Pezzer catheter is introduced into the bladder (Fig. 14-68, D).

4. The incision is closed snugly about the catheter with ab-

sorbable sutures to render the closure watertight about the cystostomy tube. The muscle, fascia, and subcutaneous tissue are closed with absorbable suture and the skin with staples or nonabsorbable material. The cystostomy tube is further secured to the skin with a no. 0 or 2-0 nonabsorbable suture to prevent it from being inadvertently dislodged from the bladder. A drain such as a Jackson-Pratt may be left in the prevesical space.

5. The wound is dressed and the cystostomy tube connected to a straight urinary drainage system.

TRANSURETHRAL RESECTION OF BLADDER TUMORS

Bladder lesions may be removed using a standard resectoscope, working element, loop, and a Foroblique telescope, which is passed through the urethra into the bladder. A 24 Fr cystoscope sheath with a catheterizing bridge and biopsy forceps may be used to remove bladder tumors located at the very top or dome of the bladder (Fig. 14-69). Transitional cell carcinoma of the bladder is one of the most difficult lesions to track because it can occur wherever there is transitional cell lining of the urinary tract. Bladder cancer has a tendency to recur in other areas of the bladder even after complete resection of the original lesions.

Usually the surgeon removes not only the bladder lesion but also a portion of the muscle of the bladder underlying the lesion so the pathologist can determine if any tumor has invaded the muscle. Also, random biopsies of the normal bladder lining are taken because transitional cell carcinoma in situ may be found on microscopic examination.

Lesions that deeply invade the muscle must be treated with an open surgical procedure, such as a partial cystectomy or total cystectomy.

Procedural considerations

The resection technique, setup, and preparation of the patient are similar to those for transurethral resection of the prostate with a few exceptions. A general, spinal, or regional anesthetic is administered. If the surgeon has any questions about lesions existing in the upper urinary tract, a retrograde pyelogram is done.

Sterile water is recommended as an irrigating solution in transurethral resection of bladder tumors. Because few vessels are uncovered during this short resection procedure, water absorption with hemolysis and systemic complications such as hyponatremia do not occur. In addition, there is a tendency for cancer cells released during the procedure to absorb water, causing them to rupture and lyse rather than remain viable and capable of implanting in the raw surface of the bladder created by the surgery.

On completion of the procedure a large catheter, usually a 24 Fr, is passed into the bladder and connected to drainage.

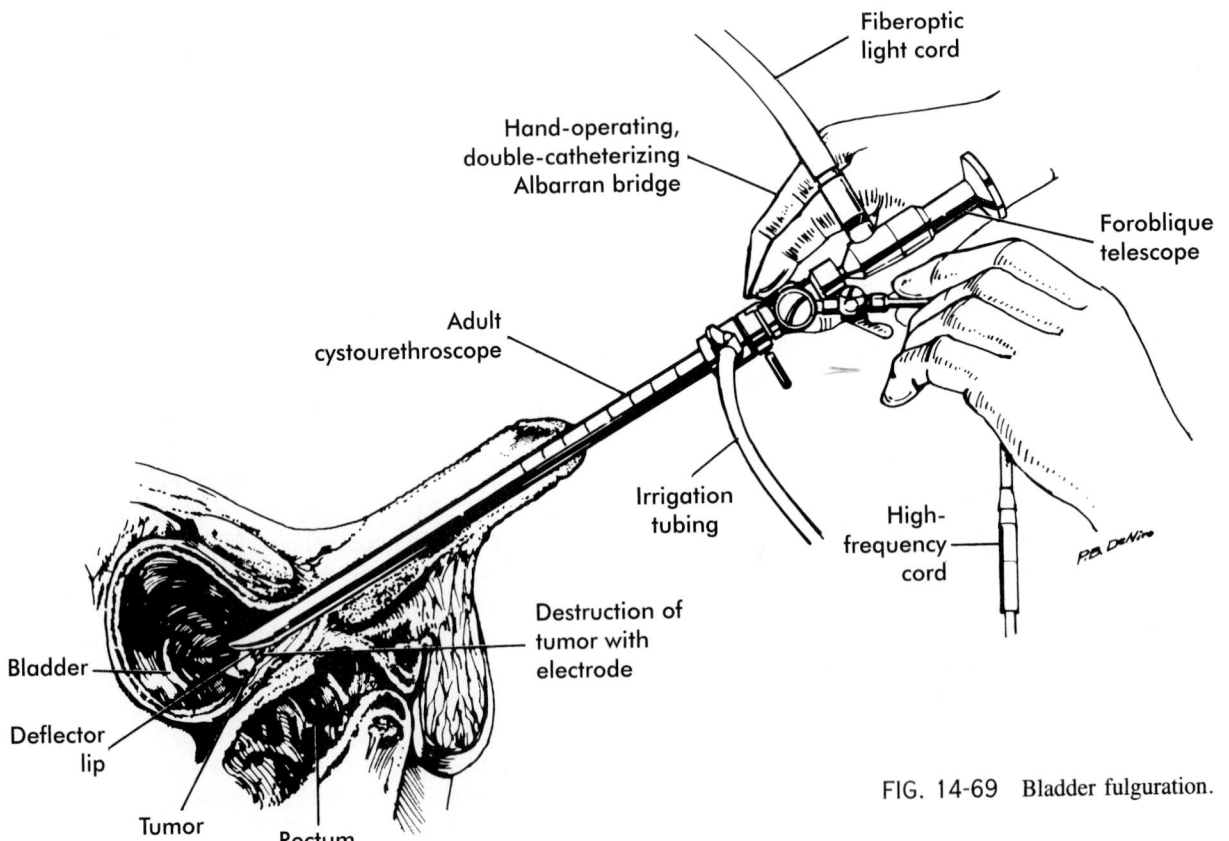

FIG. 14-69 Bladder fulguration.

TRANSURETHRAL LASER TREATMENT OF BLADDER TUMORS

The Nd:YAG laser is used to destroy small recurrent bladder tumors and may be used to coagulate the tumor bed of larger bladder tumors resected with an electrosurgical loop. It produces a powerful, highly focused beam of light in the near infrared range that is transmitted to the tumor site through a flexible glass fiber. This laser fiber is passed through the catheter channel of a cystoscope, and the fiber is directed by a deflecting laser bridge (Fig. 14-70). The advantages of the Nd:YAG laser in the eradication of bladder tumors are that bleeding is minimized, only sedation is required, operating time is short, there is minimal damage to healthy tissue, and there is no need for postoperative drainage of the bladder by a urethral catheter.

TROCAR CYSTOSTOMY

Trocar cystostomy consists of draining the bladder by puncture with a needle or trocar and inserting a catheter.

Procedural considerations

A minor set of instruments is required, along with the following available accessory items:

1 Silver probe	Catheters, as required,
1 Grooved director	or
1 Anthony suction tube and tubing	Cystostomy kit, pre-packaged
1 Trocar	

A local anesthesia setup may be used.

Operative procedure

The skin at the site of the puncture is nicked with a scalpel, and the trocar is inserted into the bladder. The trocar obturator is withdrawn, the bladder is drained through the

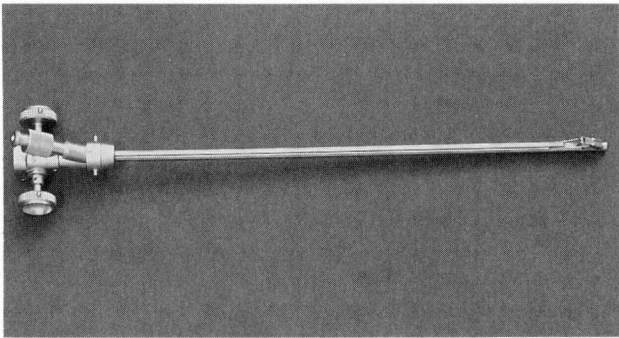

FIG. 14-70   Laser bridge, laser fiber deflected, Foroblique telescope, 21 Fr cystoscope sheath.
Courtesy Circon Corp., Santa Barbara, Calif.

trocar by suction, and a catheter is passed through the trocar cannula into the bladder. The cannula is carefully withdrawn, and the catheter is sutured to the wound edges. The wound is dressed.

SUPRAPUBIC CYSTOLITHOTOMY

Suprapubic cystolithotomy is the removal of calculi from the bladder. Obstructions, such as prostatic enlargement or foreign bodies, are common causes of bladder calculi and may be corrected at the time of surgery.

Procedural considerations

The instrument setup for open bladder operations is used, plus the following:

2 Millin T-shaped stone forceps	1 Lewkowitz lithotomy forceps
2 Millin capsule forceps	

Operative procedure

The surgical approach is similar to that described for suprapubic cystotomy. When the bladder is opened, calculi are identified and extracted. If indicated, bladder outlet obstruction is repaired.

REPAIR OF VESICAL FISTULAS

Vesical fistulas occurring between the bladder and the intestines or vagina may be repaired surgically. Vesicointestinal fistula may be caused by ulcerative colitis, diverticulitis, or neoplasms of the colon or rectum.

Vesicovaginal fistula may be a complication of radiotherapy for cervical cancer or endoscopic procedures involving surgery of the trigone or vesical neck. Such fistulas are also caused by obstetric injuries and hysterectomies.

Procedural considerations

The instrument setup is as described for open bladder operations. An intestinal resection setup (see Chapter 10) is also necessary for vesicointestinal fistulas. For vesicovaginal fistulas, vaginal preparation and a colporrhaphy set (see Chapter 13) with colostomy or ileostomy instruments are used.

Operative procedure

A colostomy proximal to the fistula may be performed to protect the repaired segment of bowel. The communicating area of bladder and bowel is totally resected. Generally, an end-to-end bowel resection is performed after excision of the involved intestinal segment. The bladder is then repaired in three layers.

If the fistula is at the dome of the bladder, the approach will be extraperitoneal. A suprapubic tube is usually left in the bladder in these cases. If the fistula is in the trigone of the bladder, a vaginal approach may be employed.

BLADDER NECK OPERATION (Y-V–PLASTY)

A bladder neck operation is an open plastic revision of a strictured bladder neck. A Y-V–plasty is performed to overcome contracture of the bladder neck caused by primary or secondary stricture.

Procedural considerations

The patient is placed in a modified Trendelenburg position. Epidural, spinal, or general anesthesia may be used. Instrumentation is as for open bladder operations.

Operative procedure

1. The bladder is approached through a transverse Pfannenstiel incision in the same manner as in retropubic prostatectomy. A self-retaining retractor is employed to achieve exposure.
2. Fine traction sutures on small, fine, cutting-edge needles (cleft palate type) are placed at the base and on either side of the urethra to start the pattern for the plastic dissection.
3. With the aid of the traction sutures and an Allis forceps, the anterior bladder wall, bladder neck, and urethra are visualized. A Y incision is made in the anterior bladder wall with its distal end extending through the vesical neck and the prostate at the 12 o'clock position (Fig. 14-71, A). Bleeding vessels in the wall of the bladder and bladder neck are ligated. The broad-based V flap is developed, and the length of the Y arm is determined by how far the stricture extends beyond the vesical neck.
4. The apex of the V is mobilized so it fits into the leg of the Y incision (Fig. 14-71, B). In this manner the vesical outlet is greatly increased in diameter. A catheter is placed in the urethra as a guide. A suture is taken through the apex of the V and into the prostatic urethra to the base of the Y and tied. The closure of the plastic repair is completed with mattress sutures on atraumatic needles (Fig. 14-71, C).
5. A cystostomy tube is placed in the bladder, and the bladder and abdominal wall are closed in the usual manner for cystostomy.

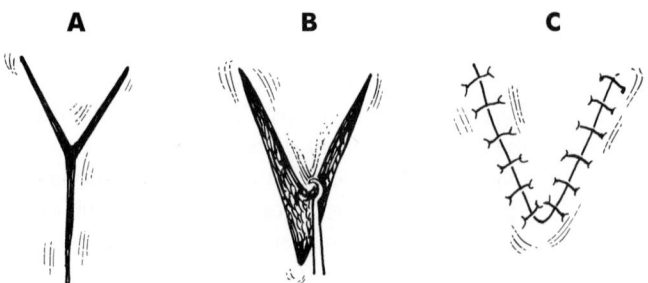

FIG. 14-71   Classic Y-V–plasty incision in bladder neck.

VESICOURETHRAL SUSPENSION (MARSHALL-MARCHETTI-KRANTZ CYSTOURETHROPEXY)

The Marshall-Marchetti operation is the traditional retropubic vesicourethral suspension and requires elevation of the pubococcygeal muscle surrounding the urethra and bladder neck for the correction of stress incontinence caused by an abnormal urethrovesical angle.

Modifications of the Marshall-Marchetti-Krantz include the Burch retropubic colposuspension and the fascial sling procedure.

Procedural considerations

The patient is usually placed in a moderate Trendelenburg position, frog-legged, with supports under each knee to allow for intraoperative vaginal manipulation. Abdominal and vaginal preps are required. A Foley catheter is inserted into the urethra at the beginning of surgery. This procedure is often combined with an abdominal hysterectomy. Surgeon and assistant double-glove for vaginal manipulation.

The basic laparotomy set and abdominal hysterectomy instruments (see Chapter 13), if needed, are used, plus the following:

1 Mason-Judd bladder retractor	2 Extra-long needle holders, retropubic needle holders, or Heaney needle holders
Nonabsorbable sutures, no. 0 or 1, swaged to 5/8-circle needles	

Operative procedure

1. A Foley catheter is inserted in the bladder through the urethra. A suprapubic transverse incision is made to expose the prevesical space of Retzius. The bladder retractor is positioned with small, moist laparotomy pads in place.
2. The bladder and urethra are freed from the posterior surface of the rectus muscle and symphysis pubis by gentle blunt manipulation.
3. The assistant places two fingers into the vagina, lifting the urethra upward against the symphysis pubis to facilitate ease of repair of the periurethral musculofascial structures.
4. A heavy, nonabsorbable atraumatic suture on a Heaney needle holder is placed through the supporting fascia of the vaginal wall on each side of the urethra. The suture is passed through the symphysis pubis, providing support to the urethra and bladder neck.
5. Generally, a row of three heavy, nonabsorbable sutures is placed on each side of the urethra, the most proximal being located just at the vesical neck.
6. The area is drained, and the wound is closed in layers and dressed.
7. The vagina may be packed with 2-inch packing, which should be removed after 24 to 36 hours. The Foley catheter is connected to a closed urinary drainage system.

TRANSVAGINAL BLADDER NECK SUSPENSION (RAZ PROCEDURE)

Vesical neck suspensions have distinct advantages over traditional open retropubic urethrovesical suspensions. The incision is superficial, the bladder and bladder neck are not dissected, and the paraurethral tissues that suspend the vesical neck are buttressed vaginally.

The original vesical neck suspension for urinary stress incontinence was developed by Pereya. This method involves insertion of the Pereya needle (Fig. 14-72, *A*) blindly through a small suprapubic stab wound. The paraurethral tissues are suspended with no. 30 stainless steel wire.

Stamey modified this technique and developed the first endoscopic vesical neck suspension by using the cystoscope to place sutures, buttressed by Gore-Tex or Dacron bolsters, exactly at the vesical neck.

Raz modified the Stamey method by placing sutures lateral to the urethra and bladder neck, lowering the risk of postoperative bladder neck obstruction. The Raz procedure has become the most popular technique for simple bladder neck suspension.

Other urethrovesical suspensions for stress incontinence, without an accompanying cystocele, include the Winter procedure and the Gittes procedure. Variations of these techniques for the patient with an accompanying cystocele include the Raz Sling procedure (vaginal wall sling) and the pubovaginal sling procedure.

Procedural considerations

The patient is placed in the lithotomy position. Although the procedure is not lengthy, care must be taken to ensure proper body alignment and avoid pressure areas when positioning the patient. The legs, positioned in stirrups, are extended to promote a flat lower abdomen. The buttocks must be at the edge of the lower hinge of the OR bed for placement of the weighted vaginal retractor. A lumbar sup-

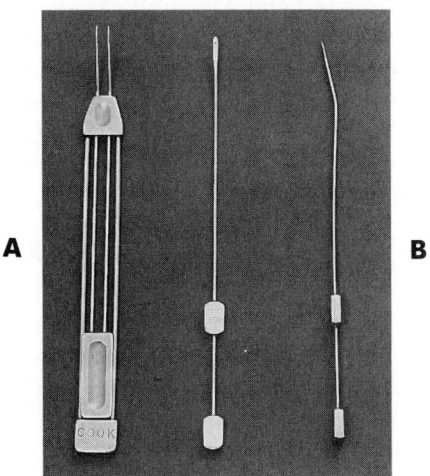

FIG. 14-72   **A,** Litvak Pereyra ligature needle, 28 cm long. **B,** Stamey needles. Used in conjunction with the treatment of female urinary incontinence.

Courtesy Pilling Co., Fort Washington, Pa.

port may help alleviate undue stress on the lower back and sacrum. After preoperative hair removal, the entire perineum, vagina, and suprapubic area are prepped. A drape is placed across the rectum to isolate it from the surgical field. Necessary instrumentation includes the following:

Vaginal instrument set	Asepto syringe
Cystoscopy setup	Vaginal packing
Pereya needles, or Stamey needles: straight, 15 degrees, and 30 degrees (Fig. 14-72, *B*), or	Nonabsorbable monofilament suture ties, no. 2
Double-prong ligature carriers	Gore-Tex bolsters, 4 mm (optional)
Martin needles, no. 7	Antibiotic irrigation (often gentamicin)
Foley catheter, 14 Fr, 5 ml (optional)	Indigo carmine (for IV administration)
Cystocath or Stamey-Malecot suprapubic catheter, no. 12 or 14	Triple sulfa or antibiotic vaginal cream

Operative procedure

1. The labia minor are sutured laterally to expose the vaginal introitus.
2. The weighted speculum is placed in the vagina.
3. A suprapubic catheter is generally placed through a stab wound in the usual manner. A Foley catheter is placed intraurethrally and the bladder drained.
4. With gentle traction on the intraurethral Foley, the anterior vaginal wall is palpated to locate the bladder neck.
5. Injectable 0.9% saline, often mixed with a local anesthetic for bleeding and pain management, is injected into the anterior vaginal wall to aid in tissue dissection.
6. An inverted U incision is made with the legs of the U distal to the bladder neck and the base of the U midway between the bladder neck and external urethral meatus.
7. The vaginal tissue is dissected laterally from the legs of the U toward the pubic bone over the periurethral fascia. Using sharp dissection with scissors, the retropubic space is opened. All adhesions within the space and along the urethral length are released with blunt finger dissection.
8. Bilaterally, helical stitches of heavy nonabsorbable monofilament suture material, on a Mayo needle, are placed vaginally to incorporate the urethropelvic fascia (at the medial edge of the retropubic space) with the pubocervical fascia and anterior vaginal wall.
9. A 3-cm transverse suprapubic incision is made above the superior margin of the pubic bone to the level of the rectus fascia.
10. The Pereya or Stamey needle of choice, or a double-prong ligature carrier, is inserted into the suprapubic incision and through the rectus fascia just above the symphysis pubis. The needle is guided through the rec-

tus fascia into the vaginal incision to meet the surgeon's index finger in the retropubic vaginal space.

11. The ligatures are transferred to the suprapubic wound with the ligature carrier and pulled upward.
12. The Foley is removed and the cystoscope inserted to determine bladder patency.
13. The vaginal incision is closed with a continuous locking stitch of no. 2-0 absorbable suture. A Sultrin-impregnated vaginal packing is placed.
14. The suspension sutures are tied separately with multiple knots and are then brought across the midline and tied together.
15. The skin is closed, following irrigation, with no. 4-0 subcuticular absorbable suture.
16. Steri-Strips and a small gauze dressing are placed over the abdominal wound and the cystocath secured and connected to drainage.

BLADDER AUGMENTATION

Augmentation enterocystoplasty, augmentation cystoplasty, clam cystoplasty, ileocystoplasty, and sigmoidocystoplasty are various terms for procedures employed to surgically enlarge the bladder capacity. The segment of bowel used is reformed into a semispherical (clam) shape to decrease peristaltic contractions and is anastomosed to the opened bladder dome. The result is a low-pressure reservoir that provides improved bladder capacity and urinary compliance.

A wide range of conditions previously treated with urinary diversion may now be successfully managed with this technique. Indications include reflex incontinence unresponsive to medical management, a small bladder capacity, detrusor hyperactivity with compromised bladder function, chronically contracted bladder as resulting from radiation or repeated infections, and neuropathic bladder combined with recurrent urinary tract infections or compromised renal function.

Intermittent catheterization and bladder irrigations are necessary postoperatively. The patient must be able and willing to learn to perform these procedures and accept this alteration in life-style.

Procedural considerations

Almost all segments of bowel as well as the stomach have been employed for bladder augmentation. Selection depends on anatomic factors, functional characteristics, and surgeon's preference. In some cases ureteral reimplantation or associated bladder outlet procedures are deemed necessary. They should be incorporated to achieve a one-stage procedure.

The patient is in the supine position and under general anesthesia. The female patient may be in a frog-leg or lithotomy position, particularly if an outlet procedure is to be performed. A nasogastric tube is inserted following induction. The entire abdomen and genitalia are prepped and draped into the operating field.

A Foley catheter is inserted in the sterile field, and the bladder is filled to capacity once the abdomen has been entered. Basic laparotomy and intestinal instruments are required.

Operative procedure

1. A supraumbilical to symphysis midline abdominal incision is made. The peritoneal cavity is exposed utilizing a Bookwalter or similar retractor.
2. The intestines and stomach are examined and the appropriate segment for reconstruction is chosen (Fig. 14-73, *A*).
3. A sagittal bladder incision is made from 2 cm cephalad to the bladder neck anteriorly and across the anterior bladder wall, the peritonealized dome surface, and the posterior bladder wall to 2 cm above the posterior interureteric ridge. This causes the bladder to be bivalved in a clam shape design.
4. Traction sutures are placed bilaterally along the bladder incision. The length of the incision is measured to correlate with the corresponding segment of bowel or stomach. Average length required is 25 cm.
5. The segment to be used is mobilized and the mesentery is closed cephalad so the segment is on the retroperitoneum. The segment is left attached to its mesentery to maintain blood supply (Fig. 14-73, *B*).
6. The isolated segment is opened, trimmed and detubularized. It is then doubly folded and sutured to form a cup patch (Fig. 14-73, *C*).
7. Anastomosis is accomplished with a running, intermittent locking, absorbable suture, beginning at the posterior apex and running up each side. With one third of the attachment complete, sutures are then placed at the anterior apex and run bilaterally to meet cephalad (Fig. 14-73, *D*).
8. Integrity of the anastomosis is checked by again filling the bladder and observing for leaks.
9. A routine abdominal closure is performed and dressings applied.
10. The nasogastric tube stays in place for 3 postoperative days. The Foley catheter will remain for 7 to 14 days. Some surgeons may choose to place a suprapubic catheter instead of a Foley.

IMPLANTATION OF A PROSTHETIC URETHRAL SPHINCTER

This procedure is usually done as a last measure in patients with stress incontinence where other modalities have failed. Problems with the device have included foreign body reaction, persistent urethral pressure causing urethral erosion, and fluid hydraulic failure.

Procedural considerations

The artificial sphincter unit has an abdominally placed, pressure-regulated reservoir that maintains a constant, predetermined pressure on the periurethral cuff. Because of the

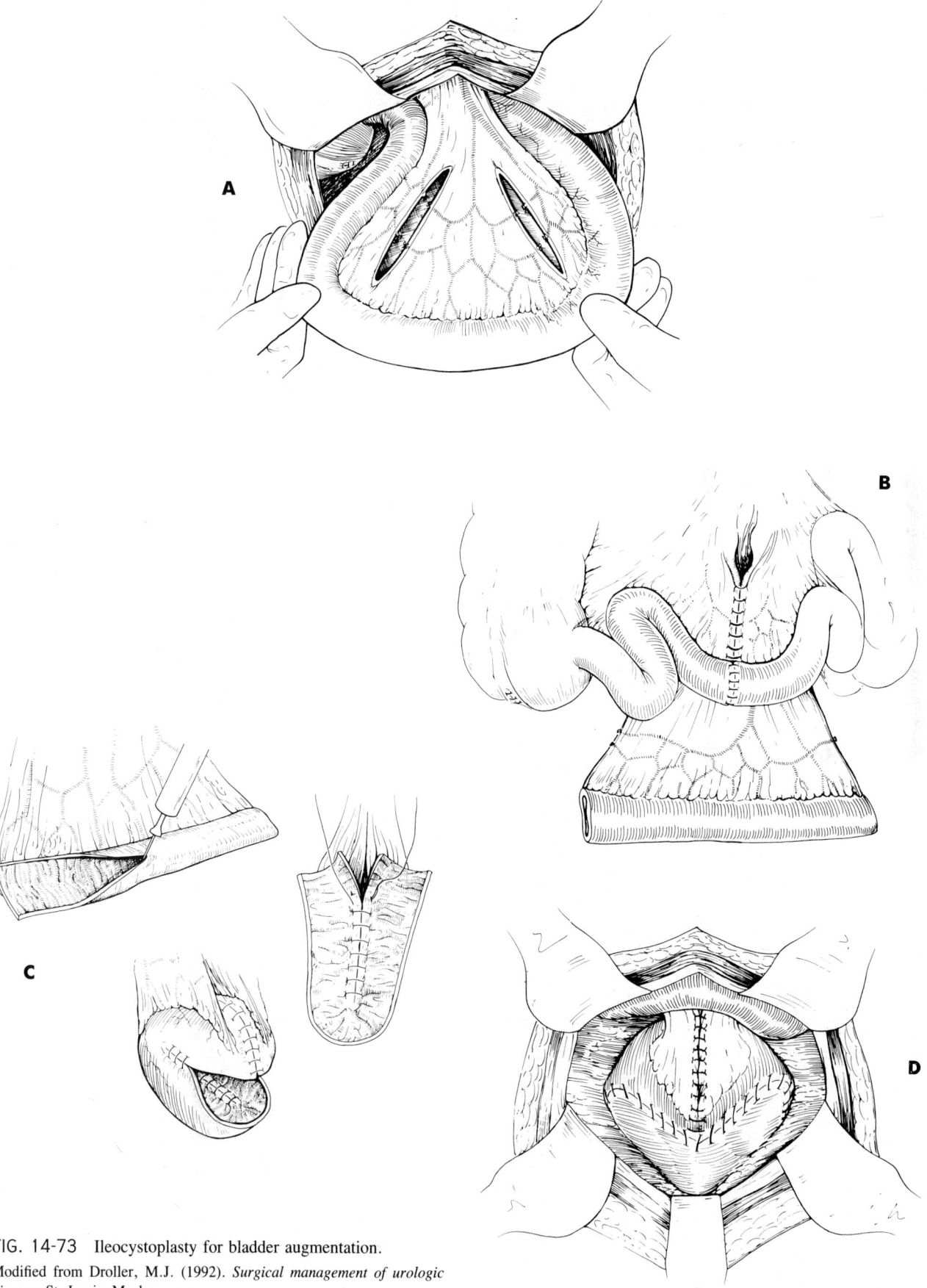

FIG. 14-73 Ileocystoplasty for bladder augmentation.

Modified from Droller, M.J. (1992). *Surgical management of urologic
disease*. St. Louis: Mosby.

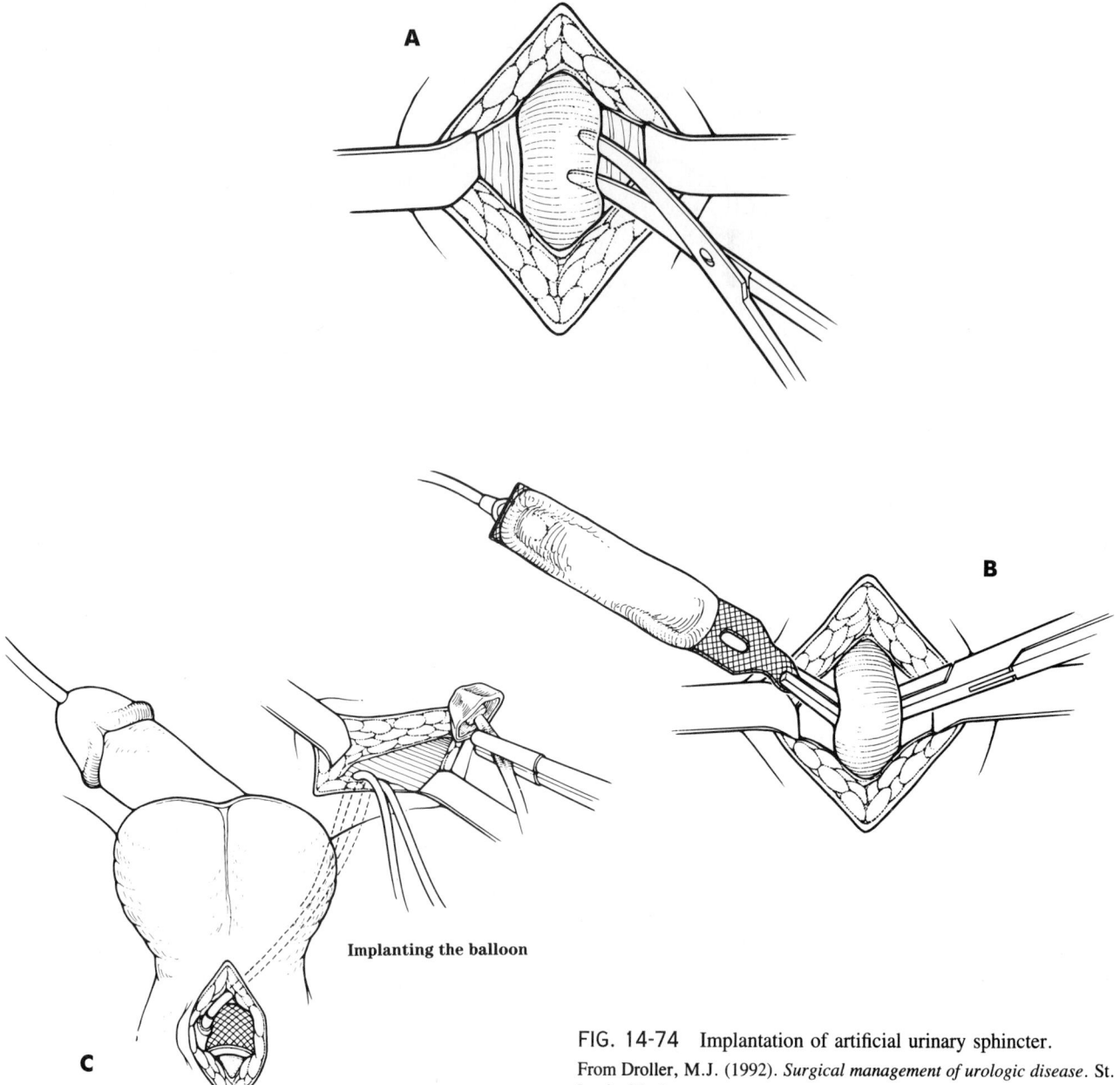

Implanting the balloon

FIG. 14-74   Implantation of artificial urinary sphincter.
From Droller, M.J. (1992). *Surgical management of urologic disease*. St. Louis: Mosby.

connection between the reservoir and cuff, any increase in intraabdominal pressure transmits more fluid into the cuff. This connection allows for a compensatory increase in urethral resistance during coughing or straining.

The scrotal or labial pump shifts the fluid into the cuff to the reservoir to allow bladder emptying. The fluid reenters the cuff through a resistor in about 60 to 120 seconds. The locking button in the AMS 800 artificial sphincter unit traps fluid in the reservoir to allow activation of the cuff.

Standard laparotomy and lithotomy setups are required, as well as the sphincter components, 12.5% Hypaque, and an antibiotic solution, as used with a penile implant. The patient is placed in a modified lithotomy position.

Stricture disease is more commonly found in the male population, and the most common cuff placement is around the bulbous urethra. Bladder neck placement of the cuff is generally reserved only for females.

Operative procedure (bulbous urethral cuff)

1. Perineal and transverse suprapubic incisions are made.
2. The bulbous urethra is mobilized through a midline perineal incision (Fig. 14-74, *A*).
3. A 2-cm space is created beneath the bulbocavernous muscle and around the bulbous urethra. The cuff, tab end first, is placed around the bulbous urethra (Fig. 14-74, *B*).

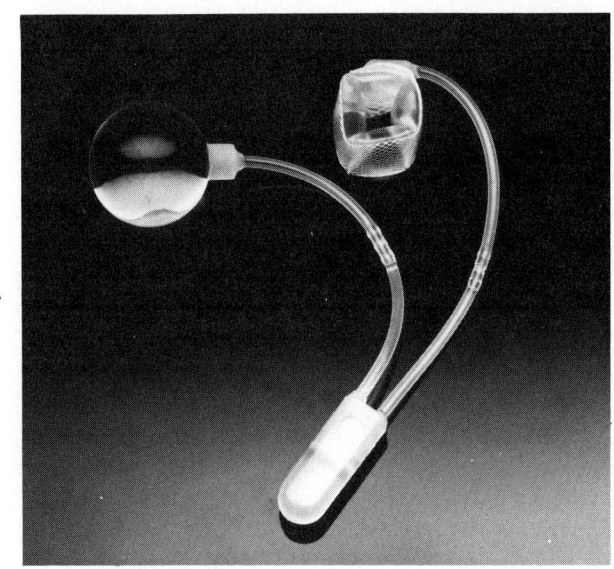

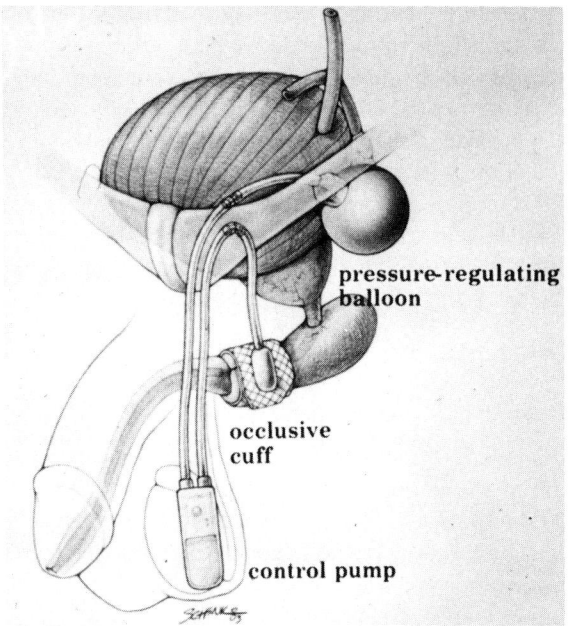

FIG. 14-75 **A,** AMS Sphincter 800. **B,** Final placement of artificial urinary sphincter.
A courtesy American Medical Systems, Minnetonka, Minn; **B** modified from Droller, M.J. (1992). *Surgical management of urologic disease.* St. Louis: Mosby.

4. The reservoir is placed beneath the rectus muscle through the suprapubic incision (Fig. 14-74, *C*).
5. The pump is introduced through the suprapubic incision and transferred to the scrotum through a subcutaneous tunnel created between the two incisions.
6. The reservoir, cuff, and pump are connected and filled with 12.5% Hypaque to the appropriate volume (Fig. 14-75).
7. The wound is closed and dressed with gauze sponges. A urethral catheter is usually not inserted.

RADICAL CYSTECTOMY AND PELVIC LYMPHADENECTOMY

Cystectomy is the total excision of the urinary bladder and adjacent structures along with pelvic lymph nodes. Cystectomy is a surgical consideration when a vesical malignancy has invaded the muscular wall of the bladder or when frequent recurrences of widespread papillary tumors do not respond to endoscopic or chemotherapeutic management. The patient should be medically able to withstand surgery with the expectation of reasonable longevity. Total cystectomy necessitates permanent urinary diversion into an ileal or colonic conduit. Conservative measures such as radiotherapy or chemotherapy may be used when the neoplasm is far advanced.

In a male patient the prostate gland, seminal vesicles, and distal ureters are removed with the bladder and its peritoneal surface. In a woman the bladder, urethra, distal urethra, uterus, cervix, and proximal third of the vagina are removed.

Procedural considerations

The patient is placed in the supine position. Instruments are as described for major abdominal procedures. For a male patient, if the prostate and seminal vesicles are to be removed, prostatectomy instruments should be added. For a female, vaginal and abdominal hysterectomy as well as plastic surgery instruments should be added (see Chapters 13 and 23).

Operative procedure

1. A midline incision from the epigastrium to the symphysis pubis, curving to the left of the umbilicus, is generally preferred.
2. The incision is deepened, the rectus muscles retracted laterally, and the peritoneum opened. At this point, long instruments are necessary.
3. Abdominal exploration and pelvic lymphadenectomy with frozen sections are performed to rule out metastatic disease.
4. In a male patient the bladder dome is lifted at its peritoneal surface. Dissection proceeds laterally on either side with ligation of the major vesical arteries. The bladder is then retracted to expose the prostate and seminal vesicles, which are dissected free in continuity with the bladder. The vas deferens is divided and the urethra cut at the level of the pelvic diaphragm.
5. The surgical specimen consisting of the bladder, distal ureters, prostate, seminal vesicles, and distal vas is removed en bloc. The urethra is ligated with absorbable suture.

6. Lap pads are placed in the denuded pelvis, and pressure is applied to reduce blood loss from oozing.

7. Urinary diversion by isolated ileal or colonic conduit may be performed or continent urinary diversion may be considered. Direct anastomosis of the ureters to the colon may be performed by ureterosigmoidostomy.

8. The surgical approach for total cystectomy in the female patient is as described for the male patient, but the urethra is removed in continuity with the bladder and internal reproductive organs.

BLADDER SUBSTITUTION (SUBSTITUTION CYSTOPLASTY)

Right colocystoplasty

Following supratrigonal resection of the bladder the right colon makes an ideal replacement reservoir with a direct enteric-to-proximal membranous urethral anastomosis. This procedure has become more functionally effective with the use of intermittent self-catheterization and selective implantation of a prosthetic urinary sphincter.

The ideal candidate for a right colocystoplasty following cystectomy for carcinoma is a male with a normal urethra, a proximally located, well-differentiated bladder tumor, absence of carcinoma in situ, and proof that the prostatic urethra is free from disease. High-dose radiation offers appreciable risks for postoperative complications and is contraindicated with enterourethral anastomosis.

Ileocecal bladder substitution

Over the last 30 years attempts at bladder replacement with an ileal segment of bowel have yielded disappointing results. There has been a high incidence of recurrent carcinoma, renal damage, incontinence, and postoperative strictures and fistulas. The ileum has been used as a reservoir to restore urinary continuity because it possesses a low intraluminal pressure. However, the short mesentery does not always permit the bowel to reach the urethra. The results with the current antireflux techniques are not consistently successful.

Although most patients have attained daytime urinary control, the majority still have problems with enuresis. Deteriorization of the upper urinary tract is a known risk with this procedure, and therefore ileocecal substitution is met with mixed reactions and recommendations.

Sigmoidocystoplasty

Because of its ease of construction, bladder proximity, decreased obstruction from mucus, and large capacity, the sigmoid colon has been appealing to many surgeons in their attempt to create a new bladder. More efficient emptying with a larger reservoir capacity seems to occur with a sigmoid replacement. Results yield higher intraluminal pressures, more effective urinary flow rates, and less nocturnal incontinence than with ileal segments.

Ileoascending cystoplasty

In an effort to improve the intestinal reservoir's capacity and antirefluxing effectiveness, the use of the ascending colon as a continent reservoir was introduced in 1965. This technique has a number of anatomic advantages over other methods of bladder replacement. The segment used can include the hepatic flexure and proximal transverse

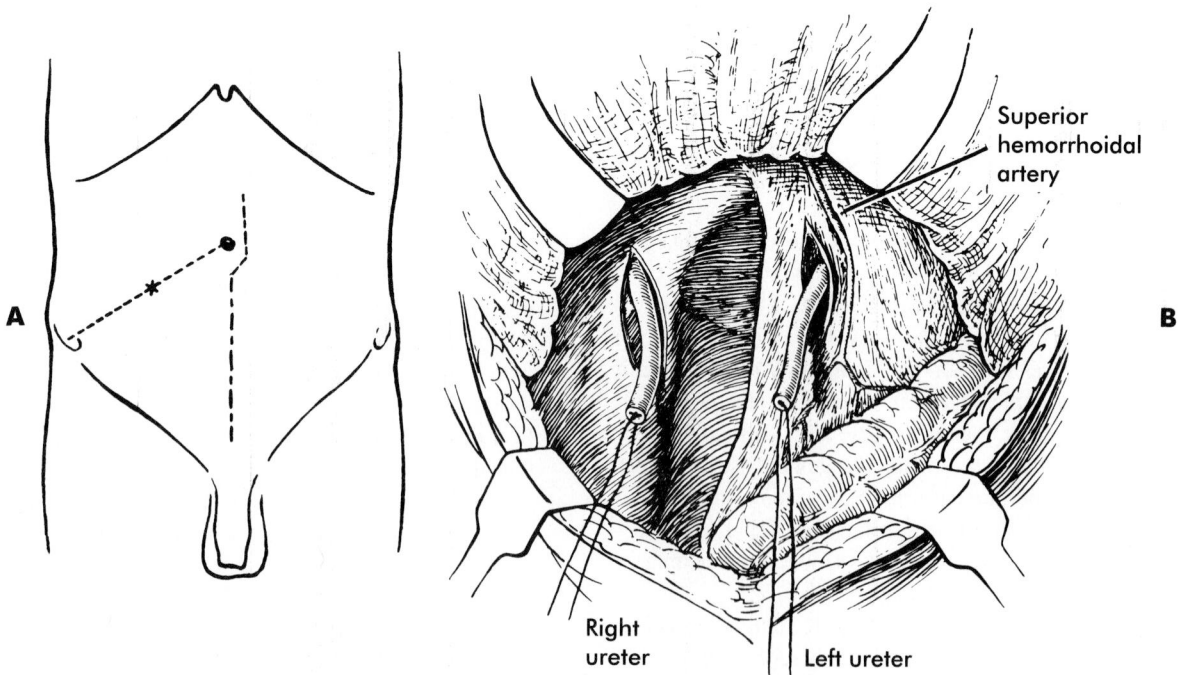

FIG. 14-76 Major steps of operation for ileal conduit, urinary diversion.
Modified from Campbell, F.M., & Harrison, J.H. (1970). *Campbell's urology*. Philadelphia: W.B. Saunders.

colon. A large-capacity reservoir is obtained, and colonic incision or tailoring is not required to achieve an appropriate shape. It easily reaches any site within the pelvis and can be anastomosed directly to the urethra without tension.

CUTANEOUS URINARY DIVERSIONS
Ileal conduit

The ileal conduit, a type of cutaneous urinary diversion, is one method by which the urine flow is diverted to an isolated loop of bowel. One end of the isolated loop is brought out through the skin so the urine can be collected in a pouch, which is intermittently emptied. The stoma sites should be carefully selected preoperatively by the surgeon and enterostomal therapist. The selected site, usually in the right lower quadrant of the abdomen (Fig. 14-76, *A*), is marked with a fine needle dipped in methylene blue to prevent erasure during skin preparation. The surgeon's goal is to create a round, protruding stoma without wrinkles in the skin to prevent urine leakage under the collecting device. Puckering around the stoma is minimized by using a subcuticular technique when suturing the stoma in place.

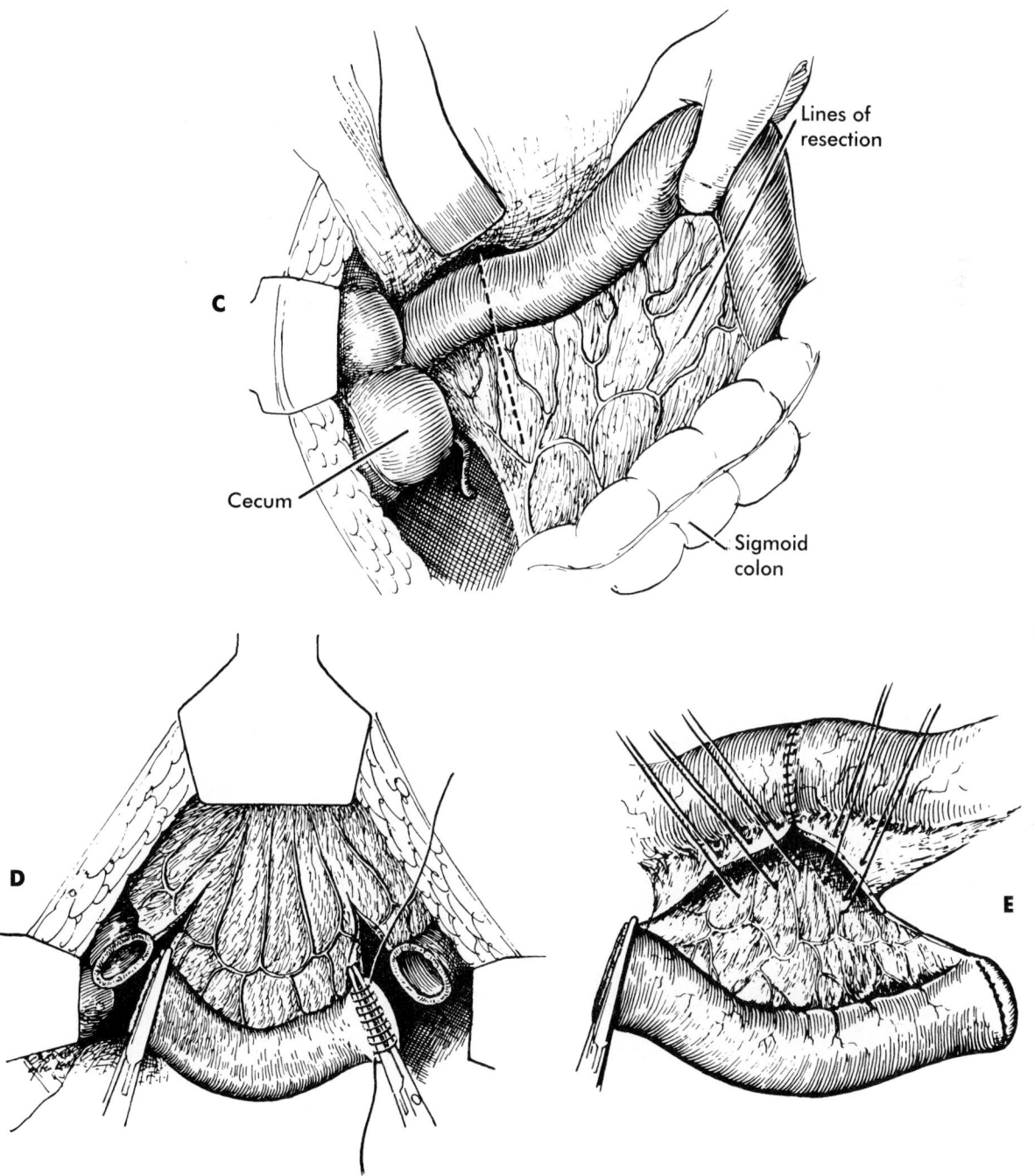

FIG. 14-76, CONT'D   Major steps of operation for ileal conduit, urinary diversion.

Continued.

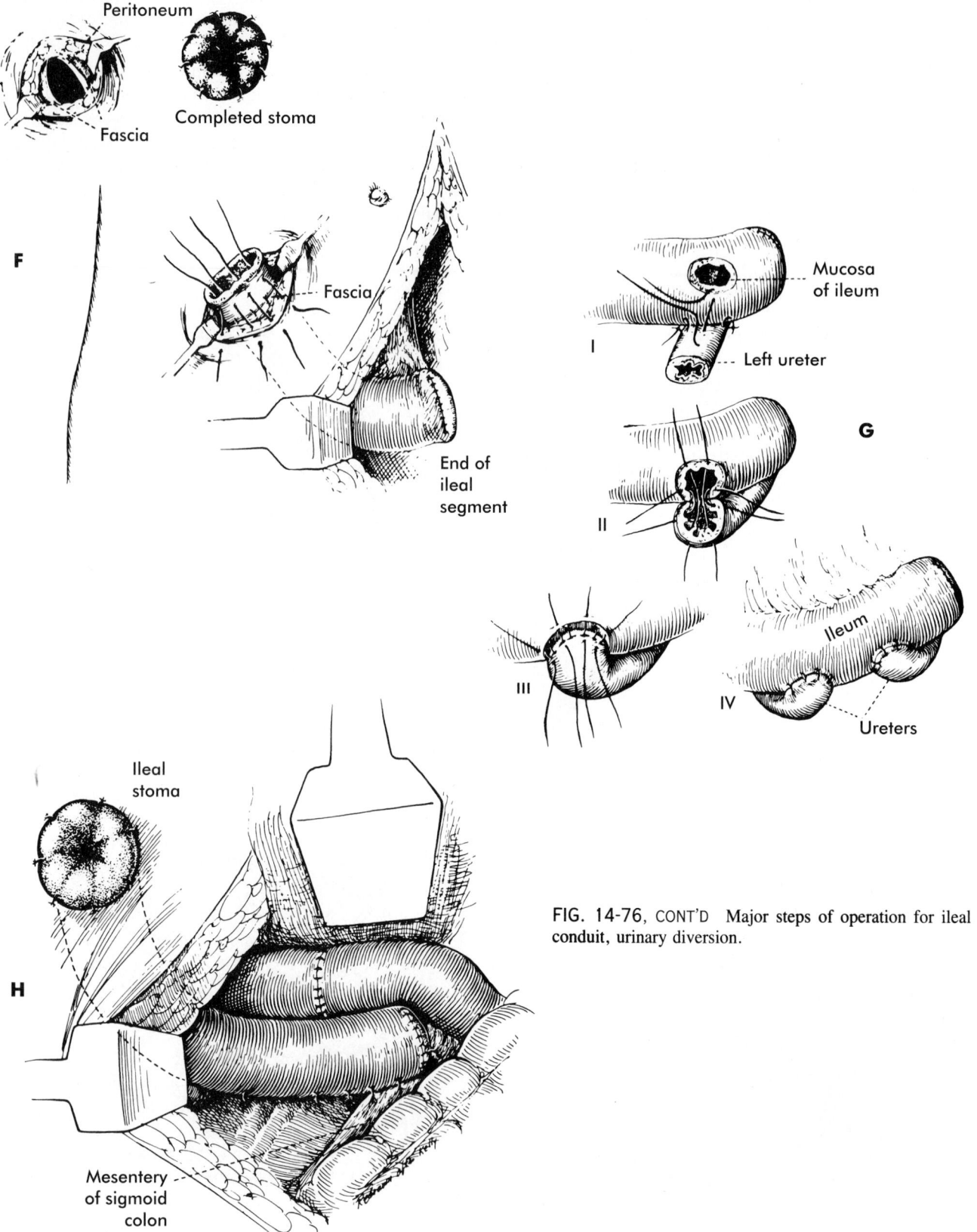

Peritoneum

Completed stoma

Fascia

F

Fascia

End of ileal segment

Mucosa of ileum

Left ureter

I

II

G

III

IV

Ileum

Ureters

FIG. 14-76, CONT'D   Major steps of operation for ileal conduit, urinary diversion.

Ileal stoma

H

Mesentery of sigmoid colon

Procedural considerations

The patient is placed in the supine position. The ureters are isolated at the pelvic brim. A cystectomy, prostatectomy, or hysterectomy may also be done at the time of the surgery.

Operative procedure

1. The bladder is decompressed with a catheter. The abdomen is entered through a midline abdominal incision. A self-retaining abdominal retractor is placed so the viscera are excluded from the region of dissection.
2. The ureters are identified and mobilized by severing them 1 to ½ inch from the bladder (Fig. 14-76, *B*). A retroperitoneal tunnel is made so that the left ureter lies close to the right ureter.
3. The distal ileum and mesentery are inspected to identify the bowel's blood supply. A drain is passed through the mesentery, midway between the two main arterial arcades adjacent to the ileum at the proximal and distal ends of the selected segment. This segment usually comprises 15 to 20 cm of the terminal ileum, a few centimeters from the ileocecal valve (Fig. 14-76, *C*).
4. Care is exercised to preserve the ileocecal artery and adequate circulation to the isolated ileal segment. The peritoneum is incised over the proposed line of division of the mesentery. Intestinal clamps are placed across the ileum, and the bowel is divided flush with the clamps. By gastrointestinal technique (see Chapter 10) the proximal end of the isolated ileal segment is closed first with a layer of absorbable sutures and then with a second layer of interrupted no. 2-0 nonabsorbable sutures. The proximal and distal segments of ileum are reanastomosed end-to-end in two layers (Fig. 14-76, *D*).
   NOTE: The advent of stapling devices has allowed a modification of the standard intestinal anastomosis. Stapling devices, with absorbable staples, are available for use in ureterointestinal procedures.
5. The mesenteric incision is closed with interrupted nonabsorbable sutures (Fig. 14-76, *E*).
6. The closed proximal end of the conduit segment is fixed to the posterior peritoneum (Fig. 14-76, *F*). The ureters are implanted in the ileal segment by fine instruments and no. 4-0 absorbable ureteral sutures on atraumatic needles (Fig. 14-76, *G*). The peritoneum and muscle of the abdominal wall lateral to the original incision are separated by blunt dissection. The abdominal opening for the stoma is made. The distal opening of the ileal conduit is then drawn through a fenestration in the muscle, fascia, and skin. The ileum is fixed to the fascia with quadrant sutures of no. 2-0. A rosebud stoma is constructed at the same time the ileum is sutured to the skin with subcuticular suture (Fig. 14-76, *H*). Ureteral stents are usually left in the stoma, and a urinary collecting pouch is placed over the rosebud stoma to collect urine. The wound is drained with two Jackson-Pratt drains. The abdominal incision is closed with no. 0 nonabsorbable suture. The skin is reapproximated with skin staples.

In cases that do not involve bladder cancer, a surgeon may choose to leave the bladder in situ rather than subject a debilitated patient to further surgery. In certain cases of extensive bladder carcinoma the surgeon may elect to treat the patient with radiation in an attempt to decrease the size of the tumor and "sterilize" the regional lymph nodes before performing a cystectomy.

Sigmoid conduit

Nonrefluxing, tunneled, ureteral anastomoses have been successfully achieved utilizing the sigmoid colon. A right paramedian incision is made and the stoma is located in the left lower quadrant of the abdomen. The redundant portion of the sigmoid colon is used for the conduit. The procedure and construction of the stoma are similar to that for the ileal conduit.

Transverse colon conduit

This method also provides a nonrefluxing urinary diversion. Patients that have had previous abdominal irradiation or surgery that has affected viable ureteral length may benefit from this approach. Operative technique is similar to that for the ileal conduit.

Ileocecal conduit

Ileocecal vessels provide an abundant blood supply to the bowel. These vessels are also easily mobilized, allowing for a viable nonrefluxing system. The most important and unique step to this method of conduit construction is reinforcement of the ileocecal valve by intussusception at the ileocecal junction. The balance of the procedure remains similar to the other techniques discussed.

CONTINENT URINARY DIVERSIONS

All continent urinary diversions provide an easily catheterized stoma and a nonrefluxing ureteral anastomosis. They may potentially be anastomosed to the proximal urethra, thus forming an orthotopic bladder. The Kock pouch, the right colocystoplasty and the Camey version of the ileocystoplasty have been modified for anastomosis to a urethral stump, or the prostatic capsule, resulting in effective continent bladder replacement. "Le bag" was developed specifically for orthotopic bladder replacement.

Kock pouch

A section of ileum proximal to the ileocecal valve is harvested and formed into a U configuration. The legs of the U are sewn together at the antimesenteric border. The intestine is opened adjacent to the serosal suture at the antimesenteric border and the back wall of the pouch is reinforced with absorbable suture.

Nipple valves are created proximally and distally by intussusception of the bowel into the reservoir cavity. Once the nipples are fixed to the sidewall of the reservoir with absorbable suture or polyglycolic staples, the anterior wall is closed. The ureters are anastomosed to the afferent limb of the pouch, preventing reflux. The efferent limb is drawn through the stoma site and anchored to the abdominal wall fascia.

Indiana pouch

This technique is a modification of the original ileocecal diversion. Surgery proceeds as for any diversionary procedure. The ileocecal valve is reinforced with nonabsorbable suture. Two rows of nonabsorbable suture are used to then imbricate the ileal segment, which serves as a catheterizable limb once it is brought to the skin level as a stoma. The cecal segment is detubularized by incising along the taenia and anastomosing the distal edge horizontally to the proximal portion. It becomes the reservoir.

"Le bag"

"Le bag" requires ascending colon and terminal ileum for its construction. Blood supply to the reservoir is provided by the ileocecal artery. The selected length of bowel is opened along its antimesenteric border, folded, and the free borders of the ileum and colon are sewn together. The pouch is rotated 180 degrees into the pelvis. The urethral remnant is anastomosed through a residual opening left in the pouch. The ureters are reimplanted through a small opening in the anterior suture line.

SURGERY OF THE URETERS AND KIDNEYS

Stones, infections, and tumors are the most common causes of urinary tract obstruction necessitating surgery to prevent renal obstruction and subsequent failure. Obstruction may also result from congenital malforma-

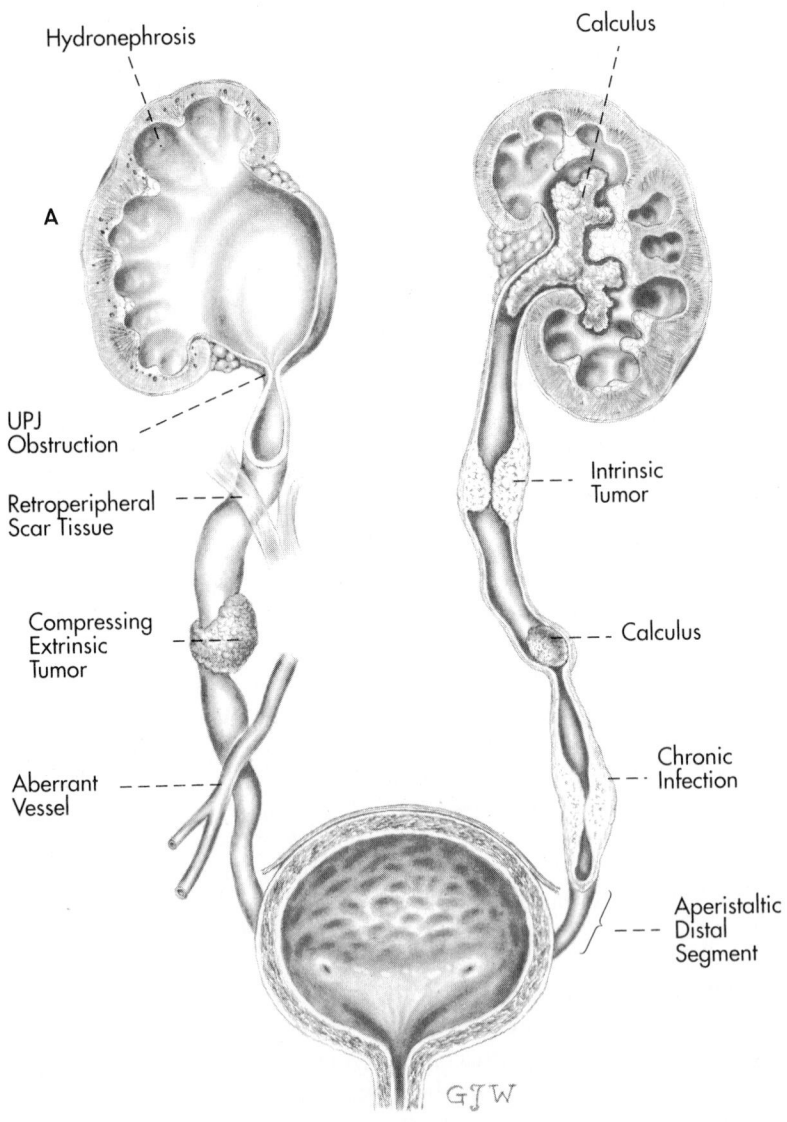

FIG. 14-77 Some common causes of urinary tract obstruction.
From Gray, M. (1992). *Genitourinary disorders*. St. Louis: Mosby.

tions or previous operations on the urinary tract (Fig. 14-77).

Although the causes of many kidney stones are obscure, certain conditions such as obstruction, stasis, and imbalance of metabolism predispose to their formation. Stones consist of various elements: calcium oxalate, calcium phosphate, magnesium ammonium phosphate, uric acid, calcium carbonate, and cystine. Stones removed during surgery are subjected to chemical analysis. These specimens should be submitted in a dry jar. Fixative agents such as formalin invalidate the results of the analysis.

Stones in the renal pelvis may fall into the ureteropelvic junction and obstruct the flow of urine. However, calculi less than 1 cm in diameter may pass down the ureter and lodge at a more distal location, such as where the ureter crosses the iliac vessels or at the ureterovesical junction. A stone may remain in a renal calyx and continue to enlarge, eventually filling the entire renal collecting system (staghorn calculus). Hydroureteronephrosis, infection, and destruction of renal parenchyma frequently result from unrelieved obstruction.

Hypothermia is useful in renal stone surgery as a means of prolonging the safe period of renal ischemia during extensive parenchymal manipulation. This method is also employed for surgery of the renal artery. Several methods enable renal cooling: ice slush or cold saline solution, surface cooling coils, perfusion of cold solutions through the renal artery, or a variation of these basic techniques, for example, perfusion of the renal pelvis with saline that has been cooled by a coil immersed in ice slush.

PROCEDURAL CONSIDERATIONS

Saline slush for renal surgery may be prepared in several ways:

1. Sterile Mason jars are filled with sterile normal saline solution and double-wrapped in sterile plastic bags. Each bag is individually wrapped and secured with a twist tie. The Mason jars are placed in a bucket of ice, to which 2 pints of isopropyl alcohol and two boxes of salt are added and mixed, for 2 to 3 hours. When the saline is ready for use, the circulating nurse removes the wrapped Mason jar from the ice, opens the plastic bags by sterile technique, and presents the Mason jar to the scrub nurse. The scrub nurse shakes the contents of the Mason jar to cause crystallization of the saline. The slush is removed from the Mason jar with a sterile spoon.
2. A rigid plastic container of 1000 ml of normal saline or lactated Ringer's solution may be placed on its side in a freezer several hours before surgery. To prevent the solution from solidifying, the container should be rotated one half turn every 20 to 30 minutes. Sterile slush may then be poured directly into a sterile basin as required.
3. A refrigeration unit that produces sterile slush provides a cost-effective, time-saving alternative to the other methods of slush preparation.

Surgical approach in renal surgery depends on the patient's condition, the amount of exposure needed, and the surgical procedure to be performed. For renal masses attention is directed toward control of the vascular pedicle. For this reason patient position and surgical exposure are of prime consideration. There are three principal surgical approaches to the kidney (Fig. 14-78):

1. The simple flank or transabdominal incision is most frequently used and may include removal of the eleventh or twelfth rib. The incision begins at the posterior axillary line and parallels the course of the twelfth rib. It extends forward and slightly downward between the iliac crest and the thorax (Fig. 14-78, *A*).
2. For the lumbar incision, the patient is placed in a supine position with bolsters under the flank and lower thorax. This effectively places the flank in an oblique position, causing the abdominal viscera to fall away from the operative incision. This approach is used for renal neoplasms and affords an excellent approach to the renal pedicle (Fig. 14-78, *B*).
3. The thoracoabdominal exposure is employed primarily for large upper pole renal neoplasms. The tenth and eleventh ribs are usually removed, and the chest cavity is opened, collapsing the lung. The leaves of the diaphragm are separated to expose the kidney. A large retractor, such as a Finochietto, and chest drains are required (Fig. 14-78, *C*).

SURGERY OF THE URETER

Ureterostomy (ureterotomy) is opening the ureter for continued drainage from it into another body part. Cutaneous ureterostomy is diversion of the flow of urine from the kidney, through the ureter, away from the bladder, and onto the skin of the lower abdomen (Fig. 14-79). A suitable urinary collecting device is placed over the ureteral stoma to keep the patient dry.

Ureterectomy is complete removal of the ureter. This procedure is generally employed in collecting system tumors and includes nephrectomy and the excision of a cuff of bladder.

Ureteroureterostomy is segmental resection of a diseased portion of the ureter and reconstruction in continuity of the two normal segments.

Ureteroenterostomy is diversion of the ureter into a segment of the ileum (ureteroileostomy, or more commonly ileal urinary conduit) or into the sigmoid colon (ureterosigmoidostomy). Ureteroneocystostomy (ureterovesical anastomosis) is division of the distal ureter from the bladder and reimplantation of the ureter into the bladder with a submucosal tunnel.

Reconstructive operations may be indicated because of a pathologic condition of the bladder or lower ureter that interferes with normal drainage. Conditions requiring urinary diversion or reconstruction of the urinary tract include malignancy, cystitis, stricture, trauma, and congenital ureterovesical reflux. Invasive vesical malignancy requiring

A Flank approach   **B** Lumbar approach   **C** Thoracoabdominal approach

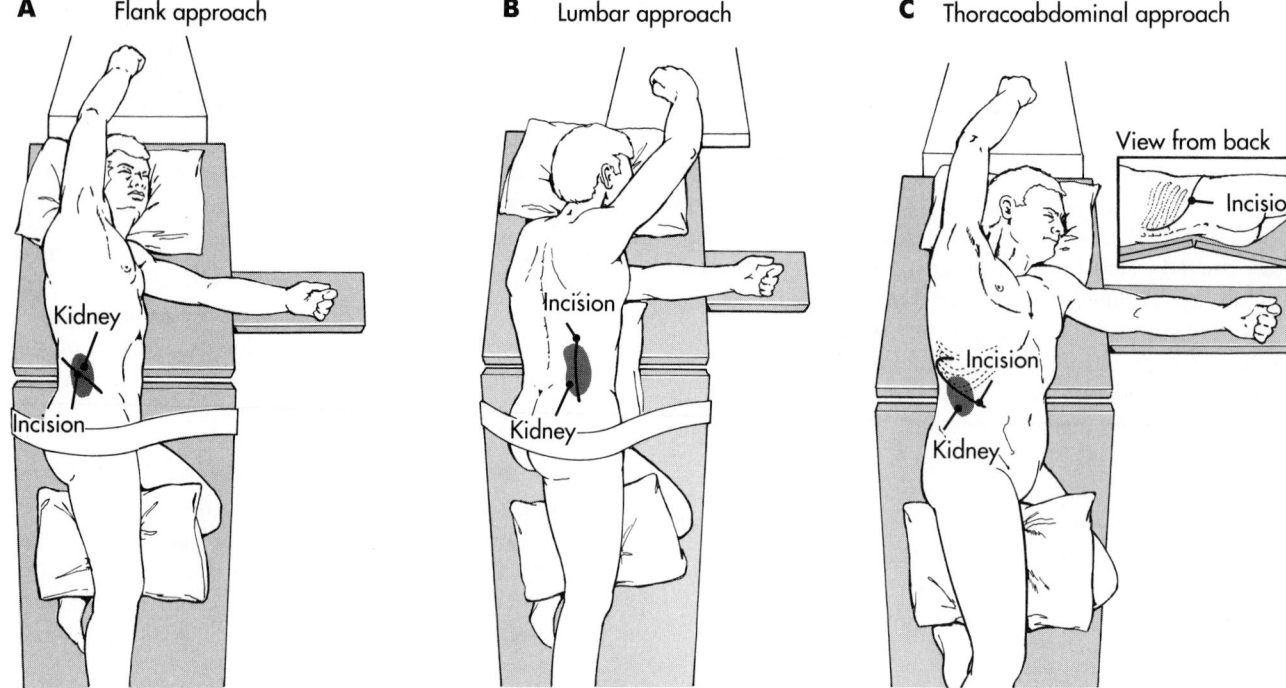

FIG. 14-78 Principal surgical approaches to the kidney.
From Brundage, D. (1992). *Renal disorders*. St. Louis: Mosby.

surgical removal of the bladder necessitates urinary diversion.

Ureterocutaneous transplant, ureterosigmoid anastomosis, and ileal conduit are urinary diversionary procedures performed when the bladder is no longer functioning as a proper urine reservoir. Etiologic factors causing irreparable vesical dysfunction are chronic inflammation, interstitial cystitis, neurogenic bladder, exstrophy, trauma, tumor, and infiltrative disease (amyloidosis). Ureterolithotomy is incision into the ureter and removal of an obstructing calculus.

Procedural considerations

The site of the incision and position of the patient depend on the nature of the proposed surgery. The patient may be placed in the supine position for abdominal surgery, in modified Trendelenburg's position for low abdominal or pelvic surgery, or in the lateral position for high or midureteral obstructing calculi.

Instruments include the nephrectomy set, plus plastic instrumentation for pyeloplasty. Additional instruments may be required, depending on the type of operation and the surgical approach used.

Operative procedures
Ureteral reimplantation

1. The ureter is exposed through the desired incision, which is determined by the location of the pathology.

A ureteral catheter, passed retrograde, may be used to facilitate identification and isolation of the ureter. The ureter is identified and dissected free with long forceps and scissors.
2. The ureter is picked up with the fine traction sutures, freed from the surrounding tissues, and severed at the desired level.
3. The distal end of the ureter is ligated, and the proximal stoma is transferred to the site of anastomosis. The anastomosis is accomplished with fine dissection instruments and fine atraumatic sutures.
4. A soft splinting stent is usually left in place until healing has taken place and free drainage is ensured.
5. The wound is closed in layers and dressed in the routine manner.

Ureterocutaneous transplant (anastomosis)

The surgical approach is the same as for a low ureterolithotomy.

1. The ureter is divided as far distally as possible.
2. The severed ureter is passed retroperitoneally through the lower abdominal wall and is sutured to the skin with an absorbable, everting suture of no. 4-0 on an atraumatic needle to form a stoma. The ureter is handled gently with plastic instruments, fixation forceps, and iris scissors.
3. A small Silastic stenting catheter is passed up into the

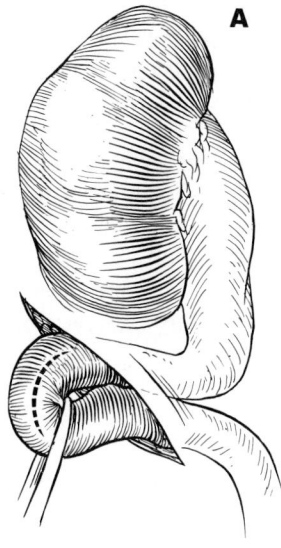

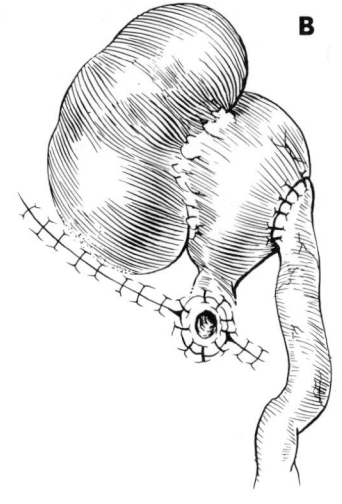

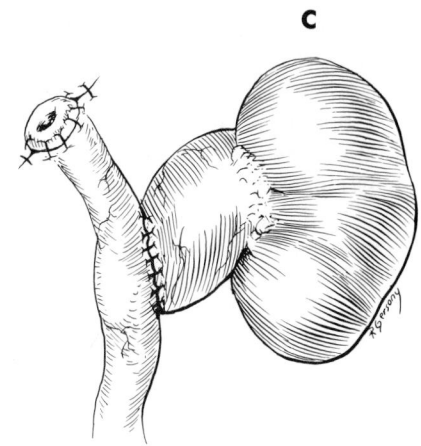

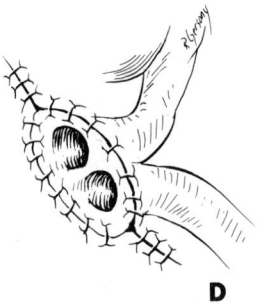

FIG. 14-79 Methods of urinary diversion.
Modified from Droller, M.J. (1992). *Surgical management of urologic disease*. St. Louis: Mosby.

ureter and is left in situ for 48 to 72 hours, during which time ureteral edema subsides. The patient will require a urine-collecting device after surgery.

Ureterosigmoid anastomosis

1. The peritoneal cavity is entered in the routine manner through a lower left paramedian incision. The major portion of the large bowel is protected with moist packs. Deep retractors are placed in position, and with long forceps and scissors the posterior peritoneum is incised.
2. The ureters are identified and divided close to the bladder. The ureters are mobilized and brought through the posterior peritoneal incision to lie near the sigmoid. Traction sutures and smooth tissue forceps are used to handle the ureters.
3. The sigmoid colon is mobilized to prevent tension on the ureteroenteric anastomosis. The sigmoid colon is sutured with no. 3-0 nonabsorbable material to the pelvic peritoneum at a point where the ureter falls easily on the bowel. Using a scalpel with a no. 15 blade, the surgeon makes an incision into the taenia of the sigmoid down to the mucosal layer. The edges of the taenia are undermined to create two parallel flaps.
4. The ureter is laid on the bowel mucosa, and a small slit

is made through the mucosa into the lumen of the colon.
5. With fixation forceps and iris scissors the ureter is beveled to lie flat in the tunical incision. The distal ureter is anchored to the bowel mucosa with no. 4-0 absorbable ureteral sutures on atraumatic needles. The other ureter is anastomosed in the same manner in a position slightly above the first.
6. The tunicae are then loosely reapproximated over the ureter with no. 4-0 absorbable sutures, creating an antireflux anastomosis.
7. The posterior peritoneum is closed with absorbable sutures. Drains are brought out retroperitoneally. The incision is closed, and the wound is dressed.

Ureterolithotomy

A kidney, ureter, and bladder x-ray film should be taken immediately before surgery to determine the exact location of the stone. The surgeon may also schedule a cystoscopic examination preoperatively and may attempt to remove the calculus endoscopically if the stone is in the most distal portion of the ureter.

The location of the calculus determines the surgical approach. A calculus high in the ureter requires a flank incision with possible removal of the twelfth rib; a more distal ureteral calculus requires a lower abdominal incision. Both of these have been described previously in some detail.

1. After exposure of the ureter, the calculus may be kept stationary with Babcock clamps or vessel loops applied above and below the calculus.
2. With a no. 15 blade, the incision in the ureter is made directly over the calculus. The calculus may then be easily removed with a Randall stone forceps.
3. A 10 Fr catheter is passed proximally up and distally down the ureter while irrigating with saline to check for ureteral patency and to dislodge any remaining fragments of calculus.
4. The ureter is closed with no. 4-0 or 5-0 absorbable sutures. All urologic stones should be placed in dry receptacles and sent to the chemistry laboratory for analysis.
5. Either of the approaches described requires routine layer surgical closure.

SURGERY OF THE KIDNEY

Nephrotomy is incision into the kidney, usually over a collecting system containing a calculus.

Pyelotomy is incision into the renal pelvis used as an access to stones in the renal pelvis or collecting system.

Pyelostomy is an opening made in the renal pelvis for temporarily or permanently diverting the flow of urine.

Nephrostomy is creation of an opening into the kidney to maintain temporary or permanent urinary drainage. A nephrostomy is used to correct an obstruction of the urinary tract and to conserve and permit physiologic functioning of renal tissue. It is also used to provide permanent urinary drainage when a ureter is obstructed or temporary urinary drainage immediately following a plastic repair on the kidney or renal pelvis.

Pyelolithotomy is removal of a calculus through an opening in the renal pelvis.

Procedural considerations

Patient preparation and instrument setup are as described for ureteral surgery.

Operative procedures
Pyelotomy or pyelostomy

1. The pelvis of the kidney is incised with a small scalpel blade.
2. Fine traction sutures may be placed at the edges of the incision for gentle retraction while the pelvis and calyces are explored.
3. In pyelostomy a small Malecot or Foley catheter is placed through the incision into the renal pelvis.
4. Pyelotomy should be used only for very short periods of renal drainage because tubes tend to dislodge easily from the renal pelvis.

Nephrostomy

1. A curved clamp or stone forceps is passed through a pyelotomy incision into the renal pelvis and then out through the substance of the renal parenchyma via a lower pole minor calyx.
2. The tip of a Malecot, Foley, or Pezzer catheter is drawn into the renal pelvis, and the pyelotomy incision is sutured closed.
3. The distal end of the nephrostomy tube is brought out through a separate stab incision in the flank. A drain is placed at the level of the pyelotomy incision, and all layers are closed in the regular manner.

Operations to remove renal calculi
Pyelolithotomy and nephrolithotomy

1. The renal pelvis is opened (Fig. 14-80, *A*), and the pelvic calculus is gently removed.
2. The pelvis and collecting systems are thoroughly irrigated with saline using an Asepto syringe to dislodge the small remaining calculi and remove them from the kidney.
3. Nephrolithotomy or extended pyelolithotomy is employed when calculi are locked in the calyceal system and cannot be removed through a pyelotomy incision. In such cases the renal parenchyma above the calculus is incised and the calculus removed. In many instances such a situation is associated with a calyceal diverticulum (Fig. 14-80, *B*).
4. After removal of the calculus the collecting system is closed and the renal cortex reapproximated with deep hemostatic no. 2-0 absorbable sutures.
5. A nephroscope is sometimes used to localize and remove calyceal calculi (Fig. 14-81). It is also useful in staghorn calculi nephroscopy to remove residual fragments in the pelvic portion of the calculus.
6. An incision in the renal pelvis may be closed with no. 4-0 absorbable atraumatic sutures.
7. The renal fossa is drained and closed, as for nephrectomy. Reinforced absorbent dressings are useful because generally some urinary leakage occurs for 3 to 4 days after surgery.

Percutaneous nephrolithotomy and litholapaxy

Percutaneous nephrolithotomy and litholapaxy facilitate the removal or disintegration of renal stones using a rigid or flexible nephroscope (see Fig. 14-81) passed through a percutaneous nephrostomy tract. Accessory instrumentation, such as the ultrasound wand (sonotrode), electrohydraulic lithotriptor probe, Candela laser fiber, stone basket, and stone grasper, is passed through the lumen of the nephroscope to achieve the desired result.

Ideally the patient is in good health and nonobese, and the calculus is no larger than 1 cm in diameter, free floating, radiopaque, and solitary. However, advances in technology complemented by the experience gained by the uro-

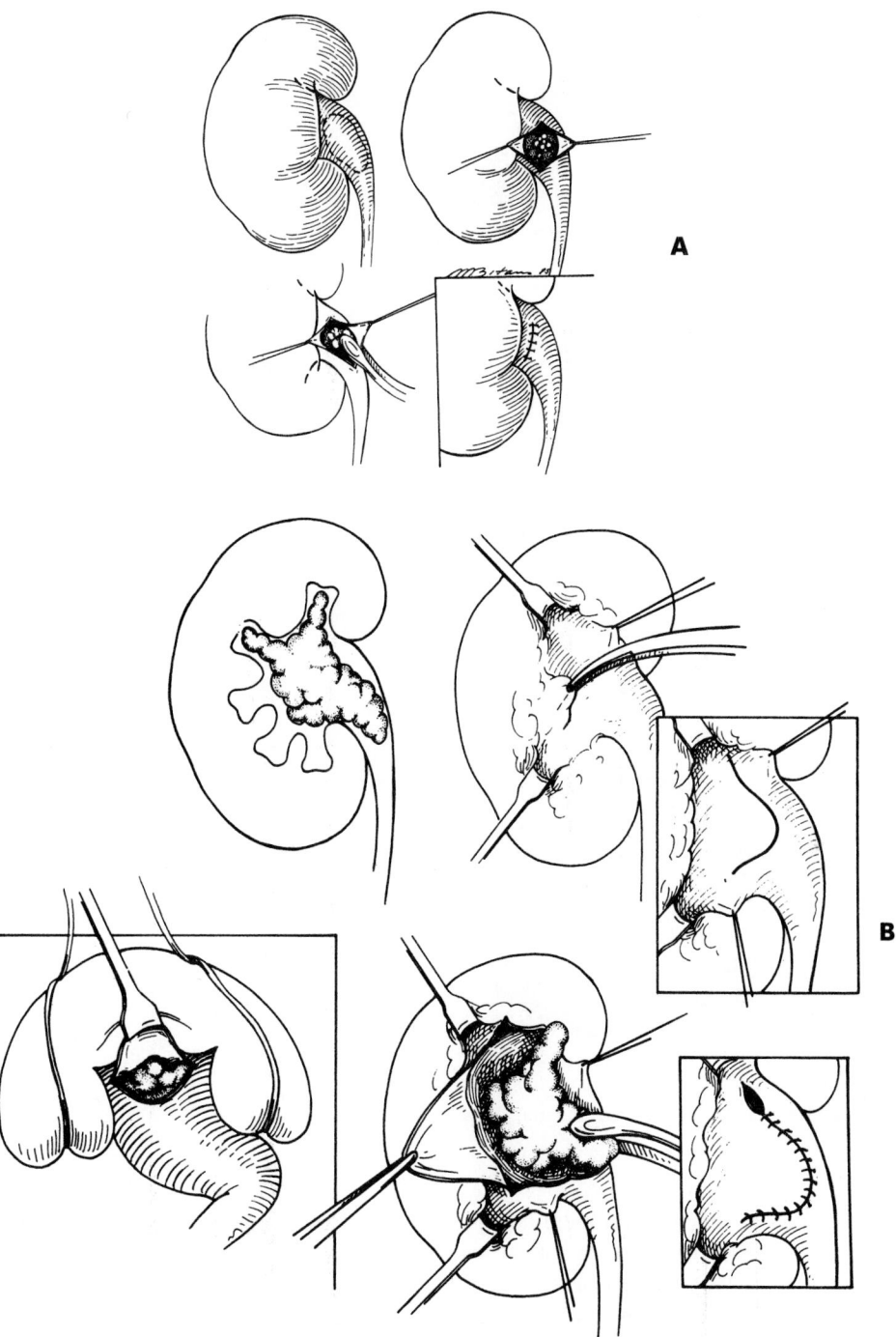

FIG. 14-80   Pyelolithotomy. **A,** Technique of simple pyelolithotomy. **B,** Technique of extended pyelolithotomy.

From Gillenwater, J.Y. (1991). *Adult and pediatric urology.* St. Louis: Mosby.

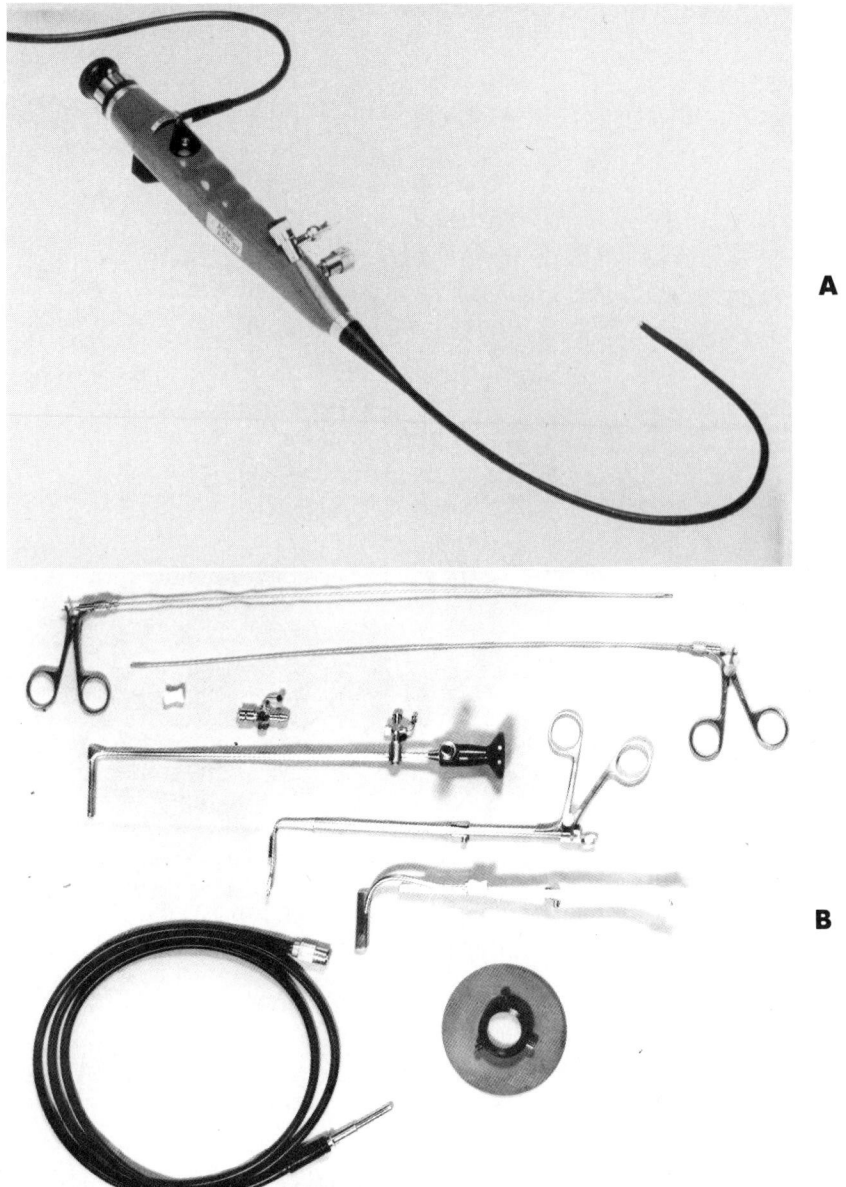

FIG. 14-81   **A,** Flexible percutaneous nephroscope. **B,** Rigid nephroscope and accessories.
A courtesy Circon Corp., Santa Barbara, Calif.

radiology team have allowed patients with more complex problems to be managed in this manner. The patient may or may not have had previous renal surgery or stone recurrence and may have an established nephrostomy tract.

Creation of the nephrostomy tract and removal of the stone can be accomplished by three different methods. Proper placement of the nephrostomy wire can decrease the operating time significantly. In the one-step procedure creation of the nephrostomy tract, tract dilatation, and stone removal are completed in a single session. The radiologist and urologist are both present, and the patient is managed with intravenous sedation. This method is generally preferred unless there are contraindications.

In the immediate two-step procedure the radiologist places the nephrostomy tube under radiographic guidance and the urologist removes the stone later the same day or the next morning. The second step is usually done in the operating room with the patient under general anesthesia.

In the delayed two-step procedure the nephrostomy tract is established with the patient under local anesthesia. The patient is discharged the following day with a 22 or 24 Fr nephrostomy tube connected to drainage. The patient is readmitted to the hospital 5 to 7 days later for the percutaneous removal of the calculus under general anesthesia.

Of basic concern during the operative phase are the patient's position and body temperature, the potential for sudden and rapid blood loss, the type of anesthesia to be given, medications required during surgery, and catheter management during and after the procedure. The patient's position, which may be prone or up to 30 degrees prone-oblique, and the draping procedure depend on whether the surgery is done in the radiology department or the operating room and the type of x-ray equipment that will be used. Postoperatively the patient may exhibit edema and bruising around the eyes and through the facial area as a result of the position required for this procedure and ESWL. It is important to alert the patient and the family to this possibility during preoperative teaching.

Extracorporeal shock wave lithotripsy

A noninvasive approach to urolithiasis management is the use of the extracorporeal shock wave lithotriptor (ESWL). This device disintegrates kidney stones by introducing shock waves through a liquid medium into the body. Immediately before the procedure an x-ray examination is made to pinpoint the position of the kidney stones. The anesthetized patient, often under epidural anesthesia, is then positioned and strapped to a gantry and lowered into a lithotriptor tube filled with specially treated water. Precise adjustments of the gantry are made to position the patient so the kidney stone is in the external focus of the ellipsoidal reflector.

Alternatively, second-generation ESWL units use water-filled cushions adjacent to the kidney area. An x-ray image intensifier with two monitors is used to visualize the kidney stone at the focal point of the shock wave. After every 100 shocks, fluoroscopy is used to locate remaining stone particles. Adjustments are made, and the patient is repositioned before further treatments. Immediately after the procedure and following placement of a ureteral stent to en-

sure patency of the ureter, x-ray examination is performed to determine the size and location of stone fragment (gravel).

ESWL is often used in conjunction with percutaneous nephrolithotomy, surgery, and transurethral ureteropyeloscopy if the patient does not pass the gravel.

Candela laser lithotripsy

Laser lithotripsy has become an exciting alternative to ESWL and EHL over the past 2 years. The Candela laser is a tunable pulse-dyed laser system that has the ability to disintegrate stones without damaging soft tissue (Fig. 14-82). The technique may be used during a ureteropyeloscopy or nephroscopy.

It may also be employed to manage ureteral calculi instead of ureterolithotomy. When the laser probe is discharged in direct contact with the calculus, a plasma (ionized gas) coats the stone's surface. This plasma expands with repeated firings, creating a shock wave that fractures the stone. Normal saline is used for continuous irrigation throughout the procedure. It is not necessary to immobilize the calculus. All persons in the room wear yellow to orange goggles. All laser precautions apply (see Chapter 31).

Reconstructive surgery of the kidney

Pyeloplasty is revision or plastic reconstruction of the renal pelvis. Pyeloplasty is done to create a better anatomic relationship between the renal pelvis and the proximal ureter and to allow proper urinary drainage from the kidney to the bladder. A temporary nephrostomy is usually included in such surgery to protect the plastic reconstruction of the ureteropelvic junction. Usually tissue healing has occurred in 10 to 12 days, and the nephrostomy tube is removed once ureteral patency is demonstrated.

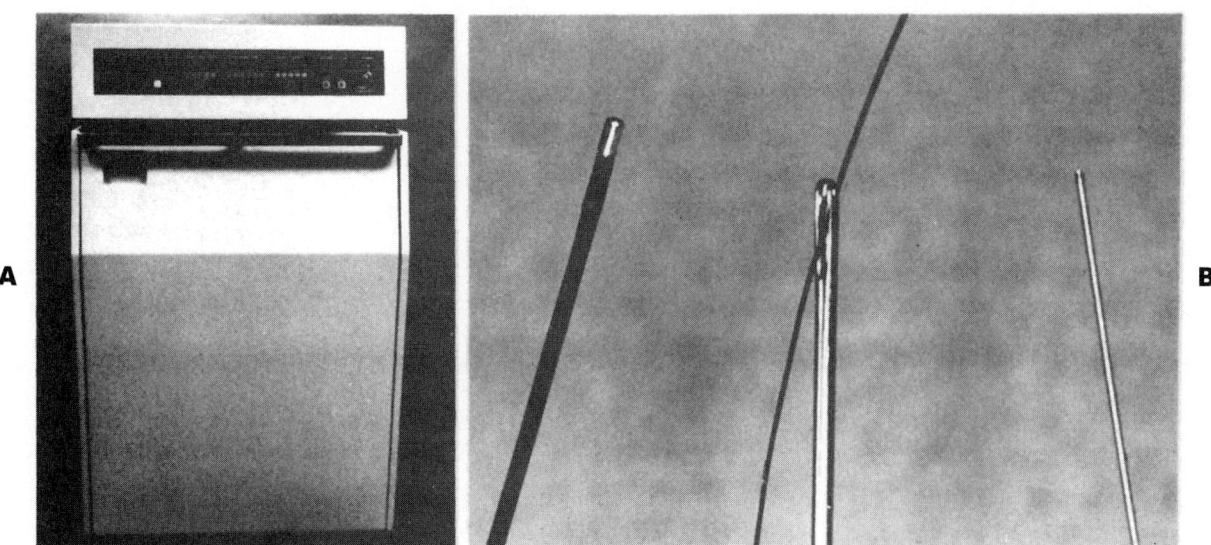

FIG. 14-82 **A,** Candela laser unit. **B,** Fiber tips.
From Gillenwater, J.Y. (1991). *Adult and pediatric urology*. St. Louis: Mosby.

Ureteroplasty is reconstruction of the ureter distal to the ureteropelvic junction.

Foley Y-V pyeloureteroplasty is combined correction of the redundant renal pelvis and resection of a stenotic portion of the ureteropelvic junction (Fig. 14-83).

Procedural considerations

The instrument setup is as described for nephrectomy, plus the following:

1 Schnidt gall duct forceps, small
1 Metzenbaum dissecting scissors, small, straight, and fine
1 Metzenbaum dissecting scissors, small, curved, and fine
1 Iris scissors, curved
2 Vascular tissue forceps, plain, 7 inches
2 Vascular tissue forceps with teeth, 7 inches

2 Vascular needle holders, 7 inches
12 Mosquito hemostats, straight and curved, 5 inches
Ureteral stent for splinting
Red rubber catheters, 8 and 10 Fr
5 Randall stone forceps
Absorbable sutures, fine, on atraumatic needles

Operative procedure

1. The kidney and upper ureter are exposed, as described for nephrectomy, by the desired surgical approach.
2. The renal pelvis and ureter are incised, trimmed, and shaped to the desired contour with fine forceps and scissors (Fig. 14-83, A). A caliper and a ruler may be used for establishing more precise relationships when plastic repair is undertaken. Anchoring sutures or vessel loops may be used for traction during reconstruction of the renal pelvis. All suture material used in such repairs is absorbable.
3. The Foley Y-V-plasty technique may be followed as shown in Fig. 14-83. It converts a Y-shaped surgical incision of the renal pelvis into a V by drawing the apex of the arms of the Y to the foot of the Y with absorbable sutures (Fig. 14-83, B). This provides a larger funnel-shaped ureteropelvic junction (Fig. 14-83, C). Interrupted no. 4-0 or 5-0 absorbable sutures are used in the repair (Fig. 14-83, D).
4. A Silastic tubing may be used to stent the repaired pelvis until adequate healing has occurred. A nephrostomy tube is also placed within the pelvis to divert urine safely while the edema in the area of the plastic repair resolves.
5. A drain is placed where the pelvis was reconstructed, and the surgical incision is closed in layers.

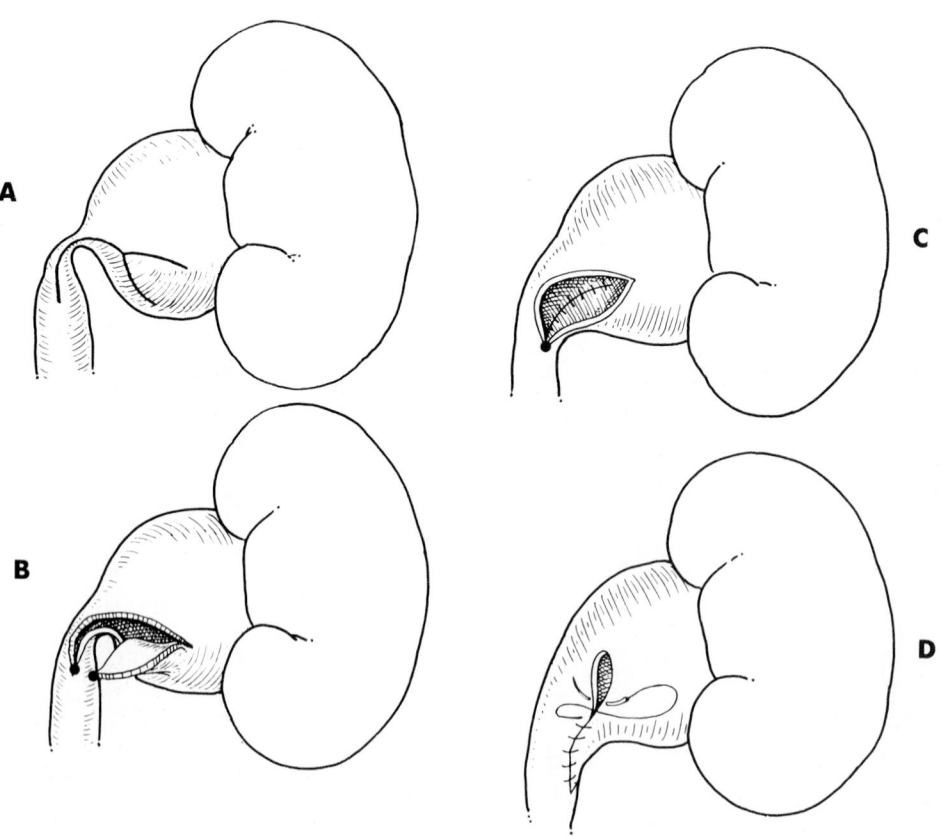

FIG. 14-83 Foley Y-V–plasty repair.
Modified from Droller, M.J. (1992). *Surgical management of urologic disease.* St. Louis: Mosby.

Operations to remove the kidney
Nephroureterectomy

Nephroureterectomy is removal of a kidney and its entire ureter. This procedure is indicated for hydroureteronephrosis of such a degree that reconstructive repair is impossible. It is also employed for collecting system tumors of the kidney and ureter.

Procedural considerations. This procedure often requires two separate incisions: a flank incision to facilitate exposure and delivery of the kidney, and a lower hemisuprapubic incision to free the lower portion of the ureter from the bladder. Another approach is extension of incision anteriorly with the patient positioned semilateral and fully prepped and draped to access the flank and lower abdomen. Only one instrument set is required, but a second skin preparation setup and set of sterile drapes may be necessary.

An alternative to open nephroureterectomy is laparoscopic nephroureterectomy.

Operative procedure

1. The patient is placed in a lateral position. The kidney and upper ureter are exposed and nephrectomy is performed as described below. The kidney is placed in a plastic bag to prevent possible spillage of tumor cells. The ureter is not cut at this time but is mobilized as far distally as possible.
2. The operating room bed is adjusted so surgery on the lower ureter may proceed. The abdomen is prepped, sterile drapes are applied, and an abdominal incision is made to expose the lower ureter and bladder on the operative side. These structures are identified and mobilized. The ureter and a small cuff of the bladder

are removed in continuity, and the bladder is repaired with a single layer of no. 2-0 absorbable interrupted sutures.
3. The ureter and cuff of bladder may be pulled superiorly into the flank incision, where the intact kidney and ureter may be removed from the surgical field.
4. A 18 or 20 Fr Foley catheter is left in the bladder, and a drain is placed behind the bladder. Both incisions are closed in sequence in the usual manner.

Nephrectomy

Nephrectomy is the surgical removal of a kidney. It is performed as a means of definitive therapy for a number of renal problems, such as congenital ureteropelvic junction obstruction with severe hydronephrosis, renal tumors, renal trauma, calculous disease with infection, cortical abscess, pyelonephrosis, and renovascular hypertension.

The advent of innovative technology in the 1990s now allows a unique approach to nephrectomy—laparoscopic nephrectomy.

Procedural considerations. In routine renal surgery the patient is placed in the lateral position with the loin directly over the kidney rest. The operative flank is uppermost, with the patient's back brought to the edge of the OR bed. The upper arm is supported on an overhead arm support, and the lower arm is flexed at the elbow so that the hand rests on or under the head pillow. The patient's legs are positioned by placing a pillow between them and flexing the lower leg at the knee. The upper leg remains extended. The kidney rest is then raised, and when the desired bed flexion is achieved, 3-inch adhesive tape is used to stabilize the patient throughout surgery. Routine skin preparation and draping procedures are carried out.

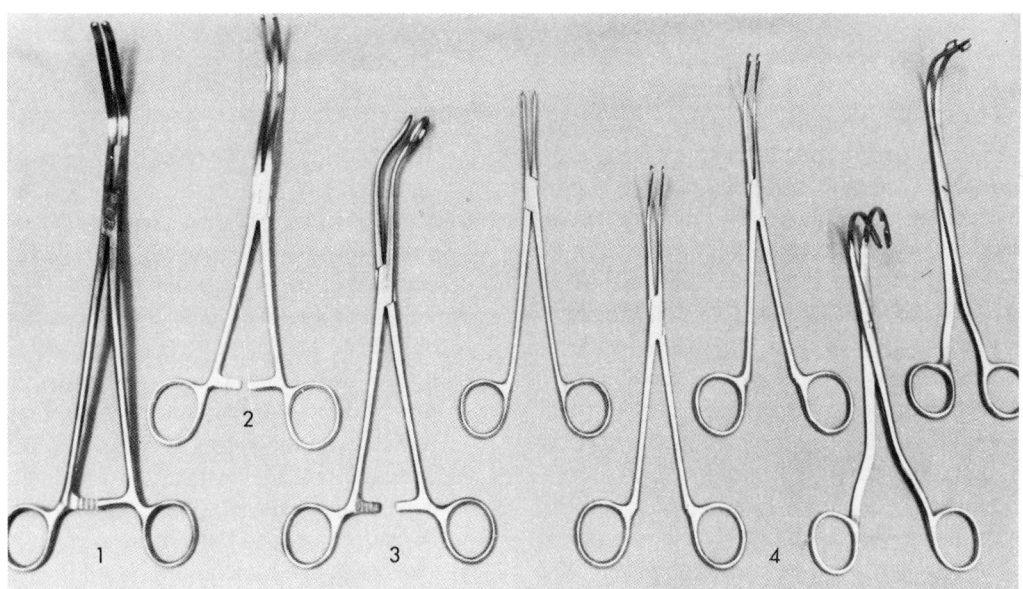

FIG. 14-84   Kidney instruments. *1,* Satinsky pedicle clamp; *2,* Mayo pedicle clamp; *3,* Lewkowitz lithotomy forceps; *4,* set of five **Randall** stone forceps.

The nephrectomy setup includes routine laparotomy setup, kidney instruments (Fig. 14-84), and the following:

2 Satinsky, Herrick, or Mayo pedicle clamps
1 Lewkowitz lithotomy forceps
5 Randall stone forceps, varied sizes
1 Silver probe (Bakes dilators may be used)

Rubber catheter, 8 or 10 Fr
Asepto syringe
Pezzer or Malecot catheter
Closed wound drainage system
Vessel loops

In certain nephrectomies the chest or the gastrointestinal tract may be opened. If the chest is opened, appropriate instruments and postoperative chest drains are needed. When the gastrointestinal tract is opened, precautions must be taken in the anastomosis and closure techniques. For rib resection the following instruments are added to the nephrectomy setup:

1 Finochietto rib retractor, large
1 Matson costal periosteotome
1 Alexander costal periosteotome
2 Doyen rib raspatories, right and left

1 Bethune rib cutter
1 Double-action duckbill rongeur
1 Bailey rib approximator
1 Langenbeck periosteal elevator

If the laparoscopic method is chosen, the approach may be transabdominal or retroperitoneal. Transabdominal is the most common approach. Indications for laparoscopy are generally for benign disease, although more radical surgeries have been accomplished in this manner. Preoperative workup is similar to any renal surgery with the addition of a full mechanical antibiotic bowel prep.

Although surgery time is much lengthier (an average of 5½ hours), postoperative recovery, analgesia requirements, and total hospital stay have lessened dramatically.

The procedure always includes cystoscopy with placement of a renal balloon catheter, a ureteral catheter, and a Foley urethral catheter under C-arm fluoroscopy. Indigo carmine is injected into the skin overlying the renal pelvis.

There should always be an open setup available in the event laparoscopy is unsuccessful. The patient is initially placed on a bean bag in the supine position. The contralateral arm is padded with thick foam from the shoulder to the fingertips. Following endotracheal intubation and placement of pneumatic compression stockings, a nasogastric tube and electrosurgical dispersive pad are placed. The patient is prepped and draped in the usual manner for thoracoabdominal surgery. Extra draping materials are utilized when the patient is repositioned.

A standard laparoscopy instrument and equipment setup that includes three 5-mm trocars, a Veress needle, and two 12-mm trocars is used. Additional instrumentation needed includes:

Flexible cystoscope
0.035 Bentson guidewire
Occlusion balloon catheter, 7 Fr, 11.5 mm
Stopcock, one-way
1-ml syringe and 25-gauge needle
0.035 Amplatz stiff guidewire
Sidearm adaptor
16 Fr Foley catheter and drainage bag
Indigo carmine
Standard laparoscopy instrumentation and equipment

Nonabsorbable monofilament suture, no. 2, on cutting needle
Irrigator/aspirator
1-L bag saline with 5000 U heparin and 500 mg cefazolin sodium (Ancef)
1-L pressure bag to pressurize irrigant to 250 mm Hg
Knife blade, no. 12 or 11
Clip appliers, 10 mm
Entrapment sack
Tissue morcellator

Operative procedures
Open lateral approach

1. The incision is carried through the skin, fat, and fascia. Bleeding vessels are clamped with hemostats and ligated.
2. The external oblique, internal oblique, and transversalis muscles are sequentially exposed and incised in the direction of the initial skin incision.
3. If necessary, a rib or ribs (eleventh or twelfth) may be resected to provide better access to the kidney. The periosteum is stripped with an Alexander costal periosteotome and Doyen rib raspatory.
4. A scalpel and heavy scissors may be used to cut through the lumbocostal ligaments. The rib is grasped with an Oschner clamp and cut with rib shears, removing the portion necessary to expose the kidney.
5. Gerota's fascia is identified and incised with Metzenbaum scissors. The incision is extended, and the kidney and perirenal fat are exposed by blunt and sharp dissection.
   NOTE: All perirenal fat that is removed during surgery may be saved in a small basin of normal saline. Perirenal fat may be used later as a bolster to stop bleeding.
6. The ureter is identified, separated from its adjacent structures, doubly clamped, divided, and ligated with absorbable no. 0 material.
7. The kidney pedicle containing the major blood vessels is isolated and doubly clamped; each vessel is triply ligated with heavy nonabsorbable ties. Each vessel is then severed, leaving two ligatures remaining on the pedicle, and the kidney is removed (Fig. 14-85).
8. The renal fossa is explored for bleeding and necessary hemostasis achieved. The fossa is then irrigated with normal saline, and the irrigant is removed by suction.
9. The fascia and muscles are closed in layers with interrupted, absorbable sutures. If necessary, retention sutures may be used in obese or chronically ill individuals in whom wound healing may be a problem. The

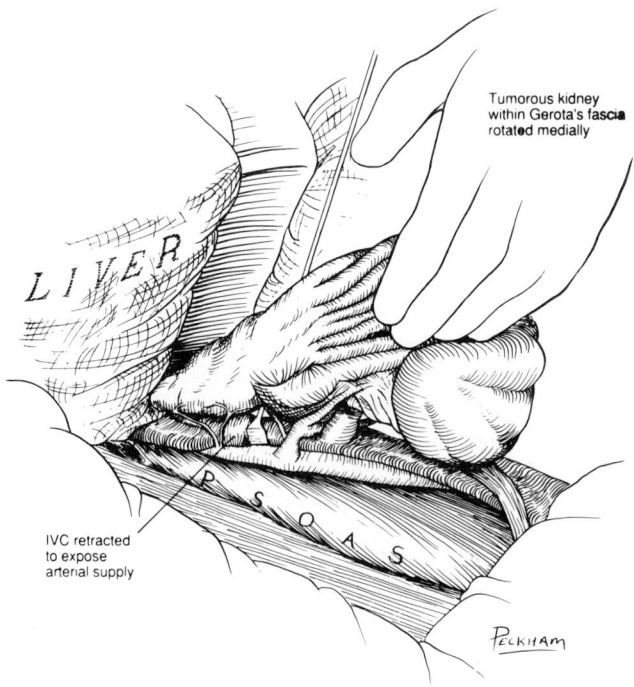

FIG. 14-85 Nephrectomy.

From Droller, M.J. (1992). *Surgical management of urologic disease*. St. Louis: Mosby.

Tumorous kidney within Gerota's fascia rotated medially

LIVER

PSOAS

IVC retracted to expose arterial supply

PECKHAM

skin edges are approximated with interrupted sutures or with skin staples.

10. The wound is dressed in a standard manner.

Laparoscopic approach

1. With a no. 12 or 11 blade a small transverse incision is made at the umbilical level.

2. The Veress needle is inserted, the location is tested with saline in the usual manner, and the abdominal cavity is inflated with CO_2 until a pressure of 20 mm Hg is obtained.

3. A nick is made in the rectus fascia with the scalpel, and the 12-mm trocar replaces the Veress needle. Towel clips are used on each side of the incision to stabilize the abdominal wall.

4. The OR bed is rotated to a 30-degree Trendelenburg's position, and the laparoscope is inserted.

5. A second 12-mm trocar is placed immediately below the costal margin in the midclavicular line.

6. The third 5-mm trocar is inserted 2 cm below the umbilicus in the midclavicular line.

7. The patient is rolled to a lateral decubitus position. The arm on the operative side is brought across the patient's chest and secured to an ether screen or Allen arm support. The legs are checked for proper flexion and padding, and the bean bag is inflated.

8. The last two 5-mm trocars are placed, one in the anterior axillary line at a level with the umbilicus and one

immediately subcostal in the anterior axillary line. All trocars are then withdrawn until 2 to 3 cm of each sheath protrudes into the abdomen. The monofilament suture secures the side arm ports to the patient's skin.

9. The ascending or descending colon is completely mobilized with electrosurgical scissors and deflected medially. The retroperitoneum is opened.

10. Through gentle motion of the ureteral catheter the ureter is identified and dissected. A Babcock clamp is placed around the dissected ureter for retraction.

11. The ureter is dissected until the lower pole of the kidney is visualized. Any veins encountered are clipped twice proximally and twice distally. The kidney is cleared of surrounding tissue and freed laterally and superiorly. Gerota's fascia is entered to free the adrenal gland and exclude it from the dissection.

12. The renal artery and vein are identified and cleared to create a 360-degree window around each vessel. The clip applier is inserted through the 12-mm port. Two clips are placed on the specimen side and three clips are clamped to the stump side of both vessels. The vessels are sharply incised.

13. Two pairs of clips are placed proximally and distally on the ureter and it is sharply incised. The specimen end is grasped and the kidney moved into the upper abdominal quadrant.

    NOTE: If nephroureterectomy is to be performed, the ureter is freed and skeletonized to the ureterovesical junction and removed en bloc with the kidney.

14. The entrapment sack is introduced through the 12-mm port. With graspers the bottom of the sack is pulled into the abdomen until the sack neck clears the end of the port and unfurls.

15. The sack is opened and the ureteral stump with attached kidney is placed in the sack. The drawstrings are pulled tight, closing the mouth of the sack.

16. The patient is returned to the supine position and the sack strings are extracted through the umbilical port. The port is removed and the neck of the sack brought to lie on the abdominal surface under laparoscopic observation. The tissue morcellator is inserted into the sack and the kidney is morcellated under suction in a clockwise fashion.

17. The abdominal cavity is exited in the standard manner. Fascial layers at the 12-mm trocar sites are closed with no. 2-0 absorbable suture in a figure-of-eight pattern. Subcuticular closure of no. 4-0 absorbable suture is done on all port sites. Steri-Strips, Telfa, and Tegaderm complete the dressings.

18. The nasogastric tube is removed in the operating room and the Foley catheter is removed on the first postoperative day. Oral intake may begin 6 hours postoperatively. The compression stockings are removed when the patient is ambulatory. Most patients leave the hospital in 4 days, return to work in approximately 2 weeks, with full convalescence in 3 weeks.

Heminephrectomy

Heminephrectomy is removal of a portion of the kidney. It is usually indicated for conditions involving the lower or upper pole of the kidney, such as calculous disease, or trauma limited to one pole of a kidney. In rare instances in which a patient has only one kidney, such surgery may be used for renal neoplasms to avoid the need for dialysis and subsequent renal transplantation.

Procedural considerations. The setup is as described for nephrectomy with the addition of vascular clamps and bulldog clamps.

Operative procedure

1. The kidney and its pedicle should be completely mobilized as described for nephrectomy.
2. The main vessels may be temporarily occluded for only 20 to 30 minutes, after which progressive renal damage may occur. Local hypothermia may be indicated to prolong ischemic operating time.
3. The renal capsule is incised and stripped back. A wedge of kidney tissue containing the diseased or damaged cortex is excised. Interlobar fat or arcuate and interlobular arteries are clamped with Hopkins' clamps and suture ligated with no. 4-0 absorbable suture on urologic needles.
4. The open collecting system is reapproximated with a continuous no. 4-0 suture.
5. Perirenal fat is placed in the area in which tissue was excised, and the renal parenchyma is reapproximated with horizontal mattress sutures. If possible, the renal capsule is reapproximated with a continuous no. 2-0 suture.

Radical nephrectomy

Radical nephrectomy is excision of kidney, perirenal fat, adrenal gland, Gerota's capsule (fascia), and contiguous periaortic lymph nodes. This procedure is performed for parenchymal renal neoplasms. A lumbar, transthoracic, or transabdominal approach to the kidney is performed, depending on the size and location of the lesion. The transthoracic or transabdominal approach is preferred because the blood vessels of the kidney can be more easily reached and ligated before the tumor is mobilized, thus decreasing the possibility of tumor embolization into the bloodstream.

Procedural considerations. The setup is as described for nephrectomy.

Operative procedure

1. In general, the procedure is as described for nephrectomy with two exceptions: (a) the renal pedicle is ligated before the kidney is mobilized, and (b) Gerota's capsule is not incised but is removed en block with the kidney.
2. Involved lymph nodes surrounding the renal pedicle are excised.

3. A chest tube is inserted if the transthoracic approach is used.

Kidney transplant

Kidney transplant entails transplantation of a living related or cadaveric donor kidney into the recipient's iliac fossa (Fig. 14-86). It is performed in an effort to restore renal function and thus maintain life in a patient who has end-stage renal disease.

Transplant from a living donor. The kidney donor must be in perfect health. ABO (blood typing) and histocompatibility (HLA tissue typing) along with a negative white cell (lymphocyte) crossmatch determine donor-recipient compatibility. It is not necessary to match the Rh factor. Once the donor has been chosen, a complete workup that includes history and physical exam as well as chest films, ECG, CBC, BUN/creatinine, blood chemistry profiles, coagulation studies, and viral titers is done. Renal function is assessed with three creatinine clearances, urinalysis, and urine cultures followed by IVPs and excretory urography. A flush aortogram assesses the vascular anatomy, and renal angiography pinpoints the kidney of choice while ruling out the presence of renal lesions. A kidney with a single renal artery is preferred, but kidneys with double and triple arteries may be used if necessary. If there is a family history of diabetes, a 5-hour glucose tolerance test is also performed.

The ideal living donor is an identical twin, although any immediate family member (usually a sibling or parent) may be a donor if the person is medically acceptable. The donor is given an intravenous solution of 1000 ml of 5% dextrose in lactated Ringer's on the evening before nephrec-

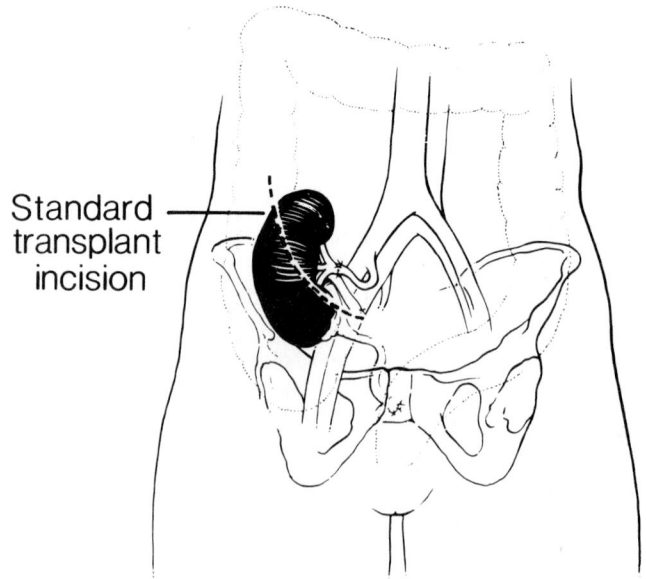

Standard transplant incision

FIG. 14-86   Transplanted kidney in recipient's iliac fossa.
From Droller, M.J. (1992). *Surgical management of urologic disease.* St. Louis: Mosby.

tomy. This is followed with 500 ml of 5% dextrose in water over the next 10 to 12 hours. The morning of surgery, about 45 minutes before transport to the operating room, the patient is given 12.5 g of mannitol to ensure diuresis during the induction of anesthesia.

Procedural considerations. Two adjacent operating rooms are prepared for the procedures; surgery on the donor and recipient proceeds simultaneously.

A Foley catheter is inserted and left in the donor's bladder to measure urinary output and prevent bladder distention from the increased urine production induced by diuretics. The donor is placed in the lateral position, prepared from midchest to midthigh, and draped in the usual manner, exposing the flank area.

Required instruments and equipment are identical to those for the nephrectomy setup plus the following for the sterile perfusion table:

1 IV pole	1 Needle catheter (Medicut), 18 gauge
Electrolyte solution (in iced basin until needed)	6 Mosquito hemostats
2 Intravenous extension tubes, sterile	2 Vascular forceps, fine, 3 inches
1 Kidney basin with cold (4° C) intravenous saline solution	1 Metzenbaum scissors, fine
	1 Suture scissors
1 Stopcock, three-way	1 Kelly hemostat

An electrolyte solution of Ringer's lactate that contains procaine and heparin is commonly used to perfuse the harvested kidney. Collins' or Sachs' solution may be used to perfuse cadaveric kidneys following harvest but should never be used to perfuse a kidney from a living donor because of the potential effect of elevated potassium in the recipient owing to residual perfusate in the kidney.

Operative procedure

1. The donor nephrectomy procedure is as described for nephrectomy; however, the ureter and renal vein and artery require meticulous dissection.
2. Maximum length of the ureter is achieved by dividing it at or below the pelvic rim if possible. To preserve adequate ureteral vascularization, the surgeon is cautious not to skeletonize the ureter.
3. Particular care must be taken to remove the maximum length of the renal vein and artery. To obtain the maximum length of the right renal vein sometimes requires partial occlusion of the inferior vena cava with a Satinsky clamp and dissection of a portion of the inferior vena cava. This is best done after the ureter has been freed. Repair of the inferior vena cava is made with a continuous no. 4-0 or 5-0 vascular suture.
4. Five minutes before the surgeon clamps the renal vessels, 5000 units of heparin sodium and 12.5 g of mannitol are systemically administered to the patient to prevent intravascular clotting and maximize diuresis. Im-

mediately after the kidney is removed from the donor, 50 mg of protamine sulfate is given intravenously to reverse the heparinization. Furosemide, mannitol, and intravenous fluids are administered to the donor to maintain adequate urinary output from the donor's remaining kidney.

5. Gentle handling of the kidney is essential. Team members must prevent undue traction on the vascular pedicle, which may induce vasospasm and reduce perfusion of the kidney.
6. To reduce warm ischemia time, the surgeon double-clamps the vein and the artery, excises the kidney, and immediately places it in cold saline solution on a sterile back table where the kidney is flushed with the designated electrolyte solution. Warm ischemia time (from the clamping of renal vessels to a point at which the kidney is perfused with cold electrolyte solution) should be kept to a minimum to prevent acute tubular necrosis and to maintain maximum renal function after transplantation. Mosquito clamps and fine vascular forceps are used to expose the renal artery to permit insertion of a needle catheter, for example, a Medicut. The cold electrolyte solution passes through the intravenous tubing and the needle catheter, flushing any remaining donor's blood from the kidney. This also decreases the kidney's metabolic rate by lowering its temperature. Flushing time is usually 2 to 5 minutes. After flushing, trimming the vessels of adventitia may be necessary to facilitate the vascular anastomosis to the recipient's iliac vessels.
7. The kidney, in cold saline solution, is covered with sterile drapes and taken by the surgeon to the room in which the recipient's iliac vessels have been exposed.
8. Wound closure for the donor is as described for nephrectomy.

Transplant from a cadaveric donor. The ideal cadaveric donor is young, free from infection and cancer, normotensive until a short time before death, and under hospital observation several hours before death. Permission to harvest the donor kidney must be obtained from the family and the medical examiner after brain death has been unequivocally established. Awareness of existing state legislation in this complex area is advisable.

The donor goes through a complete evaluation including physician consultations and lab studies. The patient's medical history is reviewed for any possible contraindications such as chronic organ donor disease, ongoing systemic infection, intravenous drug abuse, malignancy, heart or lung disease, trauma to the donor organ, and HIV positivity. Lab studies include blood typing, urinalysis, urine and blood cultures, BUN, serum creatinine, CBC, hepatitis B antigen evaluation, venereal disease, and HIV. Evaluation of arterial blood gases, electrolyte values, and liver enzymes is also necessary.

Preoperative management of the cadaver donor is vital to the success of the transplant. Organ perfusion, oxygenation, and hydration must be maintained. Arterial blood gas evaluation determines ventilatory support, and dopamine may be administered if fluids alone are not able to maintain an adequate systolic blood pressure. Urine output is monitored, and antibiotics may be administered to combat and prevent infection.

Procedural considerations. After brain death has been established, the donor is taken to the surgical suite with respiratory and cardiac function maintained mechanically. The donor is placed in the supine position and is prepared for a laparotomy. Anticoagulant and alpha-adrenergic blocking agents are administered systemically during the procedure. Adequate renal perfusion and function are maintained with intravenous fluids and diuretics.

Instruments and equipment are the same as for the nephrectomy setup, excluding the rib instruments and adding the following:

1 Metzenbaum scissors, 9¼ inches	4 Vascular needle holders, 2 short and 2 long
1 Suture scissors, 9¼ inches	1 Sternal saw or Lepshey knife and mallet
1 Metzenbaum scissors, fine	4 Umbilical tapes
1 Suture scissors, fine	Electrolyte solution (lactated Ringer's, Sachs, or Collins), cold, in iced basin until needed
2 Vascular forceps, fine	
3 DeBakey forceps, 4, 7, and 10 inches	
12 Dean hemostatic forceps	1 IV pole
12 Mosquito hemostats	2 Intravenous extension tubes, sterile
6 DeBakey clamps, angled	1 Kidney basin with cold (4° C) intravenous saline solution
Clip appliers with medium and large clips	
6 Bulldog clamps	1 Stopcock, three-way
4 Vascular clamps, angled, large	1 Needle catheter (Medicut), 18 gauge
2 Deaver retractors, extra-wide	1 Centimeter ruler
	1 Electrosurgical unit
2 Harrington splanchnic retractors, small and large	Perfusion machine or kidney transplant equipment and ice

Operative procedure

1. A midline incision is made from the xiphoid process to the symphysis pubis with bilateral supraumbilical transverse extensions through the skin, subcutaneous layer, fascia, and muscle.
2. Hemostasis is obtained with clamps, ties, suture ligatures, and electrocoagulation.
3. The kidney, renal vessels, and ureter are carefully dissected with Metzenbaum scissors, DeBakey forceps, and Dean hemostatic forceps.
4. Heparin sodium, 15,000 units, is given intravenously 5 to 10 minutes before the renal vessels are clamped.
5. The usual method of resection is en bloc resection (harvesting of donor kidneys) (Fig. 14-87), which involves the removal of sections of the inferior vena cava and

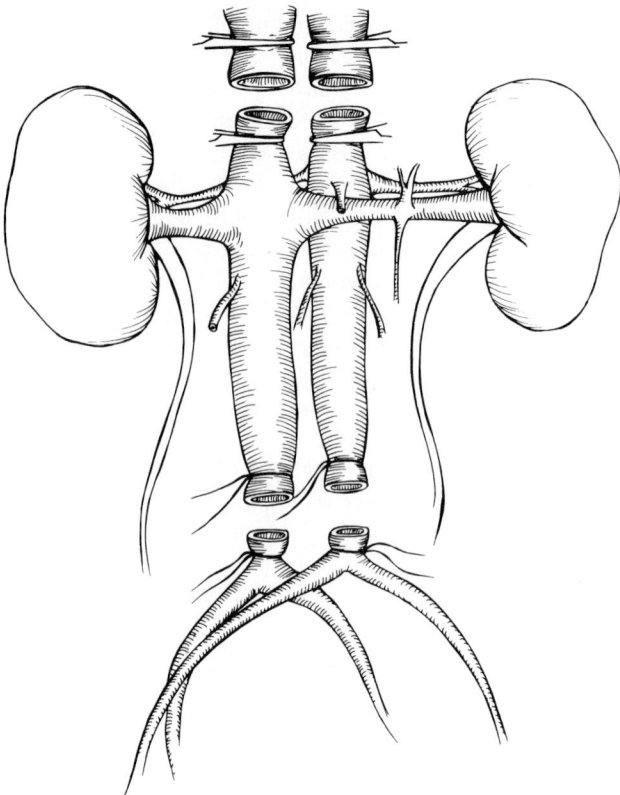

FIG. 14-87   En bloc resection.

aorta with both kidneys in continuity. An incision is made along the route of the small bowel mesentery up to the esophageal hiatus. The entire gastrointestinal tract, spleen, and inferior portion of the pancreas are mobilized by dividing the celiac axis and the superior mesenteric artery, exposing the entire retroperitoneal region. The inferior vena cava and aorta are clamped below the renal vessels with vascular clamps, and the vessels are divided. Lumbar tributaries are secured with metal clips and are divided. The kidneys and ureters are freed from their surrounding soft tissues. The ureters are divided distally at the pelvic brim. The suprarenal aorta and inferior vena cava are clamped and divided at the level of the diaphragm, close to the bifurcation. The vessels and kidney are severed from the surgical field, and the aorta and vena cava are ligated.

6. After removal of the kidneys, immediate perfusion with cold (4° C) electrolyte solution is carried out as in step 5 for a donor kidney.
7. The kidneys are placed in a container of cold saline solution and surrounded by saline slush in an insulated carrier or placed on a hypothermic pulsatile perfusion machine for transport (Fig. 14-88). A new preservative solution developed at the University of Wisconsin is being used in many institutions. It contains hydroxylathyl starch, providing a better metabolic substrate for organ metabolism. The cold ischemia time has been

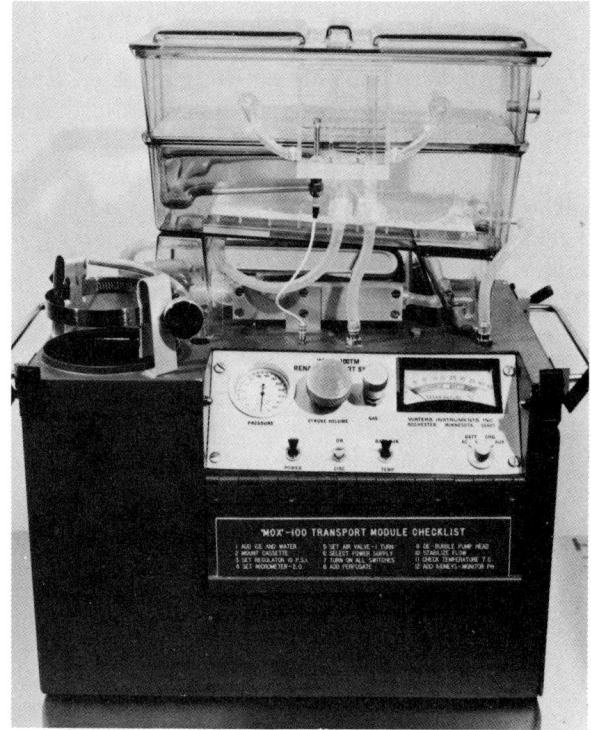

FIG. 14-88 Waters hypothermic, pulsatile perfusion machine for transport of donor organs.

dramatically increased with this solution, allowing more time for transport.

8. While kidney perfusion is begin, the abdominal lymph nodes and spleen are removed for use in tissue typing.
9. The incision is closed with interrupted sutures.
10. Artificial life-support systems are terminated.

Transplant recipient. Each potential recipient is judged individually in regard to kidney transplantation. Most persons below the age of 55 years are acceptable; older patients are less tolerant of postoperative complications. Contraindications for renal transplantation include (1) systemic disease that precludes major surgery, (2) oxalosis (a metabolic disorder), (3) a positive HLA cytotoxic antibody screen, and (4) active cancer. If required, a patient may need to undergo bilateral nephrectomy before renal transplantation for uncontrollable hypertension or kidney infections, and for reflux when there is a significant history of infections. Occasionally a large polycystic kidney may need to be removed to create a space for the new kidney. Splenectomy may be performed at this time to improve leukopenia and enhance the effects of myelosuppressive and immunosuppressive drugs.

The transplant recipient requires optimal nutritional support and adequate dialysis. All potential sources of infection must be treated. Most commonly these include teeth, bladder, nasal sinuses, and skin. The patient may need a short hemodialysis to control fluid overload or electrolyte imbalances. A repeat cytotoxic crossmatch with fresh serum specimens should follow hemodialysis. Preoperative antibiotics are commonly administered. Other important diagnostic tools for preoperative evaluation are chest films, abdominal ultrasound, voiding cystourethrogram, liver function studies, hematology, and serum values for screening hepatitis, HIV, and viral diseases.

Procedural considerations. The patient is placed in the supine position. A Foley catheter with an attached Silastic stenting catheter is inserted in the bladder by sterile technique. From 50 to 75 ml of antibiotic solution is instilled in the bladder through a sterile catheter tip syringe, allowed to remain for 20 minutes, and drained. The patient is prepped from nipples to knees and is draped in the routine manner.

Instruments and equipment required are the routine laparotomy setup, plus the following:

1 Metzenbaum scissors, 9¼ inches	3 Bulldog clamps, straight
1 Suture scissors, 9¼ inches	2 Harrington splanchnic retractors, small and large
1 Metzenbaum scissors, fine	4 Vascular needle holders, 2 long and 2 short
1 Suture scissors, fine	
1 Potts scissors, angled	2 Asepto syringes
3 DeBakey forceps, 4, 7, and 10 inches	1 Centimeter ruler
2 Vascular forceps, fine, 3 inches	1 Needle catheter (Medicut), 18 gauge on 10-ml syringe
12 Dean hemostatic forceps	1 Closed wound drainage system
12 Mosquito hemostats, straight	Electrosurgical unit
6 Mosquito hemostats, curved	1 Pediatric feeding tube, 5 Fr
6 DeBakey clamps, angled	1 Stockinette, 3 × 10 inches
2 Clip appliers with medium and large clips	Heparin sodium solution (1:1000)
3 Bulldog clamps, curved	Intravenous saline solution, cold (4° C)

Operative procedure

1. A curved right lower quadrant incision is made through the skin, subcutaneous layer, fascia, and muscle. Bleeding is controlled with clamps, ties, and electrocoagulation.
2. The inferior epigastric vessels are divided between suture ligatures. A retroperitoneal dissection is performed by mobilizing the peritoneum superiorly and medially. A Balfour self-retaining retractor is placed in the wound for exposure, and a wide Deaver retractor is inserted to reflect the peritoneum superiorly and medially.
3. With the use of the 9¼-inch Metzenbaum scissors and the DeBakey forceps, dissection is made along the entire length of the hypogastric artery and the external

and common iliac arteries to the bifurcation of the aorta, continuing down the internal iliac artery. The internal iliac artery is ligated distally and divided, with proximal control maintained by a vascular clamp. The iliac vein is dissected free by ligating and dividing the internal iliac venous branches with no. 3-0 nonabsorbable sutures or ligating clips. In more recent years there has been a tendency to dissect only the hypogastric artery and that portion of iliac vein to be anastomosed.

4. The donor kidney is brought into the operative field and placed in cold (4° C) intravenous saline solution.

5. Mosquito hemostats, 4-inch DeBakey forceps, and curved and straight fine scissors are used to make the necessary alterations on the donor kidney vessels to facilitate the anastomoses.

6. The donor kidney is returned to the cold intravenous saline solution until the time of the anastomosis.

7. Two angled DeBakey vascular clamps are placed on the internal iliac vein. A no. 11 blade is used to make a 1-cm incision in the iliac vein between the clamps. The vessel is rinsed with heparin sodium solution (10 units/ml) in the Asepto syringe. Angled Potts scissors are used to extend the incision to accommodate the donor renal vein.

8. The donor kidney is placed in the 3 × 10 inch, cold saline–soaked stockinette, with the renal vessels exiting from a hole in the side. Use of the stockinette prevents direct contact with the kidney and therefore trauma. The renal vein is anastomosed to the side of the recipient's iliac vein with no. 5-0, double-armed, vascular sutures. In like manner the renal artery is anastomosed end-to-end with the proximal portion of the internal iliac artery using no. 5-0 vascular sutures. The vessels are irrigated proximally and distally with heparin sodium solution by using the 10 ml syringe attached to the Medicut catheter before placing the final sutures.

9. The stockinette is removed for adequate visualization of the entire kidney.

10. The angled DeBakey clamps are removed from the venous vessels, and the anastomosis is checked for leakage. Immediately afterward, the clamps on the internal iliac artery are released, and the anastomosis is checked. Meticulous inspection is made of the hilum and surface of the kidney for bleeding and infarction. Diuretics are given intravenously as needed.

11. Attention is now directed to the ureter and bladder. Two long Allis forceps are used to grasp the anterior bladder wall. Using a scalpel with a no. 10 knife blade, a 4-cm incision is made anteriorly. Two narrow Harrington retractors and one narrow Deaver retractor are inserted in the bladder for exposure. The ureter is passed through the bladder wall and tunneled suburothelially for 2 to 2.5 cm. The spatulated end of the ureter is then sutured into the bladder urothelium with four to six no. 4-0 or 5-0 atraumatic absorbable sutures, creating a ureteroneocystostomy.

12. A 5 Fr pediatric infant feeding tube is passed through the ureteroneocystostomy, up to the renal pelvis, and out through the urethra with the Foley catheter. This stenting catheter will remain in place for 36 to 48 hours to ensure ureteral patency during a period in which ureteral edema may occur.

13. Retractors are removed, and the bladder is closed in three layers:
    a. Continuous no. 4-0 absorbable suture for urothelial closure
    b. Interrupted no. 2-0 absorbable suture for closure of bladder muscles
    c. An imbricating layer of no. 2-0 nonabsorbable material to bury the suture line

14. The bladder is irrigated with an antibiotic solution to check for leaks.

15. The renal anastomoses are again checked for bleeding.

16. Three metal clips are placed on the superior, inferior, and lateral aspects of the kidney to radiographically measure renal size and determine postoperative swelling.

17. Retractors are removed from the incision.

18. Closed wound suction drains are inserted into the wound, brought through the skin laterally, and secured with no. 2-0 nonabsorbable suture on a cutting needle.

19. Muscle and fascial layers are closed with a single layer of no. 0 nonabsorbable sutures on a large atraumatic needle. The subcutaneous layer is closed with no. 3-0 absorbable sutures on an atraumatic needle. Skin closure is accomplished with skin staples.

20. Dressings are applied.

21. The bladder is irrigated with 50 to 75 ml of antibiotic solution to prevent infection and free any blood clots.

ADRENALECTOMY

Adrenalectomy is partial or total excision of one or both adrenal glands. It may be performed for several reasons: hypersecretion of adrenal hormones, neoplasms of the adrenal gland, secondary treatment of neoplasms elsewhere in the body that depend on adrenal hormonal secretions, such as carcinoma of the prostate and breast, and pheochromocytoma.

Care of the patient with pheochromocytoma carries with it particular concerns for the perioperative nurse. These patients are subject to extreme elevations in blood pressure, often accompanied by tachycardia, and hypovolemic states that can induce vascular collapse. If an adrenal tumor is being excised, early ligation of the adrenal vein is crucial in avoiding a sudden blood pressure elevation from the manipulation of the gland. Following tumor removal there will be a marked drop in blood pressure that can be minimized by maintenance of blood volume and administration of norepinephrine. With bilateral adrenalectomy, cortisone replacement must be instituted.

PROCEDURAL CONSIDERATIONS

For unilateral adrenalectomy the patient may be placed in the lateral or supine position (see Chapter 4). More often, however, both glands are explored, and the supine or prone position is selected. The prone position is especially useful for known pathology, such as aldosteronism, localized benign lesions, solitary adenomas of Cushing's disease, and debilitated patients with an advanced neoplasm.

Lateral approach

The setup for a lateral approach is as described for nephrectomy, including rib resection instruments, vascular instruments, and vessel clips and appliers.

Abdominal approach

The setup for an abdominal approach is as described for laparotomy, including vascular instruments, extra-long scissors, tissue forceps, Rochester-Pean forceps, Mixter forceps, and needle holders. Penrose tubing is needed for retraction. Vessel clips and appliers may also be needed, as well as various sizes of nonabsorbable braided sutures.

Posterior approach

The setup for the posterior approach is as described for the lateral approach.

The patient is placed prone in a 35-degree jackknife position with the kidney rest under the inferior margin of the anterior rib cage. Both arms should be extended cephalad with adequate support under each shoulder.

OPERATIVE PROCEDURES

Lateral approach

1. A flank, thoracolumbar, or transthoracic incision is performed as described for nephrectomy. The rib underlying the chosen approach is resected or deflected for optimum exposure of the upper pole of the kidney. Entry is between the eleventh and twelfth ribs in a flank approach, the tenth and eleventh ribs in a thoracolumbar approach, and the ninth and tenth ribs in a transthoracic approach.
2. An opening is made through the transverse fascia with scissors. The pleura and diaphragm are protected with moist packs, and Gerota's capsule is incised to expose the kidney and adrenal gland.
3. The gland is identified and dissected free from the upper pole of the kidney by scissors and Babcock forceps. The blood supply of the gland is identified, clamped or clipped, and divided. Bleeding vessels are ligated. To release the gland, the left adrenal vein, a branch of the left renal vein, is separated by clamping and cutting. The right adrenal vein, a tributary of the vena cava, is also

divided. Fine vascular sutures may be required to repair inadvertent injury to the vena cava.
4. When hemostasis has been ensured, the wound is closed sequentially in layers: muscle, fascia, subcutaneous tissue, and skin.

Abdominal approach

1. The abdominal wall is incised with an upper abdominal incision, and the peritoneal cavity is opened and explored. Bleeding vessels are clamped and ligated.
2. The abdominal wound is retracted, and the surrounding organs are protected with moist laparotomy packs. Instruments and sutures as described for routine laparotomy are used.
3. The retroperitoneal area near the diaphragm is opened on the left side, exposing the renal fascia.
4. The renal fascia is opened to reveal the left kidney and adrenal gland.
5. The adrenal gland is freed from the kidney by sharp and blunt dissection, and all bleeding vessels are clamped and ligated with no. 3-0 nonabsorbable sutures.
6. After all bleeding is controlled, the kidney is gently replaced in the renal fascia, which is closed with interrupted no. 0 absorbable sutures.
7. The peritoneum is closed over the left kidney and renal fascia.
8. The abdominal retractors are rearranged to give access to the peritoneum over the right kidney and adrenal gland. Care must be taken to prevent trauma to the liver.
9. The same procedure is repeated on the right side, taking care to clamp and ligate the short adrenal vein.
10. The abdomen is inspected for bleeding vessels, which are clamped and ligated.
11. The wound is closed as in laparotomy.

Posterior approach

1. An incision is made over the eleventh or twelfth rib. The periosteum is elevated, avoiding the nerve and vessels on the inferior margin. The diaphragm and pleura are displaced superiorly and the appropriate rib resected.
2. Hemostasis is maintained with electrocoagulation.
3. Gerota's fascia is incised, and through sharp and blunt dissection the posterior aspect of the upper pole of the kidney is exposed.
4. The upper pole is mobilized and a padded retractor deflects the kidney downward for the approach to the adrenal gland.
5. The suprarenal fat is meticulously dissected.
6. Vessel clips are utilized for control of smaller vessels.
7. Dissection continues superiorly, laterally, and inferiorly while the integrity of the hilum of the adrenal is maintained.

8. With right-angle clamps the adrenal vein and artery are freed, divided, and ligated with no. 0 or 2-0 braided nonabsorbable ties.

9. Babcock clamps are employed for manipulation and removal of the adrenal gland.

10. Bleeding is controlled and the wound inspected for injury to renal structures. Gerota's fascia is closed with interrupted absorbable sutures. The wound is closed in the standard fashion and dressed.

BIBLIOGRAPHY

Barry, M.J. (1993). Epidemiology and natural history of benign prostatic hyperplasia. In H. Lepor & R.K. Lawson, *Prostatic diseases,* Philadelphia: W.B. Saunders.

Benign Prostatic Hyperplasia: Diagnosis and Treatment guideline. (1994). Rockville, Md: Agency for Health Care Policy and Research.

Blanford, N.L. (1993). Renal transplantation: A case study of the ideal. *Critical Care Nurse, 13* (1), 46-55.

Blasko, J.C., et al. (1989). *Transperineal ultrasound-guided implants of the prostate.* Seattle: Publisher. Abstract presented at AUA Annual Conference.

Brundage, D.J. (1992). *Renal disorders.* St. Louis: Mosby.

Clayman, R.V., et al. (1992). *Laparoscopy.* Washington, D.C.: Publisher. Abstract presented at AUA Annual Conference.

Cooner, W.H., Eggers, G.W., & Lichtenstein, P. (1988). Prostate cancer: New hope for early diagnosis. In *Ultrasonography in urology.* New York: NYU Medical Center.

Droller, M.J. (1992). *Surgical management of urologic disease.* St. Louis: Mosby.

Gillenwater, J.Y., Grayhack, J.T., Howards, S.S., & Ducken, J.W. (1991). *Adult and pediatric urology.* St. Louis: Mosby.

Glenn, J.E. (1991). *Urologic surgery.* Philadelphia: J.B. Lippincott.

Goldstein, I. (1987). Penile revascularization. *Urology Clinics of North America, 14* (4).

Gray, H. (1991). *Anatomy descriptive and surgical.* St. Louis: Mosby.

Gray, M. (1992). *Genitourinary disorders.* St. Louis: Mosby.

Horne, M.M., & Swearingen, P.L. (1993). *Pocket guide to fluid, electrolyte, and acid base balance.* St. Louis: Mosby.

Huffman, J.L., Bagley, D.H., & Lyon, E.S. (1988). *Ureteroscopy.* Philadelphia: W.B. Saunders.

Montague, D.K., et al. (1988). *Disorders of male sexual function.* Chicago: Year Book Medical Publishers.

Moore, S., Newton, M., Grant, E., & Keetch, D. (1993). Treating bladder cancer: New methods, new management. *American Journal of Nursing. 93* (5), 32-39.

Pagana, K.D., & Pagana, T.J. (1992). *Diagnostic and laboratory test reference.* St. Louis: Mosby.

Petrou, S.P., and Barrett, D.M. (1992). *The expanded role for the artificial urinary sphincter.* Washington, D.C.: Publisher. Abstract presented at AUA Annual Conference.

Phipps, W.J., Long, B.C., & Woods, N.F. (1991). *Medical-surgical nursing.* St. Louis: Mosby.

Reddy, P.K., et al. (1988). Balloon dilatation of the prostate for treatment of benign hyperplasia. *Urology Clinics of North America, 15* (3).

Smith, J.A., Stein, B.S., & Benson, R.C. (1989). *Lasers in urologic surgery.* St. Louis: Mosby.

Smith, S.E., Brumm, J., & Crim, B.J. (1991). Transplantation—A donation to life: Organ procurement. *Today's O.R. Nurse, 13* (12), 5-8.

Tanagho, E.A., & McAninch, J.W. (1991). *Smith's general urology.* Norwalk, CT: Appleton & Lange.

Thibodeau, G.A. (1990). *Anthony's textbook of anatomy and physiology.* St. Louis: Mosby.

Uroplasty TCU dilatation catheter: Clinical evaluator's manual. (1989). San Clemente: Advanced Surgical Intervention.

Walsh, P.C., et al. (1992). *Radical prostatectomy and cystoprostatectomy.* Washington, D.C.: Publisher. Abstract presented at AUA Annual Conference.

15

THYROID AND PARATHYROID SURGERY

JANE HERSHEY JOHNSON

The thyroid gland functions primarily to secrete thyroxine (T_4) and triiodothyronine (T_3), which regulate energy metabolism and play an important role in regulating growth and development. Calcitonin is also produced by the thyroid gland and is involved with the regulation of calcium homeostasis. Thyroid-stimulating hormone (TSH) from the pituitary gland controls the production and secretion of thyroid hormones. The production and release of TSH are regulated by the thyrotropin-releasing hormone (TRH) from the hypothalamus.

Iodine is necessary for synthesis of thyroid hormones. Ingested iodides are absorbed from the small intestines into the circulatory system, from which they are sequestered by the thyroid gland. Iodides are converted into thyroid hormones, some of which are stored in the gland as thyroglobulin or are secreted into the blood as thyroid hormone. After removal of the thyroid gland synthetic oral thyroxine may be administered to help maintain a more normal metabolic rate for body processes.

Thyroid surgery was not considered safe until the late nineteenth century, when it was perfected by Theodor Kocher and Theodor Billroth. Since 1941 thyroidectomy as treatment of thyroid mass (goiter) has been reduced with the use of radioactive iodine and antithyroid drugs to decrease the activity of the gland. Diseases of the thyroid gland that require surgical intervention are primarily nodules of the thyroid and diffuse toxic goiters associated with hyperthyroidism.

Benign nodules are classified as adenomas, colloid nodules, thyroiditis, and cysts. Approximately 11,000 new cases of malignant lesions of the thyroid are diagnosed each year in the United States, and 1000 people die annually from thyroid cancer in this country. Malignant tumors are classified as papillary and mixed papillary-follicular (70%), follicular and Hürthle cell (15%), medullary (10%), anaplastic (5%), and lymphoma, sarcoma, & metastatic carcinoma (<1%). Thyroid cancer is more commonly seen after 25 years of age with a female predominance of about 3:1. Patients who received low-dose external radiation to the head and neck area as a child or who have a family history of medullary cancer of the thyroid are at risk for developing thyroid cancer (Research Highlight 15-1).

Diseases of the thyroid are usually manifested by alterations in hormonal secretion, enlargement of the thyroid, or both. Three forms of treatment are available: antithyroid drugs, radioactive iodine, and surgery. Before undergoing surgery, patients usually have their hyperthyroid state controlled with antithyroid drugs and radioiodine. Patients thus treated are restored to a euthyroid state and do not exhibit the common symptoms of rapid pulse, tremors, and nervous symptoms often associated with hyperthyroidism.

The parathyroid gland secretes parathyroid hormone (PTH). PTH and vitamin D are responsible for regulating

---

☀ RESEARCH HIGHLIGHT 15-1

Patients receiving neck irradiation for malignant disease may later develop thyroid diseases. This study employed a rigorous review of records of 1787 patients with Hodgkin's disease, 1677 of whom received thyroid irradiation. The patients were followed for a mean of 9.9 years. Analysis indicated that 573 patients had clinical or biochemical signs of thyroid disease. Hypothyroidism was present in 513 patients; 30 patients developed Graves' disease (a 7.2 to 20.4 greater risk than in healthy persons); six patients had silent thyroiditis with thyrotoxicosis. Of the 44 patients with thyroid nodules, six had papillary or follicular cancer (15.6 times greater than expected). This study emphasizes the high risk of thyroid disease after patients are treated with radiation therapy for Hodgkin's disease. Perioperative patient education should include the need for continued clinical follow-up in this patient population to detect the frequent occurrence of thyroid dysfunction, especially hypothyroidism.

Hancock, S.L., Cox, R.S., & McDougall, I.R. (1991). Thyroid diseases after treatment of Hodgkin's disease. *New England Journal of Medicine, 325,* 599-605.

calcium and phosphorus concentrations. Removal of all parathyroid tissue can result in severe tetany or death. The primary disease attributed to the parathyroid glands is hyperparathyroidism, which results in elevation of serum calcium. Symptoms of hyperparathyroidism include bone disease, renal calculi, pancreatitis, peptic ulcer, listlessness, weakness, and depression. Surgical intervention is indicated when symptoms occur, calcium levels are greater than 11.0 mg/dl, or renal function is impaired.

The diagnosis of hyperparathyroidism is being made more frequently with the increased use of diagnostic tests that include multiphasic screening of blood calcium. Manifestations may be quite subtle; many patients with mild hypercalcemia (serum calcium levels 10.5 to 11 mg/dl) are without any apparent symptoms.

SURGICAL ANATOMY

THYROID GLAND

The thyroid gland is a highly vascular organ situated in the anterior neck. It consists of right and left lobes united by a middle portion, the isthmus. The isthmus is situated near the base of the neck, and the lobes lie below the larynx and beside the trachea. The upper pole of the gland is hidden beneath the upper end of the sternothyroid muscle. The lower pole extends to about the level of the sixth tracheal ring. The posterior surface of the isthmus is adherent to the anterior surface of the tracheal rings, and the gland is enclosed by the pretracheal fascia (Fig. 15-1, *A*).

Blood supply to the thyroid is from the external carotid arteries via the superior thyroid arteries and from the subclavian arteries via the inferior thyroid arteries. The thyroid gland is drained by three pairs of veins (superior, middle, and inferior thyroid veins) that extend from a plexus formed on the surface of the gland and on the front of the trachea. The capillaries form a dense plexus in the connective tissue around the follicles.

Nerve supply to the thyroid gland is derived from the cervical sympathetic trunk. On each side the superior laryngeal nerve lies in proximity to the superior thyroid artery. The recurrent laryngeal nerve that supplies the vocal cord ascends from the mediastinum and is in close associ-

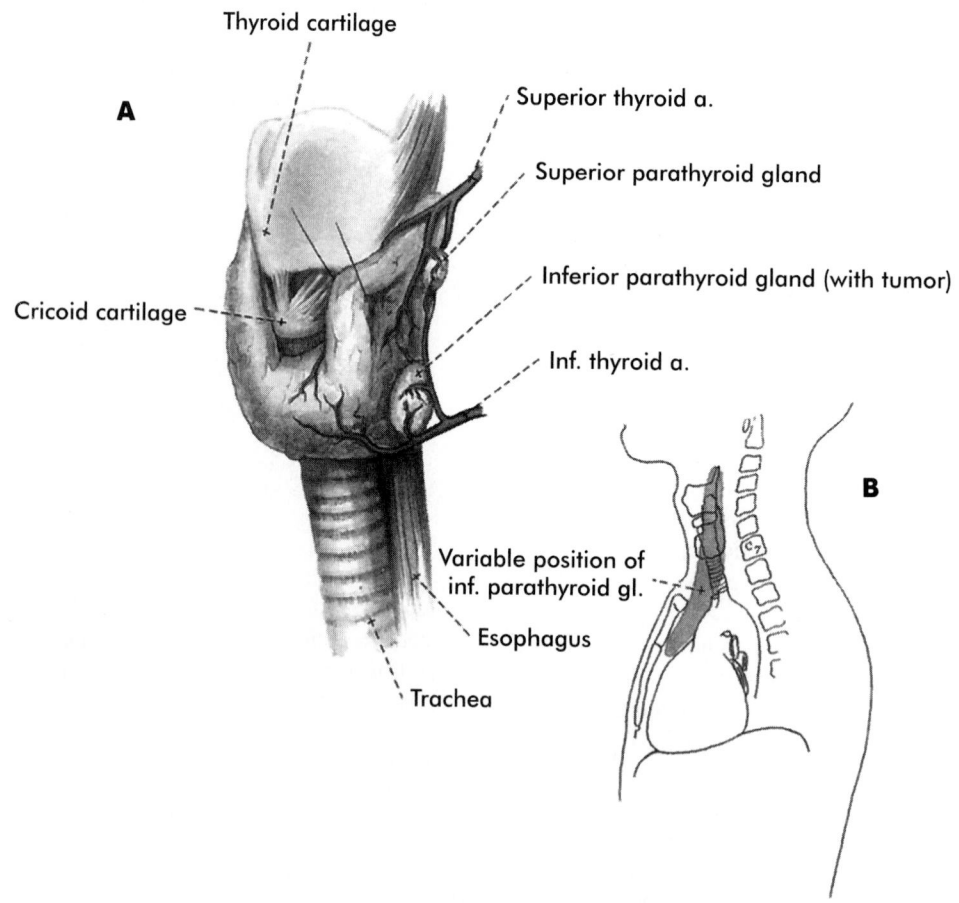

FIG. 15-1 **A,** Thyroid and parathyroid glands. Note their relation to each other and to trachea. **B,** Note the shaded area for varied locations of inferior parathyroid glands.

From Healy, J., & Hodge, J. (1990). *Surgical anatomy* (2nd ed.). Philadelphia: B.C. Decker.

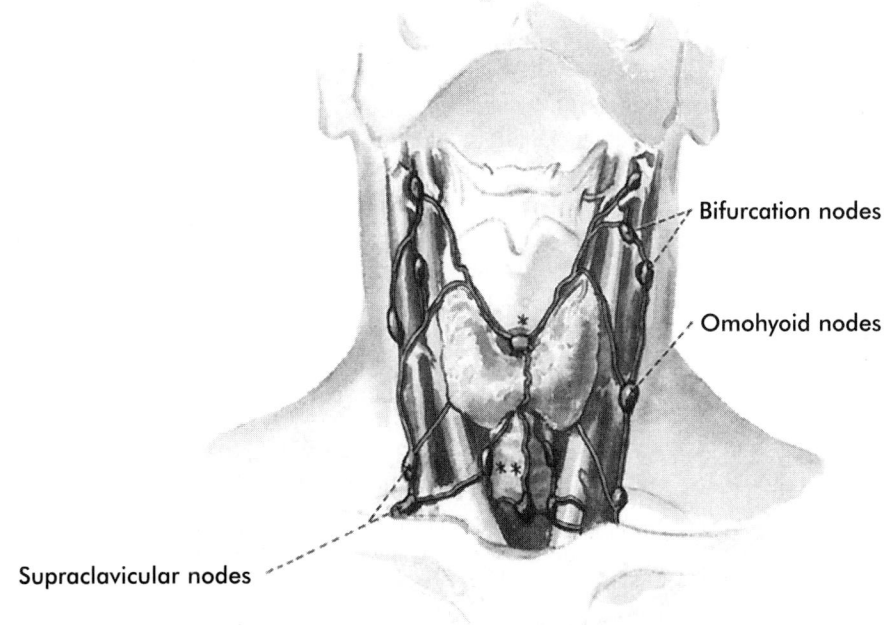

Bifurcation nodes

Omohyoid nodes

Supraclavicular nodes

*Prelaryngeal node (Delphian)
**Pre- and paratracheal nodes

FIG. 15-2 Lymphatics draining the thyroid gland.
From Healy, J., & Hodge, J. (1990). *Surgical anatomy* (2nd ed.). Philadelphia: B.C. Decker.

ation with the tracheoesophageal sulcus and the inferior thyroid artery. Sympathetic and parasympathetic nerves enter the gland, probably exerting their influence primarily on blood flow.

Lymphatic drainage of the thyroid gland is usually to the prelaryngeal (delphian), bifurcation, omohyoid, pretracheal, paratracheal, and supraclavicular nodes but may also drain directly into the deep cervical nodes, the thoracic duct, or the right lymph duct (Fig. 15-2).

PARATHYROID GLAND

The parathyroid glands consist of at least four small, red-brown to yellow-tan, ovoid masses of tissue lying behind or, rarely, within the thyroid gland inside the pretracheal fascia. The upper pair of glands lies behind the superior pole of the thyroid; the lower pair lies near the lower pole of the thyroid (see Fig. 15-1, *A*). Aberrant nodules of parathyroid tissue may be found outside the pretracheal fascia as low as the superior mediastinum, especially within the thymus (Fig. 15-1, *B*). Each parathyroid gland measures 5 to 7 mm × 3 to 4 mm × 0.5 to 2 mm and weighs an average of 30 to 40 mg. The upper glands are generally smaller than the lower ones.

Upper or superior parathyroid glands receive blood from a branch of the superior thyroid artery. Lower or inferior parathyroid glands receive blood from the superior branch of the descending inferior thyroid artery. Venous blood returns via tributaries of the thyroid veins. Lymphatic drainage of the parathyroid glands is the same as for the thyroid

gland. The parathyroid gland's nerve supply is from the cervical sympathetic trunks.

PERIOPERATIVE NURSING CONSIDERATIONS

ASSESSMENT

Preoperatively the patient with hyperthyroidism most likely has undergone appropriate drug therapy that has returned the thyroid hormone levels and metabolic state to normal. Nonetheless, the perioperative nurse should assess the patient for the presence of any symptoms that may relate to accelerated metabolism. They include irritability, hyperexcitability and exaggerated emotional responses, an abnormally elevated resting pulse, weight loss with fatigue and weakness, elevated systolic blood pressure, and cardiac symptoms such as palpitations or atrial fibrillation. The patient's cardiac and respiratory rate, muscle strength, elimination patterns, history of weight loss and heat intolerance, and emotional status should be noted. The patient may be anxious about the disease state and the success of surgery and may express concern regarding surgery in the area of the neck and its cosmetic results. Patients who are concerned about body image should have the opportunity to discuss these issues with the perioperative nurse. Skin integrity should be determined; patients with hyperthyroidism may have finely textured skin and edema in the lower extremities, placing them at risk for skin breakdown.

In addition to clinical signs and symptoms, results of diagnostic tests should be reviewed. Tests performed most commonly prior to thyroid surgery include measurements of T_3 and T_4 and radioisotope or ultrasonic scans, as well as a current electrocardiogram (ECG). Common laboratory and diagnostic tests and their normal adult ranges follow.

Direct and indirect measures of T_4 and T_3

Thyroid function tests are interpreted in light of the patient's clinical presentation. They complement the findings of physical examination.

Serum thyroxine (T_4): normal 5 to 10 μg/dl
Serum triiodothyronine (T_3): normal 110 to 230 ng/dl
Free thyroxine index (FTI, FT_4): normal 0.8 to 2.4 ng/dl[*]
Free FT_3, index: normal 0.25 to 0.65 ng/dl

Resin T_3 uptake (RT_3U): normal 25% to 35%[*]
Radioactive iodine uptake (RAIU): normal 24 hours, 8% to 30% absorbed[*]
Serum thyroid-stimulating hormone (TSH): normal 2 to 10 μmU/ml[*]

TRH testing is no longer needed to demonstrate thyrotroph suppression for mild or subclinical hyperthyroidism and for assessment of levothyroxine sodium suppressive therapy because of the availability of sensitive TSH assays (Research Highlight 15-2).

[*]Variations with different labs.

RESEARCH HIGHLIGHT 15-2

Ross and colleagues compared the measurement of TSH levels using the new chemiluminescent assay and the immunoradiometric assay. A group of 145 patients with TSH levels below 0.08 mU/L using the immunoradiometric assay had sera analyzed with the chemiluminescent assay. The new chemiluminescent TSH assay yielded an eight-to-tenfold increased sensitivity over the immunoradiometric assay. The increased sensitivity resulted in a better ability to distinguish hyperthyroidism from euthyroidism and to distinguish the degree of thyrotroph suppression in subclinical hyperthyroidism. An important clinical implication is the ability to diagnose subclinical hyperthyroidism and prevent the potential adverse consequences, especially on the skeleton.

Ross, D., Ardisson, L., & Meskell, M. (1989). Measurement of thyrotropin in clinical and subclinical hyperthyroidism using a new chemiluminescent assay. *Journal of Clinical Endocrinology and Metabolism, 69* (3), 684-688.

Assessment of thyroid anatomy

In addition to palpating the thyroid gland for size, contour, consistency, nodes, and fixation, health care professionals use scans to yield evidence of thyroid anatomy.

Thyroid isotope scan

Normal scans show normal size, shape, position, and function of the thyroid, with no areas of decreased or increased uptake. Nodules that are warm or hot are functioning and may indicate a benign adenoma or localized toxic goiter. Cold nodules are nonfunctioning and could indicate a cyst, carcinoma, nonfunctioning adenoma or goiter, lymphoma, or localized area of thyroiditis.

Ultrasonic scan

Normal scans indicate normal size, shape, and position of the thyroid gland. The ultrasonic scan is valuable in differentiating cystic from solid thyroid nodules.

Parathyroid assessment

Tests used in the diagnosis of hyperparathyroidism are serum parathormone (normal <2000 pg/ml; value varies with laboratory) and serum calcium (9 to 10.5 mg/dl) done at the same time. Thallium-technetium scan or ultrasound of the parathyroids can indicate the presence of adenoma(s) or hyperplasia.

Preoperative patient education should include an explanation of perioperative events, discussion of the incision site, type of dressing to be used, and explanation of the closed-wound suction drainage system, if its use is anticipated. The patient should also be instructed in ways to support the neck postoperatively to prevent strain on the incision line.

Hyperparathyroidism causes an imbalance in the level of serum calcium and a decrease in the level of serum phosphate. Nursing diagnoses and care planning will be based on these imbalances and the severity of the associated symptoms. Some patients are asymptomatic; other patients have symptoms that manifest themselves as disturbances in the renal, gastrointestinal, cardiovascular, musculoskeletal, or central nervous system.

Assessment should include determining whether the patient is apathetic or emotionally irritable; whether there is muscle weakness and fatigue; skeletal pain or tenderness; nausea; vomiting; constipation; peptic ulcer disease; cardiac dysrhythmia; or renal damage, stones, or disease. If any of these signs or symptoms are present, the plan of care should be adjusted. Otherwise, perioperative nursing management of the patient undergoing parathyroidectomy is essentially the same as for thyroidectomy. In the early postoperative period for both thyroidectomy and parathyroidectomy the patient should be closely observed for any signs of tetany.

NURSING DIAGNOSIS

Nursing diagnoses related to the care of patients undergoing thyroid and parathyroid surgery might include the following:

- Impaired swallowing related to mechanical obstruction (enlarged thyroid preoperatively; edema postoperatively)
- Ineffective thermoregulation related to altered metabolic rate
- Body image disturbance related to surgical scar in prominent location
- Ineffective airway clearance related to obstruction (enlarged thyroid preoperatively; edema postoperatively)
- Impaired gas exchange related to postoperative bleeding or swelling or inability to move secretions

OUTCOME IDENTIFICATION

Outcomes identified for the selected nursing diagnoses could be stated as the following:

- Patient will maintain normal swallowing.
- Patient will maintain normal body temperature.
- Patient will verbalize decreased disturbance in feelings related to body image.
- Patient will maintain a patent airway.
- Patient will maintain effective gas exchange.

PLANNING

Because a potential problem for patients with hyperthyroidism is thyroid storm (thyrotoxic crisis) the perioperative nurse must be prepared to respond quickly. It can occur in patients who are partially controlled or who are untreated for their hyperthyroidism. Thyrotoxic crisis can be precipitated by a stressful event such as surgery. By planning a quiet, calm atmosphere and helping the patient relax, the perioperative nurse can reduce the risk of thyroid storm. Collaborating with the surgical and anesthesia team, the perioperative nurse can plan for the appropriate interventions to assist in reducing body temperature and heart rate, provide oxygen and intravenous solutions, and administer medications as prescribed in the event thyrotoxic crisis occurs.

A typical care plan for a patient undergoing thyroid and parathyroid surgery follows.

IMPLEMENTATION

Positioning

After the patient is properly anesthetized, the position is changed to a modified dorsal recumbent, with an inflatable pillow or rolled sheet placed between the scapulae to extend the neck and raise the shoulders. The head is stabilized by placement on a foam headrest. If an inflatable pillow is used, it should be placed (uninflated) before the patient is anesthetized and then inflated. Some surgeons prefer to keep the legs level and elevate the back of the OR bed until distended neck veins disappear. Others position the patient in the reverse Trendelenburg's position. The latter necessitates the use of a padded footboard to keep the feet in proper alignment and prevent the patient from sliding down on the bed. The arms are positioned at the sides with the elbows adequately protected by the lift sheet or elbow guards.

Skin preparation

The operative area, including the chin and anterior neck region, lateral surfaces of the neck, from the earlobes down to the outer aspects of the shoulder, and the upper anterior chest region to the nipples, is prepared with an antimicrobial solution. Appropriate precautions must be taken to prevent solution from pooling under the neck or in the axillary area. The patient is draped with sterile towels and a fenestrated sheet. A sterile towel or lap sponge may be placed on each side of the neck to prevent pooling of blood under the neck during surgery.

The surgeon marks the incision site with a marking pen or with the pressure of a full-length fine silk tie to help ensure a wound line that blends with the patient's neck creases and skin lines.

Instrumentation

A standard instrument setup for thyroid surgery includes the following:

Soft tissue/plastic surgery instruments

2 Knife handles, no. 3	2 Vascular needle holders, 7 inch
2 Adson tissues forceps, 1 Brown and 1 regular with teeth	2 Plastic needle holders, 5 inch
2 Tissue forceps, 5 ½ inch, smooth and with teeth	1 Fine curved Metzenbaum scissors
10 Straight mosquito hemostats	2 Mayo scissors, curved and straight
10 Curved mosquito hemostats	2 Suction tips, Frazier no. 10 and Yankauer
6 Curved hemostats	2 Skin hooks
2 Kelly clamps	2 Double hooks
4 Allis tissue forceps	2 Medium dull rake retractors
4 Kocher clamps	2 Gelpi retractors
2 Small right angle clamps	2 Vein retractors
2 Regular right angle clamps	2 Senn retractors
4 Schnidt clamps	2 Small dull Weitlaners
	2 Richardson retractors, shallow

Special or thyroid instruments

4 Lahey vulsellum clamps	1 Mahorner retractor (self-retaining thyroid retractor)
2 Greene retractors or loop retractors	

EVALUATION

Evaluation of intraoperative interventions determines effectiveness of positioning aids and pressure-relief devices, drip towels to collect excess prep solutions, and other interventions based on the patient's special needs. The report to PACU personnel includes the surgical procedure, anesthesia given, location of drain, if any, dressing used, condition of skin postoperatively, and any other information specific to the patient's nursing diagnoses. Documentation

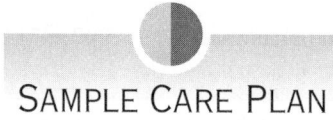

SAMPLE CARE PLAN

NURSING DIAGNOSIS: Swallowing, impaired, related to mechanical obstruction (enlarged thyroid preoperatively; edema post-operatively)

OUTCOME: Patient will maintain normal swallowing.

INTERVENTIONS:

Keep suction line and suction catheter ready until patient is discharged from OR.

Monitor for and report difficulty in swallowing.

Gently suction oropharyngeal secretions as required.

Keep vein open postoperatively until patient can swallow without difficulty.

NURSING DIAGNOSIS: Ineffective thermoregulation related to altered metabolic rate

OUTCOME: Patient's body temperature will be maintained within normal range.

INTERVENTIONS:

Monitor patient's temperature; report abnormalities.

Provide light covers if temperature elevated or patient states he or she is warm.

Change linens preoperatively and postoperatively if wet from perspiration.

Avoid using plasticized drapes.

NURSING DIAGNOSIS: Body image disturbance related to surgical scar

OUTCOME: Patient will verbalize decreased disturbance in feelings related to body image.

INTERVENTIONS:

Explain that incision is made in natural fold of skin.

Explain how techniques used for surgical closure minimize scarring.

Instruct patient in postoperative turning measures that decrease strain on suture line.

Suggest that jewelry, scarves, and certain necklines can be used to cover scar until normal fading occurs.

NURSING DIAGNOSIS: High risk for ineffective airway clearance related to obstruction secondary to enlarged thyroid (preoperatively) or edema (postoperatively)

OUTCOME: Patient's airway will remain patent.

INTERVENTIONS:

Position patient so that enlarged gland does not obstruct airway. Head of transport vehicle may need to be elevated preoperatively.

Assist anesthesia personnel during induction.

Monitor respiratory rate and signs of respiratory distress (stridor, wheezing, dyspnea, labored respirations).

Observe dressing and neck area (front, sides, and back) for signs of edema or bleeding (postoperatively).

NURSING DIAGNOSIS: High risk for impaired gas exchange related to post-operative bleeding/swelling or inability to move secretions

OUTCOME: Patient's gas exchange will remain effective.

INTERVENTIONS:

Monitor respiratory status and results of pulse oximetry.

If patient is extubated in OR, be prepared to assist anesthesia personnel; closely observe for respiratory stridor or respiratory obstruction (recurrent laryngeal nerve injury). Tracheostomy may be required; trach tray should be available.

Assess color of nailbeds.

Monitor surgical site for swelling and bleeding.

Suction patient as required to remove secretions.

Monitor patency of surgical drain.

is according to hospital protocol. It should reflect achievement of patient outcomes related to planned interventions; these should also be included in the nursing report to PACU personnel. For the nursing diagnoses selected for the patient undergoing thyroid or parathyroid surgery the following outcomes would be communicated:

- Patient maintained normal swallowing.
- Patient maintained normal body temperature.
- Patient verbalized decreased disturbance in feelings related to body image.
- Patient maintained a patent airway; there was no edema at the surgical site or signs of respiratory distress.
- Patient maintained adequate gas exchange; O_2 saturation remained normal. The patient was extubated without incident.

SURGICAL INTERVENTIONS

TOTAL THYROIDECTOMY, SUBTOTAL THYROIDECTOMY, AND THYROID LOBECTOMY

Thyroidectomy is removal of the entire thyroid gland; subtotal thyroidectomy leaves the posterior portions of each lobe intact to protect the recurrent laryngeal nerves and the integrity of the parathyroid glands; thyroid lobectomy is removal of a lobe of the thyroid gland. The purpose of surgical intervention relates to the patient's medical diagnosis.

Hyperthyroidism (Graves' disease) is associated with diffuse, bilateral enlargement of the thyroid gland. Hashimoto's thyroiditis is thought to be an autoimmune disease, and nontender enlargement of the gland occurs. Surgery is performed to relieve tracheal obstruction. Nontoxic nodular goiter does not produce an excess of hormones and is noninflammatory in character; thyroid tissue proliferates in an attempt to produce the minimal hormonal requirement. Surgery may be indicated to relieve tracheal or esophageal obstruction or to rule out a malignant nodule of the thyroid gland. Total thyroidectomy is done for malignant tumors.

Procedural considerations

These patients need an environment that is calm and quiet to reduce the risk of overstimulation, which could result in thyroid crisis.

Operative procedure

1. A transverse incision is made through the skin and first layer of the cervical fascia and platysma muscle, approximately 2 cm above the sternoclavicular junction (Fig. 15-3).
2. Flaps may be held away from the wound with stay sutures inserted through the cervical fascia and platysma muscle.

3. The upper skin flap is undermined to the level of the cricoid cartilage; the lower flap is then undermined to the sternoclavicular joint with a knife, fine curved scissors, tissue forceps, and gauze sponges. Bleeding vessels are clamped with hemostats and ligated with fine, nonabsorbable sutures.
4. The fascia in the midline is incised between the strap (sternohyoid) muscles with a knife (Fig. 15-4, *A*); the sternocleidomastoid muscle may be retracted with a loop retractor; the strap muscles may be divided between clamps, using Kochers or hemostats and a knife. The divided muscles are retracted from the operative site with retractors, thereby exposing the diseased lobe. This maneuver is necessary only for markedly enlarged lobes. Usually the strap muscles may be retracted to provide adequate exposure.
5. The inferior and middle thyroid veins are clamped, divided with Metzenbaum scissors, and ligated with fine nonabsorbable sutures (Fig. 15-4, *B*).
6. The lobe is rotated medially, and the loose areolar tissue is divided posteriorly and medially toward the tracheoesophageal sulcus with hemostats and Metzenbaum scissors. Small sponges are used for blunt dissection. Bleeding is controlled by hemostats and ligatures, as well as by electrosurgery. The recurrent laryngeal nerve is identified and carefully preserved (Fig. 15-5, *A*).
7. The thyroid lobe is pulled downward, and the avascular tissue between the trachea and upper pole of the thyroid is dissected by means of Metzenbaum scissors.
8. The superior thyroid artery is secured with two or three curved hemostats or right-angle clamps; the artery is ligated and divided and then is transfixed with nonabsorbable sutures.

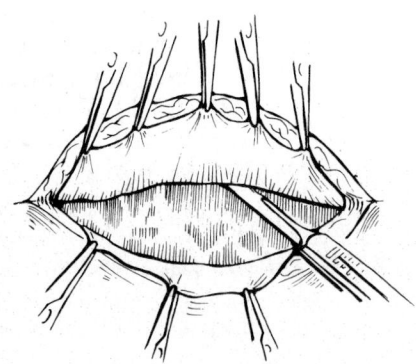

FIG. 15-3 Beginning of thyroidectomy. Skin flaps are created by dissection deep to platysma muscle and cervical fascia.

9. The inferior thyroid artery is identified and ligated by means of fine forceps, sutures, and scissors (Fig. 15-5, *A*). The thyroid lobe is then dissected away from the recurrent nerve with Metzenbaum scissors and hemostats. Bleeding vessels are clamped with hemostats and ligated with fine nonabsorbable sutures.

10. The lobe is elevated with Lahey vulsellum clamps; it is freed from the trachea with fine scissors, forceps, knife, and hemostats. The fibrous bands attached to the trachea and cricoid cartilage are divided.

11. The isthmus of the gland is elevated with fine forceps and divided between hemostats with scissors. If a pyramidal lobe is present, it is removed from its attachment to the gland to its termination in the neck, which may reach the hyoid bone.

12. The cut surface of the opposite lobe requires careful hemostasis. A running suture may be utilized for this purpose as well as to reapproximate it to the pretracheal fascia.

13. The strap muscles, if severed, are approximated with interrupted absorbable or nonabsorbable sutures. A drain may be inserted in the thyroid bed and brought

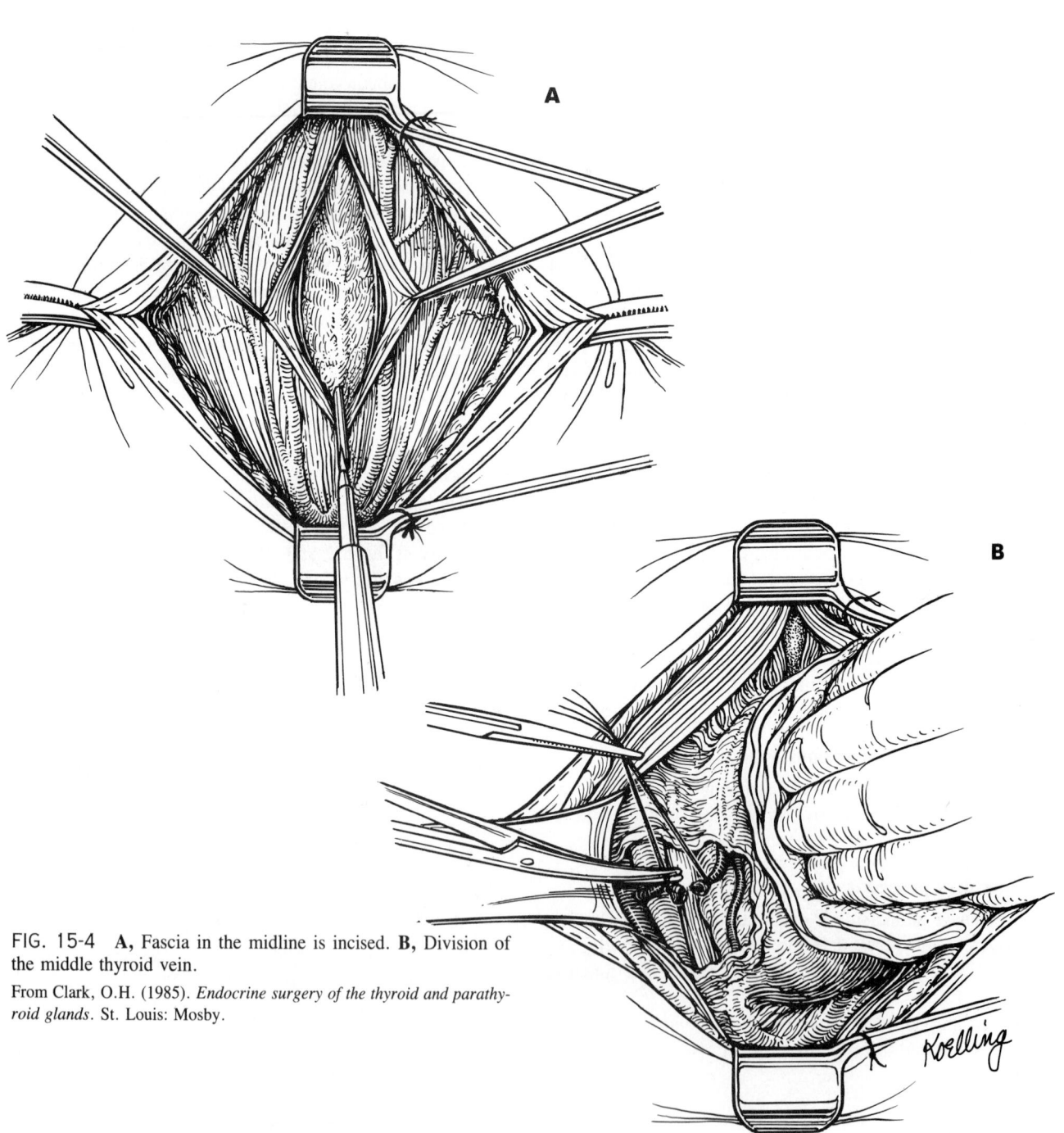

FIG. 15-4   **A,** Fascia in the midline is incised. **B,** Division of the middle thyroid vein.

From Clark, O.H. (1985). *Endocrine surgery of the thyroid and parathyroid glands*. St. Louis: Mosby.

out between the strap muscles and sternocleidomastoid muscle. Many surgeons prefer to drain the wound laterally through the sternocleidomastoid muscle and the lateral extremity of the incision in the belief that this will produce better healing and cosmetic results. However, drainage is not always necessary.

14. The edges of the platysma muscle are approximated (Fig. 15-5, *B*). The skin edges are then approximated with subcuticular, fine absorbable sutures.

15. Wound closure tapes (e.g. Steri-Strips) are applied to the wound edges and gauze dressings are placed on the wound with minimal tape.

SUBSTERNAL OR INTRATHORACIC THYROIDECTOMY

Extensions of enlarging goiters into the substernal and intrathoracic regions may be seen. They may cause tracheal and esophageal obstruction, in which case they are usually excised surgically. Longer instruments are usually required. Splitting the sternum is rarely necessary.

THYROGLOSSAL DUCT CYSTECTOMY

Thyroglossal duct cystectomy is complete excision of all portions of the cyst and duct, as well as a portion of the hyoid bone, which contains the duct, to avoid recurrent cys-

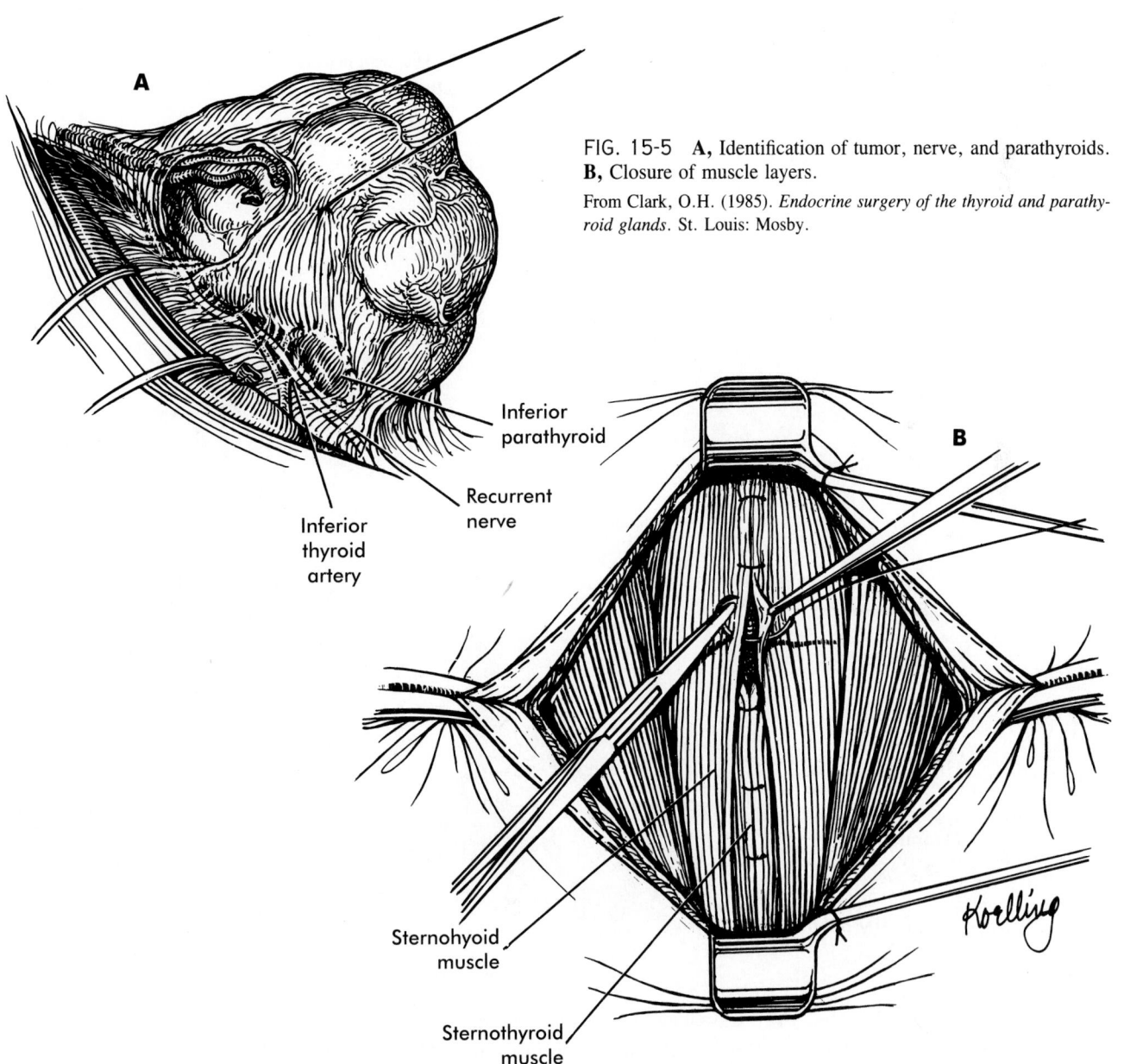

FIG. 15-5   **A,** Identification of tumor, nerve, and parathyroids. **B,** Closure of muscle layers.

From Clark, O.H. (1985). *Endocrine surgery of the thyroid and parathyroid glands.* St. Louis: Mosby.

Inferior parathyroid

Recurrent nerve

Inferior thyroid artery

Sternohyoid muscle

Sternothyroid muscle

tic formation and to prevent infections. The thyroglossal duct is an embryologic structure present during the descent of the thyroid gland into the anterior neck. When present in an adult, it exists as a pretracheal cystic pouch attached to the hyoid bone, with or without a sinus tract to the base of the tongue at the foramen cecum (Fig. 15-6).

Procedural considerations

The perioperative nursing assessment should be appropriate to the patient's age, since the patient is frequently a child or teenager (see Chapter 28 for a detailed discussion of the younger patient's needs). Reassurance and information regarding the procedure should be given.

A thyroidectomy setup, plus the following instruments, is used:

1 Probe
1 Periosteal elevator, small
1 Duckbill rongeur, small
1 Bone cutter, small
1 Syringe, 5 ml, with appropriate needle
Methylene blue dye for injection

Operative procedure

1. After the head is extended and the chin is elevated, an incision is made between the hyoid bone and the thyroid cartilage through the subcutaneous tissue.
2. The platysma muscle is incised, and the flaps are raised as described previously.
3. The strap (sternohyoid) muscles are separated in the midline.
4. Sharp and blunt dissection is used to mobilize the cyst and duct, up to the attachment to the hyoid bone. The hyoid bone is transsected twice with bone-cutting forceps, and the segment of bone and cyst is freed from adjacent structures.
5. The cephalic part of the duct is identified, a transfixion suture is passed through it, and the duct is transsected. (Methylene blue dye injection is used occasionally to visualize the whole tract.)
6. The cyst is removed. The strap muscles are closed with interrupted, fine nonabsorbable sutures. A drain may be placed. The skin is closed with subcuticular, fine absorbable sutures.

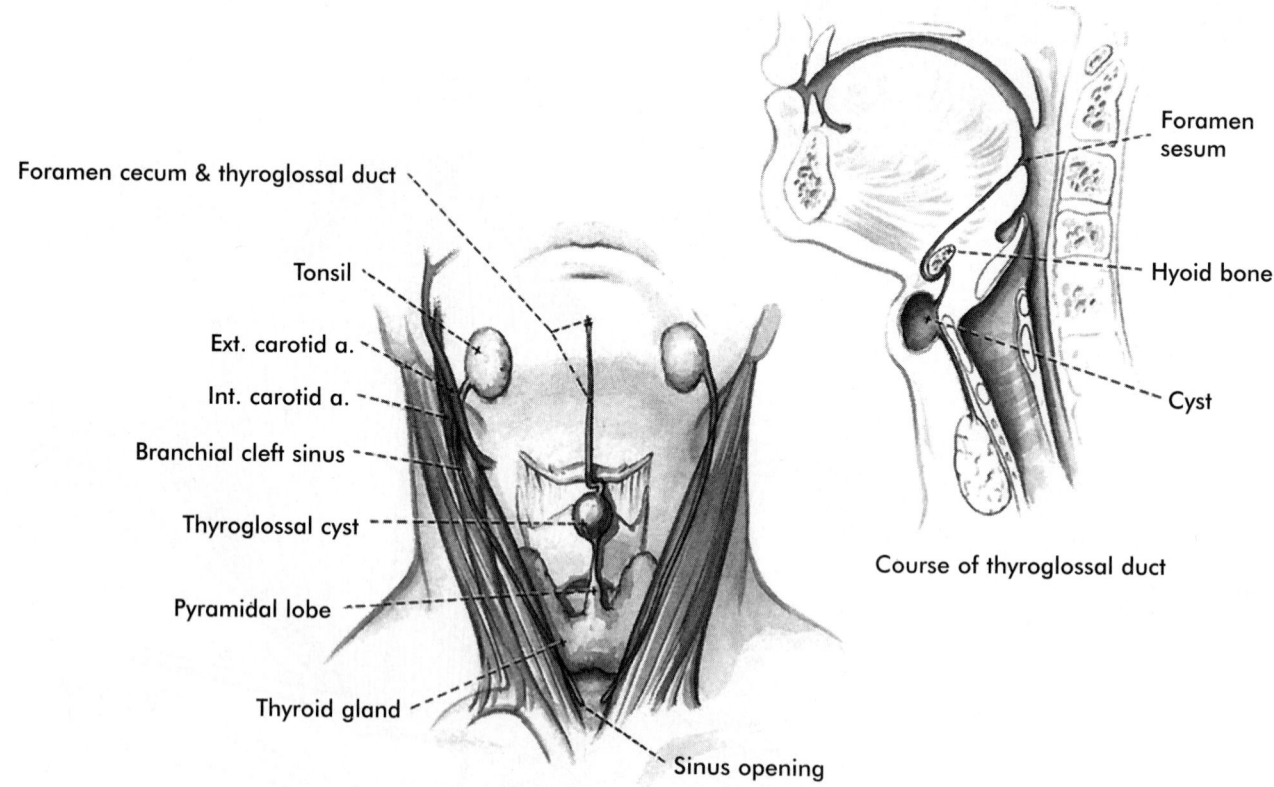

FIG. 15-6 Thyroglossal cyst showing both anterior and lateral views.
From Healy, J., & Hodge, J. (1990). *Surgical anatomy* (2nd ed.). Philadelphia: B.C. Decker.

PARATHYROIDECTOMY

Parathyroidectomy is excision of one or more parathyroid glands. Normal or atrophic glands are not removed. The presence of adenomas (hypersecreting neoplasms), hyperplasia, or carcinomas requires surgical excision. In the last case, resection of lymph nodes is essential, although metastasis may also occur by way of the bloodstream. After local excision, a metastasis may cause hypersecretion of parathormone.

Procedural considerations

The instrument setup is identical to that for thyroid operations, with the addition of numerous specimen containers that are necessary for the multiple biopsies used to determine the presence or absence of parathyroid tissue.

Operative procedure

1. See approach to the thyroid gland, described previously.
2. With the thyroid gland visible, a thorough exploration of the "normal" locations of the four parathyroid glands is conducted. Meticulous hemostasis by means of mosquito hemostats and fine ligatures is a prerequisite to location and identification of these small glands.
3. The thyroid gland is gently rotated anteriorly to provide access to the posterior thyroid sulcus, where the parathyroid glands are almost always found. Identification of the parathyroid vascular pedicle as it leaves the superior thyroid artery is an excellent means of locating the upper glands. Metzenbaum scissors, mosquito hemostats, and Kitner (peanut) sponges are used in the dissection.
4. Attention is directed toward the posterior lateral surface of the thyroid lobe or just beneath the lower thyroid pole, where the lower parathyroid glands are frequently found. Finding the vascular pedicle from the inferior thyroid artery may aid in identification. Occasionally the lower pair is found in the thymic capsule or tissue, in which case a portion of the thymus is resected.
5. Should one of the parathyroid glands evidence disease, it is resected by clamping the vascular pedicle with mosquito hemostats, dividing with small scissors or knife, and ligating with a fine nonabsorbable suture. The question of how much parathyroid tissue to remove is controversial and relates to whether single or multiple glands are involved, regardless of their size and appearance. A portion of one gland must remain to prevent complications. NOTE: A current concept or alternative for multiple gland involvement is to excise all four glands, transplanting a portion of one in an accessible site such as the neck or forearm for later removal if hypercalcemia recurs. This eliminates reexploration and potential injury to the recurrent laryngeal nerve.
6. The neck region is explored for aberrant parathyroid tissue, which is also resected (Fig. 15-1, *B*).
7. The remainder of the operation is the same as that described for the thyroid gland.

BIBLIOGRAPHY

Abernathy, C., & Harken, A. (1991). *Surgical secrets.* Philadelphia: Hanley & Belfus.

Atkinson, L. (1992). *Berry & Kohn's operating room technique.* St. Louis: Mosby.

Bagdade, J. (1992). *Year book of endocrinology.* St. Louis: Mosby.

Berkovitz, B., & Moxham, B. (1988). *A textbook of head and neck anatomy.* Barcelona: Wolf Publishing.

Cameron, J. (1992). *Current surgical therapy* (4th ed.). St. Louis: Mosby.

Edis, A., Ayala, L., & Egdahl, R. (1984). *Manual of endocrine surgery* (2nd ed.). New York: Springer-Verlag.

Farrar, J. & Toff, A.D. (1991). Iodine-131 treatment of hyperthyroidism: Current issues. *Clinical Endocrinology, 35,* 207-212.

Fischer, J. (1993). *Surgical basic science.* St. Louis: Mosby.

Galloway, J., et al. (1991). Changing trends in thyroid surgery. *American Surgeon, 57,* 18-20.

Hancock, S.L., Cox, R.S., & McDougall, I.R. (1991). Thyroid diseases after treatment of Hodgkins's disease. *New England Journal of Medicine, 325,* 599-605.

Healy, J., & Hodge, J. (1990). *Surgical anatomy* (2nd Ed.). Philadelphia: B.C. Decker.

Kaplan, E. (1986). Surgical endocrinology. In Polk, H., et al. (Eds.). *Basic surgery* (3rd ed.). Norwalk, CT: Appleton-Century-Crofts.

Kneedler, J., & Dodge, G. (1987). *Perioperative patient care, the nursing perspective* (2nd ed.). Boston: Blackwell Scientific Publications.

Lewis, S., & Collier, I. (1992). *Medical-surgical nursing* (3rd Ed.). St. Louis: Mosby.

Martinelli, A., & Fontana, J. (1990). Thyroid storm: Potential perioperative crisis. *AORN Journal, 52* (2), 305-313.

Pagana, K., & Pagana, T. (1992). *Mosby's diagnostic and laboratory test reference.* St. Louis: Mosby.

Robbins, J., et al. (1991). Thyroid cancer: A lethal endocrine neoplasm. *Annals of Internal Medicine, 115,* 133-147.

Ross, D., Ardisson, L., & Meskell, M. (1989). Measurement of thyrotropin in clinical and subclinical hyperthyroidism using a new chemiluminescent assay. *Journal of Clinical Endocrinology and Metabolism, 69* (3), 684-688.

Rothrock, J. (1990). *Perioperative nursing care planning.* St. Louis: Mosby.

Sabiston, D. (1991). *Textbook of surgery* (14th ed.). Philadelphia: W.B. Saunders.

Thibodeau, G. (1990). *Anthony's textbook of anatomy and physiology* (13th ed.). St. Louis: Mosby.

16

BREAST SURGERY

ROSEMARY ANN ROTH

Surgical procedures on the breast are commonly performed in all hospitals and free-standing surgical centers. Most procedures are performed to establish a definitive diagnosis when cancer is a possibility or to treat a breast cancer.

The possibility of and actual occurrence of breast changes, either benign or malignant, are some of the most emotionally upsetting health problems confronting women. Breast cancer is the leading cause of cancer-related death in women after 55 years of age. The probability of developing breast cancer increases with age. Estimates predict that 1 in 9 women in the United States will develop breast cancer during her life. This risk is increased if a woman's mother, sister, or daughter has had breast cancer, especially if the cancer developed before menopause.

Changing hormone levels from puberty throughout the remainder of life affect breast tissue in its physical and microscopic characteristics. In association with these changes, numerous aberrations and tumors can occur.

Operative procedures on the breast may be indicated in the presence of disease or as a result of other physical or psychologic patient considerations. Reconstructive surgery of the breast is discussed in Chapter 23.

SURGICAL ANATOMY

The breasts are bilateral mammary glands that lie on the pectoralis major fascia of the anterior chest wall. They are surrounded by a layer of fat and are encased in an envelope of skin. The breasts extend from the second to the sixth rib and horizontally from the lateral edge of the sternum to the anterior axillary line. The largest part of the mammary gland rests on the connective tissue of the pectoralis major muscle and laterally on the serratus anterior (upper outer quadrant of the breast), with a normal globular contour occurring as a result of the fascial support (Cooper's ligaments). An elongation of mammary tissue normally extends laterally on the pectoralis major toward the axilla and is known as the tail of Spence (Fig. 16-1).

Each breast is made up of 12 to 20 glandular lobes that

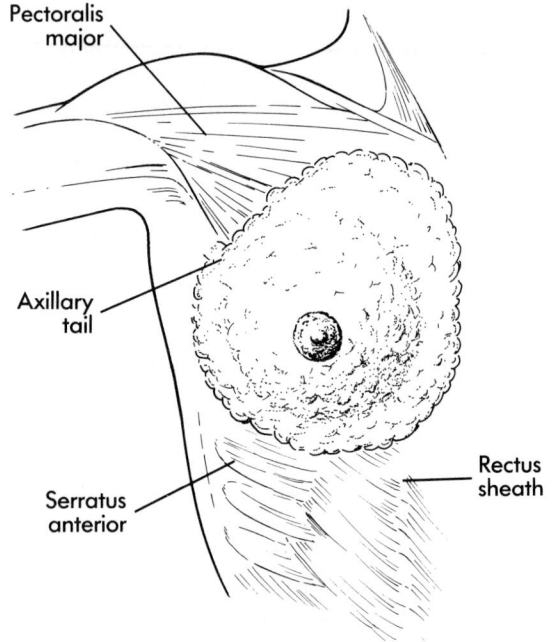

FIG. 16-1 Normal distribution of mammary tissue of adult female breast.
From Isaacs, J.H. (1992). *Textbook of breast disease*. St. Louis: Mosby.

are separated by connective tissue. Each lobe drains by a single lactiferous duct that opens on the nipple. The nipple, located in the fourth intercostal space, forms a conical projection into which the ducts open independent of each other on the surface. A pigmented circular area called the areola surrounds the nipple. Smooth muscle fibers of the areola contract to allow for nipple projection.

Three major arterial systems (Fig. 16-2) generously supply the mammary glands with blood. The main sources are branches of the internal mammary and the lateral branches of the anterior aortic intercostal arteries, all of which form an extensive network of anastomoses over the breast. A third source is the pectoral branch, deriving from a branch of the axillary artery. The veins that mainly drain the breasts

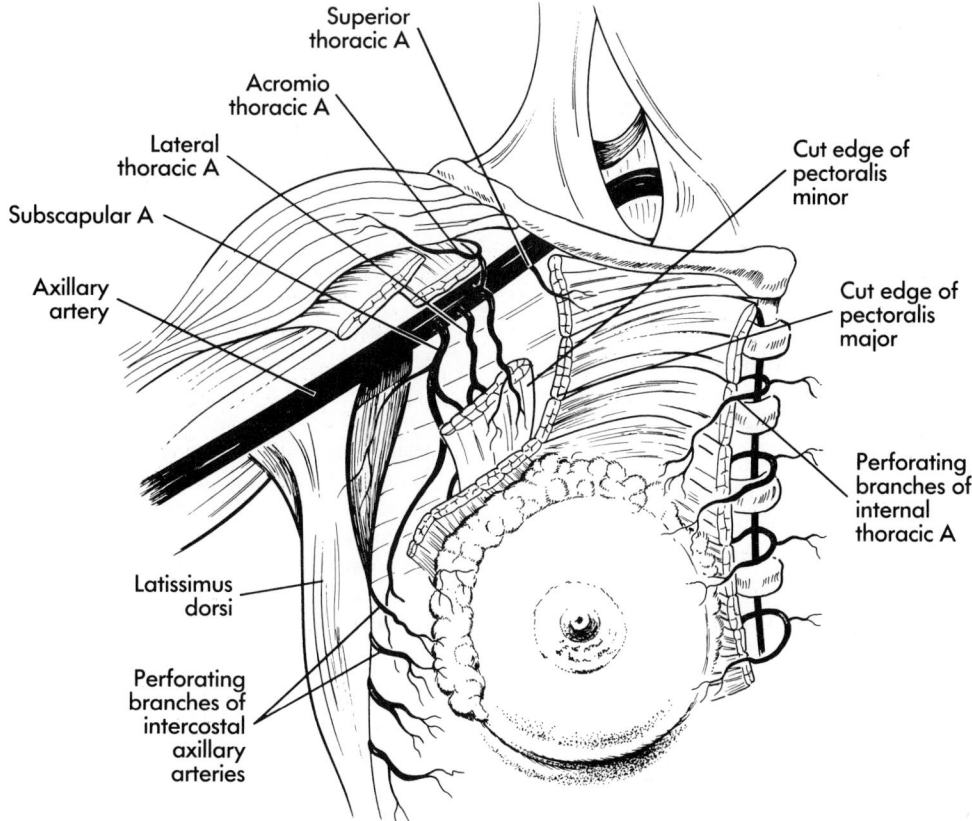

FIG. 16-2   Distribution of axillary and thoracic lymph nodes.
From Isaacs, J.H. (1992). *Textbook of breast disease*. St. Louis: Mosby.

follow the course of the arteries. The superficial veins frequently become dilated during pregnancy.

The lymph drainage system generally follows the course of the vessels. The lymphatics drain into two main areas represented by the axillary nodes and the internal thoracic chain of nodes (Fig. 16-3). The internal thoracic nodes are few but are responsible for most of the lymph drainage from the inner half of the breast. Thus one can see how the lymph system could be a channel for the spread of malignant disease from the breast to associated areas of the chest wall or to the axilla.

The sensory nerve supply is mainly from the anterior cutaneous branches of the upper intercostal nerves, the third and fourth branches of the cervical plexus, and the lateral cutaneous branches of the intercostal nerves.

Occasionally, developmental errors of the breast occur. Additional nipples or extramammary tissue in the axilla or over the upper abdomen may be present. The preferred treatment of these supernumerary structures is excision. Absence of one or both nipples may also occur and may be associated with absence of the underlying pectoral muscle and chest wall. The mammary glands are affected by three types of physiologic changes: (1) those related to growth and development, (2) those related to the menstrual cycle,

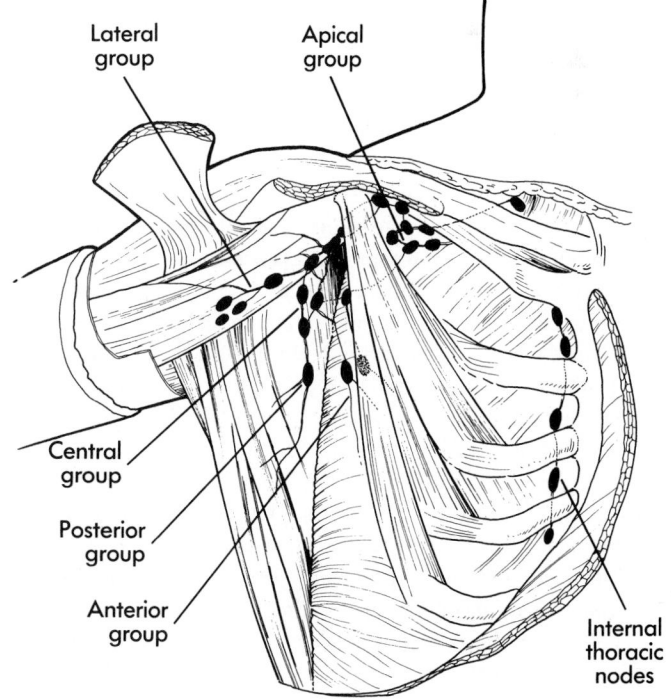

FIG. 16-3   Normal arterial blood supply of the breast.
From Isaacs, J.H. (1992). *Textbook of breast disease*. St. Louis: Mosby.

and (3) those related to pregnancy and lactation. The mammary glands are present at birth in both males and females. Hormonal stimulation, however, produces the development and function of these glands in females. Estrogen promotes growth of the ductal structures, whereas progesterone promotes lobular development.

BENIGN LESIONS OF THE BREAST

A fibroadenoma, affecting primarily young women under 30 years of age, is usually a solitary nodule. These masses are small, painless lesions that are well delineated and relatively mobile. They grow very slowly and are generally discovered by accident.

Fibrocystic change in the breast is an all-encompassing term used to describe many different breast changes. This descriptive term should be discouraged and the more specific diagnosis used. Examples of benign lesions that are generally considered under this category are multiple lesions of fibrous disease, intraductal papilloma, cysts, and solid masses. These changes affect almost all women at some time in their lives. Frequently pain is present, which calls attention to the problem and may increase during the premenstrual phase.

Nipple discharge is more commonly associated with benign lesions than with cancer. A postmenopausal woman who has some duct ectasia or who has borne children can manually produce nipple discharge. Discharge is usually significant only if it is spontaneous and persistent. Chronic unilateral nipple discharge, especially if bloody, should prompt an investigation for occult carcinoma.

BREAST CANCER

Breast cancer primarily affects women. Until it can be prevented, early detection is the greatest hope for cure. All women should practice monthly self-examination to detect palpable lesions and immediately report any changes or masses to a physician. External physical changes, such as dimpling of the skin, can also indicate the presence of a benign or malignant pathologic process.

Benign breast lesions, such as fibrocystic changes and fibroadenomas, are the most common lesions excised. The older the patient, the more likely that a mass is malignant. The most common form of breast cancer is infiltrating ductal carcinoma.

The cause of breast cancer is still unknown. Many factors, including environmental, dietary, and familial influences, have been suggested as contributors to its development (Research Highlight 16-1). Whatever the cause, its incidence is definitely increasing. The previously held belief that breast cancer spreads by direct extension from the initial site in the breast to adjacent lymph nodes may not always be correct. Breast cancer may be a systemic condition at the time of diagnosis. Distant metastases may have already occurred without adjacent lymph node involvement

RESEARCH HIGHLIGHT 16-1

In this study the relationship between intake of dietary fat as a factor in increasing the risk of breast cancer and the intake of dietary fiber as a factor in decreasing the risk of breast cancer were explored. A prospective group study of 89,494 women in the Nurses' Health Study who were between the ages of 34 and 59 was conducted. Data gathered over an 8-year period in the 1980s regarding dietary intake formed the baseline for food intake. Follow-up questionnaires were conducted every 2 years to collect data on potential risk factors, disease, and new onset of cancer. The results indicated that there was no positive association between either total fat intake and breast cancer or any protective effect from dietary fiber. Nonetheless, the researchers noted that fat intake earlier in life could have an effect similar to that positively associated with eating animal fat and risk of colon cancer. Perioperative nurses may consider counseling patients to consume low-fat diets due to those risks.

Willet, W., et al. (1992). Dietary fat and fiber in relation to risk of breast cancer. *Journal of the American Medical Association, 268* (15), 2037-2043.

at the time of its palpable detection. This theory could explain why the radical breast surgery of the past, which involved removal of all axillary and thoracic lymph nodes, did not greatly lower mortality. Survival from breast cancer is best when detected early, reducing axillary lymph node involvement and improving long-term survival. Tumor size can usually be correlated with involvement of lymph nodes. The larger the tumor, the more likely that lymph nodes are involved.

Less radical surgery is the treatment of choice today. Surgical excision of the tumor, the use of radiation therapy alone, and a combination of surgery and radiation therapy have become viable alternatives. The use of adjuvant chemotherapy is definitely recommended for premenopausal women with axillary node metastasis. There have been studies and a National Institutes of Health recommendation that similar therapy can be beneficial in node-negative breast cancer patients.

Imaging methodologies, such as mammography and ultrasonography, have helped in the detection of breast masses too small for clinical detection. Ultrasonography differentiates between solid & cystic lesions. An alternate approach to determine if a mass is solid or a cyst is the use of fine-needle aspiration (FNA). A 22- or 25-gauge needle attached to a 20-ml syringe is inserted by the physician into the mass, and a small amount of the contents is aspirated. Cytologic studies of the aspirate can assist in evaluation of

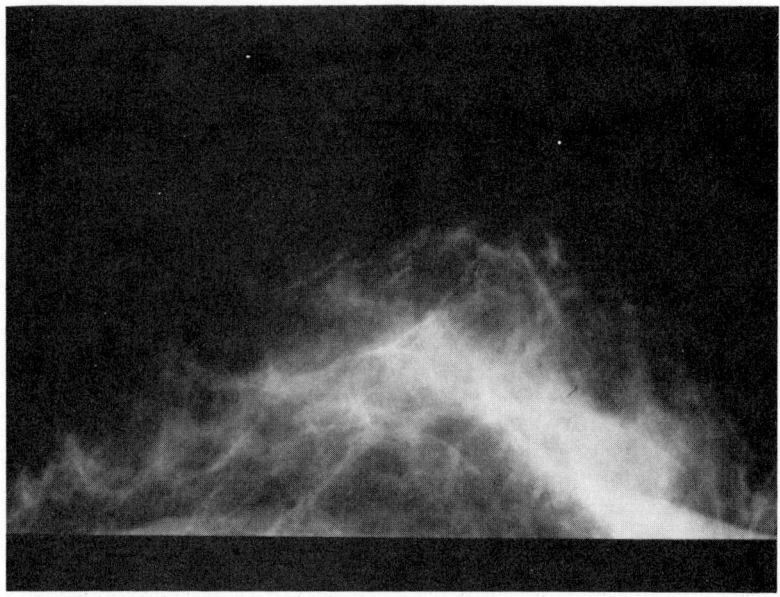

FIG. 16-4 Mammogram. Craniocaudad view of normal breast.
Courtesy Wende W. Logan, M.D., Rochester, N.Y. and the Breast Clinic of Rochester.

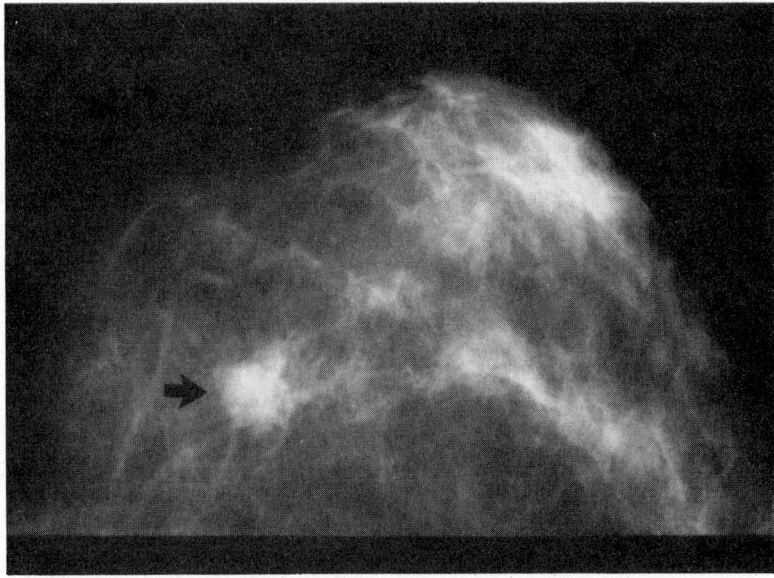

FIG. 16-5 Mammogram. Craniocaudad view of breast. *Arrow* indicates unpalpable lesion of about 1.5 cm.
Courtesy Wende W. Logan, M.D., Rochester, N.Y. and the Breast Clinic of Rochester.

the mass. Some health care facilities are capable of using mammography and stereotactic instrumentation to conduct FNA on nonpalpable lesions.

The best available screening mechanism for occult and palpable lesions is x-ray mammography (Fig. 16-4). Mammograms can detect abnormal-appearing densities and clusters of calcium deposits that are clinically nonpalpable (Fig.

16-5). These masses may be only 3 to 10 mm in diameter.

In mammography the entire breast is visualized by directing x-ray beams in several planes through the breast, yielding craniocaudad and other views (Fig. 16-4). Mammograms should be analyzed by a trained radiologist, who sends the report to the referring physician. In some instances, such as when the lesion is too small to palpate,

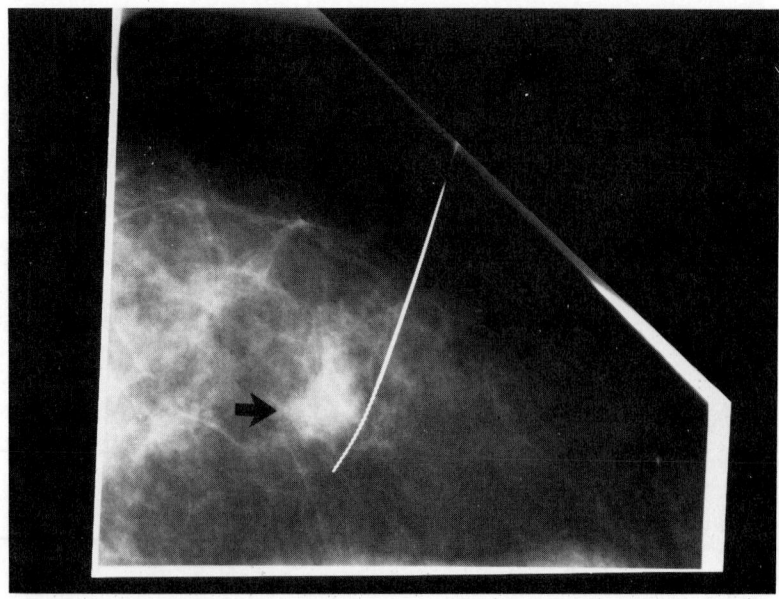

FIG. 16-6   Mammogram section. Craniocaudad view of breast. *Arrow* indicates lesion localized by wire before surgical excision.

Courtesy Wende W. Logan, M.D., Rochester, N.Y. and the Breast Clinic of Rochester.

mammograms are done immediately before surgery. The lesions, previously detected by mammogram, are localized by the insertion of a needle(s) or a wire within a needle. The needle(s) may be left in place or removed after insertion of the wire (Fig. 16-6). Once the suspect area is identified, the needle or wire is taped in place, and the patient is sent to the operating room for surgical biopsy. After biopsy, the specimen can be sent back for mammography validation of the correct surgical excision of the questionable breast tissue prior to the pathologic examination.

The accuracy of mammography depends on careful x-ray technique and breast size, structure, and density. Radiation dosage varies with individuals and techniques. As a result of improvement in radiologic techniques, the radiation exposure in a mammogram is very low. The benefits of this screening mechanism far outweigh the minute risks of radiation exposure.

Surgical treatment ranges from removal of only the tumor to modified radical mastectomy involving the breast and axillary lymph nodes. The choice of operation depends on the size, site, and the stage of the disease. Radiation therapy, chemotherapy, or hormonal therapy may be used in conjunction with surgery or as alternative treatment methods.

Techniques have been developed that determine the ability of breast cancer to bind with estrogen and progestins. This positive binding capability identifies the patient with a hormone-dependent tumor. About two thirds of all breast cancers are positive for estrogen binding, and the majority of these tumors are also positive for progestins. The presence of receptor sites is conducive to hormone manipulation. The use of antiestrogen tamoxifen, in addition to surgery and chemotherapy, increases disease-free survival in premenopausal and postmenopausal women with positive binding for estrogen. Tumors excised at surgery are evaluated for their estrogen and progestin-binding abilities.

Breast cancer is usually staged to measure the extent of the disease and to classify patients for possible treatment modalities. The TNM classification has been adopted as a mechanism to clinically stage this disease (Box 16-1). The results of staging are used in designing the treatment plan.

PERIOPERATIVE NURSING CONSIDERATIONS
ASSESSMENT

A patient undergoing breast surgery can be extremely apprehensive about the possibilities of having a malignancy, losing a body part, facing a negative reaction from her spouse and family, and experiencing a change in self-image (Research Highlight 16-2). During a preoperative interview the perioperative nurse should assess the patient's level of anxiety and possible causes, such as the possibility of the diagnosis of cancer. Identification of the patient's fears and concerns helps the nurse in planning appropriate nursing interventions (Research Highlight 16-3). The patient should identify the breast that is affected and, if possible, the quadrant of the breast mass. The nurse should assess the patient's understanding of the proposed surgical procedure.

BOX 16-1

The TNM Staging System for Breast Cancer

STAGE I

$T^1N^0M^0$

Tumor size less than 2 cm

May extend into pectoral fascia or muscle

No distant metastasis

No positive nodes

STAGE II

$T^2N^0M^0$ or $T^1N^1M^0$ or $T^2N^1M^0$

Tumor size 2 to 5 cm

May or may not extend into pectoral fascia or muscle

No distant metastasis

Mobile axillary nodes

DEFINITIONS

T = primary tumor

T^4 = tumor extension to the chest wall or skin

N = regional lymph nodes

N^0 = no growth

N^1 = movable nodes with tumor growth

N^2 = homolateral axillary nodes fixed to one another or other structures and containing growth

STAGE III

$T^1N^1M^0$ or $T^2N^1M^0$ or $T^{1-3}N^2M^0$ or $T^3N^0M^0$

Tumor size greater than 5 cm

May or may not extend into pectoral fascia and muscle

Skin edema, infiltration, or ulceration may be present

Nodes fixed to skin, deeper structures, supraclavicular nodes

No distant metastasis

STAGE IV

Any TN^3 any M or T^4 any N any M

Any TN plus M^1

N^3 = homolateral infraclavicular or supraclavicular nodes containing growth

M = distant metastasis

M^0 = absent

M^1 = present, includes skin beyond the breast

Modified from Stein, P., & Zera, R. (1991). *AORN Journal, 53,* 4. Copyright © 1991, Association of Operating Room Nurses. Reprinted with permission.

Reinforcement of knowledge or correction of misunderstandings is possible only if the nurse identifies the patient's current level of knowledge.

Discharge planning should begin as soon as the patient is informed of the necessity for surgery or when the nurse first meets the patient. Information about appropriate exercises, prosthetic devices, reconstructive techniques, and available community support groups should be given to the patient. The perioperative nurse provides or reinforces information based on clinical nursing judgment and the patient's desire for information, readiness to learn, and anxiety level.

NURSING DIAGNOSIS

Based on the nursing assessment, the perioperative nurse utilizes nursing diagnoses to develop a plan of care. Nursing diagnoses related to the care of patients undergoing breast surgery might include:

- Anxiety related to the fear of cancer
- Body image disturbance related to loss of body part
- Anticipatory grieving related to potential loss of body part

---

RESEARCH HIGHLIGHT 16-2

In this study data were collected from 257 women who had undergone one of four of the most common types of treatment for breast cancer: mastectomy, mastectomy with delayed reconstruction, mastectomy with immediate reconstruction, and conservative breast surgery. The purpose of the study was to compare body image, described as a mental picture of the physical self, which includes one's perceptions about physical appearance, state of health, skills, and sexuality, in women in the four treatment groups. The results of the study indicated that there were significant differences in body image related to the type of surgical treatment. Women who underwent conservative breast surgery reported greater satisfaction with body image than those treated by mastectomy or mastectomy with reconstruction. The author underscored the importance of nursing interventions, which not only concerned themselves with the patient's physical recovery from surgery, but also with her potential disturbances in body image.

Mock, V. (1993). Body image in women treated for breast cancer. *Nursing Research, 42* (3), 153-157.

RESEARCH HIGHLIGHT 16-3

In this study 48 women who were diagnosed with early-stage breast cancer were interviewed during the time the physician had suggested they think over their treatment options. Audiotapes of the interviews, which requested each participant to simply think aloud their decision process, were analyzed. Five indicators of decision behavior were identified: (1) perceived salience of alternatives (extent to which participant was aware of and attracted to a treatment alternative on the basis of information from the physician), (2) decision conflict (the participant considered more than one option and was motivated to take or avoid action, such as seeking additional information), (3) information seeking (participant was unable to discriminate between alternatives), (4) risk awareness (participant considered various risks of alternative treatments to assist in decision-making), and (5) deliberation (participant sought and evaluated information on alternatives).

Based on a qualitative analysis of these indicators, the researcher classified predominant decision behaviors as Deferrer (41%), Delayer (44%), and Deliberator (15%). Participants who were in the Deferrer group made quick decisions, frequently based on physician recommendation. The Delayer group allowed themselves consideration of at least two treatment options. The Deliberators appeared to use a decision style that considered each option in terms of its attributes. No conclusions were drawn about a best process for decision making. Further study is required to determine the influence, if any, on the process used to decide treatment option and the regret or satisfaction with the decision over time. In addition, the perioperative nurse should further explore what types of decision support and differential information needs are required by different decision-making behaviors.

Pierce, P.F. (1993). Deciding on breast cancer treatment: A description of decision behavior. *Nursing Research, 42* (1), 22-27.

• High risk for injury related to use of electrosurgery
• Knowledge deficit related to unfamiliarity with perioperative routines

OUTCOME IDENTIFICATION

Outcomes identified for the selected nursing diagnoses could be stated as the following:

• Patient will verbalize decreased anxiety.
• Patient will discuss feelings regarding the potential outcome of the surgical procedure.

• Patient will experience no untoward injury from electrosurgery.
• Patient will verbalize understanding of the perioperative routines.

PLANNING

Utilizing nursing diagnoses, the perioperative nurse can individualize the plan of care for each patient and allow for communication with other colleagues on the patient care team. The plan of care for a patient undergoing breast surgery can include nursing interventions that allow the patient freedom to express concerns, that answer specific questions, and that discuss breast reconstruction options, as appropriate. The Sample Care Plan shows some examples.

The perioperative nurse needs to develop criteria to measure achievement of the outcomes. A patient experiencing decreased or relief of anxiety would be evidenced by verbalization of anxiety, relaxed facial and body structures, and vital signs within normal range for the patient.

IMPLEMENTATION

Before surgery the perioperative nurse should procure the necessary medical and surgical supplies and equipment for the intended operation. Mammogram films should be available in the OR for the surgeon's review. A breast biopsy under local anesthesia will require local anesthetics, adjunct sedation, and monitoring equipment (ECG, pulse oximeter, blood pressure apparatus). Patient allergies should again be reviewed and the patient closely observed for allergic or toxic reactions to local anesthetics. For a mastectomy extra sponges are often needed. An electrosurgical unit or a surgical laser is used to provide both hemostasis and tissue dissection. The incision site is usually drained postoperatively with a closed-wound suction device. Ensuring the availability of supplies before the procedure allows the nurse to remain with, monitor, and observe the patient.

During the intraoperative phase the patient is placed on the OR bed in a supine position with the operative side near the edge of the bed. The arm on the involved side is carefully extended on a padded armboard at no greater than 90 degrees to prevent brachial plexus injury. Depending on the location of the lesion and the planned surgery, a small pad can be placed under the operative side to facilitate exposure of the incision area. Positioning the OR bed in slight Fowler's with a lateral tilt away from the surgeon can also facilitate exposure.

Skin preparation depends on the location of the lesion and the surgery intended. Skin preparation solutions vary, depending on the surgeon's preference. For a breast biopsy the area prepared is usually the affected breast and the immediate surrounding skin. For a mastectomy the area prepared can extend from above the clavicle to the umbilicus and from the opposite nipple to the bedline of the operative side, including the axilla, and possibly the upper arm on the operative side. Some surgeons caution against vig-

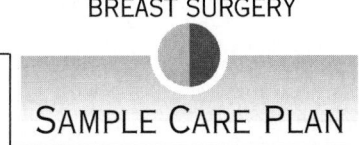

SAMPLE CARE PLAN

NURSING DIAGNOSIS: Anxiety related to fear of cancer or surgical intervention
OUTCOME: Patient will verbalize decreased anxiety.
INTERVENTIONS:
Allow time for patient's questions.
Assess verbal and nonverbal signs of anxiety.
Encourage ventilation of concerns and fears.
Provide emotional support and comfort measures (warm blankets, touch as appropriate).
Maintain quiet environment.
Demonstrate warmth, calmness, and acceptance of the patient's anxiety.
Instruct the patient in relaxation techniques such as rhythmic breathing or guided imagery.
Record patient's reactions.

NURSING DIAGNOSIS: Body image disturbance related to loss of body part
OUTCOME: Patient will discuss feelings regarding outcome of the surgical procedure.
INTERVENTIONS:
Allow patient to discuss concerns about her sexual attractiveness and perceived loss of femininity.
Discuss available resources and options (external prosthesis, alternatives in garments and dress, reconstructive surgery, as appropriate). Make referrals to nurse on discharge unit as indicated.
Maintain the patient's privacy.

NURSING DIAGNOSIS: Anticipatory grieving related to potential loss of body part
OUTCOME: Patient will discuss feelings regarding the proposed outcome of the surgical procedure.
INTERVENTIONS:
Allow ventilation of feelings.
Clarify misconceptions.

Promote an environment of support, respect, and comfort.
Refer to other professionals as appropriate.
Explore realistic alternatives and breast reconstruction.

NURSING DIAGNOSIS: High risk for injury related to use of electrosurgery
OUTCOME: Patient will experience no untoward injury from electrosurgery.
INTERVENTIONS:
Position the dispersive pad as close to the operative site as possible.
Select a site that is clean and dry, with good muscle mass; note the condition of the skin.
Protect pad from fluids and contact with metal objects.
Turn electrosurgical unit on after dispersive pad and active electrode are connected.
Set power setting as low as possible to achieve desired effect.
Use holster for active electrode on the sterile field.
Check dispersive pad contact and all connections after changes in position or requests to increase power.
Evaluate the condition of the skin upon removal of the dispersive pad.

NURSING DIAGNOSIS: Knowledge deficit related to unfamiliarity with perioperative routines
OUTCOME: Patient will verbalize understanding of the perioperative routines.
INTERVENTIONS:
Assess the patient's experience with previous surgical procedures.
Provide clear and concise explanations of all nursing interventions.
Explain roles of the health care team members.
Encourage questions.

orous scrubbing of the surgical site to prevent possible seeding of cancer cells from the main mass. The surgeon may request that only an antiseptic solution be applied to the breast.

Surgical draping should allow exposure of the affected breast. For a mastectomy the arm on the operative side should be draped free using a stockinette and drapes that allow free movement of the arm to facilitate access to the axilla. If a breast biopsy is to be immediately followed by a modified radical mastectomy, the surgeon may prefer to repeat the skin preparation and surgical draping before proceeding with the definitive surgery. Breast biopsy instruments include the following:

Cutting instruments

2 Knife handles, no. 3, with no. 10 or no. 15 blades

1 Set of intraductal probes
2 Skin hooks

Holding instruments

6 Hemostats
4 Kelly hemostats
4 Allis forceps

4 Towel clamps
2 Tissue forceps with teeth

Exposing instruments

2 Muscle retractors, small
2 Rake retractors, small

2 Mayo scissors, 1 straight and 1 curved
1 Tissue scissors

Suturing items

1 Needle holder
2 Packages of sutures, 1 absorbable and 1 non-absorbable, with swaged-on cutting needles

Instruments and supplies for a modified radical mastectomy include:

Cutting instruments

2 Knife handles, no. 3, with no. 10 and no. 15 blades

2 Mayo scissors, 1 straight and 1 curved
1 Tissue scissors, regular

Holding instruments

16 Hemostats (number will vary with size of breast)
6 Kelly hemostats
12 Allis forceps
8 Lahey clamps
6 Kocher hemostatic forceps

8 Towel clamps
2 Tissue forceps with teeth
2 Tissue forceps without teeth
2 Adson forceps with teeth

Exposing instruments

2 U.S. Army retractors
4 Richardson retractors, 2 small and 2 medium
4 Rakes, four-prong, 2 small and 2 medium

2 Skin hooks
3 Berens skin-flap retractors

Suturing items

2 Needle holders
Suture material, with swaged-on cutting needles

Accessory items

Closed wound suction device
Electrosurgical unit or laser

Marking pen
Suction tip and tubing
Skin stapler

During implementation of the plan of care, the perioperative nurse continues to collect data, continuously reassesses the patient's needs and the needs of the surgical team, provides nursing interventions, and documents care delivered. Formats for documenting perioperative patient care vary from institution to institution. However, documentation of patient problems and nursing interventions addressing these problems is important for any surgical patient. For the patient undergoing breast surgery, consideration should be given to documenting the patient's level of anxiety, the surgical position and accessory positioning devices used, the location of the electrosurgical dispersive pad, unit settings and identification number, results of perioperative monitoring, medications administered by the perioperative nurse or from the sterile field, and any drains inserted in the surgical wound.

EVALUATION

Evaluation of the patient before discharge from the operating room includes both general observation parameters important for every surgical patient and specific evaluation of the goals of the plan of care. The patient's skin at dependent pressure sites, skin preparation sites, and the dispersive pad placement site should be assessed. Whether the dressing is intact and the wound suction device is properly functioning should be noted. The report to the nurse in the PACU should include any unusual events or patient problems during surgery, the incorporation of any drains in the wound, and the achievement of identified patient outcomes. These outcomes, based on the nursing diagnoses selected, should be a part of documentation as well as the nursing report.

SURGICAL INTERVENTIONS

BIOPSY OF BREAST TISSUE

Biopsy of breast tissue is removal of suspicious tissue for pathologic examination. In a needle biopsy a disposable cutting type of needle is introduced and advanced into the breast mass to entrap a core or plug of tissue. The needle is withdrawn, and the tissue specimen is sent for diagnostic examination. In an incisional biopsy a portion of the mass is surgically excised using a curved incision line. The tissue is sent for pathologic examination. In an excisional biopsy the entire tumor mass is excised from adjacent tissue for examination as with incisional biopsy.

Biopsy is indicated in the presence of a tumor mass detected by palpation, mammography, nipple discharge, or skin changes. Fibroadenoma, an isolated cyst, or intraductal papilloma may be encountered. Definitive surgical treatment is contraindicated in the absence of a formal biopsy.

Procedural considerations

The biopsy procedure has little risk and is usually done with the patient under local anesthesia. The short delay between biopsy and further treatment does not adversely affect survival. However, when an extensive surgical procedure is anticipated, general anesthesia is preferred. In this instance the patient has given consent to proceed with the more definitive surgery.

Operative procedure

1. An incision in the direction of the skin lines or along the border of the areola is made over the tumor mass. The circumareolar incision gives the best cosmetic effect.
2. Gentle traction is applied to the mass with holding forceps. If the lesion is small, the entire mass and an edge of normal tissue are removed by sharp dissection. If a large lesion is present, a small incisional biopsy of the main mass is done. The specimen should not be placed in a formalin solution if a frozen section is to be done at the time of surgery. Exposure to formalin prevents this type of pathologic examination. The tissue specimen is examined by a frozen section to determine immediate diagnosis while the patient is still anesthetized. If a 48-hour permanent section is required, the patient will be scheduled at a later time for any further surgery that may be necessary.
3a. If the lesion is benign, the subcutaneous breast tissue of the wound is approximated with an absorbable suture. The skin is closed with fine sutures or skin staples, and a firm pressure dressing is applied.
3b. If the lesion is malignant, the incision is tightly closed with a continuous locking suture on a cutting needle.
4. If a more extensive operation is required, it may be performed immediately. The team members regown and glove; the operative site is again prepped and draped. A separate sterile setup and set of instruments for a more radical procedure are then used.

INCISION AND DRAINAGE FOR ABSCESS

Incision of an inflamed and suppurative area of the breast is performed for drainage of abscess. Breast abscesses occur most frequently during the first 4 weeks of breastfeeding. Staphylococcal or streptococcal organisms enter the breast through abraded or lacerated nipple surfaces or through the lactiferous ducts. Chronic abscesses are rare. Free drainage is required with the association of an abscess around the nipple or in breast tissue.

Procedural considerations

The condition is very painful and may require surgery under general anesthesia. Instruments are the same as for a biopsy.

Operative procedure

1. Generally, a radial incision extending outward from the nipple or a circumareolar incision is preferred. A short incision in the thoracomammary fold may be used for deep breast abscesses in the lower or outer quadrant.
2. After skin incision, the wound is deepened until pus is encountered.
3. A curved hemostat is directed into the cavity to determine the extent of the abscess. Culture specimens for aerobic and anaerobic organisms are usually taken.
4. Loculations are broken up by exploring the cavity with the index finger.
5. The opening is enlarged to ensure adequate drainage, the cavity is irrigated with warm saline solution, and bleeding vessels are ligated with absorbable sutures or coagulated.
6. The wound is drained or loosely packed with gauze. Healing occurs by granulation.

SEGMENTAL RESECTION (LUMPECTOMY, QUADRANT RESECTION, WEDGE RESECTION)

Segmental resection is removal of the tumor mass with at least a 1-inch margin of surrounding tissue. A segmental resection combined with an axillary node dissection and irradiation in stages I and II breast cancer appears to provide results equal to a more radical procedure. If one or more axillary nodes are involved, chemotherapy is also recommended.

Procedural considerations

Instruments required are as described for a modified radical mastectomy. In patients with large breasts, increased bleeding may occur, requiring additional hemostatic clamps.

Operative procedure

The procedure is as described for excisional biopsy.

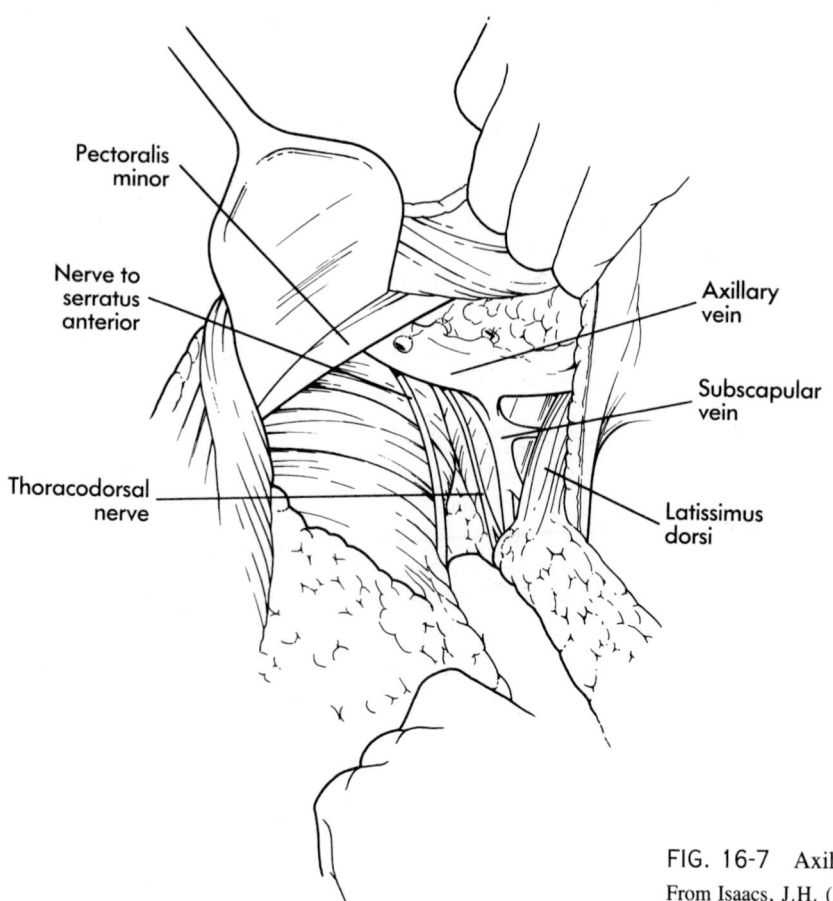

Pectoralis
minor

Nerve to
serratus
anterior

Thoracodorsal
nerve

Axillary
vein

Subscapular
vein

Latissimus
dorsi

FIG. 16-7   Axillary dissection.
From Isaacs, J.H. (1992). *Textbook of breast disease.* St. Louis: Mosby.

AXILLARY NODE DISSECTION

Axillary node dissection (Fig. 16-7) is the removal of the axillary nodes through an incision in the axilla. An axillary dissection is usually done through an incision separate from that for other breast operations. The removal and examination of the axillary nodes allow staging (see Box 16-1) of the disease. Adjunct treatment can be more accurately planned when the pathologic stage is known.

Procedural considerations

The patient is placed supine on the OR bed with the operative side near the bed edge. The arm on the operative side is extended to less than 90 degrees on an armboard. The skin is prepped and draped as previously described.

Operative procedure

1. An incision is made slightly posterior and parallel to the upper lateral border of the pectoralis major muscle, or transversely across the axilla.
2. The fascia is incised over the pectoralis muscle. The pectoralis minor muscle is exposed. Major blood and lymphatic vessels are clamped and ligated. The use of electrosurgery is avoided around the axillary vessels and nerves.
3. The tissue over the axillary vein is incised.

4. The lymph nodes between the pectoralis major and pectoralis minor muscles are removed. Care is taken not to injure the medial and lateral nerves of the pectoralis major muscle.
5. The axillary fat and lymph nodes are freed from the axillary vein and chest wall. The long thoracic nerve is identified along the chest wall near the axillary vein, and the thoracodorsal nerve posteriorly is dissected free from the specimen. The nerves are spared to preserve muscle function.
6. The fat and nodes are removed. The incision is closed with sutures and staples, and a dressing is applied. A suction drain is usually placed through a separate stab incision for lymphatic drainage.

SUBCUTANEOUS MASTECTOMY (ADENOMAMMECTOMY)

Subcutaneous mastectomy is removal of all breast tissue with the overlying skin and nipple left intact. Subcutaneous mastectomy is recommended for patients who have central tumors of noninvasive origin, chronic cystic mastitis, hyperplastic duct changes, or multiple fibroadenomas, or who have undergone a number of previous biopsies. Breast reconstruction may be undertaken at the time of mastectomy or at a later date.

Procedural considerations

The patient is positioned as for a biopsy. A modified radical mastectomy instrument set is required. If reconstruction is to be undertaken, appropriate equipment and supplies (see Chapter 23) are also required.

Operative procedure

1. An incision is usually begun in the inframammary crease and may be made on the medial or the lateral aspect of the breast. Some surgeons initially remove and preserve the nipple aerola complex by employing lateral extensions of wide periareolar incisions.
2. Blunt dissection is performed to elevate the breast from the pectoral fascia.
3. The breast tissue is removed from the skin with an attempt made to remain in a plane between the subcutaneous tissue and the breast. Dissection is carried out toward the axilla; with care, 90% or more of the breast tissue can be removed, including the tail of Spence. Some lymph nodes in the axillary area also may be removed. Bleeding vessels are clamped and ligated.
4. A decision is made at this time as to whether to proceed with reconstruction. If the subareolar tissue shows no signs of tumor, as verified by a pathologist, the areolar complex is placed on a deepithelialized dermal bed.
5. A closed wound suction catheter may be inserted. The wound is closed, and a light pressure dressing is applied.

SIMPLE MASTECTOMY (TOTAL MASTECTOMY)

Simple mastectomy is removal of the entire involved breast without lymph node dissection. A simple mastectomy is performed to remove extensive benign disease, if malignancy is believed to be confined only to the breast tissue, or as a palliative measure to remove an ulcerated advanced malignancy.

Procedural considerations

The patient is positioned as for a biopsy. A modified radical mastectomy instrument set is required.

Operative procedure

1. Through a transverse elliptical incision (Fig. 16-8, *A*), using a knife and curved scissors, the skin edges are freed from the fascia. Bleeding vessels are clamped with hemostats and ligated with sutures or electrocoagulated.
2. The skin edges of the wound can be protected with warm, moist laparotomy pads; the breast tissue is grasped with Allis forceps and is dissected free from the underlying pectoral fascia with curved scissors and knife.
3. The tumor and all breast tissue are removed. Bleeding vessels are clamped and ligated or electrocoagulated.
4. A closed wound drainage catheter is inserted and anchored to the skin with a fine suture. The wound is closed with fine sutures or staples; a dressing is applied.

MODIFIED RADICAL MASTECTOMY

Modified radical mastectomy is performed following a tissue biopsy with a positive diagnosis of malignancy and involves removal of the involved breast and all axillary contents (all three levels of nodes—axillary, pectoral, and superior apical). The underlying pectoral muscles are not removed before or after removal of axillary nodes. A modified radical mastectomy is done to remove the involved area with the hope of decreasing the spread of the malignancy. This surgery's elliptic incision with lateral extension toward the axilla gives a good cosmetic result for plastic surgery reconstruction (see Chapter 23), provides good arm movement because the pectoralis muscles are not removed, and usually does not require a skin graft.

Procedural considerations

The patient is placed supine on the operating room bed with the operative side near the bed edge. The arm on the operative side is extended to less than 90 degrees on a padded armboard. The skin is prepared and draped as previously described. Instruments and supplies for a modified radical mastectomy are required (p. 566).

Operative procedure

1. An oblique elliptic incision with a lateral extension toward the axilla is made through the subcutaneous tissue (Fig. 16-8, *A*). The bleeding points are controlled with hemostats and ligatures or electrocoagulation.
2. The skin is undercut in all directions to the limits of the dissection by means of a no. 3 knife handle with a no. 10 blade and curved scissors. Knife blades need to be changed frequently to ensure precise dissection.
3. The margins of the skin flaps are covered with warm, moist laparotomy pads and held away with retractors. The fascia and breast are resected from the pectoralis major muscle (Fig. 16-8, *B*) starting near the clavicle and extending down to the midportion of the sternum. The pectoralis muscle is left intact.
4. The intercostal arteries and veins are clamped and ligated.
5. The axillary flap is retracted for a complete dissection of the axilla. Careful attention is directed to preventing injury to the axillary vein and medial and lateral nerves of the pectoralis major muscle.
6. The fascia is dissected from the lateral edge of the pectoralis muscle (Fig. 16-8, *C*). Ligation of the vessels is preferred in the axilla and adjacent to the sternum. The fascia is then dissected from the serratus anterior muscle. The thoracic and thoracodorsal nerves are preserved (Fig. 16-8, *D*).
7. The breast and axillary fascia are freed from the latissimus dorsi muscle and suspensory ligaments (Fig. 16-8, *E*). The specimen is then passed off the field.
8. The surgical area is inspected for bleeding sites, which are ligated and electrocoagulated. The wound is irrigated with normal saline. Closed wound suction cath-

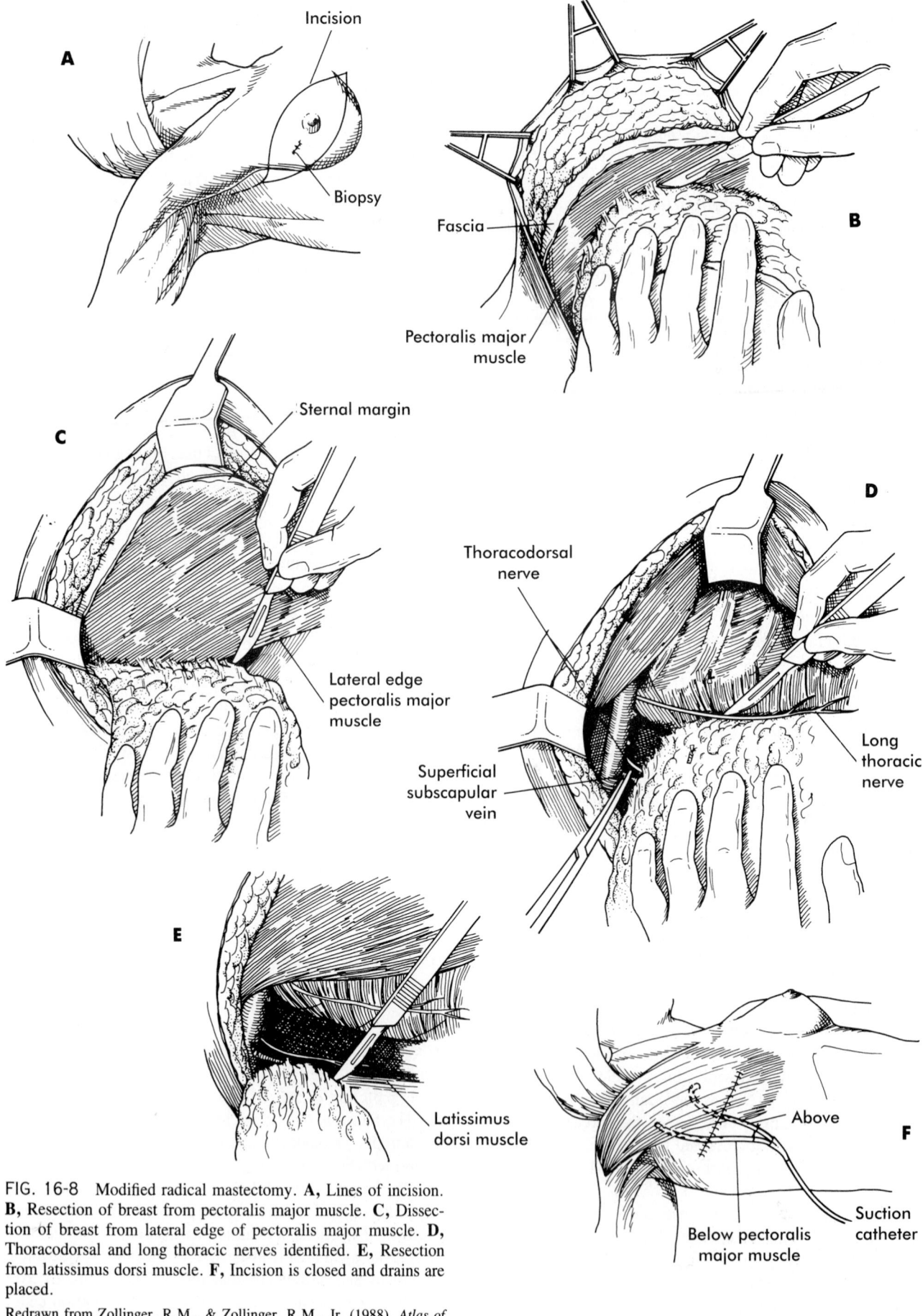

FIG. 16-8 Modified radical mastectomy. **A,** Lines of incision. **B,** Resection of breast from pectoralis major muscle. **C,** Dissection of breast from lateral edge of pectoralis major muscle. **D,** Thoracodorsal and long thoracic nerves identified. **E,** Resection from latissimus dorsi muscle. **F,** Incision is closed and drains are placed.

Redrawn from Zollinger, R.M., & Zollinger, R.M., Jr. (1988). *Atlas of surgical operations* (6th ed.). New York: Macmillan.

eters are inserted into the wound through stab wounds and secured to the skin with a nonabsorbable suture on a cutting needle (Fig. 16-8, *F*).

9. A few absorbable sutures may be used in the subcutaneous tissue to approximate the skin flaps. The incision is closed with interrupted nonabsorbable sutures or staples.

10. The dressing can be a simple gauze dressing, a bulky dressing held in place by a Surgi-Bra, or a gauze or elastic bandage wrap.

BIBLIOGRAPHY

Brown-Daniels, C., & Blasdell, A., (1990). Early breast cancer: Today's treatment options. *American Journal of Nursing, 11,* 28.

Breast cancer. (1992). *Seminars In Oncology, 19,* 217.

Breast cancer. (1993). *Abstracts of Clinical Care Guidelines, 5* (1), 1.

Conn, R. (editor). (1991). *Current diagnosis.* Philadelphia: W.B. Saunders.

Gray, H. (1989). *Anatomy of the human body* (30th ed.). Philadelphia: Lea & Febiger.

Isaacs, J. (editor). (1992). *Textbook of breast disease.* St. Louis: Mosby.

Mock, V. (1993). Body image in women treated for breast cancer. *Nursing Research, 42,* 153.

Pierce, P. (1993). Deciding on breast cancer treatment: A description of decision behavior. *Nursing Research, 42,* 22.

Sabiston, D.C., Jr. (editor). (1991). *Davis-Christopher textbook of surgery: The biological basis of modern surgical practice* (14th ed.). Philadelphia: W.B. Saunders.

Schwartz, S., et al. (1989). *Principles of surgery* (5th ed.). New York: McGraw-Hill.

Stein, P., & Zera, R. (1991). Breast cancer. *AORN Journal, 53,* 938.

Thibodeau, G.A. (1990). *Anthony's textbook of anatomy and physiology* (13th ed.). St. Louis: Mosby.

Way, L.W. (editor). (1990). *Current surgical diagnosis and treatment* (8th ed.). Norwalk, Conn: Appleton & Lange.

Willet, W., et al. (1992). Dietary fat and fiber in relation to risk of breast cancer. *Journal of the American Medical Association, 268,* 2037.

Winchester, D.P. (1986). The relationship of fibrocystic disease to breast cancer. *Bulletin of the American College of Surgeon, 71,* 29.

Zollinger, R.M., & Zollinger, R.M., Jr. (1993). *Atlas of surgical operations* (7th ed.). New York: Macmillan.

17

OPHTHALMIC SURGERY

ELAINE THOMSON-KEITH

In the time of Hippocrates, eye surgery was confined to operations on the eyelid. Until the early twentieth century, little progress was made. Since then, significant advances have taken place in ophthalmology and anesthesia. With the implementation of aseptic technique, introduction of antibiotics, and improvements in management of the surgical patient, ophthalmic surgery, like other surgical specialties, has expanded its horizons dramatically.

Innovative developments in laser applications and microsurgical technology challenge the nurse who assists in the care of the ophthalmic patient. The perioperative nurse who practices in ophthalmologic surgery must combine the art and science of nursing with up-to-date knowledge and finely tuned, highly technologic skills. In the last decade advances in surgical techniques and improved anesthetics, along with increasing pressures to contain health care costs, have created another major change in the management of patients who undergo ophthalmic surgery. Except for a small percentage of patients who have complex procedures or medical problems that contraindicate early discharge, patients today who have eye surgery do so on an ambulatory basis. Only patients with the most difficult procedures require hospitalization postoperatively, and many of those patients have operations on the day of admission. Therefore preoperative preparation, and in most cases discharge teaching, occurs in a limited period and is coordinated by the perioperative nursing team. The success of the surgical intervention depends, to a degree, on the knowledge and skill of that team as they develop and implement a perioperative plan of care. Recent studies examined during the development of Clinical Practice Guidelines for Cataract in Adults (AHCPR, 1993) support the important role the surgical team plays in positive outcome attainment.

Care for the patient in the perioperative period is focused on assisting the patient and significant other in establishing and sustaining biophysical, psychosociocultural, and spiritual equilibrium. Application of scientific principles, along with an understanding of the planned surgical intervention, is necessary to effectively identify the extrinsic and intrinsic stressors of the patient's perioperative environment. The perioperative nurse helps the patient manage these identified stressors so that equilibrium is established and sustained (Phippen, 1993).

SURGICAL ANATOMY

A working knowledge of the anatomic structures involved in ophthalmic surgery is necessary to facilitate selection of instrumentation and equipment for the procedure. The surgical team must also use this knowledge to understand the surgeon's plan of treatment and prepare the patient appropriately.

BONY ORBIT

The two orbital cavities are situated on either side of the midvertical line of the skull between the cranium and the

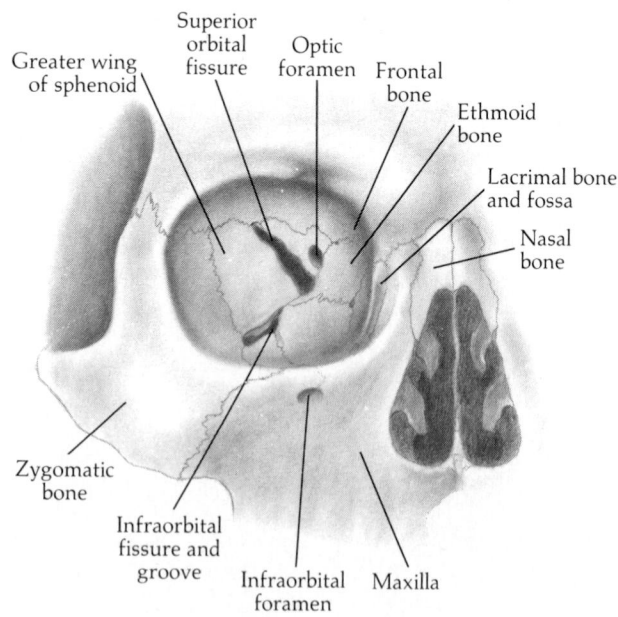

FIG. 17-1 Bony orbital cavity.

From Thompson, J.M., et al. (1993). *Mosby's clinical nursing* (3rd ed.). St. Louis: Mosby.

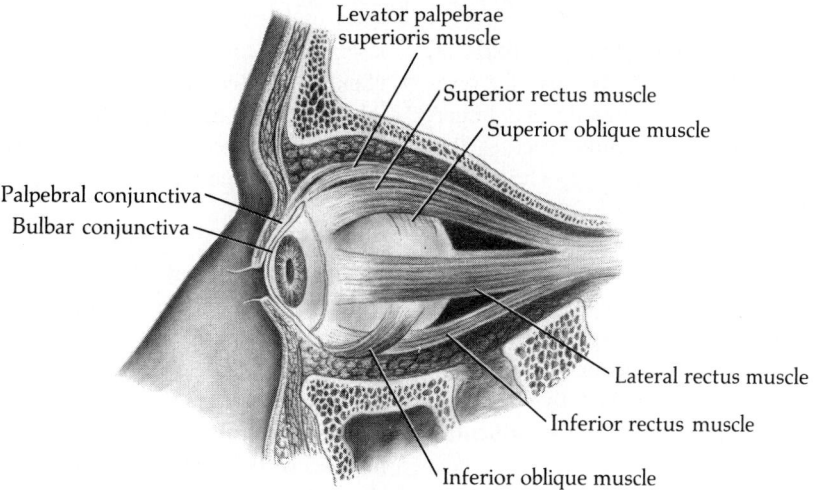

FIG. 17-2 Diagrammatic section of orbit.

From Thompson, J.M., et al. (1993). *Mosby's clinical nursing* (3rd ed.). St. Louis: Mosby.

skeleton of the face. Above each orbit are the anterior cranial fossa and the frontal sinus; medially, the nasal cavity; below, the maxillary sinus; and laterally, from behind forward, the middle cranial and temporal fossa (Fig. 17-1).

The seven bones that form the orbit are the maxilla, palatine, frontal, sphenoidal, zygomatic, ethmoid, and lacrimal bones. The margins of the bony orbit may be divided into four continuous parts: supraorbital, lateral, infraorbital, and medial.

The orbit can be considered a four-sided pyramid, with its base directed forward, lateral, and slightly downward and its apex facing posterior. The periosteum of the orbital walls is continuous with the dura mater.

The orbit is essentially a socket for the eyeball and the muscles, nerves, and vessels necessary for proper functioning of the eye (Fig. 17-2). The orbit is also a distribution center for certain vessels and nerves that supply the facial areas around the orbital aperture.

CONJUNCTIVA AND LACRIMAL APPARATUS

The conjunctiva is a thin, transparent mucous membrane that lines the back surface of the eyelids and the front surface of the globe. The conjunctiva forms a sac (conjunctival sac) that is open in front. The opening is called the palpebral fissure. When the eye is closed, the fissure becomes a mere slit.

The conjunctiva is divided into a palpebral and a bulbar part. The palpebral portion lines the back of the eyelids and contains the openings (puncta) of the lacrimal canaliculi, which establish a passageway between the conjunctival sac and the inferior meatus of the nose. The bulbar part of the conjunctiva is transparent, allowing the sclera, or white of the eye, to show through. The central portion of the bulbar conjunctiva is continuous at the limbus with

the anterior epithelium of the cornea.

The lacrimal apparatus consists of the lacrimal gland and its ducts, the lacrimal passages, the lacrimal canaliculi and sac, and the nasal lacrimal duct. The lacrimal gland produces tears and secretes them through a series of ducts into the conjunctival sac. The tears then make their way inward to the puncta, from which they are conducted by the canaliculi to the lacrimal sac and finally pass into the nasal duct. When the lacrimal glands secrete too profusely, the normal drainage process becomes insufficient and overflow tearing results (Fig. 17-3).

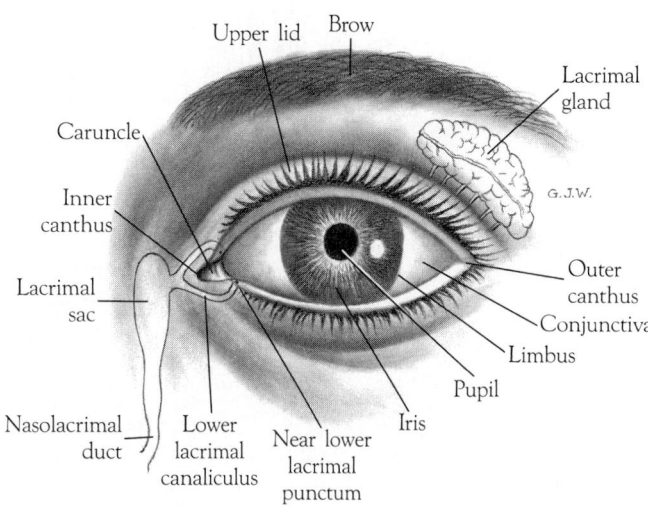

FIG. 17-3 Lacrimal apparatus, external view.

From Thompson, J.M., et al. (1993). *Mosby's clinical nursing* (3rd ed.). St. Louis: Mosby.

EYELIDS

The eyelids are two movable musculofibrous folds in front of each orbit that protect the globe and the eye from light. The upper eyelid is more mobile and larger than the lower. The upper and lower lids meet at the medial and lateral angles (canthi) of the eye. The palpebral fissure, as previously mentioned, is located between the margins of the two eyelids. When the eye is closed, the cornea is completely covered by the upper eyelid. The eyelids are closed by the orbicular muscle of the eye, which is a circular muscle that acts as a sphincter. When the fibers contract, the eyes close. The upper lid is opened by the levator muscle, which is innervated by the third cranial nerve, as well as by relaxation of the orbicular muscle.

Each eyelid consists of several layers. From front to back these are the skin, subcutaneous tissue that contains lymphatics, and muscles. Dense fibrous tissue, called tarsal cartilage, forms the framework of the lids. The tarsus is anchored to the walls of the orbit by the medial and lateral palpebral ligaments.

The free margins of each eyelid possess two or three rows of hairs called cilia, or eyelashes. Posterior to the lashes is a row of glandular orifices of the meibomian glands. Near the medial edges the free margin of each eyelid presents an opening called the punctum lacrimale. The eyelids distribute all adnexal secretions, thereby keeping the cornea moist and washing away any dust.

MUSCLES

The extrinsic ocular muscles of the eyeball are the four rectus and two oblique muscles. These six striated muscles are inserted into the sclera by tendons. Except for the inferior oblique muscles, they arise from the back of the orbit. All the muscles are supplied by cranial nerves: third (oculomotor), fourth (trochlear), and sixth (abducens). The muscles work in pairs. Movements of the eyes are brought about by an increase in the tone of one set of muscles and a decrease in the tone of the antagonistic muscles. According to the position of the recti muscles in the eyes, they are referred to as the superior rectus, inferior rectus, medial rectus, and lateral rectus. The oblique muscles insert on the back of the eye and are designated the superior oblique and inferior oblique.

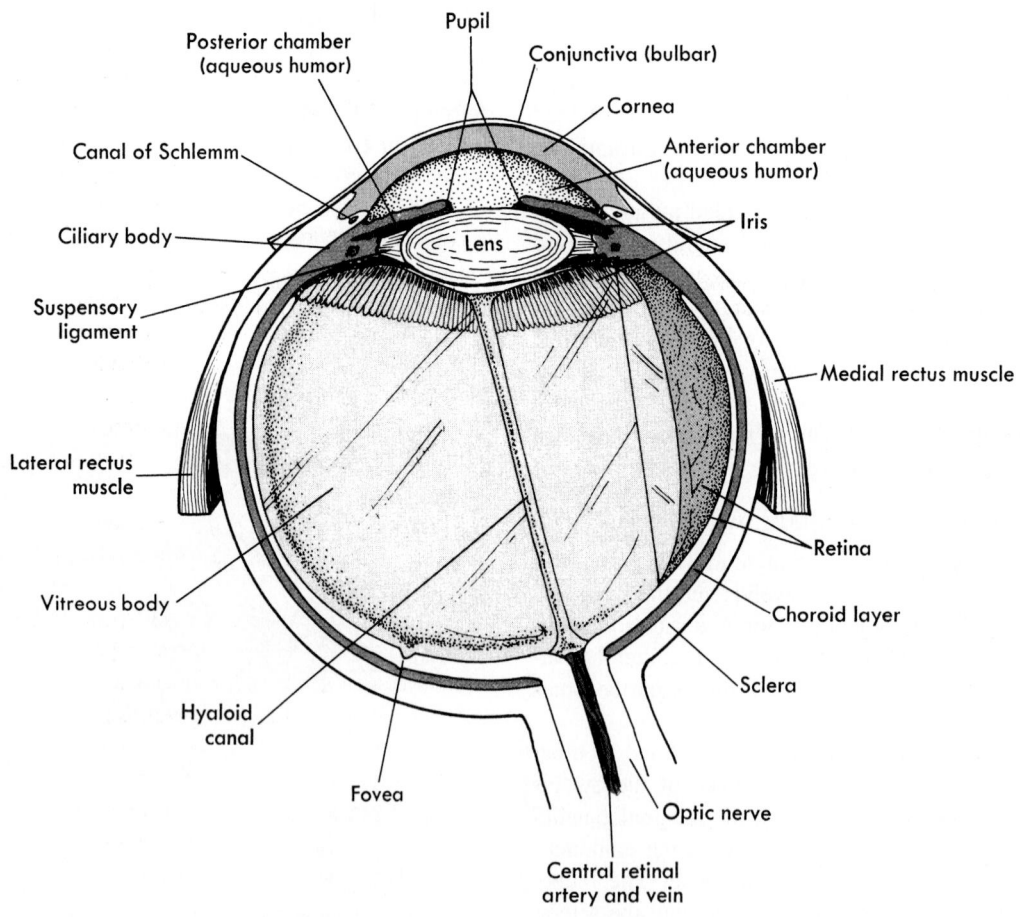

FIG. 17-4 Horizontal section through left eyeball.

From Phipps, W.J., et al. (1995). *Medical-surgical nursing* (5th ed.). St. Louis: Mosby.

GLOBE

The eyeball (globe) is supported in the orbital cavity on a cushion of fat and fascia. It is composed of three layers surrounding a fluid-filled center and occupies less than one third of the orbit. The external, corneal-scleral layer is fibrous and protects the other two; the middle, vascular, pigmented layer comprises the iris, ciliary body, and choroid; and the internal layer is the sensory retina. The fluid contents, which give the eye its globular shape, are aqueous humor (anterior) and vitreous humor (posterior to the lens). The lens, suspended behind the pupillary opening of the iris, and the cornea, combined with the aqueous and vitreous, form the refractive media of the eye (Fig. 17-4).

External layer (corneal-scleral)

The *cornea* is the anterior, transparent, avascular part of the external layer. It is crescent shaped and joins the sclera at a transitional zone called the limbus. The cornea is composed of five layers: the epithelium, Bowman's membrane, stroma (substantia propria), Descemet's membrane, and endothelium (Fig. 17-5). The epithelium consists of five or six constantly renewing cell layers and many nerve endings,

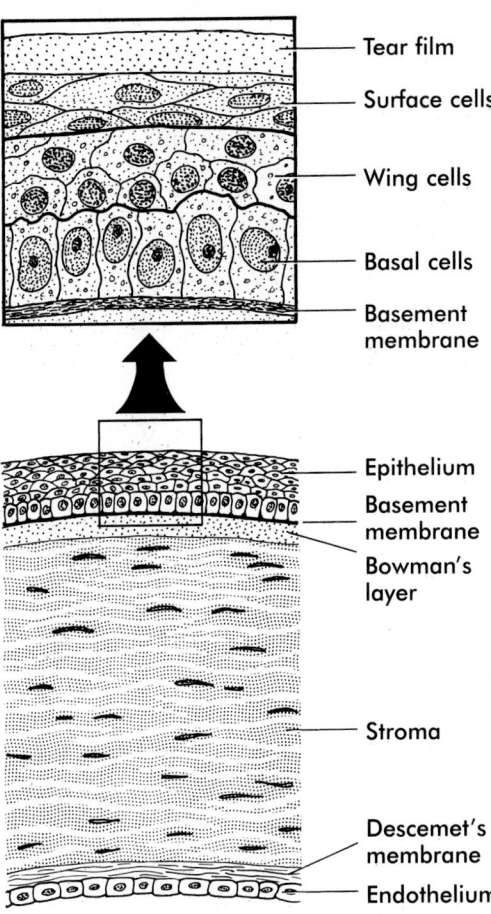

FIG. 17-5 Cornea is composed of five layers: the epithelium, Bowman's membrane, stroma (substantia propria), Descemet's membrane, and endothelium.

Labels for figure:
- Tear film
- Surface cells
- Wing cells
- Basal cells
- Basement membrane
- Epithelium
- Basement membrane
- Bowman's layer
- Stroma
- Descemet's membrane
- Endothelium

which account for corneal sensitivity. Bowman's membrane is composed of connective tissue fibers and forms a barrier to trauma and infection. If damaged, it does not regenerate, and a permanent scar is left. The stroma accounts for 90% of the corneal thickness and is composed of multiple lamellar fibers. The endothelium is a single layer of hexagonal cells that do not regenerate. These cells are responsible for the proper state of dehydration (deturgescence) that keeps the cornea clear. Damage to these cells causes corneal edema and loss of transparency (Fig. 17-6). The cornea serves as a window through which light rays pass to the retina. The branches of the ophthalmic division of the fifth cranial nerve supply the cornea. Descemet's membrane is a thin layer between the endothelial layer of the cornea and the substantia propria. This membrane may become inflamed (descemetitis) or protrude (descemetocele).

The *sclera* is the posterior opaque part of the external layer. A portion of the sclera can be seen through the conjunctiva as the white of the eye. The sclera is made up of collagenous fibers loosely connected with fascia, which receives the tendons of the muscles of the globe. The sclera is pierced by the ciliary arteries and nerves and posteriorly by the optic nerve (see Fig. 17-4).

Middle layer

The middle covering of the eye comprises the choroid, ciliary body, and iris from behind forward. The choroid contains many blood vessels and is the main source of nourishment of the receptor cell and pigment epithelial layer of the retina (see Fig. 17-4).

The *ciliary body* consists of an extension of the choroidal blood vessels, a mass of muscle tissue, and an extension of the neuroepithelium of the retina. It extends 6 to 6.5 mm from the root of the iris to the ora serrata (Fig. 17-7). The anterior 2 mm of the ciliary body is called the pars plicata, and the posterior 4 to 5 mm is the pars plana (Fig. 17-8). The ciliary muscle effects accommodation. The neuroepithelium is secretory in nature and is responsible for the formation of the aqueous humor.

The *iris*, a thin membrane, is the anterior portion of the middle layer and is situated in front of the lens. The peripheral border of the iris is attached to the ciliary body, whereas its central border is free. The iris aperture is located slightly nasal to its center, known as the pupil (see Fig. 17-4). The iris divides the space between the cornea and the lens into an anterior and a posterior chamber. Both chambers are filled with aqueous humor.

The iris with its many striations regulates the amount of light entering the eye and assists in obtaining clear images. The iris moves by means of smooth muscle fibers within the connective tissue. The sphincter pupillae muscle contracts the pupil, and the dilator pupillae dilates it. As more light strikes the eye, the sphincter constricts the pupil.

Internal layer

The innermost layer, sometimes called the nervous cov-

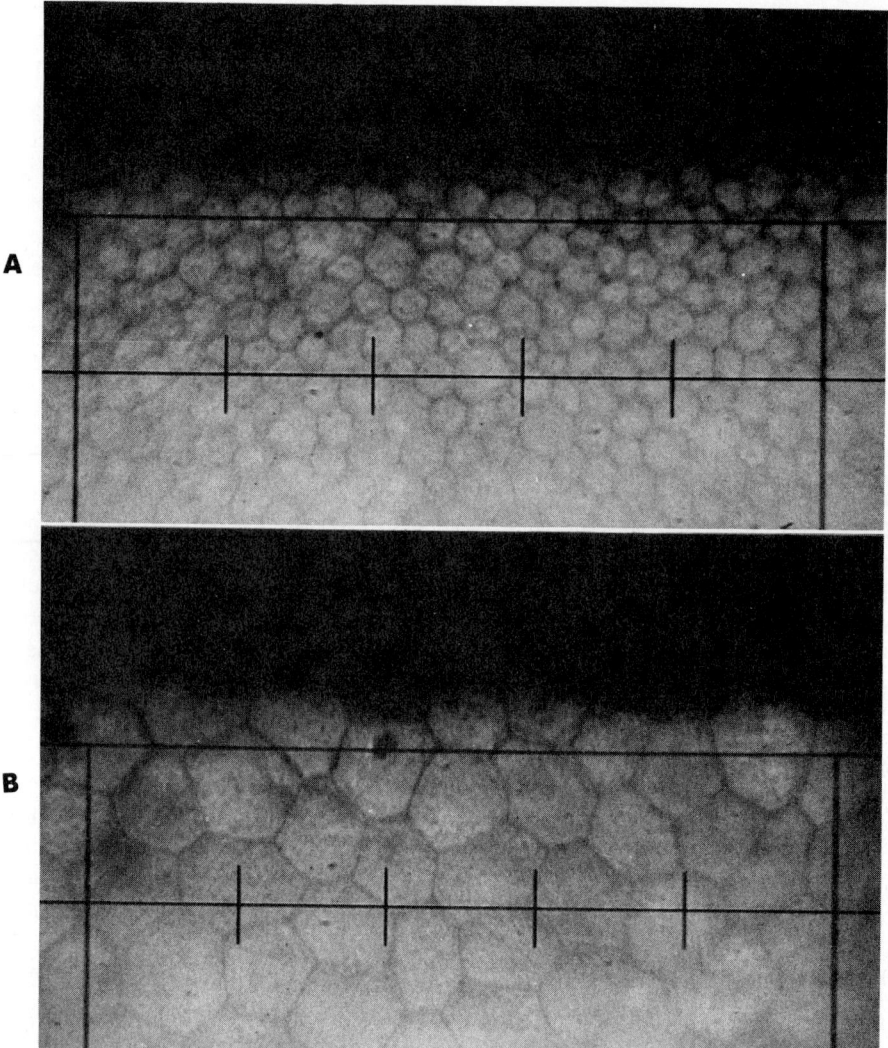

FIG. 17-6 Endothelial cells. **A,** Normal. **B,** Abnormal.
Courtesy Lorraine Koury, Argon Ophthalmic Laboratory, Inc., Portland, Ore.

ering, is the retina, a thin transparent membrane extending from the ora serrata to the optic disk (Figs. 17-4 and 17-9). This network of nerve cells and fibers receives images of external objects and transfers the impression via the optic nerve, optic tracts, lateral geniculate body, and optic radiations to the occipital lobe of the cerebrum. The nerve fibers from the retina converge to become the optic nerve, which enters the eyeball almost at its posterior point, slightly to the inner side. The point at which the nerve enters the eyeball is called the optic disk. In field testing this is the anatomic blind spot.

The retina is composed of many layers. The pigment epithelium is a single layer of epithelial cells on the external side of the retina through which oxygen and other nutrients are diffused from the choroid. The other nine layers of the retina consist of photoreceptor cells (rods and cones) and sensory neurons (bipolar cells and ganglion cells) (Fig. 17-10). The photoreceptors within the retina respond to light energy and initiate the neural response, which is eventually interpreted in the occipital cortex. The point of highest resolution is the foveal pit, which exists in the center of the area that takes on a yellow hue after death (macula lutea).

An inverted image of the object being viewed is focused on the retina. The nerve fibers leaving the retina by the way of the optic nerve travel to the lateral geniculate body of the thalamus. The fibers nasal to the foveal pit cross in the optic chiasma to go to the contralateral geniculate body. Thus all fibers composing the same half of the visual field project to the same geniculate body, from which fibers project to the ipsilateral occipital cortex for interpretation.

REFRACTIVE APPARATUS

The refractive apparatus consists of the cornea, the aqueous humor, the lens, and the vitreous body (see Fig. 17-4).

The *cornea* has the greatest refractive power of the oc-

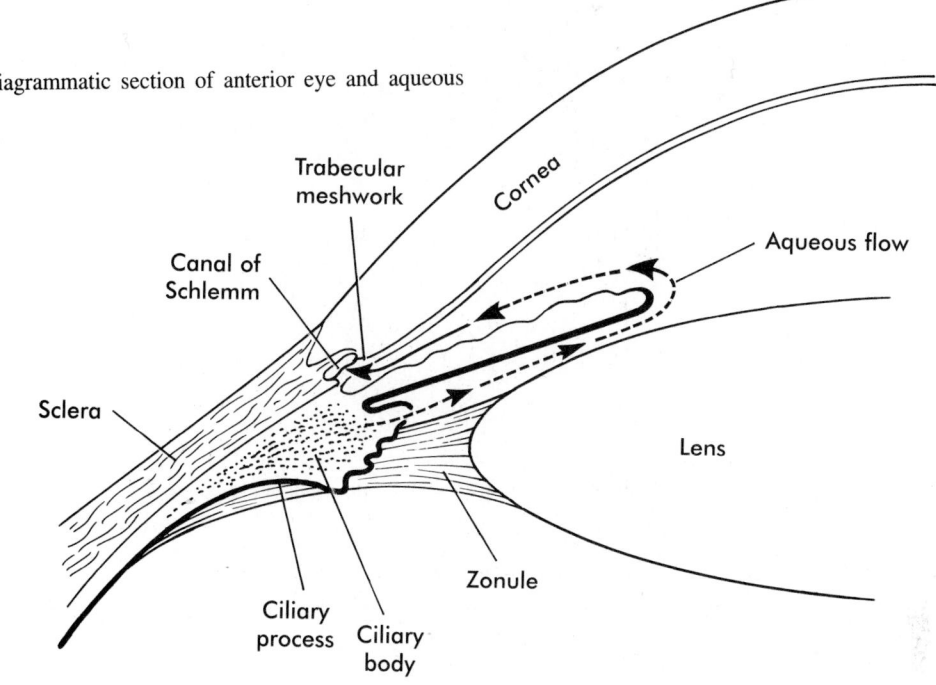

FIG. 17-7 Diagrammatic section of anterior eye and aqueous circulation.

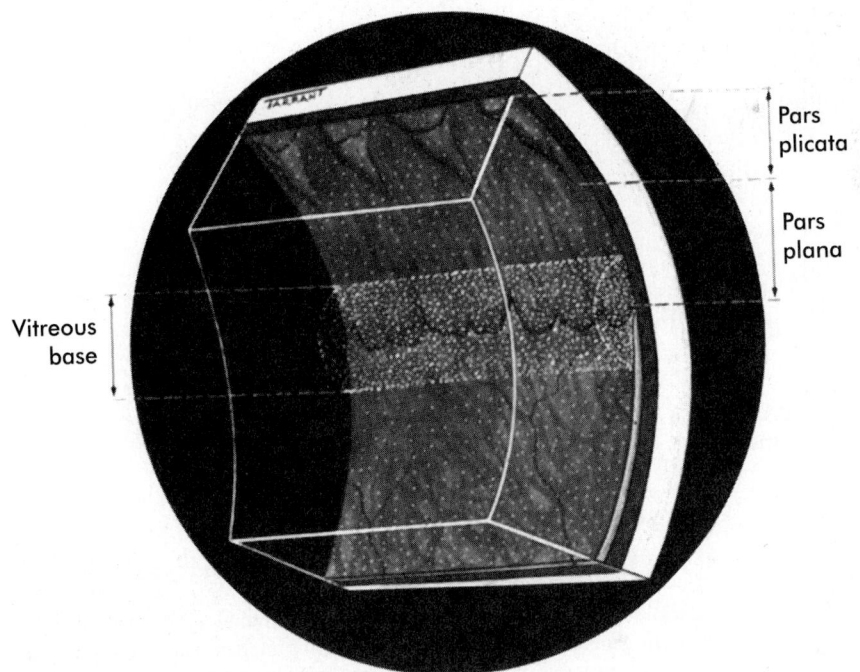

FIG. 17-8 Anatomy of pars plana.
From Kanski, J.J. (1984). *Clinical ophthalmology*. London: Butterworth & Co.

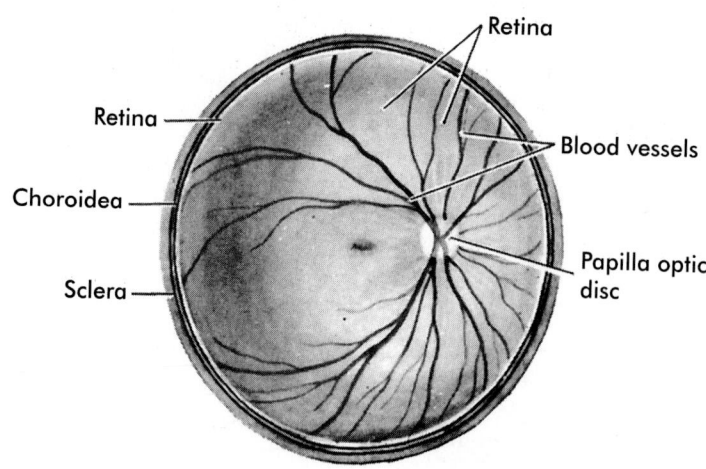

FIG. 17-9   Normal fundus of eye seen through ophthalmoscope.

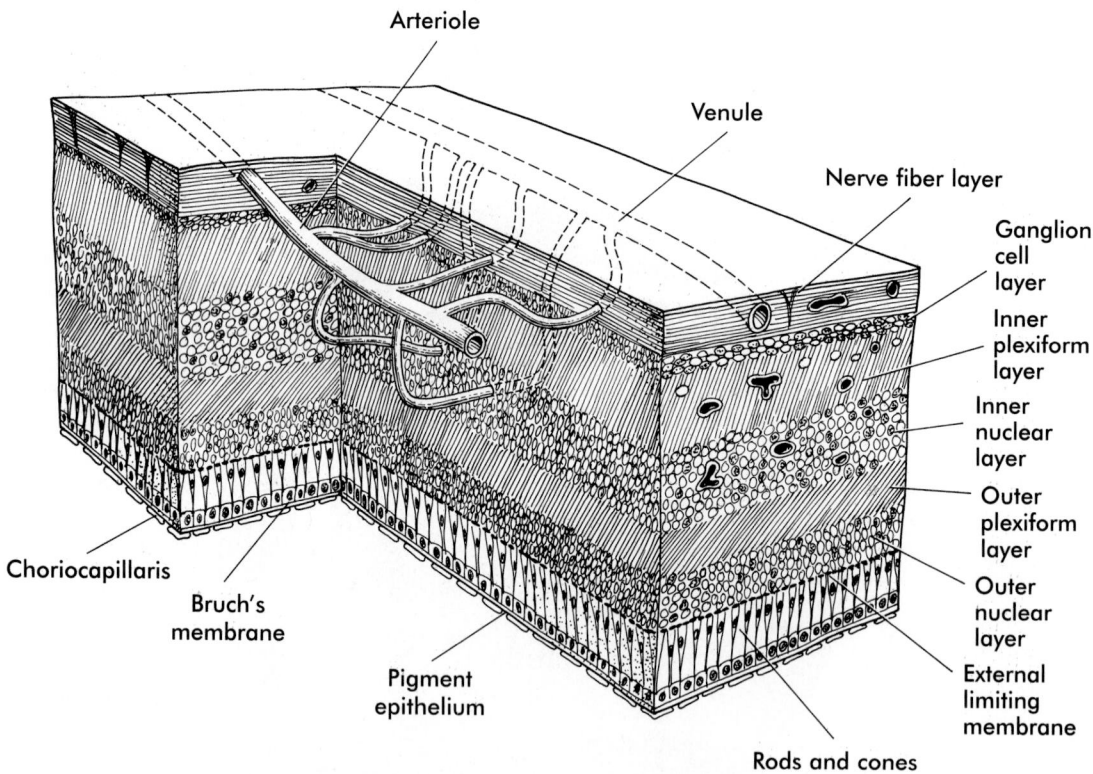

FIG. 17-10   Retinal arterioles provide two major capillary layers in retina: one in nerve fiber layer and one in inner nuclear layer. In general, diseases affecting primarily arteries, such as vascular hypertension, involve capillary network in nerve fiber layer, whereas predominantly venous diseases, such as diabetes mellitus, involve layer of capillaries in inner nuclear layer. Outer receptors, together with their cell bodies in outer nuclear layer and portion of outer plexiform layer, are nurtured by choriocapillaris of the choroid. Both systems are necessary to function of retina.

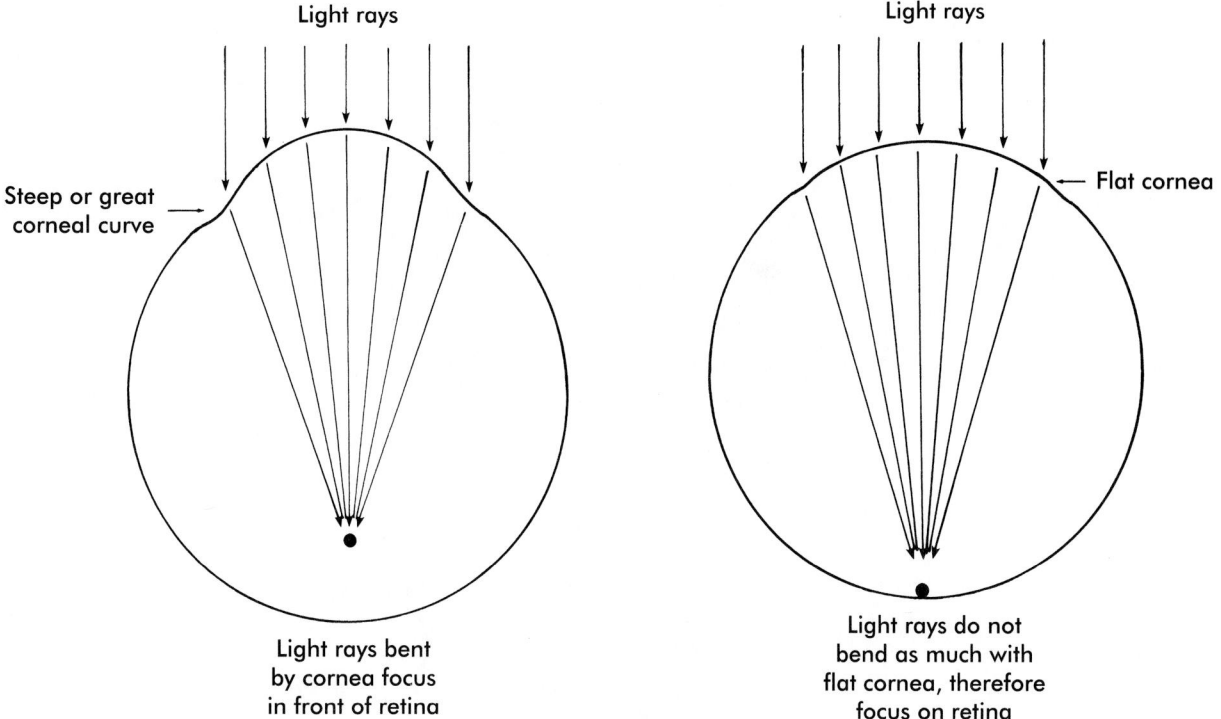

FIG. 17-11   Variations in the curvature of the cornea change its refractive power.

ular structures. Variations in the curvature of the cornea change its refractive power (Fig. 17-11).

The *lens* of the eye is biconvex and has a diameter of 1 cm (see Figs. 17-4 and 17-7). It is suspended behind the iris and connected to the ciliary body by zonular fibers. Its anterior and posterior surfaces are separated by a rounded border, the equator. The crystalline lens does not shed cells. As it grows, the cells are compressed and harden. The lens can expand and retract by means of the zonular fibers (accommodation); this accommodative power is lost with the aging process, as the lens loses its elasticity when the cells harden. This is the reason many older persons need bifocals. Eventually the hardening causes opacity of the lens—a cataract.

The *vitreous body* is a glasslike, transparent, gelatinous mass composed of 99% water and 1% collagen and hyaluronic acid. It fills the posterior four fifths of the eyeball and is adherent to the retina at the vitreous base.

The central components of a light wave enter the eyes perpendicularly, and a light wave enters at the sides obliquely. For clear vision the oblique rays must converge and come to a focus with the central rays on the retina. Light rays from an object pass through the system of refractory devices—the cornea, aqueous humor, lens, and vitreous—and are refracted so that the rays strike the macular area.

NERVE AND BLOOD SUPPLY

The optic nerve (second cranial nerve) extends between the posterior eyeball and the optic chiasma (Fig. 17-12). This nerve carries visual impulses, as well as the sensations of pain, touch, and temperature, from the eye and its surrounding structures to the brain. The third cranial nerve (oculomotor) is the primary motor nerve to all rectus muscles except the lateral rectus, which is innervated by the sixth cranial nerve (abducens). The fourth cranial nerve (trochlear) innervates the superior oblique muscle.

The ophthalmic artery, the main arterial supply to the orbit and globe, is a branch of the internal carotid artery. It divides into branches supplying the globe, muscles, and eyelids. The central retinal artery and central retinal vein travel through the optic nerve and provide an independent circulation for the inner retina.

PERIOPERATIVE NURSING CONSIDERATIONS

ASSESSMENT

Patients entering the hospital or ambulatory unit for eye surgery exhibit many emotions and reactions, such as hostility, anger, fear, grief, and helplessness. Of prime concern to most is the success of the surgical procedure. Patients undergoing eye surgery vary from infants with congenital conditions to geriatric patients whose conditions are a result of the aging process. With the increase in ambulatory surgery, the perioperative nursing staff must be prepared to not only meet the specific needs of each patient when providing care but also prepare the patient for home care.

Preparation is begun in the physician's office or clinic.

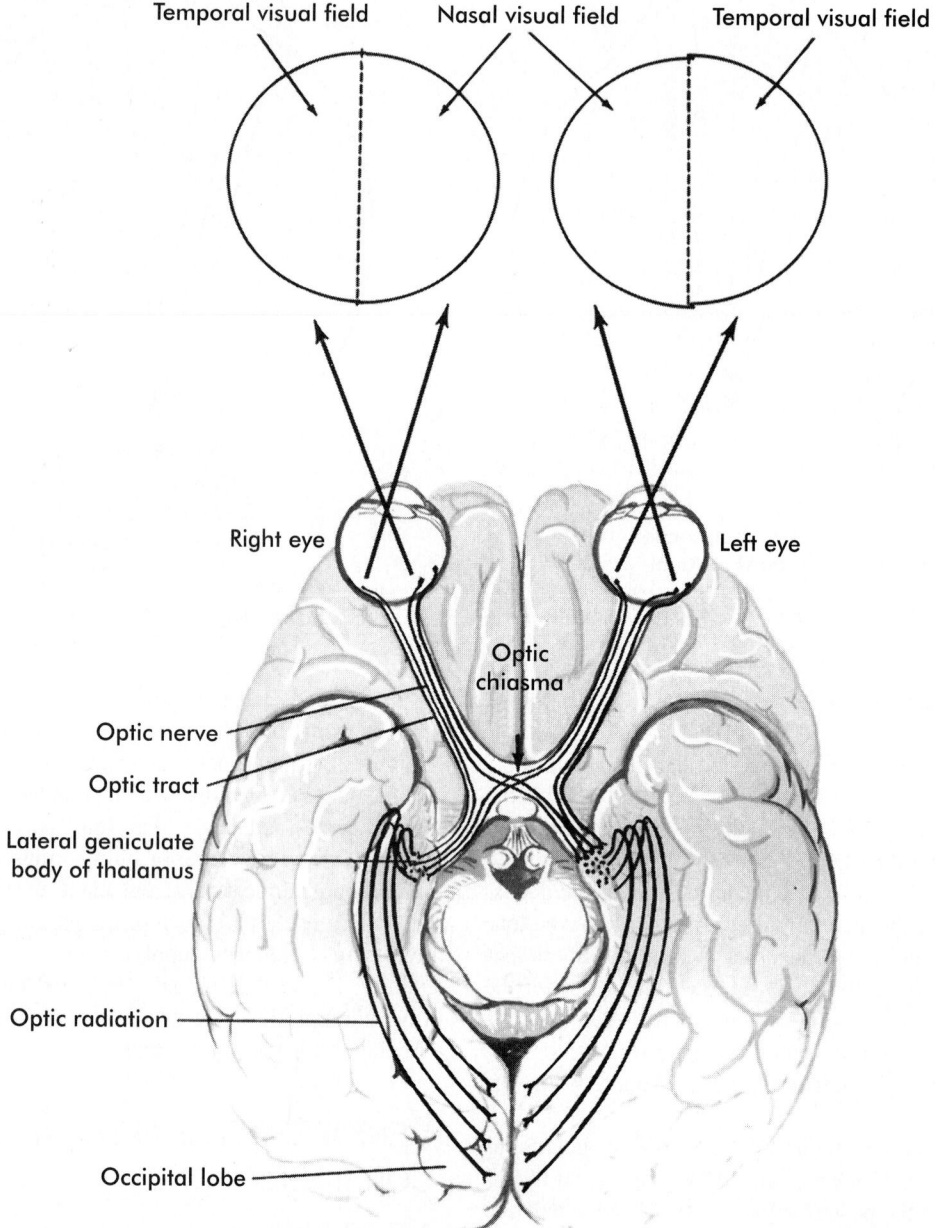

FIG. 17-12 Visual pathways. Note structures that compose each pathway: optic nerve, optic chiasma, lateral geniculate body of thalamus, optic radiations, and visual cortex of occipital lobe. Fibers from nasal portion of each retina cross over to opposite side at optic chiasma, hence terminating in lateral geniculate body of opposite side. Location of lesion in visual pathway determines resulting visual defect. For example, destruction of an optic nerve produces permanent blindness in same eye, and pressure on optic chiasma (by pituitary tumor, for instance) produces bitemporal hemianopsia, or more simply, blindness in both temporal visual fields because it destroys fibers from nasal sides of both retinas.

Modified from Thibodeau, G.A. (1990). *Anthony's textbook of anatomy and physiology* (13th ed.). St. Louis: Mosby.

Communication with the physician's office to coordinate patient preparation and teaching increases the efficiency and effectiveness of preoperative procedures.

On the patient's admission to the unit, a staff member should fully orient the patient to the physical surroundings. It may be helpful to walk with the patient to familiarize him or her with areas of the room and nursing unit. Constant description and reinforcement are important to the visually impaired. Subtle changes, such as approaching the patient from the nonaffected side, increase the patient's independence, facilitate care, and decrease the possibility of startling the patient. Consistency in nursing personnel helps the patient recognize familiar voices and faces. It is preferable to have all ophthalmic patients in one area to decrease the risk of cross-contamination and to provide specialized care. Many patients are no longer admitted to a nursing unit, but are admitted through an ambulatory admission area adjacent to the surgical suites. This presents a challenge to all involved staff to collaborate and communicate effectively, so that continuity of patient care is not jeopardized.

The nursing assessment is designed to bring to light *pertinent* information and must be carried out in a comprehensive, yet efficient, manner. A standard set of parameters should provide enough information to facilitate appropriate care in the event of an emergency. The priority of data collection depends on the patient's condition. Biophysical information, including height, weight, and vital signs; biopsychosocial factors, which include support systems, fears and anxiety; along with environmental, education, and self-care needs are assessed. The general health history includes current medication therapy and whether the patient has brought medications along. Because ocular problems may be directly related to other diseases, the medical history is very important. Additional discharge planning factors are also explored.

Data may be collected from family or significant others, or directly from physicians or their office staff. All information should be documented so that it is readily available to others. An ocular history, which includes the patient's primary problem, history of the present condition, nature of symptoms, and visual limitations imposed on the patient by the disease or condition, is collected. An external examination of the eye, including lids, lashes, conjunctiva, and lacrimal apparatus, should be performed to detect any deviations from normal. The corneal reflex should be tested and the cornea inspected for superficial irregularities. Pupil size and contour, as well as pupillary reaction, both direct and consensual, should be noted. Anterior chamber depth should be checked with oblique illumination to alert staff members to the potential for angle closure with dilatation of the pupil (Fig. 17-13).

Function of the extraocular muscles should be determined. Movement should be synchronous, and visual lines should meet on a fixed object. Documentation of this examination must be descriptive, accurate, and concise. It is of value later in assessing the outcome of the procedure.

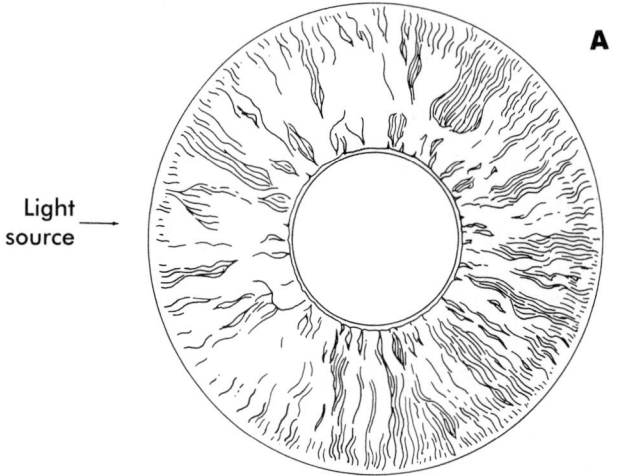

Deep anterior chamber

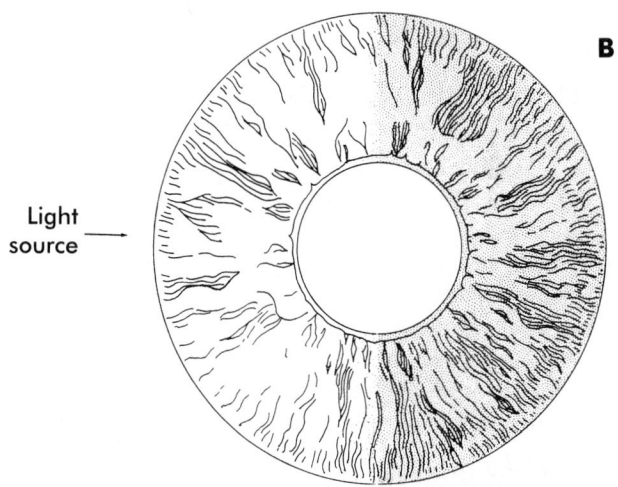

Shallow anterior chamber

FIG. 17-13 Oblique illumination of cornea. **A,** Normal anterior chamber depth (entire iris illuminated). **B,** Shallow anterior chamber (half of the iris is in shadow).

The following observations should be obtained or confirmed during perioperative nursing assessment:

- General appearance of the eye (swelling, redness, skin condition around eyes)
- Symptoms of irritation (itching, burning)
- Position of eyelids, condition of upper and lower lid surfaces, eyelid spasm
- Visual acuity, pupillary dilatation (note whether pupils are equal, round, reactive to light, and accommodative), visual fields
- Extraocular muscle movement
- Drainage from eye (note type and amount)
- Vital signs (obtain and record)
- Restlessness, discomfort, anxiety (observe for and note)
- Limitations in mobility, if any, should be noted

- Current and significant past medical problems (eye disease, diabetes, cardiovascular disease, hypertension, allergies)
- Current medication history

Laboratory studies

The results of laboratory studies, as applicable to the individual patient, should be reviewed during perioperative nursing assessment. Deviations from normal should be noted and recorded.

- Blood sugar (80 to 110 mg/dl) may be higher or lower depending on intake; critical levels are <50 and >400 mg/dl in adult males, and <40 or >400 mg/dl in adult females
- Serum potassium (adults/elderly: 3.5 to 5 mEq/L) and other electrolytes (calcium: total 9 to 10.5 mg/dl, ionized 4.5 to 5.6 mg/dl; sodium: 136 to 145 mEq/L)
- Serum enzymes and other blood work (CBC, coagulation studies)

Electrocardiogram and chest x-ray

In older adults, reports of prescribed chest x-rays and/or an ECG should be on the patient record. The older adult is more predisposed to respiratory infection from less elastic alveoli, decreased heart size unless there is enlargement associated with hypertension or heart disease, and ECG changes secondary to cellular alteration, conduction system fibrosis, and neurogenic changes.

After the assessment information has been compiled, nursing diagnoses are identified and the plan of care for the entire perioperative period is developed.

NURSING DIAGNOSIS

Nursing diagnoses related to the care of patients undergoing ophthalmic procedures might include the following:

- Knowledge deficit related to diagnosis, surgical intervention, and home care management
- Visual sensory or perceptual alteration related to surgical intervention
- Anxiety related to surgical intervention and its outcome
- High risk for injury related to increased intraocular pressure
- High risk for infection related to surgical intervention

OUTCOME IDENTIFICATION

Outcomes identified for the selected nursing diagnoses could be stated as:

- Patient and/or significant other will verbalize knowledge of the diagnosis, planned intervention, and requirements for home care maintenance prior to discharge.
- Patient will demonstrate ability to cope with visual sensory/perceptual alteration safely during the postoperative period.
- Patient will verbalize concerns and fears and utilize
- Patient will identify activities that increase intraocular pressure, and avoid during postoperative period.
- Patient will be free from signs and symptoms of postoperative infection.

PLANNING

Care plans are the framework for organizing activities in the perioperative period. Although ophthalmic surgery is often perceived as minor due to the small incision site and because many procedures generally are not lengthy, the perioperative nurse must be fully prepared for potential complications or emergencies. Patients who are admitted for ophthalmic surgery often have complex medical histories. Following a review of the patient record, supplemented by a patient or family interview or collaboration with colleagues, data collected are incorporated into a perioperative plan for patient care. A typical plan of care for the patient undergoing ophthalmic surgery follows.

IMPLEMENTATION
Patient/family education

Implementation of the care plan actually begins during the patient interview. Planning to meet the patient's educational needs should play an equal role with meeting other needs. Review and reinforcement of information initially provided in the physician's office ensure consistency in teaching. Written material and audiovisual media (television, films, pictures, and slides) may be used to enhance patient education programs but do not eliminate the need for direct interchange with patients or feedback from them. Family members or friends should be included to add support and increase understanding of the planned surgery (Research Highlight 17-1). The ophthalmic patient should be informed of the purpose and desired results of preoperative eyedrops and sedation. An explanation of what to expect from the anesthetic decreases the patient's anxiety level and enables the patient to cooperate better. The perioperative nurse should discuss the activities and routines of the intraoperative period. A brief description of the operating room and its equipment, on the patient's arrival in the surgical suite, helps allay the patient's fears.

The patient should be informed of what to expect immediately after surgery so that the postoperative recovery period is less stressful. Reassurance is especially important for patients whose eyes will be patched postoperatively. Thorough preoperative preparation of the patient, and in most cases the family who will assist with care at home in the postoperative period, plays a vital role in the successful outcome of the surgical procedure.

Managing and monitoring patient safety needs

General duties of the perioperative nursing team are discussed in previous chapters. However, some considerations are specific to the ophthalmic patient. Because many ophthalmic procedures are performed under local anesthesia, the circulating nurse or an additional perioperative nurse,

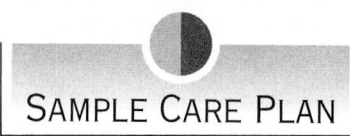

NURSING DIAGNOSIS: Knowledge deficit related to diagnosis, surgical intervention, and home care management

OUTCOME: Patient and/or significant other will verbalize knowledge of the diagnosis, the planned surgical intervention, and requirements for home care maintenance.

INTERVENTIONS:

Determine the patient's understanding of the diagnosis, the planned intervention, and the type of anesthesia to be administered.

Clarify misconceptions and provide additional explanations (or refer to appropriate member of health care team).

Explain sequence of perioperative events and what to expect in the operating room in terms that the patient can understand.

Review postoperative limitations to self-care activities.

Provide and review written instructions (in large letters) regarding medications, including specific techniques for instilling eyedrops and ophthalmic medications, applying compresses (as necessary), and applying appropriate eye dressing or protective shield.

Supervise patient practice with prescribed self-care activities (for example, instillation of medications).

NURSING DIAGNOSIS: Visual sensory/perceptual alteration related to surgical intervention

OUTCOME: Patient will cope with visual sensory/perceptual alteration safely.

INTERVENTIONS:

Introduce self and other team members so that patient can recognize voices.

Familiarize and orient patient to immediate surroundings; continuously reorient patient.

Approach patient from unaffected side.

Offer reassurance, explanations, and understanding.

Prior to discharge, review and have patient list safety measures to prevent falls and other injuries.

Refer patient to appropriate agency if home assistance is required.

NURSING DIAGNOSIS: Anxiety related to surgical intervention and its outcome

OUTCOME: Patient will verbalize concerns and fears and utilize coping mechanisms.

INTERVENTIONS:

Allow patient time to verbalize concerns.

Assist patient to identify source of anxiety.

Help the patient identify existing personal strengths and external resources.

Encourage independence by allowing patient to assist with plan of care; involve patient in identifying diversional activities.

Observe the patient's facial expressions, body posture, and vital signs.

Broadly classify the patient's level of anxiety based on nursing observation (low, moderate, high).

Offer comfort measures (for example, warm blankets).

Provide emotional support; reinforce information the patient has been previously given.

Use touch (as appropriate) to communicate reassurance.

Control environmental stimuli in the operating room.

NURSING DIAGNOSIS: High risk for injury related to increased intraocular pressure

OUTCOME: Patient will identify activities that increase intraocular pressure.

INTERVENTIONS:

Monitor the presence of, or an increase in, eye pain, pain around orbit, blurred vision, reddened eye, abdominal pain, nausea, vomiting, neurologic changes, and changes in visual fields; initiate appropriate action.

Instruct the patient to refrain from excessive exertion, such as crying, coughing, straining, overlifting, bending, rubbing the eyes, and blowing the nose.

Discuss methods to facilitate bowel elimination (diet, appropriate exercise, stool softeners if prescribed.)

NURSING DIAGNOSIS: High risk for infection related to surgical intervention

OUTCOME: Patient will be free from signs and symptoms of postoperative infection.

INTERVENTIONS:

Preoperatively, note whether the patient has a preexisting infection, is immunocompromised, or has other conditions that compromise resistance to infection.

Maintain an aseptic perioperative environment.

Adhere to good handwashing practices.

Determine and record the wound classification.

Postoperatively, monitor vital signs, fluid balance, and presence of pain.

Instruct the patient in self-care, including postoperative antibiotic therapy, if prescribed.

Teach the patient to wash hands prior to the instillation of any ophthalmic medications.

Instruct the patient to watch for redness, pain, swelling, drainage, and changes in visual acuity postoperatively, and report these problems promptly to the physician.

☀
RESEARCH HIGHLIGHT 17-1

Gallagher conducted a pilot case study to provide background for planning research studies on adaptation behaviors of sighted persons who experience loss of vision. The case study was conducted on one 25-year-old woman who had had lost her sight 2 years before the interviews. The Jalowiec Coping Scale (JCS), a self-report measure, was used. In addition, two semistructured interviews and a summation interview were conducted. The subject also kept a tape-recorded log for a period of 6 weeks. Triangulation technique was used to test for validity and reliability. Conclusions of this preliminary study support the assumption that loss of eyesight produces the same staged coping behaviors of grieving that move the individual from denial to acceptance. The study also found that there appears to be a lack of knowledge and understanding regarding the abilities or feelings of the visually impaired, and thus an inability to interact with them appropriately.

Gallagher, C. (1991). The young adult with recent vision loss: A pilot case study. *The Journal of the American Society of Ophthalmic Registered Nurses, Inc., 26* (1).

---

if available, must be prepared to monitor the patient and provide supportive care. Ophthalmic patients, like other surgical patients, have increased sensitivity to noise and activities within the room. The room should be kept quiet and peaceful to decrease anxiety and increase cooperation, thereby reducing the need for heavy sedation.

Additional patient safety needs must also be managed by both scrub nurse and circulating nurse. Foreign substances must not be introduced intraocularly. Lint-free barriers should be used to create the sterile field on the instrument table; gloved hands must be wiped with moistened towels to remove starch powder particles before the procedure begins. The portion of an instrument used in an intraocular wound should not be touched by gloved hands, and debris should be cleansed from instruments with cellulose sponges. All solutions on the sterile field must be clearly labeled, and intraocular solutions must be separated from those not used intraocularly. The entire surgical team must be knowledgeable about their roles and be prepared to function quickly in the event of a complication.

Members of the perioperative nursing team have several important responsibilities in the admission of the patient to the operating room and in the preparation of the room and the equipment. Technologic advances in ophthalmic surgery require that perioperative nurses have familiarity with equipment and check each piece carefully before the patient arrives in the operating room.

Scrupulous attention to aseptic technique and perioperative nursing measures designed for safety and comfort of the patient are of prime importance. The duties of the perioperative nursing team include the following:

1. Identifying the patient by name if awake; seeking patient cooperation and confidence by speaking softly, distinctly, and confidently; and endeavoring to keep the patient quiet and relaxed by staying close by and establishing contact by touch
2. Checking the patient's name on the wristband with the name on the chart and the name on the surgical schedule, and verbally confirming it with the patient
3. Reviewing the surgeon's preoperative orders and nurses' notes to determine if the correct operative eye has been prepared (including verification of operative eye and dilatation, if appropriate) and other procedures have been carried out according to hospital policies
4. Reaffirming preoperative orders with the surgeon
5. Preparing the operating room bed and making sure all the necessary attachments are in readiness
6. Starting an intravenous drip, placing the blood pressure cuff and pulse oximeter, recording the baseline blood pressure and heart rate, and attaching the cardiac monitor
7. When the patient is not managed with monitored anesthesia care (MAC), an oxygen cannula should be available for administration of oxygen if needed.

Ophthalmic pharmacology

Medications used in the perioperative period are extremely important to the outcome of the procedure and the safety of the patient. Drugs for diagnosing and treating eye disorders are potent. One error could result in total, irreversible blindness.

The patient's medical and ocular histories determine the selection of an appropriate ophthalmic agent. This information should be included in the patient's initial nursing assessment. The following established protocols for each medication administration greatly reduce the possibility of medication errors:

1. The perioperative nurse must be knowledgeable about the specific medication ordered, including purpose, strength, action, duration, adverse reactions, route of administration, and contraindications.
2. Expiration dates should be checked prior to medication administration.
3. The medication label must be checked during preparation and again immediately before administration. This precaution is especially important because many ophthalmic drugs are distributed in single-dose units that closely resemble one another.
4. The patient must be positively identified, and the site of the administration must be clearly translated from the physician's orders. The abbreviations OD, OS, and OU indicate right eye, left eye, and both eyes, respectively.
5. The precise dosage of medication must be given at its scheduled time to enhance its effectiveness.
6. Hand washing between patients when administering

eyedrops is imperative, and universal precautions should be followed.

The patient should be made aware of the expected effect of each medication to be able to evaluate its effectiveness, detect signs and symptoms of adverse reactions, and know when to notify the physician concerning problems. The patient should also be well informed of the special considerations associated with specific medications so that appropriate safety precautions can be taken. An example is protection of the cornea after application of a topical anesthetic. Selection of specific medication is influenced by the physician's education and experience and the patient's disease condition. Following is a classification of ophthalmic medications and specific examples of use.

Dilating drops

Dilating drops (mydriatics and cycloplegics) are used to dilate the pupil for objective examination of the retina, testing of refraction, or easier removal of the lens. Mydriatic drugs dilate the pupil but permit the patient to focus. The most commonly used mydriatic is phenylephrine 2%, 5%, or 10% (Neo-Synephrine).

A cycloplegic drug dilates the pupil and also inhibits focusing of the eye. This type of drug aids refraction procedures. Commonly used cycloplegics are tropicamide (Mydriacyl) 1%, atropine 1%, and cyclopentolate 1% (Cyclogyl). Atropine has a long-lasting effect.

Constricting drops

Miotic drugs increase contraction of the sphincter of the iris, thus causing the pupil to contract and constrict. Commonly used miotics are pilocarpine 1% to 4% and phospholine iodide 0.012% to 0.25%. In addition to their action on the pupil, miotics improve the ease with which the aqueous fluid escapes from the eye, thereby resulting in a decrease in intraocular pressure. Miotics are used in the treatment of glaucoma.

Phospholine iodide is usually discontinued before intraocular surgery is performed. Phospholine iodide, isoflurophate (DFP, Floropryl), and demecarium bromide (Humorsol) are irreversible anticholinesterase drugs and may cause prolonged apnea when used in conjunction with succinylcholine (Anectine).

Pilocarpine is sometimes used postoperatively following the extraction of a cataractous lens to cause sustained pupillary contraction and maintain position of the pupil over the implanted lens.

Acetylcholine (Miochol) is the natural cholinergic transmitter released by the parasympathetic nerves to the iris sphincter. It is relatively unstable in solution and is often used intraocularly to produce rapid pupillary contraction (constriction), especially after the insertion of an artificial lens, or pseudophakia. Acetylcholine is prepared immediately before use. Carbochol (Isopto Carbochol) is used to manage narrow- and wide-angle glaucoma. Recent studies (Silverstone et al., 1989) indicate significantly less elevation in intraocular pressure postoperatively when carbochol 0.01% (Miostat) is used in place of acetylcholine intraoperatively.

Corticosteroids

A great number of corticosteroid preparations exist. Corticosteroids are used to inhibit the normal inflammatory response to noxious stimuli. They reduce the resistance of the eye to invasion by bacteria, viruses, and fungi. An active infection is therefore an important contraindication to therapy with cortisone and its derivatives in the treatment of allergic eye conditions and chronic inflammations.

Hyperosmotic agents

Hyperosmotic drugs increase the osmolarity of the serum and, by the effect of the induced osmotic pressure gradient, shrink the vitreous body and reduce the intraocular pressure. These drugs are used routinely in the preoperative medication of patients undergoing ophthalmic surgery, as well as therapeutically in cases of uncontrolled glaucoma (usually angle-closure glaucoma).

The commonly used agents may be divided into those given orally (glycerol and isosorbide) and those given parenterally (mannitol and urea). Acetazolamide (Diamox) may be given by either route, depending on the circumstance. Hyperosmotic drugs by their nature induce diuresis; perioperative nursing personnel must be aware of this and have urinals, bedpans, and sterile urethral catheters available.

Antibiotics, lubricants, and stains

The method or route of administration of an antibiotic agent depends on the location of the problem. Selection of the drug is based on the nature and sensitivity of the organism isolated, the physician's clinical experience, the sensitivity and response of the patient, and the disease. Topical antibiotics are used in the treatment of lid and surface infections and often employed prophylactically to prevent infection. Bacitracin and neomycin sulfate are commonly used antibiotic ointments. Systemic administration of an antibiotic is prescribed for an infection in the posterior portion of the eye or orbit. An infection of this nature can threaten sight. Selection of the specific antibiotic follows the previously mentioned criteria.

Ophthalmic lubricants are used for corneal protection in situations such as faulty lid closure, complications of lacrimal gland disease, and prominence of the corneal surface in thyroid disease. Methylcellulose 0.5% is considered an excellent ophthalmic lubricant.

Fluorescein sodium is a dye and topical stain commonly used for diagnostic purposes. An intravenous preparation of the dye is used in fluorescein angiography to diagnose retinal pathology. Fluorescein strips or solution is used to stain the cornea in evaluating disruption of the corneal epithelium. The use of fluorescein strips is preferred to the use of solution because the solution can easily become contaminated. In its dilute form, fluorescein is yellow-green and temporarily stains the areas of denuded corneal epithelium.

Intraoperative medications

Several drugs used by the ophthalmologist are prepared by the perioperative nurse immediately before use during the procedure.

Sodium hyaluronate (Healon, Amvisc, Viscoat) functions as a lubricant and as a viscoelastic support, maintaining a separation between tissues. It is used in intraocular procedures to protect the corneal endothelium and as a tamponade and vitreous substitute during surgery of the retina and vitreous.

5-Fluorouracil (5-FU), an antimetabolite, previously injected into the subconjunctiva of postoperative glaucoma patients to inhibit scar formation, more recently has been applied intraoperatively, requiring special precautions (Langseth, 1993).

Mitomycin is another antimetabolite used to inhibit scar formation. It is a vesicant and should be carefully monitored for side effects.

Anesthesia

Local or local standby (monitored anesthesia care) anesthesia is preferred for most eye surgery. Consideration must be given to the patient's age, systemic condition, and discharge plan in determining whether to use preoperative sedation. The circulating nurse assembles the sterile local anesthesia setup as required by the surgeon before the patient enters the operating room, checking to ensure correct medications, proper concentrations and dosages, and needles and syringes of appropriate sizes and gauges.

Sedation, when indicated, may be prescribed and managed by either the surgeon or the anesthesiologist. The perioperative nurse, however, is often accountable for monitoring the patient's response to the sedation and the local anesthetic in the perioperative period.

Local and topical anesthetics

Tetracaine (Pontocaine) in a 0.5% solution and proparacaine hydrochloride (Ophthaine) in a 0.5% solution are two commonly used topical anesthetics. They have a rapid onset (5 to 20 seconds) and a moderate duration of action (10 to 20 minutes).

Cocaine 1% to 4% has a rapid onset and a moderate duration. It must never be injected. Cocaine produces excellent surface anesthesia but induces loosening of the corneal epithelium.

Epinephrine 1:1000 solution is a vasoconstrictor that may be applied topically to mucous membranes to decrease bleeding.

Lidocaine 1% to 2% is a commonly used medication for infiltration anesthesia or nerve blocks. It has rapid onset, a fairly long duration of action, and good diffusion proper-

ties. Allergic reactions are rare, and cross-sensitivity with other local anesthetic agents is unusual. Marcaine in a 0.25% to 0.75% solution is often used in combination with lidocaine because of its long duration.

Epinephrine in a 1:50,000 to 1:200,000 solution may be combined with injectable local anesthetics such as lidocaine to prolong anesthesia and reduce bleeding. Epinephrine in a 1:1000 solution is not used with local anesthetics because it can cause cardiac dysrhythmias. Local anesthetics should not be mixed far in advance of the time of intended use since they may deteriorate, and the reduced affect could result in discomfort for the patient.

Hyaluronidase (Wydase) is an enzyme that is commonly mixed with anesthetic solutions (75 units/10 ml) to increase diffusion of the anesthetic through the tissue and thus improve the effectiveness of the nerve block. It is contraindicated when the skin is inflamed or a malignancy of the skin is suspected.

The three methods of administration are instillation of eyedrops, infiltration, and block or regional anesthesia.

Instillation of eyedrops (Fig. 17-14). With the patient's face tilted upward, the first drop is placed in the lower cul-de-sac, and the succeeding drops (number depends on the type of operation to be performed) may be placed from above, with the patient looking downward and the upper lid raised. Gentle retraction of the lower lid is necessary for placing eyedrops in the lower cul-de-sac. Care should be taken to avoid placing eyedrops directly onto the cornea. The natural blinking of the lids distributes the drug evenly on the eye surface, regardless of where the drop is placed. When a toxic drug is instilled, the inner corner of the eyelids should be dried of excessive fluid with a tissue or clean cotton ball after each drop to minimize systemic absorption of the drug. The tip of any drug applicator must not touch the patient's skin or any part of the eye.

Infiltration method. The surgeon injects the anesthetic

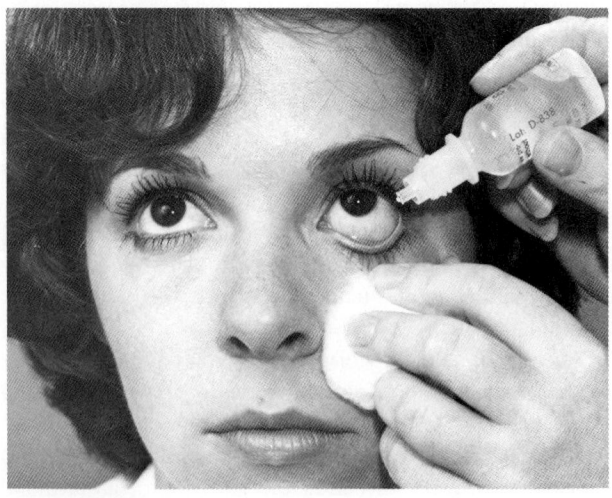

FIG. 17-14   Proper position of head for instillation of eyedrops. Gentle retraction of lower lid is necessary for drop to be placed in lower cul-de-sac.

solution beneath the skin, beneath the conjunctiva, or into Tenon's capsule, depending on the type of surgery.

Block or regional anesthesia. Retrobulbar anesthesia is injection of anesthetic solution into the base of the eyelids at the level of the orbital margins or behind the eyeball to block the ciliary ganglion and nerves (Fig. 17-15). For eyelid repairs the solution is injected through the upper or lower lid. For operations on the lacrimal apparatus the anesthetic is injected at the level of the anterior ethmoidal foramen to anesthetize the internal and external nasal nerves. Retrobulbar injection is usually performed 10 to 15 minutes before surgery to produce temporary paralysis of the extraocular muscles.

In the Van Lint block method procaine or another local anesthetic is injected into the orbicular muscle where it reaches the ends of the facial nerve (Fig. 17-16, *A*). The O'Brien akinesia technique requires blocking of the facial nerve just anterior to the tragus of the ear (Fig. 17-16, *B*). These blocks are used to prevent squeezing of the lids during ocular procedures.

General anesthesia

Youth, dementia, severe anxiety, specific systemic diseases, known sensitivity to local anesthetics, and long duration of the operative procedure are among the conditions that may dictate use of general anesthesia.

Positioning and prepping the patient

Positioning the patient for ophthalmic surgery generally requires additional devices for stabilizing the head, protecting bony prominences, and providing appropriate alignment to prevent peripheral neurovascular injury. The safety needs of the patient are related to age, size, and risk factors for discomfort. If the patient is to be sedated, ask him if he is comfortable and reassure him that there are ways to make him more comfortable. Some elderly patients prefer to not discuss their discomfort for fear of being bothersome (Yamada, 1993). Although the majority of procedures are carried out with the patient supine, there may be a need for special positioning if a patient must be turned during a vitrectomy procedure to repair a giant retinal tear.

In addition, since most ocular surgery is carried out with the use of a microscope, a special wrist rest to stabilize the surgeon's hands is used. This should be attached to the bed and secured approximately 2.5 cm below the lateral canthus prior to draping the patient.

The operative site is prepared under aseptic conditions. Topical anesthetic drops are administered first, if the patient is to be given a local anesthetic. A sterile prep tray containing sterile normal saline solution, irrigation bulb, basins, cotton sponges, cotton-tipped applicators, towels, and antimicrobial skin disinfectant is prepared.

The clipping of eyelashes or shaving of eyebrows is not usually done. When eyelashes are clipped, it is done before the skin preparation. A thin film of water-soluble lubricant is smoothed over the cutting surfaces of a curved

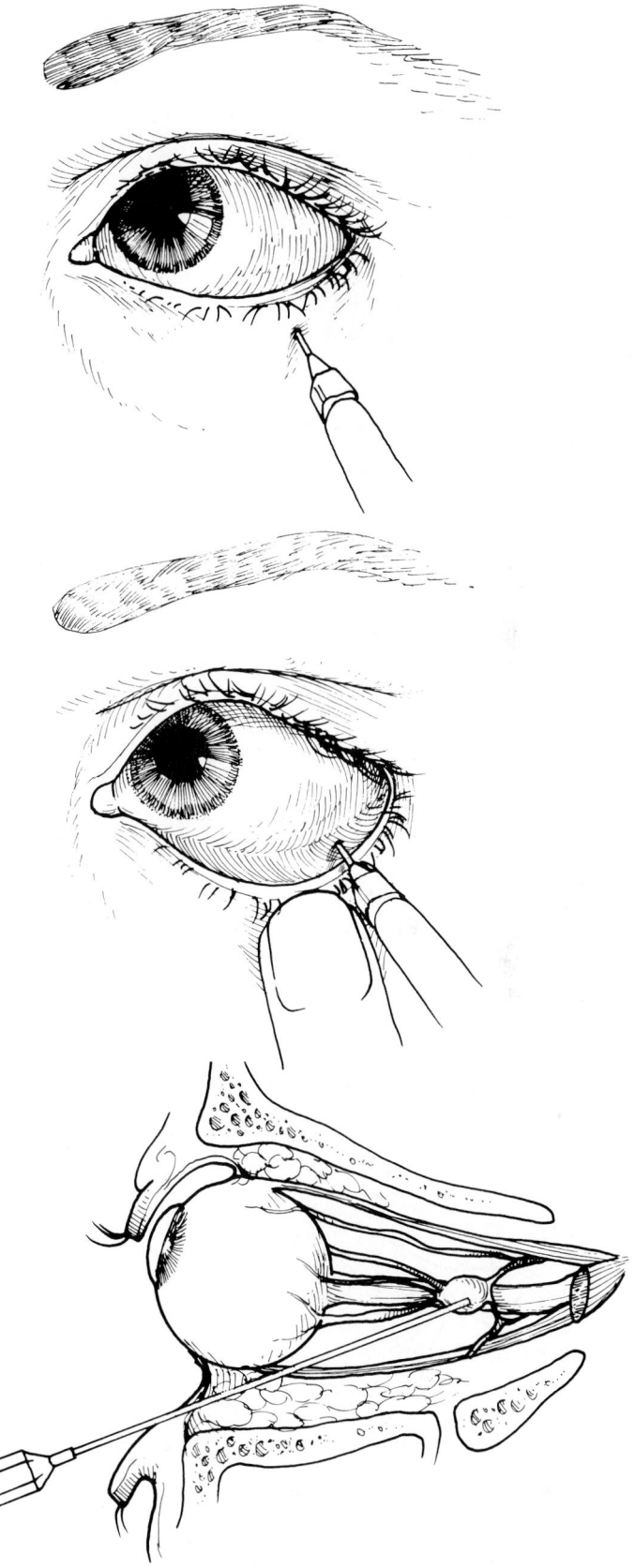

FIG. 17-15 Retrobulbar block for regional anesthesia.

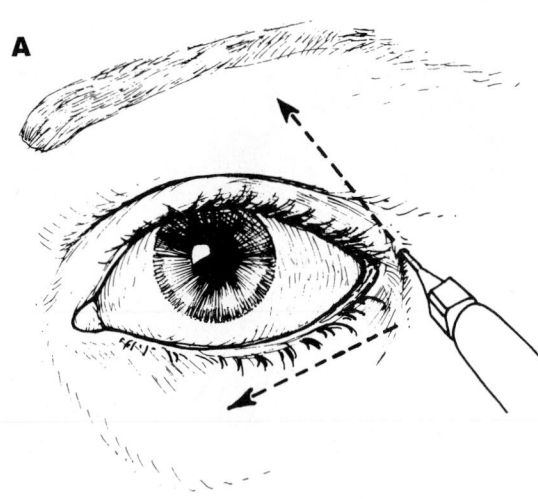

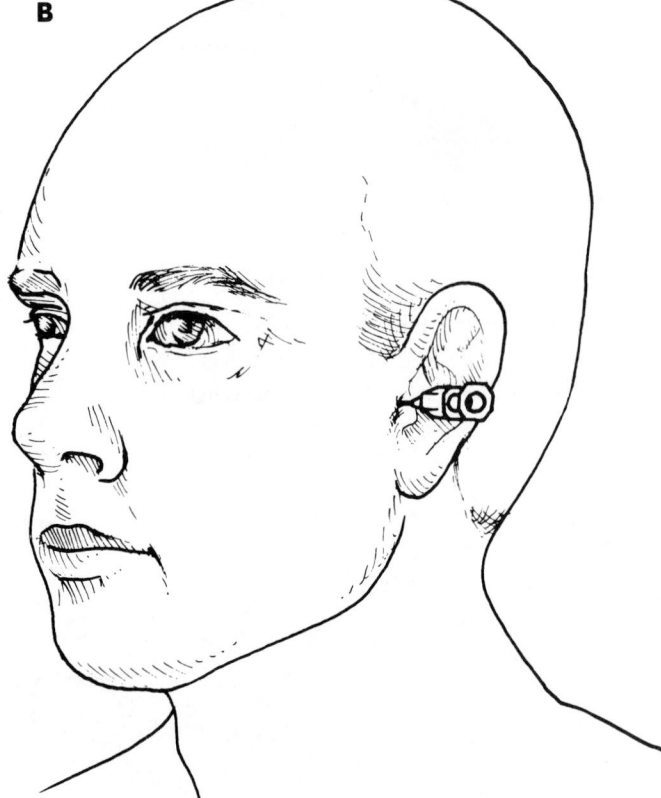

FIG. 17-16 **A,** Van Lint block. **B,** O'Brien akinesia blocking of facial nerve.

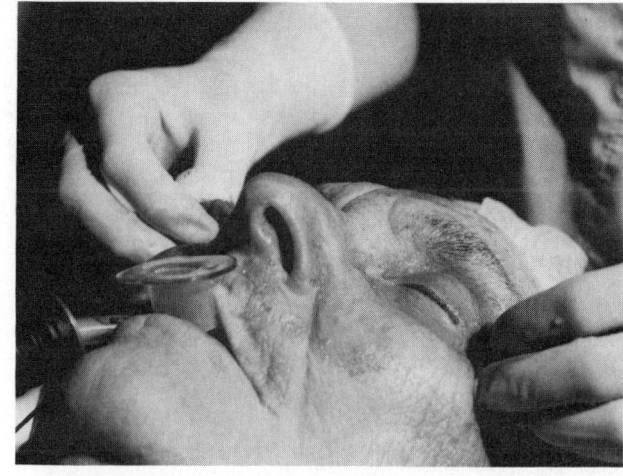

FIG. 17-17   Prepping procedure for eye surgery.

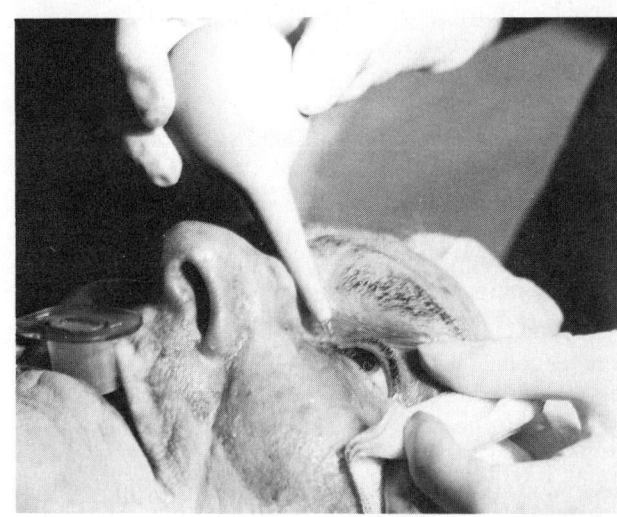

FIG. 17-18   Bulb syringe and normal saline solution are used to irrigate eye during prepping procedure. Direction of solution flow is always to outer, lateral side of face.

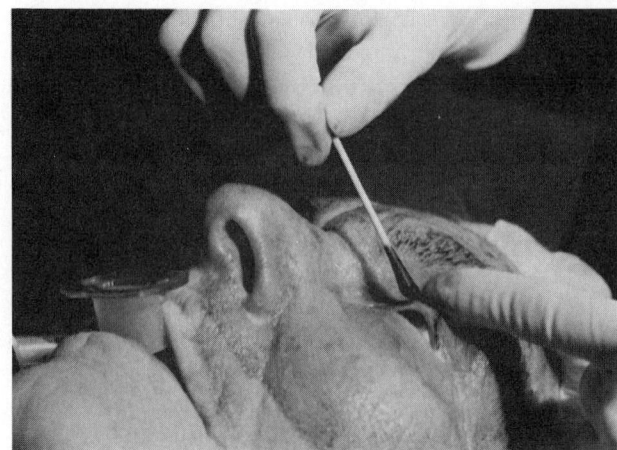

FIG. 17-19   Eyelid is everted when lid margins are cleaned.

RESEARCH HIGHLIGHT 17-2

Povidone-iodine solution has been shown to be
effective in removing surface microbes, but the effect
of irrigation on surface flora is unclear. Boes and
colleagues conducted a study to determine the
effectiveness of 5% povidone-iodine and saline
irrigation on reduction of perilimbal flora. Cultures
were grown from specimens taken from the perilimbal
conjunctiva in 100 eyes prior to preparation for
surgery. Cultures were again prepared after
instillation of povidone-iodine solution and after saline
irrigation. Bacteria were isolated in cultures from
75% of the eyes prior to preparation for ophthalmic
surgery. After povidone-iodine instillation, bacteria
were isolated from 28%, and after saline irrigation
from 24% of the eyes. Fifty-one of the culture-positive
eyes became negative after povidone-iodine instillation,
whereas only four culture-negative eyes became
culture positive. Twenty-three culture-positive eyes
became negative and 19 culture-negative eyes became
positive after saline irrigation. The researchers
concluded that 5% povidone-iodine was an effective
antimicrobial agent, whereas saline irrigation was not
significantly effective in removing perilimbal flora.

Boes, D., Lindquist, T., Frische, T., & Kalina, R.
(1992). Effects of povidone-iodine chemical preparation
and saline irrigation on the perilimbal flora.
Ophthalmology, 99 (10), 1569-1574.

eyelash scissors so the free lashes adhere to the blades rather
than fall into the eyes or onto the face.

Eye preparation includes cleansing the eyelids of the operative eye(s), lid margins, lashes, eyebrows, and surrounding skin with an appropriate antimicrobial solution (Fig. 17-
17). Care is taken to prevent the solution from entering the
patient's eyes and ears. The eyes are then irrigated with normal saline solution using an irrigating bulb (Fig. 17-18).
Some surgeons now use 5% povidone iodine (Research
Highlight 17-2). To clean the lid margins, evert the lids and
clean with cotton-tipped applicators moistened with antimicrobial skin disinfectant (Fig. 17-19). When toxic chemicals or small particles of foreign matter must be removed,
the eyes are irrigated with tepid sterile physiologic saline
solution. The conjunctival sac is thoroughly flushed, using
an irrigation bulb or an Asepto syringe.

Draping

The local anesthetic may be injected before completion
of the draping procedure. Aseptic principles for draping a
patient for an operation are discussed in Chapter 3. Special
concerns for eye surgery draping include eliminating lint
and fiber particles and providing adequate air exchange for
patients receiving local anesthetics. A method of draping
is shown in Fig. 17-20. This method eliminates the need to
lift the patient's head while draping and facilitates drape
removal at the end of the procedure.

Another method of draping is shown in Fig. 17-21. In
this method (1) the head is draped with a double thickness
half sheet and two towels; (2) a large folded sheet is used
to cover the patient and operating room bed; and (3) a fenestrated plastic eye sheet is placed over the operative site.

Instrumentation

Rapid progress in ophthalmic surgical techniques and instrumentation has contributed to almost unbelievable results
for eye patients. Exacting performance of eye instruments
is crucial to the success of operations.

Basic eye instruments are shown in Fig. 17-22. Ophthalmic forceps, called fixation forceps, are used to hold tissue
firmly in place or provide traction before incision. They
have an angled tooth that overlaps for secure fixation (Fig.
17-23). Several styles are available, and selection depends
on the surgeon's preference. Suturing forceps, used to pick
up wound edges for dissection or suturing, are single-
toothed forceps with the teeth at a right angle to the shank
of the forceps (Fig. 17-24). Suturing forceps are available
in many styles with varying sizes of teeth, such as a Castroviejo 0.12 mm or 0.5 mm. Utility or dressing forceps,
commonly called fine serrated forceps (Fig. 17-25), are
used for gentle handling of delicate tissue. There are fine
serrations on the straight shank. A variety of ophthalmic
forceps are designed for specific use with different tissues
of the eye. Some of those most commonly used are illustrated in Fig. 17-26.

Increased use of the microscope has brought changes in
the design of ophthalmic instruments. Many microsurgical
instruments were shortened to fit within a surgeon's hand
web-space because of preference and facility of movement.
Special surface finishes are used to reduce light reflection.
Instruments are designed with round handles for smoother
motion and rotation under the microscope.

Care and handling

To maintain the quality and precision of all ophthalmic
instruments, including microsurgical instruments, strict criteria for care and handling must be followed. Storage cases
protect instrument tips and cutting surfaces. The instruments should be inspected under magnification when purchased and before and after each use, observing for burrs
on tips, nicks on cutting surfaces, and alignment of jaws.
Eye instruments should be cleaned during use with nonfi-
brous sponges to avoid damaging delicate instrument tips.
Personnel handling instruments should know the name and
purpose of each instrument. Tissue can be damaged by the
use of an inappropriate instrument, and instruments can be
damaged by inappropriate use. After use, the instruments
should be cleaned and thoroughly dried before storage.

It is recommended that microsurgical instruments undergo ultrasonic cleaning with distilled water and an appropriate cleansing agent. They can be individually hand held

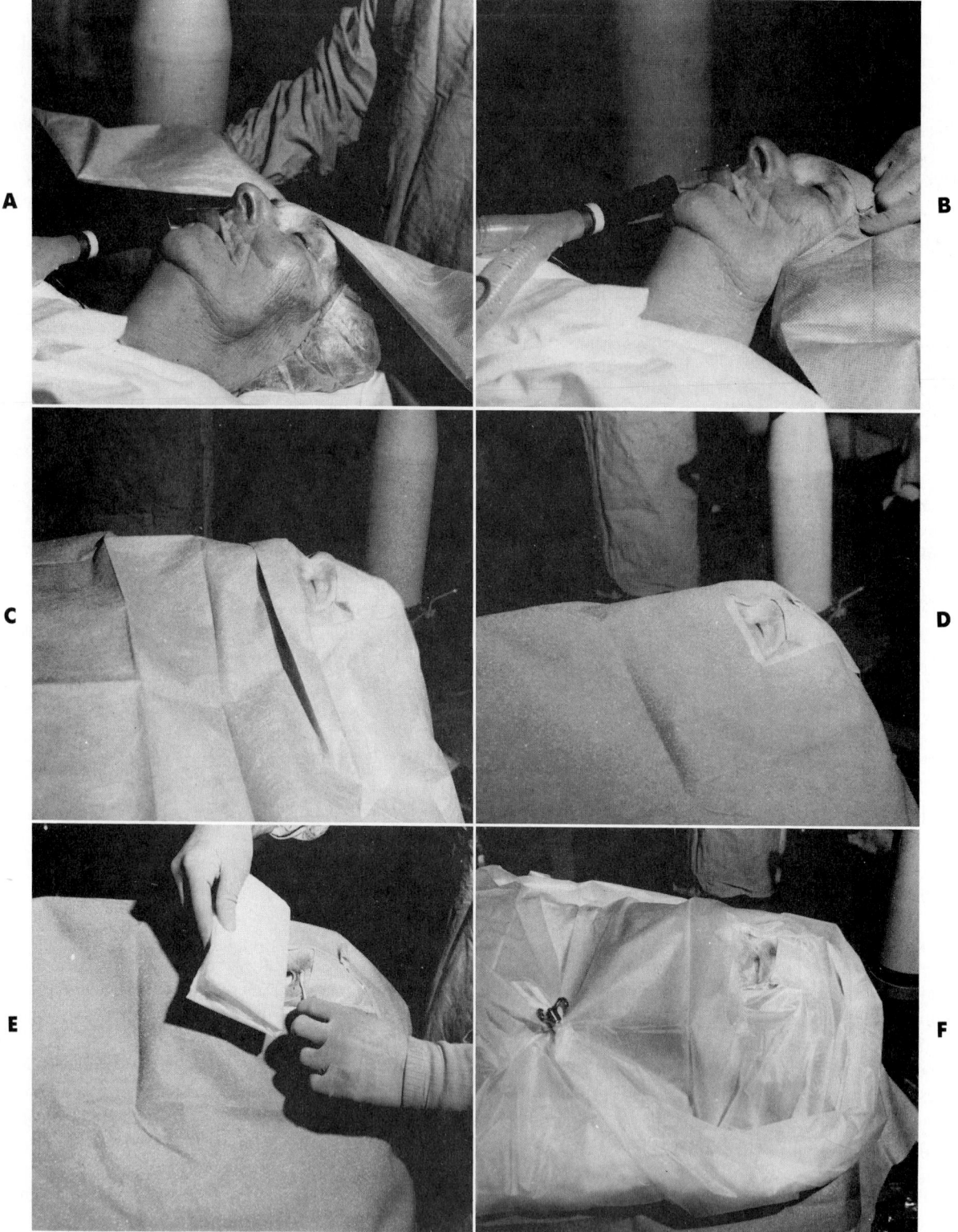

FIG. 17-20 Method of draping. **A,** With both hands under cuff of head drape, scrub nurse places adhesive strip above brow line. **B,** Adhesive strip is secured along side of patient's head anterior to ears. **C,** Adhesive towel drape is placed over patient's nose for general anesthesia. **D,** Split sheet is used to cover operating room bed and to isolate operative eye. **E,** Clear plastic adhesive drape is placed over operative eye. **F,** Drape is secured to collect irrigation fluid.

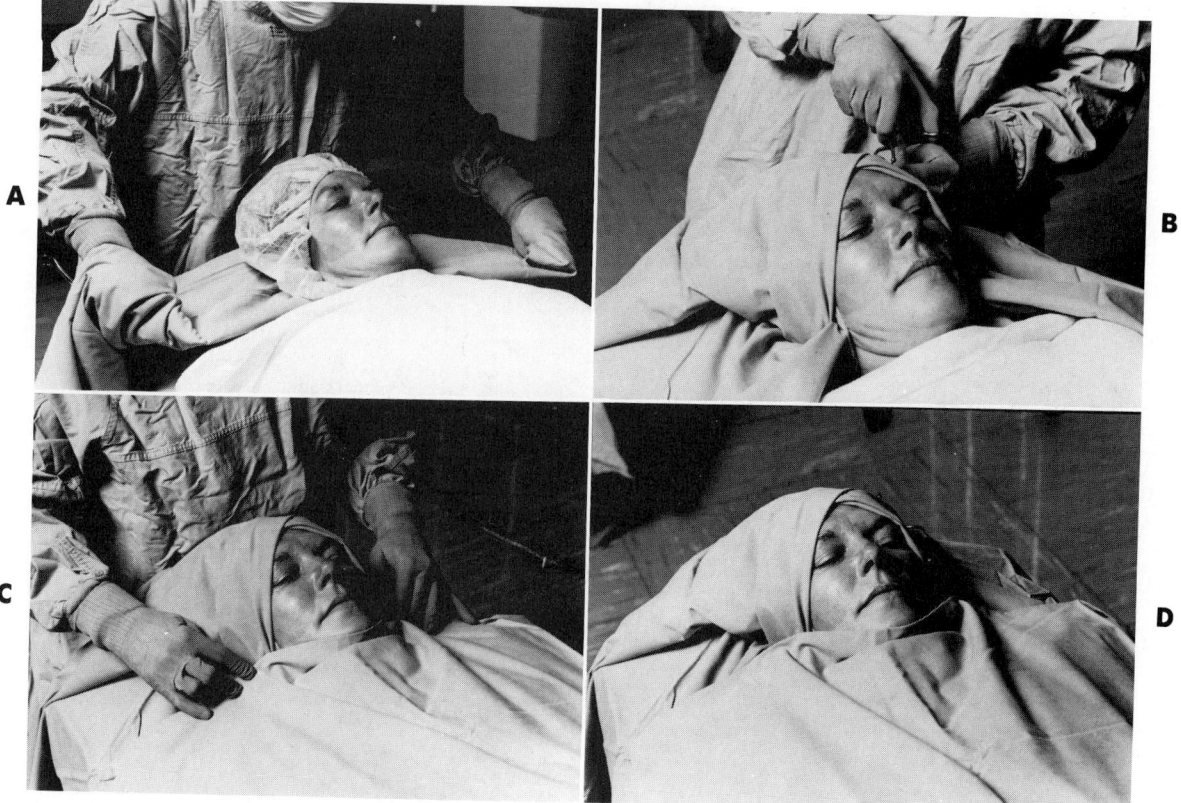

FIG. 17-21 Alternative method of draping eye surgery patient. **A,** Double-thickness half sheet and two towels are placed under head. **B,** Towel is secured around head covering ears and hair. **C,** Patient and operating room bed are covered with large folded sheet. **D,** Patient under local anesthetic is now ready for fenestrated plastic drape, completing procedure.

or immersed together in the ultrasonic cleaner as long as they are not touching each other. Instruments should be rinsed with distilled water and thoroughly dried. A hot air blower (never a towel) should be used for drying instruments. Instrument lubricant should not be used on irrigating cannulas because residue can be introduced into the eye and cause damage.

In addition to basic care and handling, a routine preventive maintenance program should be established for sharpening, realigning, and adjusting the precision eye instruments. Keeping an instrument in good repair is much less expensive than buying a new one.

Basic setup

Each ophthalmic operating room should have a sufficient number of basic, standard eye surgery setups, which can be supplemented to meet specific needs (Fig. 17-27). Instruments routinely needed for the type of operation and each surgeon's preferences should be kept on file.

Operating microscope

During the past 10 years there has been a dramatic increase in the number of microsurgical procedures in vari-

ous surgical disciplines. Although the operating microscope is employed in many types of surgical procedures, its major use is in ophthalmology. Because of the demand for use of the operating microscope and its special adaptations, perioperative nurses must understand the basic principles of operation and care of this important piece of surgical equipment.

Basic principles

To facilitate understanding of the functions of the operating microscope, a few basic optical principles are defined and explained. A microscope is a monocular or binocular instrument with a close-up lens for magnification. Binoculars are two telescopes mounted side by side that give stereoscopic vision. The length of the binoculars is condensed by the use of prisms.

Magnification is the process by which the apparent size of an image is increased. Magnification of an image is increased by moving the object closer to the eye or by using optical aids such as telescopes, binoculars, or microscopes that increase image size on the retina without reducing the eye-to-object distance. The amount of image increase becomes the magnification value of the optical aid.

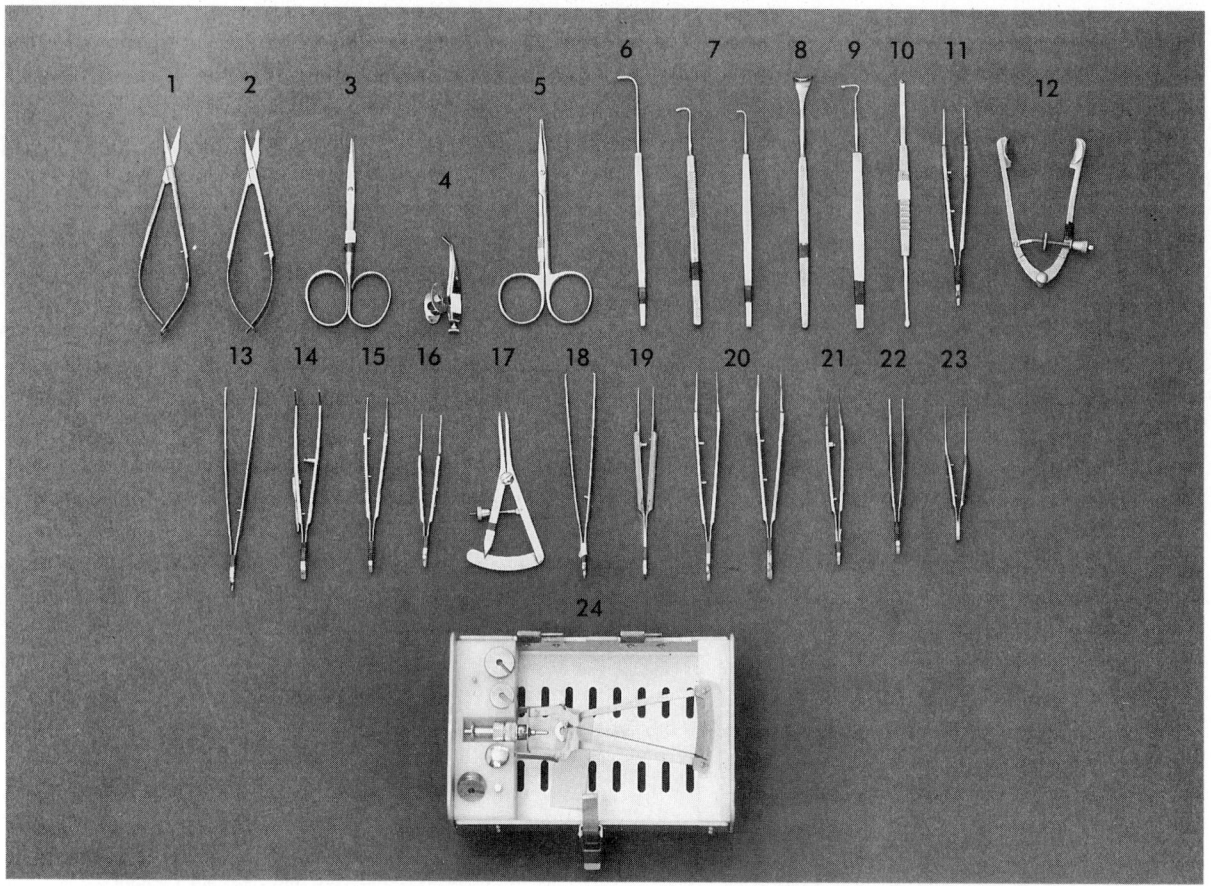

FIG. 17-22   *1*, Westcott scissors, sharp; *2*, Westcott scissors, blunt; *3*, iris scissors; *4*, Barraquer iris scissors; *5*, Stevens tenotomy scissors; *6*, Gass retinal detachment hook; *7*, muscle hooks; *8*, Demarres lid retractor; *9*, Green muscle hook; *10*, scleral depressor; *11*, Castroviejo suturing forceps; *12*, Lancaster eye speculum; *13*, fixation forceps; *14*, Jameson recession forceps; *15*, O'Brien tying forceps; *16*, Bishop-Harmon suturing forceps; *17*,Castroviejo caliper; *18*, O'Brien fixation forceps; *19*, Harper tying forceps, sraight; *20*, Castroviejo suturing forceps, 0.12 and 0.5 mm; *21*, angled McPherson suturing forceps; *22*, Bishop-Harmon suturing forceps; *23*, Colibri corneal forceps; *24*, Schiotz tonometer.

Illumination is the source of light used to view an object. The microscope illuminator is the light source used to throw light downward to illuminate the surgical area. The most common type of microscope illumination used today is coaxial illumination. Light from the illuminator bulb is routed near the viewing axis of the microscope and projected down through the objective lens (Fig. 17-28, *A*). Coaxial illumination can be transferred through a fiberoptic cable or from an incandescent bulb housed near the objective lens of the microscope. This type of shadow-free illumination provides a bright circular spot that is uniformly illuminated even in deep and narrow wounds. Fiberoptic illumination increases the diameter of the illuminated field and the light intensity.

Principal parts of the microscope are the eyepieces, binocular tubes, magnification changer, objective lens, illumination cord, beam splitter, and X-Y coupling (Fig. 17-28, *B*).

The eyepieces, or oculars, are the lenses through which a surgeon views the microsurgical field. Eyepieces are interchangeable and are available in four magnifying powers: 10×, 12.5×, 16×, and 20×. The working distance and the size of the surgical field determine the powers of the objective and the ocular lens, respectively. The objective lens is the lens attached to the bottom of the microscope, and the working distance is the distance between the objective lens and the operative field. For instance, in a procedure with long working distances and small surgical

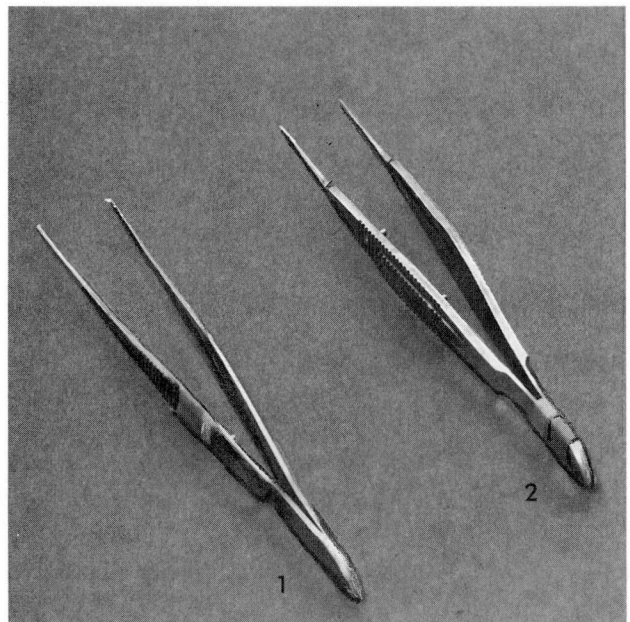

FIG. 17-23 Fixation forceps. *1,* O'Brien fixation forceps; *2,* Castroviejo fixation forceps, 0.3 mm.

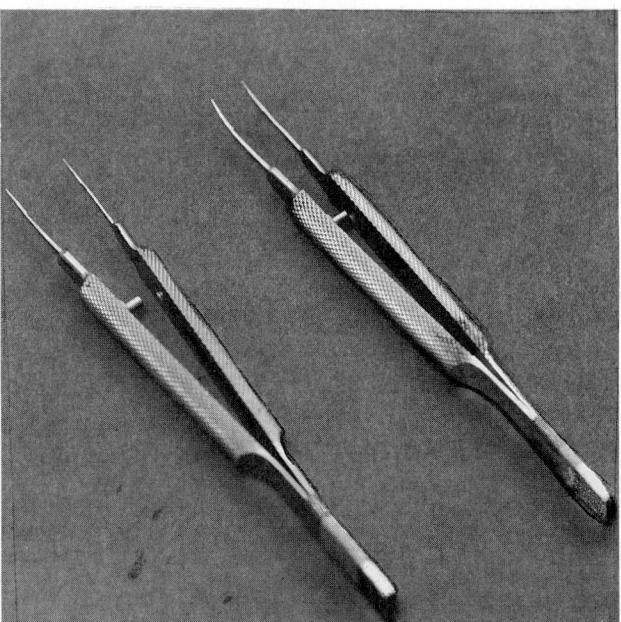

FIG. 17-24 Suturing forceps.

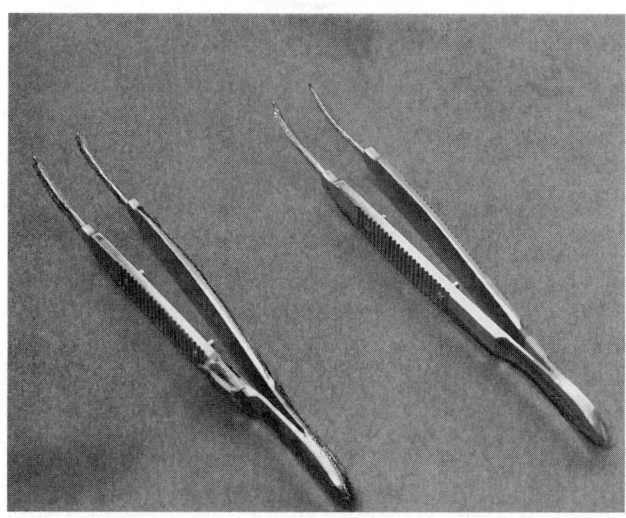

FIG. 17-25 Utility tying forceps, commonly called "fine serrated" forceps.

fields, a 20× ocular lens and a 300-mm objective lens might be used. This combination is commonly employed in neurosurgery. A procedure with shorter working distance and needing less magnification for a relatively large surgical field, such as an ophthalmic procedure, might require a 12.5× ocular lens and a 150- or 175-mm objective lens.

To focus the microscope, the user sets the spherical diopter adjustment on the oculars to correspond to his or her individual eyeglass correction and works without eye-glasses. The oculars can be adjusted to accommodate corrections of −9 to +9 diopters (D). Users who have astigmatism should wear their eyeglasses and set the oculars at zero.

The oculars fit into binocular tubes containing prisms that reduce the focal length of the microscope. The binocular tubes permit the distance between the oculars to be adjusted to fit the pupillary distance of the user (the distance between the pupils of the user's eyes), ensuring stereoscopic vision.

The magnification changer allows change in the magnification of a basic optical system. Two types of changers used on microscopes are the revolving telescope type, in which miniature telescopes of differing powers are rotated into position via knobs on the microscope body, and the zoom type, which is a motorized system of shifting lens elements to vary magnification, operated with a hand switch or foot control.

The magnification changer is a part of the microscope body, which is attached to a support that allows the instrument to be tilted. The lower end of the microscope body has a threaded mount for the objective lens. The diopter power of the objective lens determines the focal length and therefore the working distance of the microscope.

On the upper portion of the microscope body is a dovetail receptacle for attaching accessories. A beam splitter fits into the receptacle, permitting the attachment of binocular and monocular observation tubes and documentation accessories such as cameras and video equipment. A beam splitter has two-way mirrors or prisms that divert or split the

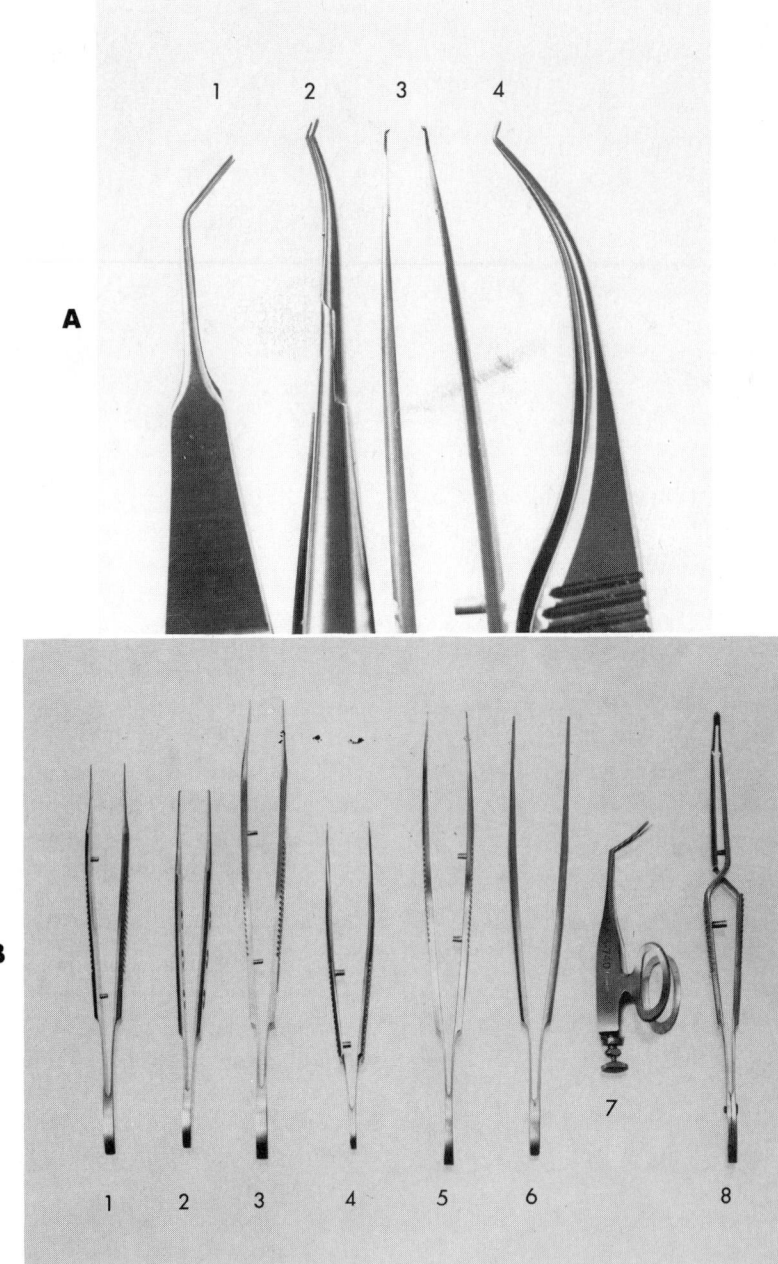

FIG. 17-26   Ophthalmic forceps. **A,** Tissue forceps modified for specific tissue. *1,* Kelman-McPherson angled tissue forceps with teeth; *2,* Corneoscleral forceps; *3,* Castroviejo corneal forceps; *4,* Colibri corneal forceps, 0.12 mm (may be used for iris). **B,** *1,* Castroviejo fixation forceps, 0.5 mm., *2,* Bishop-Harmon suturing forceps; *3,* Castroviejo suturing forceps, *4,* Colibri corneal forceps; *5,* Castroviejo-Colibri corneal forceps; *6,* Kelman-McPherson tying forceps; *7,* capsule forceps; *8,* Castroviejo cross action capsule forceps.

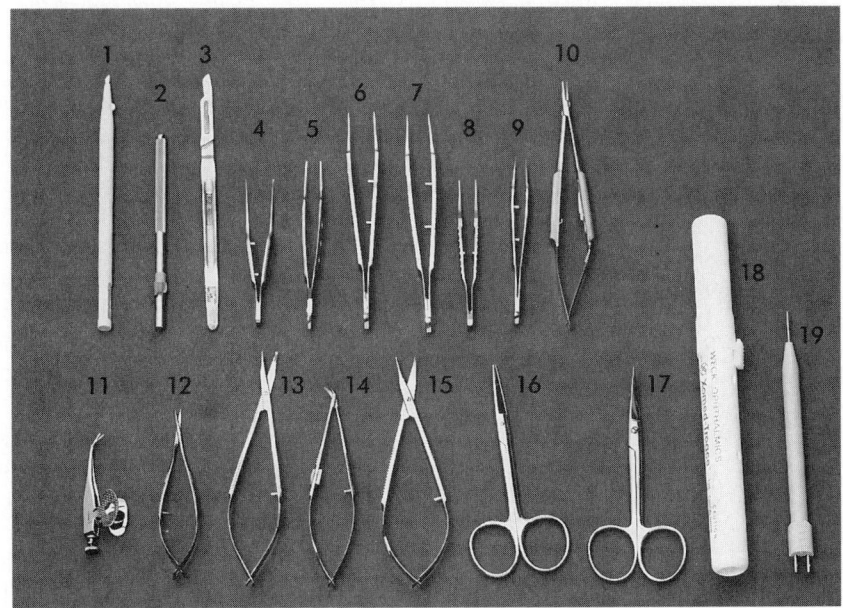

FIG. 17-27 Basic eye instrument setup. *1*, Super blade (disposable); *2*, Beaver knife handle; *3*, No. 9 Bard-Parker knife handle; *4*, Colibri corneal forceps; *5*, Bishop-Harmon suturing forceps; *6*, Castroviejo suturing forceps, 0.5 mm; *7*, Castroviejo suturing forceps, 0.12 mm; *8*, Castroviejo tying forceps; *9*, Kelman-McPherson suturing forceps; *10*, Harper needle holder *11*, Barraquer iris scissors; *12*, Vannas iridocapsulotomy scissors; *13*, Westcott tenotomy scissors; *14*, *Castroviejo corneal scissors; 15*, Westcott stich scissors; *16*, Knapp strabismus scissors; *17*, iris scissors; *18*, eye cautery, disposable; *19*, bipolar eraser tip eye cautery, disposable.

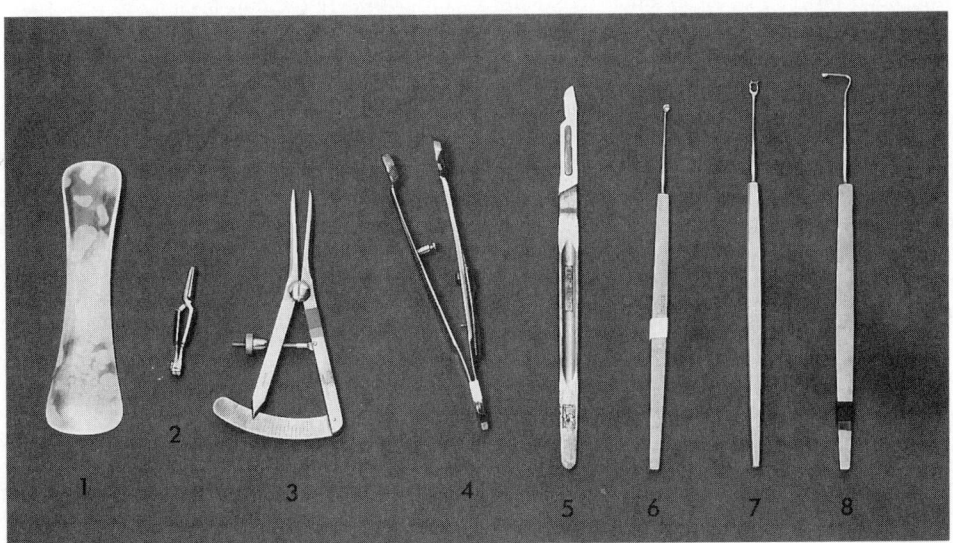

FIG. 17-28 Instruments for surgery of the eyelids and conjunctiva. *1*, Jaeger lid plate; *2*, serrefine; *3*, caliper; *4*, Green chalazion clamp; *5*, No. 9 Bard-Parker knife handle with no. 15 blade; *6*, chalazion curette; *7*, retractor; *8*, muscle hook.

optical image in several directions. This allows for attachment of binocular observation tubes, necessary for surgical assistants, and cameras or video equipment. With use of a beam splitter at least 50% of available light is diverted away from the surgeon's oculars. However, the human eye is usually versatile enough to adjust to lower light levels. Adequate lighting is essential for photographic systems, which may in some instances require a beam splitter that diverts as much as 70% of the available light. The X-Y coupling enables the operator to move the microscope head diagonally and accurately over the operative field. The choice of microscope accessories varies according to requirements of the procedure and the surgeon's preferences.

Many methods of mounting the operating microscope are used, including manually operated floor stands, motorized floor stands, and ceiling- or wall-mounted suspension systems with either manual or electromechanical height adjustment.

Care and maintenance

Proper care and maintenance of the operating microscope are essential to ensure optimal function and durability of this sophisticated, expensive piece of equipment. Procedures include (1) inspection and cleaning of all external lens surfaces before use; (2) checking all power controls including illumination intensity, magnification changer, focus, and X-Y coupling to ensure proper functioning before use; (3) checking the needed accessories such as objective lens and power, beam splitter, cameras, observer tubes, and filters; and (4) cleaning and covering after use.

Care of optics

Before and after each procedure, all external lens surfaces should be cleaned and inspected. Internal surfaces are checked for cleanliness and damage. Scratched or damaged optical systems must be repaired or replaced.

The following procedure is used for cleaning lens surfaces:

1. Loose particles (lint or dust) are removed with a soft, clean camera lens brush or with a rubber bulb syringe. When a bulb syringe is used, the bulb is held about 1 cm from the surface and squeezed briskly, directing the air toward the lens surface.
2. Blood, water, and irrigating solutions are removed with a cotton-tipped applicator or cotton ball moistened with distilled water. A circular motion is used, beginning at the center of the optic and working toward the outer edge (lens paper may also be used). The surface is dried with a cotton-tipped applicator or cotton ball in the same manner.
3. Oil or fingerprints are removed with a cleaning solvent of commercially prepared lens cleaning solution or with 50% denatured alcohol. The lens is wiped with a lightly moistened cotton-tipped applicator or cotton ball in a circular motion. The process is re-

peated until the surface is clean and free from streaks.

Solvents should be used sparingly. Excessive fluid may destroy the cemented surfaces of the lens.

Cleaning

The external surfaces of the microscope should be cleansed after use and before storage. The cleaning procedures are as follows:

1. The external surfaces are washed with a clean, damp cloth moistened with a mild soap or disinfecting solution.
2. The surfaces are wiped dry with a lint-free cloth.
3. The function of each moving part is inspected during the cleaning process. The coupling joints can be greased with petrolatum jelly if necessary. The lamp cables should be free from kinks. A new bulb should be used for each procedure expected to be over 4 hours in duration. Fiberoptic cables should not be bent or kinked. Tips of the fiberoptic cables are cleaned with cotton-tipped applicators.
4. The carriage is moved to its lowest position. The locks on the arm are loosened, and the ocular systems are moved toward the base.
5. Dust caps are placed over the eyepieces and a dust cover over the microscope head. The microscope is ready for storage.

Proper care and preventive maintenance add years of service to an operating microscope. Checking the microscope before use and being knowledgeable about proper function of the microscope and its accessories are responsibilities of the perioperative nurse.

Ophthalmic sutures

Sutures used in ophthalmic surgery are very fine, and range in size from 4-0 to 10-0. Fine eye sutures produce minimum reaction and discomfort for the patient. They should be handled as little as possible to avoid weakening and fraying. Surgical gut and collagen suture, which is packaged in solution, should be rinsed before use to prevent introducing irritants into the eye. Ophthalmic needles are also very delicate and must be handled with extreme care. Before use, needles must be inspected for evidence of burrs.

Ophthalmic dressings

At the completion of the operation the operative eye area is cleansed with saline sponges. Antibiotic ointment may be thinly spread over the skin and eyelashes to prevent adhesion of the bandage. This is frequently done after plastic procedures on the lids or lacrimal ducts. Dressings are applied to prevent palpebral movements, protect the operative wound from dust and external contaminants, and absorb any blood and tears produced.

The initial dressing, usually an eye pad, is commercially

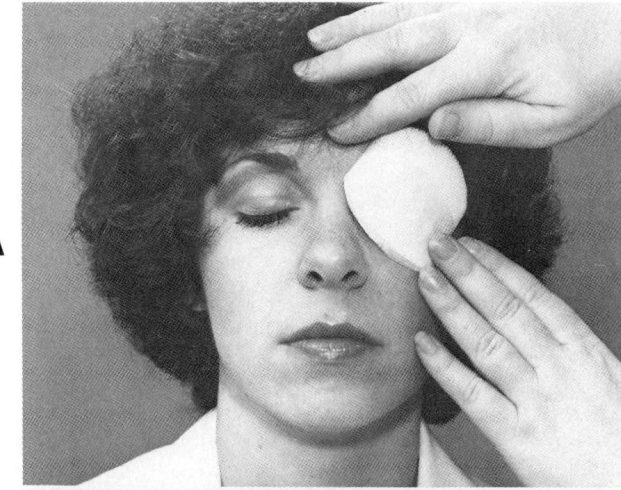

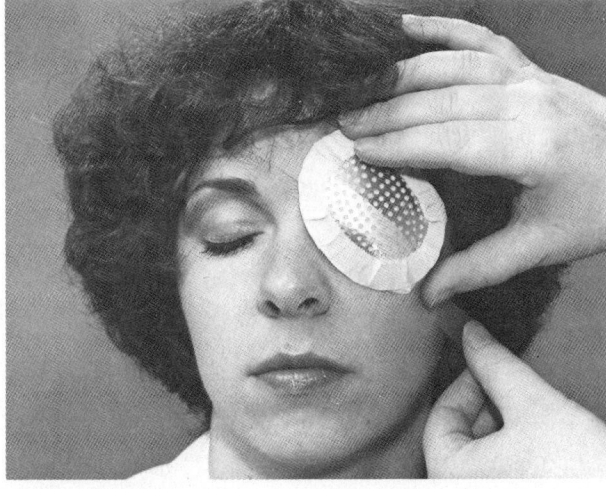

FIG. 17-29 **A,** Eye dressing is held in place by plastic, paper, or cellophane strips. Lids are gently closed before patch is applied. **B,** Protection of wound is provided by application of metal shield over dressing.

prepared and sterilized. The eye dressing is held in place with plastic, paper, or cellophane strips (Fig. 17-29, *A*). After intraocular operations, when external pressure on the eyes might be harmful, the initial dressing is covered with a protector such as a perforated aluminum plate, convex flexible celluloid plate, or another variety of shield (Fig. 17-29, *B*).

A pressure bandage may be used when a compression affect is desired. A gauze roller bandage is applied over the initial dressing, encircling the head.

EVALUATION

Before the patient is transported to the PACU or observation unit, his or her general condition is evaluated. The general appearance of the skin is assessed, with areas around the face and bony prominences noted for redness and other changes from the preoperative condition.

If the procedure was lengthy and osmotics were given, the patient may be catheterized while still anesthetized. A report to the receiving nurse in the PACU or observation area should include postoperative positioning requirements, potential problems specific to the patient, and preoperative anxiety level and utilization of coping mechanisms. Most patients have one or both eyes patched, and the sensory deficit should be noted. Documentation of all postoperative observations is important.

Evaluation should address whether the patient met the desired perioperative nursing outcomes; the patient's responses may be documented as outcome statements. The following examples are based on the nursing diagnoses identified in the care plan on p. 583.

- The patient and/or significant other verbalized knowledge regarding the diagnosis, planned intervention, and requirements for home care maintenance.
- The patient safely coped with visual sensory and perceptual alterations.
- The patient verbalized concerns and fears and utilized coping mechanisms.
- The patient identified activities that may increase intraocular pressure.
- The patient will remain free from signs and symptoms of postoperative infection.

SURGICAL INTERVENTIONS

SURGERY OF THE EYELIDS

The procedures most commonly performed on the eyelids are for treatment of chalazion, entropion, ectropion, excisional biopsy, and repair of traumatic injuries.

Removal of chalazion

Removal of a chalazion is the incision and curettage of a chronic granulomatous inflammation of one or more of the meibomian glands in the tarsal plate of the eyelid.

Procedural considerations

The patient is prepared as described for general ophthalmic surgery. This procedure is most commonly done with local anesthesia.

Operative procedure

1. The affected lid is everted with a chalazion clamp (Fig. 17-30) to expose the chalazion.
2. A cruciate incision is made on the inner lid surface, using a sharp knife; corners of the tarsal plate are resected (see Fig. 17-30).
3. The contents of the chalazion are removed with a chalazion curette. The eye is dressed and patched.

Canthotomy

Canthotomy is lengthening the opening (slit) between the eyelids before cataract surgery when exposure of the globe is inadequate or when correction of ankyloblepharon or blepharochalasis is necessary.

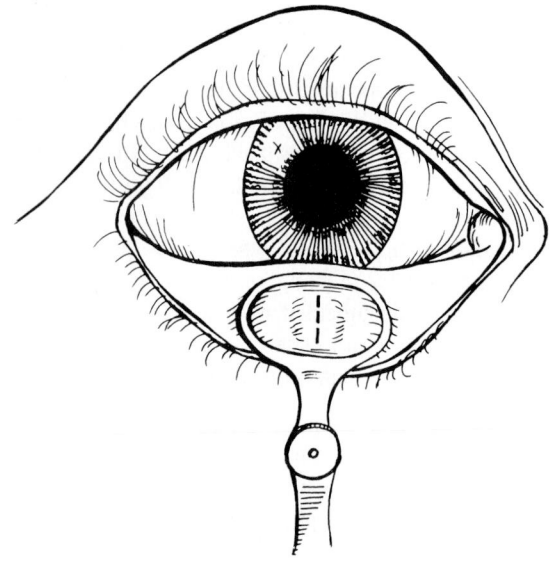

FIG. 17-30   Clamp everts eyelid during surgery for chalazion. Incision has been made on inner lid surface to avoid scarring. Viscous contents of chalazion will be removed with curette.

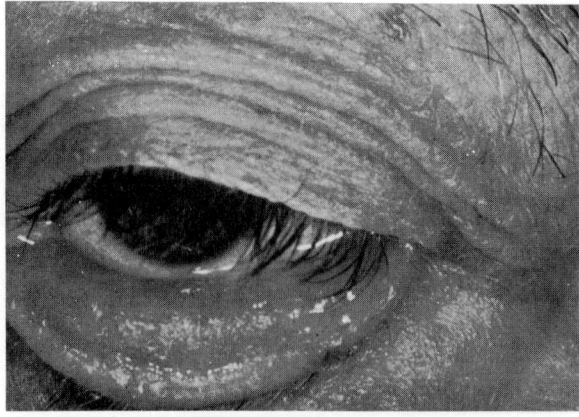

FIG. 17-31   Ectropion, or turning out of lid, is most commonly caused by senile relaxation of eyelid framework.
From Saunders, W.H., et al. (1979). *Nursing care in eye, ear, nose, and throat disorders*, (4th ed.). St. Louis: Mosby.

Procedural considerations

The patient is prepared as described for general ophthalmic surgery. This procedure is most commonly done with local anesthesia.

Operative procedure

1. A hemostat is clamped over the full thickness of the outer canthus and left in place for 60 seconds.
2. The skin and conjunctiva are incised. For canthoplasty, the adjacent bulbar conjunctiva is dissected, and its borders and those of the skin are sutured together with fine silk sutures.
3. The affected eye is dressed and patched.

Surgery for positional defects of the eyelids

Several techniques are available to treat faulty position of the eyelids. Plastic surgery is effective in the treatment of entropion, ectropion (Fig. 17-31), and blepharochalasis of the eyelids.

Plastic repair of entropion

Plastic repair of entropion is surgical correction of muscular fibers of the lid, everting the lid margins and eyelashes. Entropion (turning inward of the lid) usually affects the lower lid but may affect the upper lid. It seldom occurs in persons under 40 years of age. The two types are spastic and cicatricial. Spastic entropion results from degeneration of facial attachments between the pretarsal muscle and the tarsus, which permits the pretarsal muscle to override the lid margin during contraction. Cicatricial entropion is a complication of either the upper or lower tarsus and its conjunctiva, turning in the lashes (trichiasis) so they rub on the cornea.

Procedural considerations. A local or general anesthetic may be used, and usually a pressure dressing is required.

Operative procedure. Entropion treatment involves either removing a base-down triangle of skin, muscle, and tarsus and suturing the edges together to evert the lid margin, or exposing the orbicular muscle, dividing it, and suturing it to the lower border of the tarsus.

Plastic repair of ectropion

Plastic repair of ectropion is an operation to shorten the lower lid in a horizontal direction. Ectropion (sagging and eversion of the lower lid), usually bilateral, is common in older persons. Ectropion may be caused by the relaxation of the orbicular muscle. Symptoms are tearing, conjunctival infection, and irritation. Minor ectropion may be treated by electrosurgical penetrations through the conjunctiva. Surgery is indicated when facial paralysis is permanent or when scarring follows lacerations, lesions, or penetrating injuries and the cornea becomes exposed, resulting in ulceration and photophobia.

Operative procedure. Correction of cicatricial ectropion is accomplished either by mobilization of the surrounding skin or by free grafting. Many procedures have been devised, such as the Wharton Jones V-Y procedure, free whole skin graft, and epidermis graft. The operation includes removal of scar tissue and approximation of layers, small sliding grafts from the immediate area by means of Z-plasty or V-Y incision if loss is minimal, and free graft from the upper lid for the lower lid by means of tarsorrhaphy.

The Kuhnt-Szymanowski procedure is performed to treat senile or complete atonic ectropion. The external two thirds or the entire lid is split, the tarsoconjunctival triangle is resected, and the wound is closed by means of sutures in such a manner that a new canthus is produced (Fig. 17-32).

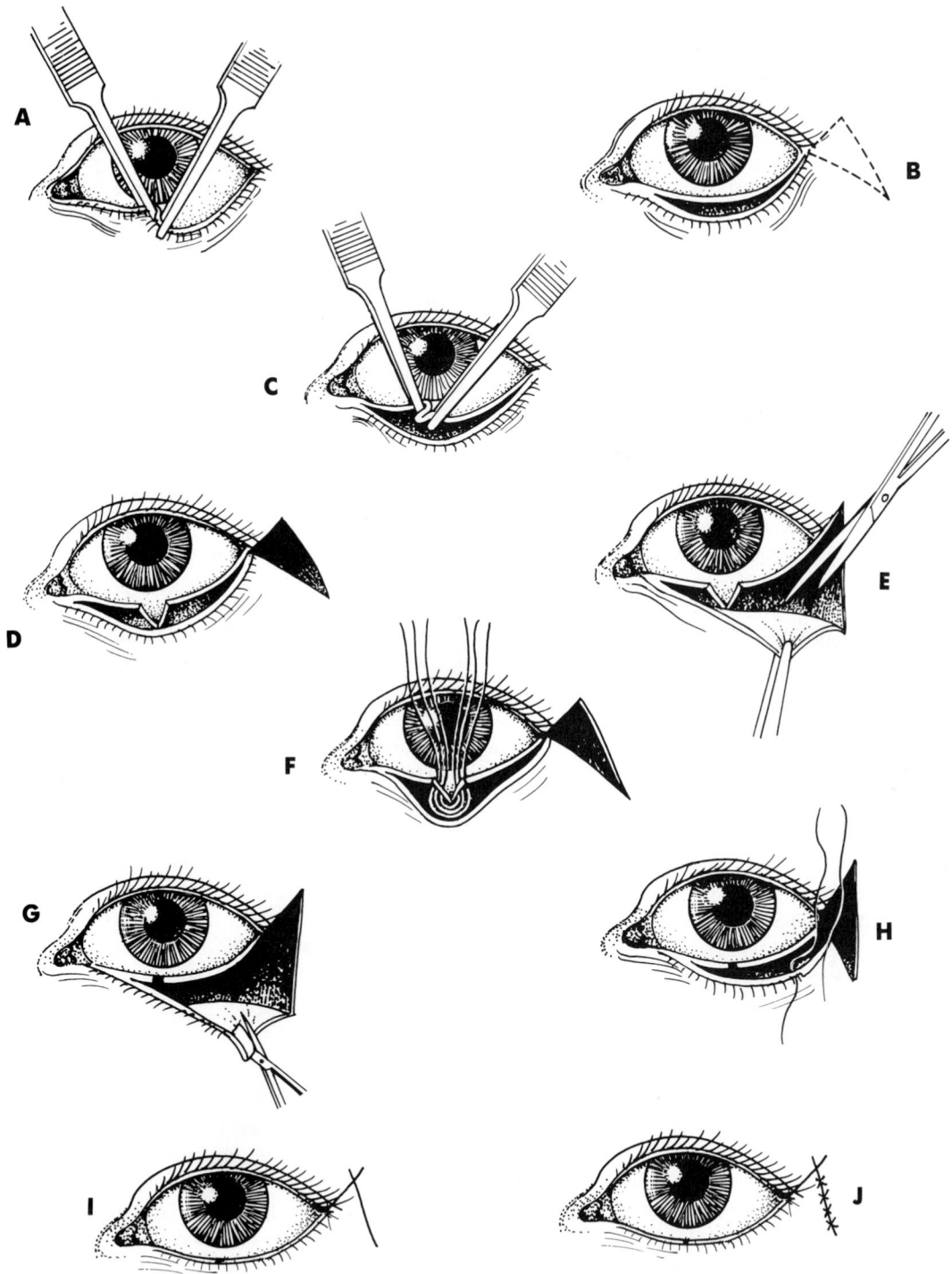

FIG. 17-32 Kuhnt-Szymanowski operation for atonic ectropion. **A,** Lower lid picked up with two smooth forceps, and amount of lengthening needed gauged. **B,** Lateral skin triangle marked, and lid split. **C,** Lateral triangle resected, and amount of tarsoconjunctiva to be excised gauged. **D,** Tarsoconjunctival triangle receded. **E,** Skin-muscle lamina dissected free. **F,** Tarsal wound closed. **G,** Excess cilia resected. **H,** Sutures placed to form a new canthus. **I,** Sutures tied. **J,** Final closure done.

Plastic repair for blepharochalasis

Plastic repair for blepharochalasis is removal of redundant skin of the upper eyelids. Blepharochalasis causes the upper lids to hang down over the eyes, sometimes obscuring vision. It may occur in older persons who have lost normal elasticity of the skin of the upper lids or in persons who have suffered from persistent angioneurotic edema with stretching of the skin of the eyelids.

Operative procedure. An elliptic segment of skin of the upper lid is removed by a plastic surgical technique.

Surgery for unilateral or bilateral ptosis

Drooping of the upper lid may be congenital, acquired, or senile. In congenital ptosis there usually is weakness of the superior rectus muscle. Acquired ptosis is generally caused by laceration of the third cranial nerve, the levator muscle, or both. Tumors may cause ptosis. Senile ptosis is the result of poor muscle tone of the levator.

The objective of ptosis surgery is to achieve a perfect cosmetic result by creating a good upper lid fold with elevation of the lid. The many surgical procedures that have been devised are based on advancement of the levator muscle, the frontalis muscles, or the superior rectus muscle. These muscles are the elevating forces of the upper lids. Some of the techniques involve resection of the levator (Iliff method), use of the superior rectus muscle (Berke method), or modification of other methods such as the Motais, Crawford frontalis collagen sling procedure, and Silver-Hildreth method.

Iliff method (resection of the levator)

The Iliff method is creation of an effective upper lid by shortening the levator muscle and reapproximating the conjunctiva and muscles to reestablish the correct relationship of the involved structures. General anesthesia is preferred.

Operative procedure. The procedure is as follows:

1. The upper lid is everted over the lid clamp. With sharp-pointed scissors, two buttonhole incisions are made through the conjunctiva, medial and lateral to the superior edge of the tarsus.
2. Blunt scissors are directed through the buttonhole incisions and spread open to enlarge the incisional opening. As the scissors are withdrawn, the angular, rubber-shod, jawed ptosis clamps are positioned to contain the conjunctiva, superior edge of the tarsus, superior arcuate artery, aponeurosis of the levator, and orbital septum.
3. Another incision is made with scissors distal to the clamp and through all structures held by the clamp.
4. The orbital septum is freed from the clamp. Structures between the orbital septum and the levator are dissected by means of blunt instruments.
5. Traction is applied to the clamp. Double-armed absorbable no. 4-0 sutures are inserted from the cut tarsal edge through all structures held by the clamp. The tissues distal to the suture line are excised.

6. The free end of each of the double-armed, sutures is passed through the orbital septum, between the skin and tarsus, and brought out through the skin at cilia margin.
7. Sutures are tied over a silicone strip or small beads. Redundant skin is invaginated with a peg to form a good lid fold.
8. The eye is closed by fastening a single suture that is passed through the skin of the lower lid to the forehead by means of an adhesive strip. Bland eye ointment is applied, and eye pads are secured by means of nonallergenic adhesive tape.

Silver-Hildreth Supramid suspension

The Silver-Hildreth method is attachment of the lid to the frontalis muscle by Supramid sutures anchored in the periosteum. This procedure may be done in the total absence of levator and superior rectus action.

Operative procedure. The procedure is as follows:

1. An incision is made in the lid fold, exposing the tarsus. An incision is made over the eyebrow centrally to the frontalis muscle.
2. A double-armed 4-0 Supramid suture is woven through the tarsus.
3. The needles are removed from the suture, and the suture is threaded on a Wright fascia needle.
4. The fascia needle is passed under the skin of the lid through the periosteum of the orbital rim and out through the brow incision. This is repeated so both ends of the suture are in the brow incision.
5. The suture is tied as it lies on the frontalis muscle.
6. The skin is closed with a nonabsorbable, subcuticular, continuous no. 6-0 suture.
7. The conjunctival sac is filled with antibiotic ointment. A double-armed, nonabsorbable (often silk) no. 4-0 suture is passed through the center of the lower lid margin and fastened to the brow with adhesive tape, thus covering the exposed cornea. A pressure dressing is applied.

Excisional biopsy

Excisional biopsy is removal of lesions, either neoplastic (benign or malignant) or viral in nature, for diagnostic examination. Basal cell carcinomas account for 95% of neoplastic lesions of the lid; the treatment of choice is excisional biopsy. Viral lesions such as papilloma and molluscum contagiosum are also treated in this way.

Operative procedure

Through-and-through excision of skin, muscle, tarsus, and conjunctiva is followed by careful structural closure of anatomic spaces.

Surgery for traumatic injuries

Lacerations of the lids, including damage to the inferior canaliculus, are repaired surgically.

Operative procedure

Paramount for success is the careful approximation of the borders of the lid margin and the ends of a torn canaliculus.

Lacerations of the lid margin are closed with a nonabsorbable (often silk) no. 5-0 suture to align the gray line of the lid that lies between the lash follicles and the orifices of the meibomian glands. Once this anatomic line has been approximated, all other sutures are placed, maintaining the approximation.

If the canaliculus has been lacerated, a pigtail probe is passed through the uninvolved punctum, through the sac, and carefully through the proximal and distal ends of the lacerated structure to emerge from the involved punctum. A Supramid no. 4-0 suture is hooked onto the probe and, by reversing the previous procedure, is pulled out of the uninvolved punctum, thus establishing continuity of the system. Accurate plastic closure of the lid defect is then carried out.

Blepharopigmentation and eyebrow enhancement

In a microsurgical procedure neutral pigments are permanently implanted intradermally between the eyelashes (blepharopigmentation) or in the eyebrows (eyebrow enhancement) to improve their appearance. This is a cosmetic procedure performed in an ambulatory surgery facility or physician's office. It was developed as an enhancement for scant eyebrows or in some cases replacement for eyeliner, particularly for individuals with allergies to cosmetics, contact lens wearers, visually impaired persons, and patients with limited dexterity.

Procedural considerations

Patients may need ice packs or sedation before infiltration of local anesthetic to reduce discomfort. The eyelids and brows are prepared as described for eye surgery, ensuring that the lid margins and lashes are cleaned thoroughly. A thin film of clear antibiotic ointment is placed on the lids to prevent staining of the superficial layers of the eyelid skin. Postoperatively, cold compresses or ice packs are applied to reduce edema and ecchymosis.

Operative procedure (Fig. 17-33)

1. A slow regional injection with a 1½-inch, 27- to 30-gauge needle is used to introduce the local anesthetic.
2. Sterile pigment is injected within the dermis of the lid at a depth no less than 0.5 mm and no greater than 1.5 mm, using a disposable electric needle.
3. At the completion of the procedure, the skin is cleansed with saline to remove superficial pigment. Antibiotic ointment is placed in each eye.

SURGERY OF THE CONJUNCTIVA

The conjunctiva of the eye is a transparent and elastic membrane that lines the inner surface of the eyelids and covers the sclera. Traumatic lacerations caused by injury as well as deficits resulting from excision of tumors, cysts, nevi, or pterygiums can usually be repaired by simple undermining and suturing.

Pterygium excision

A pterygium is a fleshy, triangular encroachment onto the cornea. Pterygiums tend to be bilateral. When a pterygium encroaches on the visual axis, it is removed surgically.

Operative procedure

The major steps in the McReynolds technique are illustrated in Fig. 17-34. A pterygium can also be excised totally and the limbus treated with an eye cautery or electrocoagulation. The conjunctiva can then be closed, or the sclera can be left bare.

Excisional biopsy

Any suspect lesion of the conjunctiva can be removed by simple elliptic excision and sent for pathologic examination. The conjunctiva may or may not be closed, depending on the surgeon's particular technique.

Reformation of the cul-de-sac (mucous membrane graft)

Reformation of the cul-de-sac involves the application of a mucous membrane graft to the conjunctiva to correct motility or exposure problems.

Various conditions and injuries, such as infections, trachoma, and chemical burns, can cause severe scarring and contractures of the conjunctiva and the underlying tissues, which may lead to problems with motility or exposure. Simple dissection is usually unsatisfactory. The patient generally requires extra mucous membrane, which may be obtained from excess conjunctiva from the opposite eye, if available, or as a mucous membrane graft from the oral cavity.

Operative procedure

1. A local anesthetic solution is injected into the mucous membrane of the lower lid or the lateral wall of the mouth with a separate set of instruments.
2. An elliptic incision is made with a no. 15 knife blade. (If the incision is made into the lateral wall, the opening of the parotid duct must be avoided.)
3. A thin, full-thickness layer of the mucous membrane is removed by sharp dissection. A second method is the use of an electric Castroviejo dermatome. The mucous membrane is then obtained from the lower lip.
4. The wound is approximated with nonabsorbable (often silk) no. 4-0 suture.
5. The mucous membrane graft is placed in a Neosporin solution, the surgeon regowns and regloves, and another set of sterile instruments is used for reconstruction of the cul-de-sac.

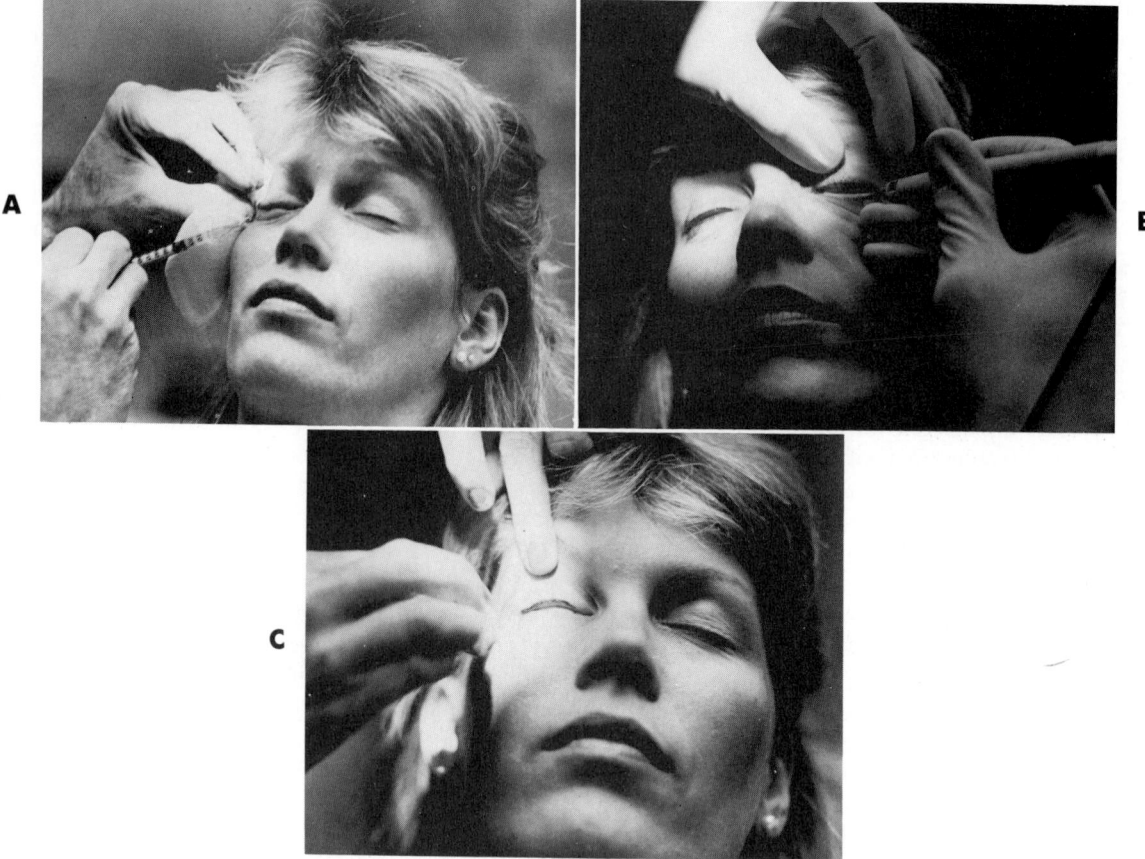

FIG. 17-33 Blepharopigmentation. **A,** Infiltration of local anesthetic into eyelids. **B,** Injection of pigment with electric needle in dermis of eyelid along eyelash margins. **C,** Completion of blepharopigmentation to upper eyelash margin.

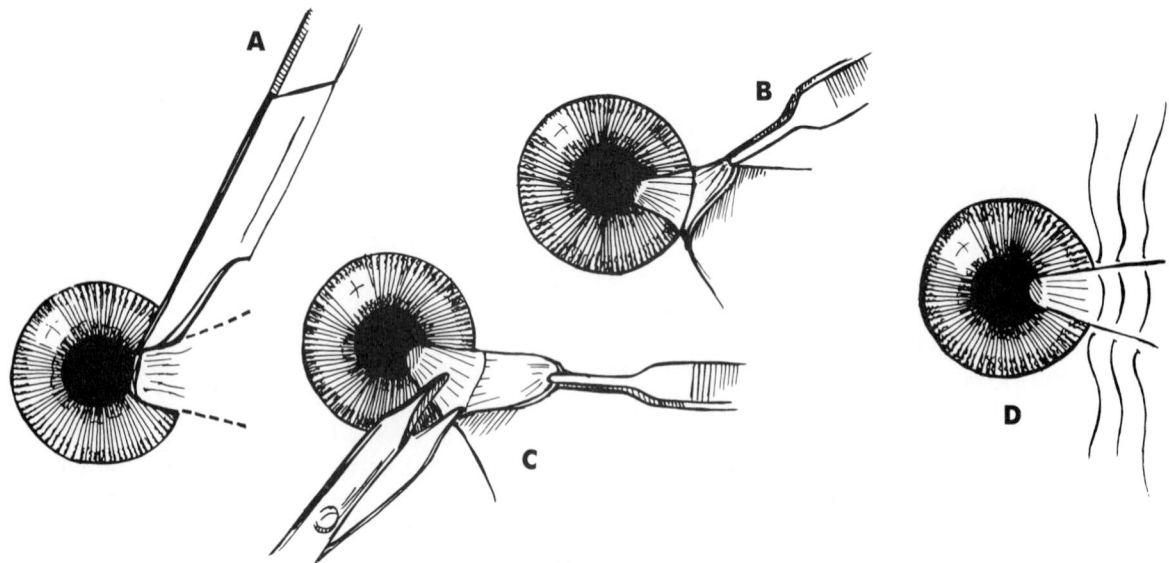

FIG. 17-34 McReynolds technique for pterygium repair. **A,** Cornea around head of pterygium is incised. **B,** Pterygium flap is dissected upward, leaving clear cornea. **C,** Lower margin of pterygium is dissected, and whole pterygium is freed from sclera. **D,** Sutures are placed for closure of conjunctiva.

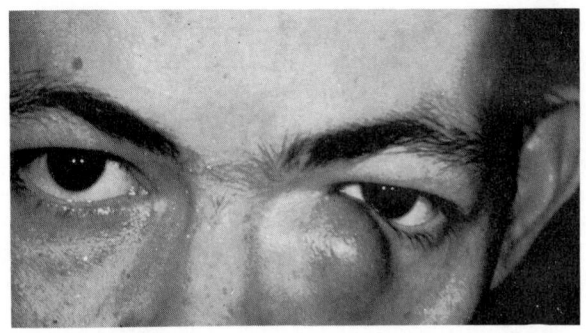

FIG. 17-35 Chronic infection of lacrimal sac (dacryocystitis) causes swelling of inner lower corner of eye socket.

From Saunders, W.H., et al. (1979). *Nursing care in eye, ear, nose, and throat disorders*, (4th ed.). St. Louis: Mosby.

SURGERY OF THE LACRIMAL GLAND AND APPARATUS

Surgery of the lacrimal gland and apparatus is usually performed for treatment or diagnosis of tumors of the lacrimal fossa or to correct deficient drainage with overflow of tears. Chronic dacryocystitis in adults (Fig. 17-35) requires dacryocystorhinostomy because of resistant obstruction of the nasolacrimal duct. Dacryocystorhinostomy is also performed when the lower canaliculus is patent but the tear duct is blocked, causing epiphora (abnormal overflow of tears) that the patient cannot tolerate. This deformity frequently follows a malunited fracture of the medial wall of the orbit. Dacryocystorhinostomy creates a new, large opening between the lacrimal sac and the nose. Instrumentation for surgery of the lacrimal system is shown in Fig. 17-36.

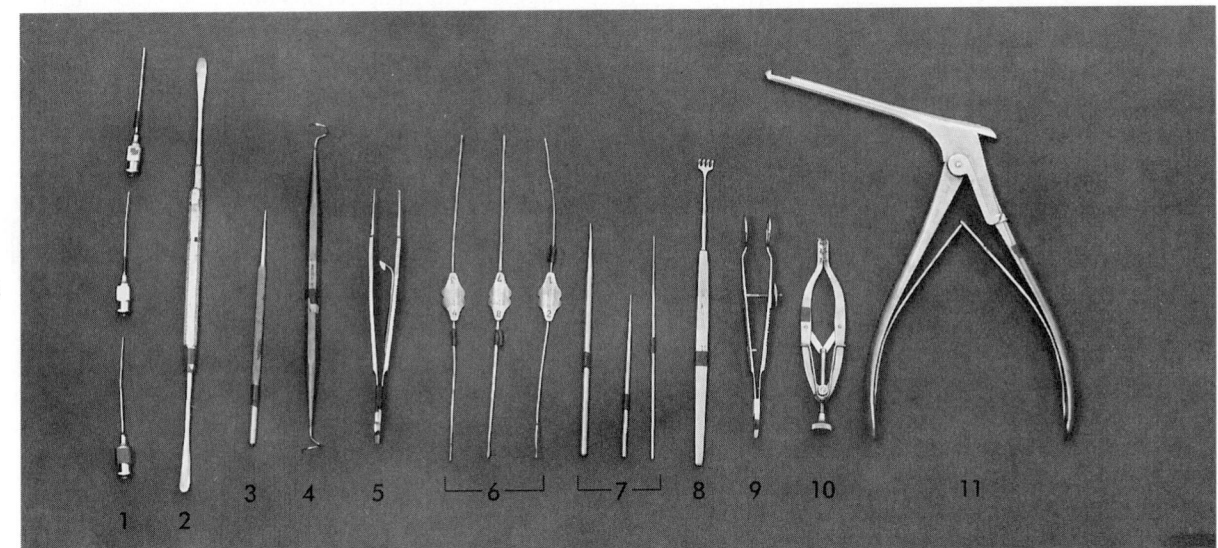

A

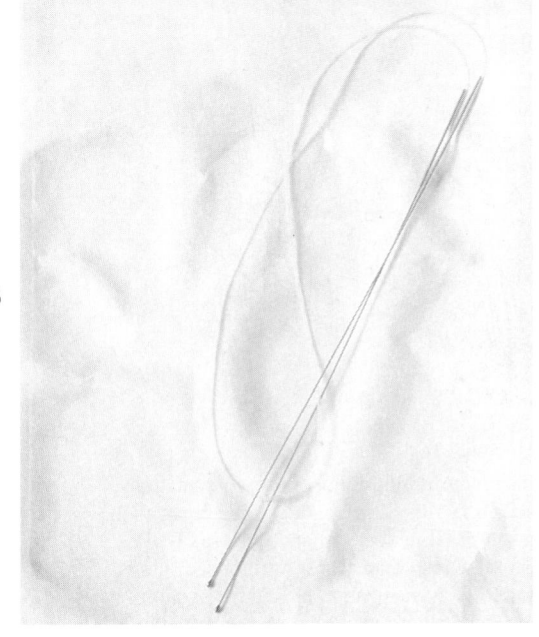

B

FIG. 17-36 **A,** Instruments for surgery of the lacrimal system. *1,* lacrimal cannulas; *2,* Freer elevator; *3,* Muldoon dilator; *4,* Worst pigtail probe; *5,* Castroviejo suturing forceps; *6,* Bowman lacrimal probes; *7,* Nettleship-Wilder lacrimal dilators; *8,* lacrimal sac retractor; *9,* Erhardt lid clamp; *10, lacrimal sac retractor; 11,* small Kerrison rongeur. **B,** Quickert canaliculus probe.

Surgery of the lacrimal fossa

Surgery of the lacrimal fossa is performed for biopsy of any structure in the lacrimal fossa and possible removal of the lacrimal gland (extirpation) to eliminate excessive tearing.

Operative procedure

1. The lacrimal fossa, which is in the upper temporal quadrant of the orbit, may be approached directly through the lid or through the conjunctiva by everting the upper lid. The lacrimal gland is divided into a palpebral and an orbital part by the orbital septum. All drainage ducts go through the palpebral portion; surgery on this part alone affects tearing because, although the orbital part is intact, no access to the eye is available.
2. Routine surgical closure procedures are followed.

Probing

The opening of the lacrimal drainage system posterior and inferior to the inferior nasal conchae is closed in approximately 35% of newborns. In most cases this closure opens spontaneously within the first 2 or 3 months of life. When the lacrimal drainage system does not open spontaneously, an acute infectious process involving the lacrimal drainage system becomes obvious. The infectious process is treated with antibiotics, followed by probing. In a child under 6 months of age, the probing procedure may be done with mummification, using topical anesthesia. After this age the procedure is done with general anesthesia.

Operative procedure

1. Manipulation is done through the upper punctum and canaliculus to prevent trauma to the inferior part of the system, which carries 90% to 95% of the total secretions.
2. The upper punctum is dilated first with a sterile safety pin and then with a punctum dilator. A lacrimal probe is then passed through the upper punctum and canaliculus into the sac, where resistance is met from the lacrimal bone. The probe is rotated 90 degrees, passed through the bony canal, and forced through the imperforate opening into the nose. A small amount of blood may be regurgitated at this time. The procedure may be repeated with a larger probe.
3. With a blunt lacrimal needle, a fluorescein solution is irrigated through the punctum to ensure the patency of the system.

Dacryocystorhinostomy

Dacryocystorhinostomy is the establishment of a new tear passageway for drainage directly into the nasal cavity.

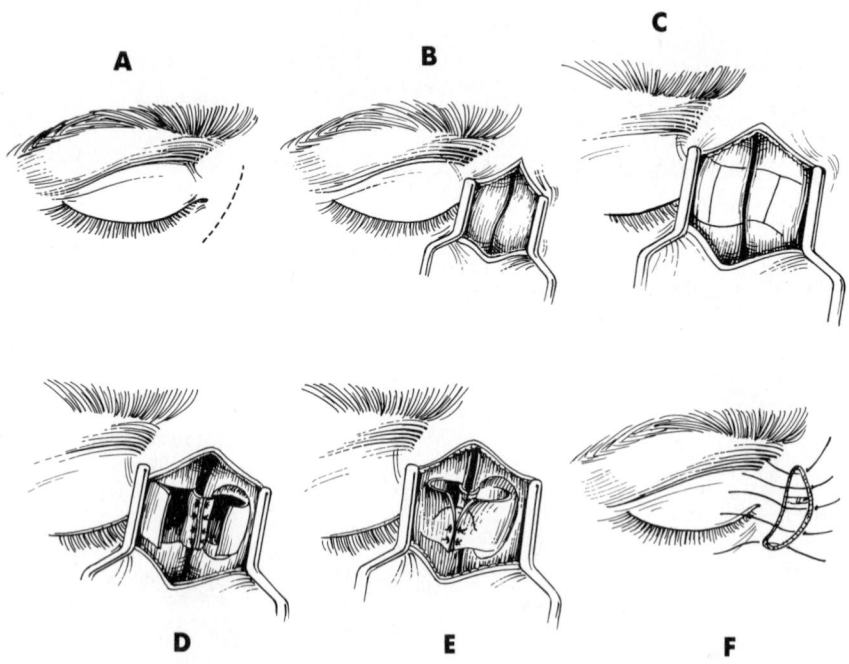

FIG. 17-37 Dacryocystorhinostomy. **A,** Skin incision for dacryocystorhinostomy or dacryocystectomy. **B,** Lacrimal sac and lacrimal bone exposed. **C,** Opening made in lacrimal bone and lacrimal crest, with *dotted lines* indicating incision to be made in wall of sac and in nasal periosteum and mucosa. **D,** Posterior flap of wall of sac sutured to posterior flap of nasal mucosa. **E,** Anterior flap of wall of sac sutured to anterior flap of nasal mucosa. (Drawing is somewhat distorted for visualization of relative positions.) **F,** Reattachment of medial canthal ligament, and wire sutures in position for closure of skin incision.

Procedural considerations

The nasal cavity is anesthetized topically with cocaine just before surgery, and a general anesthetic is administered in the operating room. The patient is prepared as described for eye surgery.

Operative procedure (Fig. 17-37)

1. An incision is made on the nasal side of the orbital rim. With blunt-pointed, curved, or flat scissors, a knife, retractors, and forceps, dissection is carried down to the periosteum, which is separated from the bone with elevators.
2. Through the lower canaliculus the sac is probed, identified, and displaced laterally.
3. The anterior lacrimal crest is perforated with a power saw, dental drill, or mallet and chisel. The hole is enlarged with rongeurs. During this time the cornea is protected by a metal retractor or plastic contact lens.
4. Irregular fragments of bone and fibrous tissue are removed, and hemostasis is obtained with bone wax if necessary.
5. The lacrimal sac and nasal mucosa are incised with H incisions with the long line vertical.
6. The mucous membrane of the nose is sutured to that of the lacrimal sac with no. 4-0 absorbable sutures. A probe is passed through the nostril into the base of the wound to test the opening from the sac into the nose. A

French catheter may be passed from the nose and sutured into the roof of the sac with no. 4-0 absorbable sutures. It remains in place until the sutures absorb, thereby acting as a stent about which epithelial union between the lacrimal and nasal mucosa can occur.

7. The interior flap of mucous membrane from the nose and sac is sutured with interrupted, absorbable no. 4-0 sutures. Skin margins are approximated and closed with nonabsorbable no. 6-0 sutures. Interpalpebral sutures are placed to maintain position of the eyelids under the dressing. Antibiotic ointment is usually applied, and eye pads and hypoallergenic transparent tape are used to dress the wound. A 4 × 4 gauze sponge may be taped under the nostrils.

SURGERY FOR STRABISMUS

Strabismus (squint) is the inability to direct the two eyes at the same object because of lack of coordination of the extraocular muscles. Corrective surgery is performed to change the relative strength of individual muscles and therefore improve coordination (Fig. 17-38). The deviation of the eye may be inward, outward, upward, or downward. The amount of deviation is a measurement of the angle formed by the visual axis of the two eyes. The lateral rectus muscle abducts the eye, the medial rectus muscle adducts it, and the other ocular muscles have both primary and secondary functions in elevation, depression, intorsion, and extorsion, according to the position of the eye.

Two basic surgical approaches are used to correct strabismus: strengthening is usually accomplished by a resection procedure, and weakening is usually done with a recession procedure. Operating on three or more muscles, in two stages, may be necessary. To some extent the type of strabismus influences the type of surgery. Instrumentation for strabismus surgery is illustrated in Fig. 17-39.

Resection

Resection is removal of a portion of muscle and attachment of cut ends (see Fig. 17-38).

Procedural considerations

Suture material varies according to the surgeon's preference, but usually the suture is on a spatula needle. The patient is prepared as described previously for eye surgery; local or general anesthesia is used. Perioperative nurses should be aware that tension or traction on ocular muscles can precipitate bradycardia.

Operative procedure

1. A speculum is inserted, and the conjunctiva is incised at one border of the muscle to be resected.
2. The muscle insertion is hooked with a muscle hook, and the conjunctiva over the insertion is opened.
3. Double-armed sutures are passed through the muscle belly at the desired position of shortening, and the muscle is incised anterior to this suture.

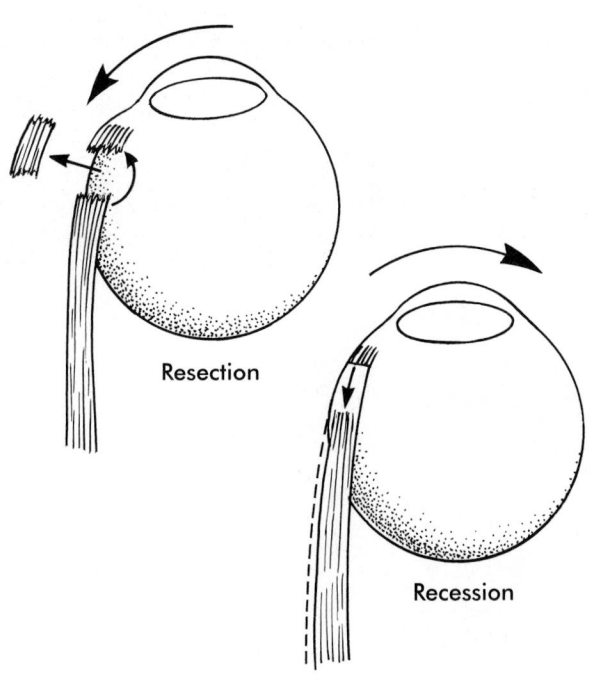

Resection

Recession

FIG. 17-38 In surgery for strabismus, *resection* of part of ocular muscle tendon rotates eye toward operated muscle, whereas *recession* moves muscle tendon backward on eye, permitting eye to rotate away from operated muscle.

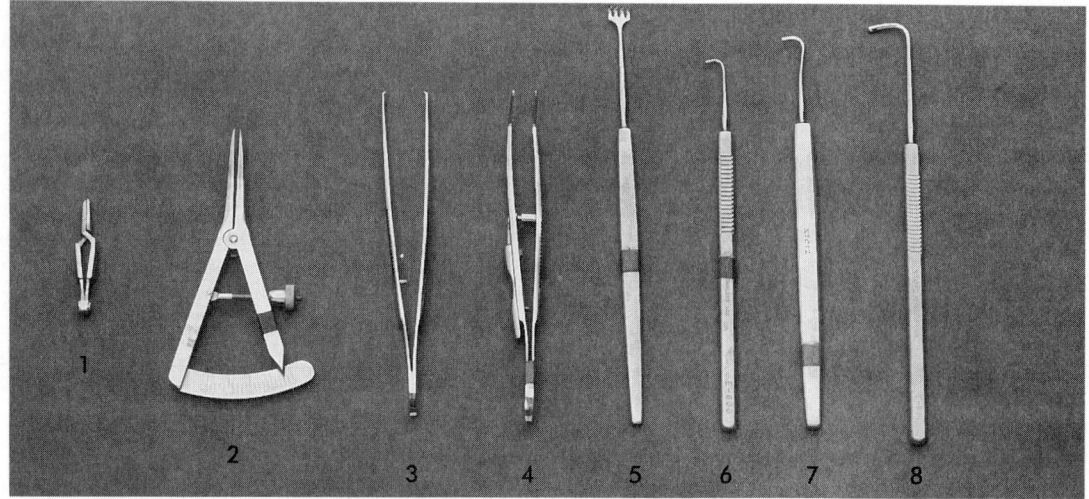

FIG. 17-39   Instruments for surgery of eye muscles. *1,* Serrefine; *2,* Castroviejo caliper; *3,* O'Brien fixation forceps; *4,* Jameson recession forceps; *5,* lacrimal sac retractor; *6 to 8,* von Graefe strabismus hooks, small, medium, and large.

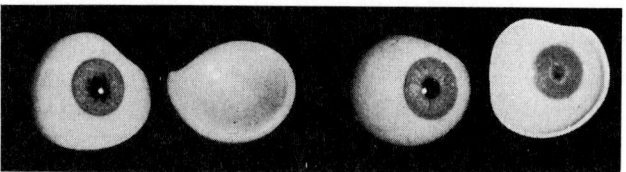

FIG. 17-40   Artificial eyes. Shell prosthesis is seen at right.

From Allen, J.H. (Ed.). (1963). *May's manual of the diseases of the eye* (23rd ed.). Baltimore: Williams & Wilkins.

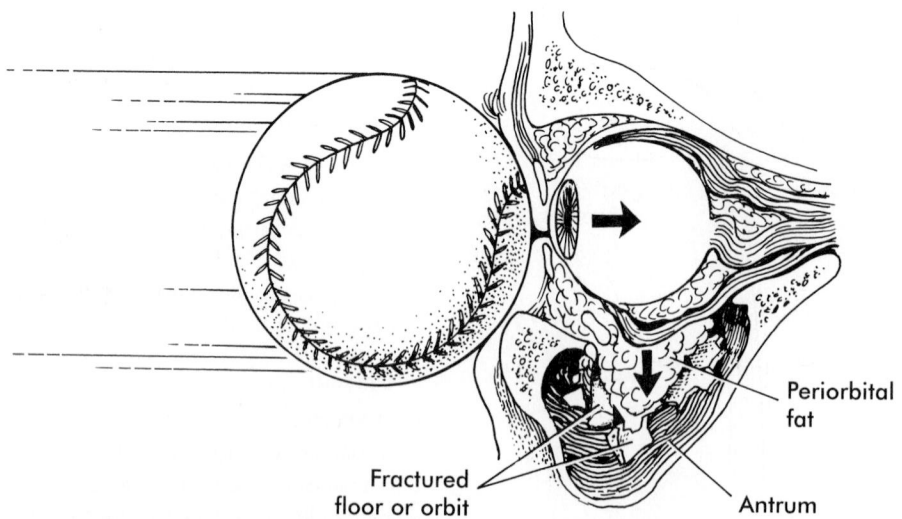

FIG. 17-41   Ball has struck rim of orbit and has pressed orbital contents backward, displacing fragments of bone into maxillary sinus. Inferior rectus muscle is incarcerated in fracture. Inferior oblique muscle may also be involved.

4. The stump of the muscle is excised from the insertion, and the muscle is then sutured to the insertion using the double-armed suture.
5. The conjunctiva is closed with an absorbable suture.

Recession

Recession is severance of the muscle from its original insertion with reattachment more posteriorly on the sclera (see Fig. 17-38).

Operative procedure

1. The insertion of the muscle is exposed as described previously.
2. Sutures are passed through the muscle tendon at its insertion into the globe, and the tendon is severed distal to the suture.
3. With calipers, marks are made on the globe at the desired distance behind the insertion, and the muscle is anchored to the globe at that point.
4. The conjunctiva is closed with absorbable suture.

Myectomy

Myectomy is a method of weakening the action of a muscle. This may be done as a lengthening procedure such as a Z marginal tenotomy or myectomy or an intersheath tenotomy of the superior oblique tendon, or it may be a complete severance of a muscle, such as an inferior oblique myectomy procedure.

Operative procedure

1. The involved muscle is isolated.
2. Cuts from opposite sides of the muscle are made through approximately three fourths of the width of the muscle, effectively lengthening the muscle.
3a. In the case of the superior oblique muscle, the tendon sheath is opened and graded sections of tendon are excised, according to the needs of the patient.
3b. Myectomy of the inferior oblique muscle is done in a graded manner by placing two Kelly hemostats across the muscle belly lateral to the inferior rectus muscle and excising the isolated strip muscle. The ends of the muscle are cauterized and released. Because of the peculiar anatomy of this muscle, lateral discontinuity weakens but does not paralyze it.

Tuck

A tuck is a method of shortening a muscle and thus strengthening it. Tucking is performed primarily on the superior oblique muscle.

Operative procedure

1. An incision is made in the conjunctiva, medial to the superior rectus muscle.
2. The Fink-Scobie hook is passed posteriorly into the orbit, and the superior oblique muscle is hooked and brought into the incision.

3. The Fink tucker is placed over the tendon, and a graded doubling of the tendon, like looping a rope, is completed.
4. A double-armed Supramid suture is passed through the base of the loop, effectively shortening the muscle.
5. The tip of the loop is sutured to the sclera. (Surgeons commonly attempt to tuck the muscle lateral to the superior rectus muscle.)
6. The conjunctiva is closed with absorbable sutures.

SURGERY OF THE GLOBE AND ORBIT

Rupture of the eyeball may be direct at the site of injury or, more frequently, indirect from an increase in intraocular pressure that causes the wall of the eyeball to tear at weaker points such as the limbus. When the intraocular contents have become so deranged that useful function is prohibited or the blind eye becomes painful, removal of the eye contents (evisceration procedure) or of the entire eyeball (enucleation) is indicated. If either procedure is required, an inert globe may be implanted as a space filler and to aid in the movement of a prosthesis (artificial eye) (Fig. 17-40).

Fractures of the walls of the orbit (Fig. 17-41) may be caused by direct blows or by extension of a fracture line from adjacent bones (Figs. 17-41 and 17-42). Isolated orbital floor, or blowout, fractures usually follow injury to the region of the eye by an object the size of an apple or an adult's fist. Orbital contents herniate into the maxillary sinus, and the inferior rectus or inferior oblique muscle may become incarcerated at the fracture site. A Caldwell-Luc

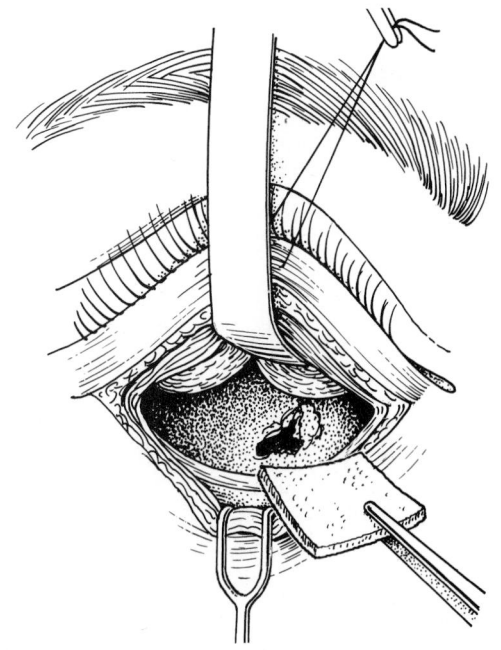

FIG. 17-42 *Cross-hatched area* shows blowout fracture site. Autogenous graft from iliac crest is held by forceps ready to be placed over fractured site. Graft usually does not require suturing.

antrostomy (see Chapter 19) may be done with reduction of the fracture from below, or the fracture site may be approached directly through the lower lid along the orbital floor and the prolapsed tissue reduced, the orbital floor reduced, and the orbital floor defect bridged with a graft of bone, cartilage, or plastic material. Instrumentation for surgery of the globe and orbit is illustrated in Fig. 17-43.

Repair of lacerations

The preferred method of closing corneal lacerations is with direct appositional suturing viewed through an operating microscope. No. 10-0 suture is generally used.

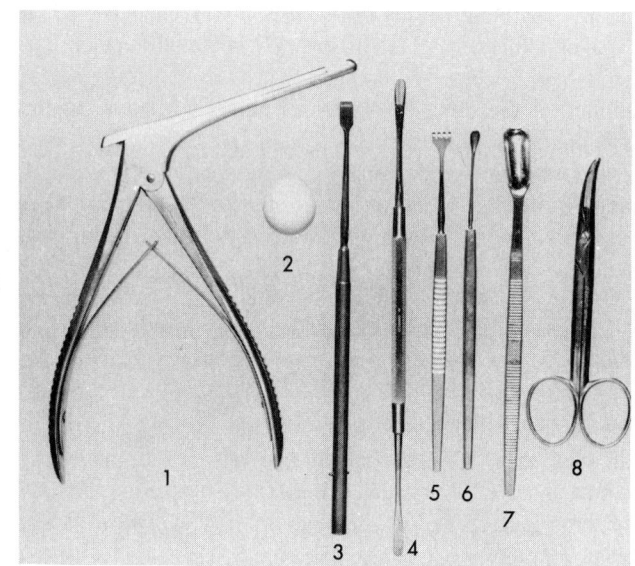

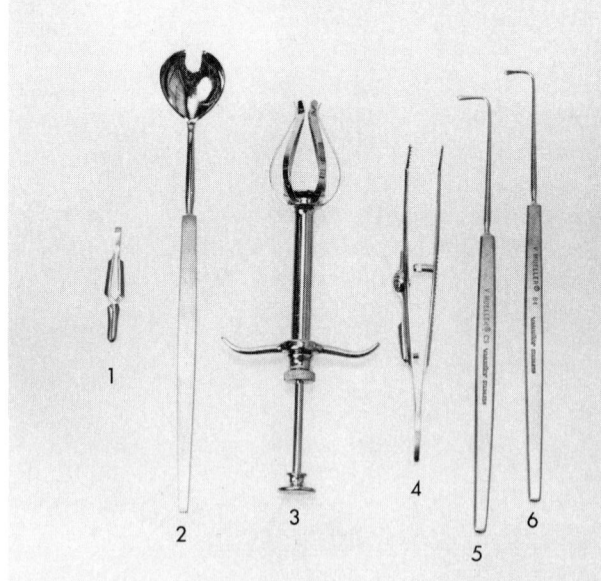

FIG. 17-43 Instruments for surgery of globe or orbit. **A,** *1,* Kerrison rongeur; *2,* orbital implant or sphere; *3,* lacrimal chisel; *4,* Freer elevator; *5,* lacrimal sac retractor; *6,* exenteration spoon; *7,* Arruga orbital retractor; *8,* enucleation scissors. **B,** *1,* Serrefine; *2,* Wells evisceration spoon; *3,* sphere introducer and holder; *4,* Jameson recession forceps; *5* and *6,* von Graefe muscle hooks.

Tissue adhesives, that is, cyanoacrylate monomers, are being used experimentally. The tissue adhesive is applied to well-dried tissue that has been properly oriented anatomically. It polymerizes and seals the wound on contact with the tissue. The tissue adhesive is supplied in packaged sterile vials (Co-Apt).

Culture specimens are usually obtained at the time of surgery. Antibiotics are injected subconjunctivally before the dressings are applied.

Enucleation

Enucleation is removal of the entire eyeball.

Operative procedure

1. A speculum retractor is introduced into the palpebral fissure.
2. The conjunctiva is divided around the cornea with sharp and blunt dissection.
3. The medial, lateral, inferior, and superior rectus muscles are divided, leaving a stump of medial rectus muscle. The globe is separated from Tenon's capsule with blunt-pointed, curved scissors, retractors, hemostats, and forceps.
4. The eye is rotated laterally by grasping the stump of the medial rectus muscle.
5. A large, curved hemostat is passed behind the globe, and the optic nerve is clamped for 60 seconds. The hemostat is removed, the enucleation scissors are passed posteriorly, and the optic nerve is transected. The oblique muscles are severed as the eye is lifted out of the socket by the stump of the medial rectus muscle.
6. The muscle cone is packed with saline sponges to obtain hemostasis.
7. The muscle cone is filled with an implant, and Tenon's capsule and conjunctiva are carefully closed. Hydroxyapatite spheres are frequently placed for later use, which will allow synchronous movement.
8. A socket conformer is placed in the cul-de-sac.
9. A pressure dressing is applied.

Evisceration

Evisceration is removal of the contents of the eye, leaving intact the sclera and the attached muscles.

Operative procedure

1. The conjunctiva is not separated from the sclera as it is for enucleation. A sharp-pointed knife is inserted through the limbus anterior to the iris.
2. The contents of the eye (iris, vitreous, lens) are removed.
3. The choroid adhering to the sclera is removed with curettes.
4. Bleeding is controlled with delicate hemostatic forceps, electrocoagulation, and sutures.
5. A plastic implant is placed within the empty shell.
6. The conjunctival and scleral edges are brought together

with nonabsorbable no. 4-0 or 5-0 sutures, and a pressure dressing is applied.

Repair of fracture of the orbit (blowout)

A fractured orbit (see Fig. 17-42) is repaired by means of graft or realignment of contents of the orbit.

Procedural considerations

The setup is as for dacryocystorhinostomy, plus a graft set (for implantation of an autogenous graft or synthetic graft materials of various sizes and thicknesses) and a flexible, narrow-width retractor. The patient is prepared as described for eye surgery. A general anesthetic is usually administered.

Operative procedure

1. The maximum ocular rotation is tested by exerting traction with a forceps on the tendon of the inferior rectus muscle to determine if the inferior muscle sling is trapped in the fracture.
2. To distribute tension over the lower lid and stretch the orbicular muscle, a traction suture is inserted through the lower lid margin.
3. With a no. 3 knife handle and no. 15 blade the lower lid is incised in the lid fold above the orbital rim.
4. The skin is separated from the orbicular muscle, and the orbital septum is identified by blunt dissection. Dissection is continued down to the periosteum of the orbital rim by means of scissors, loop retractors, elevators, and forceps.
5. The periosteum of the orbital rim is incised with a no. 15 blade. With periosteal elevators the floor of the orbit is exposed and explored. When the fracture site is identified, bone spicules are removed, and the herniated contents are freed from the maxillary antrum. The contents of the orbit are elevated by means of narrow-width, flexible retractors. A no. 4-0 traction suture is placed around the tendon of the inferior rectus muscle.
6. An autogenous graft is taken from the iliac crest, or an alloplastic material of proper size is used to repair the bony defect. The material may or may not be anchored to the orbital rim by wire sutures.
7. The periosteum is carefully closed with no. 4-0 absorbable sutures.
8. The skin is closed with no. 6-0 nonabsorbable sutures, and a pressure dressing is applied. Interosseus wiring may be carried out for fractures of the frontozygomatic junction. In addition, oculoplastic surgery has been greatly enhanced by the use of microplates and screws to stabilize fractures involving the fragile facial and orbital bones.

Exenteration

Exenteration is removal of the entire orbital contents, including periosteum, for certain malignancies of the globe or orbit.

Procedural considerations

Considerations are as described for fracture of the orbit. General anesthesia is usually administered.

Operative procedure

1. Depending on circumstances, exenteration of the eye may or may not include the removal of the lids. An incision is made down to the orbital rim, through the periosteum, and around the entire orbit.
2. With periosteal elevators the periosteum is freed from the orbital walls and the apex of the orbit.
3. The optic nerve is clamped, and the entire contents of the orbit are removed en bloc.
4. Hemostasis is obtained by the use of electrocoagulation and bone wax.
5. A skin graft or temporal muscle implant may be used to fill the orbital cavity, but this is not usually done. In most cases iodoform gauze is used to fill the cavity, a pressure dressing is put in place, and the cavity is allowed to granulate.

SURGERY OF THE CORNEA

Surgery of the cornea is indicated for a variety of conditions in which cosmetic, therapeutic, restorative, and refractive outcomes are desired. New technology has been responsible for the introduction of procedures that offer more choices for restoration of vision.

Instrumentation for corneal transplants (lamellar and penetrating), as well as for repair of lacerations and removal of foreign bodies of the cornea, is shown in Fig. 17-44.

Corneal transplant (keratoplasty)

A corneal transplant is grafting of corneal tissue from one human eye to another (Figs. 17-45 and 17-46). Keratoplasty may be classified as (1) lamellar (partial-thickness) graft, (2) penetrating (whole-thickness) graft, (3) keratectomy (peeling of the cornea), and (4) tattooing (simulation of a pupil), which is rarely done. A corneal transplant is performed when the patient's cornea is thickened and opacified. The transparency of the cornea may be impaired as a result of infection, thermal or chemical burns, or certain diseases of unknown cause. A corneal transplant is done to improve vision when the basic visual structures of the eye, that is, the retina and optic nerve, are functioning properly.

Corneas are obtained from recently deceased persons. Eye banks help coordinate services for such operations.

Operative procedures
Penetrating keratoplasty (performed with operating microscope)

1. The eye speculum is put in place, and superior rectus and inferior rectus bridle sutures are placed if a Flieringa ring is not to be used. If a ring is used, it is sutured in place with four no. 5-0 Dacron sutures.
2. The eye from the eye bank is removed from its container and may be washed in Neosporin solution, or a corneo-

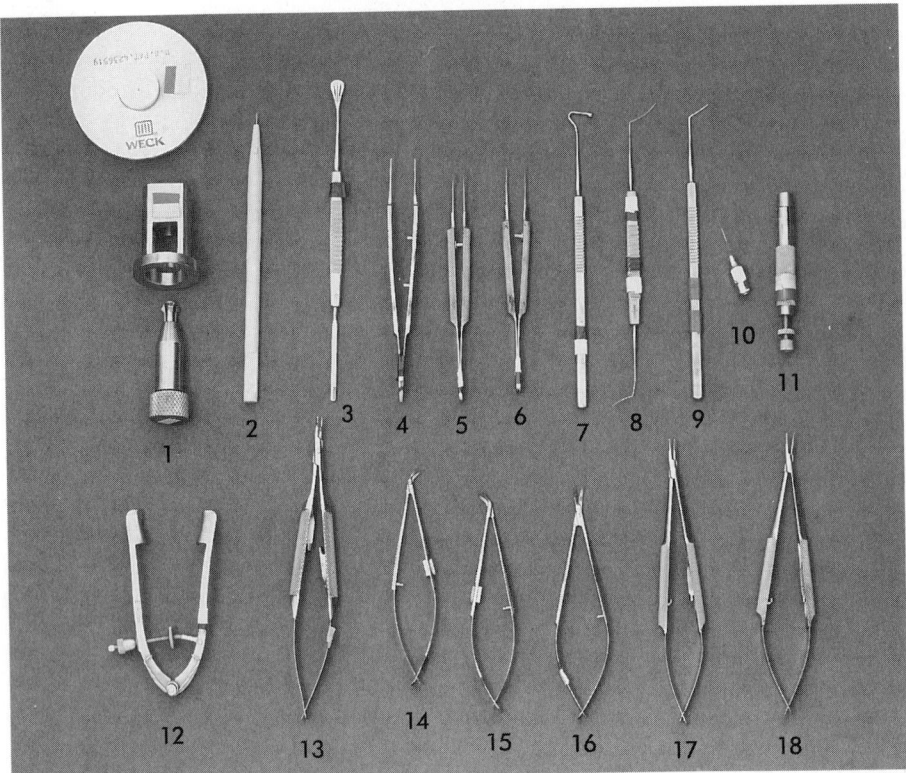

FIG. 17-44   Instruments for corneal transplant and other procedures on the cornea. *1,* Universal trephine handle with Cottingham punch; *2,* Super blade; *3,* Paton spatula; *4,* Castroviejo suturing forceps,
0.12 mm; *5,* Bishop-Harmon forceps; *6,* Colibri corneal forceps; *7,* Green strabismus hook; *8,* Castroviejo cyclodialysis spatula; *9,* Troutman corneal dissector; *10,* air cannula, 27-gauge; *11,* Castroviejo
trephine; *12,* Lancaster eye speculum; *13,* Barraquer curved micro needle holder; *14* and *15,* Troutman-
Castroviejo corneal scissors, right and left; *16,* Castroviejo corneal scissors; *17,* straight micro needle
holder; *18,* corneal scleral scissors.

scleral button that has been stored in tissue culture medium or that has been frozen (and is thawed) is removed
from its container.

3. The donor eye from the eye bank is then wrapped in a
surgical dressing for stabilization. The cornea is excised
from the donor eye by means of a corneal trephine cataract knife, corneal scissors, and forceps after the epithelium is removed with a sponge. The graft is placed,
epithelial side down, in a Petri dish containing saline-
moistened gauze (see Fig. 17-45). Some surgeons pre-
place sutures in the graft. Others place the corneoscleral
button epithelial (outside) surface down on a sterile Teflon block. The corneal trephine is then used as a punch,
and the donor button is pressed out centrally. A drop of
culture medium may be used to cover the donor button
until it is implanted.

4. The section of cornea removed from the recipient's eye
may be the same size as the graft taken from the donor's eye or may be up to 0.5 mm smaller. The anterior
chamber is entered with one of a variety of cataract
knives, and the button is excised with corneal scissors.

(If a reusable trephine is used, care must be taken to
close the guard on the trephine after use to prevent damage to the cutting surface.)

5. Peripheral iridectomies or iridotomies may be performed
at this time at the surgeon's discretion, or a cataract extraction may be completed if the lens is opaque.

6. The graft is placed into the opening of the recipient's
eye and anchored in place by means of four single-armed
sutures placed at the four cardinal meridians, viewed
through an operating microscope. The graft is sutured
to the host with either continuous or interrupted no. 10-0
nylon sutures (see Fig. 17-46).

7. Air or sodium hyaluronic acid (Healon) may be injected
into the anterior chamber of the recipient's eye to keep
the iris from adhering to the suture line. Mydriatic or
miotic solutions are used at the surgeon's discretion.

8. A subconjunctival injection of antibiotic solution or a
topical application of antibiotic drops may be used at
the completion of the procedure. Antibiotic ointment is
applied, followed by an eye patch and a metal or plastic shield.

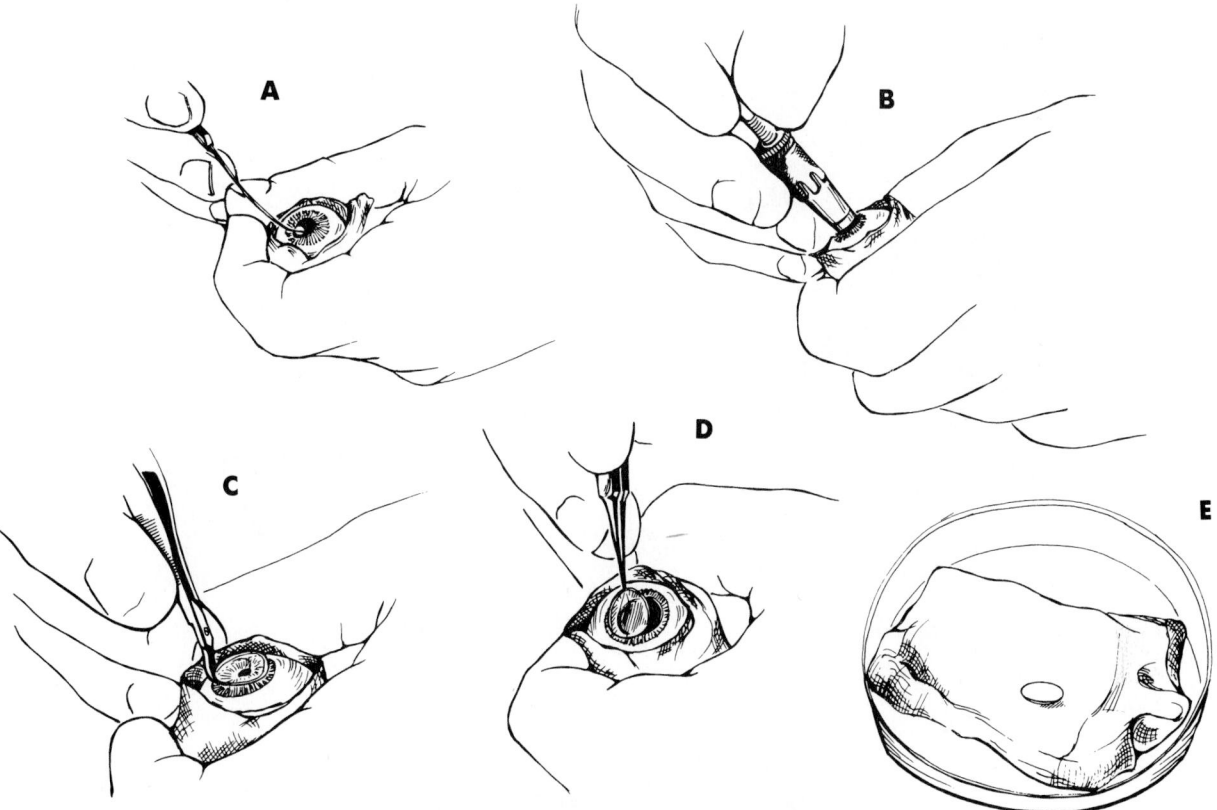

FIG. 17-45 **A,** Epithelium from donor cornea is being removed by abrading with iris spatula. Donor eye is wrapped in smooth gauze dressing. **B,** Donor eye is firmly grasped in surgeon's left hand, and corneal trephine is centered on donor eye. With twisting motion, cornea is cut through its entire thickness. **C,** Corneal scissors are used to cut any areas of corneal tissue that have not been penetrated by trephine. **D,** Corneal button is removed with fine forceps, with care taken not to touch endothelial surface. **E,** Donor corneal button is stored on moistened gauze pad, endothelial side up in covered Petri dish to preserve moisture.

Lamellar keratoplasty

1. The eye speculum and superior rectus and inferior rectus bridle sutures are placed if needed.
2. The eye from the eye bank is removed from its container and washed in Neosporin solution.
3. The eye is wrapped in a surgical dressing. A groove is made at the desired depth in the cornea with the trephine. The Castroviejo keratome is set at the desired depth, and the lamellar sheet of cornea is removed and placed in a Petri dish.
4. The recipient cornea is grooved with the same trephine to the appropriate depth. Using the operating microscope, the surgeon performs a lamellar resection, that is, removes the anterior part of the cornea at a predetermined depth with a Gill knife, Beaver knife blade no. 64, or other corneal splitter.
5. The donor tissue is sutured in place with a continuous 10-0 nylon suture.
6. A mydriatic agent and subconjunctival or topical antibiotics may be used.
7. The eye is patched.

Eye bank procedure

Donor eyes are removed immediately after death in accordance with legal regulations. The eye bank may be a central community agency or may be owned and operated by a hospital. The bank generally supplies the containers for eyes and sets forth regulations for the procedure. The enucleations are usually done in the hospital morgue under aseptic conditions. A special consent form is required and should be signed by the authorized next of kin and by a hospital representative designated by institutional policy.

Procedural considerations

The eyes are washed and irrigated in the routine manner of preparation for eye surgery. The sterile field, drapes, and instruments are essentially the same as those for an enucleation on a living patient.

Operative procedure

1. Eye specimen bottles are labeled for right and left eyes. The speculum is inserted, and after routine enucleation the donated eye is placed in the sterile specimen bottle

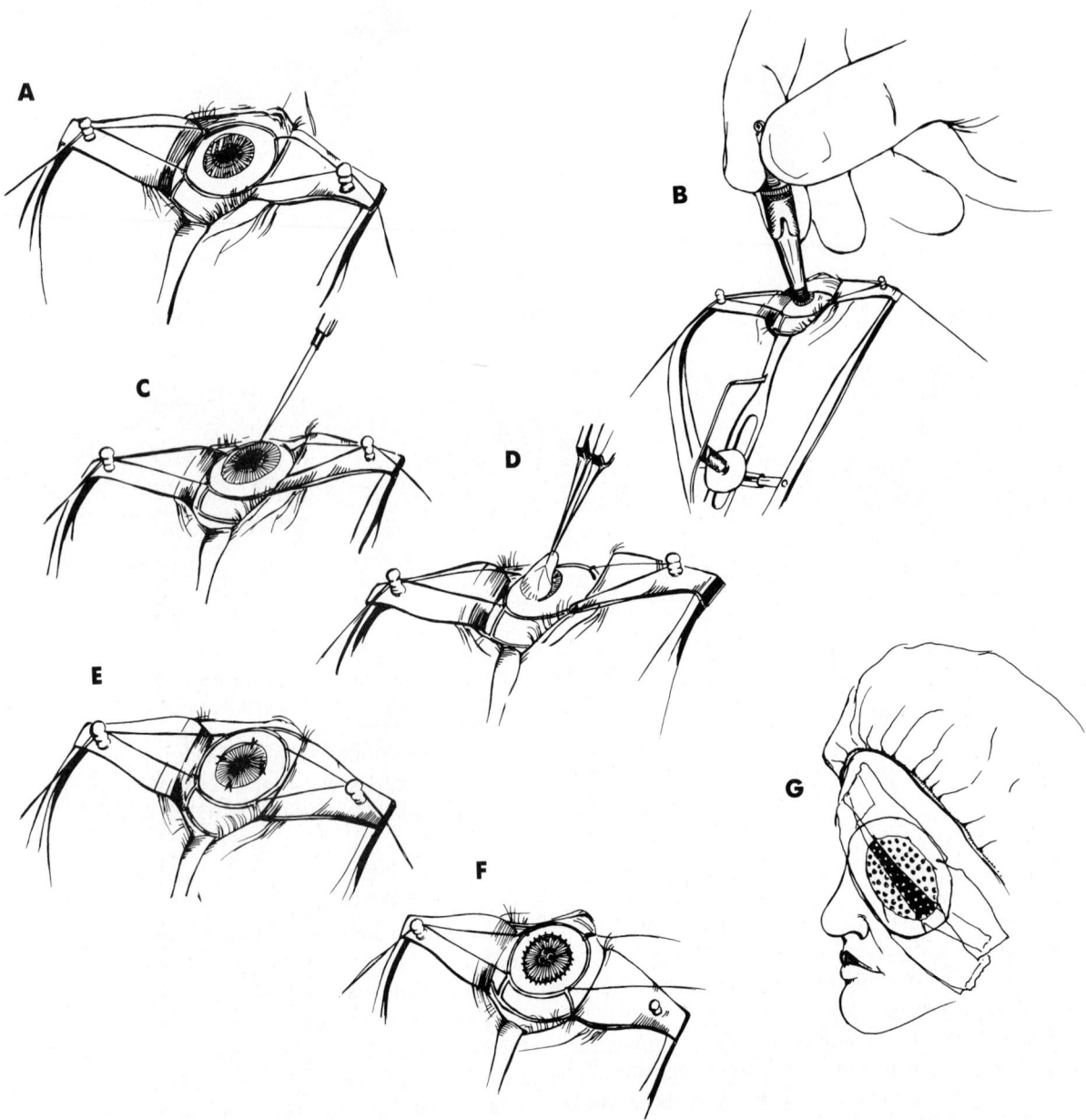

FIG. 17-46 **A,** Eye of patient who will undergo combined procedure including corneal transplantation and cataract extraction. Double Bonaccolto-Flieringa fixation ring is sutured in place with no. 5-0 Dacron sutures posted over solid-bladed eye speculum. **B,** Corneal trephine is placed on recipient cornea, and partial penetration is made approximately three fourths through stroma. **C,** Anterior chamber is entered through groove with Wheeler knife. Remainder of button is excised with right and left Katzin corneal microscissors. **D,** Corneal button is removed. **E,** Donor button sutured in place with four no. 8-0 black silk sutures. **F,** Cornea sutured in place with continuous no. 10-0 suture, with air in anterior chamber. **G,** Patient postoperatively with Fox shield properly applied on bony margins.

with the cornea up. The eye is supported on a sponge that has been soaked in saline solution. An antibiotic solution may be placed on the cornea. The eye sockets are packed with cotton, and the lids are closed.

2. Specimen bottles are sealed with tape and labeled with the donor's name, time and cause of death, time of enucleation, and date.

3. Appropriate specimens may be placed in tissue culture medium for short-term storage (72 hours) or frozen for long-term storage after the necessary manipulation.

Keratorefractive procedures

Keratorefractive procedures are corneal procedures designed to correct myopia, astigmatism, and aphakia. Many of these procedures are still in the developmental stages and are considered investigational. They include radial kerato-

tomy, keratomileusis, epikeratophakia, and keratophakia. These procedures require reshaping the cornea with relaxing incisions or cryolathing corneal tissue to change the refractive power of the cornea. Clinical trials have been conducted utilizing various technologies with excimer laser ablation over the past several years.

Radial keratotomy

Radial keratotomy is a series of precise, partial-thickness radial incisions in the cornea from a 3-mm or larger central optical zone to the limbus. These incisions result in a flattening of the cornea, which reduces the refractive error.

Radial keratotomy was first performed by Sato in Japan in 1953. In 1972 the procedure was studied and modified by the Russian physicians Fyodorov and Durnev, who in 1974 began investigation of the procedure in humans, us-

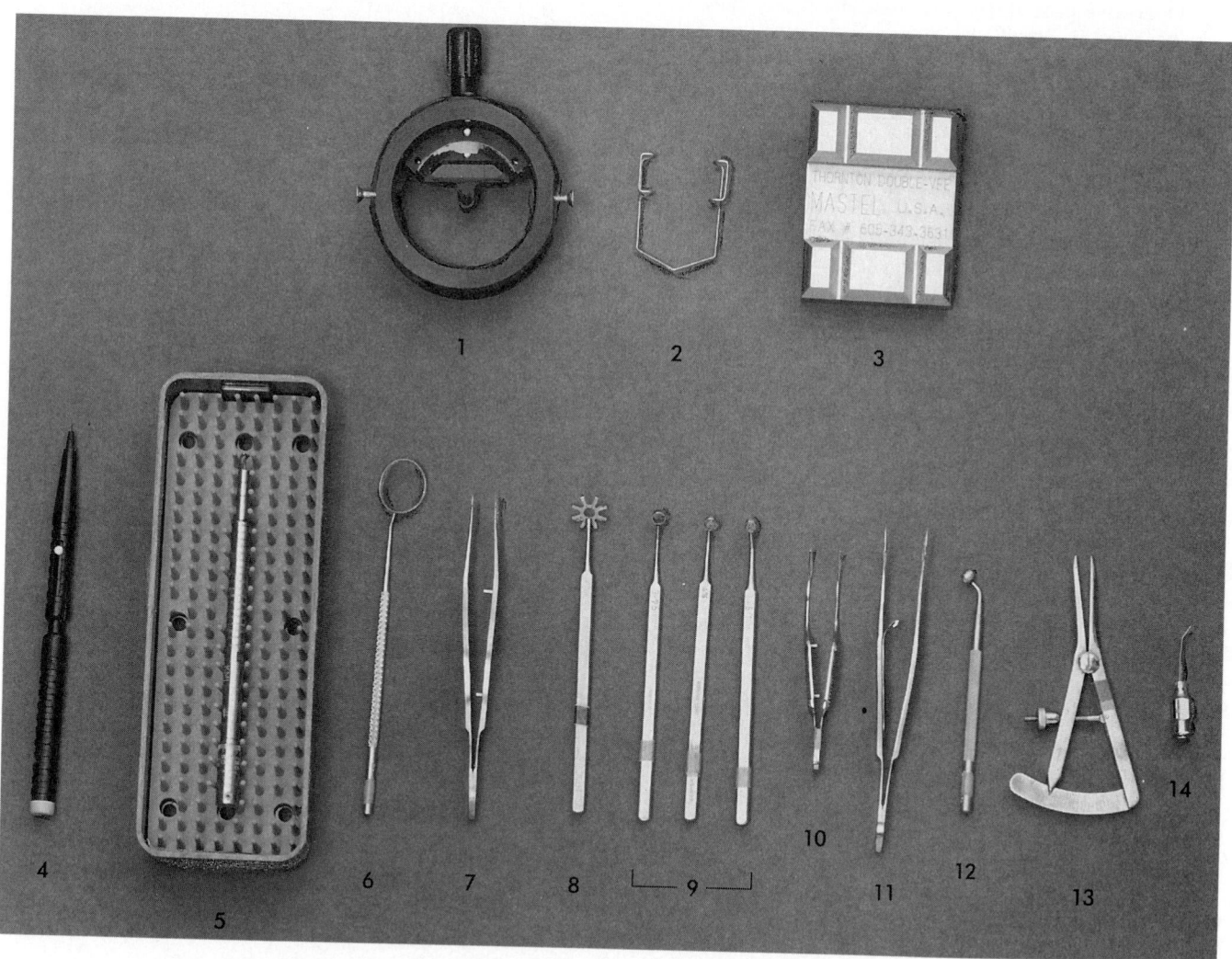

FIG. 17-47   Radial keratotomy instrumentation. *1,* Fixation device (to be attached to microscope) for patient to focus to mark optical zone; *2,* Barraquer wire speculum; *3,* Bores corneal knife gauge; *4,* Katena micrometer XTAL sapphire knife; *5,* Storz micrometer diamond knife; *6,* incision depth gauge; *7,* Rubman-Bores corneal fixation forceps; *8,* Bores corneal marker for eight radial incisions; *9,* Hoffer corneal markers with cross-hairs; *10,* Castroviejo-Colibri very delicate forceps, 0.12 mm; *11,* Bores incision spreading forceps; *12,* elliptical optic center marker; *13,* Castroviejo caliper; *14,* air cannula, 27-gauge.

ing anterior radial corneal incisions. In 1978, after review of the 4 years of data collected in Russia, Bores introduced radial keratotomy in the United States. Since then, modifications in the procedure have improved the predictability of results. Studies to ascertain the long-term results continue.

Radial keratotomy is a procedure for an adult who has at least −2 D of myopia and whose eyes are otherwise healthy. Preoperative measurement of corneal curvature (keratometry), corneal thickness (ultrasonic pachymetry), and refractive error is required to assist in the determination of optical zone diameter and depth of incisions.

Procedural considerations. The surgery is performed as an ambulatory procedure with local and topical anesthetics. The patient is prepared as for routine ophthalmic surgery.

Operative procedure. The procedure is as follows:

1. As the patient focuses on the fixation device attached to the objective lens of the operating microscope, the visual axis is marked (see Fig. 17-47).
2. The blade depth is set on the micrometer of the surgical knife (diamond, sapphire, or steel) and double-checked against a micrometer gauge (Fig. 17-47).
3. The surgeon fixates the globe with double-toothed Bores fixation forceps to decrease rotation.
4. Radial incisions are made from the margin of the optical zone to the limbus (Fig. 17-48). The numbers and depth are determined by the amount of correction desired.
5. The depth of the incisions is checked to verify uniformity.
6. The incisions are irrigated with balanced salt solution (BSS). An antibiotic solution is instilled and an eye patch applied.

Epikeratophakia

Epikeratophakia is a form of refractive keratoplasty for the correction of aphakia, myopia, and keratoconus. A piece of donor corneal tissue is shaped to a specific diopter power on a cryolathe. This tissue is sutured to the recipient cornea to change the corneal curvature and thus the refractive power of the cornea. The patient's central cornea is not surgically invaded, and the donor tissue can be removed with no residual visual effects. Epikeratophakia is therefore reversible. Lyophilized (freeze-dried) tissue lenticles are available from a few sources.

Operative procedure. The procedure is as follows:

1. The preshaped donor tissue (lenticle) is rehydrated in BSS containing 100 µg/ml of IV gentamicin for 20 minutes before application onto the recipient's eye.
2. The lenticle is placed on a Teflon block and kept moist with BSS.
3. Anesthesia is administered.
4. The lid speculum is placed between the lids.

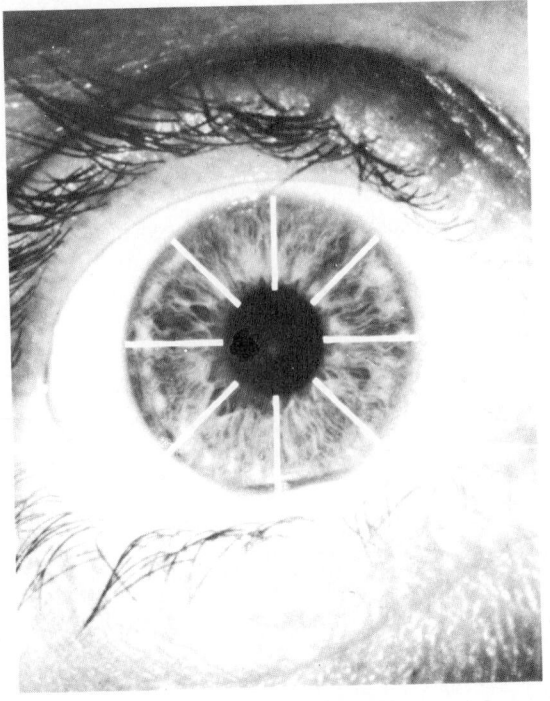

FIG. 17-48 Location of incisions in radial keratotomy. Central 3- to 4-mm optical zone of cornea is not incised, and incisions do not extend beyond corneoscleral limbus. Four, eight, or 16 radial incisions are made.

From Newell, F.W. (1992) *Ophthalmology: Principles and concepts* (7th ed.). St. Louis: Mosby.

5. A topical anesthetic (cocaine 4%) is instilled in the operative eye.
6. The visual axis of the recipient eye is marked by the surgeon.
7. A cellulose sponge is used to scrape off the patient's corneal epithelium. The debris is thoroughly removed by irrigation and aspiration. (All epithelial cells must be removed to prevent them from growing in the interface between the lenticle and the recipient cornea in the postoperative period.)
8. A circular keratotomy of 0.25- to 0.30-mm depth is made with a trephine. Again the wound is irrigated and aspirated to remove debris thoroughly.
9. A wedge-shaped annulus of the anterior stroma for 360 degrees on the inner aspect of trephine mark is removed with scissors and forceps.
10. The lenticle is positioned and sutured into place with no. 10-0 nylon interrupted sutures.
11. Suture knots are rotated and buried under the surface of the recipient side of the trephine cut.
12. A bandage contact lens is positioned on the eye. The prescribed drugs (usually an antiinflammatory agent and an antibiotic) are injected or instilled. The eye is patched; a shield is secured in place.

SURGERY OF THE LENS
Cataract extraction, generally with operating microscope

A cataract extraction is removal of the opaque lens from the interior of the eye. The lens consists of 65% water, 35% protein, and a trace of other body minerals. The disorders of the lens are opacification and dislocation, resulting in blurred vision without pain or inflammation. Cataracts (opacification) vary in degree of density, size, and location and are usually caused by aging or trauma.

Two basic methods, intracapsular and extracapsular extraction, are usually employed to remove the lens. The intracapsular method of cataract removal consists of removing the lens within its capsule. In the extracapsular method the anterior portion of the capsule is first ruptured and removed, and the lens cortex and nucleus are expressed from the eye, leaving the posterior capsule behind. Restoration of functional vision is necessary after removal of the crystalline lens. At present four options are available for correction of aphakia (absence of the lens). A patient can be fitted with aphakic spectacles 4 to 8 weeks after lens extraction. These corrective lenses are acceptable only for binocular aphakia. They distort peripheral vision and produce a significant change in image size. Contact lenses are also used to correct aphakia. They offer an excellent option for visual correction and can be used for monocular aphakia. A third option is epikeratophakia. This procedure can be considered for patients with low endothelial cell counts. The fourth option for visual correction following lens removal, and the one most commonly used today, is the implantation of an artificial lens made of polymethyl methacrylate (PMMA). New designs and new implant materials challenge perioperative nursing personnel to keep abreast of constant changes in techniques for intraocular lens (IOL) implantations.

The IOLs offer many advantages to patients. They are used for monocular aphakic correction. Rehabilitation times for patients are shortened. The IOLs may be placed in the anterior chamber, iris plane, or posterior chamber. Iris plane or iris-fixated lenses are seldom used today. Posterior lenses can be implanted only when the cataract was removed by extracapsular lens extraction (ECCE). This is the most physiologic position for an artificial lens and has led to a return to ECCE, which is now the most common method of lens extraction. Anterior chamber lenses are used after intracapsular lens extraction (ICCE) and for secondary lens implantation.

The IOLs are available in various powers at 0.5-D steps. The necessary power is determined by measuring the curvature of the patient's cornea (keratometry) and the axial length (length from cornea to retina). A mathematical formula is then used to calculate the correct lens power.

In recent years sutureless cataract techniques have become increasingly popular because of rapid visual rehabilitation. A 5-mm incision 3 mm posterior and parallel to the

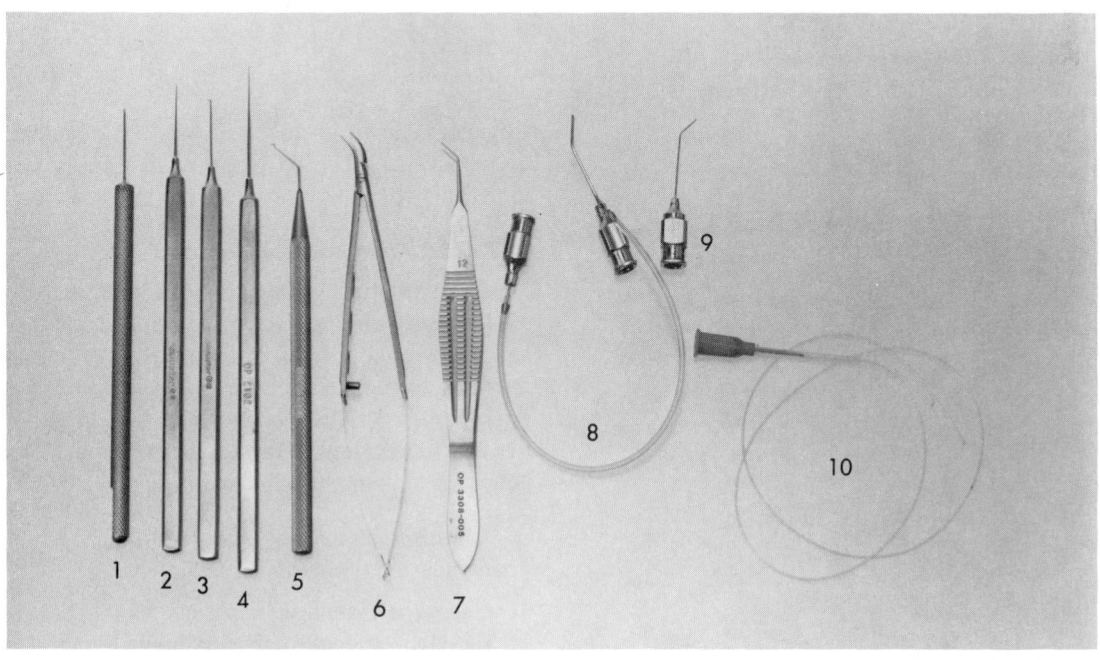

FIG. 17-49 Instrumentation for intraocular lens implantation. *1,* Round-handled Sinsky lens microhook; *2,* Sinsky lens microhook; *3,* Kugler cloverleaf lens manipulator; *4,* Bonn iris hook; *5,* Fenzl lens hook; *6,* Shepard lens-holding forceps; *7,* Castroviejo corneoscleral suturing forceps with angled tip; *8,* Morrison irrigation and aspiration cannula; *9,* air or Healon cannula; *10,* disposable Kelman anterior chamber maintainer.

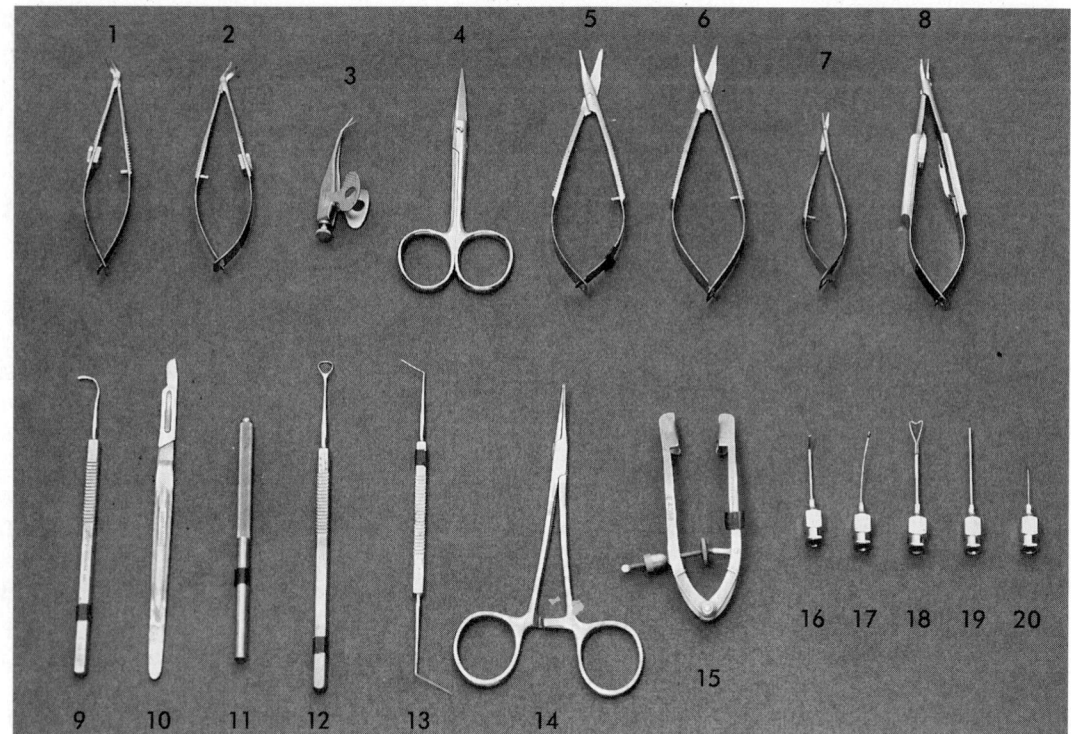

FIG. 17-50   Instrumentation for lens procedures. Forceps used are shown in Figs. 17-22 through 17-27. *1* and *2*, Troutman-Castroviejo corneal scissors; *3*, Barraquer iris scissors; *4*, Knapp straight iris scissors; *5*, Westcott stitch scissors; *6*, Westcott tenotomy scissors; *7*, Vannas iridocapsulotomy scissors; *8*, curved Barraquer needle holder; *9*, Green strabismus hook; *10*, no. 9 Bard-Parker knife handle with no. 15 blade; *11*, Beaver knife handle; *12*, lens loop; *13*, Castroviejo cyclodialysis spatula; *14*, Hartman mosquito hemostat; *15*, Lancaster eye speculum; *16*, Healon cannula; *17*, olive-tip irrigating cannula; *18*, irrigating vectis loop; *19*, lacrimal irrigator; *20*, air cannula.

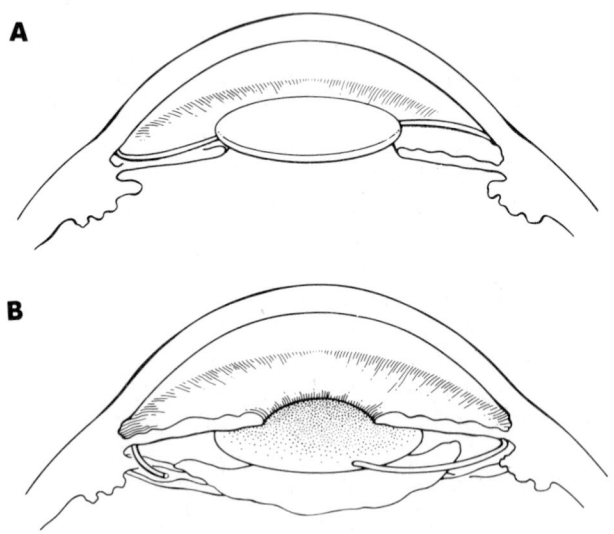

FIG. 17-51   **A,** Anterior chamber intraocular lens that is held in position with loop of nylon (haptics) placed in anterior chamber angle. **B,** Posterior chamber lens placed in lens capsule from which most of anterior portion has been excised.

From Newell, F.W. (1992) *Ophthalmology: Principles and concepts* (7th ed.). St. Louis: Mosby.

surgical limbus is entered with a 3-mm keratome and phacoemulsification carried out. The incision is then opened to 5.1 mm to allow for insertion of the IOL.

Procedural considerations

Instrumentation varies with surgeon's preference (Fig. 17-49) but usually includes forceps to insert the lens and lens haptics and a hook to aid in rotating and positioning the lens. Instrumentation for lens procedures is shown in Fig. 17-50, and IOLs are shown in Fig. 17-51. Perioperative nursing personnel must be familiar with institutional policies pertaining to IOLs and their use.

Operative procedures
Intracapsular method

1. A speculum is placed in the eye to hold the lids apart.
2. The globe is held by transfixion with a nonabsorbable no. 4-0 suture, which is inserted under the tendon of the superior rectus muscle and clamped to the drape. A conjunctival flap, either limbal or fornix based, may be prepared with the use of the scissors. Some surgeons do not dissect a flap.

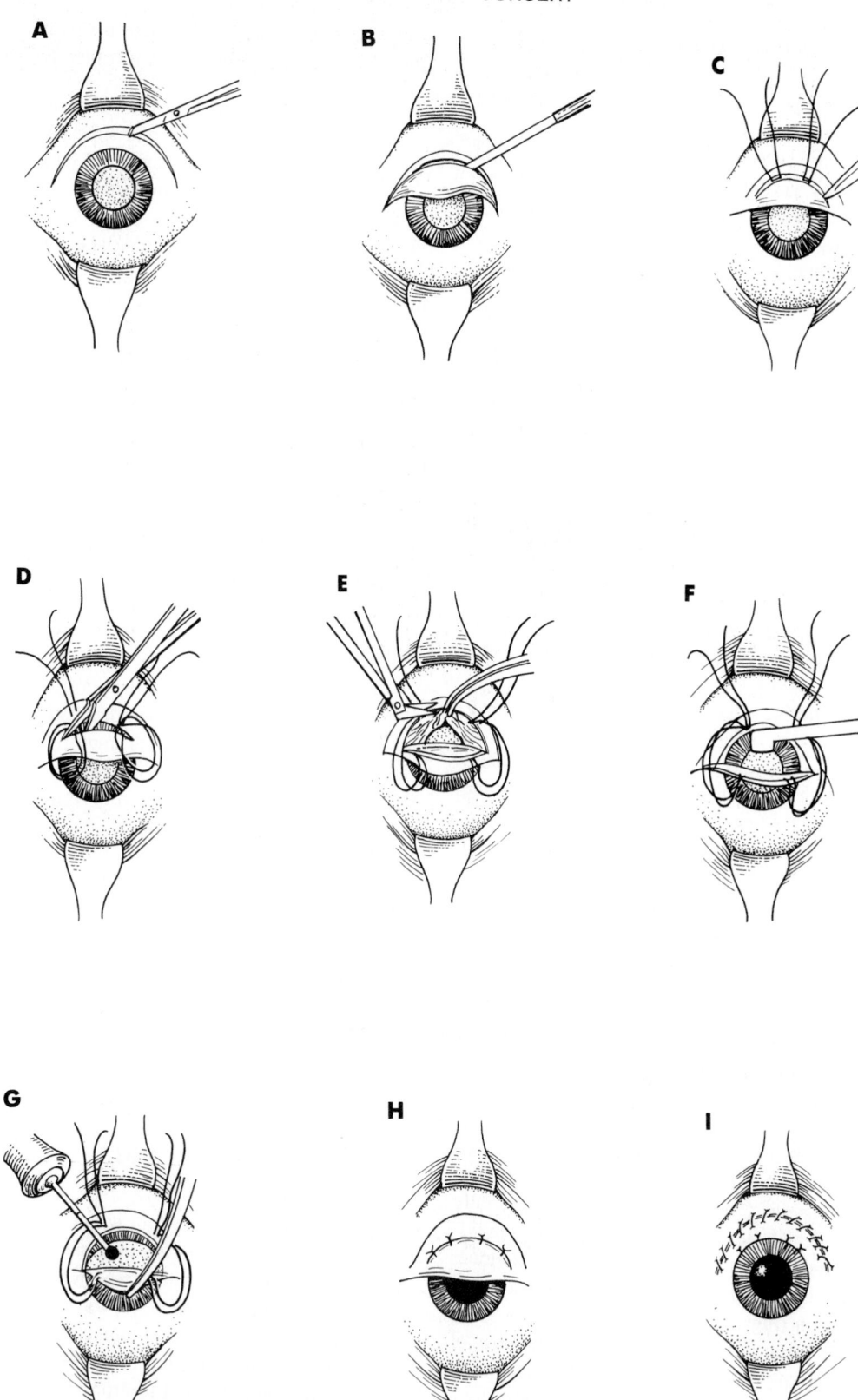

FIG. 17-52   Intracapsular lens extraction. **A,** Preparation of conjunctival flap with scissors. **B,** Non-penetrating (partial-thickness) incision made at limbus or in cornea. **C,** Corneoscleral sutures are placed. **D,** Limbal incision completed with scissors. **E,** Peripheral iridectomy is performed. **F,** Iris retractor in place for delivery of lens. **G,** Lens grasped and pulled slowly from eye with cryostat unit. **H,** Corneo-scleral sutures tied. **I,** Conjunctival flap reapproximated and sutured.

3. Bleeding points are coagulated by means of a bipolar unit, which provides maximum coagulation with minimum tissue necrosis. Partially penetrating incisions (grooves) are made at the limbus or in the cornea.

4. Corneoscleral or corneocorneal sutures are passed through the lips of the wounds. These sutures are looped out of the groove and set in an orderly manner around the margins of the incision.

5. With the keratome, or knife, the anterior chamber is entered, and the limbal wound is enlarged with corneal scissors.

6. A peripheral iridectomy or sector iridectomy is performed. Alpha-chymotrypsin (Zolyse) is injected through the iridectomy. The lens is grasped, in most cases with a cryoextractor, and extracted slowly from the eye.

7. The pupil is usually constricted with acetylcholine (Miochol) or carbachol (Miostat) if an IOL is inserted.

8. The corneoscleral sutures are tied, and the conjunctival flap is reapproximated with either absorbable or nonabsorbable sutures of the desired size.

9. Pilocarpine 2% or atropine 1% may be applied topically. Antibiotics may be used topically or subconjunctivally. The eye is dressed and patched.

10. If, at any time during the operation, vitreous gel is extruded from the eye, a partial vitrectomy is performed to prevent vitreous from becoming incorporated into the wound, which can lead to various postoperative complications. The first step usually involves an attempt to aspirate liquefied vitreous from the eye with a 19-gauge blunt needle on a 2-ml syringe. Once this is accomplished, solid vitreous may be removed by the use of Weck-Cel sponges and scissors (Westcott) or by using any of the various vitrectomy instruments available.

Extracapsular method. The standard procedure for ECCE is similar to an intracapsular extraction up to step 6, removal of the lens. At this point the capsule of the lens is opened by means of a cystotome or capsule forceps; the lens nucleus is removed by expression and a lens loop; the lens cortex is removed by irrigation and aspiration using a coaxial cannula system. Cycloplegic agents are generally used. The remainder of the procedure is as outlined previously for intracapsular extraction. If a posterior chamber IOL is used, the pupil is constricted with acetylcholine after the lens insertion (Fig. 17-52).

Phacoemulsification. Over the past years a number of microsurgical techniques have been developed for lens removal through a small incision. Basically, each technique involves opening the lens capsule and using ultrasonic energy to fragment the hard lens material, which can then be aspirated from the eye. The subsequent description and illustrations relate to the use of the Alcon Series 10,000 phacoemulsification unit (Fig. 17-53, A). All perioperative personnel using specialized instruments and equipment must have thorough knowledge of their operation, as well as possible problems and actions to correct them (17-53, B).

1. After a superior rectus bridle suture is placed, a small limbal-based flap is dissected superiorly.

2. The surgical limbus is cleaned by sharp dissection with a Beaver knife blade. Hemostasis is obtained with a disposable eye cautery.

3. A 3-mm incision is made into the eye with either a keratome or a sharp microknife.

4. The lens capsule is opened with a cystotome or capsule forceps. The anterior chamber may be kept formed with air or irrigating solution.

5. The lens nucleus is loosened from the cortex with the cystotome or a blunt cyclodialysis spatula.

6. The ultrasonic handpiece is checked by the physician for appropriate vacuum control. *This check should be made before any handpiece is introduced into the eye.*

7. The ultrasonic handpiece is introduced into the eye. Three positions are possible for the operation of the foot pedal under the surgeon's control: (1) irrigation alone; (2) irrigation and aspiration; and (3) irrigation, aspiration, and ultrasonic power. As the surgeon manipulates the handpiece and operates the footpedal to emulsify the lens nucleus, the perioperative nurse is responsible for operating the other controls and monitoring the function of the instrument.

8. When the lens nucleus has been emulsified and removed, the lens cortex is removed with the 0.3-mm aspiration-irrigation handpiece.

9. If an IOL is to be implanted, the wound is extended to accommodate the lens diameter, the IOL is inserted, and acetylcholine may be introduced to constrict the pupil.

10. A peripheral iridectomy may be performed.

11. The corneoscleral wound is closed with 7-0 or 8-0 absorbable suture, a 10-0 nonabsorbable suture, or a combination of both.

12. The conjunctival flap is closed.

13. The eye is appropriately dressed.

SURGERY FOR GLAUCOMA

Iridectomy

Iridectomy is removal of a section of iris tissue. Peripheral iridectomy is done in the treatment of acute, subacute, or chronic angle-closure glaucoma when extensive peripheral anterior synechiae have not formed. This operation is performed to reestablish communication between the posterior and anterior chambers, thus relieving pupillary block and permitting the iris root to drop away from the trabecular meshwork to reestablish the outflow of aqueous fluid through Schlemm's canal.

Procedural considerations

Instrumentation for glaucoma surgery is shown in Fig. 17-54.

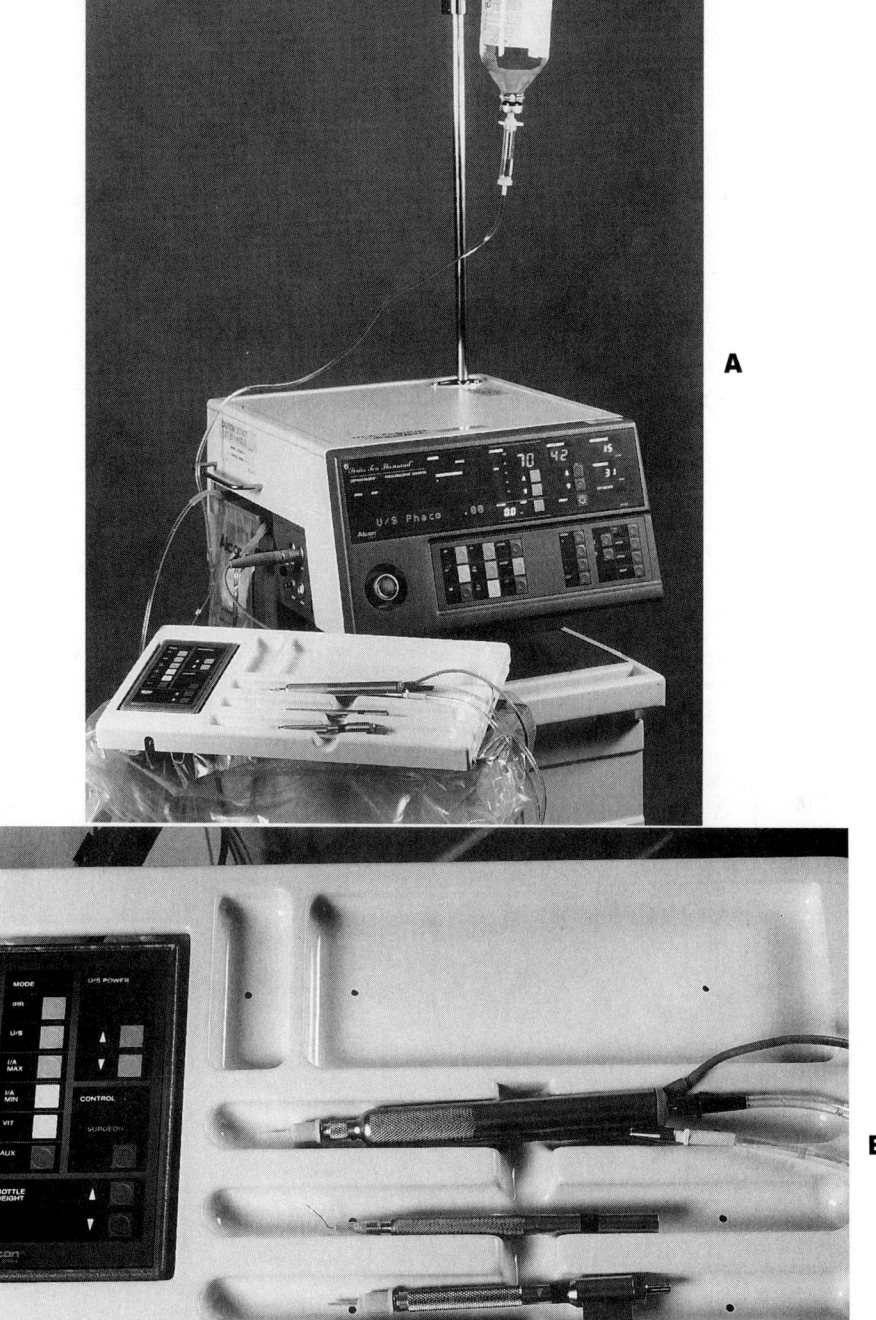

FIG. 17-53 **A,** Alcon Phaco Emulsifier Aspirator Series 10,000. **B,** Instrument tray shows; Phaco hand-piece; cystotome handle; irrigation and aspiration (I&A) handpiece; remote control.

Courtesy Visual Communications, The Methodist Hospital, Houston, Tex.

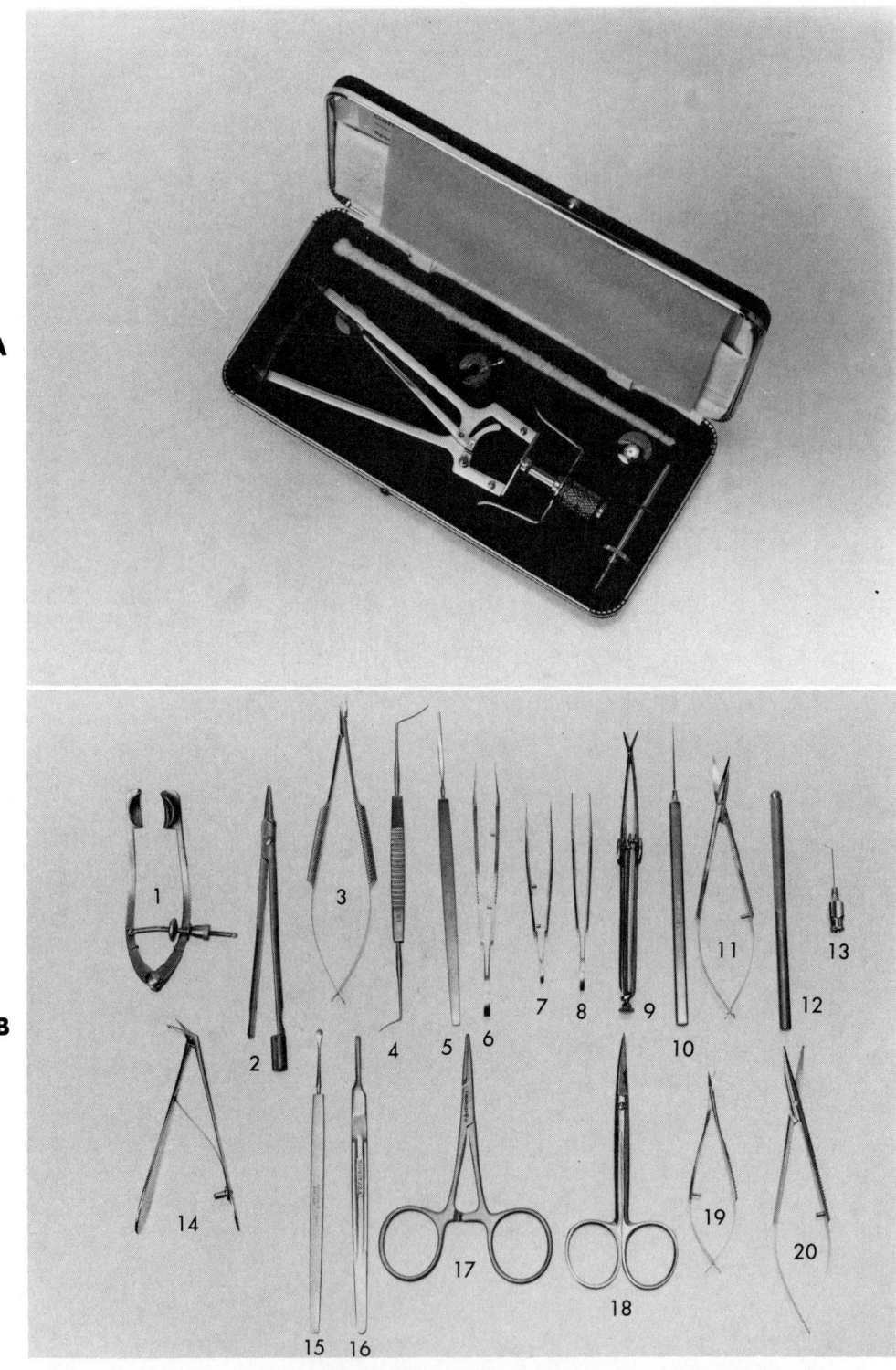

FIG. 17-54   Instrumentation for glaucoma surgery. **A,** Schiotz tonometer to measure intraocular pressure (may be autoclaved). **B,** *1,* Lancaster eye speculum; *2,* blade breaker; *3,* Barraquer curved needle holder; *4,* Castroviejo cyclodialysis spatula; *5,* Wheeler iris spatula; *6,* Castroviejo 0.12-mm suturing forceps; *7,* Colibri corneal forceps; *8,* Bishop-Harman tissue forceps; *9,* deWecker iris scissors; *10,* Bonn iris hook; *11,* Westcott stitch scissors; *12,* Beaver knife handle; *13,* air injection cannula; *14,* Holth scleral punch; *15,* Gill corneal knife; *16,* no. 9 Bard-Parker knife handle; *17,* Hartman mosquito hemostat; *18,* Knapp strabismus scissors; *19,* Vannas iridocapsulotomy scissors; *20,* Westcott tenotomy scissors.

Operative procedure

1. The speculum is introduced. The globe is fixed with a no. 4-0 suture passed under the superior rectus tendon with fixation forceps and needle holder. The suture is fastened to the drape with a hemostat.
2. A small peritomy is performed at the superior limbus. The corneoscleral junction is scraped clean of epithelium. With a Beaver knife handle and no. 64 blade a limbal groove is made down to Descemet's membrane.
3. The anterior chamber is entered with a no. 15 blade. Pressure is placed on the posterior lip of the wound to prolapse the iris. The iris is grasped, and either a peripheral or sector iridectomy is performed. The iris is stroked back into position by external manipulation with a spatula over the cornea.
4. The wound is closed with absorbable suture. Subconjunctival antibiotics may be administered, and an eye dressing applied.

Elliot trephination

Elliot trephination is the formation of a drainage channel to the subconjunctival space in the treatment of chronic glaucoma. The object of Elliot trephination is to establish a route of aqueous drainage to the subconjunctival space for absorption. The operation is done primarily for open-angle glaucoma. Postoperatively the aqueous matter escapes through the scleral hole into the subconjunctival space, where it is absorbed into the bloodstream.

Operative procedure

1. A superior rectus bridle suture of no. 4-0 silk is placed and clamped to the drape.
2. Two milliliters of saline (with the possible addition of 1 drop of 1:1000 epinephrine) are injected superiorly beneath Tenon's capsule to dissect a flap from the underlying sclera.
3. The conjunctiva is incised to the sclera. The flap is dissected anteriorly into clear cornea.
4. With the conjunctival flap raised by means of forceps, the trephine is applied at the corneal limbus.
5. After completion of trephination, the scleral disk is cut at its hinge if it is not free.
6. An iridectomy is performed with iris forceps and de-Wecker scissors.
7. The operative area is cleansed of blood, and the conjunctival flap is resutured with a no. 6-0 or 7-0 nonabsorbable suture. Cycloplegic agents are administered. The eye is dressed with a patch and a metal guard.

Anterior and posterior lid sclerectomies

Anterior and posterior lid sclerectomies are performed to provide a drainage channel to the subconjunctival space in the treatment of chronic glaucoma.

Operative procedure

1. The procedure is as described for Elliot trephination through the dissection of the conjunctival flap (steps 1 to 3).
2a. For *thermal sclerectomy* a scleral flap is made approximately 3 mm from the limbus with a Beaver no. 64 blade. The disposable eye cautery with a transilluminating head is used to outline the anterior chamber. The eye cautery is used to apply heat energy to the posterior wound edge under the scleral flap. The anterior chamber is entered with a clean sweep of the cautery. The iris usually prolapses spontaneously, or an iris forceps is used to grasp the iris, and a peripheral or radial iridectomy is performed.
2b. For *punch sclerectomy* an incision is made into the anterior chamber at the anterior or posterior margin of the limbus after the anterior chamber has been outlined with a transilluminator. A punch is introduced, and sections of either the anterior or posterior lip are removed, depending on which incision has been made. An iridectomy is performed.
3. A careful closure of conjunctiva and Tenon's capsule is accomplished with no. 6-0 nonabsorbable suture, leaving both ends free.
4. Air is introduced under the flap with a blunt 30-gauge needle on a 2-ml syringe.
5. The conjunctival flap is closed with a continuous suture. The free ends may be used to delimit the bleb. Atropine sulfate 1% is dropped on the eye, and an eye dressing is applied.

Cyclodialysis

Cyclodialysis is the formation of a communication between the anterior chamber and the space located between the sclera and the choroid. This reduces aqueous secretion and thus induces lower pressure; absorption into the suprachoroidal space is increased. Cyclodialysis is usually reserved for treatment of glaucoma associated with peripheral anterior synechiae.

Operative procedure

1. A superior rectus bridle suture of no. 4-0 silk is put in place and clamped to the drape.
2. In one of the superior quadrants between the rectus muscles, the conjunctiva is incised and dissected from the sclera. An incision is made through the sclera to the suprachoroidal space with the use of a Beaver no. 64 blade.
3. A cyclodialysis spatula is introduced through the scleral opening, and the anterior chamber is entered in the region of the iris root; the ciliary body is thus detached from the sclera by means of the spatula. The scleral incision is closed.
4. The conjunctiva is closed with fine sutures. A dressing is applied.

RESEARCH HIGHLIGHT 17-3

Of the devices used to increase aqueous drainage from the anterior chamber, the Molteno implant has become one of the most widely used. Melamid and Fiore summarized reports of clinical trials comparing results following one-stage–one-plate and two-stage–two-plate Molteno implants. Antifibrolytic therapy was used in approximately half the patients. Evaluation and conclusions drawn from eight separate studies in which a total of 569 eyes were treated were reported in terms of intraocular pressure control, technique, and major complications. Modifications of the Molteno implant have increased the success rate from 50% to 75% of procedures in 1977 to a success rate of 83% to 90% of cases in 1990. The latter study showed a mean postoperative intraocular pressure of 12.75 mm Hg with a two-plate implant compared to 25 mm Hg with a single-plate implant. Use of two plates in a two-stage operation with subconjunctival antifibrolytic therapy (5-FU), injection of hyaluronic acid, and use of a needle tract to provide an opening into the anterior chamber have enhanced the success rate of the procedure in refractory glaucoma. The researchers conclude that the Molteno implant is a useful adjunct to treatment of refractory glaucoma.

Melamid, S., & Fiore P.M. (1990). Molteno implant surgery in refractory glaucoma. *Survey of Ophthalmology,* 34(6), 441-448.

Trabeculectomy and drainage implants

The term *trabeculectomy* is a misnomer because it implies that part of the trabecular meshwork is removed during surgery. Any of the previously described operations for glaucoma may be called a trabeculectomy, with the addition of the dissection of a partial-thickness, limbal-based scleral flap before the anterior chamber is entered. This scleral limbal flap may or may not be loosely sutured before the conjunctival flap is closed. In recent years several types of drainage devices have been implanted into the posterior subconjunctival space with varying success when filtering procedures have been unsuccessful. The most widely used at present is the Molteno implant. Complications have been reduced through modifications in design and technique (Research Highlight 17-3). Adjunctive medical therapy to decrease postoperative fibrosis includes application of an antimetabolite-soaked sponge (5-fluorouracil, Mitomycin) placed under the conjunctival flap. The sponge is left in place for 3 to 5 minutes, and then the site is irrigated vigorously with copious amounts of BSS.

Procedural considerations

Because 5-FU is an antimetabolite, nursing precautions for handling hazardous waste must be carried out. The circulating nurse must wear gloves while drawing up the 5-FU from the vial to transfer to the operative field. All items used with the medication should be disposed of as hazardous waste. Instruments that come in contact with 5-FU should be washed separately (Langseth, 1993). Mitomycin is another antimetabolite used in some settings and should be handled in a similar manner.

Goniotomy

Goniotomy is the opening of a congenital membrane from the iris surface to Schwalbe's line, allowing aqueous humor to reach the trabecular meshwork in cases of congenital glaucoma.

Operative procedure

1. The patient is anesthetized without intubation.
2. An examination is performed. Corneal clarity and size, intraocular pressure, microscopic examination of the anterior segment (including gonioscopy), and examination of the posterior pole of the eye (especially the optic disk) are recorded.
3. The patient is intubated, if indicated, and prepped and draped.
4. A pediatric eye speculum and superior and inferior rectus bridle sutures are placed.
5. Under microscopic control with an appropriate gonioprism in place, the Maumenee irrigating knife is introduced through the temporal limbus. The anterior chamber is kept formed by constant irrigation through the knife. The anterior chamber is crossed, and the membrane covering the iris and angle structures is cut without damaging the trabecular meshwork. The knife is removed.
6. Air may be introduced into the eye, and a suture may be used.
7. A cycloplegic agent may be used topically.
8. The eye is dressed.

Laser therapy

Argon or Nd:YAG laser therapy is being used to treat acute (angle-closure) glaucoma and open-angle glaucoma. Laser therapy is a fairly uncomplicated ambulatory procedure in which a slit lamp is used for delivery of the laser beam. Laser treatment of glaucoma is a noninvasive procedure and, if successful, may eliminate the need for more invasive surgical procedures.

Laser trabeculoplasty

Laser trabeculoplasty is treatment for open-angle glaucoma by the placement of laser burns in the posterior part of the trabeculum, anterior to the scleral spur, to cause the surface of the trabecular meshwork to contract. This theoretically pulls open the adjacent intertrabecular spaces, resulting in increased aqueous outflow.

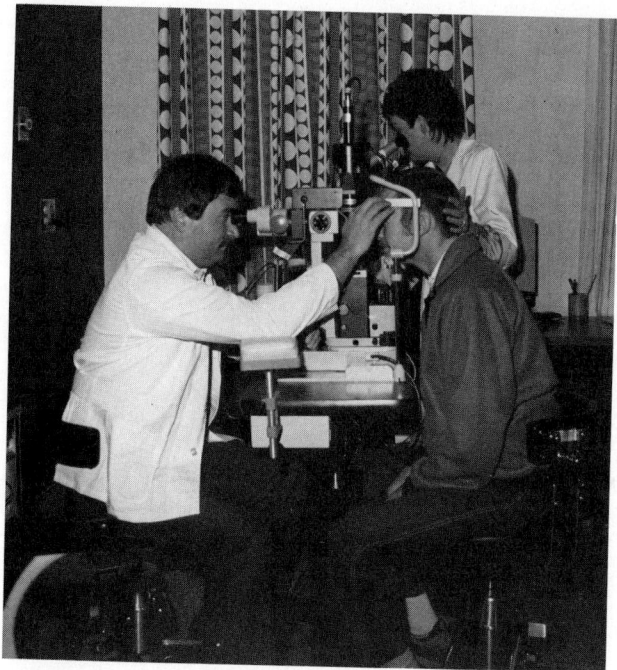

FIG. 17-55   Patient positioned at argon laser slit lamp for treatment of glaucoma.

Procedural considerations

Preoperative sedation is usually unnecessary. A topical anesthetic such as proparacaine is used. Intraocular pressure is measured preoperatively. Laser precautions are initiated (see Chapter 31).

Operative procedure for argon laser trabeculoplasty

1. One or two proparacaine (for example, Ophthaine) drops are instilled in the operative eye.
2. The patient is positioned at the laser slit lamp (Fig. 17-55).
3. A three-mirror Goldmann lens is placed, allowing visualization of the chamber angle and retraction of the eye lid. The perioperative nurse assists in this placement.
4. A landmark is selected as a starting point and laser treatment is begun, using a 50-μmm spot size for 0.1 second at 850 mW power. The laser "burns" are placed in the midtrabecular meshwork, pigmented zone, to yield about 20 burns in each quadrant for a total of 70 to 90 burns. The power should be titrated to the threshold of whitening or tiny bubble formation.
5. One hour after completion of the treatment the intraocular pressure should be measured, and topical prednisolone or dexamethasone drops should be instilled.
6. The procedure may be performed in two treatment segments rather than completed in one.

Argon laser iridotomy

Argon laser iridotomy is the placement of penetrating ar-

gon laser burns in the peripheral iris to create an opening, allowing aqueous humor to flow from the posterior chamber into the anterior chamber and out through Schlemm's canal to treat angle-closure glaucoma.

Procedural considerations

The operative considerations are as for laser trabeculoplasty.

Operative procedure

1. Topical anesthetic drops of proparacaine or an equivalent are instilled.
2. The patient is positioned at the laser slit lamp.
3. The Abraham lens is placed in the operative eye.
4. An iris crypt or "thin" area of iris is selected.
5. Initial burns are placed in a circle to put the iris on a stretch using 200-mm spot size for 0.1 second at 200 to 300 mW power. (Usually six to eight burns accomplish this.)
6. Penetrating burns are placed as needed to make an adequate opening (usually 10 to 30 applications) using 50-mm spot size for 0.1 to 0.2 second at 600 to 1000 mW power.
7. Prednisolone or dexamethasone eyedrops are instilled into the operative eye.

Cyclocryotherapy

Cyclocryotherapy of glaucoma decreases aqueous secretions by ablation of the secretory ciliary epithelium by employing a retinal cryoprobe to freeze a portion of the ciliary body.

Procedural considerations

The procedure is usually performed with topical anesthesia and retrobulbar injection. The patient is prepared as for ophthalmic surgery.

Operative procedure

1. A topical anesthetic is applied, and retrobulbar injection of a local anesthetic drug is done.
2. A lid speculum is placed in the operative eye.
3. The globe is fixed with forceps, and the retinal cryoprobe is placed about 5 mm from the limbus to prevent freezing the cornea and damaging the trabecular meshwork.
4. The upper half of the ciliary body is treated with six applications of the cryoprobe for 60 seconds each at −70°C.
5. Lid closure is verified. The corneal surface is protected with an eye patch.

SURGERY FOR RETINAL DETACHMENT

Retinal detachment is a separation of the neural retinal layer from the pigmented epithelium layer of the retina. Retinal detachment may occur because of the presence of

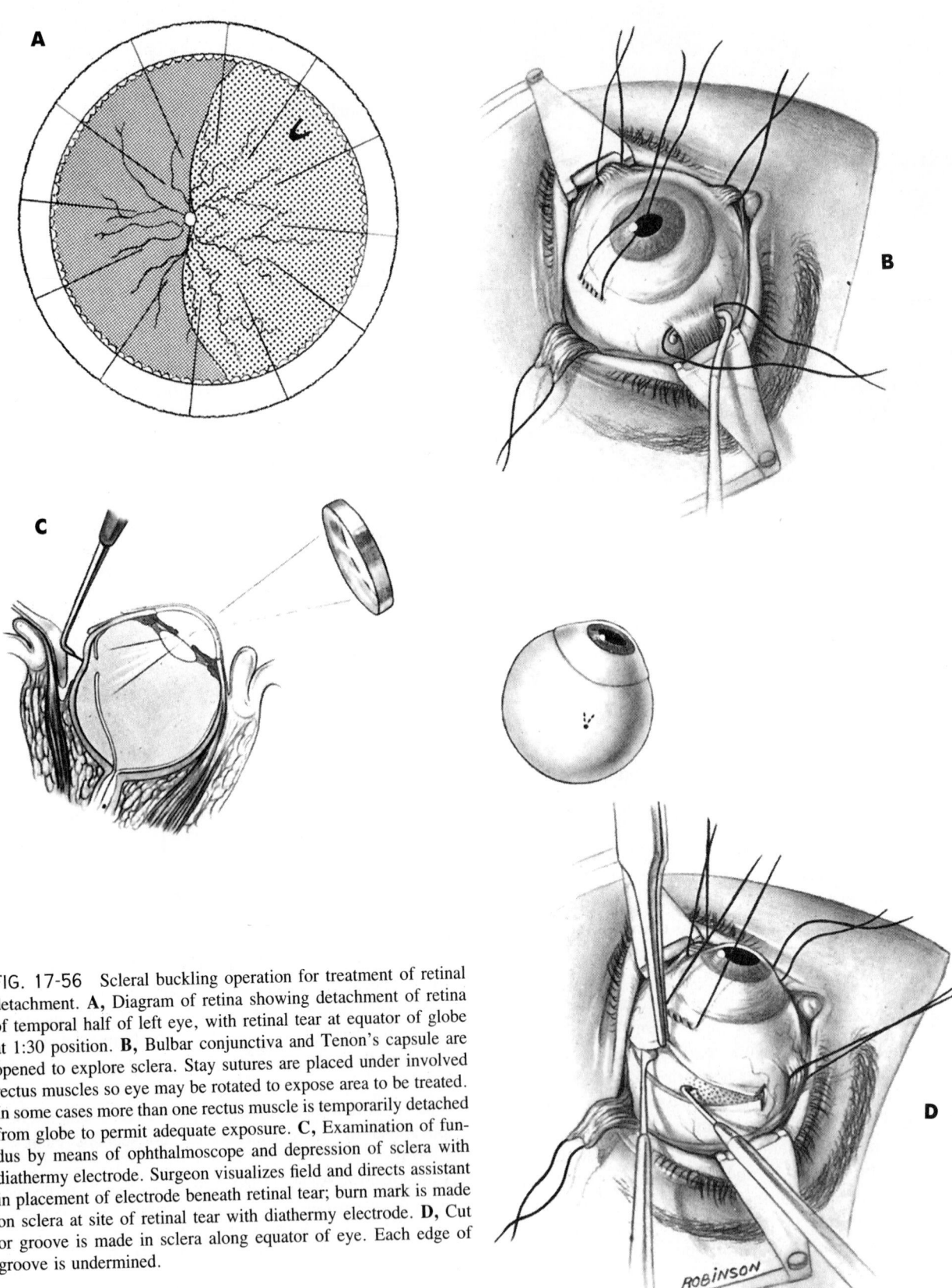

FIG. 17-56   Scleral buckling operation for treatment of retinal detachment. **A,** Diagram of retina showing detachment of retina of temporal half of left eye, with retinal tear at equator of globe at 1:30 position. **B,** Bulbar conjunctiva and Tenon's capsule are opened to explore sclera. Stay sutures are placed under involved rectus muscles so eye may be rotated to expose area to be treated. In some cases more than one rectus muscle is temporarily detached from globe to permit adequate exposure. **C,** Examination of fundus by means of ophthalmoscope and depression of sclera with diathermy electrode. Surgeon visualizes field and directs assistant in placement of electrode beneath retinal tear; burn mark is made on sclera at site of retinal tear with diathermy electrode. **D,** Cut or groove is made in sclera along equator of eye. Each edge of groove is undermined.

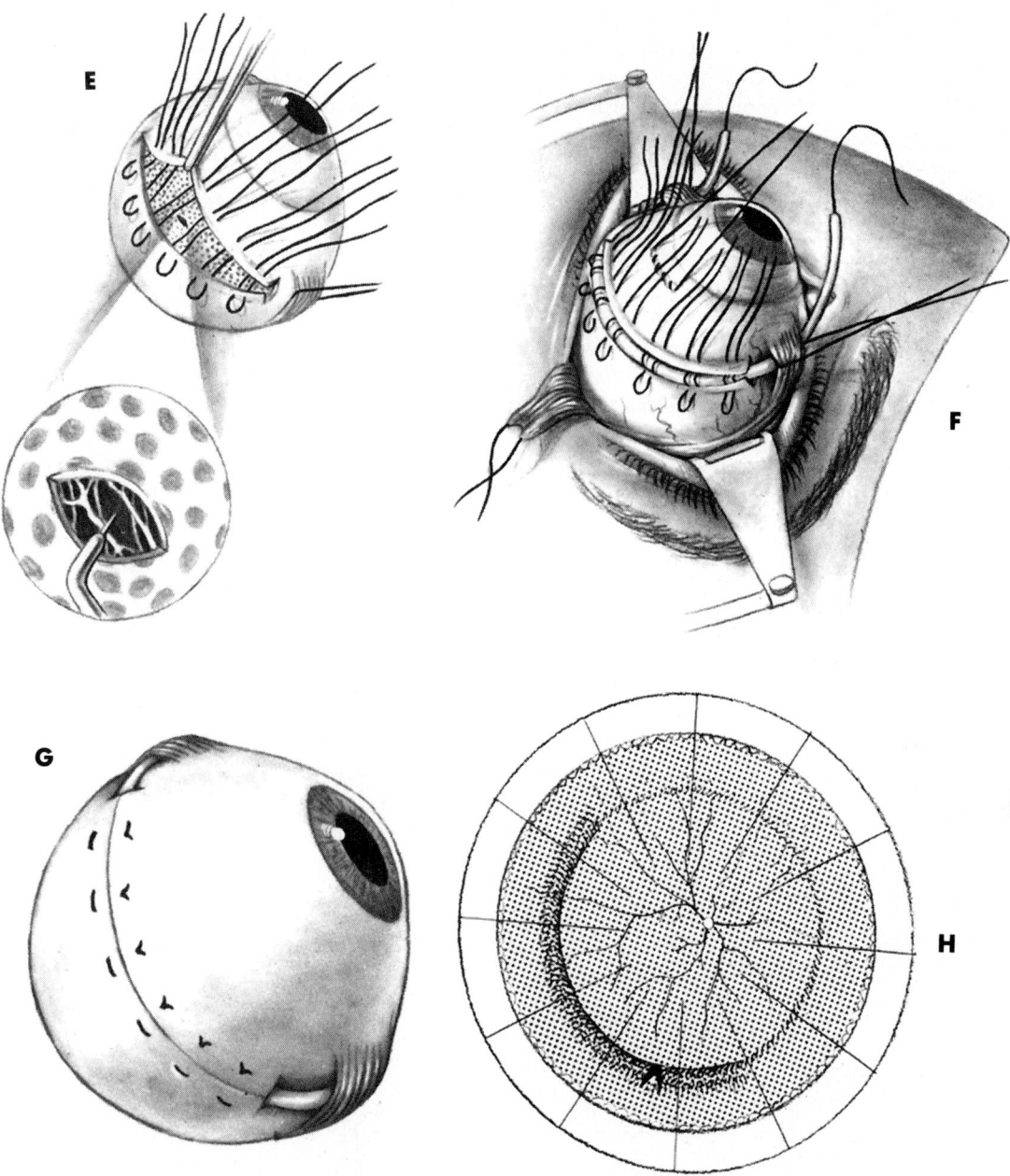

FIG. 17-56, CONT'D   E, Mattress sutures of surgeon's preference are placed across scleral groove. Small incision is made through remaining layer of sclera down to choroid. Choroid is punctured with fine electrode to allow subretinal fluid to drain. F, No. 40 Silastic band is laid in bed of scleral groove under mattress sutures. When retinal tears are large, silicone patch may be placed under band. G, Edges of scleral groove are closed over Silastic band. H, Diagram of fundus with retina in place and 1:30 position retinal tear on buckle. Diathermy reaction is seen on buckle from 12 o'clock to 5:30 positions.

From *Advancing with surgery*, Somerville, N.J., Ethicon, Inc.

intraocular neoplasms originating in the retina or choroid (exudative type) or, more commonly, as a result of retinal tears or holes associated with injury, degeneration, or rhegmatogenous detachment.

Retinal detachment usually causes the sudden onset of the appearance of floating spots before the eye, resulting from freeing of pigment or blood cells in the vitreous. The vitreous humor of the eye is a gelatinous liquid possessing an ultrastructure of fine protein fibers in a network arrangement, with some attachment to the retina. Fluid from the vitreous cavity may seep through the retinal tears and separate the retinal components. The detachment progresses as the liquid seeps behind the retina. The part of the retina that has separated from its nutritional source becomes damaged and relatively nonfunctional.

Prompt treatment of retinal detachment is aimed at preventing permanent loss of central vision. Reattachment of the retina can be accomplished only by surgery. Repair is done from outside the globe. The surgery involves sealing off the area in which the tear or hole is located and may include drainage of the subretinal fluid (Fig. 17-56).

Surgical procedures performed in the treatment of reti-nal detachment include scleral buckling using episcleral and intrascleral techniques with diathermy or cryotherapy. Cryosurgery or light coagulation may be used alone or in combination with a buckling procedure. Instrumentation for retinal surgery is shown in Fig. 17-57.

In the treatment of retinal detachment, the aim is to return the retina to its normal anatomic position. The purpose of surgery for retinal detachment is to cause an intrusion or push into the eye at the site of the pathologic cause. Treatment by diathermy or cryotherapy causes an inflammatory reaction that leads to a permanent adhesion between the detached retina and underlying structures.

Procedural considerations

The patient is prepared as for general ophthalmic surgery.

Operative procedures

A detailed drawing of the retina is made before surgery and is displayed in the operating suite. On the basis of this drawing, the conjunctiva is opened to a previously determined extent, that is, 90 degrees for a simple horseshoe

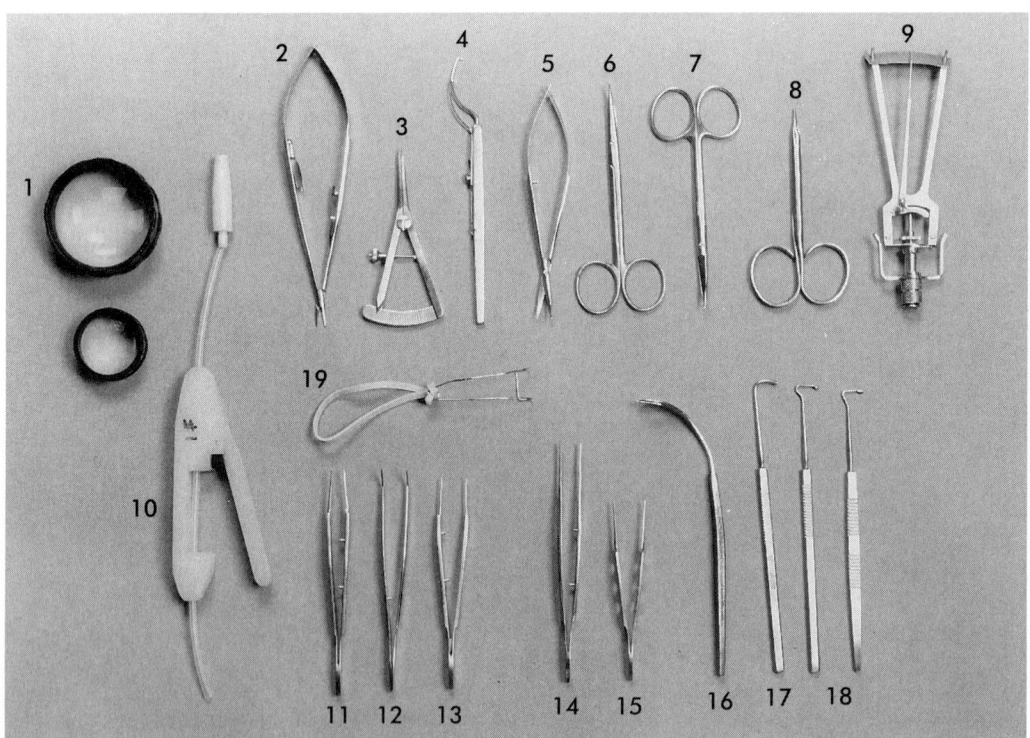

FIG. 17-57   Instruments for retinal surgery. *1,* 20 D and 30 D Nikon lenses; *2,* Castroviejo needle holder; *3,* Castroviejo caliper; *4,* Gonian marker; *5,* Westcott blunt scissors; *6,* tenotomy scissors; *7,* utility scissors; *8,* straight Stevens scissors; *9,* Schiotz tonometer; *10,* irrigating tip (Baylor); *11,* 0.5 forceps; *12,* angled Nugent forceps; *13,* tying forceps; *14,* smooth Bonaccolto forceps; *15,* Bishop forceps with teeth; *16,* Schepens retractor; *17,* cannulated muscle hook; *18,* muscle hooks.

Courtesy Visual Communications, The Methodist Hospital, Houston, Tex.

tear or 360 degrees for an aphakic detachment. With the indirect ophthalmoscope the abnormality is localized under direct visualization, and nonpenetrating diathermy marks are made over the site by indentation.

Episcleral technique

1. Cryotherapy is applied to the pathologic areas under direct visualization (an iceball is seen to form in the proper areas until all of the lesion has been treated).
2. If a localized plombage (push) is to be used, Dacron sutures are set in the sclera surrounding the lesion and tied over Silastic sponges, causing the outer shell of the eye to be pushed toward the elevated retina. If an encircling band is to be used, belt loops are made in the sclera in four quadrants with nos. 64 and 66 Beaver blades. A no. 40 Silastic band is passed 360 degrees around the eye through the belt loops, and a self-holding Watzke sleeve or sutures are applied to the band to maintain a predetermined circumference. This causes a 360-degree constriction of the outer coats into the eye.
3. If drainage of subretinal fluid is desired, under direct visualization an area is chosen in which a significant fluid level exists under the retina, and a diathermy mark is made on the sclera. The sclera is split to the choroid, and a preplaced suture is inserted. A small amount of diathermy is applied to the choroid bed. A needle is then used to puncture the choroid into the subretinal space to permit drainage of fluid. The preplaced suture is tied.

Scleral resection

An incision is made into the sclera, and a scleral flap is dissected both anteriorly and posteriorly from the original incision. Diathermy can be used in this bed, or cryotherapy can be used under direct visualization. Preserved eye bank sclera or a groove piece no. 20 may be sutured into the bed, using a no. 4-0 Supramid suture or no. 5-0 Dacron sutures with or without an encircling band as previously described. Drainage of subretinal fluid may be accomplished as previously described. Air or other replacement or ballast fluids may be introduced into the eye after the drainage of subretinal fluid. This is usually done through the pars plana under direct visualization.

A culture may be taken at the end of the surgery, and a subconjunctival injection of an antibiotic, steroid, or both may be given unless contraindicated. The conjunctiva is closed with a selected suture material, and the eye is patched.

VITRECTOMY

Vitrectomy is narrowly defined as removal of all or part of the vitreous gel (body). In the broader clinical sense of the term, it also includes the cutting and removal of fibrotic membranes, removal of epiretinal membranes, and electrocoagulation of bleeding vessels. In its normal state the vitreous gel of the eye is transparent. In certain disease states bleeding from damaged or newly formed vessels may cause the vitreous to become opaque, which may severely decrease vision. In addition to the patient's inability to see, the ophthalmologist is unable to visualize the retina and therefore treat the underlying pathologic condition before permanent damage can occur. In these cases vitrectomy is indicated to allow the patient to see and the surgeon to institute treatment if indicated.

Certain ophthalmic diseases are associated with the formation of membranes, which may block the visual axis and cause decreased vision. Contraction of these membranes may produce traction-type or rhegmatogenous retinal detachment. In these cases vitrectomy is indicated to relieve the underlying pathologic processes leading to decreased vision.

The main indications for vitrectomy in the anterior segment are the following:

1. Vitreous loss during cataract extraction
2. Opacities in the anterior segment
3. Complications associated with vitreous in the anterior chamber
4. Miscellaneous causes, such as hyphema, pupillary membranes, and residual soft lens material

The main indications for posterior segment vitrectomy via the pars plana are the following:

1. Vitreous opacities, long-standing
2. Advanced diabetic eye disease
3. Severe intraocular trauma
4. Retained foreign bodies
5. Proliferative vitreoretinopathy
6. Retinal detachment from giant tears
7. Endophthalmitis
8. Diagnostic vitreous biopsy

Procedural considerations

The procedure varies according to the location of the pathologic condition (anterior or posterior segments), the instrumentation available, and the surgeon's preference. A pathologic condition in the anterior segment can be ap-

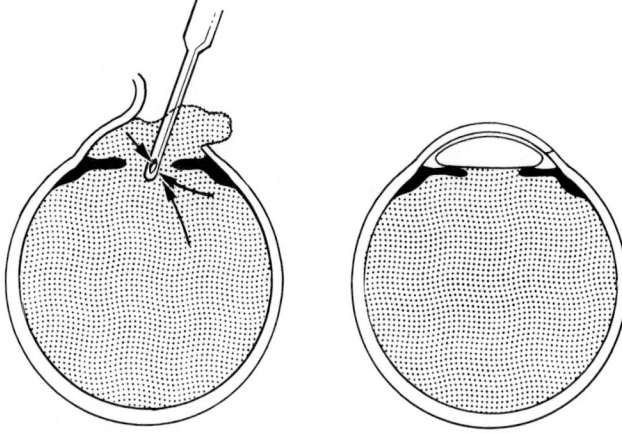

FIG. 17-58   Diagram of management of vitreous loss at time of cataract extraction.

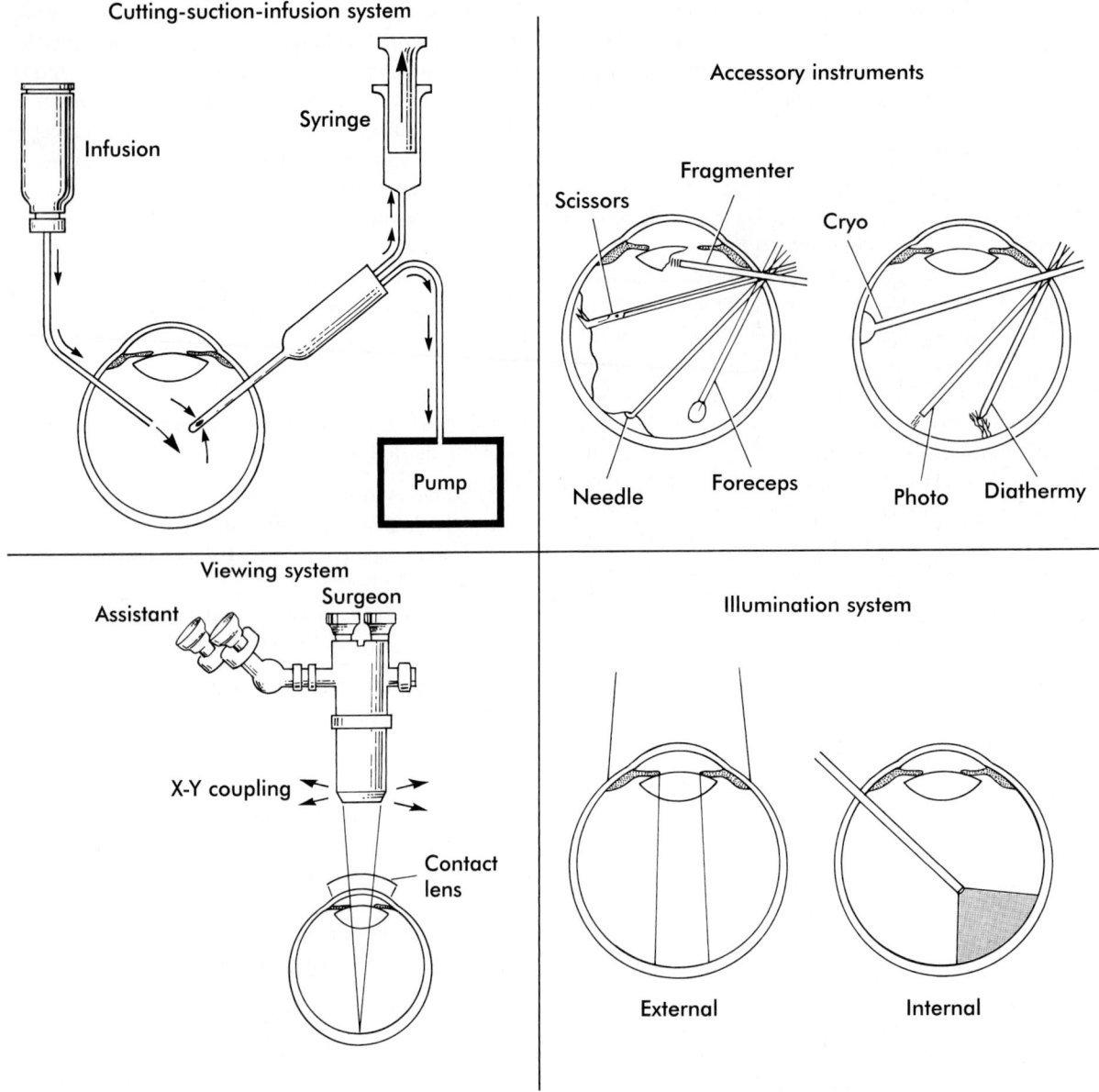

FIG. 17-59   Vitrectomy procedures require the following: *1*, cutting-suction-infusion system; *2*, accessory instruments; *3*, viewing system with **X-Y** coupling; and *4*, illumination system.

proached through a limbal incision, as in lens extraction with vitreous loss (Fig. 17-58); through "open sky," after trephine incision for penetrating keratoplasty; or through the pars plana. A pathologic condition in the posterior segment is usually approached through the pars plana.

Vitrectomy is a microsurgical procedure requiring a viewing system (operating microscope with an **X-Y** coupling, zoom lens, and fine focus), an illumination system, a cutting-suction-infusion system, and accessory instruments (Fig. 17-59).

The infusion system consists of a 500-ml bottle of buffered BSS, such as BSS Plus, a standard intravenous administration set, and an infusion needle or sleeve (Fig. 17-

60), or it may be part of a one-time use, single multifunction handpiece (Fig. 17-61). The level of intraocular pressure can be varied by elevating or lowering the infusion bottle in relation to the patient's eye.

The suction and cutting systems vary in sophistication, but all cutters engage tissue into a port and then cut it by shearing action between the edges of a moving and a nonmoving part. Guillotine cutters have a linear, to-and-fro action, whereas reciprocating or oscillating cutters rotate in a clockwise-counterclockwise fashion. Suction is operated with a pump controlled by a foot switch to maintain the level of aspiration. An endolaser or indirect laser delivery system is usually available for photocoagulation (Fig. 17-

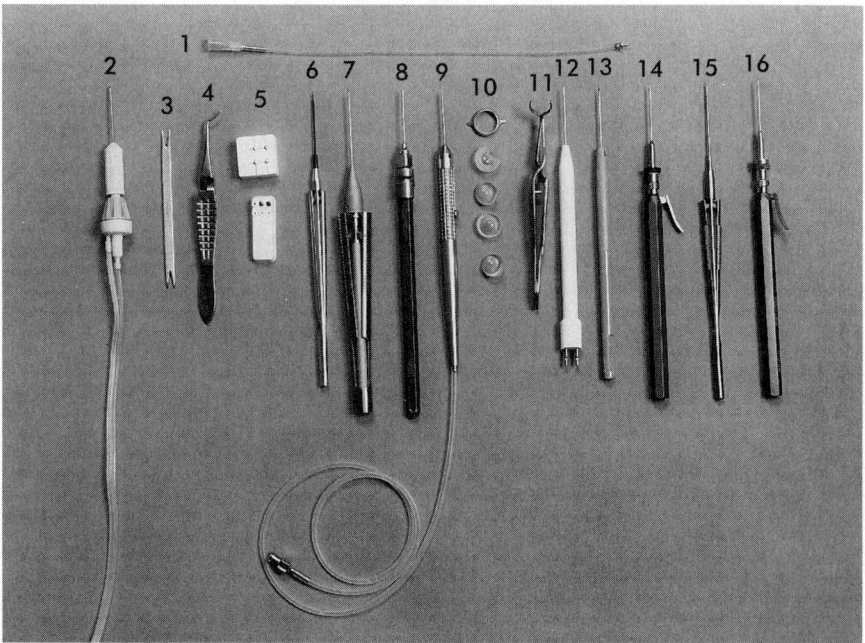

FIG. 17-60   Accessory instruments for vitrectomy; *1*, 4-mm infusion cannula; *2*, variable port vitrector *3*, 3.5- and 4-mm premeasured calipers; *4*, scleral plug holder; *5*, scleral plugs in tablets; *6*, Lambert subretinal forceps; *7*, Thomas subretinal handle; *8*, Charles vacuum cannula; *9*, Flynn needle; *10*, Landers lenses and ring; *11*, Landers lens holder; *12*, wet field endocautery; *13*, MVR blade; *14*, Grieshaber side-gripping forceps; *15*, D.O.R.C. end-gripping forceps; *16*, Grieshaber vertical cutting scissors.

Courtesy Visual Communications, The Methodist Hospital, Houston, Tex.

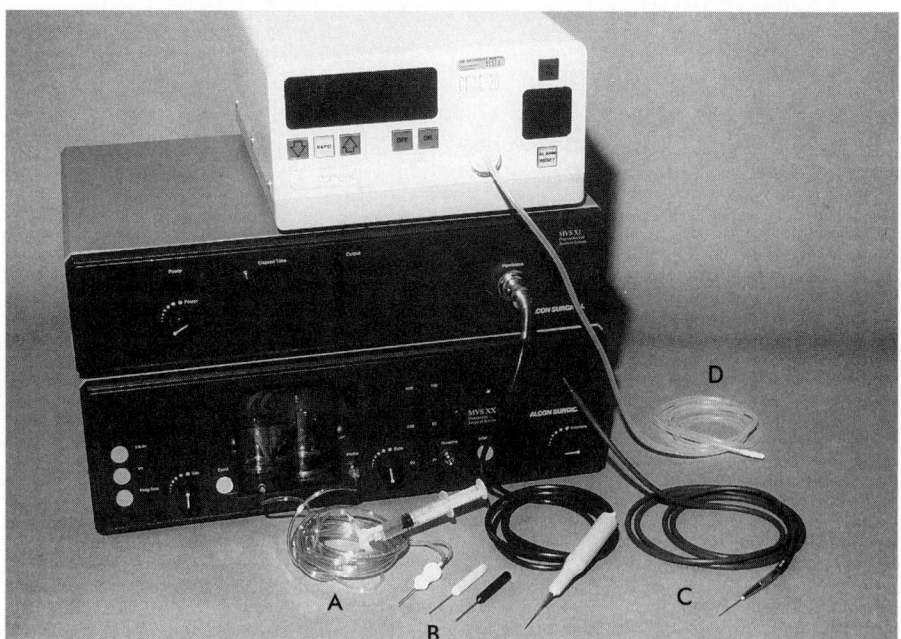

FIG. 17-61   *Top*, Trek air exchange unit. *Bottom*, Alcon surgical vitrectomy and fragmentation units showing accessories from left to right: *a*, vitrectomy tubing with disposable handpiece; *b*, extrusion handpieces; *c*, fragmentor handpiece, fiberoptic light pipe (endoilluminator).

Courtesy Visual Communications, The Methodist Hospital, Houston, Tex.

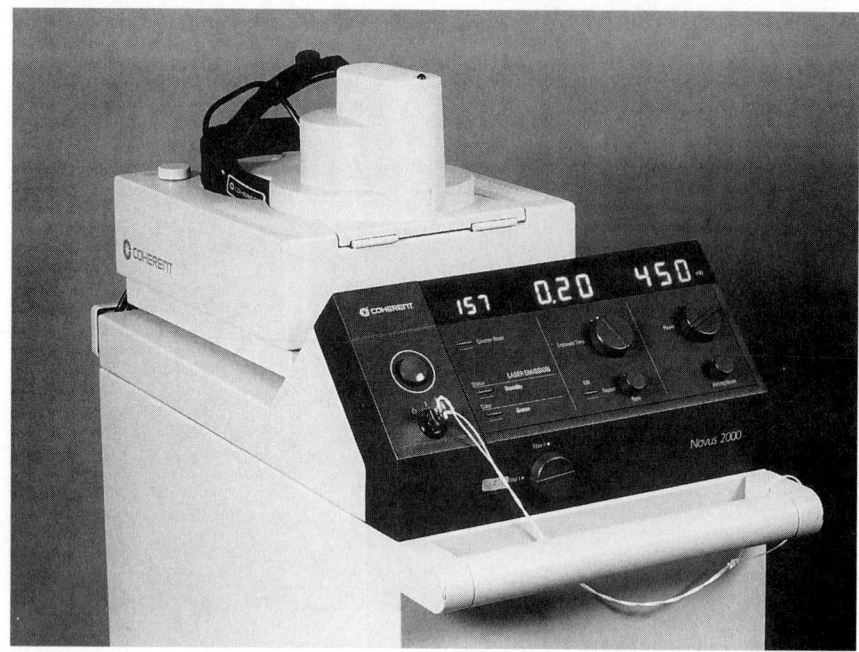

FIG. 17-62 Argon laser with indirect ophthalmoscope.
Courtesy Visual Communications, The Methodist Hospital, Houston, Tex.

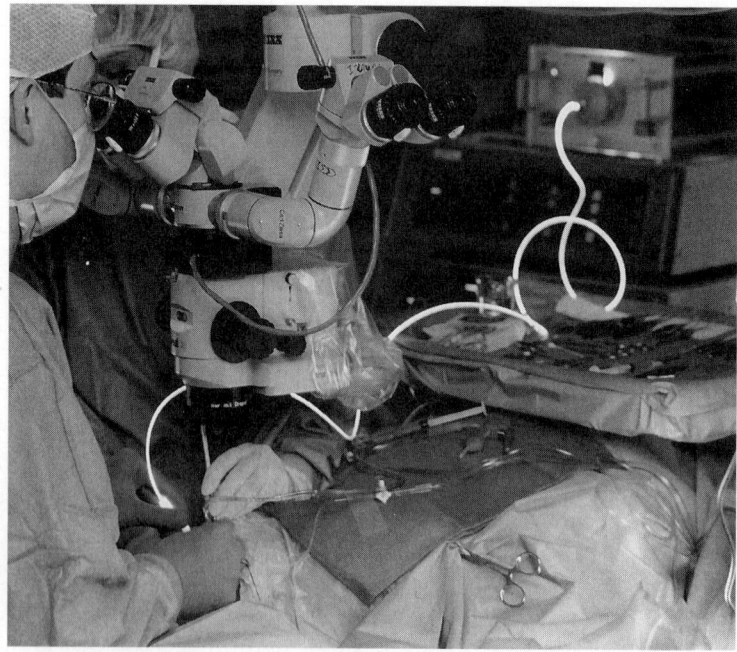

FIG. 17-63 Surgical field during vitrectomy procedure showing position of instrumentation: surgeon looks through the operating microscope while illuminating the retinal layer and vitreous with a fiberoptic light pipe. When the microscope is not draped, sterile plastic bags are used to adjust the lenses. The scrubbed personnel and surgeon must be especially vigilant to avoid contamination.
Courtesy Visual Communications, The Methodist Hospital, Houston, Tex.

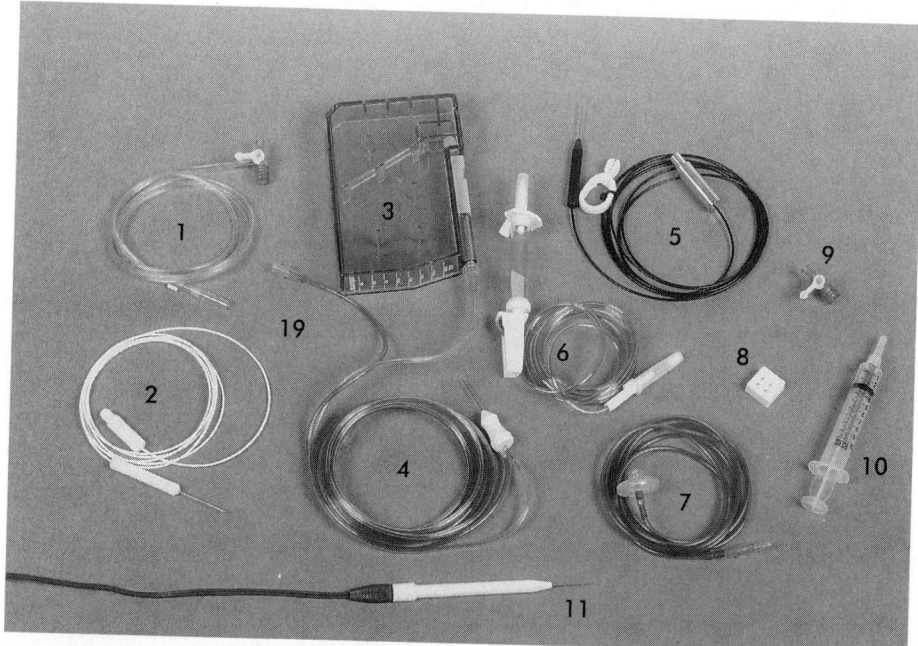

FIG. 17-64 Disposable vitrectomy accessories: *1,* Tubing with three-way stopcock for fragmentor extrusion; *2,* fiberoptic light pipe; *3,* collection cassette connected to vitrectomy tubing and probe *(4); 5,* endolaser probe; *6,* infusion tubing; *7,* air pump tubing; *8,* scleral plugs; *9,* three-way stopcock; *10,* syringe; *11,* wet field cord with hemostatic eraser.
Courtesy Visual Communications, The Methodist Hospital, Houston, Tex.

62). Illumination for vitrectomy is external, using the operating microscope for anterior segment vitrectomy, and internal, using a fiberoptic light pipe (endoilluminator) (Figs. 17-61 and 17-63). Replacement of the vitreous with air is facilitated with a special air exchange unit (see Fig. 17-61). Other substances under study for intraocular tamponade are perfluoropropane gas (C_3F_6), sulfur hexafluoride gas (SF_6), liquid perfluorocarbons, and silicone oil. Accessory instruments (Fig. 17-64) usually have a 20-gauge diameter so they can be interchanged throughout the procedure. Accessory instruments include the following:

Hooks, picks, and scissors for dissection of membranes	Flute needles for evacuating pools of blood or for fluid-gas exchange
Foreign body microforceps	Subretinal forceps
Intraocular cryoprobe for cryocoagulation	(Figs. 17-65, *A,* and 17-66)

To prepare for a vitrectomy procedure, the perioperative nurse must know the location of the problem, how the surgeon plans to address the problem (route of entry into the eye—anterior or posterior, open sky or closed), instrumentation to be used, and anticipated extent and length of the procedure.

Instrument and equipment functioning should be thoroughly checked before bringing the patient into the operating room. When a lens extraction procedure is planned, vitrectomy instrumentation should be ready in the event of ac-

cidental vitreous loss. When preparing for pars plana vitrectomy in the posterior segment, the perioperative nurse must be aware that a combined scleral buckling procedure may be necessary.

For repair of a giant retinal tear a special OR bed may be used, allowing the patient to be turned to a prone position after the vitrectomy procedure for exchange of fluid and air or a special gas to tamponade the retina. In recent years studies have been carried out using perfluorocarbons and other materials to provide retinal tamponade. These techniques allow repositioning and tamponade of the retina without the need for extremely awkward and uncomfortable positioning that was previously mandated (Research Highlight 17-4). Vitrectomy procedures vary in length from less than 1 hour to over 6 hours. When a long procedure is anticipated, care must be taken to protect the patient's skin and reduce pressure areas. A foam mattress pad, heel and elbow protectors, and elasticized stockings may be used. When the patient is positioned for vitrectomy, the head should be higher than the heart, the cheeks higher than the forehead, and the neck extended. A wrist support may be placed around the patient's head to support the surgeon's wrist during manipulation of the intraocular instruments.

While draping, the perioperative nurse should provide for removal of infusion fluid from the operative field and take care to protect electrical foot switches from fluid damage. Instrumentation for scleral buckle and vitrectomy is shown in Figs. 17-60 to 17-67.

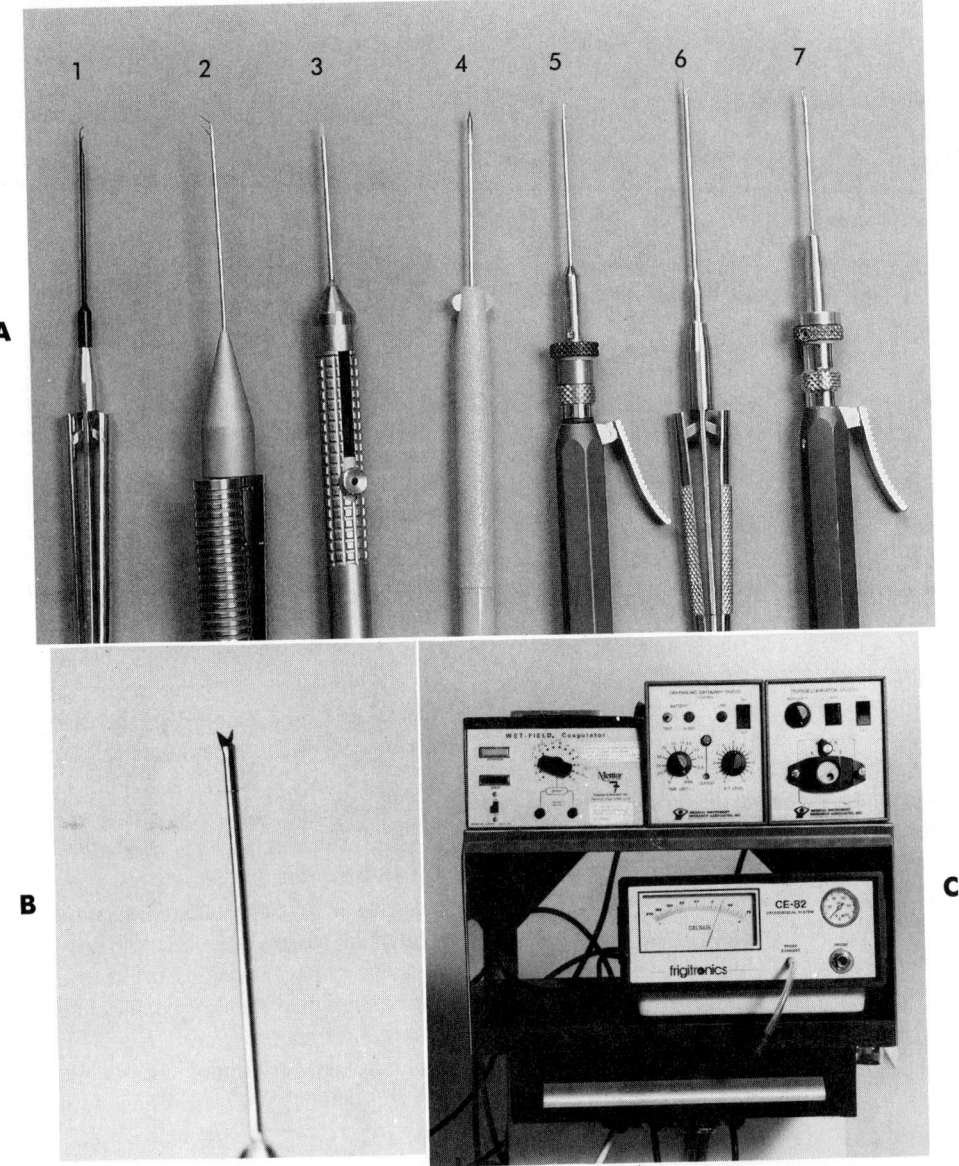

FIG. 17-65 **A,** Delicate tips of ophthalmic instrumentation. *1,* Lambert subretinal forceps; *2,* Thomas subretinal forceps; *3,* Flynn needle; *4,* MVR blade; *5,* Grieshaber side-gripping forceps; *6,* D.O.R.C. end-gripping forceps; *7,* Grieshaber vertical cutting scissors. **B,** Accessory instruments are extremely delicate, as shown in the Grieshaber vitreous scissors, and require careful handling. **C,** Power sources for accessory instruments: wet field bipolar coagulator, ophthalmic diathermy, and Frigitronics cryosurgical system.

A Courtesy Visual Communications, The Methodist Hospital, Houston, Tex.

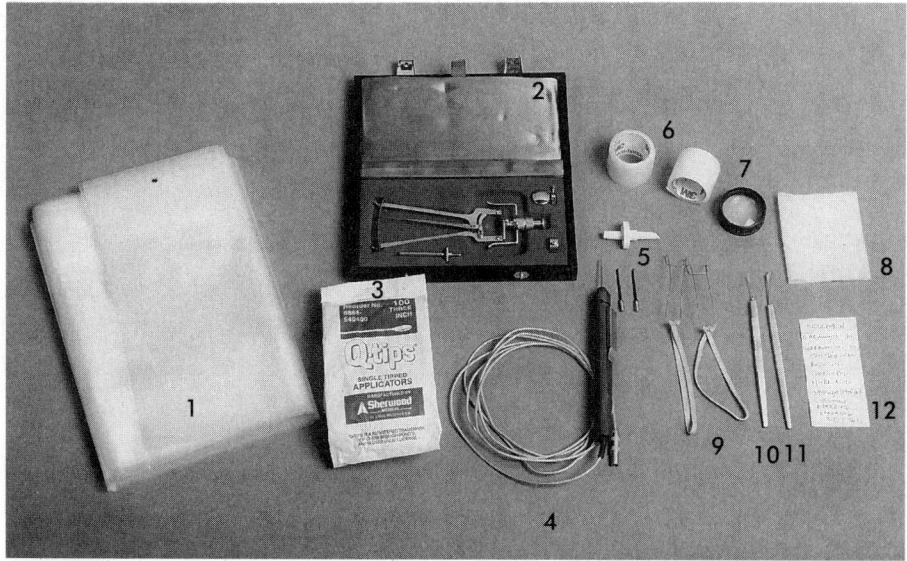

FIG. 17-66 Supplies for scleral buckle or vitrectomy. *1*, Plastic bag; *2*, tonometer; *3*, applicators; *4*, diathermy cord and tips; *5*, adapter for irrigating fluid; *6*, transpore tape; *7*, 30 D Volk lens; *8*, lens paper; *9*, Jaffe lid specula rubber bands; *10*, Ziegler knife; *11*, scarifier; *12*, labels.

Courtesy Visual Communications, The Methodist Hospital, Houston, Tex.

RESEARCH HIGHLIGHT 17-4

Multiparticipant group studies (eye centers in the United States) were conducted in two phases from September 1985 through October 1990. The first phase compared the effectiveness of sulfur hexafluoride (SF_6) gas and silicone oil as an intraocular tamponade in 101 randomized patients without prior vitrectomy and with severe proliferative vitreoretinopathy (PVR). Silicone oil was found to be superior to SF_6 gas in the treatment of retinal detachments with PVR.

The second phase of the study randomized 132 eyes without prior vitrectomy and 139 with previous vitrectomy, and compared results following intraocular tamponade with perfluoropropane (C_3F_8) gas to silicone oil in the treatment of PVR. No significant difference in the outcome was found. Both silicone oil and perfluoropropane gas produced superior results to those obtained with SF_6 gas. Additional studies to confirm the persistence of keratopathy and the incidence of recurrent retinal detachment upon removal of the silicone oil are planned.

Lean, J., et al. (1992, June). Vitrectomy with silicone oil or sulphur hexafluoride gas in eyes with severe proliferative vitreoretinopathy: Results of a randomized clinical trial. *Archives of Ophthalmology, 110,* 770-779.
McCuen, B., et al. (1992, June). Vitrectomy with silicone oil or perfluoropropane gas in eyes with severe proliferative vitreoretinopathy: results of a randomized trial. *Archives of Ophthalmology, 110,* 780-792.

Operative procedures
Anterior vitrectomy for accidental vitreous loss during cataract extraction (Fig. 17-68)

1. A vitreous cutter is placed in the eye through the cataract wound. Infusion may be through the handpiece or separately.
2. The cutter is placed in the middle of the pupil, posterior to the iris, and enough vitreous is removed to ensure that no vitreous remains in the anterior chamber and that the iris has fallen back into normal position.
3. The pupil is constricted with acetylcholine. The anterior chamber may be filled with air.
4. The procedure is completed as for lens extraction.

Anterior vitrectomy for anterior segment opacities, hyphema, pupillary membranes, and residual soft lens material (Fig. 17-68)

1. Appropriate fixation sutures or a lid speculum is placed.
2. An incision is made at the limbus either through clear cornea or under a conjunctival flap. One to three incisions are made, depending on the vitreous cutter chosen and the technique.
3. If a multifunction probe is not used, an infusion cannula is placed in one incision and the vitreous cutter in another. A third incision may be used for an accessory instrument. The vitreous is removed.
4. The incisions are closed.
5. The eye is patched.

Pars plana vitrectomy (Fig. 17-69)

1. A lid speculum and appropriate fixation sutures are placed.

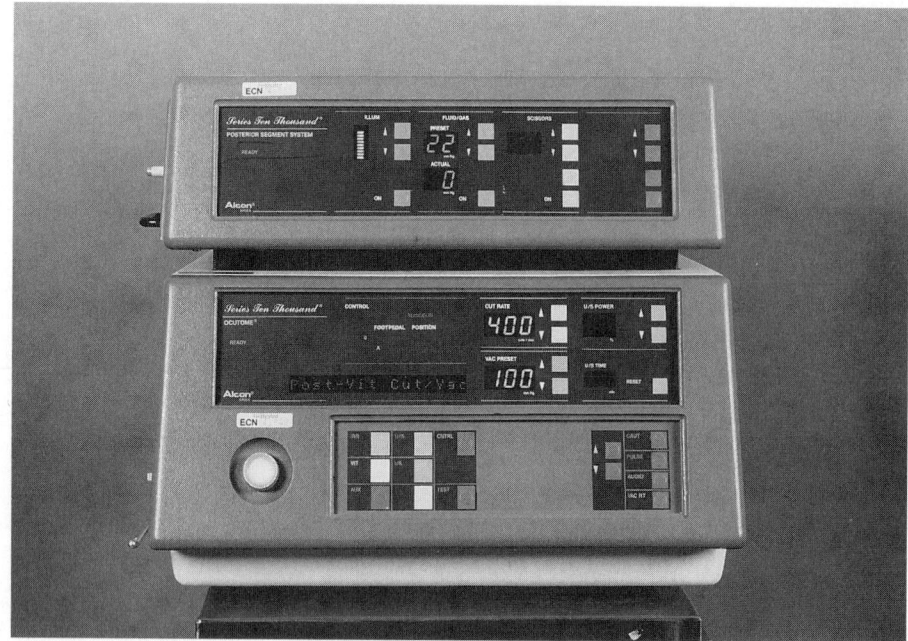

FIG. 17-67   Alcon series 10,000 Vitrector.
Courtesy Visual Communications, The Methodist Hospital, Houston, TX.

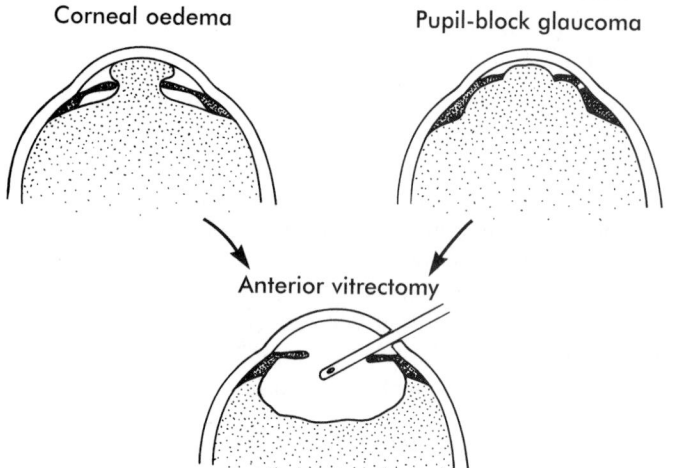

FIG. 17-68   Anterior vitrectomy procedure for complications of vitreous in anterior chamber.

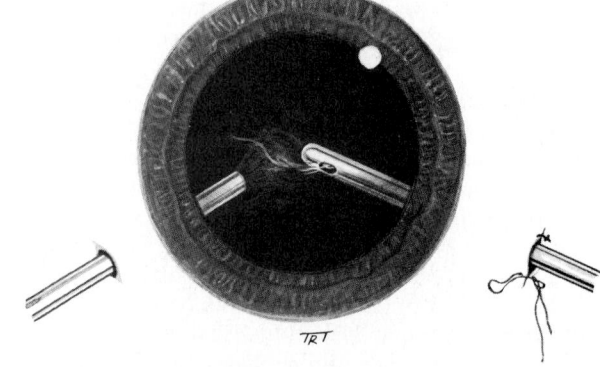

FIG. 17-69   Introduction of cutter and fiberoptic light pipe through pars plana for posterior vitrectomy.

From Kanski, J.J. (1984). *Clinical ophthalmology*. London: Butterworth.

2. Three incisions are made through the pars plana; one for infusion, one for endoillumination, and one for a vitreous cutter or other instrumentation.
3. The infusion line is sutured in place with a purse-string suture of no. 5-0 Dacron. The line is checked to ensure proper placement.
4. The operating microscope is aligned, and a fundus lens is fixed on the anterior surface of the cornea.
5. The infusion rate, cutting rate, and aspiration rate are set on the machine console. The vitreous is removed under direct visualization.

6. Once the medium has been removed and the retinal condition visualized, the necessary injections or treatment(s) are completed to provide retinal tamponade with vitrectomy instruments or accessories. A scleral buckling procedure may also be performed.
7. The pars plana incisions are closed, and the conjunctival incision is sutured. Cultures from the vitreous washings are taken, if necessary.
8. Subconjunctival injections of steroids or antibiotics are given if necessary, the eye is patched, and an eye shield is secured in place.

LASER PHOTOCOAGULATION AND CRYOTHERAPY TREATMENTS

In addition to intraocular photocoagulation with argon laser or cryocoagulation used during vitrectomy procedures, argon laser photocoagulation can be delivered through a slit lamp to the retina as a noninvasive, ambulatory procedure to treat flat retinal holes or tears, sites of potential pathologic conditions, and vascular proliferative diseases, such as diabetic retinopathy.

Operative procedures
Laser treatment

1. The patient's pupil is dilated, and a retrobulbar anesthetic may be used.
2. Proparacaine drops are instilled into the operative eye.
3. A three-mirror Goldmann or similar lens, which has been lubricated, is placed on the cornea, and the patient is positioned at the laser slit lamp.
4. The proper spot size, power setting, and duration of exposure are set.
5. Laser burns are placed in the prescribed areas.
6. The patient's eye is irrigated with physiologic saline solution to remove the viscous lens lubricant.
7. The eye is patched as necessary.

An Nd:YAG laser is also used for lysis of vitreous strands or bands and to open opaque posterior capsules. The procedure is similar to argon laser treatment in its delivery through a slit lamp. A Peyman lens for a specific depth is selected and used in place of the Goldmann lens when cutting vitreous strands. No lens or anesthetic is needed to open posterior capsules. The patient is positioned at the laser slit lamp, and pulsed laser applications using 1 to 3 mJ of power are used to open the posterior capsule.

Cryocoagulation

Cryocoagulation through the conjunctiva may be used to treat some pathologic conditions of the retina when a more invasive procedure is unnecessary or the area is not accessible with a laser.

1. The operative eye is anesthetized with local anesthetic injections and topical drops.
2. A lid speculum is placed in the operative eye.
3. The globe is positioned with a fixation forceps, and the pathologic area is localized with the indirect ophthalmoscope.
4. The retinal cryoprobe is applied to the external surface of the globe in the area of the pathologic condition, and the area is treated.
5. The eye is patched.

REFERENCES

Cataract Management Guideline Panel. (1993). *Cataract in adults: Management of functional impairment* (Clinical Practice Guideline, No. 4). Rockville, Md: U.S. Dept. of Health and Human Services, Public Health Service, Agency for Health Care Policy and Research. (AHCPR Pub. No. 93-0542. Feb. 1993, 40-43).

Langseth, F. (1993) The use of 5-fluorouracil in glaucoma filtration surgery. *The Journal of the American Society of Ophthalmic Registered Nurses, 23* (20), 11-13.

Lean, J., et al. (1992). Vitrectomy with silicone oil or sulphur hexafluoride gas in eyes with severe proliferative vitreoretinopathy; results of a randomized clinical trial. *Archives of Ophthalmology, 110* (9), 770-779.

McCuen, B., et al. (1992). Vitrectomy with silicone oil or perfluorpropane gas in eyes with severe proliferative vitreoretinopathy: results of a randomized clinical trial, *Archives of Ophthalmology, 110* (9), 780-792.

Melamid, S., & Fiore, P. (1990). Molteno implant surgery in refractory glaucoma. *Survey of Ophthalmology, 34* (6), 441-447.

Phippen, M., Wells, M., & Martinelli, A. (1993). *A conceptual model for perioperative nursing practice.* Philadelphia: W.B. Saunders.

Silverstone, D.E., Hufnagle, T., & Miller, J.M. (1989). *Effect of carbochol and acetylcholine on the corneal endothelium and IOP in cataract surgery.* Paper presented at the American Academy of Ophthalmology, New Orleans.

Yamada, S et al. (1993). An eye on comfort: positioning a patient for ophthalmic surgery. *Journal of Ophthalmic Nursing Technology, 12* (2), 75-78.

BIBLIOGRAPHY

Atkinson, L.J. (1992). Berry and Kohn's operating room technique (7th ed.). St. Louis: Mosby.

Annand, F. (1992). A challenge for the 1990's: Patient education. *Journal of Ophthalmic Nursing and Technology, 11* (5), 206-210.

Barnhart, E.R. (1993). *Physicians' desk reference for ophthalmology,* (17th ed.). Oradell, N.J.: Medical Economics Company.

Boyd-Monk, H., & Steinmetz, C. (1987). *Nursing care of the eye.* Norwalk, Conn.: Appleton & Lange.

Elfervig, L., (1993). Eye care and AIDS prevention for ophthalmic medical personnel. *Journal of Ophthalmic Nursing and Technology, 12* (3), 117-121.

Goldblum, K. (1992). Knowledge deficit in the ophthalmic patient. *Nursing Clinics of North America, 27* (3), 715-725.

Hagan, J., & Wyatt, B. (1993). Preoperative evaluation and workup of the cataract and intraocular lens implant patient. *Journal of Ophthalmic Nursing and Technology, 12* (3), 123-128.

Hannon, V. (1993). Cataract surgery. *Journal of Ophthalmic Nursing and Technology, 12* (1), 13-17.

Kanski, J. (1989). *Clinical ophthalmology* (2nd ed.). London: Butterworth.

Lambrix, K.K. (1987). Epikeratophakia. *AORN Journal, 46* (2), 218-236.

Langseth, F. (1988). Transscleral cyclophotocoagulation: A laser treatment for glaucoma. *AORN Journal, 48* (6), 1122-1127.

Langseth, F. (1991). Levator aponeurosis surgery: Surgical correction for blepharoptosis. *AORN Journal, 54* (4), 731-741.

Martinelli, A. (1991). Glaucoma. *AORN Journal, 54* (4), 743-759.

Mailhot, C., & Slezak, L. (1993). *Ophthalmology surgery: Advanced training for operating room clinical specialities.* Garden Grove CA, Medcom.

Nelson, L.B., Calhoun, J., & Harley, R. (1991). *Pediatric ophthalmology.* Philadelphia: W.B. Saunders.

Occupational exposure to bloodborne pathogens. (1992). Washington, DC: U.S. Department of Labor, Occupational Safety and Health Administration. (OSHA 3127 1-30)

Obstbaum, S. (1991). Small incision surgery: Wound construction and closure. *Journal of Cataract and Refractive Surgery, 17* (Suppl. 1991). 659-748.

Pagana K., & Pagana, T. (1992). *Mosby's diagnostic and laboratory test reference*. St. Louis: Mosby.

Paige, B. (1992). The excimer laser: Program implementation and nursing implications. *Journal of Ophthalmic Nursing and Technology, 11* (6), 251-255.

Plona, R., & Schremp, P. (1992). Nursing care of patients with ocular manifestations of human immunodeficiency virus infection. *Nursing Clinics of North America, 27* (3), 793-805.

Rakel, B. (1992). Interventions related to patient teaching. *Nursing Clinics of North America, 27* (2), 397-405.

Rankin, S., & Duffy, K. (1990). *Patient education issues: Principles and practices*. Philadelphia: J.B. Lippincott.

Reeves, W. (1993). Surgical experience of the ophthalmic patient. *Journal of the American Society of Ophthalmic Registered Nurses, 28* (1), 16-22.

Ruehl, C., & Schremp, P. (1992). Nursing care of the cataract patient. *Nursing Clinics of North America, 27* (3), 727-743.

Servidido, C., & Abramson, D. (1992). Choroidal melanoma. *Nursing Clinics of North America, 27* (3), 777-790.

Smith, S. (1992). Diabetic retinopathy. *Nursing Clinics of North America, 27* (3), 745-759.

Smith, S. (1992). *Standards of ophthalmic nursing practice*. San Francisco: American Society of Ophthalmic R.N.'s (ASORN) in conjunction with American Academy of Ophthalmology.

Spadoni, D., & Cain, C.L. (1988). Laser blepharoplasty: The transconjunctival method. *AORN Journal, 47* (11), 1184-1194.

Spaeth, G. (1990). Ophthalmic surgery: Principles and practice (2nd ed.). Philadelphia: W.B. Saunders.

Stein, H., Shott B., & Stein, R. (1988). The ophthalmic assistant: Fundamentals and clinical practice (4th ed.). St. Louis: Mosby.

Steur, K. (1991). Facial fractures: Diagnosis to discharge. *AORN Journal, 54* (4), 774-792.

Thomson-Keith, E. (1991). *Care of the ophthalmology patient*. Denver: The Association of Operating Room Nurses, Inc.

Vaughan, D., Asbury, T., & Riordan-Eva P. (1992). *General ophthalmology* (13th ed.). Los Altos, Calif.: Appleton & Lange.

18

OTOLOGIC SURGERY

PATRICIA S. COUTELLIER

New concepts and procedures related to otologic surgery are being introduced, and older procedures are constantly being refined. Antibiotics, the operating microscope, delicate instruments, improvements in implantable prosthetic devices, and better understanding of the anatomy and physiology of the ear enable the otologic surgeon to perform procedures that improve patients' hearing and balance and to have greater control over diseases of the middle ear and mastoid. Surgical treatment for sensorineural hearing loss, or Ménière's disease, can be offered to patients who are afflicted by intolerable tinnitus or vertigo severe enough to be disabling. Surgical treatment aimed at correcting hearing losses resulting from conduction apparatus abnormalities includes stapedectomy and ossicular replacement procedures. New hope for deaf patients has been found in the area of cochlear implantation. Technologic advancements have contributed significantly to improved outcomes for patients with otologic problems.

The Latin word *audire* means to hear; thus, the word *auditory* refers to the sense of hearing. The physical nature of sound results from the compression and rarefaction of pressure waves and moving molecules, but the sensations humans actually experience are the product of complex mechanical, electrical, and psychologic interactions in the ear and central nervous system. The study of the ear and its diseases is known as otology, derived from the Greek word *otos,* meaning ear.

The ear is a complex mechanism that receives sound waves, discriminates their frequencies, and then transmits this information to the central nervous system for interpretation. When a person falls asleep, hearing is the last sense to disappear; when a person awakens, it is the first sense to return. An additional function of the human ear is the maintenance of body equilibrium.

For a person to hear, the following sequence takes place:

1. The sound waves collect in the auricle.
2. The waves pass into the external canal and cause the eardrum to vibrate.
3. The ossicles, arranged in a lever system, respond to the vibration. First the malleus moves, and then this movement is transmitted to the incus, which in turn transmits it to the stapes. The amplification occurs because the area of the eardrum or tympanic membrane is much greater than the stapes footplate, thereby concentrating the sound in the cochlea.
4. The small footplate of the stapes delivers the sound to the inner ear by rocking the oval window.
5. Sound pressure, delivered through the oval window into the cochlea, sends a fluid wave through the perilymph, which in turn deflects the membranes of the endolymphatic compartment.
6. The receptors of hearing (hair cells) are distorted, causing the mechanical waves to be transformed into electrochemical impulses.
7. The fluid wave is damped and absorbed at the round window membrane.
8. These impulses are sent by way of the acoustic nerve to the brainstem (pons) and then are relayed to the temporal cortex of the brain, where they are interpreted as meaningful sound.

The amplitude of the air waves that strike the tympanic membrane determines the loudness or intensity of the sound. In dealing with hearing loss, the loudness is measured in decibels (dB). It is a logarithmic method of dealing with large numbers; the decibel is a ratio, not an absolute value, that compares the relationship between two sound intensities and the smallest perceptible change in loudness that the human ear can hear. Hearing loss is expressed by recording auditory acuity for each frequency in decibels.

SURGICAL ANATOMY

The ear is a sensory organ that functions in the identification, localization, and interpretation of sound, as well as in the maintenance of equilibrium. Anatomically, it is divided into the external, middle, and inner ear (Fig. 18-1).

The external ear, including the auricle (or pinna) and external auditory canal, is composed of cartilage covered with skin. The auricle, extending slightly outward from the

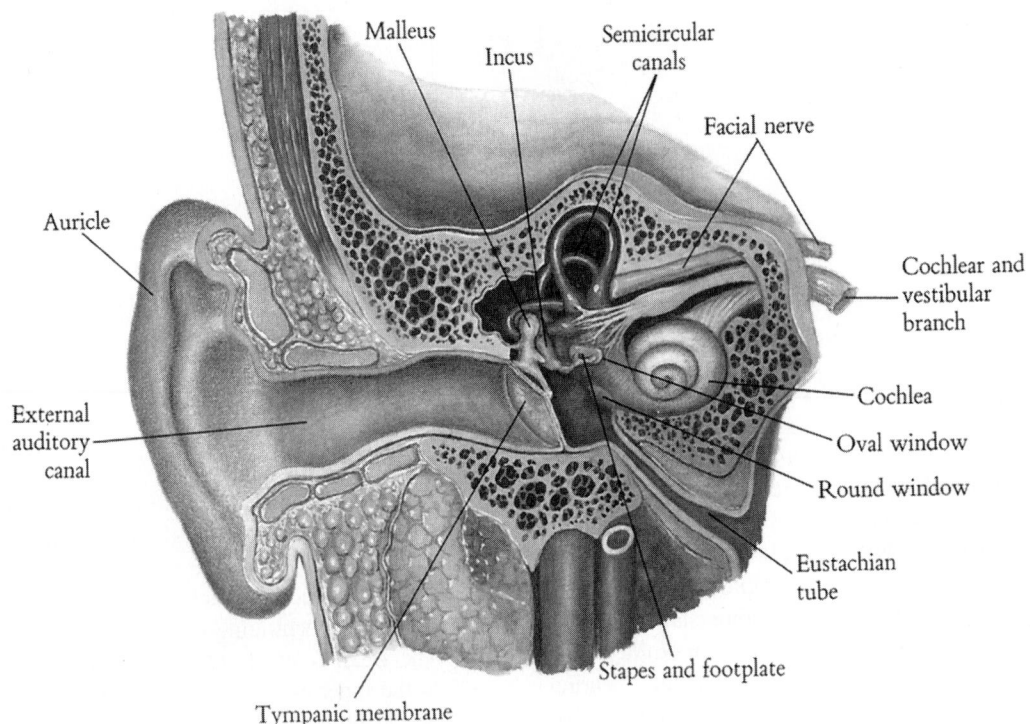

FIG. 18-1 Schematic drawing of external ear, middle ear, and inner ear.

From Seidel, H.M., et al. (1991). *Mosby's guide to physical examination* (2nd ed.). St. Louis: Mosby.

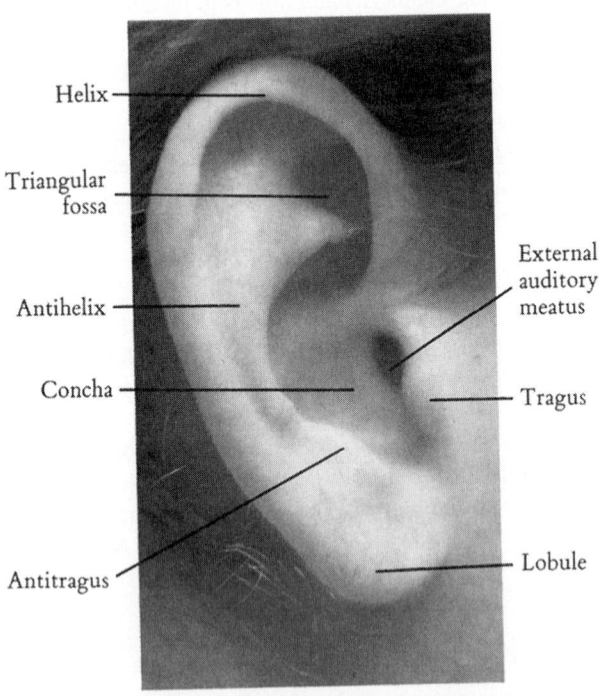

FIG. 18-2 Anatomic structures of auricle. Helix is prominent outer rim, whereas antihelix is area parallel and anterior to helix. Concha is deep cavity containing the auditory canal meatus. Tragus is protuberance on antihelix opposite tragus. Lobule is soft lobe on bottom of auricle.

From Seidel, H.M., et al. (1991). *Mosby's guide to physical examination* (2nd ed.). St. Louis: Mosby.

skull, is positioned on a nearly vertical plane. Note its structural landmarks in Fig. 18-2.

The external auditory canal, an S-shaped pathway leading to the middle ear, is approximately 2.5 cm in length in adults (Fig. 18-1). Its skeleton of bone and cartilage is covered with very thin, sensitive skin. This canal lining is protected and lubricated with cerumen, secreted by the sebaceous glands in the distal third of the canal.

The middle ear is an air-filled cavity in the temporal bone. It contains the ossicles, which form a chain that conducts vibrations from the eardrum across the middle ear into the oval window, the opening in the inner ear. The malleus, resembling a hammer, consists of a head, neck, handle, and short process (Fig. 18-3). The handle and short process of the malleus are attached to the undersurface of the eardrum and join it to the second bone in the series, the incus. The incus, which resembles an anvil, consists of a body and long and short processes (Fig. 18-3). The long crus of the incus is in contact with the third and innermost bone, the stapes. Resembling a stirrup, the stapes consists of a head, neck, anterior and posterior crura, and footplate that fits into the oval window (Fig. 18-3).

The tensor tympani and stapedius muscles attach to the ossicles. The tensor tympani muscle draws the drum inward to increase its tension, whereas the stapedius muscle draws the stapes away from the oval window to dampen intense and potentially damaging vibrations passing through the ossicles into the inner ear. The middle ear and mastoid are

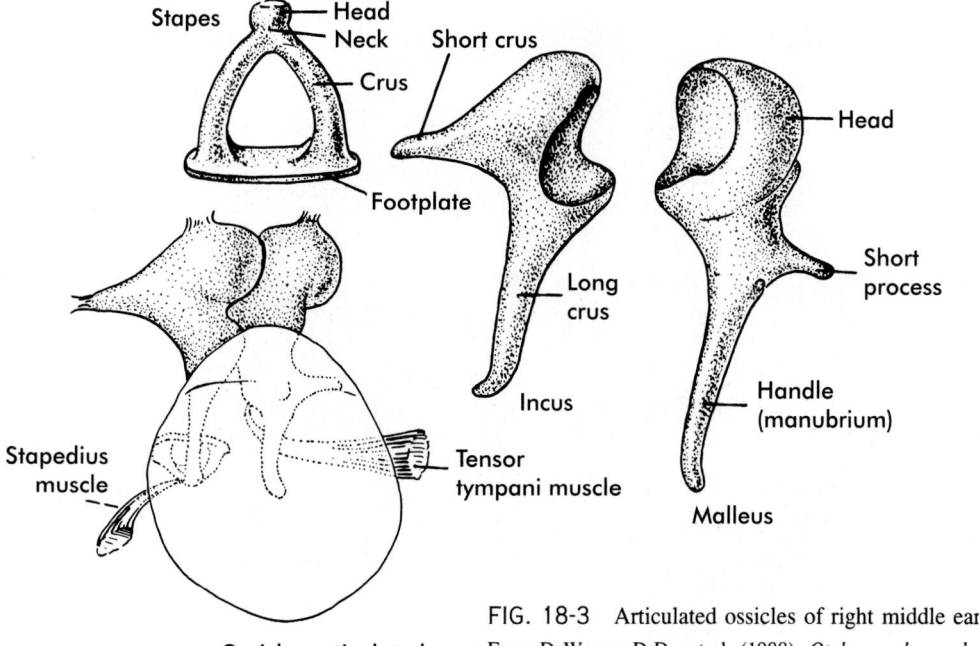

FIG. 18-3   Articulated ossicles of right middle ear.

From DeWeese, D.D., et al. (1988). *Otolaryngology—head and neck surgery* (7th ed.). St. Louis: Mosby.

supplied with blood from the branches of the internal and external carotid artery systems.

The middle ear mucosa produces a small amount of mucus, which is rapidly cleared by the ciliary action of the eustachian tube, a cartilaginous and bony passageway between the nasopharynx and the middle ear. This passage opens briefly to equalize the middle ear pressure with that of atmospheric pressure when swallowing, yawning, or sneezing.

The inner ear is a membranous curved cavity inside a bony labyrinth consisting of the vestibule, semicircular canals, and cochlea. The cochlea, a coiled structure containing the organ of Corti, transmits sound impulses to the eighth cranial nerve. The semicircular canals contain the end organs for vestibular function.

HEARING

Hearing is an interpretation of sound waves by the brain. Sound waves travel through the external auditory canal and strike the tympanic membrane, setting it in vibration. The malleus, attached to the tympanic membrane, begins vibrating, as do the incus and stapes, which are attached to the malleus on the other side (Fig. 18-4). The vibrations are passed to the oval window of the inner ear in which the stapes is inserted. From here they travel via the fluid of the cochlea to the round window, where they are dissipated. Vibrations in the membrane cause the delicate hair cells of the organ of Corti to strike against the membrane of Corti, stimulating impulses in the sensory endings of the auditory division of the eighth cranial nerve. These impulses are transmitted to the temporal lobe of the brain for interpretation. Sound vibrations may also be transmitted by bone directly to the inner ear. A cross-section of the external, middle, and inner ear in relation to other structures of the head and face are shown in Fig. 18-5.

PERIOPERATIVE NURSING CONSIDERATIONS

ASSESSMENT

A thorough nursing history is necessary to properly assess the health status of patients with otologic dysfunctions. The assessment should include a review of the following:

1. Environmental hazards such as exposure to loud, continuous noise (factory, airport, rock music, shooting ranges, jackhammers)
2. Ototoxic drugs taken including salicylates, aminoglycosides, furosemide, streptomycin, quinine, and ethacrynic acid.
3. Symptoms of dizziness or vertigo, including:
   a. Time of onset, duration of attacks
   b. Description (to-and-fro movement or rotary motion—room moving around patient or patient rotating), change of sensation with positional change of the head and neck
   c. Associated symptoms of nausea and vomiting with or without tinnitus, hearing loss, and visual changes; unsteadiness, loss of balance, or falling

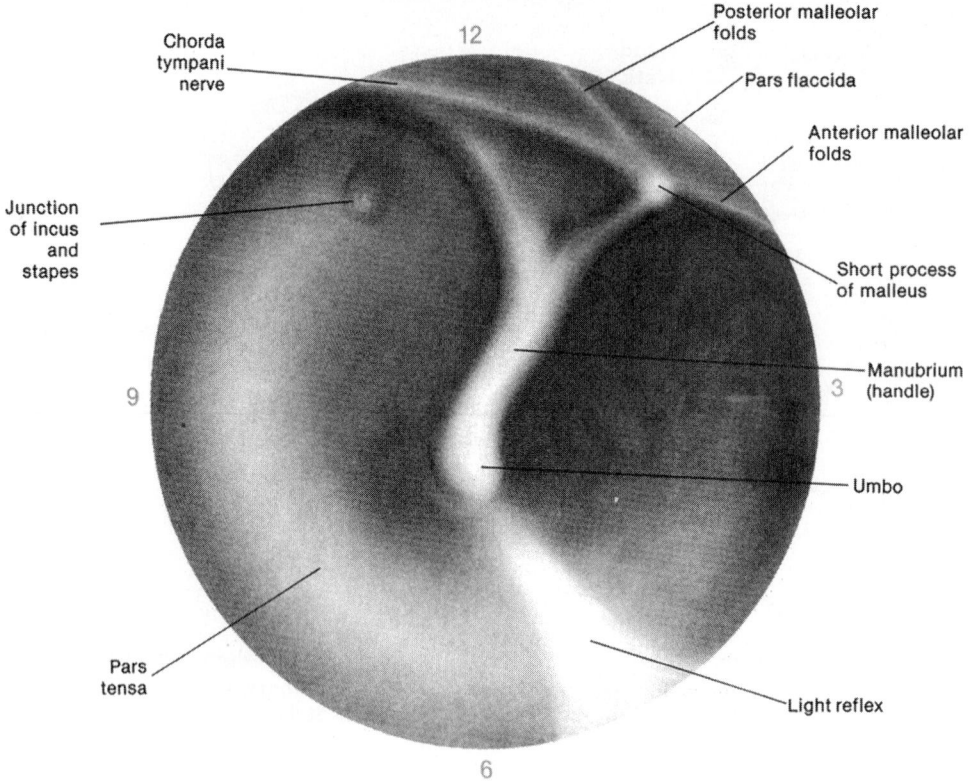

FIG. 18-4   Structural landmarks of tympanic membrane.

From Seidel, H.M., et al. (1991). *Mosby's guide to physical examination* (2nd ed.). St. Louis: Mosby.

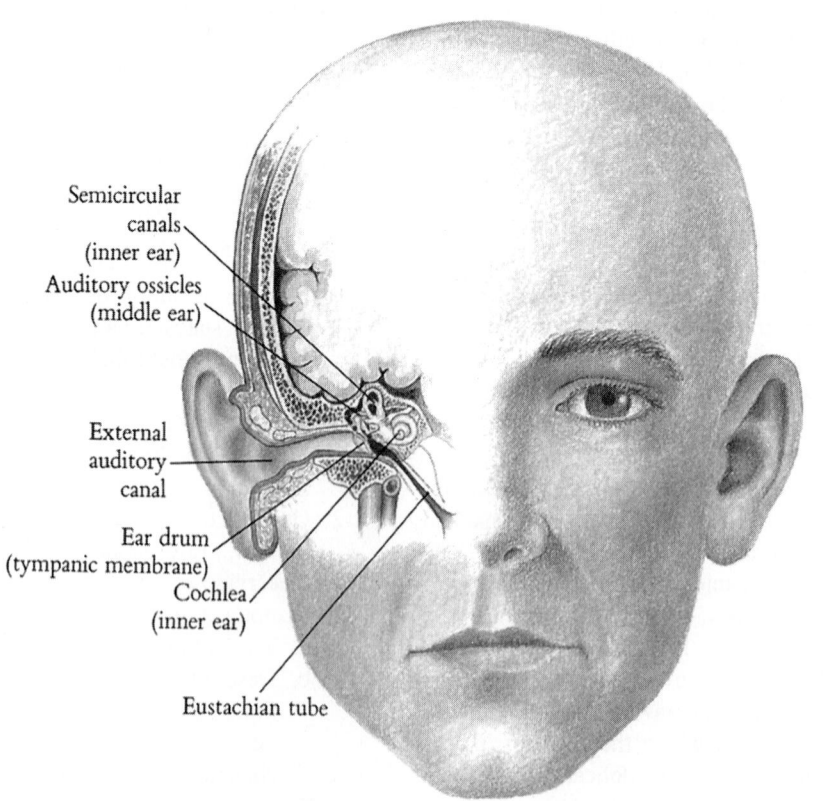

FIG. 18-5   Cross-section of external, middle, and inner ear in relation to other structures of head and face.

From Seidel, H.M., et al. (1991). *Mosby's guide to physical examination* (2nd ed.). St. Louis: Mosby.

4. History of earache, including:
   a. Onset, duration, pain, fever, discharge (serous mucoid, purulent, sanguinous)
   b. Concurrent upper respiratory tract infection, frequent swimming, trauma to the head, related complaints in the mouth, teeth, sinuses, or throat
   c. Associated symptoms: reduced hearing, ringing in the ear, vertigo
   d. Method of ear cleaning
5. Hearing loss in one or both ears, including:
   a. Onset: instant (may indicate vascular disruption), over a few hours or days (may indicate viral infection), slow or gradual
   b. Behaviors in infants and children: no reaction to loud or strange noises, no babbling after 6 months of age, no communicative speech and reliance on gestures after 15 months of age, inattention to children the same age
   c. Optimal hearing: on telephone, in quiet or noisy environment; wearing of hearing aid
   d. Speech preference: soft or loud; monotonous tone or erratic volume
   e. Adaptive responses: lip reading, sign language, written communication, physical disability that interferes with adaptation such as problems operating a hearing aid
   f. Interference with daily life due to hearing loss (such as inability to hear traffic, television, alarms, telephone, and conversation)
6. Medical history: frequent ear problems during childhood; surgery; antibiotic use, dosage, and duration; trauma to head, physical limitations such as arthritis and back or neck problems
7. Family history: hearing problems or hearing loss, Ménière's disease
8. External ear examination, including size, shape, symmetry, landmarks, color, position, and presence of deformities, lesions, and nodules
9. Facial or abducens nerve involvement: inability to look downward, nystagmus, facial asymmetry, and facial paresis

Many diagnostic procedures are performed on the otologic patient prior to the patient's arrival in the operating room. Studies of greatest significance to the perioperative nurse and those which the nurse should be responsible for having in the operating room prior to the procedure include the following:

Audiogram

An audiogram records a measurement on a grid that plots frequency on the X axis and hearing level on the Y axis. The typical frequency range is from 250 to 8000 Hz, with vertical lines denoting octave and some half-octave frequencies. Hearing level (HL) is listed in decibels (dB) and is based on national standards appropriate for the test measurement. An example of the standard audiogram form is given in Fig. 18-6, and the set of symbols that is commonly used to record thresholds is shown in Fig. 18-7. The appropriate symbol is recorded on the form at the intersection of frequency and the measured threshold. If no response is observed, an arrow pointing down at a 45-degree angle is plotted at the limits of the instrumentation. The audiogram determines whether the client has normal hearing, conductive hearing loss, or sensorineural hearing loss.

Magnetic resonance imaging (MRI)

MRI is the use of powerful magnetic and radio frequency waves to reproduce details of the human body with no known risk to patients; it uses no radiation. MRI is used in otology for imaging the brain and internal auditory canals. This test may be contraindicated for patients with implantable metal objects such as inner ear implants, since the magnet could move the implant and cause injury to the patient.

Computed tomography (CT scan)

CT scans are x-ray studies with or without instilled contrast medium and computer technology to produce a sequential series of positive images of transverse sections of cranial bones and tissue. In otology this test may be used to show the relationship of mass to ossicles and other bony structures of the ear.

NURSING DIAGNOSIS

Examples of nursing diagnoses that pertain to many patients having otologic surgery include the following:

- Sensory/perceptual alteration (auditory)
- Powerlessness due to hearing deficit
- High risk for injury, related to sensory deficit
- Body image disturbance related to neurologic deficit and removal of hair

OUTCOME IDENTIFICATION

Outcomes identified for the selected nursing diagnoses for patients undergoing otologic surgery could be stated as:

- Patient will demonstrate improved self-expression and decreased frustration with communication.
- Patient will be able to identify factors that can be controlled personally or by family, nursing staff, or surgical team.
- Patient will be free from injury at completion of perioperative experience.
- Patient will discuss feelings regarding outcome of the surgical procedure.

PLANNING

Plans for patient teaching should be implemented preoperatively and should include the following:

1. The patient should be advised that the ear canal should be kept dry for 10 days to 3 weeks after surgery if the procedure is being performed through the ear canal. The patient should also be told that some

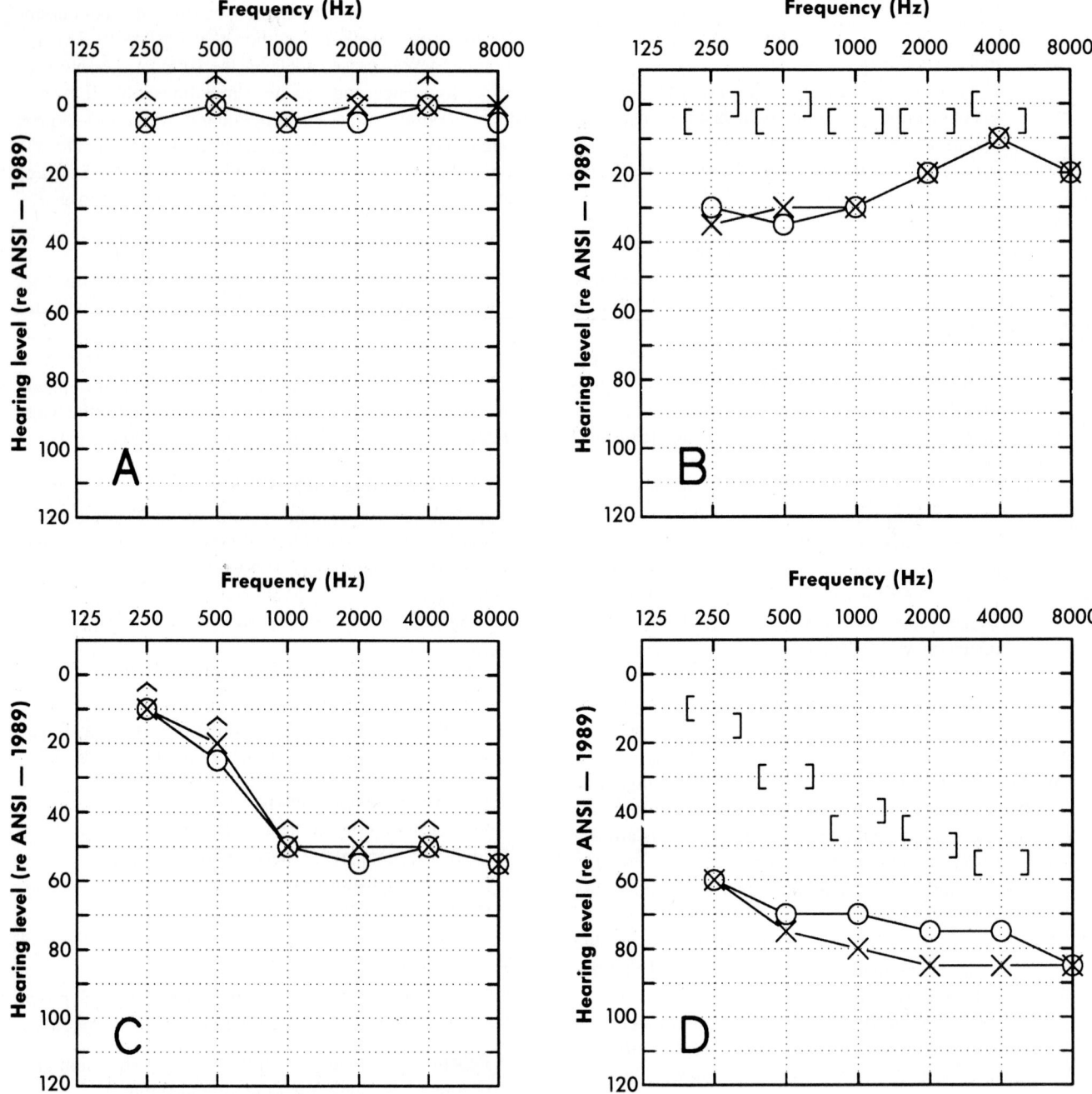

FIG. 18-6   Representative audiograms. **A,** Normal hearing bilaterally. **B,** Bilateral symmetric low-frequency conductive hearing loss. **C,** Bilateral symmetric high-frequency sensorineural hearing loss. **D,** Bilateral moderate to severe mixed hearing loss.

From Cummings, C.W., et al. (1993). *Otolaryngology—head and neck surgery* (7th ed.), (Vol. 4). St. Louis: Mosby.

hair may be shaved from around the ear, depending upon the procedure.
2. The patient should be cautioned not to lie on the operated ear for the first 24 hours after surgery. The head of the bed should be elevated 30 degrees during this period.

3. The patient should be told that vertigo may occur after surgery and that in that case the patient should obtain assistance to get out of bed. Moving slowly and smoothly may alleviate these unpleasant sensations. If the symptoms persist or are severe, antimotion drugs may be necessary.

Response

Modality	Ear		
	Left	Unspecified	Right
Air conduction—earphones			
Unmasked	X		O
Masked	□		△
Bone conduction—mastoid			
Unmasked	>	∧	<
Masked	]		[
Bone conduction—forehead			
Unmasked		∨	
Masked	Γ		⌐
Air conduction—sound field	⚹	$	Ø
Acoustic-reflex threshold			
Contralateral	⊃		⊂
Ipsilateral	⊢		⊣

FIG. 18-7 Symbols used to represent different threshold responses on the audiogram.

From Guidelines for audiometric symbols. (1990, April) *ASHA*, (Suppl. 2), 25-30. Reprinted with permission of American Speech-Language-Hearing Association, Rockville, Md.

4. The patient should be cautioned against deep coughing or nose blowing. If sneezing is unavoidable, both the nose and the mouth should be kept open. These points are important and should be reinforced; strict adherence may prevent dislodgment of a graft or prosthesis.

5. The patient should be made aware that hearing may be diminished during the immediate postoperative period. The nurse should emphasize that this condition is temporary and that the hearing will usually improve gradually.

6. The patient should be reminded not to swim or dive during the first month after surgery. In addition, the patient should be cautioned not to drive during the first postoperative week. Air travel is also not advised during the first postoperative week; after that, it may be allowed only in an airliner with a pressurized cabin.

7. If an upper respiratory tract infection or any other change in physical status occurs, such as foul smelling drainage from the ear, increasing pain, fever, bleeding or a discharge of clear fluid from the ear or nose, the patient should consult the physician immediately.

The Sample Care Plan addresses the needs of the patient undergoing otologic surgery.

IMPLEMENTATION

The age group of patients requiring surgical intervention for otologic conditions ranges from pediatric to adult. The following nursing interventions should be instituted for these patients:

1. Consider the child's fears about surgery, separation from parents, and pain. Provide calm, careful, and comforting nursing behaviors to reduce the child's resistance behaviors and fear in the operating room. Verify that the child has maintained an NPO status.

2. Preoperative teaching through the use of pictures and play is very helpful in assisting the child to overcome fear. Initiate teaching as appropriate for age and developmental status. Allow the child to bring a security object (teddy bear, favorite doll) to the OR as a comfort measure (according to institutional policy). It is also beneficial to have the security object in the child's arms on awakening in the PACU.

   Preoperative teaching may include the recommendation that hair be shampooed the night before surgery. The sequence of perioperative events should be explained. It is important, at the outset, to explain to the patient that hearing acuity may not return immediately. For the patient receiving a local anesthetic, carefully review the patient's need to remain immobile during the procedure. Explain perioperative monitoring devices and accessories (electrosurgical unit, drills) that may be used if the patient will be awake.

3. The nurse should remain with the child throughout the induction phase of anesthesia. If institutional policy permits, parents may also be present during the induction, and the nurse should offer support and explanation to them at this time.

4. If the adult patient uses a hearing aid, it should be worn to surgery and it may be properly dispositioned at the time of, or after, anesthesia induction. If local anesthesia is used, the hearing aid in the unaffected ear should remain in place. Documentation of the hearing aid disposition is essential.

5. Patients with impaired hearing acuity need to be protected from injury. The environment should be controlled, since excess stimulation, loud conversations, and use of the intercom interfere with the patient's ability to hear and comply with instructions and explanations. If hearing loss is uncompensated, a paper and pencil may be used as a means of communication.

6. Patient monitoring for local anesthesia may be performed by the perioperative nurse for stapedectomy or tympanoplasty procedures. Monitor the patient according to institutional protocol.

7. Hair will need to be secured with a shower cap; shaving may be indicated depending on the surgical

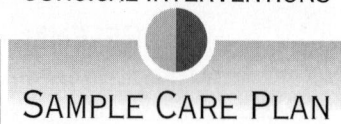

SAMPLE CARE PLAN

NURSING DIAGNOSIS: Sensory/perceptual alteration (auditory)

OUTCOME: Patient will demonstrate improved self-expression and decreased frustration with communication.

INTERVENTIONS:

Identify a method by which patient can communicate basic needs.

Promote continuity of care to reduce frustration.

Identify factors that promote communication.

Allow patient to wear hearing aid to the OR.

Speak slowly and deliberately into the dominant ear.

NURSING DIAGNOSIS: Powerlessness due to hearing deficit

OUTCOME: Patient will be able to identify factors that can be controlled personally or by family, nursing staff, or surgical team.

INTERVENTIONS:

Increase effective communication between patient and health care personnel regarding the surgical intervention.

Allow patient to assume position of comfort.

Offer emotional support.

Ensure privacy.

Provide patient and family opportunities to express their feelings.

Provide and reinforce information given to patient.

Keep needed items within reach during postoperative period.

NURSING DIAGNOSIS: High risk for injury related to sensory deficit

OUTCOME: Patient will be free from injury at completion of perioperative experience.

INTERVENTIONS:

Speak clearly and deliberately to patient and confirm that patient has heard and understood communications.

Provide adequate assistance during movement onto OR bed and positioning.

Complete all transfer and positioning maneuvers slowly.

Identify physical limitations and position or support patient accordingly to provide optimal comfort during the procedure.

Control excess stimulation and noise level in OR

NURSING DIAGNOSIS: Body image disturbance related to neurologic deficits and removal of hair

OUTCOME: Patient will discuss feelings regarding outcome of the surgical procedure.

INTERVENTIONS:

Allow patient to discuss concerns about removal of hair and potential for facial weakness or paralysis.

Discuss available resources and options (use of wig, wearing of head scarf, acoustic neuroma support group, as appropriate). Make referrals to nurse on discharge unit as indicated.

---

approach. Skin preparation should be carried out carefully to protect the eyes and prevent pooling of solution.

8. Special equipment and supplies vary depending on the ear procedure. An ear instrument tray, microsurgical ear instruments, suction, microscope, appropriate head and scope drapes, drills, items for local anesthesia, selected prostheses, irrigating accessories, electrosurgical unit, topical hemostatic agents, antibiotic ointment, and local anesthetic agents will be needed. A nerve stimulator or nerve integrity monitor may be requested.

9. Thermal warming blankets and warm intravenous and irrigating solutions assist in maintaining normothermia. Warm irrigation is essential during local procedures to reduce the risk of inducing dizziness.

10. Sequential compression hosiery may be utilized per physician request to decrease the risk of deep venous thrombosis and pulmonary embolism during long surgical procedures such as acoustic neuroma resection.

11. Note the serial number and lot numbers of otologic implants according to institutional policy.

12. The laser may be used. Initiate and document laser safety precautions (see Chapter 31).

13. Discharge teaching and planning may be initiated by the perioperative nurse. Precautions and restrictions in ear and dressing care, nutritional, fluid, and activity needs, signs and symptoms to report to the physician (elevated temperature, pain, drainage, loss of hearing acuity), and medications (antibiotics, antiemetics, analgesics) should be reviewed.

Positioning

Depending on the type of microscope and OR bed used, the patient may be placed on the bed in the opposite direction from the normal supine position, with the patient's head at the foot of the bed. This positioning facilitates proper placement of a microscope mounted on a floor stand, as well as allowing adequate space for the surgeon and assistant to be positioned on sitting stools near the surgical site. The OR bed should be prepared with the mattress and sheets taped securely to its frame to prevent the patient and mattress from sliding during lateral rotation of the bed. The patient should be positioned with the operative side as close to the edge of the bed as possible. This positioning gives the surgeon access in viewing all areas of the middle ear and mastoid. The patient is secured on the OR bed with one or more belts to ensure safety when the bed is laterally rotated during the procedure. A test rotation may be performed prior to draping the patient to ensure that the patient is adequately secured. If the patient has neck or back problems caused by arthritis or other conditions, special padding or supports should be provided.

Quiet and immobility of the patient are necessary in otologic surgery. In some procedures, such as myringotomy with the patient under local anesthesia, an attendant should hold the patient's head firmly in position. For other operations, such as stapedectomy, the patient's head may be immobilized and supported in a foam headrest. Several types of commercial foam headrests are available for this use. Other options include an ophthalmic headrest with a crescent-shaped pad, a headrest with a horseshoe-shaped pad, and a headrest with skull pins such as the Mayfield (used in certain neurotology procedures). The headrest used is determined by the otologic procedure being performed and surgeon preference.

Preparation of the operative site

For most otologic procedures the hair is removed and skin shaved at least 1 inch from the site of the proposed incision. The hair is removed primarily from the area above the ear for an endaural approach and behind the ear for a postauricular approach. The underhair is shaven while the top hair is maintained for postoperative cosmetic esthetic image enhancement. A commercial adhesive may be applied to the skin and the hair draped out of the operative field with tape or adhesive drapes.

A povidone-iodine solution is used to prep the exposed auricle and the periauricular skin. The meatus is cleansed with cotton applicators. The surgeon should determine if the external ear canal is to be filled with the prepping solution. A skin degreaser may be used to dry the ear canal. The face may be prepped on the operative side to permit observation of facial nerve stimulation.

Facial nerve monitoring

Audible facial nerve monitors are now used in many otologic cases when the facial nerve is at risk. Electrodes are placed in the facial muscles prior to draping the patient if monitoring is to be accomplished. Muscle-relaxing anesthetic agents must be avoided in these cases.

For some cases intraoperative hearing assessment may be necessary. This may be performed with a conventional audiometer if the patient is awake (that is, under a local anesthesia). If general anesthetics are in use, hearing may be assessed using auditory brainstem response (ABR). This requires a technician or audiologist to assist in the monitoring. Because these personnel might not be accustomed to sterile protocol in the operating room, instruction and assistance must be given by the nursing team.

Draping

The draping procedure is usually based on the surgeon's preference. Typically, for major otologic procedures commercially available adhesive drapes are applied around the ear to keep the patient's hair out of the surgical field (the surgeon may choose to expose a portion of the face on the affected side to observe facial nerve movement.) A disposable, antistatic, adhesive drape may be applied under the drape towels or over the towels and body drape.

A fenestrated drape is unfolded over the patient and the head of the bed, with the operative site in view through the opening. Many disposable drapes have an adhesive tape which may then be used to secure the sheet to the patient. A fluid collection pouch that is attached to suction is use-

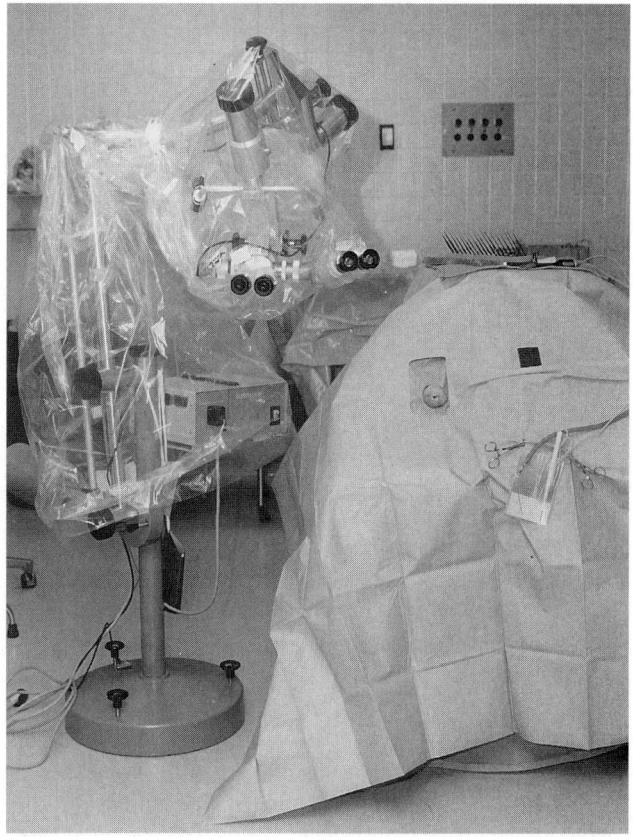

FIG. 18-8 Draped microscope in place over patient in preparation for stapedectomy. Suction, tubing, and drill are assembled in position ready for use.

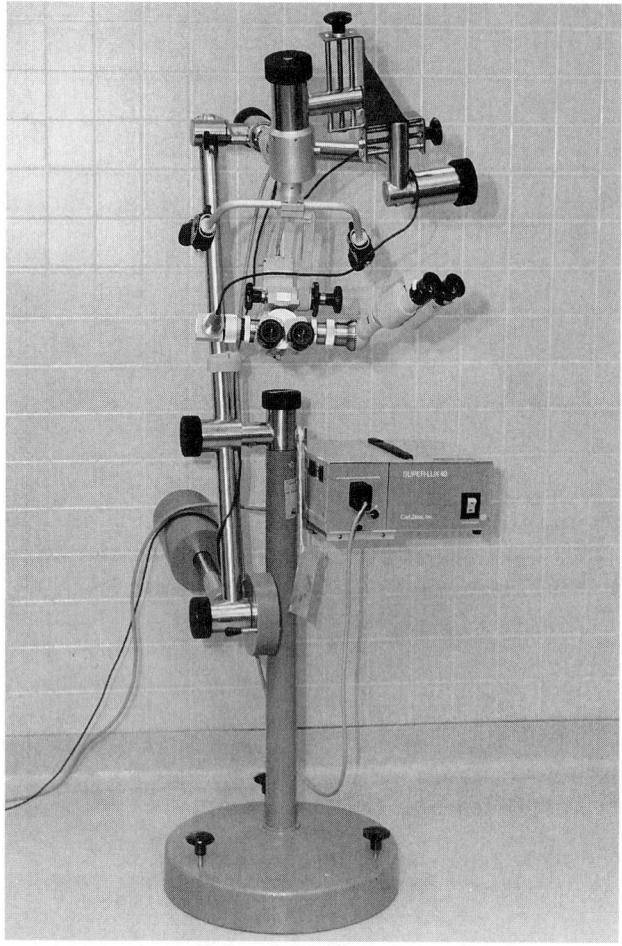

FIG. 18-9 Operating microscope used during various otologic procedures. Lens system allows magnification of 6 to 40 times without change in distance between microscope and ear. Xenon light provides excellent visualization.

ful if drilling and irrigation are planned during a mastoidectomy.

The draped Mayo stand with sterile instruments and the draped operating microscope are positioned over the patient (Fig. 18-8).

Instrumentation

A standard ear surgery setup for otologic procedures (excluding myringotomy) includes an ear, nose, and throat (ENT) drape pack, a basin set, a skin prep set, instruments, ear prostheses if needed, and OR bed accessories. A microscope (Fig. 18-9) and a variety of drills should be available, based on the type of surgical procedure being performed.

The scrub nurse usually stands near the instrument table and passes the instruments in such a manner that the surgeon does not have to turn away from the microscope. Middle ear instruments (Fig. 18-10) are passed with the tips pointing downward and are placed with slight pressure into

the web of the surgeon's hand between the thumb and index finger (as one would place a pencil ready for use). The surgeon can sense the instrument and close the fingertips on the instrument without needing to visualize it. Likewise, middle ear forceps (Fig. 18-11) are passed with the scrub nurse holding onto the shaft of the forcep just above the fingerloops. The forceps are delivered to the surgeon by providing slight pressure of the fingerloops against the palmar surface of the hand. The scrub nurse holds the instrument in this position until the surgeon adjusts the index finger and thumb into the fingerloops of the instrument. All microsurgical instruments should be handed on an exchange basis to prevent costly damage to instruments from inadvertent falls. After each use, microsurgical instruments should be wiped free of debris using a commercially available foam rubber sponge wipe.

Suction tips are passed in the same fashion as the middle ear instruments and should be irrigated clean after each use with a control syringe filled with water.

A universal set of ear surgery instruments can be used for all middle ear procedures. When an endaural approach is required, only endaural retractors must be added to the universal set. The set includes the following items:

2 Towel clamps, non-perforating, 5¼ inches
6 Towel clamps, non-perforating, 3 inches
2 Knife handles, no. 3, with no. 15 blades
8 Mosquito hemostats, curved, 5 inches
2 Rochester-Pean forceps, curved, 6¼ inches
1 Metzenbaum scissors, short, curved
1 Metzenbaum scissors, short, straight
1 Plastic scissors, sharp, curved
1 Plastic scissors, dull, curved
1 Foam upper lateral scissors
1 Bellucci scissors
1 Mayo scissors, straight
2 Brown needle holders
1 Malleus nipper (Fig. 18-12)
1 House-Dieter malleus nipper
1 Bayonet tissue forceps, short (Fig. 18-12)
2 Adson tissue forceps with teeth

2 Frazier suction tips (Fig. 18-12)
4 Baron suction tips, nos. 5 and 7 Fr., 2 each (Fig. 18-12)
2 House suction tips
4 Rosen suction tips
1 Dean elevator
1 Endaural speculum (Fig. 18-12)
6 Ear specula, assorted sizes (Fig. 18-12)
1 Shea speculum holder (Fig. 18-12)
2 Senn retractors
2 Rake retractors, dull
2 Saunders-Paparella self-retaining retractors, two-pronged (Fig. 18-12)
2 Schuknecht self-retaining retractors, three-pronged (Fig. 18-12)
2 Wullstein self-retaining retractors, three-pronged (Fig. 18-12)
1 Small Richardson retractor
1 Ruler
2 Lempert mastoid curettes (Fig. 18-12)
8 Medicine cups
2 Rubber ear syringes

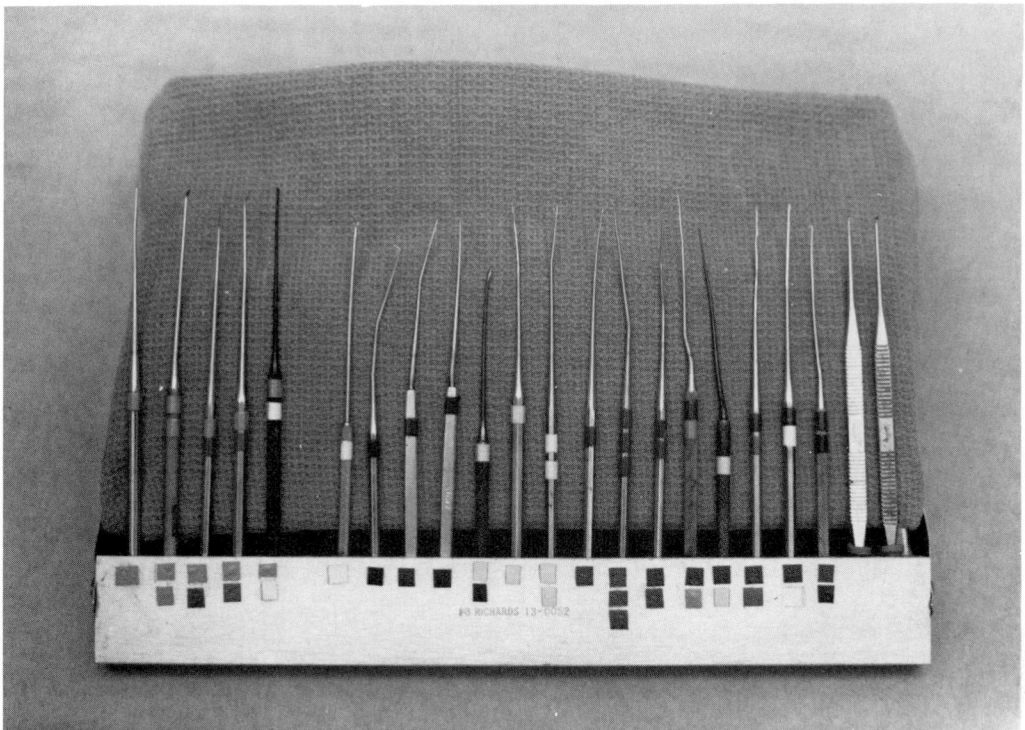

FIG. 18-10 Microsurgical middle ear instruments in protective rack, including various types of knives, hoes, needles, and hooks. The delicacy of these instruments requires protection of tips.

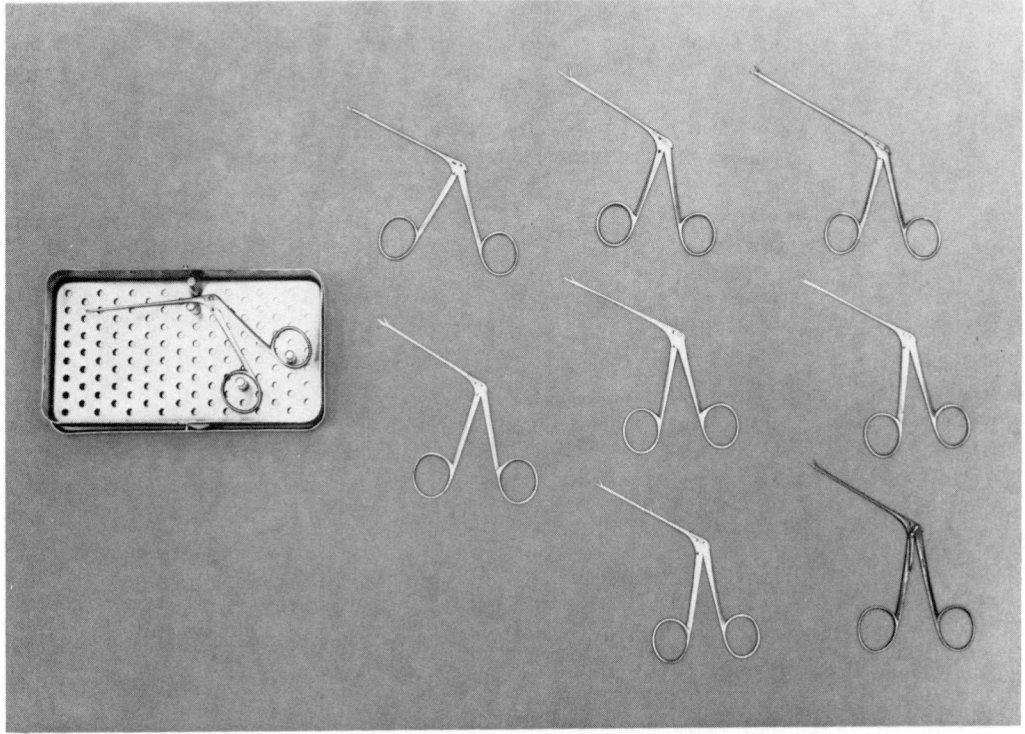

FIG. 18-11 Microsurgical middle ear forceps, including various sizes of cup forceps and alligator forceps.

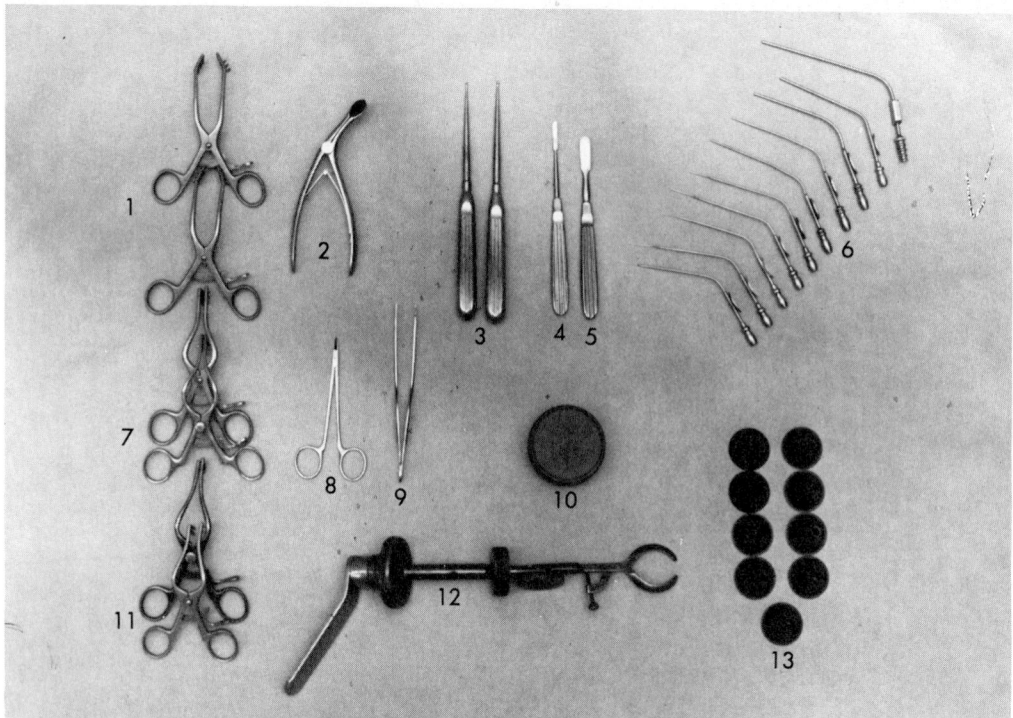

FIG. 18-12 Otologic instruments used for middle ear procedures. *1*, Schuknecht self-retaining retractors; *2*, endaural speculum; *3*, Lempert mastoid curettes; *4*, Joseph elevator; *5*, Dean elevator; *6*, suction tips of assorted sizes; *7*, Wullstein self-retaining retractors; *8*, malleus nipper; *9*, bayonet tissue forceps; *10*, cutting block; *11*, Saunders-Paparella self-retaining retractors; *12*, Shea speculum holders; *13*, ear specula of assorted sizes.

1 Cutting block
Microsurgical middle
   ear forceps
   (Fig. 18-11)
Cup forceps, large
Cup forceps, standard
Cup forceps, miniature
House alligator forceps,
   smooth
Alligator forceps, min-
   iature
Alligator forceps, large
Wire crimping forceps
Microsurgical middle
   ear instruments (usu-
   ally in protective
   rack) (Fig. 18-10)
Myers-Schlosser canal
   knife
Lancet-Bellucci canal
   knife
House sickle knife
House incal-stapedial
   knife
Austin right-angle knife
Billeau earloop
Hough drum scraper

Oval window rasp
Strut introducer, as
   needed for specific
   prostheses
Gilford duckbill
Hough hoe, 90-degree
Hough excavator hoe
House-Barbara straight
   needle
Rosen Needle
McGee footplate hooks,
   assorted lengths
House crura hooks, as-
   sorted lengths
Saunders stapes hooks,
   assorted lengths
Schuknecht hooks, as-
   sorted lengths
Paparella curettes

Accessory items

Suction tubing
Drill (Fig. 18-13)
Operating microscope
   with sterile cover
   (Fig. 18-8)
Electrosurgical unit

Nerve integrity monitor-
   ing system (for facial
   nerve monitoring)
Argon laser or CO_2 la-
   ser (used in laser
   stapedotomy and
   acoustic tumor sur-
   gery)
Bipolar coagulator

Sequential compression
   hosiery
Thermal warming blan-
   ket
Video camera system
   (desirable for those
   assisting and observ-
   ing)

Care and handling of otologic instruments

The basic principles of care, handling, and sterilization of instruments are discussed in Chapter 3. Delicate instruments should be handled individually. To prevent damage, they should not be put into a large basin of cleaning solution or allowed to come into contact with each other. They should be washed, rinsed, and dried individually. A soft-bristled toothbrush can be used to clean the instruments, and care should be used to prevent damage to their tips. Fine, delicate instruments for tympanoplasty and stapedectomy procedures should be kept in a special instrument rack. This type of metal tray separates instruments from one another, protects them from damage, and facilitates handling during surgery. The instruments should be arranged in the rack with consideration given to grouping like items

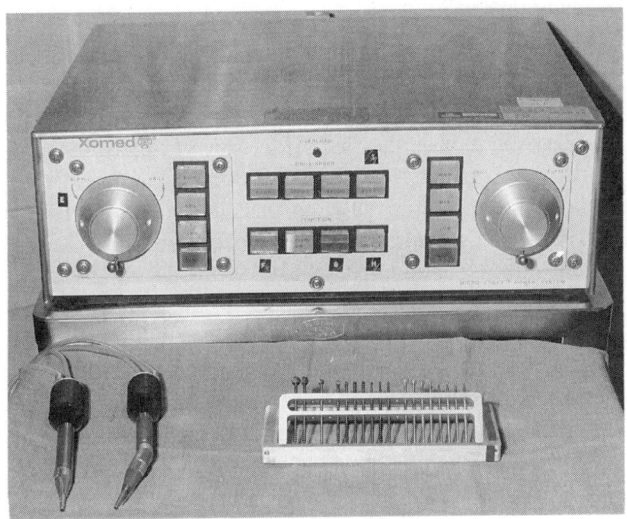

FIG. 18-13 XOMED MPS surgical drill system with straight and angled handpieces; the burr rack contains a variety of burrs of different sizes and shapes with carbide and diamond cutting surfaces.

Courtesy XOMED Inc., Jacksonville, Fla.

together on the rack such, as knifes, hoes, needles, and hooks. Color-coded taping of the instruments and the instrument rack is helpful in maintaining the order of the instruments and aids in the ease and speed of the scrub nurse identifying and delivering the instruments to the surgeon.

Operating microscope

The operative site is viewed by means of a microscope, which illuminates and magnifies the small, delicate anatomic structures encountered in otologic surgery. Several kinds of operating microscopes (Fig. 18-9) with different attachments are available for otologic surgery. The microscope may be a floor- or ceiling-mounted model. Optimal light for an otologic microscope is provided by a xenon or halogen light source. Numerous types of monocular and binocular heads are available for the microscope. These heads may be fixed in a straight or angled plane, or they may be designed to be adjustable in an inclinable plane. For operations through an ear speculum the microscope provides direct light and permits the surgeon to select a magnification of 6, 10, 16, 25, or 40. A common eyepiece magnification for an otologic microscope is 12.5 and a usual objective (lens) is a 250f or 300f. The total magnification is determined by multiplying the magnification of the eyepiece times that of the microscope body times that of the objective. The surgeon usually selects the type of head and objective to be used according to personal preference. Video equipment may be attached to the microscope, which allows other team members to follow the procedure and to anticipate the necessary instrumentation. Before lenses are put into the microscope, they should be checked to ensure

that they are free from lint, dust, fingerprints, and soil. The surgeon adjusts the microscope before it is draped for surgery and manipulates it during the procedure. The microscope is draped with a sterile cover (Fig. 18-8).

Care should be taken when removing the drapes from the microscope to avoid discarding the eyepieces with the drapes or dropping them on the floor. Eyepieces have been lost or damaged in this manner, necessitating costly repair or replacement.

When the microscope is not in use, it should be kept in a storage area that is away from traffic, free from dust, and properly ventilated. Ideally, a set of eyepieces should be left in the scope to prevent the inside of the scope from becoming dusty. The microscope may also be covered with either a protective cover or a plastic bag.

Specula

Varying sizes of specula are needed to fit the different sizes and shapes of the ear canals encountered.

Needles and syringes for local anesthesia

Local anesthesia is preferred for some operations and is given by block injections (see Chapter 6). For stapes surgery the initial local anesthetic, such as a solution of lidocaine with epinephrine, is injected with a 27-gauge, 1½-inch needle attached to a 3-ml syringe with a Luer-Lok.

Knives

For myringotomy a sharp knife in perfect condition is needed. Disposable myringotomy knives are used only once. Nondisposable myringotomy knives should be sharpened after each use. Prepackaged, sterile, disposable myringotomy sets are available from several manufacturers and are now widely used. They are relatively inexpensive and provide good instrumentation for the surgeon. For stapes surgery the circumferential knives with blades facing to the right and others to the left are designed for various purposes: (1) to make the primary incision, (2) to elevate the periosteum, (3) to elevate the fibrous annulus, (4) to separate the incudostapedial joint, and (5) to dissect or resect scar tissue or the stapedial tendon.

Scissors

Mayo and Metzenbaum scissors are used in otologic surgery, depending on the tissue to be excised. Delicate scissors with angular blades or crossover blades (Bellucci or Jacobsen type) are used in middle ear operations to incise and divide the stapedial tendon or scar tissue bands.

Drills and burrs

Electric or air-driven drills or ototomes and burrs are used to remove bone. Cortical and hard cellular bone may be removed by means of an electric drill with a rotating type of burr. For stapes procedures, several microburrs are needed.

The drill may be fitted with either the straight or angled handpiece in various circumstances (Fig. 18-13). A complete selection of bits, from round cutting burrs to diamond polishing burrs (Fig. 18-13), should be available. The purpose of cutting burrs is to remove the bone quickly from areas not close to vital structures. Conversely, diamond or polishing burrs are used on bone around vital structures because these burrs remove the bone more slowly and transfer less heat to surrounding bone.

The scrub nurse must be familiar with the various drill systems available. Some surgeons believe that the air-powered systems offer more speed and torque. Others think that the electric-powered drills offer equal torque yet better control of the drill tip. Knowledge of the method of burr seating, cleaning, maintenance, and sterilization of the drill system is imperative to ensure its maximum use.

During surgery the surgeon holds the handpiece in the same manner as a pen and uses the sides of the burr as the cutting edge. A wire brush may be sterilized and used by the scrub nurse to keep the burrs clean and free from bone bits during the procedure. At the end of the procedure the burrs should be thoroughly cleaned, inspected for nicks or other damage, and discarded if necessary. Because of the speed and torque of the drill, continuous irrigation is necessary to minimize the transfer of heat from the burr to surrounding bone and structures. Some surgeons prefer to have the scrub nurse irrigate as they suction and drill; others choose a suction irrigator that allows them to control the amount and direction of the irrigation as they drill and suction away debris.

Bone curettes

Various types of bone curettes are used to remove soft or thin bone or substance on the dura, on the sinus wall, or in the vicinity of the facial nerve. Curettes must be sharp. For stapes surgery strong shank curettes are needed to remove the annulus and posterior canal wall bone or bridge.

Dissecting forceps

In radical mastoidectomy and tympanoplasty several types of grasping and cutting alligator forceps are needed for manipulation within the canal and the middle ear (Fig. 18-11).

Suction tips

For mastoidectomy and tympanoplasty procedures several patent suction cannulas with or without attached irrigators are needed. Adequate suctioning must be available at all times.

For stapes surgery the tips of the suction apparatus must be available in various gauges (18, 20, 22, and 24) and equipped with finger valves to vary the degree of suction (Fig. 18-12). These fine-needle suction tips must be flushed frequently during the procedure with sterile water to prevent clogging.

Coagulation tips

In radical mastoidectomy, tympanoplasty, and stapes procedures electrocoagulation is used to control oozing. In stapes surgery a monopolar or bipolar insulated suction tip may be used to coagulate small bleeding vessels at the margin of the incision. This tip is attached to the active electrode of a delicate coagulating machine. The objective is to control oozing and prevent blood from entering the middle ear during suctioning.

Continuous irrigation equipment

Irrigation of the operative field is done frequently with sterile warm saline, Tis-U-Sol, or Ringer's solution, suctioning apparatus, and bulb syringes to prevent clogging of the burr and to remove bone dust in areas where osteogenesis is to be avoided.

Synthetic materials to control bleeding

Absorbable gelatin sponge (Gelfoam) plugs or pledgets may be placed against the bone. Bone wax may be used in some cases; however, it is a foreign body, and absorbable substances are preferred.

Anesthesia

Ear procedures in children are done with general anesthesia; adults may receive local or general anesthetics. For procedures such as modified radical mastoidectomy and tympanoplasty a general anesthetic with endotracheal intubation is used. A local block anesthetic such as lidocaine with epinephrine or a general anesthetic may be administered for stapes surgery.

Complications can result from the accumulation of nitrous oxide in closed spaces in the body because nitrous oxide diffuses into and out of body cavities faster than nitrogen does. During middle ear surgery, middle ear pressure may rise, which indicates that tympanic membrane rupture has occurred. Dislodgement of the tympanic membrane graft may follow the development of negative middle ear pressure on the discontinuation of nitrous oxide after the closure of the previously open middle ear.

Lasers

The role of the carbon dioxide laser in otology and neurotology includes its use in stapedotomy and intracranial tumor removal. This is delivered through a micromanipulator. Likewise, the use of the argon laser in middle ear and stapedectomy surgery has been shown to be a useful tool. The argon beam may be delivered via a hand-held probe.

EVALUATION

Intraoperative nursing care should be evaluated at the completion of the surgical procedure before the patient is transported to PACU or the nursing unit (if a local anesthetic has been given). If the patient has had a local anesthetic, the nurse will have had the opportunity to evaluate the patient throughout the procedure. The patient can communicate any discomfort during the procedure and indicate any instructions not heard, such as when the surgeon asks, "Can you hear my voice?" or "Are you comfortable?"

During evaluation, the perioperative nurse determines if the patient met the outcomes in the nursing care plan. Some outcomes can be reached during the preoperative and intraoperative phases of care; they are evaluated prior to the patient's discharge from the operating room. Others require ongoing monitoring and measurement in the postoperative phase. Part of the nursing report to the PACU or nursing unit should include the outcomes of care provided:

- The patient will express himself or herself effectively and with minimal frustration.
- The patient will identify factors that can be controlled personally or by family, nursing staff, or surgical team.
- The patient is free from injury.
- The patient will discuss feelings regarding outcome of the surgical procedure.

SURGICAL INTERVENTIONS

INCISIONAL APPROACHES

The majority of otologic procedures are performed either through the ear canal (endaural) or from behind the ear (postauricular) approach.

The endaural approach may be used for repair of small perforations or stapes work.

The postauricular approach is utilized for mastoidectomies and a modified postauricular approach for cochlear implants or translabyrinthine removal of acoustic tumors.

The middle fossa approach may be used for excision of small acoustic tumors or vestibular nerve sections. This may be a verticle incision above the ear toward the vertix.

The postaural incision may be used to expose the mastoid process. It follows the curve of the postaural fold, beginning at the upper attachment of the auricle and continuing behind the postaural fold downward to the tip of the mastoid process.

For stapes surgery a circumferential incision is made in the posterior half of the canal, starting at the inferior aspect of the annulus and ending posterior to the short process of the malleus.

For myringotomy a circumferential (posteroinferior) incision is made. It provides for wide drainage and removal of pus or fluid under pressure from the middle ear.

OTOLOGIC PROCEDURES

Myringotomy

Myringotomy is the incision of the tympanic membrane. It is performed to treat otitis media in the presence of an exudate. Serous otitis media can be very difficult to diagnose because it is asymptomatic in pediatric patients. The only symptom may be conductive hearing loss.

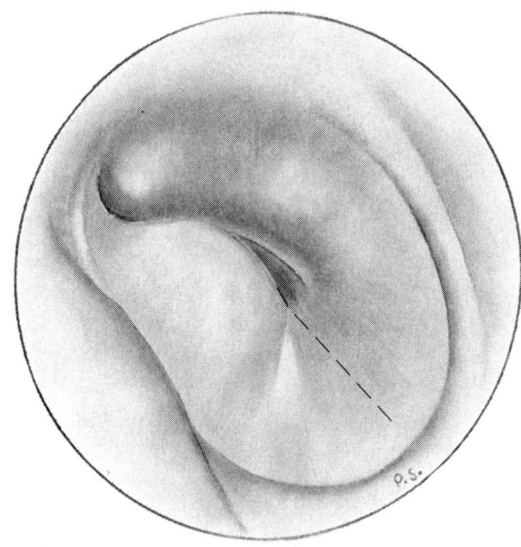

FIG. 18-14   In purulent otitis media, pus under pressure pushes eardrum outward, resulting in bulging tympanic membrane. *Dotted line* represents radial myringotomy incision.

Modified from DeWeese, D.D., & Saunders, W.H. (1982). *Textbook of otolaryngology* (6th ed.). St. Louis: Mosby.

Serous otitis media is very common in children between the ages of 6 months and 2 years. About 50% to 60% of children in this age group have effusion in the middle ear in the first 2 years of life. The incidence may again peak between the ages of 4 and 6 years; 30% of children in this age group have fluid in the middle ear with hearing loss at some time.

About 95% of children with serous otitis media have spontaneous resolution. Hearing loss is the main concern when fluid is present in the middle ear. This hearing loss could affect language development and IQ level if fluid persists for a long time. The accepted practice is removal of the fluid and placement of ventilating tubes in the eardrum if the fluid persists more than 8 to 12 weeks and is accompanied by hearing loss.

Otitis media is primarily a pediatric problem, but adult cases are seen. It may respond to one treatment only to return and require another type of therapy. Tympanic fibrosis is common in adults and is a result of repeated infections that have occurred in childhood. Acute otitis media is a collection of infected pus in the middle ear. The patient may have severe pain and bulging of the tympanic membrane (Fig. 18-14). Failure to respond to oral antibiotics and analgesics or other complications such as facial nerve paralysis or labyrinthitis may require a myringotomy. By release of the pus or fluid, hearing is restored and the infection can be controlled. The procedure may be performed for chronic serous otitis media in which the presence of fluid in the middle ear produces a hearing loss. Frequently,

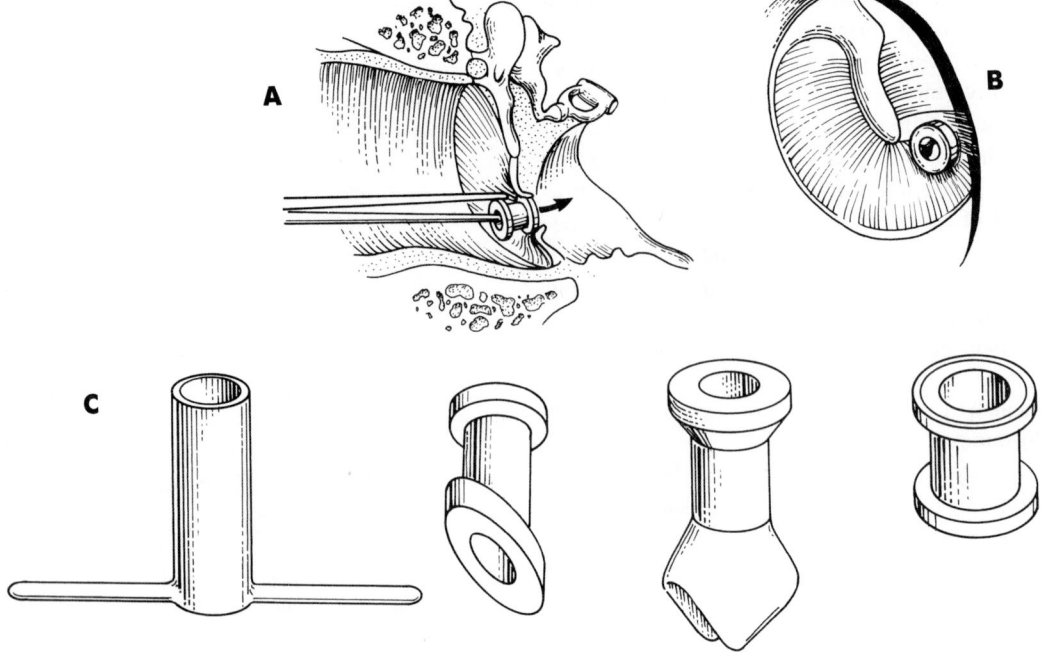

FIG. 18-15 **A,** Tube (placed on end of alligator forceps) being inserted into tympanic membrane. **B,** Tube in place. **C,** Several types of plastic tubes that may be inserted into tympanic membrane. Purpose of tubes is to aerate middle ear and reduce middle ear infections.

From Saunders, W.H., et al. (1979). *Nursing care in eye, ear, nose, and throat disorders* (4th ed.). St. Louis: Mosby.

tubes are inserted into the tympanic membrane (Fig. 18-15) to allow ventilation of the middle ear. Care must be taken to avoid getting water in the ears while the tubes are in place. Myringotomy is usually performed on an ambulatory surgery basis.

Procedural considerations

Myringotomy is considered a clean procedure. The patient is usually not prepped or draped. The surgeon may wear gown and gloves or gloves only, depending on the policy related to universal precautions at the institution in which the procedure is performed. The instrument setup includes the following:

1 Myringotomy knife	Aural specula, assorted
2 Aural applicators,	sizes
metal	Rosen needle
1 Hartmann aural for-	1 Suction tip and tubing
ceps, delicate type	1 Culture tube
3 Buck ear curettes	Cotton, absorbent

Several disposable myringotomy sets are available commercially. They are relatively inexpensive and afford an expedient procedure.

Operative procedure

1. With microscopic visualization, the aural speculum is inserted in the ear canal. The excess cerumen is removed with a wire loop curette or Toby forceps. With a sharp myringotomy knife a small, curved or radial incision is made in the anterior inferior quadrant of the pars tensa (Fig. 18-14).
2. A culture may be taken to determine the type of organism present.
3. Pus and fluid are suctioned from the middle ear.
4. A tube may be inserted into the incision with alligator forceps or a tube inserter.
5. Antibiotic drops may be instilled following the positioning of the tube.

Several types of disposable myringotomy tubes are available for implantation, depending on the length of time the surgeon wishes the tube to remain in place (Fig. 18-15). Once the tube falls out, the tympanic membrane incision usually heals.

Tympanoplasty

Tympanoplasty was first performed in the early 1950s. The success rate of the procedure at that time was about 30%. With progress in surgical technique and use of the operating microscope, antibiotic therapy, and better grafting tissue, the success rate soon grew to 90% to 95%.

Tympanoplasty is a surgical procedure performed on the middle ear structures, including the eardrum and ossicles, which usually leads to improved hearing and prevention of recurrent infection.

Perforation of the eardrum (tympanic membrane) is the most common serious ear injury necessitating surgical intervention. Perforations may result from (1) direct injury (for example, cotton applicators, pencil), (2) blow to the ear, (3) tears from temporal bone fractures, and (4) lightning injury. Early diagnosis is the key to proper management.

Conductive hearing loss is caused by an obstruction in the external canal or middle ear, which impedes the passage of sound waves to the inner ear. It may be due to disease of the middle ear or tympanic membrane. Occasionally the tympanic membrane does not heal following myringotomy.

Ossicular discontinuity may result from chronic otitis media, trauma, or cholesteatoma, a skin cyst that erodes bone. Various methods and materials are being used in constructing a closed, air-contained middle ear cavity and restoring a sound-pressure transforming action. Among these materials are homografts and Teflon, Plasti-Pore, silicone, hydroxyapatite, and metal prostheses.

Procedural considerations

The ear is prepped and draped as previously described. An endaural or postauricular approach may be used. Both these approaches provide similar functional results. The procedure is most often performed with the patient under local anesthesia.

Operative procedure

1a. When an *endaural approach* is used, the ear speculum is introduced into the external meatus of the ear canal, and the microscope is brought into place. The surgeon injects local anesthetic into the external meatus and external auditory canal and postauricularly, using a 1- or 3-ml syringe. Lidocaine (Xylocaine) with epinephrine is generally used unless the patient's general medical condition necessitates a substitute. The purpose of the injection of local anesthetic is twofold: to make the operation painless and to reduce the amount of bleeding. A tympanomeatal incision is then made, using a sharp round knife.

1b. When a *postauricular approach* is used, the surgeon injects local anesthetic (lidocaine with epinephrine) postauricularly using a 3-ml or 5-ml syringe. An ear speculum is introduced, and the microscope is brought into place. The surgeon injects local anesthetic into the external auditory canal using a 1-ml syringe. The microscope head is moved from directly over the patient's ear. The skin incision is made behind the fold of the ear with a no. 15 knife blade. The bleeding vessels are coagulated. An incision is made in the periosteum down to the bone, and the periosteum is elevated from behind the incision with a Lempert elevator.

2. At this point the temporalis fascia is usually harvested to provide the graft material for the repair of the tympanic membrane. Lidocaine with epinephrine may be injected under the fascia to separate it from the temporalis muscle. A narrow Shambaugh elevator or duck-bill elevator is used to separate the fascia. Small, sharp scissors or a knife blade serves to remove the amount of fascia needed. The fascia is trimmed of excess tissue with small, sharp scissors and either laid flat or molded onto an ear speculum. Some surgeons prefer to thin the fascia by using a House Gelfoam press. The fascia is then set aside to dry while the tympanic membrane is prepared.

3. The canal skin may be elevated from the canal with a duckbill elevator, Rosen needle, gimmick, or similar microinstrument, or it may be removed, depending on the size and location of the tympanic membrane perforation.

4. The edges of the tympanic membrane are prepared for the graft by removing all epithelium from the drum surrounding the perforation, usually with a sickle knife, Rosen needle, 45- or 90-degree pick, or cup forceps.

5. If an edge of the perforation or tympanic membrane cannot be visualized because of the bony canal, the surgeon uses a microcurette or drill to remove the overhang of bone.

6. The middle ear is explored with a pick or similar instrument, and any epithelium present is removed with an alligator or cup forceps. The ossicular chain is tested for mobility. Each ossicle is inspected to ensure that it is intact and mobile.

7. If the malleus or incus is diseased or eroded, it may be removed and replaced with a partial ossicular replacement prosthesis (PORP). Ossicles that are removed may be reshaped with the aid of a drill and small burr, and replaced. If all ossicles are diseased or eroded, they may be removed and replaced with a total ossicular replacement prosthesis (TORP). This step is accomplished with microinstrumentation such as Bellucci scissors, cup forceps, malleus nipper, incudostapedial joint knife, sickle knife, picks, and Rosen needle.

8. Once confident that the middle ear has been explored and corrected, the surgeon prepares the graft for insertion. The edges are trimmed with a no. 15 knife blade or sharp scissors. The surgical site is suctioned with a microsuction. Hemostasis may be achieved by applying very small, epinephrine-soaked Gelfoam balls with an alligator forceps. Radiopaque microcottonoids are available for use in hemostasis if necessary.

9. Different tissues, such as temporalis fascia, or loose connective tissue, tragus perichondrium, and vein grafts, have been used for a tympanoplasty procedure. The most common tissue used is temporalis fascia. Most surgeons prefer to use autograft tissue, although homograft tympanic membranes have also been used. The risk of transmission of infectious disease has reduced homograft use. For easier manipulation, the graft may be dipped in water, saline, or a Tis-U-Sol solution before its insertion with alligator forceps. A gimmick, sickle knife, pick, Rosen needle, or similar

microinstrument is used to position the graft into place. Small pledgets of absorbable gelatin sponge may be packed around the graft to ensure support and position. Some surgeons prefer to pack the middle ear before the graft insertion to provide support.

10. The external ear canal is packed with moistened absorbable gelatin sponge pledgets or antibiotic ointment.
11. The incision is closed with suture of the surgeon's preference.
12. A pressure dressing may be applied for the first 24 hours to prevent dislodgement of the new graft. This dressing usually consists of fluffed gauze placed around the ear and an elastic gauze wrapped around the affected ear and the head.

Mastoidectomy

Mastoidectomy is the removal of the diseased bone of the mastoid process, along with the cholesteatoma present in the middle ear and mastoid. Cholesteatoma is the result of accumulation of squamous epithelium and its products in the middle ear and mastoid. It occasionally forms a cystlike mass. As it expands, it is destructive to the middle ear and mastoid. As a result, the diseased bone (ossicles and mastoid bone) must be removed to prevent recurrence of the cholesteatoma.

There are three types of mastoidectomy. A *complete mastoidectomy* is removal of the diseased bone of the mastoid while the ossicles, eardrum, and canal wall are left intact. The complete mastoid procedure is performed to eradicate chronic infections unresponsive to antibiotics or for removal of cholesteatoma. A serious surgical accident that can occur during a complete mastoid procedure is injury to the facial nerve. Other complications include injury to the sigmoid sinus, inner ear balance or hearing mechanisms, and dura.

A *modified radical mastoidectomy* is removal of the diseased bone of the mastoid along with some of the ossicles and the canal wall. The eardrum and some of the ossicles remain, thus leaving a mechanism for the patient to hear. A *radical mastoidectomy* is the removal of the canal wall

along with the ossicles and eardrum. The radical mastoidectomy is rarely performed today. With either the modified radical or radical mastoidectomy a meatoplasty is performed to enlarge the ear canal opening. This facilitates cleaning the mastoid bowl that has been created.

Procedural considerations

General anesthesia is usually selected, but local anesthesia can be used. The patient is prepped and draped as for a tympanoplasty. An endaural or postauricular incision may be used (Fig. 18-16), but most surgeons believe that the postauricular incision offers better exposure to all areas of the mastoid and middle ear. A drill is used to remove diseased bone and tissue while the surgeon continually observes for anatomic structures, such as the facial nerve, within the mastoid.

Operative procedure

1 to 6. These steps are as for tympanoplasty.
7. The mastoid bone is drilled initially with a large cutting burr, usually under direct vision. As the mastoid cavity is created, the scrub nurse should be able to anticipate changes needed in burr size. Once the vital structures have been identified, diseased bone is usually removed from them by use of diamond burrs of the appropriate size. The surgeon may interrupt drilling to explore areas of the mastoid with a pick, Rosen needle, mastoid searcher, gimmick, or other microinstrument to identify surrounding structures.
8. On completion of the mastoidectomy the surgeon focuses on the middle ear. Diseased ossicles are removed, middle ear mucosa is inspected and removed if necessary, and all evidence of cholesteatoma is removed. Depending on the extent of the disease and the reliability that the patient will be available for follow-up, the surgeon then reconstructs the ossicular chain or prepares the cavity created by a radical mastoidectomy. Some surgeons do not reconstruct at the time of mastoidectomy but follow the patient for a specified time. If cholesteatoma does not recur during that pe-

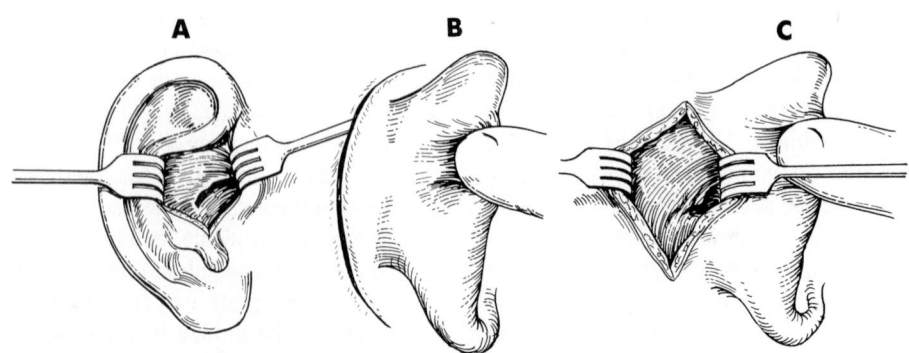

FIG. 18-16   Mastoidectomy incision. **A,** Endaural. **B,** Postauricular. **C,** Postauricular incision retracted.

riod, the patient receives a reconstructive procedure to restore hearing.

9. The mastoid cavity and middle ear may be packed with absorbable gelatin sponge. The external auditory canal may be packed with absorbable gelatin sponge or antibiotic ointment.

10. The incision is closed with suture of the surgeon's preference.

11. A pressure dressing is applied and kept in place for the first 24 hours. This dressing usually consists of fluffed gauze around the ear and plain or elastic gauze wrapped around the head and affected ear. A commercially available product known as a Glasscock dressing may be used for this purpose (Fig. 18-17).

Stapedectomy

Stapedectomy is removal of the stapes for treatment of otosclerosis and replacement with a prosthesis to restore ossicular continuity and improve hearing.

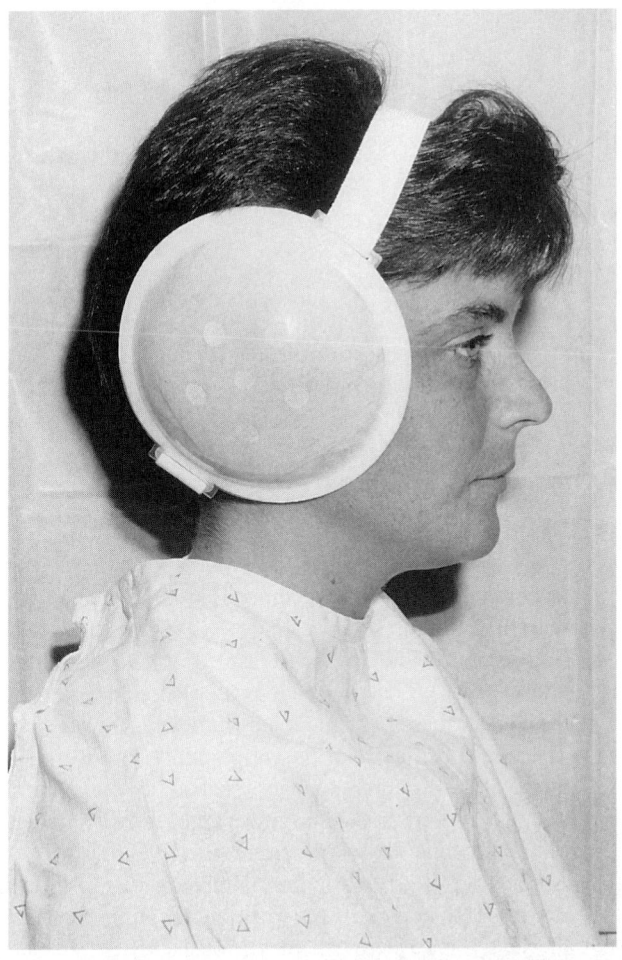

FIG. 18-17 Completed Glasscock dressing following mastoidectomy. Telfa and fluffed gauze bandage comprise primary dressing. Rigid ear cup and Velcro adjustable nonelastic strap comprise the protective exterior dressing.

Courtesy Oto-Med Inc., Lake Havasu, Ariz.

Otosclerosis is the overgrowth of bone around the stapes footplate, resulting in immobility of the footplate. Sound waves cannot be transmitted adequately through the oval window and round window to be changed into electrochemical impulses in the cochlea.

There are two types of procedures for replacing the immobile stapes. In *stapedotomy* the footplate of the stapes is not removed; only the superstructure is removed. A hole is made in the stapes footplate, and the prosthesis is secured laterally to the long process of the incus and positioned medially over the hole created in the footplate. In *stapedectomy* the entire stapes (superstructure and footplate) is removed, a graft is placed over the oval window, and a prosthesis is attached laterally to the long process of the incus and positioned medially on the graft over the oval window.

Procedural considerations

Various materials are used as the prosthesis for the stapes; the most common are stainless steel and Teflon (Fig. 18-18). The prosthesis of choice is determined by the surgeon.

The scrub nurse must be aware of each step in the procedure and hand the instruments to the surgeon expediently. Because the oval window is left uncovered, some perilymph may leak from the inner ear into the middle ear. This leak subjects the patient to the possible complication of a sensorineural hearing loss postoperatively or, more seriously, a "dead ear."

Microsuctions (18 to 25 gauge) are used in this procedure because other suction tips are too large and may suction perilymph from the oval window as well as promote bleeding in the middle ear.

Following the incision and reflection of the flap, footplate hooks are used because the tips on picks are so large and long that they may cause damage rather than assist in the procedure.

Operative procedures
Stapedectomy

1. A temporalis fascia, fat, perichondrium, or vein graft may be harvested before the procedure. This graft is used to cover the oval window. Depending on the surgeon's graft preference, the ear, hand, or a portion of the abdomen may be prepped for the graft.

2. The ear speculum is introduced, and the microscope is brought into position. The ear canal is cleansed of wax and debris and may be gently washed with Tis-U-Sol and suctioned with a Baron or microsuction tip.

3. The surgeon injects lidocaine with epinephrine into the ear canal.

4. An ear speculum is inserted, the tympanomeatal flap is created (using a flap knife, roller knife, or sickle knife), and the tympanic membrane is reflected forward (using duckbill elevators or a drum elevator), exposing the middle ear (Fig. 18-10).

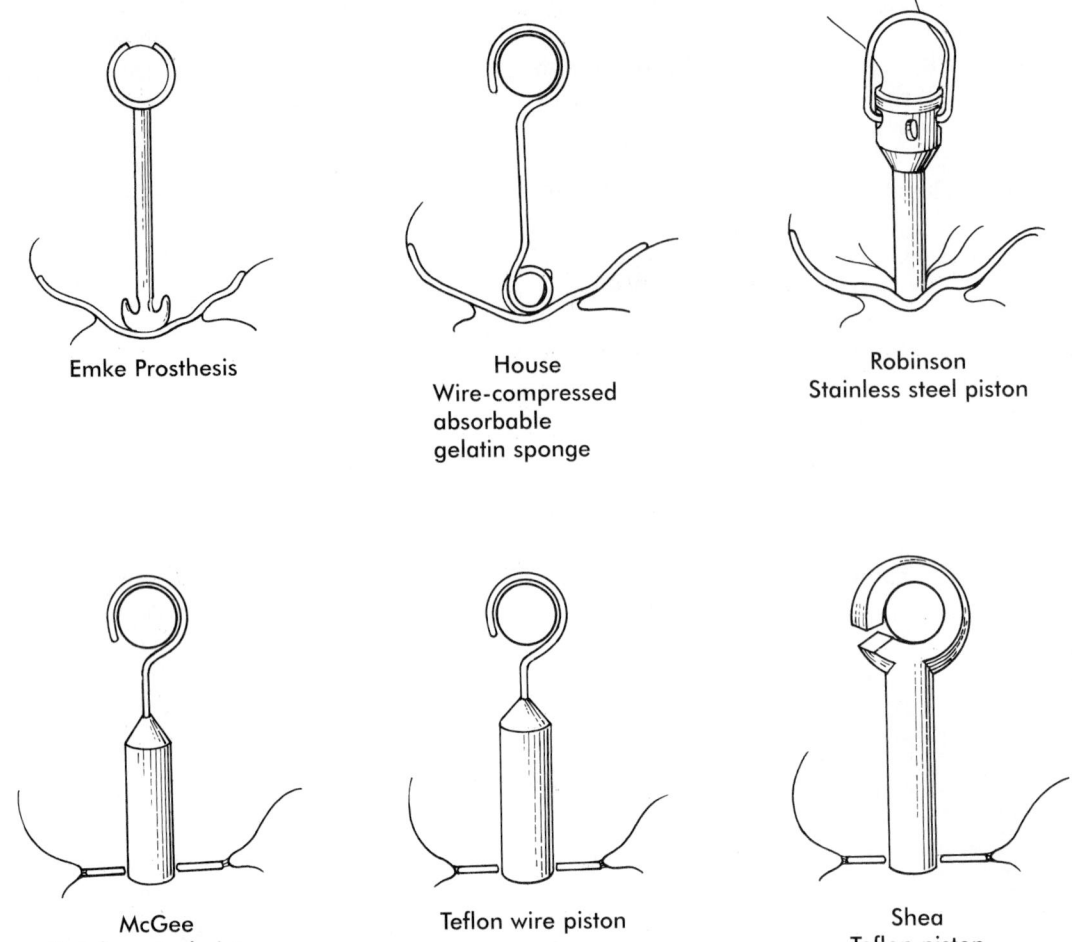

Emke Prosthesis

House
Wire-compressed
absorbable
gelatin sponge

Robinson
Stainless steel piston

McGee
Stainless steel piston

Teflon wire piston

Shea
Teflon piston

FIG. 18-18   Stapedectomy prostheses. Top three diagrams show various prostheses used after the footplate has been removed. Bottom three diagrams indicate that the footplate had been "drilled" to precisely accept a prefabricated piston.

5. If visualization of the ossicles is inadequate owing to the overhang of bone, the surgeon may use microcurettes or a drill to remove enough bone to allow proper visualization. The surgeon usually attempts to save the chorda tympani nerve because it controls taste from the anterior two thirds of the tongue. If this nerve obstructs the view of the stapes, it may on rare occasion be sacrificed for exposure.

6. The surgeon may measure the distance from the incus to the stapes footplate at this time or after the removal of the stapes. It is accomplished with a measuring stick and done to ensure the proper fit of the prosthesis.

7. The incudostapedial joint is disarticulated to allow fracture and subsequent removal of the stapes, usually accomplished through the use of a House or Guilford-Wright joint knife but a laser (CO_2 or argon) may be utilized. A comparison of argon laser stapedectomy to traditional fenestration techniques is described in Research Highlight 18-1.

8. Both crura of the stapes are lasered or fractured laterally, usually with a footplate pick or Rosen needle, and the superstructure is removed with alligator forceps. The surgeon may take this opportunity to ensure hemostasis using tiny sponges soaked in epinephrine along with a microsuction tip. The laser helps coagulate middle ear vessels, thus improving hemostasis.

9. An opening is created in the footplate with a laser or a sharp footplate pick. If the footplate is extremely thick, the laser or a microdrill may be used. If a stapedectomy is to be carried out, each half of the footplate is then removed using a Hough hoe, footplate pick, or footplate hook.

10. The oval window is then inspected, and the graft is placed over the oval window with alligator forceps or

RESEARCH HIGHLIGHT 18-1

Rauch and Bartley conducted a retrospective review of all stapedectomies performed at the Massachusetts Eye and Ear Infirmary over 13 months to compare the results of argon laser stapedectomy to conventional footplate fenestration techniques. Although the procedure was new and unfamiliar to the surgical staff, the complication rate was lower with the argon laser than with footplate fenestration by traditional pick or drill techniques. The incidence of footplate fracture or removal preventing use of a small fenestra technique was five times as likely to occur with traditional instruments as with the argon laser ($p <$ 0.025). In revision stapedectomy sensorineural hearing loss was four times as likely to occur with traditional instruments as with the argon laser ($p \leq$ 0.05). The argon laser did not alter the operating time. Though not ideal for every case, the argon laser endoootoprobe offers the surgeon a significant new tool to improve the outcome in stapes surgery.

Rauch, S.D., Bartley, M.L. (1992). Argon laser stapedectomy: comparison to traditional fenestration techniques. *American Journal of Otology, 13* (6), 556-560.

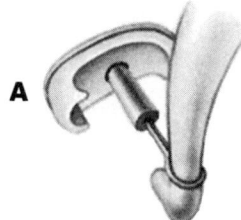 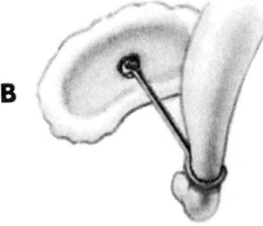

FIG. 18-19 **A,** Placement of wire piston firmly crimped about incus. **B,** Total stapedectomy after placement of perichondrium over oval window. Wire loop prosthesis is crimped and placed against oval window membrane.

From DeWeese, D.D., et al. (1988). *Otolaryngology—head and neck surgery* (7th ed.). St. Louis: Mosby.

a pick. The edges of the graft are smoothed and positioned with a Hough hoe, pick, or gimmick.

11. The prosthesis is passed on alligator forceps to the surgeon, who introduces it into the middle ear with the shaft of the prosthesis resting against the oval window graft.

12. The wire is positioned over the long process of the incus (Fig. 18-19) by using picks, Hough hoes, or footplate hooks. Once it is in proper position, the surgeon crimps the wire onto the long process of the incus and thus ensures its attachment.

13. The surgeon may test the patient's hearing by softly whispering to the patient (if the procedure is performed under local anesthesia) or by touching the malleus with a pick and observing for mobility of the malleus, incus, and stapes prosthesis (if performed under general anesthesia).

14. Tiny squares of moistened, compressed, gelatin sponge may then be placed around the base of the prosthesis to ensure its stability. Alligator forceps, picks, gimmick, and similar instruments may be used for this step in the procedure.

15. The tympanomeatal flap is returned to its original location, using a drum elevator, duckbill elevator, or Rosen needle, and the external ear canal may be packed with an antibiotic gel or ointment or a moistened compressed gelatin sponge.

16. Cotton is placed in the concha of the ear and a Band-Aid or small dressing is usually applied to the graft site.

Stapedotomy. The stapedotomy procedure is similar to stapedectomy but has these differences:

1. No graft is taken before the procedure.
2. The footplate is not removed. A hole is made in the footplate, using the CO_2 or argon laser or drill bits of increasing size. The prosthesis is inserted when the perforation in the footplate is the appropriate size.
3. Following positioning and crimping of the prosthesis, either a moistened, compressed, gelatin sponge or a few drops of the patient's blood may be placed around the junction of the prosthesis and the footplate to ensure stability of the prosthesis.

The scrub and circulating nurses must be knowledgeable in the operation, safety, and procedure for use of the laser if the surgeon elects to perform stapedotomy with a laser (see Chapter 31).

Ossicular reconstruction

Ossicular reconstruction is commonly performed for the replacement of the incus portion of the ossicular chain. There are many surgical techniques for ossicular reconstruction. Autografts of ossicles taken from the patient's ear may be used, but they must be reshaped to reestablish the ossicular chain. Preserved homografts are less popular than in the past, since patients are refusing to even consider these grafts due to the risk (albeit very low) of transmission of infectious disease.

About 50% to 60% of ossicular problems are related to the incus, and 10% affect the stapes as a result of otosclerosis. Malleus dysfunction accounts for 10% of ossicular problems and is mainly due to the formation of cholesteatoma. The balance of ossicular problems may be a combination of the above.

Alloplastic materials have been produced and improved upon for use in ossicular reconstruction. This material is used in the manufacturing of partial and total ossicular reconstruction prostheses.

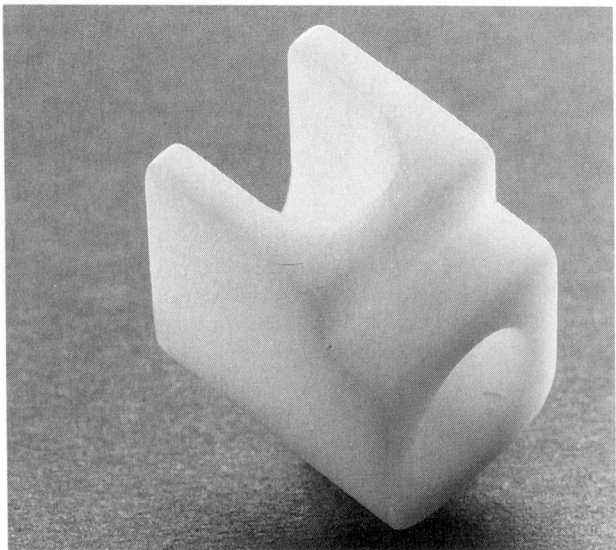

FIG. 18-20 Applebaum incudostapedial joint prosthesis, made of hydroxyapatite, used to reconnect the incus and stapes in cases where there is erosion of long process of incus.

Courtesy Smith and Nephew, Richards, Memphis, Tenn.

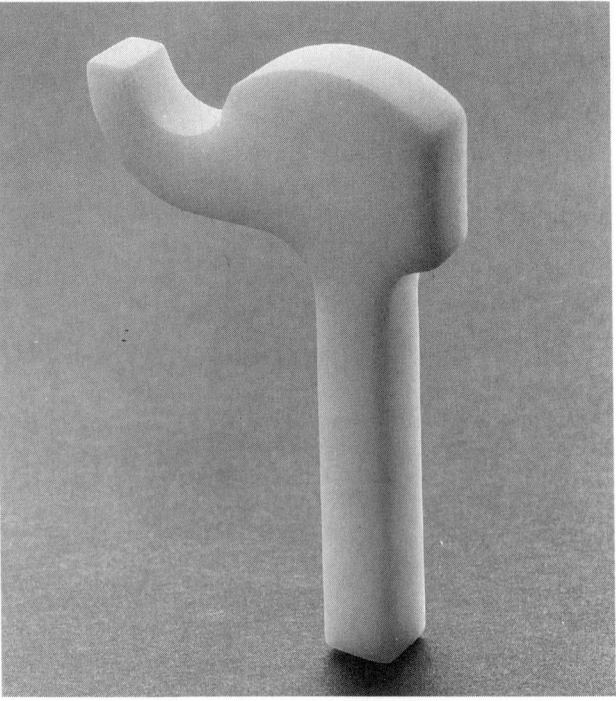

FIG. 18-21 Wehrs incus-stapes prosthesis, partial ossicular replacement prosthesis (PORP) made of hydroxyapatite, used to connect undersurface of malleus to center of stapes footplate.

Courtesy Smith and Nephew, Richards, Memphis, Tenn.

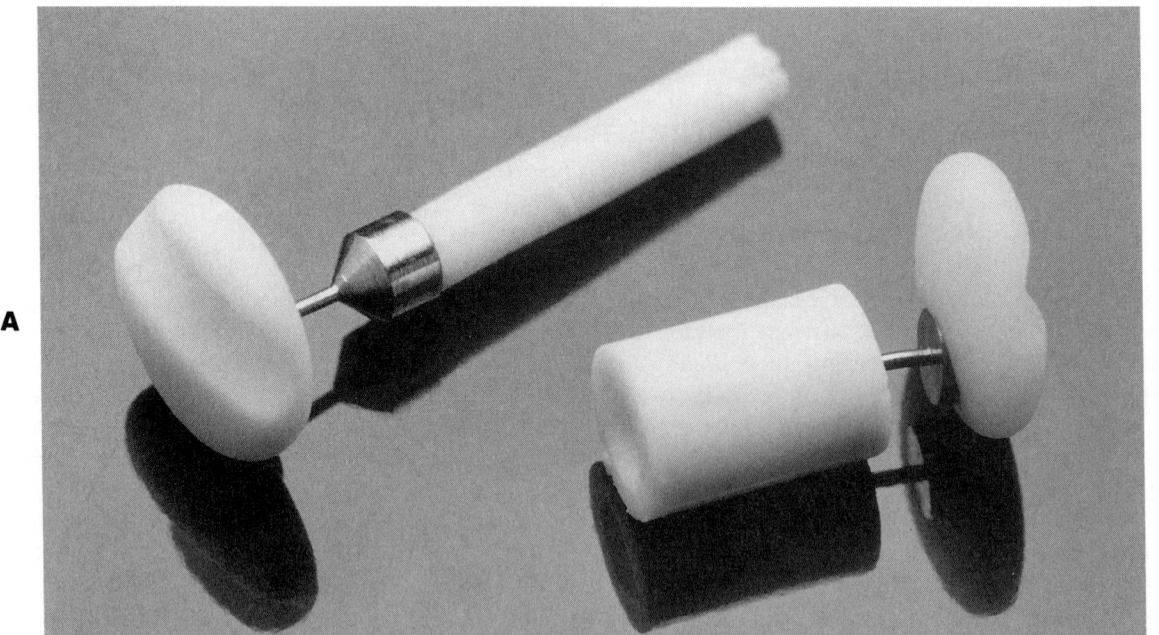

FIG. 18-22 **A,** Causse Flex hydroxyapatite offset total ossicular replacement prosthesis (TORP). **B,** Causse Flex hydroxyapatite offset partial ossicular replacement prosthesis (PORP).

Courtesy Microtek Medical, Inc., Columbus, Miss.

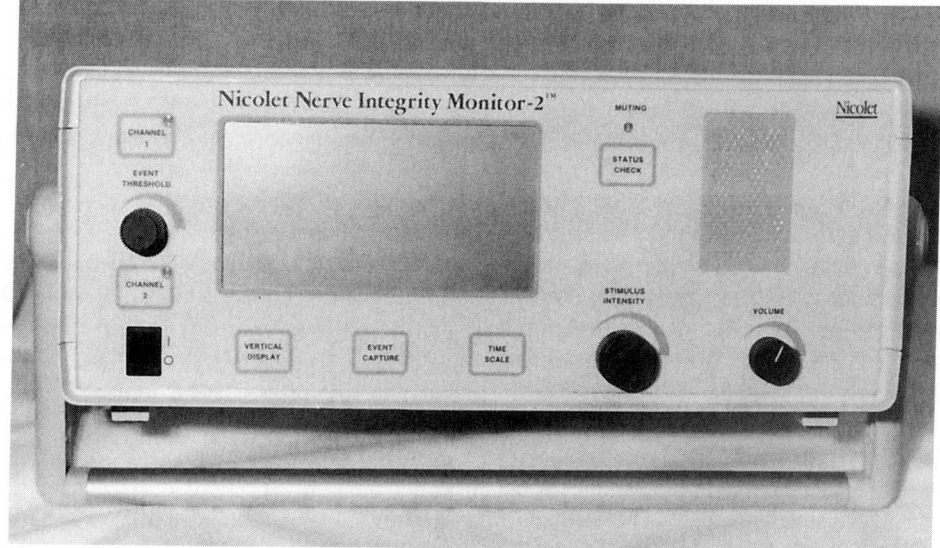

FIG. 18-23   Nerve integrity monitor system for intraoperative facial nerve monitoring. Courtesy XOMED, Inc., Jacksonville, Fla.

Hydroxyapatite is currently utilized in a number of prostheses because its mineral content is very similar to bone and it is well tolerated by the middle ear, thereby decreasing extrusion rates over other materials. Because it is brittle, it is often combined with other materials to make it more easily trimmed for a precise fit in the middle ear (Figs. 18-20 to 18-23).

Procedural considerations

The patient is prepped and draped as for stapedectomy.

Operative procedure

The procedural steps are similar to those for stapedectomy except that the stapes footplate is not removed or opened.

Endolymphatic shunt

An endolymphatic shunt procedure is the creation of an opening into the endolymphatic sac and the insertion of a shunt to allow drainage of excess endolymph into the cerebrospinal fluid or into the mastoid cavity. In Ménière's disease the endolymphatic sac cannot resorb endolymph, resulting in an overaccumulation. This surplus leads to vertigo, in which patients feel a spinning sensation. Movement usually increases the vertigo, which may be accompanied by severe nausea and vomiting. The vertigo attacks occur unpredictably and may last from several minutes to several hours. Most patients with Ménière's disease complain of tinnitus, pressure or fullness in the affected ear, and a fluctuating hearing loss that begins in the lower frequencies. Diagnostic audiometry reveals the hearing loss to be sensorineural. The vertigo may be so severe that it disrupts the patient's life-style. On a medical regimen of tranquilizers, diuretics, vasodilators, and a low-sodium diet, approximately 85% of patients are able to adequately control their symptoms. For those whose symptoms persist, surgical intervention is recommended.

Procedural considerations

Preoperative assessment by the perioperative nurse confirms that the patient's electrolyte levels (especially potassium) are adequate and provides a basis for the support system to be carried out intraoperatively and postoperatively. Because Ménière's disease may develop bilaterally in 20% of patients, conservative therapy is often employed.

The patient is prepped and draped as for a mastoidectomy.

Operative procedure

1 to 7. These steps are as for mastoidectomy.
8. Drilling with a diamond burr over the posterior fossa dura is continued until the endolymphatic sac is identified.
9. An incision is made into the lateral wall of the sac with a microknife such as a sickle, Beaver blade, or Ziegler. An incision is then made through the medial wall, exposing the subarachnoid space.
10. A shunt (commercially prepared tube, Silastic tubing, or Silastic sheeting) is inserted with microforceps and is manipulated into place, usually with microinstruments such as a Rosen needle, fine pick, or gimmick. When the shunt is designed to drain into the mastoid, only the lateral wall of the sac is incised.

11. The incision is closed with suture of the surgeon's preference.
12. A pressure dressing is applied to the affected ear.

Labyrinthectomy

Labyrinthectomy is a procedure that destroys the membranous labyrinth to relieve the patient of severe vertigo. The procedure is usually performed when the disease is unilateral, a shunt has been ineffective, and the patient's hearing is poor. Because the inner ear is destroyed, the patient may be very dizzy for several days until the brainstem begins to compensate for the destroyed labyrinth. The operation also leaves the ear deaf.

Procedural considerations

This procedure may be performed on the patient via the transmastoid or transtympanic approach. The patient is prepped and draped as described for tympanoplasty.

Operative procedures
Transmastoid approach

1 to 7. These steps are as for mastoidectomy.
8. A hole is drilled into the horizontal semicircular canal with a small diamond burr.
9. The membranous labyrinth is removed with a fine pick or hook and microsuctions. Streptomycin-soaked absorbable gelatin sponge may be placed in the inner ear to ensure destruction of all nerve elements.
10. The hole may be covered with bone or temporalis muscle or fascia.
11. The incision is closed with suture of the surgeon's choice.
12. A pressure dressing is applied.

Transtympanic approach

1 to 9. These steps are as for stapedectomy.
10. The incus is separated from the malleus, usually with a pick, and removed with alligator or cup forceps.
11. The membranous labyrinth is removed by means of picks and microsuctions. Streptomycin-soaked absorbable gelatin sponge is introduced into the inner ear.
12. Moistened absorbable gelatin sponge may be placed in the oval window and middle ear space.
13. The tympanomeatal flap is returned via a gimmick, drum elevator, picks, or Rosen needle.
14. The external auditory canal may be packed with absorbable gelatin sponge or a rosebud pack as described for the tympanoplasty procedure.
15. An external pressure dressing of elastic gauze is applied.

Vestibular neurectomy

A vestibular neurectomy may be done by any of 3 routes; the retrolabyrinthine, the suboccipital (or retrosigmoid), or the middle cranial fossa approach. Described below is the retrolabyrinthine approach; the other approaches are described in following sections. In vestibular neurectomy the vestibular portion of the eighth cranial nerve (acoustic nerve) is transected, but the cochlear portion is left intact to relieve the patient of severe vertigo. Vestibular neurectomy is performed when a patient has adequate hearing and a labyrinthectomy is not indicated.

Procedural considerations

The patient's abdomen or lateral thigh is prepped and draped for the purpose of obtaining fat or a segment of muscle and fascia to be used for obliteration of the mastoid cavity at the end of the procedure. If the abdomen is used, most surgeons prefer to take fat from the left side to avoid future confusion with an appendectomy scar. Setups for the graft and neurectomy procedure are separate to avoid cross-contamination. The graft may be taken before the procedure or after the vestibular nerve has been transected, depending on the surgeon's preference. The patient is prepped and draped as for tympanoplasty.

Operative procedure

1. Lidocaine with or without epinephrine is injected subcutaneously using a 3- or 5-ml syringe.
2. A retrolabyrinthine U-shaped incision is made slightly posterior to the area of the postauricular incision used in other otologic surgery.
3. An incision is made in the mastoid muscles with a no. 10 or 15 blade. These muscles are elevated with a Lempert, Joseph, or similar elevator.
4. A self-retaining retractor is inserted after the muscles and periosteum are elevated.
5. The surgeon begins drilling, usually with a large cutting burr, and continues until a complete mastoidectomy is performed. The sigmoid sinus and posterior and inferior semicircular canals are skeletonized with a diamond burr. The posterior fossa bone is removed, exposing the posterior fossa dura. During the drilling process burr sizes and types (cutting and diamond) may be changed as vital structures are identified. The scrub nurse must ensure that irrigation and suction are adequate. The surgeon may pause during the drilling to verify vital structures with a microinstrument such as a Rosen needle, gimmick, pick, or searcher.
6. The posterior fossa dura is incised with a sickle or Ziegler microknife. Hemostasis may be achieved by the use of bipolar forceps, a moistened absorbable gelatin sponge covered by a cottonoid, or Surgicel. Cottonoids, Surgicel, and gelatin sponge may be loaded onto bayonet forceps before the forceps are placed in the surgeon's hand or may be introduced into the field by the scrub nurse with the use of bayonet forceps while the surgeon controls another bayonet forceps.
7. As exploration and dissection of the cochleovestibular nerve are carried out, cottonoids may be used to cover vital structures and thus maintain orientation.

The vestibular portion of the eighth cranial nerve (acoustic) is identified by the surgeon and transsected with microscissors or a microknife.

8. Hemostasis is achieved by the methods mentioned in step 6.
9. The dural incision is closed with suture of the surgeon's preference, usually no. 4-0 silk or nylon on a very small needle.
10. Fat from the abdomen or fascia and muscle from the lateral aspect of the thigh are packed over the closed dural incision, and the skin incision is closed.
11. A pressure dressing of elastic gauze is applied.

Facial nerve decompression

Facial nerve decompression is a procedure designed to identify and relieve an area of compression of the facial nerve. The most common form of facial paralysis is Bell's palsy. It provokes more controversy regarding proper management than any other disorder of the facial nerve. The cause is unknown, although clinical and laboratory evidence suggests a virus of the herpes simplex group. The patient experiences multiple problems such as decreased tearing, inability to close the affected eye, and drooping of the affected corner of the mouth with pooling of oral secretions. Preoperatively the eye is protected by ointments and the eyelid is taped closed, or an adhesive bubble is placed over the eye to trap moisture. This protection is continued into the postoperative period unless a tarsorrhaphy (suturing the eyelid closed) is performed intraoperatively. The patient is taught to place food at the back of the tongue on the unaffected side to assist in mastication. Tilting the head to the unaffected side while eating decreases the pooling of oral secretions and drooling. The patient must be taught proper mouth care because the pooling of oral secretions may lead to dental caries or gingivitis. This regimen is continued until the nerve manifests its regeneration by the return of facial movement. The facial nerve may be decompressed via a translabyrinthine approach when trauma has destroyed the hearing and caused facial nerve paralysis. The narrowest segment of the bony canal compressing the facial nerve is deep in the temporal bone and may also be approached through the middle cranial fossa approach when hearing is to be preserved. Both approaches may be useful under selected circumstances.

Transmastoid, translabyrinthine approach
Procedural considerations. The patient is prepped and draped as described for tympanoplasty.
Operative procedure

1 to 7. These steps are as for mastoidectomy.
8. Following complete mastoidectomy, the dissection is carried out by the use of cutting and diamond burrs until the internal auditory canal and the posterior fossa bone are removed.
9. The bone immediately over the facial nerve is removed by the use of nerve excavators and picks.

10. The facial nerve sheath is incised with a facial nerve knife, neurectomy knife, sickle knife, neurectomy scissors, or micropicks. The incision and decompression are carried out from the stylomastoid foramen to the brainstem.
11. Hemostasis is achieved by the use of moistened absorbable gelatin sponge, cottonoids, Surgicel, bipolar forceps, or a combination.
12. The incision is closed with suture of the surgeon's preference.
13. A pressure dressing of elastic gauze is applied.

Middle cranial fossa approach
Procedural considerations. The patient's hair is shaved almost to the midline on the affected side. Povidone-iodine is usually used for the prep, which includes the portion of the head that has been shaved, the affected side of the face, and the neck. Lidocaine with or without epinephrine is usually injected subcutaneously above the ear to assist in hemostasis.
Operative procedure

1. The temporalis muscle is incised and elevated with a Lempert, Shambaugh, or similar elevator.
2. Hemostasis is achieved by clamping and tying vessels or with electrocoagulation.
3. A square of bone is drilled from the temporal bone to expose the middle cranial fossa dura. (The bone is saved for replacement at the end of the procedure.)
4. A self-retaining retractor with a blade for retraction of the middle fossa (for example, a Fisch middle fossa retractor or House-Urban retractor) is inserted.
5. The microscope is brought into place, and the dura is elevated from the floor of the middle fossa with a Freer elevator, a gimmick, or similar instruments.
6. Once hemostasis is achieved and the blade is inserted over the dura to expose the middle fossa, drilling may proceed.
7. When the bone becomes quite thin, the surgeon may remove the remaining bone with excavators to avoid damaging the nerve sheath.
8. The facial nerve sheath is incised with a facial nerve knife, neurectomy knife, neurectomy scissors, or microknife.
9. The retractor is removed when hemostasis is achieved, and the bone flap is replaced.
10. The temporalis muscle is approximated and sutured. The incision is closed with suture of the surgeon's preference.
11. A pressure dressing of elastic gauze is applied.

Damage to the facial nerve from trauma, infection, or tumors may be treated surgically by these approaches. Facial nerve grafting requires the use of a separate setup for obtaining a nerve for grafting and microinstrumentation for handling the nerves as well as suturing them. Microsutures such as nos. 8-0 to 11-0 are used.

Removal of acoustic neuroma (vestibular schwannoma)

An acoustic neuroma arises from the Schwann cells of the vestibular portion of the eighth cranial (acoustic) nerve and are therefore more appropriately termed vestibular schwannomas. These tumors are benign but may grow to a size that produces symptoms of cerebellar and brainstem origin.

Vestibular schwannoma was a rare clinical finding in the past. With the extension of life expectancy and improved diagnostic technology, the diagnosis of these tumors has become more frequent. Brainstem auditory evoked response is a highly sensitive noninvasive test for this tumor. If this test yields suspicious findings, an MRI of the brain and internal auditory canals is performed.

Depending on the rate and direction of tumor growth, symptoms may include hearing loss, tinnitus, vertigo, headaches, double vision, diplopia, decreased corneal reflex, decreased blink reflex, impaired taste, reduced lacrimation, facial paralysis, diminished gag reflex, vocal cord paralysis, atrophy or fasciculation of the tongue, weakness of the sternocleidomastoid and trapezius muscles, disturbance in balance and gait, hydrocephalus, lethargy, confusion, drowsiness, and coma. Most patients complain of only a unilateral tinnitus and hearing loss, the main symptoms of a possible acoustic neuroma.

Several centers have developed great expertise in acoustic neuroma surgery, which requires the combined team of an otologist and a neurosurgeon.

Procedural considerations

The translabyrinthine approach for the removal of an acoustic tumor has increased in popularity over the past decade. It reduces mortality and morbidity and offers a good chance of saving the facial nerve, if the tumor has not directly invaded it. The patient should be informed preoperatively about the presence of a Foley catheter, arterial line, temperature probe, shaved head, and graft site incision during the postoperative period. Postoperative complications may include a cerebrospinal fluid leak, vertigo, facial nerve weakness or paralysis, and wound infection. These patients require considerable postoperative teaching in preparation for discharge. Areas addressed in discharge instructions include activity, oral care, diet, medication, return office visit, eye care, and graft site and suture line care. Emotional support is vital because of the severity of the disease, the operative procedure, and the altered body image patients experience as a result of removal of their hair and facial

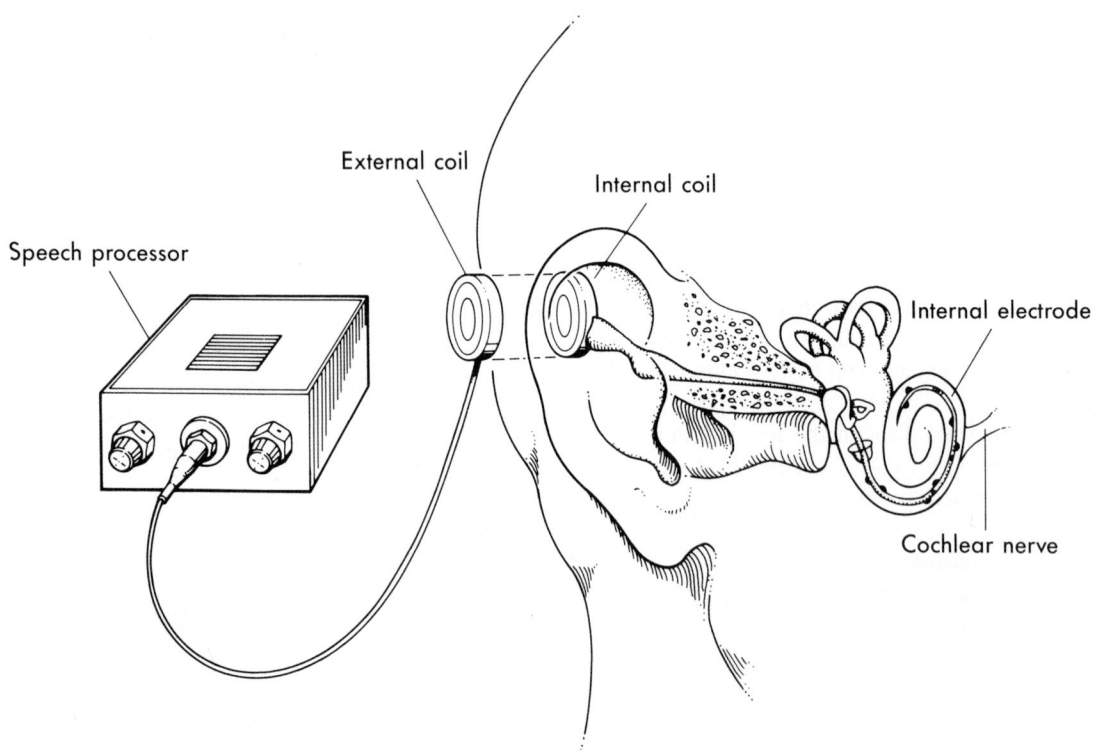

FIG. 18-24 Cochlear implant system. Sound is transformed into electrical signal in speech processor. Signal is transmitted from external to internal induction coil, which is connected to electrode implanted near cochlear nerve.

From Cummings, C.W., et al. (1993). *Otolaryngology—head and neck surgery* (7th ed.), (Vol. 4). St. Louis: Mosby.

weakness or paralysis. Members of the national support group, the Acoustic Neuroma Association, may be of assistance.

The patient's hair is shaved to the midline of the affected side. Some patients prefer to have the entire head shaved to facilitate wearing a wig. The options should be presented preoperatively to enable the patient to make a decision before surgery.

The patient is prepped and draped as described for labyrinthectomy. Lidocaine with or without epinephrine may be injected subcutaneously behind the ear. A facial nerve monitor is routinely utilized in the excision of cerebellopontine angle tumors (Fig. 18-24).

Sequential compression hosiery is used intraoperatively and for the first 24 to 46 hours postoperatively or until the patient is ambulatory to decrease the risk of deep venous thrombosis and pulmonary embolism.

Operative procedure

1. A postauricular incision is made slightly longer and wider than the incision in mastoidectomy. The periosteum is elevated from the mastoid bone with a Lempert, Shambaugh, or similar elevator.
2. Self-retaining retractors are inserted, and the cortical mastoidectomy is begun with a large cutting burr.
3. The microscope is brought into position, and the attic is opened to visualize the ossicles. The sigmoid sinus, middle fossa dura, and superior petrosal sinus are left with a thin covering of bone. The semicircular canals are exposed. The incus is removed with alligator or cup forceps and suction.
4. The semicircular canals are excised with the drill. The utricle and saccule are removed, and the aqueduct of the vestibule is drilled out.
5. On completion of the drilling, the remainder of bone is removed with nerve excavators, Fisch dissectors, or picks from the dura of the internal meatus, posterior fossa, middle fossa, and petrosal angle. The wedge of bone between the facial and superior vestibular nerves (Bill's bar) is removed.
6. The dura is opened with microscissors or a dura knife. Dissection of the tumor ensues with a gimmick, Freer microelevator, microinstrument, and bipolar forceps (with or without suction, depending on the surgeon's preference). Hemostasis is frequently achieved through the use of a moistened absorbable gelatin sponge, cottonoids, Surgicel, and a bipolar coagulator.
7. When the tumor has been removed by the use of pituitary cup forceps, long alligator forceps, and similar instruments, hemostasis is achieved.
8. Graft material is obtained to pack the mastoid cavity created from the drilling. It may be fat, fascia, or muscle. The packing is performed meticulously to avoid a cerebrospinal fluid leak postoperatively.
9. On completion of the packing, the wound is closed with suture of the surgeon's choice.
10. A thick pressure dressing, consisting of gauze for absorbency and elastic gauze for pressure, is applied.

The patient is placed in an intensive care setting for close observation for 24 hours. Initial postoperative nursing care includes monitoring of neurologic and routine vital signs, monitoring of facial nerve function on the affected side, observation of the dressing for drainage, close monitoring of temperature, monitoring of intake and output, observation and testing of nasal drainage to determine cerebrospinal fluid leak, positioning, deep breathing by the patient (coughing is discouraged because of the possibility of dislodging the graft), administering medications for pain and nausea, antibiotics, and stool softeners (to prevent straining, which might dislodge the graft), and providing emotional support to the patient. Early ambulation is advised to maintain proper circulation and avoid pulmonary complications, which could lead to coughing and subsequent dislodgment of the graft. While the patient's opposite vestibular system is compensating for the removed system, the patient needs assistance in moving and ambulating. The family is advised to help as needed, while allowing the patient to move at his or her pace to avoid sudden vertigo and nausea.

If facial function is altered on the affected side because of manipulation, edema, or surgical excision, the patient must use supportive measures until adequate function returns. These include lubrication, covering, and inspection of the eye to avoid corneal injury, frequent brushing and rinsing of the oral cavity to prevent dental caries from the pooling of secretions on the affected side, a semisoft to soft diet to allow the patient more ease in directing the food toward the back of the unaffected side of the mouth, and tilting the head toward the unaffected side. The soft diet and head tilting are designed to decrease the collection of food and the spillage of food from the affected side yet allow the patient to maintain dignity while eating.

Cochlear implantation

Cochlear implantation is the placement of an electrode into the snail-shaped cochlea of the inner ear for stimulation of remaining nerves in the otherwise profoundly deaf patient. Approximately half a million people in the United States have complete deafness. Cochlear implantation seems to be beneficial for a certain segment of that group. The most important prerequisite for candidacy is little or no benefit from the use of conventional hearing aids. Adults who become profoundly deaf after acquiring language skills are candidates. Children who are either congenitally deaf or acquire deafness prior to age 18 years are cochlear implant candidates. The acquisition of language skills prior to deafness is not a necessary requirement for children to be candidates. Appropriate auditory training and psychologic counseling are needed following appropriate selection of candidates.

Technologic advancements have given the deaf patient

new hope in the area of cochlear implantation. The device is implanted in the cochlea, with the receiver resting in the mastoid. As the device receives sound through the receiver, it emits electrical impulses through the transmitter into the cochlea and along the acoustic nerve. These impulses are interpreted as sound in the temporal cortex of the cerebrum. The patient must be taught to interpret these sounds through extensive training.

Risk of meningitis or infection is rare, but these patients should be followed closely postoperatively.

Operative procedure

1. A U-shaped incision is made, creating a skin flap well behind the mastoid. The flap, including the temporalis muscle, is elevated, exposing the underlying bone. The site of the internal coil is identified, and with a special drill a circular depression in the squamous portion of the temporal bone is made to house the internal coil.
2. A mastoidectomy is accomplished with preservation of the bony ear canal and opening of the facial recess.
3. The coil is secured in the depressed area in the temporal bone, and the electrode is introduced through the facial recess and through a cochleostomy into the cochlea. It is secured in place with a piece of temporalis fascia.
4. The wound is closed. The patient is observed for 6 to 8 weeks until complete wound healing has occurred. Then the external device is applied over the internal coil. This allows transmission of an electrical signal, picked up at an ear level microphone and processed in a microprocessor worn on the body.

Computerized facial nerve monitoring

Technology enables the surgeon to monitor movement and function of the facial nerve intraoperatively. This monitoring decreases trauma to the facial nerve during tumor dissection and assists the surgeon in determining the point of surgical intervention in idiopathic facial nerve palsy.

The mechanism of hearing can also be tested during surgical intervention to determine the effectiveness of a procedure and thus predict the patient's postoperative result.

Implantable hearing aids

A good deal of research in the development of implantable hearing aids is going on in different parts of the world. At the present time conductive hearing aids are available for a small percentage of the hard-of-hearing who have conductive hearing loss due to chronic ear disease and cannot benefit from a hearing aid. Implantable hearing aids for sensorineural hearing loss are the challenge of the future.

BIBLIOGRAPHY

Benumof, J.L., & Saidman, L.J. (1992). *Anesthesia and perioperative complications*. St. Louis: Mosby.

Cummings, C.W., et al. (1993). *Otolaryngology—head and neck surgery* (7th ed.), (Vol. 4). St. Louis: Mosby.

DeWeese, D.D., et al. (1988). *Otolaryngology—head and neck surgery* (7th ed.). St. Louis: Mosby.

Pagana, K.D., & Pagana, T.J. (1992). *Mosby's diagnostic and laboratory test reference*. St. Louis: Mosby.

Rauch, S.D., & Bartley, M.L. (1992). Argon laser stapedectomy: Comparison to traditional fenestration techniques, *American Journal of Otology, 13(6)*, 556-560, 1992.

Rothrock, J.C. (1990). *Perioperative nursing care planning*. St. Louis: Mosby.

Seidel, H.M., et al. (1991). *Mosby's guide to physical examination* (2nd ed.). St. Louis: Mosby.

Smith, M.F.W., & McElveen, J.T., Jr. (1992). *Neurological surgery of the ear*. St. Louis: Mosby.

19

RHINOLOGIC AND SINUS SURGERY

BRENDA C. KERSTEN

R hinologic surgery is performed to treat internal and external injuries and malformations and to provide for effective functioning of the respiratory system.

Sinus surgery has changed significantly during the past several decades, primarily due to the evolution and refinement of endoscopic sinus surgery. In 1901 Hirschmann used a modified cystoscope to examine the sinuses. The value of paranasal sinus endoscopy was debated through the 1920s, with Zarniko questioning whether the endoscope was a worthwhile diagnostic tool or just an interesting toy. After the Second World War, maxillary sinus endoscopy gained the support of individuals in a number of countries, although it still did not achieve widespread acceptance. In the 1950s Hopkins made fundamental improvements in the optics of endoscopy, including a light source that was separate from the instrument, excellent resolution with high contrast, a large field of vision despite the small diameter of the endoscope, and perfect fidelity of color.

Thanks to these new endoscopes, which met the highest technical requirements, endoscopy of the upper airways has enjoyed worldwide popularity since the early 1970s. Although initially the maxillary sinus was the focus of diagnostic interest, endoscopy was soon extended to the other paranasal sinuses. The Hopkins rod rigid nasal endoscopes made it possible to examine in detail the clefts and recesses of the nose. Today the nasal endoscopic examination, in combination with tomography, allows the identification of small, circumscribed changes in the paranasal sinuses. These small changes are frequently of considerable pathophysiologic significance.

SURGICAL ANATOMY

The nose is covered with skin and is supported internally by bone and cartilage. The two external nares provide openings through which air can enter and leave the nasal cavity. These openings contain internal hairs that help prevent coarse particles sometimes carried by air from entering the nose.

The nose is divided into the prominent external portion and the internal portion known as the nasal cavity (Fig. 19-1). The chief purpose of the nose is the preparation of air for use in the lungs.

The external nose projects from the face. The upper portion of the external nose is formed by the nasal bones and the frontal process of the maxillae, and the lower portion is formed by a group of nasal cartilages and connective tissue covered with skin (Fig. 19-2). The nostrils and the tip of the nose are shaped by the major alar cartilages. The nares are separated by the columella, which is formed by the lower margin of the septal cartilage, the medial parts of the major alar cartilages, and the anterior nasal spine, all of which are covered by skin. The nasal cavity is a hollow space behind the nose that is divided medially into right and left portions by the nasal septum.

The nasal septum is composed of three structures: the nasal cartilage, the vomer bone, and the perpendicular plate of the ethmoid bone. The septum is covered by mucous membrane on either side. A deviated or fractured septum may be repaired surgically by mobilization of the fracture or removal of the deformed cartilage or bone.

The internal portion, or nasal cavity, is divided by the nasal septum into two parts at its midline. The nasal cavity communicates with the outside by its external openings, called the nares. The nares open into the nasopharynx through the choanae. The nasal cavity is also associated with each ear by means of the eustachian tube and with the paranasal sinuses (frontal, maxillary, ethmoidal, and sphenoidal) through their respective orifices (meatuses). The nasal cavity also communicates with the conjunctiva through the nasolacrimal duct. The nasal cavity is separated from the lingual cavity by the hard and soft palates (see Fig. 19-1) and from the cranial cavity by the ethmoid bone. It is held together by periosteal covering over bone and by perichondrium, which extends over the cartilages. The turbinate bones of the nasal structure are arranged one above the other, separated by grooves and meatuses. These act as drainage passages of the accessory sinuses and are known as the sphenoethmoidal recesses and the superior, middle, and inferior meatuses, respectively (Fig. 19-3).

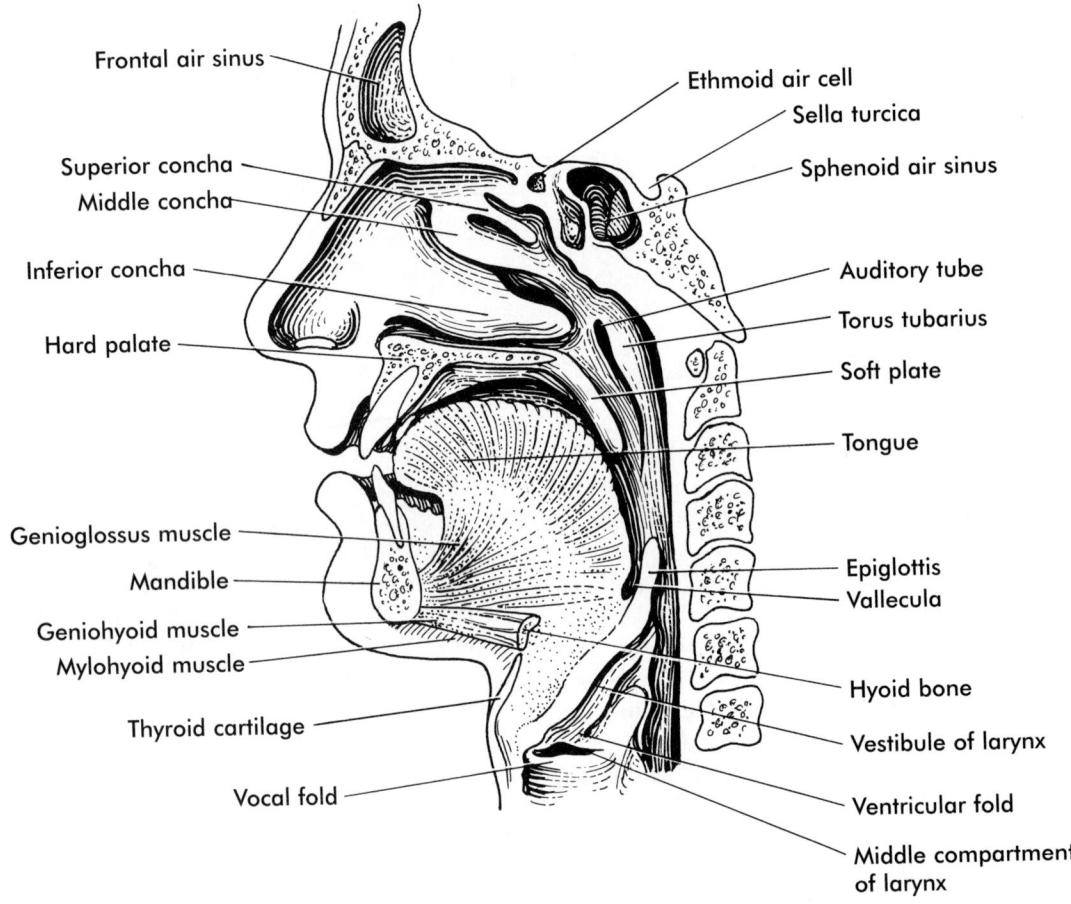

FIG. 19-1   Sagittal section of face and neck.

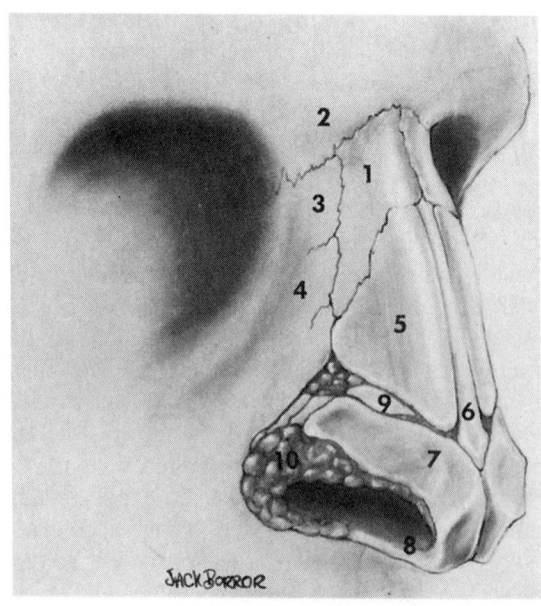

FIG. 19-2   Nasal bony framework. *1,* Nasal bone; *2,* frontal bone; *3,* lacrimal bone; *4,* maxillary bone; *5,* upper lateral cartilage; *6,* nasal septum; *7,* lower lateral cartilage, lateral crus; *8,* lower lateral cartilage, medial crus; *9,* sesamoid cartilage; *10,* fibrofatty tissue.

From Saunders, W.H., et al. others. (1979). *Nursing care in eye, ear, nose and throat disorders.* St. Louis: Mosby.

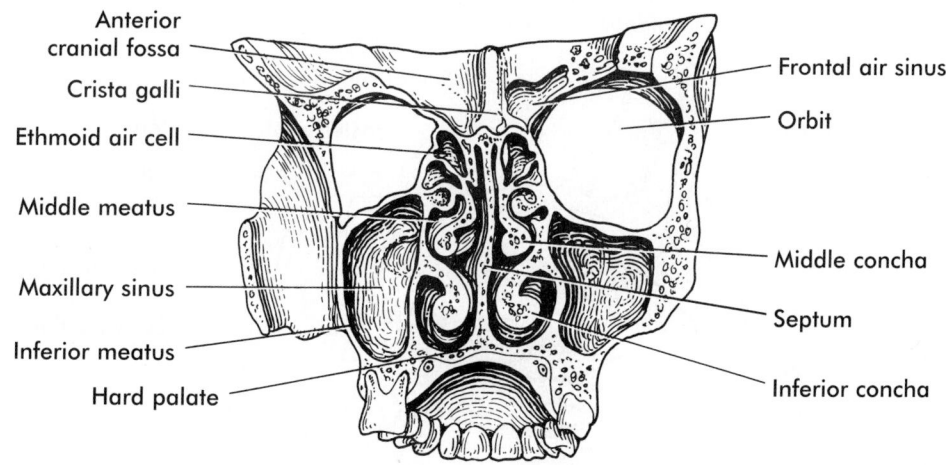

FIG. 19-3   Vertical section through nose. Plane of section passes slightly oblique through left first molar tooth and behind second right premolar tooth. Posterior wall of right frontal sinus removed.

The nasal sinuses serve as air spaces and communicate with the nasal cavity through the meatuses. Anteriorly, on each side of the skull, the frontal sinus, the anterior ethmoidal sinus, and the maxillary sinus (antrum of Highmore) drain into the middle meatus; posteriorly the ethmoidal and the sphenoidal sinuses drain into the superior meatus and the sphenoethmoidal recess. A passageway for the flow of air is provided by the irregular air spaces between these structures. Because of their shape, the air is forced to flow in thin air waves.

The sensory nerve supply of the nasal cavity is derived from the trigeminal nerve.

The nose and sinuses receive their blood supply (Fig. 19-4) from the branches of the internal maxillary, anterior ethmoid, sphenopalatine, nasopalatine, pharyngeal, and posterior ethmoid arteries. Masses of communicating veins lie below the epithelial layer of the turbinate bones, and the veins just beneath the skin anastomose freely. Dilatation of the superficial veins may cause the turbinate bones to swell, whereas contraction of these vessels may cause the bones to shrink.

PERIOPERATIVE NURSING CONSIDERATIONS

ASSESSMENT

As with any operation performed with the patient under local anesthesia for which the patient's understanding and cooperation are important, the purpose and nature of the endoscopic and nasal procedure must be explained in a manner that is understandable. The patient's physician will have earlier discussed the indications and the purpose of the procedure. Tomograms or CT scans are helpful in showing the relationship between the diseased ethmoid and other paranasal sinuses and for pointing out the potential technical difficulties and the risks inherent because of the proximity of the neighboring structures. These relationships can be shown to the patient to facilitate understanding the steps and sequence of the surgical intervention, and the approximate length of the procedure, since the patient is often a conscious participant.

Apart from the physician obtaining an informed consent, the patient, who is receiving local anesthesia with sedation, must be informed that after premedication has been administered, he or she will become very drowsy, but will not be asleep, and consequently will be aware of most of the events taking place. Patients should be informed that they will be aware that their nose is being operated upon but will not feel pain. It is inevitable that there will be some blood loss, but the loss of blood is almost invariably small and should not affect the patient in any way. Patients should always be sufficiently awake to tell the surgeon if they wish to expectorate. Patients should always be reminded to indicate promptly if they do not feel well, become nauseated, or feel faint. In this way the patient is motivated to be a participant in the procedure.

The perioperative nurse must collect comprehensive baseline data during preoperative assessment of the patient to facilitate accurate monitoring during the surgical procedure. That assessment should include vital signs, allergies, skin condition, sensory deficits, central nervous system problems, and mental status of the patient. Close attention should be paid to any past drug reactions experienced by the patient, especially if related to the administration of local anesthetics. Questions about previous dental experiences involving this type of anesthesia and the patient's tolerance to it can provide a clue to how the patient will react to the anesthetic agents.

Cardiac status should be noted because many surgeons use epinephrine as an additive to the local anesthetic. The epinephrine acts as a vasoconstrictor and reduces the blood

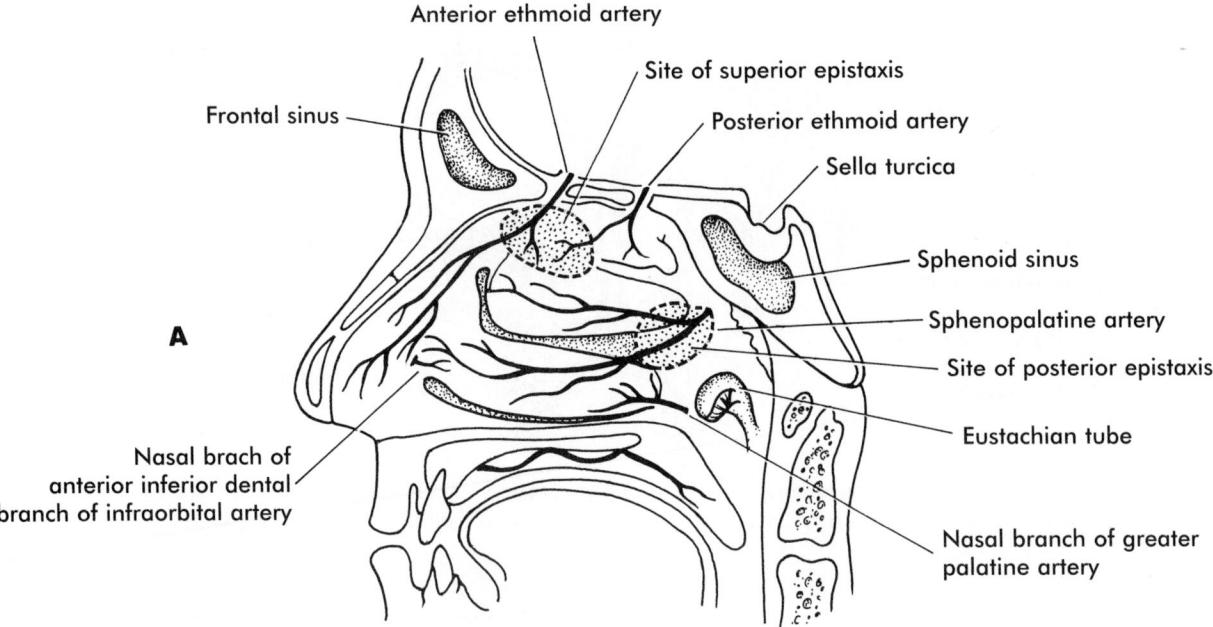

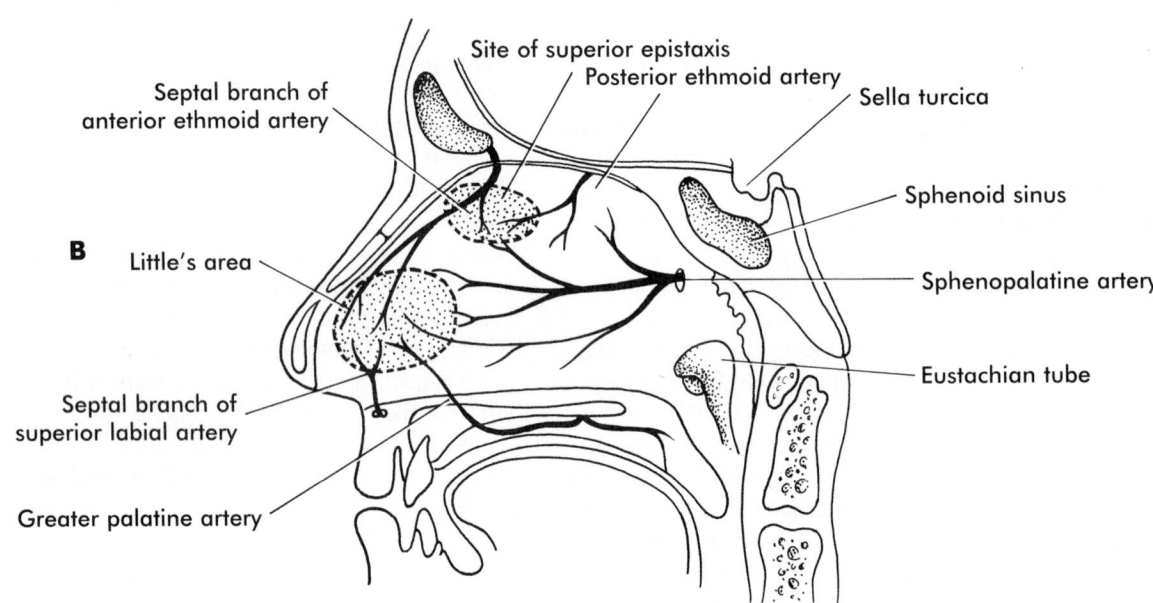

FIG. 19-4 **A,** Blood supply of lateral nasal wall. **B,** Arteries of nasal septum.

loss during surgery but may also contribute to cardiac dysrhythmias. In addition, cocaine is often preoperatively administered intranasally to afford the patient more comfort during injection of local anesthetic and to achieve local vasoconstriction. Respiratory patterns and any respiratory conditions, such as asthma, should be noted. Physical limitations of the patient can determine additional aspects that should be included in the intraoperative care of the patient.

NURSING DIAGNOSIS

Nursing diagnoses appropriate to patients undergoing rhinologic or sinus surgery are as follows:

- Sensory/perceptual alterations (olfactory and gustatory) related to nasal packing postoperatively
- High risk for pain related to local anesthesia
- Anxiety related to fear of the unknown
- High risk for infection related to surgical site

OUTCOME IDENTIFICATION

Outcomes identified for the selected nursing diagnoses could be stated as:

- The patient will verbalize understanding of anticipated postoperative alteration in the senses of smell and taste.

- The patient will demonstrate effective coping with the physical and psychologic effects of pain.
- The patient's anxiety will be reduced or controlled.
- The patient will experience no signs or symptoms of infection postoperatively.

PLANNING

Planning of the patient's care is based on the preoperative assessment, identified nursing diagnoses, and expected outcomes as well as the nurse's knowledge of the scheduled surgical procedure and associated events, such as the administration of local anesthesia. Development of a meaningful care plan enables the perioperative nurse to meet the patient's needs effectively during surgical intervention.

Supplies necessary to ensure comfort of the patient should be obtained. They may include a foam headrest, a pillow for under the knees, and warm blankets.

Preparation of the operating room includes checking the availability and functional capability of suction, the surgeon's headlight, the pulse oximeter to measure oxygen saturation, oxygen administration equipment, a cardiac monitor, and a blood pressure cuff.

Because local anesthesia is frequently utilized for nasal surgical procedures, the nurse must be prepared to react quickly to signs of allergic reactions or toxic responses. Symptoms of adverse drug reactions include changes in skin such as rash or itching, restlessness, unexplained anxiety or fearfulness, diaphoresis, complaints of blurred vision, tinnitus, dizziness, nausea, palpitation, disturbed respiration, pallor or flushing, and syncope. Emergency drugs, suction apparatus, and resuscitation equipment should be readily available. The risks of local anesthesia are less than those of general anesthesia. Intraoperative pain has an important warning function that contributes greatly to the avoidance of injury to the roof of the ethmoid, the orbit and the optic nerve. Another important feature is that local anesthesia ensures that the surgical team exerts the greatest care and proceeds as atraumatically as possible. Even the well-sedated patient will not tolerate roughness under local anesthesia. The postoperative recovery time is clearly shorter after local anesthesia. General anesthesia should be reserved only for the exceptional patient. If general anesthesia must be used, the nose is prepared in the same way as for local anesthesia, except that topical phenylephrine may be used instead of topical epinephrine for hemostasis during the surgical procedure.

The Sample Care Plan on p. 670 addresses the needs of patients undergoing rhinologic or sinus surgery. It is especially important that preoperative diagnostic scans are displayed in the operating room so that the surgeon can see them by simply raising his or her eyes from the patient. Even after the most thorough preoperative study of the diagnostic scans, there are frequently situations where another review provides additional information for the surgeon and nurse.

IMPLEMENTATION

For most procedures the patient is placed on the OR bed in a supine position. The hair in the nostrils may be clipped with fine, curved scissors. An antibiotic ophthalmic ointment may be put into the eyes of the patient undergoing general anesthesia to protect them from the prep solutions. The patient under local anesthesia should be instructed to keep eyes closed. The person prepping should use the utmost care not to get prepping solutions in the patient's eyes. The face may be cleansed with povidone-iodine.

Prepping and draping of the patient are usually done before injection of the local anesthetic. However, the surgeon may request that the topical anesthetic be placed on the prep table so the nose may be topically anesthetized for a period before the anesthetic injections are started. This allows the topical anesthetic to take effect earlier and affords more vasoconstriction and comfort for the patient. Some surgeons also request that the local anesthetic be placed on the prep table so it can be injected before the skin is prepared. The circulating or monitor nurse should observe any changes in the vital signs of the patient. The amount of both topical and local anesthetic agents used and any additions to the local anesthetics, such as epinephrine, should be recorded on the appropriate records. Several principles of nursing care are basic to all types of nasal surgery. The following information should be given to the patient.

1. Some discomfort may occur during the initial administration of a local anesthetic. If the surgeon uses a topical anesthetic (usually cocaine) as the first phase of anesthesia, it is applied to the nose with applicators. The patient may find the applicators or packing uncomfortable or may have the urge to sneeze. These sensations disappear as the anesthetic takes effect. The needle may cause momentary discomfort, and a burning sensation may occur as the anesthetic is injected. If the surgeon uses epinephrine with the local agent, the resulting weak, quivery feeling and the increased heart rate are effects of the epinephrine and disappear after a few minutes. The patient's cardiac status should be noted at this time.
2. Certain procedures may be performed on entry to the operating room or holding area in accordance with operating room policies, for example, insertion of intravenous lines, application of monitoring devices, and oxygen administration.
3. During the surgical procedure the patient feels the surgeon working and may feel pressure at some point, but should *not* feel pain. The patient should let the surgeon know if any discomfort is felt during the procedure, and more anesthetic can be given.
4. After surgery the head of the bed is elevated to facilitate breathing and drainage.
5. A nasal pack will probably be inserted, and there

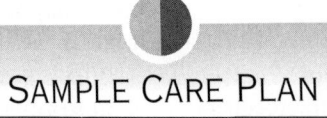

SAMPLE CARE PLAN

NURSING DIAGNOSIS: Sensory/perceptual alterations (olfactory and gustatory) related to nasal packing postoperatively

OUTCOME: The patient will verbalize understanding of the anticipated alteration in the senses of smell and taste.

INTERVENTIONS:

Explain to the patient that a "moustache" dressing will be in place postoperatively and that it will greatly interfere with the sense of smell.

Inform the patient that the sense of taste will also be altered, as with having a head cold.

Assure the patient that these alterations are usually temporary.

Encourage the patient to maintain proper dietary intake even if the food does not smell or taste as it should.

NURSING DIAGNOSIS: High risk for pain related to local anesthesia

OUTCOME: The patient will verbalize knowledge of the physical and psychologic responses to surgical pain.

INTERVENTIONS:

Explain to the patient that some initial discomfort (for example, pinprick, followed by slight burning, then numbness) may be felt during the administration of the local anesthetic.

Inform the patient prior to the injection of the local anesthetic; provide support and reassurance as needed.

Describe the sequence of events to the patient to prevent unrealistic expectations.

Observe for, document, and report any changes in the patient's vital signs (blood pressure, heart rate and rhythm, respiratory rate, and oxygen saturation), skin condition, and mental status.

Be aware of the maximum recommended dosage of local anesthetics (see Chapter 2) and be alert for signs of allergic reactions or toxic responses.

Ask the patient whether he or she is experiencing any pain; communicate the presence of pain sensation to the surgeon.

NURSING DIAGNOSIS: Anxiety related to fear of the unknown

OUTCOME: The patient will verbalize knowledge of the steps of the perioperative process.

INTERVENTIONS:

Using a teaching guide such as a photo album, inform the patient and family of what the preop holding area, OR, and PACU look like. Explain the function of each.

Explain all activities performed by the nursing staff and provide the rationale for each.

Assure the patient that he or she will be informed before any procedure is done.

Provide time for the patient to express fears and concerns.

NURSING DIAGNOSIS: High risk for infection related to surgical site

OUTCOME: The patient will be free from signs and symptoms of infection.

INTERVENTIONS:

Review chart for recent lab results and vital signs.

Obtain baseline data (skin integrity, color).

Maintain aseptic technique and handwashing practices.

Provide antibiotic ointment for packing, as prescribed.

Explain the importance of the moustache dressing. Demonstrate correct procedure for moustache dressing change.

Educate patient and family regarding reportable signs and symptoms of infection.

If antibiotic therapy is prescribed, explain medication regimen and potential adverse drug effects.

may be some difficulty in swallowing. When the patient attempts to swallow, a sucking action occurs in the throat because the packing does not allow air passage through the nose, thereby creating a partial vacuum.

6. Measures to maintain oral hygiene are frequently offered and encouraged because of the postoperative mouth breathing.
7. Some bruising and swelling can be expected after surgery but gradually subside.
8. Forceful nose blowing must be avoided for a time to prevent movement of the rearranged nasal structures.
9. The sense of smell is diminished for a time after surgery but gradually returns.
10. Some numbness may be noticed postoperatively, but this gradually disappears.
11. A moderate amount of discomfort should be expected after surgery; medication is prescribed for this.
12. The procedure for changing the moustache dressing

that is in place postoperatively to absorb any drainage should be reviewed with the patient.
13. Potential complications of bleeding, cerebrospinal fluid leak, and visual or tear duct problems should be reviewed with patients.

Draping

The patient is draped as follows:

1. A small sheet with two towels on top of it is placed over the head of the bed and under the patient's head (head drape).
2. The uppermost towel is brought around the head, including the hairline.
3. The ends of the uppermost towel are secured with a towel clamp, and the free ends are tucked under the patient's head.
4. A split sheet is applied.
5. Moist gauze pads, tape, Band-Aids, or a towel can be placed over the patient's eyes to protect them from injury by instruments and from nasal drainage.

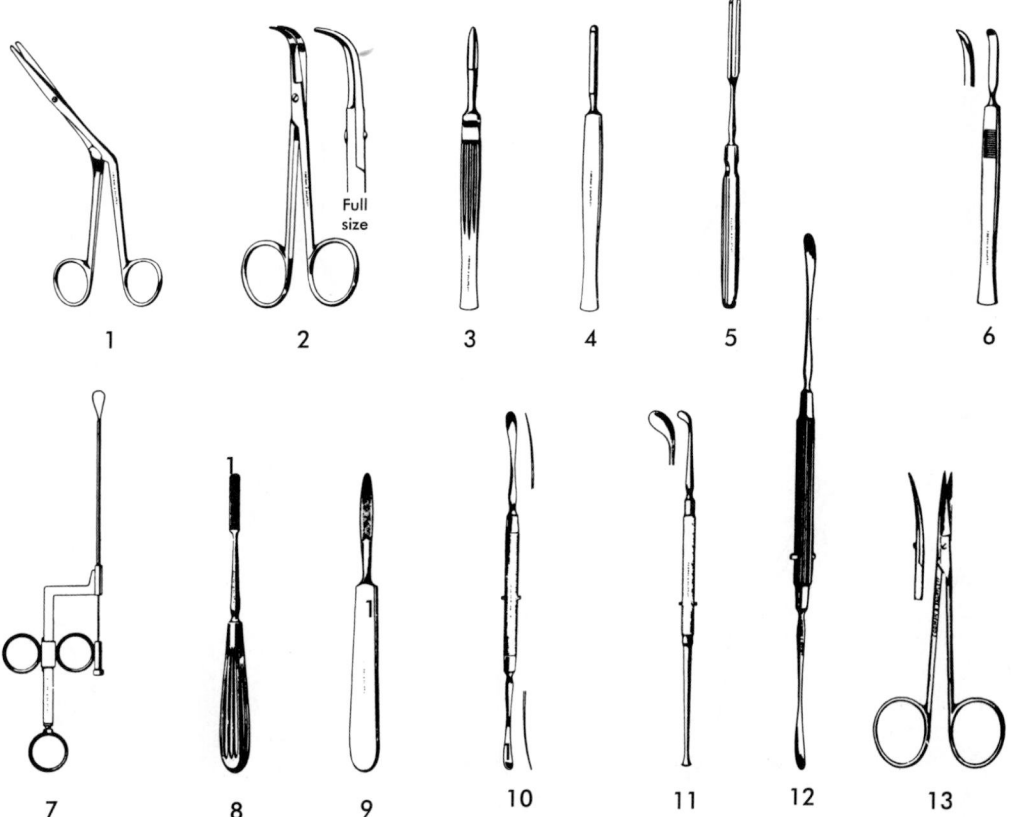

FIG. 19-5 Cutting instruments for operations on external nose and nasal cavity. *1,* Nasal scissors, angled; *2,* Fomon upper lateral scissors; *3,* cartilage knife, beveled blade; *4,* cartilage knife, straight; *5,* cartilage knife, swivel blade; *6,* cartilage nasal knife, curved; *7,* nasal snare; *8,* nasal rasp, narrow; *9,* nasal rasp; *10,* double-ended elevator; *11,* golf stick elevator-dissector; *12,* Freer dissecting elevator; *13,* iris scissors, straight and curved.

Courtesy Codman & Shurtleff, Inc., Randolph, Mass.

Instrumentation

Sterile instruments, supplies, and other items required for rhinologic surgery include the following:

Local anesthesia setup

Cocaine crystals, 4 grains
Cocaine topical solution, 4% or 10%
Lidocaine 1% or 2% (usually with epinephrine 1:100,000)
Luer-Lok syringes, 10 ml
Needles, 27-gauge (1 ½ inches) and 30-gauge (1 inch)

Bayonet tissue forceps
Metal applicators
Cotton balls
X-ray detectable cottonoids ½ inch by 3 inches, with attached strings

Supplies

1 ENT drape pack
1 Split sheet (if not included in the pack)
1 Gauze packing (plain or petrolatum) ½ inch by 72 inches

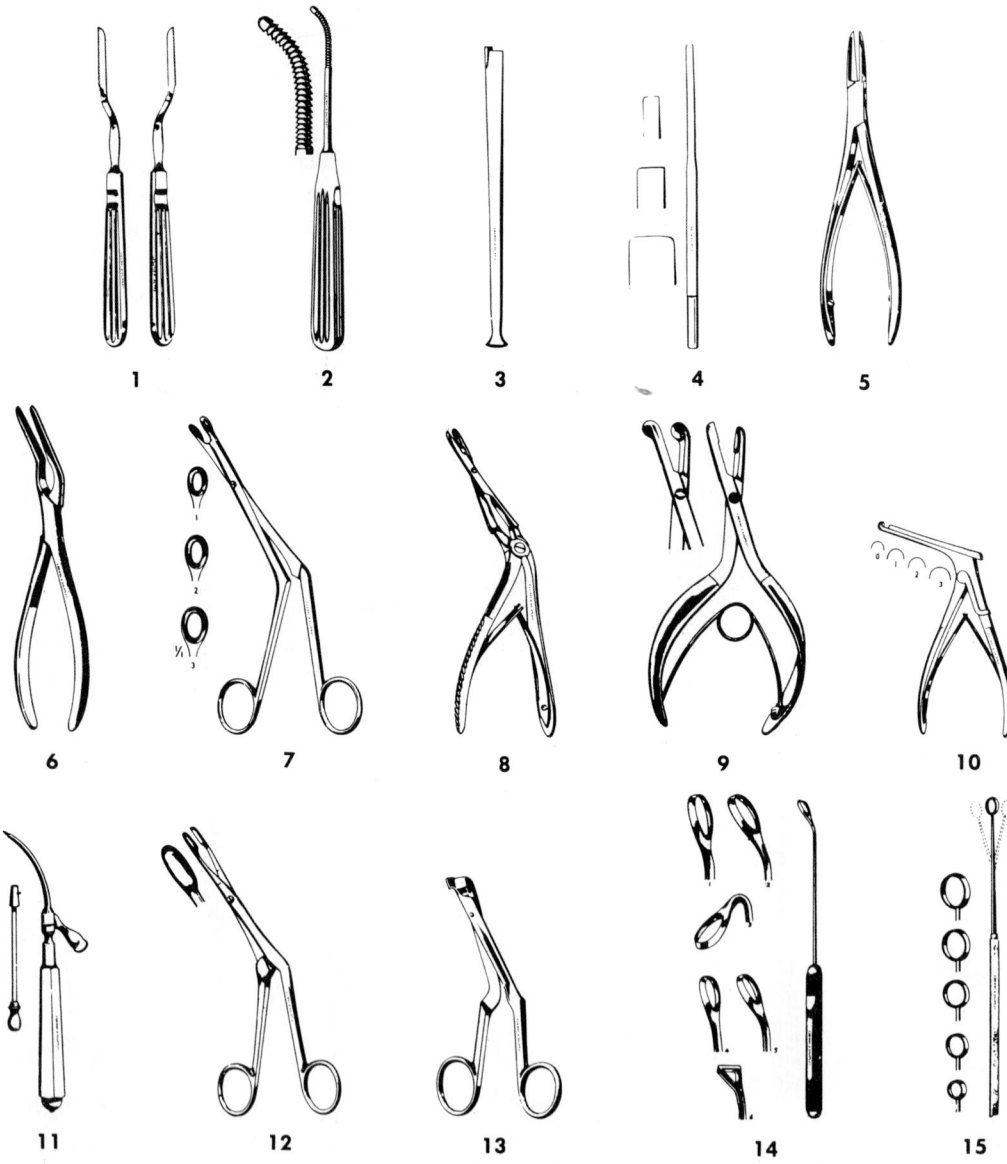

FIG. 19-6   Cutting instruments for operations on external nose and nasal cavity, continued. *1*, Freer nasal saws, right and left; *2*, reamer; *3*, nasal chisel with guard; *4*, osteotome, narrow widths; *5*, nasal bone cutter; *6*, Asch septum forceps; *7*, Bruening septum forceps; *8*, double-action nasal rongeur; *9*, McCoy septum forceps; *10*, Kerrison rongeur; *11*, antrum trocar and stylet; *12*, septum-cutting forceps; *13*, septal ridge-cutting forceps; *14*, Coakley ethmoidal sinus curettes; *15*, Myles antrum ring curettes.

Courtesy Codman & Shurtleff, Inc., Randolph, Mass.

10 X-ray detectable ½-inch by 3-inch cottonoids with attached strings
3 Medication cups
1 Marking pen
1 Package of labels
1 Basin set
Gloves
2 Gowns
1 Skin prep tray
1 Tube of antibiotic ointment or cream
1 Headlight

Cutting instruments (Figs. 19-5 and 19-6)

2 Knife handles, no. 3 or no. 7, for intranasal procedures with no. 15 blades
1 Myles septum-cutting forceps
1 Ballenger swivel knife
1 Freer septum knife
1 Septal forceps
1 Kerrison rongeur
1 Freer septum chisel
1 Freer dissecting elevator
1 Ballenger nasal gouge
1 Knight scissors
1 Fomon scissors
1 Joseph knife (sharp)
1 Joseph knife (blunt)
1 McKenty knife
1 Button knife
1 Maltz rasp
1 Glabella rasp
1 Fomon rasp
2 Freer nasal saws (right and left)
2 Neivert osteotomes (right and left)
2 Narrow osteotomes
1 Bone cutter
2 Jansen-Middleton forceps (open and closed)
6 Coakley curettes (assorted shapes and angles)
1 Suture scissors

Holding and clamping instruments

5 Towel clamps
2 Kelly hemostats, straight
1 Mayo forceps, curved
2 Bayonet tissue forceps
1 Adson tissue forceps

Exposing instruments (Fig. 19-7)

2 Killian nasal specula
1 Cottle nasal speculum
4 Skin hooks (two single and two double)
Retractors, assorted sizes

Suturing items

1 Needle holder, small
1 Jacobson bayonet needle holder (for intranasal procedures)
Suture of the surgeon's preference

Accessory items (Fig. 19-8)

1 Ruler
3 Frazier suction tips (various sizes)
1 Suction tubing
Obturators for suction tips
1 Mallet
1 Yankauer suction tube
1 Caliper
1 Antrum suction tip

Postoperative care of instruments

Care of the instruments used in nasal surgery follows the general care regimen of all other surgical instruments. Chisels, gouges, and other cutting instruments should be inspected carefully for any nicks and for dullness and sent for repair as needed. Using damaged instruments may cause tissue damage in succeeding procedures. Rasps and files

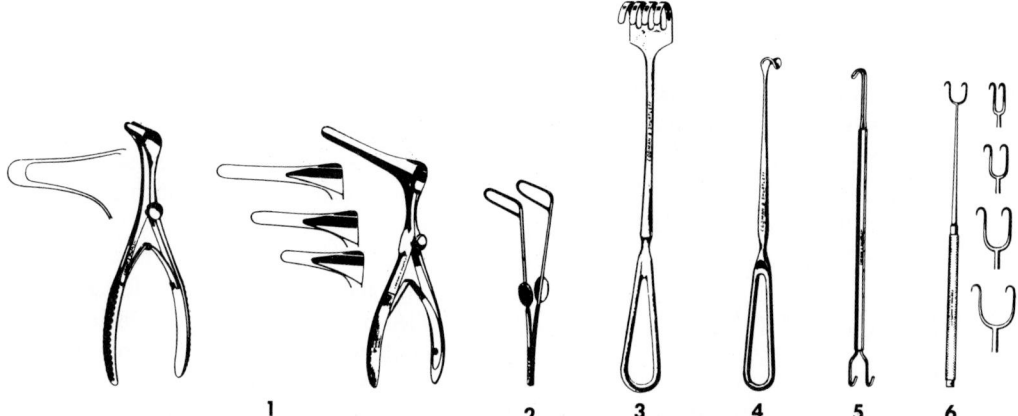

FIG. 19-7 Exposing instruments for operations on external nose, nasal cavity, and sinuses. *1,* Vienna and Killian nasal specula; *2,* Bosworth nasal wire speculum; *3,* Volkmann rake retractor; *4,* Cushing vein retractor; *5,* one- and two-pronged retractor, double-ended; *6,* two-pronged retractors, sharp, various sizes.

Courtesy Codman & Shurtleff, Inc., Randolph, Mass.

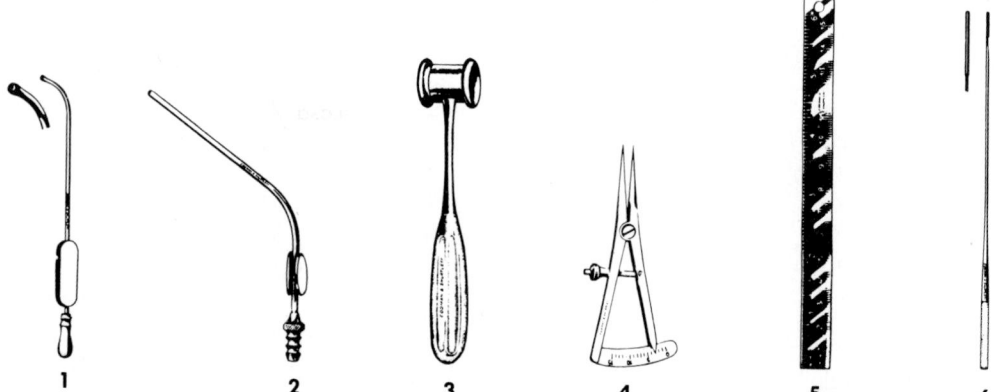

FIG. 19-8 Accessory instruments for operations on external nose and nasal cavity. *1,* Antrum suction tip; *2,* Frazier suction tip; *3,* metal mallet; *4,* caliper; *5,* ruler; *6,* nasal applicator.
Courtesy Codman & Shurtleff, Inc., Randolph, Mass.

should be thoroughly cleaned and all bone debris removed. Special attention should also be given to suction tips. Lenses on headlights used during the procedure should be checked for cleanliness. Spatter on lenses should be removed according to the manufacturer's instructions.

EVALUATION

The patient should be assessed postoperatively for any difficulties in breathing. Nasal packing inhibits breathing; however, the patient should be able to breathe normally through the mouth. Reddened or bruised areas related to positioning should be noted and treatment begun. The amount of drainage present on the moustache dressing should be noted. The head of the PACU bed should be elevated before transport to the unit. A thorough report is called to PACU and any variances reported and documented. Goals of the nursing care plan are reviewed and may be communicated and documented as outcome statements:

- The patient verbalized understanding of anticipated postoperative alteration in the senses of smell and taste.
- The patient demonstrated effective coping with the physical and psychologic effects of pain.
- The patient's anxiety was reduced or controlled.
- The patient will experience no signs and symptoms of infection postoperatively.

SURGICAL INTERVENTIONS

RHINOLOGIC SURGERY

Submucous resection of the septum, or septoplasty

A septoplasty is straightening of either the cartilaginous or osseous portions of the septum that lie between the flaps of the mucous membrane and the perichondrium. When the nasal septum is deformed, fractured, or injured, normal res-

piratory function and nasal drainage may be impaired. Deviations of the septum involving cartilage, bony parts (spurs), or both may block the meatus and compress the middle turbinate on that side, thereby resulting in an obstruction of the sinus opening. Septal deviations tend to produce sinus disease and nasal polyps.

The objective of a submucous resection is to establish an adequate partition between the left and right nasal cavities, thereby providing a clear airway through both the internal and external cavities of the nose.

Procedural considerations

The setup is as described in the general preparation for nasal surgery.

Operative procedure

1. The nostril is opened with a speculum. An incision is made through the mucoperichondrium of the septum with a knife having a no. 15 blade. The tissues are separated and elevated with a Freer elevator (Fig. 19-9).
2. The cartilage is incised with a knife, and the mucous membrane is elevated with a septal elevator; deviated cartilage and bony, thickened structures are trimmed or removed with a septum punch and a nasal cutting forceps.
3. The bony septal spurs are trimmed by means of a chisel, gouge and mallet, or punch forceps. Bleeding is controlled by using ½-inch by 3-inch x-ray detectable cottonoids with attached strings soaked in a topical hemostatic agent; suctioning is used to expose the field.
4. The perpendicular plate of the ethmoid as well as the vomer may be removed by means of a suitable septum-cutting forceps (see Fig. 19-6).
5. The incision may be sutured with absorbable no. 4-0 atraumatic suture on a small straight needle.

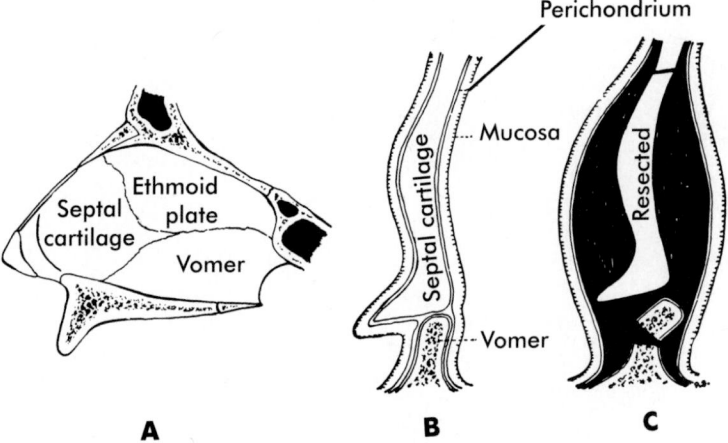

FIG. 19-9 **A,** Primary components of septum. Incision line is for Killian type of submucous resection. **B,** Septum with deviated cartilage and spur at junction of vomer and septal cartilage. **C,** Resection of obstructive parts after careful elevation of mucoperichondrium and mucoperiosteum.

From DeWeese, D.D., & Saunders, W.H. (1982). Textbook of otolaryngology (6th ed.). St. Louis: Mosby.

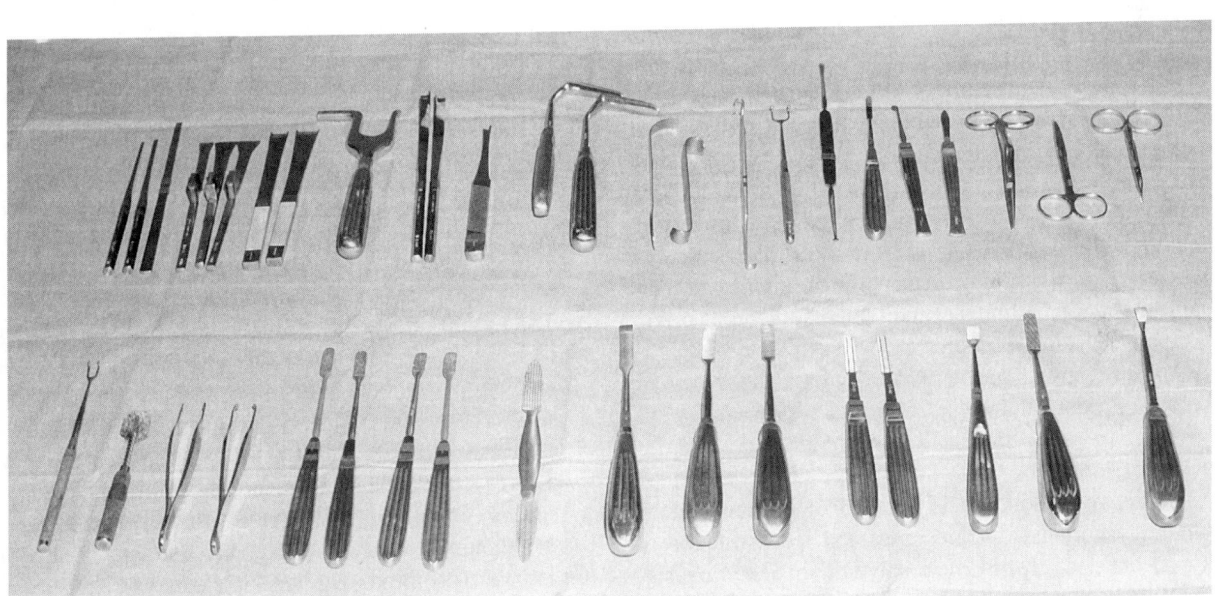

FIG. 19-10 Rhinoplasty instruments. *Top row,* 2-mm osteotome; 3-mm osteotome; 4-mm Cottle osteotome; 10-mm Rubin osteotome; 14-mm Rubin osteotome; 16-mm Rubin osteotome; 10-mm Cinelli osteotome; 14-mm Cinelli osteotome; Rubin nasofrontal osteotome; right curved guarded chisel; left curved guarded chisel; Parkes lateral osteotomy chisel; two Aufricht nasal retractors (long and short); Parkes nasal retractor; S-shaped blade retractor; Cottle knife guard and retractor; Fomon ball retractor; Cottle elevator; Joseph periosteal elevator; Freer septum knife; Joseph nasal scissors; Fomon dorsal scissors; Stevens tenotomy scissors. *Bottom row,* Double-pronged skin hook; wire brush; Adson-Brown tissue forceps; Beásley Babcock tissue forceps; four diamond rasps (two straight, two curved); converse rasp; Aufricht glabellar rasp; Parkes rasp (one fine, one medium); two Maltz rasps; Lewis rasp; rasp, straight fine; Glabella rasp.

Courtesy The Ohio State University Medical Center, Columbus, Ohio.

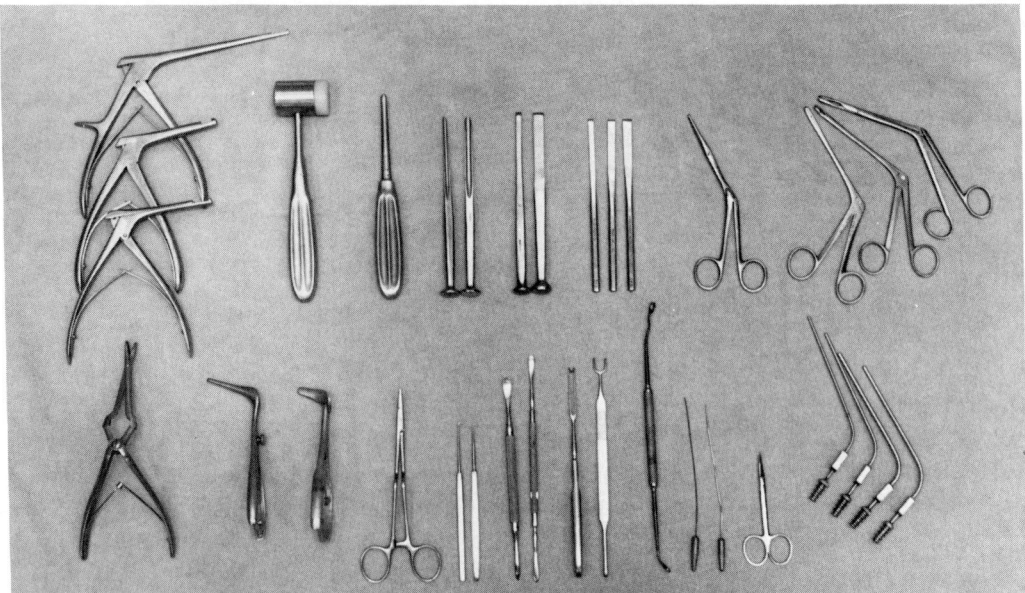

FIG. 19-11 Nasal instruments. *Top row, left to right,* Kerrison rongeurs, 2, 4, and 6 mm; mallet; septal displacer; gouges; small chisels; small osteotomes; Knight nasal scissors; Knight polyp forceps, small, medium, and large. *Bottom row, left to right,* Jansen-Middleton forceps; medium and short nasal specula; Jacobson-Bayonet needle holder; single skin hooks; Alberg periosteal elevator; Freer elevator; Ballenger swivel knife; Cottle knife guard/retractor; Faulkner antrum curette (double ended); University of Iowa cotton applicators; Knapp scissors, light curve; Frazier suction tips, sizes 1, 2, 3, and 4.

6. Nostrils are packed with gauze impregnated with antibiotic ointment or cream to keep the septal flaps in a midline position. Some surgeons use mattress sutures that provide a patent airway while maintaining support for the septum. Nasal tampons may be used instead of packing. The face is cleansed with moist and dry compresses. A moustache dressing may be applied. External dressings or splints depend on the surgeon's preference, as does application of a small ice bag to the nose. A surgical glove filled with ice is an excellent ice bag because it is small and lightweight.

Corrective rhinoplasty

A corrective rhinoplasty is removal of the hump, narrowing and shortening of the nose, and reconstruction of the tip of the nose. It may help solve the patient's physiologic or appearance problems.

Procedural considerations

The patient's face is prepped as described in the general preparation for nasal surgery. The patient is usually placed in a supine position. The rhinoplasty and nasal instruments are shown in Figs. 19-10 and 19-11.

Operative procedure

1. A hemitransfixion incision is made through the skin of one nostril with a knife and no. 15 blade. A nasal speculum, sponges, and skin hooks can be used for exposure.
2. The skin of the nose is undermined by elevators, knives, and scissors. The periosteum and periochondrium are freed with elevators and a periosteal dissector.
3. The nasal bones may be fractured with either a straight or curved osteotome or a saw. The upper lateral cartilage may be trimmed with a no. 15 blade or plastic scissors. The dorsal hump can be taken down with an osteotome. A cartilaginous hump can be taken down with a no. 15 blade. The septal cartilage may be removed by means of a cutting forceps, such as the Jansen-Middleton. Bony spurs can be taken down with the mallet and osteotome. The field is cleared by suctioning.
4. The edges of the cartilages are trimmed by means of scissors or a no. 15 blade.
5. To prevent or control infection and the formation of a hematoma, the blood is suctioned from the nose, and the wound is cleansed. A drainage port is often made in the mucoperichondrial flap to allow for drainage.
6. The cartilage and bones are molded into proper position. The hemitransfixion incision is sutured with absorbable sutures. Dressings with a pressure splint are applied. A moustache dressing may be secured below the nares to absorb any bleeding. The head is elevated, and ice packs may be applied to the eyelids.

SINUS SURGERY

Intranasal antrostomy (antral window)

An intranasal antrostomy is an opening made in the lateral wall of the nose under the inferior turbinate. This procedure is now rarely indicated but may be used for patients with ciliary dyskinesia such as immotile cilia syndrome.

Procedural considerations

The setup is as described in the general preparation for nasal surgery. Instrumentation includes the following:

5 Towel clamps
2 Nasal specula
4 Dean applicators
1 Metal tongue depressor
1 Yankauer suction tube
2 Antrum suction tips
1 Universal handle with punches
1 Dean antrum rasp, concave
2 Dean antrum rasps, left and right
2 Wiener rasps, dull and sharp
6 Coakley curettes
1 Freer elevator
1 Dean elevator
2 Bayonet forceps
1 Suture scissors
2 Knife handles, no. 7, with no. 15 blades
1 Polyp forceps
1 Nasal snare with wires
2 Syringes, 10 ml

Operative procedure

1. When the patient has been anesthetized, prepped, and draped, the inferior turbinate is explored with bone-cutting forceps, elevators, and dissectors (see Figs. 19-5 and 19-6).
2. An opening is made into the maxillary sinus (see Fig. 19-3) beneath the inferior turbinate by means of a gouge, perforator, or rasp (see Fig. 19-5). The opening is enlarged with cutting forceps and antrum punches. Accessory polyps and degenerate mucosa are removed with a snare, polyp forceps, and suction.
3. The sinus can be irrigated with saline solution and suctioned. The sinus is packed with gauze impregnated with antibiotic ointment or cream. The face is cleansed, and a drip pad (moustache dressing) is applied under the nostrils.

Nasal polypectomy

A nasal polypectomy is the removal of polyps from the nasal cavity (Fig. 19-12). The tissues become edematous, resulting in the formation of polyps that obstruct the free passage of air and make breathing difficult.

Procedural considerations

For polyps arising from the border of the middle turbinate, the instruments are as described for submucous resection. An intranasal setup is used if the polyps arise above

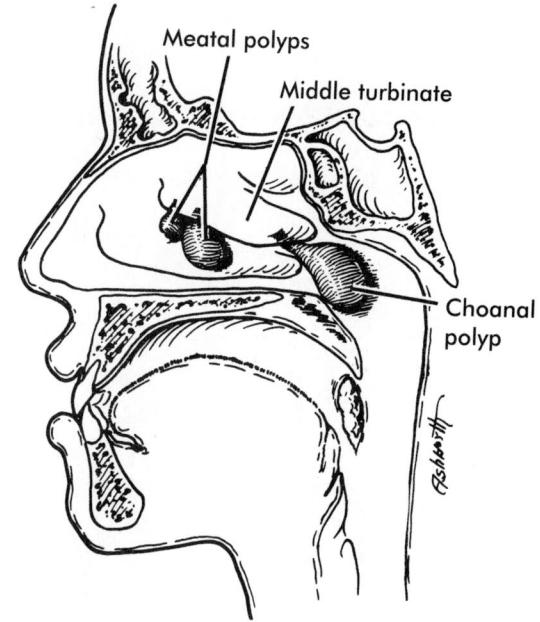

FIG. 19-12 Nasal polyps. Choanal polyp is usually single and originates in maxillary sinus; however, most polyps are found in middle meatus.

From DeWeese, D.D., & Saunders, W.H. (1982). *Textbook of otolaryngology* (6th ed.). St. Louis: Mosby.

or from the semilunar hiatus. In some cases polyps are removed in conjunction with a Caldwell-Luc operation, ethmoidectomy, enlargement of the frontal sinus, or opening of the sphenoidal sinus.

Operative procedure

The operation is as described for the intranasal antrostomy or other types of operations on the sinuses with removal of the polyps and degenerated tissue.

If the intranasal approach is used, local and topical anesthetics are applied to shrink the mucosa and ensure vasoconstriction. The polyps are removed with a nasal snare, hemostasis is obtained, and the nose is packed with an antibiotic-impregnated gauze. A drip pad or moustache dressing is then applied under the nostrils.

Radical antrostomy (Caldwell-Luc)

A radical antrostomy entails an incision into the canine fossa of the upper jaw and exposure of the antrum for removal of bony diseased portions of the antral wall and contents of the sinus (Fig. 19-13), or establishment of drainage by means of a counteropening into the nose through the inferior meatus. In the presence of pus in acute sinus disease the mucous membrane may become thickened and polyps may form, resulting in an obstruction of the nasal cavity and external passageway. In such cases the patient suffers from nasal catarrh, headaches, and cough. Chronic sinusitis may be associated with asthma. The purpose of a

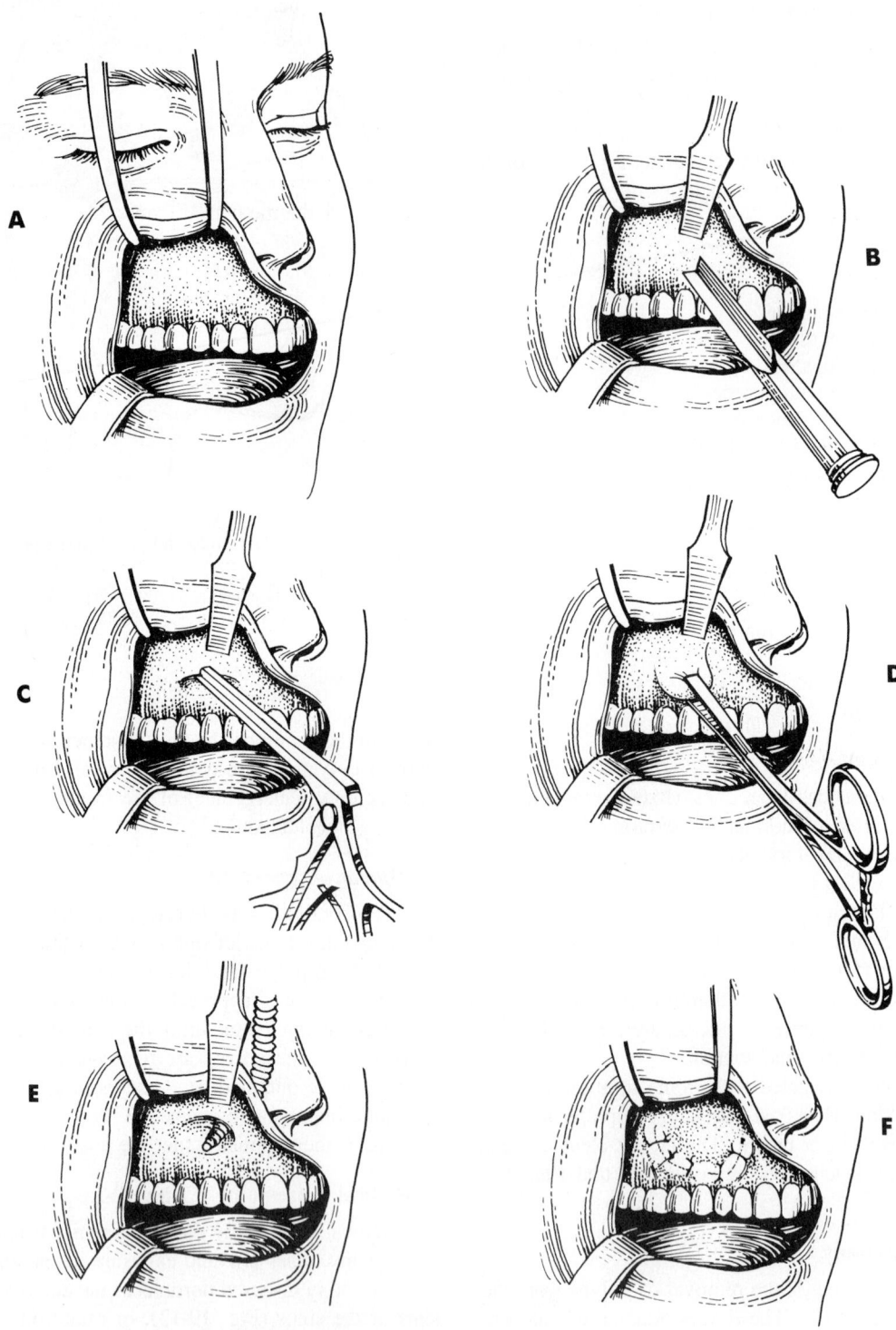

FIG. 19-13 Caldwell-Luc operation. **A,** Incision. **B,** Flap retracted and perforation made in canine fossa. **C,** Perforation enlarged with Kerrison rongeur. **D,** Removal of diseased antral membrane. **E,** Rasp used to make nasoantral window. **F,** Incision closed.

radical antrostomy is to establish a large opening in the nasoantral wall of the inferior meatus, which ensures adequate gravity drainage and aeration and permits removal, under direct vision, of all diseased tissues in the sinus.

Procedural considerations

The setup is as described for intranasal antrostomy, plus the following:

2 Jansen-Middleton septum-cutting forceps
2 Kerrison rongeurs, upbiting and straight
1 Ferris-Smith forceps
1 Killian dressing forceps
1 Weil nasal forceps
1 Ethmoid curette
2 Caldwell-Luc retractors
1 Mallet
2 Kelly hemostats
2 Allis forceps
8 Towel clamps
1 Adson tissue forceps with teeth
1 Adson-Brown tissue forceps
2 Single skin hooks
2 Double skin hooks
2 Freer elevators (sharp and dull)
1 Pennington elevator
1 Ball-ended elevator
1 Ballenger V-shaped chisel
1 Knight nasal scissors
1 Takahashi forceps
2 Ethmoid forceps, straight and upbiting
1 Metzenbaum scissors
2 Mayo scissors, curved and straight
2 Scissors, curved, small, blunt and sharp
1 Suture scissors
2 Knife handles, no. 3 and no. 7, with no. 15 blades
2 Straight chisels, 2 mm and 4 mm

The patient is usually given a general anesthetic.

Operative procedure (see Fig. 19-13)

1. The upper lip is elevated with a Caldwell-Luc retractor, and a transverse incision is made in the gingivolabial sulcus just above the teeth; the incision is carried down to the underlying bone. Periosteum and soft tissue are elevated with dissectors and periosteal elevators.
2. The thin bony plate is perforated with a chisel, the antrum is entered, and its opening is enlarged with nasal rongeurs. The anterior angle of the sinus may be opened by enlarging the window with Jansen-Middleton septum-cutting forceps, double-action rongeurs, and Kerrison rongeurs.
3. The mucous membrane of the antrum is removed with Coakley curettes and Takahashi forceps.
4. Nasoantral drainage may be established by removal of a portion of the nasoantral wall below the inferior turbinate by means of cutting forceps and rasps.
5. The nose and sinus are packed with antibiotic or petrolatum-impregnated gauze.

6. The labial incision may be sutured with absorbable no. 3-0 atraumatic suture on a small, curved needle. The patient's face is cleansed and dried. If iodoform packing is used, the patient should be warned that there may be a foul taste in the mouth postoperatively.

Endoscopic sinus surgery

Endoscopic sinus surgery involves the endoscopic resection of inflammatory and anatomic defects of the sinuses. The amount of disease resected is much less than that removed by the more traditional methods.

The purpose of endoscopic sinus surgery is to ensure adequate ventilation and to restore mucociliary clearance in the sinuses. If there is contact between the mucosa and the sinuses, mucociliary clearance is inhibited and secretions are retained in the sinus, which predisposes the patient to sinus infections. Endoscopic sinus surgery can bring relief to patients with chronic sinus problems. This procedure is preferred to the Caldwell-Luc procedure because there is decreased morbidity and provides for a more physiologic type of drainage.

Candidates for endoscopic sinus surgery are patients who have had recurrent acute or chronic sinusitis that is refractory to antibiotic therapy. Chronic sinusitis can be caused by anatomic deformities or an allergy history. Immunologic abnormalities, fluctuations in hormone levels, and environmental factors may also contribute to chronic sinusitis. Pa-

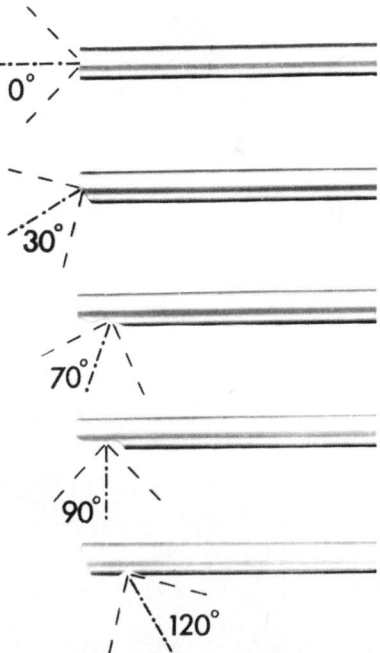

FIG. 19-14 Schematic drawing shows direction of view with different endoscopes. Angle of deflection is always relative to long axis of endoscope at its tip.

From Stammberger, H. (1991). *Functional endoscopic sinus surgery.* Philadelphia: B.C. Decker.

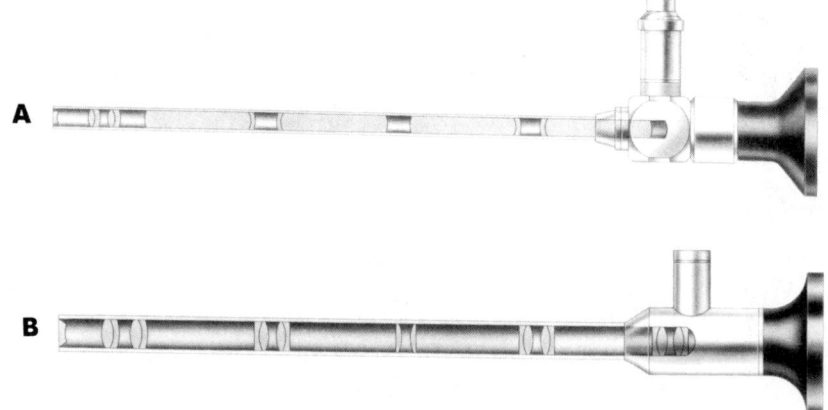

FIG. 19-15   Longitudinal section through endoscope with traditional lens arrangement **(A)** and with Hopkins rod lens system **(B).** In contrast to single lens or group of lenses in traditional system, Hopkins system uses quartz rod lenses. These give greater clarity, more brightness, and wider angle with scope of smaller diameter.

From Stammberger, H. (1991). *Functional endoscopic sinus surgery.* Philadelphia: B.C. Decker.

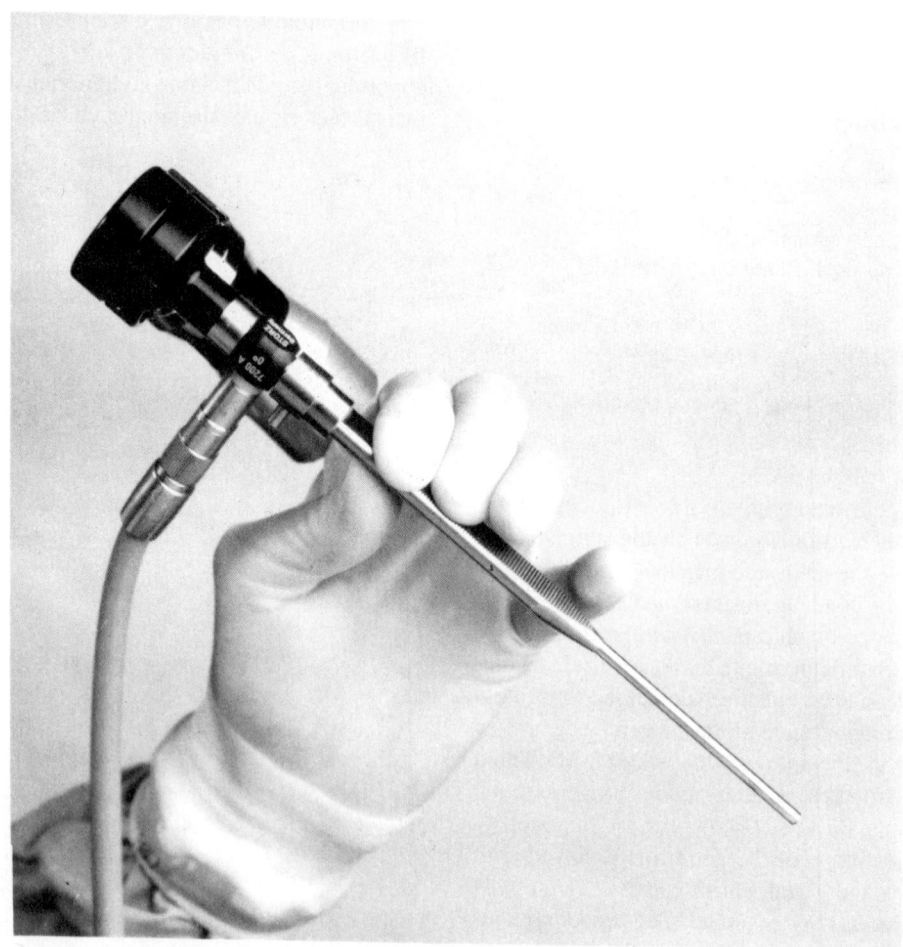

FIG. 19-16   Flat handle for endoscope prevents bending, provides good grip and precise orientation, and contributes to motion-free photography.

From Stammberger, H. (1991). *Functional endoscopic sinus surgery.* Philadelphia: B.C. Decker.

tients who are considered candidates for endoscopic sinus surgery undergo an office endoscopic exam preoperatively. During this procedure none of the sinus cavities is opened. These patients must also have CT scans done to determine the areas affected by the sinusitis.

Procedural considerations

The endoscopic sinus surgery instruments enable the physician to view the patient's anatomy, diagnose disease processes, and remove and confirm pathology while the patient is under either local or general anesthesia. These instruments are of delicate nature and should be cared for in an appropriate manner.

Endoscopes have different directions of view—0, 30, 70, 90, and 120 degrees (Fig. 19-14)—and may have either the traditional lens arrangement or the Hopkins rod lens system (Fig. 19-15). The 0-degree endoscope (straight forward anterior view) is the standard scope for surgical procedures. The majority of surgical procedures are performed under the guidance of the endoscope. Because of its direct forward-looking orientation, this is the only endoscope whose long axis always points in the direction in which one looks (that is, directly along the axis of the shaft). This allows the most precise orientation. Combined with a flat handle (Fig. 19-16), it can be held securely and permits easy, motion-free phogography and video documentation. The 0-degree 4-mm nasal endoscope is also useful in maxillary sinus endoscopy for orienting the trocar sheath precisely toward the area from which a biopsy is to be taken or mucous membrane removed.

The 30-degree 4-mm diameter telescope also allows a forward view and can be introduced without difficulty. This endoscope is the diagnostic instrument of choice, and because of the orientation of its lens it allows a careful inspection of the middle meatus, the sphenoethmoidal recess, and the entire epipharynx. It is also used in maxillary sinus endoscopy, where its wide-angle view is particularly useful.

This endoscope is also very useful for working in the frontal recess. It may be used in combination with a round handle (see Fig. 19-17), which facilitates rotation of the endoscope around its long axis, between the fingers. The round handle makes these maneuvers much easier.

The 70-degree angled 4-mm endoscope is used primarily for diagnostic purposes and in some special surgical situations, particularly in the frontal recess and in manipulations in the maxillary sinus, through an enlarged ostium. This endoscope does not allow a view along the shaft of the scope, and consequently great care and experience are necessary in avoiding contact with the mucous membranes and injury during its introduction. It is frequently helpful to introduce a trocar sheath over a 0- or 30-degree endoscope to the position to be inspected with the 70-degree scope. The trocar sheath is then held fixed in this position and the 70-degree endoscope is introduced through the sheath, placing it in the required position and avoiding mucosal contact during the introduction.

The 120-degree endoscope is used only during maxillary sinus endoscopy, for instance, to inspect the anterior wall of the sinus through a trocar sheath introduced through the canine fossa. The use of handles with the slender endoscopes facilitates a more precise manipulation of the instrument and also avoids the risk of bending or kinking.

In addition to endoscopes, other instruments and equipment are utilized in endoscopic sinus surgery:

Suction tips (Figs. 19-18 and 19-19)
Maxillary sinus trocar (Fig. 19-20)
Freer-type suction elevator (Fig. 19-21)
Sickle scalpel (Fig. 19-22)
Biopsy forceps (Figs. 19-23 to 19-25)
Blakesley-Weil forceps (Figs. 19-26 to 19-29)
Forceps, delicate, upward bent (Fig. 19-30)
Struycken modified nasal cutting forceps (Fig. 19-31)
Endoscopic scissors (Fig. 19-32)
Bent spoon (Fig. 19-33)
Stammberger-Ostrum backward-cutting antrum punch (Fig. 19-34)
Flat handle for endoscope (Fig. 19-16)
Round handle for endoscope (Fig. 19-17)
Acrylic cup for antifog solution (Fig. 19-35)
Fiberoptic light cords
Fiberoptic light source
Video monitor

Text continued on p. 689.

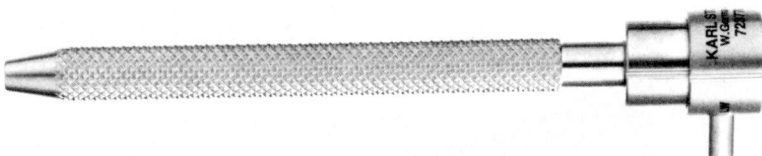

FIG. 19-17 Round endoscope handle facilitates rotation of endoscope around its longitudinal axis. Knurled handle also promotes good grip and precision of movement while preventing endoscope shaft from bending.

From Stammberger, H. (1991). *Functional endoscopic sinus surgery.* Philadelphia: B.C. Decker.

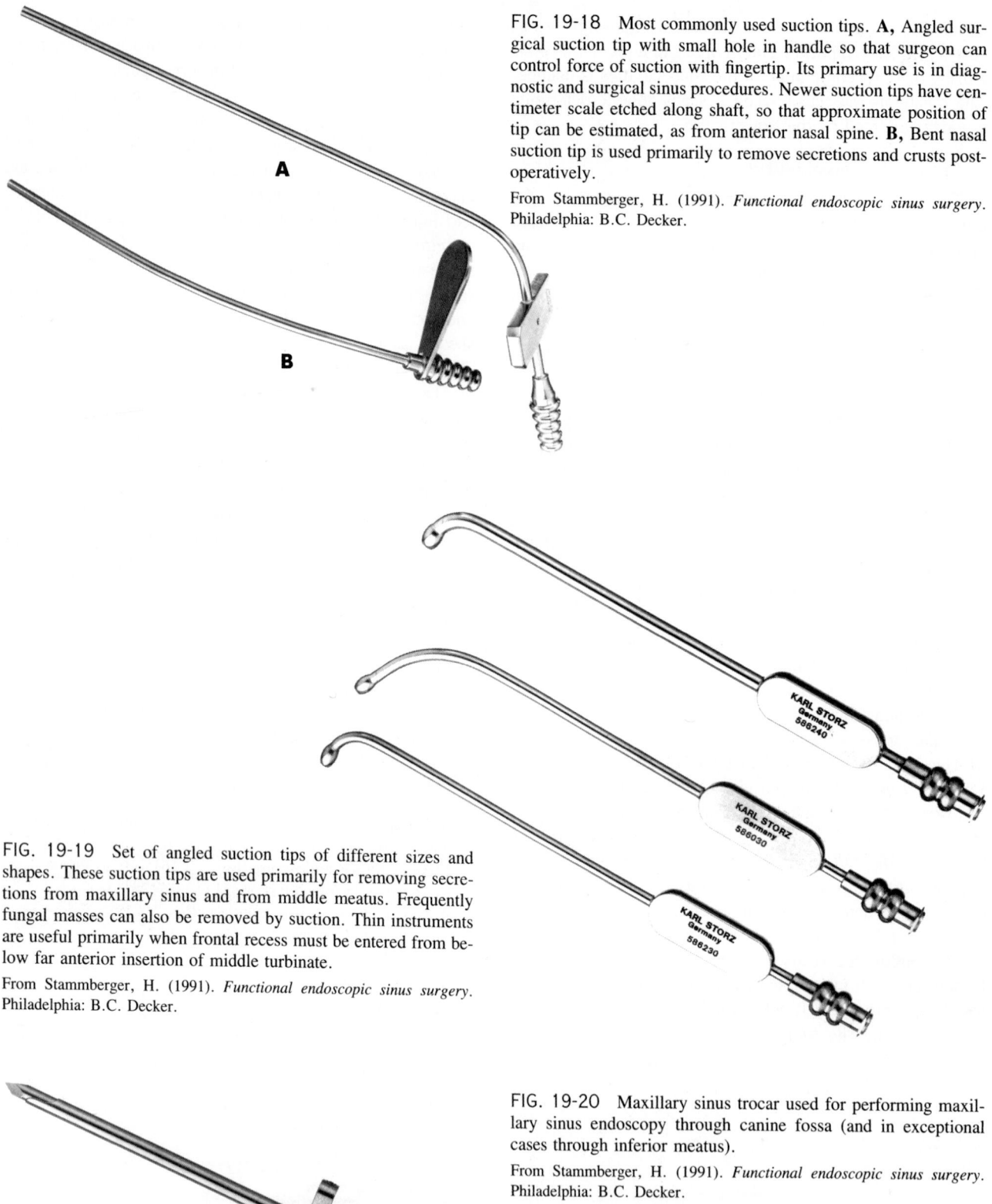

FIG. 19-18 Most commonly used suction tips. **A,** Angled surgical suction tip with small hole in handle so that surgeon can control force of suction with fingertip. Its primary use is in diagnostic and surgical sinus procedures. Newer suction tips have centimeter scale etched along shaft, so that approximate position of tip can be estimated, as from anterior nasal spine. **B,** Bent nasal suction tip is used primarily to remove secretions and crusts postoperatively.

From Stammberger, H. (1991). *Functional endoscopic sinus surgery.* Philadelphia: B.C. Decker.

FIG. 19-19 Set of angled suction tips of different sizes and shapes. These suction tips are used primarily for removing secretions from maxillary sinus and from middle meatus. Frequently fungal masses can also be removed by suction. Thin instruments are useful primarily when frontal recess must be entered from below far anterior insertion of middle turbinate.

From Stammberger, H. (1991). *Functional endoscopic sinus surgery.* Philadelphia: B.C. Decker.

FIG. 19-20 Maxillary sinus trocar used for performing maxillary sinus endoscopy through canine fossa (and in exceptional cases through inferior meatus).

From Stammberger, H. (1991). *Functional endoscopic sinus surgery.* Philadelphia: B.C. Decker.

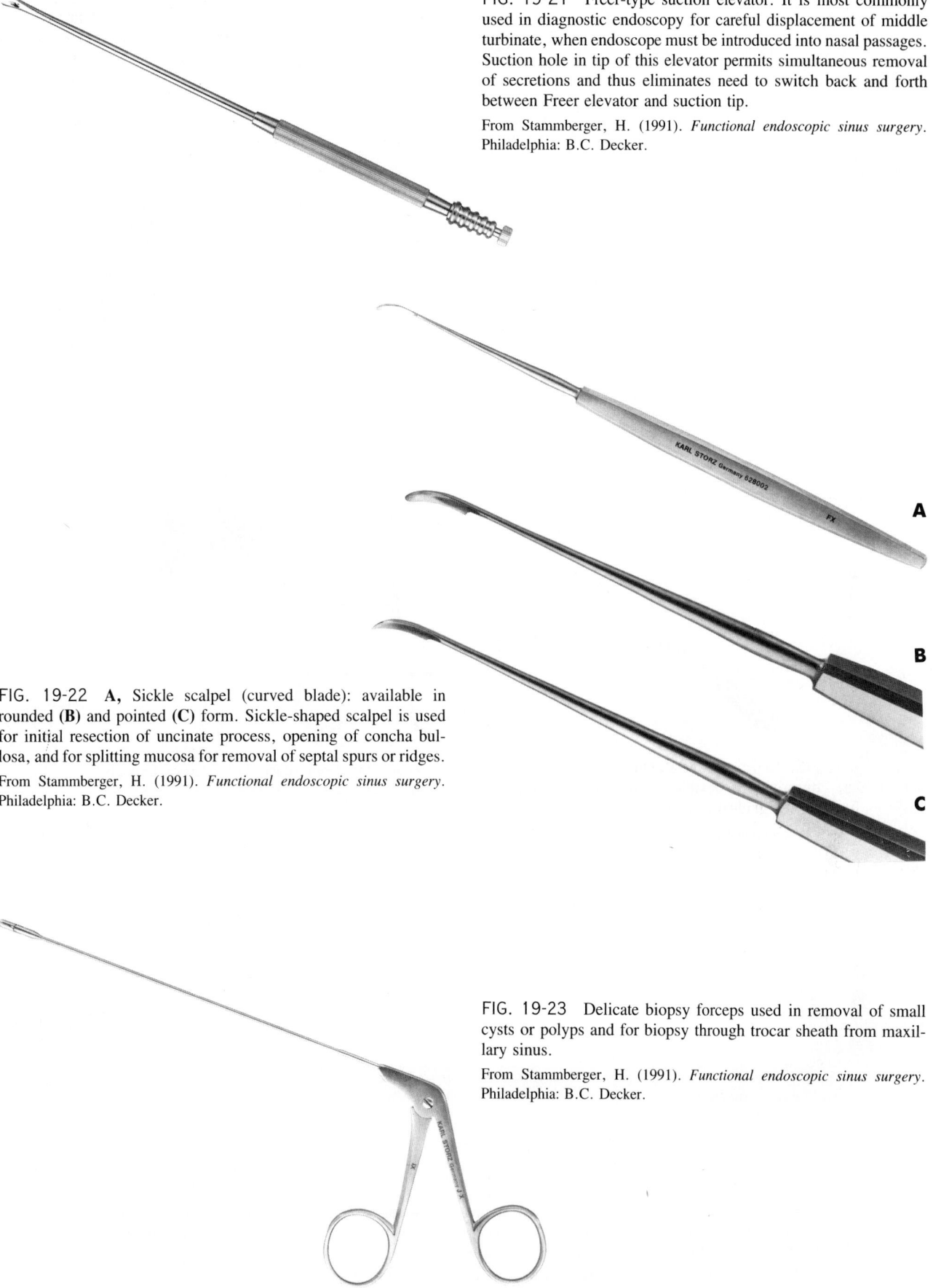

FIG. 19-21   Freer-type suction elevator. It is most commonly used in diagnostic endoscopy for careful displacement of middle turbinate, when endoscope must be introduced into nasal passages. Suction hole in tip of this elevator permits simultaneous removal of secretions and thus eliminates need to switch back and forth between Freer elevator and suction tip.

From Stammberger, H. (1991). *Functional endoscopic sinus surgery.* Philadelphia: B.C. Decker.

A

B

C

FIG. 19-22   **A,** Sickle scalpel (curved blade): available in rounded **(B)** and pointed **(C)** form. Sickle-shaped scalpel is used for initial resection of uncinate process, opening of concha bullosa, and for splitting mucosa for removal of septal spurs or ridges.

From Stammberger, H. (1991). *Functional endoscopic sinus surgery.* Philadelphia: B.C. Decker.

FIG. 19-23   Delicate biopsy forceps used in removal of small cysts or polyps and for biopsy through trocar sheath from maxillary sinus.

From Stammberger, H. (1991). *Functional endoscopic sinus surgery.* Philadelphia: B.C. Decker.

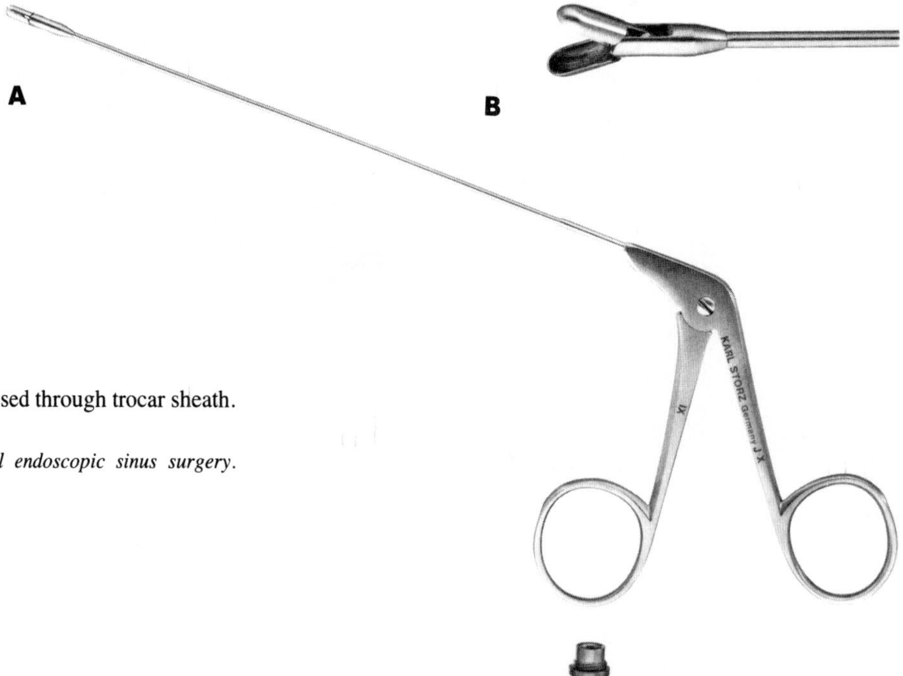

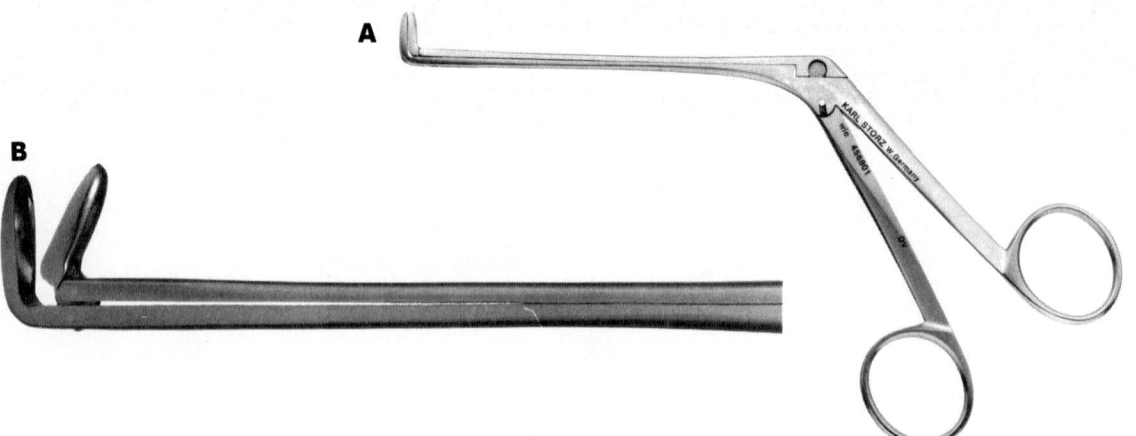

FIG. 19-24 **A,** Biopsy forceps to be used through trocar sheath.
B, Close-up view of forceps mouth.

From Stammberger, H. (1991). *Functional endoscopic sinus surgery.*
Philadelphia: B.C. Decker.

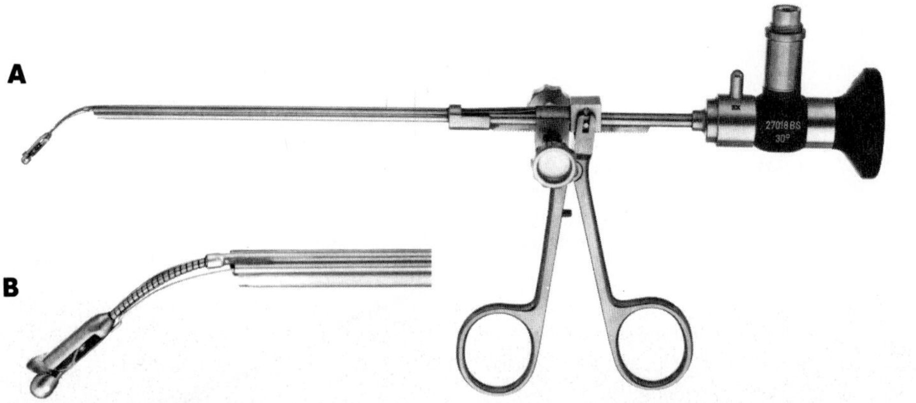

FIG. 19-25 **A** and **B,** Optical biopsy forceps with 2.7-mm 30-degree endoscope. For insertion through trocar sheath, flexible part of forceps is maximally retracted. After insertion, flexible forceps can be advanced gradually downward into visual field of 30-degree lens.

From Stammberger, H. (1991). *Functional endoscopic sinus surgery.* Philadelphia: B.C. Decker.

FIG. 19-26 **A,** Blakesley-Weil forceps. Jaws flex at right angle. **B,** Jaws, which are shown in detail, are also available in 4-mm longer version. Forceps are used to prepare roof of ethmoid, for work in frontal recess and in maxillary sinus, through enlarged ostium.

From Stammberger, H. (1991). *Functional endoscopic sinus surgery.* Philadelphia: B.C. Decker.

A

B

C

D

E

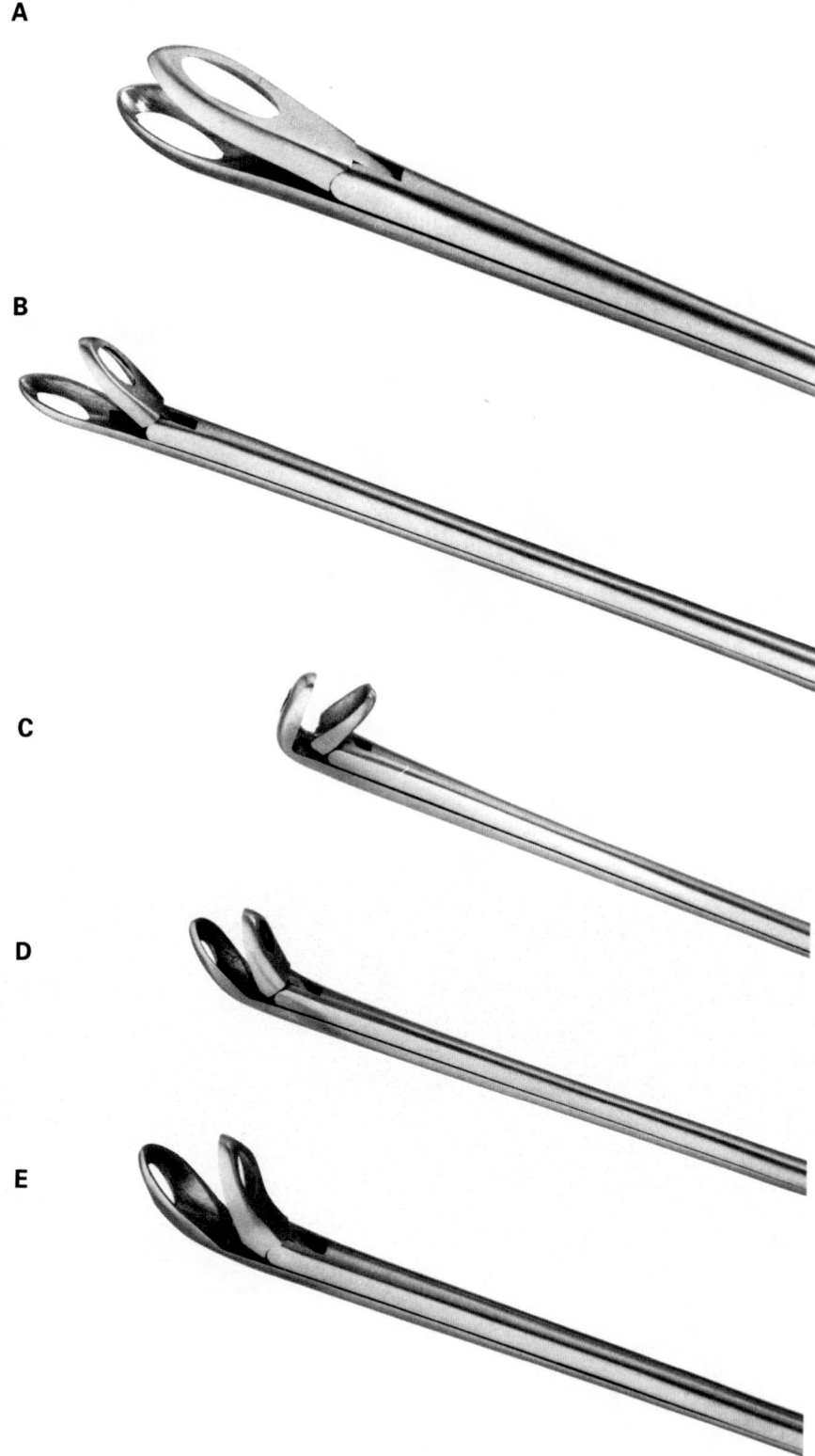

FIG. 19-27   Blakesley-Weil forceps (**A**) is available in variety of sizes and shapes. Most procedures are performed with delicate Blakesley-Weil forceps in its straight form (**B**) and in its flexed form (**D** and **E**). Large form (**C**) is used very rarely, as in cases of excessive polyposis, when all finer bony structures have been destroyed by chronic inflammation or by pressure from polyps. This instrument is too large for most other purposes.

From Stammberger, H. (1991). *Functional endoscopic sinus surgery*. Philadelphia: B.C. Decker.

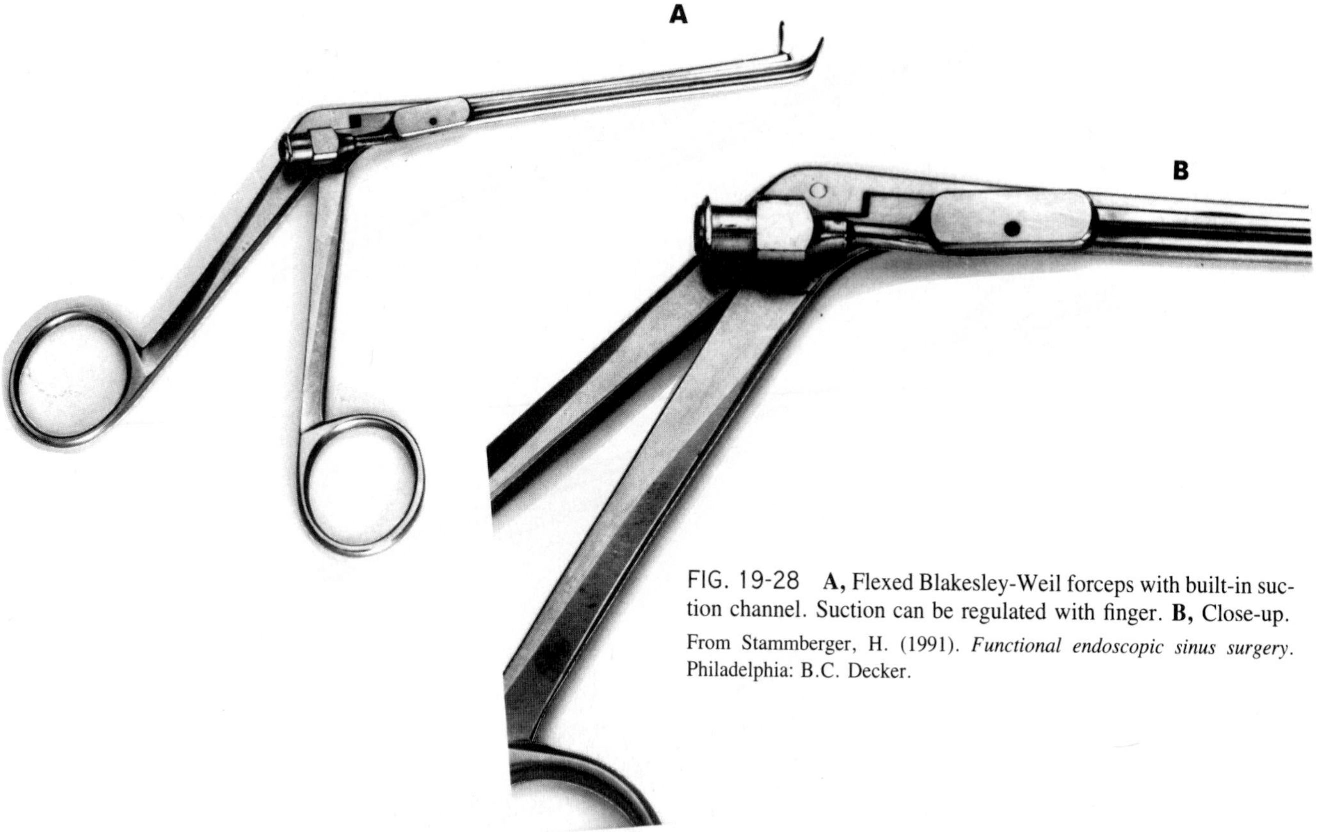

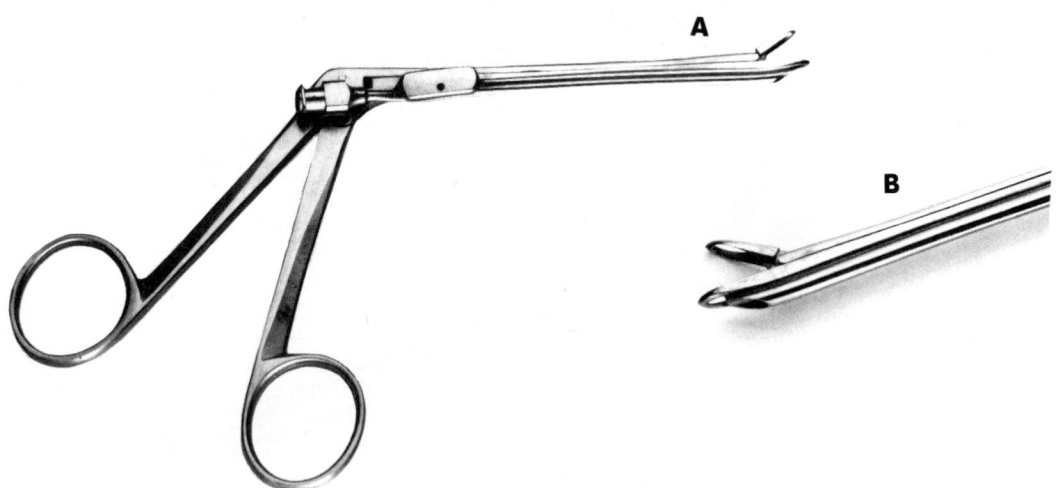

FIG. 19-28 **A,** Flexed Blakesley-Weil forceps with built-in suction channel. Suction can be regulated with finger. **B,** Close-up.

From Stammberger, H. (1991). *Functional endoscopic sinus surgery.* Philadelphia: B.C. Decker.

FIG. 19-29 **A,** Straight, delicate Blakesley-Weil forceps with built-in suction channel. **B,** Close-up.

From Stammberger, H. (1991). *Functional endoscopic sinus surgery*. Philadelphia: B.C. Decker.

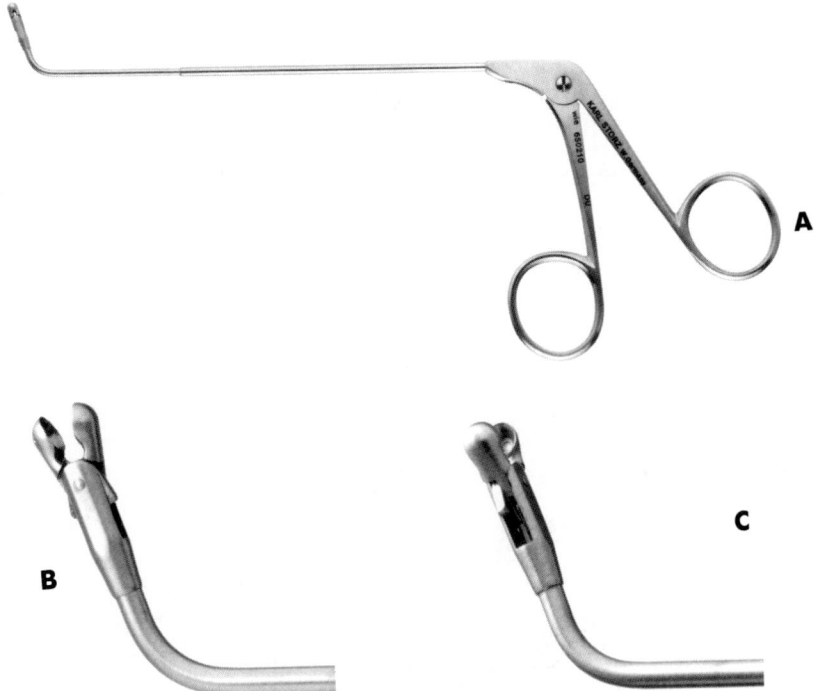

FIG. 19-30 **A,** Upward bent, delicate forceps. **B,** Jaws close longitudinally. **C,** Jaws close crosswise. These forceps are useful for manipulations in frontal recess in combination with 30- or 70-degree lenses. They are also suitable for manipulations in maxillary sinus, such as removal of small polyps or opening of cysts through natural ostium.

From Stammberger, H. (1991). *Functional endoscopic sinus surgery*. Philadelphia: B.C. Decker.

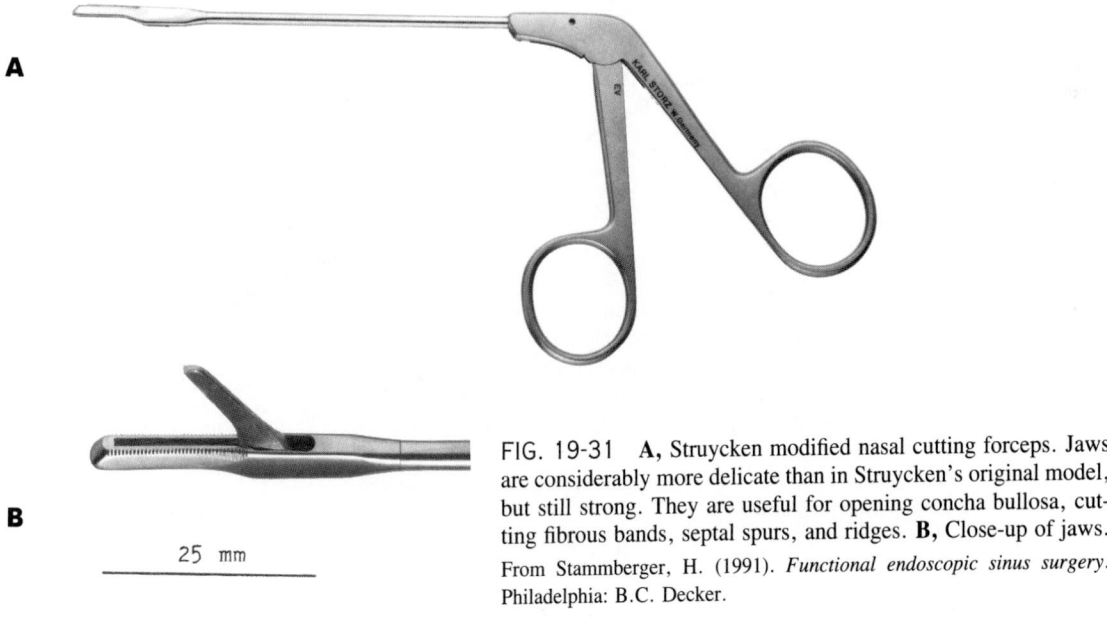

FIG. 19-31 **A,** Struycken modified nasal cutting forceps. Jaws are considerably more delicate than in Struycken's original model, but still strong. They are useful for opening concha bullosa, cutting fibrous bands, septal spurs, and ridges. **B,** Close-up of jaws.

From Stammberger, H. (1991). *Functional endoscopic sinus surgery*. Philadelphia: B.C. Decker.

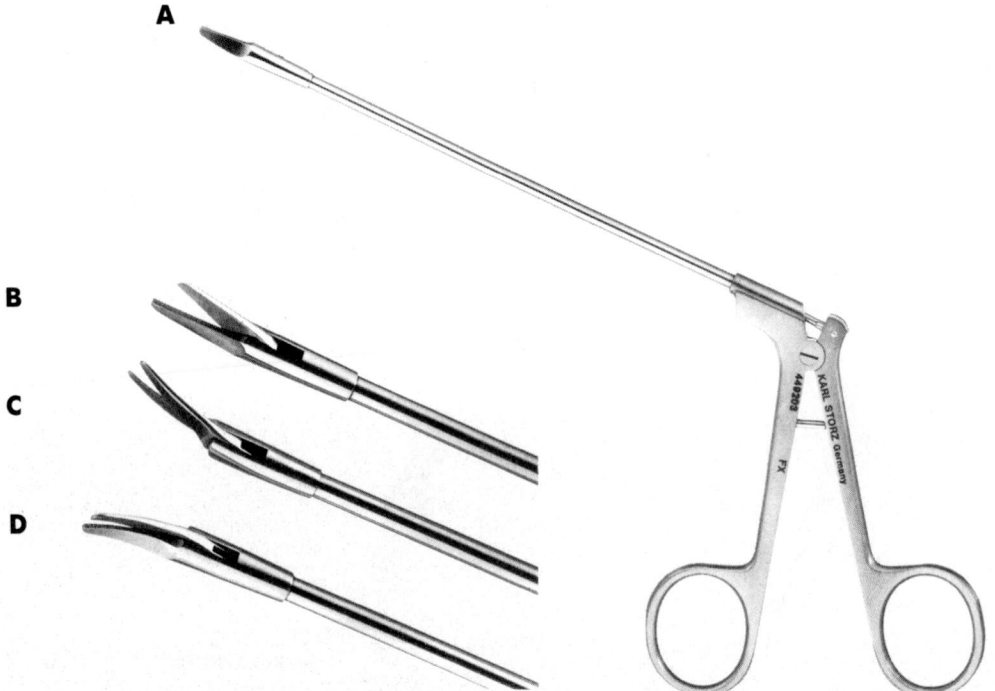

FIG. 19-32 **A,** Set of scissors for endoscopic use. **B,** Straight jaws angled to right **(C)** and to left **(D).** This set of scissors is useful for opening concha bullosa, resecting stalks of coarse single or recurrent polyps, and for cutting fibrous strands and synechiae.

From Stammberger, H. (1991). *Functional endoscopic sinus surgery*. Philadelphia: B.C. Decker.

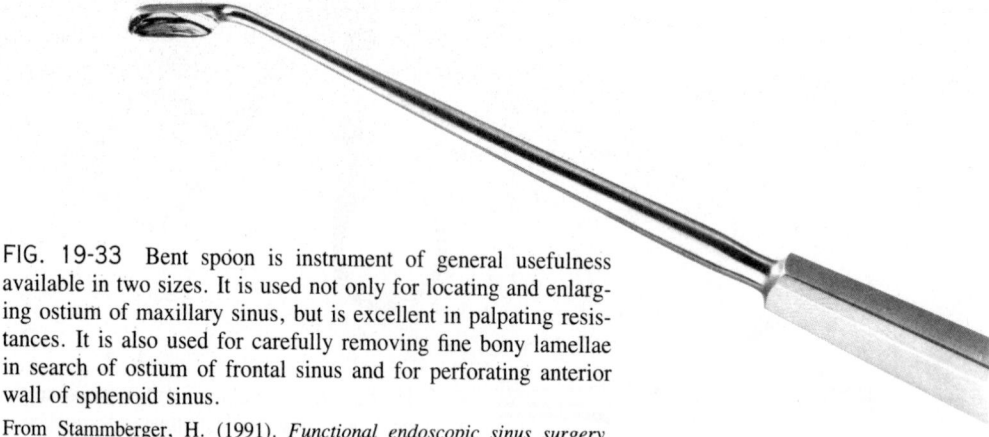

FIG. 19-33 Bent spoon is instrument of general usefulness available in two sizes. It is used not only for locating and enlarging ostium of maxillary sinus, but is excellent in palpating resistances. It is also used for carefully removing fine bony lamellae in search of ostium of frontal sinus and for perforating anterior wall of sphenoid sinus.

From Stammberger, H. (1991). *Functional endoscopic sinus surgery*. Philadelphia: B.C. Decker.

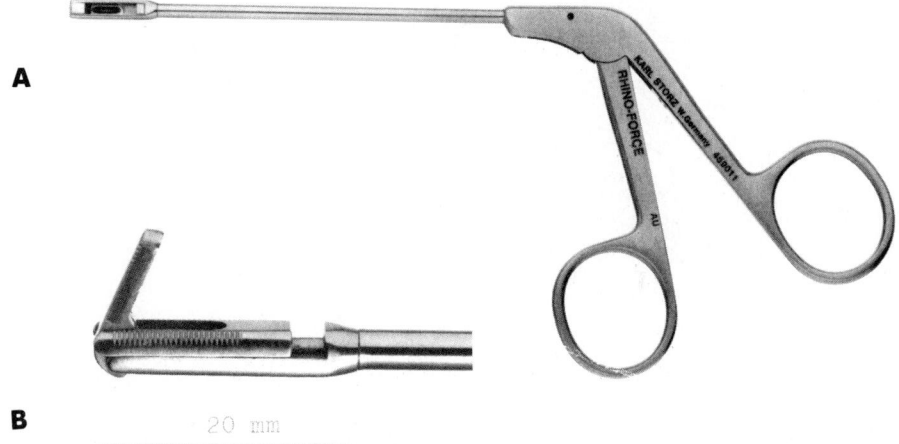

FIG. 19-34   **A,** Stammberger-Ostrum backward cutting antrum punch. **B,** Close-up of jaws. These back-biting forceps are available in two models (sideward cutting to right and left). They are used for enlargement of ostium of maxillary sinus at expense of anterior fontanelles and for retrograde resection of uncinate process.

From Stammberger, H. (1991). *Functional endoscopic sinus surgery*. Philadelphia: B.C. Decker.

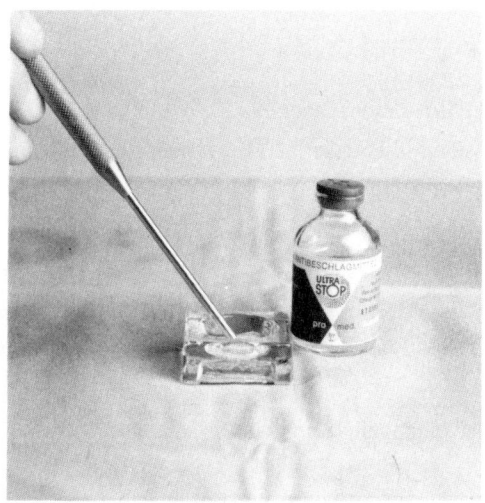

FIG. 19-35   Acrylic cup used for application of antifog solution to distal lens of endoscope. Bottom of cup is covered with layer of cotton to protect lens. Few drops of antifog solution are usually sufficient for entire procedure.

From Stammberger, H. (1991). *Functional endoscopic sinus surgery*. Philadelphia: B.C. Decker.

The light source and video monitor for trainees and observers are located at the head of the OR bed (Fig. 19-36). When photography or videotaping is planned, the light source is placed behind the surgeon to allow the cable to run in a straight line. This is particularly important to prevent kinking and possible damage to the delicate fiberoptics.

Some light sources are very noisy because of their built-in cooling fans. The patient should be cautioned about this noise, which is generated directly alongside the head.

This procedure may be done with the patient under local anesthesia and IV sedation. The patient is placed in a supine position. The face and throat are prepped, and the patient is draped as for other nasal procedures.

Operative procedure

1. The surgeon may apply topical anesthesia followed by the local anesthesia.
2. Before being introduced initially into the nose, the endoscopes should be wiped with a thin film of antifog solution. Before each subsequent introduction, the lens is treated with antifog solution that is not wiped off, but left as a thin layer on the lens.
3. The natural ostium of the maxillary sinus is enlarged to provide for physiologic drainage through the middle meatus (see Fig. 19-3).
4. The diseased tissue is visualized through a 0-, 30-, 70-, or 120-degree endoscope. Straight or angled forceps may be used to remove only the diseased tissue (Fig. 19-37).

A   **B**

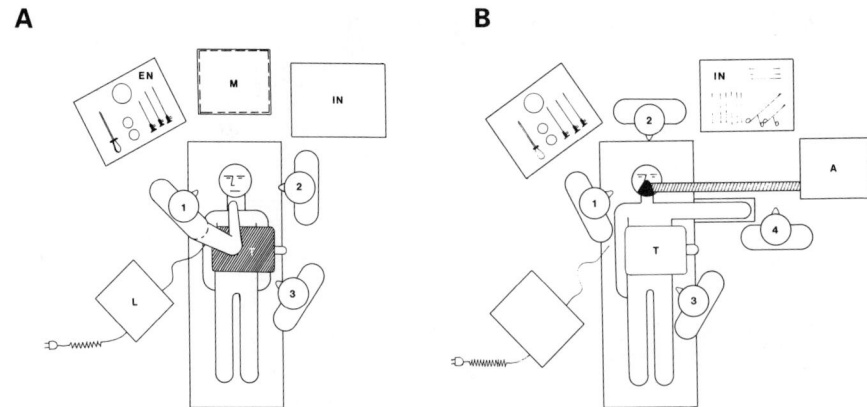

FIG. 19-36 **A,** Position of patient for functional endoscopic sinus surgery with patient under topical and local infiltration anesthesia. *1,* Surgeon; *2,* scrub nurse; *3,* assistant; *L,* light source; *EN,* movable table with endoscope and accessories; *M,* video monitor, alternate location for light source; *IN,* movable instrument table; *T,* Mayo stand to hold suction tips and other equipment and serve as armrest for surgeon. **B,** Position of patient and arrangement of equipment for endoscopic sinus surgical procedure to be performed with patient under general anesthesia. *1,* Surgeon; *2,* scrub nurse; *3,* assistant; *4,* anesthesiologist; *T,* Mayo stand for instruments and armrest; *IN,* movable instrument table; *A,* anesthesia machine and its connections.

From Stammberger, H. (1991). *Functional endoscopic sinus surgery*. Philadelphia: B.C. Decker.

5. If an anterior ethmoidectomy is indicated, the endoscope is inserted through the middle meatus (see Fig. 19-3) into the frontal recess, and the ethmoidectomy is performed.

6. Due to the small incisions made, no sutures are required.

7. Antibiotic ointment is applied intranasally using a 10-ml syringe with a small catheter on the end to ensure proper placement.

8. Nasal packing is not required. A moustache dressing is applied (see Research Highlight 19-1).

Frontal sinus operation (external approach)

A frontal sinus operation involves making an incision through the anterior wall of the floor of the frontal sinus for removal of diseased tissue, cleansing of the sinus cavity, and drainage. In acute frontal sinusitis, in which the patient suffers from persistent headaches and edema of the upper eyelid, and in cases in which medical therapy has failed, surgical treatment may be indicated. Drainage of the frontal sinus may be performed by a simple trephine opening through the floor of the sinus. In the presence of chronic suppuration with repeated acute attacks of frontal sinusitis, surgery may be done to remove the diseased lining of the sinus and to reconstruct the nasofrontal duct, thereby ensuring adequate drainage.

Procedural considerations

The setup is as described for intranasal antrostomy, plus the following items:

1 Power saw with oscillating blade
2 Brawley or Spratt frontal rasps
1 Potts or Cushing nerve hook, blunt
2 Cushing forceps, straight, fine
2 Adson tissue forceps
Dural hooks
Raney clip appliers and clips

The patient is given a general anesthetic. The surgical approach depends on the preference of the surgeon and the patient. If a coronal incision is to be made, the hair should be shaved from the hairline to slightly past the crown of the head. If a brow incision is to be made, no shaving is necessary. Fat may be taken from the abdomen for subsequent use in obliterating the sinus space.

The patient's eyes are usually protected during the procedure with tarsorrhaphies (suturing the eyelids closed), sterile ocular occluders, or tape. The patient's head and face are prepped with a povidone-iodine scrub and solution.

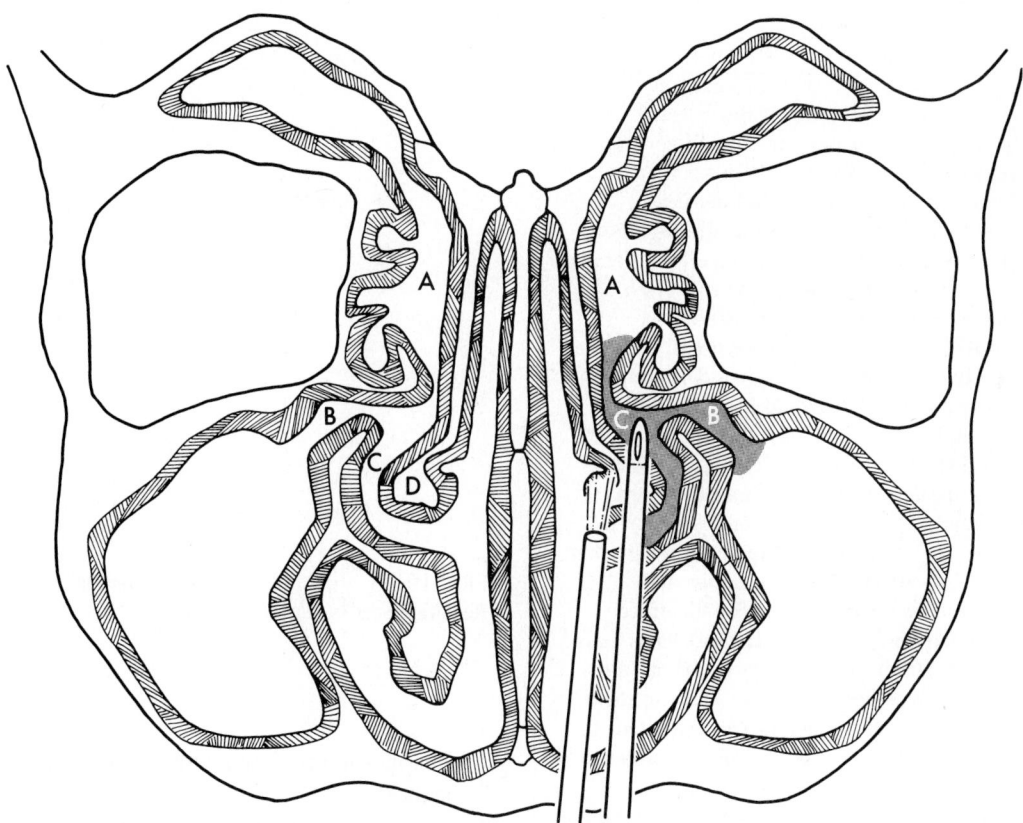

FIG. 19-37 Surgery is performed using endoscope and forceps via intranasal approach. Diseased tissue is being removed from shaded areas depicting *(A)* ethmoid sinus area, *(B)* maxillary sinus ostia, and *(C)* middle meatus. *(D),* Middle turbinate is unaffected.

From Thawley, S.E., & Garrett, H. (1988). Endoscopic sinus surgery; an outpatient procedure that minimizes tissue removal. *AORN Journal, 47,* 902. Copyright © AORN, Inc., 10170 East Mississippi Avenue, Denver, CO 80231.

Operative procedure

1a. When a *coronal* approach is used, the incision is made in the scalp skin from ear to ear, well behind the hairline. The edges of the skin are compressed by the application of Raney clips. The flap is reflected to expose the upper portion of the nose, thus exposing the anterior of the sinus.

1b. When a *brow* approach is used, the incision is made in the superior margin of the eyebrow(s), hemostasis is obtained, and the flap is elevated, exposing the anterior sinus wall.

2. A template (steam-sterilized radiologic outline of the frontal sinus) is placed over the sinus and marked on the pericranium with a marking pen.

3. The pericranium is elevated.

4. An oscillating saw is used to cut through the bone overlying the frontal sinus. An elevator may be used to free the bone from the sinus.

5. The mucosa of the sinus is removed in its entirety through the use of elevators and a drill.

6. Absorbable gelatin sponge or a fat graft taken from the abdomen is placed in the sinus to obliterate the space.

7. The bone flap is replaced, and the pericranium is repositioned and sutured.

8. The skin incision is closed with suture of the surgeon's preference.

9. A pressure dressing of elastic gauze is applied for 48 to 72 hours.

Potential postoperative complications include osteomyelitis, meningitis, cerebrospinal fluid leak, abscess, and stenosis of the nasofrontal duct.

Frontal sinus trephination

Frontal sinus trephination is the creation of a hole in the frontal sinus to drain pus or fluid accumulation. This procedure is performed for early signs of frontal sinusitis. After the procedure the patient should be observed for signs of intracranial involvement.

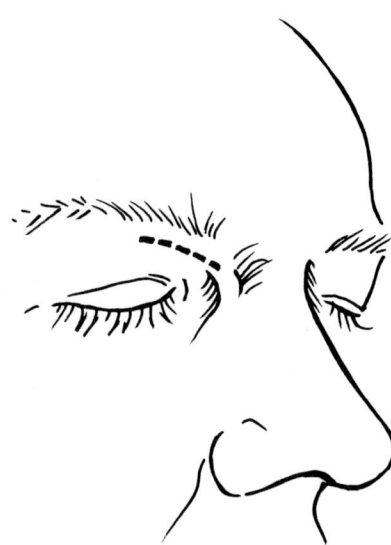

FIG. 19-38   Incision to expose ethmoidal and frontal sinuses. Resulting scar is almost invisible.

Procedural considerations

The patient's face is prepped with a povidone-iodine scrub and solution. The face is draped as previously described. The skin under the eyebrow is injected with local anesthesia with or without epinephrine.

Operative procedure

1. The incision is made medially below the eyebrow, along the same contour of the brow (Fig. 19-38).
2. The periosteum is elevated from the bone, and a small diamond or cutting burr is used to create a hole into the sinus.
3. Cultures are generally taken before the aspiration of the pus present in the sinus.
4. A large Silastic or Teflon tube or a large catheter is placed through the incision into the sinus to facilitate postoperative irrigation.

5. The incision is closed with suture of the surgeon's preference.
6. A small dressing is usually applied to absorb drainage from the incision and catheter.

Ethmoidectomy

An ethmoidectomy is the removal of the diseased portion of the middle turbinate, removal of ethmoidal cells, and removal of diseased tissue in the nasal fossa through a nasal or an external approach. The purpose of an ethmoidectomy is to reduce the many-celled ethmoidal labyrinth into one large cavity to ensure adequate drainage and aeration.

Procedural considerations

The setup for the nasal approach is as described for intranasal antrostomy; for the external approach the setup is as described for the frontal sinus operation.

Operative procedure

For the nasal route the procedure is similar to intranasal antrostomy described previously. For the external route, the procedure is similar to the frontal sinus operation described previously.

Sphenoidectomy

A sphenoidotomy is the creation of an opening into one or both of the sphenoidal sinuses by the intranasal or external ethmoidectomy approach. In surgical treatment of sinusitis of the sphenoidal sinus, visualizing the cavity is difficult because of its depth. Surgery of the sphenoidal sinus is usually performed intranasally or through an external ethmoidectomy approach.

Procedural considerations

The setup is as described for intranasal antrostomy, with the addition of long, sphenoid curettes, antrum rasps, and antrum punches.

Operative procedure

The operation is as described for intranasal antrostomy.

Turbinectomy

Anterior inferior turbinectomy is removal of the anterior end of the inferior turbinate. *Inferior turbinectomy* is removal of the greater part of the lower border of the hypertrophied inferior turbinate. *Anterior middle turbinectomy* is removal of the anterior end of the middle turbinate body. In all cases turbinectomy may include removal of polyps (see Fig. 19-12). A turbinectomy is preferred to provide adequate ventilation and drainage and relieve pressure against the floor of the nose.

Procedural considerations

The setup is as described for intranasal antrostomy.

Operative procedure

The nose is packed with petrolatum-impregnated gauze on all sides of the turbinate. An incision is made. The affected turbinate is amputated and removed, the polyps are removed, and the cavity is packed, as described for intranasal antrostomy.

Outfracture of turbinates

Turbinate outfracture is similar to turbinectomy, except that the turbinate is infractured and then outfractured by the use of a septal displacer. Unipolar cautery may also be used in conjunction with outfracturing.

Repair of nasal fracture

Repair of a nasal fracture involves manipulation and mobilization of nasal bones. When the nose is struck by a direct frontal blow, usually both nasal bones are fractured, displaced outward, and depressed into the ethmoidal sinus (see Fig. 19-3). The septal cartilages are displaced. Prompt reduction should be done.

Procedural considerations

The patient is placed on the OR bed in a supine position, and a topical anesthetic may be applied. The setup includes a topical anesthesia set, plus a rubber-covered Salinger elevator or Asch septum-straightening forceps, a straight hemostat, petrolatum-impregnated gauze packing, a plastic mold or aluminum splint, and adhesive tape.

Operative procedure

A rubber-shod narrow forceps is inserted into the nostril; the nasal bones are elevated and molded into place by external manipulation.

BIBLIOGRAPHY

Association of Operating Room Nurses. (1994). Recommended practices for monitoring the patient receiving local anesthesia. In *AORN standards and recommended practices for perioperative nursing*. Denver: The Association.

Cummings, C.W., Frederickson, J.M., Jarker, L.A., Krause, C.J., & Schuller, D.E. (1993). *Otolaryngology head and neck surgery*, Vol. 1. St. Louis: Mosby.

Jeppesen, F. (1986). *Septo and rhinoplasty: A step by step instruction*. Copenhagen: Munksgaard.

Rice, D., & Schaeffer, S.D. (1988). *Endoscopic paranasal sinus surgery*. New York: Raven Press.

Rothrock, J.C. (1991). *Perioperative nursing care planning*. St. Louis: Mosby.

Sessions, D.G., Cummings, C.W., Weymuller, E.A. Jr., Makielske, K.H., & Wood, P. (1992). *Atlas of access and reconstruction in head and neck surgery*. St. Louis: Mosby.

Stammberger, H. (1991). *Functional endoscopic sinus surgery*. Philadelphia: B.C. Decker.

20

LARYNGOLOGIC AND HEAD AND NECK SURGERY

SUE SILCOX

Patients undergoing laryngologic or head and neck surgical procedures present a challenge to the perioperative nurse. These patients have physical as well as psychosocial needs. They may be experiencing upper airway insufficiency upon arrival to the operating room or have an altered airway postoperatively. Head and neck surgery patients must cope with an altered body image in addition to the altered upper airway. Postoperative bleeding can create feelings of panic and suffocation. The perioperative nurse must quickly assess, plan, and implement actions to ensure an adequate airway, as well as reassure the patient and explain the actions and expected outcomes.

These patients range from pediatric to geriatric, thus imagination and creativity are vital components of the perioperative nurse's armamentarium in assessing the patient's comprehension of the anticipated surgical procedure.

Patients undergoing head and neck surgical procedures for malignancy frequently manifest these characteristics:

- Elderly
- History of tobacco use
- History of alcohol intake or abuse
- History of systemic disease (cardiovascular)
- Nutritionally deficient
- Frightened or angry (due to attempting to cope with permanently altered life-style)

The perioperative nurse is responsible for assessing, planning, and implementing care for these patients intraoperatively and providing support for them postoperatively as they learn to cope with an altered body image and an altered life-style.

SURGICAL ANATOMY

OROPHARYNX

The throat includes the structures of the neck in front of the vertebral column; these are the mouth, tongue, pharynx, tonsils, larynx, and trachea.

The mouth extends from the lips to the anterior pillars of the throat. The portion of the mouth outside the teeth is the buccal cavity, and that on the inner side of the teeth is the lingual cavity. The tongue occupies a large portion of the floor of the mouth. The hard and soft palates form the upper and posterior boundaries of the oral cavity, separating it from the nasal cavity and the nasopharynx. The soft palate emerges from the posterior border of the hard palate to form the uvula, a fingerlike movable projection. The uvula joins the base of the tongue anteriorly and the pharynx posteriorly.

The pharynx serves as a channel for both the digestive and respiratory systems. It is situated behind the nasal cavities, mouth, and larynx. The food and air passages cross each other in the pharynx, a funnel-shaped structure, wider above and narrower below, about 12 cm in length. It is composed of muscular and fibrous layers and is lined with mucous membrane. It is associated above with the sphenoidal sinus and the basilar part of the occipital bone, and it joins the esophagus below. Seven cavities communicate with the pharynx: the two nasal cavities, the two tympanic cavities, the mouth, the larynx, and the esophagus. The cavity of the pharynx may be subdivided from above downward into three parts: nasal, oral, and laryngeal. Infection can spread from the pharynx to the middle ear through the eustachian tube.

The nasopharynx communicates with the oropharynx through the pharyngeal isthmus, which is closed by muscular action during swallowing. The oropharynx and the laryngopharynx cannot be closed off from each other; both serve respiratory and digestive functions.

The pharynx comprises three groups of constrictor muscles (Fig. 20-1). Each muscle fits within the one below, and each inserts posteriorly in the median line with its mate from the opposite side. The constrictor muscles provide constriction of the pharynx for swallowing. Between the origins of the constrictor muscle groups are so-called intervals through which ligaments, nerves, and arteries pass.

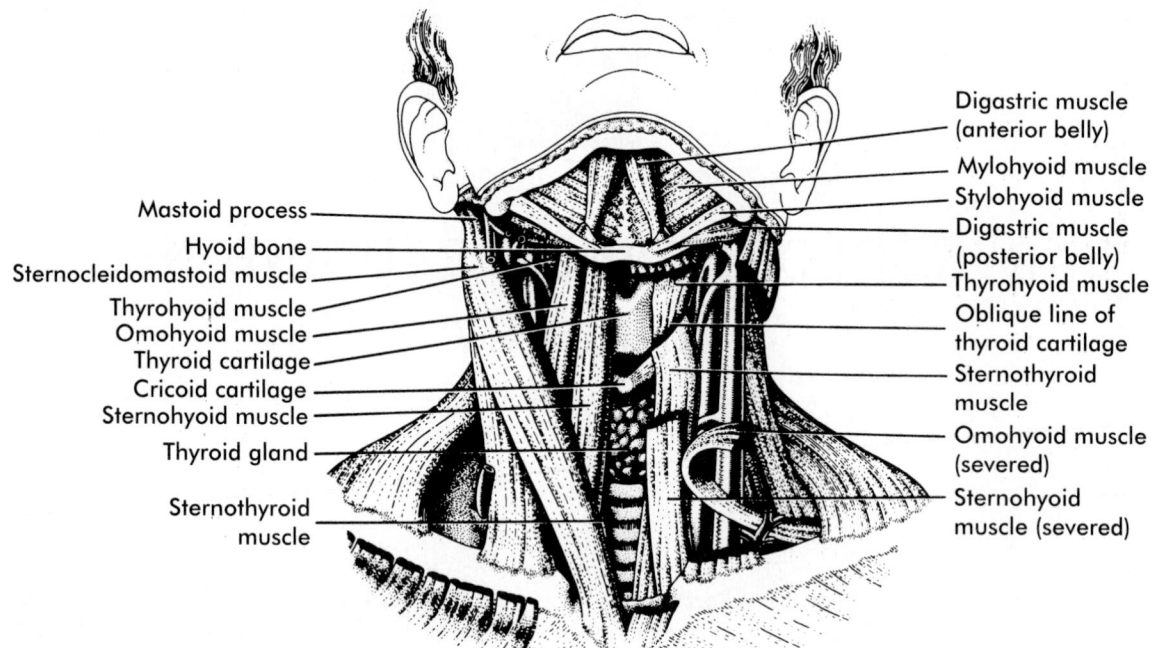

FIG. 20-1　Extrinsic muscles of the larynx.
From Marino, L.B. (1981). *Cancer nursing*. St. Louis: Mosby.

The recurrent laryngeal nerve is closely associated with the lower portion of the pharynx.

The tonsils are situated one on each side of the oropharynx, lodged in a tonsillar fossa that is attached to folds of membrane-containing muscle. One pair, the palatine tonsils, are the only lymphatic organs covered with stratified squamous epithelium. These tonsils may become inflamed (tonsillitis). The lateral surface of each tonsil is usually covered with a fibrous capsule. The anterior and posterior tonsillar pillars join to form a triangular fossa, with the posterior lateral aspects of the tongue at its base. The lingual tonsils are lodged in each fossa. The adenoids or pharyngeal tonsils are suspended from the roof of the nasopharynx and consist of an accumulation of lymphoid tissue.

The arteries of the tonsils enter the upper and lower poles. The tonsils are supplied with blood by tonsillar branches of the ascending palatine branch of the facial artery (branch of the external carotid artery). The external carotid artery on each side lies behind and lateral to each tonsil. The nerves supplying the tonsils are derived from the middle and posterior palatine branches of the maxillary and glossopharyngeal nerves.

LARYNX AND ASSOCIATED STRUCTURES
Larynx

The larynx is located at the upper end of the respiratory tract. It is situated between the trachea and the root of the tongue, at the upper front part of the neck. The larynx has three main functions: as a passageway for air, as a valve for closing off air passages from the digestive system and the pharynx, and as a voice box on which sound and speech depend to a degree.

The larynx is a cartilaginous box situated in front of the fourth, fifth, and sixth cervical vertebrae. The upper portion of the larynx is continuous with the pharynx above, and its lower portion joins the trachea. The skeletal structure provides for patency of the enclosed airway. The complex muscle action and arrangement of tissues within the structure provide for closure of the lumen for protection against trauma and entrance of foreign bodies and for speech.

Cartilages

The skeletal framework of the larynx consists of cartilages and membranes. Of the nine separate cartilages, three are single and six are arranged in pairs. The main cartilages of the larynx include the thyroid, cricoid, epiglottis, two arytenoid, two corniculate, and two cuneiform. The thyroid cartilage, or Adam's apple, forms the anterior portion of the voice box. The cricoid cartilage, which resembles a signet ring, rests beneath the thyroid cartilage (Fig. 20-2). The epiglottis is a slightly curled, leaf-shaped, elastic fibrous membrane. It is prolonged below into a slender process, attached in the midline to the upper border of the thyroid cartilage. When the cricothyroid muscle contracts, it pulls the thyroid cartilage and the cricoid cartilage, thereby tightening the vocal cords and, if unopposed, closing the glottis. The arytenoid cartilages, which rest above the signet ring portion of the cricoid cartilage, support the posterior portion of the true vocal cords.

Laryngeal ligaments

The extrinsic ligaments of the larynx are those connecting the thyroid cartilage and epiglottis with the hyoid bone and the cricoid cartilage with the trachea (Fig. 20-3). The intrinsic ligaments of the larynx are those connecting several cartilages of the organ to each other. They are considered the elastic membrane of the larynx.

The mucous lining of the larynx blends with the fibrous tissue to form two folds on each side of the larynx. The upper set is known as the false cords. The lower set is called the true vocal cords because they are primarily concerned with the speaking voice and protection of the lower respiratory channels against the invasion of food and foreign bodies.

Laryngeal muscles

The laryngeal muscles perform two distinct functions: the extrinsic muscles open and close the glottis, and the intrinsic muscles regulate the degree of tension on the vocal cords. The spoken voice also depends on the sphincter action of the soft palate, tongue, and lips. The muscle action of the larynx permits the glottis to close either voluntarily or involuntarily by reflex action. The closure of the inlet by this mechanism protects the respiratory passages. The closure of the glottis and the action of the vocal cords are precisely coordinated to produce the voice.

Two branches of the vagus nerve supply the intrinsic muscles. The recurrent laryngeal nerve branch of the vagus is the important motor nerve of the intrinsic muscles of the larynx. The sensory nerve, which is derived from the branches of the superior laryngeal nerve, supplies the mucous membrane of the larynx. When both the recurrent laryngeal nerves become divided or paralyzed, the glottis remains closed so tightly that air cannot be drawn into the lungs. As a lifesaving measure an endotracheal or tracheostomy tube is inserted immediately.

The larynx derives its blood supply from the branches of the external carotid and subclavian arteries.

TRACHEA

The trachea, a cylindrical tube about 15 cm in length and 2 to 2.5 cm in diameter, begins in the neck and extends from the lower part of the larynx, on a level with the sixth cervical vertebra, to the upper border of the fifth thoracic vertebra. The tube descends in front of the esophagus, enters the superior mediastinum, and divides into right and left main bronchi. The trachea is composed of a series of incomplete rings of hyaline cartilage. The carina is a ridge on the inside of the bifurcation of the trachea. It is a landmark during bronchoscopy and separates the upper end of the right main branches from the upper end of the left main branches of the bronchi. Branches given off from the arch of the aorta—the brachiocephalic (innominate) and left common carotid arteries—are in close relation to the trachea. The cervical portion of the trachea is related anteriorly to the sternohyoid and sternothyroid muscles and to the isthmus of the thyroid gland.

SALIVARY GLANDS

The salivary glands consist of three paired glands: the sublingual, submandibular, and parotid. They communicate with the mouth and drain their secretions into its cavities. Saliva is the combined secretion of all these glands. The

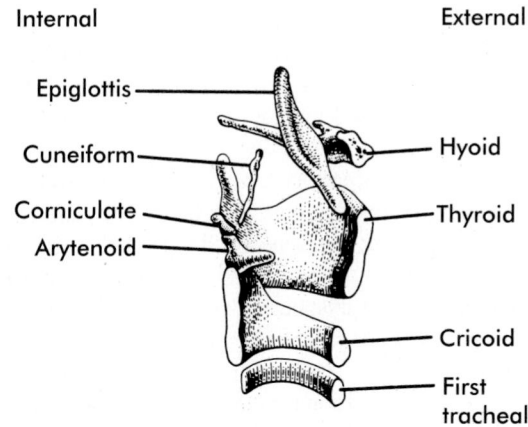

FIG. 20-2   Skeletal framework.
From Marino, L.B. (1981). *Cancer nursing.* St. Louis: Mosby.

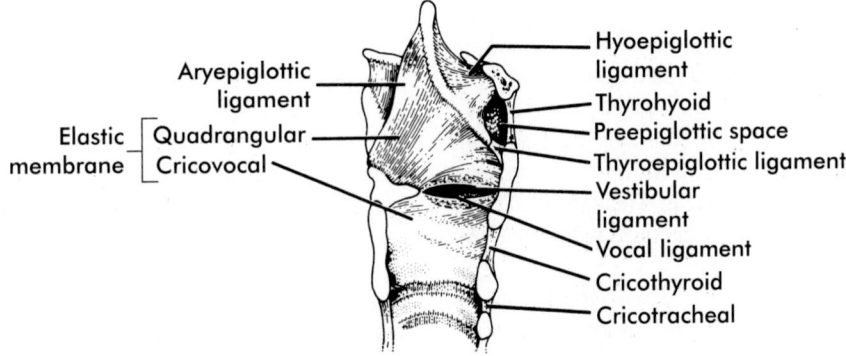

FIG. 20-3   Ligaments of larynx.
From Marino, L.B. (1981). *Cancer nursing.* St. Louis: Mosby.

salivary glands consist of tissues found in the mucosa of the cheeks, tongue, palates, floor of the mouth, pharynx, lips, and paranasal sinuses. Tumors can occur in any of these structures.

The external carotid artery supplies the salivary glands and divides into its terminal branches: the internal maxillary and superficial temporal. The superficial temporal and internal maxillary veins unite to form the posterior facial vein.

The sublingual gland lies on the undersurface of the tongue beneath the mucous membrane of the floor of the mouth at the side of the tongue, on the inner surface of the mandible. It is supplied with blood from the submental arteries, and its nerves are derived from the sympathetic nerves. The many tiny ducts of each gland separately enter the oral cavity on the sublingual fold.

The submandibular gland lies partly above and partly below the posterior half of the base of the mandible and on the mylohyoid and hyoglossus muscles. This gland is closely associated with the lingual veins and the lingual and hypoglossal nerves. The external maxillary artery lies on the posterior border of the gland. Its duct (Wharton's duct) enters the mouth at the frenulum of the tongue.

The parotid gland, the largest of the salivary glands, lies below the zygomatic arch in front of the mastoid process and behind the ramus of the mandible. This gland is enclosed in fascia, attached to surrounding muscles, and is divided into two parts—a superficial and a deep portion—by means of the facial nerve. The parotid duct (Stensen's duct) pierces the buccal pad of fat and the buccinator muscle, finally opening into the oral cavity opposite the crown of the upper second molar tooth. The superficial temporal artery and small branches of the external carotid artery arise in the parotid gland behind the neck of the mandible.

GENERAL STRUCTURES OF THE NECK

The general topography of the organs lying in front of the prevertebral fascia has been described. A layer of deep cervical fascia surrounds the neck like a collar and is attached to the trapezius and sternocleidomastoid muscles. In front of the neck the deep fascial layer is attached to the lower border of the mandible.

The pretracheal fascia of the neck lies deep in the strap muscles (sternothyroid, sternohyoid, and omohyoid) and partially encloses the thyroid gland, trachea, and larynx. The pretracheal fascia is pierced by the thyroid vessels. It fuses with the front of the carotid sheath on the deep surface of the sternocleidomastoid muscle. The carotid sheath consists of a network of areolar tissue surrounding the carotid arteries and vagus nerve.

Laterally the carotid sheath is fused with the fascia on the deep surface of the sternocleidomastoid muscle; anteriorly it is fused with the middle cervical fascia along the lateral border of the sternothyroid muscle. Lying between the floor and roof of this triangular formation of muscles

are the lymph glands and the accessory nerve. Arteries and nerves traverse and pierce this triangle.

LYMPHATIC SYSTEM OF THE NECK

The lymphatic system serves both immunologic and circulatory functions. Interstitial fluid, which may contain bacteria, viruses, or tumor cells, is returned to the blood circulation via the lymphatic channels. As the lymph nodes trap the foreign matter they may become enlarged, infected, or the focus of metastatic cancer (Meyerhoff and Rice, 1992). The lymphatic drainage of the neck can be divided into superficial and deep nodes (Fig. 20-4). The nasal cavity, paranasal sinuses, and the pharynx drain into the retropharyngeal nodes. The mouth, lips, and external nose are drained by the submandibular nodes. The lymphatics of the tip and lateral aspects of the tongue drain to the submental nodes, and the posterior tongue lymphatics drain to cervical nodes (Meyerhoff and Rice, 1992).

PERIOPERATIVE NURSING CONSIDERATIONS

ASSESSMENT

The nursing history must be thorough, including definite and questionable risk factors, such as sun exposure, tobacco use, ethanol use, radiation, family history of carcinoma, and the patient's dental history. Specific factors that should be assessed include the following:

The patient's respiratory status. Note the quality and character of respirations; note the quality and character of the voice, hoarseness, "hot potato" voice, or hyponasal speech; inspiratory stridor, expiratory stridor, hemoptysis, or dyspnea; a lesion in the oral cavity, nasopharynx, or larynx; bleeding from the oral cavity or nasopharynx. Note any history of COPD.

The patient's nutritional status. Note weight loss and length of time; dysphagia.

The patient's metabolic status. Note lab values.

The patient's circulatory status. Note pedal pulses and color of the nailbeds, especially in children, elderly patients, and patients in respiratory distress. Note preoperative vital signs compared with vital signs on admission to the patient care unit; note the presence of antiembolism stockings (the perioperative nurse should ensure proper fit of these stockings when checking pedal pulses).

Infection. Note the temperature, color, and turgor of the skin over the affected site; note lesions and their characteristics.

The patient's dentition. Note dentures and their fit, lesions, loose teeth, persistent bad breath, and poor oral hygiene.

The patient's anxiety level. Note restlessness, poor eye contact, facial tension, increased perspiration; note the

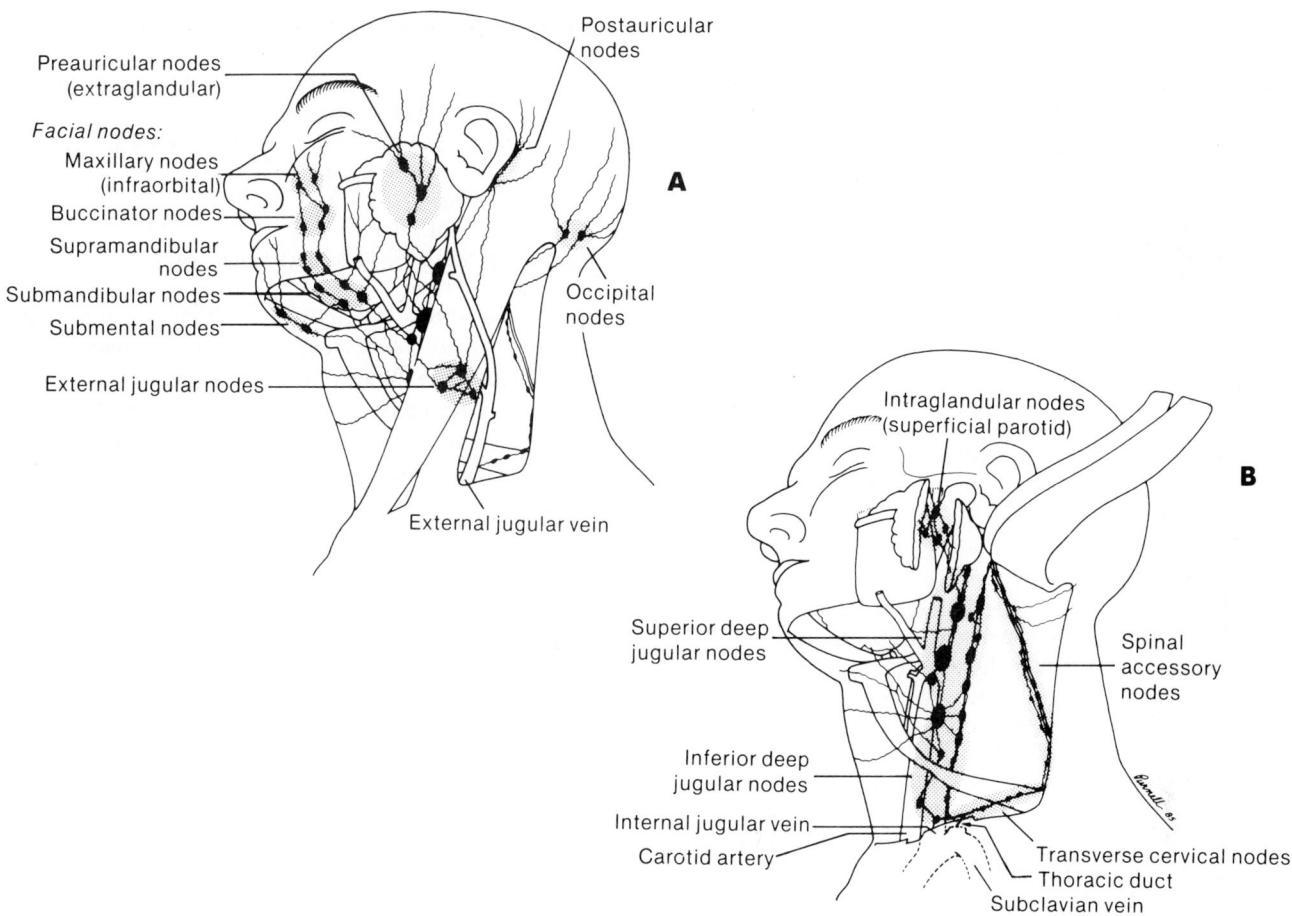

Preauricular nodes
(extraglandular)

Facial nodes:

Maxillary nodes
(infraorbital)

Buccinator nodes

Supramandibular
nodes

Submandibular nodes

Submental nodes

External jugular nodes

Postauricular
nodes

A

Occipital
nodes

External jugular vein

Intraglandular nodes
(superficial parotid)

B

Superior deep
jugular nodes

Spinal
accessory
nodes

Inferior deep
jugular nodes

Internal jugular vein

Carotid artery

Transverse cervical nodes

Thoracic duct

Subclavian vein

FIG. 20-4 **A,** Superficial cervical and facial nodal drainage patterns. **B,** Deep cervical lymphatic drainage patterns. Note that sternocleidomastoid muscle is reflected.

From Cummings, C.W., et al. (1993). *Otolaryngology—Head and neck surgery.* St. Louis: Mosby.

area around the patient's eyes for signs of crying (edema, redness).

Pain. Note location and character, odynophagia, sore throat, facial pain, otalgia; note preoperative medications and the time they were administered.

The patient's musculoskeletal system. Note problems in range of motion in all four extremities; note joint replacements, back or neck stiffness or pain, trismus.

The patient's allergies.

The patient's understanding of the surgical procedure. Note questions and give answers or ask surgeon to clarify information for the patient.

The presence of a mass. Note the length of time the mass has been evident; note if decrease in size of the mass followed antibiotic therapy; note a fixed versus mobile mass; note cranial nerve palsies involving VII, IX, X, XI, XII.

The availability of replacement blood. Note if the patient has designated donor units (the patient's blood usually will have been typed and the blood samples held, or typed and cross-matched for two units, min-

imally, depending on the anticipated extent of the procedure).

The patient's support personnel. Note family members' names and their location during the surgical procedure, introduce them to the nurse who will be in contact with them during the procedure, and establish initial communication and the intervals between which the nurse will be in contact with them regarding the patient.

Laboratory/diagnostic studies

Chest x-ray (to rule out mediastinal/pulmonary involvement and tracheal compression and to assess the patient's pulmonary status)

CT or MRI of neck (to delineate normal and abnormal soft tissue structures)

Ultrasound of mass (to determine solid versus cystic mass)

ECG

Complete blood count

RBC (may be increased with dehydration or decreased with dietary deficiencies)
  Male: 4.7 to 6.1 million/mm^3
  Female: 4.2 to 5.4 million/mm^3
  Child: 3.8 to 5.5 million/mm^3
Hemoglobin (elderly values slightly decreased; may be increased with dehydration, congestive heart failure or chronic obstructive pulmonary disease; may be decreased with cancer, nutritional deficiency or severe hemorrhage)
  Male: 14 to 18 g/dl
  Female: 12 to 16 g/dl
  Child: 11 to 16 g/dl
Hematocrit (may be increased with trauma or dehydration; may be decreased with hyperthyroidism, cirrhosis, hemorrhage, malnutrition, dietary deficiency, or in the elderly)
  Male: 42% to 52%
  Female: 37% to 47%
  Child: 31% to 43%
WBC (may be increased with infection, trauma, stress, tissue necrosis and inflammatory process; may be decreased with dietary disease, autoimmune disease and overwhelming infections)
  Adult: 5000 to 10,000/mm^3
  Child: (2 years and younger): 6200 to 17,000/mm^3
Platelet count: 150,000 to 400,000/mm^3 (may be increased with malignant disorders, cirrhosis and trauma; may be decreased with hemorrhage, liver disease, kidney disease, or systemic lupus erythematosus (SLE) (Pagana, 1992).
Urinalysis (note glucose level; if not negative, check blood glucose level)
Prothrombin time (PT), partial thromboplastin time (PTT)
  PT: 11 to 12.5 seconds (may be increased with cirrhosis, hepatitis, vitamin K deficiency, salicylate intoxication or disseminated intravascular coagulation [DIC])
  PTT: 60 to 70 seconds; APTT: 30 to 40 seconds (may be increased with clotting factor deficiencies, cirrhosis, vitamin K deficiency or DIC; may be decreased with early stages of DIC or extensive cancer) (Pagana, 1992).
Blood chemistries
  Chloride—adult/elderly: 90 to 110 mEq/L (may be increased with dehydration, kidney dysfunction or anemia; may be decreased with congestive heart failure, diuretic therapy or hypokalemia)
  Potassium—adults/elderly: 3.5 to 5 mEq/L (may be increased with acute or chronic renal failure; may be decreased with diuretic therapy, diarrhea, vomiting, or insulin, glucose or calcium administration)
  Blood urea nitrogen (BUN)—adult: 10 to 20 mg/dl (elderly may be slightly higher); may be increased with renal disease, congestive heart failure, or dehydration; may be decreased with liver failure, overhydration or malnutrition) (Pagana, 1992)
If the thyroid gland is suspect, the following tests may be indicated:
Serum calcium levels (to determine parathyroid function)—adult: 9 to 10.5 mg/dl

Serum calcitonin (to assess potential for medullary carcinoma)
Thyroid scan (to assess presence of "cold" nodule, which is often indicative of carcinoma)
Thyroid antibody tests (may show decreased levels in carcinoma): titer less than 1:100
Serum thyroxine (T$_4$): 4 to 11 mg/dl
TSH: 2 to 10 mU/ml
T$_3$ resin uptake: 25% to 35% (Pagana, 1992)

The patient should be given explanations about the operating room environment and perioperative routines to decrease apprehension. Warm blankets, thermadrapes, reassurance, and a quiet environment should be provided to ensure that the patient is comfortable, calm, and warm prior to the surgical experience.

NURSING DIAGNOSIS

Nursing diagnoses related to the care of patients undergoing laryngologic or head and neck surgery might include the following:

· Impaired gas exchange due to airway obstruction
· Anxiety related to impending surgery
· High risk for infection
· Body image disturbance
· Altered nutrition: less than body requirements
· Impaired verbal communication

OUTCOME IDENTIFICATION

Outcomes identified for the selected nursing diagnoses could be stated as:

· The patient will experience adequate gas exchange.
· The patient will demonstrate effective coping skills and a decreased level of anxiety.
· The patient will not exhibit signs of infection.
· The patient will experience a sense of self-worth and self-respect.
· The patient will maintain weight within 10 pounds of admission weight.
· The patient will establish an effective communication method with staff and family.

PLANNING

Development of a meaningful perioperative nursing care plan assists nursing personnel in meeting the needs of patients undergoing laryngologic or head and neck surgery. A Sample Care Plan for a patient undergoing laryngologic and head and neck surgery is on p. 701.

IMPLEMENTATION

The patient with a neck mass seldom undergoes surgical excision of the neck mass as a primary procedure. Endoscopic evaluation may be the initial surgical procedure, unless the primary lesion is clearly delineated.

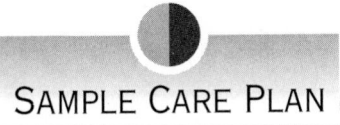

SAMPLE CARE PLAN

NURSING DIAGNOSIS: Impaired gas exchange due to airway obstruction
OUTCOME: Patient will experience adequate gas exchange.
INTERVENTIONS:
Check BP, rate and quality of respirations, rate and quality of pulse, and apical pulse preoperatively.
Auscultate chest for breath sounds preoperatively.
Elevate head of bed 45 to 60 degrees as tolerated, pre-operatively and intraoperatively.
Check arterial blood gases as ordered.
Monitor oxygen saturation perioperatively.
Administer steroids as ordered.
Monitor preoperatively for and report signs of impaired gas exchange, such as stridor, confusion, hypoxia, restlessness, and irritability.
Provide equipment, instruments, and supplies for a tracheotomy.

NURSING DIAGNOSIS: Anxiety related to impending surgery
OUTCOME: The patient will demonstrate effective coping skills and a decreased level of anxiety.
INTERVENTIONS:
Assess patient's level of anxiety (alertness, ability to comprehend, ability to perform ADL).
Maintain calm and safe environment.
Assist patient in identifying possible sources of stress.
Allow patient to ventilate and ask questions. Assess patient for recommendation of preoperative visit by patients with altered communication methods.

NURSING DIAGNOSIS: Altered nutrition: less than body requirements
OUTCOME: The patient will maintain weight within 10 pounds of admission weight.
INTERVENTIONS:
Weigh daily and record.
Monitor I & O.
Consult dietitian about formula or food selection.
Encourage full consumption of prescribed diet.

NURSING DIAGNOSIS: High risk for infection
OUTCOME: Patient will not exhibit signs of infection.
INTERVENTIONS:
Note temperature and WBC preoperatively.
Note temperature, color, and turgor of skin at operative site.
Note lesions in close proximity to surgical site.
Note patient's nutritional status.
Ensure sterile environment during surgical procedure.
Monitor traffic patterns during surgical procedure.
Monitor blood loss and fluid replacement during surgical procedure.
Note patient's temperature during surgical procedure.
Ensure that initial dressing is dry and clean.

NURSING DIAGNOSIS: Body image disturbance
OUTCOME: The patient will experience a sense of self-worth and self-respect.
INTERVENTIONS:
Encourage patient to verbalize feelings and changes related to health status and surgical procedure.
Involve family and/or significant others in initial communication with patient.
Encourage patient to ask questions.

NURSING DIAGNOSIS: Impaired verbal communication
OUTCOME: The patient will establish an effective communication method with staff and family.
INTERVENTIONS:
Agree upon a method of communication preoperatively to be used postoperatively. Suggestions include:
  a. Writing with a pen/pencil and paper, or using an erasable slate
  b. Hand signals or signs, body expressions
  c. Picture board
Provide assurance and support postoperatively, as speech pathologist initiates speech training.
Reassure patient of *some* method of communicating, postoperatively.

Positioning

Routine positioning of the laryngologic or head and neck surgical patient involves placement of the patient in a supine position on the operating room bed. A shoulder roll may be utilized for hyperextension of the neck, depending on the surgeon's preference. The headrest should allow easy movement of the head from side to side yet maintain support. The extremities are well padded at pressure points and at major nerves. A pillow should be placed under the thighs and the legs slightly frogged to decrease pressure on the patient's back; this positioning should be carried out before the patient is anesthetized to ensure comfort, with the exceptions of placement of the shoulder roll and hyperextension of the neck.

Prepping

Men should be instructed to shave the face on the morning of surgery. Further removal of hair intraoperatively depends on the site of surgery and the anticipated extensiveness of the surgical intervention. Parotid surgery may require shaving the patient's hair from just below the temple to a line even with or slightly behind the pinna of the ear. Head and neck surgery often requires removal of hair on the chest to the nipple area on both sides.

Laryngeal procedures for benign lesions do not usually involve preparation of the skin because of the intraoral approach. Head and neck procedures involve extensive preparation and usually include the entire area from the chin to the nipples. Some surgeons prefer the patient's face to be included in the prep, depending on the type of surgery anticipated and the site of the lesion. Povidone-iodine scrub and solution are generally preferred for preparation of the skin. If a flap may be raised to reconstruct a defect, saline should be available to remove the discoloration from the skin and allow the surgeon to check for flap viability.

Draping

As with prepping, draping of the patient for a laryngeal procedure for a benign lesion (intraoral approach) is minimal, with the primary focus being protection of the patient's eyes and face. This may be accomplished by (1) placing ointment in the patient's eyes, (2) taping the eyelids closed with a nonabrasive, nonirritating tape, (3) applying moist cotton balls over the tape (if use of the carbon dioxide laser is anticipated), and (4) placing self-adhering eyepads over the cotton balls. A huck towel may be placed over the patient's face to expose only the lips and chin.

Draping for head and neck procedures often varies according to surgeon preference. If the preference is to have the patient's face exposed, a commercially prepared head drape may be used. If unavailable, a head drape can be made by utilizing a sterile sheet folded in half with a sterile huck towel on the innermost side to wrap the patient's hair. A towel clamp or sterile tape can secure the head drape in place. Towels can be opened fully, crushed, and placed in the space at both sides of the patient's neck and shoulder area to prevent contact with the unsterile operating room bed linen during the procedure. The area of the endotracheal tube may be isolated by a self-adherent, clear drape. Sterile towels are utilized to drape the neck, shoulder, and chest areas. An impervious drape is used to cover the patient from the chest to the foot of the operating room bed. A split sheet may then be used to drape over the huck towels and body drape. Commercially prepared split sheets have adhesive backing along the split that facilitates adherence to the area to be draped out and decreases slippage with subsequent contamination resulting from manipulation of the head during the surgical procedure.

Instrumentation

The instrumentation used in laryngologic surgery is quite specific and is discussed with each surgical intervention. Head and neck instrumentation consists of general surgical instruments such as:

Mosquito hemostats	Adson forceps with teeth
Kelly hemostats	Vascular forceps
Crile hemostats	Towel clamps
Mayo-Pean forceps	Needle holders
Allis forceps	Yankauer suction tubes
Babcock forceps	Frazier suction tips
Thyroid tenacula	Rake retractors
Right-angle clamps	Army-Navy retractors
Skin hooks	Vein retractors
Mayo scissors	Green retractors
Metzenbaum scissors	Long tenotomy scissors

Intraoral, laryngeal, and mandibular procedures require the addition of periosteal elevators (such as Joseph, Freer, Cleoid), cartilage scissors, bone cutter, rongeurs (such as Lempert, Adson), tracheal hooks, tracheal spreader, and saws. Although a Gigli saw and handles may be used on rare occasions, technology has made the sagittal saw standard in the operating room armamentarium. Saws are either nitrogen powered or electric. The choice of power source should be a collaborative effort among the perioperative nursing staff and surgeon. A dermatome may be used if skin grafting of surgical defects or flap reconstruction is anticipated. In the case of large reconstructive surfaces, a skin mesher may be used to extend the skin graft.

Equipment

Equipment that may be utilized in head and neck surgery includes an electrosurgical unit (both monopolar and bipolar), a hypothermia-hyperthermia unit, headlights (both fiberoptic and nonfiberoptic), pulse oximeter, blood warmer, temperature recorder, and humidifier. Although the last four items of equipment are primarily the responsibility of anesthesia personnel, the circulating nurse collaborates in providing access to electrical outlets to power the equipment and participates in interventions based on the results of patient monitoring.

Lasers utilized in head and neck and laryngeal surgery include the carbon dioxide (CO_2) and Nd:YAG lasers, depending on the location and type of lesion.

The evolution of microvascular free flap surgery for head and neck reconstruction has added a host of equipment to ensure the success of the surgical procedure and the safety of the patient. This equipment includes a surgical microscope (where the assistant may work at a 180-degree angle from the surgeon), a Doppler unit (to determine the viability of blood vessels), an electromyographic nerve monitor (to determine the location and quality of nerves), and a demagnetizer (to treat microsurgical instruments).

Safety in head and neck surgery is primarily patient related with the exception of lasers, which warrant both patient and staff safety precautions (see Chapter 31). All equipment should be checked prior to use to ensure that it is in proper working condition. Visual inspection should ensure that all equipment is clean. Headlights, in particular, should be inspected for blood prior to and following each use. Personnel should be reminded to wear safety glasses for eye protection in accordance with OSHA regulations. The circulating nurse should inspect the masks of the scrub team during the procedure for contamination by blood and body fluids and assist them in changing masks as needed.

Medications

Medications used in laryngeal surgery are targeted at decreasing bleeding and edema in the airway. Typical medications include the following:

Steroids are often given intraoperatively and postoperatively but may be given preoperatively in the presence of edema or airway obstruction.

Epinephrine or phenylephrine hydrochloride may be placed topically when vocal cord lesions are excised manually or biopsy specimens are taken to identify a primary tumor site.

Lidocaine (Xylocaine) is instilled into the trachea to decrease coughing immediately prior to insertion of a tracheotomy tube.

Medications used in head and neck surgery include antibiotics and steroids. They are primarily given intravenously; however, an antibiotic may also be added to irrigating solutions. Chemotherapeutic agents are often an important aspect of adjuvant therapy for the head and neck cancer patient. The perioperative nurse should be familiar with the chemotherapeutic agents prescribed for the patient.

Patient education

Preoperative patient education includes preparing the patient for alterations in body image and function. Altered methods of communication must be discussed prior to disruption of oral or laryngeal function, allowing the patient the opportunity to practice prior to the disruption of speech.

The presence of edema, drains, nasogastric tube, Foley catheter, dressings, and altered mobility must be discussed. The operating room environment and presence of equipment should be described to the patient preoperatively to keep anxiety at a minimum. Dietary preferences and eating habits should be discussed to effectively develop a postoperative nutritional plan. Elimination habits should be discussed, if appropriate, and alternate methods presented to the patient. Any special considerations of positioning should be discussed prior to surgery.

Postoperative patient education for laryngologic and head and neck surgery includes interventions to keep the airway clear and patent (turning, coughing and deep breathing; providing a humidified environment; monitoring sputum; tracheostomy care), maintenance of adequate nutritional status to promote healing (dietary consultation; monitoring intake and weight; eating small, multiple meals and snacks), wound care (incision site care, oral hygiene, symptoms indicative of infection or potential wound breakdown), medications, activity limitations, potential complications, postoperative course, additional therapies and coping mechanisms to avoid alcohol and tobacco use, as well as the patient's altered body image. Specific patient instructions are included under Procedural Considerations.

Monitoring considerations

Intraoperative monitoring of the patient includes assessment of the circulatory, metabolic, urinary, respiratory, and musculoskeletal systems at regular intervals. Assessment of fluid volume is a collaborative effort. Blood loss and urinary output are communicated to anesthesia personnel. The perioperative nurse participates in the administration of fluid replacement therapy, assists in maintaining patency of lines, and notes the patient's response. Pedal pulses and pressure points should be checked without disturbing the surgical field or team. The scrub and circulating nurses must be aware of significant findings during the surgical procedure to anticipate changes or additional supplies and equipment needed. Communication with the patient's family or support persons is vital during the surgical procedure to decrease their anxiety.

Additional methods of monitoring the laryngologic or head and neck surgical patient include:

Pulse oximeter: usually monitored via the great toe because the BP cuff is on one arm of the patient and the arterial line and intravenous infusion line are in the other arm

Blood pressure cuff: preferably automatic because of the necessity of frequent monitoring when dissecting around vital structures in the neck

Arterial line: detects sudden changes in BP and serves as a vehicle to obtain Po_2 and Pco_2 levels

Foley catheter: monitors the patient's urinary function, especially important for the elderly or debilitated patient

Temperature monitoring: usually via rectal probe or endotracheal tube probe

Esophageal stethoscope: usually contraindicated in head and neck procedures because of the interruption of the esophagus or structures adjacent to the esophagus

Computerized anesthesia monitoring system: standardized method of ensuring the safety of the patient while the anesthetic is being administered.

Accurate and thorough monitoring is critical to safe and effective patient outcomes. Perioperative nurses should be familiar with monitoring equipment, able to interpret results, and remain responsive to implementing collaborative interventions based on those results.

EVALUATION

Postoperative evaluation includes reassessing potential patient problems identified in the preoperative assessment as well as assessing the electrosurgical dispersive pad site, surgical incision, dressing, drains, respiratory status, skin turgor, and color of the head and extremities. Preoperative assessment findings, intraoperative changes in the patient's condition, and the postoperative evaluation must be documented and communicated to ensure continuity of care and patient safety. The report should also include relevant nursing diagnoses and outcomes of care. Some nursing diagnoses may have already been resolved; others are ongoing and require continued planning and intervention during the patient's recovery from anesthesia and postoperative rehabilitation. A complete nursing report allows the PACU or ICU nurse to detect significant changes in the patient's condition in an early stage. Special considerations should also be reported, such as the necessity for flexion of the neck to avoid disruption of the suture line of the trachea in a patient who has undergone tracheal resection. Documentation should include the postoperative report given and the name of the RN to whom that report is given, prior to the patient's discharge from the operating room. Based on the nursing diagnoses selected for the patient undergoing laryngologic or head and neck surgery, the nursing report might include the following outcome statements:

- The patient's gas exchange remained normal.
- The patient demonstrated efective coping skills and a decreased level of anxiety.
- The patient will not exhibit signs of infection (ongoing).
- The patient verbalized feelings regarding disturbances in body image.
- The patient's nutritional status will be maintained (ongoing).
- The patient is able to communicate effectively (ongoing).

SURGICAL INTERVENTIONS

LARYNGOSCOPY

Laryngoscopy is direct visual examination of the interior of the larynx by means of a lighted speculum known as a laryngoscope (Fig. 20-5) to obtain a specimen of tissue or secretions for pathologic examination.

Procedural considerations

To facilitate this examination, the patient should be sufficiently relaxed by reassurance and by drug preparation if the procedure is performed under local anesthesia. Sedatives are usually ordered before surgery. Immediate preoperative assessment should include the presence of any dental appliances and condition of dental work and loose teeth. Any stiffness or immobility of the neck or shoulders should be evaluated. Respiratory problems such as asthma must receive careful attention. The patient should be cautioned about not eating or drinking after surgery until the gag reflex has returned and swallowing occurs without difficulty. Most laryngoscopies are performed with the patient under general anesthesia. Infants usually do not require an anesthetic. If an adult cannot tolerate a general anesthetic, the patient must be well-prepared preoperatively, and the application of a local or topical anesthetic of lidocaine (Xylocaine), tetracaine (Pontocaine), cocaine, or cetacaine will be performed immediately before the procedure.

The setup includes the following:

Local anesthesia setup

Gauze sponges, 4 × 4 inches
Laryngeal mirror
Cotton balls
Small cup of hot water (to warm the laryngeal mirror so it does not fog when inserted into the mouth to view the vocal cords)
Emesis basin
Syringe, 5 ml, and Abraham cannula
Medication cup
Jackson laryngeal applicating forceps
Cetacaine spray, with angulated tip, or other topical anesthetic for the oral mucosa

Instrument setup

1 Laryngoscope (surgeon's choice), size suitable to the patient (adult, child, or infant)
2 Laryngeal suction tubes
1 Light carrier, fiberoptic
2 Laryngeal biopsy forceps, 1 straight and 1 upbiting
2 Sponge-carrier forceps with extra sponges
1 Tooth guard
1 Fiberoptic light cord

Accessory items

Suction tubing	Gauze sponges
Specimen jar	Sterile towels
Basin of sterile saline	Gloves

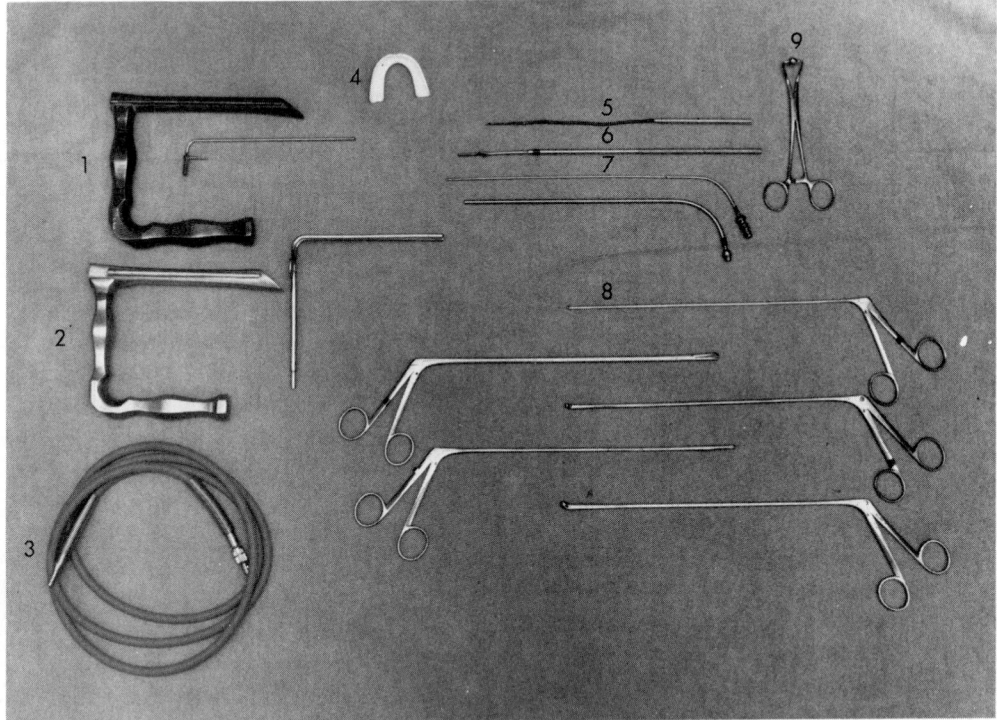

FIG. 20-5   Laryngoscopy instruments. *1*, Anterior commissure laryngoscope and light carrier; *2*, Dedo Pilling laryngoscope and light carrier; *3*, fiberoptic light cord; *4*, tooth guard; *5*, laryngeal pigtail applicator; *6*, long knife handle; *7*, laryngeal suction tubes, small and medium; *8*, assorted laryngeal cup forceps and laryngeal alligator forceps; *9*, nonperforating towel clamp.

If the surgeon wishes to perform a suspension laryngoscopy, a self-retaining laryngoscope holder is added to the instrument table. A special platform may be mounted onto the operating room bed, or a Mayo stand may be placed above the patient's chest and over the operating room bed to provide a place for the laryngoscope holder to rest. The surgeon usually expects to use the operating microscope during suspension laryngoscopy. The patient is placed in a supine position to facilitate visualization of the vocal cords. A shoulder roll should be immediately available if slight hyperextension of the neck is necessary to assist in visualization of the larynx.

Operative procedure

1. Moist gauze pads or tape should be put over the patient's eyes to protect them from the instrumentation and to prevent injury and irritation from secretions during the procedure. The head may also be wrapped in a sterile towel. Some surgeons may request a sterile drape to cover the patient.
2. The spatula end of the laryngoscope is introduced into the right side of the patient's mouth and directed toward the midline; then the dorsum of the tongue is elevated, exposing the epiglottis.
3. The patient's head is first tipped backward and then lifted upward as the laryngoscope is advanced into the larynx.

4. The larynx is examined, a biopsy is taken, secretions are aspirated, and bleeding is controlled.
5. The patient's face is cleansed. The patient is then taken to the PACU.

Microlaryngoscopy

Microlaryngoscopy facilitates improved diagnosis and allows the laryngologist to view with relative ease areas that were previously inaccessible or difficult to visualize. It may also be used for minor surgery of the larynx, especially for the removal of polyps or nodes on the vocal cords.

Procedural considerations

If the procedure is done to remove polyps or nodes from the vocal cords, the patient must be cautioned about not speaking for a while postoperatively. The patient should be provided with a pencil and paper or erasable slate to aid in communication. The patient's restriction on speaking should be noted on the nursing care plan, on the front of the chart, and on the door of the patient's room.

The basic instrument setup for laryngoscopy is used. Microlaryngeal instruments are added to the setup and include the following (Fig. 20-6):

Self-retaining laryngoscope holder
Jako microlaryngeal grasping forceps
Jako microlaryngeal cup forceps, straight and upbiting
    cups

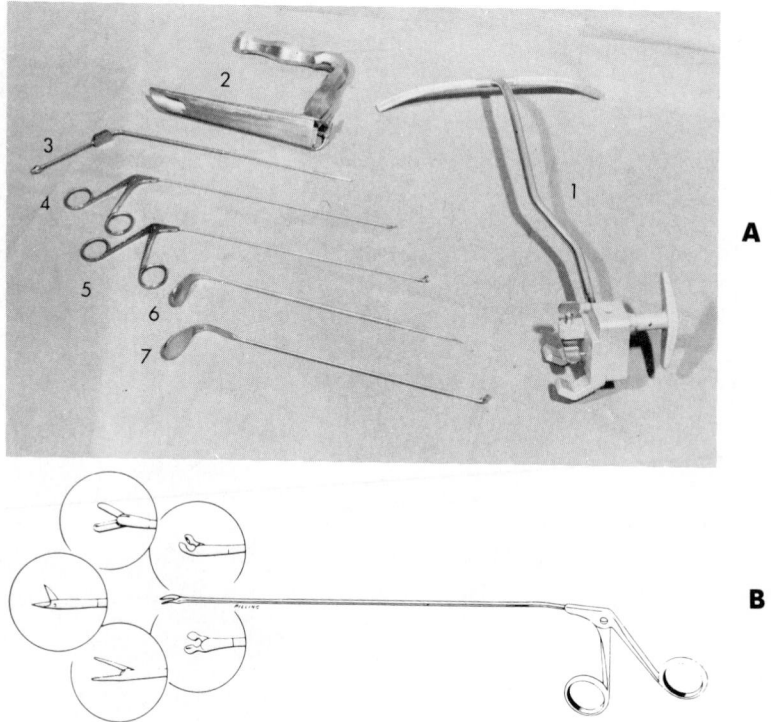

FIG. 20-6   Jako microlaryngeal instrumentation. **A,** Basic setup for microlaryngoscopy. *1,* Lewy self-retaining laryngoscope holder; *2,* Jako laryngoscope; *3,* suction tube; *4,* grasping forceps; *5,* cup forceps; *6,* probe; *7,* mirror. **B,** Closeup of working ends of instruments.

A from DeWeese, D.D., & Saunders, W.H. (1982). *Textbook of otolaryngology* (6th ed.). St. Louis: Mosby; **B** courtesy Pilling Co., Philadelphia.

Jako microlaryngeal scissors, straight, angled, and upbiting
Jako microlaryngeal knives, straight and curved
Laryngeal probe
Microlaryngeal mirror
Open-ended microlaryngeal suction tube
Laryngoscope (dual light channel)

The aforementioned instruments have a length of 22 cm to allow use with the microscope, being long enough to keep the surgeon's hands out of the visual field. The microscope is used. The head is adjusted to allow visualization of the larynx. The surgeon usually adjusts the microscope. The microscope lens should have a 400-mm focal length. Focal length is the distance from the lens to the operative area and is the point at which the field can be clearly viewed through the microscope. Beyond this point the field becomes fuzzy. The 400-mm lens gives the surgeon a 40-cm focal length, or working distance. A general rule for determining focal length of a lens is to divide the millimeter power, for example, 400 mm, by 10. In this instance it is 40 cm.

Care of endoscopic equipment

Endoscopic equipment is fragile and should be handled carefully. Rigid endoscopes should be thoroughly cleaned and lumina checked for cleanliness. Long, narrow brushes and long pipe cleaners are available for cleaning the lumen

and suction and light channels. The scopes should be dried carefully before sterilization. The light carriers are stored in the endoscopes. The endoscope should be checked for any dents, roughened edges, or deep scratches on the surface. Any of these can cause tissue damage or lead to corrosion of the instrument. Endoscopes should be handled individually.

Fiberoptic equipment is also fragile. The light cables should be handled with care and not allowed to drop or swing free while being carried. This can break the filaments inside the cords, rendering them unusable. Most cables can be autoclaved, but according to manufacturer's instructions only. They should be coiled loosely when not in use, and care should be taken not to put anything heavy on top of the cables. Kinking and sharp bending of the cables must be avoided.

The main advantage of fiberoptics is that the light, although very bright, remains cool when used for a relatively long time. A simple test for the integrity of the cable is to hold one end of the cable to a bright light and inspect the opposite end. Dark spots are an indication that some of the fibers are broken. If more than 25% of the fibers are broken, the cable should be sent for repair, or replacement should be considered.

Telescopes for rigid equipment, as used for bronchoscopy, should also be handled carefully to prevent damage. The telescope should be cleaned carefully, thoroughly dried, and returned to its case for protection during storage. Telescopes may be sterilized, but strict adherence to manufacturer's instructions must be followed. Gas sterilization is the method of choice. If a telescope is dropped or hit against another object, it should be sent to the manufacturer for examination and repaired if required. Suction tubes should be flushed thoroughly with running water. An instrument-cleaning solution may also be used for this purpose. The lumen should be cleaned with a long pipe cleaner to remove remaining debris. The tube is then rinsed again, and the lumen dried with a clean, dry pipe cleaner. The suction tube should be inspected for dents or nicks, especially on the end, to prevent damage to delicate tissues.

Biopsy forceps should be thoroughly cleaned, and the edges of the cups inspected for chips or nicks. They should also be checked periodically for sharpness. If the forceps are dull, nicked, or chipped, tissue will be torn or ripped instead of cut cleanly when a specimen is taken, resulting in more bleeding than usual. It is a good practice to rotate the use of biopsy forceps regularly depending on the frequency of use. All forceps should be thoroughly cleaned, dried, and inspected for damage after use and should be sent for repair if necessary.

Proper care of endoscopic equipment can extend the service life of these instruments indefinitely.

Carbon dioxide laser surgery of the larynx

The advent of the CO_2 laser added a new dimension to the laryngologist's treatment of lesions of the larynx and vocal cords. This laser is efficient and has a high power output. It uses a combination of carbon dioxide, nitrogen, and helium gases that becomes energized to a high degree by an electric current. As the energy level subsides, light beams are produced and are reflected off the mirror-lined walls of the laser tube. These beams eventually form a single beam of light that has a high intensity in the ultraviolet range and is therefore invisible to the eye. For this reason a red beam from a helium-neon laser is added to the CO_2 dioxide beam so it can be properly aimed at the affected tissue. The beam destroys tissue at a precise point with minimal destruction of the surrounding tissue. It is especially useful in surgeries such as removal of webs in the larynx, vocal cord papillomas, and carcinoma in situ of the larynx, as well as benign endobronchial lesions.

Procedural considerations

The basic setup for laryngoscopy and microlaryngoscopy is used. All instrumentation used for laser laryngoscopy should be ebonized. General anesthesia is usually given. The operating microscope with a 400-mm lens is used, with the laser micromanipulator attached to the microscope head (Fig. 20-7). The manufacturer's instructions for attaching it must be followed. The beam should also be tested for proper working order. Signal lights on the console illuminate if any malfunction occurs in the equipment or if the gas supply is low. Extreme care should be used when handling this delicate equipment.

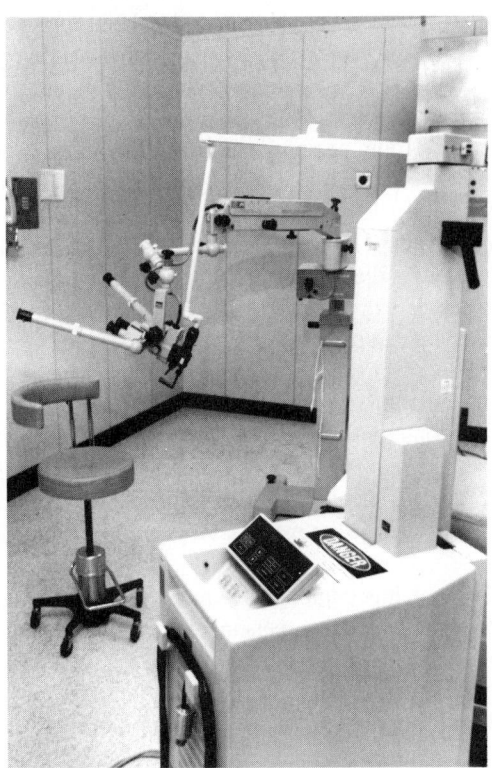

FIG. 20-7   Operating microscope with laser micromanipulator attached.

Precautions

1. Laser light is reflected by shiny surfaces or absorbed by moisture. Because silicone, latex, and red rubber endotracheal tubes are combustible, they must be protected by being carefully wrapped with adhesive sensing tape. In addition, saline-soaked gauze or cottonoid patties with strings are placed just above the tube cuff. These precautions eliminate the possibility of the tube or cuff being punctured or set afire by a stray laser beam. A safer alternative is the use of copper (Carden), stainless steel (Porch), or commercially prepared laser-retardant endotracheal tubes and a jet ventilation system.

2. Because the laser beam can destroy tissue, the patient's healthy tissue must be protected. This is best done by covering the areas such as the eyes, the oral cavity, and the peritracheal area with wet gauze pads or cottonoid patties. Cottonoid patties covering the balloon on the endotracheal tube are effective in preventing rupture of the cuff. *It is imperative that all gauze pads or patties be kept wet during the surgery to prevent damage to healthy tissue from stray or reflected beams of light.* Moisture is the most effective barrier to stop the laser energy from penetrating healthy tissue or igniting materials in the area. Should the endotracheal tube be ignited for some reason (not a common occurrence but the most dangerous of complications) during the procedure, a ventilating bronchoscope, grasping forceps of some type, and a tracheostomy tray should be available. A syringe con-

taining sterile saline with a red rubber (open-ended) catheter attached, as well as an Asepto containing sterile saline must be on the surgical setup as the primary action in the event a fire occurs.

3. Operating room personnel must wear eyeglasses or special plastic protective goggles when the CO_2 laser is in use. Contact lenses do not protect the eyes from stray laser beams. The corneas are especially vulnerable to stray laser radiation and must be protected. If the corneas are left unprotected and energy is absorbed, corneal opacification can result.

4. Signs indicating that a laser is in use should be placed on the operating room door during the procedure to keep extra people out of the room while the laser is used.

5. If the laser equipment does not test properly before the procedure, it should be checked by biomedical engineering personnel or the manufacturer before being used.

The use of this equipment requires thorough education of perioperative nursing personnel, anesthesia staff, and surgeons. The teaching should include the assembly and disassembly of the equipment, proper techniques for the immediate preoperative testing of the equipment, precautions that must be taken while in use, and a basic explanation of the principles of laser use (see Chapter 31). These points should be clearly understood by all involved to prevent any undue tissue damage to the patient or injury to personnel.

BRONCHOSCOPY

The trachea, bronchi, and lungs are visualized directly with a rigid or flexible bronchoscope that has a fiberoptic lighting system. A rigid scope gives a larger viewing area, whereas a flexible scope is easily inserted into the patient and manipulated. Bronchoscopy is fully described in Chapter 24. The Nd:YAG laser may be utilized for lesions of the trachea or bronchi, depending on the type of lesion.

ESOPHAGOSCOPY

Esophagoscopy is the direct visualization of the esophagus and the cardia of the stomach. This procedure is utilized to observe the area for extension of tumor, remove tissue and secretions for study, or observe for primary tumor site.

Procedural considerations

Esophagoscopy facilitates the diagnosis of esophageal carcinoma, diverticula, hiatal hernia, stricture, benign stenosis, or varices. Patients with suspected obstruction, symptoms of bleeding, or regurgitation may require endoscopy. The Nd:YAG laser may be utilized in the treatment of some of these lesions. Esophagoscopy may also be used for therapeutic manipulations, such as removal of a foreign body or insertion of an esophageal bougie.

Before the esophagoscopy a member of the surgical team may be designated responsible for holding and moving the patient's head throughout the procedure. The movement of

the patient's head during the procedure ensures the examination of all areas of the esophagus because it is not a rigid structure like the bronchus.

The setup includes the following:

Esophagoscopes, desired type, size and length (Figs. 20-8 and 20-9)
Suction tubing
Fiberoptic light source and light cords
Bougies, if desired
Forceps, desired type and length
Specimen containers
Water-soluble lubricating jelly
Gauze sponges
Basin with sterile saline
Suction tubes (velvet-eye tips to avoid suctioning the mucosa of the esophagus into the tip)

Operative procedure

1. The fiberoptic light carrier is inserted into the esophagoscope, and a fiberoptic light cord is attached. A thin layer of lubricant is applied to the scope. The scope is passed into the mouth. The tongue, epiglottis, laryngeal inlet, and cricopharyngeal lumen are identified. The person holding the patient's head may tip the head backward while extending the neck anterior. Usually the esophagoscope is passed to the right side of the tongue and the patient's head is turned slightly to the left.

2. When the scope has passed the inferior constrictors, the patient's head is moved in various directions so that all areas of the esophageal wall may be examined.

3. Specimens of secretions from the esophageal lumen may be obtained with an aspirating tube and suctioning ap-

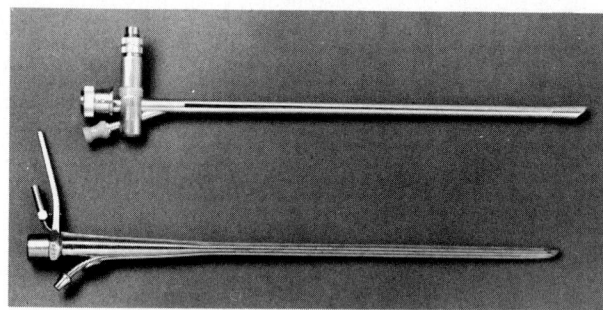

FIG. 20-8   Pediatric and adult esophagoscopes.

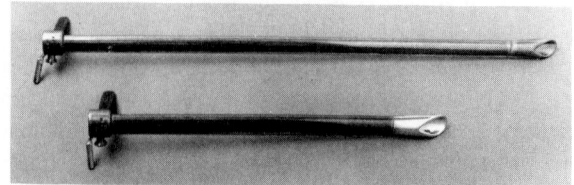

FIG. 20-9   Jesberg adult esophagoscopes.

paratus. In some cases saline may be injected through the esophagoscope's aspirating channel and the fluid withdrawn immediately for histologic study. A biopsy of tissue may be taken using forceps of the surgeon's preference. Following biopsy, the area is assessed for bleeding, and the esophagoscope is then removed.

TRIPLE ENDOSCOPY

When laryngoscopy, bronchoscopy, and esophagoscopy are performed on a patient, the procedure is termed *triple endoscopy*. The order in which the procedures are performed depends on the surgeon's preference. The purpose of triple endoscopy is usually diagnostic. While inspecting for a malignancy, the surgeon views the structures, takes specimens for biopsy, and possibly makes smears or washings of the suspect areas.

TONSILLECTOMY AND ADENOIDECTOMY

The palatine tonsils and adenoids are removed by sharp or blunt dissection. Enlarged tonsils and adenoids are usu-

ally associated with difficulty in breathing and hearing, chronic colds, enlarged glands of the neck, otitis media, and pressure on the eustachian tubes caused by adenoiditis. Rheumatism, bronchitis, and hearing loss may be associated with diseased tonsils.

Special preoperative teaching and orientation sessions for pediatric patients have decreased the stress of the perioperative period for children undergoing this surgery. During these sessions parents are instructed in the essentials of postoperative care.

Procedural considerations

The patient is anesthetized and may be placed in slight Trendelenburg's position. The neck is hyperextended by placing a roll under the shoulders. A small headrest may be necessary if the patient's head is unstable. Typical draping includes application of a head drape and an impervious sheet over the patient. The instruments and supplies required include the following (Fig. 20-10):

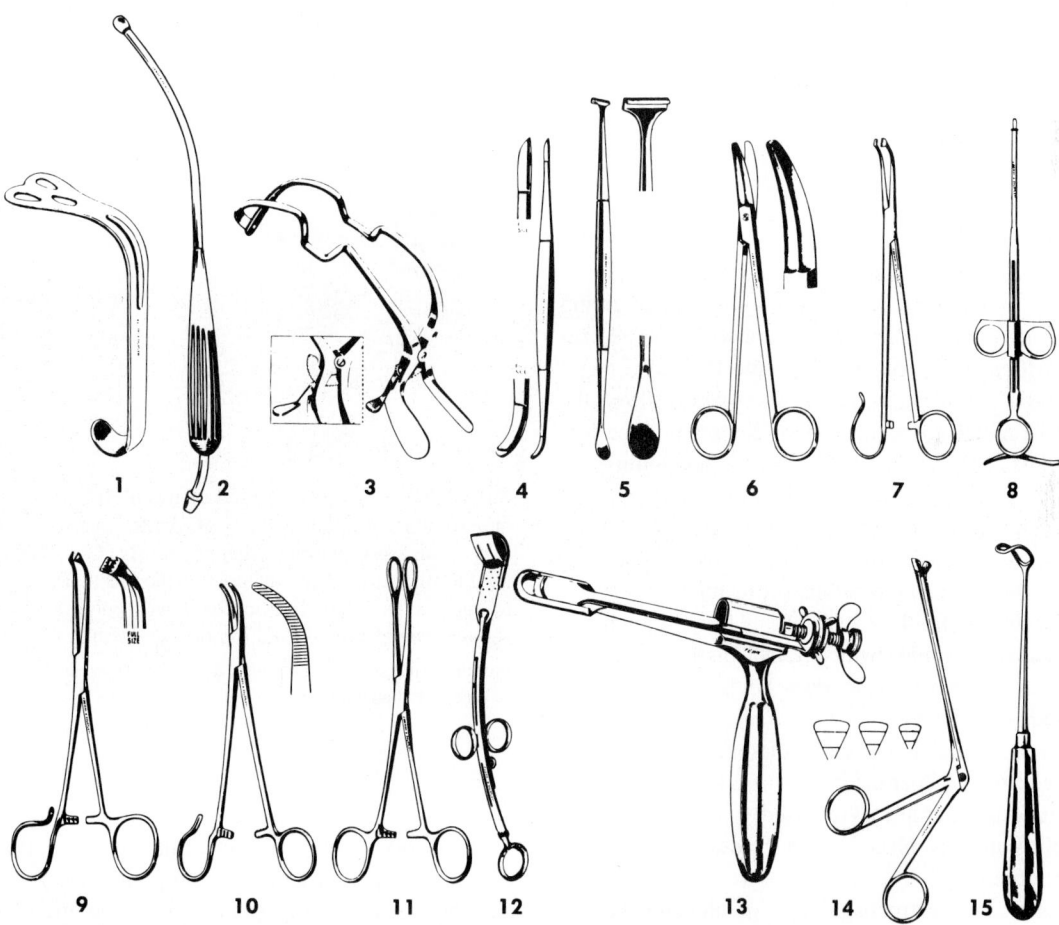

FIG. 20-10   Instruments for tonsillectomy and adenoidectomy. *1*, Tongue depressor; *2*, Yankauer suction tube; *3*, Jennings mouth gag; *4*, tonsil knife; *5*, Hurd dissector and pillar retractor; *6*, Boettcher tonsil scissors; *7*, White tonsil-grasping forceps; *8*, Eves tonsil snare; *9*, Allis-Coakley forceps, curved; *10*, Dean hemostatic forceps; *11*, Ballenger sponge-holding forceps, serrated jaw; *12*, LaForce adenotome; *13*, Daniel tonsillectome; *14*, adenoid punch; *15*, Barnhill adenoid curette.

Courtesy Codman & Shurtleff, Inc., Randolph, Mass.

1 Knife handle, no. 7 with no. 12 blade
1 Tonsil knife
1 Tonsil snare with additional wires
1 LaForce or Sluder tonsil guillotines, if desired
1 Metzenbaum scissors, curved, 7½ inches, or Boettcher scissors
1 Mayo scissors
Adenoid curettes, assorted sizes
1 Adenoid punch
LaForce adenotomes, assorted sizes
1 Hurd dissector and pillar retractor
2 Sponge-holding forceps
1 Towel clamp
2 Tonsil-grasping forceps, straight and curved
2 Dean hemostatic forceps
Jennings mouth gag, suitable size
Self-retaining mouth gag with tongue blades, if desired
1 Uvula or palate retractor
1 Tongue depressor
1 Needle holder, 7 inches
1 Yankauer suction tube with suction tubing
Tonsil sponges of assorted sizes
Gauze sponges
Basin set
Cold sterile saline solution
Electrosurgical handpiece, with suction attached
Electrosurgical unit
Headlight of surgeon's preference

Operative procedure

1. A general anesthetic is used, an endotracheal tube is inserted, the mouth is retracted open with a self-retaining retractor, and the tongue is depressed with a blade retractor. Efficient suction is most important. The metal suction tube is introduced gently and passed along the floor of the mouth, over the base of the tongue, and into the pharynx. During the procedure the suctioning ensures adequate exposure of the operative site and prevents blood from reaching the lungs or stomach.

2. The tonsil is grasped with a pair of tonsil-grasping forceps, and the mucous membrane of the anterior pillar is incised with a knife; the tonsil lobe is freed from its attachments to the pillars with a tonsil dissector, curved scissors, and gauze sponges on a holder. The tonsil is withdrawn with forceps.

3. The posterior pillar is cut with scissors, and the tonsil is removed with a snare (Fig. 20-11). In some cases a tonsil guillotine clamp may be used.

4. A tonsil sponge is placed in the fossa with sponge-holding forceps.

5. The vessels are electrocoagulated, or bleeding vessels are clamped with tonsil forceps and tied with slipknot absorbable no. 0 ligatures, and the free ligature ends are cut.

6. The adenoids are removed with an adenotome or curette. Bleeding is controlled by pressure with tonsil sponges, sometimes soaked in a hemostatic solution. (The ade-

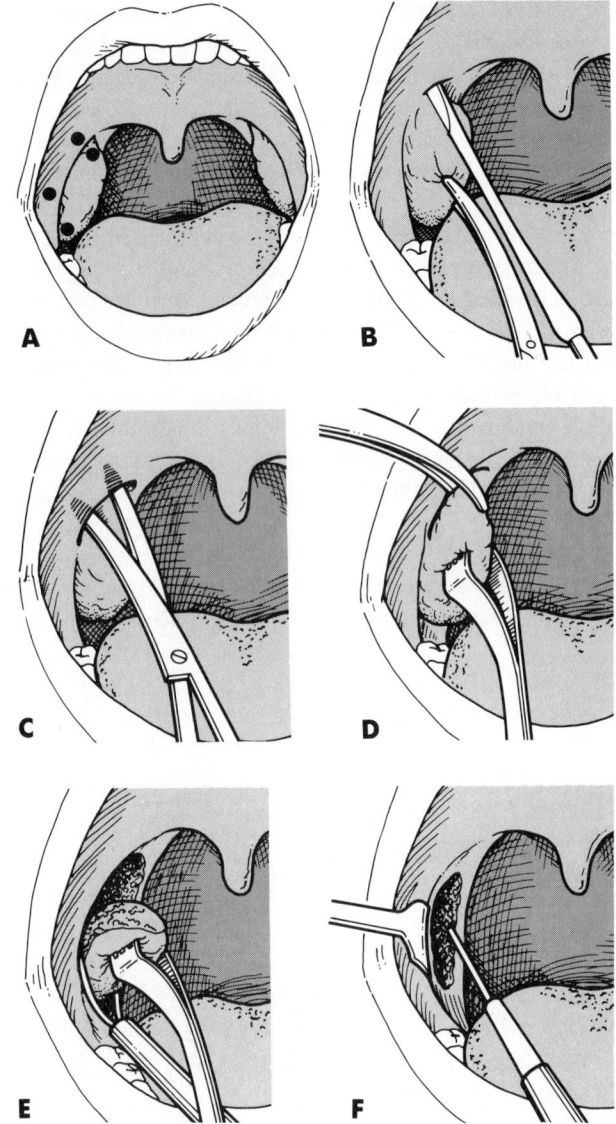

FIG. 20-11 Surgical method of tonsillectomy. **A,** Local anesthesia infiltration points. **B,** Tonsil knife is used to make an incision at the tonsil anterior pillar superiorly. **C** and **D,** Scissors are used to dissect the superior pole of the tonsil. **E,** A snare is used to separate the tonsil from the lower pole. **F,** Hemostasis is achieved by electrocoagulation or tying of bleeding vessels.

From Luckmann, J., & Sorenson, K.C. (1987). *Medical-surgical nursing* (3rd ed.). Philadelphia: W.B. Saunders.

noidectomy may be performed prior to the tonsillectomy, depending on surgeon preference.)

7. The fossa is carefully inspected, and any bleeding vessels are cauterized or clamped and tied. Retractors and endotracheal tube are removed, the patient's face is cleaned, and the head is turned to one side. The patient is placed in the semirecumbent (Fowler) position or on one side, horizontally, to prevent aspiration of blood and venous engorgement postoperatively.

SURGERY OF THE ORAL CAVITY

Benign or malignant lesions of the tongue, floor of the mouth, alveolar ridge, buccal mucosa, or tonsillar area are excised. Benign or small malignant tumors of the oral cavity may be excised without neck dissection. In the presence of tongue cancer without evidence of metastasis, a prophylactic neck dissection may be performed in an effort to control a cancerous growth in the upper jugular chain of the neck.

In the treatment of carcinoma of the floor of the mouth with involvement of the mandible, a portion of the tongue is removed in a combined operation—a radical neck dissection and resection of both the mandible and the tongue. When the primary intraoral lesion is confined to the tongue, a neck dissection and a hemiglossectomy are performed without resection of the mandible. In the presence of a lesion of the tonsil or an extensive lesion at the base of the tongue with pharyngeal wall involvement, a resection of the ascending ramus of the mandible is necessary, and portions of the base of the tongue, pharyngeal wall, and soft palate are removed to secure an adequate margin of normal tissue around the lesion.

Psychologic preparation of the patient is extremely important, since these procedures may be done for a minor lesion in the oral cavity or they may be the first part of much more extensive surgery in the head and neck area. A supportive and accepting family is most important to the patient at this time because of the possibility of disfigurement after surgery.

Procedural considerations

The patient is placed in a supine position with shoulders elevated. Generally, endotracheal anesthesia is used, and a pharyngeal pack of moist gauze may be inserted in the mouth. Instruments and supplies include the following items:

2 Knives, no. 3 and no. 7, with no. 10 and no. 15 blades
1 Metzenbaum scissors, curved, 7 ¼ inches
1 Mayo scissors, straight
1 Mayo scissors, curved
1 Suture scissors
4 Foerster or Ballenger sponge-holding forceps
6 Towel clamps
2 Tissue forceps without teeth, 5 ½ inches
2 Tissue forceps with teeth, 5 ½ inches
2 Adson forceps
2 Brown-Adson forceps
2 Nasal dressing forceps (bayonet style)
4 Allis forceps, 3 and 4 teeth
6 Mayo-Pean forceps, curved, 6 ½ inches
3 Mayo-Pean forceps, curved, 9 ¼ inches
6 Crile hemostats, straight
2 Rochester-Carmalt forceps, 8 inches
3 Tonsil artery forceps
1 Metal anesthesia tube
1 Mouth gag
2 McBurney retractors

3 Bosworth tongue depressors
1 Cheek retractor
2 Parker retractors
1 Cushing loop retractor
1 Nerve hook
1 Crile-Wood needle holder, 8 inches
1 Crile-Wood needle holder, 5 ½ inches
Absorbable suture, no. 2-0 and no. 3-0, for ligatures
Nonabsorbable suture, no. 3-0, taper point needles
Nonabsorbable suture, no. 4-0 atraumatic on cutting-edge needles
1 Catheter, whistle-tipped, with open end, 14 Fr
2 Yankauer suction tubes and tubing
1 Tracheostomy instrument set
1 Local anesthesia set for nerve block, if desired
1 Minor throat pack, including gauze compresses and tonsil sponges
1 Minor neck drape pack
Tracheostomy tubes, assorted sizes
1 Syringe, 10 ml
Electrosurgical unit

Operative procedure

Although the procedure may be scheduled as a local excision, frequently lesions of the oral cavity require more extensive excision. The setup should be designed to include the instruments for a neck dissection, or they should be readily available. For some tumors of the oral cavity a tracheostomy is performed to ensure an airway after surgery. An Nd:YAG laser may be used to excise locally confined lesions of the oral cavity.

EXCISION OF THE SUBMANDIBULAR GLAND

This operation is performed to remove mixed tumors and multiple calculi associated with extensive chronic inflammation. An incision is made in the neck beneath the chin to remove the gland and tumor.

Procedural considerations

The patient is placed on the operating room bed in a supine position, with the affected side uppermost, and prepped as for neck surgery. The instruments include a minor neck dissection setup. A set of lacrimal probes should also be added to the instrument setup if exploration of the submandibular (Wharton's) duct is necessary during surgery. The circulating nurse must ensure that no local anesthetic is delivered to the sterile field if identification of major nerves is anticipated.

Operative procedure

1. A small skin incision is made below and parallel to the mandible, extending forward to beneath the chin (Fig. 20-12, *A*). The platysma is incised with scissors; the skin flaps and undersurface of the platysma and cervical fascia covering the gland are undermined with fine hooks, tissue forceps, and Metzenbaum scissors (Fig. 20-12, *B*).

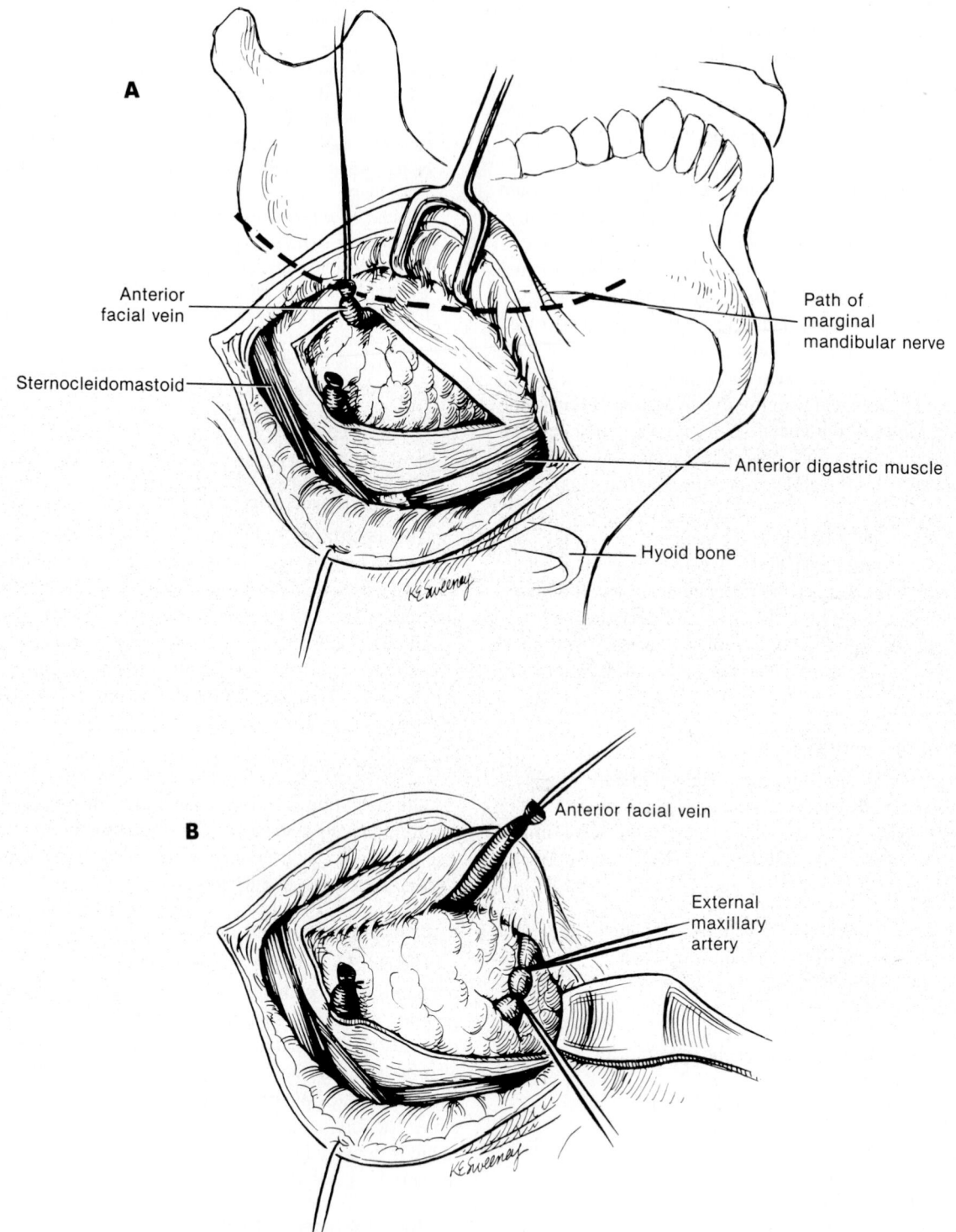

FIG. 20-12 Excision of submandibular gland. **A,** Submandibular incision, made in a natural skin crease 3 to 4 cm inferior to mandible. Marginal mandibular nerve generally lies just superficial to anterior facial vein. **B,** External maxillary artery is identified on submandibular gland.

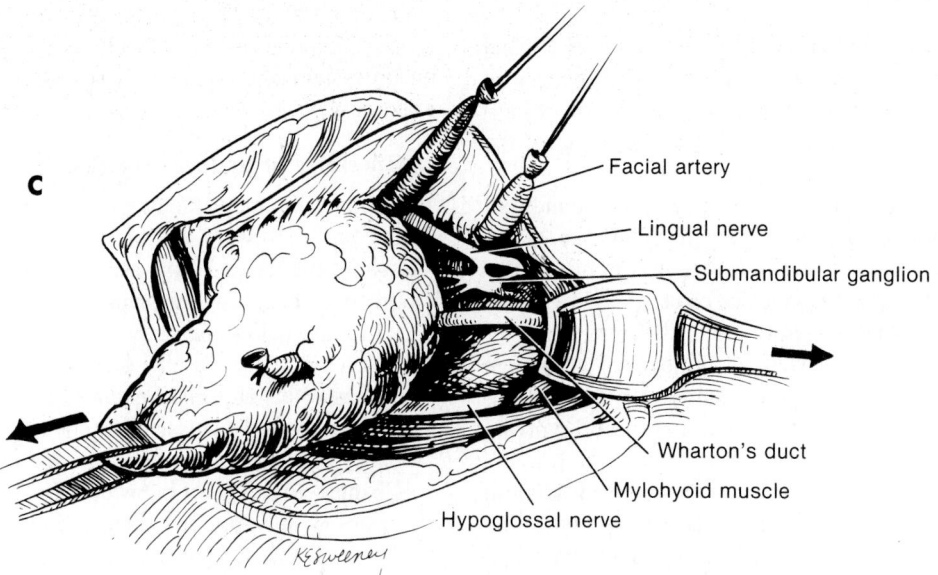

C

Facial artery

Lingual nerve

Submandibular ganglion

Wharton's duct

Mylohyoid muscle

Hypoglossal nerve

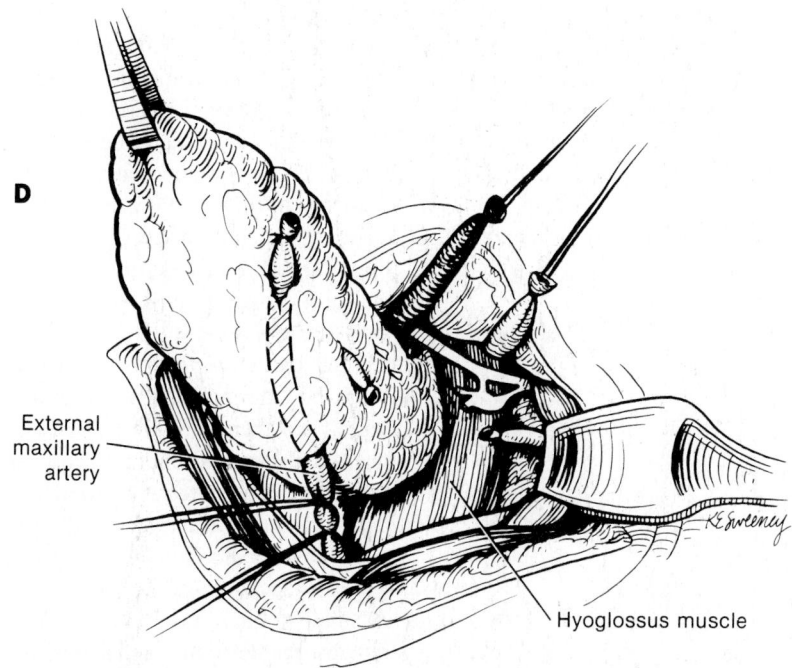

D

External
maxillary
artery

Hyoglossus muscle

FIG. 20-12, CONT'D   **C,** Mylohyoid is retracted anteriorly and gland posteriorly. This exposes lingual nerve, submandibular ganglion, and Wharton's duct. **D,** Hypoglossal nerve, running between hyoglossus and mylohyoid muscles. External maxillary artery must be divided a second time.

From Cummings, C.W., et al. (1993). *Otolaryngology—Head and neck surgery*. St. Louis: Mosby.

2. The mandibular branch of the facial nerve is retracted away with a small loop retractor.
3. The submandibular gland is elevated from the mylohyoid muscle (Fig. 20-12, *C*). The edge of the muscle is retracted to expose the lingual veins and nerve and the hypoglossal nerve.
4. The gland is freed by blunt dissection, and the submandibular duct is clamped, ligated, and divided.

5. The external maxillary artery is clamped, ligated, and divided. The submandibular gland is removed (Fig. 20-12, *D*).
6. The wound is closed with interrupted absorbable sutures. The skin edges are approximated with nonabsorbable sutures. A drain is inserted in the submandibular bed and secured to the skin. Dressings are applied.

PAROTIDECTOMY

The tumor and a portion of or the entire parotid gland are removed through a curved incision in the upper neck and behind the lobe of the ear or through a Y type of incision on both sides of the ear and below the angle of the mandible.

The majority of benign tumors of the salivary glands occur in the parotid gland. These benign tumors are of the same types as are those found in soft tissues in other parts of the body. In the parotid gland the closeness of the facial nerve makes removing the entire tumor difficult. (Fig. 20-13). Parotidectomy is indicated for removal of all benign and some malignant tumors, for inflammatory lesions, for vascular anomalies, and for metastatic cancer involving lymph nodes overlying the gland.

If the removal of malignant tumors involves adjacent structures, such as the mandible or cheek, the operation may become a radical removal of the involved structures. The patient must be aware of the possible complication of facial nerve weakness or paralysis.

Procedural considerations

The patient is placed on the operating room bed in a supine position with the entire affected side of the face uppermost. The entire side of the face, the mouth, the outer canthus of the eye, and the forehead are prepped and left exposed.

The instrument setup is a neck dissection set. A nerve

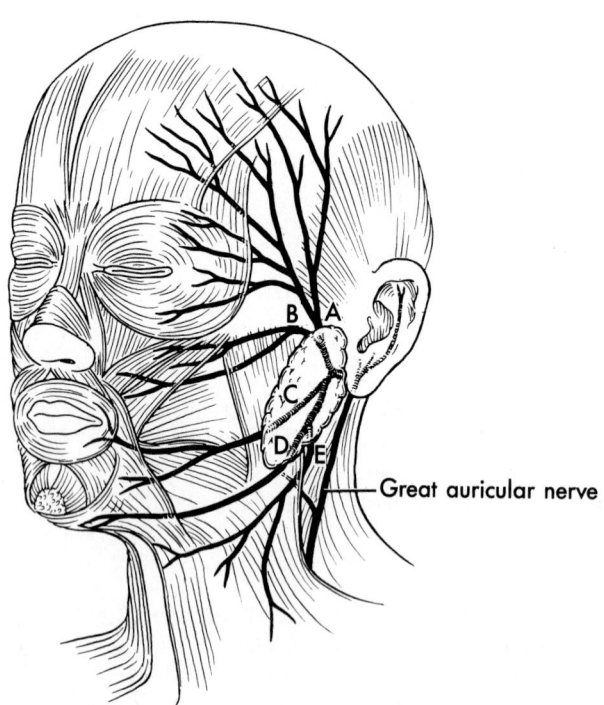

FIG. 20-13   Branches of facial nerve: *A*, temporal; *B*, zygomatic; *C*, buccal; *D*, mandibular; *E*, cervical.

From Cummings, C.W., et al. (1993). *Otolaryngology—head and neck surgery*. St. Louis: Mosby.

stimulator should be available for use. A set of lacrimal probes should be included in the setup if exploration of the ductal system of the parotid is necessary during the course of surgery.

Operative procedure (Fig. 20-14)

1. The incision may extend from the posterior angle of the zygoma downward in front of the tragus of the ear and behind the lobule of the ear backward over the mastoid process, then downward and forward on the neck parallel to and below the body of the mandible. (A chin incision may also be used.) Bleeding vessels are controlled by hemostats and fine ligatures, or by cautery.

2. With fine-toothed tissue forceps and scissors the skin flaps are elevated as described for thyroidectomy (see Chapter 15). The skin wound edges are retracted by means of silk sutures fastened to clamps.

3. The upper portion of the sternocleidomastoid muscle is exposed and retracted, the auricular nerve is identified, and the lower part of the parotid gland is elevated with curved hemostats.

4. The superficial temporal artery and vein and external jugular vein are identified by means of blunt dissection.

5. The parotid tissue is dissected from the cartilage of the ear and the tympanic plate of the temporal bone. The temporal, zygomatic, and mandibular and cervical branches of the facial nerve are identified and preserved.

6a. The *superficial portion* of the parotid gland containing the tumor is removed. In some cases the entire superficial portion is removed, followed by ligation and division of the parotid duct.

6b. When the *deep portion* of the parotid gland must be removed, the facial nerve is retracted upward and outward, and then the parotid tissue is removed from beneath the nerve. Kocher retractors are used to retract the mandible. The external carotid artery is identified. In many cases the internal maxillary and superficial temporal arteries are clamped, ligated, and divided.

7. The wound is closed in layers with absorbable suture. A small drain is inserted, the skin is closed with fine nonabsorbable suture, and a pressure dressing is applied.

TRACHEOSTOMY

Tracheostomy is opening of the trachea and insertion of a cannula through a midline incision in the neck, below the cricoid cartilage. It is used as an emergency procedure to treat upper respiratory tract obstruction and as a prophylactic measure in the presence of chronic lung disease or sleep apnea in which an obstruction could occur. A prophylactic tracheostomy is performed at the time of surgery to permit easy and frequent aspiration of the tracheobronchial tree secretions and diminish the dead space that exists from the opening of the mouth down to the supraclavicular region. The creation of a new clearance (tracheostomy) nearer to the functional areas in the lung provides for a greater volume of air for the patient with a partly destroyed lung. An-

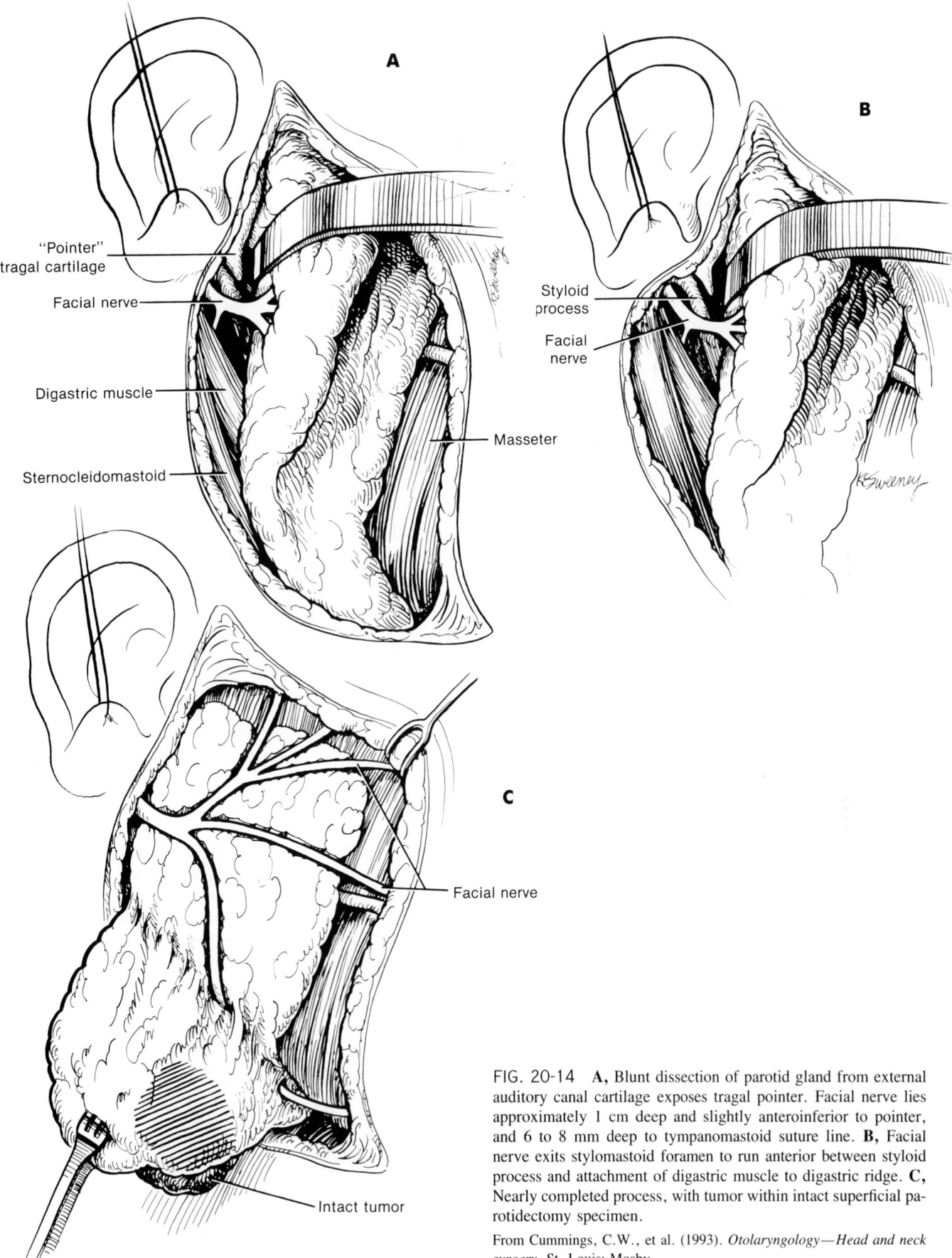

"Pointer"
tragal cartilage

Facial nerve

Digastric muscle

Sternocleidomastoid

Masseter

A

Styloid
process

Facial
nerve

B

Facial nerve

C

Intact tumor

FIG. 20-14 **A,** Blunt dissection of parotid gland from external
auditory canal cartilage exposes tragal pointer. Facial nerve lies
approximately 1 cm deep and slightly anteroinferior to pointer,
and 6 to 8 mm deep to tympanomastoid suture line. **B,** Facial
nerve exits stylomastoid foramen to run anterior between styloid
process and attachment of digastric muscle to digastric ridge. **C,**
Nearly completed process, with tumor within intact superficial parotidectomy specimen.

From Cummings, C.W., et al. (1993). *Otolaryngology—Head and neck
surgery*. St. Louis: Mosby.

esthesia may be maintained through a prophylactic tracheostomy.

The patient's psychologic status should be carefully evaluated because of the altered body image and physical status, which may be either temporary or permanent, depending on the disease entity involved. Tracheostomy care should be explained carefully and thoroughly so the patient will understand why it must be done so frequently, especially the suctioning of the tube. Reinforcement should be given about the ability to communicate with others by means of a pencil and paper or message board. As recovery progresses, the patient can be shown how to occlude the opening of the tube for brief periods to be able to speak a few words. If a tracheostomy tube with a disposable inner cannula is inserted, the circulating nurse must ensure that the patient has replacement cannulas in the event occlusion or blockage occurs in the immediate postoperative period.

Procedural considerations

The patient is placed in a supine position, with the shoulders raised by a rolled sheet to hyperextend the neck and head. The neck is prepped, and sterile drapes are applied. Along with a basic minor drape pack, the following instruments and supplies should be included:

2 Knife handles, no. 3 with no. 10 and no. 15 blades
1 Metzenbaum scissors, curved
1 Mayo scissors, straight
1 Suture scissors
2 Allis forceps, straight
1 Needle holder
2 Tissue forceps with fine teeth
2 Tissue forceps without teeth
2 Adson forceps
4 Towel clamps
2 Sponge-holding forceps
4 Mosquito hemostats, straight
4 Kelly hemostats, curved
1 Mayo-Pean forceps, curved
2 Crile hemostats, curved
2 Volkmann rake retractors
2 Army-Navy retractors
2 Frazier skin hooks
1 Jackson tracheal hook
1 Tracheal dilator
1 Cushing nerve hook
2 Brophy tenaculum hooks
Absorbable no. 3-0 sutures
Absorbable no. 3-0 atraumatic sutures on fine, ½-circle, taper-point needles
Nonabsorbable no. 2-0 atraumatic sutures on ⅜-circle, cutting-edge needles
2 Catheters, whistle-tipped, open-ended, 14 Fr
1 Yankauer suction tube
1 Frazier suction tip
1 Suction tubing
Tracheostomy tubes (Fig. 20-15), appropriate for age and size of patient

Cardiac arrest setup, oxygen, and thiopental sodium (Pentothal) setup
Local anesthesia set

Operative procedure

1. A vertical or transverse incision may be used. A vertical incision is made in the midline from approximately the cricoid cartilage to the suprasternal notch. When a transverse incision is made, it extends approximately one fingerbreadth above the suprasternal notch parallel to it and from the anterior border of one sternocleidomastoid muscle to the opposite side. Soft tissues and muscle are divided, and the isthmus of the thyroid gland that joins both lobes of the gland in the midline over the trachea is retracted in an upward direction with retractors, resulting in exposure of the underlying tracheal rings, usually the third and fourth (Fig. 20-16, *A*). In some cases two curved clamps may be inserted through this incision across the isthmus and the isthmus transsected (Fig. 20-16, *B*). The transsected ends of the isthmus are secured with absorbable sutures.

2. Lidocaine 1% (1 or 2 ml) may be instilled into the trachea to reduce the coughing reflex when the tube is inserted. Air is first drawn into syringe to ensure that the needle point is located in the lumen. With a knife and no. 15 blade, an incision is made in the trachea directly across the two tracheal rings. The cut ends of the cricoid cartilage are elevated with a hook (Fig. 20-16, *C*).

3. A tracheostomy tube is inserted into the trachea (Fig. 20-16, *D*), the obturator is quickly removed, and the trachea is suctioned with a catheter.

4. The wound edges are lightly approximated with nonabsorbable no. 2-0 sutures, or the wound edges are allowed to fall together around the tube. One or two skin sutures are inserted above the tube. The lower angle of the wound may be left open for drainage.

5. The tracheostomy tube is held in place with tapes tied with a square knot to the side of the neck. The inner cannula is then inserted. A gauze dressing split around the tube is applied to the wound.

6. An additional tracheostomy tube of the same size should be kept adjacent to the patient at all times, in the event the tube becomes dislodged or plugged with secretions. This practice expedites changing the tracheostomy tube with minimal potential for complications to the patient.

UVULOPALATOPHARYNGOPLASTY (UPPP)

UPPP is primarily performed to relieve obstructive sleep apnea and snoring. Two or more of the following indications are reason to perform the operation.

1. An O_2 saturation that drops below 80
2. Apnea index worse than 20
3. Significant daytime sleepiness
4. Heroic snoring, producing social or marital problems
5. Cardiac arrhythmias, other than tachycardia, or bradycardia during sleep

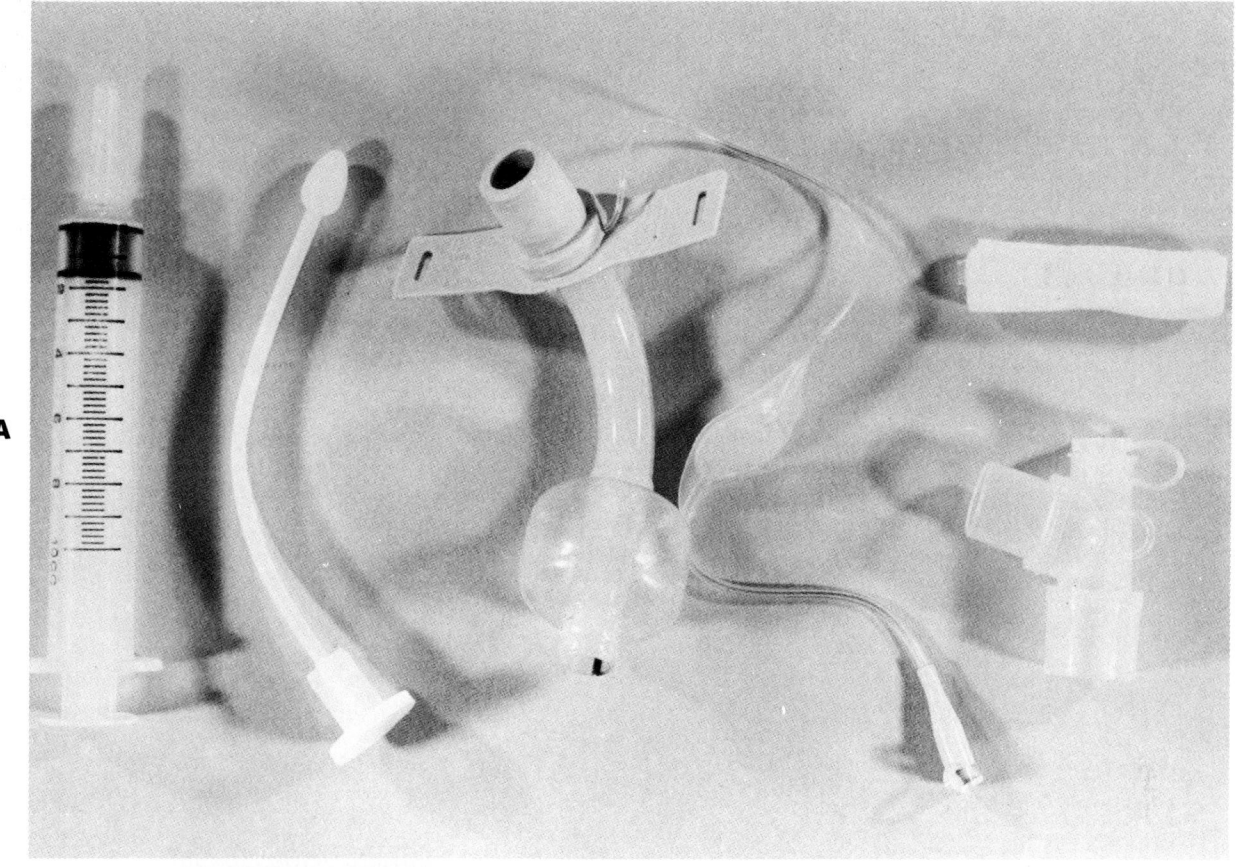

A

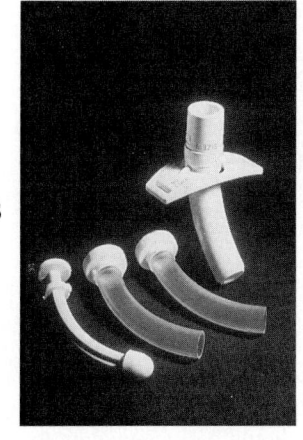

B

FIG. 20-15 **A,** Portex tracheostomy tube with cuff inflated, obturator, syringe, adapter, and neck ties. **B,** Uncuffed tracheostomy tube with disposable inner cannula.

B From Sigler, B.A., & Schuring, L.T. (1993). *Ear, nose, and throat disorders.* St. Louis: Mosby.

Procedural considerations

A tracheostomy may be performed in conjunction with UPPP because of postoperative edema with subsequent airway obstruction. The tracheostomy tube is removed and the incision closed when the danger of postoperative edema and bleeding has passed (if the surgical procedure is successful). Because some of these patients are obese (causing the tissue of the pharynx to sag during sleep), preoperative planning should include obtaining an assortment of tracheostomy tubes, including extralong tubes, before the start of the procedure. Care must be taken in positioning the obese

patient to ensure proper body alignment. Emergency tracheostomy or bronchoscopy should be planned, in the event of airway obstruction following anesthetic induction. The surgeon may choose to administer local anesthesia with anesthesia personnel monitoring the patient, and then induce general anesthesia after an adequate airway is established. A tonsillectomy is performed (if they are present) along with the UPPP. Instrumentation and positioning are similar to those discussed under tracheostomy and tonsillectomy, with the exception noted previously of the need to properly position the obese patient.

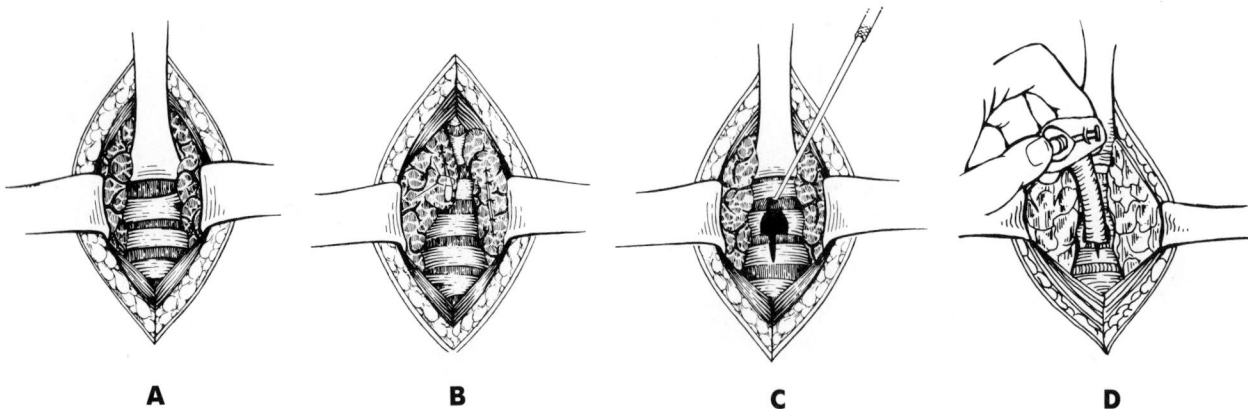

A   **B**   **C**   **D**

FIG. 20-16   Operative technique for elective tracheostomy. **A,** Retractor exposing trachea by drawing isthmus of thyroid upward. **B,** Alternative method to that shown in **A.** Isthmus of thyroid is divided to expose trachea. **C,** Two tracheal rings are cut, and upper ring is partially resected. Tracheal hook pulls trachea from depth of wound nearer surface. **D,** Insertion of tube.

Modified from DeWeese, D.D., & Saunders, W.H. (1982). *Textbook of otolaryngology* (6th ed.). St. Louis: Mosby.

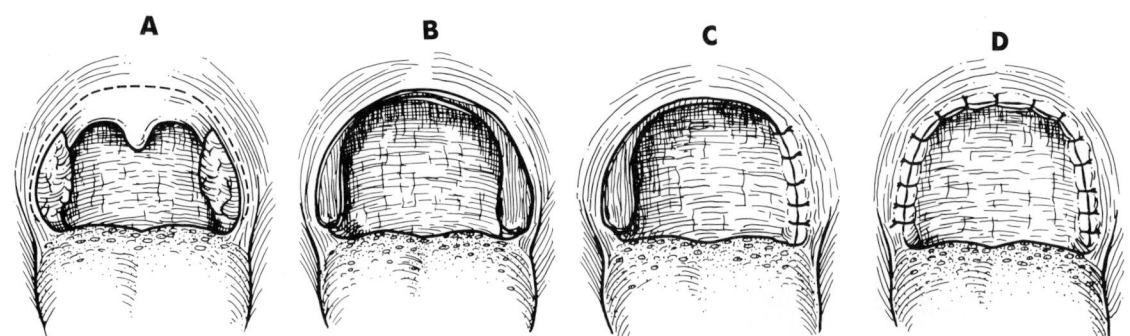

A   **B**   **C**   **D**

FIG. 20-17   Technique of palatopharyngoplasty as advocated by Simmons et al.

From Luckmann, J., & Sorenson, K.C. (1987). *Medical-surgical nursing* (3rd ed.). Philadelphia: W.B. Saunders.

Operative procedure

1. The mouth gag (usually self-retaining) is inserted.
2. The tissue to be resected may be outlined by an electro-surgical blade. A no. 3 knife handle with no. 15 blade or a no. 7 knife handle with a no. 12 blade may be used to make the incision in the soft palate and anterior to the tonsillar pillar (if the patient has not previously had a tonsillectomy), or posterior to the tonsillar pillars if the patient has had a tonsillectomy (Meyerhoff and Rice, 1992) (Fig. 20-17).
3. The tissue is resected via Metzenbaum scissors and long forceps with teeth or by hand-controlled electrosurgical pencil.
4. Larger blood vessels may be clamped until the tissue is removed, or a suction coagulator or hand-controlled electrosurgical pencil may be used to obtain hemostasis as the tissue is excised.

5. Once the tissue is removed and hemostasis is obtained, absorbable sutures are used to approximate the edges of the mucosa. Depending on the surgeon's preference, no. 2-0 and 3-0 absorbable suture should be available. Needle holders should be long enough to allow the surgeon ease in delivering the atraumatic needle to the edges of the mucosa.
6. The oral cavity should be rinsed of blood and debris, and the incision inspected prior to patient discharge from the operating room.

Care should be taken when inspecting the incision in the postoperative period not to disturb the incision with a tongue blade, if one is used to provide access for inspection. The patient must not be provided with a straw for fluid intake because it might disturb the suture line. Gentle oral cavity rinsing is recommended several times daily to decrease the chance of postoperative infection and to increase patient comfort.

LARYNGOFISSURE

Laryngofissure is opening the larynx for exploratory, excisional, or reconstructive procedures.

Procedural considerations

A laryngofissure is performed whenever access to the intrinsic larynx is necessary. The thyroid cartilages are split in the midline, and the true vocal cords and false vocal cords are incised at the midline anteriorly. A neck dissection instrument set is required, plus an oscillating power saw.

Operative procedure

1. A tracheostomy is performed, and an endotracheal tube inserted. A general anesthetic is administered. (This procedure may also be done with the patient under local anesthesia.)
2. A transverse incision is made through the skin and first layer of the cervical fascia and platysma muscles, approximately 2 cm above the sternoclavicular junction or in the normal skin crease. The upper skin flap is undermined to the level of the cricoid cartilage, and the lower flap is undermined to the sternoclavicular joint.
3. Bleeding vessels are clamped with mosquito hemostats and ligated. The strap muscles are elevated and incised in the midline.
4. The thyroid cartilages are cut with an oscillating saw, and the true vocal cords are visualized through an incision into the cricothyroid membrane. The true vocal cords are divided in the midline (anterior commissure), and the interior of the larynx is exposed.
5. The tracheostomy tube must be left in place after surgery to ensure an airway.

LARYNGEAL FRAMEWORK SURGERY

Procedures such as thyroplasty (types I to IV) are designed to improve the quality of the voice without disturbing the mucosa and underlying structures of the vocal cords (see Research Highlight 20-1).

PARTIAL LARYNGECTOMY

Partial laryngectomy is removal of a portion of the larynx. It is done to remove superficial neoplasms that are confined to one vocal cord or to remove a tumor extending up into the ventricle on the anterior commissure or a short distance below the cord. Cancers confined to the intrinsic larynx (Fig. 20-18, *A*) are generally a low-grade malignancy and tend to remain localized for long periods. The patient should be prepared for an altered voice quality postoperatively.

Procedural considerations

The patient is placed in the supine position. The operative site is prepped and draped as described for thyroidectomy (see Chapter 15), or for head and neck procedure. The setup for partial laryngectomy includes a neck dissection

---

RESEARCH HIGHLIGHT 20-1

Research is currently being carried out to study the action of the structures that move the vocal cords as well as the mechanism of vocal cord vibration. Past procedures have been performed on the vocal cords and adjacent structures to correct immobility, altered mobility, and poor voice quality. Current procedures are targeting the laryngeal framework for correction of position, movement, and tension of the vocal cords to obtain the optimum voice quality for the patient, without disturbing the vocal mucosa. These procedures involve the patient undergoing local anesthesia so that voice quality can be determined at the time of surgery. A combined external (the area over the thyroid cartilage) and internal approach (via a flexible laryngoscope) is used to adequately assess vocal cord movement as the procedure is performed. Preoperative and postoperative assessment of vocal cord movement can be done in the surgeon's office by video stroboscopy.

Isshiki, N. (1991). Laryngeal framework surgery. *Advances in Otolaryngology—Head and Neck Surgery,* *5,* 37-57.

---

setup, Freer or Cottle periosteal elevator, oscillating saw, tracheostomy tubes, and an electrosurgical unit.

Operative procedure

1. A tracheostomy is performed as previously described, and an endotracheal tube is inserted.
2. A vertical incision or a thyroid incision with elevation of a flap may be employed (Fig. 20-18, *B*).
3. The sternothyroid muscles are separated in the midline and retracted by means of Green retractors.
4. The fascial covering over the thyroid cartilage is incised with a knife, and with a Freer periosteal elevator the perichondrium is elevated from the cartilage on the side of the tumor.
5. The thyroid cartilage is divided longitudinally in the midline by means of an oscillating saw.
6. The cartilages are retracted, and the cricothyroid membrane is incised with a knife. A blunt-nosed laryngeal scissors is introduced between the vocal cords to divide the mucosa of the anterior wall of the glottis.
7. The divided cartilages are retracted with Kocher retractors to expose the interior of the larynx. A small, moist gauze pack may be placed in the trachea to prevent aspiration of blood or mucus. A small amount of a topical anesthetic may be applied to the larynx to prevent laryngeal muscular spasm. The extent of the intrinsic laryngeal tumor is determined.
8. With a small periosteal elevator, the mucosa on the involved side of the larynx is freed; the false cord and mucosal layer of the region are lifted by means of a

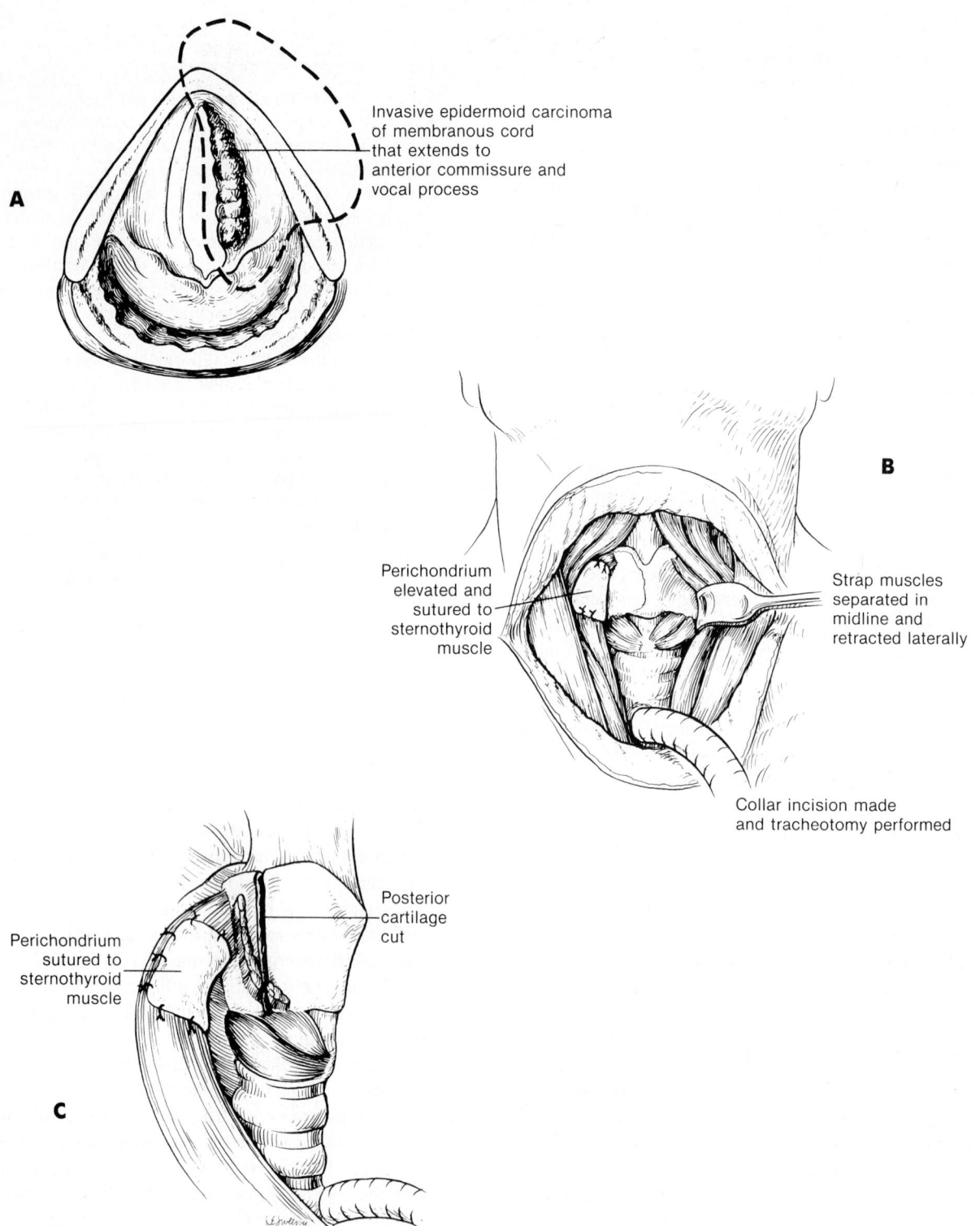

A, Invasive epidermoid carcinoma of membranous cord that extends to anterior commissure and vocal process

B, Strap muscles separated in midline and retracted laterally

Perichondrium elevated and sutured to sternothyroid muscle

Collar incision made and tracheotomy performed

Posterior cartilage cut

Perichondrium sutured to sternothyroid muscle

FIG. 20-18 Standard hemilaryngectomy. **A,** Broken lines outline full extent of resection in standard hemilaryngectomy for invasive epidermoid carcinoma of membranous cord that extends to anterior commissure and vocal process. **B,** Neck flap is elevated after collar incision is made and tracheotomy performed. Strap muscles are separated in midline and retracted laterally. On side of lesion, perichondrium is elevated and its attachment to sternothyroid muscle maintained. **C,** External perichondrium is sutured to overlying sternothyroid muscle, and it is retracted laterally to expose posterior border of thyroid cartilage so posterior cartilage cut can be made approximately 5 mm from edge.

From Cummings, C.W., et al. (1993). *Otolaryngology—Head and neck surgery*. St. Louis: Mosby.

periosteal elevator and hooks. The involved cord is excised with straight scissors (Fig. 20-18, *C*).

9. In some cases the thyroid cartilage may be removed with a knife and straight scissors. Bleeding is controlled with hemostats, fine absorbable ligatures and sutures, and electrocoagulation.

10. The gauze pack is removed from the trachea. The perichondrium is approximated with absorbable no. 2-0 sutures. The strap muscles are approximated in the midline with absorbable no. 2-0 sutures. The platysma and the skin edges are approximated separately with fine nonabsorbable sutures.

11. A tracheolaryngeal tube is left in place and removed at a later date when the airway is adequate. Dressings are applied to the wound and around the tube.

SUPRAGLOTTIC LARYNGECTOMY (FIG. 20-19)

Supraglottic laryngectomy is excision of the laryngeal structures above the true vocal cords.

Procedural considerations

Supraglottic laryngectomy is indicated in cancer of the epiglottis and false vocal cords. It is designed to remove the cancer, yet preserve the phonatory, respiratory, and sphincteric functions of the larynx. A neck dissection is almost always performed. The patient will have to undergo swallowing therapy postoperatively to learn how to decrease the incidence of aspiration. The instrument setup is as described for neck dissection.

Operative procedure

The procedure is similar to that described for partial laryngectomy, with the exception of use of an oscillating saw.

TOTAL LARYNGECTOMY

Total laryngectomy is complete removal of the cartilaginous larynx, the hyoid bone, and the strap muscles connected to the larynx and possible removal of the preepiglottic space with the lesion. A wide-field laryngectomy is done when there is a loss of mobility of the cords and to treat cancer of the extrinsic larynx and hypopharynx (Fig. 20-20). Malignant tumors of the extrinsic larynx are more anaplastic and tend to metastasize. When laryngeal carcinoma involves more than the true cords, a prophylactic (preventive) radical neck dissection is done to remove the lymphatics.

Laryngectomy presents many psychologic problems. The loss of voice that follows total laryngectomy is traumatic for the patient and family. The patient may be taught to talk either by using esophageal voice or with an artificial larynx. Esophageal voice is produced by the air contained in the esophagus rather than by that in the trachea. Speech requires a sounding air column. With instruction and practice, the patient is able to control the swallowing of air into the esophagus and reintroduction of this air into the mouth with phonation. The sounding air column is then transformed into speech by means of the lips, tongue, and

teeth. A tracheoesophageal fistula facilitates insertion of a Blom-Singer duckbill prosthesis for purpose of speech (Fig. 20-21, *A*). This fistula may be created during the initial surgical procedure, or at a later date when healing has occurred (Fig. 20-21, *B*).

Because the stump of the trachea is brought out to the skin of the neck to form a stoma, all the patient's breathing is done directly into the trachea and no longer through the nose and mouth. This air is no longer moistened by the nose. Drying and crusting of the tracheal secretions occur. Humidification may be provided by covering the opening with a moist gauze compress. The patient will be anxious to know about postoperative voice quality, which depends on the specific procedure performed. Table 20-1 lists surgical procedures and associated predictions of postoperative voice qualities.

Procedural considerations

The patient is placed on the operating room bed in a supine position with neck extended and shoulders elevated by a shoulder roll or folded sheet. A general anesthetic is administered. An effective suction apparatus is essential. The proposed operative site, including the anterior neck region, the lateral surfaces of the neck down to the outer aspects of the shoulders, and the upper anterior chest region, is prepped and draped in the usual manner. The instrument setup is a neck dissection set.

Operative procedure

1. A tracheostomy may be performed initially to control the airway, or it may be incorporated into the procedure, depending on surgeon preference. If performed initially, a cuffed, wire-reinforced, flexible endotracheal tube will ensure effective delivery of the anesthetic and give the surgical team flexibility as the larynx and trachea are manipulated during the surgical procedure.

2. A midline incision is made from the suprasternal notch to just above the hyoid bone. Skin flaps are undermined on each side. The sternothyroid, sternohyoid, and omohyoid muscles (strap muscles) on each side are divided by means of curved hemostats and a knife.

3. The suprahyoid muscles are severed from the portion of the hyoid to be divided. The hyoid bone is divided at the junction of its middle and lateral thirds with bone-cutting forceps. Bleeding vessels are clamped and ligated.

4. The superior laryngeal nerve and vessels are exposed and ligated on each side with long curved fine hemostats and fine ligatures.

5. The isthmus of the thyroid gland is divided between hemostats. Each portion of the thyroid gland is dissected from the trachea with Metzenbaum scissors and fine tissue forceps. The superior pole of the thyroid is retracted. The superior thyroid vessels are freed from the larynx by sharp dissection.

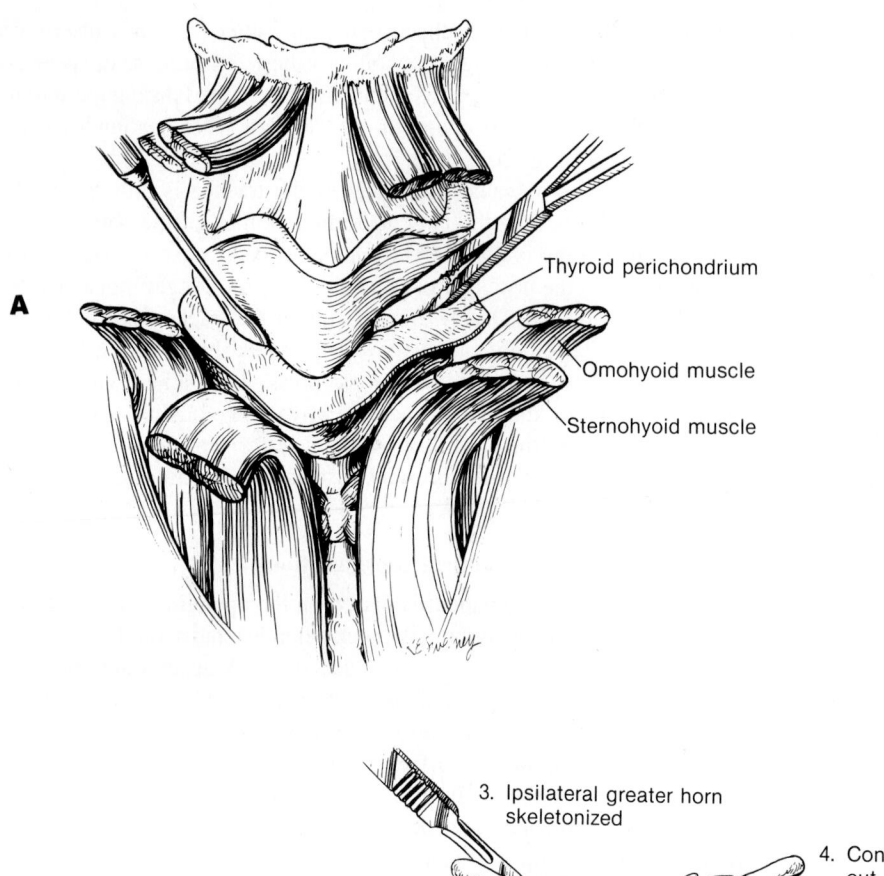

A

Thyroid perichondrium

Omohyoid muscle

Sternohyoid muscle

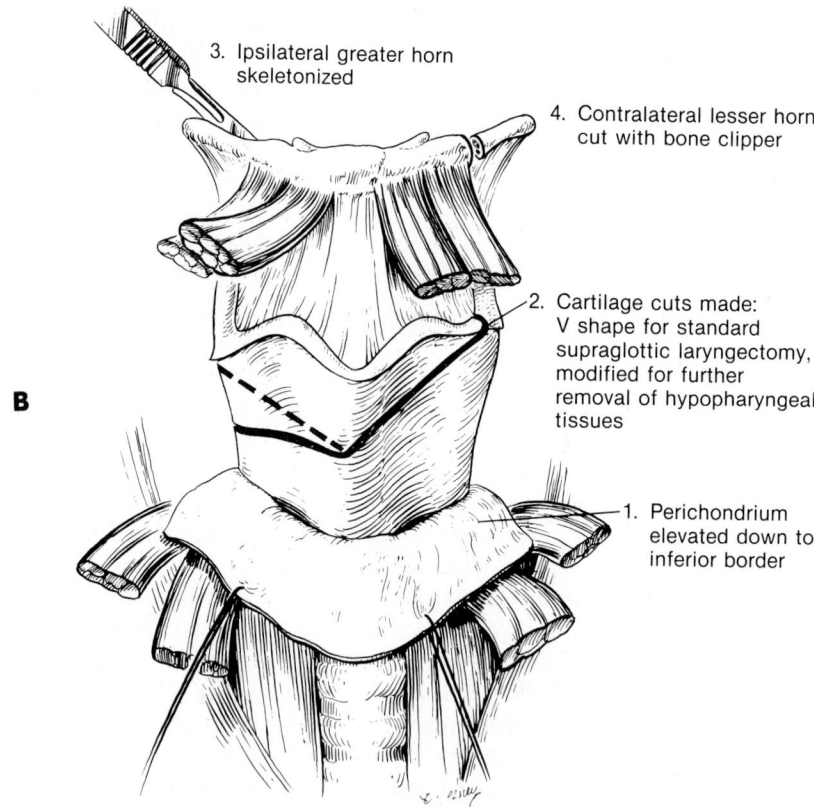

3. Ipsilateral greater horn
skeletonized

4. Contralateral lesser horn
cut with bone clipper

B

2. Cartilage cuts made:
V shape for standard
supraglottic
laryngectomy,
modified for further
removal of hypopharyngeal
tissues

1. Perichondrium
elevated down to
inferior border

FIG. 20-19 Supraglottic laryngectomy. **A,** Strap muscles are cut just above thyroid cartilage, and thyroid perichondrium is incised along superior border of thyroid cartilage. Thyroid cartilage perichondrium is carefully elevated and dissected inferiorly by first using "peanut" and then Freer elevator. **B,** Thyroid cartilage perichondrium elevation is completed down to inferior border, and then cartilage cuts are made. V shape is outlined for standard supraglottic laryngectomy. This may be modified for further removal of hypopharyngeal tissues according to size of lesion. Ipsilateral greater horn is skeletonized, and contralateral lesser horn is cut with bone clipper.

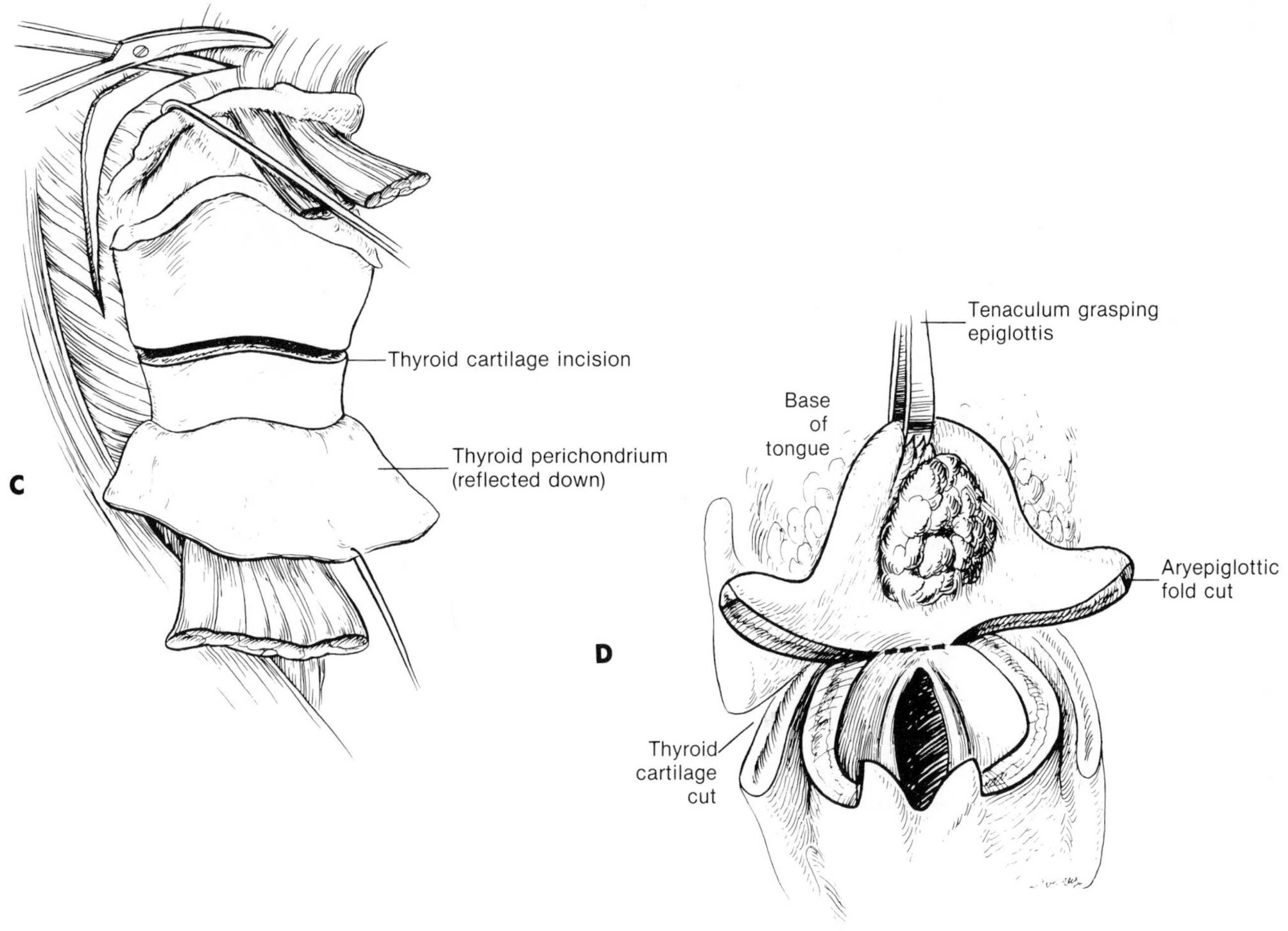

C

Thyroid cartilage incision

Thyroid perichondrium
(reflected down)

Tenaculum grasping
epiglottis

Base
of
tongue

Aryepiglottic
fold cut

D

Thyroid
cartilage
cut

FIG. 20-19, CONT'D **C,** Piriform fossa and vallecula are then entered on side of lesion, while greater horn of hyoid bone is retracted for exposure. **D,** Epiglottis is grasped with tenaculum, and scissors are used to cut through aryepiglottic fold in front of arytenoid and down into ventricle. Once both supraglottic cuts have been made through aryepiglottic folds, intervening tissues are cut to join up with thyroid cartilage cuts.

From Cummings, C.W., et al. (1993). *Otolaryngology—Head and neck surgery*. St. Louis: Mosby.

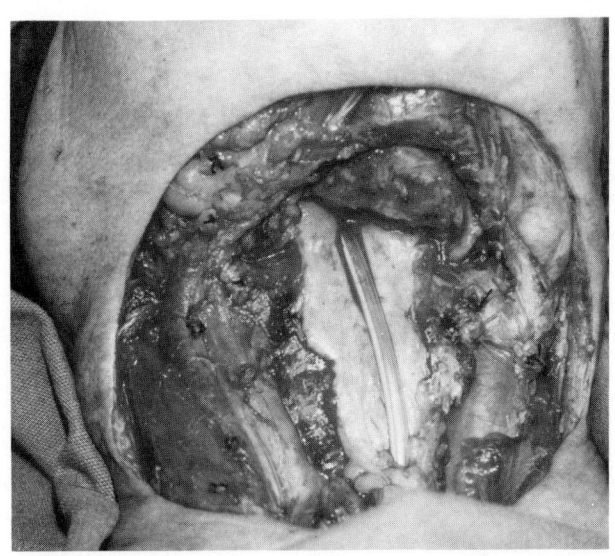

FIG. 20-20 Wide-field laryngectomy defect for radiation recurrent tumor, including anterior neck skin, thyroid, sternomastoid, and selective neck node resection.

From Cummings, C.W., et al. (1993). *Otolaryngology—Head and neck surgery*. St. Louis: Mosby.

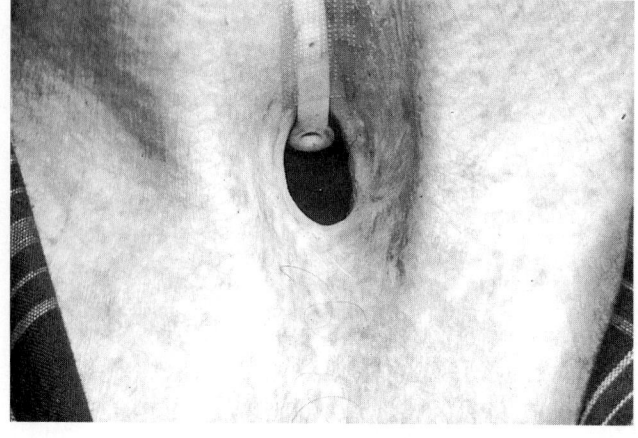

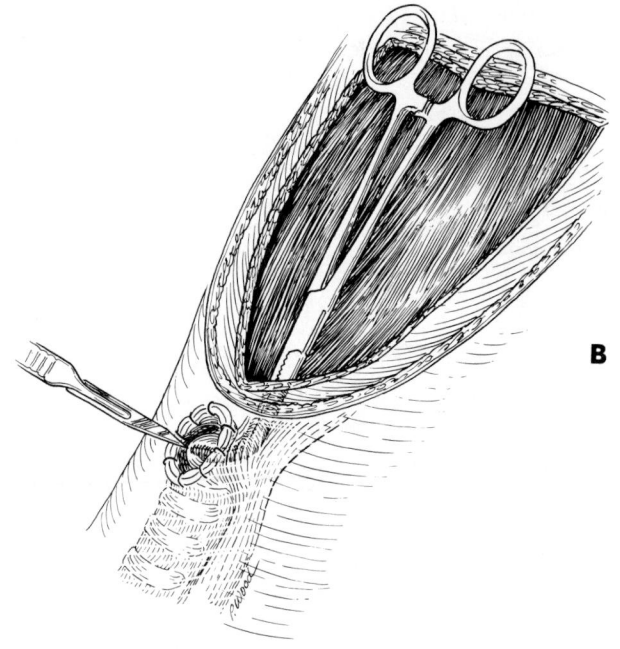

FIG. 20-21 A, Speech valve in place. **B,** Primary tracheo-esophageal puncture technique. Note preliminary repair of stoma to allow accurate positioning of puncture site prior to pharyngeal closure. Feeding tube (14 Fr) is inserted through puncture down esophagus to the stomach.

A From Sigler, B.A., & Schuring, L.T. (1993). *Ear, nose and throat disorders.* St. Louis: Mosby; **B** from Cummings, C.W., et al. (1993). *Otolaryngology—Head and neck surgery.* St. Louis: Mosby.

TABLE 20-1

Surgical procedures for laryngeal carcinomas and predictions of vocal quality after surgery

Structures removed	Structures left	Postoperative condition
TOTAL LARYNGECTOMY		
Hyoid bone	Tongue	Loses voice
Entire larynx (epiglottis, false cords, true cords)	Pharyngeal walls	Breathes through tracheostomy stoma
Cricoid cartilage	Lower trachea	No problem swallowing
Two or three rings of trachea		
SUPRAGLOTTIC OR HORIZONTAL LARYNGECTOMY		
Hyoid bone	True vocal cords	Normal voice
Epiglottis	Cricoid cartilage	May aspirate occasionally, especially liquids
False vocal cords	Trachea	Normal airway
VERTICAL (OR HEMI) LARYNGECTOMY		
One true vocal cord	Epiglottis	Hoarse but serviceable voice
One false cord	One false cord	Normal airway
Arytenoid	One true vocal cord	No problem swallowing
Half thyroid cartilage	Cricoid	
LARYNGOFISSURE AND PARTIAL LARYNGECTOMY		
One vocal cord	All other structures	Hoarse but serviceable voice; occasionally almost normal voice
		No airway problem
		No swallowing problem
ENDOSCOPIC REMOVAL OF EARLY CARCINOMA		
Part of one vocal cord	All other structures	May have a normal voice
		No other problems

From Saunders, W.H., et al. (1979). *Nursing care in eye, ear, nose, and throat disorders* (4th ed.). St. Louis: Mosby.

6. The larynx is rotated. The inferior pharyngeal constrictor muscle is severed from its attachment to the thyroid cartilage on each side.
7. The endotracheal tube is removed. The trachea is transsected just below the cricoid cartilage over a Kelly or Crile hemostat previously inserted between the trachea and esophagus. The upper resected portion of the trachea and the cricoid cartilage are held upward with Lahey forceps. A balloon-cuffed wire-reinforced endotracheal tube with a Murphy eye is inserted in the distal trachea.
8. The larynx is freed from the cervical esophagus and attachments by sharp and blunt dissection. A moist pack is placed around the endotracheal tube to help prevent leakage of blood into the trachea.
9. The pharynx is entered. In most cancers of the intrinsic larynx the pharynx is entered above the epiglottis. The mucous membrane incision is extended along either side of the epiglottis; the remaining portion of the pharynx and cervical esophagus is dissected well away from the tumor by means of fine-toothed tissue forceps, Metzenbaum scissors, knife, and fine hemostats. The specimen is removed en masse.
10. A nasal feeding tube is inserted through one naris into the esophagus; closure of the hypopharyngeal and esophageal defect is begun with continuous, inverting fine sutures of absorbable no. 3-0. The nasal tube is guided down past the pharyngeal suture line.
11. The pharyngeal suture line is reinforced with interrupted sutures; the suprahyoid muscles are approximated to the cut edges of the inferior constrictor muscles.
12. The diameter of the tracheal stoma is increased by means of a knife and heavy scissors. The two portions of the thyroid behind the tracheal opening are approximated with interrupted nonabsorbable sutures, thereby obliterating dead space posterior to the upper portion of the trachea.
13. A closed wound drainage system is used, and the suction drains are appropriately placed.
14. The edges of the deep cervical fascia and the platysma are closed separately.
15. A laryngectomy tube of desired size is inserted into the tracheal stoma; a pressure dressing is applied to the wound and neck. (A cuffed tracheostomy tube may be inserted for 24 to 48 hours postoperatively until edema subsides; then it is replaced with a laryngectomy tube.)

RADICAL NECK DISSECTION

In a radical neck dissection the tumor, surrounding structures, and lymph nodes are removed en masse through a Y-shaped or trifurcate incision in the affected side of the neck. This procedure is done to remove the tumor and metastatic cervical nodes present in malignant lesions, as well as all nonvital structures of the neck (Fig. 20-22, *A*). Metastasis occurs through the lymphatic channels by way of the bloodstream. Diseases of the oral cavity, lips, and thyroid gland may spread slowly to the neck. Radical neck surgery is done in the presence of cervical node metastasis from a cancer of the head and neck that has a reasonable chance of being controlled.

A prophylactic neck dissection implies elective radical neck surgery when there is no clinical evidence of metastatic cervical cancer.

Procedural considerations

The patient is placed on the OR bed in a supine position. General endotracheal anesthesia is administered before the patient is positioned for surgery.

During the operation the anesthesiologist works behind a sterile barrier, away from the surgical team. The patient's head is moderately extended with the entire affected side of the face and neck facing uppermost. During surgery the face of the patient is turned away from the surgeon. The preoperative skin prep is extensive. The patient's neck is draped, leaving a wide operative field. If a skin graft is to be harvested to cover and protect the carotid artery (such as when a patient has received extensive previous or preoperative radiation therapy), the thigh area is also prepped and draped with sterile towels in readiness for obtaining a dermal graft before closure of the neck wound. It is usually more convenient to use the thigh on the same side as the neck dissection.

The instrument setup includes the following:

50 Mosquito hemostats, curved
8 Allis forceps
8 Kelly hemostats
8 Pean forceps
4 Thyroid tenacula
4 Babcock forceps
2 Right-angle clamps
Needle holders, assorted
12 Towel clamps
2 Tonsil suction tubes
1 Trousseau tracheal dilator
2 Rake retractors
2 Army-Navy retractors
2 Richardson retractors
2 Vein retractors
4 Skin hooks, 2 single and 2 double
1 Gelpi retractor
4 Knife handles, no. 3, with no. 10 and no. 15 blades
1 Tracheal hook
2 Mayo scissors, straight and curved
2 Metzenbaum scissors
2 Scissors, small, curved, sharp and blunt
4 Tissue forceps, 2 with and 2 without teeth
2 Adson tissue forceps
2 Brown-Adson tissue forceps
1 Periosteal elevator
2 Freer elevators
1 Bayonet forceps
Brown or Stryker dermatome (if a skin graft is anticipated)

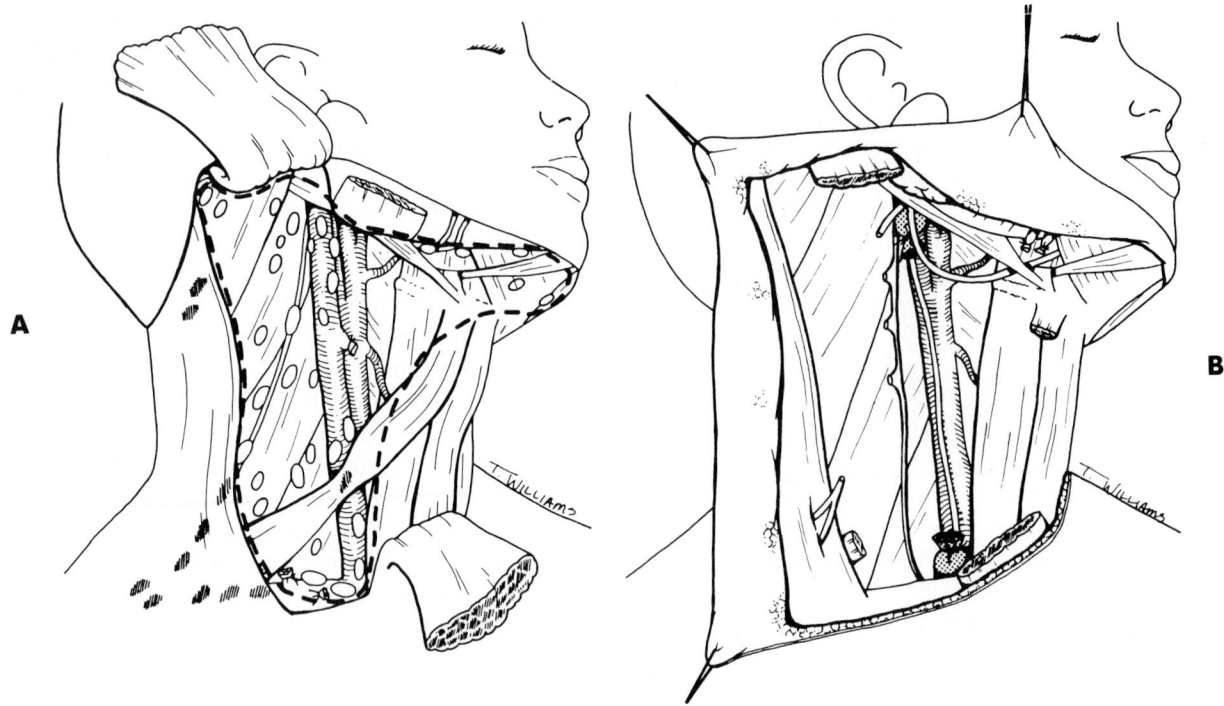

FIG. 20-22   Radical neck dissection. **A,** Diagramatic outline of extent of operation. **B,** Diagramatic representation of operation.

From Cummings, C.W., et al. (1993). *Otolaryngology—Head and neck surgery*. St. Louis: Mosby.

Operative procedure

1. One of several types of incisions may be used, including the Y-shaped, H-shaped, or trifurcate incision (Fig. 20-23).

2. The upper curved incision is made through the skin and platysma with a knife, tissue forceps, and fine hemostats; ligatures are used for bleeding vessels. The upper flap is retracted; then the vertical portion of the incision is made, and the skin flaps are retracted anteriorly and posteriorly with retractors. The anterior margin of the trapezius muscle is exposed by means of curved scissors. The flaps are retracted to expose the entire lateral aspect of the neck. Branches of the jugular veins are clamped, ligated, and divided.

3. The sternal and clavicular attachments of the sternocleidomastoid muscle are clamped with curved Pean forceps and then divided with a knife. The superficial layer of deep fascia is incised. The omohyoid muscle is severed between clamps just above its scapular attachment.

4. The internal jugular vein is isolated by blunt dissection and then doubly clamped, ligated with medium silk, and divided with Metzenbaum scissors. A transfixion suture is placed on the lower end of the vein.

5. The common carotid artery and vagus nerve are identified. The fatty areolar tissue and fascia are dissected away, using Metzenbaum scissors and fine tissue for-

ceps. Branches of the thyrocervical artery are clamped, divided, and ligated.

6. The tissues and fascia of the posterior triangle are dissected, beginning at the anterior margin of the trapezius muscle and continuing near the brachial plexus and the levator scapulae and the scalene muscles. During the dissection, branches of the cervical and suprascapular arteries are clamped, ligated, and divided.

7. The anterior portion of the block dissection is completed. The omohyoid muscle is severed at its attachment to the hyoid bone. Bleeding is controlled. All hemostats are removed, and the operative site may be covered with warm, moist laparotomy packs.

8. The sternocleidomastoid muscle is severed and retracted. The submental space is dissected free of fatty areolar tissue and lymph nodes from above downward.

9. The deep fascia on the lower edge of the mandible is incised; the facial vessels are divided and ligated.

10. The submandibular triangle is entered. The submandibular duct is divided and ligated. The submandibular glands with surrounding fatty areolar tissue and lymph nodes are dissected toward the digastric muscle. The facial branch of the external carotid artery is divided. Portions of the digastric and stylohyoid muscles are severed from their attachments to the hyoid bone and on the mastoid. The upper end of the internal jugular vein is elevated and divided. The surgical specimen is removed (Fig. 20-22, *B*).

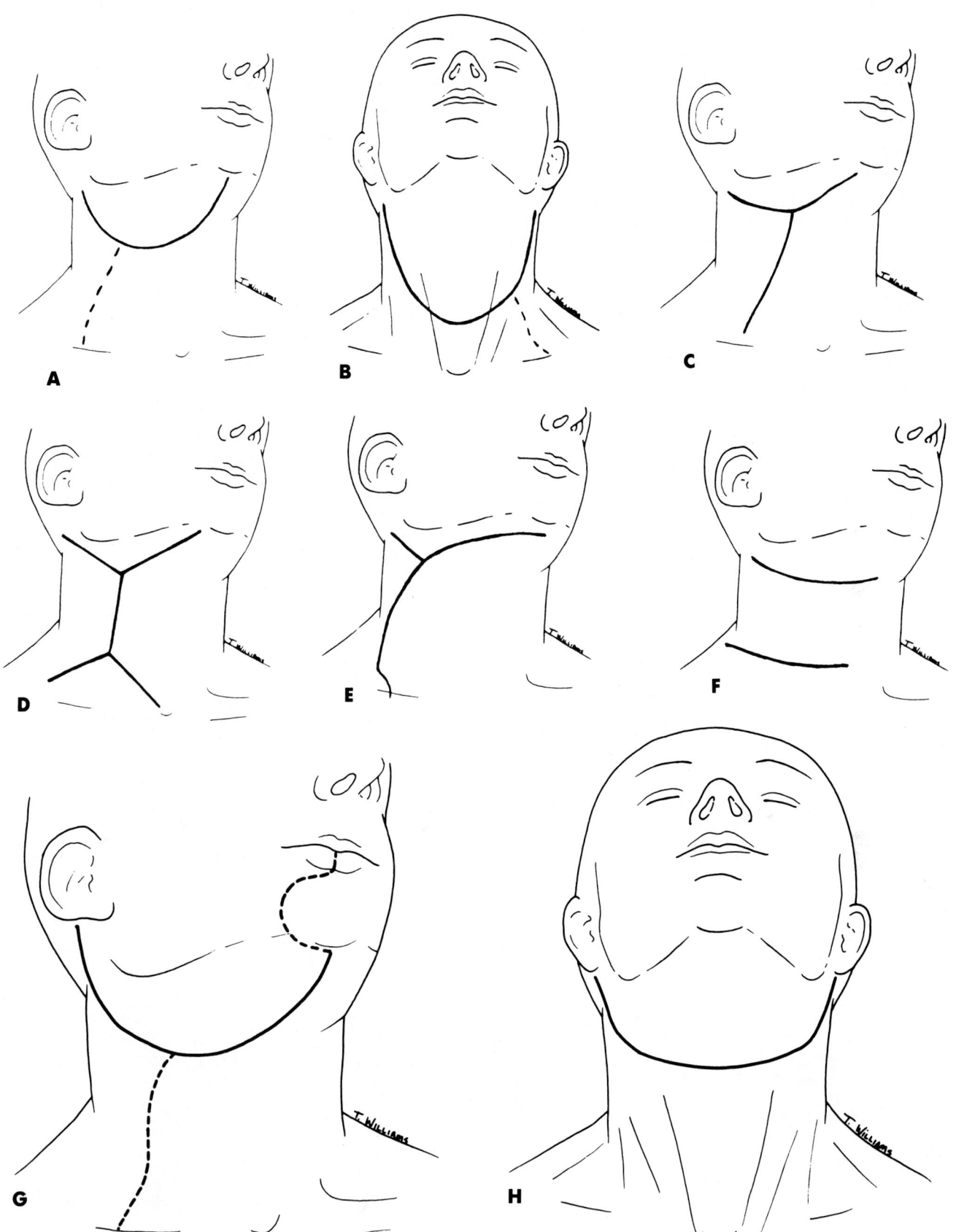

FIG. 20-23   Neck dissection incisions. **A,** Latyschevsky and Freund. **B,** Freund. **C,** Crile. **D,** Martin.
E, Babcock and Conley. **F,** MacFee. **G,** Incision used for unilateral supraomohyoid neck dissection. **H,**
Incision used for bilateral supraomohyoid neck dissection.

From Cummings, C.W., et al. (1993). *Otolaryngology—Head and neck surgery*. St. Louis: Mosby.

11. The entire field is examined for bleeding and then irrigated with warm saline solution. If necessary, a skin graft is placed covering the bifurcation of the carotid artery extending down approximately 4 inches, and sutured with no. 4-0 absorbable on a very small cutting needle. Closed wound suction drains are placed in the wound.

12. The flaps are approximated with interrupted, fine nonabsorbable sutures or with skin staples. A bulky pressure dressing may be applied to the neck, depending on surgeon preference.

MODIFIED NECK DISSECTION (FIG. 20-24)

Modified neck dissection is removal of neck contents with the exception of the sternocleidomastoid muscle, internal jugular vein, and eleventh cranial nerve.

Procedural considerations

When performed by an experienced surgeon, this type of neck dissection can facilitate removal of a tumor and lymph nodes suspected of metastases and allow the patient a minimal defect and unimpaired shoulder function. With radical and modified neck dissection, the surgeon and radiologist may decide on a course of postoperative radiation therapy or chemotherapy. The decision depends on the type and location of tumor, stage of disease, and condition of the patient.

RECONSTRUCTIVE PROCEDURES

Head and neck surgical procedures to remove malignant tumors are reconstructed depending on the surgical defect. The wound may be closed primarily, or local flaps and split-thickness skin grafts (as with facial and intraoral defects) or full-thickness skin grafts (as in nasal and facial defects) may be used. Regional flaps (such as the pectoralis major musculocutaneous flap), microvascular tissue transfer (such as the radial forearm flap, free jejunal flap, and rectus abdominis flap), or microvascular osteocutaneous flaps (such as the iliac crest flap) may be utilized to restore function as well as cover defects. Combinations of the above grafts and

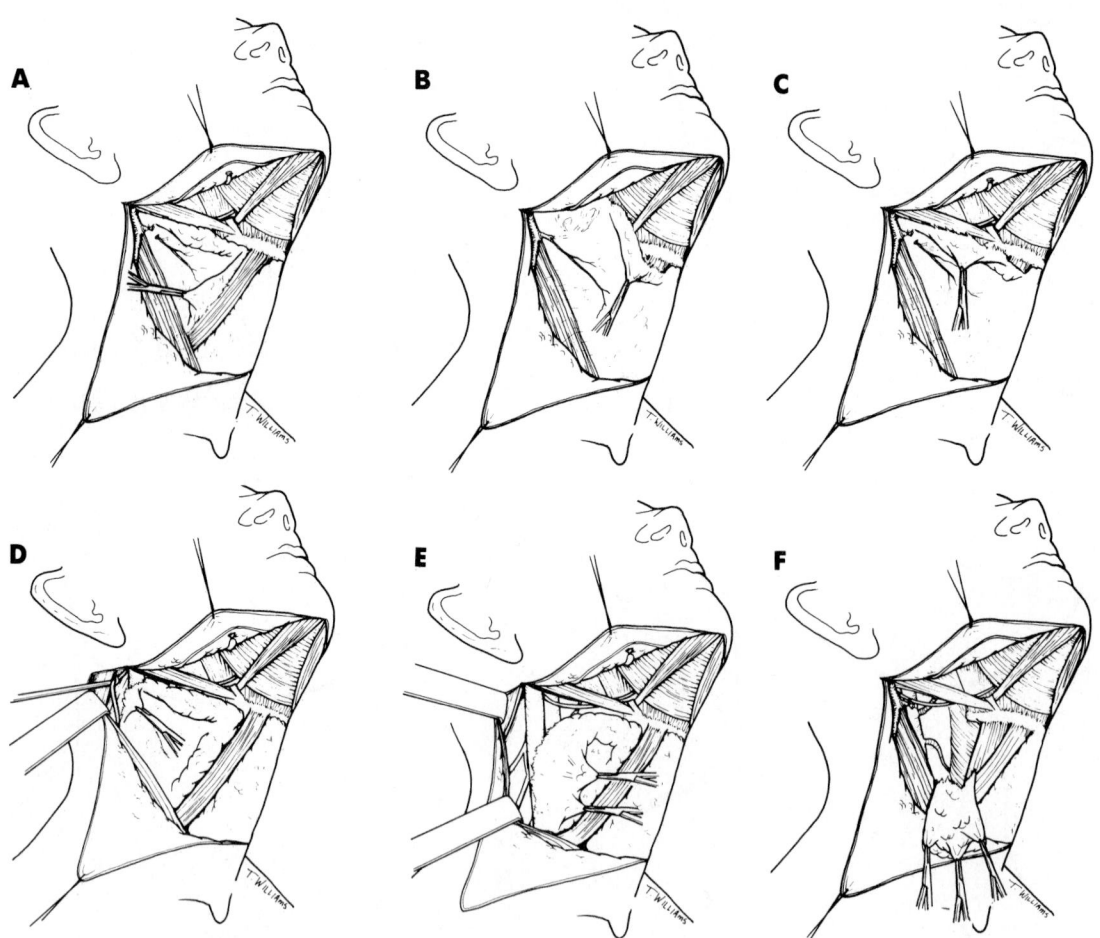

FIG. 20-24 Steps of modified radical neck dissection with preservation of spinal accessory nerve, internal jugular vein, and sternocleidomastoid muscle.

From Cummings, C.W., et al. (1993). *Otolaryngology—Head and neck surgery*. St. Louis: Mosby.

flaps are often necessary when large defects are created.

Microvascular flaps extend surgical and anesthetic time significantly, since veins and arteries are microscopically connected, nerve grafts may be used, and bone must be connected with the use of plates and screws.

The use of a Doppler unit (intraoperatively and postoperatively) and thorough nursing assessment skills are paramount in detecting occlusions or spasms of the vessels and subsequent survival of the transplanted flap.

REFERENCES

Isshiki, N. (1991). Laryngeal framework surgery. *Advances in Otolaryngology—Head and Neck Surgery, 5*, 37-57.

Meyerhoff, W.L., & Rice, D.H. (1992). *Otolaryngology—Head and neck surgery*. Philadelphia: W.B. Saunders.

Pagana, K.D., & Pagana, T.J. (1992). *Diagnostic and laboratory test reference*. St. Louis: Mosby.

BIBLIOGRAPHY

Banis, J.C. Jr., & Swartz, W.M. (1990). Refinements in free flaps for head and neck reconstruction. *Clinics in Plastic Surgery, 17*, 673-682.

Cannon, C.R. (1990). Patient-controlled analgesia (PCA) in head and neck surgery. *Otolaryngology—Head and Neck Surgery, 103*, 748-751.

Crumley, R.L. (1990). Teflon versus thyroplasty versus nerve transfer: A comparison. *Annals of Otology, Rhinology and Laryngology, 99*, 759-763.

Cummings, C.W., et al. (1993). *Otolaryngology—Head and neck surgery*. St. Louis: Mosby.

Davis, J.P., Nield, D.V., Garth, R.J., & Breach, N.M. (1992). The latissimus dorsi flap in head and neck reconstructive surgery: A review of 121 procedures. *Clinics in Otolaryngology, 17*, 487-490.

Flood, T.R., & Hislop, W.S. (1991). A modified surgical approach for parapharyngeal space tumors; Use of the inverted 'L' osteotomy. *British Journal of Oral and Maxillofacial Surgery, 29*, 82-86.

Freeman, M.S. (1990). Incision planning and basic soft-tissue surgery. *Otolaryngology Clinics of North America, 23*, 865-874.

Friberg, D., & Lundberg, C. (1990). Antibiotic prophylaxis in major head and neck surgery when clean-contaminated wounds are established. *Scandinavian Journal of Infectious Diseases Supplement, 70*, 87-90.

Gavilan, J., Gavilan, C., & Herranz, J. (1992). Functional neck dissection: Three decades of controversy. *Annals of Otology Rhinology and Laryngology, 10(1)*, 339-341.

Govila, A. (1990). Nonmicrosurgical transfer of the radial forearm flap for head and neck reconstruction. *Annals of Plastic Surgery, 24*, 109-116.

Habel, G., Oregan, B., & Carter J. (1991). Free jejunal transfer in oral reconstruction. *British Journal of Oral and Maxillofacial Surgery, 29*, 159-163.

Hayashi, A., & Maruyama, Y. (1991). Subclavicular approach in head and neck reconstruction with the latissimus dorsi musculocutaneous flap. *British Journal of Plastic Surgery, 44*, 71-74.

Helmus, C., Grin, M., & Westfall, R. (1992). Same-day-stay head and neck surgery. *Laryngoscope, 102*, 1331-1334.

Hickey, S.A., Buckley, J.G., Mitchell, D.B., & O'Connor, A.F. (1990). Securing of suction drains in head and neck surgery [Letter]. *Journal of Laryngology and Otology, 104*, 69-70.

Isaacson, G., Kim, J.H., Kirchner, J.C., & Kirchner, J.A. (1990). Histology of Isshiki thyroplasty type I. *Annals of Otology, Rhinology and Laryngology, 99*, 42-45.

Isshiki, N., Kojima, H., & Sawada, M. (1991). Special instruments for laryngeal framework surgery. *Annals of Otology, Rhinology and Laryngology, 100*, 728-730.

Kroll, S.S., Reece, G.P., Miller, M.J., & Schusterman, M.A. (1992). Comparison of the rectus abdominis free flap with the pectoralis major myocutaneous flap for reconstructions in the head and neck. *American Journal of Surgery, 164*, 615-618.

Mahieu, H.F., & Dikkers, F.G. (1992). Indirect microlaryngostroboscopic surgery. *Archives of Otolaryngology—Head and Neck Surgery, 118*, 21-24.

Maragos, N.E. (1991). Phonosurgery—a classification. *Otolaryngology—Head and Neck Surgery, 104*, 282-283.

McCaffrey, T.V. (1992). Head and neck cancer surgery. *Current Opinions in Oncology, 4*, 499-503.

Miller, M.J., Swartz, W.M., Miller, R.H., & Harvey, J.M. (1991). Cost analysis of microsurgical reconstruction in the head and neck. *Journal of Surgical Oncology, 46*, 230-234.

Rebeiz, E., April, M.M., Bohigian, R.K., & Shapshay, S.M. (1991). Nd:YAG laser treatment of venous malformations of the head and neck; An update. *Otolaryngology—Head and Neck Surgery, 105*, 665-661.

Robbins, K.T., Favrot, S., Hanna, D., & Cole, R. (1990). Risk of wound infection in patients with head and neck cancer. *Head and Neck, 12*, 143-148.

Schusterman, M.A., & Horndeski, G. (1991). Analysis of the morbidity associated with immediate microvascular reconstruction in head and neck cancer patients. *Head and Neck, 13*, 51-55.

Shaha, A.R. (1990). Extended neck dissection, *Journal of Surgical Oncology, 45*, 229-233.

Shestak, K.C., Myers, E.N., Ramasatry, S.S., Johnson, J.T., & Jones, N.F. (1992). Microvascular free tissue transfer for reconstruction of head and neck cancer defects. *Oncology, 6*, 101-10.

Sigler, B.A., & Schuring, L.T. (1993). *Ear, nose and throat disorders*. St. Louis: Mosby.

Silcox, S. (in press). ORL patient. In K.L. Saleh (Ed.), *Core curriculum for post anesthesia nursing practice* (3rd ed.). Philadelphia: W.B. Saunders.

Snow, G.B., Patel, P., Leemans, C.R., & Tiwari, R. (1992). Management of cervical lymph nodes in patients with head and neck cancer. *European Archives of Otorhinolaryngology, 249*, 187-194.

Sullivan, P.K., Fabian, R., & Driscoll, D. (1992). Mandibular osteotomies for tumor extirpation: The advantages of rigid fixation. *Laryngoscope, 102*, 73-80.

Tabet, J.C., & Johnson J.T. (1990). Wound infection in head and neck surgery: Prophylaxis, etiology and management. *Journal of Otolaryngology, 19*, 197-200.

Watkinson, J.C., & Breach, N.M. (1991). Free flaps in head and neck reconstructive surgery: A review of 77 cases. *Clinical Otolaryngology, 16*, 350-353.

Woo, P. (1990). Laryngeal framework reconstruction with miniplates. *Annals of Otology, Rhinology and Laryngology, 99*, 772-777.

21

ORTHOPEDIC SURGERY

BRENDA GREGORY DAWES AND DAVID MICHAEL SILEO

The word *orthopaedia,* derived from the Greek *orthos,* meaning straight, and *paidios,* meaning child, was first used by Nicholas Andre in 1741 as the title for a book dealing with the prevention and correction of skeletal deformities in children. Orthopedic surgery has been defined by the American Board of Orthopaedic Surgery (1982) as "the medical specialty that includes the investigation, preservation and restoration of the form and function of the extremities, spine and associated structures by medical, surgical and physical methods."

Orthopedic surgery is an ever-changing field that is a challenge for the perioperative nurse. Technologic advances in the multitude of systems and hardware utilized have resulted in improved treatment of orthopedic disorders. In addition to understanding anatomic and physiologic responses, the perioperative nurse should have a general understanding of the concepts of these systems and the purpose they serve to provide the most safe and efficient care. A knowledge of the principals of bone fixation and healing, and the relationship of bone and soft tissues will provide a strong basis to ensure continued understanding of the care required for the orthopedic patient. Using the nursing process provides a systematic approach when providing the unique care required in orthopedics.

SURGICAL ANATOMY

ANATOMIC STRUCTURES

The 206 bones of the body form the appendicular or axial framework that supports soft tissues, provides storage areas and reservoirs for minerals, and serves as a site for formation of blood cells (Fig. 21-1). The skeletal system is composed of varied elements including bone, muscle, and associated structures.

Bone remains in a constant state of formation and resorption, preventing development of excessive thickness or thinness. These processes are related to individual metabolism and absorption of calcium, vitamin D, and phosphorus. Levels of minerals affect disease processes, causing bone changes. A layer of connective tissue called periosteum covers all bone.

Muscles are masses of tissue that cover bones and provide movement to the skeletal system. Muscles interact with nerves, minerals, skin, and other connective tissue to contract and extend. Individual muscles are short or long and vary in diameter, depending on their position on a specific bone.

Ligaments, tendons, and cartilage also form the skeletal structures. Ligaments are bands of dense connective tissue that hold bone to bone. They provide stability to a joint by encircling or holding ends of bone in place. Tendons are tough, long strands of fibers that form the ends of muscles. They transmit forces to bone or cartilage without being damaged. Cartilage is a layer of elastic, resilient supporting tissue found at the ends of the bones. It forms a cap over the bone end to protect and support the bone during weight-bearing activities and provides a smooth gliding surface for joint movement. Cartilage is aneural, alymphatic (without nerves or lymph tissue), avascular, and high in water content (Mourad, 1991). The lack of vascularity and loss of water from cartilage during a lifetime are causes of resulting degenerative disease such as arthritis. Weight bearing and joint movement keep cartilage from becoming thin or damaged and helps prevent degenerative conditions (Thibodeau and Patton, 1994).

Joints are articulations where bones are joined to one another or where two surfaces of bones come together. Joints are classified by the type of material between them or according to movement. Material between joints is fibrous, cartilaginous, or synovial. The type of movement is synarthrotic (immovable), amphiarthrotic (slightly movable), or diarthrotic (freely movable). Synarthrotic joints are connected by fibrous tissue or ligaments. such as the suture-type joints holding the bones of the skull, and connections between two bones such as the radius and ulna. Amphiarthrotic joints are connected by cartilage. Joints of this type include the symphysis pubis, intervertebral joints, and manubriosternal joint. The majority of joints are diarthrodic; these are the only joints with one or more ranges of motion. These joints are lined with a synovial membrane and are called synovial joints. Examples include the knee, cervical vertebrae 1 and 2, the radius articulating on the

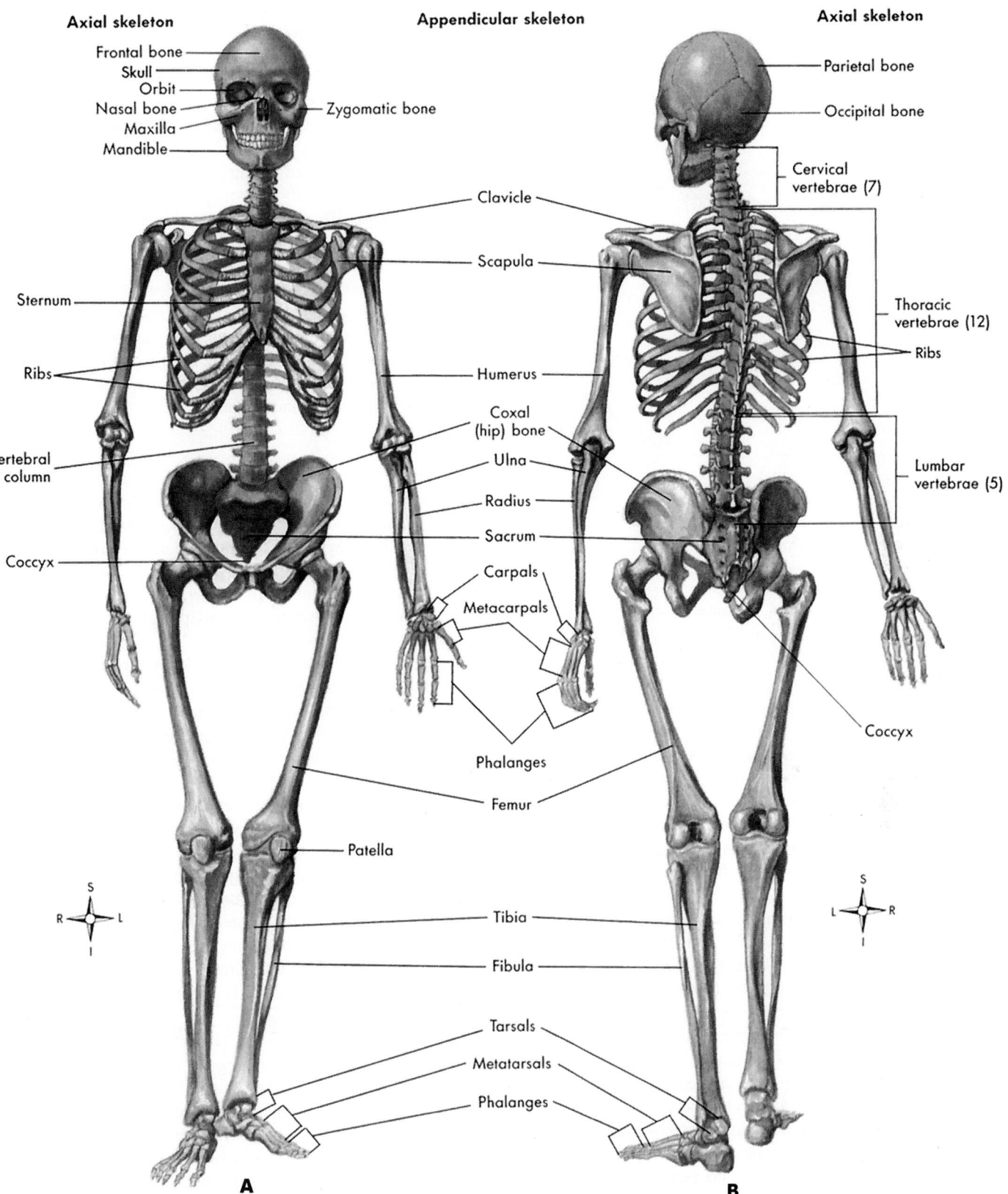

FIG. 21-1   Human skeleton, anterior and posterior views. Number in parentheses indicates number of bones in that unit.

From Thibodeau GA and Patton K: *Anatomy and Physiology,* ed 2, St. Louis, 1993, Mosby.

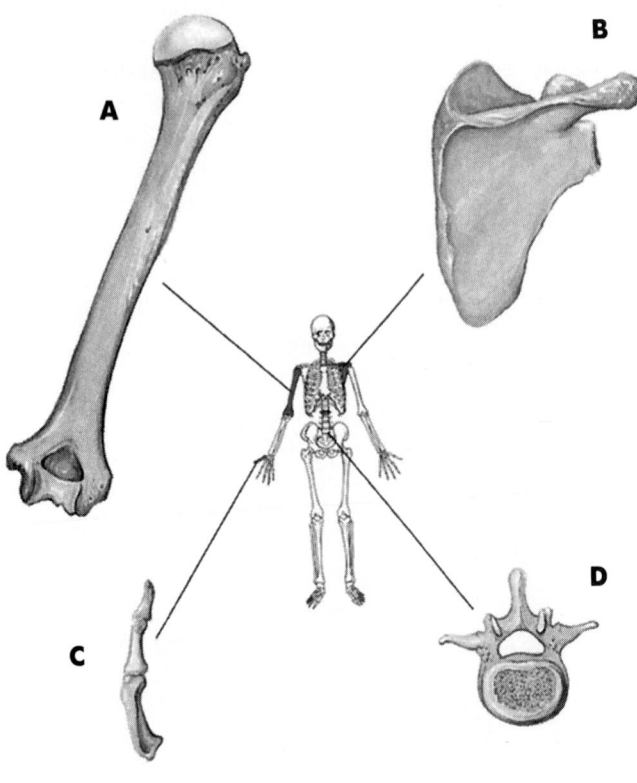

FIG. 21-2   Types of bones. Examples of bone types include **A,** Long bones (humerus); **B,** Flat bones (scapula); **C,** Short bones (phalanx); and **D,** Irregular bones (vertebra).

From Thibodeau GA and Patton K: *Anatomy and Physiology,* ed 2, St. Louis, 1993, Mosby.

wrist bones, the hip, and the shoulder.

There are two types of bone tissue: cortical and cancellous. Cortical bone is the hard bone forming the outer shell—the main supporting tissue. Cancellous bone is soft and spongy, located at the ends of long bones, iliac crest, tibia, and sternum. It contains the red bone marrow for hemopoiesis.

Bones are divided according to their shape: long, short, flat, irregular, and round (Fig. 21-2). Long bones are present in the limbs and consist of a shaft and two ends; the ends generally flare out, are covered with articular cartilage, and provide a surface for articulation and musculotendinous attachment. Short bones, such as the carpals and tarsals (in the wrist and midfoot), are present when the structure is strong but limited movement is required. Flat bones are scapula, sternum, and pelvic girdle. Irregular bones are found in the skull and vertebral column. Round (sesamoid, resembling a sesame seed) bones are found within tendons. The patella is the largest sesamoid bone. Most sesamoid bones are small and located between the metacarpal and proximal phalanx in the thumb.

Long bones are divided into three sections: the shaft, or diaphysis, and two ends, or epiphyses. The shaft is composed of compact bone. The epiphyses flare out and consist of cancellous bone. They are covered by cartilage, which provides a cushion and offers protection during weight bearing and movement. Until skeletal maturity a line of cartilage called the epiphyseal plate separates the epiphysis from the diaphysis. Fractures in this region suffered by children can be devastating because often they lead to malformation and permanent limb shortening.

Trabeculae are located within cancellous bone and consist of an interconnecting network of bone oriented along the lines of stress. These structures are important for weight bearing, providing strength to withstand stress placed upon the bone. The periosteum is a thin outer covering of bone containing nutrient arteries for nourishment of bone cells. Disruption of these periosteal vessels after bone trauma can influence the ability of bone to heal. The haversian system consists of thousands of microscopic units found in the cortical bone. These units of matrix cells, canals, and conduits allow flow of nutrients and facilitate calcium absorption.

VERTEBRAE

Vertebrae form the longitudinal axis of the skeleton. The vertebral bodies are connected by several cartilagenous joints, which enable the vertebrae to flex, extend, or rotate while being held together. The bodies of adjacent vertebrae are connected by intervetebral disks and ligaments. The ligamenta flava bind the laminae of adjacent vertebrae together. Other ligaments connect the spinous processes and vertebral bodies.

Seven cervical vertebrae form the skeletal framework of the neck. Twelve thoracic vertebrae support the thoracic region, and five lumbar vertebrae support the small of the back. Below the lumbar vertebrae lie the sacrum and coccyx. Each of these bones is formed by the fusion of vertebrae.

The vertebral column is curved. Following birth, there is a continuous posterior convexity. As development occurs, secondary posterior concavities develop in the cervical and lumbar regions, resulting in improved balance.

Each area of the vertebral column has specific bony structures. General features include a body (except the first two cervical vertebrae) on the anterior part. Posterior vertebrae consist of a neural arch formed by pedicles and laminae and the spinous or transverse processes.

SHOULDER AND UPPER EXTREMITY

The clavicle, which is a long, doubly curved bone, serves as a prop for the shoulder and holds it away from the chest wall. The clavicle rests almost horizontally at the upper and anterior part of the thorax, above the first rib. It articulates medially with the manubrium of the sternum and laterally with the acromion of the scapula and is tethered to the underlying coracoid process of the scapula by the coracoclavicular ligaments.

The scapula (shoulder blade) is a flat, triangular bone that forms the posterior part of the shoulder girdle, lying

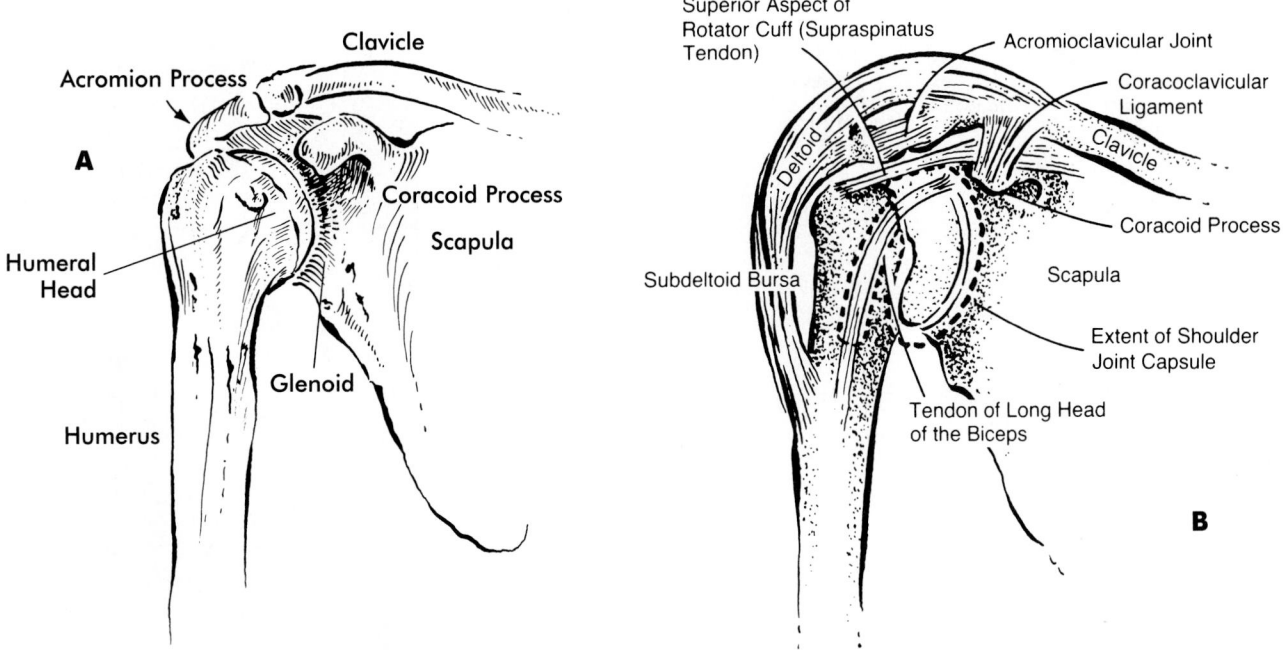

FIG. 21-3 Shoulder. **A,** Joint showing anterior view. **B,** Girdle showing articulations.
Redrawn from Lewis RC: *Primary care orthopedics,* New York, 1988, Churchill Livingstone.

superior and posterior to the upper chest. The glenoid cavity on the lateral side of the scapula provides a socket for the humerus (the bone of the upper arm), and the acromion process articulates with the clavicle medially. The scapula is attached to the thorax by muscles.

The shoulder girdle is made up of three articulations: the glenohumeral, coracoclavicular, and acromioclavicular (ac) joints (Fig. 21-3). The glenohumeral joint has a multidirectional range of motion, whereas the latter two joints have limited motion. The acromiocalvicular joint, located at the top of the shoulder, is the articulation between the outer end of the clavicle and a flattened articular facet situated on the inner border of the acromion. The muscles immediately surrounding the shoulder joint are the supraspinous, infraspinous, teres minor, and subscapular muscles; together they are referred to as the rotator cuff. These muscles stabilize the shoulder joint while the entire arm is moved by the powerful deltoid, pectoralis major, teres major, and latissimus dorsi muscles. The shoulder girdle strength and stability are maintained by the soft tissue integrity, not the bony structures. Pathology in this area can be the result of bone, soft tissue, or combined injury.

The humerus is the longest and largest bone of the upper extremity. It is composed of a shaft and two ends. The proximal end, or head, has two projections, the greater and lesser tuberosities (Fig. 21-4). The circumference of the articular surface of the humerus is constricted and is termed the anatomic neck. The anatomic neck marks the attachment to the capsule of the shoulder joint. The constriction

below the tuberosities is called the surgical neck and is the site of most fractures.

The greater tuberosity is situated at the lateral side of the humeral head. Its upper surface has three impressions where the supraspinous, infraspinous, and teres minor tendons insert. The lesser tuberosity is situated in front of the neck and has an impression for the insertion of the tendon of the subscapular muscle. The attachment sites for the rotator cuff, the tuberosities, are separated from each other by a deep groove (bicipital groove) in which lies the tendon of the biceps muscle of the arm. The tendon of the pectoralis major inserts on the lateral margin of the bicipital groove, and the latissimus dorsi and teres major insert on the medial margin.

The distal humerus flattens and ends in a broad articular surface. The surface is divided into the medial and lateral condyles, which are separated by a slight ridge. On the lateral condyle the rounded articular surface is called the capitellum; it articulates with the head of the radius. On the medial condyle the articular surface is termed the trochlea, which articulates with the ulna.

The ulna is located medial to the radius. The proximal portion of the ulna, the olecranon, articulates with the trochlea of the humerus at the elbow. The radius rotates around the ulna. At the proximal end is the head, which articulates with the capitellum of the humerus and the radial notch of the ulna. The tendon of the biceps muscle is attached to the tuberosity just below the radial head. The distal end of the radius is divided into two articular surfaces. The distal

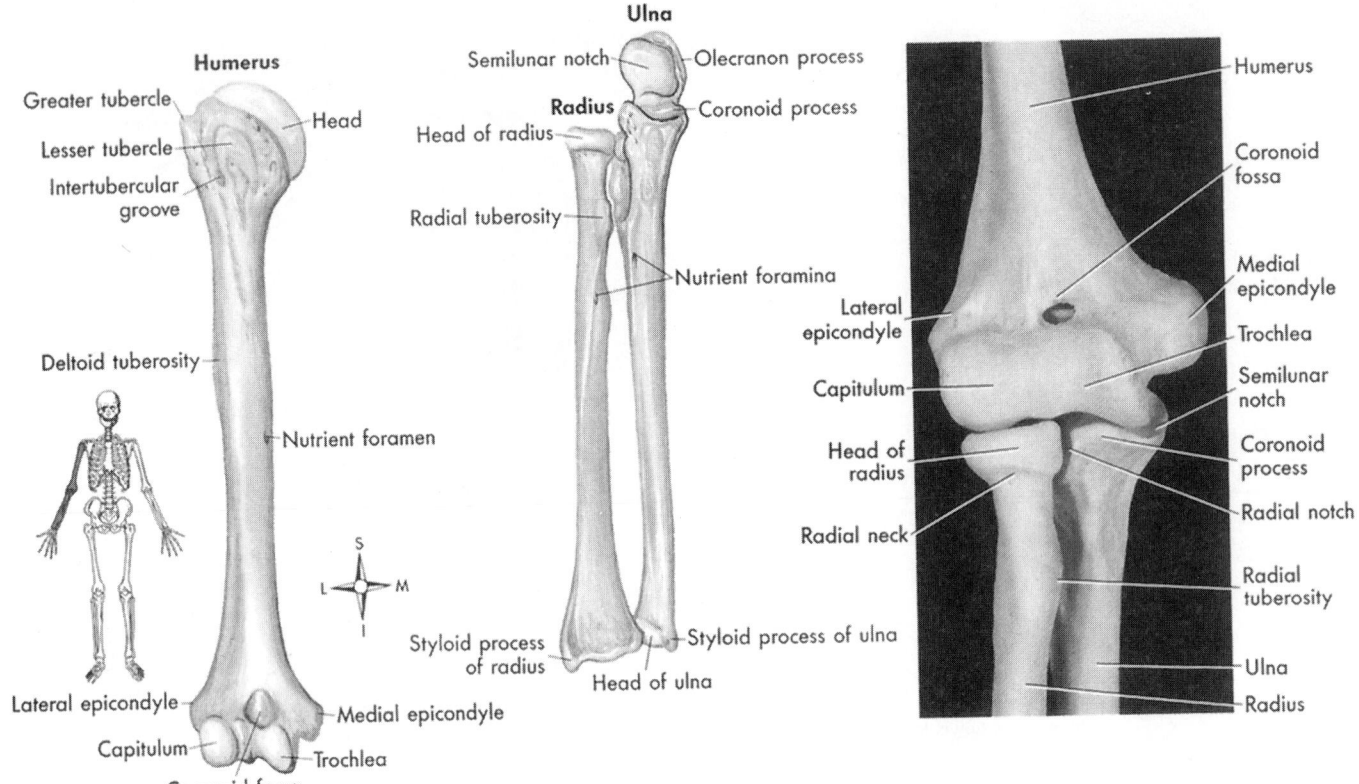

FIG. 21-4   Bones of the arm anterior view showing the humerus, radius, and ulna.
From Thibodeau GA and Patton K: *Anatomy and Physiology,* ed 2, St. Louis, 1993, Mosby.

surface articulates with the carpal bones of the wrist, and the surface on the medial side articulates with the distal end of the ulna.

WRIST AND HAND

The skeletal bones of the wrist and hand consist of three distinct parts: (1) the carpals, or wrist bones; (2) the metacarpals, or bones of the palm; and (3) the phalanxes, or bones of the digits (Fig. 21-5).

There are eight carpal bones arranged in two rows. The distal row, proceeding from the radial to the ulnar side, includes the trapezium, trapezoid, capitate, and hamate; the proximal row consists of the scaphoid, lunate, triquetrum, and pisiform. Functionally, the scaphoid links the rows as it stabilizes and coordinates the movement of the proximal and distal rows. Each carpal bone consists of several smooth articular surfaces for contact with the adjacent bones, as well as rough surfaces for the attachment of ligaments. The five metacarpal bones (long bones) are situated in the palm. Proximally they articulate with the distal row of carpal bones, and distally the head of each metacarpal articulates with its proper phalanx. The heads of the metacarpals form the knuckles. The phalanges, or fingers, consist of 14 bones in each hand, two in the thumb and three in each finger. Each phalanx consists of a shaft and two ends.

PELVIS, HIP, AND FEMUR

The pelvis (Fig. 21-6) is a stable circular base that supports the trunk and forms an attachment for the lower extremities. It is a massive irregular bone created by the fusion of three separate bones. The largest and uppermost of the three bones is the ilium; the strongest and lowermost is the ischium, and the anteriormost is the pubis. Together this construct provides stability to the entire pelvis.

The hip, a ball and socket joint, is formed by the acetabular portion of the innominate (coxal) bone and the proximal end of the femur (Fig. 21-7). The hip joint is surrounded by a capsule, ligaments, and muscles, to provide stability. The iliofemoral ligament connects the ilium with the femur. The ischiofemoral and pubofemoral ligaments join the pubic bone to the femur.

The acetabulum is a deep, round cavity that articulates with the head of the femur. The proximal end of the femur consists of the femoral head and neck, the upper portion of the shaft, and the greater and lesser trochanters (Fig. 21-8).

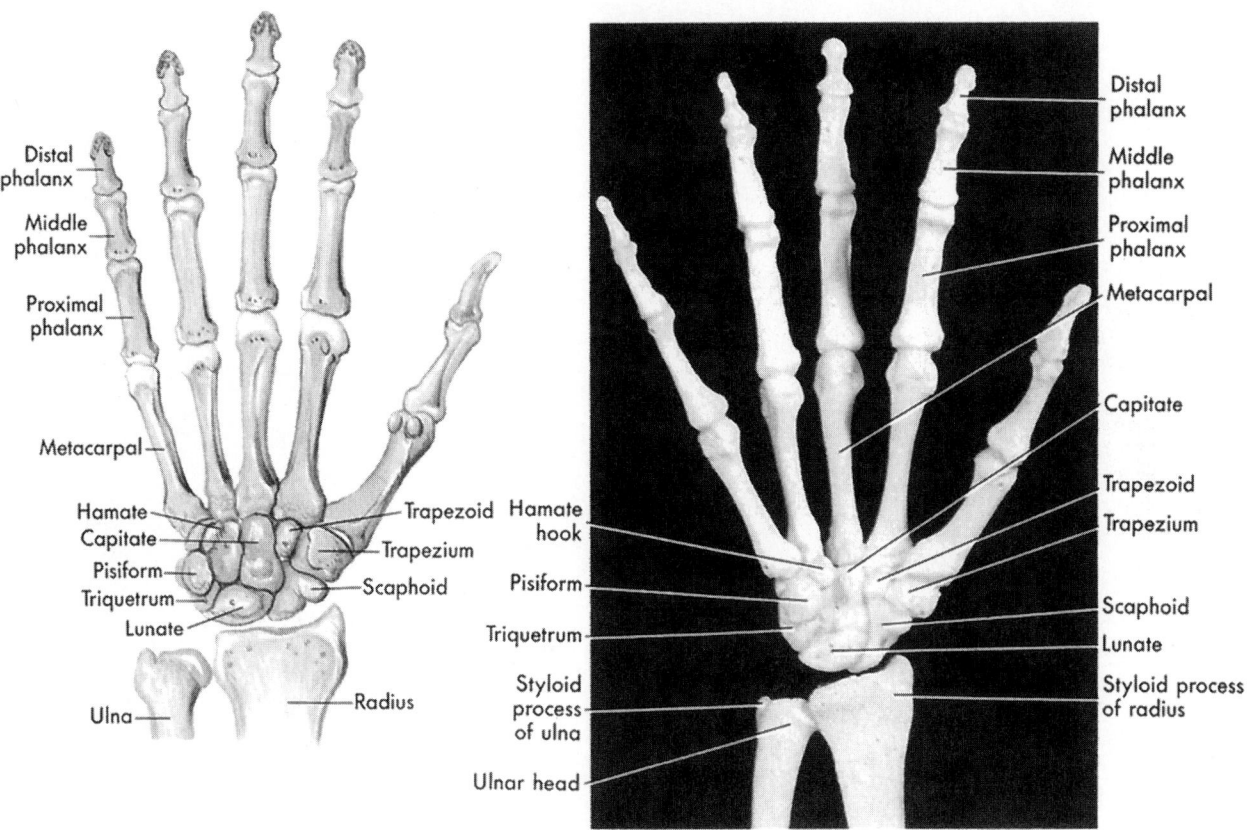

FIG. 21-5   Bones of the wrist and hand, palmar view.
From Thibodeau GA and Patton K: *Anatomy and Physiology*, ed 2, St. Louis, 1993, Mosby.

The greater trochanter is a broad process that protrudes from the outer upper portion of the shaft and projects upward from the junction of the superior border of the neck with the outer surface of the shaft. It serves as a point of insertion for the abductor and short rotator muscles of the hip.

The lesser trochanter is a conical process projecting from the posterior and inferior portion of the base of the neck of the femur at its junction with the shaft. It serves as a point of insertion for the iliopsoas muscle. The lower end of the femur terminates in the two condyles. Anteriorly the condyles are separated from one another by a smooth depression, called the intercondylar or patellar groove, forming an articulating surface for the patella. Posteriorly they project slightly, and the space between them forms the intercondylar fossa, a supporting structure for neurovascular structures.

The upper or condylar end of the tibia presents an articular surface corresponding with those of the femoral condyles. The articular surface of the two tibial condyles forms two facets, which are deepened by the semilunar cartilage into fossae for the femoral condyles.

KNEE, TIBIA, AND FIBULA

The knee joint (Fig. 21-9) consists of two articulations. One articulation is between each condyle of the femur and the tibial plateau and the second is between the patella and femur. These areas are subject to degenerative changes, often requiring reconstructive surgery. The bones of the knee joint are connected by extraarticular and intraarticular structures. The extraarticular attachments are the capsule, quadriceps muscle, and two collateral ligaments. The intraarticular ligaments are two cruciate ligaments and the attachments of the menisci.

The patella, or kneecap, is anterior to the knee joint in the intercondylar groove of the distal femur. It is a sesamoid bone contained within the quadriceps tendon. The anterior surface of the patella is united with the patellar tendon as the tendon originates and inserts above and below the knee joint. The posterior surface of the patella articulates with the femur.

The capsule of the knee joint is attached proximally to the femoral condyles, and it is attached distally to the condyles of the tibia and to the upper end of the fibula. The

Text continued on p. 740.

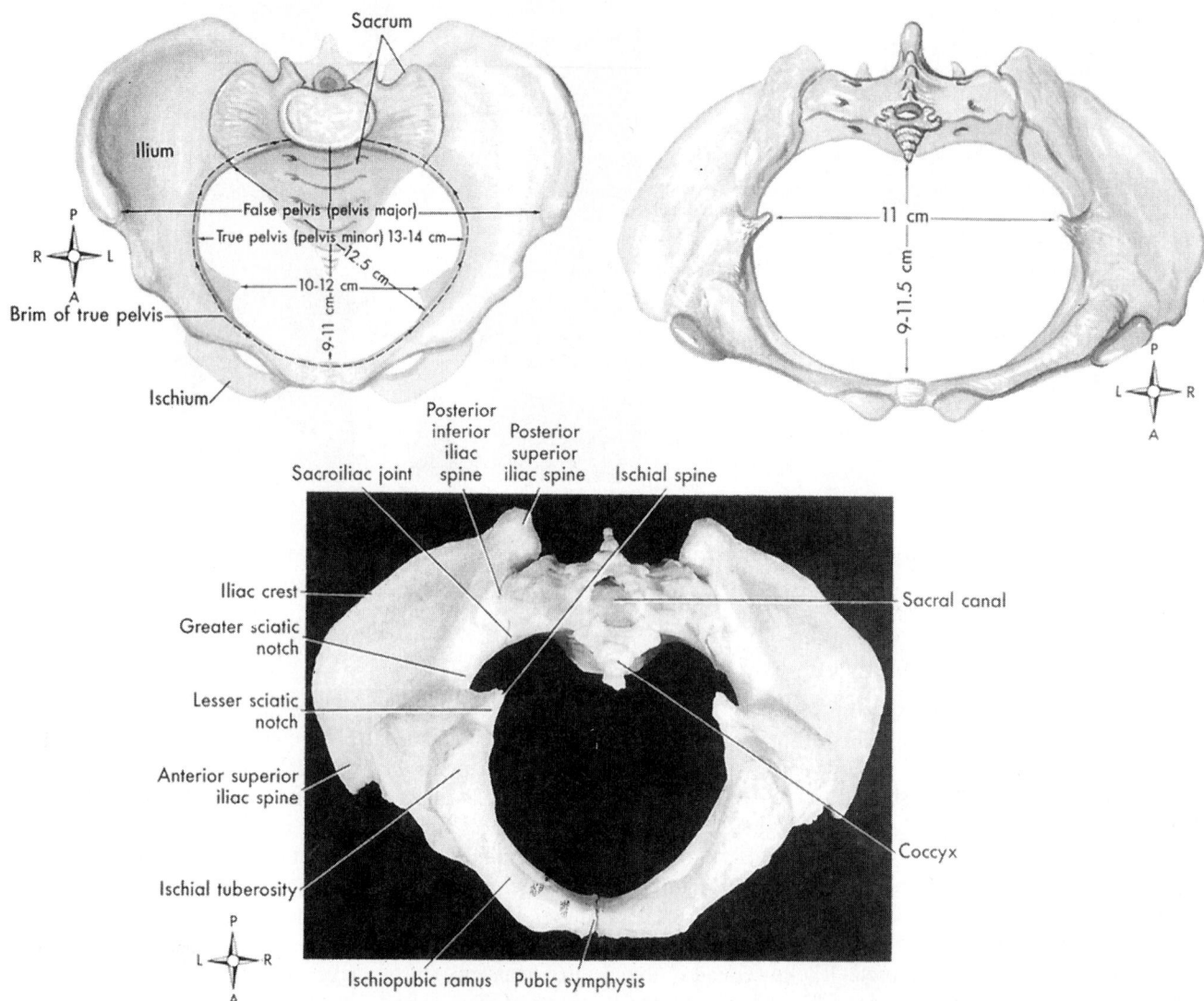

FIG. 21-6   Pelvis, superior view.

From Thibodeau GA and Patton K: *Anatomy and Physiology,* ed 2, St. Louis, 1993, Mosby.

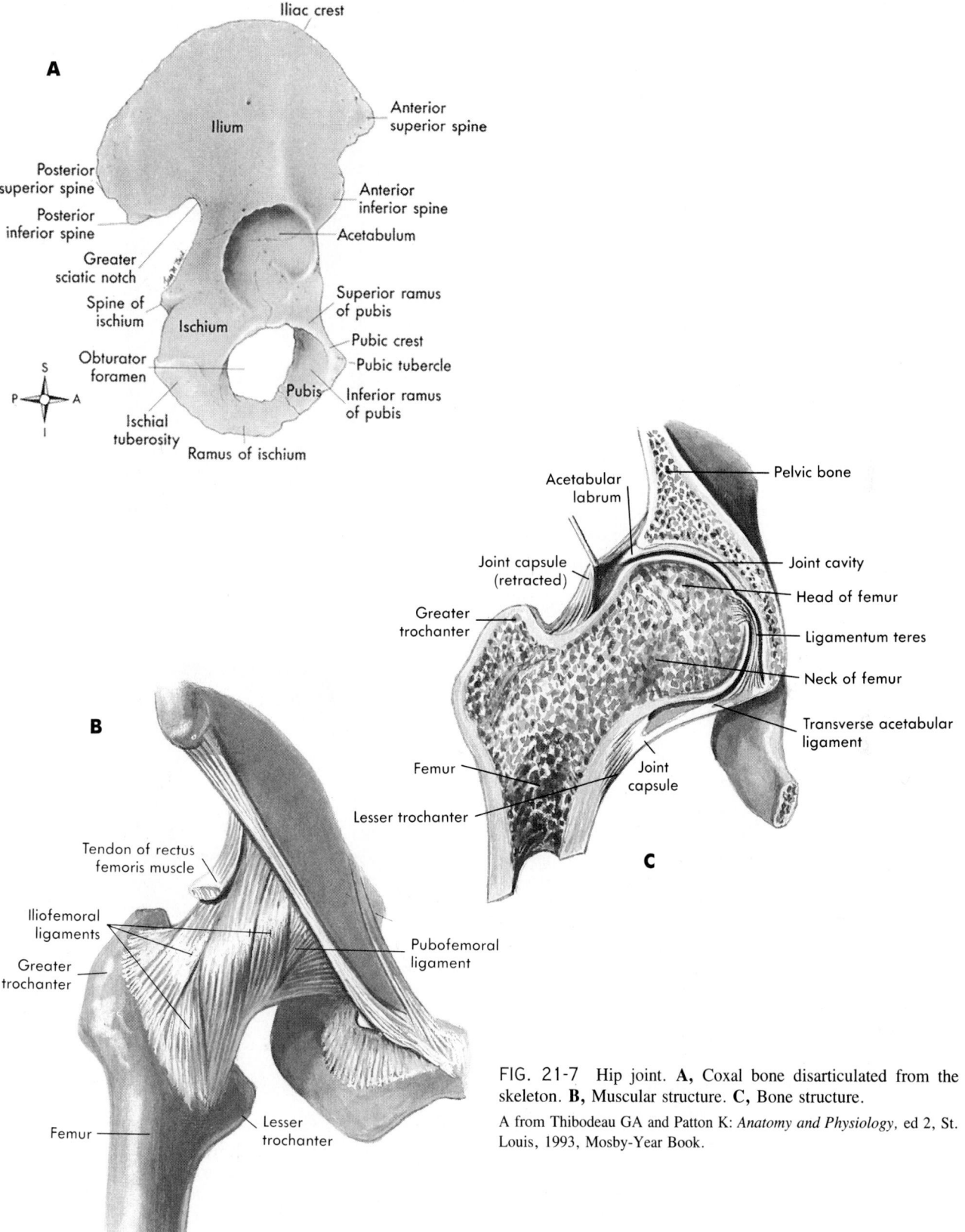

FIG. 21-7 Hip joint. **A,** Coxal bone disarticulated from the skeleton. **B,** Muscular structure. **C,** Bone structure.

A from Thibodeau GA and Patton K: *Anatomy and Physiology,* ed 2, St. Louis, 1993, Mosby-Year Book.

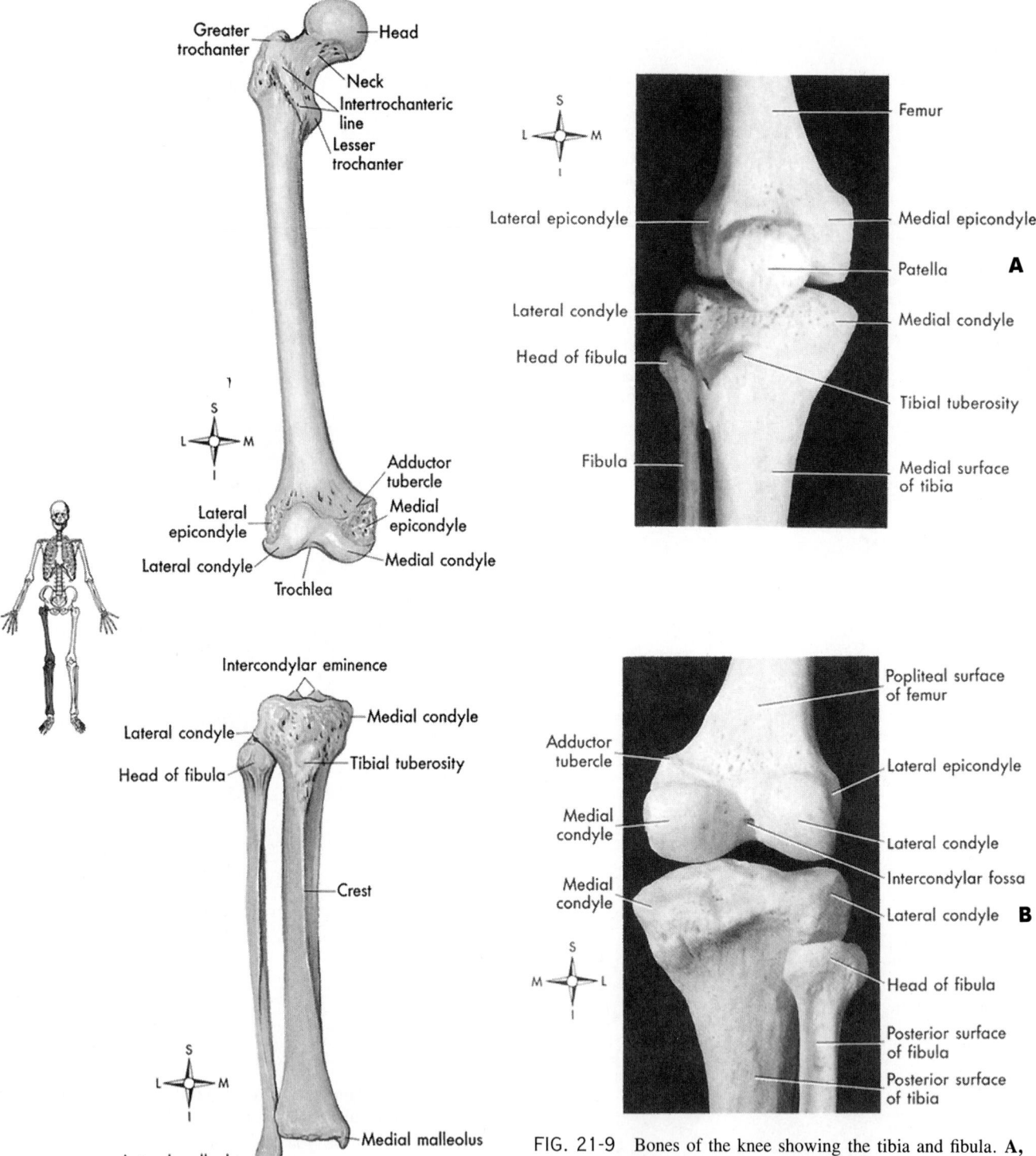

FIG. 21-8 Bones of the upper and lower leg.

From Thibodeau GA and Patton K: *Anatomy and Physiology,* ed 2, St. Louis, 1993, Mosby-Year Book.

FIG. 21-9 Bones of the knee showing the tibia and fibula. **A,** Anterior aspect and **B,** Posterior aspect.

From Thibodeau GA and Patton K: *Anatomy and Physiology,* ed 2, St. Louis, 1993, Mosby-Year Book.

A

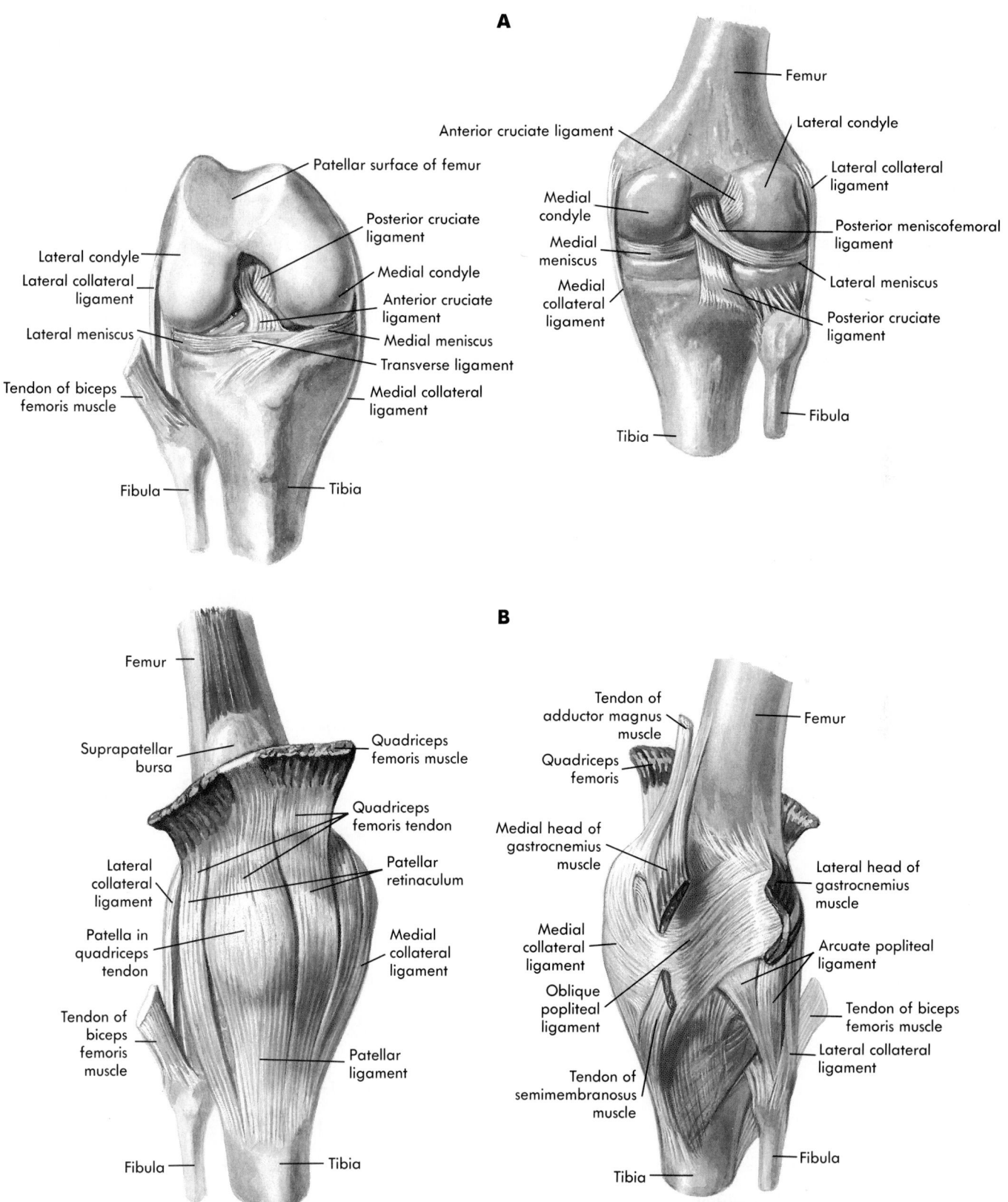

Patellar surface of femur

Posterior cruciate ligament

Lateral condyle

Lateral collateral ligament

Lateral meniscus

Tendon of biceps femoris muscle

Fibula

Tibia

Medial condyle

Anterior cruciate ligament

Medial meniscus

Transverse ligament

Medial collateral ligament

Femur

Anterior cruciate ligament

Lateral condyle

Lateral collateral ligament

Medial condyle

Medial meniscus

Medial collateral ligament

Posterior meniscofemoral ligament

Lateral meniscus

Posterior cruciate ligament

Tibia

Fibula

B

Femur

Suprapatellar bursa

Quadriceps femoris muscle

Quadriceps femoris tendon

Patellar retinaculum

Lateral collateral ligament

Patella in quadriceps tendon

Medial collateral ligament

Tendon of biceps femoris muscle

Patellar ligament

Fibula

Tibia

Tendon of adductor magnus muscle

Quadriceps femoris

Femur

Medial head of gastrocnemius muscle

Lateral head of gastrocnemius muscle

Medial collateral ligament

Oblique popliteal ligament

Arcuate popliteal ligament

Tendon of biceps femoris muscle

Lateral collateral ligament

Tendon of semimembranosus muscle

Tibia

Fibula

FIG. 21-10   Knee joint. **A,** Bony structure. **B,** Superficial aspect.

capsule is reinforced in front by the patellar and quadriceps tendon, on the sides by the medial and lateral collateral ligaments, and posterior by the popliteus and gastrocnemius muscles.

The cruciate ligaments (Fig. 21-10), consisting of two fibrous bands, extend from the intercondylar fossa of the femur to attachments anterior and posterior to the intercondylar surface of the tibia.

The menisci are interposed between the condyles of the femur and those of the tibia (Fig. 21-10). Each meniscus is attached to the joint capsule. The ends of the cartilage are attached to the tibia in the middle of its upper articular surface. These structures are almost totally avascular, and degenerative changes are usually permanent.

Synovial membrane lines the capsule of the joint and covers the infrapatellar fat pad, parts of the cruciate ligaments, and portions of the bone. The portion of the knee joint cavity that extends upward in front of the femur is called the suprapatellar pouch or bursa.

The tibia is the larger and stronger of the lower leg bones. The fibula is smaller and located more lateral. The fibula articulates at the proximal end with the lateral condyle of the tibia. The proximal end of the tibia articulates with the femur to form the knee joint. Distally, the tibia articulates with the fibula and with the talus, forming the ankle joint.

ANKLE AND FOOT

The ankle is a hinge joint, formed by the distal end of the tibia, lateral malleolus, and medial malleolus of the fibula. These structures form a mortise for the reception of the upper surface of the talus and its facets. The talus is an irregular bone consisting of a body, neck, and head. The bones are connected by ligaments, which spread out from the malleoli to be attached to the calcaneus and navicular bones (Fig. 21-11). The joint is surrounded by a thin capsule.

The bony framework of the foot (Fig. 21-12) comprises seven tarsal bones, five metatarsal bones, and 14 phalanges. The calcaneus forms the heel and gives support to the talus. The cuboid bone articulates proximally and posteriorly with the calcaneus and distally with the fourth and fifth metatarsals and the third cuneiform bones.

The navicular bone articulates with the cuneiform bones, which lie side by side in front of the scaphoid. The metatarsal bones articulate proximally with the tarsal bones and distally with the bases of the first phalanges of the corresponding toes. There are two phalanges for the great toe and three for each of the other toes.

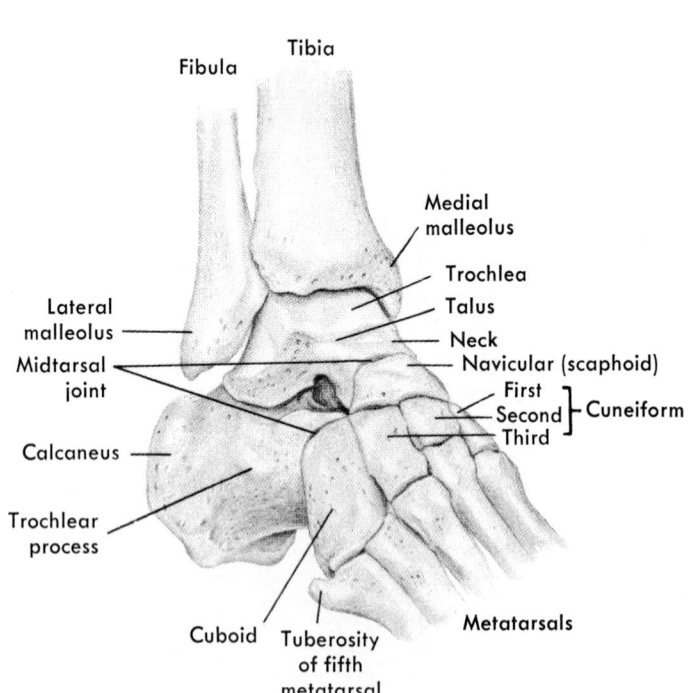

FIG. 21-11   Anatomy of ankle.
Courtesy Zimmer, Inc., Warsaw, Ind.

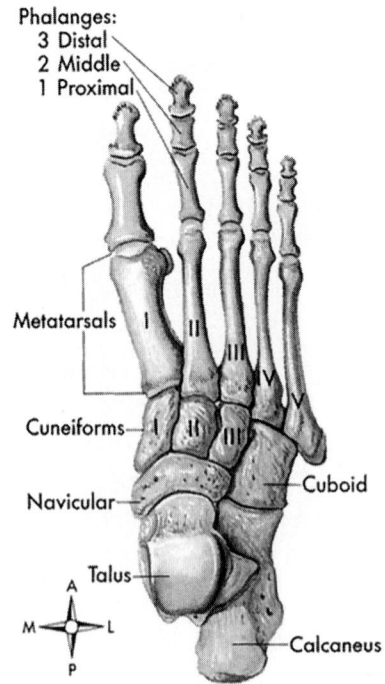

FIG. 21-12   Bones of the foot viewed from above.

From Thibodeau GA and Patton K: *Anatomy and Physiology,* ed 2, St. Louis, 1993, Mosby.

PERIOPERATIVE NURSING CONSIDERATIONS

ASSESSMENT

Assessment of the perioperative orthopedic patient is ongoing, beginning with the initial patient contact. Familiarity with orthopedic procedures and anticipated patient outcome improves the ability to gather appropriate information and complete the nursing process. The nursing assessment is also enhanced by obtaining patient specific information from the physician. The informed consent provides information to confirm the posted procedures and verify the operative site. The consent may have been obtained before admission to the surgery suite and should be reviewed for accuracy and completeness.

The assessment is completed by reviewing the medical history and physical to determine the problem and onset. The patient's medical record also contain results of radiographic studies, lab data, and other findings. The nursing history is obtained by observation and interview to determine physical, psychosocial, and other needs. The patient should be assessed for range of motion, neurovascular status, and general condition. The patient understanding of the surgical procedure and postoperative rehabilitation is determined and patient education reinforced.

Assessment information helps determine specific needs related to surgical positioning, skin preparation, equipment, instrumentation, and supplies. Environmental controls are also considered, including room temperature, traffic flow, lighting, and personnel attire.

Information should be communicated with technical and anesthesia team members and persons in other disciplines. The information collected helps the perioperative nurse plan and coordinate activities, facilitate a smooth transition, and reduce operative time.

NURSING DIAGNOSIS

Nursing diagnosis related to the care of patients undergoing orthopedic surgery might include the following:

- Anxiety
- High risk for peripheral neurovascular function
- High risk for injury
- Impaired gas exchange
- High risk for infection

OUTCOME IDENTIFICATION

Outcomes identified for the patient with orthopedic trauma undergoing surgical repair include:

- The patient will verbalize understanding, fears, and apprehension.
- The patient will be protected from peripheral neurovascular injury.

- Injury will be prevented during the perioperative period.
- The patient will maintain adequate ventilation and oxygen exchange.
- The patient will not experience postoperative infection.

PLANNING

The care of surgical patients undergoing any type of surgery requires planning for routine procedures that are always followed and anticipating the unexpected. The perioperative nurse should be consistent and systematic in the planning process to expedite actual steps required to facilitate the surgical procedure. Care of the orthopedic patient presents unique challenges due to the psychosocial, physical, and technical patient needs. Planning includes attention to environmental, positioning, transfusion supplies, equipment, and instrument needs in addition to practices that will prevent complications (Brown and Seltzer, 1991; Chapman, 1993).

The optimal environment is comfortable for the patient and surgical team. The patient should feel relaxed and secure enough to allow the surgical team to become his or her advocates during the procedure. Physical preparation of the environment changes with individual patients. At the time the procedure is posted in the operating room, traffic flow is considered to determine room location. The temperature is selected for the procedure considering patient age, attire worn by the operative personnel (body exhaust suits), or use of polymethyl methacrylate (PMMA), or bone cement. The physical environment and surroundings are prepared to be free from physical hazards including electrical cord placement. Patient and personnel safety and infection control measures are a priority when planning.

Equipment and instrumentation needed for the procedure are planned before patient arrival in the operating room, particularly because orthopedic procedures vary significantly due to the patient physical condition or age. It may be necessary to communicate with the product representative to facilitate obtaining items needed for the procedure. Planning should include personnel familiarization with equipment and instrumentation.

Procedural information should be reviewed to plan positioning and protective measures. Aseptic technique is a routine in the perioperative environment and should be considered a priority when caring for the orthopedic patient (Research Highlight 21-1). Osteomyelitis is an infection of the bone that can go unrecognized for a long time and requires expensive, intensive treatment. Osteomyelitis can lead to severe bone loss and possible loss of a limb. Preventive measures, including administration of antibiotics within 1 hour of the surgical incision, have been demonstrated to be efficacious in preventing wound infection (Drez, Finney, and Roberts, 1991).

Operating room equipment such as defibrillators and resuscitative equipment must always be available, functional,

RESEARCH HIGHLIGHT 21-1

Extensive methods have been introduced as operative practices to decrease postoperative infection in orthopedics. Antibiotic prophylaxis, use of ultraclean air, and body exhaust suits are common practice in orthopedic surgery. The results of infection following large joint replacement have been studied; the risk in elective procedures not requiring implants has been studied less. Data on wound infection are believed to be underreported due to differences in recording infection or the presentation of an infection several weeks postoperatively. In a study of a series of 1207 elective orthopedic procedures it was found that the inpatient risk of infection varied by procedure. The greater risk occurred with revision total knee, ankle fusion, subtalar fusion, primary total knee replacement, spinal fusion, and revision total hip replacement. Revision surgery carried an approximate threefold risk over primary procedures. Patients undergoing spinal and hindfoot fusion suffered considerable morbidity as a consequence of infection.

Taylor, G.J.S., Bannister, G.C., and Calder, S. (1990). Perioperative wound infection in elective orthopaedic surgery. *Journal of Hospital Infection, 16,* 241.

RESEARCH HIGHLIGHT 21-2

Improved medications and delivery methods make pain relief safe and effective. Pain management guidelines for patients emphasize patient specific analgesia plans, frequent pain assessment and documentation, and aggressive use of pharmacologic and nonpharmacologic therapy. A plan should be developed with the patient before surgery that considers the patient's health, personal preferences, and attitude about pain control and narcotics. Patient education should include family members. Emphasis should be placed on the need to reduce pain to a tolerable level; elimination of pain may not be realistic. Pain management is a collaborative effort by medical, nursing, and pharmacologic personnel.

Agency for Health Care Policy and Research. (1992). *Clinical practice guideline: Acute pain management.* Rockville, Md.: U.S.D.H.H.S.

and familiar to staff. This includes supplies needed for emergency treatment of a patient condition, such as malignant hyperthermia or unanticipated blood loss. Orthopedic procedures may also require a change in the plan of care in the event of a fracture, damage to vascular integrity, or other change in the patient condition, requiring an understanding of methods and equipment needed to manage these situations.

The nursing process requires continual feed back and modifications. An effective plan entails communication, safety, optimal environment, and effective human resource. A typical care plan for the patient undergoing orthopedic surgery follows.

IMPLEMENTATION

Implementing care of the orthopedic surgical patient requires an understanding of anatomic, physiologic, psychologic, and technical patient needs. Orthopedic surgical procedures demand special equipment, instruments, and psychomotor skills that are different from those required by other specialties. Implementation includes an understanding of the procedures, patient needs, perioperative practices, and methods of improvising to protect the patient while delivering care.

Patient education

Patient education begins with the first patient contact, usually during the visit to the surgeon or nurse practitio-

ner. The practice of preoperative teaching requires innovative techniques including videos, patient brochures, and other teaching aids. This information is reinforced immediately before surgery. The trend toward same day surgery and "A.M. admits" further challenges the perioperative skills required to complete a patient assessment and preoperative teaching. Assessment of the patient's level of understanding enhances the ability to reinforce teaching appropriately and address any unresolved issues. Patients must be provided with the opportunity to ask questions and demonstrate psychomotor skills required during the rehabilitation process.

Explanation about the intraoperative phase, including personnel and the environment, positioning required, and procedures such as regional anesthesia or application of the tourniquet, should be given to the patient. The patient may be alert during the procedure, therefore noise due to power equipment and activities that will occur should be explained. Immobilization devices such as splints, casts, braces, and drains are demonstrated and explained. Pain management techniques should also be discussed (Research Highlight 21-2).

Positioning and positioning aids

The orthopedic patient requires proper positioning on the OR bed or specialty bed to provide adequate exposure of the operative area, maintain body alignment, minimize strain or pressure on nerves and muscles, allow for optimal respiratory and circulatory functions, and provide adequate stabilization of the body. Selection of position depends on several factors, including the type of procedure, location of the injury of lesion, and surgeon preference. The guidelines for placing the patient in the supine or recumbent po-

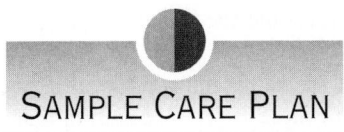

SAMPLE CARE PLAN

NURSING DIAGNOSIS: Anxiety
EXPECTED OUTCOME: The patient will verbalize fears and apprehension related to their pending surgery.
INTERVENTIONS:
Encourage verbalization of feelings, expression of fear and stimulate questions about procedure, anticipated outcome, and postoperative rehabilitation.
Explain routine activities and encourage questions.
Empower the patient and encourage participation in activities.
Demonstrate respect and attend to patients needs.
Remain with patient; ensure other personnel are introduced.
Discuss concerns with the family and seek information to understand the patient's needs.

NURSING DIAGNOSIS: High risk for peripheral neurovascular function.
EXPECTED OUTCOME: The patient will be protected from peripheral neurovascular injury related to positioning, use of equipment or prolonged surgical time.
INTERVENTIONS:
Complete a preoperative assessment including visualization of skin color, pulses.
Position in proper body alignment considering range of motion and extremities free from constriction.
Protect neurovascular structures and prevent pressure that might impede these areas by properly padding bony prominence and pressure points.
Provide padding (air mattress or gel pads) when long surgical times are expected or patients are predisposed to peripheral vascular compromise.
Anticipate needs to minimize surgical time.

NURSING DIAGNOSIS: High risk for injury
EXPECTED OUTCOME: Injury will be prevented during the perioperative period due to extremity and joint immobility or improper use of equipment or instrumentation.
INTERVENTIONS:
Assess range of motion; identify the areas at risk for injury due to immobilization.
Use proper lifting and transfer techniques when transferring the patient to and from the OR bed.

Ensure personnel with knowledge of the patient's condition and equipment are available to supervise and assist with transfer of the patient.
Use proper restraint devices to protect patients from falls or movement of the extremities.
Avoid extending or flexing extremities beyond range of motion when there is resistance.
Use positioning devices, such as pillows, to maintain position.
Insert a catheter as appropriate using sterile technique; monitor output during the procedure.

NURSING DIAGNOSIS: Impaired gas exchange
EXPECTED OUTCOME: The patient will maintain optimal ventilation and oxygen exchange, with minimal adverse effects related to positioning or blood loss.
INTERVENTIONS:
Obtain preoperative evaluation of the patient's pulmonary status.
Ensure full chest excursion when positioning, particularly the lateral and prone positions.
Monitor vital signs, pulse oximetry, and blood loss.
Complete a vascular assessment (pulse and color check) preoperatively and compare to postoperative status.

NURSING DIAGNOSIS: High risk for infection
EXPECTED OUTCOME: The patient will not experience postoperative infection.
INTERVENTIONS:
Change the plan of care for high-risk patients as anticipated following assessment.
Implement aseptic practices for skin preparation, draping of the patient and equipment, opening supplies, and equipment for the procedure moving throughout the operating room.
Initiate antibiotic therapy preoperatively and/or intraoperatively per physician orders.
Implement procedure specific precautions such as using body exhaust systems and pulsatile lavage.
Anticipate equipment needs and prepare for the procedure.
Sterilize instruments according to policy and procedure and the manufacturer guidelines.
Handle implants cautiously.

sition are followed, with modifications to facilitate the specific orthopedic procedure.

Procedures are performed in lateral, prone, or modified positions resulting in use of devices to support these positions that could have a untoward effect. Patients undergoing a surgical procedure risk neuromuscular and skin injury. Preoperative assessment should be thorough to plan the position, taking into consideration the anticipated postoperative status (Walsh, 1991). Neurovascular compromise, impaired chest excursion, and the danger of falls are considerations when positioning to protect the patient throughout the procedure. The safety strap is not always adequate security, and other methods should be selected. The surgeon is responsible for selecting the position and ensuring that adequate exposure can be obtained. The operating room staff should understand the meaning of terms such as flexion, extension, abduction, and adduction when positioning a patient. Personnel should understand the function of the orthopedic surgical table and attachments. Attachments such as the leg attachment for arthroscopy, three-point positioner for lateral position, and positioning devices for shoulder procedures should also be familiar. The prin-

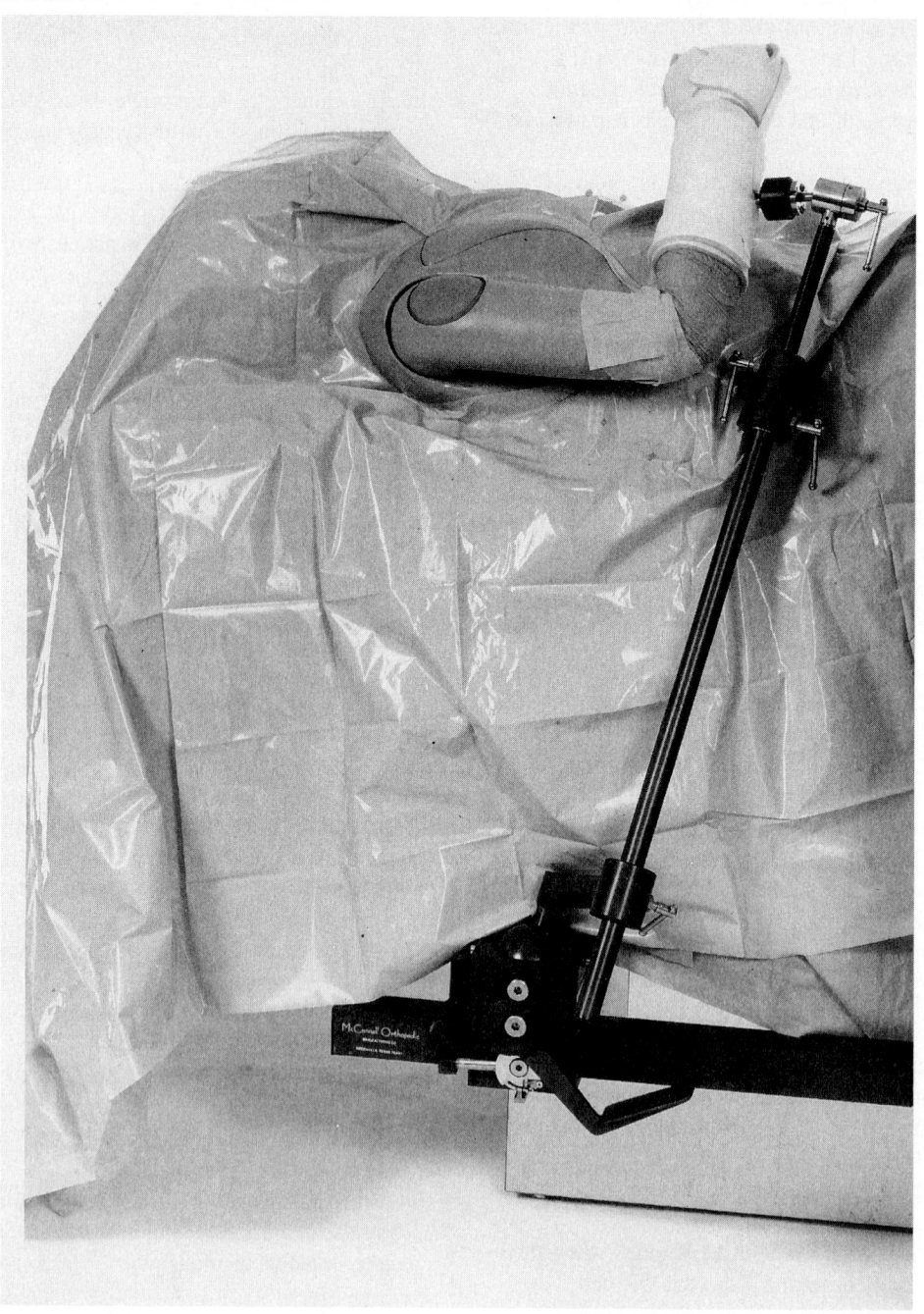

FIG. 21-13   Shoulder positioner, attached to the bed, allows distraction of the joint for visualization.
Courtesy McConnell Orthopaedic Manufacturing Co., Greenville, Tex.

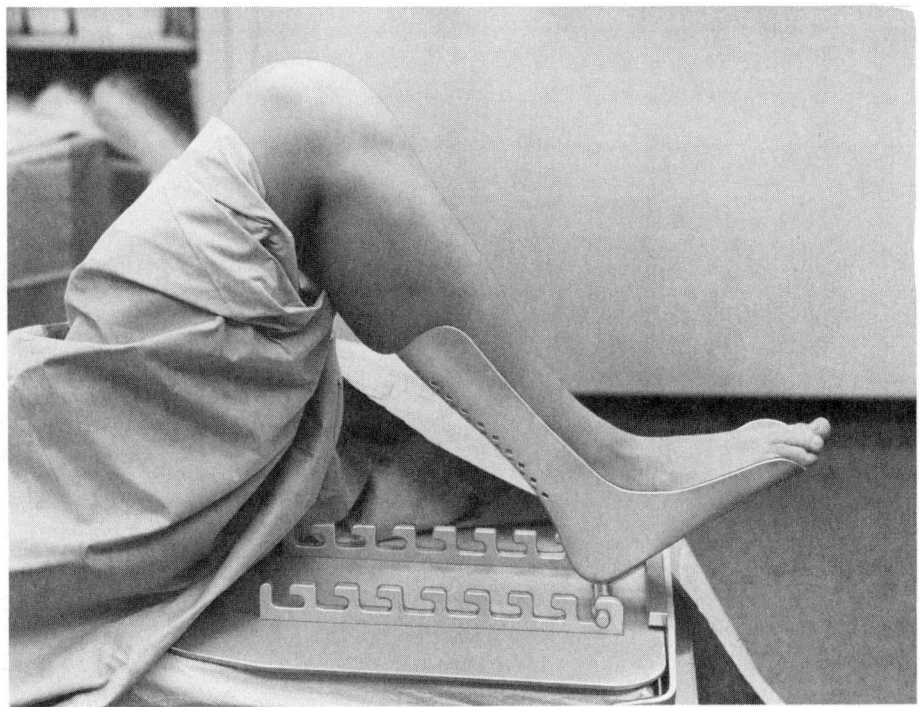

FIG. 21-14 Alvarado knee holder used during total joint procedures to position the extremity for exposure.
Courtesy Zimmer, Inc., Warsaw, Ind.

ciples of positioning and the different types of positions used in orthopedic surgery are described and illustrated in Chapter 4.

Many orthopedic operations require a device for holding the extremities. Various holders are available for holding both upper and lower extremities. Positioners used intraoperatively can be sterilized for the procedure, resulting in the ability to reposition as needed throughout the procedure. These types of positioners include the McConnell shoulder positioner (Fig. 21-13), Alvarado foot holder (Fig. 21-14), and ankle distractor (Fig. 21-15). Many other orthopedic positioning devices are available for procedures.

The lateral position is sometimes used for a total hip arthroplasty. Anterior and posterior supports are positioned at the umbilicus and lumbar region, respectively. These are secured to the bed and hold the patient in the lateral position. A vacuum bean bag can also achieve this position. Holding devices are padded and the patient is evaluated to ensure undue pressure is avoided. Pressure points on the lateral skull, ear, axilla, hip, knee, and ankle should be adequately padded. The anterior iliac crests, knees, anterior aspect of the ankle joint, ears, and eyes are critical areas to assess and protect from pressure. The feet are placed in the neutral position to prevent excessive plantar flexion or dorsiflexion. A conscientious effort should be made to avoid leaning on the patient to prevent injury.

The patient is positioned prone for surgery on the posterior aspect of the body, including the back, or posterior portion of the shoulder, arm, or leg. Surgery on the Achilles tendon and posterior iliac bone graft harvesting are often approached in this position. This position presents a challenge for the anesthesia team to monitor and manage the airway because of the potential for impairment of chest excursion and gas exchange. Extremities need to be brought through a normal range of motion when transferring and positioning into the prone position. Vascular integrity is always verified before moving and repeated after the patient is positioned.

The prone position is often attained with the use of adjunctive frames, such as the Wilson, Hastings, Canadian, Relton-Hall, and Andrews frames, or the Andrews bed (Fig. 21-16). Each frame has qualities that meet the patient or physician needs. The Hastings and Andrews frames and Andrews bed maintain the patient in a modified knee-chest position. The frames require assembly and are labor intensive when positioning; some can be used only with certain beds. The Andrews bed is similar to the frame but has the attachments built in and is used only for providing this position.

On a fracture table (Fig. 21-17), generally used for femoral neck and shaft fixation, the patient is placed in supine position to allow exposure to the surgical site and maintain alignment. The legs are positioned on outriggers, allowing access by the image intensifier to obtain multiple radiographic views. Applying or releasing traction can be done to reduce the fracture or aid in intramedullary surgical techniques. Like all positioning devices, the fracture table must be set up by experienced personnel and padded adequately.

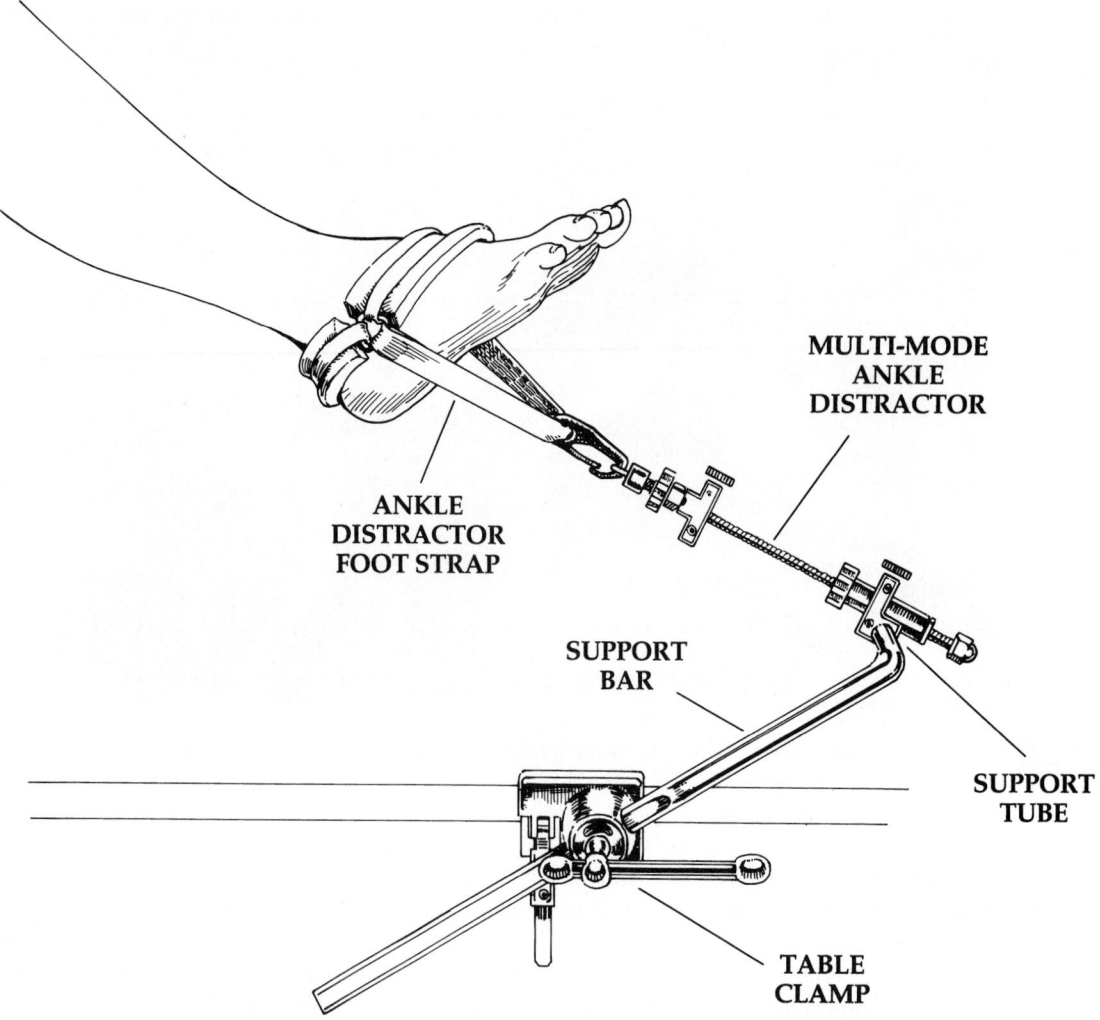

MULTI-MODE
ANKLE
DISTRACTOR

ANKLE
DISTRACTOR
FOOT STRAP

SUPPORT
BAR

SUPPORT
TUBE

TABLE
CLAMP

FIG. 21-15   Ankle distractor, noninvasive, for distraction of the joint and visualization.
Courtesy Acufex Microsurgical, Inc., Mansfield, Mass.

There are several moving parts, which can lead to injury if not operated properly.

Surgical prep

A primary concern in orthopedic surgery is the prevention of infection. The orthopedic surgical prep must be meticulously carried out using aseptic technique. Physicians often instruct patients to complete a scrub prep before arrival at the operating room with an antibacterial cleanser. The surgical prep for the orthopedic patient can include removal of hair from the surgical site followed by an intraoperative skin prep. Traumatic injury requires precautions during the skin prep to prevent further injury caused by solution contact with membranes or injury to the bone and soft tissue from movement.

Studies have shown that surgical shave preps could increase the possibility of infection caused by abrasion and cutting of the skin. If hair removal from the incisional site is necessary, it should occur immediately before surgery, using clippers or a depilatory. If the hair removal requires use of a razor, the site can be lubricated using soap before shaving (AORN, 1994).

Skin preparation is completed to remove transient microorganisms from the operative site. The site should be prepared with a broad-spectrum antimicrobial agent. The scrub prep might include using soap and water to remove superficial oil and skin debris. Povodine-iodine solutions are used to scrub the surgical area. The prep is applied using sterile gloves and supplies, proceeding from the incision site to the periphery. Pooling of the prep solution beneath the patient or tourniquet must be avoided (AORN, 1994). Excess solutions should be allowed to dry before draping. The groin and anal areas should be isolated when the surgical site is on the upper third of the leg.

Devices such as leg stirrups may help in supporting an extremity to complete a circumferential prep. When multiple extremities or other areas, such as a bone graft site, are prepped, cross-contamination of previously prepped areas must be prevented. Knowledge of aseptic technique and the ability to organize the activity are important in proper preparation of the surgical site.

Draping

Application of sterile drapes is the final step in preparing the patient for the operation. Extremities are covered with a cloth or impervious (waterproof) stockinette, a cylindrical drape that is rolled up the arm or leg. Strike-through must be prevented by using impervious sheets when a large amount of fluid is utilized, such as during arthroscopy and wound irrigation. Prefabricated disposable drapes with fenestration for the upper and lower extremity are available.

Disposable or reusable drapes may be used for orthopedic procedures, considering the ability to implement aseptic technique. Iodophor-impregnated adhesive drapes can be used to isolate the surrounding area from the incisional site. It has been reported that these drapes wall off the incisional area from the rest of the field, but there is also concern that a dark, moist area is created (Kneedler and Dodge, 1983).

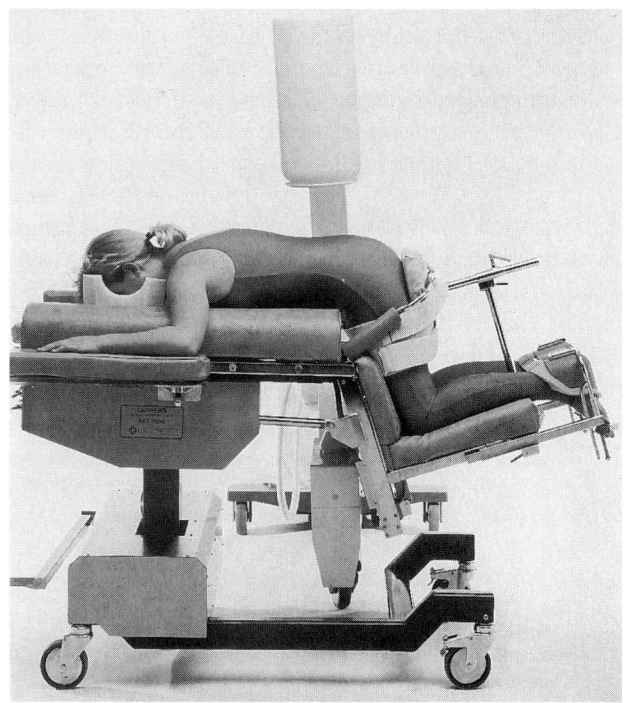

FIG. 21-16   Andrews bed used for prone positioning.
Courtesy OSI, Hayward, Calif.

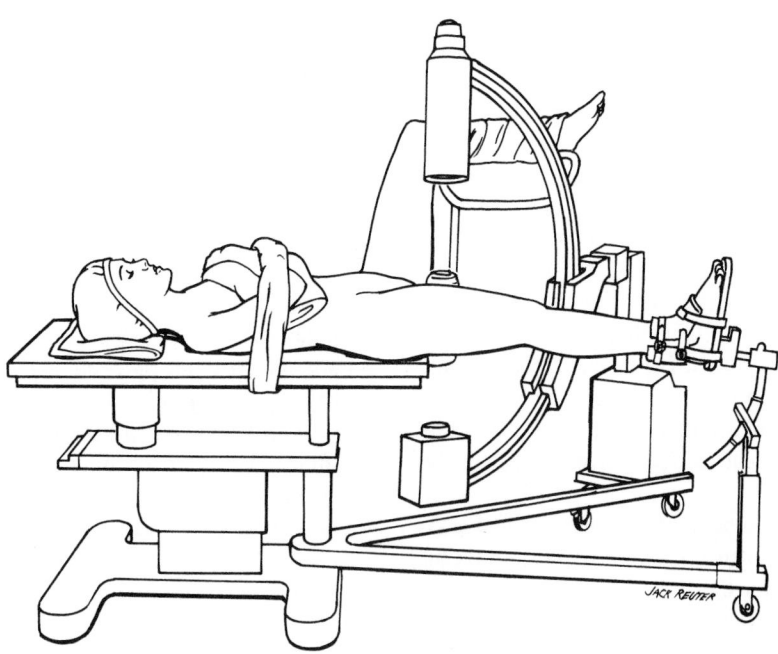

FIG. 21-17   Patient positioned on the orthopaedic fracture bed for femoral neck, femoral shaft fixation, or tibial fixation with image intensifier in position.
From Gregory B: *Perioperative Nursing Series: Orthopaedic Surgery,* St. Louis, 1994, Mosby.

Equipment and supplies

Orthopedic operating rooms require a variety of special equipment and accessories in addition to routine operating room equipment. Nitrogen, battery, and electric power equipment are commonplace in the modern orthopedic operating room. Video equipment, pneumatic tourniquets, laminar air flow systems, x-ray equipment, lasers, and special orthopedic tables are included in the operative armementarium. Manufacturers' pamphlets with illustrations and directions on equipment use and sterilization should be readily available for reference. Quality assurance programs should be in place to ensure continuous monitoring of function.

Radiographic intervention

Radiographic intervention is widely used in orthopedic surgery. Many procedures require portable x-ray or fluoroscopy for confirmation of results. The fluoroscopy, also known as image intensifier, allows the team to view the progression of the procedure. Fluoroscopy confirms fracture reduction or intramedullary reaming of the humerus, femur, or tibia. Radiographic equipment is operated by a technician. An understanding of equipment placement, function, and safety precautions is necessary. The operating room nurse is responsible for communicating with the radiology personnel concerning the procedure, aseptic technique, and traffic flow in the operating room. X-ray cassettes brought onto the sterile field are draped with a sterile plastic cover. Lead aprons and thyroid shields are to be worn by all personnel in close proximity to the x-ray equipment, and personnel should be monitored for exposure to radiation. Patients should be covered with lead aprons or protective devices in the appropriate areas if interference with the operative site can be avoided.

Pneumatic tourniquets

Pneumatic tourniquets are frequently used for procedures involving the extremities (Fig. 21-18). A tourniquet is a cylindrical bladder inflated by compressed gas or ambient air. It will produce a relatively bloodless surgical field with circumferential pressure on arterial and venous circulation. The limb is exsanguinated by elevating it or wrapping it distal to proximal with an Ace or Esmarch rubber bandage before incision. The majority of tourniquets used today are run by a microprocessor for regulation of pressure and time settings. Auditory and visual feedback is provided for the user.

Tourniquet safety should be a priority; the surgical team should understand recommended parameters and precautions. Safety guidelines for the use of tourniquets include preventive measures and evaluation (AORN, 1994). Preoperative assessment of the patient includes determining predisposition to contraindications for use, including compartment syndrome, McArdle's syndrome, hypertension, or other vascular problems. If the tourniquet must be used for patients with these conditions, guidelines for tourniquet use

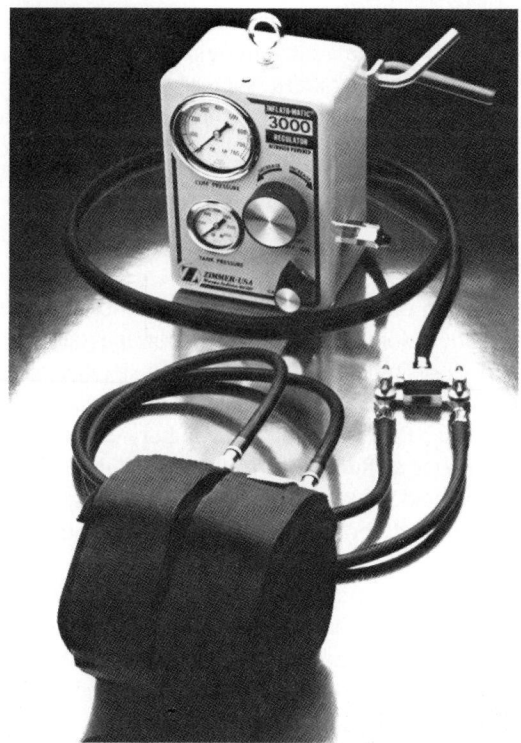

FIG. 21-18   Pneumatic gauge and tourniquet cuff.
Courtesy Zimmer, Inc., Warsaw, Ind.

must be observed. The tourniquet equipment should be checked for proper function, and personnel should be familiar with operation of equipment.

The exact pressure of inflation has not been determined. Inflation pressures are established based on the systolic blood pressure, age of the patient, and circumference of the extremity. Tourniquet inflation should be kept to a minimum. It is recommended in the average, healthy 50-year-old to apply continuous tourniquet pressure less than 1 hour on the upper extremity and 1½ hours on the thigh (Crenshaw, 1992).

The tourniquet should be placed in a location to eliminate compression on bony structures and superficial neurovascular structures. The cuff should be positioned as high as possible without pinching skin folds. Webril or stockinette is wrapped around the extremity and kept free of wrinkles and gathers beneath the cuff. Cuffs should overlap a minimum of 3 and maximum of 6 inches; excess overlap can pinch skin folds. A short tourniquet can predispose loosening after inflation. Care must be taken to ensure the line from the air supply to the cuff is not kinked.

Tourniquet equipment should be checked periodically and serviced when problems arise. Injury from tourniquets may result from inadequate precautions, faulty preparation, or use of inaccurate equipment. The gauges and other related equipment can be checked with commercially available test equipment. The patient evaluation requires immediate assessment of the extremity following removal of the

A   B   C

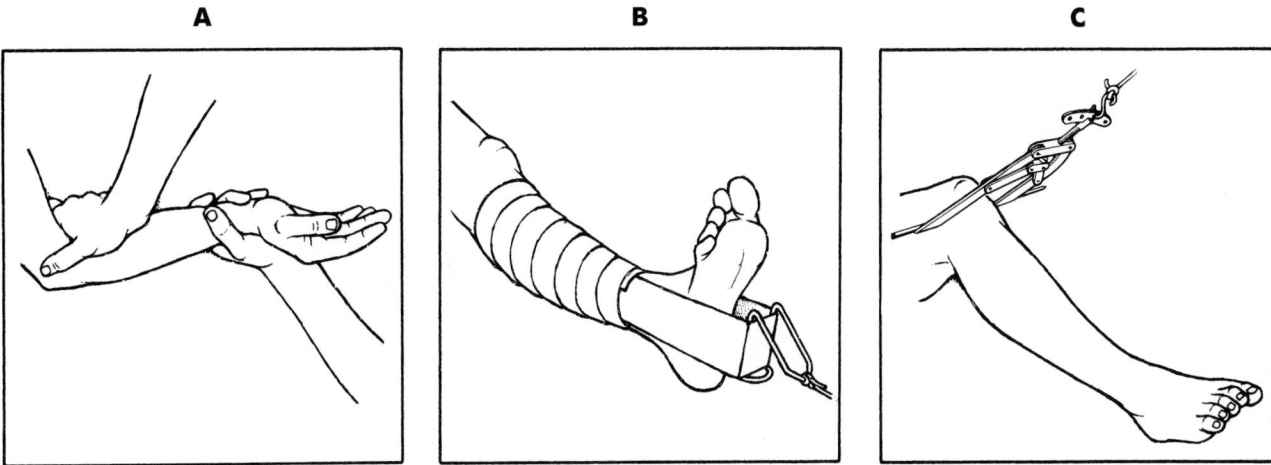

FIG. 21-19   Traction techniques including **A,** Manual, **B,** Skin and **C,** skeletal.
Courtesy Zimmer Traction Handbook, 1989, Zimmer, Inc.

tourniquet. Abnormal findings need to be reported to the surgeon and documented.

Traction

Traction is used preoperatively, intraoperatively, or postoperatively for prevention or reduction of muscle spasm, immobilization of a joint or body part, reduction of a fracture of dislocation, and treatment of joint pathology. Traction alignment must be constant.

Various traction techniques can be utilized, including manual, skin, and skeletal (Fig. 21-19). In manual traction the hands are the force pulling on the bone being realigned. Skin traction uses strips of tape, moleskin, or elastic bandage applied directly to the skin. Common forms of skin traction are Buck's extension and Russell traction. Skeletal traction applies forces directly to the bone using pins. Manual and skin traction can be done in the emergency room or patient room, whereas skeletal traction is done primarily in the emergency room preoperatively or in the operating room.

Skeletal traction is often used in conjunction with the fracture table using the traction attachment to aid in reduction of long bone fracture. Postoperatively the patient may be confined to bed with balanced skeletal traction using a Thomas splint (Fig. 21-20) and a Pearson attachment. Some cervical spine fractures or injuries may require Crutchfield or Gardner-Wells tongs inserted directly in the skull to stabilize the vertebrae and reduce spinal cord damage or further injury. Application of skeletal traction requires the use of sterile supplies, including a traction bow, pins, and drill (Fig. 21-21).

Traction frames are placed on the postoperative bed to accommodate traction immediately. Nursing care of the patient in traction should include ensuring the traction is continuous and skin tapes or skeletal pins secured. Neurovas-cular status should be checked routinely, including skin color, pulse, temperature, and sensation. Changes from baseline or normal need to be reported. Supplies and frames should be available and assembled before transferring the patient to the postoperative bed.

Postoperative immobilization

Postoperative immobilization may require use of a cast, splint, or other supplies designed for the anatomy. A cast is a method of immobilizing a fractured bone during healing. The forces of distraction, rotation, and malalignment are overcome with the application of a cast. Closed reduction with a cast may be possible, which minimizes the disadvantages and complications of open reduction, such as infection and tissue damage.

Casting is accomplished primarily with plaster or synthetic materials, such as fiberglass. Plaster is less expensive, with a greater weight-to-strength ratio (it requires greater weight of plaster to produce the same strength when using fiberglass). Plaster casts may be burdensome to some patients if too heavy. They are routinely used as the primary cast following surgical procedures and are replaced later with a lighter fiberglass cast to promote patient mobility.

Casting material sets up and hardens rapidly once activated with water, making it imperative to be prepared with all necessary materials. Webril or stockinette should be applied to the extremity under the cast to protect the skin from thermal injury while the plaster sets as well as undue abrasion and pressure. The plaster must be prepared, applied and handled carefully and safely.

Types of casts are shown in (Fig. 21-22). A short arm cast is applied from below the elbow to the knuckles following wrist fractures. A long arm cast is carried from above the elbow to the knuckles, immobilizing forearm or

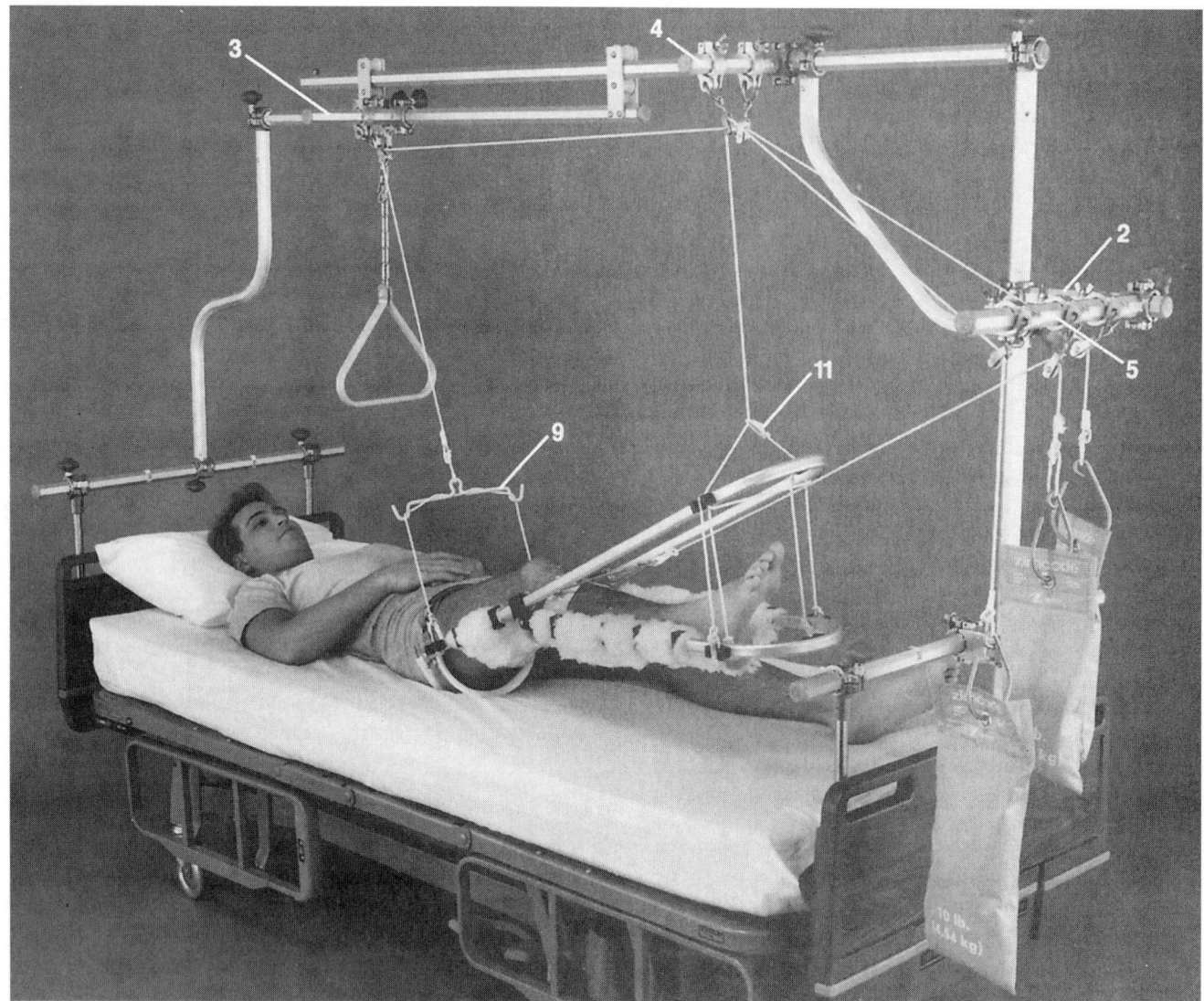

FIG. 21-20 Thomas splint balanced suspension.
Courtesy Zimmer Traction Handbook, 1989, Zimmer, Inc.

elbow fractures. The short leg cast is applied from below the knee to the toes to immobilize the ankle and foot. The long leg cast is utilized for fractures involving the femur, tibia, fibula or complicated ankle fractures. The femoral cast brace is used in the treatment of femoral shaft fractures. A snug-fitting thigh cast and short leg cast are hinged at the knee joint. The cast brace is generally used after 4 to 6 weeks of skeletal traction following initiation of callus formation at the fracture site. A cylinder cast incorporates the leg from the groin to the ankle and is applied when complete knee immobilization is required. This is often required after surgery involving soft tissue reconstruction around the knee.

The hip spica cast is used when complete leg immobilization is desired. The trunk, affected side, and unaffected side may all be incorporated into the cast. Spinal immobi-

lization is accomplished with a body jacket.

Splints are also employed for postoperative immobilization but are not cylindrical and allow for swelling. Closer observation of the surgical area is possible with the use of splints.

Another immobilization device is the abduction pillow (Fig. 21-23), used after total joint replacement. This prevents leg adduction, internal rotation, and hip flexion, which could dislocate the hip. Further discussion of this and other devices is included in the section on surgical interventions.

Lasers

Lasers accomplish cutting and coagulating using minimally invasive techniques. Laser application has been increasing in the field of orthopedics. Their use mandates

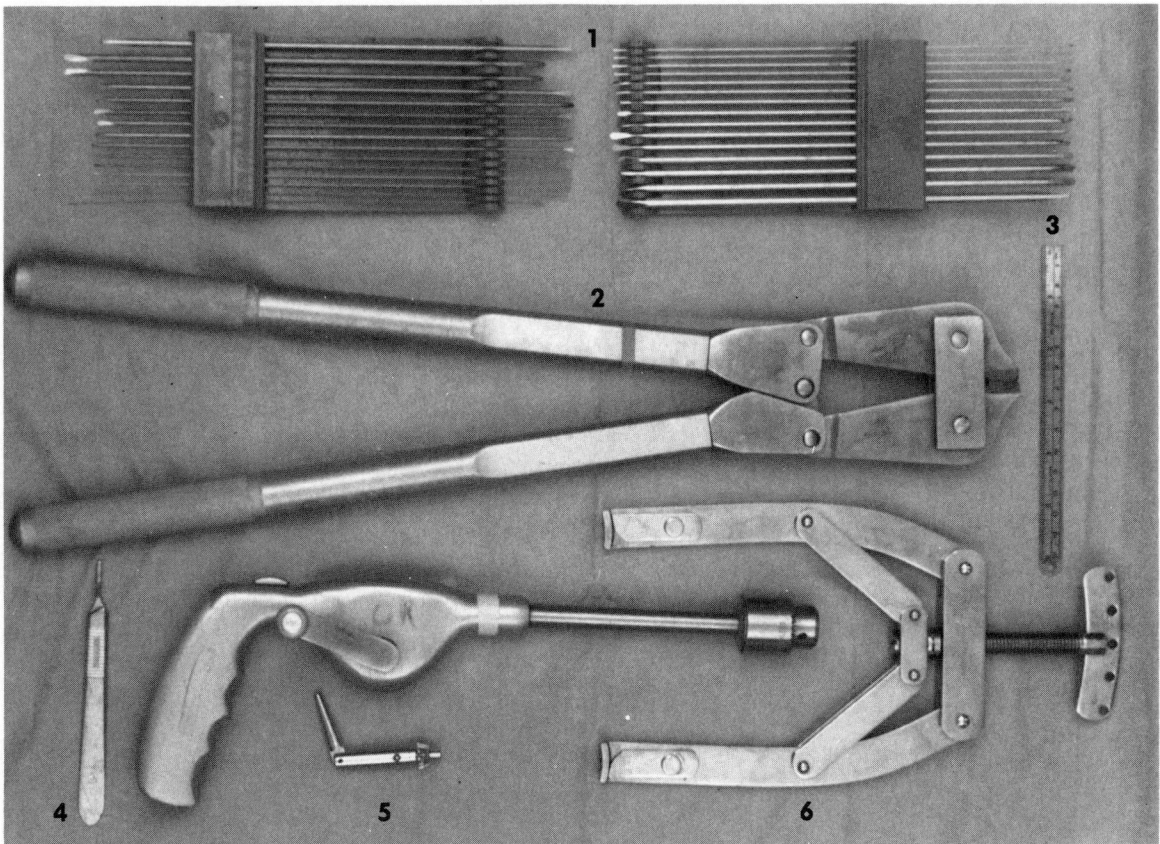

FIG. 21-21 Instruments for insertion of skeletal traction: *1*, Kirschner wires and Steinman pins; *2*, Bolt cutter; *3*, Ruler; *4*, Knife handle (using no. 15 blade); *5*, Hand drill with chuck key; *6*, Traction bow.

safety precautions, certification, patient consent, and protective attire. Laser types include carbon dioxide, holmium, neodymium:YAG, KTP, erbium, and excimer. Laser technique differs for use on bone, muscle, tendon, and cartilage. Lasers have been used successfully for osteotomy, revision arthroplasty (removal of PMMA), nerve and tendon repair, arthroscopy, and diskectomy (Sherk, 1990).

Airflow control

Airflow control in the orthopedic operating room has been a concern due to the need to prevent introduction of microorganisms. Postoperative infections may result from airborne bacteria or transient bacteria from the patient or surgical team. Laminar airflow is a system designed to provide highly filtered air and continuous air exchange for reducing airborne bacteria. Body exhaust suits (Fig. 21-24) are also used as defense airborne bacteria. Aseptic practices and conscientious behaviors in operating rooms using conventional airflow can be used to maintain low rates of wound infections. The addition of other protective measures should be weighed to determine the benefit and outcome (McQuarrie, Glover, and Olson, 1990).

Postoperative management equipment

Postoperative management equipment used for the patient is planned during the preoperative period. Special equipment may include continuous passive range of motion machines, pain management techniques, compression devices, and blood salvage. Continuous passive range of motion (CPM) machines (Fig. 21-25) are frequently used following total knee arthroplasty, surgical repair of supracondylar fractures, total elbow arthroplasty, total shoulder arthroplasty, femoral shaft fracture fixation, and, less frequently, in total hip arthroplasty. It is also used following rotator cuff repair and removal of loose bodies. CPM stimulates the healing effect on articular tissues including cartilage, tendon, and ligaments. The benefits of CPM include inhibition of adhesion formation and joint stiffness, decreased pain and swelling, early functional range of motion, and decreased effects of immobilization (Smith, 1990). It does not interfere with healing incisions over the moving joint. The device is applied early in the postoperative period (Research Highlight 21-3).

Pain management may include insertion of an epidural catheter or use of the patients controlled analgesia (PCA) pump. The PCA pump administers a predetermined intra-

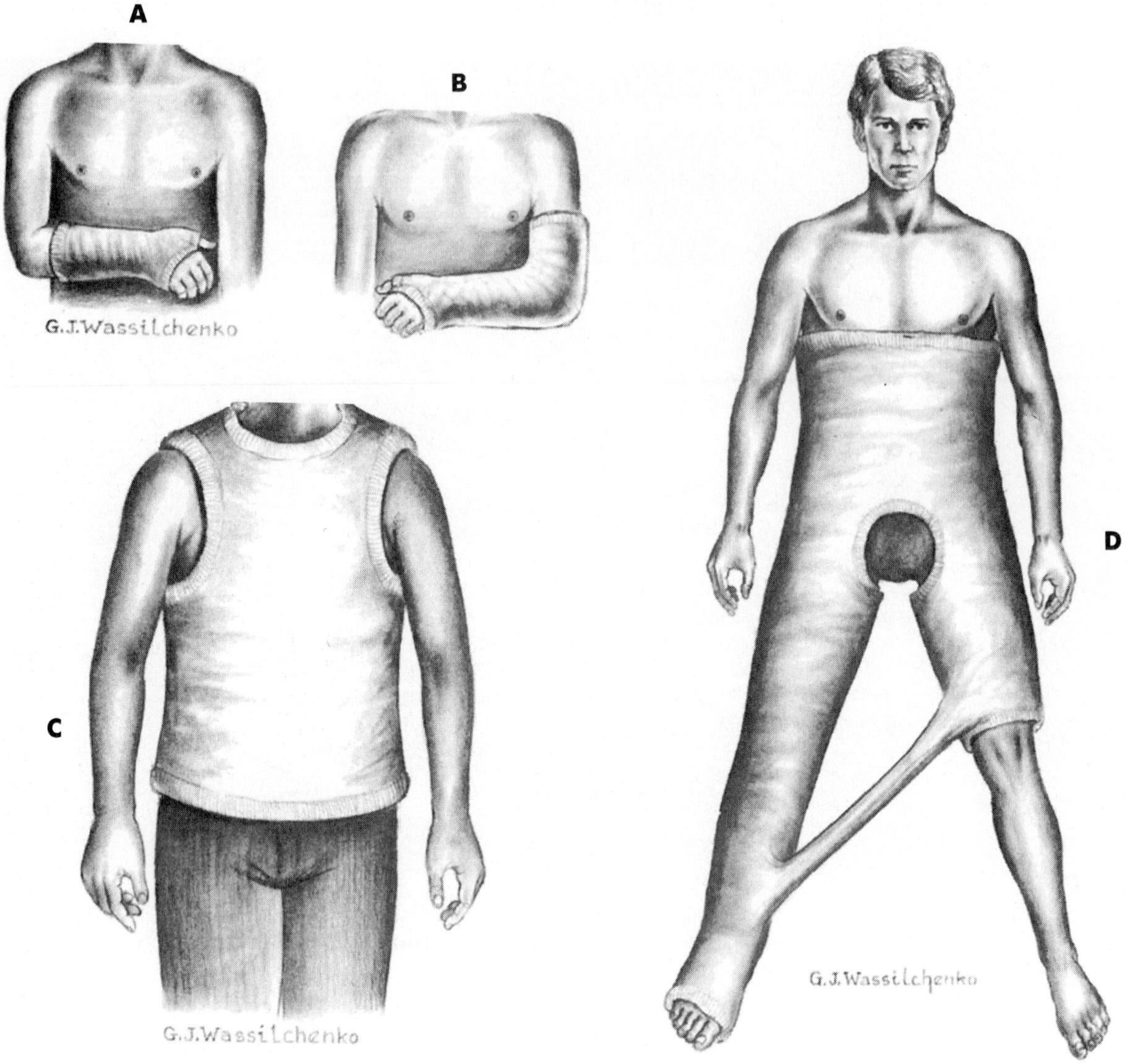

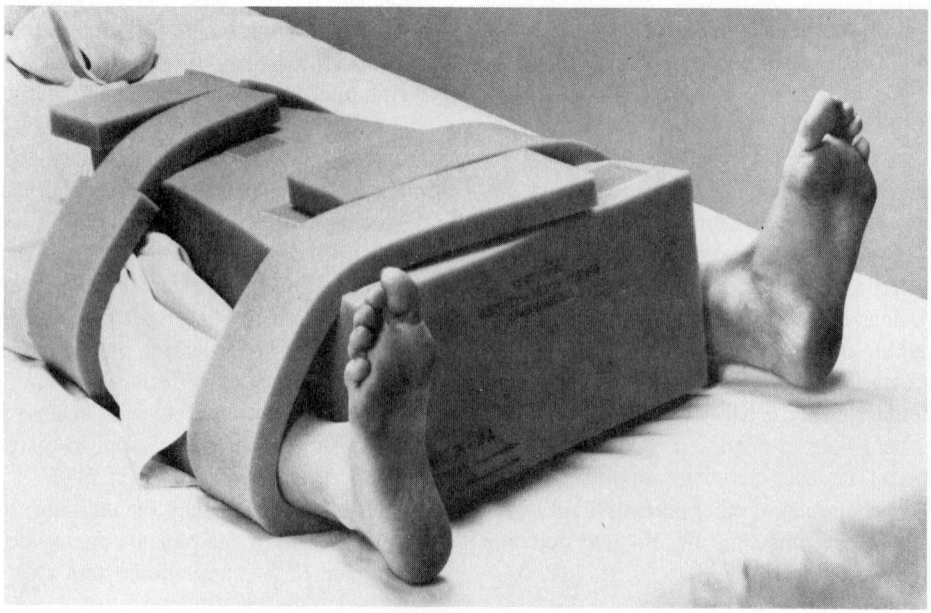

FIG. 21-22 Types of casts. **A,** Short arm cast. **B,** Long arm cast. **C,** Plaster body jacket cast. **D,** One and one-half hip spica cast.

From Thompson JM et al: *Mosby's manual of clinical nursing*, ed 2, St. Louis, 1989, The CV Mosby Co.

FIG. 21-23 Abduction pillow aids in immobilizing hip joints after surgery.

Courtesy of Span & Aids, McGaw Park, Ill.

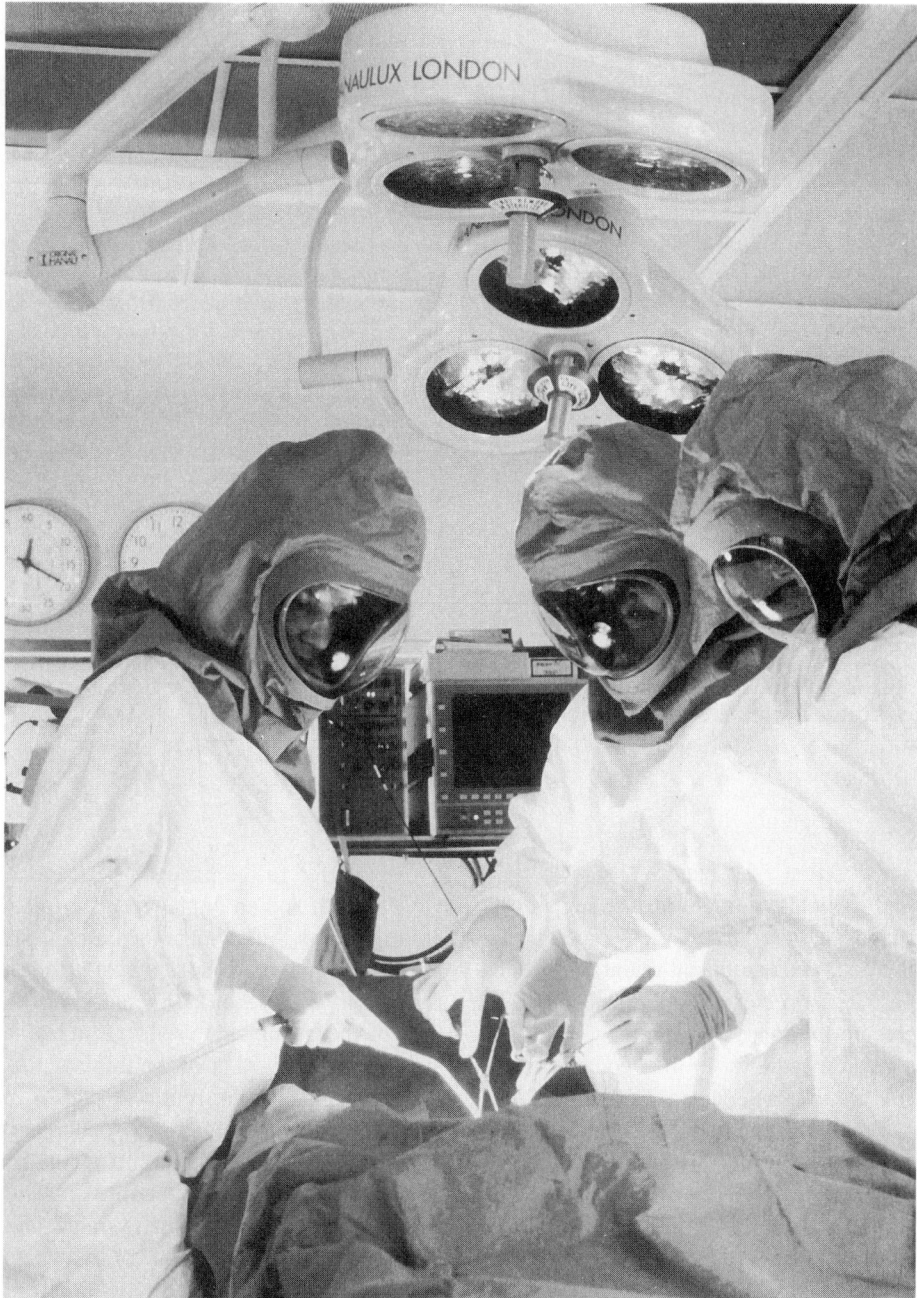

FIG. 21-24   Body exhaust system.
Courtesy DePuy, Inc., Warsaw, Ind.

venous dose of narcotic substitute for pain relief. It allows a continuous of analgesic and bolus administration when the patient believes this is necessary. The advantages include rapid pain relief, increased patient satisfaction, and often less use of medication than with traditional intramuscular analgesia.

Management of fluid and electrolyte balance may include use of intraoperative autologous transfusion or postoperative blood salvage (Research Highlight 21-4). A potential problem with salvage of large amounts of blood is depletion of clotting factors; therefore coagulation problems should be identified. Postoperative blood salvage is accomplished with a closed drainage system. It requires an understanding of the system for safe use.

Instruments and accessory items

Orthopedic surgical procedures require an extensive inventory of instruments and implants. Successful management and optimal patient care are dependent on a well-stocked inventory of the specific instruments required to im-

---
※

RESEARCH HIGHLIGHT 21-3

Seventy-four patients were assessed following total knee arthroplasty to determine the role of this therapy in postoperative rehabilitation, considering the benefits of early use on the outcome. Complication rates were also compared. Patients in the CPM group were found to have a lower incidence of complications, especially wound healing and thromboembolic disease. Analgesic use was reduced. Leg raising was achieved slightly earlier, but the long-term review of range of motion was equal. It was concluded that CPM was effective in improving many results but not effective in improving the ultimate range of motion of the knee following arthroplasty. (Wasilewski, Woods, Torgerson, Healy 1990).

Wasilewski, S.A., et al. (1990). Value of continuous passive motion in total knee arthroplasty. *Orthopedics, 13*.

※

RESEARCH HIGHLIGHT 21-4

Complications of bloodborne disease and related complications have increased the emphasis on use of autologous blood transfusion techniques. Autologous blood is considered the safest type of blood transfusion, eliminating risk of infection and alloimmunization. Autotransfusion programs include autologous deposit, immediate preoperative plasma and platelet collection, intraoperative salvage, and use of postoperative blood salvage. It has been suggested that preoperative blood volume calculations and hemoglobin concentrations would enable a cautious approach to transfusion. Studies comparing use of autoreinfusion devices may be costly and increase potential risks to the patient.

Evans, R.L, et al (1993). The efficacy of postoperative autotransfusion in total joint arthroplasty. *Orthopaedic Nursing, 12:3*. Faris, P.M. et al. (1991). Unwashed filtered shed blood collected after knee and hip arthroplasties: A source of autologous red blood cells. *The Journal of Bone and Joint Surgery*, 73-A (8), 1169-1177. Tate, D.E. & Freidman, R.J. (1992). Blood conservation in spinal surgery: Reveiw of current techniques. *Spine*, 17(12), 1450.

plant and apply hardware. Revision surgery requires that the operating staff is prepared with the appropriate tools and extractors needed to remove an old implant and an understanding of equipment use.

Implant inventories

Implant inventories consist of plates and screws, intramedullary nails and rods, total joint implants, and a host of accessory items. Consideration is given to surgeon preference, patient population, and equipment initial cost when selecting stock items. These items must be stocked in a timely fashion to prepare for consecutive implant use.

Strict guidelines are now required by the Food and Drug Administration (FDA) in proper documenting and tracking of implant devices. The documentation should include but

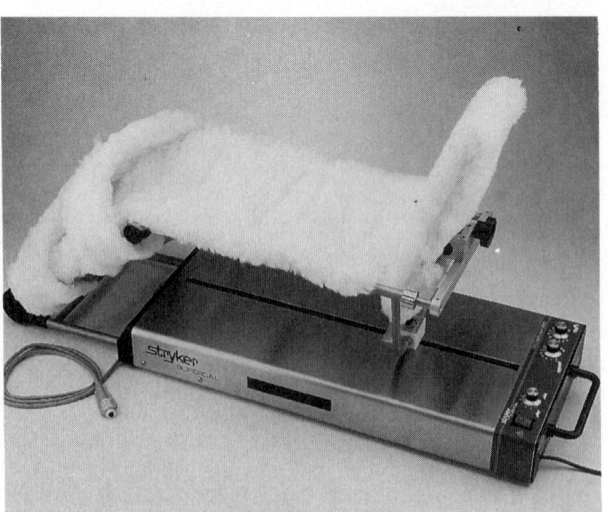

FIG. 21-25   Continuous passive motion machine used for passive range of motion.

not be limited to the patient's permanent record, the operative record, and an implant registry maintained by the operating rooms. Many manufacturers now include mailers to return information to the company for data collection. Information to be recorded includes the lot and serial numbers of those implants used, the manufacturer, size, type, and anatomic position of the implant.

Many implants are routinely part of modern orthopedic inventory. Inventories should be organized by manufacturer, type of implant (total hip versus knee), and comparative sizes. There are numerous implant systems in stock in operating rooms, and many more that may come in to the hospital on a loaner or consignment basis. Staff must be familiar with the varied types and refer to manufacturer information pertaining to each implant. Practices should ensure the correct implant is opened on the operative field to prevent unnecessary expense or error in placement.

Many different alloys are used in the manufacturing of implants. However, the implantation of devices with different metallic composition must be avoided to prevent galvanic corrosion; internal fixation implants used during an orthopedic procedure should be of the same metal. Screws, for example, should be of the same composition as the metal plate affixed to the bone. Alloys most frequently used include stainless steel, cobalt-chromium, and titanium-vanadium-aluminum.

Internal fixation devices should never be reused due to resulting imperfections, scratches, and weakening of the implant. Literature refers to the effect of scratches and abrasions on the strength of an orthopedic implant, and to the

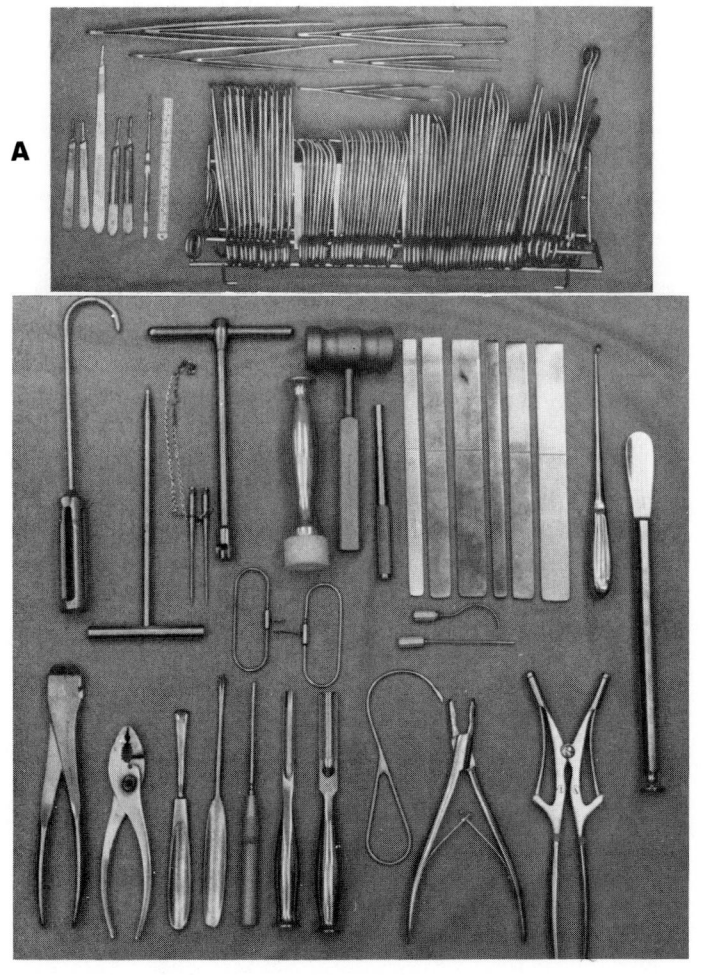

FIG. 21-26 Instrumentation used for hip procedures includes **A**, *Left to right* top: St. Mary's retractors. *Middle:* Adson-Beckman retractor, Aufranc femoral neck retractors (superior and inferior), *Bottom:* Richardson, Army-Navy, Hohmann retractor (narrow, blunt and sharp, broad and extrabroad sharp), Volkman (sharp, blunt) Weitlaners, initial incision with blades and ball-and-chain retractors. **B,** *(left to ride) Top:* Bone hook, femoral head extractor, pin retractors with T-handle extractor, femoral prosthesis driver, mallet, bone tamp, osteotomes (curved, straight) no. 2 angled Brun curette. *Middle:* Gigli saw handles, small wire passers, (curved, straight) Watson-Jones gouge (hip skid). *Bottom:* Pin cutter, pliers, Langenbeck periosteal elevators (wide, narrow), navicular gouge, Smith Peterson gouge (3/8, 5/8), Charnley trochanteric wire passer, Adson-cranial rongeur, Harris wire tightener.

potential for increased corrosion where scratches occur (Gustilo, 1993). These imperfections are inevitable with use. Bending implants to conform to the contour of the bone should be avoided whenever possible to prevent loss of strength. When bending is necessary, the proper bending press should be used. Once an implant is bent, it should not be reshaped or straightened or it might weaken the implant.

Orthopedic equipment and implants require special care, storage, and handling. When possible, implants should be individually wrapped and processed. Most implants today, excluding some plates and screws, are separately packaged by the manufacturer. During sterilization, implants should not be placed in a position in which knocking or bumping might occur. Appropriate sterilizing cases and trays should be used, and implants should be sterilized according to the manufacturer's instructions. An internal fixation device that has become damaged as a result of improper storage or handling must be discarded.

The orthopedic operating room nurse should have a working knowledge of the general types and sizes of implants that might be selected. Radiographs are often templated preoperatively, providing a general idea of the size of the implants needed.

Orthopedic instrumentation

Orthopedic instrumentation varies from very small to large instruments. Some procedures require multiple containers. Organization of instrument sets for multiple uses prevents the need for duplication and requires thoughtful consideration of anatomic and physiologic needs. When preparing for a procedure the nurse should open the minimum of instruments, yet be prepared for unexpected or untoward events. Careful planning and preparation of instrumentation will ensure efficient utilization of time and equipment.

Instruments that do not function properly (as a result of dullness, poor adjustment, lack of lubrication, damage, improper fit, or incomplete cleaning) are primary sources of complaints and problems in the operating room. Instrument maintenance is vital to ensure availability for the procedure and ease in completion. Instruments should be used for the intended purpose during the procedure. Movable parts should be lubricated after each cleaning and checked for cracks or damage following each use. The perioperative nurse is responsible for instrument maintenance and familiarity with sterilization and packaging procedures.

The following basic bone instrument sets should be available in the orthopedic operating room. Soft tissue in-

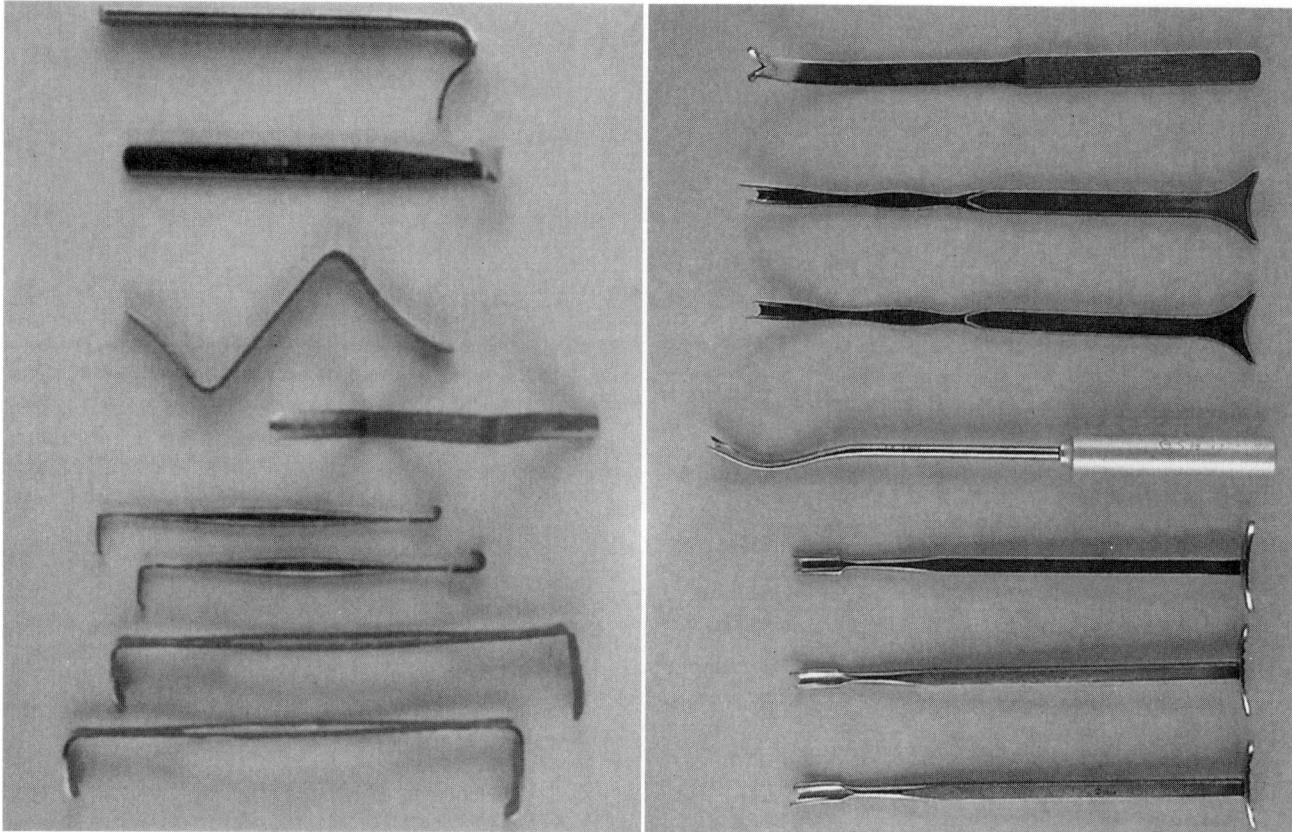

FIG. 21-27   Instrumentation used for procedures on the knee *top to bottom* **A**, 2 Blount knee retractors; 2 Doane knee retractors; 2 Miller-Senn retractors; 2 Army-Navy retractors **B**, 3 Smillie cartilage knives (left, right, straight); 1 Downing cartilage knife (meniscectomy knife); 2 Smillie cartilage knives (top, bottom); 1 McKeever cartilage knife;

strument sets appropriate for the size of the anatomic site are used for procedures not requiring bone instruments or in addition to the sets. Additional instruments and special equipment are mentioned in the section on surgical intervention.

> *Incision hip set:* total hip arthroplasty or fractures of the neck and proximal femur (Fig. 21-26)
>
> *Total knee set:* total knee arthroplasty or supracondylar and distal femoral fractures (Fig. 21-27)
>
> *Shoulder set:* shoulder arthroplasty and other shoulder procedures (Fig. 21-28)
>
> *Large bone set:* bone work on the large bones including hip, knee, upper arm, and elbow (Fig. 21-29)
>
> *Extremity or small bone set:* bone work on the hand or foot (Fig. 21-30)
>
> *Fusion/bone graft instruments:* additional instruments necessary for an autograft (Fig. 21-31)

Powered surgical instruments

Powered surgical instruments (Fig. 21-32) used in the operating room have eliminated the need for many hand-operated tools, thereby reducing operative time and improving technical results. They are available as air, battery, or electrical driven equipment. Fingertip control provides the surgeon speed and power. Variable speed saws, drills, and reamers offer wide flexibility but require an understanding of compatibility between equipment. These instruments are extremely powerful and high speed. Power equipment has a safety control that prevents inadvertent activation, which should be engaged when passing the instrument to the surgeon. Power equipment should not be rested on the patient when not in use.

While using power instruments, it is important to be aware of the manufacturer's recommended cleaning and lubricating instructions. With proper care, powered tools have a long life span and many uses.

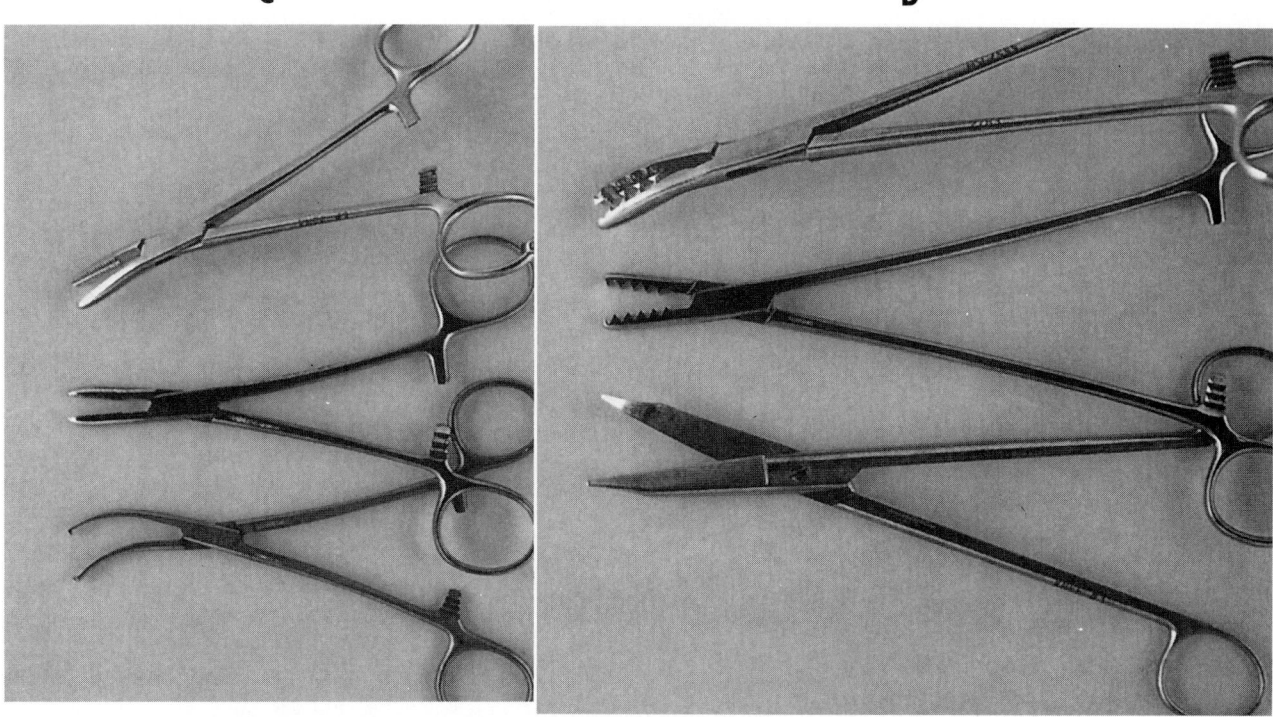

FIG. 21-27 cont'd.   Knee instruments used for procedures on the knee.

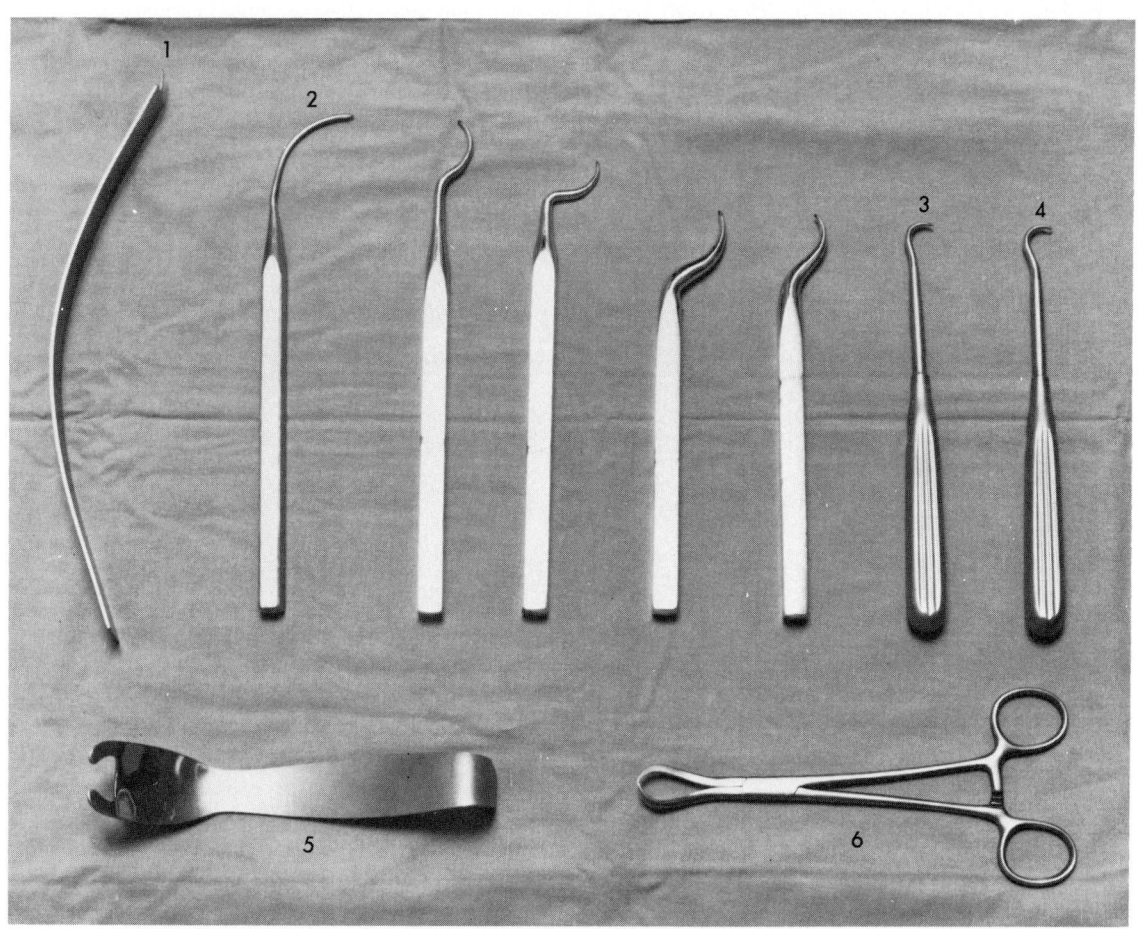

FIG. 21-28   Bankart instruments. *1*, Rowe capsule retractor (pitch fork); *2*, Five Rowe glenoid punches; *3*, Curved awl; *4*, Ligature retriever; *5* Humeral head retractor; *6*, Glenoid reaming forceps.

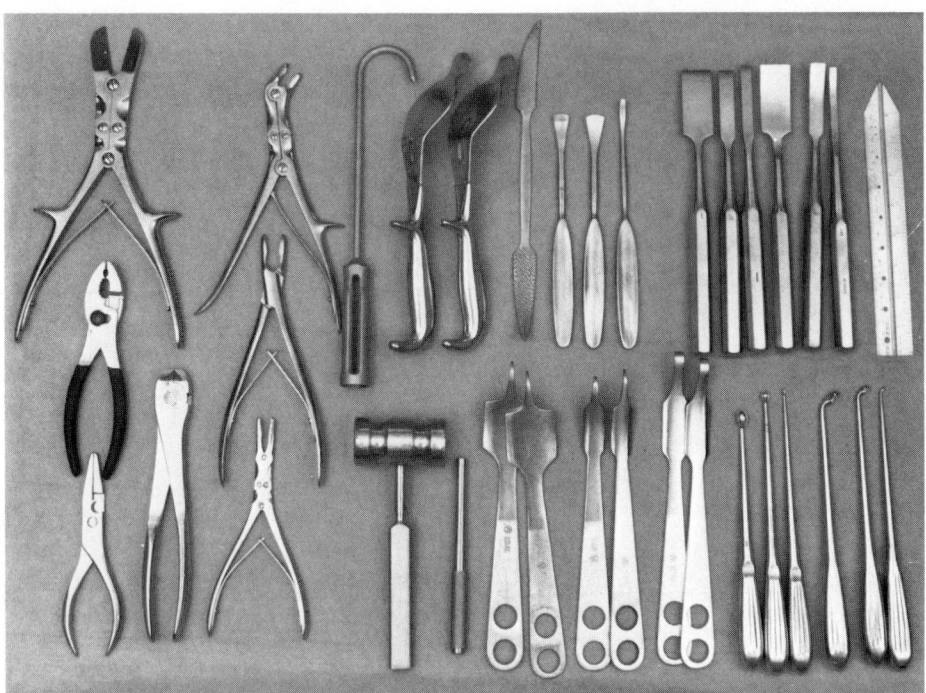

FIG. 21-29   Large bone set: *(left to right) Top:* Stille-Liston bone-cutting forceps, Stille-Leur rongeur, bone hook, Bennett retractors, rasp, Langenbeck periosteal elevators (wide and narrow), Cushing periosteal elevators, osteotomes (straight, curved) ruler, *Middle:* pliers, Adson-cranial rongeur, *bottom:* needle-nosed pliers, pin cutter, Zaufal-Jansen rongeur, mallet, bone tamp, Hohmann retractors (wide sharp, narrow sharp and blunt), curettes (straight, curved).

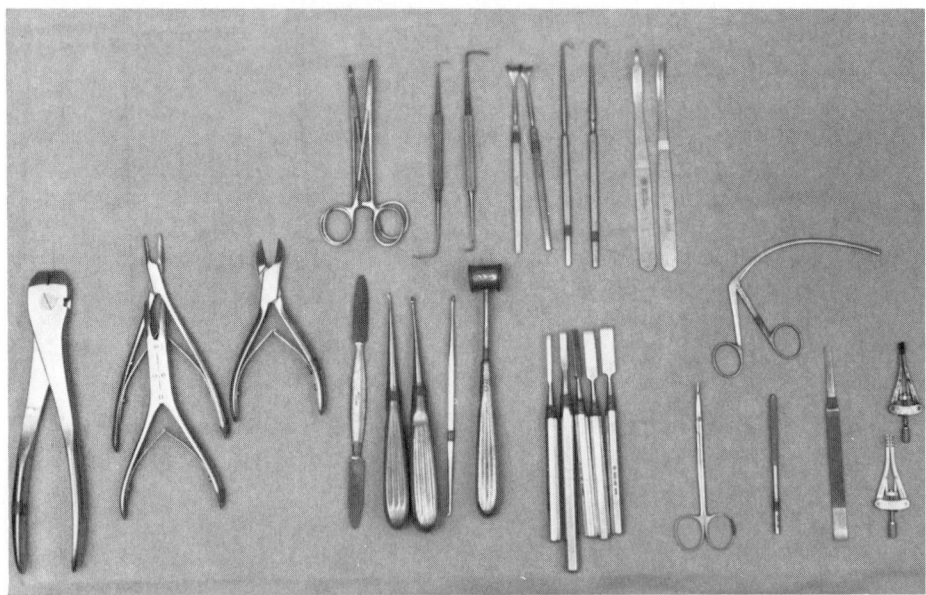

FIG. 21-30   Extremity or small bone set *(left to right) Top:* baby Mixters, Ragnell retractors, Alm retractors, Volkman hooks, mini Hohmann retractors. *Bottom:* pin cutter, Lempert and Carroll rongeurs, Liston bone cutter, bone rasp, small curettes, fine double-ended curette, small mallet, Hoke osteotomes, Litler scissors, tendon passer, Beaver blade handle, Carroll elevator, Miltex self-retaining retractors.

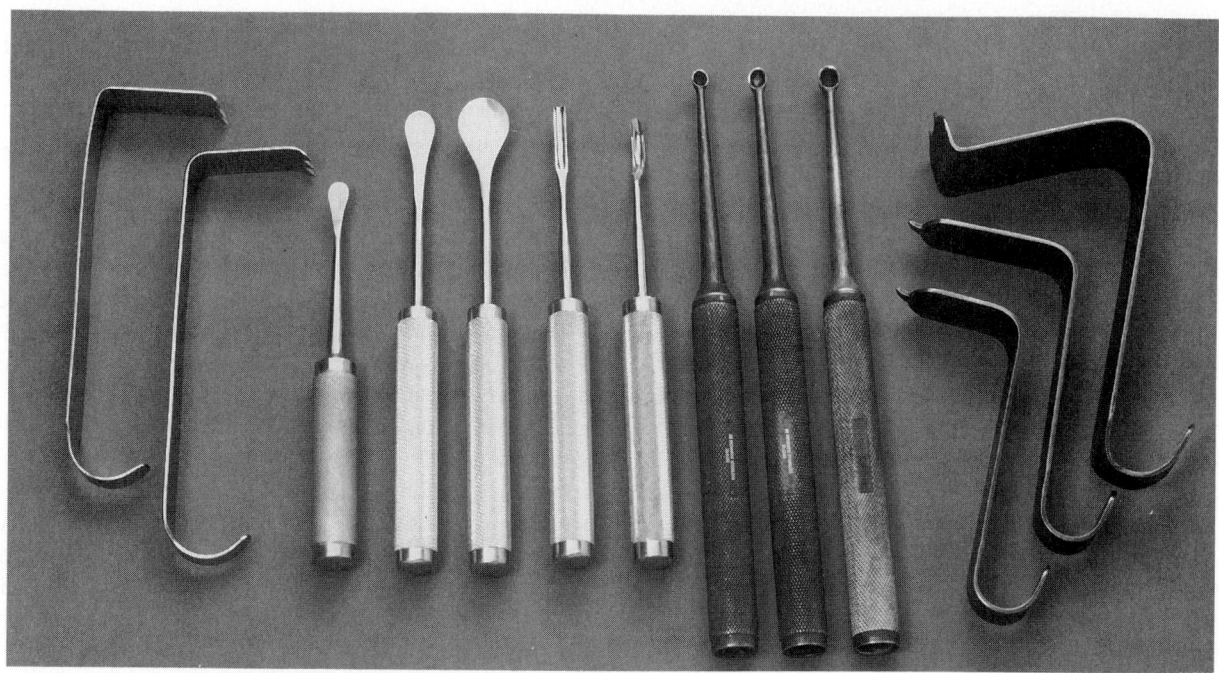

FIG. 21-31 Fusion/bone graft instruments. *Left to right:* Hibbs retractors, Cobb periosteal elevators, Cobb gouges, McElroy curettes, spinal retractors and iliac graft retractor.

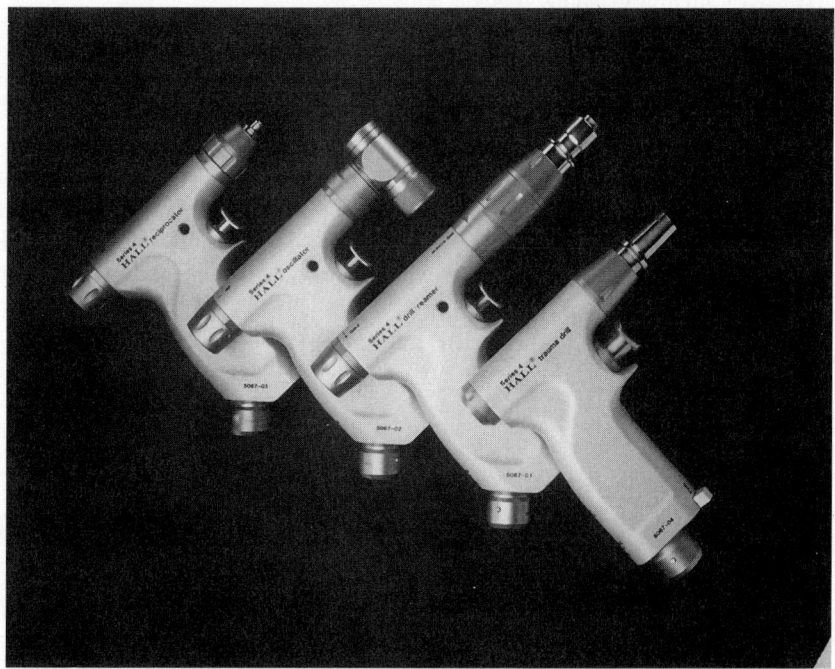

FIG. 21-32 Pneumatic powered surgical instruments for large bone procedures: reciprocating saw, the oscillating saw, the drill/reamer and the trauma drill.

Courtesy Hall Surgical Division, Carpinteria, Calif.

Suture material

Suture material requires increased tensile strength and minimal degradability for the type of tissue. Tendons and ligaments are fibrous, avascular tissues, resulting in a slower healing process that tissues rich in blood supply. Absorbable suture may be used for sewing tendon or ligaments to bone. Nonabsorbable suture, including polyester and surgical steel, are also used. For various ligament replacement grafts a harvested tendon may be customized with multiple strands of suture material, increasing tensile strength and length of time until fibrous union occurs.

Polymethyl methacrylate

Polymethyl methacrylate (bone cement) (PMMA) is a polymer consisting of a liquid and powder component which react and cure after being mixed together. Bone cement chemically resembles Plexiglas, with barium added to make it radiopaque. The resultant fumes when bone cement is mixed can be noxious and possibly harmful to persons in close proximity. Many special hoods and mixing devices are available to minimize staff exposure to the fumes.

Adverse effects of PMMA are hypotension, cardiac arrest, cerebral vascular accident, pulmonary embolus, and thrombophlebitis (Howmedica, 1979). Cardiac arrest and death are less common but have resulted following insertion of bone cement. This has been attributed to pressurization of the cement in the canal and also a chemical/blood reaction that the patient may suffer. Research remains to be done to discover the cause of adverse reactions. Patient care should include monitoring for side effects. Cement and preparation techniques are mentioned later in the chapter.

Medications

Medications delivered in the operating room require the same precautions as other specialty areas. Antibiotics, hemostatics, and antibacterial agents are used commonly. Antibiotics are delivered both intravenously and locally in the irrigation. The intravenous antibiotic of choice is a recent generation cephalosporin. Various antibiotics utilized in the irrigation include polymixin and bacitracin. Irrigation may also be delivered using pulsatile lavage, with antibiotics added to the solution. Hemostatic agents may include Gelfoam, thrombin, Avitene, and bone wax. Antibacterial ointments are impregnated in gauze dressing (Xeroform) or applied before the application of the dressing. Other medications used during orthopedic procedures include steroids, local anesthetics, and normal saline.

Protective measures

Protective measures are taken in the perioperative environment during procedures or when handling patient-exposed trash, linen, or instruments. Frequent use of radiography also requires use of leaded aprons, gloves, thyroid shields, and other devices for the personnel or patient. Orthopedic procedures require caution due to the use of fluids for irrigation or bloody procedures. Personnel protective measures include handling items (blades, sharp instruments, and bone) cautiously to prevent inadvertent punctures or cuts and wearing protective eyewear and cover attire, including gowns and boots. Sharp bone edges are also a hazard, and can puncture latex gloves and skin. Double gloving or use of protective gloves should be employed to protect the patient and personnel. Nonlatex gloves have been developed for personnel with sensitivity to latex.

EVALUATION

Evaluation is an ongoing process, occurring throughout the procedure. The perioperative nurse evaluates the patient considering the nursing diagnosis and attainment of outcomes. This part of the nursing process provides feedback as to the effectiveness of the plan and implementation and alterations needed for improving patient care.

The evaluation process validates nursing care. Was the patient protected from peripheral neurovascular injury? Was he or she free from injury? Was adequate oxygenation maintained? Does the patient have more questions pertaining to the recovery phase? The answers will dictate whether there is a need to maintain or modify the plan. The evaluation information is shared with the nurse caring for this patient postoperatively to provide continuity of care.

The following outcomes should be accomplished for the orthopedic patient:

- The patient demonstrated verbal and nonverbal cues, indicating that the level of apprehension was minimized as the procedure progressed.
- The patient was free from peripheral neurovascular compromise on discharge to the postoperative area as evidenced by presence of pulses, warmth of the extremity, capillary refill of the fingers, toes of the affected extremity, intact movement, and sensation.
- The patient was free from injury due to transfer, positioning, and untoward events during the operative phase as evidenced by maintenance of skin integrity and absence of reddened areas.
- The patient maintained adequate ventilation/perfusion as evidenced by blood gases and arterial saturation during the operative procedure, vital signs within normal limits, and hemorrhage not present.
- The patient was free from infection as evidenced by temperature within normal limits, incision site clean and dry without visual signs of infection.

Bone healing processes

The healing process involves several stages (Fig. 21-33). When a bone is damaged, such as during a surgical procedure or fracture, bleeding occurs. The amount of extravasated blood depends on the vascularity of the fracture site. The blood exudate infiltrates the surrounding area, where a clot is formed. Fibroblasts invade the hematoma and form a fibrin meshwork.

As osteoblasts invade the fibrin meshwork, blood vessels develop to build collagen. After several days, calcium

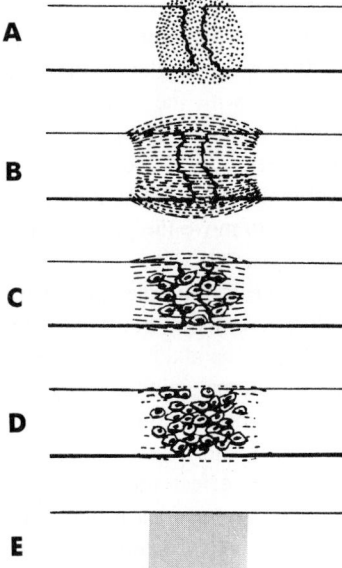

FIG. 21-33   Bone healing process: **A,** Hematoma formation. **B,** Fibrin network formation. **C,** Invasion of osteoblasts. **D,** Callus formation, and **E,** remodeling.

From Phipps WJ, Long BC, and Woods NF: *Medical-surgical nursing,* St. Louis, 1987, The CV Mosby Co.

deposits may form in the granulation tissue. These deposits eventually form new bone, known as callus. Within the callus, cartilage cells develop a temporary semirigid tissue that helps stabilize the bone fragments. The callus is immature bone that is remodeled by new connective tissue cells (osteoblasts) of the periosteum and the inner membrane of the bone cavity. Through this process, mature bone is formed, excess callus is reabsorbed, and trabecular bone is laid down.

After several months, depending on the age and physical condition of the individual, the bone becomes firmly united, although the ossification process is not yet completed. Complete union of the fractured bone or joint is determined by means of clinical and radiologic examination.

Healing of bone is classified by degree. Nonunion signifies that the process of healing has ended without producing bony union. Delayed union signifies that healing has not occurred within the average time. The average time depends on many factors, and delayed unions must not be considered nonunion until the healing process has ceased without bony union. Malunion signifies that the fracture has united with deformity sufficient to cause impairment of the function or a significant angulation of the extremity.

Diseases of skeletal tissue

Bone diseases can be metabolic, infectious, or degenerative. Metabolic diseases are disorders of bone remodeling. The most common are osteoporosis, osteomalacia, and Paget's disease. The most common infectious process is os-

teomyelitis. Degenerative musculoskeletal conditions are associated with aging. Osteoarthritis is the most common degenerative change.

Osteoporosis is one of the most common and serious of bone diseases. Over a million fractures occurring each year are attributed to osteoporosis; 40% are vertebral fractures, 20% are femoral (hip) fractures, and 15% are distal forearm fractures (Licata, 1988). It is characterized by excessive loss of calcified matrix, bone mineral, and collagenous fibers, causing a reduction of total bone mass. Decreasing levels of estrogen and testosterone in the older adult result in reduced new bone growth and maintenance of existing bone. Inadequate intake of calcium or vitamin D; lack of weight-bearing activities, exercise, and physical inactivity; smoking; and caffeine intake are other contributing factors. Osteoporotic bone is porous, brittle, and fragile, fracturing easily under stress. This results in susceptibility to spontaneous fractures and pathologic curvature of the spine.

Osteomalacia is a metabolis bone disease characterized by inadequate mineralization of bone due to vitamin D deficiency, which leads to reduced absorption of calcium and phosphorus. A large amount of osteoid does not calcify in patients with this disease. Risk factors for development of osteomalacia include malabsorption problems, vitamin D and calcium deficiencies, chronic renal failure, and inadequate exposure to sunlight. Treatment includes dietary supplements and exposure to sunlight.

Paget's disease is a disorder affecting older adults. It is characterized by proliferation of osteoclasts and compensatory increased osteoblastic activity, resulting in rapid, disorganized bone remodeling. The bones are weak and poorly constructed.

An infectious musculoskeletal condition affecting the bone and marrow is osteomyelitis. The infection may develop from bloodborne pathogens deposited at the site. *Staphylococcus aureus* accounts for 90% of the osteomyelitic infections; streptococci cause the second largest number (Mourad, 1991). The infection develops as pathogenic organisms become trapped in small arteries and capillaries in the metaphyseal area. As the organisms proliferate, they block blood flow, causing an area of the bone to become necrotic. Osteomyelitis most frequently develops from hematogenous spread, or the extension of another infection. This may occur in the presence of strep throat, urinary tract infection, or skin ulceration. Osteomyelitis may result from gross bone contamination or improper technique. A gunshot wound or compound fracture may cause gross bone contamination. A breakdown in aseptic technique, sterility, or inappropriate traffic patterns may also result in osteomyelitis. High-risk patients such as the debilitated, diabetic or poorly nourished experience increased susceptibility.

Osteoarthritis is a condition noted by degenerative changes in articular cartilage. It is a condition of older adults, and the most common form of arthritis. Overuse has been indicated as contributing to the presence of osteoarthritis, particularly in joints with repetitive movement. It is a result of progressive deterioration of the cartilage within the joint, varying for different persons. The major weight-bearing joints such as the hip, lumbar spine, and knee are the most commonly affected, but the glenohumeral joint, elbow, wrist, ankle, and fingers are all affected. It is characterized by deterioration and atrophy of articular cartilage and formation of new bone at the joint surfaces. Radiologically, osteophyte formation, joint space narrowing, and possible sclerosing of subchondral bone surfaces may be present.

Complications

Complications of surgical procedures may result in prolonged recovery or inability to return to previous levels of function. The most common orthopedic complications that might occur include compartment syndrome, thromboembolism, fat embolism, and infection.

Compartment syndrome is a condition of increased venous pressure caused by constriction of edematous tissues within a muscle compartment. The constriction is caused by unyielding fascial coverings over muscles. Venous pressure increases, causing ischemia. Ischemia longer than 6 hours can lead to permanent tissue damage, and the pressure must be released. Compartment syndrome may be a result of traumatic injury or ischemic contracture caused by constriction of a cast. Compartment syndrome associated with fractures of the extremity should be treated at the time of fracture stabilization. Slit catheter monitoring may be used to determine precise pressure. The patient's extremity is prepped and a fasciotomy completed.

Thromboembolism is one of the most common complications occurring after skeletal trauma and elective musculoskeletal surgery. The occurrence is correlated with age, obesity, the extent and duration of the musculoskeletal procedure, degree and length of immobilization, a history of thromboembolic disease, and severity of the underlying systemic disease. Prevention includes maintenance of fluid and electrolyte balance and prevention of shock. Adequate hydration must replace lost blood or fluids. Preoperatively it is important to plan the procedure to minimize surgical time; anticoagulant therapy may be necessary.

Pulmonary embolism is a fatal complication of orthopedic procedures. Symptoms include apprehension, dyspnea, tachycardia, and rales. The relationship to deep venous thrombosis makes early recognition and preventive measures important.

Wound infection can be evaluated as a result of the orthopedic condition being treated or complication following a musculoskeletal procedure. Patient-dependent factors include nutritional status, immunologic status, and infection at a remote site (caries, urinary tract). Postoperatively, infections may present as persistent, unexplained pain, effusion, erythema, wound drainage, or failure to heal. Superficial infections can progress to deep infections and result in osteomyelitis or septic arthritis.

Orthopedic trauma

Multiple trauma is a phenomenon drastically effecting the cost of health care in dollars and human suffering. Trauma is on the rise with the increased mobility of our society and social factors such as drinking and driving. Multiple trauma patients can arrive in the operating room a short time after initial field stabilization and transport. It is sometimes necessary to move the patient directly to the operating room.

Care of the orthopedic multiple trauma patient requires management different from that of a routine orthopedic procedure. Along with basic and advanced cardiac life support and stabilization of internal injuries, there is a great need for immediate stabilization of long bones, pelvic, and spinal fractures.

Many complications affect the outcome if a multiple trauma patient is not treated in a proper and timely fashion. Adult respiratory distress syndrome and fat embolism correlate with the time and type of treatment of long bone fractures. Statistically it has been shown that morbidity, pulmonary complications, and stabilization are significantly increased when treatment is delayed. Some studies report 2% to 3% complications with early treatment versus 38% when treatment is delayed (Gustilo, 1993). Following hemodynamic stability and resolution of life-threatening conditions, stabilization of long bone, spine, and pelvic fractures should be undertaken.

Bone banking

Programs have developed for acquisition, sterilization, and storage of bone allograft. The American Association of Tissue Banks (AATB) accredits and periodically inspects bone banking programs to ensure that specific guidelines are followed in the retrieval, processing, storage, and distribution of bone allograft. Accredited programs comprise a national tissue network that provides hospitals and surgeons with various types of high-quality allograft tissue.

Patients who consent to donate are thoroughly screened. Screening procedures include HIV and hepatitis testing. A detailed medical and social history is obtained. The harvesting process must be completed using sterile technique. Culture specimens are taken and sent to the institution that performs further testing. Once the tissue is determined acceptable, it is returned to the bone bank for storage. Frozen allografts are stored in plastic or cloth wraps to ensure sterility and prevent grafts from drying out. Allografts are frozen until use. Vacuum-sealed freezers are monitored with an alarm that sounds if the temperature rises above $-70°$ C. Tissue maintained at $-70°$ C or colder may be stored for up to 5 years before expiration (American Association of Tissue Banks, 1987; Buckham, 1991). When requested for a procedure, the bone allograft is delivered to the field, slightly thawed, cultured, and washed with an antibiotic solution. Banked bone is available in many shapes of cortical and cancellous tissue (Fig. 21-34).

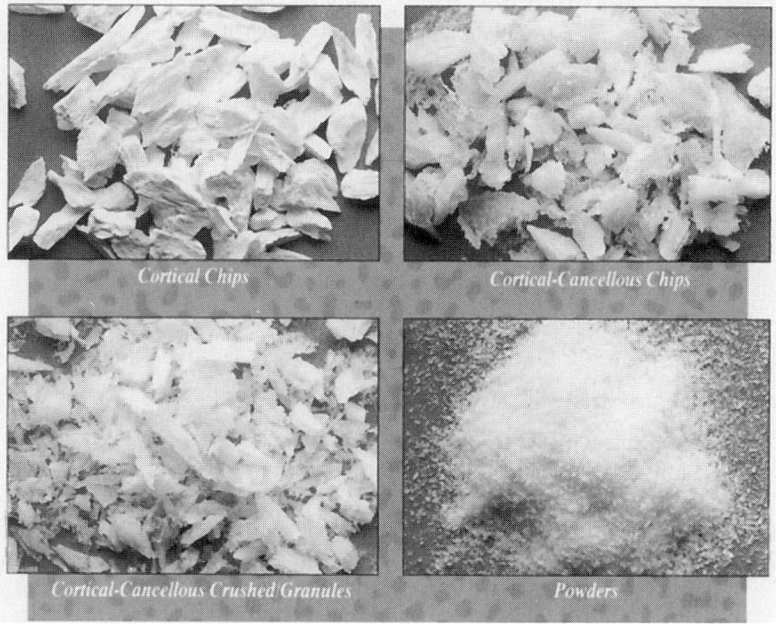

FIG. 21-34   Demineralized bone showing cortical and cancellous bone in chips, granules, and powder.
Courtesy Osteotech, Shrewsbury, N.J.

Records are maintained on both donors and recipients. Donor records provide the donor identification, medical history (with circumstances of death if applicable), lab results, and graft description. Recipient records include recipient identification, surgeon and organization implanting the graft, surgical procedure, culture results, and any adverse reactions. Like other implants, the recipient's operative record should include the name of the bone bank from which the allograft was received, type of allograft, tissue number, and expiration date if applicable.

Bone banking has drastically improved results when faced with the reconstruction of the acetabulum or other supporting structures that will support implant fixation. Entire segments of bone in the form of the shaft or joint are used when there is great bone loss due to trauma and oncologic conditions.

Surgical Interventions

BONE GRAFTING

Bone grafting may be used to fill cavities following removal of large amounts of bone that might result in instability, to fill bony defects, and to promote union of fractures at the time of open reduction. The type of graft to be used depends on the location of the fracture or defect, the condition of the bone, and the amount of bone loss due to injury. Bone graft may be used for procedures involving revision of joints if there is significant bone loss due to resorption or mechanical destruction following removal of bone cement.

Bone graft may be the patient's own bone (autogenous) or bone obtained from a tissue bank (homogenous). Autogenous bone grafts are often harvested from the iliac crest, where there is cortical and cancellous bone. Various harvesting techniques are used. Struts of cortical bone from the iliac crest can be fashioned to the desired shape and used in areas needing structural strength. The amount of cancellous bone is plentiful. It is used to promote bone growth in areas of defect. Local bone graft material may be taken from the site of injury. Homogenous allografts are used when bone is not available from the patient due to lack of sufficient quantity or because a secondary procedure is undesirable for the patient.

Procedural considerations. Cancellous grafts may be taken from the ilium, olecranon, or distal radius; cortical grafts may be taken from the tibia, fibula, or ribs. When the recipient site of an autogenous graft is diseased, instruments used for the recipient site must be separated from donor graft site instruments. The operating team must change their gowns and gloves to take the bone graft, and again follow the procedure to prevent cross-contamination. The patient is positioned to allow exposure to the surgical site. A sandbag may be placed beneath the area for easier anatomic location and access.

The instrumentation for taking a bone graft includes soft tissue instruments and a bone graft set (Fig. 21-31) and might include the following:

Power saw and drill
    with graft site attach-
    ments
Wound drain

Operative procedure—harvest of bone graft. A cancellous bone graft consists of spongy bone usually taken from the anterior or posterior crest of the ilium. A cortical bone graft, consisting of hard, dense bone, is removed from the crest of the ilium or the tibia. The location of the crest of the ilium is subcutaneous, allowing exposure without difficulty.

1. An incision is made along the border of the iliac crest, and the muscles on the outer table of the ilium are stripped, elevated, and retracted.
2. Strips of the iliac crest can be removed with an osteotome or oscillating saw.
3. A cortical window may also be made in the outer table, and the cancellous bone chips obtained with curettes or gouges.
4. The deep and superficial layers may be drained to evacuate blood and assess any further bleeding.
5. The wound is closed in layers and a pressure dressing applied.

ELECTRICAL STIMULATION

Electrical stimulation is artificially applied electrical current that induces or influences osteogenesis. Three types of stimulators (Fig. 21-35) are available for treatment of nonunion, including invasive (implantable), semiinvasive (percutaneous), and noninvasive (capacitance coupling). The bone stimulator of choice depends on the patient, pathologic condition, and physician comfort with the device.

The bone growth stimulator is used in patients with high risk of nonunion. It can be used to provide electrical stimulation for treatment of nonunion, delayed union, congenital pseudarthrosis, and bone defects. It may be used with or without internal fixation devices, external fixation devices, or bone grafting. Patients who have undergone previous surgery, who have sustained significant tissue loss, or in whom bone grafting is contraindicated are candidates. Along with their use in accelerating fracture healing, bone growth stimulators have been successfully used in an infected nonunion after débridement because the electrical stimulation retards bacterial growth. The normal range of electrical current is 18 to 22 µA. Electrical stimulation requires long periods of immobilization of the site. This prolonged immobilization may impede rehabilitation.

Procedural considerations. Instructions for implanting and components selected vary according to the type. The position of the patient depends on the implant site.

A soft tissue set is used in addition to the following:

Implant instrumentation, monitor, and implant of the surgeon's choice	Curettes Rasp Power drill and drill bits
Osteotomes	

Operative procedure

1. The surgical site is exposed and débrided as necessary. A stimulator may be implanted following the surgical procedure.
2. A slot is fashioned spanning the nonunion site.
3. A second incision is made about 8 to 10 cm from the first one and dissected. Before implanting the genera-

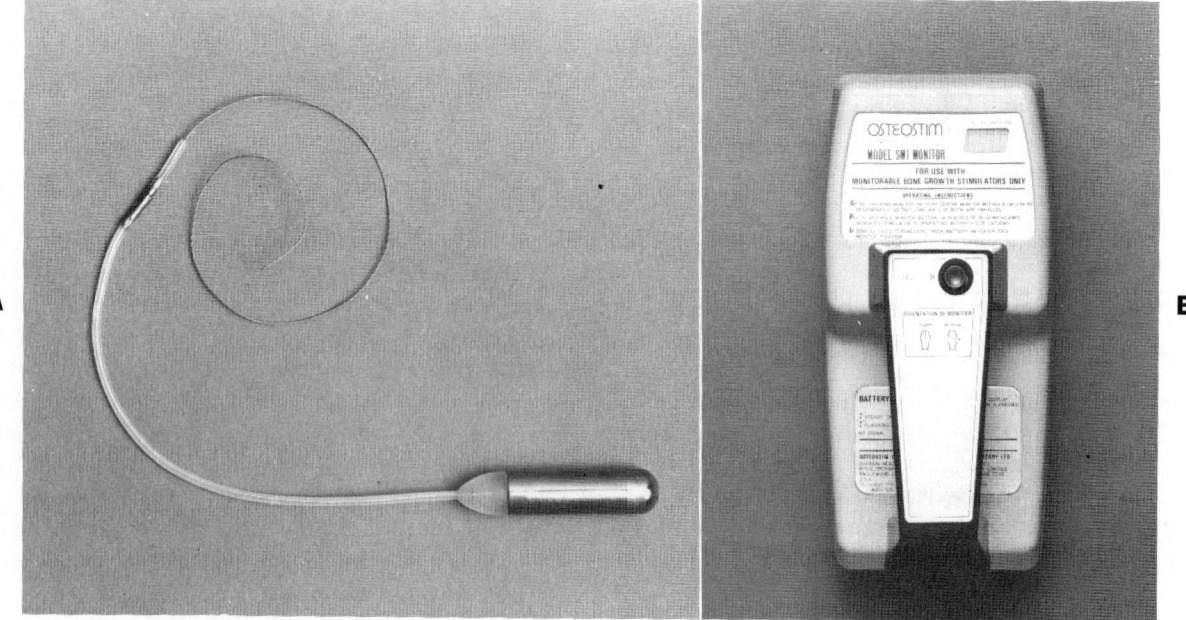

FIG. 21-35 Bone stimulator used following procedures to induce bone formation. **A,** Bone growth stimulator cathode and lead. **B,** Monitor for bone growth stimulator.

Courtesy Orthopaedic Division of Telectronics Proprietary, Ltd., Englewood, Colo.

tor, it is imperative that hemostasis be obtained. The use of electrosurgical equipment may interfere with function of the bone growth stimulator.

4. A subcutaneous channel for the cathode is created, using blunt or mechanical dissection.

5. The long cathode lead is guided through the channel.

6. The generator is carefully implanted near the skin surface. The generator should be inserted in soft tissue, not against bone or metal fixation devices; it should not create a bulge beneath the skin.

7. The electrical coils are placed in the prepared bone slot in equal lengths above and below the fracture site.

8. Cancellous bone grafts are placed between the coils if large bony defects are being treated.

9. Routine closure of the subcutaneous and skin tissue is carried out.

10. Once union has occurred (5 to 6 months), the generator is removed. The stimulator can be removed using local anesthesia with minimal instrumentation.

FRACTURES AND DISLOCATIONS

A fracture is a break in the continuity of a bone. The care of fractured bones or dislocation of a joint is complicated when there is trauma to the soft tissues, including muscles, nerves, ligaments, and blood vessels.

Types

Fractures are classified into two main groups: closed fractures and compound or open fractures. Closed fractures are those in which there is no communication between the bone fracture and the skin surface. Incomplete closed fractures are those in which the whole thickness of the bone is not broken but is bent or buckled, as in greenstick fractures, which occur in children before puberty. Open fractures exist when the break in the bone communicates with a wound in the skin. These fractures are usually considered contaminated, requiring measures to control potential infection.

There are many varieties of fracture architecture (Fig. 21-36), including (1) transverse fracture, in which the frac-

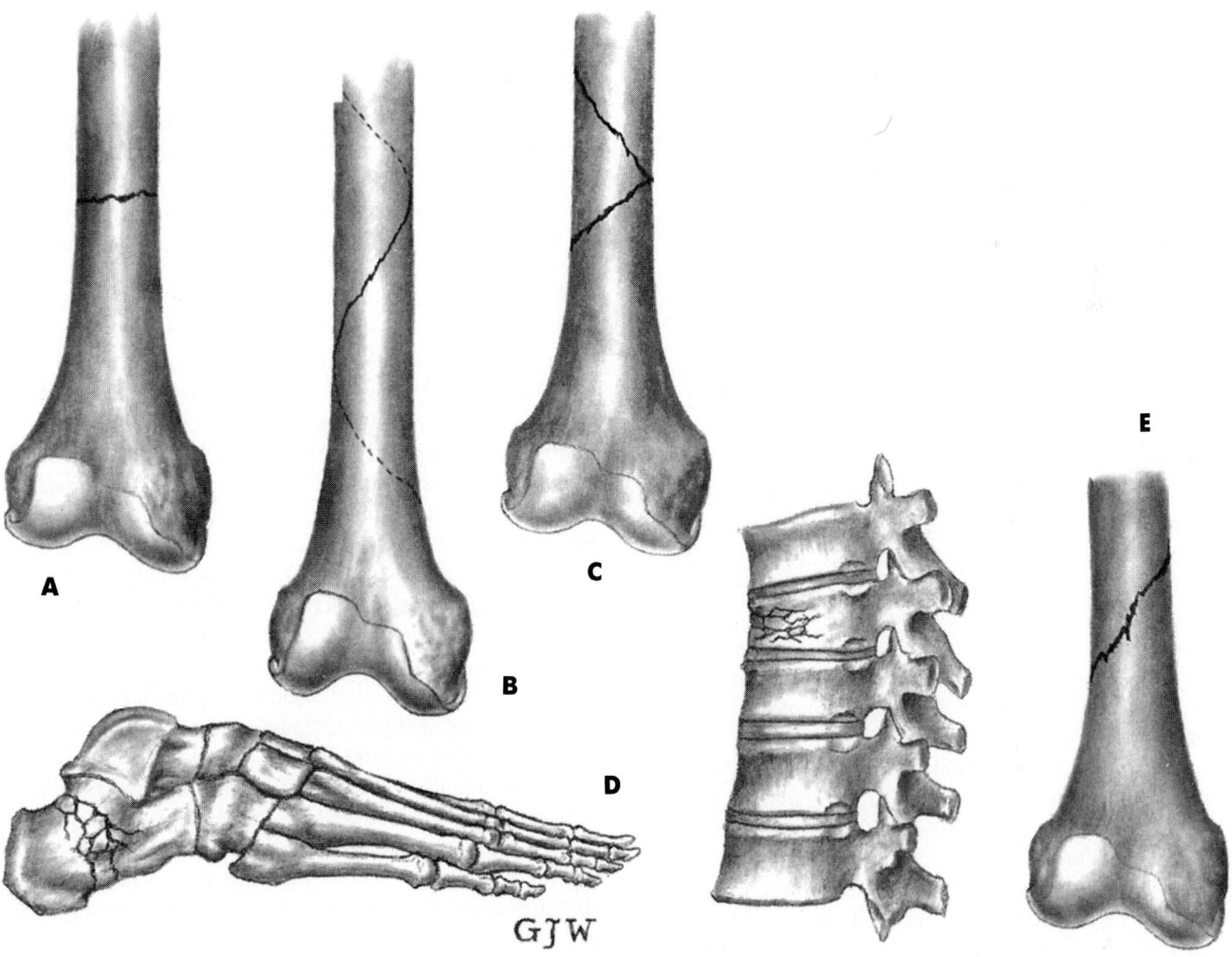

FIG. 21-36 Fracture types. **A,** Transverse. **B,** Longitudinal or Spiral. **C,** Comminuted. **D,** Compression. **E,** Oblique. Fracture types may be open or closed.

From Gregory B: *Perioperative Nursing Series: Orthopaedic Surgery,* St. Louis, 1994, Mosby.

ture line runs at a right angle to the longitudinal axis of the bone; (2) longitudinal fracture, which runs along the length of the bone; (3) oblique fracture and spiral fracture, in which bone is twisted apart (similar except that oblique is shorter than spiral); (4) communicated fracture, in which the bone fragments splinter into more than two pieces; (5) compression fracture, in which one fragment is driven into the other end and is relatively fixed in that position; and (6) pathologic fracture in which a bone will fracture easily because it is weakened by disease. A fracture in the shaft of a long bone is described as being in the proximal, middle, lower third or at the junction of these two divisions. A fracture of one of the bony prominences of the end of a long bone is described as a fracture of that prominence by name. Examples include a fracture of the olecranon, medial malleolus, or lateral condyle of the femur.

An epiphyseal separation occurs when a fracture passes through or lies within the growth plate of a bone. When this occurs in a child with immature bone, retardation of limb length and growth may occur. These injuries require immediate and expert treatment.

An *avulsion fracture* results in a ligamentous attachment remaining intact on a separated bone fragment. This may occur following joint dislocation or rotational injury, such as the femoral condyle separating from the tibial plateau. A *dislocation* is a complete displacement of one articular surface from another. This injury can disrupt neurovascular structures and often requires immediate attention. A *subluxation* is a partial dislocation, often indicated by ligamentous instability.

Principles of treatment

The purpose of fracture treatment is to reestablish the length, shape, and alignment of the fractured bones or joints and restore anatomic function. Acute fracture treatment is necessary to alleviate neurovascular compromise. The surgical team should consider the following principles when providing care for the patient: (1) the patient (extremity, fracture site) must be handled gently; (2) initial general medical treatment must be provided; (3) equipment and personnel must be readily available to treat impending or existing shock and control hemorrhage; (4) principles of aseptic technique must be maintained; (5) positioning must allow adequate circulatory and respiratory function with adequate exposure; and (6) patient comfort must be considered.

The primary goal in treatment of an upper extremity fracture is to preserve mobility and restore range of motion, enabling the individual to perform skilled and delicate work. In fractures of a lower extremity the objectives of surgery are to restore alignment and length and provide stability of the extremity for weight bearing.

In the presence of open fractures involving soft tissues, several associated conditions may arise, including (1) secondary hemorrhage, (2) infection, (3) severe damage to soft tissues, (4) damage to blood vessels and nerves, and (5) Volkmann's contracture.

Basic treatment techniques
Closed reduction

Fractures may be treated by closed reduction, or manipulating the fragments into position without incising the skin. This is the treatment of choice when possible to decrease the opportunity for infection, improve results (including bone union of the fracture), and minimize the recovery period. Significant bone comminution, periosteal damage, or soft tissue entrapped within the fracture site may result in complications.

Procedural considerations. The choice of anesthesia depends on the site of fracture and patient condition. A closed reduction can be performed with (1) infiltration of local anesthetic agent into the fracture site, (2) intravenous regional anesthesia, (3) regional or spinal nerve block, or (4) general anesthesia. Closed reduction may take place before an open procedure to reduce the fracture site. Skeletal traction may also be applied to the fracture site (Fig. 21-37), requiring a surgical skin prep and application of drapes. The appropriate casting or brace materials should be readily available to prevent loss of fracture reduction. Supplies should be available in the event it is necessary to open the fracture site and apply fixation.

Operative procedure

1. The fragments are manipulated into alignment by the surgeon using manual traction. Reduction is confirmed using radiography (x-ray or fluoroscopy).
2. After reduction has been obtained, the fracture is immobilized with casting material or bracing technique.

External fixation

This method of fracture management provides rigid fixation and reduction with the ability to manage severe soft tissue wounds. Because of the increased chance of infection in patients with an open fracture, external fixation is often the preferred treatment. Advantages of external fixation include the absence of casting material, fracture stabilization at a distance from the injury site, ability to perform subsequent procedures such as skin grafts or vascularized grafts, minimal joint interference, early mobilization, and the ability to use internal fixation or other skeletal fixation devices at the same time or sequentially.

Indications for external fixation include (1) severe open fractures, (2) highly comminuted closed fractures, (3) arthrodesis, (4) infected joints, (5) infected nonunion, (6) fracture stabilization to protect arterial or nerve anastomosis, (7) major alignment and length deficits, (8) congenital deformities, and (9) static contractures. External fixation provides a bridge between fracture reduction and insertion of an internal fixator such as intramedullary nail, allowing time for vascular recovery. Internal fixation can take place at a later date.

Many improvements have been made in the design and articulations of external fixation devices. The fixators can be applied to most anatomic sites. The available external fixators vary greatly in design; however, all contain three

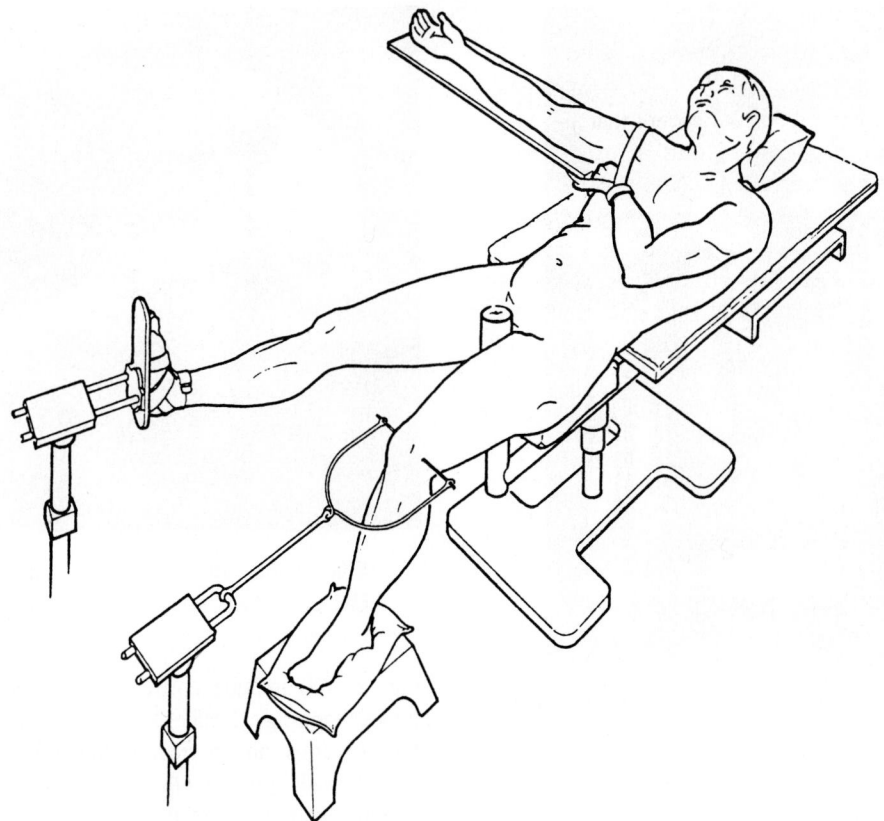

FIG. 21-37　Application of skeletal traction with the patient positioned supine on the fracture table.

From Gustilo RB, Kyle RF, Templeman D: *Fractures and dislocations,* vol 2, St. Louis, 1993, Mosby.

main components: (1) bone-anchoring devices (threaded pins, Kirschner wires), (2) longitudinal supporting devices (threaded or smooth rods), and (3) connecting elements (clamps and partial or full rings). Improvements have resulted in use of lightweight, stronger materials, which are radiopaque, to use as connecting rods. This also prevents postoperative radiographic interference when viewing the fracture site for progress in healing.

The Ilizarov device uses principles of tension-stress and distraction to correct bone defects and limb length discrepancies. It is not routinely used for acute fracture fixation; however, the principles and technique are similar. Limb length may be adjusted with gradual bone distraction of bone ends, stimulating new bone formation.

Procedural considerations. External fixators are applied with the patient under general or regional anesthesia using sterile technique. Radiographic imaging ensures fracture reduction following closed manipulation, and proper pin placement. The incision site is small to allow introduction of pins. Irrigation and débridement at the fracture site and surrounding soft tissue may be necessary if there is soft tissue damage.

A soft tissue set appropriate for the operative site will be required in addition to the following:

Fixation device of choice with instrumentation: Torus (Fig. 21-38), AO/ASIF (Fig. 21-39), Ilizarov (Fig. 21-40), AO/ASIF pelvic fixator (Fig. 21-41), wrist external fixator (Fig. 21-42)
Power drill

Pulsatile lavage with 3000 ml normal saline solution
Periosteal elevator
Pin cutter, appropriate for the pin size
Gauze wrap and povidone ointment or antibiotic-impregnated dressing

Operative procedure—application of a unilateral frame

1. The fracture is reduced manually.
2. The skin is incised over an area free from neurovascular structures.
3. Blunt dissection to the bone or with the elevator may be necessary.
4. A drill sheath is used to protect surrounding soft tissue while predrilling the cortex.
5. Hand or low-speed power drilling is used to insert the half pins above and below the fracture.
6. Universal joints are slipped over the pins and joined with a connecting rod.

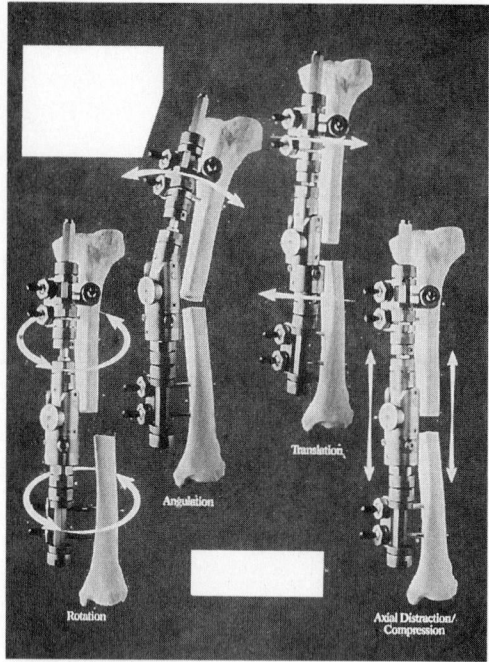

FIG. 21-38   Torus external fixator positioned on a long bone.
Courtesy Zimmer, Inc., Warsaw, Ind.

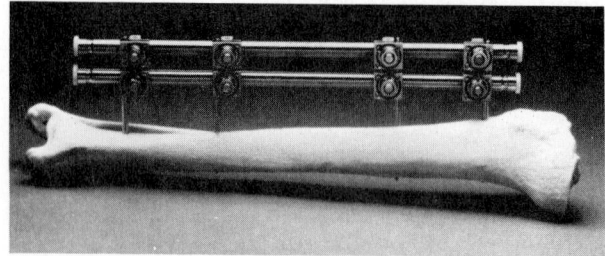

FIG. 21-39   AO/ASIF fixator tubular external fixation device.
Courtesy Synthes U.S.A., Paoli, Pa.

7. The frame is tightened using the appropriate wrenches.
8. X-ray or fluoroscopy is utilized to confirm reduction and alignment.
9. The pin sites are covered with an antibacterial agent and dressed with sterile gauze.

Internal fixation

Internal fixation is often the treatment of choice for correction of fractures of long bones or those in the hip region. Application of compression plates and screws, and insertion of pins, intramedullary rods, nails, or wiring are methods of internal fixation. Fractures of most anatomic parts can be repaired using internal fixation.

There are many principals and techniques when utilizing internal fixation of fractures. Three types of screws

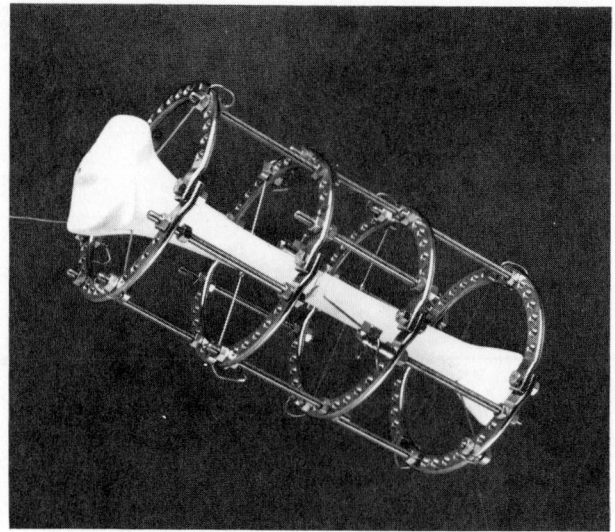

FIG. 21-40   Ilizarov tibial external fixator device.
Courtesy Richards Medical Co., Memphis, Tenn.

(Fig. 21-43) include cortical, cancellous, lag, pretapped, and self-tapping. Cortical bone screws have threads that are close together and narrower than other types of threads. These threads run along the entire length of screw and transfix bone, gaining purchase (grab) of bone cortex.

Cancellous bone screws feature threads that are broader and farther apart than those of cortical screws. Cancellous screws are used in cancellous bone, which is less dense than cortical bone; the bone accumulates within the threads to provide the purchase for fixation. Like cortical screws, cancellous screws can traverse fracture sites and hold plates onto bone. The screw does not completely cross the bone, and one end remains buried. Cancellous screws are commonly used when fractures occur at the condylar ends of the shaft.

Plating of a fracture may occur with or without dynamic compression (Fig. 21-44). Dynamic compression uses screw and plate geometry to apply forces at the fracture site. Semitubular plates are less rigid and do not have the ability to produce dynamic compression. This type of plate is utilized in the forearm and fibula, where weight bearing, which could break the plate, is not a factor.

Closed method. The fracture is reduced using closed reduction methods of manipulation and traction, then aligned with percutaneous insertion of pins, intramedullary nails, or rods. Pins can be placed percutaneously (Fig. 21-45) to fix fractures involving the digits, the wrist, and the foot. A rod or nail is placed percutaneously in a large bone such as the humerus or femur (Fig. 21-46). Improved instrumentation and the use of fluoroscopy have made closed reduction with internal fixation a safe and effective practice. Closed reduction is, however, a misnomer, since small openings in the soft tissue and bone are made to facilitate introduction of the devices. These incisions are considerably smaller then those created when repairing the fracture

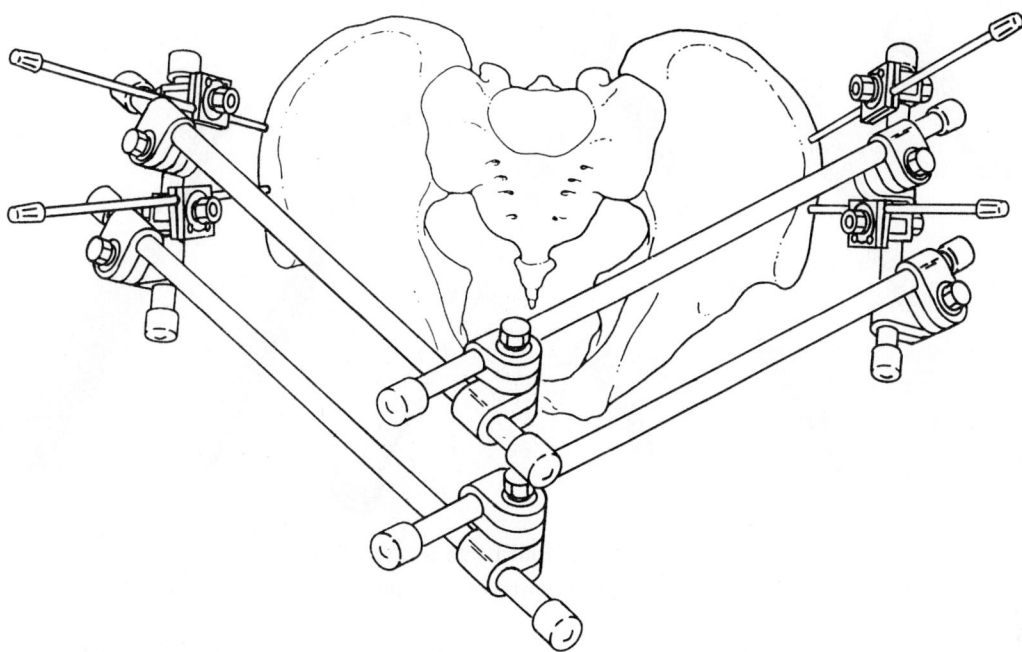

FIG. 21-41   AO/ASIF pelvic external fixator, double frame using tube to tube clamps.
Courtesy Synthes U.S.A., Paoli, Pa.

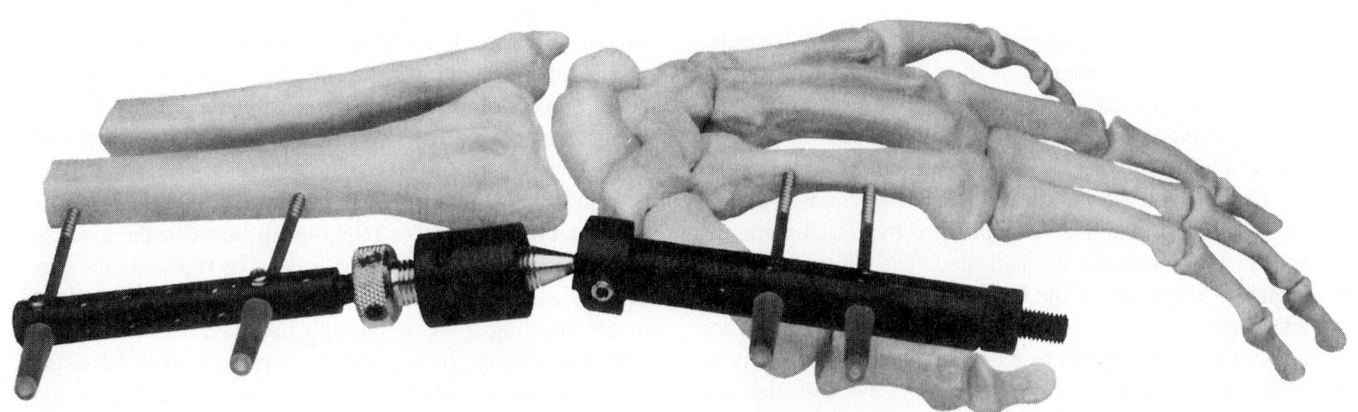

FIG. 21-42   Clyburn dynamic wrist external fixator.
Courtesy Zimmer, Inc., Warsaw, Ind.

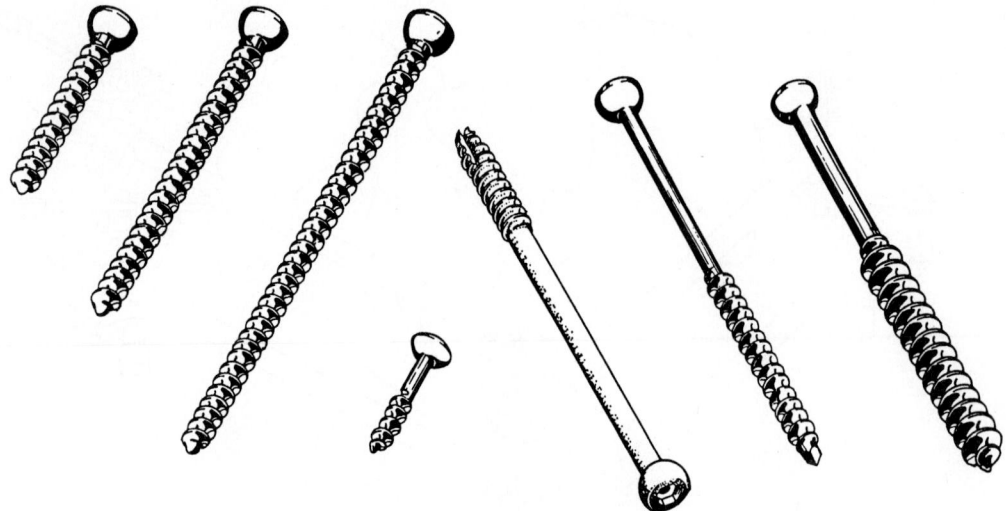

FIG. 21-43   Types of screws used for fixation with or without plating systems.
From Gustilo RB, Kyle RF, Templeman D: *Fractures and dislocations,* vol 1, St. Louis, 1993, Mosby.

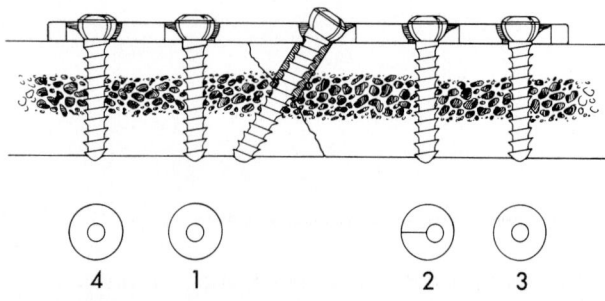

FIG. 21-44   Plating a closed forearm fracture using dynamic compression showing final position of the screw insertion.

Illustration by Beverly Kessler courtesy LTI Medica and The UpJohn Co. Copyright 1982, Learning Technology, Inc.

using open reduction. The advantages of closed reduction over open reduction and internal fixation are (1) a lower incidence of infection and (2) absence of additional soft tissue or vascular damage.

Open method—open reduction and internal fixation. Open reduction and internal fixation is a method of providing exposure of the fracture site and using pins, wire, screws, a plate and screw combination, rods, or nails to correct the fracture (Fig. 21-47). Open reduction and internal fixation is used when satisfactory reduction of a fracture cannot be obtained or maintained by closed methods, and skeletal traction is not indicated. The advantage is that anatomic alignment of the fracture can usually be obtained and verified through direct observation. Fractures that are comminuted or difficult to reduce can be more effectively treated using this technique. The incidence of infection and nonunion is increased when the wound is opened.

The procedure varies for each anatomic site, utilizing the principles for specific fixation devices. Several procedures

described in the text identify steps for completion of open reduction and internal fixation. Reference examples include:

Pin fixation—application of a unilateral frame
Wire fixation—reduction of patellar fracture, tension banding of the olecranon
Screw fixation—correction of scaphoid fractures
Plate and screw fixation—repair of the comminuted distal humeral fracture
Rod or nail fixation—correction of fractures of the shaft of the humerus, femoral shaft, or tibial shaft

SURGERY OF THE SHOULDER
Correction of acromioclavicular joint separation

Acromioclavicular joint separation (Fig. 21-48) is frequently occur in athletic and occupational injuries, resulting from a force applied downward, most commonly from a fall directly to the top of the shoulder. The ligamentous support of the acromioclavicular joint and the coracoclavicular ligaments that tether the clavicle to the underlying coracoid process of the scapula are disrupted. The result is either a posterior or superior displacement of the lateral end of the clavicle.

The purpose of surgery in an acutely injured patient is to reestablish the proper relationship between the clavicle and the coracoid process. This is done by replacing the coracoclavicular ligament with heavy suture or Mersilene tape or by inserting a screw through the clavicle and into the coracoid process. It may also be necessary to stabilize the acromioclavicular joint by placing a smooth Steinman pin across the acromium and into the clavicle. Sometimes the outer third of the clavicle is also resected. If resection of the clavicle is the only treatment required, this may be com-

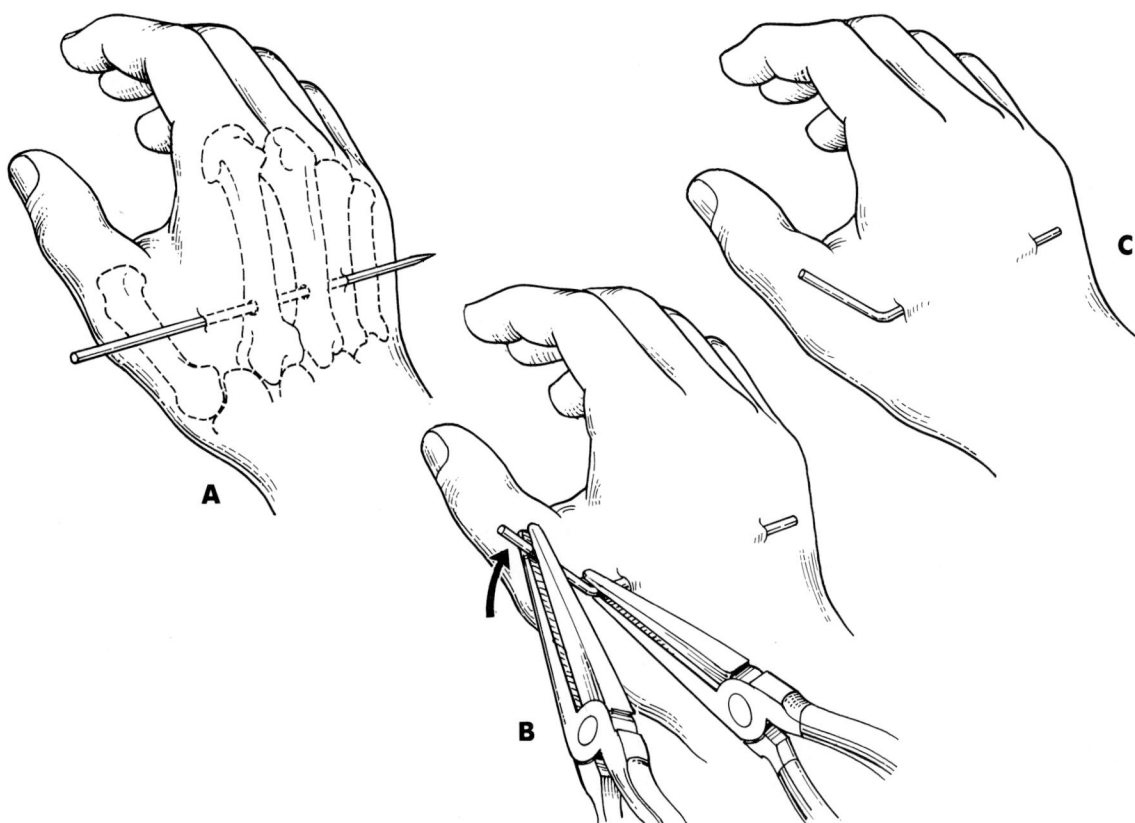

FIG. 21-45   Pin insertion placement for a wrist fracture.

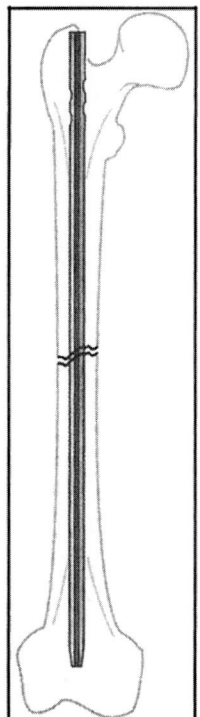

FIG. 21-46   Rod placement for femoral fracture.
Courtesy Biomet, Inc., Warsaw, Ind.

pleted arthroscopically. Shoulder arthroscopy is detailed in the arthroscopic procedures section.

Procedural considerations. The patient is placed in the supine or semisitting position with a sandbag or folded sheet under the affected shoulder. The shoulder is positioned slightly off the operating table (Fig. 21-49) to allow full range of motion. The head is turned as far as possible to the opposite side. The extremity is draped with a stockinette to the midhumeral level.

A soft tissue set and bone instrumentation specific for the shoulder (Fig. 21-50) is required, in addition to the following:

Bone screws and instru-	Free-cutting needles
mentation	Shoulder positioner
Power instruments	

Operative procedure—Weaver-Dunn procedure

1. A short curvilinear incision is made over the distal calvicle, and dissection is carried down to expose the acromioclavicular joint.
2. The coracoacromial ligament is detached from the acromium end, retaining the attachment to the coracoid end.
3. An oblique distal clavicular resection is completed using a microsagittal saw.
4. The clavicle is held in the reduced position while traction is applied to the coracoacromial ligament to de-

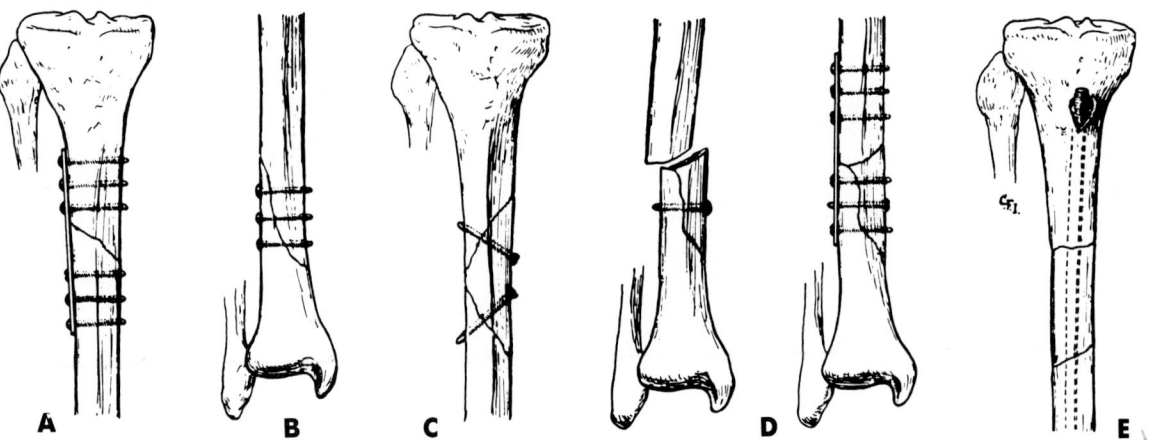

FIG. 21-47 Types of internal fixation for fracture repair. **A,** Plate and screws for transverse or short oblique fracture. **B,** Transfixion screws for long oblique or spiral fractures. **C,** Transfixion screws for long butterfly fragment. **D,** Fixation for short butterfly fragment. **E,** Medullary fixation.

From Edmonson AS, Crenshaw AH, editors: Campbell's operative orthopaedics, ed 7, St. Louis, 1987, Mosby.

termine proper ligament length. Residual tissue is resected if present.

5. Two holes are drilled in the distal clavicle.
6. Nonabsorbable suture such as Mersilene or cotton dacron is passed in a mattress fashion through the coracoidacromial ligament and through the drill holes in the clavicle.
7. With the clavicle held in reduction the sutures are snugged and tied. The ligament is secured in close relationship with the osteotomized distal clavicle. The ligament is affixed within the medullary canal.
8. The muscles are closed over the joint and the subcutaneous and skin layers approximated.
9. One or two drains are brought through separate stab wounds in the skin.
10. The dressing and immobilization sling are applied.

Correction of sternoclavicular dislocation

Traumatic dislocation of the sternoclavicular joint usually occurs from an indirect blow on the anterior shoulder while the arm is abducted. The clavicle most frequently is displaced anteriorly, but posterior or retrosternal dislocations can occur. Posterior dislocation can be more severe because injury to the trachea, esophagus, thoracic duct, and large vessels of the mediastinum is possible. Except in severe cases, dislocation of the sternoclavicular joint is treated nonoperatively with manual traction and immobilization bandages.

Clavicular fracture

Fractures of the clavicle are some of the most common bony injuries. These injuries rarely require surgical intervention. Approximately 90% of the clavicular fractures are the result of a direct blow on the clavicle or falling on the outstretched hand. The most common site of clavicular fracture is the middle third portion of the bone, mainly at the middle and outer third junction. Clavicular fractures are usually treated by immobilization in a figure-of-eight splint. The chances of nonunion are greatly increased when open reduction is used for a clavicular fracture. The outcome may result in a bony prominence, which may be disturbing to the patient; the overriding fragments are resorbed with time.

Clavicular fractures may require open reduction and internal fixation following nonunion, neurovascular compromise that cannot be resolved with reduction, distal clavicular fracture with torn coracoclavicular ligaments, or persistent wide separation of the fragments with soft tissue entrapment. Surgery is necessary when the fracture is displaced enough to cause underlying damage to the vessels and brachial plexus. Open reduction is accomplished with a tubular plate and screws or intramedullary pin fixation.

Procedural considerations. The patient is placed in the supine or semisitting position with a sandbag or folded sheet under the affected shoulder and the head turned as far as possible to the opposite side. The entire extremity is prepped and draped. The following instrument setup is required:

Soft tissue and bone set	Semitubular plate and
Bone reduction clamps	screws if plating
Reduction forceps	Steinman pins if pinning
Power drill	ning
Kirschner wires	Bone graft instruments

Operative procedure

1. A 2.5-cm incision is made over the fracture site. The incision may need to be extended for comminuted fractures.
2. Dissection is carried down to the clavicle, taking care not to strip periosteum or disrupt vessels or nerves.

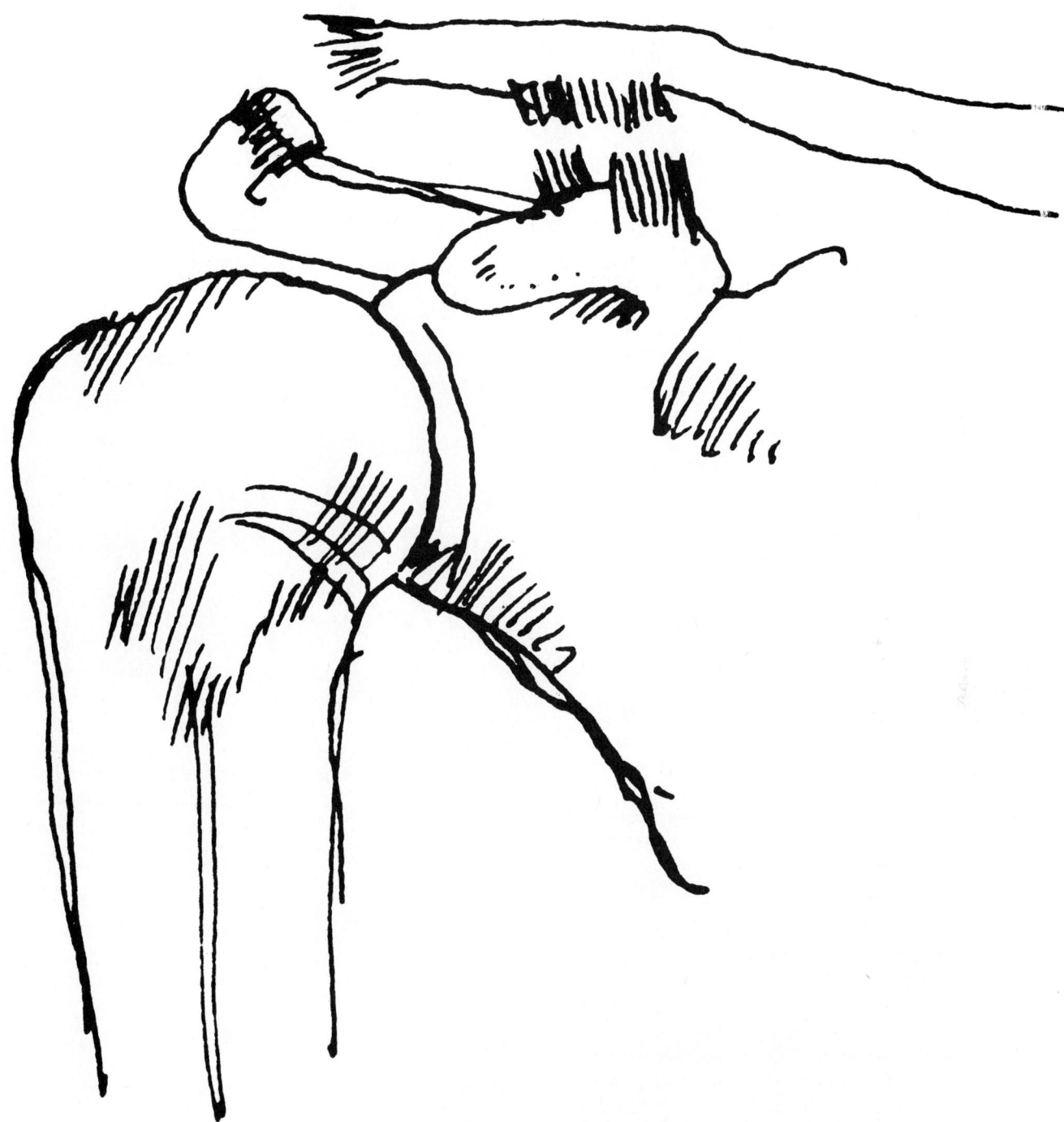

FIG. 21-48   Acromioclavicular joint separation following injury to the shoulder.
From Gustilo RB: *The Fracture Classification Manual*, St. Louis, 1991, Mosby.

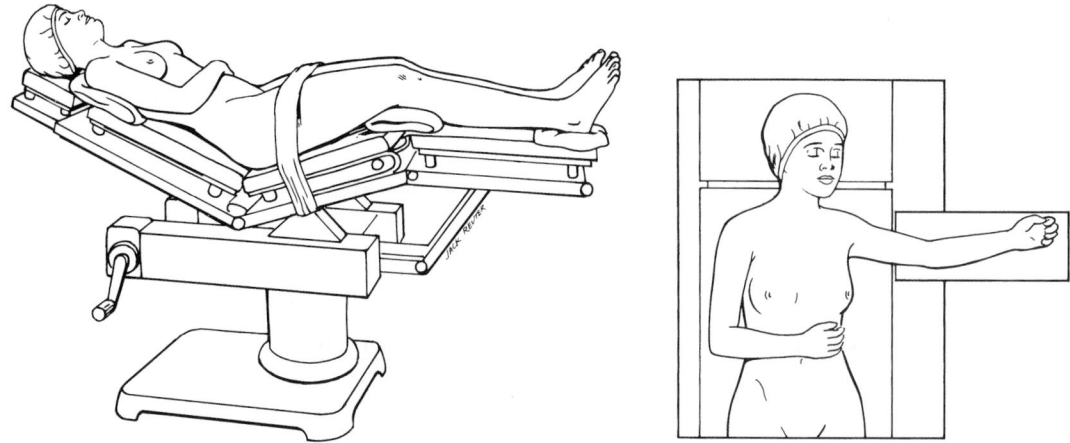

FIG. 21-49   Positioning for a surgical procedure on the shoulder with the patient in a semisitting position and support beneath the affected shoulder.

From Gregory B: *Perioperative Nursing Series: Orthopaedic Surgery,* St. Louis, 1994, Mosby.

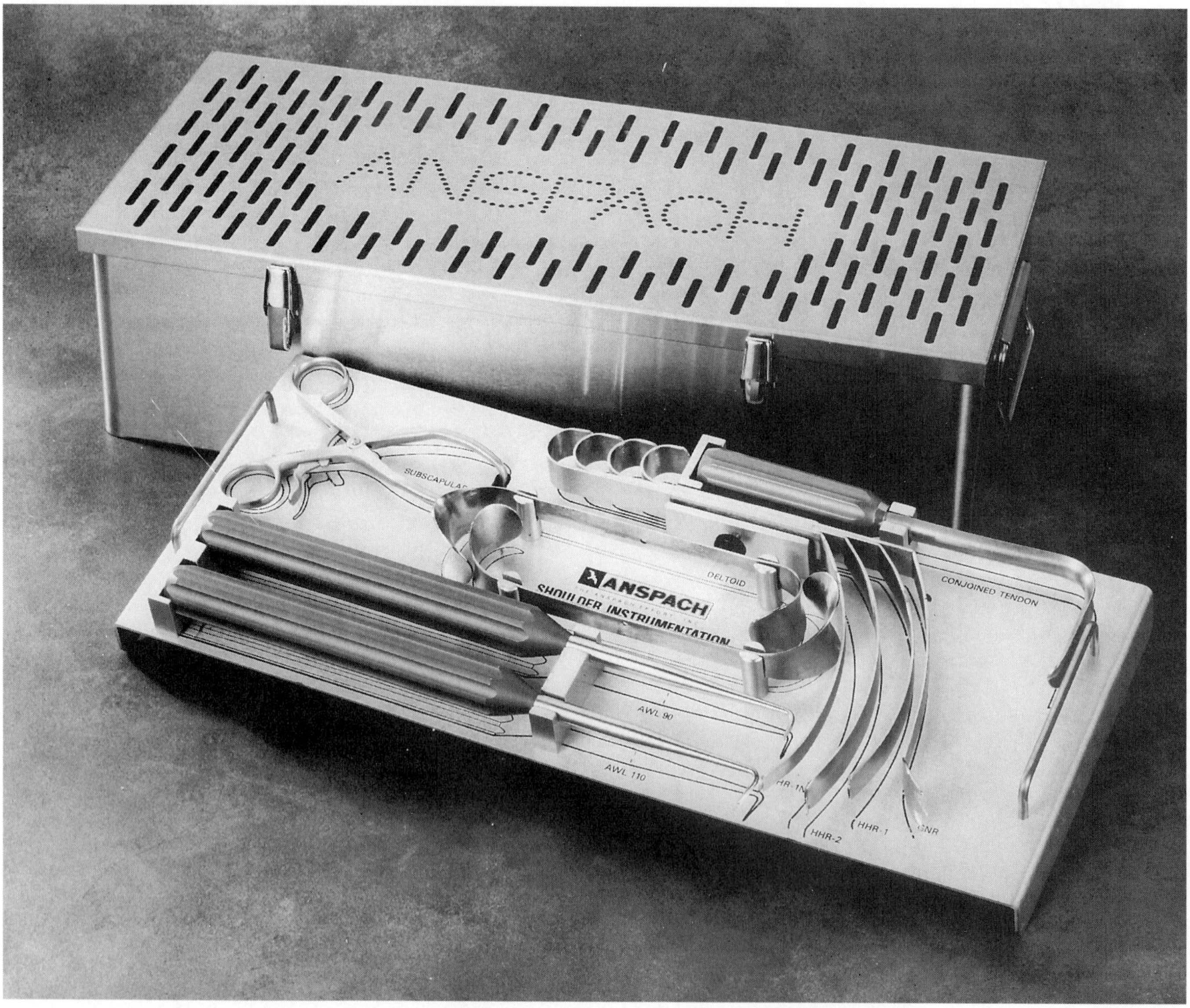

FIG. 21-50   Shoulder instrumentation set including humeral head retractors, glenoid neck retractor, modified gelpi retractors, Goulet retractors, conjoined tendon retractor, subscapularis retractor, and glenoid awl.

Courtesy The Anspach Effort, Inc., Palm Beach Gardens, Fl.

3. The fracture site is exposed and reduced, using bone-holding forceps.

4. If pinning the clavicle is to be done, a Steinman pin is passed into the medial fragment medullary canal and removed.

5. The pin is then passed in the same manner into the distal fragment.

6. The fracture is again reduced and a threaded Steinman pin is transfixed across the fracture site through both fragments.

7. If plating the clavicle is to be done, a small semitubular plate is used with at least two screw holes on each side of the fracture site.

8. The periosteum must be stripped off the clavicle sparingly but sufficiently to apply the plate to the anterior surface.

9. Extreme care must be taken when drilling screw holes to avoid damage to the subclavian vein and thoracic contents.

10. After closure an immobilization sling is applied.

Correction of rotator cuff tear

A rotator cuff tear occurs through the insertion of the tendinous fibers of the infraspinous, supraspinous, teres minor, and subscapular muscles on the humerus. Rotator cuff syndrome (impingement) involves multiple pathologic conditions. The approach to diagnosis and treatment is similar for both.

Rotator cuff tears and impingement frequently follow traumatic injury of patients with weakened tendinous fibers who have degenerative changes within the joint or in the throwing athlete, such as pitchers and football quarterbacks. Patients with rotator cuff tears are unable to initiate abduction of the shoulder because the stabilizing forces of the ruptured tendons on the humeral head are lost. Many rotator cuff tears can be treated conservatively with special splints or braces. This pathology may be seen alone or in combination with impingement from calcium deposits, tendinitis, subacromial bursitis, tenosynovitis, and other nonarticular lesions.

There are a variety of procedures that may be performed for these conditions. Methods of repair depend on the size and shape of the tear. The common goal is to restore joint stability, alleviate pain, and allow the patient to return to normal activities. In some instances a significant reduction in preinjury activity may be permanent.

Procedural considerations. If surgery is necessary, the patient is placed in the supine or semisitting position with a sandbag or folded towel under the affected shoulder. The head is tilted to the opposite side as far as possible.

A soft tissue and bone set is required in addition to the following:

Shoulder instruments	Heavy nonabsorbable
Power drill, Bur, and	suture
microsagittal saw	Shoulder positioner
Free-cutting needles	

Operative procedure

1. An anterosuperior deltoid incision is made.

2. The coracoacromial ligament is divided at the acromial attachment.

3. A subacromioplasty (resection of the under surface of the acromion) is completed. This is also primary treatment for impingement syndrome.

4. Small, simple tears can be repaired by suturing the torn edges with heavy, nonabsorbable sutures.

5. Massive tears may require attaching the torn edges to the greater tuberosity through drill holes.

6. If the defect cannot be bridged, then a flap from the subscapularis tendon can be transposed and sutured to the supraspinatus and infraspinatus muscles.

7. If impingement is involved or solely the cause of rotator pathology, other measures using the same approach are taken.

8. Calcium deposits encased in tendon are excised to alleviate mechanical obstruction or acromioplasty performed, as stated earlier in this procedure.

9. Following closure a shoulder immobilizer is applied and in place for 3 to 4 weeks.

Correction of recurrent anterior dislocation of the shoulder

The anterior fibers of the shoulder capsule are stretched and weakened as a result of frequent dislocations of the shoulder joint. More then 150 operations or modifications have been devised to treat recurrent anterior dislocation. The goals are to (1) prevent recurrence, (2) prevent surgical complications, (3) prevent creation of arthritis changes, (4) maintain joint motion, and (5) correct the problem. The surgeon will select the procedure appropriate for the patient condition that will satisfy the conditions necessary for correction of the problem. A stapling procedure was once common treatment of recurrent dislocation, but has been replaced by other practices. The common and accepted procedures are mentioned in this section.

Procedural considerations. The patient is placed in the supine or semisitting position with a sandbag or folded sheet under the shoulder. The arm is draped free so the extremity can be manipulated. An anterior curved incision or a longitudinal incision in the anterior axillary fold is made over the shoulder joint.

A soft tissue and bone set is required in addition to the following:

Shoulder instruments	Gelpi retractors
Power drill and Bur	Free-cutting needles,
Shoulder instruments	heavy suture
(Fig. 21-50)	Shoulder positioner

Operative procedures

Bankart procedure (Fig. 21-51). The attenuated anterior capsule is reattached to the rim of the glenoid fossa with heavy sutures. The glenoid fossa rim is decorticated

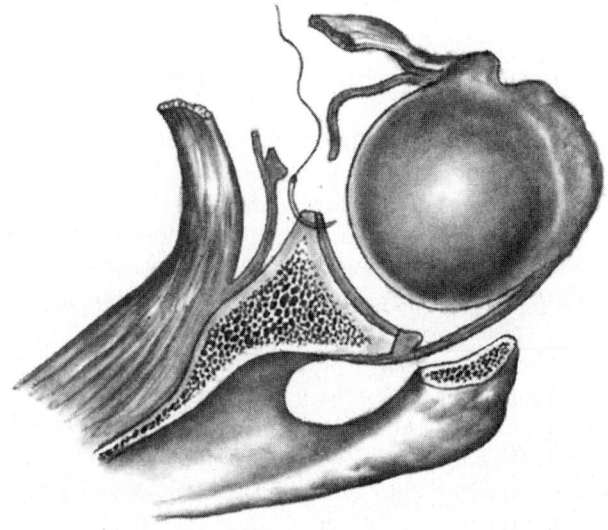

FIG. 21-51 Bankart procedure for restoration of shoulder stability; holes are made in the rim of the glenoid, and the free lateral margin of the capsule is sutured to the rim of the glenoid; the medial margin of the capsule is sutured to the lateral surface.

From Gregory B: *Perioperative Nursing Series: Orthopaedic Surgery*, St. Louis, 1994, Mosby.

with a curette to provide a raw surface to which the capsule is attached and promote adherence. Special instruments designed for the Bankart procedure are desirable. The Bankart instruments such as the curved awl and humeral head retractor facilitate the surgery. If the coracoid process is to be removed to obtain better operative exposure, a drill, bone screws, and washer should be available for reattachment. Postoperatively the extremity is immobilized in a sling or shoulder immobilizer. The patient may return to contact sports or heavy labor after approximately 6 months.

Putti-Platt procedure. The steps of the Putti-Platt are similar to those of the Bankart in that the joint capsule is sutured to the glenoid rim. Additionally, the Putti-Platt procedure requires the lateral advancement of the subscapularis. This produces a barrier against dislocation of the shoulder.

1. The subscapularis tendon is divided 2.5 cm medial from insertion.
2. The glenoid and humeral head are inspected using palpation to assess osteochondral changes.
3. The lateral portion of the subscapularis is sutured to the anterior glenoid rim.
4. The medial portion of the subscapularis is sutured to the rotator cuff at the greater tuberosity. The layers of the shoulder joint are imbricated (overlapped), a technique used often in soft tissue reconstruction.
5. The incision is closed and a shoulder immobilizer is applied. This is worn for approximately 3 weeks.
6. External rotation of the arm should be avoided immediately after the repair.

Bristow procedure. The coracoid process, along with the attached muscles, is detached and inserted onto the neck of the glenoid cavity, where it is attached with a screw through the subscapularis muscle. This stabilizes the anterior joint capsule and prevents recurrent dislocation. Disadvantages of this procedure are (1) internal rotation contracture, (2) inattention to labrum or capsule pathology, (3) potential for injury to the musculocutaneous nerve, (4) reduction of internal rotation power by shortening of the subscapularis muscle, and (5) possible limitation of external rotation. Penetration of the screw in the articular surface is another potential complication.

Correction of the humeral head fracture

Comminuted fractures of the humeral head (Fig. 21-52) with diplacement may require open reduction and internal fixation with screws or pins or closed reduction with a humeral nail or rod. However, if the fracture is badly comminuted, a prosthetic replacement is indicated. Traumatic or degenerative arthritic shoulder joints may be so painful or dysfunctional that a total shoulder joint replacement is necessary.

Extensive rehabilitation for the shoulder is required. Surgery should be performed as soon as possible. Delay can allow time for increasing scar formation, contracture of the muscles, and increasing osteoporosis of the bone fragments. The shoulder is the most difficult joint in the body to rehabilitate because it has (1) the greatest range of motion, (2) a second space beneath the acromion that must be mobilized, and (3) many muscles, weakened by trauma, that enter into complex movements.

Procedural consideration. See the section on shoulder arthroplasty.

SURGERY OF THE HUMERUS, RADIUS, AND ULNA

Fractures of the humeral shaft

Reduction of the fractured humerus is usually accomplished by closed manipulation and immobilization. When closed reduction is impossible or when nonunion of the fracture has occurred, surgery is indicated. The fracture is reduced and held with medullary fixation, compression plate, or lag screw. A rigid locking nail, with distal and proximal bone screws that will transfix the rod within the canal, control rotation of the fracture fragments, and prevent distraction at the fracture site (Fig. 21-53) may be the choice for repair. Multiple flexible nails may be used if more rigid nails are not available. Bone graft may be used, depending on both the extent of the fracture and the length of time since injury. Closed reduction versus open is the treatment of choice because the risk of nonunion and infection is minimized. Compression plating of shaft fractures is usually reserved for when other treatment has failed or with supracondylar involvement.

Procedural considerations. The patient is positioned supine with the body near the edge of the bed to facilitate moving the extremity. The extremity is prepped and draped from the middle of the chest to below the elbow. Fluoros-

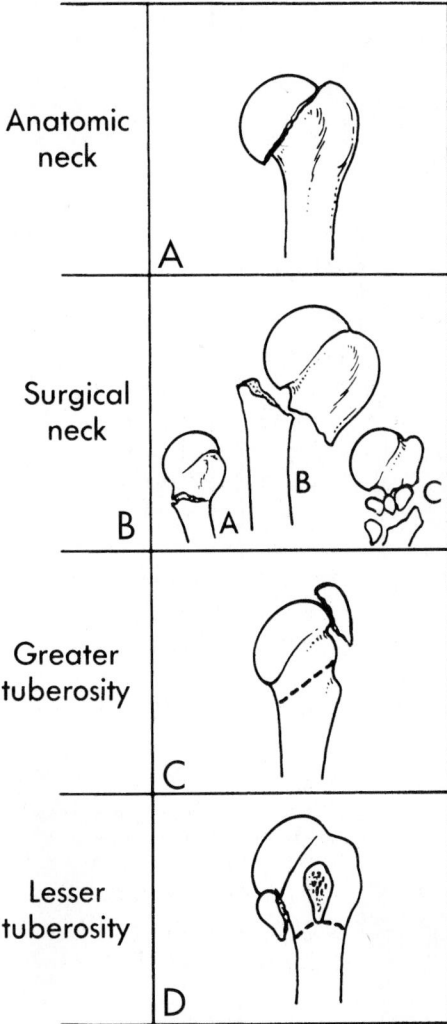

Anatomic neck

A

Surgical neck

B

A B C

Greater tuberosity

C

Lesser tuberosity

D

FIG. 21-52 Fractures and fracture dislocations relate to the pattern of displacement. Fractures can occur in two, three, or four parts.

Redrawn from Neer CS II: *J Bone Joint Surg* 52-A:1077, 1970.)

copy and permanent x-rays are required to ensure proper alignment, reduction, and placement of implants. A radiolucent table improves imaging ability.

Soft tissue and a large bone set are required in addition to the following:

Enders nails or interlocking medullary nail and associated instruments	Polymethyl methacrylate (for pathologic fractures when open reduction is needed)
Power drill	Sterile covers for use of radiograph
Traction tray	
Bone graft instruments	

Operative procedure — medullary fixation: antegrade technique

1. Proper length and alignment of the fracture must be attained with traction. Nail length should ensure proximal burying to avoid subacromial impingement and be 1 to 2 cm proximal to the olecranon fossa. A skin incision is made from the lateral point of the acromion over the tip of the greater tuberosity. The fascia is incised and the greater tuberosity palpated.

2. A small awl is inserted to enter medial to the greater tuberosity and confirmed with fluoroscopy in both AP and lateral views.

3. The awl is withdrawn; a ball-nosed reamer guidewire is inserted, advancing down the medullary canal (periodically verified with the fluoroscopy). Confirmation is made with each step to ensure the wires, reamers, or implant has not fractured through the cortex along the shaft.

4. The guide wire is advanced to within 1 to 2 cm of the olecranon fossa, avoiding distraction or shortening.

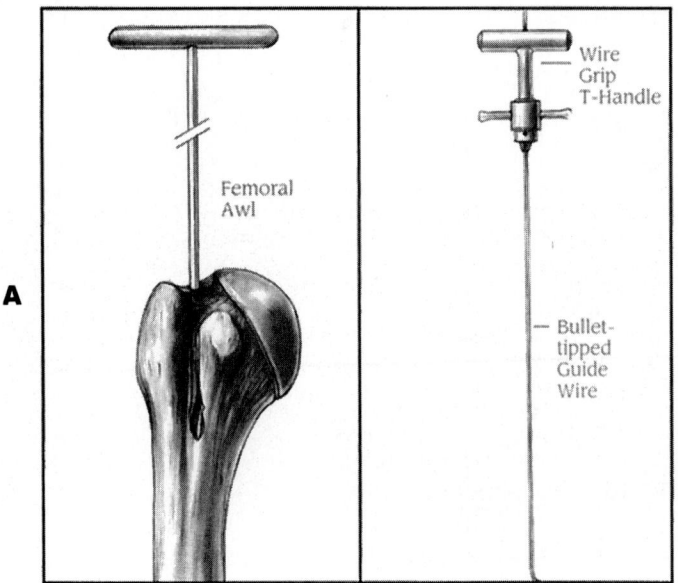

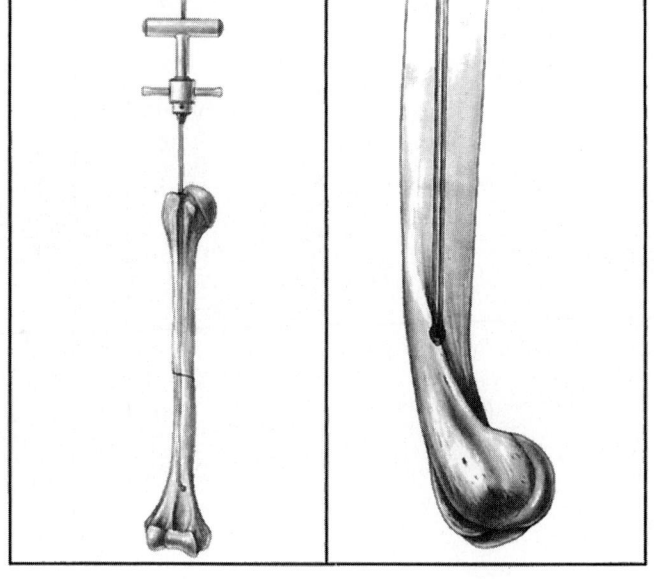

FIGURE 5 Attach Wire Grip Handle

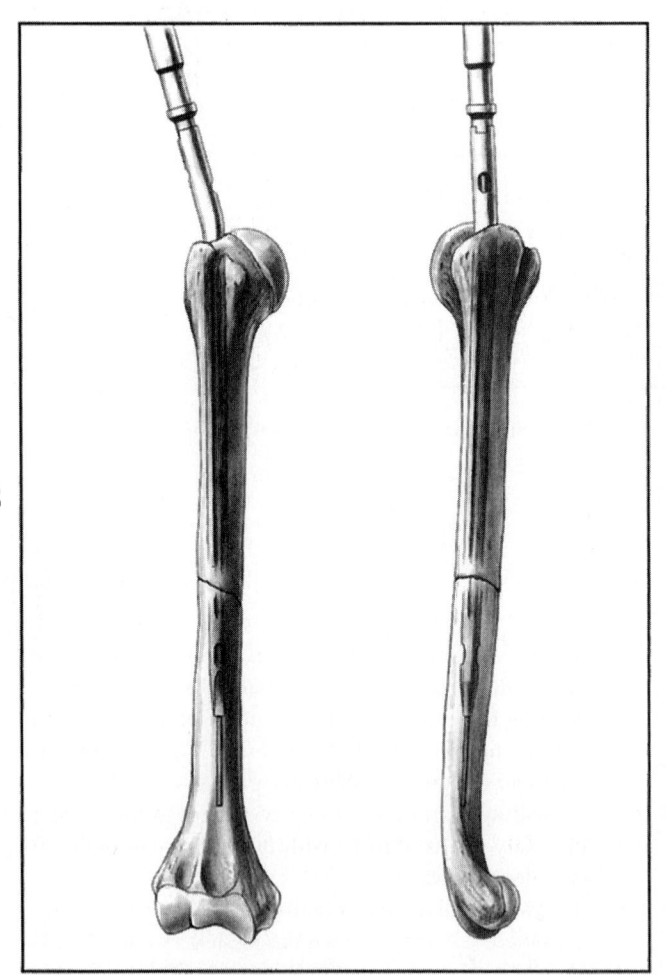

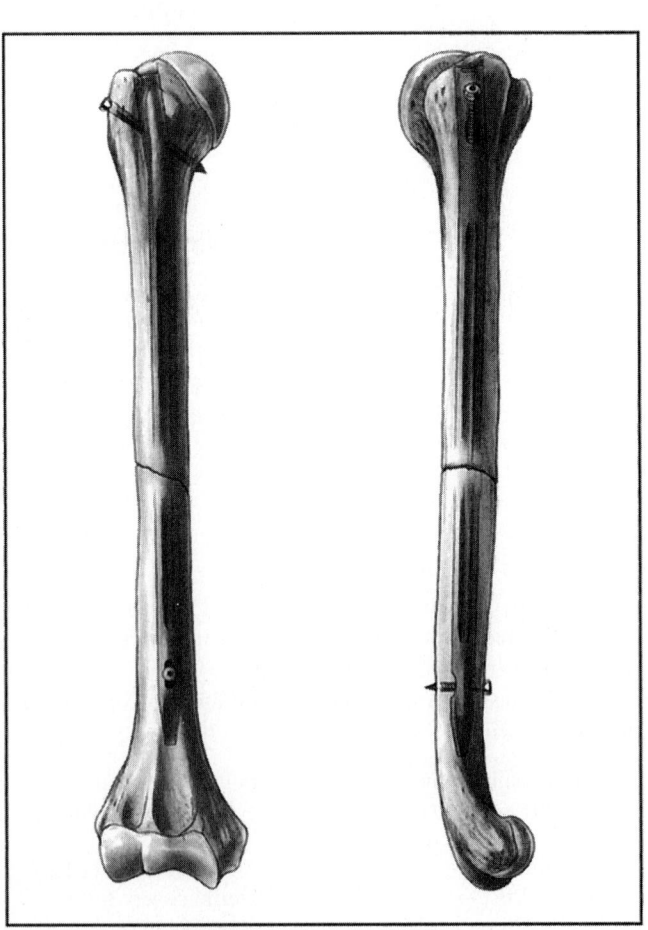

FIG. 21-53   Placement of the humeral rigid locking nail with distal and proximal screws. **A,** following incision and exposure, a femoral awl is used to make an entry portal. **B,** The guide wire is advanced into the center of the epicondylar region. **C,** Following reaming, the nail is advanced over the fracture site and seated. **D,** Proximal and distal locking takes place after determining the correct screw placement.

Courtesy Zimmer, Inc., Warsaw, Ind.

5. If Enders nails are being used, each one is advanced in the same fashion as the guide wire.

6. Nail length can be determined by using a second guide wire of the same length held against what remains extended from the humerus. The difference between the length protruding and the length remaining on the second rod is the approximate length requirement of the humeral nail. Another method utilizes a nail-length gauge that is held directly against the upper arm, viewed with fluoroscopy, and read directly on the gauge. Enders nails may be held directly against the arm and viewed with fluoroscopy to determine proper length.

7. If using Enders nails, two or three nails are driven down the shaft, across the fracture site, and into the distal fragment. Fluoroscopy is used to confirm proper placement and reduction.

8. If intramedullary nailing is to be accomplished, the humerus is reamed with a cannulated reamer down the shaft over the guide wire. Reaming of the canal is completed in 0.5-mm increments. The humerus becomes smaller in diameter. Reaming is gentle to ensure protrusion through the bone does not occur. The bone is reamed 0.5 to 1 mm larger than the selected nail diameter.

9. The medullary exchange tube is used to maintain fracture reduction.

10. The ball-tip guide wire is replaced with a non–ball-tip guide wire.

11. The medullary nail is assembled for impaction with the appropriate outrigger and drill guides.

12. The nail is guided into the proximal humerus and the humeral nail driver used to impact within the canal. Care must be taken to avoid splitting the humerus or creating a supracondylar fracture by wedging the tip of the nail.

13. As the nail approaches and crosses the fracture site, manual reduction must be maintained.

14. The proximal drill guide is attached to the nail impacter with the nail coupled; a stab wound is made in the skin, and the nail is pushed to reach the bone.

15. An 8-mm drill sleeve is inserted through the drill guide, followed by a 2.7-mm drill guide into the first guide.

16. The cortex is scored with the 2.7-mm trocar, and transfixing of the hole is completed with a 2.7-mm drill from the lateral to distal cortex.

17. The humeral screw depth gauge is inserted and read directly to determine the appropriate screw size.

18. A 4-mm fully threaded humeral screw is inserted. to the selected length. Screw position can be confirmed by inserting a guide wire down the end of the nail, where it will be impeded by the transfixing screw.

19. Fluoroscopy is used to target the distal humeral locking screw.

20. A second percutaneous access is created to the bone surface of the humerus from the anterior to posterior cortex of the bone.

21. With the free hand technique, the cortex of the bone is scored followed by the 8-mm hand-held drill sleeve and the 2.7-mm drill bit.

22. The selected size humeral screw is gauged and inserted. Placement is confirmed with fluoroscopy, and the impacter assembly is removed from the nail.

23. Full-view x-rays are obtained in both dimensions, and the wound is irrigated and closed.

Note: This describes a straightforward, uncomplicated procedure. There are many variations of approach and technique used depending on the complexity of fracture and associated injury. The fracture site may often have to be opened if it is comminuted or will not reduce properly through closed techniques. The radial nerve or other neurovascular structures may incur entrapment and trauma requiring exploration and repair.

Furthermore, this type of fixation using locked rods is preferred for this type of fracture. However, it is not the only method. Often a retrograde technique is utilized, with the patient in the prone or lateral decubitus position. The reader should note this technique, since it is used more commonly in the care of femoral shaft fractures and appears later in the chapter.

Distal humeral fractures (supracondylar, epicondylar, and intercondylar)

Distal humeral fractures are classified into several types depending on location and the presence or absence of articular involvement (Fig. 21-54). Supracondylar fractures of the humerus do not involve the articular surface and can generally be treated with closed reduction and casting. Transcondylar fractures may or may not have articular involvement, and this will accordingly dictate treatment. Intercondylar fractures involve both condyles with a communication of injury, are intraarticular, and present the greatest challenge for the surgical team. Fractures of the articular components, the capitellum and trochlea, are usually the result of a fall on an outstretched arm. The force drives the radial head to shear off the capitellum, producing an intraarticular fragment. The lateral or medial condyles and epicondyles are also subject to fracture by various mechanisms.

Patients may present with a single isolated fracture or any combination mentioned above. Neurovascular and other soft tissue trauma is considered the practitioner is deciding the type of reduction and fixation. Screws, pins, a variety of different plates, and dynamic compression technique can be used for internal fixation. Certain fixation techniques of the distal humerus may require an osteotomy of the olecranon (proximal ulna) to properly align and affix hardware (Fig. 21-55). The general goals of treating these injuries are (1) to maintain neurovascular integrity, (2) to restore normal joint articulation, (3) to preserve motion of the joint, and (4) to correct other soft tissue injuries.

Procedural considerations. Regional anesthesia can be utilized for procedures on the distal humerus. Bone graft

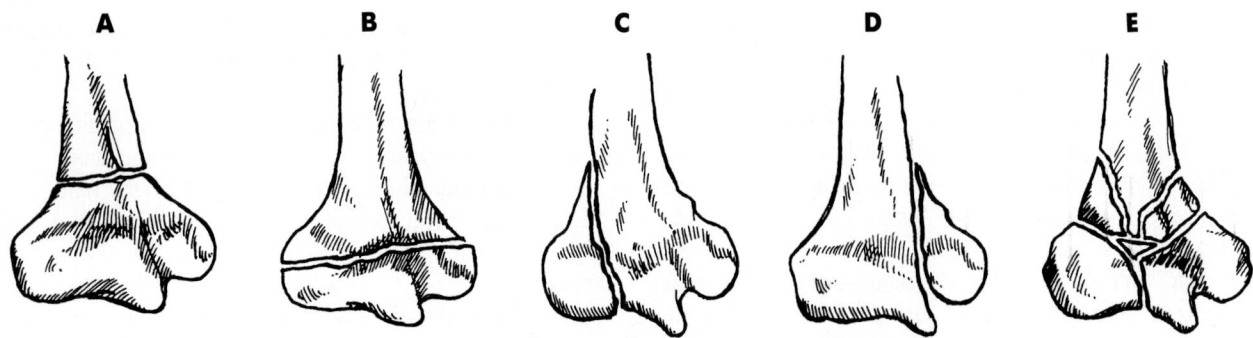

FIG. 21-54   Classification of distal humeral fractures. **A,** Supracondylar. **B,** Transcondylar. **C,** Lateral condyle with trochlea. **D,** Medial condyle. **E,** Intercondylar with comminution.

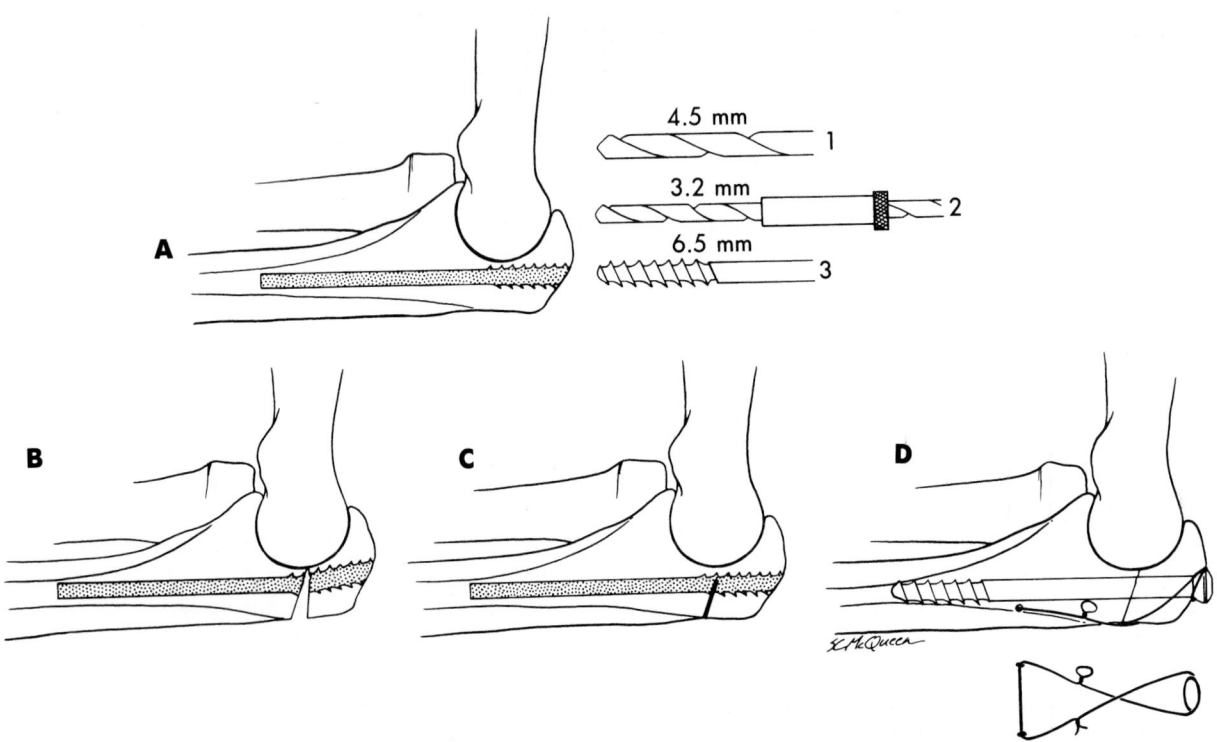

FIG. 21-55   Osteotomy of the olecranon with placement of a lag screw and tension band wire fixation.
From Crenshaw AH, editor: *Campbell's Operative Orthopaedics,* 5 vols, ed 8, St. Louis, 1992, Mosby.

harvesting may require use of general anesthesia. The patient may be prone with the elbow flexed over a small table, supine with the arm over the chest, supine with the arm on a hand table, or in the lateral position. A tourniquet is placed before the surgical prep and may be inflated during surgery as needed.

A soft tissue set, large bone set, and bone graft set are needed in addition to the following:

AO/ASIF compression   Bone-holding clamps
  sets (Fig. 21-56)   (Fig. 21-57)
Reconstruction plates   Smooth Kirschner wires
Power drill

Operative procedure—comminuted distal humeral fracture (Fig. 21-58)

1. An incision is made over the distal humeral fracture site.
2. The fracture is exposed and reduced using bone reduction clamps and temporary small smooth Kirschner wires, driving them across the fracture sites with the power drill.
3. A cancellous bone screw is placed using drill and tap to transfix from one condyle to the other. Care must be taken not to violate joint surface with the threads of the screw.

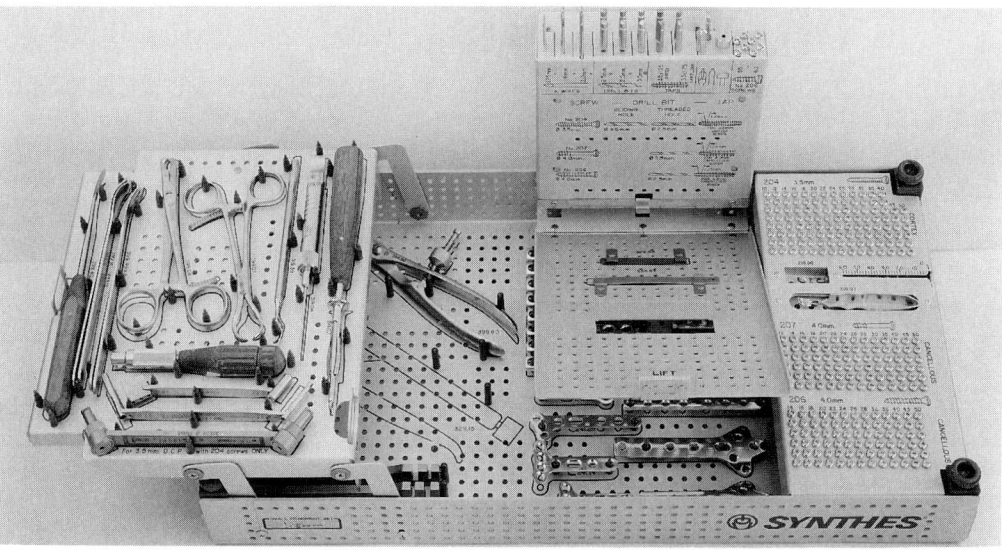

FIG. 21-56   AO/ASIF compression sets range in size for repair of fractures; small fragment set shown.
Courtesy Synthes U.S.A., Paoli, Pa.

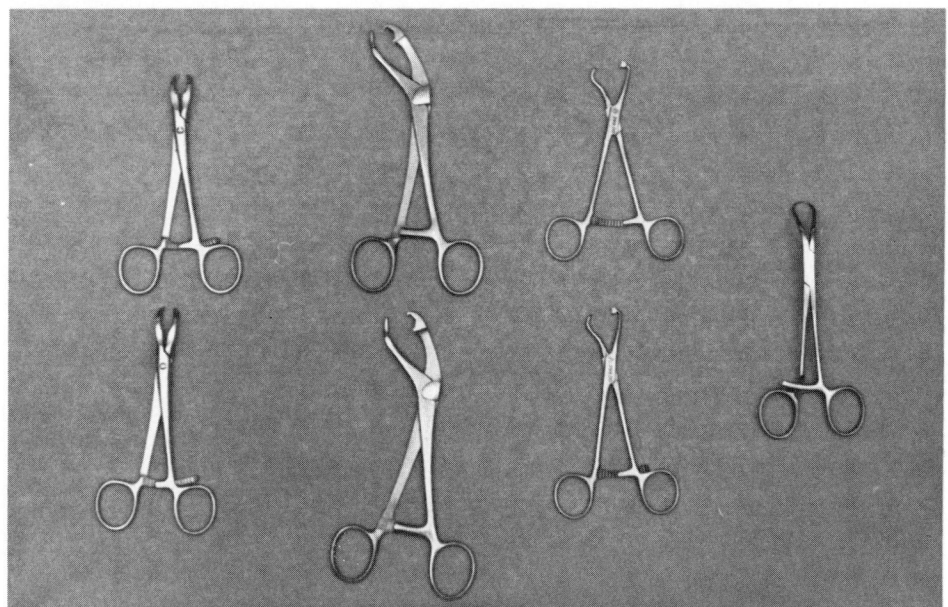

FIG. 21-57   Small bone clamps. *Left to right:* reduction, Verbrugge bone holding, plate holding, reduction with points.

4. Kirschner wires are removed if reduction is maintained.

5. A one-third semitubular or reconstruction plate is contoured to the shape of the distal humeral fracture and applied to bridge the fracture fragments.

6. Throughout the entire procedure, periodic inspection of the articular surface is completed to ensure integrity.

7. The plates are held in place by hand while the elbow is put through a range of motion. The plates should not encroach upon the olecranon or coronoid fossa (distal ulna), since this will limit flexion and extension of the arm.

8. The bone is drilled and tapped from one cortex to the other with the appropriate drill and tap.

9. The screw is inserted and seated to the bone surface on the plate. This is done for all subsequent screws, observing the fracture site and articular surface.

10. Interfragmentary screws may be used in addition to the cortical screws spanning the condyles.

11. If the olecranon was previously osteotomized for exposure, it is reattached using the tension band technique (Fig. 21-59) with a cancellous bone screw and heavy-gauge (18 or 20) wire.

12. The wound is irrigated and a drain placed as needed; the incision site is closed. A long arm posterior splint is applied.

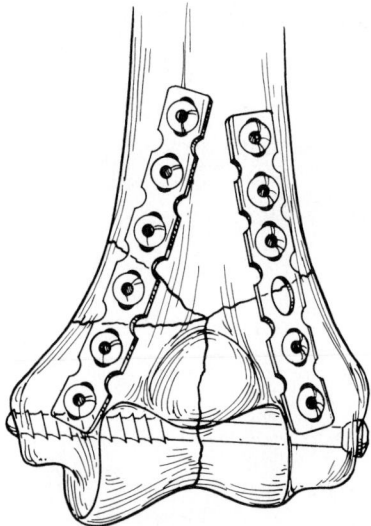

FIG. 21-58   Repair of the distal comminuted humeral fracture with 3.5 mm reconstruction plates.

From Crenshaw AH, editor: *Campbell's Operative Orthopaedics*, 5 vols, ed 8, St. Louis, 1992, Mosby-Year Book.

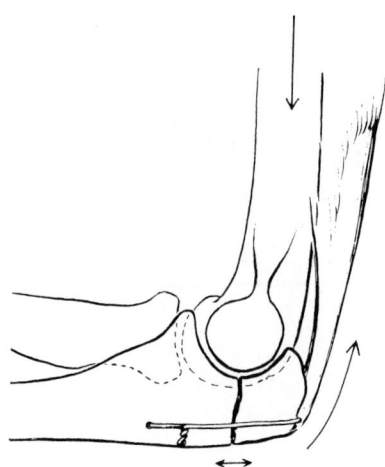

FIG. 21-59   Tension band technique used for repair of the olecranon.

From Knight RA:AAOS *Instr Course Lect* 14:123, 1957.

Olecranon fracture

If the olecranon fracture fragment is small, it may be excised and the triceps tendon reattached to the ulnar shaft. This does not result in loss of stability of the elbow joint. However, larger fragments must be reduced and held with internal fixation. The olecranon is often electively osteotomized for surgical exposure (see previous section) and repaired in the same fashion as a traumatic fracture.

Procedural considerations. The patient is placed in the prone position with the arm on an arm board or hand table.

A soft tissue set and bone set are required in addition to the following:

AO/ASIF instrumenta- tion and cancellous screws (or Steinman pins) Power drill Kirschner wires	Heavy (16- and 18- gauge) stainless steel wire (long lengths) Bone reduction clamps Wire tightener

Operative procedure—tension banding (Fig. 21-60)

1. An incision is made over the olecranon, and the fracture is exposed.
2. A drill hole is made in the distal fragment traversing the bone.
3. Stainless steel wire is passed through the drilled holes, crossed over, and pulled toward the tip of the olecranon.
4. After using the drill and tap, a cancellous bone screw is used to attach the proximal fragment to the distal, stopping short of totally seating the screw.

5. The wire is pulled and looped around the exposed shaft of the screw while reduction is maintained manually or by using a reduction clamp. The wire can be tightened using the wire tightener. The cancellous screws can be substituted by two smooth Steinman pins, bending over the exposed portion to hook the loop of wire.
6. The remaining screw is threaded into the bone; always observe the fracture site for opposition.
7. The wound is irrigated and closed. Drains are generally not necessary. A long arm posterior splint is placed.

Note: Utilizing this technique requires early active motion of the arm. Compression of the fracture site is achieved by placing the elbow through range of motion and applying force by the hardware.

Transposition of the ulnar nerve

Transposition of the ulnar nerve involves freeing the nerve from a groove at the back of the medial epicondyle of the humerus and bringing it to the front of the condyle. The ulnar nerve is frequently divided or damaged following fracture or wounds to the elbow caused by trauma. Dislocation of the elbow may also cause ulnar nerve damage. Late traumatic neuritis may occur following an old injury resulting in stretching of the ulnar nerve. The hand appears atrophied, and sensory loss is high. In severe cases a claw hand deformity occurs.

Procedural considerations. The patient is placed in the supine position with the extremity slightly flexed on a hand table or over the chest. A tourniquet is applied to the upper arm, and the entire arm (fingers to tourniquet) is prepped and draped.

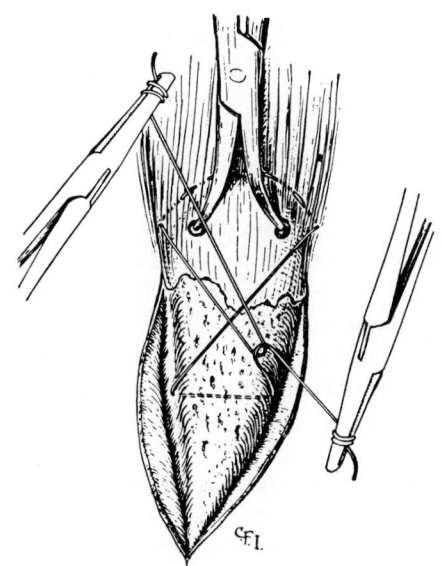

FIG. 21-60 Operative procedure: tension banding with stainless steel wire passed through drill holes; figure of eight adds stability to the fracture.

From Crenshaw AH, editor: *Campbell's Operative Orthopaedics*, 5 vols, ed 8, St. Louis, 1992, Mosby.

A soft tissue set is required. Bone instruments may be required.

Operative procedure

1. An incision is made on the lateral aspect of the elbow near the epicondyle.
2. The fascia and the flexor carpi ulnaris muscle are divided.
3. The ulnar nerve is freed and the medial intermuscular septum is dissected.
4. The nerve is then drawn anteriorly and placed deep in the brachialis flexor muscle origin.
5. The wound is irrigated and closed. A drain is not necessary. A short arm posterior splint is applied to the elbow postoperatively.

Excision of the head of the radius

Fractures of the radial head can be displaced or nondisplaced, segmental or comminuted. Complications can arise when treatment is delayed, causing limitation of motion, pain, and traumatic arthritis. A congruous radial head is essential for proper rotation of the forearm at the elbow. Consequently, in an adult it is necessary to excise the radial head if a severely comminuted fracture with angulation interferes with rotation. The radial head should never be excised in children. The outcome for the patient undergoing radial head excision may result in some permanent loss of rotation of the forearm. Noncomminuted fractures that are easily reduced can be treated using closed reduction and casting.

Procedural considerations. The patient is supine with the arm over the chest or on a hand table. A tourniquet is applied.

A soft tissue set, small bone set, and oscillating microsaw with blades are required.

Operative procedure

1. An incision is made on the shaft of the radius from 5 cm distal to the radial head extending proximally over the lateral humeral condyle.
2. Dissection is continued between the extensor carpi ulnaris and extensor digitorum muscles onto the joint capsule.
3. With the head and neck of the radius exposed through the joint capsule, the joint is irrigated to clear bone debris and blood clots.
4. The radial head is then excised just proximal to the radial tuberosity, taking care to remove all periosteum and limit new bone formation. The remaining annular ligament is also excised. The radial head can be reassembled to ensure all fragments have been retrieved.
5. The wound is closed, and a long arm posterior splint is applied with the elbow at 90 degrees.

Fractures of the proximal third of ulna with radial head dislocation (Monteggia)

This type of fracture presents with a proximal ulnar fracture and dislocation of the radial head. The fracture is rarely treated with open reduction in children. The open technique is often used to treat adults. A direct blow to the ulnar aspect or a fall while the arm is hyperextended produces this type of injury. If the open reduction approach is chosen, closed reduction of the radial dislocation is attempted and often successful. At times the annular ligament may prevent reduction of the radial head dislocation, and open reduction becomes necessary. There are various deforming forces of the forearm depending on the location of fracture in relation to the insertion of muscles. These forces are often encountered when treating forearm injuries.

Procedural considerations. The patient is placed in the supine position with or without a hand table. A tourniquet is applied and inflated as needed.

A soft tissue set and large bone set are required in addition to the following:

Power power drill	Bone reduction clamps
AO/ASIF instrumentation, plates, and screws	Bone-grasping forceps

Operative procedure—fixation with dynamic compression plate (Fig. 21-61)

1. The radial head dislocation is reduced using a closed technique.
2. An incision is made; the ulnar fracture site is dissected.
3. The periosteum is stripped and the fragments reapproximated utilizing bone reduction and grasping forceps.

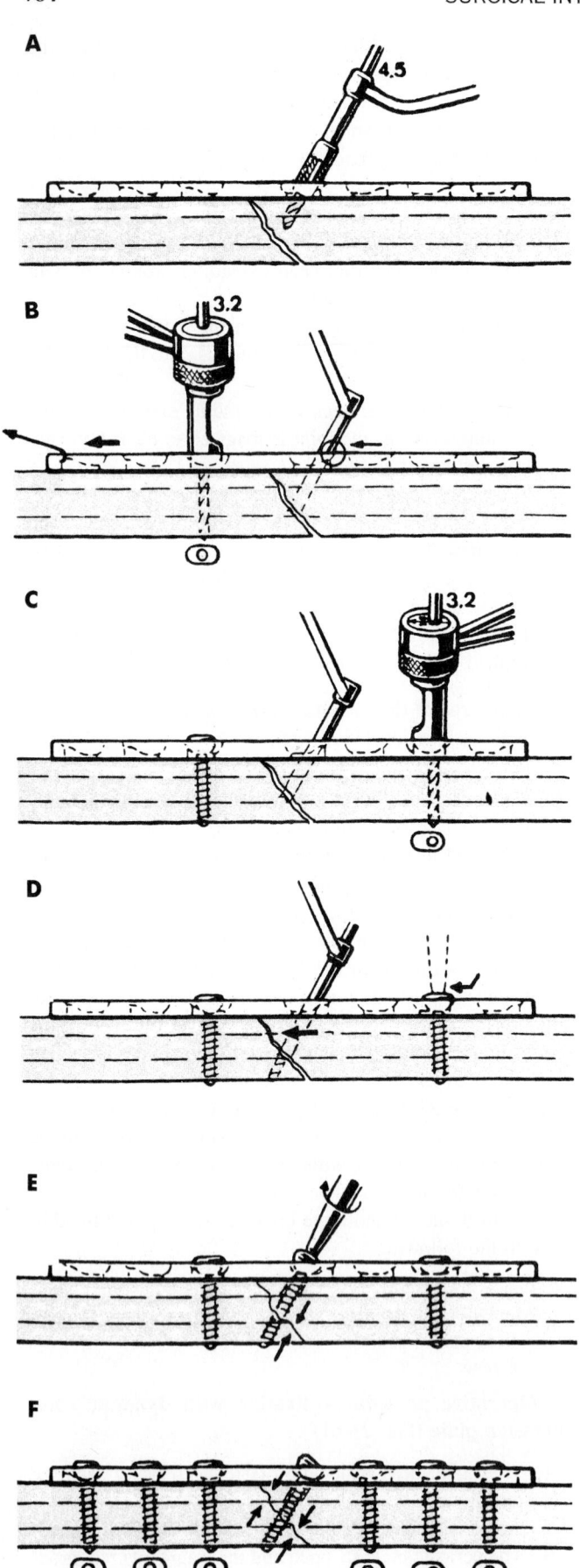

4. The bone is assessed for placement of a small or large fragment dynamic compression plate (DCP), with at least three screw holes proximal and three distal to the fracture site.

5. A concentric (neutral) hole is drilled in the ulna through one of the screw holes on the plate to the opposite cortex.

6. After gauging the hole, the selected size screw is inserted, with purchase of the opposite cortex ensured. A second screw is inserted on the opposite fragment in the neutral position.

7. On either side of the fracture site an eccentric (loading) hole is drilled in the same fashion to the opposite cortex. The hole is gauged and tapped and screw inserted.

8. The selected screw is entered eccentrically into the plate. As the screw seeks the center of the screw hole while riding the bevel of the screw hole it compresses the fracture site. This screw should be tightened down and the other screws slighted loosened.

9. The fracture site is now visualized as the action of the screw in the plate compresses the fracture site.

10. The remaining bone screws are inserted following the same procedure.

11. The wound is irrigated and closed; a drain may or may not be inserted.

12. A long arm posterior splint is placed with the arm in 110 to 120 degrees of flexion.

Note: The dynamic compression technique was developed in Europe, particularly Switzerland and Germany, and is marketed in this country under several different trade names including AO/ASIF group (Synthes), and the European compression technique (Zimmer). Fracture management in the United States often uses these guidelines and techniques. Dynamic compression plates are stockier and stronger than the semitubular plates mentioned earlier for distal humeral fractures. They are used to plate shaft fractures where stress forces on the shaft are greater and stronger plates are required. Dynamic compression plating to midshaft fractures of the femur are less common today. The insertion of rods evens the stress load of the bone. Fractures of the radius and ulna may also be treated with Rusch

FIG. 21-61 Fixation with dynamic compression plate. **A,** Gliding hole with drill bit. **B,** Fracture reduced, drill sleeve inserted and the fracture drawn together, a hole drilled and screw inserted in the neutral position to correct the fracture. **C and D,** One screw is inserted in load position (eccentric) into the other fragment; as the screw is tightened, axial compression is generated. **E,** Lag screw inserted across the fracture site and **F,** Remaining screws inserted in the neutral position.

From Muller ME, Algower M, Schneider R, and Willenegger H: *Manual of internal fixation: techniques recommended by AO-ASIF group,* ed 3, Berlin, 1990, Springer-Verlag.

rods, a device similar to Enders nails. The technique of dynamic compression plating is generally achieved in the same manner illustrated in the previous procedure when treating all shaft fractures. This technique appears later in the chapter.

Correction of Colles' fracture with external fixation

Colles' fracture is a dorsally angulated fracture of the distal radius. Most can be managed successfully with closed reduction and immobilization, but external fixation has recently gained wide popularity. Internal fixation is indicated when the distal radius is severely comminuted. In these cases Kirschner wires are used for internal fixation.

Procedural considerations. The patient is in the supine position with the arm extended on a hand table.

A soft tissue set and small bone set is required, in addition to the following:

External fixation device of choice	Small elevator
Power drill	Fluoroscopy

Operative procedure (see application of the unilateral frame)

1. Small incisions are made and two pins are placed at the bases of the second and third metacarpals.
2. Two pins are placed in the radius 8 cm from the styloid.
3. Pin placement is confirmed in both the AP and lateral views.
4. A frame is constructed incorporating all four pins.
5. Reduction of the fracture is obtained and the frame is secured (Fig. 21-42).
6. Postreduction films are taken to check alignment and pin position.

SURGERY OF THE HAND

Hand surgery has become a highly specialized area. There are numerous procedures for treating bone, soft tissue, or both that the orthopedic nurse encounters. Many of the techniques and principles applied to large bone are utilized in the treatment of hand injuries. Hand procedures range from carpal tunnel release to complex digit reimplantation.

Tourniquets are often used for hand surgery, as are regional anesthetic techniques. The operating team usually sits down at a hand table, but may move to areas such as the iliac crest for bone grafting. The scrub nurse must be organized and vigilant to control traffic around the operative area.

The instruments for hand surgery are common to orthopedics, but on a smaller scale. Many instruments and reconstruction systems have been developed primarily for hand surgery. Air or battery power drills and saws are frequently used. The surgery often requires the use of eye loupes (glasses for magnification) or the microscope.

Carpal tunnel release

Carpal tunnel syndrome results from entrapment of the median nerve on the volar surface of the wrist caused by thickened synovium, trauma, or aberrant muscles. Carpal tunnel syndrome is frequently seen in patients with rheumatoid synovitis or malaligned Colles' fracture and is associated with obesity, Raynaud's disease, pregnancy, and occupational injuries. The symptoms are pain, numbness, tingling of the fingers, and weakness of the intrinsic thumb muscles. These symptoms are usually reversible after the flexor retinaculum is incised, which relieves the compressed median nerve. Carpal tunnel release is being completed endoscopically, resulting in the release of the median nerve with minimal trauma.

Procedural considerations. The patient is placed in the supine position with the arm extended on a hand table. A tourniquet is applied to the upper arm. A hand set is required. The endoscopic approach requires use of specialized equipment for the procedure.

Operative procedure

1. A curvilinear, longitudinal volar incision is made from the proximal side of the palm, paralleling the thenar crease and extending to the crease of the wrist across the wrist joint.
2. The deep transverse carpal ligament is divided. Care must be taken to avoid damage to the median nerve. At this point the release is completed.
3. If indicated, a tenosynovectomy is completed.
4. The wound is closed, and a compression dressing and volar splint are applied.

Excision of ganglia

Ganglia are benign outpouchings of the synovium from the intercarpal joints or tendon sheaths that become filled with synovial fluid, causing pain and weakness. Ganglia are usually found on the dorsal surface of the wrist or on the tendon sheath over the metacarpophalangeal joint but are also found on the volar surface. Ganglia appear as firm masses that vary in size. They may resolve spontaneously but occasionally require excision due to discomfort or cosmetic reasons.

Procedural considerations. The patient is supine with the arm extended on a hand table. A hand set is required.

Operative procedure

1. A transverse incision is made over each ganglion.
2. Generous margins are removed around the base to prevent recurrence.
3. The wound is irrigated and closed, and a pressure dressing is applied.

Fractures of the carpal bones

Most fractures of the carpal bones are treated by closed reduction and immobilization. However, it is occasionally necessary to operate on a fracture because of acute insta-

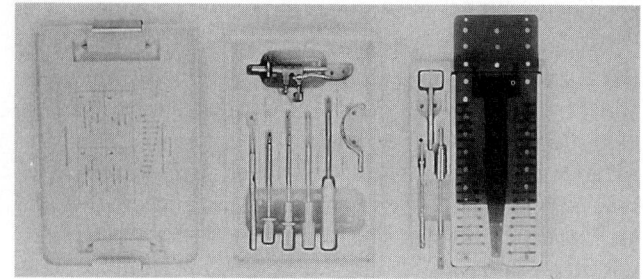

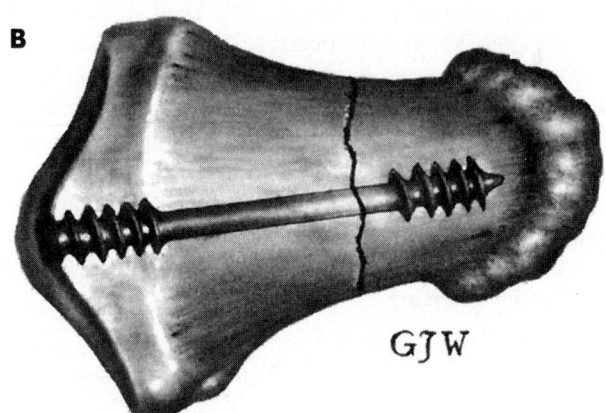

FIG. 21-62 **A,** Herbert bone screw set system and **B,** Screw placement.

A Courtesy Zimmer, Inc., Warsaw, Ind.; B from Gregory B: *Perioperative Nursing Series: Orthopaedic Surgery,* St. Louis, 1994, Mosby.

bility, delayed union, or nonunion. The scaphoid is the most commonly fractured carpal bone. Internal fixation is accomplished with Kirschner wires, small compression screws, or minifragment compression plates and screws. A bone graft from the distal radius or olecranon may be taken.

For displaced or unstable scaphoid fracture the Herbert bone screw (Fig. 21-62) has several advantages: (1) strong internal fixation, (2) compression at the fracture site with reversed threads at each end of the screw, and (3) reduced time required for external immobilization.

Procedural considerations. The patient is supine with the arm extended on a hand table. Fluoroscopy should be available.

A soft tissue and small bone set are required, in addition to the following:

Herbert screw set	Power drill
Minifragment compression set if desired	Smooth Kirschner wire

Operative procedure (Fig. 21-63)

1. An anterior incision is made over the scaphoid bone.
2. The superficial palmar branch of the radial artery is ligated and divided.
3. The flexor carpi radialis tendon sheath is incised and retracted to expose the capsule of the wrist.
4. The capsule is entered, and the scaphoid fracture is identified.

5. The fracture is reduced by manipulation and temporarily held with small Kirschner wires.
6. The scaphoid fracture is reduced and held with Herbert jig. A short drill bit and then a long drill bit are inserted to create a channel for the screw.
7. The Herbert screw is then inserted and turned until it is seated within the scaphoid.
8. Bone graft is placed around the fracture site if needed. (The loss of significant bone can often be corrected by fashioning a strut of bone from graft.)
9. The wound is irrigated and closed.
10. A splint is applied with thumb spica or long arm cast incorporating the thumb.

SURGERY OF THE HIP AND LOWER EXTREMITY
Fractures of the acetabulum

Fractures of the acetabulum usually result from high-energy injuries such as motor vehicle accidents and falls with a landing on the extended extremities. The fracture is directly related to the force transmitted to the femoral head via the greater trochanter or lower extremity. Management of these fractures can often present the orthopedic team with a complex and challenging task. Improvements in implant and instrument design, radiographic technique, and the emergence of magnetic resonance imaging and computerized tomography have revolutionized the management of these fractures. Indications for internal fixation of acetabu-

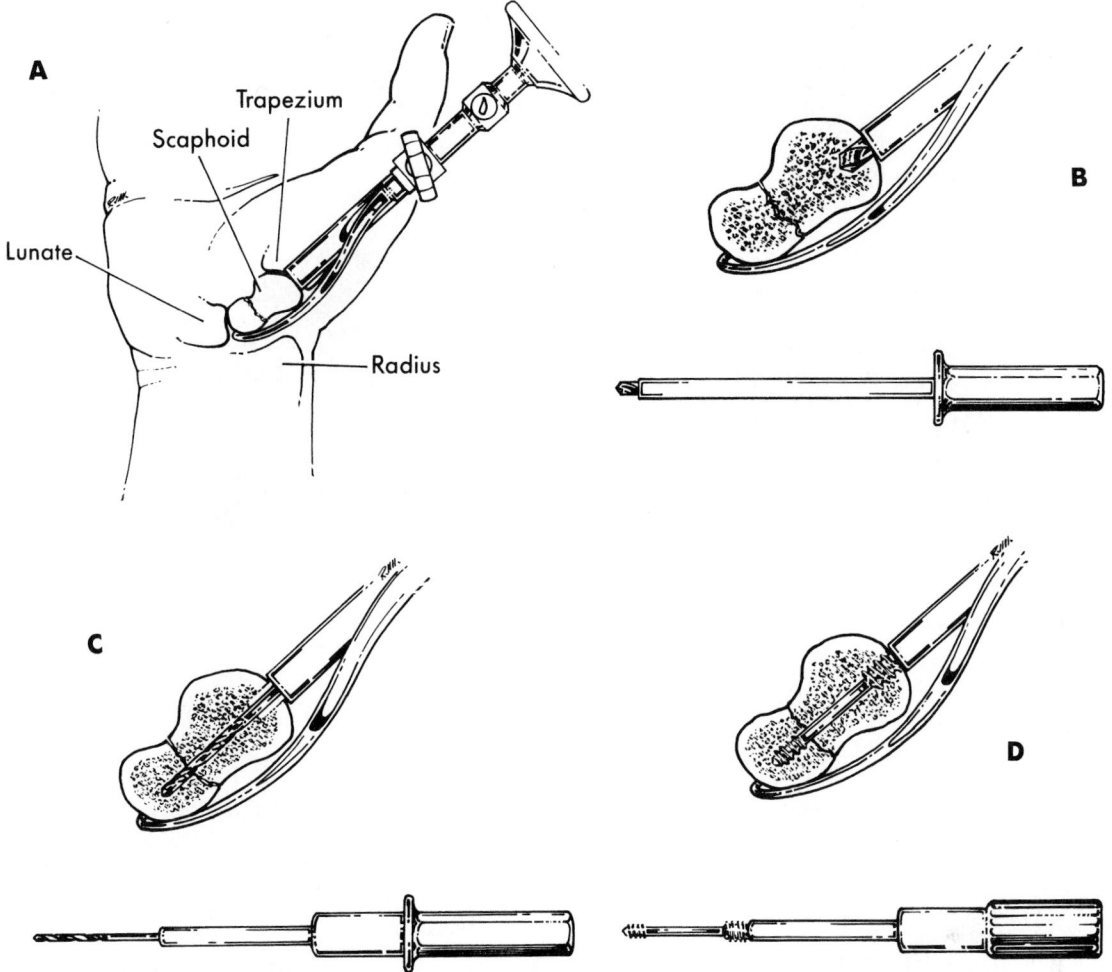

FIG. 21-63 Repair of the scaphoid. **A,** Fracture site is exposed. **B,** Alignment guide reduces the fracture and guides all subsequent instrumentation. **B,** The screw hole is drilled by hand. **C,** The tap is inserted. **D,** The Herbert bone screw is inserted through the drill guide.

Redrawn from Sprague HH and Howard FM: *Contemp Orthop* 16:18, 1988.

lar fractures include (1) greater than 2 mm of displacement, (2) presence of intraarticular loose bodies, (3) inability to reduce under closed methods, (4) unstable fractures of the posterior acetabular wall, and (5) open fractures. Internal fixation is usually delayed 3 to 10 days to allow time for the patient to be evaluated and clinically stabilized. Until internal fixation is placed, the fracture is reduced under closed methods and the patient maintained in skeletal traction. General anesthesia may be required for closed reduction and placement of skeletal traction when the acetabular fracture is severely displaced or dislocated. The fractures are divided into five basic groups: fractures of the posterior wall, posterior column, anterior wall, anterior column, and transverse fractures (Fig. 21-64). Internal fixation is accomplished with reconstruction plates and screws, total hip replacement with bone grafting (see total hip replacement), or fusion if the fracture cannot be reduced.

Procedural considerations. The surgical approach depends on the type and area of the fracture and the surgeon's preference. The patient is placed on a fracture table or stan-

dard OR bed in the lateral or supine position. General anesthesia is generally the anesthetic of choice, but this can be done solely with a regional block or concurrent epidural infusion. Procedures of this magnitude can be lengthy and involve considerable blood loss. Appropriate measures should be taken to avoid complications due to these factors. The room should remain warm, the patient protected from pressure injury, and red blood cell salvaging techniques employed.

A soft tissue set and large bone set are required in addition to the following:

Total hip set	Pelvic reduction clamps
Bone graft set	Femoral distracter
Acetabular instruments (Fig. 21-65)	Plate-bending irons
Reconstruction plates and screws, 3.5 and 4.5 mm	Kirschner wire and Steinman pins
Large fragment bone screws	Pulsatile lavage supplies with 3000 ml normal saline solution
Power drill	Fluoroscopy

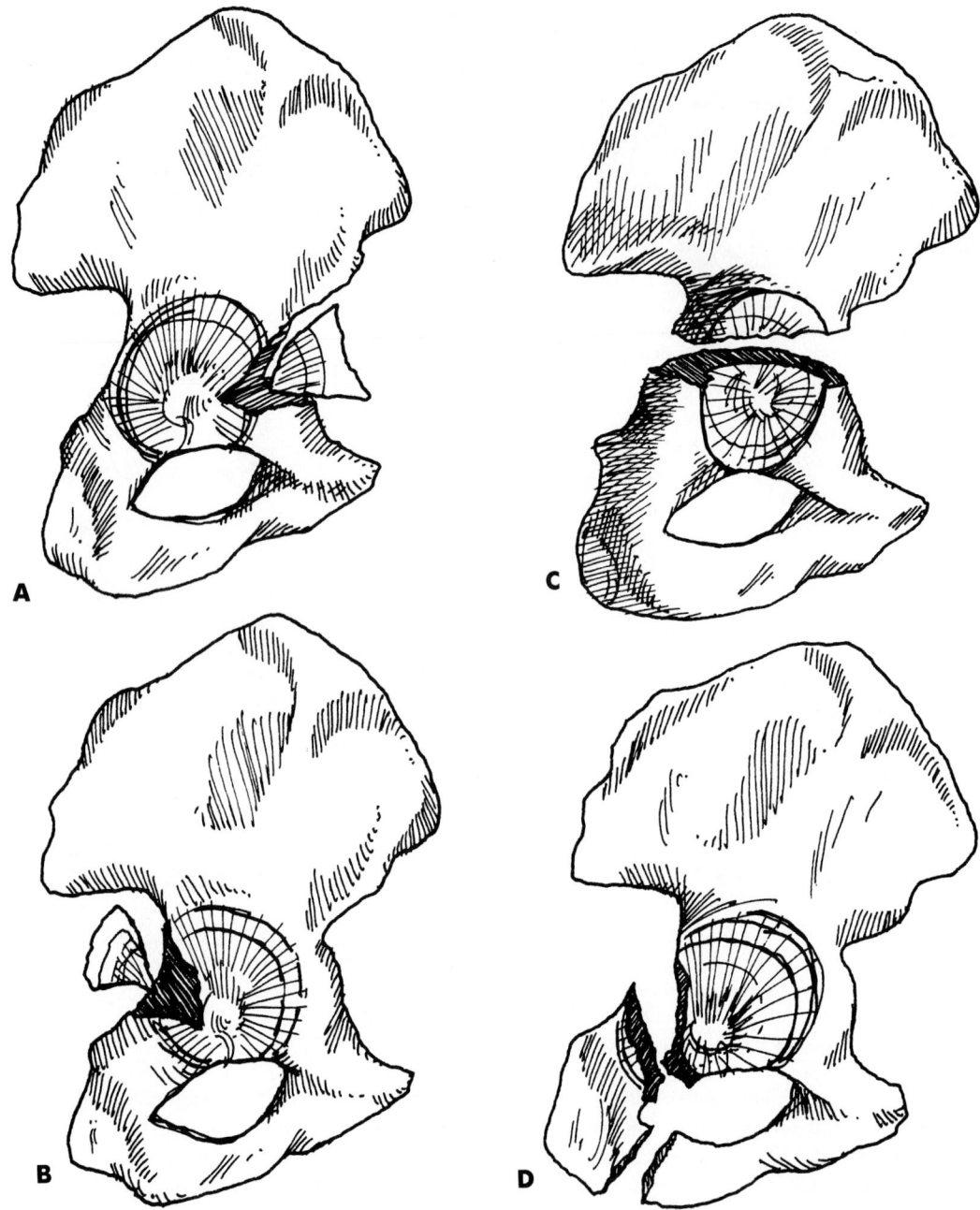

FIG. 21-64   Acetabular fractures. **A**, Anterior wall. **B**, Posterior wall. **C**, Transverse. **D**, Posterior column.

From Gustilo RB: *The Fracture Classification Manual*, St. Louis, 1991, Mosby-Year Book.

Operative procedure—posterolateral approach

1. A lateral incision is made over the acetabular fracture site.
2. The joint is opened and the femur dislocated from the acetabulum.
3. Self-retaining or hand-held hip retractors are used to maintain exposure of the acetabulum.
4. Measures such as a femoral distraction or osteotomy of the trochanter can be utilized to improve visualization and access to the fracture.
5. The fracture is reduced using bone clamps, forceps, and a ball spike.
6. Reduction is accomplished in gradual steps using Kirschner wires to hold the fragments temporarily in place.
7. Reconstruction plates are fitted and contoured to the fracture site and secured with screws.
8. Long cancellous lag screw fixation is also used to provide interfragmentary compression, particularly in column fractures.

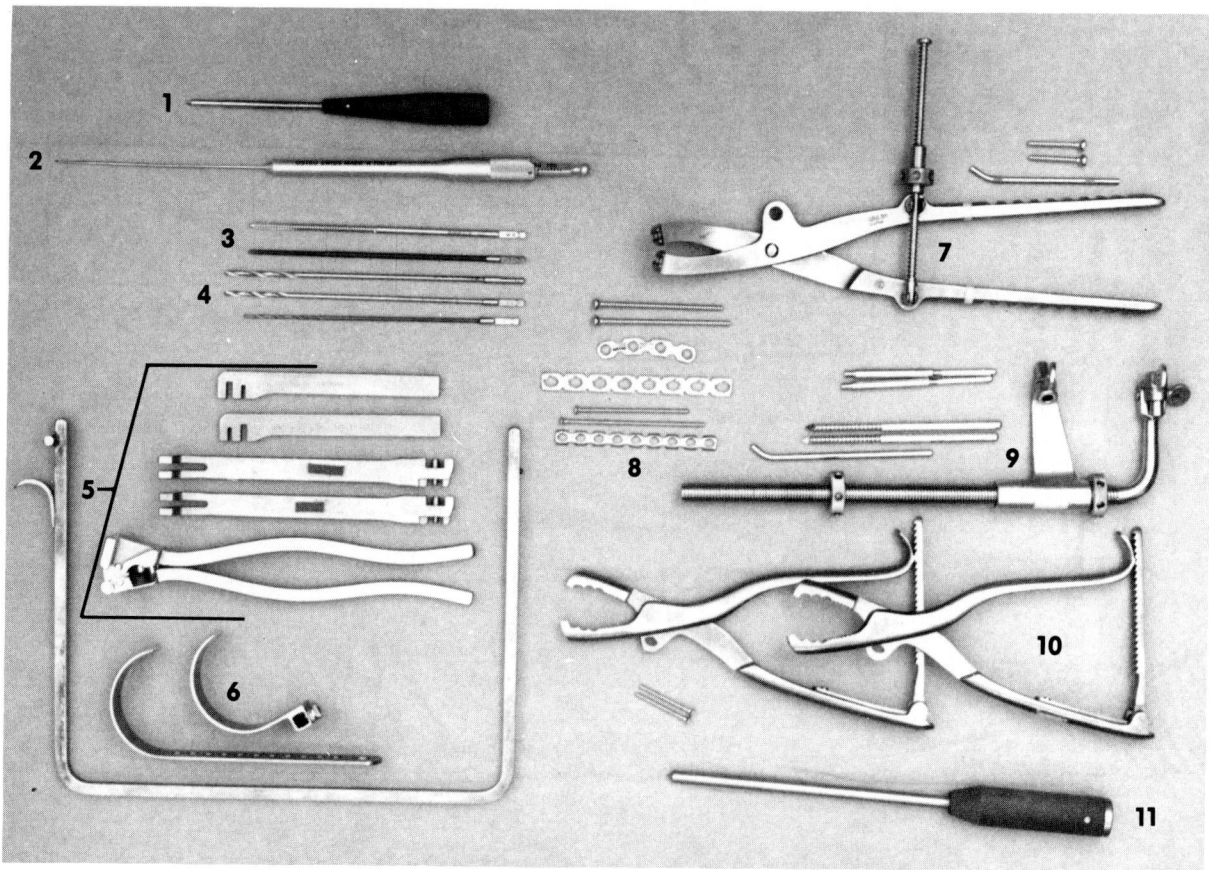

FIG. 21-65 Acetabular fracture instruments with implants: *1,* Screwdriver, small and large (not shown); *2,* Depth gauge; *3,* Tap; *4,* Drill bits; *5,* Plate bending irons; *6,* Initial incision retractor with blades; *7,* Pelvic reduction clamp with accessories; *8,* Reconstruction plates and screws; *9,* Femoral distractor and accessories; *10,* Faraboef forceps with screws; *11,* Ball spike.

9. Bone graft may be needed for additional fixation. A femoral head allograft technique is sometimes used, in which the allograft is mushroomed to create a new acetabulum.
10. The wound is irrigated with antibiotic solution delivered by pulsatile lavage, ensuring the articular surfaces are free from loose bodies.
11. The wound is closed, drains are inserted, and pressure dressings are applied.
12. The leg is maintained in abduction and external rotation with traction.

Note: If there is associated traumatic dislocation of the hip with the acetabular fracture, prompt treatment should address the dislocation. The dislocation should be reduced as soon as possible and skeletal traction inserted if needed to maintain reduction. Acetabular fractures may often accompany femoral shaft fractures, which also need to be treated concurrently with the surgeon's desired method (see femoral shaft fractures).

Hip fractures

Hip fractures are classified by anatomic location. The types of femoral neck fractures include intertrochanteric and subtrochanteric fractures (Fig. 21-66), and these can each be subclassified. Fracture dislocations also have a classification system and treatment protocol. Fractures of the greater or lesser trochanter are less common and can usually be treated nonoperatively.

Femoral neck fractures and intertrochanteric fractures commonly require open reduction and internal fixation. Neck fractures are more common in women due to several factors, including osteoporosis. Most elderly patients require a preoperative medical evaluation to define and treat anesthetic risks. However, effort should be made to correct the fracture as soon as possible to avoid complications related to immobility, skin pressure, pulmonary congestion, and thrombophlebitis. Avascular necrosis and degenerative changes can occur as a result of diminished blood supply, resulting in irreversible changes to the femoral head. Buck's traction may be placed preoperatively to reduce discomfort due to overriding of fracture fragments.

Manipulation, reduction, and internal fixation of these fractures are greatly facilitated by use of a fracture table, which also permits adequate radiographic examination to determine placement of the internal fixation. Subtrochanteric fractures are addressed in a later section on trauma.

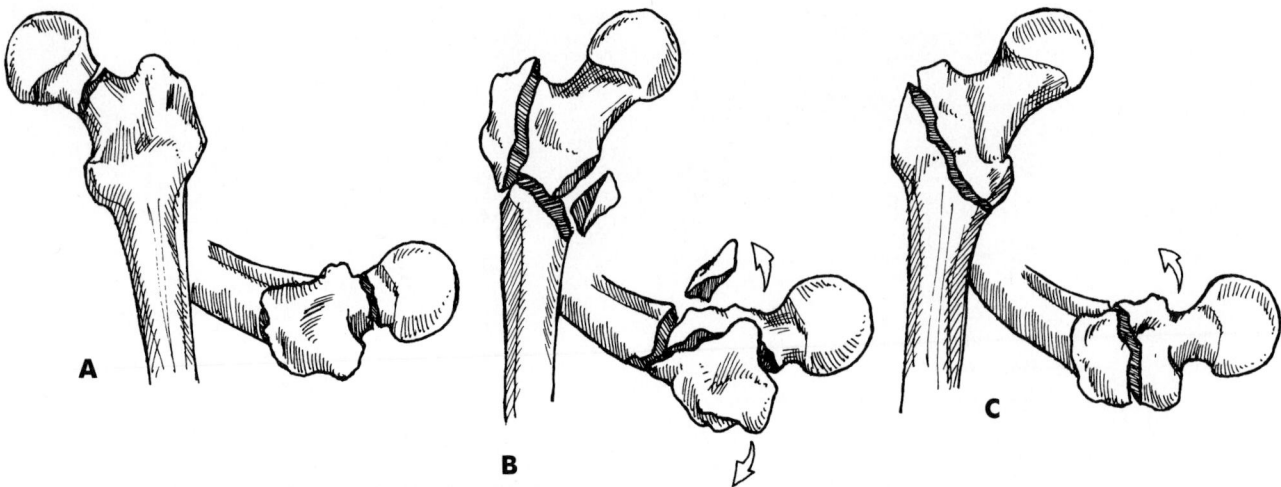

FIG. 21-66   Femoral neck fracture pathology. **A,** Intertrochanteric. **B,** Comminuted subtrochanteric.
C, Mid-cervical femoral neck.

From Gustilo RB: *The Fracture Classification Manual,* St. Louis, 1991, Mosby.

Intertrochanteric fractures

Intertrochanteric fractures most frequently occur in the older population. The fractures usually unite without difficulty. However, because the lower extremity is externally rotated at the fracture site, internal fixation is necessary to prevent malunion. Internal fixation allows patients to get out of bed earlier, thereby decreasing mortality and morbidity.

Procedural considerations. The patient is placed in the supine position on the fracture table and the fracture is reduced by manipulating the extremity and confirming with fluoroscopy (see Fig. 21-18). Various internal fixation devices, including Ambi, Freelock, DHS hip screws, and medullary fixation (see section on trauma) may be used. Success of the procedure is determined by bone quality, fragment geometry, ability to reduce adequately, implant design, and implant insertion technique. Blood loss is minimized because the hip joint is not opened.

A soft tissue and large bone set are required, in addition to the following:

Compression hip screw instrumentation	Power drill
Compression plates and screws	Bone reduction clamps
	Plate-holding clamps

Operative procedure—Ambi compression plate and lag screw (Fig. 21-67)

1. The fracture is reduced by closed reduction and maintained by adjusting the table traction.
2. Reduction is checked in both the AP and lateral views with fluoroscopy.
3. An incision is made from the greater trochanter distally to accommodate the length of the implant.
4. The dissection is completed to the fascia lata, and the vastus lateralis is exposed.
5. The reduction is visually confirmed; the guide pin is inserted after determining the angle of plate to be used. A 135-degree angle plate is commonly used.
6. The pin should be centralized in the femoral head approximately 1 cm short of the femoral articular surface. Care must be taken to not enter the joint space, since this might result in arthritic changes. Further penetration of the pin through the acetabulum and into the pelvis can potentially damage large vessels or bowel. A second pin can be used to control rotation in high neck or unstable fractures.
7. The lateral cortex is opened with the conical cannulated drill bit over the guide pin.
8. The depth gauge is placed over the guide pin. The size of the required lag screw is determined from the guide.
9. A double-barrel reamer is adjusted to correspond to the depth of the guide pin. The cortex is reamed over the guide pin to create a channel for the lag screw and barrel of the compression plate.
10. The lag screw channel is tapped to the full distance of reaming to allow proper seating of the lag screw, particularly in young patients with firm bone. Reaming depth of osteoporotic bone is reduced 5 mm and the tap depth reduced approximately 1 to 2 cm, to allow sufficient screw purchase.
11. The plate angle can be confirmed with a trial; the implants (plate and lag screw) are delivered to the back table.

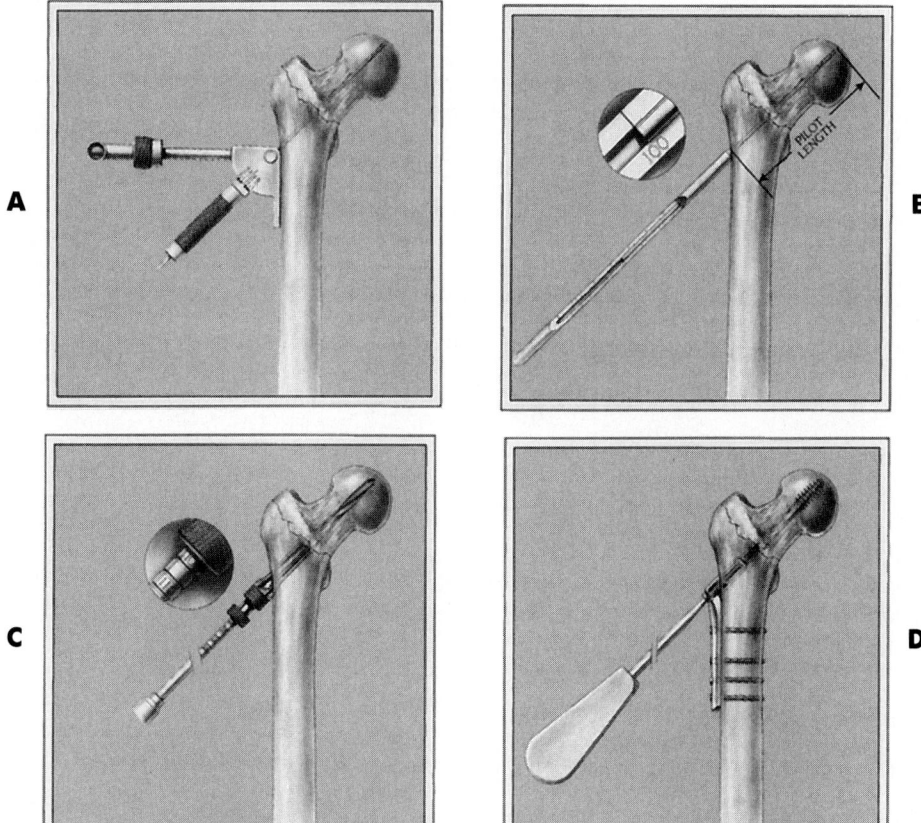

FIG. 21-67 Intertrochanteric fracture repair with compression plate. **A,** Guide pin is inserted. **B,** Depth of guide pin is obtained. **C,** The lag screw channel is reamed. **D,** The tube/plate is applied and lag screw inserted.

Courtesy Zimmer Technique Manual, Warsaw, Ind.

12. The plate, lag screw, and the insertion wrench with centering sleeve are assembled. A screw stabilizer is passed through the center of the insertion wrench and threaded into the lag screw.

13. The entire assembly is placed over the guide pin and the lag screw advanced to the desired depth, periodically verifying with fluoroscopy. Penetration of the lag screw through the femoral articular surface must be avoided.

14. The insertion wrench is disassembled, and the barrel of the compression plate is placed over the lag screw. The barrel of the plate should fully covered the lag screw. The plate is seated on the lateral femoral shaft.

15. The plate is secured to the shaft of the femur with plate-holding forceps. The guide pin is removed. At this point traction can be released to allow compression of the fracture site.

16. Screw holes are made using the drill guide and 3.5-mm drill bit. The length is determined and cortical screws inserted through the screw hole on the plate ensuring purchase on the opposite cortex of the shaft. The top screw hole on the plate can accept a 6.5-mm cancellous screw, which can be angled for better purchase in comminuted fractures.

17. Traction is released if not done previously. A compression screw is inserted into the barrel of the screw and threaded into the back of the lag screw, compressing the fracture site. The compression screw exerts a powerful force. The amount of compression applied should correlate with the quality of the bone.

18. The wound is irrigated and closed. Two suction drains may be inserted during closure. Weight bearing may begin as early as the first postoperative day.

Note: Many of the same techniques and principles of long bone fracture fixation are utilized in treatment of various types of hip fractures. The different screw types, dynamic compression, and the lag screw effect are described throughout the chapter (see ulnar fractures).

Femoral neck fractures—internal fixation

Anatomic reduction is necessary before internal fixation of femoral neck fractures because of the high incidence of associated complications, such as nonunion and avascular necrosis of the femoral head. The degree of displacement, tamponade pressure from intracapsular bleeding, and delays in reduction and fixation can affect the blood supply to the femoral head. These factors contribute to death of the femoral head and failed fixation. Growing children may sus-

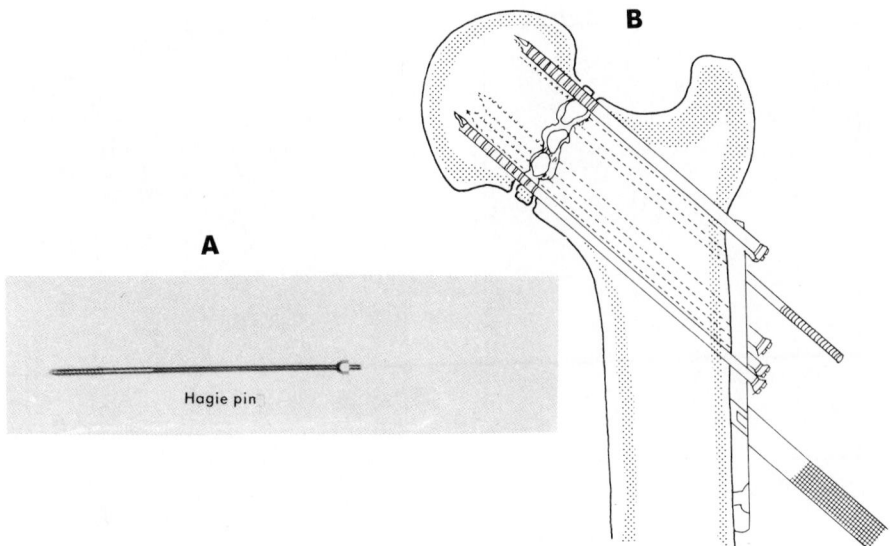

FIG. 21-68   Fixation pins including **A,** Hagie and **B,** Deyerle.

From DePalma A, editor: *Clinical orthopedics and related research,* vol 39, Philadelphia, 1965, JB Lippincott Co.

tain fractures through the epiphyseal growth plate (slipped capital femoral epiphysis). These injuries are treated by reduction and internal fixation of the femoral head, similar to the procedures used in the adult. The Garden and AO nomenclature are the most popular classifications for grading the fractures. Pins of various designs, such as Knowles (Fig. 21-68) and Hagie pins and universal cannulated screws (Fig. 21-69), are used for fixation. In cases of severe comminution or avascular necrosis of the femoral head the patient may require a prosthetic replacement (see total joint arthroplasty).

Procedural considerations. The patient is placed on a fracture table under general or regional anesthesia (spinal or epidural). Slight traction and external rotation are adjusted on the affected side. A soft tissue set and large bone set are required in addition to the following:

Fixation device of choice with instrumentation	Power drill
	Large bone-holding forceps
Kirschner wires (standard in some fixation systems)	Cobra retractors
	Fluoroscopy

Operative procedure—cannulated screw fixation

1. The fracture is exposed through a 15-cm lateral incision over the greater trochanter.
2. The dissection is carried through the subcutaneous and fascial layers; the vastus lateralis is detached anteriorly and retracted, exposing the femoral neck.
3. The femoral head is exposed using a small periosteal elevator to manipulate the head into an anatomic position.

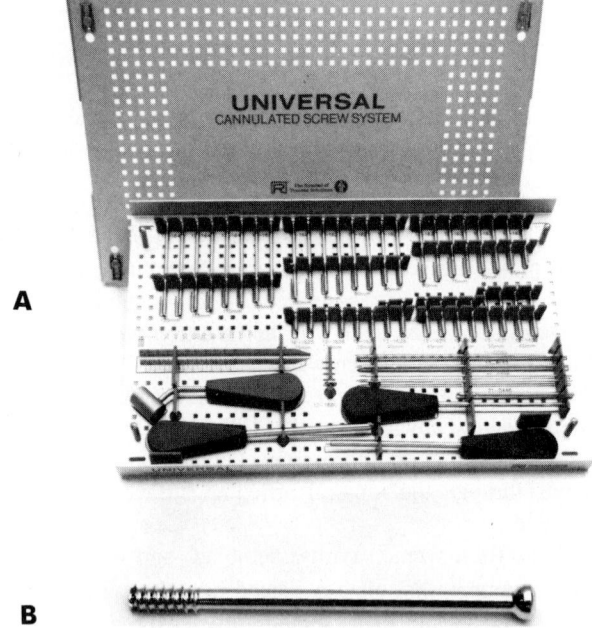

FIG. 21-69   **A,** Universal cannulated screw system. **B,** Universal cannulated screw.

Courtesy Richards Medical Co., Memphis, Tenn.

4. Two guide pins are driven into the middle of the femoral head, one anterior and one posterior, within 5 mm of subchondral bone; a third pin is placed adjacent to the medial cortex at a 135-degree angle. Care must be taken to not violate the articular surface.
5. The guide pins are measured for correct screw length and the cannulated screws are inserted over the guide pin without applying compression until all are seated.

6. Compression of the anterior screws is completed first and the posterior screws last to avoid collapse of the posterior aspect of the neck.
7. Traction is released and the fracture site visualized with fluoroscopy while the hip is rotated through a full range of motion.
8. X-rays are taken to verify the position of the screws; the wound is irrigated and closed.

Note: Screw protrusion into the joint space can be distarous to the articular surface. Radiopaque dye can be injected to rule out communication with the joint.

Femoral head prosthetic replacement—unipolar and bipolar implants

Original designs of femoral endoprostheses were indicated for displaced femoral neck fractures that led to avascular necrosis or nonunion and also were used in the young patient as an alternative to fixation of an acetabular component. The implants were a single unit including stem and head, required limited rasping and canal preparation, and could be implanted fairly quickly. Currently this procedure is accepted treatment for traumatic femoral fractures with an uninvolved acetabulum, and for select patients with osteoarthritis or avascular necrosis. Conventional designs include Austin-Moore, Thompson (Fig. 21-70) and Mueller. Two-piece modular components are also used. Many femoral head fractures are treated with total hip implants, requiring greater bone preparation and longer surgical times (see total hip arthroplasty). The acetabular side of the joint is not reconstructed if there are not deficiencies in the cup. In deciding between the endoprosthetic design and total hip reconstruction, consideration must be given to the patient's medical condition, age, and level of activity.

Current biomaterials, methods of fixation (cemented versus uncemented), prosthetic life, and modular components allow conversion of a hemiarthroplasty (reconstruction of one side of the joint) to a total hip arthroplasty, provided the femoral component is adequately fixed. Depending on the patient condition, the acetabulum may eventually require arthroplasty as a result of degenerative changes. Improved technology and surgical technique have increased the life span of implanted components. The portion of the implant that articulates within the acetabulum can be removed and replaced with a smaller femoral head. The acetabulum is then prepared for prosthetic implantation by various means of fixation. The ability to convert from hemiarthroplasty to total arthroplasty considerably reduces the amount of surgery required.

Bipolar endoprostheses (Fig. 21-71) were introduced to reduce the shear stresses affecting the acetabular surface. Bipolar design prostheses were designed to decrease motion and friction between the prosthetic head and the acetabulum that are seen with conventional (unipolar) endoprostheses. A femoral head prosthesis is snapped into a rotating polyethylene-lined cup that, when inserted, moves as one unit. Friction occurs between the ball and plastic instead of between the head and the acetabulum. This was a revolutionary design in the mechanics of hip motion and stresses. Surfacing data have some surgeons and engineers evaluating the use of bipolar versus unipolar. It is believed

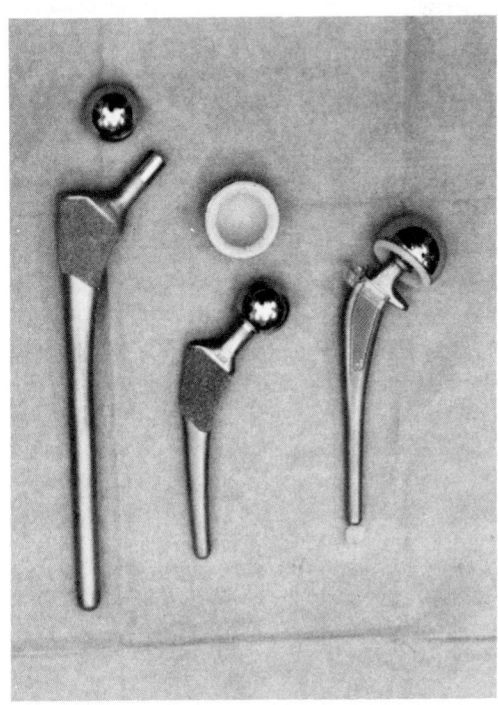

FIG. 21-71 Bipolar endoprostheses.
Courtesy Howmedica, Inc., Rutherford, N.J.

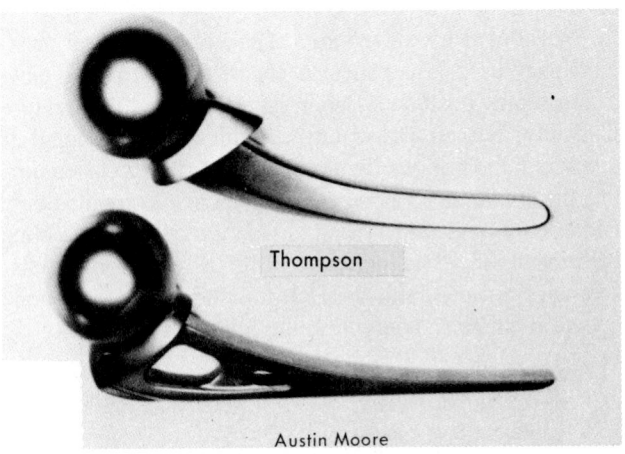

Thompson

Austin Moore

FIG. 21-70 Femoral endoprosthesis. Austin Moore and Thompson.
Courtesy Zimmer, Inc., Warsaw, Ind.

bipolar motion subsides after fibrous growth has taken place, allowing for only unipolar motion. Second, there have been cases of bone resorption and subsequent prosthetic loosening in cases in which bipolars were used. Those involved are looking at evidence of metallic head wear of the polyethylene cup creating microscopic fragmentation and a chemical lysis of bone. There has been a resurgence in the use of unipolar heads for femoral head replacement.

Procedural considerations. The patient is placed in the lateral position following the administration of general or regional anesthesia. A scrub and paint prep is done from umbilical level down to and including the foot. Instrumentation for total hip replacement should be available but not opened until inspection of the resected joint is completed to determine if a total arthroplasty is required.

The soft tissue and large bone are required in addition to the following:

Endoprosthesis instruments, trials, and implants (Fig. 21-72)	Power reciprocating saw (Fig. 21-73)
Femoral head template or caliper	Polymethyl methacrylate (if used)
	Hip "extras"

Operative procedure—modular Austin-Moore endoprosthesis

1. A linear incision is made from 5 cm below the posteroinferior iliac spine toward the posterior aspect of the greater trochanter and distally along the posterior aspect of the proximal femur for 7 mm.
2. The capsule is entered and the femoral head removed and gauged with the template. Fragments that may be loose in the acetabulum or attached to the ligamentum teres are removed.
3. A trial cup is inserted into the acetabulum and axial compression applied while clearance of lateral motion is checked.
4. The femoral neck is fashioned to achieve an accurate prosthetic fit.
5. A punch is then used to open the medullary canal from the femoral neck. The intramedullary canal is reamed and rasped to accommodate the prosthesis.
6. Once the canal is prepared, the prosthesis of choice is inserted with or without bone cement.
7. A unipolar or bipolar assembly is snapped onto the neck of the femoral stem. The height of the head determines the neck length and is selected after trial reduction.
8. The hip is reduced, and closure is accomplished in layers over suction drains.

Femoral shaft fractures—internal fixation

Fractures involving the femoral shaft are very common in today's orthopedic operating room. Prolonged immobility, complications, and disability can result if femoral shaft fractures are not managed appropriately. The femur is the largest principal load-bearing bone in the body. Fractures of the femoral shaft can be surgically treated with several techniques now available. Consideration for treatment are type and location of fracture (location on shaft), the number of segments involved, the degree of comminution (Fig. 21-74), and the activity level of the patient. Femoral shaft fractures are often associated with ipsilateral (same side) trochanteric or condylar fractures. Pathologic fractures often occur in this region.

Possible treatment methods of femoral shaft fractures are closed reduction, skeletal traction, and femoral cast bracing. External fixation has limited indications when treating fractures associated with wound infection or neurovascular compromise. It may serve temporarily until such time that internal fixation can be performed. Although plates and screws are used for femoral shaft fractures, their use is widely disputed and losing popularity. Complications such as bent or broken plates, refractures, and deep wound infections have been reported. Intramedullary fixation devices have become the preferred method of treatment. Intramedullary nails and rods increase the load sharing of the bone, making the implant less likely to fracture. Bone healing requires a load across the fracture site to promote osteosynthesis and prevent refracture. The open or closed method of intramedullary nailing can be utilized with locked and nonlocked nails. Closed methods of intramedullary fixation often minimize exposure of the surgical site and surgical time, resulting in less opportunity for infection.

Intramedullary nail and rod designs vary: (1) flexible nails like the Rusch or Ender type, (2) standard rods such as the Sampson and AO rods, and (3) interlocking nails (see humeral shaft fracture) such as the Gross-Kempf and Russell-Taylor varieties (Fig. 21-75). Closed reduction and intramedullary nailing with or without locking screws has become the method against which other methods are measured. Incidence of scarring, blood loss, and infection are all favorable. Fracture hematoma remains intact at the fracture site, which is important in bone healing, and the rate of bone union is increased.

Procedural considerations. General or epidural anesthetics are used. The patient is placed on the fracture table in the supine position, traction is applied, and the fracture manually reduced and confirmed with the fluoroscopy. If the fracture is profoundly unstable, care must be taken during manipulation to prevent neurovascular complications. For open intramedullary fixation extra retractors and bone instruments may be required to facilitate retraction and dissection. For closed reduction a soft tissue set and large bone set are required in addition to the following:

Intramedullary rod set, intramedullary nail implants, and associated instruments	Power reamer and drill
	Steinman pins
	Skeletal traction tray (Fig. 21-21)
Long guide wires for reamers	Fluoroscopy

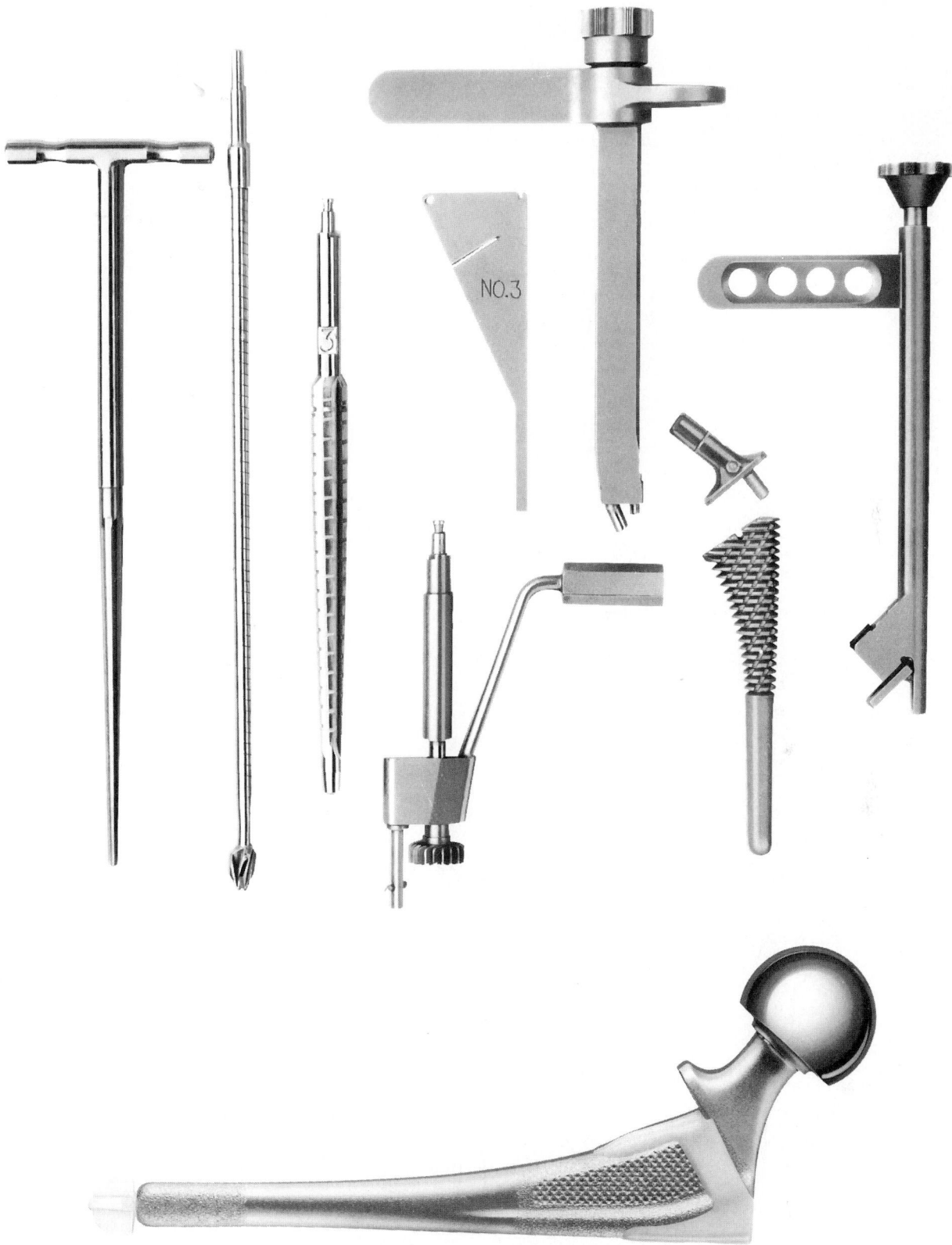

FIG. 21-72   Instrumentation for endoprosthetic implant.
Courtesy Howmedica, Inc. Rutherford, NJ

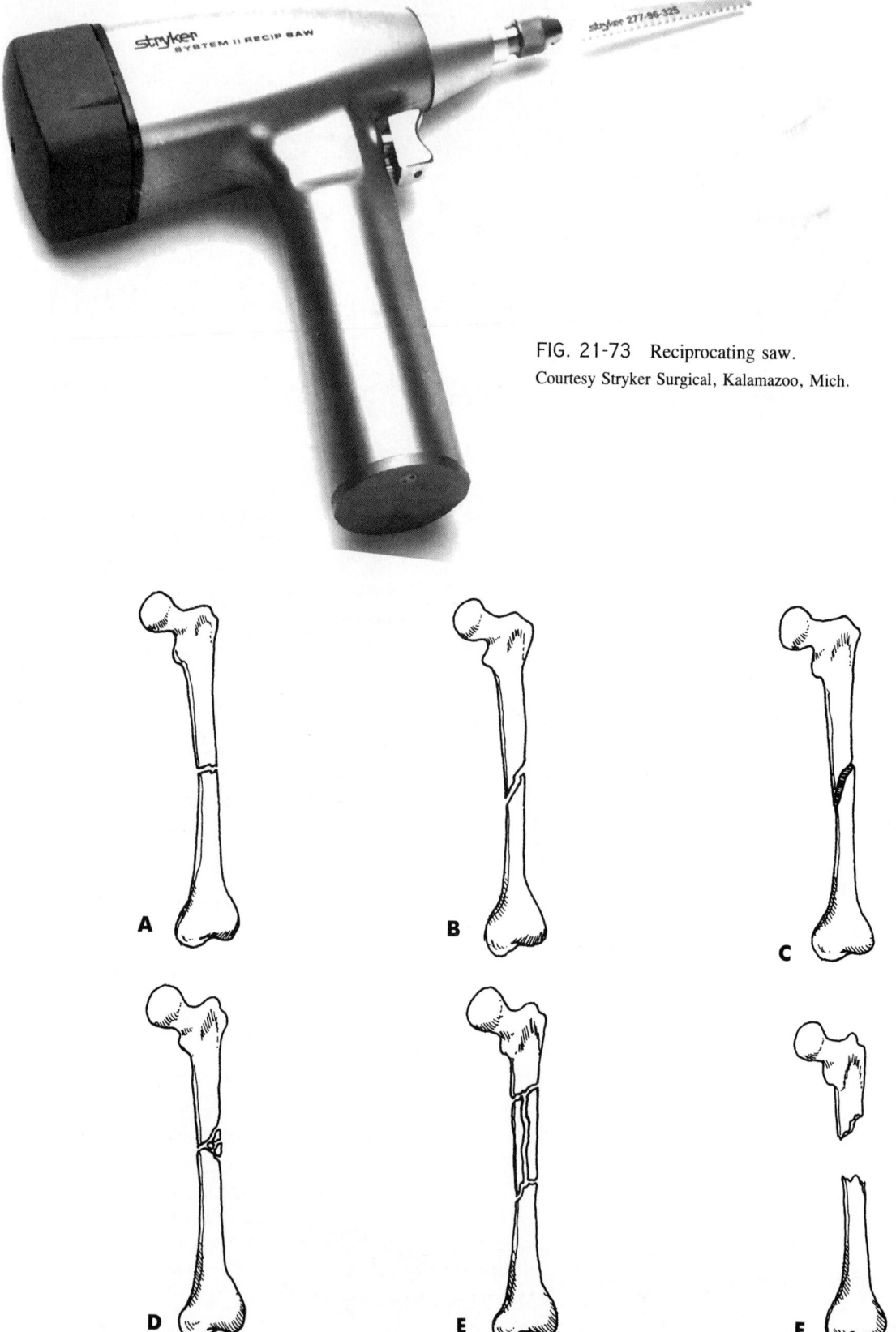

FIG. 21-73   Reciprocating saw.
Courtesy Stryker Surgical, Kalamazoo, Mich.

FIG. 21-74   Femoral shaft fractures. **A,** Transverse. **B,** Oblique. **C,** Spiral. **D,** Comminuted. **E,** Longitudinal split. **F,** Complete bone loss.
From Gustilo RB: *The Fracture Classification Manual,* St. Louis, 1991, Mosby.

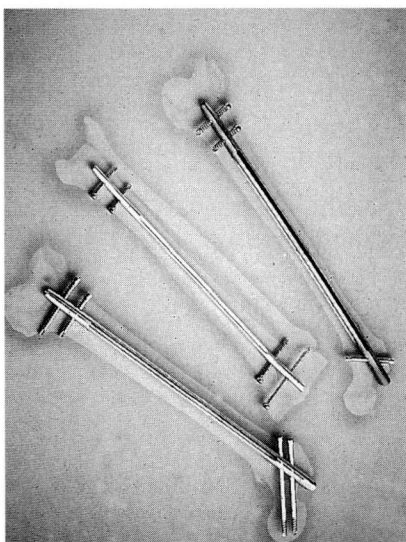

FIG. 21-75 Interlocking nails, Gross Kempf.
Courtesy Zimmer, Inc., Warsaw, Ind.

Operative procedure—Russell Taylor rod with or without locking screws

1. An incision is made over the tip of the greater trochanter and continued proximally and medially for 6 to 8 cm. The fascia of the gluteus is incised and the piriform fossa palpated.
2. With a threaded guide pin followed by an awl, the trochanteric fossa is identified and the cortex penetrated. A 3.2-mm guide rod is inserted to the level of the fracture. A curved guide pin is available for more severely displaced fractures.
3. Under fluoroscopy the guide wire is advanced across the fracture site and into the distal fragment until the ball tip of the guide wire reaches the level of the epiphyseal scar. A second guide wire is held against the portion of the guide wire extending out of the proximal femur and the length measured. That measurement is subtracted from 900 mm (total guide wire length) to determine the length of the intramedullary nail required.
4. The cannulated reamers are placed sequentially over the guide wire. The entire femur is reamed at 0.5-mm increments. The entire shaft, and especially the fracture site, should be visualized with fluoroscopy as the reamers pass.
5. The final reamer size should be verified with the reamer gauge. The femur is reamed 1 mm over the selected nail diameter. Inserting a nail in an inadequately reamed femur or inserting a nail that is too large can cause severe bone splitting and comminution.
6. The proximal screw guide/slap hammer is assembled onto the nail. The nail is oriented to match the curve of the femur.
7. Using the handle of the inserter, the rotation of the nail is controlled and the nail driven into the femur. The nail is fully seated when the proximal screw guide is flush with the greater trochanter. The inserter is disengaged from the slap hammer.
8. Using the power drill and correct drill sleeves, a 4.8-mm hole is drilled through both cortices and the depth measured directly off of the bit.
9. Through the appropriate drill sleeve, a 6.4-mm self-tapping locking screw is inserted and the drill sleeve removed.
10. Using the fluoroscopy the distal screw holes are confirmed as perfect circles on the screen. The distal targeting device is mounted on the nail followed by the left or right adapter block. The adapter block is adjusted until the calibration reads the length of the nail. The cross hairs are aligned in the adapter to the holes in the distal nail, confirming with fluoroscopy.
11. An incision is made through the adapter block over the distal femur to the lateral cortex. Following the same steps as those for placing the proximal screw, one or two distal locking screws are inserted. There are various free-hand techniques for inserting distal locking screws. Refer to the surgical technique guides.

Note: Many errors and complications, some disastrous, can occur when proceeding with intramedullary fixation. Late nailings (>12 hours) can lead to complications related to difficulties in reduction. Traction should be utilized if a delay is expected. Reamers and nail guides can perforate the cortex. Some surgeons may used an unreamed technique in large femoral canals, which alleviates the potential for reaming injuries but increases the chance for femoral fracture. Nails that insert with great difficulty may be too large for the canal and become incarcerated in the bone, requiring bone resection to remove. Nails inserted that are undersized can bend and eventually break with weight bearing. Infection in the open or closed nailing is a serious complication. The literature reports infection rates from 1.5% to 10% after open reduction and 1% in closed nailings. Safe, efficacious intramedullary nailing requires proper technique and attention to detail.

Supracondylar fractures of the femur

Fractures of the distal femur in the multiple trauma patient are treated early to promote rapid ambulation, which decreases complications due to immobility. In an effort to deliver quick fracture reduction and stabilization, many orthopedic trauma systems have been developed. Often these are the same systems used in daily orthopedic procedures with modifications to expedite implantation and fixation. Some of the intramedullary devices do not require reaming.

Procedural considerations. Initial stabilization of the patient may immediately precede the nailing procedure. Often there are other team members attending to treatment of other systems. The operating room nurse has the challenge to control traffic, coordinate team efforts, and protect the patient from increased risk of infection by the inadvertent contamination of instruments and implants. If possible, the patient is positioned on the fracture table. The affected extremity is prepped and draped following application of the tourniquet. The nail can be inserted using the closed or open technique.

The soft tissue set and large bone set are required in addition to the following:

Intramedullary rod set	Power drill
Intramedullary supra-	Guide wires
condylar nail implant	Fluoroscopy
(Fig. 21-76)	

Operative procedure—intramedullary supracondylar nail

1. The knee is flexed up to 90 degrees and an intrapatellar incision is made just large enough to pass the curved awl.
2. The awl is placed in the intercondylar notch centralized within the femur.
3. A guide pin is placed across the fracture site during fluoroscopic observation.

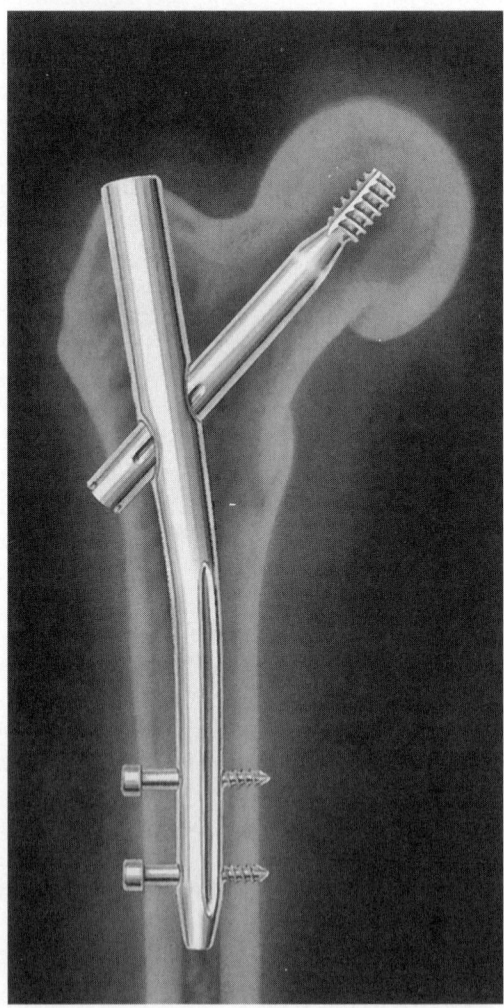

FIG. 21-76 Supracondylar nail
Courtesy Howmedica, Inc., Rutherford, N.J.

4. The entry point is reamed 1.5 mm larger than the selected nail to avoid displacing the condyles.
5. Steinman pins can be used to stabilize the fracture fragments during insertion of the nail.
6. The nail and guide bar are assembled and the nail advanced by hand into the intramedullary canal.
7. Using a mallet, nail insertion is completed until countersinking of the distal nail end 1 to 2 mm below the surface of the intercondylar notch occurs.
8. Through the holes in the guide bar, transfixing screws (5-mm cortical) are inserted to lock the rod in the same manner as other locked intramedullary nails.
9. Hardware placement is confirmed using fluoroscopy.
10. The incision site and other wounds are irrigated and closed.
11. Continuous passive motion machine should be applied immediately postoperatively.

SURGERY OF THE LOWER LEG (DISTAL FEMUR, TIBIA, AND FIBULA)

Many procedures on the lower leg use the same principles of fracture fixation already mentioned. Meticulous detail is required to ensure proper alignment and surgical result for the patient. As in the hip, fractures of the knee require secure fixation to allow bone healing, preserve motion, and provide joint mobility as early as possible. Fracture treatment for the various described injuries is based upon location and the pattern of fracture. Methods of fixation for the distal femur and tibia include pins, wire, compression plates, supracondylar plates, and cannulated screws. Multiple trauma patients with one or a combination of fractures may require more than one method of fixation. Open reduction and internal fixation must ensure anatomic restoration of the joint surface and rigid fixation, and allow early motion of the knee joint.

Most operations on the knee are performed with the patient in the supine position and the leg prepped and draped from the groin to the middle of the calf or including the entire foot. It is occasionally necessary for the surgeon to operate with the foot of the OR bed dropped and the patient's knee flexed to 90 degrees. Consequently, it is important to position the patient so the knee is at a break in the bed; if necessary the lower leg can be flexed at the knee during the operation. A tourniquet is often used.

Femoral condyle and tibial plateau fractures

Often with fractures involving the distal femur and proximal tibia the joint surfaces are involved. Anatomic alignment of the articular surfaces of the distal femur and proximal tibia is necessary to provide joint stability and decrease the chance of posttraumatic arthritis. Nonunion is the most common complication in supracondylar fractures leading to failure of surgery. As with humeral head and hip fractures, it is important that the articular surfaces are reopposed as close as possible to avoid future degenerative changes. Unfortunately, these often cannot be avoided, and patients with this type of injury are facing future joint arthroplasty

A   B   C

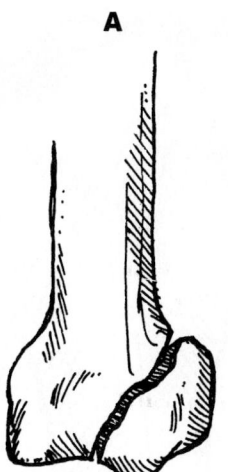 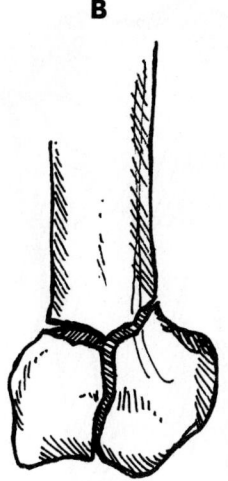 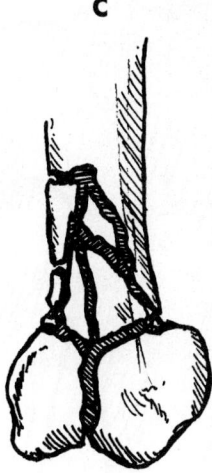

FIG. 21-77 Femoral condylar fractures. **A,** Linear. **B,** T-shaped. **C,** T-shaped with comminution.
From Gustilo RB: *The Fracture Classification Manual,* St. Louis, 1991, Mosby.

and replacement (see total joint replacement).

Distal femoral fractures result in varying degrees of comminution. Condylar fractures can be single or multicondylar, separating both condyles (Fig. 21-77). Type A fractures are extraarticular. Type B are single condyle fractures in the sagittal or coronal planes, whereas type C fractures are T and Y configurations. Type C fractures have varying degrees of shaft and condylar comminution, presenting the greatest challenge to treat.

Simple, undisplaced distal femoral fractures can be treated with closed reduction and immobilization by casting if anatomic reduction is achieved. Also, nondisplaced extraarticular fractures can be treated with a hinged cast brace. Comminuted fractures in this region can also be treated in this manner if there is minimal shortening and angulation. Traction can be used initially to augment this type of treatment. Distal femoral fractures are treated with open reduction if distal tibial traction and manipulation attempts fail. Flexible nails, blade plates, condylar compression screws, and condylar buttress plates are accepted methods of treating condylar fractures. Attention must be given to the attachment of the cruciate ligaments, which originate in the condylar notch and may require fixation of a partial or full disruption as a result of the injury (see cruciate deficient reconstruction) to the knee.

Tibial plateau fractures historically have been attributed to bumper or fender injuries, but a variety of falls or other trauma frequently is the cause. Compression force of the distal femur upon the tibia produces the varying types of plateau fractures. Commonly this occurs from abduction of the tibia while the foot is planted, driving the lateral femoral condyle into the lateral tibial plateau (also called the condyle). Several authors have developed classification systems based on fracture and dislocation patterns. The general theme of these fracture classifications can be summa-

rized by the following types (Fig. 21-78): (1) minimally displaced unicondylar fracture, (2) local compression, (3) split or wedge compression, (4) bicondylar, and (5) condylar (involving the total condyle). Fractures of the tibial plateau are often associated with dislocation, which may spontaneously reduce at the time of trauma and maintain reduction after the patient reaches the operating room.

Special attention must given to the possibility of neurovascular insult; this must be addressed immediately. Elevation and fixation of the depressed fracture is the focus for treatment of plateau fractures. As with distal femoral fractures, the articular surfaces and cruciate insertion require reapproximation and fixation. Repair to the menisci and ligaments should occur simultaneously to prevent knee instability.

Blade plates, buttress plates, and cannulated screws (Fig. 21-79) are all methods in which fractures of the tibial plateau are fixed. Bone graft from the iliac crest and fibular head autograft are often used when there is a significant amount of bone lost to comminution with proximal tibial fractures.

Procedural considerations. The patient is placed in the supine position under general or regional anesthesia. A pneumatic tourniquet is applied as high up on the femur as possible. Care must be taken to ensure the genitals are protected during the tourniquet placement. The leg is prepped, draped with a stockinette, and a window opened in the stockinette proximal and distal to the joint line.

A soft tissue set and large bone set are required, in addition to the following:

Total knee set	Power drill
Bone graft set	Steinman pins and Kirschner wires
Instruments and implants for the fixation system desired	Bone reduction clamps
	Fluoroscopy and x-ray available

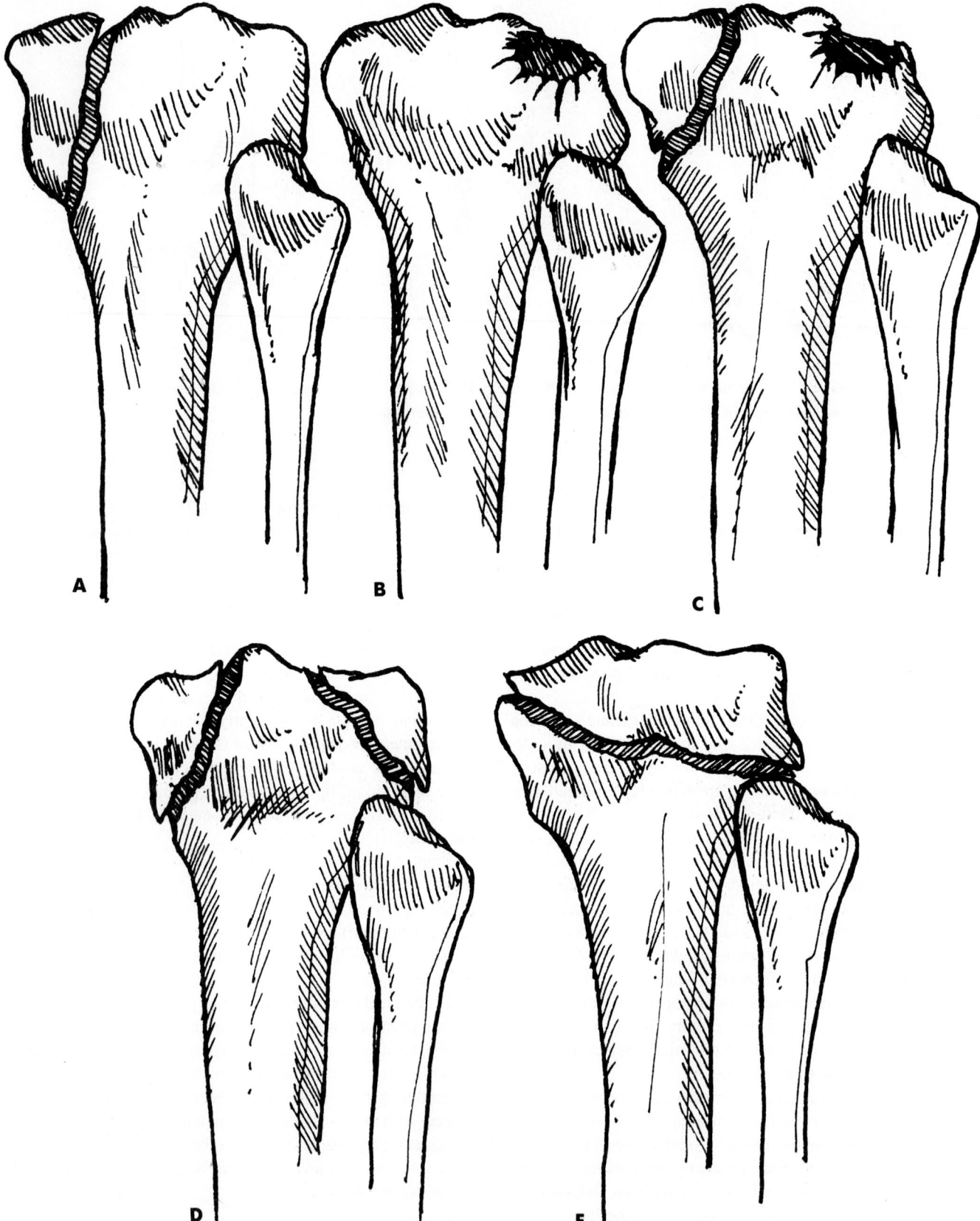

FIG. 21-78   Tibial plateau fractures. **A,** Unicondylar. **B,** Local compression. **C,** Split or wedge compression. **D,** Bicondylar. **E,** Condylar.

From Gustilo RB: *The Fracture Classification Manual,* St. Louis, 1991, Mosby.

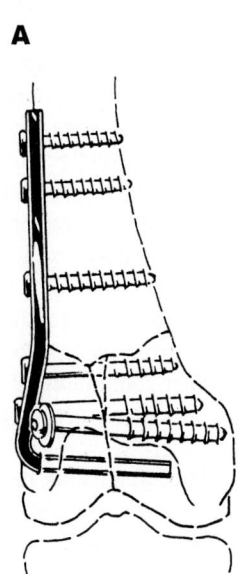 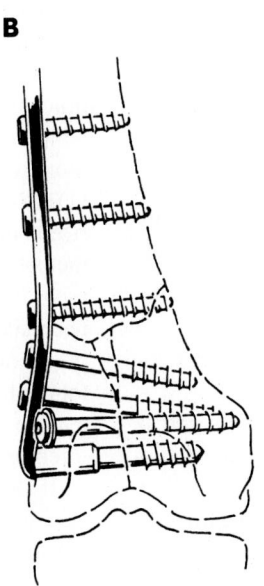 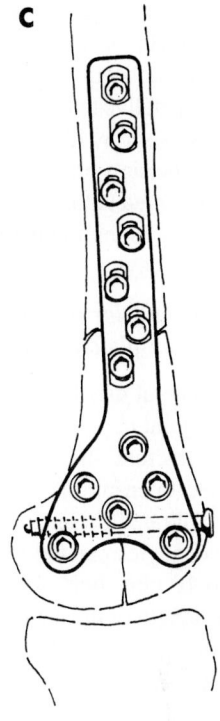

FIG. 21-79 Tibial plateau repair using **A,** Blade plate. **B,** Dynamic compression screw. **C,** Buttress plate.

From Gustilo RB: Kyle RF, Templeman D: *Fractures and dislocations,* vol 2, St. Louis, 1993, Mosby.

Operative procedures
Intercondylar fracture T type (AO blade plate)

1. A lateral incision is made from the knee joint extending proximally, long enough to allow the application of the selected plate. There will be three or four plate holes above the most proximal fracture.

2. The iliotibial band is incised and the vastus lateralis muscle dissected close to the bone, exposing the anterior surface at the femur at the fracture site. The vastus is retracted anteriorly. The quadriceps and patella are reflected medially to expose the entire distal femur. The patellar tendon attachment may be lifted from the tibial tuberosity with a plug of bone to completely retract the patella out of the field.

3. Traction is applied if the shaft of the femur is wedged between the two condyles.

4. A Steinman pin is inserted into, not through, each condyle. These pins are used as levers to manipulate and reduce the two condylar fracture fragments. Bone reduction forceps may be used to aid in reduction. Attention is given to the patellor femoral groove.

5. Multiple Kirschner wires (K-wires included with system) are used to fix the fracture fragments. One is placed transversely, across the knee joint, to serve as a guide to the condylar surface. A second wire is inserted parallel to the first at the level of the midpatella. A third is inserted transverse, 1 cm above the articular surface and parallel to the first two, serving as a guide for the blade of the plate.

6. The medial and lateral condyles are fixed with 6.5-mm cancellous bone screws. This screw requires a 4.8-mm drill bit and depth gauge. The screws are placed as anterior and posterior as possible to avoid the path of the subsequent blade plate.

7. An area exactly in the middle of the femoral condyle, anterior to the insertion of the collateral fibular ligament, is identified. Using the chisel, a path is cut for the blade of the plate transversing the femoral condyles. The chisel is inserted parallel to the third K-wire, ensuring the articular surface will not be penetrated by the plate. The blade of the plate must fall 8 to 10 mm short of the medial cortex to avoid penetration of the cortex.

8. The 95-degree condylar plate is inserted in the prepared channel and hammered down to the surface of the lateral femur. The contour portion of the plate should conform to the distal femoral shaft.

9. Through the distalmost hole in the side plate portion a cancellous bone screw is inserted to supplement fixation of the distal fragment. The plate is secured to the shaft of the femur using plate-holding forceps proximal to the fracture site. The knee is put through a range of motion. The fracture site and articular surface are visualized to ensure there is no soft tissue trapped between fragments.

10. The tension device is applied and tension is placed on the plate to compress the fracture fragments. The plate is secured to the femoral shaft with 4.5-mm cortical

bone screws. The holes are drilled to 3.2 mm and tapped bicortically with a 4.5-mm tap (see screw and plate application).

11. The patellar tendon is reattached with a 6.5-mm cancellous screw if previously removed.

12. The incision site is irrigated. The capsule is closed with interrupted suture. The remainder of the site is closed. The leg is immobilized until range of motion begins in 4 to 5 days.

Supracondylar fracture (compression plate) (see Ambi compression plate technique for femoral neck fractures)

1. The lateral distal femur is exposed above and below the knee joint.

2. The fracture site is reduced and multiple K-wires inserted to ensure fixation.

3. A calibrated Steinman pin is placed transversely across the condyles parallel to the joint line. The pin must stop 8 to 10 mm short of the medial cortex.

4. The length of the lag screw is gauged by reading directly on the calibrated Steinman pin, and adjustable double reamers are used to ream to this depth.

5. A lag screw is inserted across the condyles, followed by the compression screw.

6. The plate is secured and attached to the femoral shaft with cortical bone screws. The repair is visualized using fluoroscopy.

7. The incision site is irrigated and closed. A knee immobilizer is placed.

Medial and lateral Y-type tibial plateau fractures

1. A long anterior lateral incision starting 2.5 cm above the superiolateral aspect of the patella and tendon, proceeding distally around the patella to the anterior tibia just below the tibial tuberosity, is made. The distal tibial shaft should be exposed.

2. The level of the prepatellar bursa is identified. Blunt dissection beneath the skin is used and the proximal tibia is retracted to expose the proximal tibia from midline medially to midline laterally.

3. The patellar tendon is detached with a tibial bone plug to expose both the medial and lateral articular surface. The articular surface is reconstructed using temporary K-wires.

4. A contoured T-plate is attached to the medial aspect of the tibia using cancellous screws in the proximal portion and cortical screws in the distal portion. A smaller T-plate is inserted on the lateral side and secured in the same manner. The K-wires are removed. Care should be taken to see that the screws do not interfere with each other as they transverse from opposite sides of the tibia.

5. The patellar tendon is reattached using a 6.5-mm cancellous screw through the bone plug.

6. The wound is closed and immobilized at 30 degrees with a posterior splint.

Patellectomy and reduction of fractures patella

Patellectomy was a frequently performed procedure until the early 1970s. It is possible to excise a portion of the patella (for comminuted fracture) or the entire patella (for painful degenerative arthritis) without significantly affecting ordinary activities. Patellectomy has been shown to significantly reduce power of extension as the joint extends, which is the most important function of the knee. Furthermore, other complications associated with patellectomy are: (1) slow return of quadriceps mechanism strength, (2) quadriceps muscle atrophy, and (3) loss of knee protection from the patella. Removal of the entire patella may result in relative lengthening of the knee extensor mechanism, which necessitates imbrication of the quadriceps tendon at the time of operation to prevent a lag in knee extension. Patellectomy should be performed only when comminution is extensive and reconstruction of the articular surface (patellofemoral) is not possible.

If the fracture consists of two large fragments that can be anatomically reduced, fixation is accomplished with a tension band, a circumferential loop technique, or bone screws. Tension band wiring produces compression forces across the fracture site and results in earlier union and immediate mobility of the knee.

Procedural considerations. The patient is supine. The tourniquet is applied and the leg prepped and draped. A soft tissue set and bone set are required in addition to the following:

Power drill and bits	Heavy needle holders
18-gauge wire	Bone reduction clamp
Wire tightener	

Operative procedure

1. A transverse curved incision is made over the patella.

2. Dissection is carried down to expose the surface of the patella, the quadriceps, and patellar tendons.

3. The joint is irrigated, and the fracture is reduced with bone reduction clamps.

4. One length of wire is passed around the insertion of the patellar tendon and then around the quadriceps tendon. A second wire is passed more superficially through the bone fragments.

5. The fracture is over corrected and the wire is tightened with the wire tightener. In flexing the knee or contracting the quadriceps the condyles press against the patellar fragments, producing compression at the fracture site.

Correction of recurrent dislocation of the patella

Recurrent dislocation of the patella can be the result of violent initial dislocation, or more commonly from underlying anatomic abnormalities. The underlying condition causes an abnormal excursion of the extensor mechanism

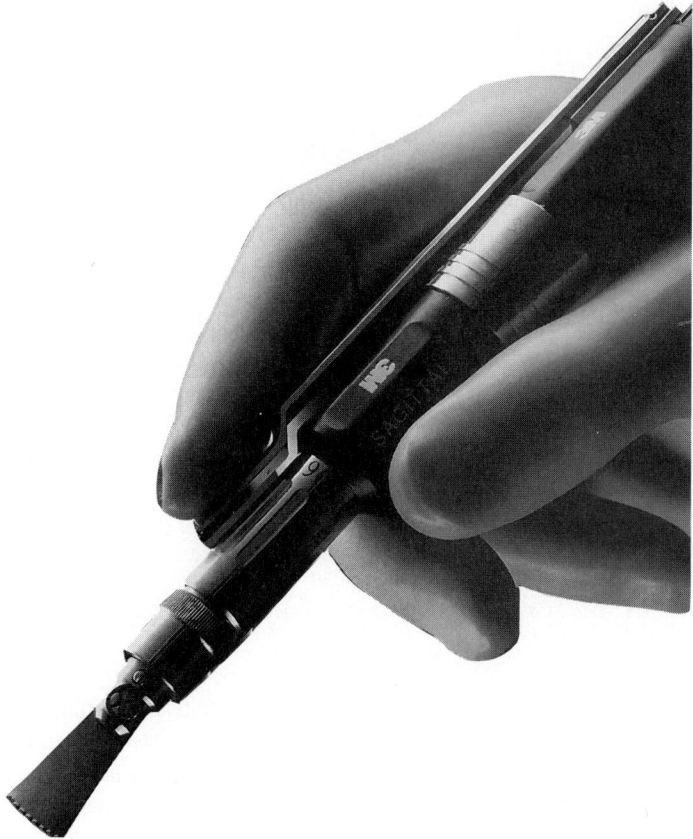

FIG. 21-80 Micro sagittal saw and various attachments.
Courtesy 3M Health Care, St. Paul, Minn.

over the femoral condyles. Dynamic forces, such as the vastus lateralis, and static forces, such as the shape of the patella, tend to displace the patella laterally. Dislocations occur when there are extreme displacing forces combined with internal rotation of the femur and flexion of the knee. If untreated, patellar dislocations will deteriorate the knee by causing abnormal patellofemoral articulation, chondromalacia, and meniscal tears.

Conservative treatment aimed at quadriceps strengthening may be indicated in some patients. Numerous operations have been designed to realign the knee extensor mechanism. All the procedures include incising the lateral quadriceps tendon and shifting the insertion of the patellar tendon medially or distally to the original insertion of the tibia.

Procedural considerations. The patient is positioned supine. The tourniquet is applied, the leg prepped and draped. A soft tissue set and bone set are required in addition to the following:

Power drill
Microsagittal saw
  (Fig. 21-80)
Osteotomes
AO drill, tap, and
  gauge for 6.5-mm
  cancellous screw

**Operative procedure—patellar realignment
(Elmslie-Trillat)**

1. A lateral parapatellar incision is made beginning proximal to the patellar pole, laterally around the patella, and extending to 2 cm distally and just lateral to the tibial tuberosity.
2. A skin flap is developed and retracted medially to expose the capsule. A medial arthrotomy is completed, the joint is inspected, and any pathology is present is repaired.
3. The lateral retinaculum is released from the vastus lateralis proximally and the patellar tendon distally.
4. Using a ½-inch osteotome the tibial tuberosity is scored medially and laterally, just below the fat pad and under the patella.
5. The osteotomy is continued using a microsagittal saw distally for 4 to 6 cm, leaving the periosteum hinged at the distalmost part of the osteotomy.
6. The entire segment, with patellar tendon attached, is displaced medially and held in place by hand while putting the knee through a range of motion. Tracking of the patella on the femoral groove is completed by systematically moving the knee medially in increments.
7. A cancellous bone bed is prepared at the point of reattachment of the tibial tuberosity.

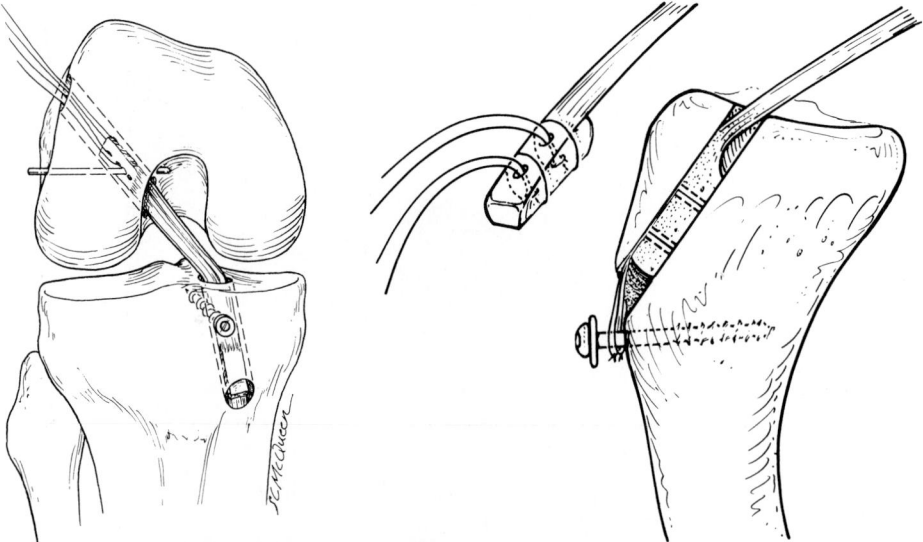

FIG. 21-81   Patellar tendon reattachment with an AO screw.

From Crenshaw AH, editor: *Campbell's Operative Orthopaedics*, 5 vols, ed 8, St. Louis, 1992, Mosby.

8. The tuberosity is displaced medially and a 6.5-mm cancellous bone screw is placed (Fig. 21-81).
9. The wound is irrigated and closed, and a long-leg cylinder cast is applied and bivalved immediately.

Repair of collateral or cruciate ligament tears

The stability of the knee depends on the integrity of the cruciate and collateral ligaments. If any of these supporting structures is damaged, an unstable knee is likely unless properly repaired. Injuries to these supporting structures are usually not isolated. More frequently several of the ligaments are injured at the same time. For example, the injury commonly referred to as the "terrible triad" includes a torn anterior cruciate ligament, torn medial meniscus, and torn medial collateral ligament.

The knee demonstrates grave disability with major ligamentous disruption. The collateral ligaments reinforce the knee capsule medially and laterally. They resist varus and valgus stresses on the knee. The cruciate ligaments control anteroposterior stability. Along with the ligaments, the muscle groups stabilize the joint and control movement. Because muscle strength is the first line of defense for the knee, damage is repaired to protect the ligaments. For optimum function of the joint, damaged structures should be reconstructed as close as possible to the original anatomic structures. If the knee is left untreated, osteoarthritis will develop.

Injury to a single cruciate ligament may not significantly compromise knee function. When combined with other injuries, surgery may be warranted. Various types of ligament grafts may be utilized to replace or augment the cruciate ligaments. Autografts, allografts, and artificial substitutes are available. Ligament substitutes act as a scaffold, stent, or augment of the torn cruciate ligaments. Scaffolds support the soft tissue initially to allow ingrowth of the host tissue. Stents protect the joint from excessive stress while the permanent ligament substitute is healing. Augmentation, such as the patient's own iliotibial band, protects the graft initially after repair of a partial tear. Synthetic ligaments, which are less popular, include carbon fiber grafts, polyglycolic acid material, Dacron, polyester, and Gore-Tex. All synthetic grafts are subject to mechanical failure from weakening with fragmentation and synovitis. These are recommended for salvage procedures only when conventional reconstruction has failed and when all other autogenous tissue is unavailable for substitution. Biologic materials from Animals, such as bovine xenografts, are also available for ligament substitution, although they are subject to increased risk of infection, synovitis, and rejection. Homogenous allografts are the substitute of choice for knee reconstruction when no autogenous graft is available from the patient. Disadvantages of homogenous allografts include long-term weakening, possible rejection, and the possibility of infectious disease transfer in tissue.

Autogenous tissues are currently the substitute of choice, with the middle third of the patellar tendon and a block of patella being the most reliable. To minimize necrosis and maintain graft strength, the fat pad with its blood supply may be preserved along with the patellar tendon. Using this graft and other soft tissue autografts, the cruciate-deficient knee is being reconstructed arthroscopically (see arthroscopy section). A combination of a torn anterior cruciate ligament, medial meniscus, and medial collateral ligament often indicates the need for an open procedure (arthrotomy). When reconstructing the cruciate ligament, it is important to have the graft biomechanically correct to maintain proper function. There are many devices and systems utilized to provide this placement assistance and gauge appropriate

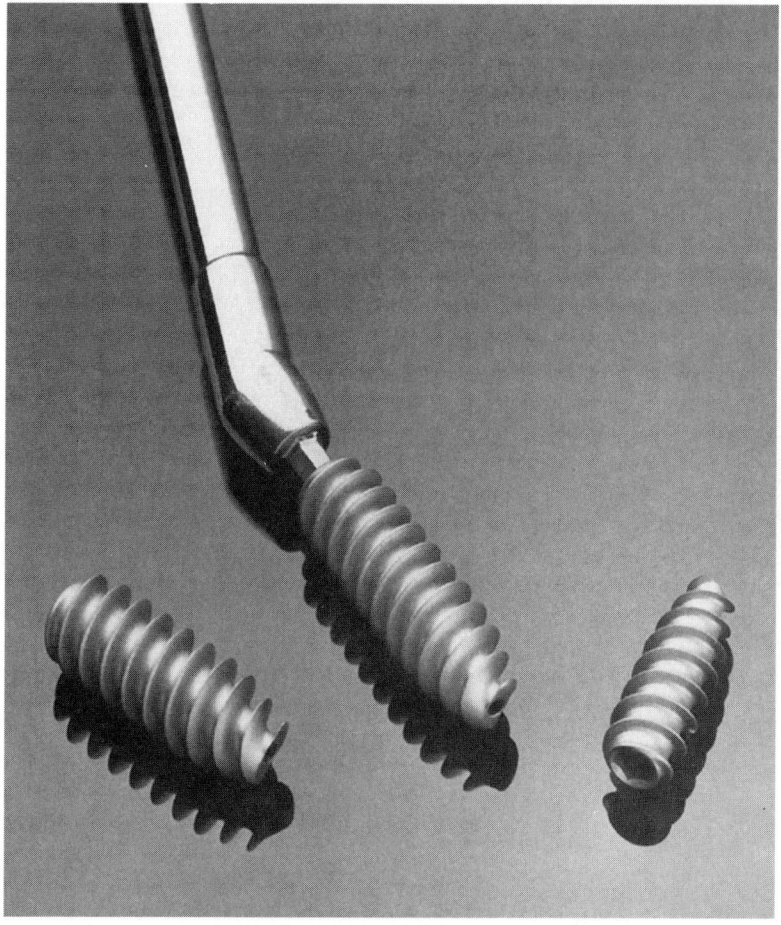

A

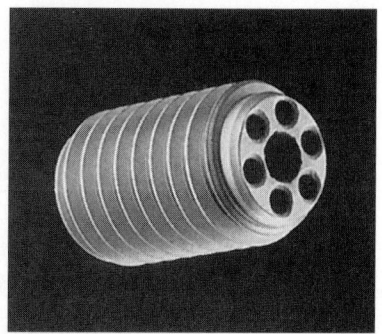

B

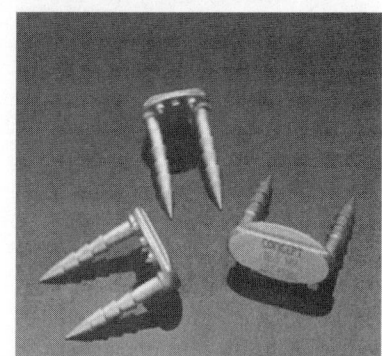

C

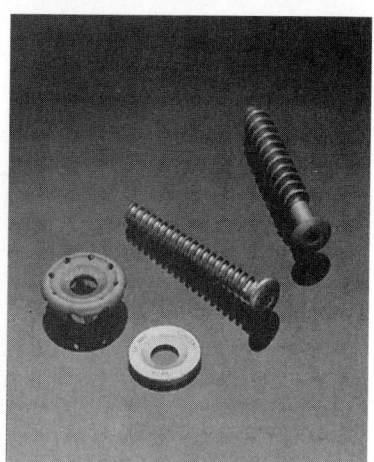

D

FIG. 21-82 Fixation devices for ligament repairs. **A,** Interference screws. **B,** endosteal fixation device. **C,** Soft tissue fixation staples. **D,** Cortical screws and washers.

Courtesy Linvatec.

graft tension. These devices are either used separately or in some combination. Though the variations are many, the principles are the same.

Procedural considerations. The patient is placed in the supine position with a tourniquet applied to the upper thigh. A surgical prep is done from the upper thigh down to and including the foot. Soft tissue instruments are required in addition to the following:

Power drill, microsagittal saw, and burrs
Fixation device of choice, including polyethylene buttons, bone staples, bone screws with spiked washers, interference screws (Fig. 21-82)
Steinman pins

Reconstruction guide (Fig. 21-83), tensometers (Fig. 21-84), and isometers of choice
Arthroscopy instruments (see Fig. 21-112)
Meniscal repair instruments

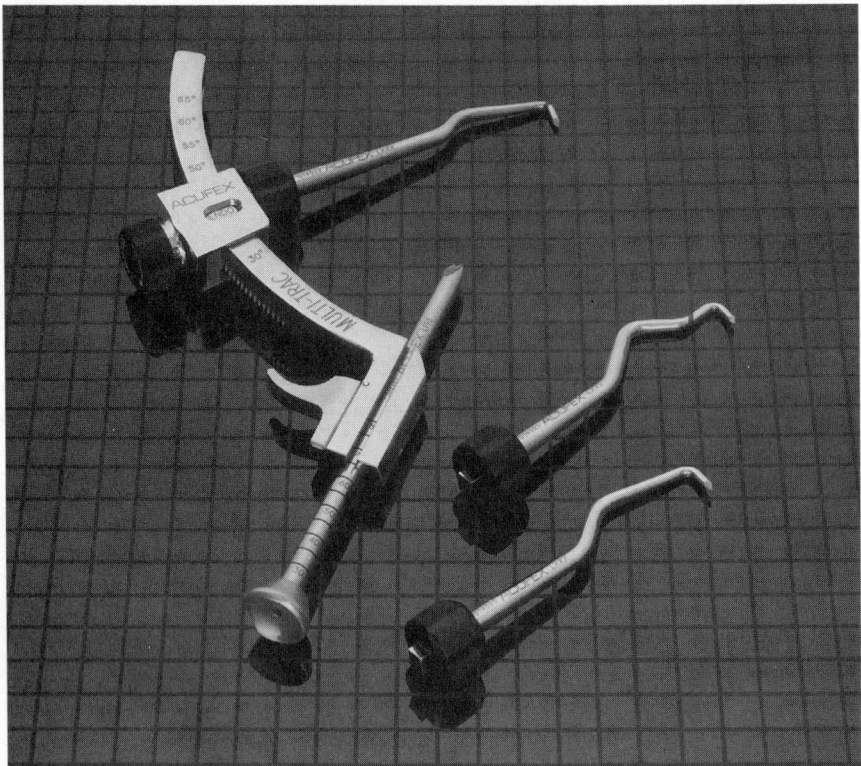

FIG. 21-83   Reconstruction guide used for ligament repair.
Courtesy Acufex Microsurgical, Inc., Mansfield, Mass.

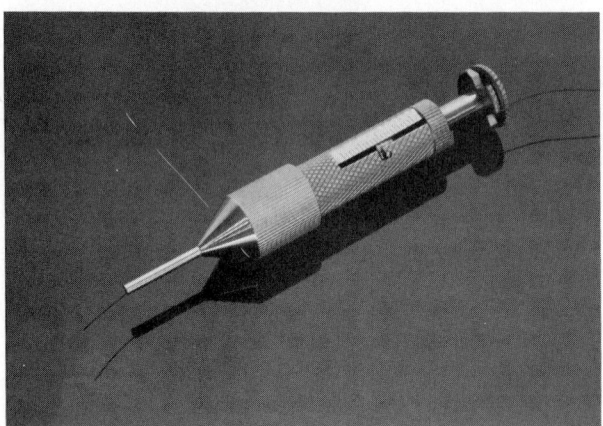

FIG. 21-84   Tension isometer used to determine isometric placement of ligament substitute.
Courtesy Acufex Microsurgical, Inc., Norwood, Mass.

Operative procedure—ruptured anterior cruciate repair (Fig. 21-85)

1. An examination under anesthesia is performed immediately after induction as the ligaments are completely lax, to evaluate the severity of the ligamentous injury.
2. A straight midline or slightly medial incision is made across the knee.
3. Meniscus tears in the vascular zone (peripheral) are repaired with arthroscopic meniscal repair instruments or cutting needles with a heavy absorbable suture to repair the meniscofemoral and meniscotibial ligaments. If the meniscus is not repairable, partial meniscectomy is performed.
4. The middle third of the patellar tendon with patellar and tibial bone plugs is harvested, using a power saw and osteotome.
5. A notchplasty is then performed, débriding and smoothing the lateral intercondylar wall with a burr and curette.
6. The femoral and tibial osseous tunnels are developed by using the ligament guide to pass guide wires from the lateral femoral condyle and tibial tubercle into the intercondylar notch at isometric points near the anatomic attachment site of the anterior cruciate ligament.
7. The pins are temporarily removed to measure isometric positioning with a tension isometer.
8. The pins are then replaced and overdrilled with cannulated drills as close to the size of the patellar tendon graft as possible. The tunnels are smoothed with a curette.
9. Sutures are placed through drill holes at both ends of the graft to pass the graft through the tunnels.
10. Once the graft is passed through the femoral and tibial osseous tunnels, it is fixed at both ends with staples, screws, or polyethylene buttons.
11. The medial collateral ligament and posterior oblique ligament are then individually repaired at their inser-

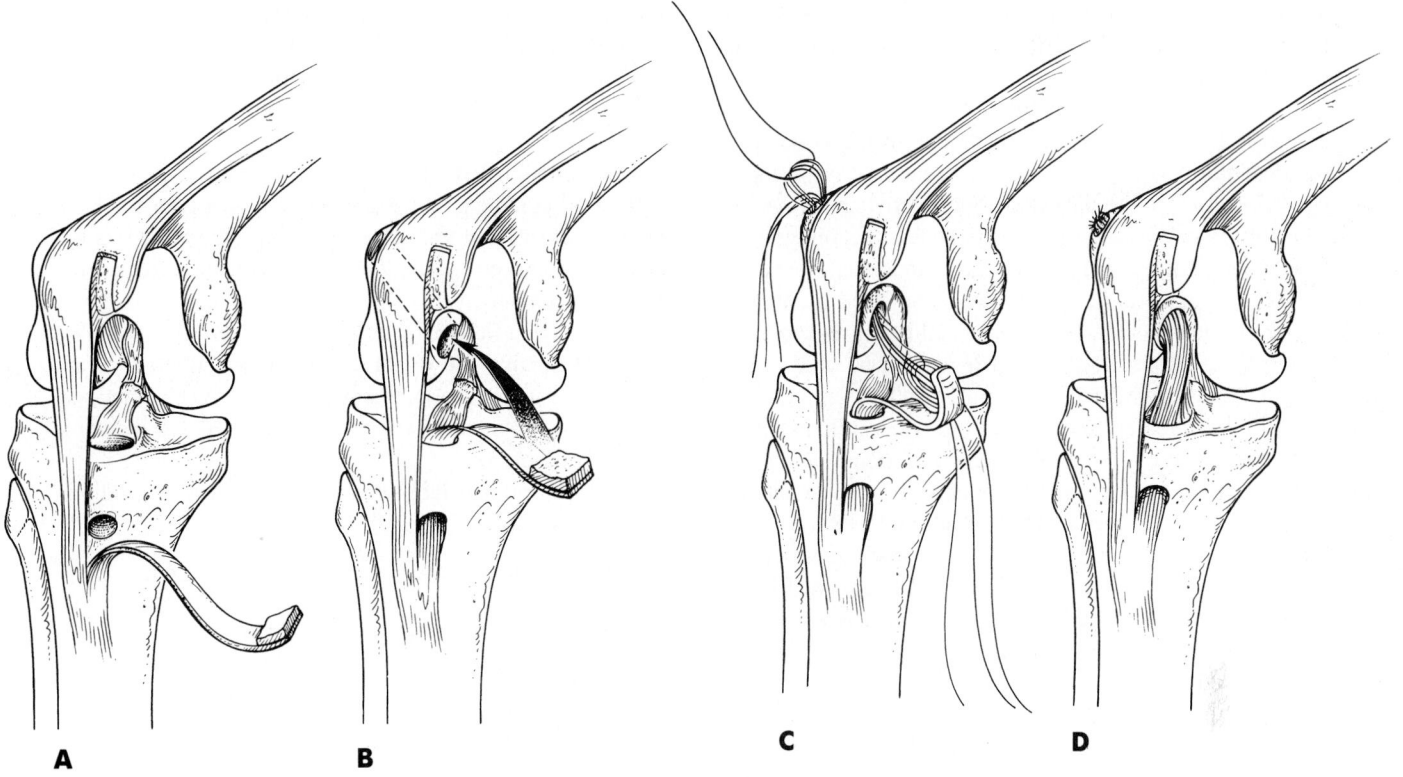

A **B** **C** **D**

FIG. 21-85 Reconstruction of anterior cruciate ligament using split patellar tendon. **A,** A piece of bone is dissected from the patellar tendon and patellar tendon split. **B,** Tendon is pulled into the knee joint. **C,** Sutures are placed through the graft and passed through lateral femoral condyle. **D,** Sutures are secured.

Redrawn from Eriksson E: *Orthop Clin North Am* 7:167, 1976.

tion sites with bone screws and spiked washers.
12. Additional extraarticular repair is done if necessary.
13. The wound is closed over intraarticular and subcutaneous drains, and a locking knee brace or cast is applied.

Popliteal (Baker's) cyst excision

Baker's cysts occur in joints, frequently affecting the popliteal fossa. Baker's cysts are frequently painful and can become very large, especially when associated with rheumatoid arthritis. Cysts in the popliteal fossa occur without a precipitating cause in children; in adults they often indicate an intraarticular disease process, such as rheumatoid arthritis, or a torn medial meniscus.

Procedural considerations. In contrast to many other operative procedures on the knee, the patient is placed in the prone position with chest rolls under the thorax during surgery.

A soft tissue set and a bone set are required.

Operative procedure

1. An oblique incision is made in the popliteal area over the mass.
2. The deep fascia is divided to expose the mass.
3. The cyst is then freed by blunt dissection and clamped at its attachment to the joint capsule.
4. The cyst is divided, and the pedicle is inverted and closed.

5. After the mass has been removed, the wound is irrigated and closed.
6. The knee is immobilized in extension with a posterior splint.

Fractures of the tibial shaft

The location of the tibia results in frequent exposure to injury. Open fractures are more common in the tibia than other major bones because on third of its surface is subcutaneous. Tibial shaft fractures are difficult to treat. The blood supply to the tibia is more precarious than that of other long bones because of its lack of enclosure by heavy muscle. The presence of hinge joints at the knee and ankle allows no adjustment for rotational deformity after fracture, so special care is required to correct during reduction and fixation. Rotational deformities are often seen; delayed union, nonunion, and infection are fairly common complications. Closed reduction and casting provide excellent healing without significant nonunion or infection. Surgical reduction and internal fixation are indicated when soft tissue is caught between fragments, initial treatment has been delayed, and a severe rotational defect is present in the segmental fracture. In general, torsional fractures seem to heal better and are more amenable to treatment than transverse fractures. This may be because of less vessel disruption within the periosteum. The important prognostic indicators are as follows: (1) the amount of initial displacement, (2) the degree of comminution, (3) the presence or absence of infection, and (4) the severity of soft tissue injury excluding infection.

External fixation of open tibial shaft fractures (see Fig. 21-39) is less commonly necessary due to the increase in intramedullary nailing without significant increase in infection. However, in the presence of gross contamination, severe soft tissue and vascular injury, bone infection, and delayed treatment, external fixation is the treatment of choice. The Ilizarov external fixation device is indicated when there is significant bone loss and limb lengthening is required. Plate and screw fixation is another method in which tibial shaft fractures can be treated. Infection and nonunion of tibial shaft fractures are twice as likely when utilizing plate and screw fixation. Plate and screw fixation is indicated when there are intraarticular fragments of the knee and ankle associated with the injury. Closed intramedullary nailing is the treatment of choice in tibial shaft fractures because infection is less likely to occur and periosteal blood supply is preserved. Interlocking nails are preferred in most cases. They can control rotation of fragments by proximal and/or distal locking. Static locking nails (locking both proximal and distal ends of the nail) are indicated for fractures with comminution, bone loss, and lengthening osteotomies. Dynamic locking nails (locking the end closest to the fracture site) are indicated for proximal or distal tibial fractures, nonunions, and malunions. Locking tibial nails include the Russell-Taylor and the Synthes AO tibial nails (see Fig. 21-75).

The key to successful treatment of open tibial fractures, as in all open fractures, is meticulous and systematic débridement of all foreign matter and devitalized tissue. Care should be taken to reduce devascularization when reducing and fixing the fracture. Systemic antibiotics and those delivered by pulse lavage will help reduce the chance of infection.

Procedural considerations. The patient is usually given general or regional anesthesia while still on the hospital bed and then transferred to the fracture table. The patient is positioned supine on the fracture table with the affected hip flexed approximately 45 degrees and the knee at 90 degrees. This provides a horizontal orientation of the tibia. Using a calcaneal traction pin or table foot holder, traction is applied and rotational alignment obtained. After rotational alignment is obtained, a tourniquet is applied and the leg is prepped and draped.

A soft tissue and large bone set is required in addition to the following:

Intramedullary reamer set (Fig. 21-86)	ing procedure only)
Intramedullary nail and insertion instruments of choice	Power drill and reamer-driver
Compression plate and screw set (open plat-	Bone reduction clamps (open nailing procedure only)

Operative procedures
Closed or open tibial intramedullary nailing (Fig. 21-87)

1. If the open technique is required, the fracture site is exposed, reduced, and irrigated as necessary. Focus is then turned toward the nailing procedure.

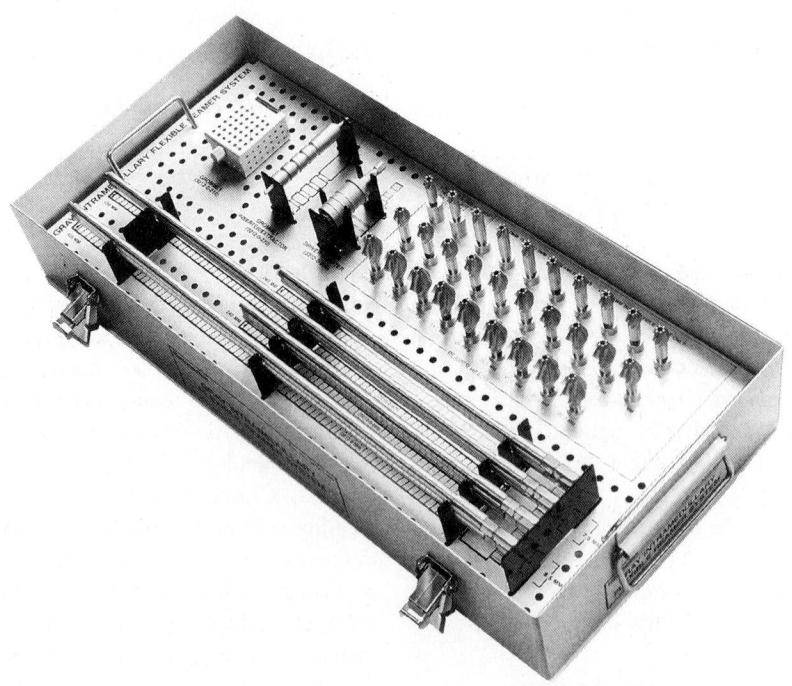

FIG. 21-86 Intramedullary flexible reamer system.
Courtesy Howmedica, Inc., Rutherford, N.J.

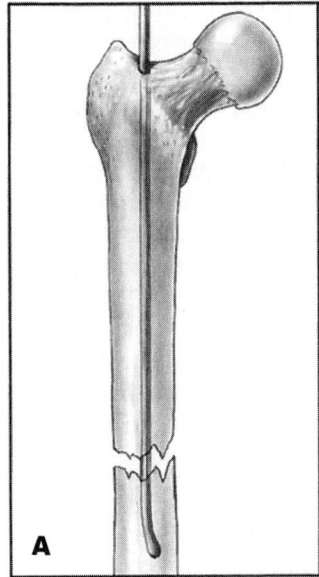

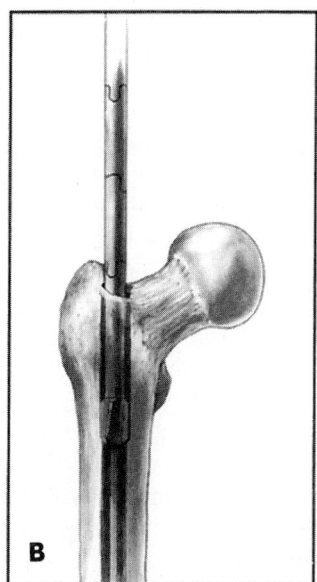

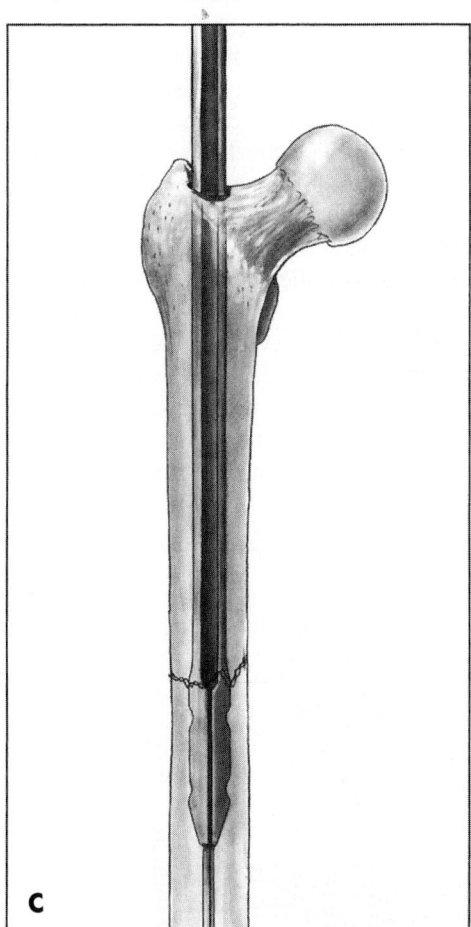

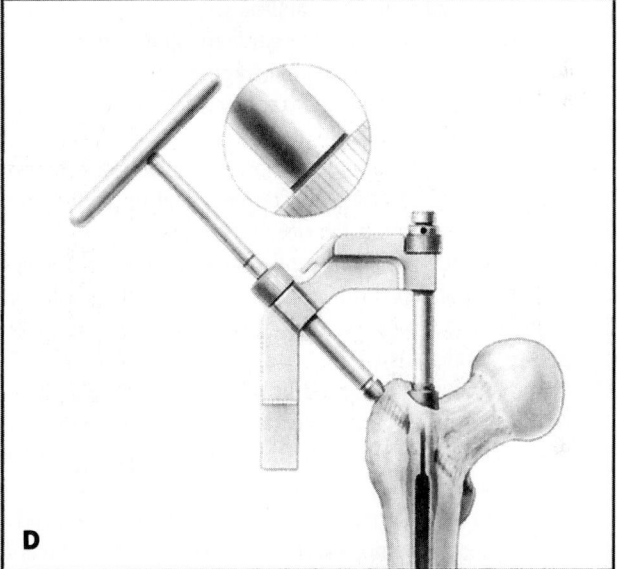

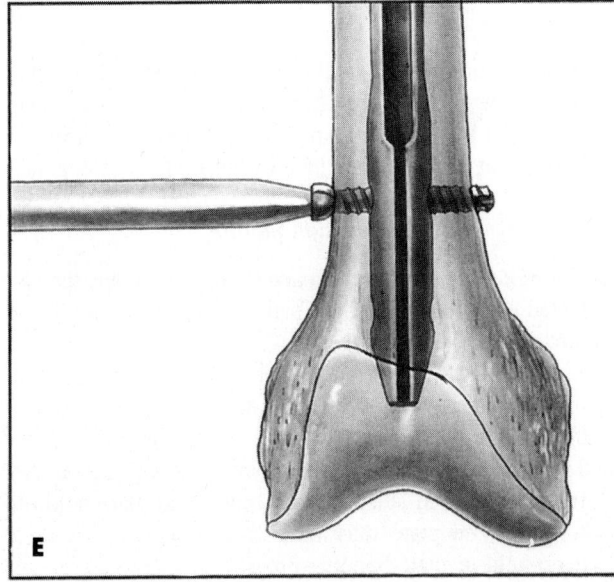

FIG. 21-87   Intramedullary nailing with **A,** Guide rod insertion.
B, Reaming over the guide rod. **C,** Driving the nail over the guide
rod. **D,** Placing proximal and distal interlocking nails.

Courtesy Zimmer Inc., Warsaw, Ind.

2. A 5-cm incision is made medial to the patellar tendon to just below the tibial tuberosity.

3. Using a curved awl, the medullary canal is opened just proximal to the tibial tuberosity.

4. A guide rod (3.2 mm) is inserted into the shaft of the tibia down to the fracture site. The proximal fragment is reduced distally and the guide rod advanced into the distal fragment. Rod types include straight guide rod for simple fractures, curved for the displaced type, and a cutting tip for an obstructed canal.

5. The length of the required nail is determined by the guide rod method (see the section on femoral nails) or by using the nail length gauge and confirming with fluoroscopy.

6. With cannulated reamers over the guide rods, the entire tibia is reamed 1 mm greater than the nail to be inserted. Inserting a nail too large for the canal can have a detrimental effect.

7. The driver, proximal drill, guide, and hexagonal bolt are assembled onto the tibial nail.

8. The nail is inserted over the guide rod and, using a mallet, driven down the proximal fragment to enter the distal fragment, crossing the fracture site. The nail is not fully seated.

9. The guide rod is removed to prevent incarceration and complete the nail seating. The proximal tip of the nail should be flush with the tibial entry site.

10. Proximal locking is accomplished with the corresponding drill and tap through the proximal drill guide for 5-mm cortical bone screws (see the section on humeral and femoral nails).

11. Distal screws are inserted utilizing the distal targeting device or the freehand technique. The 5-mm cortical bone screws are inserted, traversing the tibia through the tibial nail.

12. The wounds are irrigated. If bone graft is to be used, it is placed around the fracture site and the layers closed. Dressings are applied and cast immobilization accomplished.

Dynamization, or removal of either the proximal or distal screws, may take place after 3 months for fractures that are stable but lack callus. Dynamization produces compressive forces at the fracture, thereby generating osteogenesis.

Tibial dynamic compression plating

1. A longitudinal incision is made (to accommodate the selected plate) lateral to the tibial crest to expose the fracture site.

2. The periosteum is stripped only enough for application of the plate. Circumferential stripping can diminish blood supply.

3. The fracture is reduced, and a plate is placed across the fracture site and secured with bone- and plate-holding forceps. The plate may have to be contoured with a hand-held or plate-bending press.

4. Using the neutral drill guide a 3.2-mm bicortical hole is drilled in the plate screw hole close to the fracture site, gauged, and tapped to 4.5 mm. The first bone screw is inserted, ensuring purchase of the screw on the opposite cortex.

5. Using the load drill guide (eccentric), the second hole is drilled next to the fracture line in the opposite fragment. Drill and tap are accomplished as in the previous step. As the screw enters the bone, it will seek the center of the screw hole (the screw is eccentric and screw hole is beveled). The fracture site is brought under compression as the screws seats in the hole.

6. The wounds are irrigated. If bone graft is to be used, it is placed around the fracture site and the layers closed. Dressings are applied and cast immobilization completed.

SURGERY OF THE ANKLE AND FOOT
Ankle fractures

Ankle fractures include fractures of the medial malleolus (tibia), lateral malleolus (fibula), and posterior malleolus (posterior aspect of the articular surface of the distal tibia). They may or may not be associated with ligamentous injury. Ankle fractures can be classified in anatomic lines as monomalleolar, bimalleolar, and trimalleolar. Because medial malleolar and posterior malleolar fractures involve the distal weight-bearing articular surface of the tibia, open reduction and anatomic alignment are necessary. Fixation of the lateral malleolus is also important because it forms the ankle mortise.

Anatomic reduction prevents the occurrence of degenerative joint disease. Displaced fractures are treated with pins, malleolar or bone screws, or plates and screws (Fig. 21-88). Bimalleolar fractures may treated with closed reduction and casting, but around 10% of these develop non-

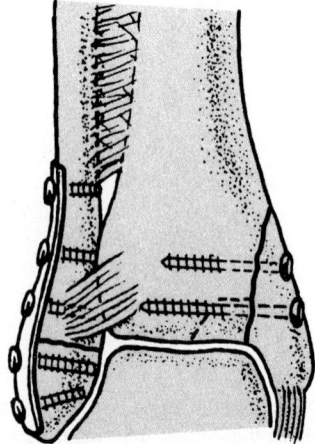

FIG. 21-88   Plate/screw placement for lateral malleolar fragment repair using one-third tubular plate.

From Muller ME, Allgower M, Schneider R et al: *Manual of Internal Fixation*, ed 3, New York, 1991, Springer-Verlag NY Inc.

union. The lateral malleolus (distal fibula) is important for lateral and rotational stability of the joint. Open reduction and internal fixation using Steinman pins or screws placed obliquely into the tibia is a common technique. Lateral or malleolar fractures can be fixed with the cancellous lag technique, overdrilling the first fragment and allowing compression of the fragments. Fracture of the lateral malleolus can also be treated with a Rusch rod, inserted through the fragment and into the fibular canal. Trimalleolar fractures require surgery more than the other variety of fractures. The posterior lip of the articulating surface of the tibia is usually involved and needs to be anatomically reduced to minimize degenerative changes.

Procedural considerations. The patient is placed in the supine position. The affected leg is prepped and draped following application of a pneumatic tourniquet. The patient is placed in the supine position. If the lateral ankle is involved, a padded sandbag is placed beneath the hip to internally rotate it.

A soft tissue set and small bone set are required, in addition to the following:

Power drill	Bone reduction clamps
AO small fragment set, plates, and screws	Steinman pins

Operative procedure—trimalleolar fracture

1. Incisions are made medial and lateral across the ankle.
2. The posterior malleolar fracture is exposed and reduced with bone-holding clamps and manipulation.
3. The fracture is temporarily held in reduction with two Kirschner wires inserted above the anterior tibial lip and directed anterior to posterior, engaging both fragments.
4. A drill hole is made anterior to posterior through both fragments. After measuring with a depth gauge, a malleolar, small cancellous, or other preferred screw is inserted through the fracture. The wires are removed.
5. The lateral malleolar fracture is then manipulated into reduction.
6. If the fracture is oblique and not comminuted, it is reduced with one or two lag screws placed anterior to posterior. If the fracture is transverse, a long screw or medullary pin is inserted across the fracture line into the canal of the proximal fragment. A small semitubular or one-third tubular plate is applied if the fracture occurs above the syndesmosis.
7. Once the posterior and lateral malleolar fractures have been fixed, the medial malleolar fracture is finally reduced using bone clamps.
8. The reduction is held with two Kirschner wires while a hole is drilled through the medial malleolus into the metaphysis of the tibia.
9. Once the appropriate length of screw is determined by a depth gauge, a malleolar screw is inserted across the fracture site. The Kirschner wires are removed.

10. If rotational stability is needed, an additional smaller screw or compression wiring is added.
11. Intraoperative x-rays are taken in AP, lateral, and mortise views.
12. The wounds are irrigated and closed, and a short or long leg cast is applied.

Triple arthrodesis

The talocalcaneal (subtalar), talonavicular, and calcaneocuboid joints must be fused in patients with marked inversion or eversion deformities of the foot. Such deformities occur in clubfoot, poliomyelitis, and rheumatoid arthritis. Occasionally this operation is necessary for patients who have pain resulting from degenerative or traumatic arthritis. This triple fusion does not interfere with flexion and extension of the foot at the ankle joint.

Procedural considerations. The patient is placed in the supine position. The surgical prep is carried out from midcalf up to and including the foot. The iliac crest area should also be prepped if bone grafting is anticipated.

A soft tissue set and small bone set are required, plus the following:

Bone graft set	Power drill and saw
AO compression plates and screws, bone staples	Kirschner wires
	Small lamina spreader

Operative procedure—anterior arthrodesis

1. An anterior or anteriolateral approach is used.
2. The articular cartilage is resected from the distal tibia, fibula, and dome of the talus.
3. Equinus, varus, or valgus deformities are corrected by removing bony wedges from the tibia and talus.
4. The fusion is supplemented using cortical bone graft from the distal tibia or iliac crest.
5. The ankle is held in 0 degrees of flexion, in 0 to 5 degrees of valgus, and slight external rotation.
6. The graft is secured to the tibia with bone screws and dead space filled with cancellous bone graft.
7. The incision site is irrigated, and dressings and a short leg cast are applied.

Bunionectomy

A bunion (hallux valgus) is a soft tissue or bony mass at the medial side of the first metatarsal head. It is associated with a valgus deformity of the great toe (Fig. 21-89). A bunion is caused by a basic structural defect of the foot, which predisposes to the development of this deformity. Ill-fitting shoes accentuate the situation and speed the development of bunions. Bunions are 40 times more common in women because of shoe styles, including high heels and pointed toes. Other factors that may contribute to this deformity are heredity, flatfeet, foot pronation, longer first toe, muscle imbalance, and inflammatory disturbances of the feet.

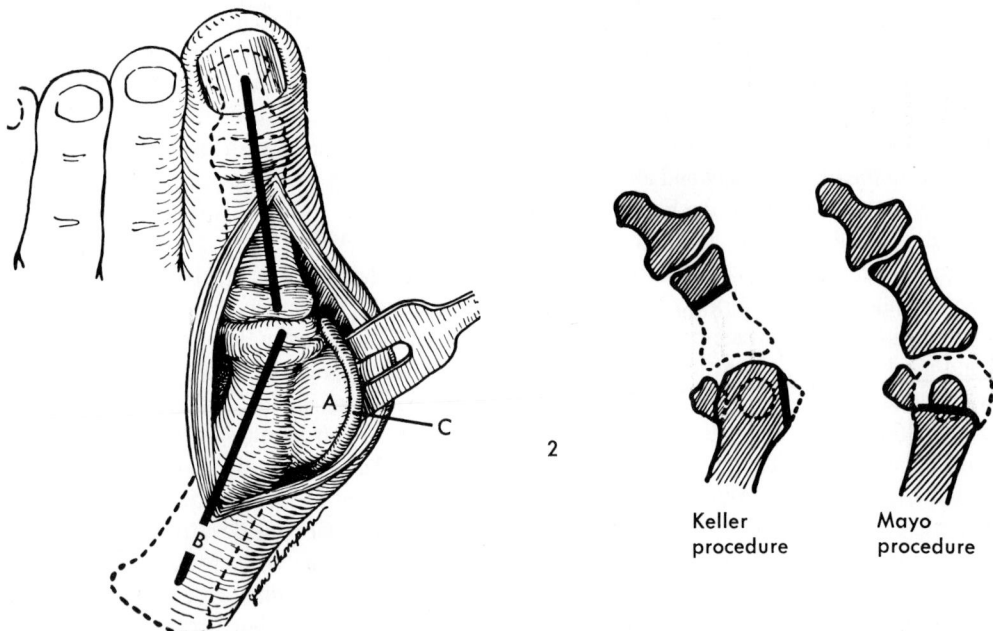

FIG. 21-89 **1,** Bunion **A,** Exostosis of metatarsal head. **B,** Hallux Valgus deformity. **C,** Overlying bursa. **2,** Operations for hallux valgus.

From Richards V: *Surgery for general practice,* St. Louis, 1956, Mosby.

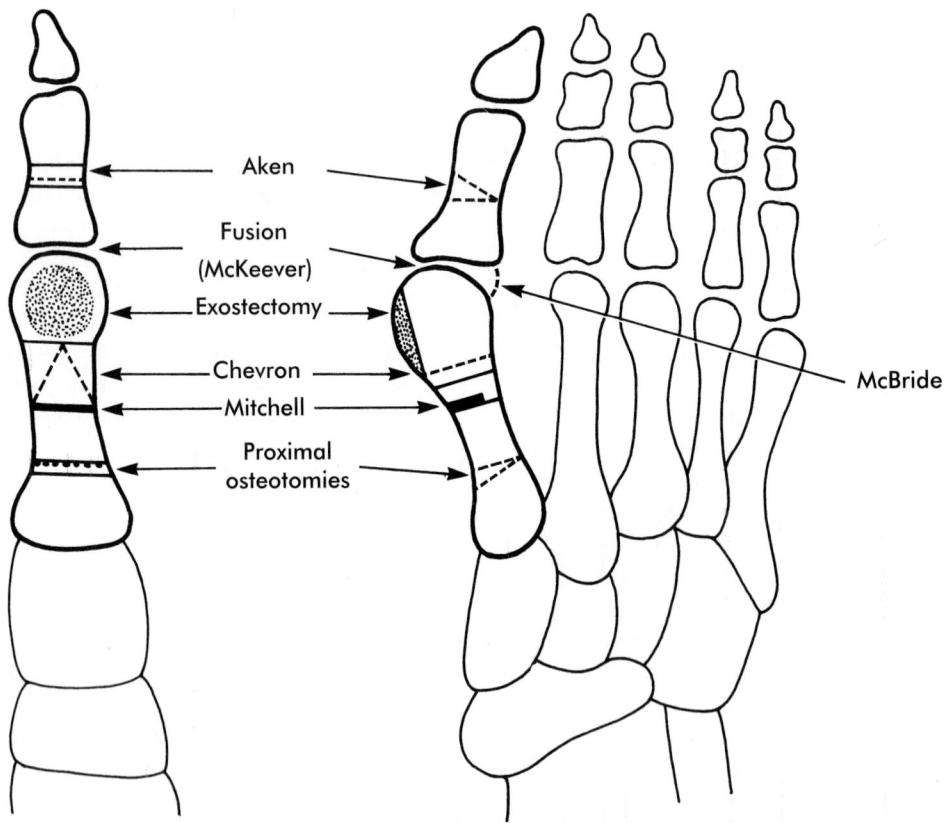

FIG. 21-90 Types of bunionectomies.

Symptoms include pain on the dorsomedial aspect of the first metatarsal head or directly over the medial exostosis, swelling of the big toe, painful plantar callus, and plantar keratosis. Discomfort to the entire foot occurs as the forefoot becomes more fatigued and symptomatic, with pain radiating to the leg and knee.

Hallux valgus is treated with a variety of surgical procedures (Fig. 21-90). All these procedures remove the exostosis and attempt to realign the great toe by removal of bone transfer of tendons, osteotomy of the first metatarsal shaft, or appropriate imbrication of soft tissue.

The goals of surgery are correction of the deformity (cosmesis), resection of the abnormal bony components (reconstruction), and normal or near-normal range of motion (function).

Procedural considerations. The patient is given general or regional anesthesia, and a tourniquet is applied to the proximal thigh. The foot and leg are prepped and then draped using a sterile stockinette.

A soft tissue set and small bone set are required, in addition to the following:

Power wire driver and   Kirschner wires
    microsagittal saw

Operative procedure

1. A dorsomedial, curvilinear incision extending from the distal portion of the proximal phalanx of the great toe to the metatarsal cuneiform joint is commonly used.
2. Dissection is carried down through the joint capsule.
3. A flap incision is made to expose the underlying bone to resect the hypertrophic bone found at the dorsomedial aspect of the first metatarsal head.
4. One third of the proximal phalanx is also resected with a power oscillating saw.
5. The wound is then irrigated and closed, and a bandage is applied to maintain the toe in the rectus position. Postoperative convalescence requires a minimum of 6 weeks.

Correction of hammer toe deformity

A hammer to flexion deformity develops at the proximal interphalangeal joint of the four lateral toes. This deformity causes painful calluses on the dorsal joints of the four lateral toes, since the cocked-up digits rub against the shoes. The deformity is treated by incising the long extensor tendon to the toes and fusing the middle joint. A smooth Kirschner wire is frequently used to stabilize the fusion and position the toe properly during the postoperative period.

Procedural considerations. The patient is placed in the supine position and the tourniquet applied. The foot is prepped and draped. A soft tissue and small bone set are required, plus the following:

Power drill   Kirschner wires

Operative procedure

1. A straight, longitudinal incision is made over the dorsomedial or dorsolateral area of the affected digits.
2. The capsular tissue of the distal third of the proximal phalanx and proximal interphalangeal joint is entered to expose the defect completely.
3. A small rongeur or microsaw is used to resect the distal third portion of the proximal phalanx.
4. Once the capital fragment is excised, the remaining portion of the distal proximal phalanx is débrided with a rongeur or rasp.
5. Digital alignment can be maintained with small Kirschner wires.
6. The wounds are irrigated and closed, and a sterile dressing and orthopedic shoe are applied for postoperative recovery.

Metatarsal fractures

Metatarsal fractures occur in various sites. These fractures have a reduced healing potential because metatarsals mainly consist of cortical bone, which lacks vascularity. Treatment is determined by the extent of the fracture; the greater the displacement, the greater the need for reduction. In general, transverse and short, oblique midshaft fractures of the metatarsals are internally fixed because of their instability and displacement. Pins, wires, screws, and plates are used for internal fixation of metatarsal fractures. The simplest method is Kirschner wire fixation.

Procedural considerations. The patient is placed in the supine position, a tourniquet is applied, and the foot is prepped and draped.

A soft tissue set and small bone set are required in addition to the following:

Power wire driver   Kirschner wires

Operative procedure

1. A small incision is made over the fracture.
2. The distal fragment is identified and retracted.
3. A smooth Kirschner wire is driven distally, exiting the skin.
4. The wire driver is then switched and attached to the end protruding from the skin.
5. The pin is then driven proximally into the canal of the proximal fragment.
6. If the fracture is more complex or comminuted, the fracture site is transfixed by crossing two Kirschner wires through the fracture.
7. The small incision is closed, and a short leg cast is applied.

Metatarsal head resection

Patients with rheumatoid arthritis frequently have dorsally dislocated toes and prominent and painful metatarsal heads on the plantar surfaces of the feet. Excision of all the metatarsal heads commonly relieves the pain and corrects an associated bunion deformity.

Procedural considerations. The patient is placed in a supine position, a tourniquet is applied, and the foot is prepped and draped.

A soft tissue set and small bone set are required in addition to the following:

Power microsagittal saw
Kirschner wires
Pliers

Operative procedure

1. A transverse plantar incision is made and tissue dissected to the metatarsal head.
2. The saw is used to excise the metatarsal head.
3. The incision is closed.

PELVIC FRACTURE AND DISRUPTION

Multiple trauma patients often present with multiple fractures that can be life threatening. Complications of pelvic fractures include injury not only to major vessels and nerves, but also to major visceral organs, such as the intestines, bladder, and urethra. Factors influencing mortality include associated visceral injury, hemorrhage, and head injury.

Pelvic classification is divided into three main groups (Fig. 21-91). Type A fractures are stable, without ring involvement (A1), and minimally displaced fractures of the ring (A2). Type B are rotationally unstable and vertically stable and are also subclassified: B1 is an open book fracture, B2 has ipsilateral lateral compression, and B3 has contralateral compression. Type C fractures are both rotationally and vertically unstable: C1 is unilateral, C2 bilateral, and C3 is associated with the acetabulum. Roentgenograms, CT scan, and MRI all prove useful in determining the type and appropriate treatment for pelvic trauma.

TYPE A	Stable
	A1-Fractures of the pelvis not involving the ring
	A2-Stable, minimally displaced fractures of the ring
TYPE B	Rotationally unstable, vertically stable
	B1-Open book
	B2-Lateral compression: ipsilateral
	B3-Lateral compression: contralateral (bucket handle)
TYPE C	Rotationally and Vertically unstable
	C1-Unilateral
	C2-Bilateral
	C3-Associated with an acetabular fracture

(From Tile M: J Bone Joint Surg 70-B: 3, 1988.)

FIG. 21-91   Classification of pelvic injuries.
From Tile M: *J Bone Joint Surg* 70-B:3, 1988.

Treatment is based on classification and may include closed manipulation and reduction or internal and external fixation. Internal and external fixation are also used concurrently in the treatment of some pelvic fractures.

Type A fractures can often be treated nonoperatively. Type B1 fractures may be treated with internal or external fixation, requiring a laparotomy with placement of two hole plates and cancellous bone screws. Type C fractures usually require open procedures to fix the fractures with plates and screws. and reduction of sacral disruptions with transiliac rods. Type C fractures may be treated with external fixation when the patient is hemodynamically unstable, and a quicker, simpler procedure is prudent.

External fixation is the most widely recommended treatment for type B fractures of the pelvis (Fig. 21-41). A technique similar to that of external fixation of extremity fractures is done in the operating room with anesthesia and sterile conditions. If external fixation is to be used, the earlier it is attempted, the greater chance of success.

Procedural considerations. This procedure is often done during other emergent and resuscitative efforts in the operating room. The operating room nurse must provide the best care under these conditions. The patient's entire pelvic area is prepped and draped. A pelvic skeleton in the room may help the team visualize maneuvers and pin placement to be attempted to complete the reduction.

A soft tissue set is needed in addition to the following:

External fixator   Power equipment

Operative procedure—AO external fixation

1. The pelvic disruption is reduced manually and confirmed with x-ray. The disruption may not be able to be completely reduced without traction using a distal femoral pin. If required, this is inserted under sterile conditions.
2. Kirschner wires are inserted percutaneously to determine the position of the pin placement, taking into consideration the inward and downward crest slope.
3. Parallel rows of pins are placed in the anterior iliac crest area. This is carried out by drilling the outer cortex and placing 5-mm half pins medially and distally. The pins should enter cancellous bone between the outer and inner table of ilium.
4. Three universal frames are placed over the pins as close to the skin as possible for maximum rigidity.
5. Optimal reduction of the fracture is visualized using x-ray. The cross bar is applied and compression and distraction maneuvers used to maintain the reduction.
6. The cross bar is removed and connecting rods applied with couplers.
7. The cross bar is reattached and joints of the frame tightened.
8. The pin sites of tented skin are released. The wounds are dressed with iodine ointment and gauze.
9. The frames are generally left in place for 8 to 12 weeks.

TOTAL JOINT ARTHROPLASTY

Arthroplasty of the joints is performed to restore motion of the joint and function to the muscles and ligaments. It is indicated in individuals with a painful, disabling arthritic joint that is no longer responsive to conservative therapy. The procedure is generally reserved for those with a less active lifestyle. The younger patient, very active older person, or laborer may better be served with a reconstructive procedure such as arthrodesis or osteotomy.

Early arthroplasty techniques utilized interpositional substances from autogenous tissue such as muscle, fat, and skin. These techniques improve results in ankylosed joints but have been ineffective in treatment of arthritic joints. Synthetic substances such as vitallium were used for interposition with the same poor results in the arthritic joint.

The modern age for total joint replacement surgery began in the 1960s with the development by Sir John Charnley of a total hip replacement arthroplasty. The components included a stainless steel femoral head and a polyethylene acetabular component, and fixation with polymethyl methacrylate revolutionized total joint replacement. Similar components for the knee soon followed. Designs were soon developed for use in the elbow, wrist, and ankle. Subsequent failure rates have all but eliminated most ankle and wrist replacements, but total hip and knee replacements are done in large numbers each year. Improvements in implant design, materials, and fixation techniques are ongoing.

Though the metals have become stronger and more wear resistant, the classic combination of metal on polyethylene is the mainstay of joint implants. Metals used in hip and knee implants include cobalt-chrome (weight-bearing femoral head) and titanium (stems of hips and tibial components). Femoral heads made of ceramic were developed in an attempt to reduce wear of the polyethylene caused by articulation. The acetabulum and tibial articulating surfaces continue to be substituted with ultra–high weight polyethylene (UHWPE), which provides superior wear and deforming characteristics.

Because of a relatively high rate of loosening of cement-fixed implants, especially in younger patients, alternative means of fixation of been developed in recent years. Some of these developments have included coating the implant with a thin layer of polymethyl methacrylate (PMMA) to enhance cement bonding. Porous-coated implants (Fig. 21-92) were developed to allow fixation by bony ingrowth onto the implant surface, and press-fit designs that achieve an interference fit within the femoral canal. Ten- and 15-year data are being evaluated on alternative method fixation with promising early results.

Bone cement, or PMMA, is another area that has received considerable attention in the search for optimal bone implant fixation. Cement seems to exhibit various degrees of porosity depending on mixing methods and cement pressurization within the canal. Bone cement must prevent motion at the implant interface. Porosity can lead to fatigue and fracture, which ultimately can lead to implant loosen-ing. PMMA, chemically similar to plexiglass, has barium sulfate added to it to make it possible to assess distribution and changes at a later time. The use of bone cement, and possibly the pressurization within the femoral canal, has been shown to cause hypotensive events in patients. These periods are transient and the actual cause is unclear. One theory is that the monomer from cement enters the circulation and causes peripheral vasodilatation and direct myocardial depression. Local tissue effects of PMMA may include (1) tissue protein coagulation caused by polymerization, (2) bone necrosis caused by occlusion of nutrient metaphyseal arteries, and (3) cytotoxic and lipotoxic effects of nonpolymerized monomer.

Despite the high rate of success of total joint implantation over the years, there are numerous potential complications. They are generally divided into medical complications, mechanical complications, and infections.

Medical complications include, but are not limited to, cardiac dysrhythmias, myocardial infarction, hemorrhage, and pulmonary emboli. Mechanical complications consist of implant breakage, loosening, and wear. Infection in the patient with a total joint implant is a catastrophic complication that usually requires additional surgery, prolonged hospitalization, and a greater economic burden.

Most surgeons recommend the routine use of antibiotics in primary and revision joint arthroplasty. Antibiotic coverage is initiated preoperatively, continued during lengthy procedures, and administered for 24 to 48 postoperatively. Pulsatile lavage systems or routine irrigation may be used to keep tissues moist, remove debris, and dilute bacteria that may be present. Additional antibiotics are added to the physiologic saline solutions used for irrigation and to PMMA; however, data do not support or dispute this practice. Results of studies vary, due to variables in settings. It is believed that standard measures, appropriate use of perioperative antibiotics, and implementation of techniques recommended in the operating room should result in wound infection rates between 1% and 1.5% (McQuarrie, Glover, and Olson, 1990).

The operating room and surrounding environment may play a role in the success or failure of total joint implantation. Airborne and contact contamination of a wound may be more significant in this procedure than others and certainly prove more catastrophic. These factors, in light of a large amount of foreign material left in a patient, make it imperative that asepsis and strict technique are observed. Draping technique, traffic control, and proper operating room attire should accompany the plan of care for the patient undergoing total joint replacement.

Total hip replacement

Total hip replacement (arthroplasty) is a common orthopedic procedure performed on older persons. It is indicated for patients with hip pain due to degenerative joint disease or rheumatoid arthritis. In the past, reconstructive surgery of the hip consisted of subtrochanteric osteotomy, cup arthroplasty, and prosthetic femoral head replacement (see the section on endoprosthesis). Since the development of the total hip arthroplasty, these procedures are rarely performed.

Total hip replacement can be cemented, noncemented, or hybrid. Hybrids involve cementing one component, usually the femoral stem, and not cementing the acetabular cup. Hybrid arthroplasty is becoming increasingly popular. Advances in cemented total hip replacement have resulted because of changes in stem design and application of cement procedures (Crenshaw, 1992). The concern of component loosening has led to the development of porous ingrowth (Fig. 21-92) and anatomic press-fit designs (Fig. 21-93). Porous-coated components contain surface pores that allow bone ingrowth resulting in attachment of the component to the bone. Press-fit (interference) femoral components involve using a larger stem than the reamed canal, providing a firm fit. Press-fit femoral components that have partial porous pads are another stem design that is utilized. When porous-coated and press-fit prostheses are cemented, the rough surfaces help to enhance cement fixa-

tion. If cement is used, enough reaming of the bone needs to be done to allow a mantle of cement to envelop the implant. When bony ingrowth implants are used, a tight fit is desired, allowing intimate contact between implant and bone.

The primary function of the femoral component is the replacement of the femoral head and femoral neck following resection. The femoral head should ultimately sit where it reproduces the center of rotation of the hip. The neck length is variable and is built in to several different heights of femoral heads that are eventually seated onto the Morse taper of the femoral stem. The version (implant rotation within the canal) is very important; too much anteversion or retroversion leaves the hip prone to dislocation. The normal position of the proximal femur is slight anteversion.

Femoral stems can be collarless or have collars that sit down on the resected femur. Collars will produce forces upon the bone and may be desired in cases of osteoporotic bone, where bone genesis may be diminished due to the disease process.

Acetabular cups have also presented challenges in trying to maintain fixation within the socket. When cement techniques of the 1970s are used, femoral loosening plateaus about 5 years following surgery (Crenshaw, 1992). Wear properties of the ultra–high molecular weight polyethylene are also a concern. For this and other reasons associated with component failure the idea of modularity was developed. Modular components (Fig. 21-94), such as a polyethylene cup that snaps into a metal acetabular shell, greatly decrease the amount of surgery needed in the case

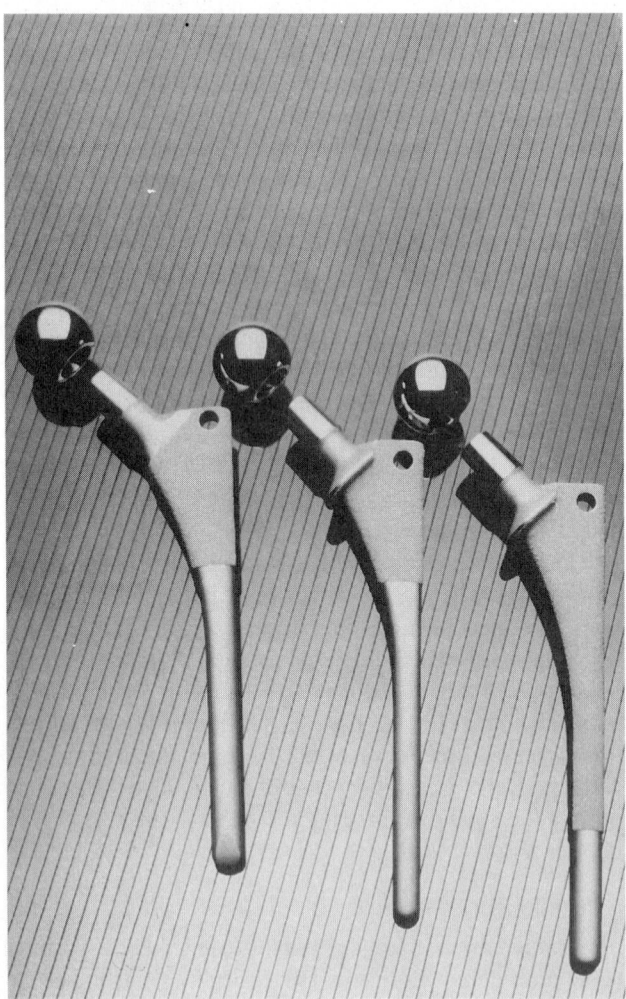

FIG. 21-92 Porous coated implants, acetabular component. Courtesy DePuy, Inc., Warsaw, Ind.

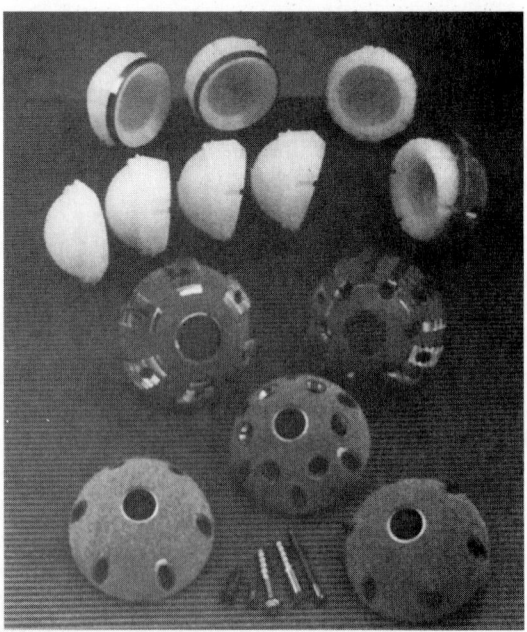

FIG. 21-93 Press-fit implants. The area is prepared to secure the implant for use without cement.

From Cameron HU: *The Technique of Total Hip Arthroplasty,* St. Louis, 1992, Mosby.

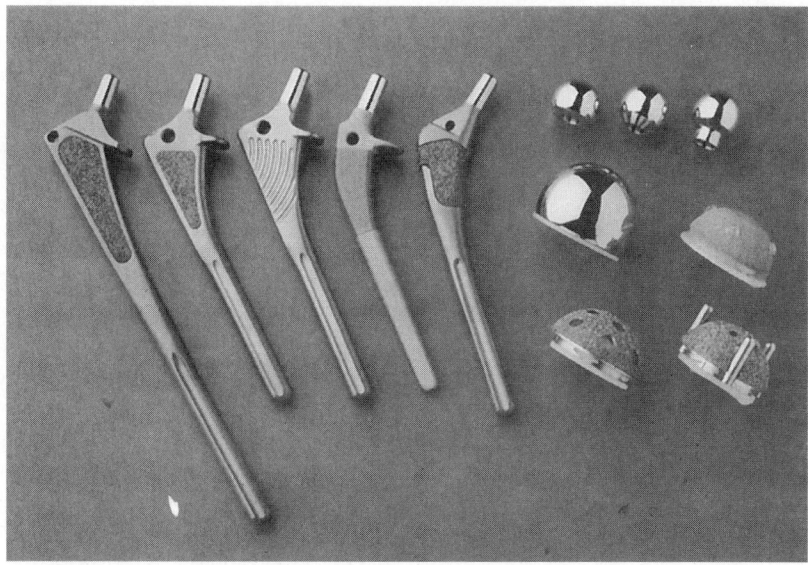

FIG. 21-94 Modular hip components that can be used independently in the event of need for only one or failure of one component.

Courtesy Zimmer, Inc., Warsaw, Ind.

of some revisions. In the case of excessive cup wear or a femoral neck length that is short, surgery is minimized with the ability to exchange the modular components without removing the implants fixed to the bone.

Acetabular cups come with a textured back for cement fixation and may have standoff pegs to allow an appropriate cement mantle. Noncemented cups may have large self-tapping threads circling the outside to bite into the subchondral bone of the resected socket; however, these are less popular because of stress risers placed on bone by the sharp edges of the threads. Others have sintered metal on the implant to promote areas where bony ingrowth can take place (interdigitation of bone). Usually the bony ingrowth implants have several screw holes to allow temporary fixation while bone healing and ingrowth take place.

No one prosthesis is suitable for every patient's needs. Modular hip systems allow the orthopedic surgeon to choose from an array of interchangeable components that have been developed. Various femoral head sizes (22 mm, 26 mm, 28 mm, 32 mm) are available to maintain proper center of rotation. Acetabular cups may be snap-fit, low profile, or deep profile, which adds additional thickness to the medial wall, where there may be significant bone loss.

With modular systems, unipolar or bipolar cups are also an option that may be used when the acetabulum is relatively normal. The unipolar and bipolar cups with appropriate head sizes are designed to fit on various modular system stems.

Custom prostheses or revision and extra long stems are available when there is significant bone loss. These implants are employed in cases of revision where fixation is needed farther down the femoral canal or in oncologic cases where tumor and corresponding bone have been resected.

Young, active individuals with strong healthy bones are ideal candidates for noncemented total hip replacement arthroplasties. Elderly patients with osteoporosis and poor quality bone are usually candidates for cemented components because their bones may lack the compressive strength to support weight-bearing forces.

Hip reconstruction (cemented)

There are numerous implants available for total hip implantation. Many of the implants can be used for the same surgical indications, and one implant may not function any better then another, provided all other conditions and techniques are the same. The instruments required to implant any one device cannot be used for another. It is very important to ensure that all of the instrumentation is available before starting surgery. Furthermore, the surgical effort should be coordinated and without disruption. Once an implant has been inserted with bone cement that has hardened, significant bone resection and loss would result if correction were necessary.

PMMA adheres to the polyethylene and metal but not to the bone. It fills the cavity and interstices of the bone and forms a mechanical bond. PMMA is manufactured as liquid monomer and a powder and is mixed under sterile conditions by the scrub nurse in the operating room at the time of implantation. It usually takes 10 to 12 minutes to harden. Because of the potential harmful effects of PMMA fumes to the nasal epithelium, an exhaust system should be used during the mixing process.

Procedural considerations. The patient is positioned in the lateral decubitus position and secured in place with anterior and posterior bolsters. This position is essential to ensure correct anatomic placement of the acetabular cup.

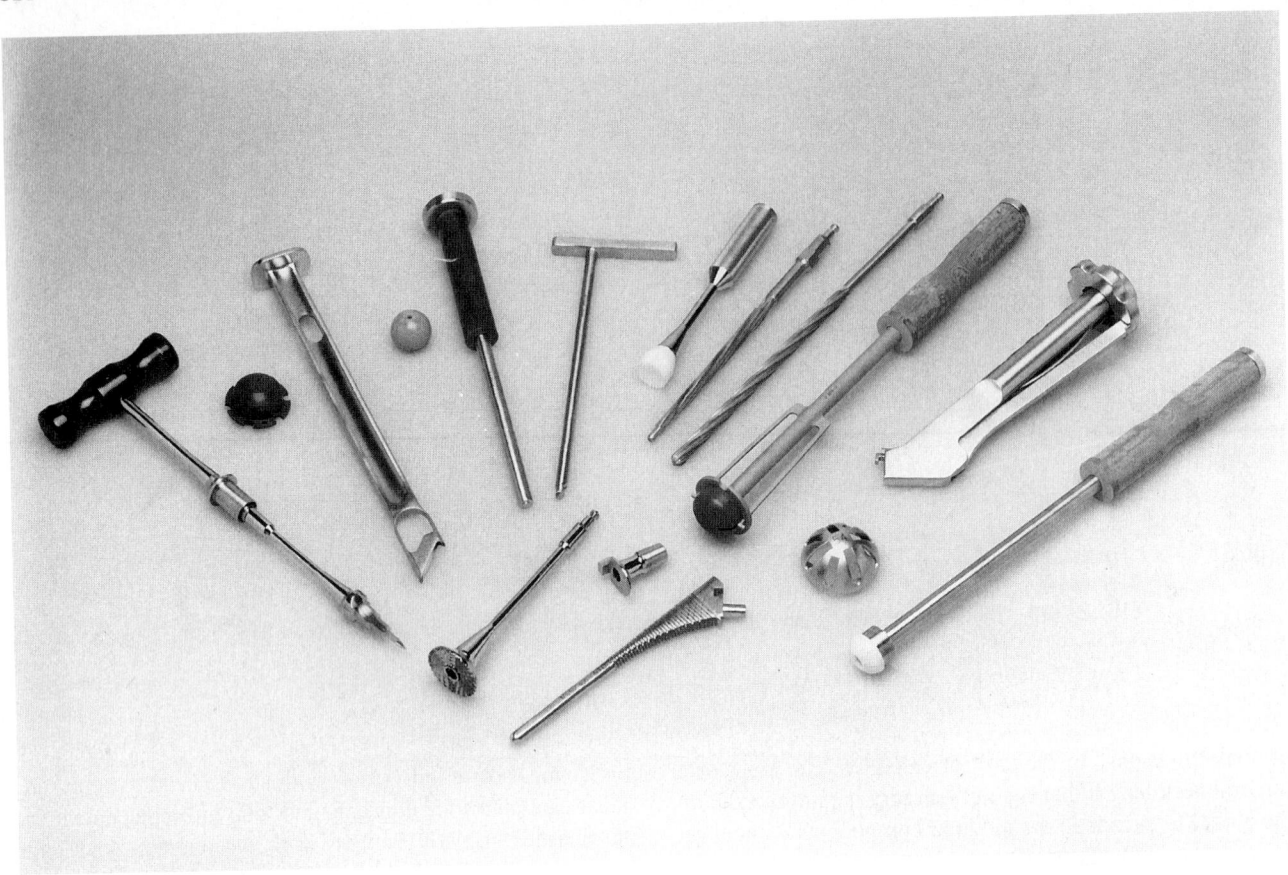

FIG. 21-95   Anatomical Medullary Locking (AML) Total Hip System, used for total hip arthroplasty.
Courtesy DePuy, Inc., Warsaw, Ind.

Bony prominences should be adequately padded. A surgical preparation is completed from the level of the umbilicus down to and including the foot, and the patient is draped. The x-rays are overlaid with the implant templates.

A soft tissue set and large bone set are required in addition to the following:

Hip retractor set
Total hip implant and corresponding instrumentation (Fig. 21-95)
Power reamer driver and reciprocating or oscillating saw
Trochanter pack (for trochanteric osteotomy) (Fig. 21-96)

Polymethyl methacrylate and supplies (Fig. 21-97)
Pulse lavage with 3000-ml bag of normal saline solution (Fig. 21-98)
Acetabular reamers (Fig. 21-99)
Femoral canal suction wicks
Cement restrictor and inserter (Fig. 21-100)

Revision of total hip arthroplasties requires the same instrumentation as cemented total hip in addition to the following:

Cement removal instrumentation (Fig. 21-101)
Revision instruments and implants

Fluoroscopy (have available)
Long (bronchoscopic) suction cannula
Headlight

Operative procedure—cemented Modular Hip System

1. A slightly curved incision is made over the greater trochanter, from a point level with the anterior iliac spine distally to 10 cm below the greater trochanter.
2. Femoral neck exposure is accomplished by putting the hip in internal rotation and extension with knee flexion, putting the rotators under tension. They are identified, tagged with suture, and released.
3. Once a capsulotomy is performed, the hip can be dislocated. Forward hip flexion, adducting the leg, and internal rotation will present the femoral head posteriorly into the surgical site.
4. The femoral osteotomy guide is placed over the lateral femur. This identifies the point on the femoral neck where the osteotomy should be made. Some femoral osteotomy guides will also gauge the neck length required. The level is marked and a femoral osteotomy is carried out with a reciprocating saw.
5. The femur is retracted to expose the acetabulum, allow completion of the capsulotomy, and expose the bony rim of the entire acetabulum.
6. The acetabulum is inspected, any osteophytes are removed, and articular cartilage is reamed with bone-conserving reamers in a circumferential manner. The smallest reamer is progressed in a graduated method 1

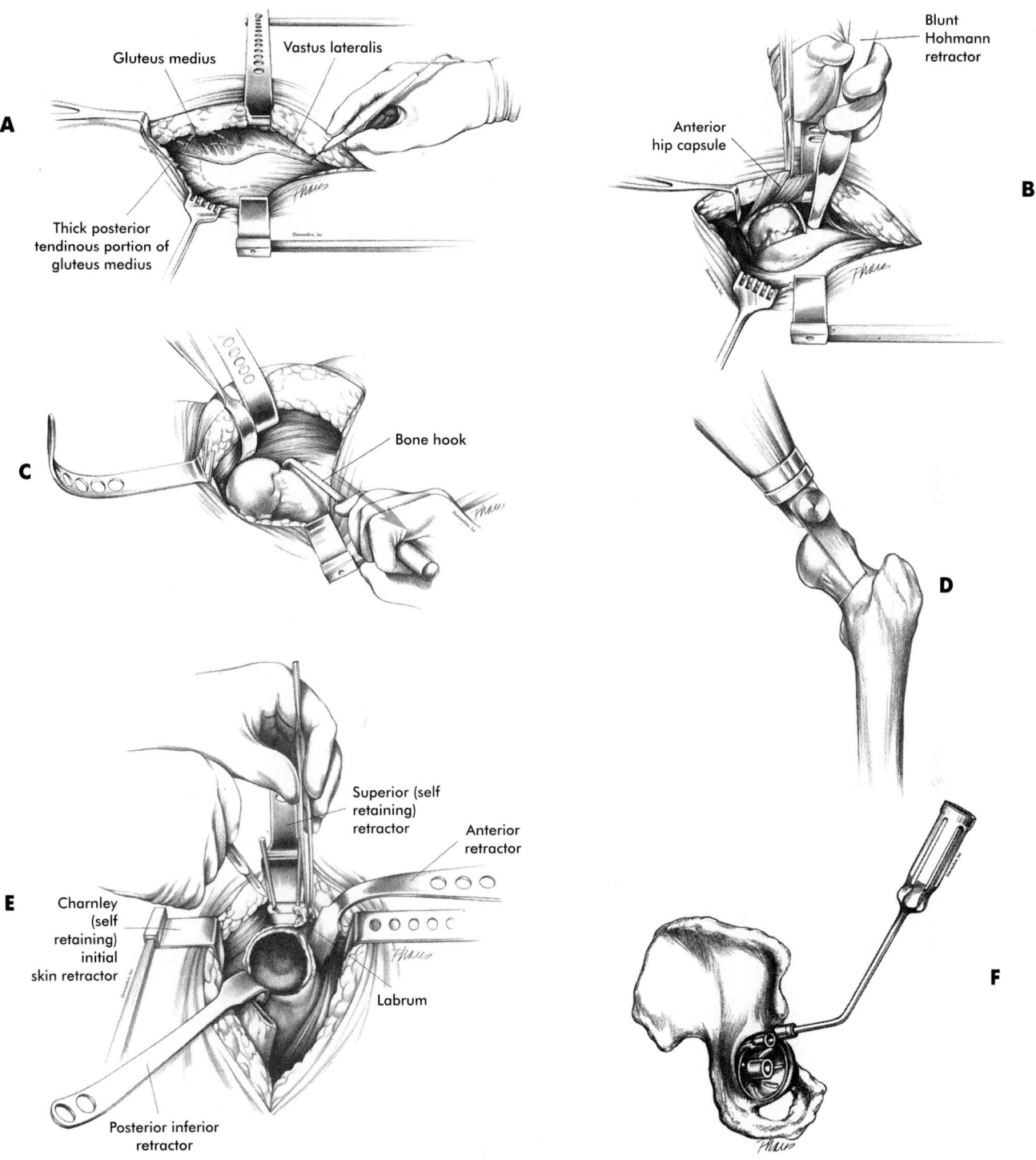

FIG. 21-96   **A,** Following the incision, the Charnley Retractor is placed, the fascia lata is incised followed by detachment of the gluteus minimus; **B,** an anterior capsulotomy is completed; **C,** the hip is flexed, adducted and externally rotated to dislocate from the acetabulum; **D,** the femoral neck is cut using an oscillating saw blade; **E,** the rim of the acetabulum is debrided of labrum, redundant capsule and marginal osteophytes; **F,** the acetabulum is reamed; following reaming the appropriate drill guide is inserted into the acetabulum.

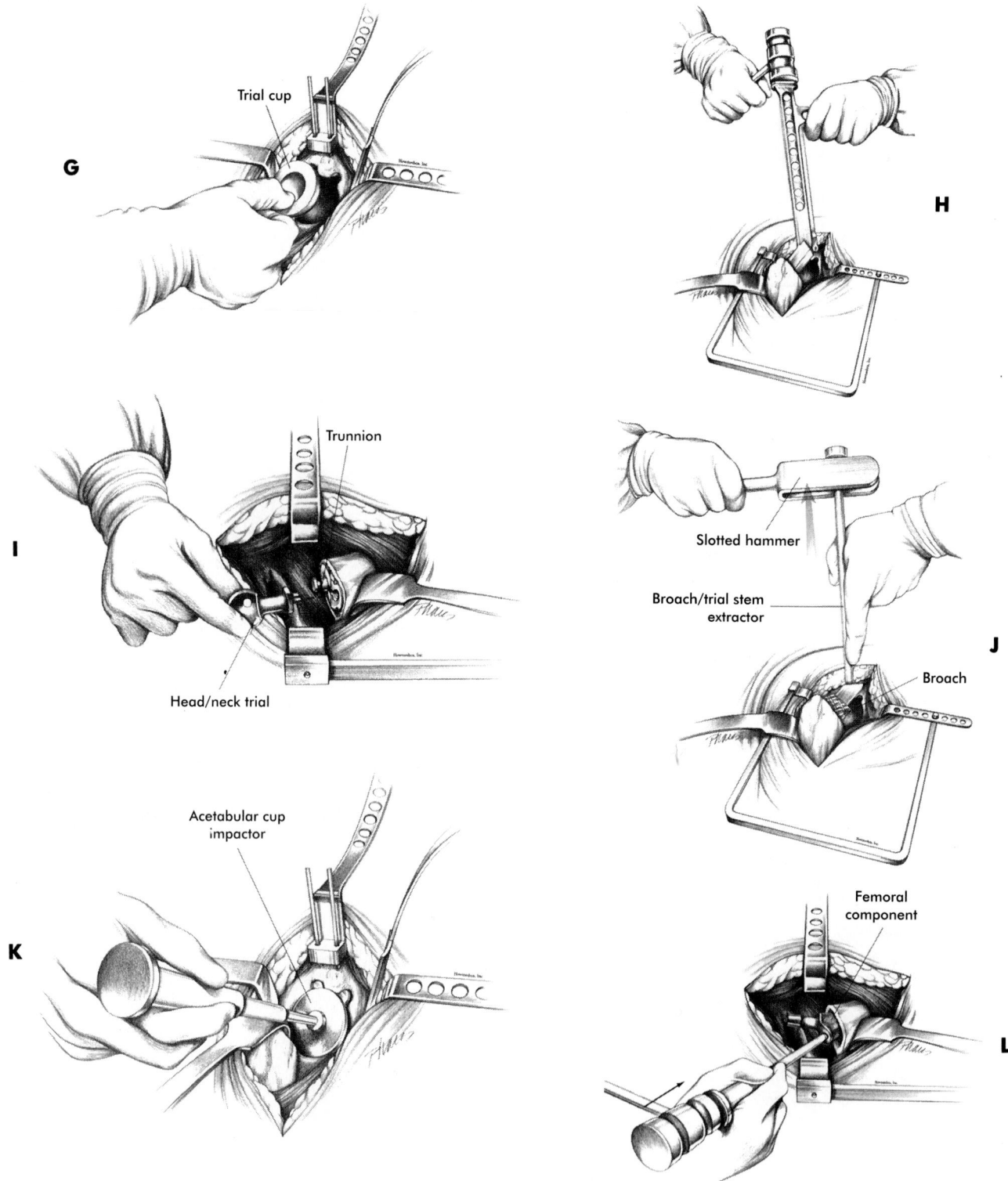

FIG. 21-96, CONT. **G,** following drilling of the holes for the acetabular fixation pegs, the trial acetabular cup is inserted; **H,** the proximal wedge of cancellous bone is removed and the appropriate size femoral broach is introduced down the axis of the femoral canal; **I,** the trial head/neck assembly is placed on broach trunnion of trial reduction; **J,** using the slotted hammer, the femoral broach is extracted; the trial acetabular cup is removed; **K,** acetabular fixation pegs are seated, the acetabular cup introduced and the component seated; **L,** the femoral canal is irrigated with pulsatile lavage and dried with suction and gauze sponges; the femoral canal is plugged and filled with methyl methacrylate; the femoral component is inserted.

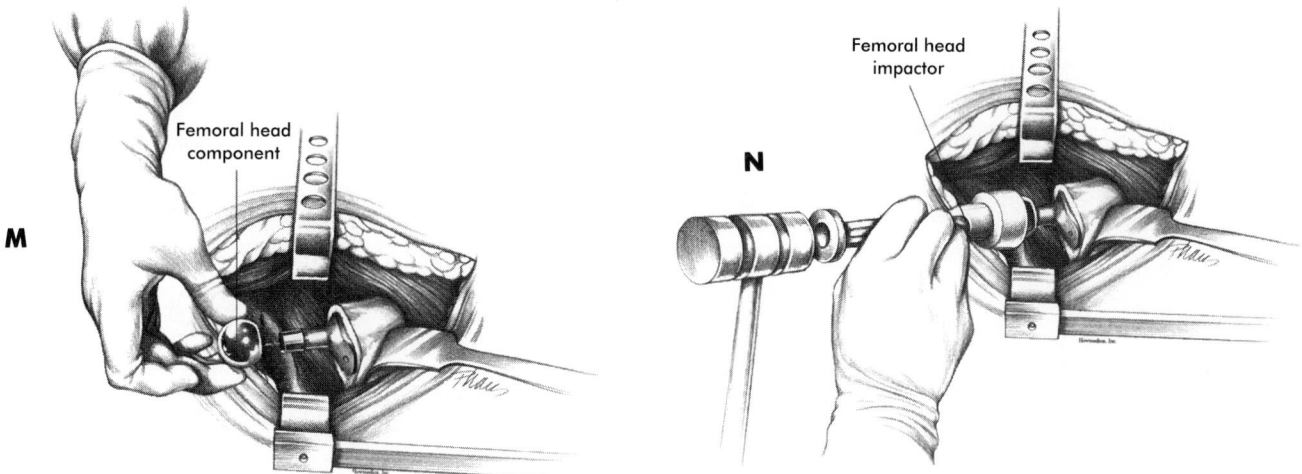

FIG. 21-96, CONT. **M**, the femoral head component is placed on trunnion; **N**, the femoral head is impacted, the femur reduced and the wound irrigated prior to closure.

(Courtesy Howmedica, Inc., Rutherford, N.J.)

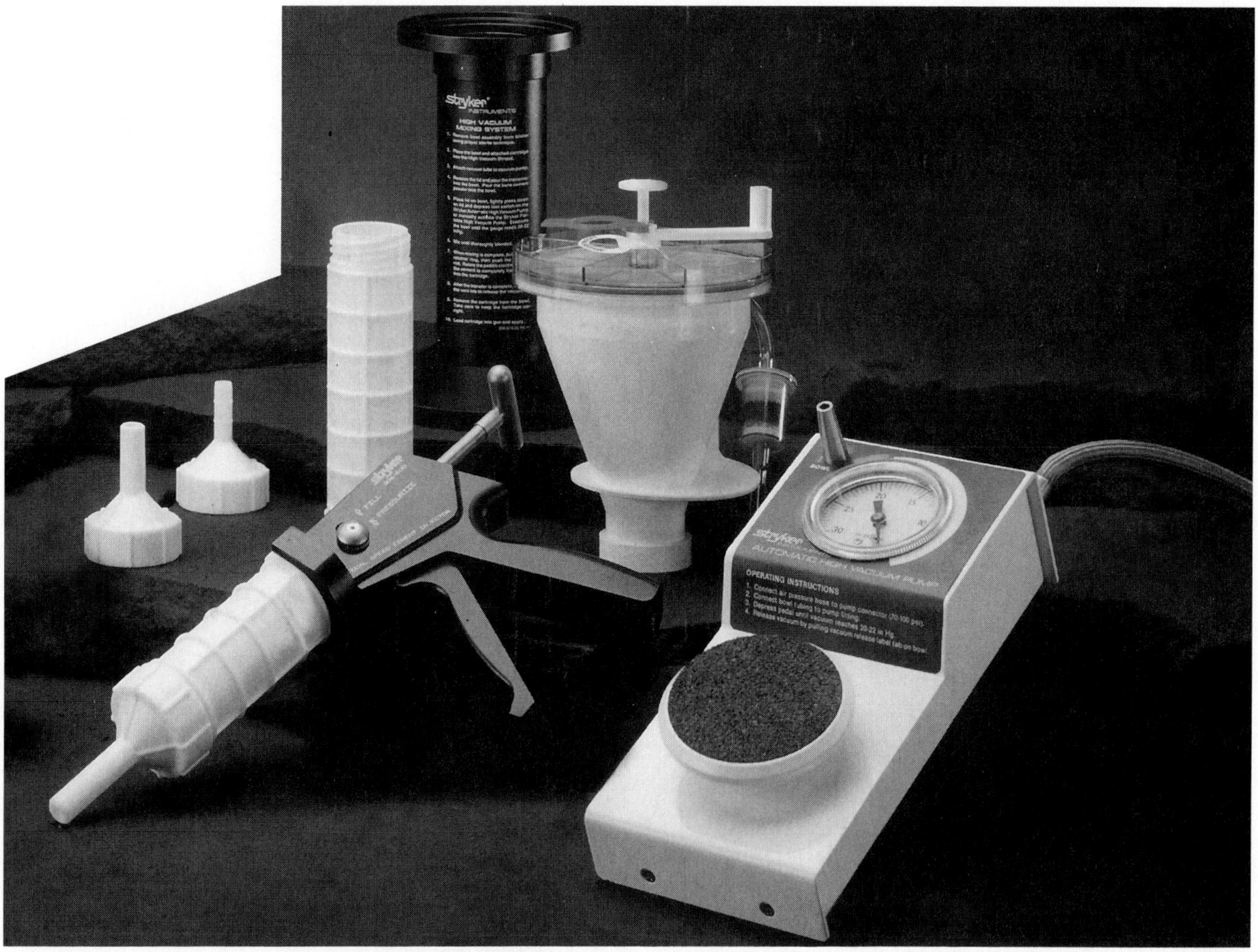

FIG. 21-97 Polymethyl methcralate and supplies for mixing and delivery in the canal.

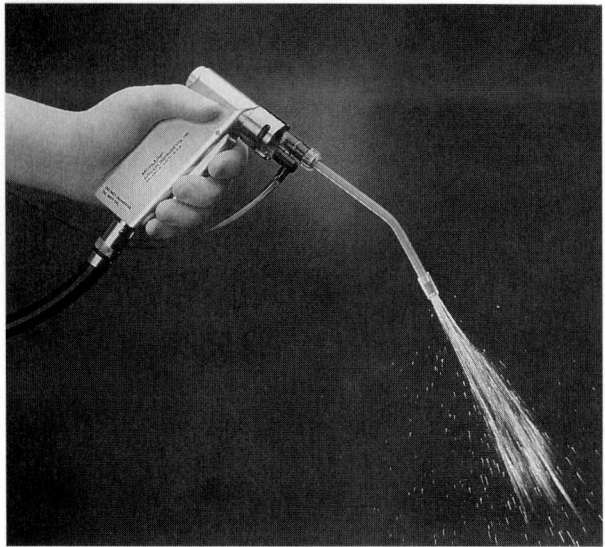

FIG. 21-98 Pulse lavage used for pressurized irrigation when irrigating surgical wounds, debriding bone during a joint replacement, debriding open fractures or traumatic wounds, irrigation of soft tissue injuries or irrigation of contaminated wounds.

Courtesy Micro-Aire Surgical Instruments, San Fernando, Calif.

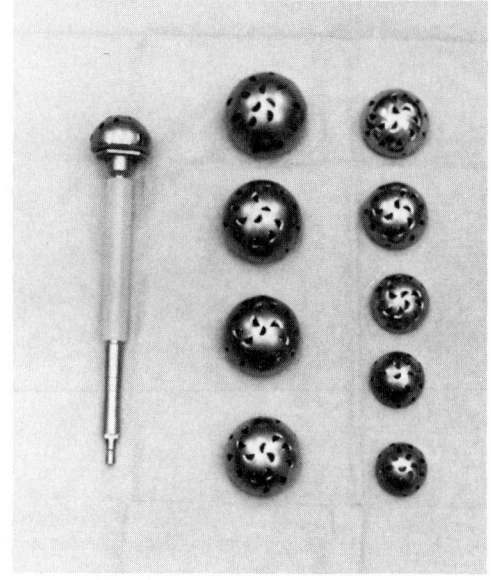

FIG. 21-99 Acetabular reamers.

Courtesy Howmedica, Inc., Rutherford, N.J.

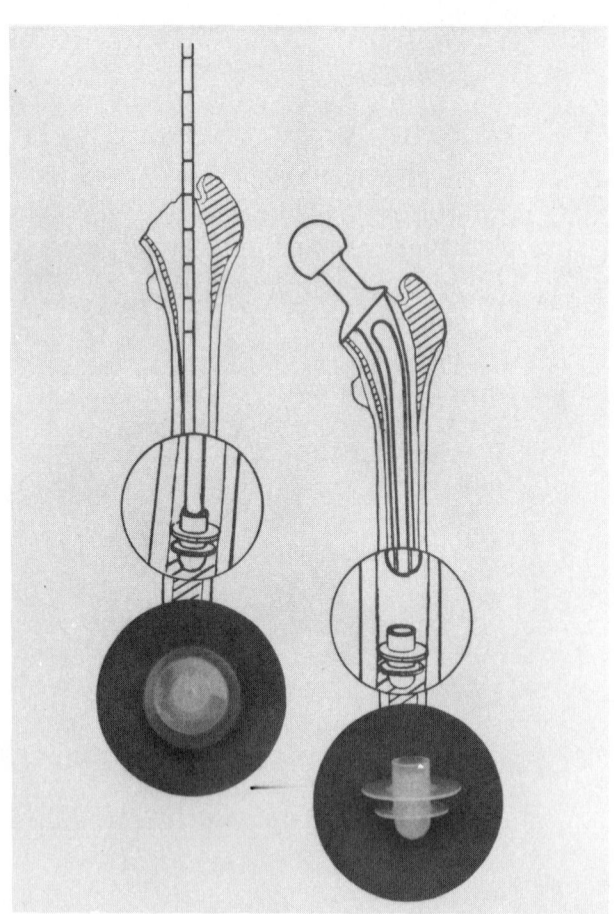

FIG. 21-100 Cement restrictor and inserter used for occlusion of the medullary canal prior to delivery of the cement.

Courtesy Richards Medical Co., Memphis, Tenn.

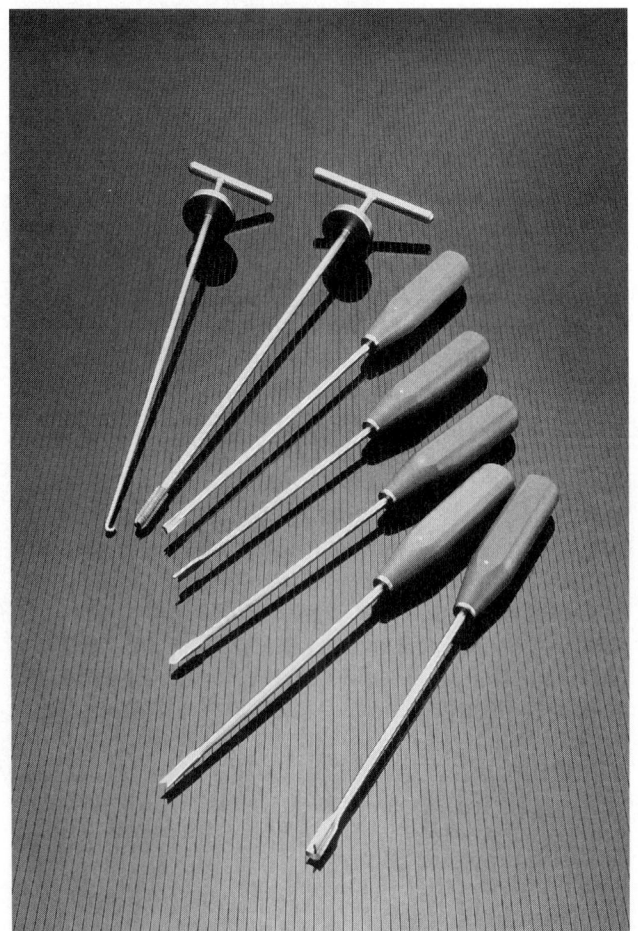

FIG. 21-101 Implant removal instrumentation for **A,** Cemented or **B,** Noncemented implants.

Courtesy DePuy, Inc., Warsaw, Ind.

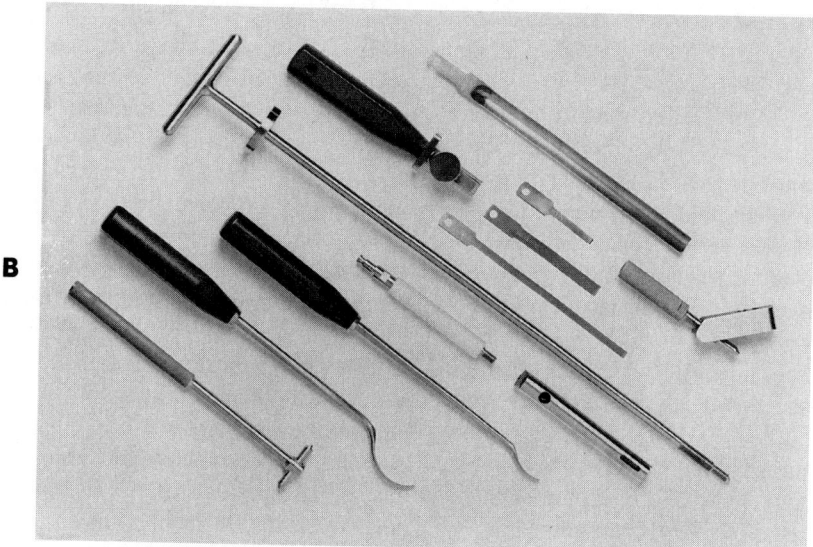

B

FIG. 21-101, CONT.   See legend, opposite page.

or 2 mm at a time until the cartilage is reamed down to expose osteochondral bone. A hemispheric shape and bleeding bone should result.

7. Remaining soft tissue is curretted from the floor of the acetabulum, and cystic areas are filled with cancellous bone from the femoral canal and packed with a bone tamp. Any other bone grafting of major bony defects is accomplished using the fixation of choice (bone screws).

8. Several 6-mm holes are drilled in the floor of the acetabulum, removing bone debris. Holes are undercut using curettes. These prepared holes act as anchoring areas for the bone cement.

9. Trial acetabular components are placed on the positioning device and positioned in the socket. The cup is assessed for size, position within the socket, and the relationship of the component compared with the bony margins of the acetabulum.

10. The prepared acetabular socket is lavaged, dried using wicks, and filled with cement that has been injected and pressurized with an injecting gun. The acetabular shell component is positioned and held motionless until the cement polymerizes. Extruded cement is trimmed from around the edge of the component. A polyethylene insert is later snapped into the shell.

11. A sponge is placed in the acetabulum to protect the component from bone debris and subsequent cement as attention is turned to the femur.

12. The proximal femur is exposed by dropping the knee toward the floor and pushing the leg proximally. The femoral canal is accessed using a box osteotome or trochanteric reamer followed by the T-handle canal reamer.

13. Beginning with the smallest broach, alternatively impact and extract in the proximal femoral canal. Progressively larger broaches are used to crush and remove

cancellous bone until cortical bone is reached. A broach that is not advancing should not be used. This could result in shattering the femur.

14. With the final broach seated to the desired depth in the canal, the neck is prepared with a calcar reamer. The broach remains as the femoral trial component along with the various size head, neck, and offset trial components.

15. The trial component is removed, and the canal is lavaged and brushed to accommodate the PMMA.

16. A cement restrictor is inserted into the femoral canal. The femoral components are passed and assembled on the back table.

17. The cement is injected and pressurized within the femoral canal.

18. The femoral component, with the proximal and distal centralizers, is inserted into the canal with or without the femoral head.

19. The appropriate size of femoral head is positioned onto the stem, and reduction is carried out. The joint is taken through a range of motion to check for positioning, stability, and the limit to which dislocation occurs.

20. Depending on the surgeon and the surgical approach, the greater trochanter may or may not have been removed for exposure of the hip joint. If removed, it is reattached with 18-gauge wire.

21. The wound is closed in layers over suction drains. The skin is closed with staples, and a sterile dressing is applied to provide compression to the wound.

22. An abduction pillow or splint is placed between the patient's legs postoperatively.

Hip reconstruction (noncemented)

Fixation with a noncemented prosthesis is initially accomplished by a tight fit and intimate contact of the implants within bone of substantial strength. As with all prosthetic designs, it is essential to fill the medullary canal and wedge the prosthesis in as tightly as possible to provide temporary press-fit fixation. These prostheses closely follow normal anatomic shape. Only the instrumentation corresponding to the implant should be used. Precise machining of the femoral canal must be ensured. Acetabular components usually are fixed to the bone with screw fixation. Sufficient time is then allowed for the cancellous bone to heal by growing into the porous portions of the prosthesis.

The healing process requires the same amount of time as a long bone cortical fracture (approximately 3 months). Extreme caution is taken postoperatively to protect the operative hip from excessive compression, rotation, and shear stresses.

There are numerous noncemented implants, such as the anatomic medullary locking (AML), the Harris-Galante, Osteolock, Omnifit, and Bias long revision stems.

Procedural considerations. The position and incision are the same as for the total hip replacement (cemented). The x-rays and implant templates are placed on the view box.

Operative procedure—noncemented AML hip system (Fig. 21-96)

1. Following the incision, the capsule is entered and the femoral head is dislocated.
2. A pilot hole is established in the trochanteric fossa as an intramedullary reference point.
3. Reaming of the intramedullary canal is then performed in a progressive manner with fully fluted rigid reamers.
4. A femoral neck osteotomy is achieved by positioning an osteotomy template along the axis of the femur and cutting at the level of the collar.
5. Attention is directed to the acetabulum, which is cleared of soft tissue and reamed with hemispheric reamers.
6. Trial acetabular sizers are placed to determine correct position and size of the prosthetic component.
7. A hollow osteotome is used in the femoral canal to connect the pilot hole to the osteotomy site.
8. Femoral broaches are then inserted to enlarge the intramedullary space for trial insertion.
9. A power calcar planer may be placed over the trunion of the broach and used to contour the femoral neck.
10. A trial head and neck component is positioned onto the fitted broach, and a trial reduction is carried out.
11. If trial reduction is satisfactory, all trial components are removed.
12. The appropriate size AML acetabular component is inserted into the acetabulum, and a polyethylene insert is locked into place.
13. The femoral component is placed into the canal, and the modular head is seated on the trunion.
14. Reduction of the hip is followed by standard closure with drains.
15. Abduction of the hip is maintained postoperatively with a foam abduction pillow.

Total knee replacement

Total knee replacement (arthroplasty) is a surgical procedure designed to replace the worn surfaces of the knee joint. Success depends on patient selection, component design, surgical technique, and rehabilitation.

Patients with severe destruction of the knee joint resulting from degenerative rheumatoid or traumatic arthritis or destruction of only the medial or lateral compartments of the knee joint as a result of extreme varus or valgus deformity complain of pain and instability. Arthroplasty of the knee has been successful in relieving pain and providing stability. Complications involving the extensor mechanism is receiving increased attention as causative factor in implant failure.

Like total hip replacement, knee surface replacement began as interposition of tissue between the resected bone ends to prevent them from fusing. Several substances were used, including skin, muscle, fat, and chromatized pig bladder. In the 1920s and 1930s Campbell used free fascial transplants as interposition material and achieved limited success in ankylosed (fused) joints but not in the treatment of arthritic joints. Following the success with materials for total hip replacement, total knee replacement progressed as a mechanism used to alleviate joint pain and deformity. Most authors feel that the modern age of total knee replacement is as late as 1971, with the development of a minimally constrained prosthesis addressing biomechanical considerations.

Continued clinical analysis of various implant designs and increased knowledge of the biomechanics of the normal knee have resulted in the introduction of second-generation implants with improved geometry. Experiences with these second-generation implants led to further refinement of both instrumentation and surgical technique. Alternate fixation techniques and improvements with the conventional cement methods are both areas of current investigational efforts.

The challenge for finding the optimal knee implant is in reproducing the complicated range of motion of the knee. Motion of the knee occurs in three planes: flexion and extension, abduction and adduction, and rotation. Designs of total knees should allow preservation of the normal ligaments whenever possible, while providing soft tissue balance when necessary to maintain stability.

Total knee implants may be classified into three different categories, according to the portions of the knee to be replaced. Unicompartmental implants are used to replace just one opposing articular surface (medial or lateral) of the femur and tibia. These implants, however, have lost popularity in recent years due to biomechanical and technical pitfalls. They account for less than 10% of all total knee replacements performed in the United States (Crenshaw, 1992). Biocompartmental designs, mentioned only to demonstrate the progression of total knee design, replaced both the medial and lateral surfaces of the femur and tibia. This implant design is almost completely rejected as a technique for knee replacement. Tricompartmental implants replace not only the opposing femorotibial joint, but also the patellofemoral joint. Most of the total knee replacements completed today are of this variety.

The tricompartmental knees are further divided into three categories (Fig. 21-102). Unconstrained prostheses have very little constraint built in between the femoral and tibial

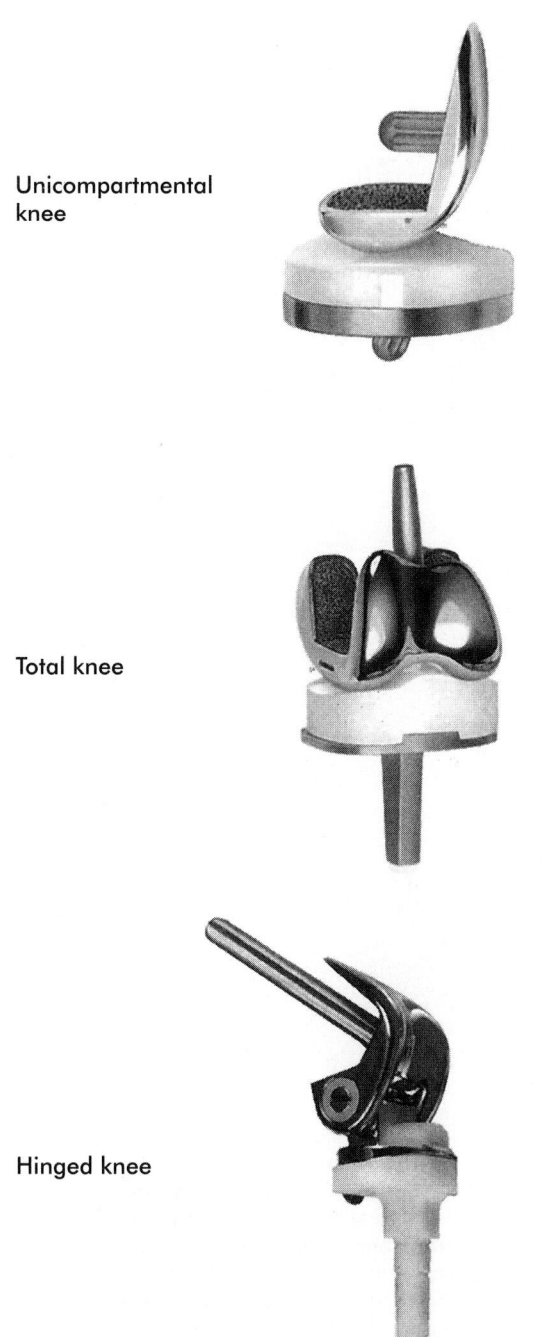

Unicompartmental
knee

Total knee

Hinged knee

FIG. 21-102 Tricompartmental knee implant. **A,** Unconstrained. **B,** Semiconstrained. **C,** Fully constrained hinge.

Courtesy Howmedica, Inc., Rutherford, N.J.

components and depend on the integrity of soft tissues to provide stability of the reconstructed joint. Where there is significant deformity and the need for soft tissue release, the surgeon may decide to use a semiconstrained prosthesis. The design of the prosthesis lends itself to more inherent stability necessitated by ligamentous deficiency. Fully constrained prostheses are linked together with pure hinges, rotating hinges, and nonhinged designs. This design is used in the presence of marked bone loss, instability, deformity, and revision surgery where there has been significant bone loss. Fully constrained prostheses do not provide a normal range of motion, which leads to excessive wear and implant loosening and breakage.

Methods of fixation of total knee implants include both cemented and noncemented techniques. The noncemented variety encompasses both porous bony ingrowth and press-fit designs. The choice of implant and method of fixation depend on the predisposition of the bone, patient age and activity level, and surgeon comfort with a particular technique. Previous designs did not allow the retention of the posterior cruciate ligament as it was resected, possibly leading to increase in joint instability. Newer designs, however, allow the posterior cruciate to be retained. Some surgeons feel the retention of the posterior cruciate ligament dictates the need for absolute ligament balancing beyond what may be possible in the reconstructed knee.

Procedural considerations. The patient is placed in the supine position. A tourniquet is applied to the upper thigh. The surgical prep is completed.

A soft tissue set and large bone set are required, plus the following:

Total knee instruments, trials, and implants	Power drill and oscillating saw
Polymethyl methacrylate and cement supplies	Pulse lavage with 3000 ml normal saline solution

Operative procedure—Miller-Galante total knee replacement (Fig. 21-103)

1. An anterior longitudinal incision is made over the knee.
2. The capsule is entered anteromedially, and the patellar ligament is elevated.
3. With exposure established, the joint is inspected, osteophytes are removed, and the patella is everted.
4. Medial and lateral tibial plateaus are now presented; with a portion of the infrapatellar fat pad excised and the tibia subluxed, the plateau surfaces can be visualized.
5. The knee is flexed to 90 degrees, a hole is drilled into the distal femoral shaft from the intercondylar notch, and the femoral intramedullary alignment guide is inserted. This is positioned on the femur so equal amounts of posterior condyle are showing.
6. The anterior femoral cutting guide is attached to the intramedullary guide to allow the tip to touch the an-

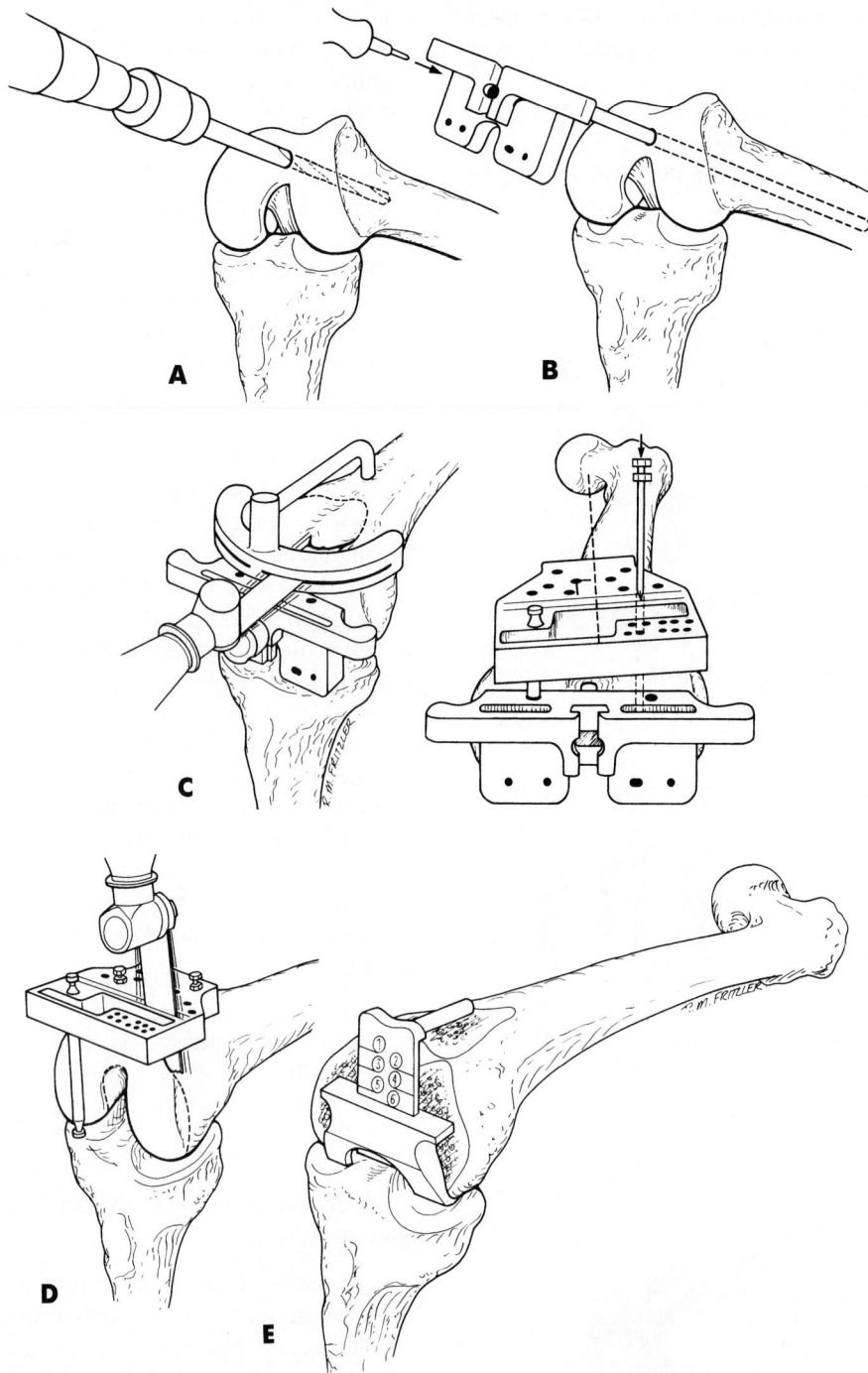

FIG. 21-103 **A,** MG II total knee implant, instrumentation, and procedure. **A,** Following exposure of the intercondylar notch, an 8 mm hole is drilled in the center of the distal femur. **B,** The femoral intramedullary alignment guide is inserted and passed up the medullary canal. **C,** Correct rotational alignment is maintained; the anterior femoral cutting guide is attached to the femoral intramedullary alignment guide. **D,** Femoral cuts are completed. **E,** The anteroposterior measuring guide is placed flat on the cut surface and femoral component size determined. **F,** Femoral holes are drilled and pegs inserted. **G,** Final femoral cuts are completed. **H,** The tibial cutting guide is selected and positioned, and an oscillating saw is used to resect the tibia. **I,** The patella is grasped with the patellar saw guide and the reciprocating saw is used to cut the patella. Following preparation of bony surface, a trial reduction is completed and component fit determined; if the implants are to be fixed with polymethylmethacrylate, surfaces are cleansed with pulsatile lavage; the tibial fixation plate is placed, followed by the femoral and patellar components.

Courtesy Zimmer, Inc., Warsaw, Ind.

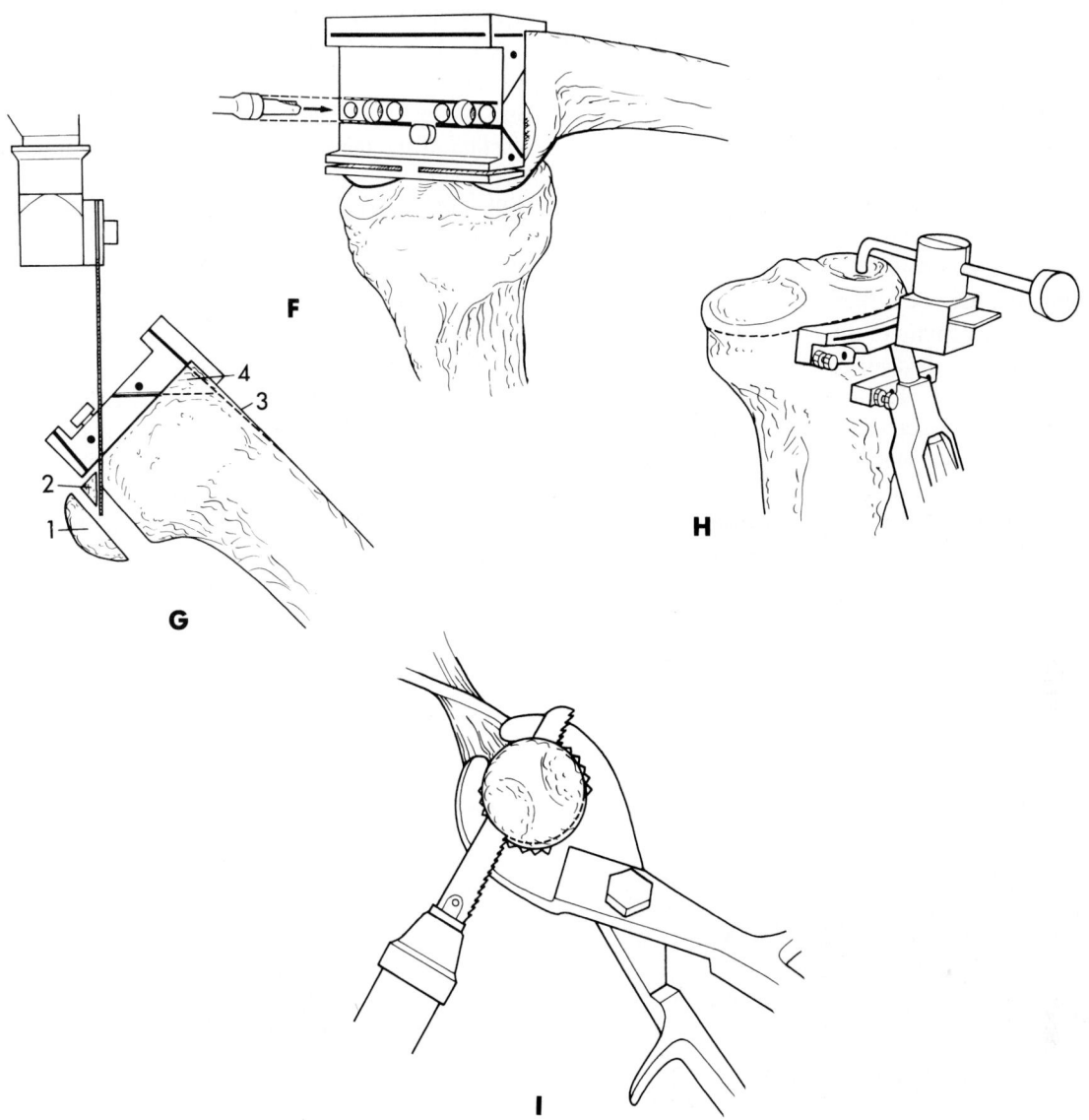

F

G

4
3

2

1

H

I

FIG. 21-103   For legend, see opposite page.

terior cortex just proximal to the condyle. The anterior femoral condyle cut is completed through the guide.

7. The distal cutting guide is attached to the intramedullary guide, the distal guide is pinned to the bone, the intramedullary guide is removed, and the distal femoral cut is completed.

8. The cutting guide is removed and the anterioposterior measuring device placed on the distal femoral cut. The femoral size is indicated on the measuring device. This provides the size of the required implant plus the size of the finishing guide.

9. The corresponding finishing guide is pinned on the distal femur, and the following cuts are made through the slots on the guide: (a) posterior condyle, (b) posterior chamber, (c) anterior condyle, and (d) anterior chamber. This fashions the distal femur for the femoral component. Attention is now turned to tibial preparation.

10. The tibial alignment guide is positioned with the distal most part over the center of the ankle and the guide parallel to the shaft of the tibia. The top of the guide is placed against the proximal bone and pinned through the pinning platform to the tibial tubercle.

11. Using the tibial depth resection guide, the amount of tibial surface to be cut is determined. The proximal tibial cut is completed using the oscillating saw through the cutting slots. Care must be taken to not transect the posterior cruciate if a sparing implant is to be used.

12. The patella is grasped with the patellar saw guide and the patella cut flat leaving adequate thickness. An anchoring hole is drilled in the center of the cut surface of the patella using the patellar drill guide.

13. Trial implants are inserted and reduction achieved. Various thicknesses of tibial surfaces can be tried until stability is demonstrated. The thickest component with

full flexion and extension should be used. Range of motion and ligament stability are checked and appropriate soft tissue releases are done if the knee is disproportionately tight.

14. The provisional tibial fixation plate that corresponds with the selected implant is pinned to the resected tibial surface. The fixation holes are drilled and a holding peg inserted. These will be the cement anchors for the actual tibial component.

15. The tourniquet may be released for reperfusion while preparing for cementing of the prosthesis.

16. Using the pulsatile lavage, surfaces are cleaned and bony debris removed. The tourniquet is reinflated.

17. The tibial plate is cemented onto the surface, followed by the femoral component. A tibial surface trial or actual implant is placed on top of the tibial plate. The leg is brought into full extension to maintain compression on both components. The patellar component is simultaneously cemented and held in place with the patellar clamp.

18. After the cement has hardened, a final inspection and range of motion are performed before irrigating and closing the wound.

19. The wound is dressed with bulky gauze and elastic bandages. The patient is placed on a CPM (see Fig. 21-25).

Total shoulder arthroplasty

Prosthetic replacement of the shoulder joint may be necessitated by traumatic injury or degenerative arthritis disease. The procedure may be a hemiarthroplasty with reconstruction of the humeral side, or total with replacement of the humeral head and glenoid (Fig. 21-104).

Shoulder motion is difficult to restore; therefore the need for rehabilitation is vital. A prosthetic implant does not solely ensure return of function, but will offer the anatomy to support exercise for restored function.

Procedural considerations. The patient is placed in a 30-degree, semisitting position with the arm on a padded armboard and draped free and the shoulder hanging slightly off the OR table to allow movement through the entire range of motion. The head is supported to avoid neck extension. A pad is placed beneath the scapula. Precautions and practice related to total joint implantation must be observed to prevent an infected joint, which can be catastrophic. When implanting a prosthesis, particularly with cement, it is imperative that all supplies be available and in the room. Inventory must be checked for a complete range of implant sizes.

A soft tissue set and large bone set are required, plus the following:

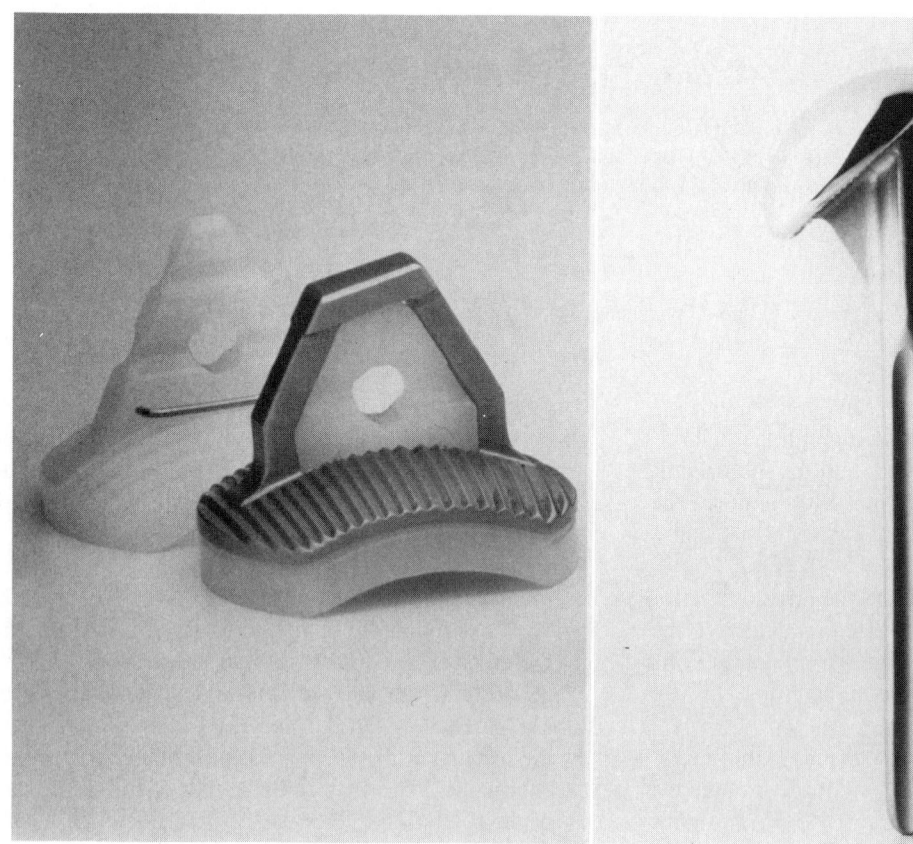
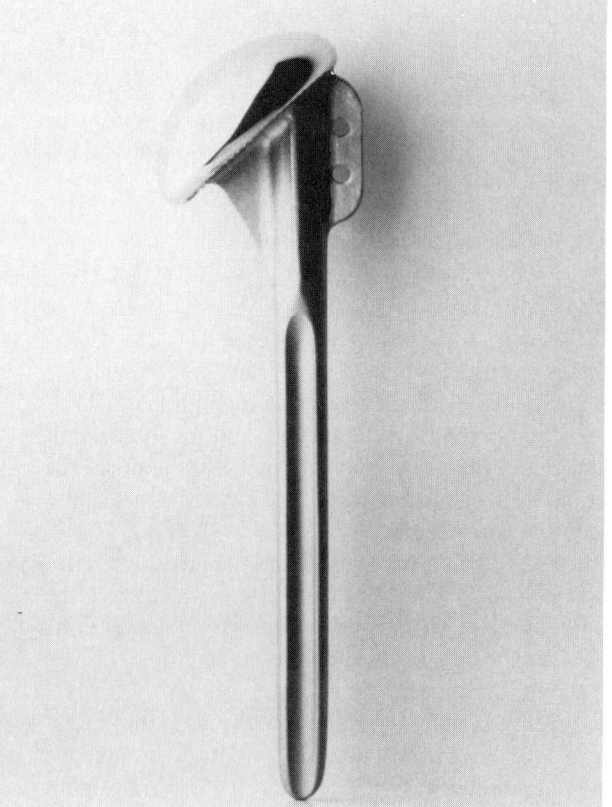

FIG. 21-104   Neer shoulder prosthesis.
Courtesy 3M Orthopedic Products, St. Paul, Minn.

Shoulder instruments
Implants and the associated instrumentation and trials
Curette set, long
Heavy-gauge wire
Power drill, reamer, and saw

Polymethyl methacrylate and cement supplies (see Fig. 21-97)
Pulsatile lavage with 3000 ml normal saline solution (see Fig. 21-98)

Operative procedure—Neer total shoulder arthroplasty (Fig. 21-105)

1. A 16-cm incision is made from the midacromion distally along the deltopectoral groove.
2. The celphalic vein is identified and the deltopectoral groove opened and retracted.
3. The deltoid attachment may be removed if the patient is large or muscular, which may affect rehabilitation.
4. The long head of the biceps is identified as the landmark between the tuberosities and rotator interval.
5. The subscapularis is elevated from the underlying capsule, divided 2 cm medial to the bicipital groove, and a stay suture placed.
6. The subscapularis is retracted medially with the lesser tuberosity, thereby exposing the joint and associated structures.
7. The capsule is exposed by elevation. An elevator is placed beneath the capsule to protect the axillary nerve. The long head of the biceps is left undisturbed and free in its groove so it will continue to function as a depressor of the head after surgery.
8. After external rotation, the fractured humeral head is removed. The incision site is irrigated to remove blood and clot from the joint.
9. The proximal humeral shaft is examined to select the appropriate size stem, available in a various lengths and diameters.
10. Marginal osteophytes are trimmed.
11. The glenoid is inspected for integrity and sized for a prosthesis if it is to be replaced.
12. A central hole for prosthesis fit is made into the glenoid with a high-speed burr and curette.
13. Stem diameter and length are estimated to check the prosthesis for fit. The largest stem diameter possible is used.
14. With the shaft held forward and upward, the intramedullary canal is located with a long curette. A ¼ -, ⅜ -, or ½-inch drill is selected to correspond to the diameter of the canal; depending on the prosthesis stem length, 5 or 6 inches down the medullary canal is drilled. Final preparation of the shaft is accomplished with the appropriately sized tapered reamer.
15. A heavy-gauge wire (no. 20) or heavy nonabsorbable suture is passed through holes that have been drilled on the tuberosities. Length of the rotator cuff is checked by pulling the tuberosities distal to the collar of the prosthesis.

16. Neck length and stability of the joint are determined before final impaction of the prosthesis.
17. A check for 35- to 40-degree retroversion is done by palpating the epicondyles at the elbow.
18. The implant is seated on the calcar with a driver and mallet, with its articular surface protected with a moist sponge. Just before final seating, further trimming of high spots with a osteotome or high-speed burr may be required. PMMA is used except in young patients, in whom a firm press-fit can be achieved.
19. Wires or sutures are passed through the holes in the neck of the prosthesis, reducing the tuberosities beneath the collar, and secured. If wires are used, they are buried in drill holes in the bone.
20. The shoulder is reduced. The interval of the rotator cuff is closed and the biceps tendon reattached if previously detached.
21. The joint is irrigated as each compartment and layer are closed.
22. A closed drainage system is inserted between cuff and deltoid, avoiding contact of the drainage tubes with the axillary artery. Routine closure is accomplished.
23. ABD pads are placed between the body and the arm. A shoulder immobilizer is used. Passive range of motion machines may be used in patients prone to adhesion or contracture. Pendulum and gentle exercise are permitted at 10 days.

Total elbow arthroplasty (Fig. 21-106)

Total elbow replacement is indicated in patients with traumatic lesions or excessive bone loss from rheumatic or degenerative arthritis, resulting in elbow instability and pain. The primary indications are pain, instability, and bilateral elbow ankylosis. Arthroplasty of the elbow is not as prevalent as arthroplasty of the shoulder, knee, or hip. The design of implants and methods of fixation for postoperative stability have presented challenges that have been overcome in arthroplasty of other joints but have remained a challenge in elbow arthroplasty. Postoperative stability of the elbow implant depends largely on the soft tissues surrounding the joint. There are devices that provide more constraint for the patient with significant soft tissue laxity or loss of bone stock. The Coonrad-Morrey, Tri-Axial, and Pritchard-Walker are just a few of the total elbow prostheses available.

The prosthesis may be used with or without PMMA, depending on the quality of the diseases bone and the design of the implant. If PMMA is not employed, bone grafting with local bone that has been resected may be used to help seat the ulnar component snugly and achieve adequate bony contact against the porous coating of the metal ulnar component. Patients with degenerative arthritis generally have better results than those with traumatic injury following elbow arthroplasty.

Infection in the presence of implants and other foreign bodies can be disastrous. Preventive measures such as pro-

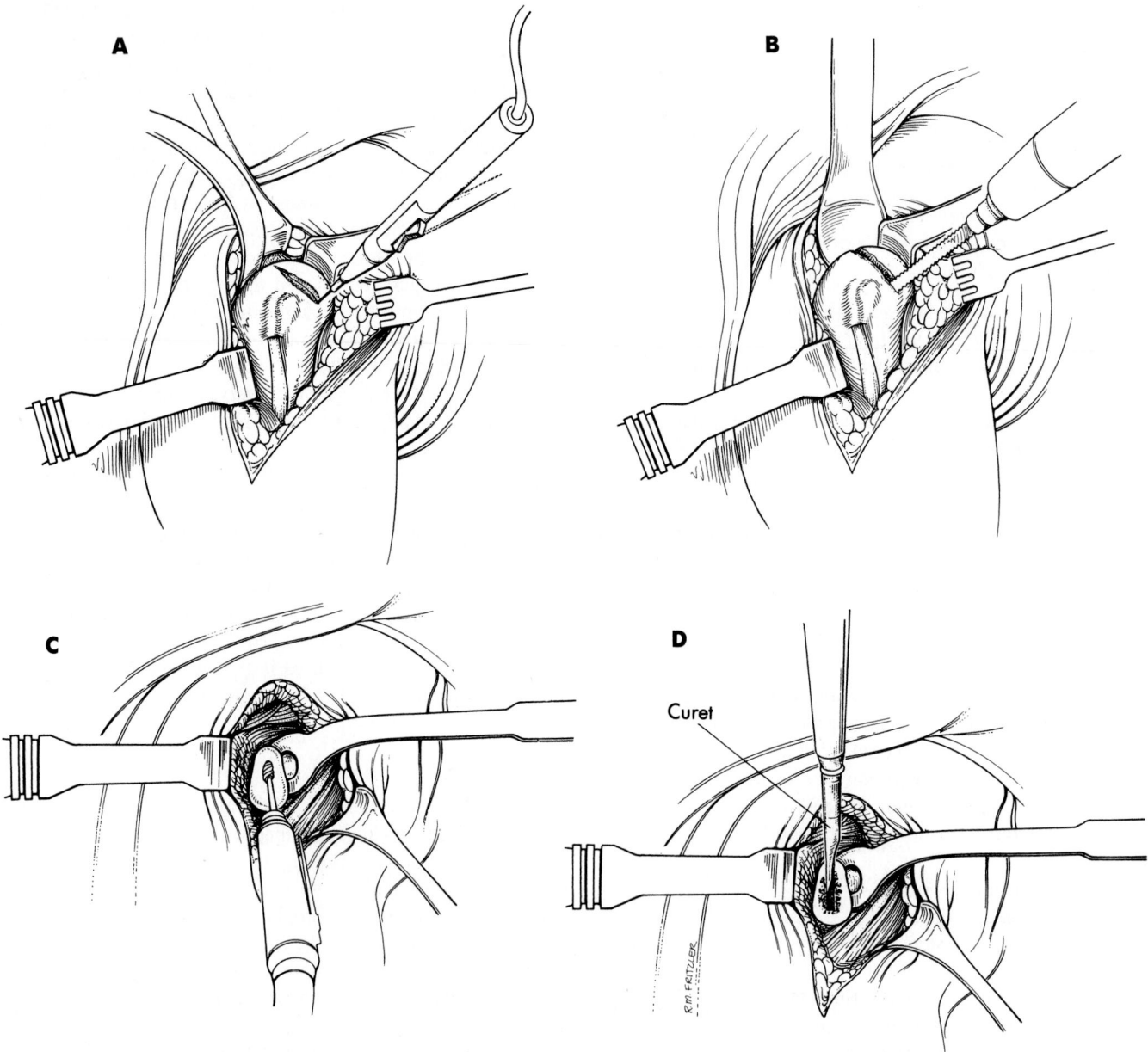

FIG. 21-105 Total shoulder arthroplasty. **A,** The patient is positioned and a deltipectoral incision is made, the capsule released. **B,** Humeral head is removed with reciprocating saw. **C,** Following exposure of the glenoid, a fenestration for the glenoid component is made. **D,** The glenoid bow curetted.

phylactic antibiotics, antibiotic irrigant, and laminar airflow might be used when available.

Procedural considerations. In the operative procedure the patient is in the supine or semi-Fowler position with the arm over the chest. A tourniquet is applied and can be inflated if needed. The arm is prepped from shoulder to fingers and draped.

A soft tissue set and small bone set are required, plus the following:

Total elbow implants and instruments
Power drill, saw, and burr
Awl
Heavy-gauge (16 and 18) wire
Wire tightener
Polymethy methacrylate and cement supplies
Pulsatile irrigation with 3000 ml normal saline solution

Operative procedure (Fig. 21-107)

1. The limb is exsanguinated and the tourniquet inflated to the desired pressure.

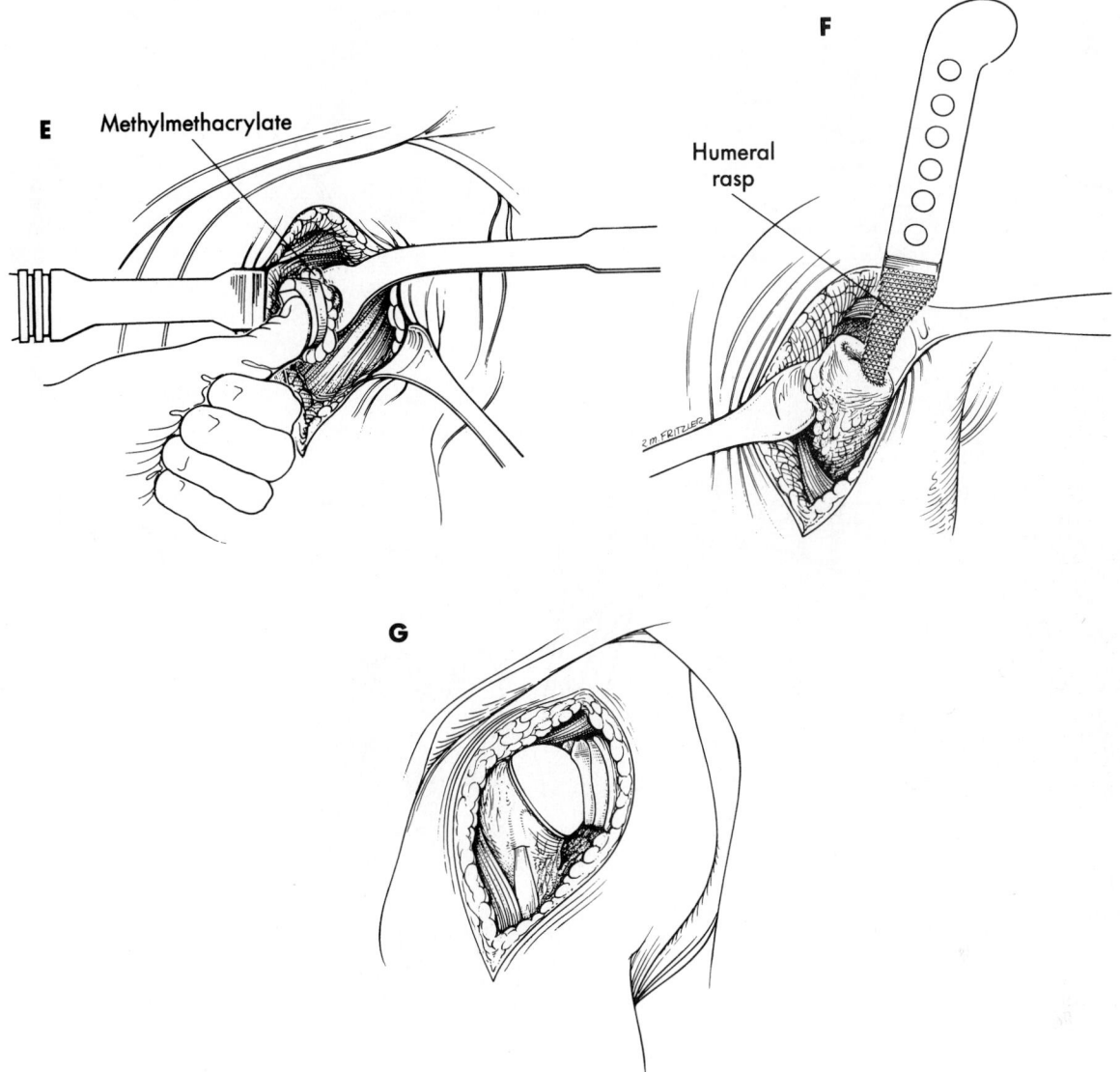

FIG. 21-105, CON'T. **E,** Cancellous bone is evacuated and cement impressed. **F,** Humeral shaft is rasped. **G,** Humeral component is inserted.

Redrawn from Gristina AG, Webb LX: *Proximal humeral and monospherical glenoid replacement: surgical technique,* Rutherford, NJ, 1983, Howmedica, Inc.

2. A midline posterior incision is made, protecting the ulnar nerve during the surgery.

3. The triceps mechanism is elevated in continuity with the periosteum and elbow joint explored.

4. The distal humerus, proximal ulna, and radial head are explored, preserving the collateral ligaments.

5. The midportion of the trochlea is removed to allow access to the distal humerus; the medullary canal is opened with a high-speed burr and the canal entered with a twist hand reamer.

6. The distal humerus is notched with the appropriate cutting guide.

7. A high-speed burr is used to burr through subchondral bone to allow access to the medullary canal of the ulna and serially ream the canal.

8. After the humerus and ulna have been prepared for insertion of the trial prosthesis, the elbow is evaluated for flexion and extension. Bony adjustments are made where necessary.

9. The canals are cleaned of all bone fragments by irrigating with pulsatile antibiotic lavage.

10. The canal is dried before implant insertion and preparation checked before mixing cement, ensuring the correct size component is available.

11. The cement is inserted into the canals followed by the prosthesis. Flexion and extension of the elbow are avoided until the cement has hardened.

12. Any bone graft that may be required is secured with wire or pins.

13. The tourniquet is deflated and hemostasis obtained.

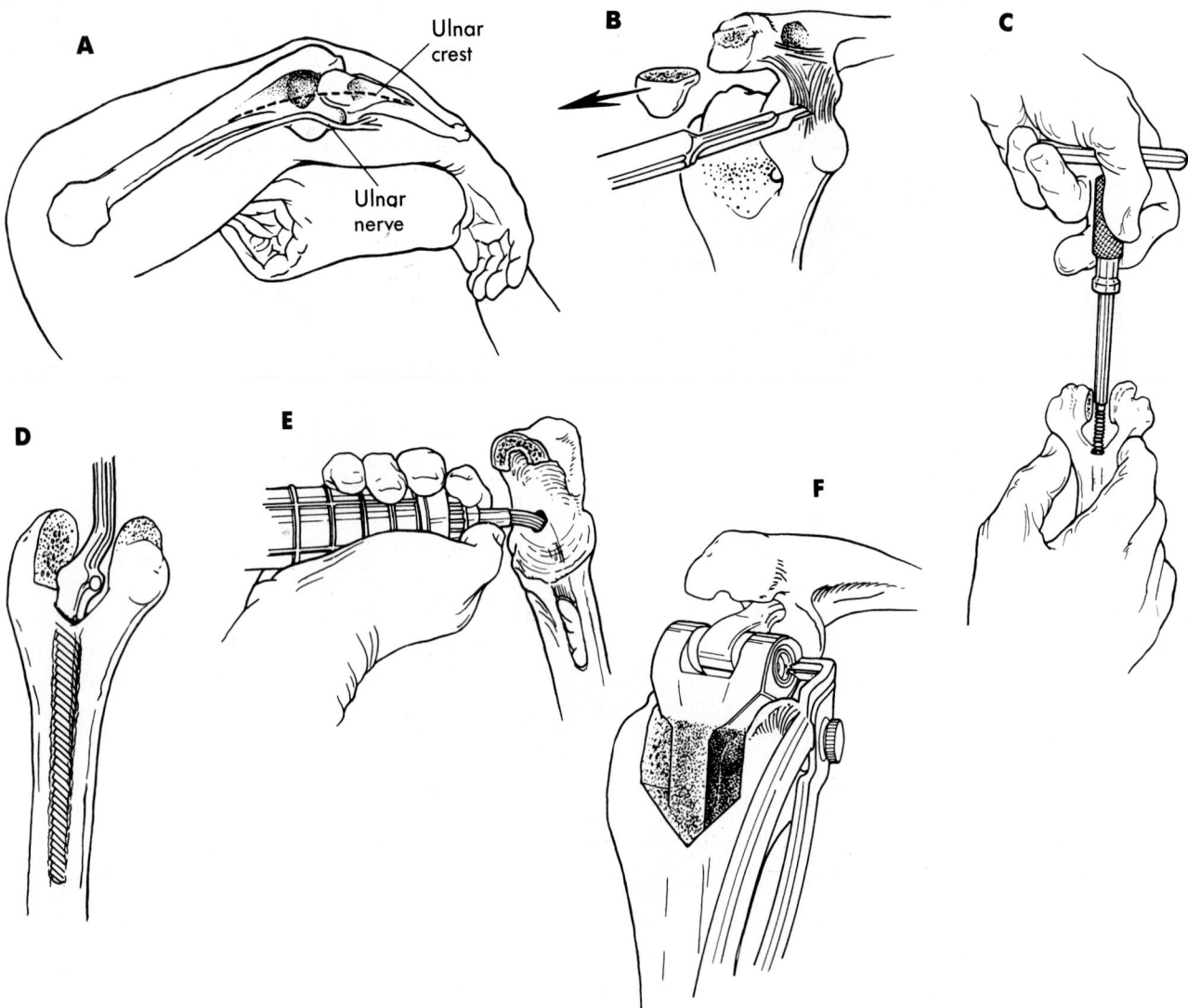

FIG. 21-106   Total elbow arthroplasty. **A,** The arm is draped free and the incision made. **B,** The tip of the olecranon is excised with an oscillating saw. **C,** The canal is identified with a Bur and the canal opened with a twist reamer. **D,** The capitellum is measured and cut. **E,** The medullary canal is cleaned, dried, and bone cement inserted. **F,** Ulnar prosthesis is inserted followed by cementing and inserting the humeral components.

Redrawn from Zimmer, Inc., Warsaw, Ind.

14. The triceps mechanism is repaired. The incision site is irrigated and closed. A drain may be inserted.
15. A long arm posterior splint is applied with the elbow at 90 degrees.

Total ankle joint replacement

Long-term results for total ankle arthroplasty, especially in the young, are extremely poor. The procedure is reserved for older or more sedentary patients, especially those with subtalar or midtarsal arthritis. Ankle arthrodesis should be considered first in joint reconstruction. Indications for total ankle arthroplasty include (1) failed arthrodesis, (2) bilateral ankle arthritis when arthrodesis has already been performed on one ankle, (3) after talectomy owing to avascu-

lar necrosis, and (4) revision of a previous arthroplasty. Total ankle replacement prostheses are made of high-density polyethylene and metal components.

Procedural considerations. The patient is positioned supine with the tourniquet placed. The leg is prepped and draped.

A soft tissue set and small bone set are required, plus the following:

Power drill and saw
Total ankle joint replacement instrumentation with implants
Polymethyl methacrylate and cement supplies
Pulse lavage with 3000 ml normal saline solution

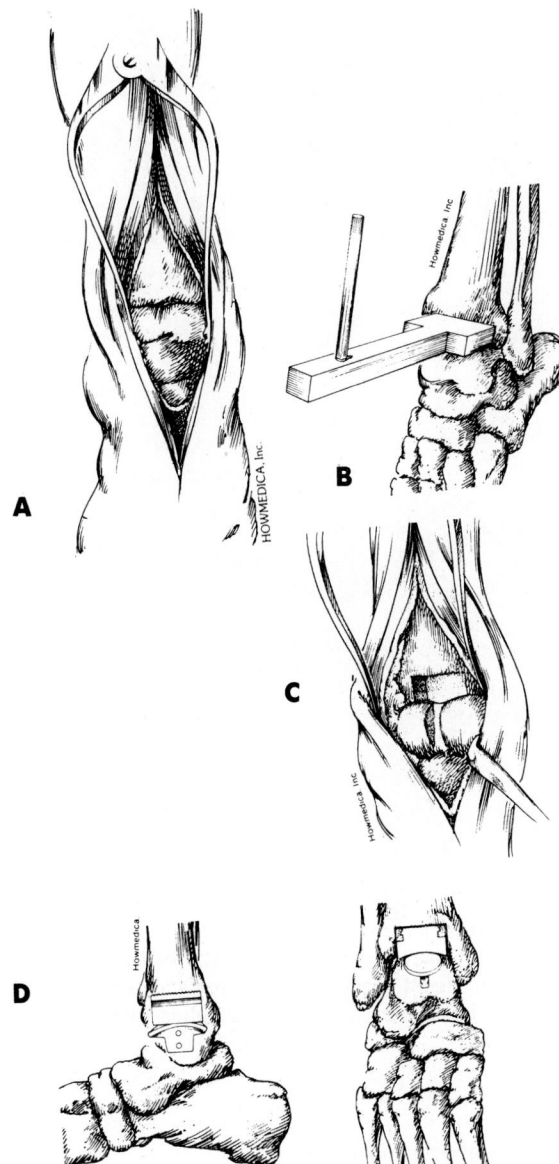

FIG. 21-107   Total ankle arthroplasty. **A,** An anterior incision is made and the tibiotalar joint and talus dome are exposed. **B,** The sizing template is used to mark the tibia. **C,** An air drill is used to create a defect and anchoring holes prepared. **D,** Trial reduction is completed and talar and tibial components cemented in place.

Courtesy Howmedica, Inc., Rutherford, N.J.

Operative procedure (Fig. 21-107)

1. An anterior incision is made over the ankle joint.
2. Exposure of the tibiotalar joint and talus dome is achieved using dissection.
3. Once the center of the talus is identified and marked, a sizing template is used to mark the tibia.
4. A 1-inch wide by ⅜-inch deep defect is made using the air drill. Anchoring holes can be made in the tibia. The template is positioned in the defect while the foot is distracted.

5. The talus is marked and a ½-inch deep by 3/16-inch groove is made with a reciprocating saw to accommodate the talar component.
6. A trial fit is carried out to ensure that the talar unit is in the center of the talus and that the tibial unit is parallel to the plane of the floor, both centered over the dome of the talus.
7. Once trial reduction is complete, the talar and tibial components are cemented into place.
8. The ankle joint is irrigated and closed, a drain inserted, and a posterior splint applied.

Metacarpal arthroplasty

Metacarpal joint replacement is most often performed in patients who have pain or a disabling deformity associated with rheumatoid or degenerative arthritis of the metacarpophalangeal or interphalangeal joints. The results of rheumatoid reconstructive surgery are generally good, and pain can be eliminated and joint alignment and joint stability restored in the majority of patients. The greatest problems following an operation are weakness of grasp and pinch and progression of the disease in adjacent joints.

Procedural considerations. The patient is placed in the supine position with the arm extended on a hand table. A tourniquet is applied, and the entire extremity is prepped and draped.

A hand set, the Swanson set, and Swanson trials and implants are required in addition to the following:

High-speed burr   Swanson burrs

Operative procedure

1. Incisions are made on the dorsum of the appropriate fingers.
2. The proximal and distal portions of the joints are excised, and intramedullary canals are reamed.
3. Trial implants are inserted to facilitate correct fit of the prosthesis.
4. Once the appropriate sized implant is determined, it is positioned into the canal, and appropriate tendon and ligament repairs are made to improve stability.
5. The joint is irrigated and closed, and a bulky dressing is applied.
6. A short arm posterior splint is applied for immobilization.

Metatarsal arthroplasty

Silastic implantation is indicated in the treatment of deformities associated with rheumatoid arthritis, hallux valgus, hallux rigidus, and a painful or unstable joint.

Procedural considerations. The patient is placed in the supine position. A tourniquet is applied, and the entire extremity is prepped and draped.

A small bone set is required, plus the following:

Swanson instruments and implants (Figs. 21-108 and 21-109)   Power wire driver, microsagittal saw, and bur

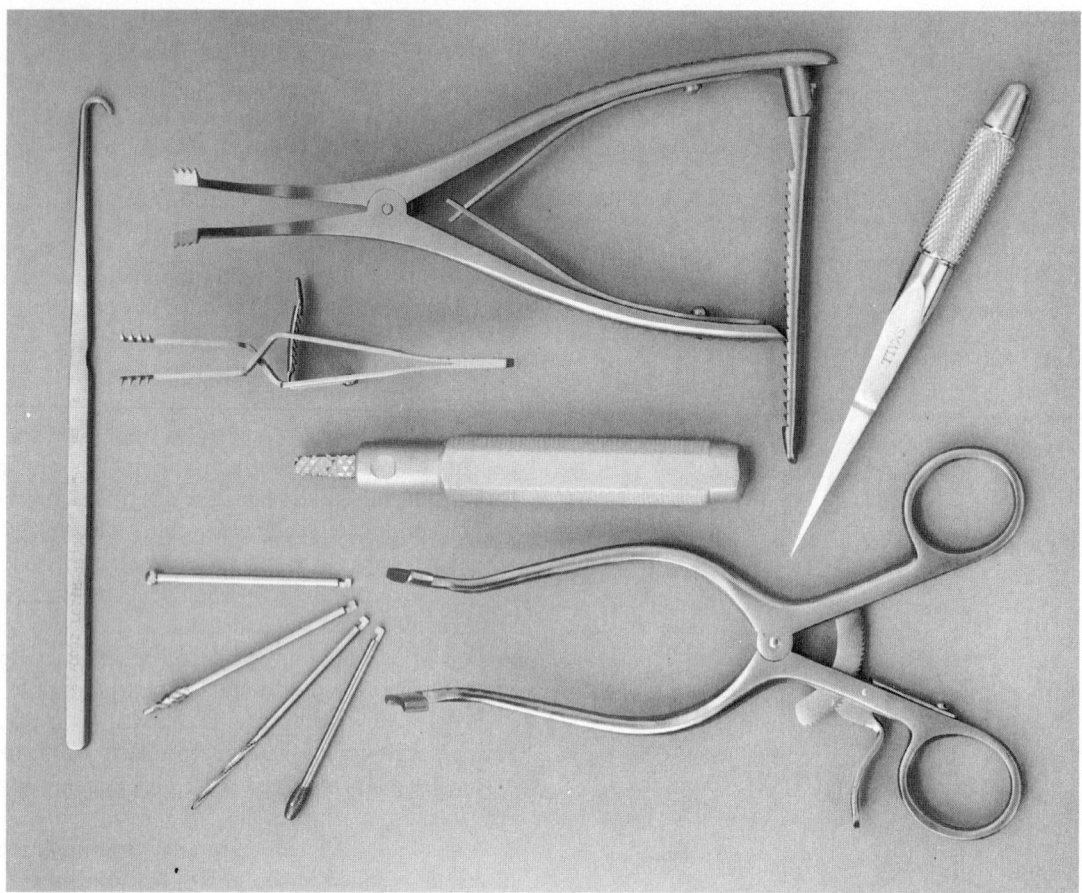

FIG. 21-108　Swanson instrumentation: 1. tendon hook 2. (from top) Inge Retractor 3. Holzheimer retractor 4. rasp. 5. burrs 6. Mertlaner swanson retractor 7. small intramedullary broach ; 2. Swanson awls (scaphoid/lunate: large, small, pointed end); 3. Swanson mallet, 4. Langenbeck (narrow) subperiosteal elevator: 5. Langenbeck (wide) subperiosteal elevator; 6. Freer-Swanson (narrow) ganglion knife; 7. Swanson elevator; 8. tendon hooks, large, medium, small.

Courtesy Dow Corning Wright, Arlington Tenn.

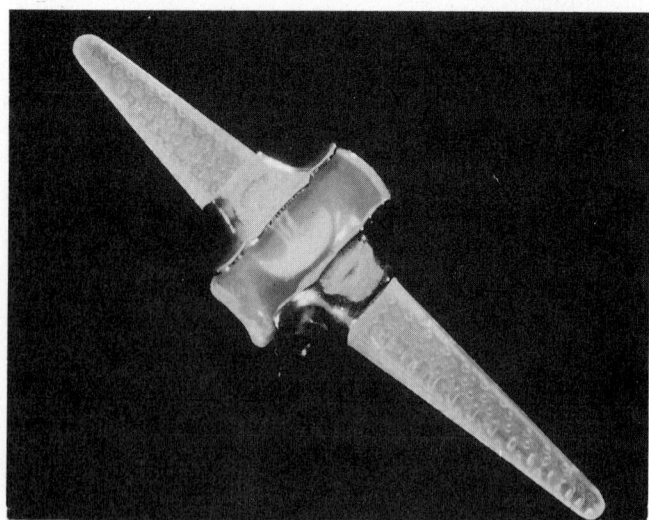

FIG. 21-109　Silastic implant for finger joint.

Courtesy Dow Corning Wright, Arlington, Tenn.

Operative procedure

1. The incision is made over the appropriate joints.
2. Resection of the proximal phalanx with removal of exostosis of the metatarsal head is carried out.
3. The medullary canal is reamed and trial implants are fitted.
4. The appropriate size metatarsal implant is determined and seated.
5. The wound is irrigated and closed.
6. A bulky compression dressing and orthopedic show are applied for early ambulation.

Congenital dislocation of the hip

A congenital dislocation of the hip is an abnormal development present at birth. It is a lateral or upward dislocation of the femoral head from the acetabulum. When alignment is disrupted, soft tissue and bony changes result in contractures of the hip muscles, a shallow acetabulum, and possibly a deformed femoral head. Treatment of congenital dislocation of the hip varies depending on the age

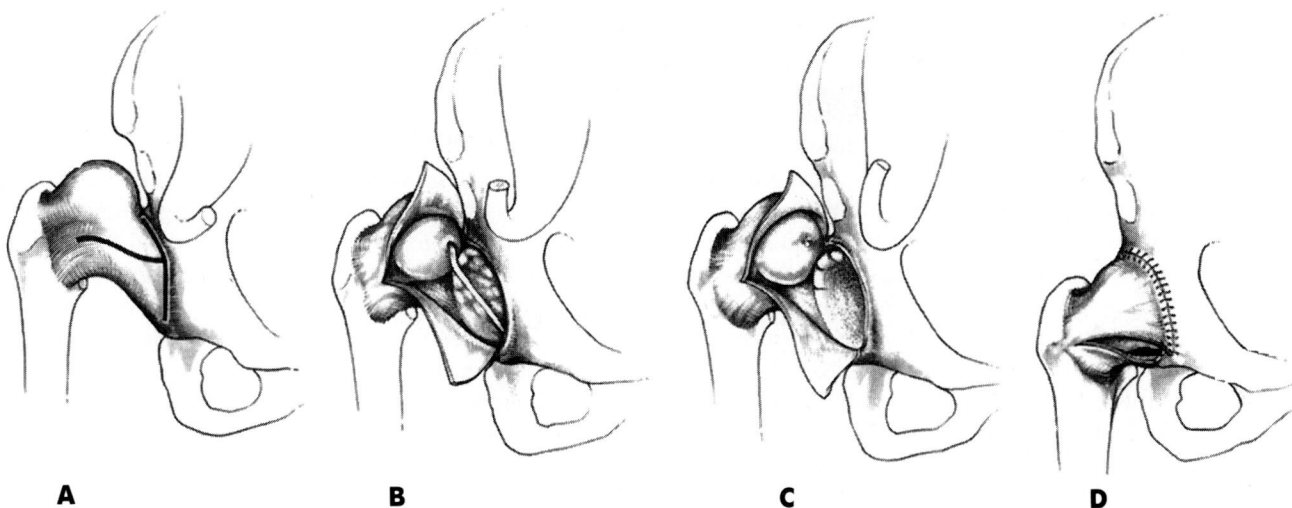

FIG. 21-110 Repair of congenital hip disorder using open reduction. **A,** T-shaped incision of capsule. **B,** Capsulotomy of the hip and locating the true acetabulum. **C,** Removal of tissue from the depth of the acetabulum and **D,** Capsulorrhaphy.

of the patient and the stability of the hip. Treatment modalities include application of a Pavlik harness, closed reduction and spica cast application, and surgical correction. Surgery involves soft tissue release and/or acetabular and femoral procedures. Many of the total hip systems have congenital dysplastic hip (CDH) implants, which allow joint reconstruction.

Procedural considerations. The patient is usually in the lateral position for these procedures. An anterior incision is usually made for open reduction, whereas a lateral incision is made for the subtrochanteric osteotomy. The surgeon's preference dictates the incision for an innominate osteotomy.

A soft tissue set and bone set (appropriate for age) are required plus the following instruments:

Total hip set	Power reamer, driver,
CDH implants and in-	and saw
strumentation	Steinman pins

Operative procedures
CDH total joint replacement. Total joint replacement is carried out in similar fashion to the previously mentioned procedures. The implant and technique do require specific technique.

Open reduction (Fig. 21-110)

1. The hip joint is opened, and the soft tissue in the acetabulum is excised.
2. The femoral head can then be reduced into the acetabulum and held by suturing the capsule.

Derotational osteotomy. A derotational osteotomy is performed when the head is improperly seated in the acetabulum.

1. The femur is placed in internal rotation and divided.
2. The distal fragment is rotated externally to place the knee and foot straight ahead.

3. If the patient is a young child, the osteotomy is frequently performed in the supracondylar region, and the patient is immobilized in a plaster spica cast.
4. For an older child, the osteotomy is frequently done in the subtrochanteric region, and the osteotomized fragments are held with an osteotomy blade plate or an intermediate compression screw. Immobilization may not be necessary.

Innominate osteotomy

1. A complete division of the wing of the ilium is made by an osteotomy from the sciatic notch to the anterior margin of the ilium, superior to the acetabulum.
2. The ilium is then wedged down to increase the depth of the acetabulum by opening the osteotomy site and inserting a bone graft.
3. The bone graft is held in place with two heavy wires.
4. Heavy suture is used to close the capsule, and a spica cast is applied for postoperative immobilization.

ARTHROSCOPY

Progress and development of arthroscopy and arthroscopic procedures has evolved, changing the approach, diagnosis, and treatment to many ailments of the joints. Arthroscopic techniques require skill and accomplishment in identifying three dimensional and spatial relationships and, most important, a sense of one's own limitation when it comes to arthroscopic versus open procedures.

The advantages of arthroscopic surgery surpass the disadvantages. Among the advantages are (1) decreased recovery and rehabilitation time, (2) smaller incisions, (3) less inflammatory response, (4) less postoperative pain, scar, and extensor disruption, (5) reduced complications, (6) reduced hospital stay and cost, and (7) easier, more rapid surgical procedures.

Disadvantages usually relate to the size and delicacy of the instruments. Maneuverability within a joint may be difficult and produce scuffing and scoring of the articular surfaces. Accomplishment of arthroscopy by the surgeon can be time consuming and the initial outlay expensive. Nursing care changes are also required.

Improvements in lens systems, fiberoptic cables, and miniaturization have made operative arthroscopy a logical extension of diagnostic arthroscopy. Surgical arthroscopy has also been aided with development of numerous second puncture instruments and devices to repair and excise deficits. There is a multitude of motorized shaving and abrader systems. Irrigation systems provide regulated distention of the knee joint by infusing normal saline or Ringer's lactate. These systems may function by gravity flow or are mechanized with microprocessors built in to monitor joint pressures and adjust accordingly. Lasers and electrosurgical units can be used in tandem with arthroscopic equipment. Integrated video systems can record and store still and video images on film, tape, or floppy disk for education and documentation.

Arthroscopy is commonly performed on the knee, shoulder, and wrist. It is used less often in the elbow, hip, and ankle. Many corrective procedures that previously required an arthrotomy or other open procedures can be completed with the assistance of the arthroscope.

Arthroscopic equipment has certain requirements for care and handling. Fiberoptics, lenses, and cameras are heat sensitive, requiring consideration for sterilization. Temperatures and moisture generated by steam autoclaves can damage materials used in video equipment or deteriorate the sealant, making the moisture accessible to the lens. Alternatives to steam sterilization of this equipment are ethylene oxide, cold sterilization, and disinfection. Each requires consideration of patient care options for consistency. Strict guidelines and aseptic technique must be followed when utilizing this method of disinfection. Equipment must be soaked according to the manufacturer's instruction, followed by complete rinsing and immersion in sterile water to prevent chemical burns (AORN, 1994). Cold water sterilizing machines can also be used to sterilize heat-sensitive equipment. The cycle time is approximately 30 minutes, and they use proven bactericidal and sporicidal detergents, allowing rapid turnover in comparison to the other methods. Another measure of protection is the use of sterile telescoping drapes for items such as camera cables and power cords.

Scopes, lenses, and fiberoptic cords used in the surgery should be handled carefully, and cords should never be kinked or twisted. When mishandled, gradual deterioration and fiber breakage occurs in the cables and light cannot be transmitted. When stored, the cords should be loosely coiled or hung.

Two types of arthroscopy may be performed: (1) *diagnostic arthroscopy* is for patients whose diagnosis cannot be determined by history or physical examination or whose arthrogram findings are insufficient to warrant surgical exploration; diagnostic arthroscopy may be performed before an anticipated arthrotomy, and surgical treatment may be modified on the basis of the findings of the arthroscopic examination; (2) *operative arthroscopy* is for patients presenting with an intraarticular abnormality or ligamentous injury.

Arthroscopy of the knee

The knee is the joint in which arthroscopy lends itself to the greatest number of diagnostic and surgical procedures. Arthroscopic surgery of the knee is indicated for diagnostic viewing, synovial biopsies, removal of loose bodies, resection of plicae, shaving of the patella, synovectomy, partial meniscectomy, meniscus repair, and anterior cruciate ligament reconstruction.

Arthroscopy may be diagnostic and be the initial step for an arthrotomy. Anesthesia for knee arthroscopy may be general, spinal, or local. Tourniquets are often placed on the thigh but are inflated only if bleeding obscures the view. If there are no contraindications, an epinephrine solution may be injected at the portal sites, or diluted into the distention fluid.

Procedural considerations. The patient is placed in the supine position on a standard OR bed. The foot end of the bed may be flexed 90 degrees. A lateral post can be attached to the operating room table at the level of the midthigh. This post can provide a method of countertraction to open the medial side of the joint, providing better visualization of structures (Fig. 21-111). The leg is prepped. The entire extremity is draped to allow complete range of motion and manipulation of the knee joint. The procedure requires specialized equipment for fluid collection and personnel protection.

Instruments and equipment needed for an arthroscopy include the following:

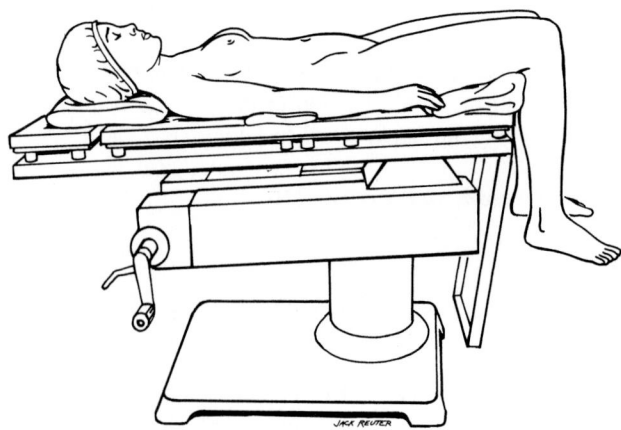

FIG. 21-111   Positioning for a knee arthroscopy to enhance visualization.

From Gregory B: *Perioperative Nursing Series: Orthopaedic Surgery,* St. Louis, 1994, Mosby.

Diagnostic arthroscopy

Arthroscopy instrumentation (Fig. 21-112)
Arthroscopes, 30 and 70 degrees (Fig. 21-113)
Inflow and egress cannulas (Fig. 21-114)
Video with camera, light source, and peripheral equipment (Fig. 21-115)
Arthroscopy pump and tubing (Fig. 21-116)
3000 ml normal saline or Ringer's lactate × 6
60-ml Luer-Lok syringes

10-ml control syringe
1½-inch 21-gauge needle
Spinal needle

Operative arthroscopy

Add the following:
Second puncture instruments
Arthroscopic anterior cruciate reconstruction guides
Meniscal repair set for meniscal repair
Arthroscopic powered shavers and abraders (Fig. 21-117)

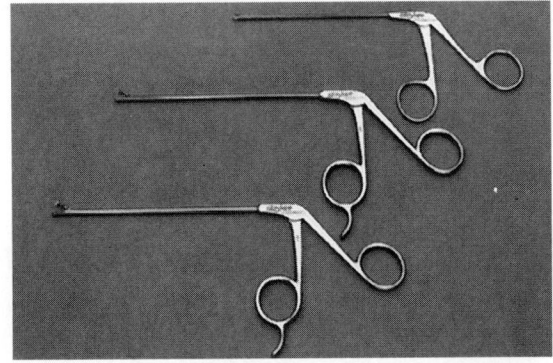

FIG. 21-112 Arthroscopy instrumentation.
Courtesy Stryker Endoscopy, Kalamazoo, Mich.

Operative procedures
Diagnostic arthroscopy

1. The anteromedial and anterolateral joint lines and portal positions are marked with a skin marker.
2. The skin areas for portal placement are infiltrated with 1% lidocaine with 1:200,000 epinephrine. If the knee has an effusion, this is aspirated with a 16-gauge needle on a 60-ml syringe, followed by a small amount of distending fluid.
3. After a small stab incision with a no. 11 knife blade, the irrigation cannula and trocar are inserted into the lateral suprapatellar pouch near the superior pole of the patella. lactated Ringer's or normal saline solution is connected to the cannula, and the joint is distended using gravity or a pressure-sensitive arthroscopy pump.
4. A stab incision is then made anterolaterally or anteromedially 2 to 3 mm above the tibial plateau or patellar tendon at the joint line. A sharp trocar and sheath are inserted through the stab wound and just through the capsule.
5. A blunt trocar is used to pass the sheath into the knee joint. The trocar is removed and a 30-degree scope is inserted into the sheath. The light source and video camera are connected to the scope.
6. The inflow may remain in the suprapatellar area and the egress tubing connected to the arthroscope, or the position may be reversed.
7. A spinal needle can be introduced under direct vision to determine the best angle for an opposite portal for insertion of probes and operative instruments. The cruciates and menisci are probed to determine integrity and tears.

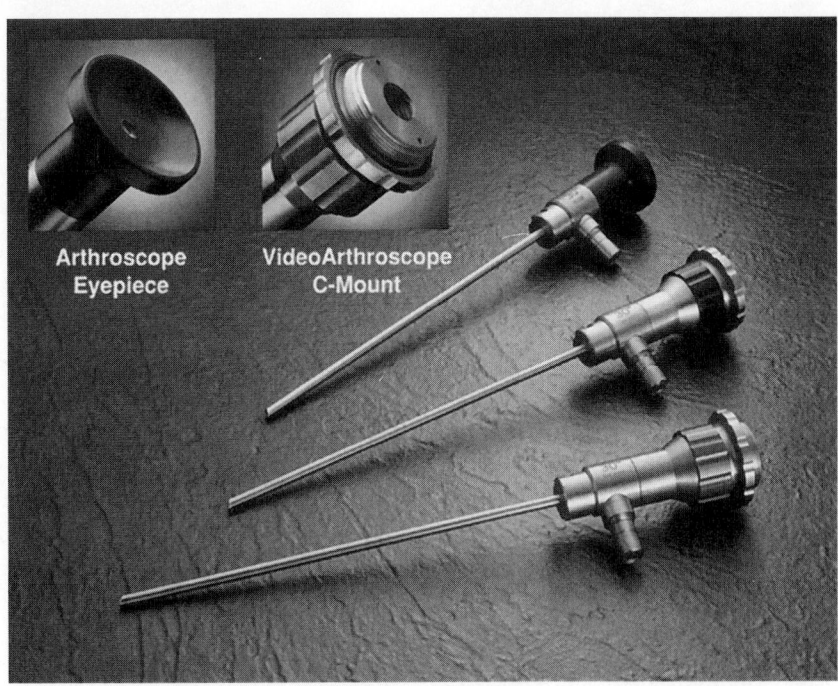

FIG. 21-113 Arthroscopes, 30 and 70 degrees with camera attachments.
Courtesy Smith + Nephew Dyonics, Andover, Mass.

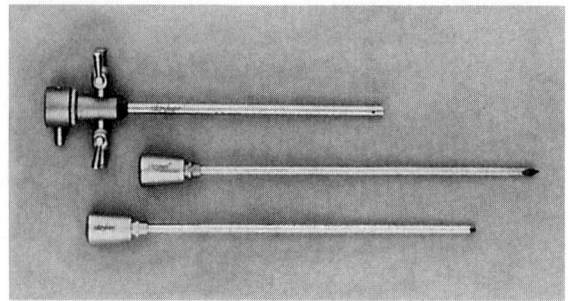

FIG. 21-114   Cannulas.
Courtesy Stryker Endoscopy, Kalamazoo, Mich.

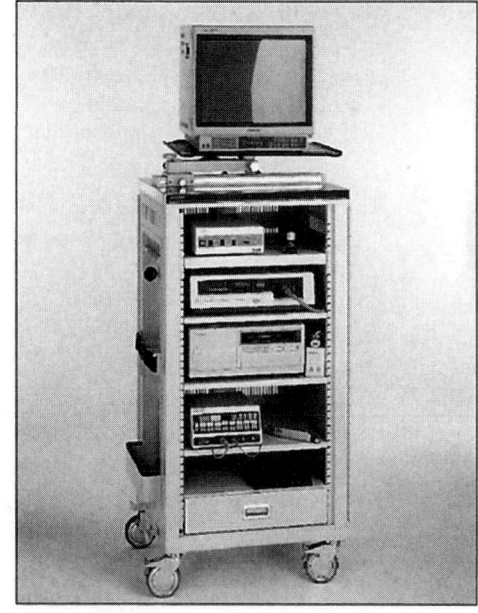

FIG. 21-115   Arthroscopy tower with video monitor, light source, camera and shaver system.
Courtesy Stryker Endoscopy, Kalamazoo, Mich.

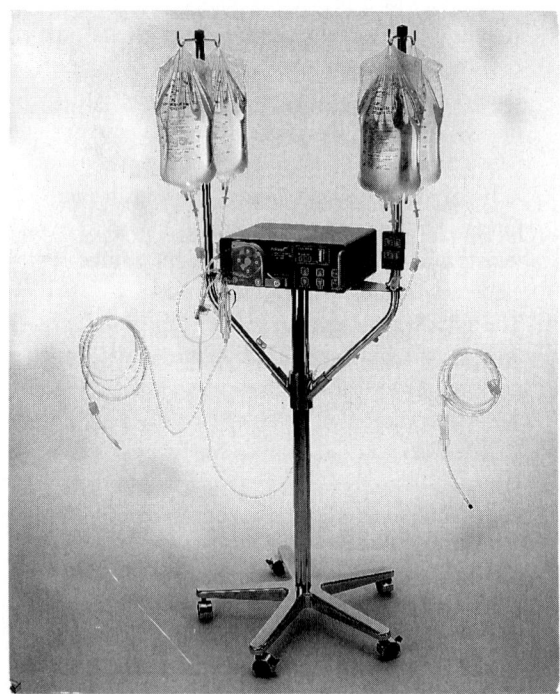

FIG. 21-116   Arthroscopy pump.
Courtesy Arthrex Inc, Naples, Fl.

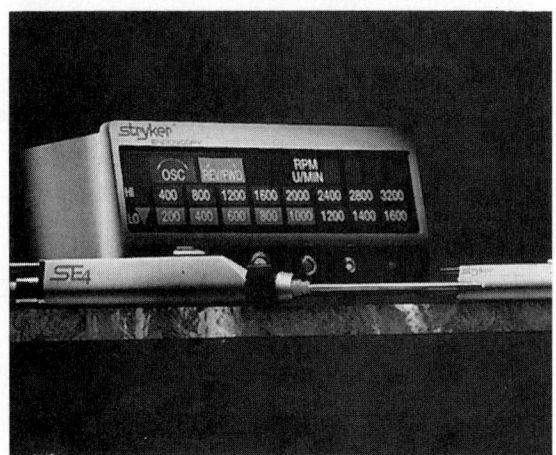

FIG. 21-117   Arthroscopic shavers.
Courtesy Stryker Endoscopy, Kalamazoo, Mich.

8. The scope is moved to the opposite portal to allow a complete examination to be performed.
9. The joint is irrigated periodically and at the end of the procedure to maintain good visualization and clear the joint of blood and tissue fragments.
10. The portals are closed with nylon or undyed Vicryl suture and ½-inch Steri-Strips.
11. Bupivacaine 0.25% (Marcaine), 30 ml, with epinephrine 1:200,000 may be injected intraarticularly to minimizing bleeding and postoperative pain.
12. Gauze dressing, Webril, and 4-inch and 6-inch elastic bandages are applied.

Operative arthroscopy. The following is a list of some of the arthroscopic operative procedures:

1. Resection of synovial plica
2. Patellar débridement
3. Excision of meniscal tears
4. Partial or total meniscectomy
5. Lateral retinacular release
6. Removal of loose body
7. Abrasion or drilling of osteochondral defects
8. Synovectomy
9. Treatment of osteochondritis dissecans
10. Meniscal repairs
11. Anterior cruciate ligament reconstruction

Arthroscopic resection and repair of meniscal tear

Menisci are important structures in the knee joint that distribute load across the joint and provide capsular stability. A tear in the meniscus is the most common knee injury requiring arthroscopic surgery (Fig. 21-118). Although both menisci can sustain tears, the medial meniscus is injured much more frequently than the lateral.

Treatment of meniscus tears is aimed at preserving the structures. Some minor tears heal with cast immobilization, but some persist and cause symptoms. In these more severe cases surgical intervention is necessary. A partial or complete meniscectomy may be necessary to alleviate troublesome symptoms such as locking, pain, and swelling. Partial meniscectomy is preferred, leaving a peripheral rim to share load bearing and stabilize the knee. Complete meniscectomy removes all of this loadbearing protection and also reduces knee stability. The goal is to leave an intact, balanced rim.

Arthroscopic meniscal repair is widely accepted as the standard of care. Arthroscopy provides much greater exposure than an arthrotomy and enables the surgeon to approach the meniscus from the inner margin where most tears begin. Suture repair is appropriate for meniscal tears occurring in the vascular zone (outer 10% to 25%), which heal predictably with repair and immobilization.

Operative procedure (Fig. 21-119)

1. Steps 1 to 9 of the diagnostic arthroscopy procedure are repeated.
2. Working and scope portals are determined. The lateral bucket handle tear is identified and displaced and reduced with a probe.
3. The attachment of the anterior horn of the meniscus is cut with a hook knife and clamped with a grasper.
4. Accessory portal is determined with a spinal needle.
5. Traction and twisting motion are maintained on the meniscal horn to present a better edge to divide the remainder of the tear. Various scissors or push knives can be used to complete resection.
6. The motorized shaver is used to trim any frayed edges of the meniscus.

7. Limited débridement of chronic tears is completed to clean the edges.
8. When the medial meniscus is to be sutured, a cannula is placed next to the inner edge of the tear. Two long meniscus stitching needles with absorbable Vicryl or PDS suture are inserted into the cannula, through the meniscus, across the tear, and through the capsule.
9. The needle tips are felt beneath the skin, and a small incision is made to pull the suture out of the joint.
10. The sutures are tied over the capsule. Positioning the cannula enables either horizontal or vertical sutures to be placed.
11. After completing partial meniscectomy or suture repair, the joint is thoroughly irrigated.
12. The incisions are closed, and the knee is lightly dressed and wrapped with Webril and elastic bandages.

Arthroscopic anterior cruciate ligament repair

The anterior cruciate ligament is an important stabilizing structure of the knee and the most frequently torn ligament. Injury is usually a result of simultaneous anterior and rotational stresses. Candidates for anterior cruciate ligament reconstruction are active individuals with instability that is sufficient to interfere with their activities and that has failed to respond to bracing, rehabilitation, exercises, and other nonoperative treatment methods. The selected treatment method depends on the classification and severity of the tear, the experience and preference of the surgeon, and whether a previous repair has failed.

Reconstruction of the anterior cruciate ligament may be intraarticular, extraarticular, or a combination of both. Arthroscopic repair causes less patellar pain and less disturbance of extensor mechanisms and therefore is becoming the treatment of choice if there is no other significant capsular instability or gross disruption of the knee joint.

Anterior cruciate ligament repair most often involves replacement of the ligament with a substitute. Substitutes include autografts, allografts, and synthetic ligaments. Autografts are currently the method of choice, with a free

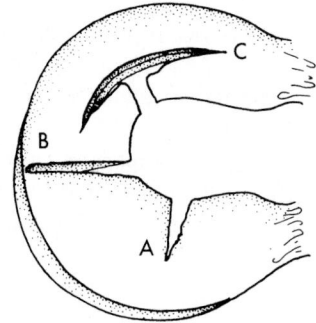

FIG. 21-118 Meniscal tear: **A,** Incomplete. **B,** Complete. **C,** Incomplete longitudinal.

From Shahriaree H: *O'Connor's textbook of arthroscopic surgery,* Philadelphia, 1984, JB Lippincott Co.

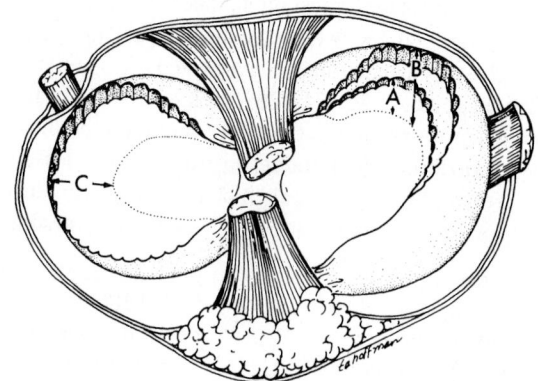

FIG. 21-119 Lateral and medial meniscal excision.

From Shahriaree H: *O'Connor's textbook of arthroscopic surgery,* Philadelphia, 1984, JB Lippincott Co.

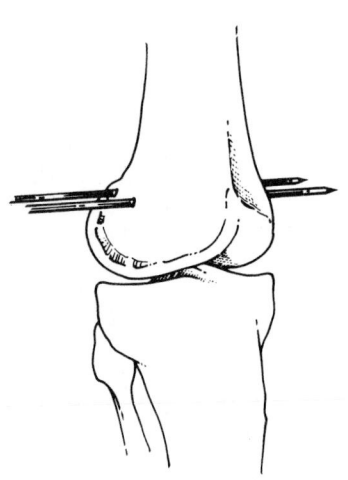
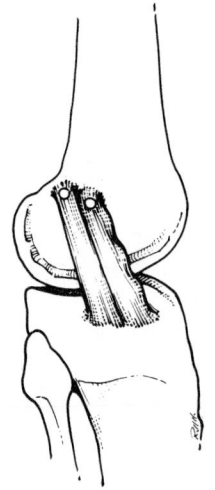
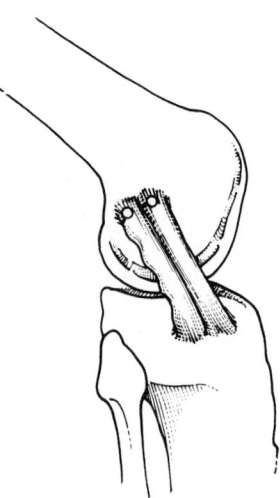

FIG. 21-120 Synthetic ligament augmentation device (LAD) routed through tibial tunnel and secured with a button, staple or screw.

From Crenshaw AH editor: *Campbell's Operative Orthopaedics*, 5 vols, ed 8, St. Louis, 1992, Mosby.

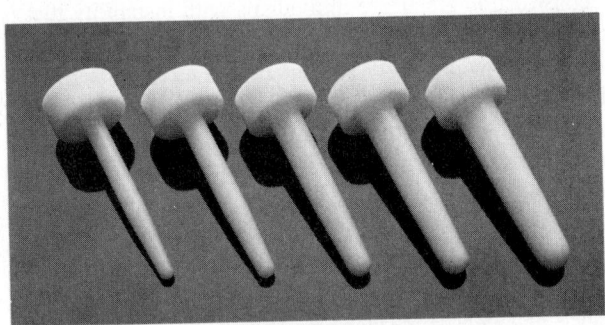

FIG. 21-121   Bone tunnel plugs.

Courtesy Acufex Microsurgical, Inc., Norwood, Mass.

central-third patellar tendon graft attached to patellar and tibial bone blocks used most often. The semitendinosus tendon and iliotibial band are sometimes used instead. Autografts may be used along or augmented. A ligament augmentation device (Fig. 21-120) strengthens the graft and protects it from rupture during early postoperative healing.

Procedural considerations. Instrumentation for an anterior cruciate ligament repair includes all instruments required for an operative arthroscopy, plus the following:

ACL reconstruction guide system	Bone tunnel plugs (Fig. 21-121)
Tension isometer	Power drill and micro-sagittal saw
Fixation of choice (bone screws, staples,	spiked washers, or interference screws) (see Fig. 21-82)

Operative procedure—patellar tendon graft

1. An exam under anesthesia is performed immediately after induction to further evaluate the stability of the knee.
2. A diagnostic arthroscopy is then carried out through the standard anteromedial and anterolateral portals.
3. Any meniscal tears or other intraarticular injuries are treated before attending to the ligament.
4. The remaining anterior cruciate ligament tissue is débrided with a full-radius resector.
5. A notchplasty is then performed, widening the intracondylar notch with a 4.5-mm arthroplasty burr, rasp, osteotome, and curettes. Notchplasty aids in arthroscopic visualization and protects the graft from abrasion and amputation.
6. After preparation of the intracondylar area, a small incision is made on the distal lateral aspect of the femur and is carried down to the flare of the lateral femoral condyle.
7. A femoral aiming device is positioned, and a guide pin is inserted from the femoral site into the posterosuperior region of the intercondylar notch at an isometric point (Fig. 21-122).
8. Another small incision is made anteriorly, below the knee and medial to the tibial tubercle.
9. The tibial aiming device is positioned and a guide pin is inserted from the anterior tibial incision into the intercondylar notch, anterior and medial to the center of the tibial anatomic attachment site of the anterior cruciate ligament (Fig. 21-123).
10. The pins are then replaced with a heavy suture passing through the femoral and tibial pin sites.

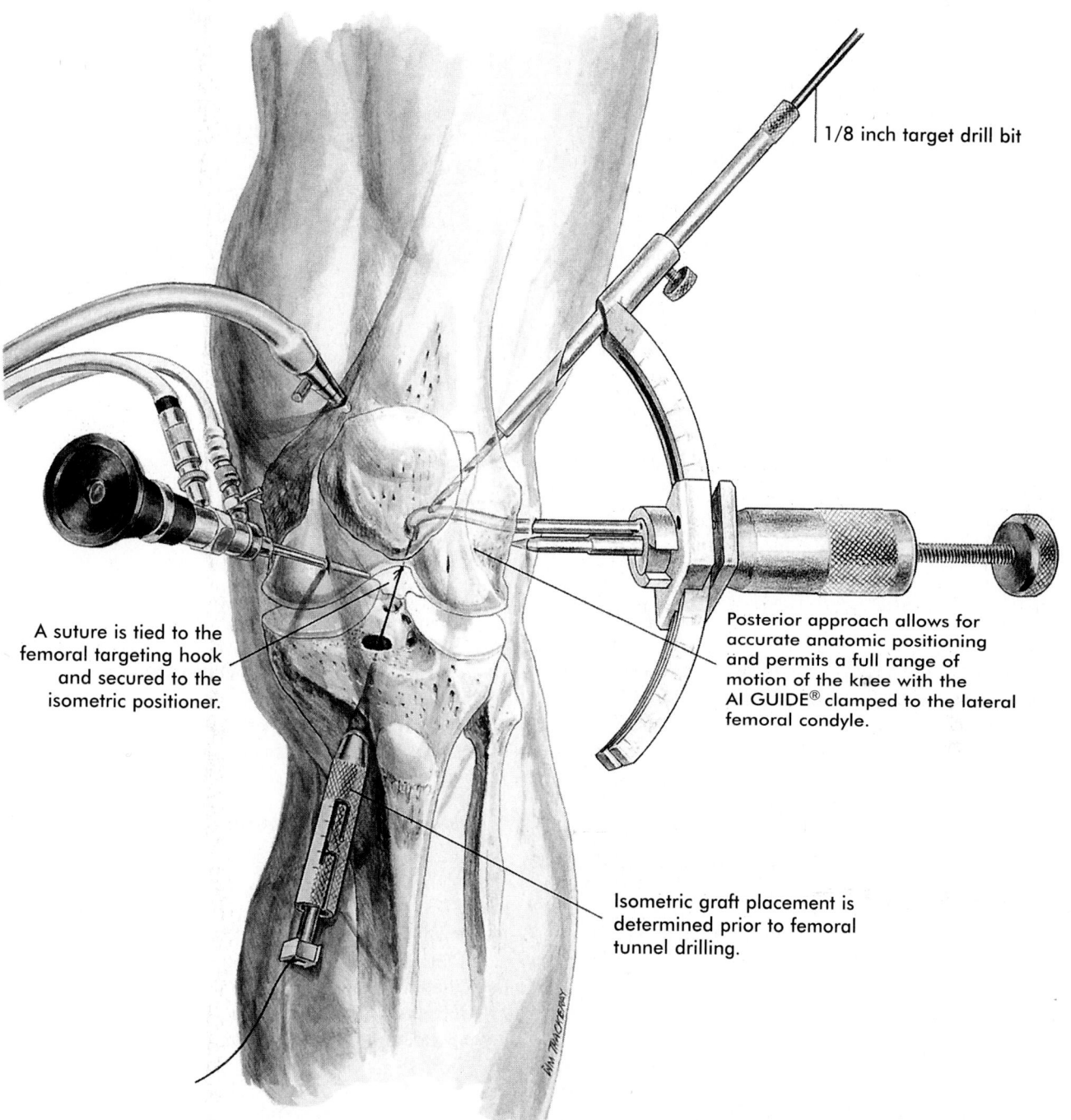

1/8 inch target drill bit

A suture is tied to the femoral targeting hook and secured to the isometric positioner.

Posterior approach allows for accurate anatomic positioning and permits a full range of motion of the knee with the AI GUIDE® clamped to the lateral femoral condyle.

Isometric graft placement is determined prior to femoral tunnel drilling.

FIG. 21-122   Femoral aiming device positioned for ACL reconstruction.
Courtesy Johnson and Johnson

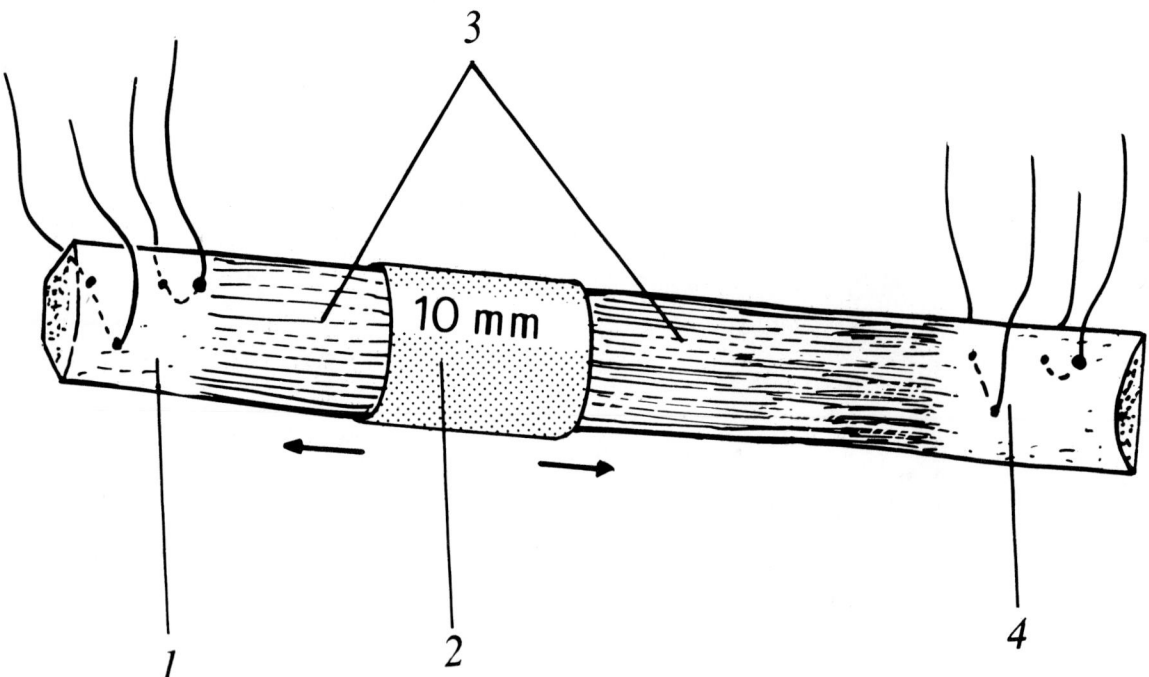

FIG. 21-123 Sizing tubes are used to determine the minimum diameter tunnel necessary for passage of the graft.

11. Isometric placement of the guide pins is checked with a tensioning device that is attached to the heavy suture. The knee is put through a range of motion to determine correct isometric measurement.
12. Once isometric positioning is determined, a longitudinal skin incision is made medial to the midline near the patellar tendon.
13. The central-third portion of the patellar tendon with tibial and patellar bone plugs is harvested with a minisaw and osteotome.
14. The graft is sized to the appropriate width, usually 10 to 12 mm, using sizing tubes (Fig. 21-123).
15. Heavy (Ethibond or Mersilene) suture is placed through drill holes made at each end of the graft in the bone plugs (Fig. 21-124).
16. The guide pins are then reinserted and overdrilled with cannulas that are close in width to the prepared graft. Overdrilling establishes the tunnels so they are in the center of the previous insertion sites of the anterior cruciate ligament.
17. The femoral and tibial osseous tunnels are smoothed with curettes, a rasp, or an abrader. If the tunnels are made before the graft is harvested, they are temporarily occluded with bone tunnel plugs (Fig. 21-121) to minimize fluid extravasation.
18. Both ends of the graft are fixed with a barbed staple,

bone screw with washer, interference screw, or ligament button (Fig. 21-125).
19. The incisions and joint are irrigated and closed.
20. A hinged knee brace is applied over the dressing. The brace allows 10 to 90 degrees of motion.

Arthroscopic posterior cruciate ligament repair

Surgical procedures for tears of the posterior cruciate ligament considered if significant disabling instability has occurred. Patients usually return to adequate function without operative treatment. The arthroscopic procedure for repair of the posterior cruciate ligament is similar to the technique used to repair the anterior cruciate ligament, except that isometric placement is posterior within the joint and the femoral attachment is proximal to the medial epicondyle.

Arthroscopy of the shoulder

Shoulder arthroscopy is a useful diagnostic and therapeutic tool in the management of shoulder disorders. It is particularly beneficial in the evaluation and management of patients with chronic shoulder problems. Arthroscopy provides extensive visualization of the intraarticular aspect of the shoulder joint. Indications for shoulder arthroscopy include removal of loose bodies, lysis of adhesions, synovial biopsy, synovectomy, bursectomy, stabilization of disloca-

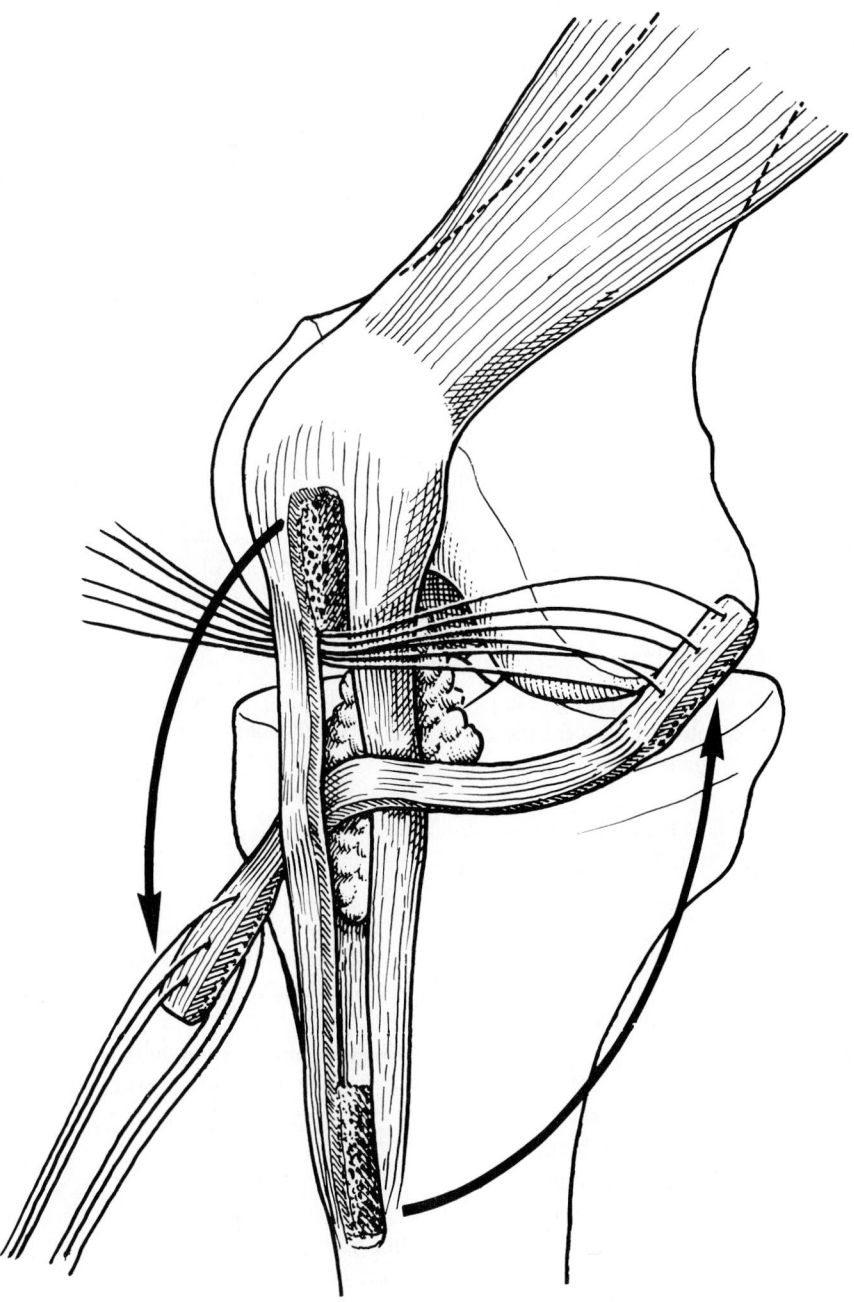

FIG. 21-124   Three drill holes are placed in each bone block of the patellar graft and a heavy suture is placed in each drill hole.

From Laurin CA, Riley LH Jr., Roy-Camille R: *Atlas of Orthopaedic Surgery, Volume 3: Lower Extremity,* 1992, Masson.

tions, correction of glenoid labrum, biceps tendon and rotator cuff tears, and relief of impingement syndrome.

Procedural considerations. The patient is placed in the lateral position. The position is maintained by using a vacuum beanbag positioning device or lateral rolls with a kidney rest. Three-inch adhesive tape is secured across the patient's hips. Proper padding of the uninvolved axilla and lower extremity is important to prevent soft tissue or neurovascular problems. The affected extremity is placed in a shoulder suspension system (see Fig. 21-13) and Buck's traction or a Velcro immobilizer is applied to the forearm to achieve adequate distraction to the glenohumeral joint. The extremity is abducted 40 to 60 degrees and forward flexed 10 to 20 degrees, with 5- to 15-pound weights placed on the pulley system. Weight may be added to further distract the glenohumeral joint.

The shoulder is prepped and draped free, permitting full range of motion during the procedure. The surgeon stands posterior to the patient.

The operative instruments and arthroscope commonly used for the knee may also be used in the shoulder, plus an 18-gauge needle, switching sticks, and a Wissinger rod. There are a variety of fixation devices (screws and tacks) that can be used to bony defects and labrum tears.

Operative procedure (Fig. 21-126)

1. An 18-gauge spinal needle is inserted through the posterior soft spot and directed anteriorly toward the coracoid process, where the surgeon's index finger has been positioned.
2. The glenohumeral joint is distended with normal saline or lactated Ringer's solution. This facilitates entry of the arthroscope.
3. Bupivacaine 0.25% (Marcaine), 2 to 3 ml, with epinephrine 1:200,000 is injected along the needle track to minimize bleeding.
4. With the needle removed, a stab incision is made with an 11 blade over the needle site.
5. The arthroscope sleeve and sharp trocar are then introduced through the posterior joint capsule.
6. Once the capsule has been penetrated, a blunt obturator replaces the sharp trocar to enter the joint.
7. The athroscope is inserted and attached to inflow and outflow tubing, the video camera, and light source.
8. Operative instruments are placed through an anterior portal that is established lateral to the coracoid process by using a Wissinger rod.
9. A third portal can be established near the anterior portal or supraspinous fossa portal. Switching sticks are used to change portals.
10. The arm is moved and rotated as needed to visualize various structures in and around the joint.
11. Glenoid tears can be repaired with the insertion of an absorbable fixation tack.
12. At the conclusion of the procedure, the joint is irrigated. The surgeon may inject a long-acting local an-

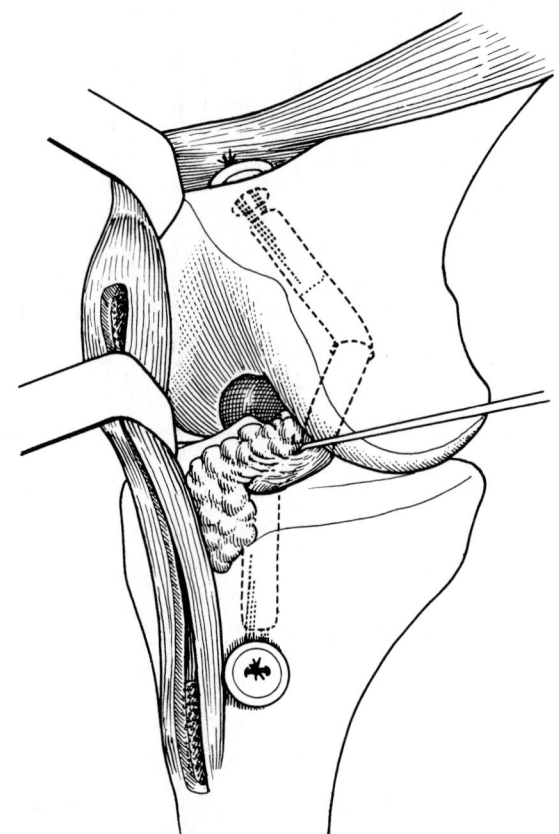

FIG. 21-125   A patellar tendon graft is affixed by tying sutures over bone buttons at the tibial and femoral drill holes.

esthetic drug into the joint and subacromial space through the portal to minimize postoperative discomfort.

13. The puncture wounds are closed and dressed with a sterile 4 × 4 gauze pad. The patient's arm is placed in a sling for recovery.

Arthroscopy of the elbow

The elbow joint is accessible to arthroscopic examination, although it requires more attention to detail than the knee because instruments must be placed through deeper muscle layers and close to important neurovascular structures.

Arthroscopy of the elbow, both diagnostic and operative, has become fairly routine. Indications for its use include extraction of loose bodies, evaluation or debridement of osteochondritis dissecans of the capitellum and radial head, partial synovectomy in rheumatoid disease, débridement and lysis of adhesions of posttraumatic or degenerative processes at or near the elbow, diagnosis of a chronically painful elbow when the diagnosis is obscure, and evaluation of fractures of the capitellum, radial head, or olecranon.

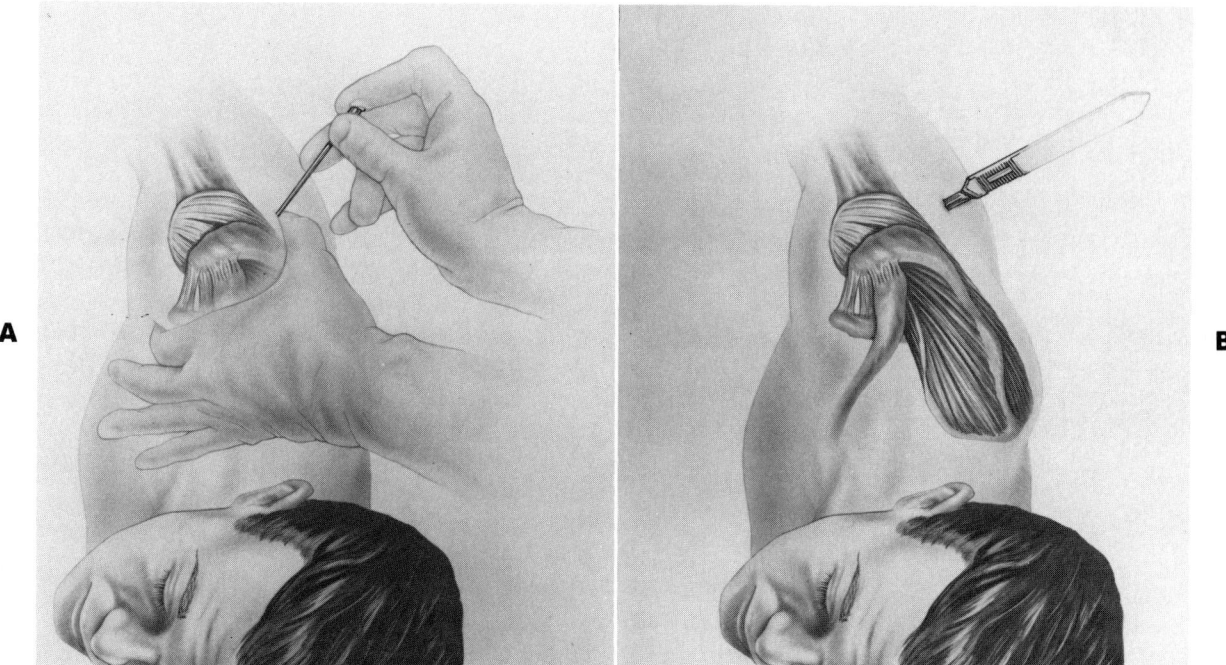

FIG. 21-126 Shoulder arthroscopy. **A,** The spinal needle is inserted for dilation of the joint if indicated. **B,** An incision is made over the glenohumeral joint.

Procedural considerations. General anesthesia is preferred to local anesthesia because it affords complete comfort to the patient and provides total muscle relaxation.

The patient is placed in the supine position. The forearm is flexed on an armboard or placed in a prefabricated wrist gauntlet connected to an overhead pulley device and tied off at the end of the OR bed. If lifted overhead, the entire arm is allowed to hang free over the side of the bed with the elbow flexed approximately 90 degrees. This provides excellent access to both the medial and lateral aspects of the elbow, allows the forearm to be freely pronated and supinated, and places the important neurovascular structures in the antecubital fossa at maximum relaxation. A tourniquet is routinely used for hemostasis. The entire arm, including the hand, is prepped and draped.

The three portals most commonly used for diagnostic and operative arthroscopy of the elbow are the anterolateral, the anteromedial, and the posterolateral.

Operative arthroscopy instruments commonly used for the knee may also be used in the elbow. However, smaller diameter scopes and instruments may be desired instead.

Operative procedure

1. The bony anatomic landmarks are outlined with a marking pen before initiation of the procedure. Lateral structures to be marked and identified are the radial head and the lateral epicondyle. The medial epicondyle is marked.
2. An 18-gauge needle is inserted anterior to the radial head from the lateral side, and the joint is distended.
3. Once joint distention has been achieved with approximately 15 to 30 ml of lactated Ringer's or normal saline solution, a stab wound incision is made with a no. 11 blade and the sharp trocar with cannula is inserted through the joint capsule.
4. The sharp trocar is replaced with the blunt obturator to provide safe entry of the cannula into the joint.
5. The scope replaces the blunt obturator and is attached to the video and light source.
6. A second and third portal are established anteromedially and posterolaterally for triangulation. With the patient's elbow flexed to 90 degrees and adequate distention maintained at the time of insertion of the instruments, the neurovascular structures are displaced anteriorly. This provides greater area above the medial and lateral humeral epicondyles in which to insert the various instruments.
7. Outflow and inflow are controlled by alternating the valve on the scope or using a separate 18-gauge needle with drainage tubing.
8. After diagnostic and operative procedures have been completed, the joint is irrigated, the puncture sites are sutured, and a compression dressing is applied with Webril and elastic bandages.

Arthroscopy of the ankle

The talocalcaneal articulations are complex and play an important role in the movements of inversion and eversion of the foot. The subtalar joints function as a single unit, but anatomically they are divided into anterior and posterior joints. The surgeon and nurse must be familiar with the extraarticular anatomy of the ankle to prevent neural or vascular damage.

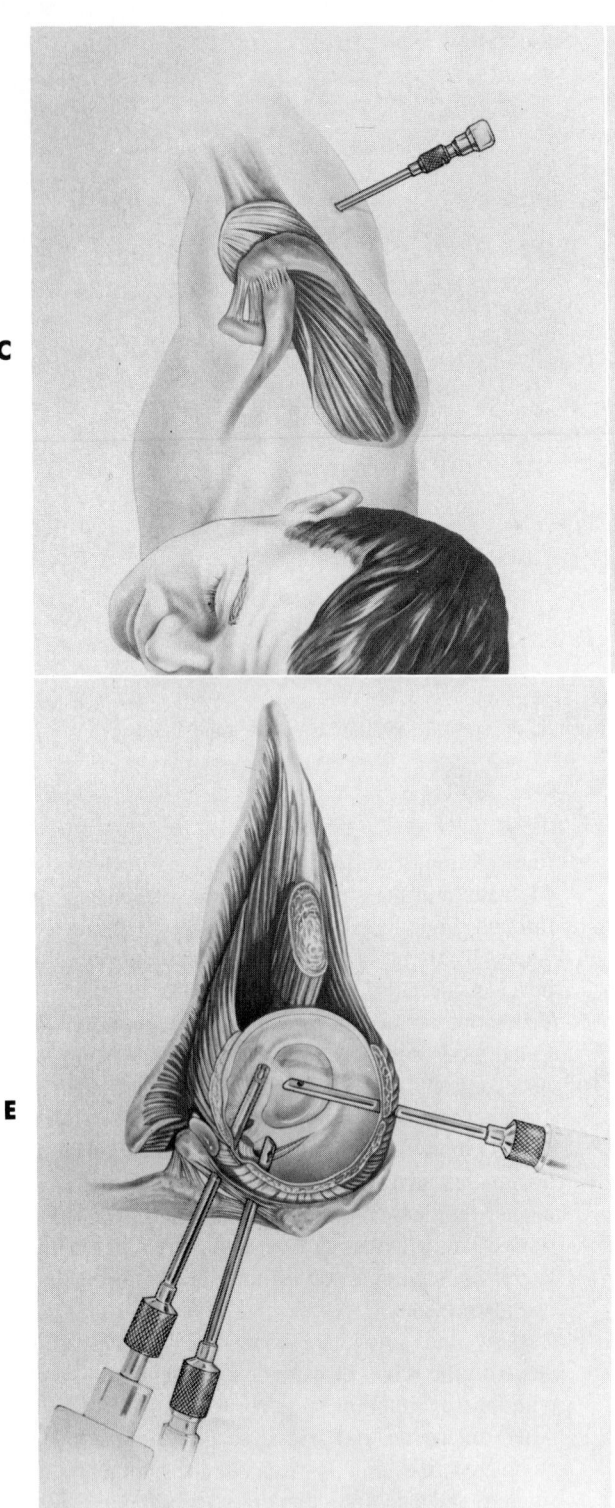

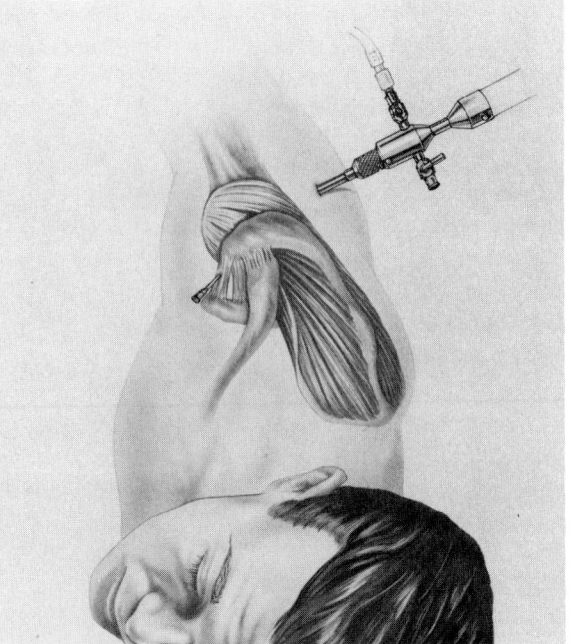

FIG. 21-126 CONT.   **C,** The arthroscope sleeve and sharp trocar are inserted. **D,** The arthroscope is inserted and attached to the inflow and outflow tubing, video camera and light source. **E,** Operative instruments are placed through the portal.

Courtesy Dyonics, Inc., Andover, Mass.

Indications for ankle arthroscopy include osteochondral fragments or loose bodies, persistent ankle pain following trauma and despite adequate conservative treatment, biopsy, posttraumatic arthritis of the ankle joint, unstable ankle before lateral ligamentous reconstruction, and osteochondritis dissecans of the talus.

Procedural considerations. General anesthesia is preferable because manipulation and distraction of the joint to obtain adequate arthroscopic viewing require muscle relaxation. The position of the patient is based on the surgeon's preference. The patient may be supine with the knee flexed approximately 70 degrees or supine with a sandbag under the buttock of the operative side. Ankle and thigh holders may be used; when better posterior visualization is necessary, a distracter may be used to increase the space between the tibia and talus (see Fig. 21-15). A tourniquet is placed around the upper thigh but is not used unless excessive bleeding, uncontrolled by irrigation, is encountered. Routine skin prepping and draping are done.

Operative instruments and the arthroscope commonly used for the knee may also be used for the ankle; however, miniaturized instruments and needle scopes for the ankle are becoming more available.

Operative procedure

1. The important extraarticular anatomic structures are outlined on the skin using a sterile marking pen.
2. Examination of the ankle joint using the anterolateral portal is then performed. The anteromedial joint line is palpated, and an 18-gauge, 1½-inch needle is inserted into the joint.
3. Sterile plastic extension tubing is attached to the needle, and a 50-ml plastic Luter-Lok syringe filled with

normal saline is connected to the tubing to distend the joint. Approximately 15 to 20 ml are needed.

4. After intraarticular injection is confirmed by the ease with which the saline can be injected and by palpation of the joint as it is distended, a small incision is made with a no. 11 blade over the site of the anterolateral portal.

5. A hemostat is then inserted and used to dissect to the capsule.

6. The sheath of the arthroscope and sharp trocar are placed into the incision, angled approximately 30 to 45 degrees laterally, and inserted with a sharp plunge as joint distention is maintained. Entrance into the joint is felt as the sleeve and trocar "pop" through the capsule and is confirmed by the rush of saline on removal of the trocar from the sheath.

7. The arthroscope is inserted into the sheath, the needle is removed, and the plastic tubing and syringe are attached to the stopcock on the arthroscope sleeve. The video camera and light source are connected to the scope. Joint distention must be maintained.

8. Triangulation through other portals is easily done by first inserting the 18-gauge needle for localization while viewing with the arthroscope. Posterior viewing is done in the same fashion except that the patient is usually placed in the prone position and instruments are inserted through the posterior portals.

9. After the procedure is completed, the joint is irrigated and wounds are closed with Steri-Strips or a single suture and covered with a dressing and short leg compression elastic wrap.

SURGERY OF THE SPINAL COLUMN
Treatment of back pain

Back pain is a natural result of degenerative and arthritic change, punctuated by protrusion or rupture of a disk. It gradually progresses but may also disappear gradually. With aging, a degenerative disk space narrowing or facet arthropathy begins to appear radiologically. The lower lumbar spine carries the burden of the body, holds a person upright, and returns the body to the vertical position from sitting, lying, or a bent-over position. Degenerative changes, ruptured disk, and facet arthropathy develop at the lowest two limb segments, where the greatest weight, torsion, and shearing stress occur. It sometimes extends into the upper and middle spine.

Cervical spine degenerative disk narrowing also develops most often at the two lowest cervical spaces, which are also the levels of greatest stress resulting from movement of the head and neck. Sometimes lumbar or cervical degenerative changes develop early from excessive repetitive movements or injury.

Back pain may be treated by injection procedures, electrodes, stimulators, braces, or traction. A natural recovery may result following 6 or 7 days of intense pain, subsiding between 6 weeks and 4 months. Motor and sensory deficits usually disappear with resolution of pain. The ability to re-

cover without surgery depends on fragment size and compression on the nerve root. Neural compression remains the major indication for disk excision.

Spinal fusion is a consideration, usually with demonstrable posttraumatic, postsurgical, rheumatoid, infectious, or neoplastic instability.

Procedural considerations. Following assessment, patient-specific care is provided. X-rays are obtained. Bilateral pulses are assessed in the extremities. Elastic wraps or stockings may be placed. Range of motion is assessed, particularly of the arms, because of the need for the extended prone position. The patient is positioned prone to eliminate lordosis, reduce venous congestion, and keep the abdomen free. A Foley catheter may be placed. The patient is positioned using chest rolls or special frames (see Fig. 21-16) following administration of general anesthesia. Depending on the extent of the procedure, blood availability may be required. The skin is prepped and the area draped. A spinal laminectomy set is used, in addition to the following:

Spinal retractor of choice	Medications such as gelfoam, thrombin, bone wax
Bipolar cautery	

Operative procedure—Laminectomy

1. A midline incision is made over the affected disk.
2. The underlying ligamentous insertion is divided and the superior lateral tip of each spinous process is exposed.
3. The muscles are dissected to permit retraction without tension.

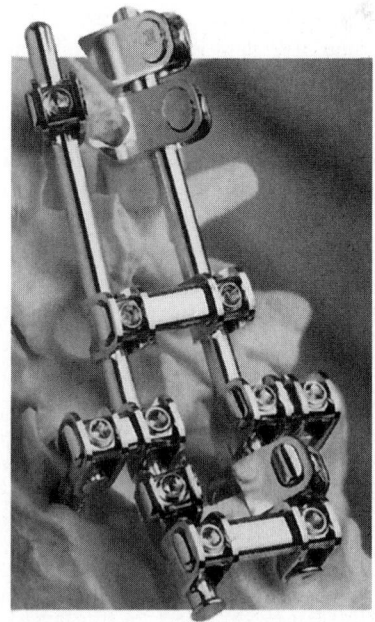

FIG. 21-127   Pedicle screw placement using the Rogozinksi system.

Courtesy Richards Medical Co., Memphis, Tenn.

4. Muscle attachments at the laminal margins are divided to expose the lamina and facet.
5. The lateral margin of dura is exposed. Bone removal is continued. The medial portion of the inferior articulating surface is excised.
6. The bone and residual ligamentum flavum is excised. The nerve root is exposed above and below the disk space. Venous bleeding is controlled with cottonoid pledgets. Veins are coagulated with monopolar or bipolar cautery. Bone wax is used to maintain a dry field.
7. Disk space is evacuated of degenerated disk material.
8. Gelfoam pledgets may be placed in the lateral epidural space in the presence of residual venous bleeding.
9. The incision is closed in layers.

Pedicle fixation of the spine

Pedicle screw fixation (Fig. 21-127) has become an increasingly popular method of surgical fixation of the spinal column. Screw fixation was initially used in an attempt to avoid postoperative external immobilization and prolonged bed rest. Pedicle screw fixation has been used most in degenerative processes, particularly iatrogenic instability following decompression, degenerative and isthmic spondylolisthesis and diskogenic disease. It is also indicated for tumor, trauma, degenerative spinal disorders, postoperative hypermobility, and infection.

Three basic approaches for fixation have been described as the procedure has evolved. Each has improved upon the first, based on anatomic placement of the screw. Positioning and placement of the screw within the spine are established following direct visualization of the pedicle.

Procedural considerations. Patient-specific considerations are given following the assessment (see laminectomy section). The patient is placed under general anesthesia and positioned prone. The skin is prepped and drapes applied.

A spinal laminectomy set is used, in addition to:

Instrumentation and implants of choice	Gelfoam, thrombin, bone wax
Spinal retractor	Power equipment
Medications such as	

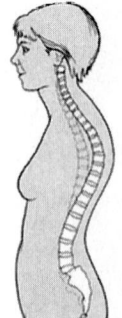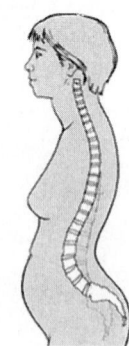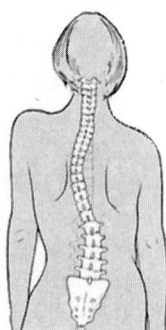

FIG. 21-128 Scoliotic deformity.

From Thibodeau GA and Patton K: *Anatomy and Physiology*, ed 2, St. Louis, 1993, Mosby.

Operative procedure

1. A standard midline incision is made. The laminectomy procedure is followed.
2. The areas of the pedicles to be fixated are located using external landmarks.
3. The posterior cortical wall at the entrance site is removed using a high-speed burr.
4. A Penfield dissector is used to identify the entrance hole through the pedicle.
5. A gearshift probe is inserted to identify the path into the vertebral body.
6. The hole is tapped (5.5 mm) and the hole widened.
7. The screw is placed. Guidelines for screw sizes are: 7 mm for S1, L5, and L4; 6.25 mm for L3 and L2; 5.5 mm for L1 and T12.
8. A posterolateral graft is performed, using graft strips from the iliac crest.
9. The plate or rod is contoured to approximate the patient's physiologic lordosis. The longitudinal device is locked onto the screws in the appropriate position.
10. A screw-plate system may require use of the oblique and transverse washers between the screw head and plate to provide a flush fit at the screw-plate interface.
11. The foramina are checked for patency before closure. The excess machined portion of the screw is cut close to the upper locking device.
12. A suction drain is placed; the wound is closed in layers.

Treatment of scoliosis

Scoliosis is a three-dimensional deformity (Fig. 21-128) with lateral deviation of the spinal column from the midline; it may include rotation or deformity of the vertebrae. Types are congenital, juvenile, adolescent, and adult. School screening programs provide quick and simple detection. For effective treatment of scoliosis, early detection is critical.

Some form of scoliosis occurs in 1 in 10 people (Dell and Regan, 1987), affecting 1 million people in the United States. Two in 100 require medical treatment. Of all treated patients, 8% are female. Scoliosis can be idiopathic (80% of the time) or congenital and may result from muscular or neurologic diseases or unequal leg lengths (Dell and Regan, 1987).

Posterior spinal fusion with Harrington rods

Posterior spinal fusion is most frequently performed in adolescence, when the laterally deviated curve is still flexible. Harrington rods are internal splints that help maintain the spine as straight as possible until the vertebral body fusion has become solid. The distraction rods are placed on the concave side of the curve, and compression rods are placed on the convex side. On the convex side of the curve, three to eight hooks are inserted in the transverse processes of the vertebrae and pulled together with a threaded rod. In

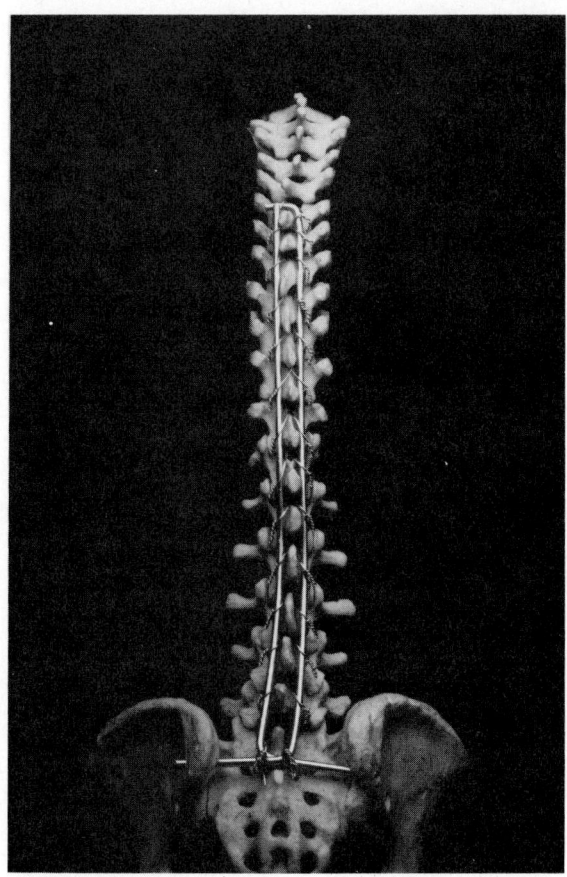

FIG. 21-129   Luque spinal system in place on a scoliotic spine.
Courtesy Zimmer, Inc., Warsaw, Ind.

this way the scoliotic deformity can be corrected as much as the flexibility of the spine allows.

The posterior elements of the vertebrae are denuded of soft tissue, and the bone graft is added. Blood loss can be expected and an accurate record of the loss must be maintained. After surgery the patient is placed in an immobilizing jacket.

Some disadvantages of the Harrington rod system over other systems are that there is only end-point fixation, rod breakage is increased, fixation is less, sagittal plane curves are difficult to manage, distraction for correction is not always desired, and the patient is required to wear a postoperative cast or brace. Other systems have evolved from the Harrington rod that are used for correction of some scoliotic deformities. It remains a viable treatment of idiopathic scoliosis.

Procedural considerations. The patient is placed in the prone position on the frame or with rolls under the chest and abdomen to facilitate respiration. Before the procedure begins, an x-ray cassette is placed under the patient so an x-ray film for accurate identification of the vertebrae to be fused can be taken during the operation. A single straight longitudinal incision is made down the midline of the back. Because of the amount of bleeding, the skin and subcuta-

neous tissues are often infiltrated with a vasoconstricting solution, such as epinephrine.

Basic spinal instrumentation and bone graft instruments are required, plus the following:

Harrington rod instrumentation
Large pin cutter (designed to cut large pins but provided with small end so it will fit in wound)

Operative procedure

1. The appropriate hooks are selected and inserted. A Harrington distraction rod of appropriate length is inserted through the two proximal self-adjusting hooks, which have been placed under the laminae.
2. A rod clamp is clamped onto the Harrington rod just below the hook, and a single regular spreader is used to obtain the first inch of distraction.
3. The Bobechko spreader is used to span over the first hook, closest to the smooth part of the rod, to apply distraction force on the most proximal hook.
4. Two C locking rings are inserted around the first ratchet immediately below the hook to prevent dislodgment of the hooks. The excessive length of protruding rod above the most proximal hook is cut off with a rod cutter. The compression is tightened.

Luque segmental spinal rod procedure

The Luque segmental method employs smooth, L-shaped, stainless steel rods, usually ³⁄₁₆ or ¼ inch in diameter, with sublaminar wires placed at every level possible (Fig. 21-129). It is more secure and longer than the Harrington rod system, and was the first system to employ multiple point fixation. Luque instrumentation applies corrective forces to the spinal segments at each level, thereby spreading the corrective forces throughout the length of the deformity. Two Luque rods are wired to both sides of the spine. The rods are contoured to achieve no more than 10 degrees of increased correction beyond that exhibited on preoperative x-ray study.

Procedural considerations. The patient is placed in the prone position on the frame or with rolls under the chest and abdomen to facilitate respiration. Patient care is provided (see section on laminectomy), including assessment of pulses. A straight midline incision is made in the back. Because of the amount of bleeding, the skin and subcutaneous tissues are often infiltrated with a vasoconstricting solution such as epinephrine.

Basic spinal instrumentation is required, plus the following:

Luque rods and instrumentation	Wire cutter
Wire tightener	Bone graft instruments

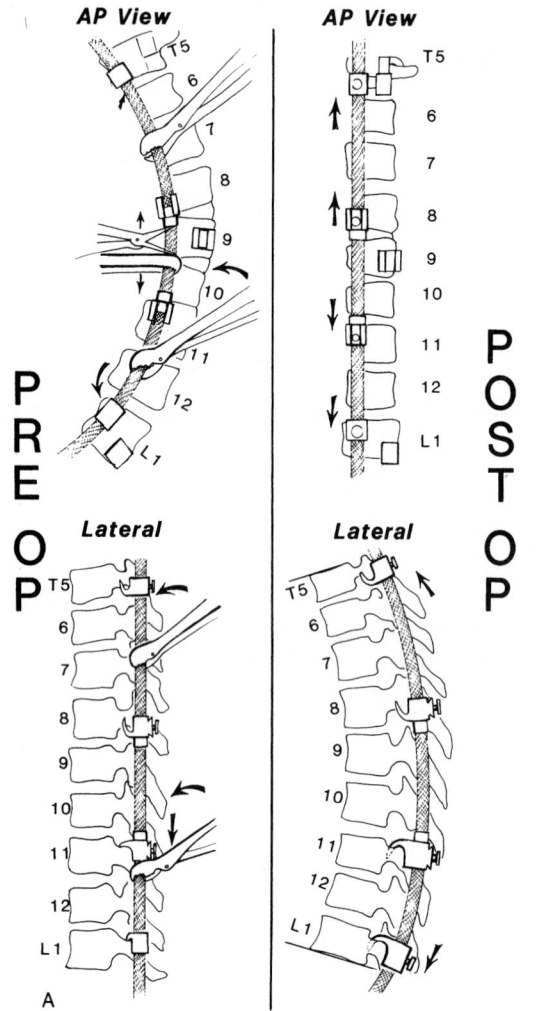

FIG. 21-130   Cotrel-Dubousset system, representing rotation of rods.

From Bradford DS et al: *Moe's textbook of scoliosis and other spinal deformities*, ed 2, Philadelphia, 1987, WB Saunders Co.

Operative procedure

1. The ligamentum flavum is detached, exposing the neural canal.
2. Doubled stainless steel suture wire is passed under the lamina. The wire loop will be cut later to form two wires at each level.
3. Total bilateral facetectomies are made, forming posterolateral troughs for subsequent bone grafts.
4. Wedge osteotomies may be necessary in severe immobile curves to avoid stretching the spinal cord during correction.
5. The wire loop is cut, resulting in two separate wires at each level.
6. Rod migration is prevented by securing the L bend to the base of the spinous process.
7. Initial placement of the convex rod is made.

8. Initial placement of the concave rod is made.
9. Transverse wiring is done to add increased stabililty to the system.
10. Stabilization of the lumbosacral joint is corrected by bending the rods distally to form sacral bars.

Cotrel Dubousset system procedure

The Cotrel Dubousset system (Fig. 21-130) provides three-dimensional correction of spinal deformities without sublaminar wiring and neurologic risks. This instrumentation permits distraction, compression, and derotation. The scoliotic curve is corrected by derotation and, at the same time, restoration of the normal sagittal contours. In addition to correction of scoliosis, the Cotrel Dubousset system can be applied to correct kyphosis or lordosis and to stabilize and rebuild the spine after tumor resection or after traumatic injury. No external support is necessary. The Cotrel Dubousset system has no ratchets or notches. It consists of metallic rods with diamond crosscut patterns on which hooks and screws can be positioned in any position, level, or degree of rotation. The rod is held in the open hooks with blockers. The rods are then interlocked by means of devices for transverse traction (DTT). The Cotrel Dubousset system was the forerunner to the systems used today, such as the Texas Scottish Rite Hospital system, and the Isola system.

Procedural considerations. The patient is placed in the prone position under general anesthesia. Patient care is provided (see laminectomy section). Basic spinal instrumentation is required in addition to the following:

Bone graft instruments
Cotrel Dubousset system and instrumentation

Operative procedure

1. Closed hooks are inserted at both ends of the surgical site, and open hooks are inserted at various levels in between.
2. Decortication and facet excision are done at the remaining interposed vertebrae levels for rod placement.
3. Bone graft is placed in the areas that will be under the rod.
4. The appropriate concave rod is bent to shape for sagittal plane correction and manipulated into the end hooks.
5. Stabilization along the length is achieved with blockers that anchor the rod into the open hooks.
6. The spine is then derotated using the rod holders. The frontal plane scoliosis curve becomes the sagittal plane kyphosis.
7. Hooks are reseated for secure fixation.
8. To correct kyphosis, the convex rod is then bent to shape and seated.

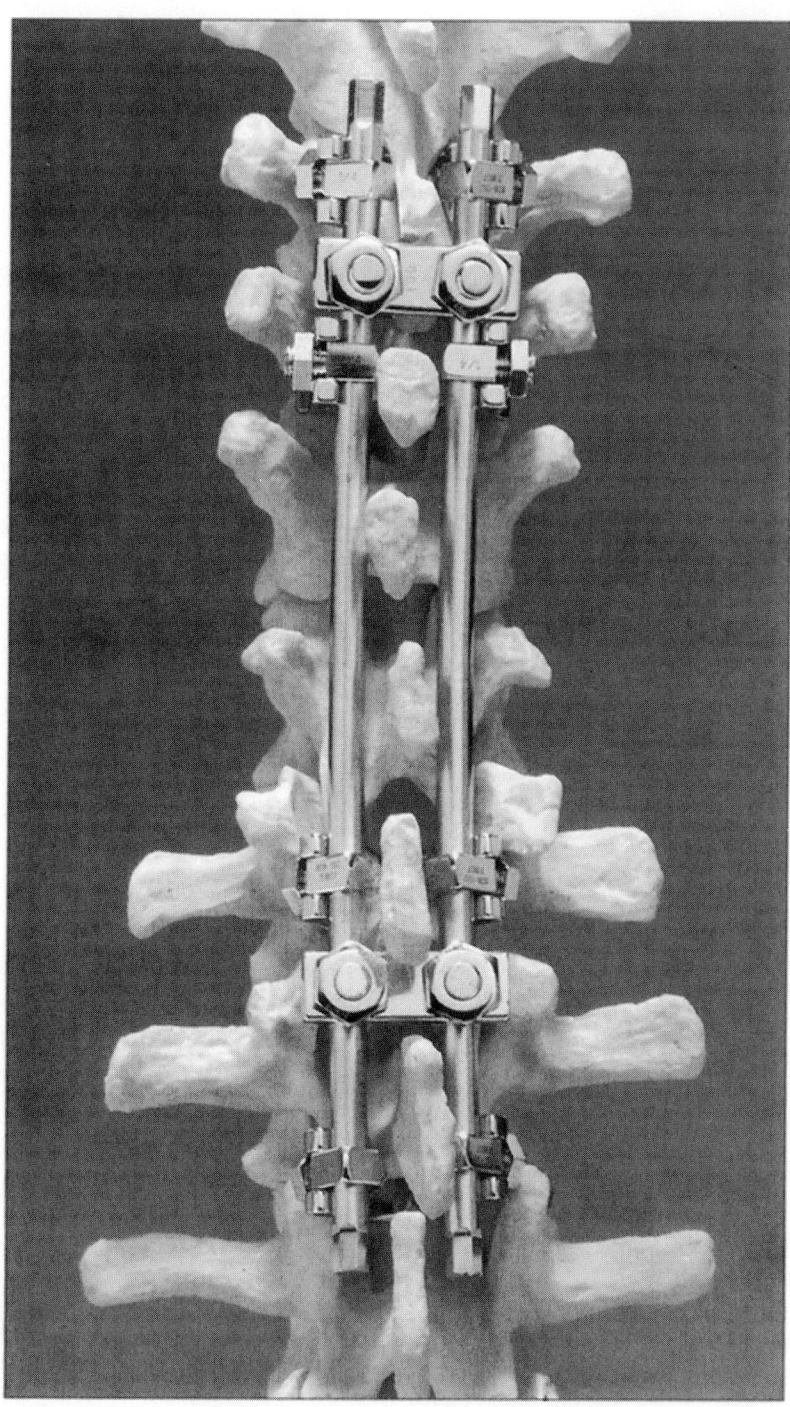

FIG. 21-131 Texas Scottish Rite System.
Courtesy Danek, Memphis, Tenn.

9. Once the rods have been placed, final stabilization is completed by applying the DTT, usually near the ends of the rods.
10. Remaining bone graft is applied to the fusion area.

Texas Scottish Rite Hospital (TSRH) crosslink system

The TSRH crosslink system (Fig. 21-131) is a multicomponent stainless steel implant used to rigidly lock spinal rods together. Locking the rods increases construction stiffness and prevents rod migration. The system was originally designed for the Luque segmental system to prevent migration between the rods and wires before complete fusion occurred. By rigidly crosslinking the rods, loss of scoliotic correction was reduced. This system can also be utilized with the Harrington and Cotrel Dubousset systems. Crosslinks are indicated when the rigidity of a spinal system alone is not sufficient to generate fusion in a reasonable amount of time.

Procedural considerations. Patient-specific considerations are given following the assessment (see laminectomy section). The patient is placed under general anesthesia and positioned prone. The skin is prepped and drapes applied.

A spinal laminectomy set is used, in addition to the following:

Instrumentation and implants of choice
Spinal retractor
Power equipment
Medications such as
    Gelfoam, thrombin,
    bone wax

Operative procedure

1. Eyebolts are placed on the spinal rods before the rods are implanted.
2. The rods are secured with hooks or wires, depending on the system used.
3. Once the rods are positioned, crossplates of varying widths accommodating different rod-to-rod distances are bolted in placed between the rods and nuts.

Anterior spinal fusion with Isola instrumentation

Isola instrumentation involves screw fixation into each vertebral body, complete disk excision and grafting, and segmental connection of the vertebral bodies. A semirigid rod connects the segments. The Isola technique is the preferred method of anterior spinal instrumentation for potential instability following multilevel resection for spinal stenosis and degenerative disease. A combination hook and screw method is utilized to provide purchase on the bone.

Procedural considerations. The patient is positioned supine, ensuring respiratory excursion is adequate. The approach to the anterior spine requires familiarity of the abdominal and vascular anatomy. The radiology team should be available both before and during the surgery for identification of proper levels to be manipulated.

A major soft tissue set and laminectomy set are required, in addition to the following:

Vascular set
Spinal instrumentation
Power equipment

Operative procedure

1. An incision is made to the fascia.
2. Electrosurgery is used through the fascia and muscle to expose the spine.
3. The muscle is elevated laterally off of the selected level to be decompressed.
4. The spinous processes are stripped of their muscular attachments.
5. The posterior elements are exposed using elevators and sponges.
6. The transverse processes are identified and exposed using electrosurgery.
7. The spinous process is cut off with a large bone cutter and the level to be decompressed is palpated.
8. The bone in the area of the stenosis is devoid using Kerrison rongeurs and the ligamentum flavum is debrided.
9. The facets of the lamina are resected, decompressing the nerve root, and foramenotomy is completed bilaterally, further freeing the nerve roots.
10. Cancellous bone screws are used to hold plates onto the lamina to hold the subsequent rod where pedicles do not remain because of resection. Pedicle hooks are used in pedicles that remain.
11. The rod-hook-plate assembly is constructed and inserted into the back after the rod is contoured.
12. The correction is performed with distraction and compression of the rod.
13. Any bone graft is placed to the appropriate area and final radiographic views observed.
14. Wound drains are inserted and the incision is closed in layers.

REFERENCES

American Association of Tissue Banks. (1987). *Technical manual for surgical bone banking*. Arlington, va.: American Association of Tissue Banks.
American Board of Orthopaedic Surgery. (1982).
Association of Operating Room Nurses. (1994). *AORN standards and recommended practices*. Denver: The Association.
Brown, M.D., and Seltzer, D.G. (1991). Perioperative care in lumbar spine surgery. *Orthopaedic Clinics of North America, 22*(2), 353-358.
Buckham, K.R. (1991). Surgical bone banking: The living donor. *Orthopaedic Nursing, 10*(2), 47-53.
Chapman, M.W. (1993). *Operative orthopedics*. Philadelphia: J.B. Lippincott.
Crenshaw, A.H. (ed.). (1992). *Campbell's operative orthopaedics*. St. Louis: Mosby.

Dell, D.D, & Regan, R. (1987). Juvenile idiopathic scoliosis. *Orthopaedic Nursing, 6*(6), 23.

Drez, D., Finney, T.P., & Roberts, T.S. (1991, February). Sepsis in orthopedic surgery. *Orthopedics, 14,* 157.

Gustilo, R., Kyle, R., & Templeman, D. (1993). *Fractures and dislocations.* St. Louis; Mosby.

Howmedica. (1979). *Surgical Simplex P.* Rutherford, N.J.

Kneedler, J., & Dodge, G. (1983). *Perioperative patient care: The nursing perspective.* St. Louis: Blackwell.

Licata, A.O. (1988). Some thoughts on osteoporosis in women. *Cleveland Clinic Journal of Medicine, 55*(3), 233.

McQuarrie, D.G., et al. (1990). Laminar airflow systems: Issues surrounding their effectiveness. *AORN Journal, 51,* 1035.

Mourad, L.A. (1991). *Orthopaedic disorders.* St. Louis: Mosby.

Sherk, H.H. (1990). *Lasers in orthopaedics.* Philadelphia: J.B. Lippincott.

Smith, J.E. (1990). Applying the continuous passive motion device. *Orthopaedic Nursing, 9*(3), 54.

Thibodeau, G.A., & Patton, K.T. (1993). *Anatomy and physiology* (2nd ed.). St. Louis: Mosby.

Walsh, C.R. (1991). Collaborative practice: A coordinated approach to patient care. *Orthopedic Nursing, 10,* 52.

BIBLIOGRAPHY

Barrett, J., and Bryant, B.H. (1990, August). Fractures: Types, treatment, perioperative implications. *AORN Journal, 52,* 350.

Buckham, K.R. (1989, October). Surgical bone banking: Recommendations for setting up a program. *AORN Journal, 50,* 4.

Gaehle, K., et al. (1991, September). Adult lumbar scoliosis: Treatment with combined anterior-posterior spinal fusion. *AORN Journal, 54,* 546.

Good, L.P. (1992). Compartment syndrome: a closer look at etiology and treatment. *AORN Journal, 56.*

Green, S.A. (1989). Ilizarov methods: Innovations from a Siberian surgeon. *AORN Journal, 49,* 215.

Hales, A.L. (1989). Arthroscopically assisted anterior cruciate ligament reconstruction. *AORN Journal, 49,* 234.

Hampel, G. (1988). Closed interlocking nailing in the lower extremity. *AORN Journal, 47,* 1203.

Hester, R., & Nelson, C. Current concepts review: Methods to reduce intraoperative transmission of blood-borne disease. *The Journal of Bone and Joint Surgery, 73-A,* 1108.

Johnson, L.L. (1993). *Diagnostic and surgical arthroscopy: The knee and other joints.* St. Louis: Mosby.

Jones, L., & Brooks, J. (1990). The ABV's of PCA. *RN, 20*(5), 54.

Kneedler, J., & Dodge, G. (1983). *Perioperative patient care: The nursing perspective.* St. Louis: Blackwell.

Laurin, C., Riley, L.H., & Roy-Camille, R. (1991). *Atlas of orthopaedic surgery.* St. Louis: Mosby.

Lilliott, N. (1991). Discharge instructions: Advice for knee and shoulder arthroscopy outpatients. *AORN Journal, 54.*

Lopez, J.O., and Silva, I. (1988). Shoulder arthroscopy: A diagnostic and therapeutic tool. *AORN Journal, 48,* 1078.

Malawer, M.M., et al. (1991). Postoperative infusional continuous regional analgesia. A technique for relief of postoperative pain following major extremity surgery. *Clinical Orthopaedics and Related Research, 266,* 277.

Monk, H.L. (1993, April). Fractures are never simple. *RN.*

Musclow, E.C. Bone and tissue banking from Czitrom A.A. & Gross A.E. ed (1992). Allografts in Orthopaedic Practice. Baltimore: Williams and Wilkins.

Pagana, K.D., & Pagana, T.J. (1992). *Diagnostic and laboratory test reference.* St. Louis; Mosby.

Phipps, W.J. et al. (1995). *Medical-surgical nursing: Concepts and clinical practice* (5th ed.), St. Louis: Mosby.

Renshaw, T.S. (1988, April). The role of Harrington instrumentation and posterior spine fusion in the management of adolescent idiopathic scoliosis. *Orthopedic Clinics of North America, 19,* 257.

Rosman, M., and Brown, K. (1991). Preoperative Ilizarov frame construction for correction of ankle and foot deformities. *Journal of Pediatric Orthopaedics, 11,* 238.

Slye, D. (1991, March). Orthopedic complication, compartment syndrome, fat embolism syndrome, and venous thromboembolism. *Orthopaedic Nursing, 26,* 113.

Tate, D.E., Friedman, R.J. (1992). Blood conservation in spinal surgery: Review of current techniques. *Spine , 17*(12), 1450.

Taylor, G.J.S., Bannister, G.C., & Calder, S. (1990). Perioperative wound infection in elective orthopaedic surgery. *Journal of Hospital Infection, 16,* 241.

Wasilewski, S.A., et al. (1990, March). Value of continuous passive motion in total knee arthroplasty. *Orthopedics, 13.*

Woodin, L.M. (1993, August). Cutting postop pain. *RN.*

22

NEUROSURGERY

RUTH E. VAIDEN

Perioperative nurses must understand the structure and function of the nervous system to provide intelligent, safe, humanistic care for neurosurgical patients. From a range of variables of normal development, they must identify those critical for each patient and recognize and respond to a variety of dependency needs, such as the normal response to preoperative sedation, as well as pathologic conditions such as paralysis, aphasia, and coma. Based on an understanding of the many pathologic conditions that result in surgical intervention, they must plan and manage complex patient care. They must be familiar with the use, care, working order, and safety factors of sophisticated instrumentation. They need to appreciate the limitations and stresses facing neurosurgeons. Anticipating and responding to potential complications inherent in specific patients, procedures, and neurosurgical emergencies require great speed but the same care and precision as elective situations. Basic general information to assist perioperative nurses to function effectively in their own clinical settings is presented here.

SURGICAL ANATOMY

The nervous system, the most complex and least understood of body systems, has been divided in various ways to simplify study. Structural divisions are the central nervous system (brain and spinal cord) and the peripheral nervous system (cranial and spinal nerves).

Nervous system tissue is composed of neurons and neuroglial cells that support the neurons. The brain and spinal cord are protected by bony structures. The cranial nerves originate within the brain and emerge through openings in the skull to run peripherally. The spinal nerves that emerge from the spinal cord through the vertebral foramina also run peripherally. In this chapter, therefore, peripheral nerves are those outside the cranial cavity and vertebral canal.

The nervous system is divided functionally into voluntary and autonomic (involuntary) systems. The nervous system functions as the communication system for the rest of the body. The functions of all body systems are dependent,

in part, on nervous system function. In turn, the nervous system is directly dependent on circulatory system function for life-sustaining glucose and oxygen. Nervous system functions include orientation, coordination, conceptual thought, emotion, memory, and reflex response.

Within the framework of neurosurgical techniques, logical divisions of the nervous system are the head, or cranium; the back, or spine; and the peripheral nerves. These subdivisions lend themselves to meaningful discussion of supporting structures, body positions, instrumentation, and other considerations useful to the nurse providing care for neurosurgical patients during the intraoperative phase of care.

HEAD

Scalp layers of the head (Fig. 22-1) include skin, subcutaneous tissue, galea, and occipitofrontal musculature. Scalp skin is thick. The subcutaneous tissue, which is exceptionally dense, tough, and vascular, is firmly attached to the galea. Most of the blood vessels lie superficial to the galea. The subgaleal space contains loose areolar tissue that permits mobility of the scalp. It is in this bloodless plane that the standard craniotomy scalp flap is hinged. The pericranium, or outer periosteum of the skull, separates the galea from the cranium.

The arterial supply of the scalp comes from the external carotid artery through the superficial temporal, posterior auricular, occipital, frontal, and supraorbital branches. Most veins roughly follow the course of the arteries, except emissary veins that drain directly through the skull into the intracranial venous sinuses. Unlike the arteries, the surface veins of the brain have many large anastomoses. The scalp, the extracranial arteries, and portions of the dura mater are the only pain-sensitive structures that cover the brain. The brain itself is insensate.

The skull is formed by 24 bones, joined by serrated bony seams called sutures. Eight bones form the walls of the cranial cavity, which houses the brain. There are four single bones—frontal, occipital, ethmoid, and sphenoid—and four paired bones—temporal and parietal (Fig. 22-2). The

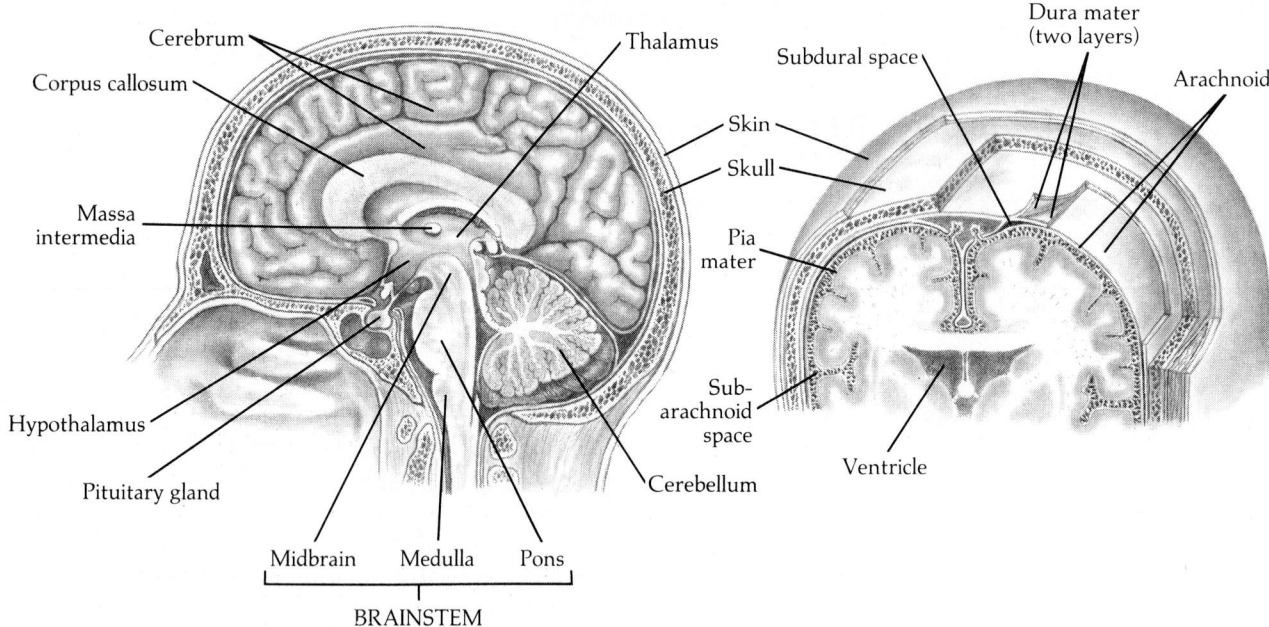

FIG. 22-1   Scalp is composed of following layers: skin, subcutaneous tissue, galea, and periosteum of skull. Skull bone has three tables: outer, diplöe or spongy layer, and inner. Dura mater lies beneath skull and completely encapsulates brain. Other structures are identified for reference and are described in text.

Modified from Anthony, C.P., & Kolthoff, J.N. (1983). *Textbook of anatomy and physiology* (11th ed.). St. Louis: Mosby.

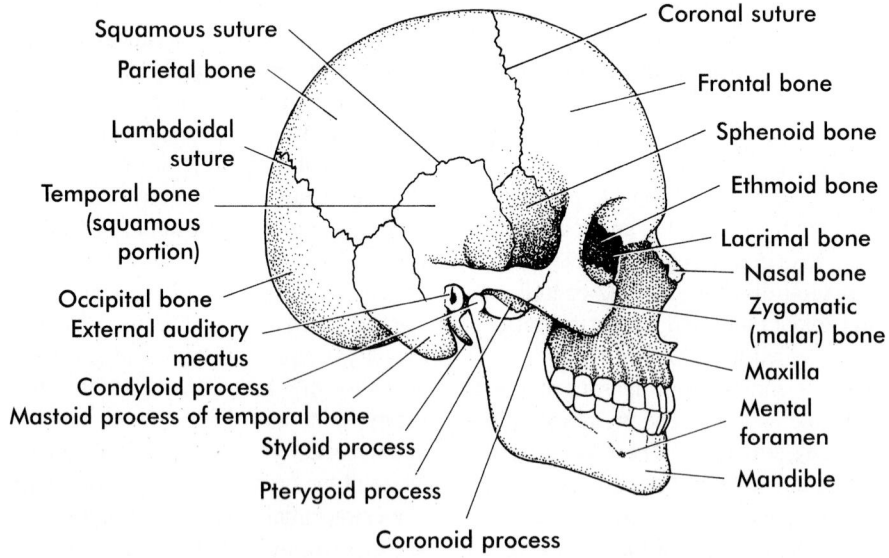

FIG. 22-2   Skull viewed from right side.

From Anthony, C.P., & Kolthoff, N.J. (1975). *Textbook of anatomy and physiology* (9th ed.). St. Louis: Mosby.

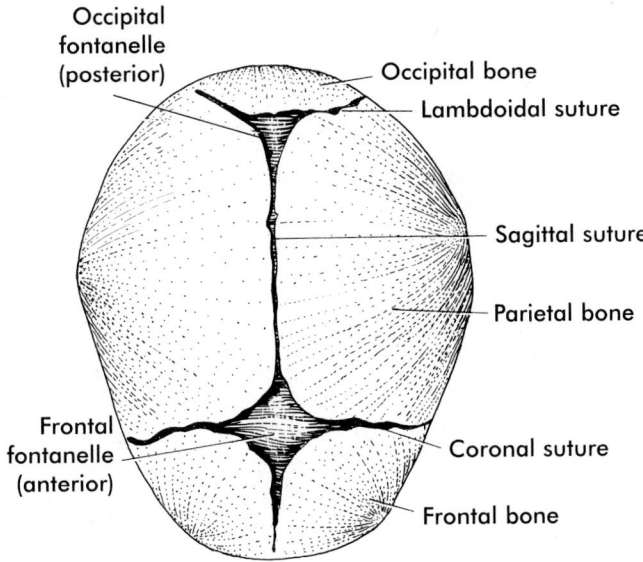

FIG. 22-3 Skull at birth viewed from above.

Modified from Anthony, C.P., & Kolthoff, N.J. (1983). *Textbook of anatomy and physiology* (11th ed.). St. Louis: Mosby.

coronal suture joins the frontal and parietal bones. The squamous sutures border the squamous part of the temporal bones. The lambdoid suture joins the occipital and parietal bones. The sagittal suture lies in the medial plane and joins the two parietal bones (Fig. 22-3).

At the top of the skull in front of and behind the parietal bones are the anterior and posterior fontanelles, which are open at birth. The posterior fontanelle is closed by 2 months and the anterior by about 18 months after birth. If the suture lines close prematurely, the skull cannot expand as the brain grows. This condition, craniosynostosis, may demand early surgical intervention.

The skull is ovoid and is wider in back than in front. The flattened, irregular bones consist of two tables of compact bone that enclose a layer of spongy bone, or *diplöe* (see Fig. 22-1).

The interior of the skull is anatomically divided into three cranial fossae: anterior, middle, and posterior (Fig. 22-4). The anterior fossa is limited posteriorly by the sphenoid ridge, along which pituitary tumors and aneurysms of the circle of Willis are generally approached. The frontal lobes and olfactory bulbs and tracts lie in the anterior fossa. The temporal lobes lie in the middle fossa, which is shaped like a butterfly. The sella turcica, formed by the sphenoid bone, is the most central part of the middle fossa and houses the pituitary gland. The floor and lateral walls of the middle fossa are shaped from the greater wings of the sphenoid bone and parts of the temporal bone, which house the internal and middle ear structures (Fig. 22-4). The posterior fossa, the largest and deepest fossa, is formed by the occipital, sphenoid, and petrous portions of the temporal

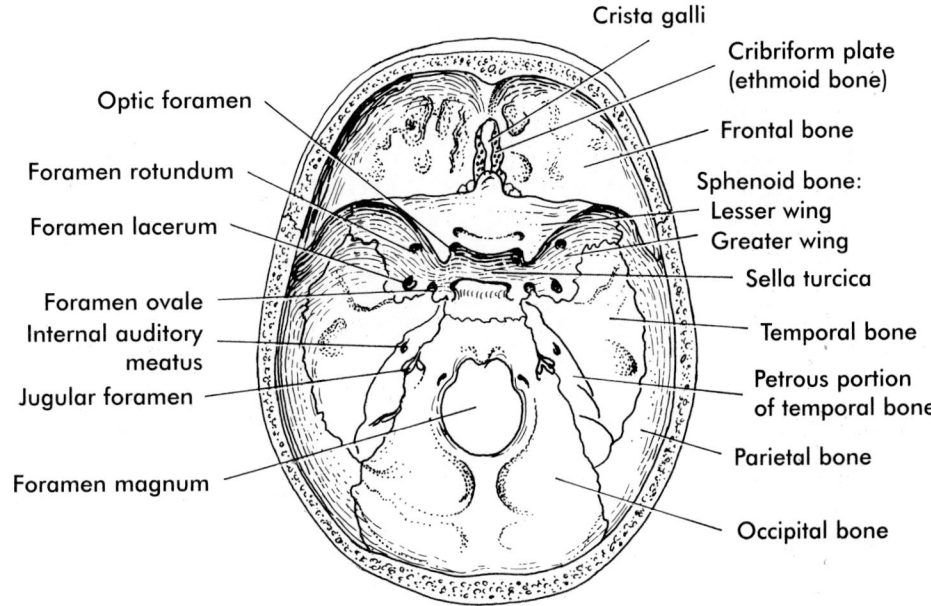

FIG. 22-4 Floor of cranial cavity.

Modified from Anthony, C.P., & Kolthoff, N.J. (1983). *Textbook of anatomy and physiology* (11th ed.). St. Louis: Mosby.

bones; the cerebellum, pons, and medulla lie here, as do many cranial nerves. The foramen magnum, the largest opening in the skull, permits the spinal cord to join the brainstem in the posterior fossa. There are numerous other openings in the base of the skull for passage of arteries, veins, and cranial nerves (see Fig. 22-4).

Between the skull and brain are the meninges, three covering membranes: the dura mater, arachnoid, and pia mater (see Fig. 22-1). The dura mater is a tough, shiny, fibrous membrane that is close to the inner surface of the skull and folds to separate the cranial cavity into compartments. The largest fold is the falx cerebri (see Fig. 22-1), an arch-shaped, vertically placed, midline structure separating the right and left cerebral hemispheres. A smaller fold of dura mater, the falx cerebelli, separates the cerebellar hemispheres vertically. A transverse fold, the tentorium cerebelli, forms the roof of the posterior fossa. The tentorium supports the temporal lobe and occipital lobes of the cerebral hemispheres. Below the tentorium lie the cerebellum and brainstem. Structures above the tentorium are referred to as supratentorial, and those below as infratentorial (Fig. 22-5). At margins of these dural folds lie large venous sinuses that drain blood from the intracranial struc-

tures into the jugular veins. Several arteries also lie within the layers of the dura. The largest is the middle meningeal, a source of serious epidural hemorrhage if torn by an overlying skull fracture. The rigid skull makes hemorrhage and swelling in the brain critical. The volume of the intracranial cavity is fixed. Increasing the intracranial contents by a hemorrhage, tumor, or edema can lead to serious intracranial pressure problems. Pressure on brain tissue may cause irreparable damage.

Beneath the dura mater is a fine membrane, the arachnoid. The outer layer of arachnoid closely approximates the dura mater. The inner layer forms innumerable weblike filaments that bridge to the surface of the brain (see Fig. 22-1). The outer surface of the arachnoid membrane adheres closely to the dura mater with no space normally between the two membranes. The inner surface is separated from the pia mater beneath it by the subarachnoid space, which is filled with cerebrospinal fluid that bathes the brain. Around the base of the brain, particularly, this space becomes enlarged to form cisterns. The major intracranial nerves and blood vessels pass through these compartments. Intracranial approaches can be charted in terms of the basal cisterns.

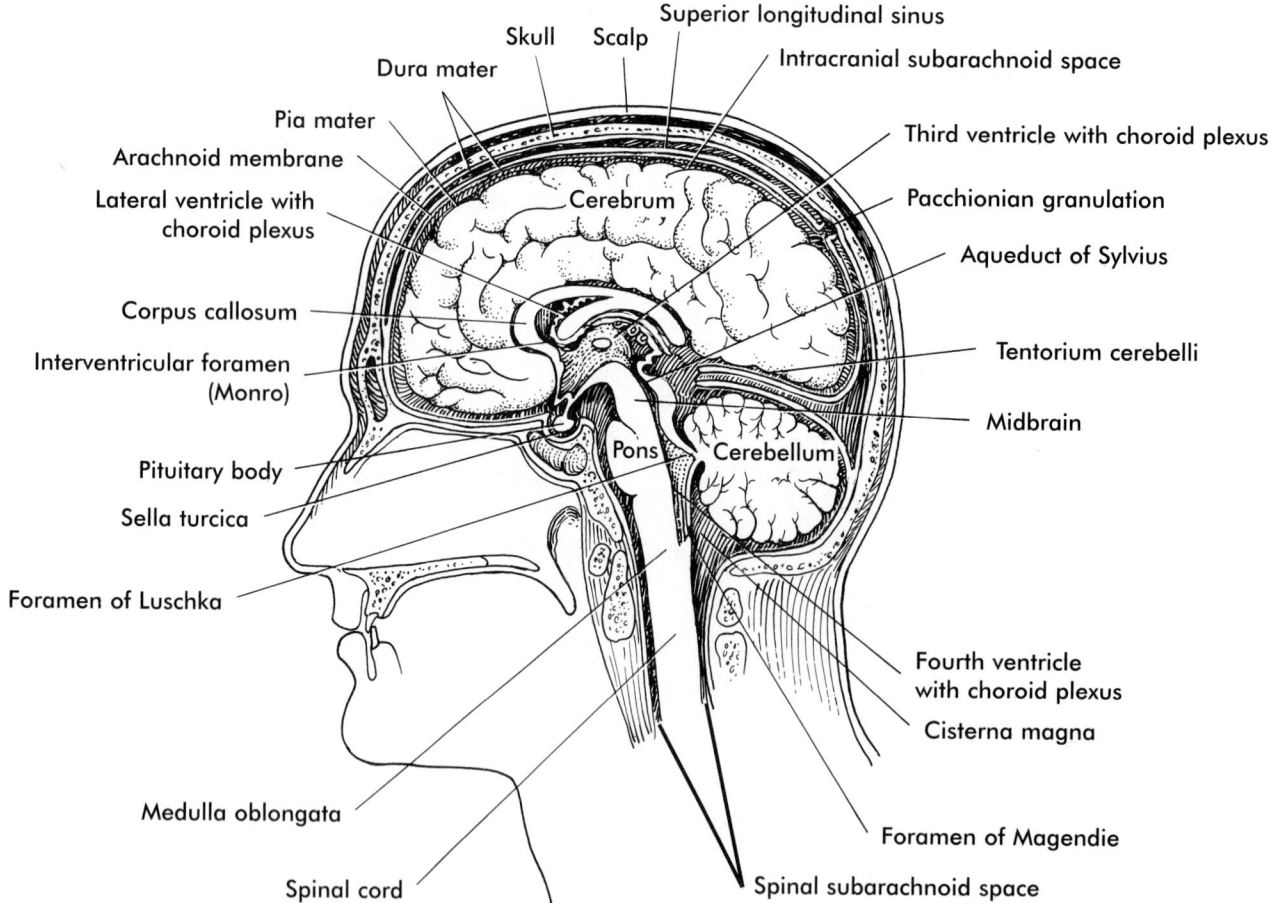

FIG. 22-5 Sagittal section of head showing cerebrospinal fluid spaces and their relationship to venous circulation and principal subdivision of the brain and its coverings.

From Conway-Rutkowski, B.L. (1982). *Carini and Owens' neurological and neurosurgical nursing* (8th ed.). St. Louis: Mosby.

The pia mater, the innermost membrane, is like gossamer and attaches to the gray matter, dipping into the sulci and gyri. The pia mater has a rich vascular network that helps form the choroid plexus of the ventricles.

The brain is divided into the cerebral cortex, basal ganglia, hypothalamus, midbrain, brainstem, and cerebellum (Figs. 22-5 and 22-6).

The right and left cerebral hemispheres are the largest parts of the brain. Each hemisphere is composed of cerebral cortex and is divided into frontal, parietal, occipital, and temporal lobes, insula, rhinencephalon, basal ganglia, and hypothalamus. The two hemispheres are divided by a longitudinal fissure and joined underneath the falx by a large transverse bundle of nerve fibers, the corpus callosum (see Fig. 22-6). Each of the cerebral hemispheres controls sensation and motor activity to and receives sensory stimuli from the opposite half of the body.

The surfaces of the hemispheres form convolutions called gyri and intervening furrows called sulci. Two sulci of anatomic importance to the surgeon are the central sulcus, or fissure of Rolando, which separates the motor from the sensory cortex, and the lateral sulcus, or fissure of Sylvius, which marks off the temporal lobe (Fig. 22-7). The insula (island of Reil) lies deep within the fissure of Sylvius and can be exposed by separating the upper and lower lips of the fissure. The frontal lobe is anterior to the fissure of Rolando and controls the higher functions of intellect and abstract reasoning. The motor cortex lies anterior to the fissure of Rolando. Destruction leads to loss of voluntary motor function on the opposite side of the body (Fig. 22-8).

Posterior to the fissure of Rolando is the parietal lobe, extending back to the parietooccipital fissure. This area contains the final receiving and integrating station for sensory impulses from the contralateral side of the body. The occipital lobe lies posterior to the parietooccipital fissure. It receives and integrates visual impulses and registers them as meaningful images (see Figs. 22-7 and 22-8).

Inferior to the fissure of Sylvius, in the middle fossa, is the temporal lobe. Lesions of the left temporal lobe in right-handed individuals and in many left-handed persons may affect the comprehension and verbalization of words, resulting in aphasia. Rhinencephalic structures, such as the anterior limbic area, may exert an inhibitory effect on brain mechanisms in the expression of emotions, such as anger. Restlessness and hyperactivity may result from lesions of this area. The rhinencephalon has many connections with the hypothalamus. Malfunctions may affect sexual behavior, emotions, and motivation. Loss of recent memory may indicate a lesion of this area.

The convoluted surface of the cerebrum consists of gray matter, the cerebral cortex, which contains the cell bodies of the many nerve pathways of the brain. The underlying

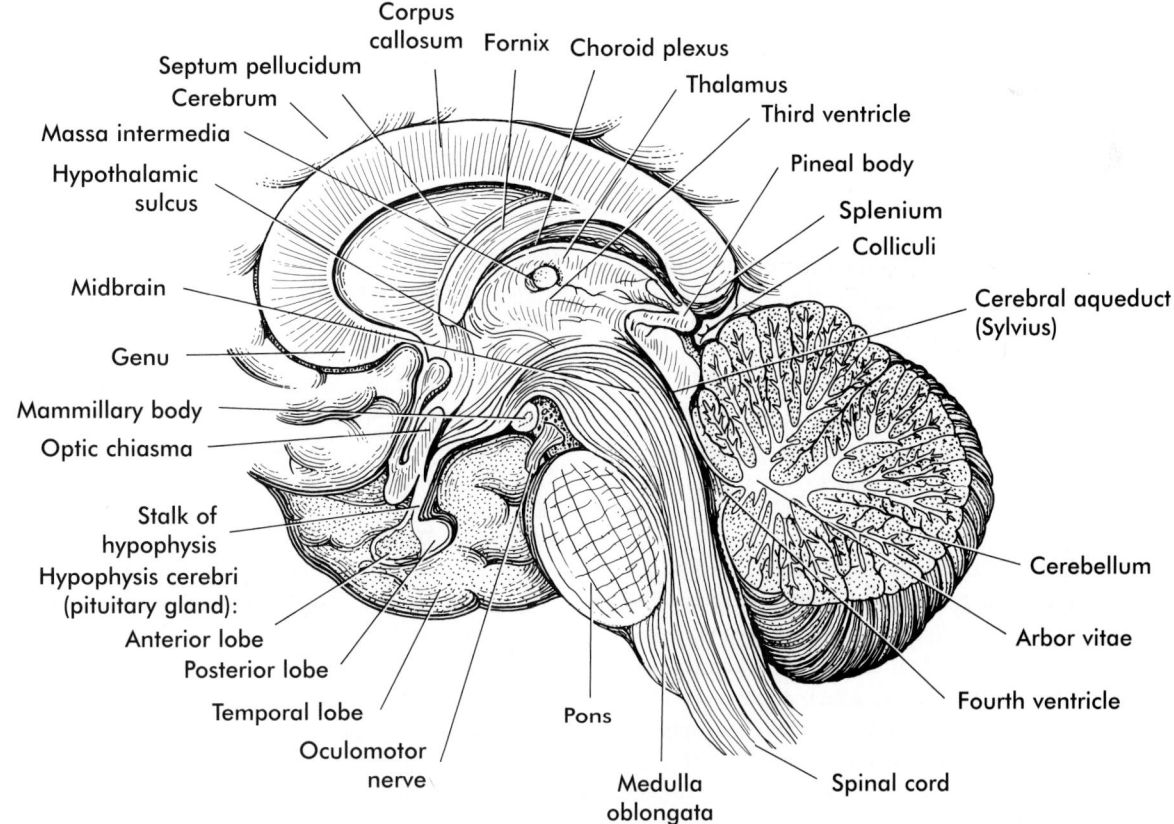

FIG. 22-6 Sagittal section through midline of brain showing structures around third ventricle including corpus callosum, thalamus, and hypothalamus.

From Anthony, C.P., & Kolthoff, N.J. (1975). *Textbook of anatomy and physiology* (9th ed.). St. Louis: Mosby.

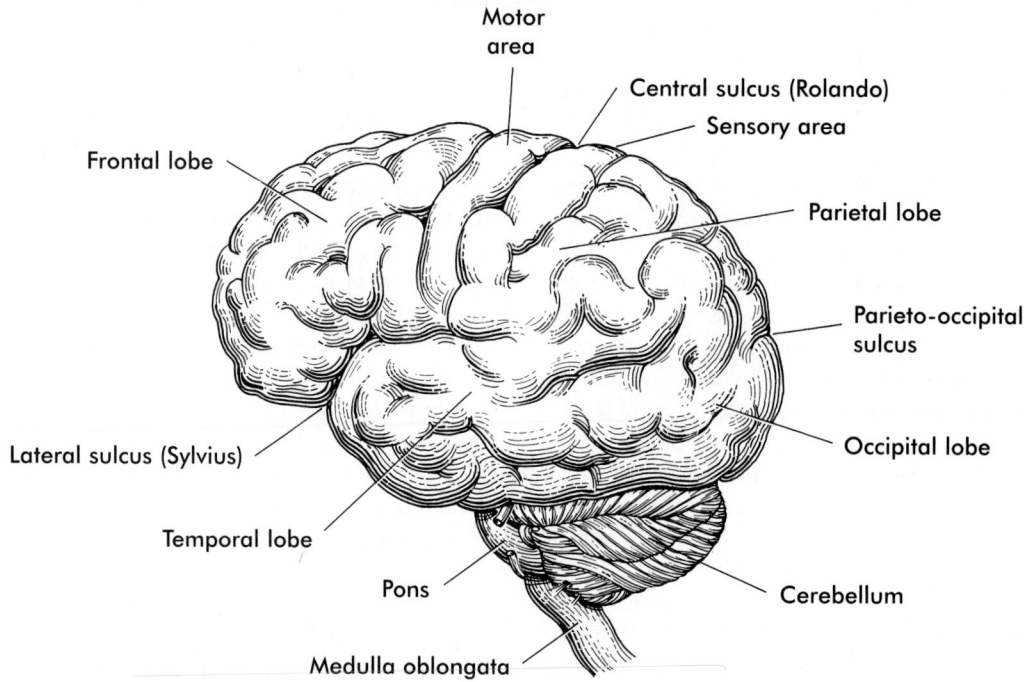

FIG. 22-7   Lateral view of cerebral hemisphere (showing lobes and principal fissures), cerebellum, pons, and medulla oblongata.

From Conway-Rutkowski, B.L. (1982). *Carini and Owens' neurological and neurosurgical nursing* (8th ed.). St. Louis: Mosby.

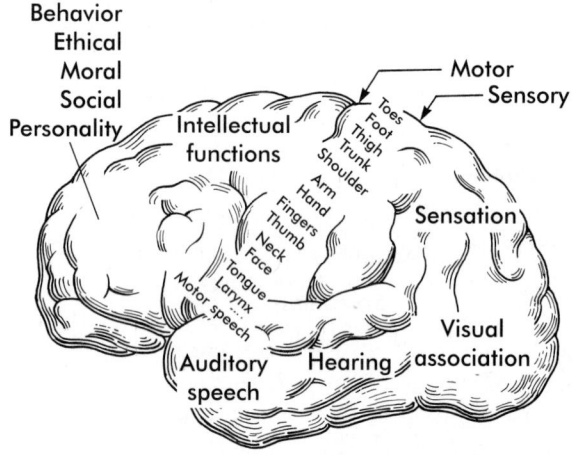

FIG. 22-8   Principal functional subdivisions of cerebral hemispheres.

Modified from Conway, B.L. (1982). *Carini and Owens' neurological and neurosurgical nursing* (8th ed.). St. Louis: Mosby.

white matter contains millions of myelinated nerve axons and is relatively avascular compared with the cortex. The nerve pathways, or fiber tracts, are of three types: (1) commissural fibers, which pass from one cerebral hemisphere to the other; (2) association fibers, which connect gyri regions and lobes longitudinally within a cerebral hemisphere; and (3) projection fibers, including the great motor and sensory systems, which run vertically to connect the cortical regions with other portions of the central nervous system.

In prefrontal lobotomy, association fibers in the frontal lobe were divided to effect changes in personality that may

be beneficial in certain psychiatric disorders. Cingulotomy, in which the cingulum is interrupted, also may be performed for treatment of these disorders.

Deep in the brain are five basal ganglia, or collections of nuclei, of the extrapyramidal system. Three of them, the caudate nucleus, putamen, and globus pallidus, collectively referred to as the corpus striatum, associate with the thalamus for motor control (see Fig. 22-6). Lesions here may cause rigidity of the skeletal muscles and various types of spontaneous tremors. The basal ganglia and thalamus can be selectively destroyed surgically in an effort to relieve the tremors and rigidity associated with multiple sclerosis, Parkinson's disease, various forms of cerebellar degeneration, and late effects of severe brain trauma. In addition to rhythmic processing of brain activity and its influence on affect and higher brain activity, the thalamus is the major relay station for incoming sensory stimuli. Many of these stimuli are subsequently relayed to a final destination in the parietal cortex. Because of its central role in perception of body sensations, surgical lesions can be made in the thalamus in an attempt to alleviate pain.

Along the floor of the third ventricle is the hypothalamus (see Fig. 22-6), which is principally concerned with the autonomic regulation of the body's internal environment and is intimately connected with the pituitary gland.

The short, stocky portion of the brain, between the cerebral hemispheres and pons, is the midbrain (see Fig. 22-5), also referred to as the mesencephalon. It is made up of the cerebral peduncles, numerous nerve tracts and nuclei, and association centers that control the majority of eye

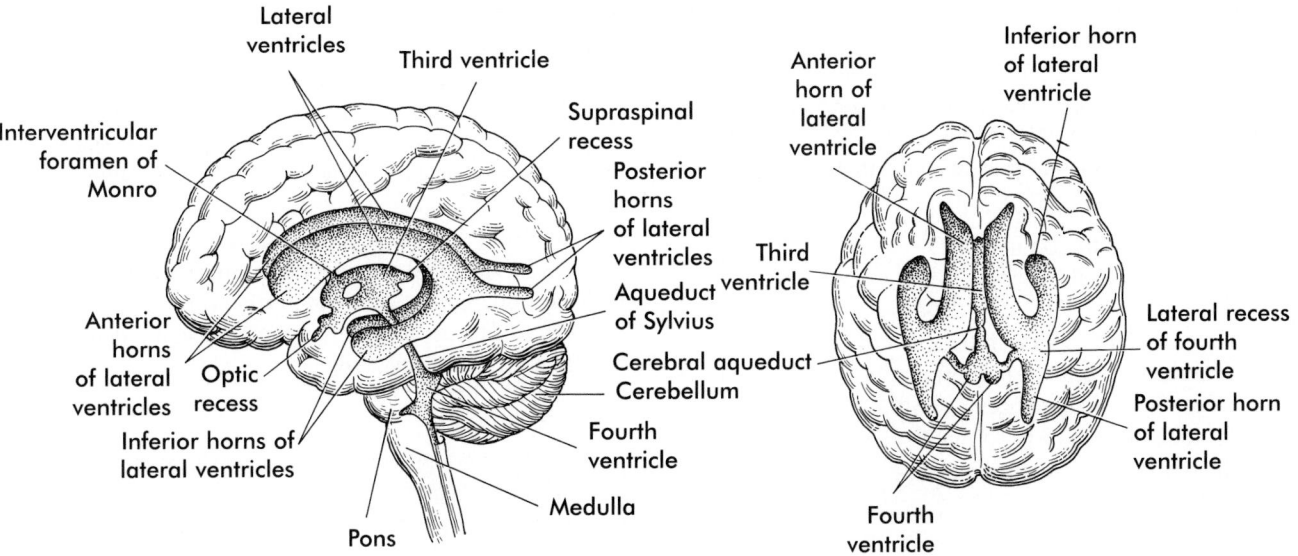

FIG. 22-9 Ventricular system showing its relationship to various parts of brain.
From Conway-Rutkowski, B.L. (1982). *Carini and Owens' neurological and neurosurgical nursing* (8th ed.). St. Louis: Mosby.

movements. The hindbrain, or brainstem, immediately below the midbrain, consists of the pons and medulla oblongata (see Fig. 22-7). The midbrain and brainstem form the floor of the fourth ventricle in the posterior fossa of the skull and contain many large efferent and afferent tracts and nuclei of most cranial nerves. The brainstem contains the cardiovascular and respiratory regulatory centers. Surgery directly on the brainstem is extremely dangerous.

The cerebellum, which occupies most of the posterior fossa, forms the roof of the fourth ventricle (see Figs. 22-6 and 22-7). It has two lateral lobes and a medial portion, the vermis. The fissures of the cerebellum are small and run transversely. The cerebellum is principally concerned with balance and coordination of movement. It has many complex connections with higher and lower centers and exerts its influence unilaterally, in contrast to the cerebral hemispheres, which act contralaterally. At least half the brain tumors in children originate in the cerebellum. In adults and children the most common surgical lesions in this area are tumors and abscesses. By splitting the vermis in the exact midline, a satisfactory exposure of tumors that lie in the fourth ventricle is obtained without sacrificing the important cerebellar functions.

Cerebrospinal fluid system

Within the brain are four communicating cavities, or ventricles, filled with cerebrospinal fluid (CSF). In the lower medial portion of each cerebral hemisphere lies a large lateral ventricle, which resembles a wishbone and is separated anteriorly from its counterpart by a thin pellucid septum (Fig. 22-9). Each lateral ventricle has a body and three horns: frontal, occipital, and temporal. Below the bodies of the lateral ventricles is a central cleft, or third ventricle. It communicates anteriorly with the lateral ventricles through the foramen of Monro and posteriorly with the fourth ventricle through the aqueduct of Sylvius, a long narrow channel passing through the midbrain. The fourth ventricle is a rhomboid cavity in the posterior fossa, between the cerebellum and the brainstem. In the roof of the fourth ventricle is the foramen of Magendie, an opening into the cisterna magna; at the lateral margins are the two foramina of Luschka, which open into the cisterna pontis.

Much of the CSF originates in the choroid plexuses of the ventricles. These are tufted, vascular structures that allow certain fluid elements of the blood to pass through their ependymal linings. Choroid plexus is found along the floor in each lateral ventricle, on the roof of the third ventricle, and in the posterior portion of the fourth ventricle. Most of the fluid is formed in the lateral ventricles and flows through the interventricular foramen of Monro to the third ventricle and through the aqueduct of Sylvius to the fourth ventricle, where it escapes into the subarachnoid space of the basal cisterns through the foramina of Magendie and Luschka. From the basal cisterns the fluid flows around the spinal cord, over the cerebellar lobes, around the medulla and the base of the brain, and over the cerebral hemispheres in the subarachnoid space. The fluid is absorbed into the venous circulation through villi of the arachnoid (pacchionian granulations) into the great dural venous sinuses, particularly the superior sagittal sinus, and by diffusion through perivascular, perineural, and periradicular channels (see Fig. 22-1).

The total amount of circulating CSF averages 125 to 150 ml in the adult. Each lateral ventricle contains 10 to 15 ml, the rest of the ventricular system contains 5 ml, the cranial subarachnoid space averages about 25 to 35 ml, and the

862　　　　　　　　　　　SURGICAL INTERVENTIONS

spinal subarachnoid space contains about 75 to 90 ml. The ventricular fluid normally has 5 to 15 mg/100 ml protein content, whereas the spinal fluid has 25 to 45 mg/100 ml. These values may be considerably elevated in pathologic conditions of the central nervous system.

The characteristics of normal spinal fluid are as follows:

- Appearance: clear and colorless
- Pressure: 70 to 200 mm H$_2$O
- pH: 7.35 to 7.4
- Specific gravity: 1.005 to 1.009
- Glucose: 50 to 75 mg/100 ml (⅔ of blood sugar)
- Chlorides: 120 to 130 mEq/L
- Cells: 0 to 10 (lymphocytes only)
- Protein: lumbar 15 to 45 mg/dl; cisternal 10 to 25 mg/dl; ventricular 5 to 15 mg/dl
- Culture: negative
- Gamma globulin: 6% to 13% of total protein

Spinal fluid bathes the brain and spinal cord, helps support the weight of the brain, and acts as a cushion for the brain and spinal cord by absorbing some of the force of external trauma. By variation in its volume, it aids in keeping intracranial pressure relatively constant. If the brain atrophies, the CSF increases in amount to fill the dead space; if the brain swells, the CSF decreases in amount to compensate for the increase in brain mass. The fluid can carry certain drugs to diseased parts of the brain. It does not, however, play a significant role in supplying nutrition to the structures that it bathes.

The rate of absorption of CSF is related to the osmotic and hydrostatic pressure of the blood. When intracranial pressure rises, an intravenous injection of hypertonic mannitol or a nonosmotic diuretic is employed to dehydrate the blood and decrease the volume of CSF.

Elevations in CSF pressure can be caused by an expanding mass within the skull, such as a tumor, hemorrhage, or cerebral edema; an increase in formation of fluid, as in meningitis, encephalitis, and other febrile conditions; an increase in venous pressure within the skull from an obstruction to normal venous drainage; a blockage of absorption by inflammatory conditions of the arachnoid and perivascular spaces; any mechanical obstruction of the ventricular or subarachnoidal fluid pathways; or problems with the absorption of CSF. Increase in CSF production or decrease in CSF absorption can lead to hydrocephalus. Hydrocephalus can be classified as either communicative (normal CSF pathways open) or noncommunicative (obstruction of CSF pathways). The appropriate surgical procedure depends on the precise type of hydrocephalus.

Blood supply

The arterial supply to the brain, which requires 20% more oxygen than any other organ, enters the cranium through the two internal carotid arteries anteriorly and the two vertebral arteries posteriorly. These communicate at the base of the brain through the circle of Willis (Fig. 22-10), which ensures continuity of the circulation if any one of the four main channels is interrupted. However, these connections are extremely variable and do not always have functional anastomoses. The main branches for distribution of blood to each hemisphere of the brain from the internal carotid arteries are the anterior and middle cerebral arteries. Each artery nourishes a specific area of the brain (Fig. 22-11). The anterior cerebral artery supplies the anterior two thirds of the medial surface and adjacent region over the convexity of the hemisphere, thus including about half of the frontal and parietal lobes. The middle cerebral artery supplies most of the lateral surface of the hemisphere, including half of the frontal, parietal, and temporal lobes. The posterior cerebral artery, which originates off the basilar artery, supplies the occipital lobe and the remaining half of the temporal lobe, principally on the inferior and medial surfaces. The brainstem and cerebellum are supplied by branches of the basilar and vertebral arteries.

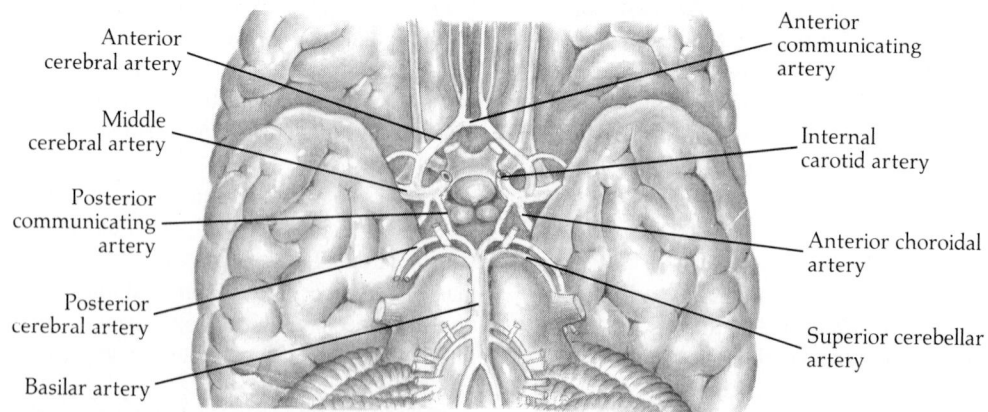

FIG. 22-10　Principal cerebral arteries and circle of Willis.
From Conway-Rutkowski, B.L. (1982). *Carini and Owens' neurological and neurosurgical nursing* (8th ed.). St. Louis: Mosby.

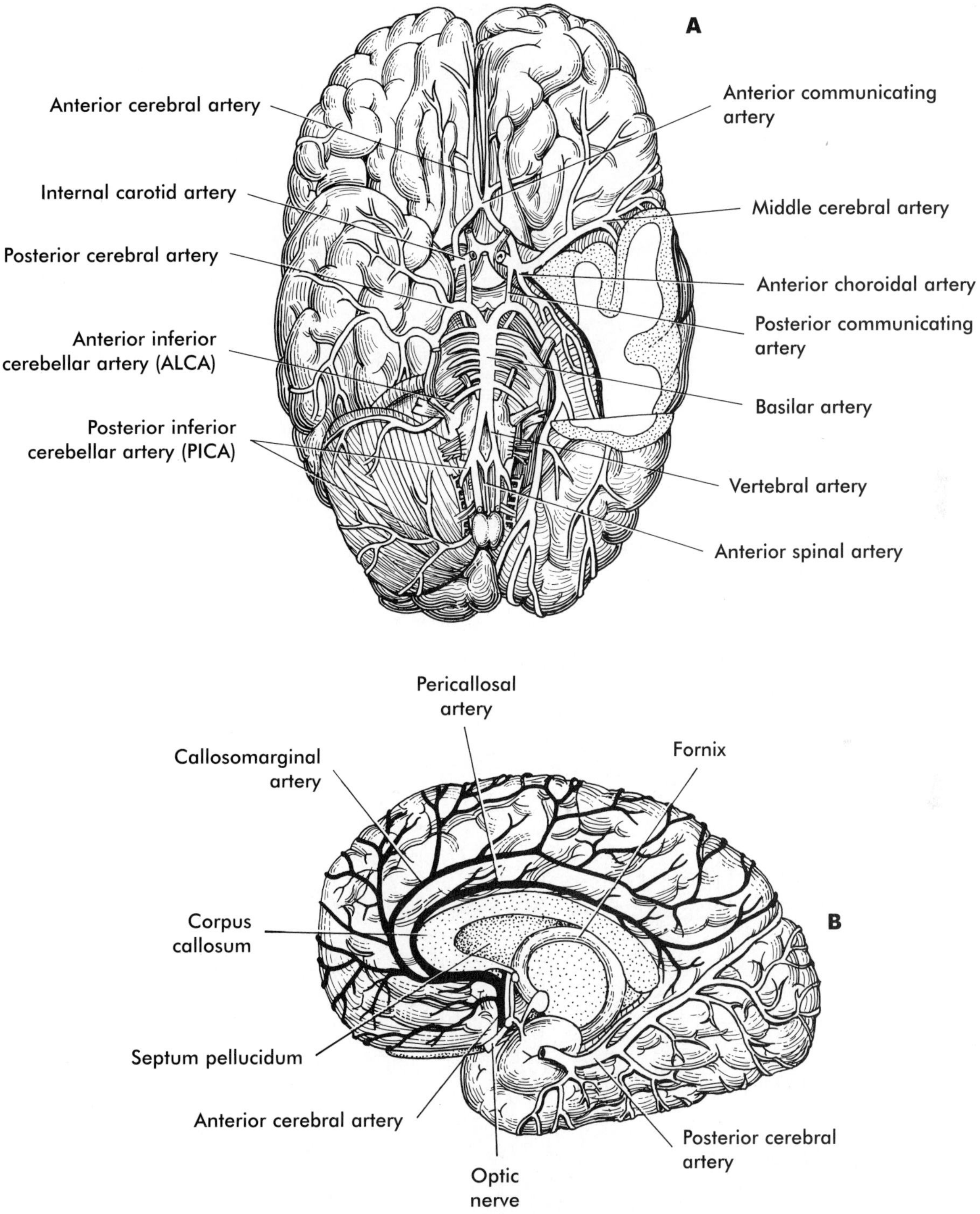

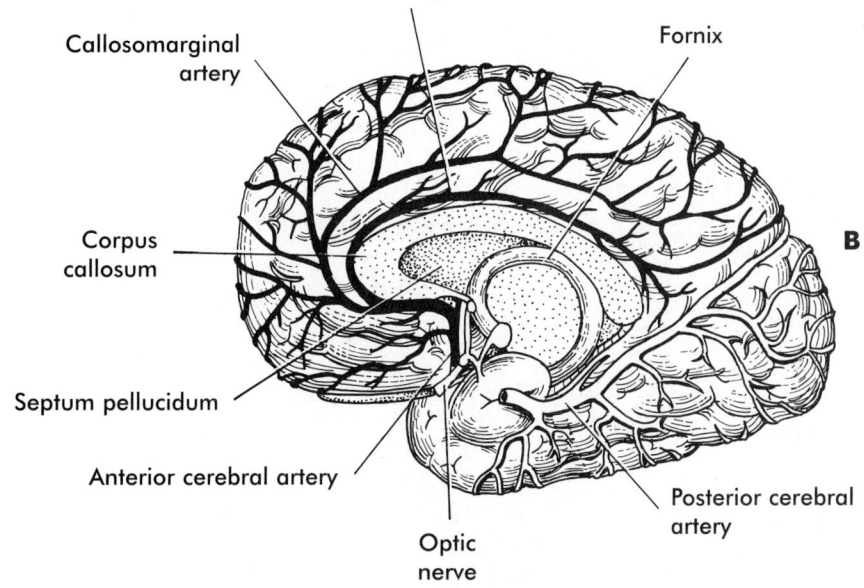

Anterior cerebral artery

Internal carotid artery

Posterior cerebral artery

Anterior inferior
cerebellar artery (ALCA)

Posterior inferior
cerebellar artery (PICA)

Anterior communicating
artery

Middle cerebral artery

Anterior choroidal artery

Posterior communicating
artery

Basilar artery

Vertebral artery

Anterior spinal artery

Pericallosal
artery

Callosomarginal
artery

Corpus
callosum

Septum pellucidum

Anterior cerebral artery

Optic
nerve

Fornix

Posterior cerebral
artery

FIG. 22-11 **A,** Arteries of the inferior surface of the brain. Left half of cerebellum and part of left
temporal lobe have been removed. **B,** Arteries of medial surface of brain. Anterior cerebral artery and its
branches are shown in black; posterior cerebral artery and its branches are shown in white.

From Nolte, J. (1988). *The human brain: An introduction to its fundamental anatomy* (2nd ed.). St. Louis: Mosby.

Continued.

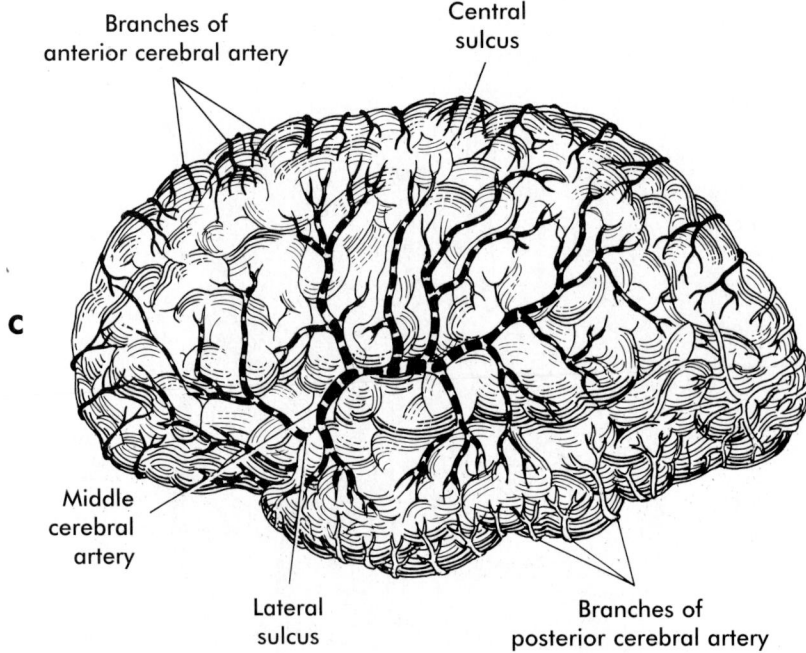

Branches of anterior cerebral artery

Central sulcus

C

Middle cerebral artery

Lateral sulcus

Branches of posterior cerebral artery

FIG. 22-11, CONT'D **C,** Arteries of lateral surface of brain. Middle cerebral artery and its branches are shown striped; small branches of anterior cerebral artery reaching around from medial surface are shown in black; those of posterior cerebral artery are shown in white.

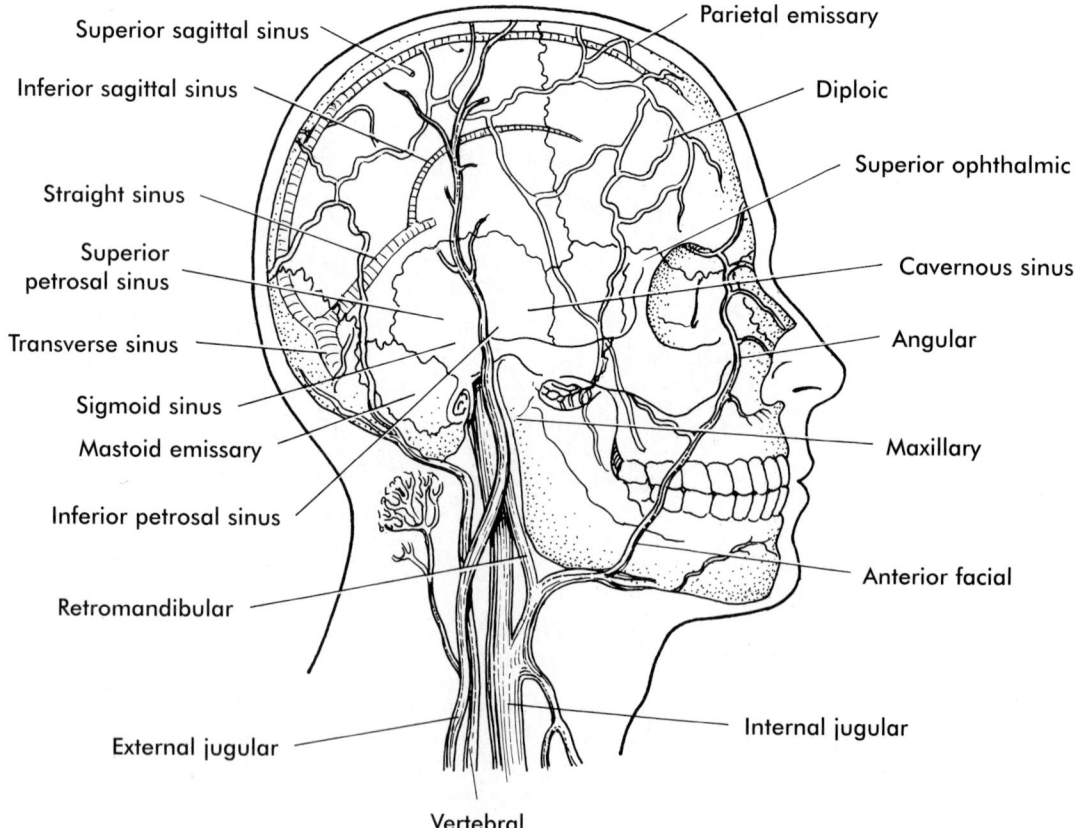

Superior sagittal sinus

Inferior sagittal sinus

Straight sinus

Superior petrosal sinus

Transverse sinus

Sigmoid sinus

Mastoid emissary

Inferior petrosal sinus

Retromandibular

External jugular

Vertebral

Parietal emissary

Diploic

Superior ophthalmic

Cavernous sinus

Angular

Maxillary

Anterior facial

Internal jugular

FIG. 22-12 Semischematic projection of large veins of head. Deep veins and dural sinuses are projected on skull. Note connection (emissary veins) between superficial and deep veins.

From Anthony, C.P., & Thibodeau, G.A. (1983). *Textbook of anatomy and physiology* (11th ed.) St. Louis: Mosby.

The circle of Willis is of particular interest surgically because of the development of aneurysms in this area. An aneurysm is a dilatation in the wall of a large artery. Aneurysms usually develop in or near the crotch of a bifurcation of the circle of Willis. It is thought that the weakness develops because of the superimposition of two lesions: a congenital absence of the media and a degeneration of the internal elastic lamina that normally strengthens the arterial wall. Erosion of the lamina results from the wear and tear of pulsatile pressure.

The most common sites of intracranial aneurysms are (1) adjacent to the anterior communicating artery, (2) at the junction of the posterior communicating artery and the internal carotid artery, (3) at the origin of the anterior cerebral arteries, (4) at the first bifurcation of the middle cerebral artery, and (5) on the basilar arteries.

The cerebral veins do not parallel the arteries as do the veins in most other parts of the body. The external cortical veins anastomose freely in the pia mater, forming larger cerebral veins, and as such they pierce the arachnoid membrane, cross the subdural space, and empty into the great dural venous sinuses. A subdural hemorrhage following head trauma may arise from disruption of these bridging vessels; an epidural hemorrhage often results from lacerations of the middle meningeal artery, a branch of the external carotid artery that supplies the dura mater. The deep cerebral veins, which drain the interior of the hemispheres, empty principally into the great vein of Galen and the inferior sagittal sinus (Figs. 22-12 and 22-13).

The blood transports oxygen, nutrients, and other substances necessary for the proper functioning of living tissue. The needs of the brain for oxygen and glucose are critical. The brain can store only small amounts of oxygen and energy-producing nutrients. Constant flow of blood to the brain must be maintained.

The brain uses oxygen in the metabolism of glucose, the chief source of energy. Protein and fat metabolism plays little part in energy production. In the face of an oxygen deficit, the survival time of central nervous system tissue is very short. In the face of low blood sugar, central nervous system function is compromised and unconsciousness results.

Generally, all factors affecting the systemic blood pressure indirectly affect the cerebral circulation. The brain normally receives 20% of the cardiac output. The cerebral blood flow is kept constant by an autoregulation phenomenon such that increases in blood pressure lead to vasoconstriction of cerebral arteries, and decreases in blood pressure cause cerebral vasodilatation to maintain a relatively constant cerebral blood flow. When the mean arterial pressure falls below 60 mm Hg, the autoregulation mechanism usually fails. Thus controlled hypotension may be safely used in intracranial surgery.

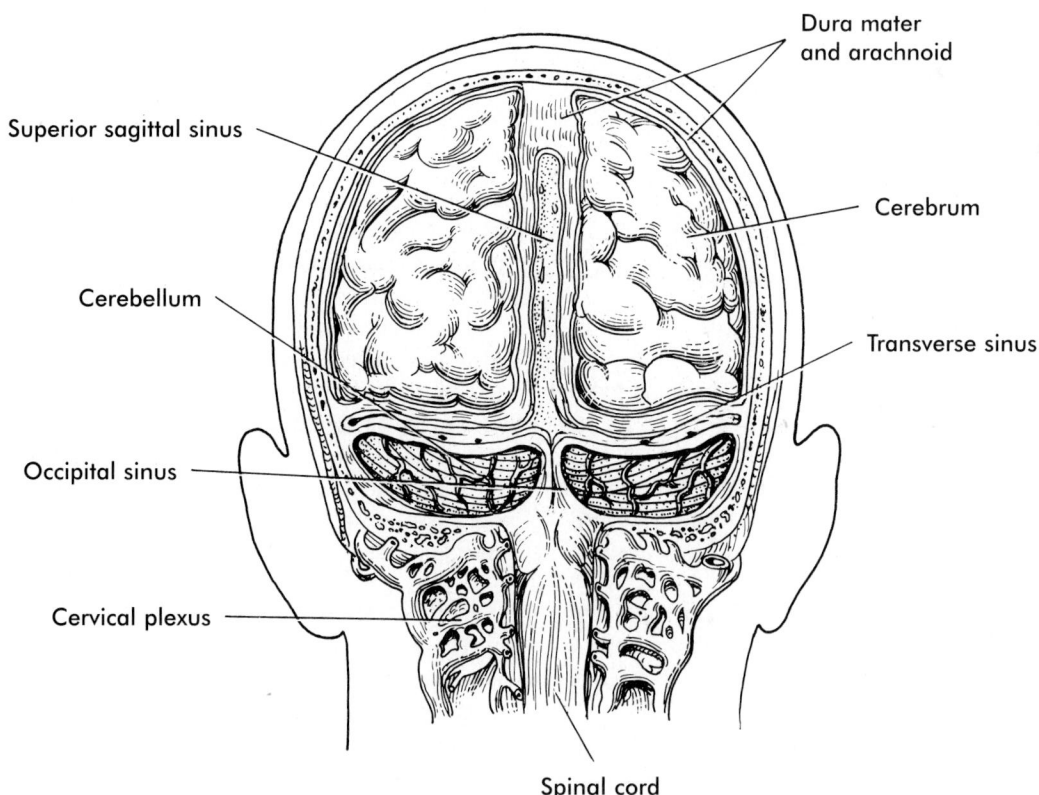

FIG. 22-13   Venous sinuses shown in relation to brain and skull.
From Anthony, C.P., & Thibodeau, G.A. (1983). *Textbook of anatomy and physiology* (11th ed.). St. Louis: Mosby.

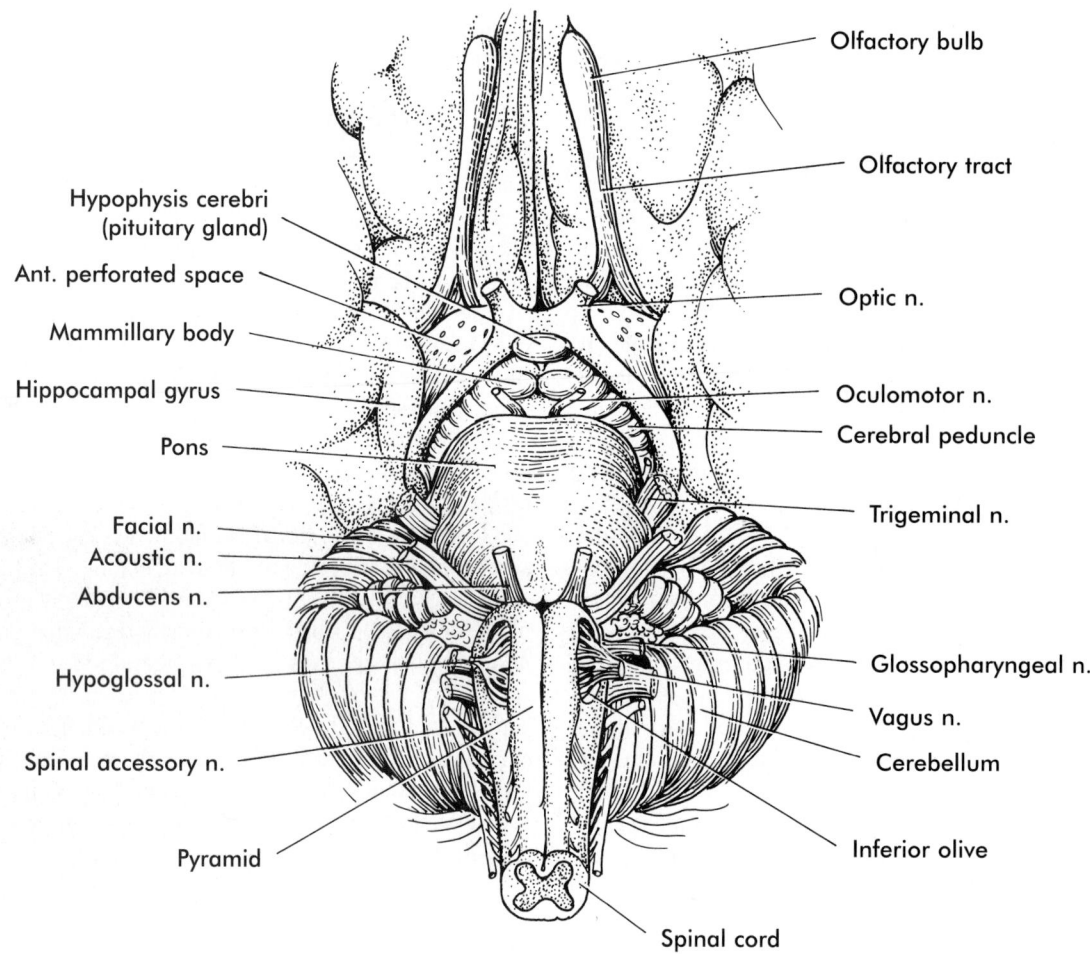

FIG. 22-14   Ventral surface of brain showing attachment of cranial nerves.
From Anthony, C.P., & Kolthoff, N.J. (1975). *Textbook of anatomy and physiology* (9th ed.). St. Louis: Mosby.

Cranial nerves

Twelve pairs of cranial nerves arise within the cranial cavity (Fig. 22-14). From a surgical standpoint, they are considered with the head.

First cranial nerve

The olfactory nerve, a fiber tract of the brain, is located under the frontal lobe on the cribriform plate of the ethmoid bone. It transmits the sense of smell. Frontal lobe tumors, fractures of the anterior fossa of the skull, and lesions of the nasal cavity may affect the olfactory nerve.

Second cranial nerve

The optic nerve is a fiber tract of the brain. Originating in the ganglion cells of the retina, it passes through the optic foramen in the apex of the orbit to reach the optic chiasma, where a partial crossing of the fibers occurs, so the fibers from the nasal half of each retina pass to the opposite side. Posterior to the chiasma, the visual pathway is called the optic tract; still farther back, it becomes the optic radiation. Lesions in various parts of this pathway produce characteristic defects in the visual fields. For example, a lesion of the chiasma usually destroys the temporal

vision of each eye (bitemporal hemianopia), whereas a lesion of the occipital lobe produces impairment of vision (homonymous hemianopia) affecting the right or left halves of the visual fields of both eyes.

Lesions that affect the optic nerve and are treated by neurosurgery include primary gliomas of the nerve, pituitary tumors that press on the optic chiasma, and occasionally meningiomas in the region of the sella turcica and olfactory groove. The optic nerves and chiasma are best exposed through a frontal craniotomy, along the floor of the anterior fossa, or through a frontotemporal approach along the sphenoid ridge.

Third, fourth, and sixth cranial nerves

These three pairs of nerves—the oculomotor, the trochlear, and the abducens, respectively—are conveniently considered together because they are the motor nerves to the muscles of the eyes. They are affected by many toxic, inflammatory, vascular, and neoplastic lesions. The third nerve may be affected by aneurysms of the internal carotid artery, and pressure against this nerve accounts for pupillary dilatation when temporal lobe herniation resulting from increased intracranial pressure is present.

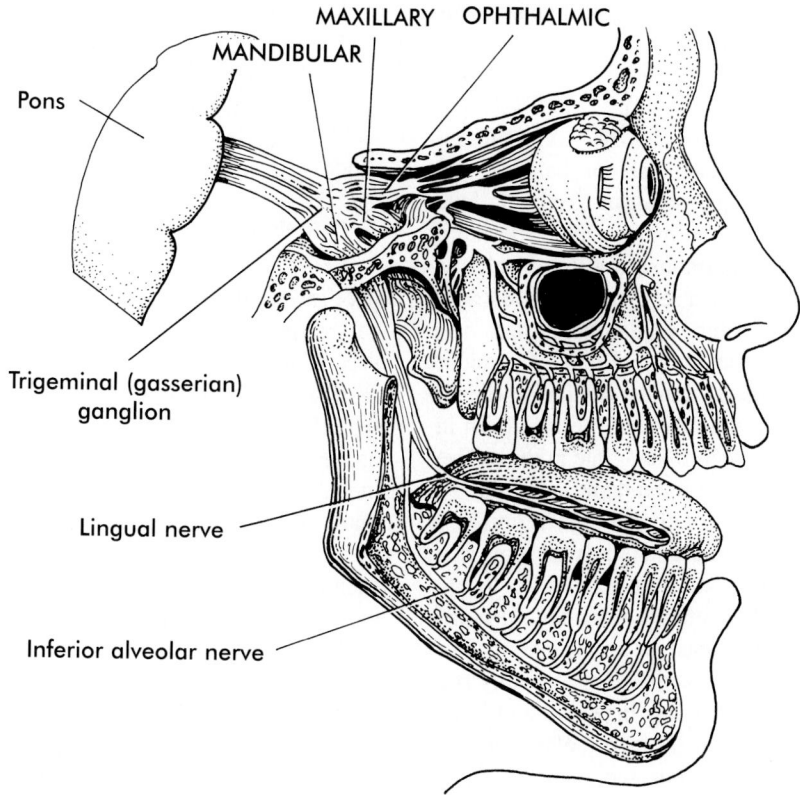

FIG. 22-15 Trigeminal (fifth cranial) nerve and its three main divisions.
From Anthony, C.P., & Kolthoff, N.J. (1975). *Textbook of anatomy and physiology* (9th ed.). St. Louis: Mosby.

Fifth cranial nerve

The trigeminal nerve has two functions: (1) sensory supply to the forehead, eyes, meninges, face, jaw, teeth, hard palate, buccal mucosa, tongue, nose, nasal mucosa, and maxillary sinus, and (2) motor innervation of the muscles of mastication. The sensory fibers that arise from cells in the gasserian ganglion travel along the medial wall of the middle cranial fossa and then extend peripherally in three divisions: ophthalmic, maxillary, and mandibular. Behind the ganglion the fibers enter the brainstem by way of the sensory root. The motor root, which originates from cells in the brainstem, follows the course of the larger sensory component (Fig. 22-15).

Trigeminal neuralgia (tic douloureux) is characterized by excruciating, piercing paroxysms of pain, affecting one or more of the major peripheral divisions. The recurrent attacks are usually brought on by stimulation of trigger zones present about the face, nares, lips, and teeth. This affliction, of unknown cause, tends to occur unilaterally and in older persons. Medical treatment is frequently unsuccessful. A great variety of neurosurgical procedures have been proposed for its control. Peripheral neurectomies of the supraorbital or infraorbital nerves may easily be performed with the patient under local anesthesia, but the effect is temporary because the nerves regenerate. Trigeminal neuralgia can also be treated by a posterior fossa approach using the operating microscope. The microscope allows decompression of the trigeminal nerve from normal surrounding blood vessels and selection of its various fibers. Sensations of pain and temperature are eliminated, and the sensation of touch and corneal reflex are preserved. Trigeminal neuralgia can also be treated by retrogasserian rhizotomy with radiofrequency current and chemical rhizolysis.

Seventh cranial nerve

The facial nerve supplies the musculature of the face and the anterior two thirds of the tongue (for taste). It originates in the brainstem, passes through the skull with the eighth nerve by way of the internal acoustic meatus, continues along the facial canal, and exits just posterior to the parotid gland. The nerve may be damaged by acoustic neurinomas, fractures at the base of the skull, mastoid infections, and surgical procedures in the vicinity of the parotid gland.

Bell's palsy, a facial lower motor neuron paralysis, can affect the seventh nerve. It may last for a few weeks to a few months, but recovery usually takes place. When permanent interruption of the nerve occurs, useful operations for restoration of function include spinal accessory-facial and hypoglossal-facial anastomosis. These operations are performed high in the neck behind the parotid gland, using the operating microscope.

Eighth cranial nerve

The acoustic nerve has two parts, both sensory—the cochlear for hearing and the vestibular for balance. The former receives stimuli from the organ of Corti, the latter from the semicircular canals. The major surgical lesion of the eighth nerve is acoustic neurinoma, a histologically benign tumor growing from the nerve sheath at its entrance into the internal auditory meatus. This tumors arises deep in the angle between the cerebellum and pons. Symptoms may include unilateral deafness, tinnitus, unilateral impairment of cerebellar function, numbness of the face from involvement of the fifth cranial nerve, and, late in the course, papilledema caused by increased intracranial pressure.

The operative approach is usually through a unilateral suboccipital craniectomy; in some instances a translabyrinth approach may be used. Great care must be taken to prevent injury to the pons, and an attempt is made to preserve the facial nerve. Ménière's disease is an affliction of the eighth nerve characterized by a recurrent and usually progressive group of symptoms including dizziness and a sensation of fullness or pressure in the ears. When medical measures fail to alleviate the problem, section of the eighth nerve may be performed; this procedure has given consistently excellent results.

Ninth cranial nerve

The glossopharyngeal nerve supplies the sense of taste to the posterior third of the tongue and sensation to the tonsils and pharyngeal region and partially innervates the pharyngeal muscles. Rarely it is involved in a painful tic similar to trigeminal tic. Its sensory component can be sectioned for this reason, to treat a hypersensitive carotid sinus, or, along with the fifth nerve, to treat painful malignancies of the face, mouth, and pharynx. The ninth nerve lies near the eighth nerve in the posterior fossa and is exposed in a similar way.

Tenth cranial nerve

The vagus nerve has many motor and sensory functions, chief among which are innervation of pharyngeal and laryngeal musculature, control of heart rate, and regulation of acid secretion of the stomach. In neck surgery the surgeon carefully avoids the recurrent laryngeal branch; in gastric surgery the surgeon may sever the vagus nerve at the lower end of the esophagus to treat a peptic ulcer. The neurosurgeon is concerned mainly with preventing damage to the vagus nerve during posterior fossa surgery.

Eleventh cranial nerve

The spinal accessory nerve is a motor nerve to the sternocleidomastoid and trapezius muscles. To restore mobility to the face, it may be anastomosed to the peripheral end of a damaged facial nerve.

Twelfth cranial nerve

The hypoglossal nerve innervates the musculature of the tongue. Its neurosurgical interest is similar to that of the spinal accessory nerve.

The contents of the cranial nerves are demonstrated in Table 22-1.

Pathologic lesions of the brain

Brain tumors are not as rare, nor is their prognosis as poor, as is often believed. Early diagnosis simplifies surgical treatment because increased intracranial pressure and severe neurologic changes are not usually present. Brain tumors are either malignant or benign, depending on the cell type. Primary tumors generally do not resemble the carcinomas and sarcomas found elsewhere in the body and rarely metastasize outside the central nervous system. If both primary and metastatic tumors of the brain and its covering membranes are included in the term *intracranial tumors,* such tumors may be classified pathologically as germ cell, mesodermal, neuroepithelial, metastatic, and miscellaneous as follows:

A. Germ cell tumors
 1. Teratoma is a congenital tumor containing embryonic elements.
 2. Germinoma is a neoplasm arising from germ cells.
 3. Embryonal carcinoma is a tumor arising from premature exoderm.
 4. Choriocarcinoma is an extremely rare, very malignant neoplasm.
 5. Craniopharyngioma occurs in children and adults and arises from the region of the pituitary stalk; it is usually cystic; calcification above the sella turcica is often seen on x-ray films. In addition to headache, vertigo, vomiting, and papilledema, diabetes insipidus and visual field changes are common.
B. Meningeal lesions
 Meningioma is a slow-growing tumor, originating in the arachnoidal tissue; it is very vascular and may adhere to the dural venous sinuses or major arteries, making its complete removal difficult.
C. Neural sheath tumor
 Neurinoma usually arises from the neurolemma sheath cells of the vestibular portion of the eighth cranial nerve within the auditory meatus, grows to fill the cerebellopontine angle, and may indent the brain stem.
D. Vascular tumors
 1. Angioma is an often congenital arteriovenous malformation.
 2. Hemangioblastoma may be solid or cystic; it is likely to occur in cerebellar hemispheres; sometimes it is present in association with angiomas of the retina and other organs.
E. Neuroepithelial tumors
 1. Gliomas
   a. Glioblastoma multiforme is an infiltrative, fast-

TABLE 22-1

Contents of the Cranial Nerves

Nerve	Functional component	Origin or termination within CNS	Peripheral sensory or motor ending
I	SVA	Olfactory bulb	Olfactory epithelium
II	SSA	Lateral geniculate nucleus and superior colliculus	Originates in ganglion cells of retina
III	(G) SE	Oculomotor nucleus	Superior, inferior, and medial recti; inferior oblique; levator palpebrae superioris
	GVE	Edinger-Westphal nucleus (part of oculomotor nucleus)	Sphincter pupillae, ciliary muscle*
IV	(G) SE	Trochlear nucleus	Superior oblique
V	GSA	Spinal and main sensory nuclei	Skin and deep tissues of head; dura mater
		Mesencephalic nucleus	Muscle spindles and other mechanoreceptors
	SVE	Trigeminal motor nucleus	Muscles of mastication, tensor tympani, and a few others
VI	(G) SE	Abducens nucleus	Lateral rectus
VII	GSA	Spinal trigeminal nucleus	Outer ear
	SVA	Solitary nucleus	Taste buds of anterior two thirds of tongue
	GVA	Solitary nucleus	Small portion of nasopharynx
	GVE	Superior salivatory nucleus	Submandibular, sublingual salivary glands; lacrimal gland*
	SVE	Facial motor nucleus	Muscles of facial expression; stapedius
VIII	SSA	Cochlear and vestibular nuclei	Organ of Corti; cristae of semicircular canals; maculae of utricle and saccule
IX	GSA	Spinal trigeminal nucleus	Outer ear
	SVA	Solitary nucleus	Taste buds of posterior third of tongue
	GVA	Solitary and spinal trigeminal nuclei	Carotid body and sinus; mucous membranes of nasal and oral pharynx and middle ear
	GVE	Inferior salivatory nucleus	Parotid gland*
	SVE	Nucleus ambiguus	Pharynx (stylopharyngeus)
X	GSA	Spinal trigeminal nucleus	Outer ear
	SVA	Solitary nucleus	Taste buds of epiglottis
	GVA	Solitary and spinal trigeminal nuclei	Thoracic and abdominal viscera; mucous membranes of larynx and laryngeal pharynx
	GVE	Dorsal motor nucleus	Thoracic and abdominal viscera*
	SVE	Nucleus ambiguus	Larynx and pharynx; heart*
Cranial XI	SVE	Nucleus ambiguus	Larynx and pharynx
Spinal XI	SVE	Accessory nucleus, cervical cord	Sternocleidomastoid; trapezius
XII	(G) SE	Hypoglossal nucleus	Muscles of tongue

From Nolte, J. (1988). *The human brain: an introduction to its functional anatomy* (2nd ed.). St. Louis: Mosby.
*Final destination after synapse in a parasympathetic ganglion.
GSA, General somatic afferent; fibers are related to receptors for pain, temperature, and mechanical stimuli in somatic structures such as skin muscles, and joints; *GVA,* general visceral afferent; fibers are related to receptors in visceral structures such as the walls of the digestive tract; *GVE,* general visceral efferent; fibers are preganglionic autonomic; *GSE,* general somatic efferent; fibers innervate skeletal muscles; *SSA,* special somatic afferent; fibers are related to the special senses of sight, hearing and equilibrium; *SVA,* special visceral afferent; fibers are related to the special senses of smell and taste; *SVE,* special visceral efferent; fibers innervate the branchiomeric muscles; muscles of the larynx, pharynx, and face are branchiomeric muscles.

growing, rapidly recurring cerebral tumor that occurs most frequently in middle age. It may invade both cerebral hemispheres by crossing in the corpus callosum. Areas of necrosis are characteristic. Astrocytomas and oligodendrogliomas may transform into this malignant tumor with time.

b. Medulloblastoma is a fast-growing, rapidly recurring tumor of the vermis of the cerebellum and fourth ventricle that usually occurs in young children. It characteristically metastasizes in the subarachnoid spaces, usually spreading to the base of the brain by this route.

c. Ependymoma occurs most frequently in children and is likely to arise in or near the ventricular walls. It commonly occurs in the fourth ventricle, where it abuts or involves vital medullary centers. It also frequently metastasizes in the subarachnoid spaces.

d. Astrocytoma usually occurs in the cerebellum of children and the cerebrum of adults. It is often cystic and discrete in children, infiltrating and ill defined in adults.

e. Oligodendroglioma is usually found in the cerebral hemispheres and is infiltrating but occasionally moderately well defined.

f. Others not mentioned include choroid plexus papillomas, pinealomas, and microgliomas.

2. Pituitary tumors

a. Chromophobe tumor is relatively common in the anterior pituitary glands of adults. It causes compression of the pituitary, adjacent optic chiasma, and hypothalamus. The latter may lead to diabetes insipidus.

b. Eosinophilic adenomas are secretory, causing an excessive amount of growth hormone in the serum.

c. Basophilic adenomas are responsible for the excessive secretion of corticotropic, gonadotropic, and thyrotropic hormones. Acromegaly or, less commonly, Cushing's syndrome may occur and cause the patient to seek help long before the tumor has expanded sufficiently to compromise the optic chiasma.

d. Prolactinoma or prolactin cell adenoma exhibits considerable differences in clinical presentation depending on the sex of the patient. In women of reproductive age the onset of amenorrhea and galactorrhea with associated infertility is an obvious sign. The diagnosis of a prolactinoma is established early in the course. In men the clinical endocrinal symptoms, which include decreased libido and impotence, are not as conspicuous and initially may be disregarded by the patient. As a result, male patients frequently do not seek medical attention until the tumors are large and have spread beyond the confines of the sella.

F. Metastatic tumors usually arise from carcinoma, more rarely from sarcoma, and occasionally from melanomas and retinal tumors. The most common sources are bronchogenic carcinoma and carcinoma of the breast.

Tumors not discussed here are eosinophilic granulomas, tuberculomas, and other granulomas; brain abscesses; colloid cysts; fibrous dysplasia; and lymphomas. A brain lesion is diagnosed by history, neurologic examination, and diagnostic studies. The manifestations of an intracranial tumor fall into two classes: those resulting from irritation or impairment of function in specific areas of the brain directly affected by the tumor and those resulting from diffuse increased intracranial pressure.

Lesions in the left frontotemporal region, where motor speech originates, lead to aphasia; occipital tumors produce hemianoptic visual defects; large frontal lobe tumors may cause striking personality changes. Cortical tumors frequently produce focal seizures of diagnostic value. The onset of epileptiform seizures in an adult is often associated with an intracranial neoplasm. Pituitary tumors characteristically press on the optic chiasma and impair the temporal vision of each eye. They disturb pituitary glandular function, resulting in hypopituitary states, pituitary dwarfism, or acromegaly. Posterior fossa tumors often manifest their presence by blocking the CSF circulation, but they may also destroy cerebellar function, resulting in incoordination, ataxia, scanning speech, and deafness.

BACK

The spinal column consists of 33 vertebrae: seven cervical, twelve thoracic, five lumbar, five sacral (fused as one), and one coccygeal (fused from four small vertebrae) (Fig. 22-16).

The first cervical vertebra, or atlas, supports the skull. The second cervical vertebra, or axis, can be identified by its odontoid process, a vertical projection extending into the foramen of the atlas like a stick in a hoop; it rests against the anterior tubercle. Ligaments hold the two together but allow considerable rotational movement.

The other cervical, thoracic, and lumbar vertebrae are more alike in structure. Each has a body, an oval block of spongy bone situated anteriorly. An intervertebral disk, a fibrocartilaginous elastic cushion, separates one body from another (Figs. 22-17 and 22-18). The spinal cord lies in a canal formed by the vertebral bodies, pedicles, and laminae. Articular surfaces or facets project from the pedicles and form joints with the facets of the vertebrae above and below. Transverse processes extend laterally and serve as hitching posts for muscles and ligaments. Spinous processes extend posteriorly (see Fig. 22-17) and can be palpated in all except obese persons. The vertebrae are held together by multiple ligaments and muscles. Motion of the spine occurs at the articular facets and through the elastic intervertebral disks (see Fig. 22-18).

The spinal cord is protected by this bony framework. The dura mater is separated from its bony surroundings by

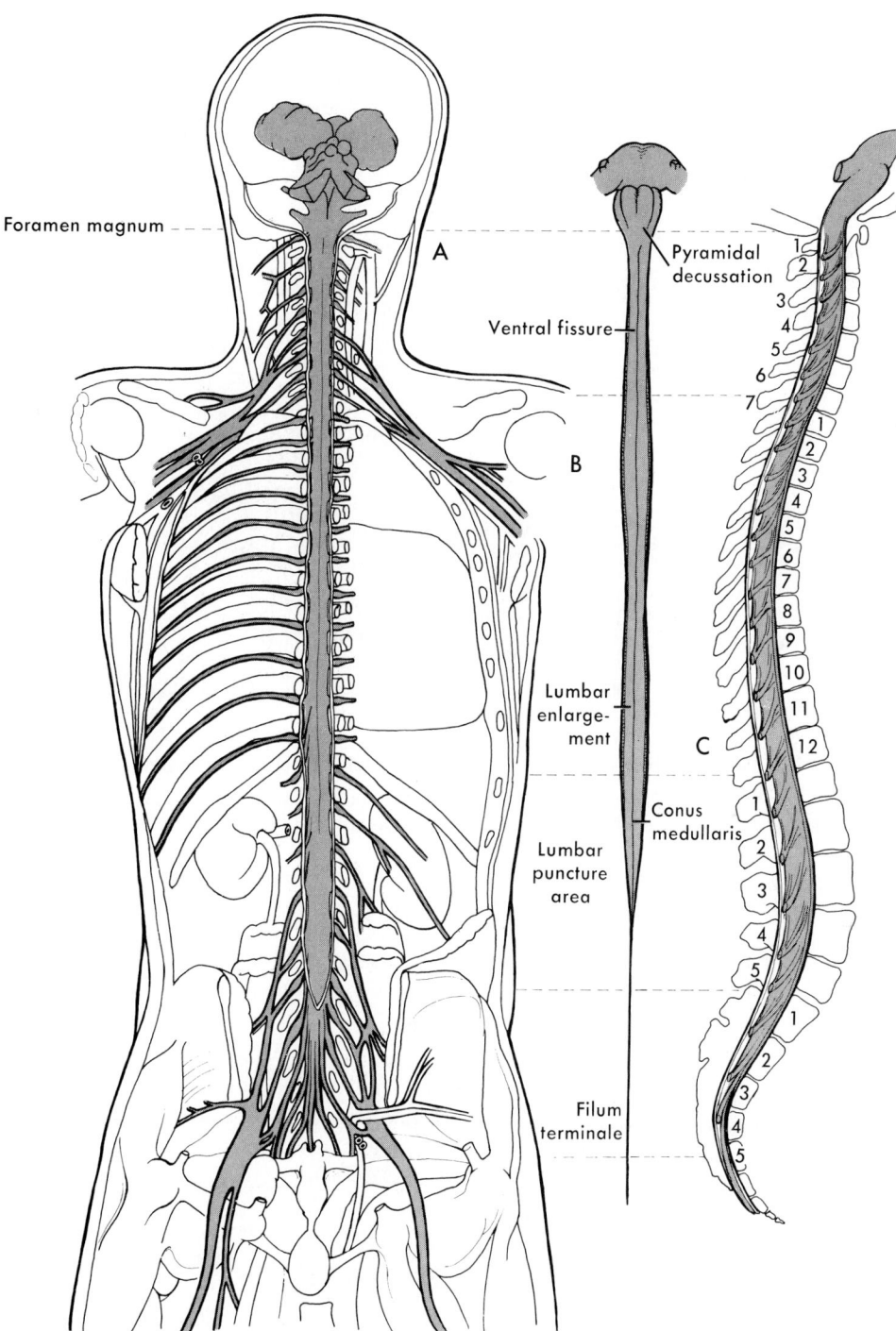

FIG. 22-16   Posterior view of brainstem and spinal cord. **A,** Torso dissected from back is shown. Dura mater has been opened and cord exposed. Levels concerned can be easily determined by referring to ribs on left side of thorax. Cord proper terminates opposite body of second lumbar vertebra (**B**) as conus medullaris. **B,** Ventral surface of cord stripped of dura mater and arachnoid. It is symmetric in structure, two halves of which are separated by ventral fissure. This fissure stops at foramen magnum. Caudally, pia mater leaves conus medullaris as glistening thread or filum terminale. **C,** Cord is exposed from lateral side. Dura mater has been opened. Since cord is shorter than canal and spinal nerves leave through intervertebral foramina, one at a time, lowest portion of canal is occupied only by a bundlelike accumulation of nerve roots—cauda equina. Caudal end of dural sac, enclosing spinal cord and cauda equina, lies somewhere between bodies of first and third sacral vertebrae. Size and position of the three views correspond, and elimination of major vertebral levels is indicated by transverse lines for all three figures.

Modified from Mettler, F.A. (1948). *Neuroanatomy* (2nd ed.). St. Louis: Mosby; from Conway-Rutkowski, B.L. (1982). *Carini and Owens' neurological and neurosurgical nursing* (8th ed.). St. Louis: Mosby.

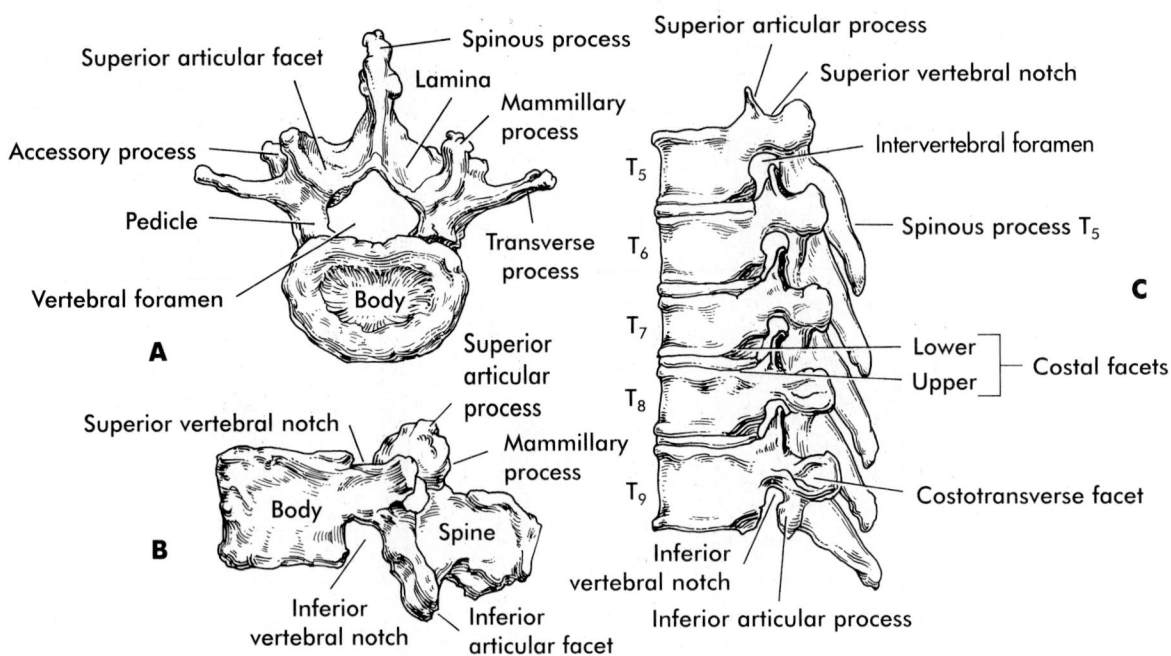

FIG. 22-17 **A,** Fourth lumbar vertebra from above. **B,** Fourth lumbar vertebra from side. **C,** Fifth to ninth thoracic vertebrae, showing relationships of various parts.

From Mettler, F.A. (1948). *Neuroanatomy* (2nd ed.). St. Louis: Mosby.

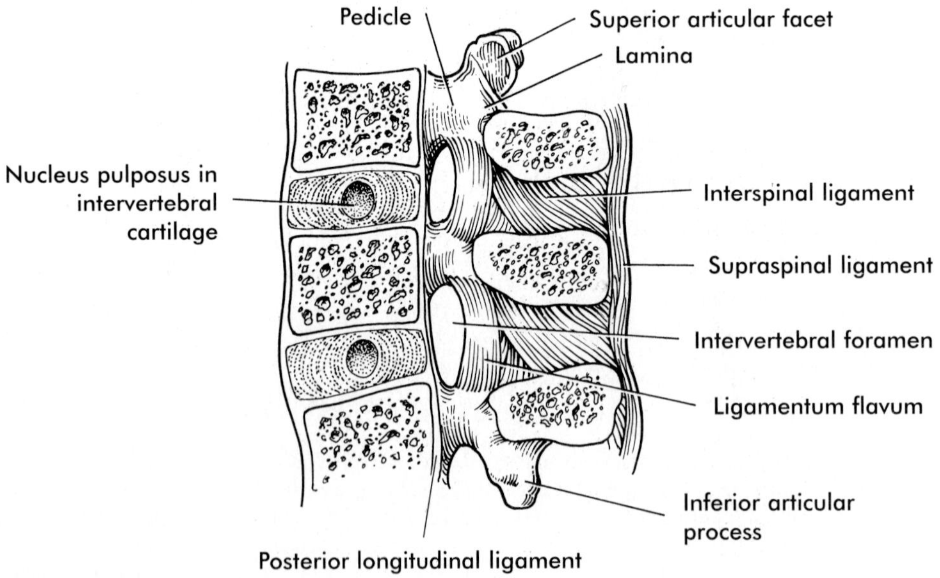

FIG. 22-18 Median section through three lumbar vertebrae, showing intervertebral disks (nuclei pulposi).

From Mettler, F.A. (1948). *Neuroanatomy* (2nd ed.). St. Louis: Mosby.

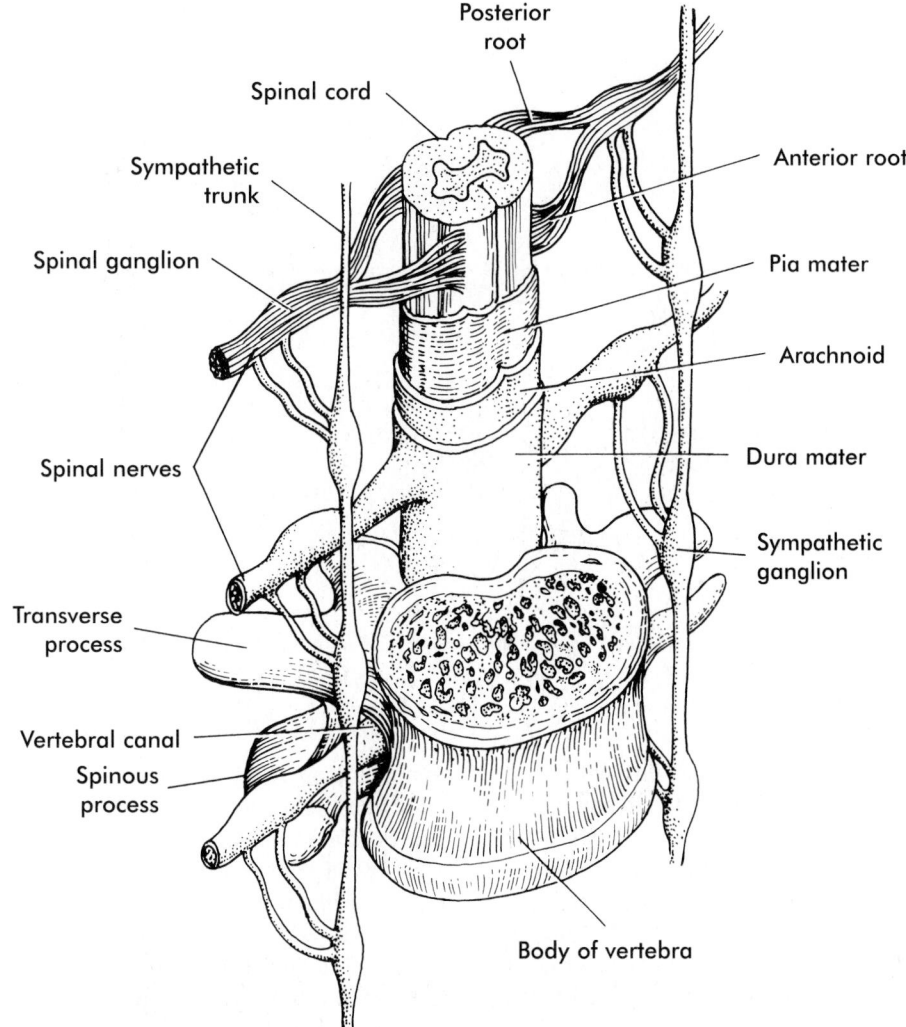

FIG. 22-19   Spinal cord, showing meninges, formation of spinal nerves, and relationships to vertebra and to sympathetic trunk and ganglia.

From Anthony, C.P., & Kolthoff, N.J. (1975). *Textbook of anatomy and physiology* (9th ed.). St. Louis: Mosby.

a layer of epidural fat. Beneath the dura mater is the arachnoid, a continuation of the same structure in the head. The subarachnoid space contains spinal fluid. A thin layer of pia mater adheres to the cord, and CSF also circulates from the fourth ventricle into the central canal of the cord.

The spinal cord is a downward prolongation of the brainstem, starting at the upper border of the atlas and ending at the upper border of the second lumbar vertebra. The cord is oval in cross-section. It is slightly flattened in the anteroposterior diameter. A cross-section looks like a gray H surrounded by a white mantle split in the midline, anteriorly and posteriorly, by sulci (Fig. 22-19).

The peripheral white matter carries long myelinated motor and sensory tracts; the central gray matter consists of nerve cell bodies and short unmyelinated fibers (see Figs. 22-16 and 22-19). The principal long pathways are the laterally placed pyramidal tracts, carrying impulses down from the cerebral cortex to the motor neurons of the cord;

the dorsal ascending columns, mediating sensations of touch and proprioception; and the anterolaterally placed spinothalamic tracts, carrying pain and temperature sensations to the thalamus, the sensory receiving station of the brain (Fig. 22-20).

At each vertebral level are two pairs of spinal nerves (see Fig. 22-19): an anterior or motor root, the cell bodies of which lie in the anterior horn of the spinal gray matter; and a posterior or sensory root, the cell bodies of which lie in the spinal ganglia in the intervertebral foramina, through which the nerves exit from the spinal canal and emerge from the cord. Each pair of roots forms one spinal nerve. The cervical nerves pass out horizontally, but at each lower level they take on an increasingly oblique and downward direction. In the lumbar region the course of the nerves is nearly vertical, forming the cauda equina (see Fig. 22-16). This phenomenon is explained by the fact that the spinal cord, which fills the entire spinal canal in the fetus, grows at a slower rate than the bony spine, thus leaving the lower

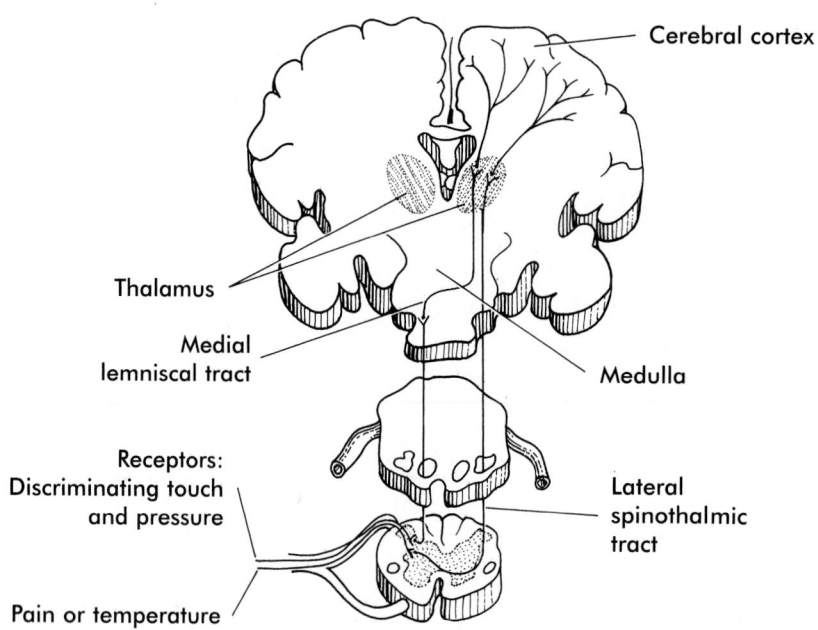

FIG. 22-20   Lateral spinothalmic and medial lemniscal neural tracts.

nerves a progressively longer course to their exit.

The vasculature of the spinal cord and vertebral column is a rich, delicate network. The arterial blood supply to the spinal cord arises from the vertebral arteries as the anterior spinal artery and the posterior spinal arteries. These vessels branch and anastomose on both sides of the cord and within the substance of the cord. They also branch into anterior and posterior radicular arteries that form spinal rami as they accompany the spinal nerve roots through the intervertebral foramina.

A series of venous plexuses surround and innervate the spinal cord at each level in the vertebral canal. They anastomose with each other and form the intervertebral veins as they exit through the intervertebral foramina with the spinal nerves to join the intercostal, lumbar, and sacral veins. The lateral longitudinal veins near the foramen magnum empty into the inferior petrosal sinus and cerebellar veins. The venous network innervates the bony structures and musculature as well as the spinal cord and nerve roots. Venous bleeding during spinal surgery is a potential problem for which the perioperative nurse must be prepared.

Pathologic lesions of the spinal cord and adjacent structures

Operations are performed to correct congenital malformations, injuries, tumors, herniated and degenerative intervertebral disks, abscesses, and intractable pain.

The most common congenital lesion encountered is a lumbar meningocele, or meningomyelocele, a failure of the union of the vertebral arches during fetal development. The fluid-filled, thin-walled sac often contains neural elements. Surgical correction is necessary when the sac lining is so thin that there is a potential or actual CSF leak. The operation consists of excising the sac wall to preserve adhering nerves, closing the dura mater, and reinforcing the closure with fascial flaps swung from the paraspinal muscles. Skin closure without tension is essential for primary healing. Large skin and subcutaneous flaps must occasionally be fashioned to ensure healing.

Injuries to the spinal cord are serious. No regeneration of destroyed or divided nerve tracts occurs. Recovery may take place with lesser degrees of injury, such as contusion or compression. Surgery can be of value in preventing further damage by débridement of penetrating wounds, removal of foreign bodies, relief of pressure on the cord or roots, open reduction of certain dislocations and fractures, and measures aimed at stabilizing the spine. In cervical injuries skeletal traction by means of tongs applied to the skull is often the preferred treatment.

Spinal cord tumors are classified according to location as extradural (outside the dura mater) or intradural (inside the dura mater). Intradural tumors may be either extramedullary (outside the cord) or intramedullary (within the cord). Extradural tumors include sarcomas and carcinomas, which may be metastatic from adjacent structures in or about the vertebrae. Other extradural lesions include Hodgkin's disease, lipomas, neurofibromas, chondromas, angiomas, abscesses, and granulomas.

Intradural tumors can be extramedullary, in which case they are usually benign and originate from the dura mater and arachnoid surrounding the cord and from the root sheaths of spinal nerves. Neurinomas are especially common in the thoracocervical area and may be part of generalized neurofibromatosis. Meningiomas also commonly occur in intradural extramedullary locations. Less frequently, lipomas or other types of tumors are found. Gliomas are the most common intramedullary tumors and have a less favorable prognosis. These tumors infiltrate the cord tissue and are much more difficult to remove than extramedullary tumors.

The majority of intradural tumors are extramedullary and benign and, if diagnosed early before severe neurologic deficits occur, offer an excellent prognosis. They manifest their presence by pain of a radicular nature and various motor and sensory disabilities below their segmental locations.

Cord tumors frequently produce spinal fluid blockage and can be pinpointed accurately with MRI, which is now the procedure of choice with or without enhancement. Intraspinal injection of contrast material (myelography) is another option. A standard laminectomy is used for exposure and removal.

The rare surgical infections of the spinal cord take the form of extradural abscesses and granulomas. Treatment consists of a combination of excision, drainage, chemotherapy, and occasionally spinal fusion.

The most frequently encountered neurosurgical problem is the herniated intervertebral disk. Because of weakness or rupture of the circular ligament (annulus fibrosus), which confines the soft center of the disk (nucleus pulposus), herniation of the latter may occur and give rise to pain from nerve root compression. When pain is severe or nerve damage excessive, surgical excision of the disk offers the most satisfactory relief. The procedure entails interlaminar exposure and piecemeal removal of the displaced nucleus. If the spine is unstable or there are other incontrovertible reasons for operative stabilization of the bony spine, a fusion of one type or another may be combined with the disk surgery (see Chapter 21).

Another method of treating disk disease is chemonucleolysis, a technique whereby primary lumbar intervertebral disk disease is treated by an intradiskal injection of chymopapain, a proteolytic enzyme in the form of a sterile lyophilized powder. However, the injection of chymopapain into the lumbar nucleus pulposus is not an innocuous procedure. Hypersensitivity to the drug and anaphylactic reactions have been reported. The patient needs to be checked for allergies to meat tenderizer, since this would demonstrate the sensitivity to the drug. Reports of transverse myelitis and subsequent paraplegia associated with chymopapain injection have raised serious questions about its use in young and otherwise healthy patients. A newer concept is that of percutaneous lumbar diskectomy, through a posterolateral approach. The method entails gaining access to the disk space through the use of an introduction system and cannulae. A 2-mm aspiration probe (called a Nucleotome) is then placed through the cannula into the disk space, and the nucleus pulposus is aspirated. Patients who have had previous surgery at the same level are not candidates for this approach.

Certain painful spinal lesions, usually of a malignant na-

ture, can be controlled by epidural opiates, temporarily or permanently with a pump, or by dividing the pain fibers supplying the affected area. It may be accomplished by sectioning the sensory roots intraspinally (posterior rhizotomy) or by incising the spinothalamic tracts (anterolateral cordotomy) that carry pain and temperature impulses. A laminectomy is necessary for exposure.

PERIPHERAL NERVES

Within the context of this discussion the peripheral nervous system includes the cranial nerves outside the cranial cavity, the spinal nerves, the autonomic nerves, and the ganglia. This division is artificial and only for the purpose of delineating surgical approaches. The cranial nerves have been described under the section on the head because all arise within the cranial cavity, and most are approached neurosurgically through the head. There are 31 pairs of spinal nerves, each pair numbered for the level of the spinal column at which it emerges: cervical one (C1) through eight (C8), thoracic one (T1) through twelve (T12), lumbar one (L1) through five (L5), sacral one (S1) through five (S5), and coccygeal one. The thoracic region is sometimes referred to as the dorsal region with D1 being synonymous with T1 and so on. The first pair of cervical spine nerves emerges between C1 and the occipital bone. The eighth cervical nerves emerge from the intervertebral foramina between C7 and T1. The first thoracic nerves emerge between T1 and T2.

In the cervical and lumbosacral regions the spinal nerves regroup in a plexiform manner before they form the peripheral nerves of the upper and lower extremities; those in the thoracic region form cutaneous and intercostal nerves. The principal nerves of the upper plexus include the musculocutaneous, median, ulnar, and radial; those of the lumbosacral plexus include the obturator, femoral, and sciatic.

Each spinal nerve divides into anterior, posterior, and white rami. Anterior and posterior rami contain voluntary fibers; white rami contain autonomic fibers. Posterior rami further branch into nerves going to the muscles, skin, and posterior surfaces of the head, neck, and trunk. Most anterior rami branch to the skeletal muscles and the skin of extremities and anterior and lateral surfaces. In the process they form plexuses, such as the brachial and sacral plexuses. Spinal nerves contain sensory dendrites and motor axons; some have somatic axons, and some have axons of preganglionic autonomic motor neurons.

The autonomic (involuntary) nervous system consists of all the efferent nerves, through which the cardiovascular apparatus, viscera, glands of internal secretion, and peripheral involuntary muscles are innervated (Fig. 22-21). A major anatomic difference between the somatic and autonomic nervous systems is that in the former an impulse from the brainstem or spinal cord reaches the end organ through a single neuron, whereas in the latter an impulse passes through two neurons—the first ending in an autonomic ganglion and the second running from the ganglion to the

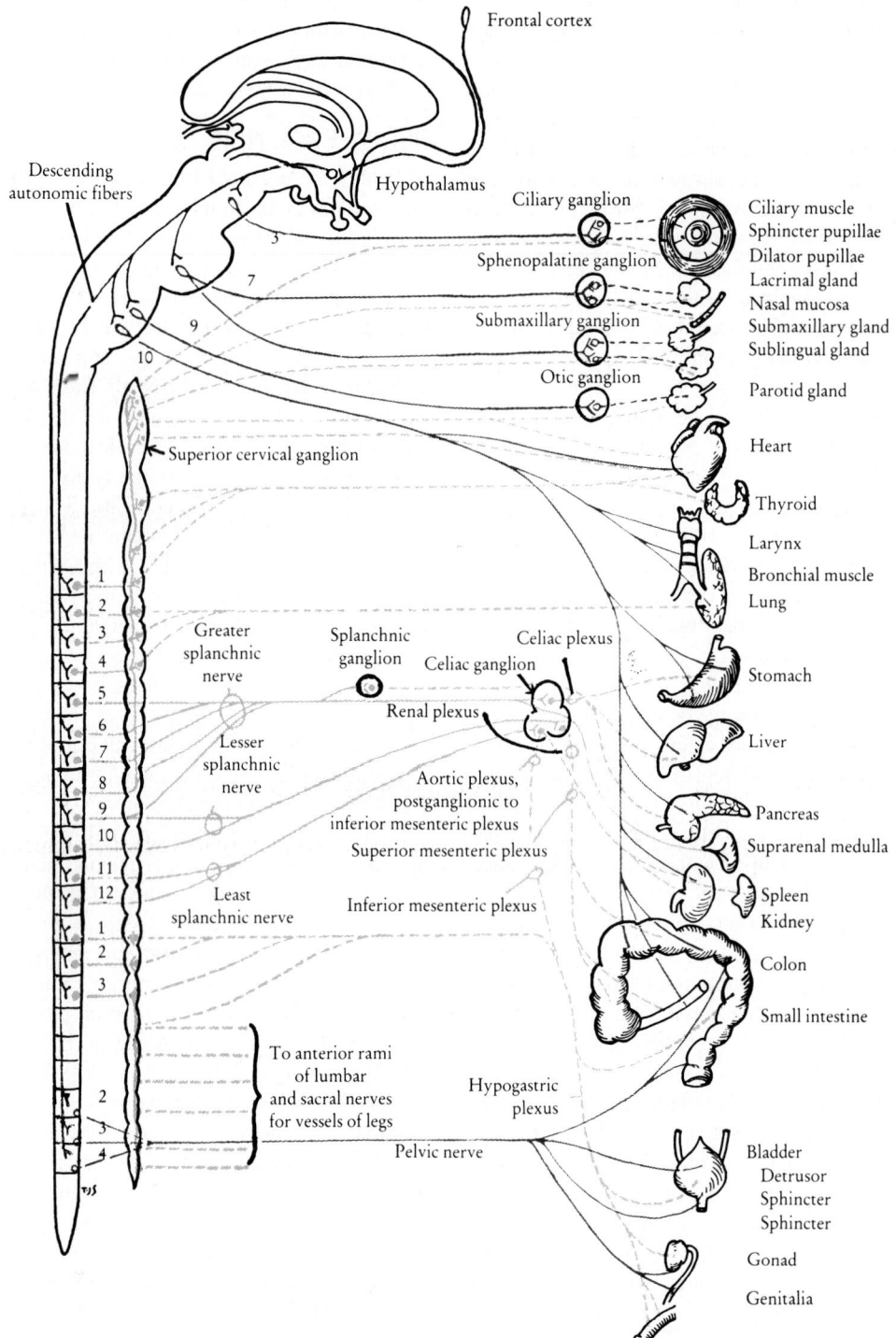

FIG. 22-21 Sympathetic division of the autonomic nervous system.

From Conway-Rutkowski, B.L. (1982). *Carini and Owens' neurological and neurosurgical nursing* (8th ed.). St. Louis: Mosby.

end organ. Some of the ganglia lie adjacent to the vertebral column to form the sympathetic trunks or chains; others are closely associated with the end organs.

The preganglionic neurons from the brainstem, which go out along the cranial nerves, and those from the second, third, and fourth sacral segments to the pelvic viscera end in ganglia in proximity to their end organs; thus their postganglionic fibers are very short. This is known as the parasympathetic, or craniosacral, division of the autonomic nervous system. The preganglionic fibers from the thoracic and lumbar spinal cord end in the paravertebral ganglia, making up the sympathetic chain, and their postganglionic fibers are relatively long. This is termed the sympathetic, or thoracolumbar, division of the autonomic nervous system.

The two divisions are distinct anatomically and physiologically. The chemical substance mediating transmission of impulses at most postganglionic sympathetic nerve endings is norepinephrine, and at all parasympathetic and preganglionic sympathetic neurons, acetylcholine.

The majority of organs have dual innervation, part from the craniosacral and part from the thoracolumbar divisions. The functions of these two systems are antagonistic. Together they work to maintain homeostasis. In general the thoracolumbar division functions as an emergency protection mechanism, always ready to combat physical or psychologic stress. The craniosacral division functions to conserve energy when the body is in a state of relaxation.

Stimuli arising from internal organs or from outside the body traverse visceral and somatic afferent nerve fibers to make reflex connections with preganglionic autonomic neurons in the brainstem and spinal cord. Such stimuli trigger activity of these involuntary systems automatically. When these automatic mechanisms break down or overact, surgery may be indicated. Thoracolumbar sympathectomy was once performed in hypertension to try to decrease blood vessel tone and lower the blood pressure. Vagotomy is done to decrease acid secretion to the stomach in peptic ulcer patients. Lumbar sympathectomy is used to relieve vasospastic disorders of the legs.

PERIOPERATIVE NURSING CONSIDERATIONS

ASSESSMENT

Communication between the perioperative nurse and surgeon, either directly or through a knowledgeable person, such as a clinical nurse specialist, operating room supervisor, privately employed nurse, RNFA, or resident who has direct communication with the surgeon, is essential for intelligently planning care for the neurosurgical patient in the operating room. Information the perioperative nurse needs before the arrival of the patient in the operating room includes the diagnosis; the diagnostic studies done and reports needed at the time of operation; the age, size, level of consciousness, physical disabilities resulting from neuropathologic conditions (as well as those from other causes), and communication problems of the patient; the specific surgical approach and body position to be used; the need for any special equipment, instruments, and supplies not ordinarily used; the amount of blood ordered and available; the method or methods planned to reduce intracranial pressure in the case of cranial surgery; the need for radiologic support during the procedure; and the planned preliminary procedures, such as carotid ligation, lumbar puncture, placement of monitoring lines, and Foley catheter insertion. This information permits the perioperative nurse to plan for needed equipment, instruments, and supplies.

Most diagnostic procedures are performed before the patient arrives in the operating room. Of greatest significance to the perioperative nurse are radiologic studies that produce either positive or negative images the surgeon can use during the operation to locate the pathologic condition. The perioperative nurse is responsible for having these images in the operating room before the procedure begins. The studies include the following:

1. *Myelography*—injection of contrast medium into the spinal subarachnoid space to demonstrate a defect by radiography.
2. *Pneumonencephalography (PEG)*—injection of air into the subarachnoid space, usually through a lumbar or cisternal puncture, to outline the ventricular system and the cranial subarachnoid space to identify deviations from normal. Because of advances in radiologic techniques, this procedure has become somewhat outdated.
3. *Ventriculography*—injection of air directly into the lateral ventricles when a block exists between the spinal canal and the lateral ventricles. Also somewhat outdated, but remains an excellent tool if CT or MRI cannot be obtained.
4. *Angiography (arteriography)*—injection of contrast medium into the brachial, carotid, vertebral, or femoral arteries to study the intracranial blood vessels for size, location, and configuration and to diagnose space-occupying lesions and vascular abnormalities.
   a. *Digital subtraction angiography (DSA)*—a computerized radiologic procedure. An intravenous rather than arterial injection is required; a contrast medium injection to allow examination of selected arterial circulation is used. DSA provides an alternative to cerebral angiography for high-risk patients by using computer technology.
   b. MR angiography—Magnetic resonance angiography may prove to be a sensitive screening procedure for carotid stenosis. It can detect dissection of cranial cervical vessels, as well as permit follow-up in a noninvasive fashion and guide treatment.
   c. *Three-dimensional computerized tomography angiography*—uses contrast-enhanced CT brain scan data to generate a three-dimensional image

of the intracranial vasculature with minimal risk to the patient.

    d. Stereoscopic display of MR angiography—recent advances in MRI permit high-resolution imaging of blood flow. Projection angiograms can be produced to overcome the tomographic nature of conventional MR scans. These angiograms are similar to plain x-ray film or digital subtraction angiograms in the demonstration of blood vessels, but the three-dimensional information inherent in them is partially lost in single projections. Stereoscopic image pairs allow the clinician to perceive the relative distance of vessels to one another. MR angiography permits perception of vascular anatomy in three dimensions.

5. *Venography*—dural sinus studies for narrowing sinuses and interference with cranial drainage, which often occur in lesions of the posterior fossa. This study has been essentially replaced with newer MRI software.

6. *Computed tomography (CT scan)*—use of x-ray studies with or without instilled contrast medium and computer technology to produce a sequential series of positive images of transverse sections of the brain and spinal cord in which differences in tissue density can be detected and deviations from normal identified. This study remains the gold standard for evaluation of acute head injury.

7. *Isotope brain scan*—injection of radioactive substance intravenously to demonstrate brain lesions.

8. *Echoencephalography*—method of recording referred ultrasound from reflecting surfaces; especially helpful in the identification of subdural hematomas. *Echo doppler*—noninvasive technique used to assess the blood flow in the carotid artery. The procedure can be done in or out of the surgical suite.

9. *Magnetic resonance imaging (MRI)*—use of powerful magnetic waves to reproduce details of the human body with no known risk to patients; uses no radiation. Advances in MRI scanning provide enhancement of the scan with the use of gadolinium. Many patients experience extreme feelings of claustrophobia during MRI.

NURSING DIAGNOSIS

Five nursing diagnoses to be considered in caring for the neurosurgical patient are as follows:

- Anxiety related to surgery/surgical outcome
- Knowledge deficit related to diagnostic tests and surgical procedures
- High risk for ineffective breathing patterns related to location of tumor, surgical position, or effects of general anesthesia
- High risk for pain related to pathophysiologic alterations
- High risk for infection related to surgical intervention

OUTCOME IDENTIFICATION

Outcomes identified for the selected nursing diagnoses could be stated as:

- The patient's anxiety will be reduced or controlled.
- The patient and/or family will verbalize knowledge regarding diagnostic and/or surgical procedures.
- The patient will maintain effective breathing patterns.
- The patient will report a reduction in pain.
- The patient will be free from signs and symptoms of infection.

PLANNING

Preparation can significantly reduce both anesthesia and intraoperative time for the patient as well as physical and psychologic stress for both the surgeon and the perioperative nurse. Planning for the patient's care in the operating room is based on the results of nursing assessment and the identification of relevant nursing diagnoses. The plan of care then identifies desired outcomes derived from the nursing diagnoses; priorities are set and nursing interventions designed to assist the patient to reach the desired outcomes. Nursing interventions identified for the patient's plan of care may include reassessment, teaching, counseling, referrals, and specific interventions to assist the patient in achieving patient care outcomes. The Sample Care Plan shown on the opposite page could be utilized by the perioperative nurse for the patient who is undergoing a neurosurgical procedure.

IMPLEMENTATION

Neuropathologic conditions requiring surgical intervention can be found in any age group. The most common problems requiring neurosurgical procedures in infants and children include meningocele, myelomeningocele, encephalocele, craniosynostosis, hydrocephalus, brain tumors, and trauma. The perioperative nurse plays a vital role in maintaining blood volume, body temperature, and fluid balance in pediatric patients. The perioperative nurse's role in maintaining blood volume includes planning for minimizing and monitoring blood loss, as well as for blood replacement. The surgeon may minimize blood loss by infiltrating the tissues at the site of incision with normal saline solution; minimizing or eliminating periosteal stripping and carefully attending to intracranial emissary veins and sinuses; and using electrosurgery and bipolar coagulation, bone wax, Gelfoam, thrombin, or Surgicel. The surgeon's preferences for instruments and supplies must be prepared and ready for use before needed. Sponges from the operative field must be continuously placed within view of the anesthesiologist or weighed as they are discarded from the field. Blood or blood products must be available in the surgical suite. A blood warmer must be ready to use as careful, accurate fluid replacement therapy is carried out. When the anesthesiologist is unable to see the operative field (which is usually the situation during *any* cranial surgery), the perioperative nurse must inform the anesthesiologist immediately of ac-

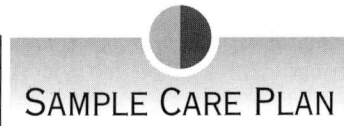

SAMPLE CARE PLAN

NURSING DIAGNOSIS: Anxiety related to surgery/surgical outcome

OUTCOME: The patient's anxiety will be reduced or controlled.

INTERVENTIONS:

Broadly classify the patient's anxiety (low, moderate, high).

Provide reassurance and explanations; repeat as necessary.

Provide ongoing opportunity for patient (and/or family) to ask questions and express fears.

Involve other support persons (social worker, case manager, chaplain) as appropriate.

Determine the patient's coping skills.

Assist the patient to utilize personally effective coping skills.

Use touch to communicate caring (as appropriate).

NURSING DIAGNOSIS: Knowledge deficit related to diagnostic tests and surgical procedures

OUTCOME: The patient and/or family will verbalize knowledge regarding diagnostic tests and/or surgical procedure.

INTERVENTIONS:

Determine patient or family knowledge level (and desire for knowledge).

Correct misinformation; refer to other health care team members as appropriate.

Identify patient or family readiness and motivation to learn.

Provide information about procedures; use understandable terms.

Explain perioperative routine; include both factual information and expected sensations associated with tests, surgical procedure, perioperative environment, and postoperative care.

Base psychoeducational interventions on individual needs.

NURSING DIAGNOSIS: High risk for ineffective breathing patterns related to location of tumor, surgical position, or effects of general anesthesia

OUTCOME: The patient will maintain effective breathing patterns.

INTERVENTIONS:

Provide appropriate positioning accessories; assist in their placement.

Monitor arterial blood gases (ABGs); interpret and report variations from expected values.

Review results of pulse oximetry for blood oxygen saturation.

Collaborate with anesthesiologist in monitoring end-tidal volume carbon dioxide.

Maintain open suction line.

Note respiratory rate, depth, and characteristics of breath sounds.

Encourage patient to cough and breathe deeply on emergence from anesthesia.

Communicate with PACU regarding postoperative requirements for ventilatory assistance.

Check airway patency frequently during transport to PACU.

NURSING DIAGNOSIS: High risk for pain related to pathophysiologic alterations

OUTCOME: The patient will report a reduction in pain.

INTERVENTIONS:

Determine effectiveness of preoperative medications; communicate ineffectiveness.

Administer additionally prescribed medications to control pain and/or anxiety; monitor patient response.

Assist patient to utilize personally effective pain control measures.

Provide physical comfort measures (such as warm blankets) and emotional support.

Explain postoperative regimens for control of pain.

NURSING DIAGNOSIS: High risk for infection related to surgical intervention

OUTCOME: The patient will be free from signs and symptoms of infection.

INTERVENTIONS:

Adhere to strict aseptic technique.

Implement environmental precautions.

Control traffic patterns.

Document wound classification.

Identify and correct breaks in technique.

Dress wound, intravenous line sites, and drain exit sites aseptically.

Monitor for postoperative indications of infection (elevated temperature; redness, swelling, warmth, or drainage at incision site; persistent incisional pain).

Provide patient or family with specific information regarding wound care and the signs and symptoms that should be reported.

tive bleeding at the operative site.

The perioperative nurse must place a warming blanket on the OR bed before the pediatric patient arrives. If the room temperature can be individually regulated, the thermostat should be set to a temperature about 22.2° C (72° F) after consultation with the anesthesiologist. The child's body and extremities can be wrapped in plastic materials. Body temperature is monitored with a rectal, intraaural, or esophageal thermistor probe. The thermistor unit must be calibrated and placed within the view of the anesthesiologist before surgery.

Some means to control and monitor fluid intake and output must be planned with the anesthesiologist and neurosurgeon: microdrip intravenous tubing or an electronic drip regulator such as an I-Vac unit may be used for regulating intravenous intake; a Foley catheter may be inserted into the bladder and attached to a urinometer and closed drainage system if the child is to undergo a prolonged procedure; output should be recorded at timed intervals decided on by the perioperative nurse and anesthesiologist and based on the child's general condition. Irrigation fluid and suction bottle contents are measured and recorded.

Parents of infants and children are usually extremely anxious, as are the families of most surgical patients. Arrangements by which families can have contact with the patient through a perioperative nurse who has direct access to the operating room during the operation and the postanesthesia recovery relieve anxiety and diminish perceived waiting time for them.

Older children, adolescents, and adults come to the operating room fearful and apprehensive about the outcome of the surgical procedure and its effect on them and their life-style. Both male and female patients are devastated by having their hair removed. During this procedure the perioperative nurse should provide psychologic support and give realistic reassurance and information to both conscious, responsive patients and patients who may be incoherent or unconscious but still hear what is going on around them and feel what is being done to them. Hair removal from the head, like all other forms of preoperative preparation, should be done as close to the time of skin incision as possible to decrease the possibility of postoperative wound infection. Some surgeons prefer complete hair removal because dressings are easier to apply, hair regrowth is more even, a better wig fit can be obtained, and it is far easier to prepare a sterile field around such an operative site. However, because of the severe disturbances in body image caused by total hair removal, an effort should be made to facilitate a compromise between patient and surgeon. Whenever possible, minimal hair removal is recommended. There may be a relationship between hair removal and postoperative recovery, especially in the areas of orientation, social interaction, and compliance. Also, when the patient's wishes are considered, the patient has a degree of control over what is happening.

An aged person undergoing neurosurgical intervention brings a potential range of problems such as hearing, sight, and mobility deficiencies unrelated to the neuropathologic condition. Responses to stimuli generally are slower in the elderly. The skin is more prone to pressure injury. The ability to heal may be impaired. More time and greater care must be taken with older patients. Communication can be established and reassurance given by touching and by being nearby while the patient is conscious. Vigilant monitoring of blood loss, temperature, and urine output is also required in caring for the older patient in the operating room. Surgery may be performed with the patient under local anesthesia, and the perioperative nurse may be responsible for monitoring vital signs, as well as for providing a human communication link for the patient. Sitting with the patient and explaining the procedure and the sensations that will be experienced makes the patient more comfortable and cooperative and diminishes fears.

Among neurosurgical patients are those who have little or no apparent loss of function, those who are coping with chronic pain and are looking forward to the operation for the relief it will bring, and those who are totally or partially dependent for everything because they are unconscious, quadriplegic, or aphasic. If pain is present, the perioperative nurse should know the type and site of the pain and aim to make the patient as comfortable as possible while conscious. If the patient is acutely and severely traumatized, the perioperative nurse must be aware of injuries other than those for which the patient is being treated neurosurgically so these injuries can be taken into consideration. A perioperative nurse with prior knowledge of a given situation is better prepared to cope with that situation and can plan individualized care based on that knowledge.

Basic neurosurgical maneuvers

Scientific advances that enable surgeons to control pain, hemorrhage, infection, and other physiologic responses have contributed largely to the neurosurgeon's ability to operate successfully on the nervous system. The extent of a modern neurosurgical operation may be determined not so much by the physiologic hazards involved as by the degree of neurologic disability that may be expected after surgery. Knowing the hazards and having everything ready in advance will enhance the ability of the surgeon to achieve a favorable outcome.

Preliminary procedures

A number of procedures or therapeutic measures may be performed by the neurosurgeon or other member of the team in a holding or induction room before positioning, prepping, and draping take place. It is important that the perioperative nurse know why these procedures are done in order to anticipate them and be prepared to facilitate them.

A Foley catheter is often inserted into the bladder to monitor urinary output during the procedure. It is essential for prolonged procedures and when mannitol is to be given intravenously, so the bladder does not become distended. A Foley catheter is also required when hypothermia or hypotension will be induced, when excessive bleeding is anticipated, and in trauma patients for continuous assessment of kidney function.

A right atrial or central venous pressure line is required for management of air embolism. An air embolus can occur in any position but there is an increased risk when the operative field is above the heart. A left atrial pressure line may also be inserted in the operating room immediately before the surgical procedure is begun.

When excessive intracranial bleeding is a possibility, the neurosurgeon may choose carotid cutdown and temporary ligation or tourniquet placement for occlusion of the carotid arteries during bleeding. Carotid cutdown is a separate surgical procedure and requires a special sterile setup, including drapes and instruments. Procedures that may require such management include intracranial vascular surgery and removal of meningiomas.

In some situations CSF drainage may be required. This can be done by placement of a ventricular cannula, such as the Scott or Seletz, or by placement of a spinal needle in the lower lumbar spinal canal. The stylet of either needle is left in place until drainage is required. The surgeon can remove the ventricular stylet, but the perioperative nurse must be able to remove the spinal needle stylet. When the lumbar puncture method is used, the patient is placed in a semilateral position and stabilized, so the patient does not roll onto the needle and the perioperative nurse can remove the stylet without contaminating it during the procedure. An extension tubing and stopcock can be attached to the needle at the time of lumbar puncture. When this is done, the tubing and stopcock are supported so traction is not put on the needle and are placed where they are accessible to the perioperative nurse or anesthesiologist. The stopcock can be opened for drainage. Another alternative to drainage is to place a lumbar drain rather than leave a hard metal needle in the back or a cannula in the brain.

Induced hypotension may be required to manage bleeding. Intracranial vascular surgery and removal of some tumors also may require induced hypotension. Sodium nitroprusside (Nipride) is an effective agent. Very little of the drug is required to produce an immediate and dramatic hypotensive state. Recovery from the effects of the drug is immediate. When mixed in solution for intravenous administration, sodium nitroprusside is unstable in light. The perioperative nurse must have a roll of aluminum foil available to cover the intravenous bottle and tubing completely when the drug is hanging and in use or ready for immediate use; an electronic device to measure and control the amount administered must also be set up.

Some surgeons prefer to use antibiotics in the immediate preoperative period. A second-generation cephalosporin, Ancef, is the most common drug of choice.

Skin preparation

Head hair is best removed after the patient has arrived in the surgery department but before arrival in an operating room. The hair is first clipped with electric clippers, which are cleaned and disinfected after each use. The hair is placed in a container, labeled with the patient's name, and kept with the patient after surgery. The scalp is then shaved, using warm, soapy water and either a straight razor or several disposable safety razors. As soon as the patient experiences any pulling, the razor blade should be changed. The perioperative nurse should explain to the patient exactly what is being done and what sensations to expect during the procedure.

For surgery on the cervical spine it is possible to secure long hair on top of the head and remove neck hair with clippers to a level even with the top of the ears or just below the occipital protuberance. Postoperatively patients with long hair can comb it down over the shaved area until the hair regrows.

Patients undergoing thoracic or lumbar spine surgery may not need to be shaved. If hair is present, it can be removed by a depilatory or clipping just before surgery.

After hair removal the skin should be inspected carefully for any signs of inflammation or infection. If any such signs are noted, they should be reported to the surgeon immediately.

An antiseptic skin prep is done after the patient is positioned and before draping. Skin prepping may be done by the perioperative nurse, surgeon, or resident. General principles and precautions cited in Chapter 3 apply to neurosurgical preparations, regardless of who performs them.

Many neurosurgeons mark the incision line with a marking pencil, a marking solution and wooden stick, or a scalpel. If a marking solution is used, indigo carmine, gentian violet, or brilliant green is recommended. Methylene blue should *never* be found in a neurosurgical operating room because it produces an inflammatory reaction in central nervous system tissue and could be disastrous if accidentally injected into the subarachnoid space, for example.

After marking, the surgeon may inject the incision site and the sites for application of towel clamps with a local anesthetic agent or with normal saline solution. Any solution will apply pressure within the tissues and decrease bleeding at the time of incision. The local anesthetic agent has the additional effect of decreasing the effect of the stimulus of the skin incision.

Positioning

The basic body positions and their modifications are used in neurosurgery. The perioperative nurse must know the position for each procedure; the hazards and precautions of each position; and the equipment, supportive positioning devices, and time necessary to place a patient in a given position (see Chapter 4). General considerations of special importance in positioning for neurosurgery include protecting the eyes from pressure, chemical burns, and corneal scratches; maintaining joints in functional alignment with no pressure or tension on superficial nerves and vessels; and checking the Foley catheter for tension and kinks to ensure drainage.

The dorsal recumbent, or supine, position or some modification of it is used for supratentorial craniotomy, subtemporal decompression, and anterior cervical fusion. The lateral position is used for thoracic and lumbar laminectomy by some surgeons and for lumbar sympathectomy. Modifications of the prone position can be used for lumbar, thoracic, and cervical laminectomy and for posterior fossa craniectomy. The sitting, or upright, position can be used for cervical laminectomy, posterior fossa craniectomy, temporal craniectomy, and ventriculography. Only specific aspects of the sitting position for neurosurgical procedures and the knee-chest position, a modification of the prone position, are covered in this chapter.

The extreme sitting, or upright, position may be the neurosurgeon's choice for infratentorial cranial surgery and posterior cervical laminectomy when acute trauma is not the cause of cervical cord disease. Advantages of this position include optimum visibility of the operative field and decreased blood loss because of the lowered arterial and venous pressures. However, hypotensive changes also pose potential problems: some patients cannot tolerate the upright position under general anesthesia; thus the patient is slowly placed in this position as the anesthesiologist monitors the blood pressure. Most patients have a drop in arterial pressure but rapidly adapt to the position; those who do not are placed in the prone position. In the sitting position the venous pressure in the head and neck may be negative, predisposing to air embolism. Other potential problems with this position include neck flexion with airway compromise and difficulty in achieving and maintaining functional alignment.

Preoperatively, elastic bandages, wrapped from the patient's toes to groin, special tensor stockings, such as TED hose, or sequential compression stockings may be applied. All these help prevent venous stasis in the lower extremities and help maintain the blood pressure. Other precautions during positioning and throughout the procedure include checking the heels, soles, and popliteal areas to prevent pressure; checking male genitals to ensure that pressure will not compromise circulation and cause necrosis, and female breasts to prevent any unnecessary pressure; preventing thighs from contacting the metal crossbar table attachment; stabilizing the head in the headrest; and stabilizing the shoulders and torso to prevent neck flexion.

Preparations should be made in collaboration with the anesthesiologist to manage air embolism if this complication should occur. The patient may be placed in a G-suit before positioning to prevent this complication. The G-suit also assists in maintaining the blood pressure. A right atrial line can be placed under direct vision fluoroscopy either in the cardiac catheterization laboratory or radiology department, before arrival of the patient in the operating room, or in the operating room, using the image intensifier. After anesthesia induction, the anesthesiologist may place an esophageal stethoscope or attach the patient to a Doppler unit to hear air entering the right atrium. The air can be withdrawn through the atrial line with a 50-ml syringe and

three-way stopcock connection. If the management of air embolism includes repositioning the patient with the surgical wound open, the repositioning must be accomplished quickly, without endangering the patient in other ways, such as contamination of the surgical wound, displacement of a joint, or dislodgement of the endotracheal tube.

The most common position for lumbar and thoracic laminectomy is prone. Both legs are wrapped with elastic bandages, or tensor hose are used to prevent venous stasis in the extremities.

Anesthesia induction and intubation take place on the transport vehicle. The patient is then placed on the OR bed in the prone position. Special bed attachment supports or a chest roll must be placed under the chest on each side from the shoulder to the iliac crest to permit lung expansion during the procedure. The bottom of the bed is dropped to about a 25-degree angle. The patient's knees are flexed, and the lower legs elevated and supported on two large pillows and the bed mattress, under which the footboard is placed at a right angle to the bed. The knees are padded with foam. The arms are flexed at the elbows and supported by pillows on wide armboards. Care is taken to prevent pressure or tension on the brachial plexus. The Wilson back frame, Kambin, or Andrews spinal frame can be used. The patient is placed prone on the frame with pillows under the legs and pillows or sheets supporting each arm. For surgery on the neck and posterior skull, the foot of the bed is not dropped; the ankles and feet are supported on a large pillow; and the arms are secured at the patient's sides, protecting the ulnar, median, and radial nerves. A horseshoe or Mayfield point headrest may be used.

The major problems encountered with the prone position include increase in venous pressure and bleeding at the operative site, peripheral venous stasis, and decrease in vital capacity. Precautions include checking female breasts, male genitals, and knees to prevent pressure on these areas; avoiding hyperextension of shoulders and pressure on the brachial plexus when turning the patient to begin positioning and during the procedure; preventing abduction of the arms and occlusion of the subclavian and axillary arteries; and protecting the eyes from pressure, corneal scratches, and chemical burns.

The knee-chest, or tuck, position is also used for lumbar laminectomy. This is a modification of the prone position, in which the patient's hips and knees are flexed so the body is supported on the thighs and lower legs, with the abdomen and chest hanging free or supported on chest rolls. The Hicks spinal surgery frame (Butt Board) may be used for the knee-chest position, as well as the Andrews spinal frame or table. Advantages of this position include decreased bleeding because of the collapse of epidural veins, better exposure resulting from hyperflexion of the spine, absence of pressure on the vena cava, and increased ease of ventilation. Operating time is usually reduced when this position is used.

Disadvantages of the knee-chest position include the difficulty of maintaining physical stability on the OR bed, hypotension, and pooling of blood in the lower extremities.

Draping

Most neurosurgeons do their own draping. Draping for some procedures is complex and requires the cooperation of surgeon, assistant, and scrub nurse. Four or more towels are placed around the operative site. They may be secured by disposable skin staples, small towel clamps, or silk sutures on a heavy cutting needle. When sutures are used, the surgeon also needs heavy, 6-inch toothed tissue forceps and suture scissors. Forceps, scissors, needle holders, and needles are discarded after towels have been secured in place.

A plastic adhesive drape may be placed either before or after the towels. The skin must be completely dry for the drape to adhere tightly to the skin.

Fluid-impervious barrier drape sheets and towels are essential. If an overhead instrument table is used, it should be covered with a sheet large enough that the front edge can be fanfolded at the front edge of the table until the table is brought forward over the patient toward the operative site. The fanfolded sheet can then be secured at the lower border of the operative site to bridge the gap between the unsterile undersurface of the table and the sterile field. Mayo stands should also be covered with effective barriers. The particulars of draping for neurosurgical procedures vary and are influenced by the patient's position, the surgeon's preferences, and what is available in each hospital. Therefore a detailed description of the draping for each procedure is not provided here. The particulars of draping for each procedure should be clearly described on the neurosurgeon's preference card. Doubts can be clarified by communication with the neurosurgeon before the operation.

As a general rule, neurosurgeons prefer to have all equipment ready before making the incision. Therefore they can be helpful to the perioperative nurse in attaching and hooking up suction tubings, electrosurgical cords, and other equipment that will be needed for the operation.

Hemostasis

Meticulous hemostasis is of particular importance in neurosurgery. The first consideration is control of hemorrhage from the highly vascular scalp. Compression of the edges of the wound with gauze sponges and fingers during the initial incision is followed by application of hemostatic clips and clamps. When clips are used, they are applied so that they include the galea and skin edge, whereas clamps are attached directly to the galea and then everted. Before the incision is made, normal saline solution or a local anesthetic agent may be injected to minimize scalp bleeding.

Bone wax, a hemostatic material described in Chapter 5, is prepared for all cranial and spinal cord operations. The surgeon firmly rubs the wax into the bleeding surface of the bone after all periosteum has been scraped off. When the skull flap has been elevated, bone wax is also rubbed

into the diplöe to control bleeding from the bone edge. During spinal surgery, bone wax is used on the cut edges of the laminae.

Electrosurgery is routine for neurosurgical procedures. Perioperative nurses must understand the uses and hazards of the electrosurgical unit and be familiar with the safety measures. Electrocoagulation may be used to stop bleeding in the galea, in the periosteum, on the surface of the dura, on the spinal cord, and in the brain. The coagulation current seals the blood vessels. The electrical current is applied to the forceps, a metal suction tip, or other instrument, which acts as a conducting tool. To be effective, the coagulating current must contact the vessel in a dry field. For this reason, suctioning is necessary to remove blood as the contact is made between the instrument carrying the current and the bleeding point.

Bipolar electrosurgical units are frequently used (Fig. 22-22). Bipolar units provide a completely isolated output with negligible leakage of current between the tips of the forceps, permitting use of coagulating current in proximity to structures where ordinary unipolar coagulation would be hazardous. Ringer's lactate or normal saline irrigation is used during bipolar coagulation to minimize tissue heating, shrinkage, drying, and adherence to the forceps. Some bipolar units have built-in irrigating systems. Need for a dispersive pad is eliminated. The use of the bipolar coagulation technique allows hemostasis of almost any size vessel encountered. Vessels as large as the superficial temporal ar-

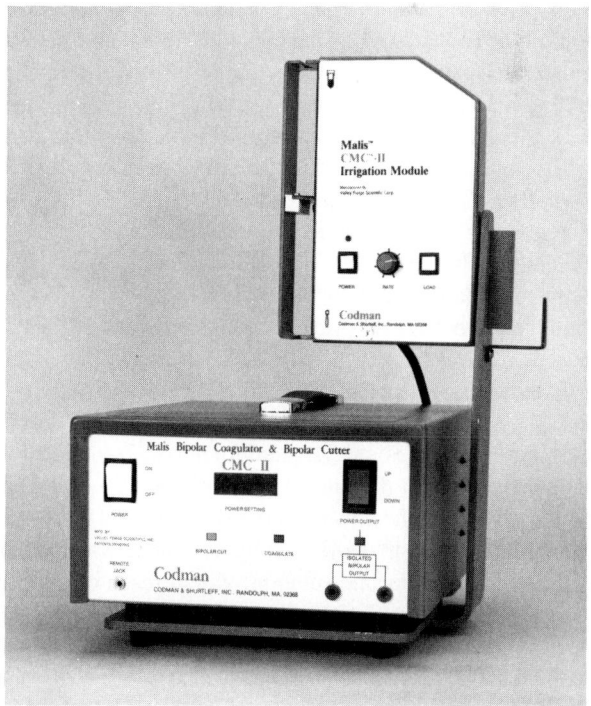

FIG. 22-22 Malis bipolar coagulator and bipolar cutter, with irrigation module.

Courtesy Codman & Shurtleff, Inc., Randolph, Mass.

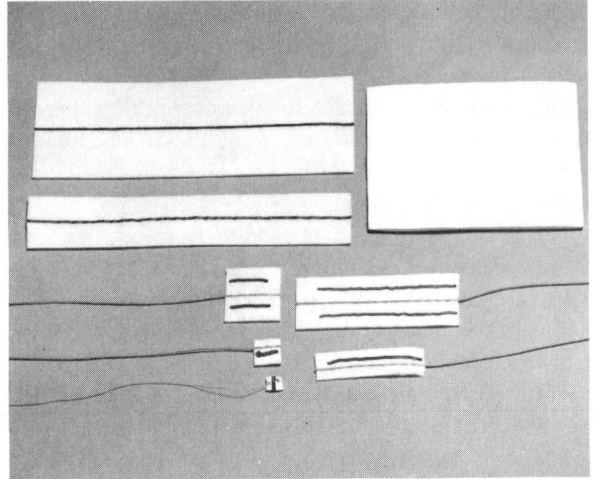

FIG. 22-23   Cottonoid strips and neuro patties.
Courtesy Codman & Shurtleff, Inc., Randolph, Mass.

tery, as well as those too small for suture or clip ligation, may be coagulated with bipolar units.

Electrosurgery is also used for cutting with a lower power setting. When the surgeon is using a cutting electrode to remove a tumor, the circulating nurse should stand by the machine to adjust the settings as needed. As the surgeon uses the cutting electrode, an assistant holds a suction tip to one side of the area of dissection to remove smoke.

Gauze sponges are used to control bleeding before the skull or spinal canal is entered. Coarse gauze sponges injure fragile tissues such as the brain and spinal cord, so wet compressed rayon cotton (cottonoid) pledgets or strips are used in place of gauze sponges to control bleeding beneath the skull and around the spinal cord. Sterile cottonoid strips and pledgets, or patties, must be available in a variety of sizes (Fig. 22-23). Strips are usually 6 inches long, although some surgeons prefer them 3 inches in length. The standard widths are ¼, ½, ¾, and 1 inch. Strips have x-ray–detectable markers or strings attached. Pledgets should have both x-ray–detectable markers and strings attached.

Standard sizes for pledgets are ¼ × ¼ inch, ½ × ½ inch, ¾ × ¾ inch, and 1 × 1 inch. All strips and pledgets must be counted. Some surgeons prefer to use Biocal or Telfa strips, which the nurse cuts to size before use. During the procedure the nurse maintains a supply of these special neurosurgical sponges, thoroughly soaked with normal saline or Ringer's lactate solution, within reach of the surgeon's forceps. They may be displayed on a waterproof surface, such as a towel; a sterile inverted metal basin (emesis basin, small bowl); a plastic drape, such as 3M or Vi-Drape; a piece of rubber clipped to a folded towel; or a patty plate, a flat piece of metal that attaches to the Mayo tray with two small towel clamps. The surgeon may prefer that the nurse keep a supply of these moist sponges on the palm or back of one hand and extend them toward the surgeon as needed. The sponges are aligned on the display surface in order of size. As soon as one is used, it is replaced. Loose, wet cotton balls may be used as a temporary pack or tamponade in a bleeding tumor bed after a tumor has been removed. The gentle pressure of the cotton balls along with time and patience on the part of the surgeon may stop bleeding not controllable by other means. The scrub nurse is responsible for counting the number of cotton balls placed in the tumor bed and ensuring that none is left behind at closure.

A variety of hemostatic clips is available and used by neurosurgeons to occlude both superficial and deep vessels. The original clip used by Cushing and later modified by McKenzie is made of silver. Newer clips such as the Samuels hemoclip and the Ligaclip are of tantalum or an alloy that is compatible with the MRI scanner. The scrub nurse removes the clips from a special cartridge with the appropriate applicator and passes them to the surgeon for application to a vessel. Such clips enable the surgeon to occlude vessels in areas difficult to reach by other means and to ligate superficial vessels of the brain before cutting them and without destroying any surrounding tissues. Clips can be obtained in a variety of sizes.

Hemostatic scalp clips include Raney, Adson, and LeRoy clips. Autoclips and Michel clips are still used occasionally (Fig. 22-24). There are also plastic disposable scalp clips of the Raney and Leroy Raney types. Each type of clip has a specific clip applier by which the clips are placed on the scalp edges. At time of closure clips are removed by a hemostat, a special clip remover, or the applier, which simultaneously serves as a remover. A minimum of two clip appliers is essential; the scrub nurse loads one clip applier while the surgeon is using the other to place the clip on the scalp. The Adson clips are loaded on the appliers from a special rack. After use they must be reshaped before replacement on the clip rack; there is a special instrument for this purpose. The Raney and Michel clips are loaded by hand. If the Raney clips are nondisposable, they are difficult to clean by hand and should be placed in a sonic cleaner or soaked in hydrogen peroxide.

Numerous special clips are used for permanent or temporary occlusion of vessels or an aneurysm neck in the surgical treatment of intracranial aneurysm. These are discussed in the Microneurosurgery section.

Neurosurgeons almost routinely use certain hemostatic agents in addition to mechanical hemostasis. Gelfoam is one of these agents. It comes in two forms: a powder and a compressed sponge. The sponge is produced in three sizes: nos. 12, 50, and 100. The sponge form can be applied to an oozing surface dry or saturated with saline solution or topical thrombin. The larger pieces of Gelfoam are cut into a variety of sizes of strips and pledgets. The surgeon's preference dictates the exact method of preparation and use. Gelfoam is absorbable and can be left in the body.

Surgicel, a rayonlike cellulose gauze, and Oxycel, an ab-

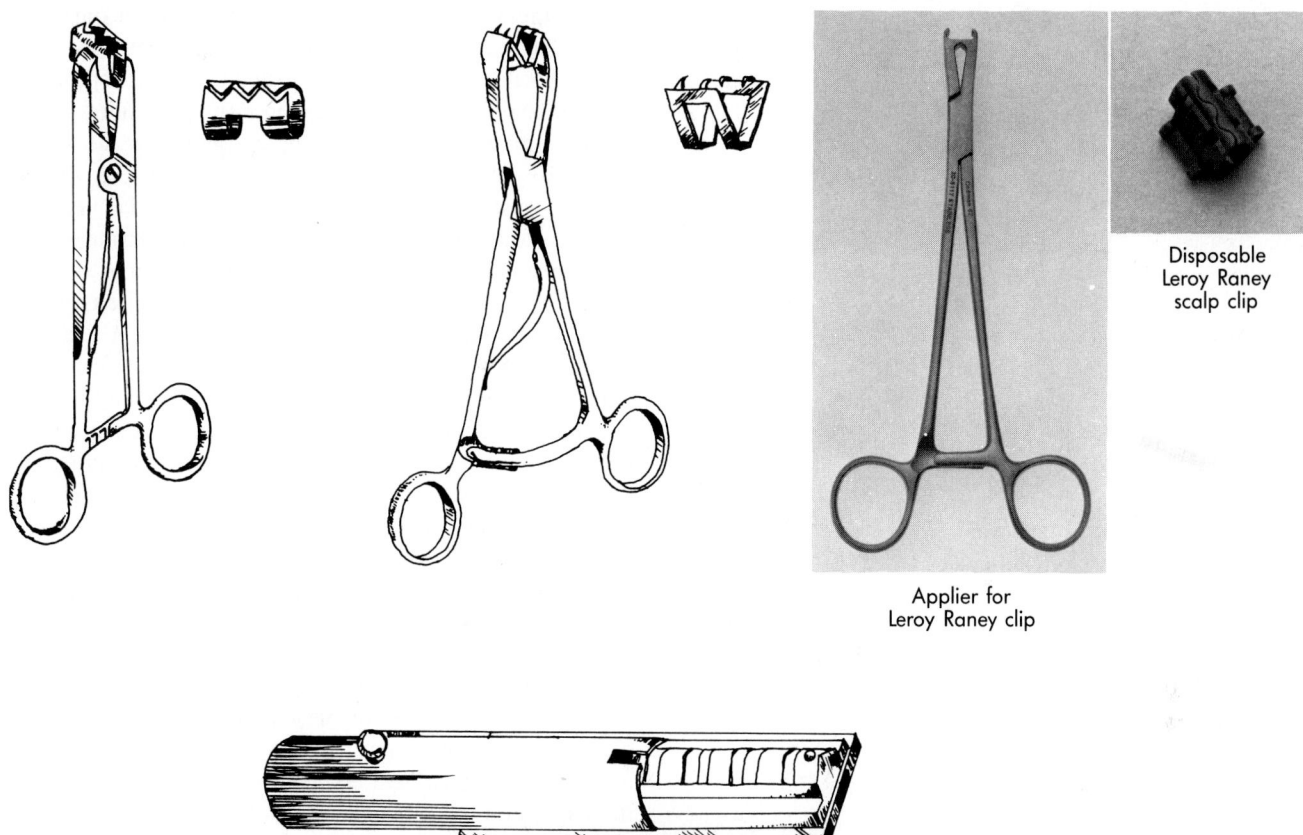

FIG. 22-24   Scalp clip appliers and clips, disposable Leroy Raney scalp clip, and applier for Leroy Raney scalp clip.

Courtesy Codman & Shurtleff, Inc., Randolph, Mass.

sorbable hemostatic agent that comes in both cotton and gauze forms, are used to control bleeding from oozing surfaces, vessels, and sinuses in the brain and spinal canal. These hemostatic substances are also cut into suitable sizes and shapes and are handed to the surgeon dry, followed by a moist cottonoid strip or patty. The hemostatic material adheres to the bleeding area as gentle pressure is applied to the cottonoid material for several minutes.

Pieces of fresh muscle tissue can be used to tamponade and control bleeding where the usual forms of hemostasis are not possible.

Most surgeons use Polyglactin, synthetic, absorbable, black braided nylon, or silk suture material for traction sutures and wound closure.

Irrigating the wound with Ringer's lactate or normal saline solution may facilitate hemostasis. This procedure definitely helps the surgeon identify active bleeding points. Two completely filled bulb or Asepto syringes should always be within reach of the surgeon. Suction is the best means of keeping the wound dry and permitting control of bleeding. Therefore suction and irrigation are used together.

Metal suction tips, such as the Cone, Sachs, Frazier, Bucy, and Adson (Fig. 22-25), are used because they not only keep the wound dry but also can be used to conduct coagulation current from a monopolar unit to the bleeding point. The Bucy-Frazier tip is insulated and attached to both suction and electrosurgical units to become the active coagulating electrode. Use of the suction-coagulation unit is limited to areas in which gross coagulation can be done safely, for example, during the opening phase of a surgical procedure.

Suction can be used to remove necrotic or traumatized brain tissue or soft brain tumors rapidly after a sample has been obtained for pathologic examination. It is also useful in evaluating abscess cavities, removing fluid from a ventricle or the subarachnoid space, holding a solid tumor during its removal, and applying compression to a bleeding vessel.

Many neurosurgeons irrigate surgical wounds with an antibiotic solution before wound closure. The antibiotic must be mixed with irrigation solution according to the surgeon's preference so it is ready for use when needed. Gelfoam may be soaked in antibiotic solution before use.

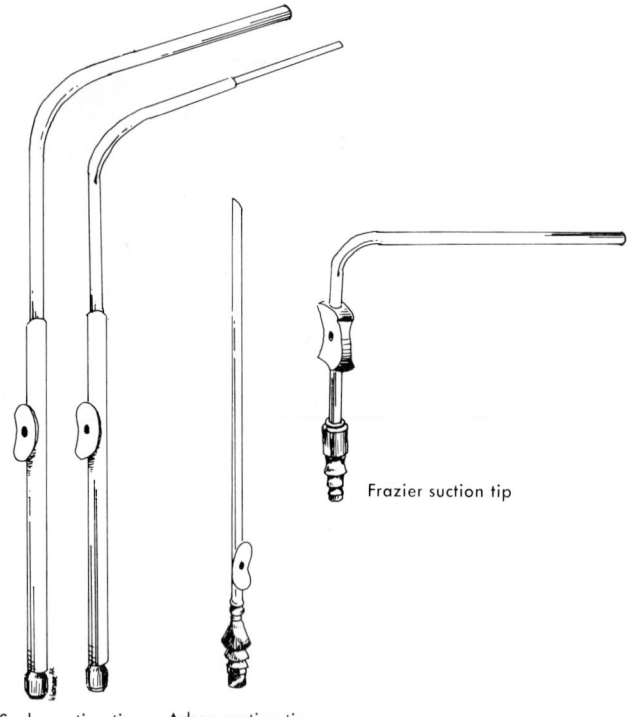

Sachs suction tips   Adson suction tip

Frazier suction tip

FIG. 22-25   Suction tips.

Equipment

An operating room used for neurosurgical procedures should be large enough to accommodate the equipment needed for procedures done by the neurosurgeons on the hospital staff. The emphasis of this discussion is equipment that is *necessary* for neurosurgery in any setting.

Essential built-in equipment includes a minimum of eight electrical outlets per wall, four overhead spotlights, six single or three double x-ray view boxes, and four wall or ceiling vacuum suction outlets capable of high negative pressure. Other equipment that can be built in if the situation demands includes a two-way telephone communication line, a ceiling-mounted operating microscope with camera, a closed-circuit television unit with monitor, an electrocardiogram-electroencephalogram monitor with readouts, and a wall or ceiling source of nitrogen or compressed air to operate air-powered equipment. Additionally, many operating rooms now have computer consoles for three-dimensional reformation and stereotaxis, EMG, evoked potentials, and spinal cord monitoring. Consideration must be given to enough room for the equipment in the rooms that are designated for neurosurgery.

Some basic mobile equipment is needed for any setting in which neurosurgery is done. An OR bed and complete set of bed attachments and neurosurgical headrests are essential. The best headrest is one that can be adapted for use in any body position, such as the Amsco multipoise, the Gardner, and the Mayfield skull clamp (Fig. 22-26, *B*).

Each of these headrests has a three-pin suspension and skull clamp that attaches to a headrest bed attachment for secure fixation of the skull during the operation. This is especially useful when the patient is placed in a sitting position. Two or three sterile pins are placed in the head after the insertion sites are prepared with an antiseptic, such as an iodophor. The headrest skull clamp is first attached to the pins and then to the bed attachment. Precautions during insertion of the pins include avoiding the frontal sinuses, superficial temporal arteries, and the eyes. Other headrests, such as the Light-Veley or Multipoise (Fig. 22-26, *A* and *B*), that are of more limited use may be preferred by the individual neurosurgeon. In many instances, especially for supratentorial craniotomy, the head can be stabilized by a rubber doughnut. A mobile cart should be used for storage of the neurosurgical headrests and bed parts, as well as any other positioning devices and aids used by the neurosurgeon.

One special neurosurgical overhead instrument table, such as the Mayfield table (Fig. 22-27), is preferable, but two large Mayo trays can be used for any neurosurgical procedure. One large instrument back table is a must. It should be at least 6 to 8 inches higher than the standard table because the scrub nurse must frequently work on a high lift to see the operative field and perform effectively. The extra height of the back table enables the perioperative nurse to maintain a sterile field and to work more comfortably.

Eight to 10 footstools are needed. They can be arranged side by side or on top of each other for the safety, efficiency, and comfort of the personnel. Kickbuckets are needed for trash and sponges. Also useful are two small utility tables for preparation and special equipment and supplies.

A cooling-heating unit with two blankets, such as the K-thermia unit, should be available for use. An electronic temperature monitoring device with esophageal, intraaural, and rectal probes is essential.

Other essential equipment includes a monopolar electrosurgical unit, a bipolar electrosurgical unit, at least one fiberoptic headlight, and one fiberoptic light source for lighted retractors and telescopes, if they are used. Also needed is an operating microscope such as the Zeiss or Storz, a tank of nitrogen, if not built in, with a special pressure gauge for operating air-powered instruments, four pressure bags and bulb pumps for infusion of blood, two blood-warming units, one or two electronic intravenous rate control units such as I-Vac units, a solution warmer, and a nerve stimulator. A cryosurgical unit, an image intensifier, and a stereotaxic apparatus may be needed if the surgical procedure requires them. A laser, ultrasonic surgical aspirator, and intraoperative ultrasound should be available (Fig. 22-28).

Instrumentation

Scientific developments in other fields have been applied to the health care delivery system in general. Some of the

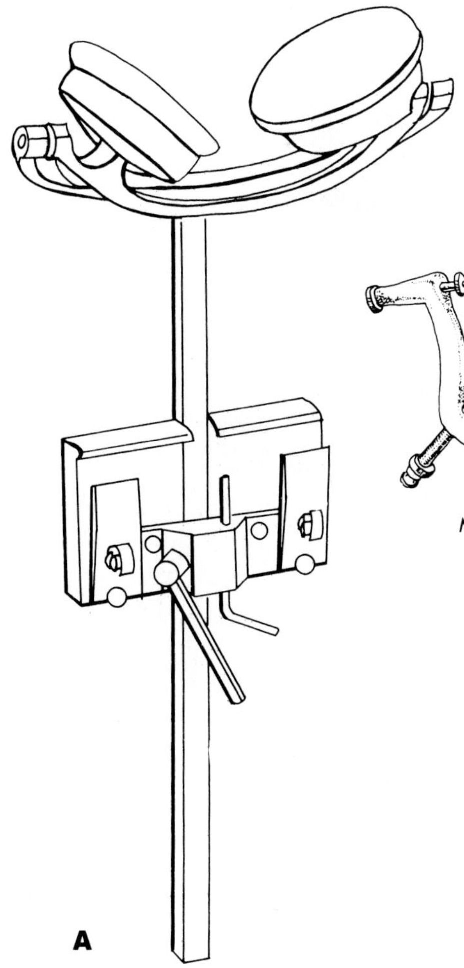

FIG. 22-26 **A,** Light-Veley headrest. **B,** Three-pin suspension skull clamps for stabilizing head during neurosurgical procedures. **C,** Mayfield headrest.

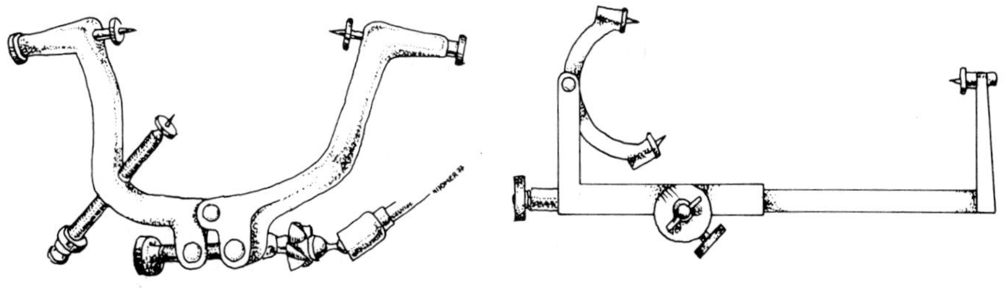

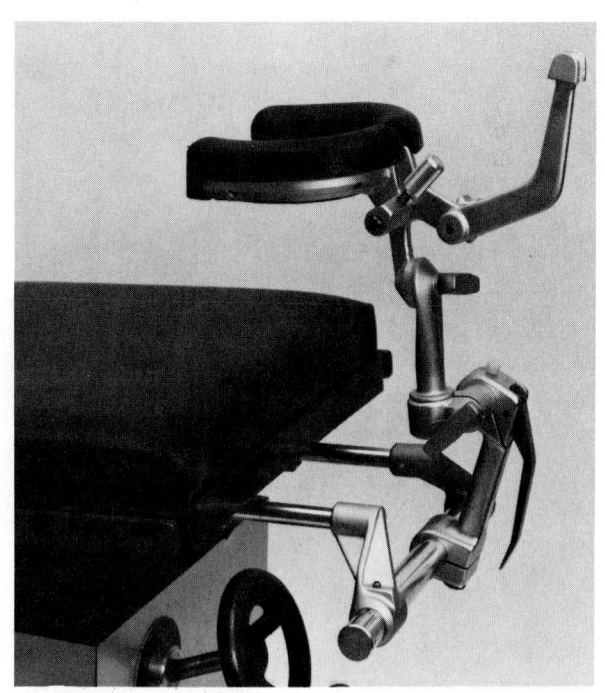

Multipoise skull clamp

B

Gardner skull clamp

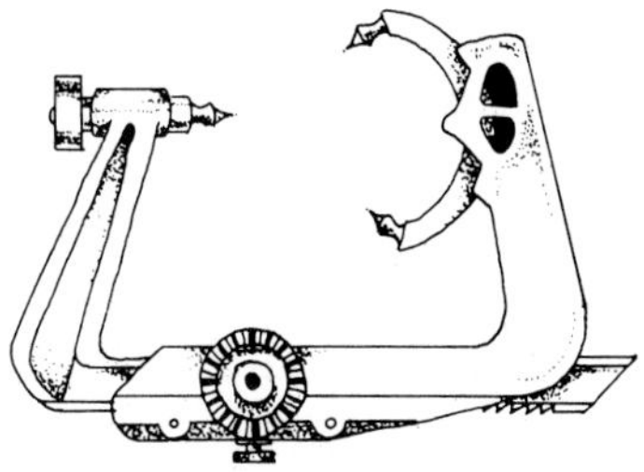

Mayfield skull clamp

A

C

developments with application to neurosurgery in the forms of specialized instrumentation and equipment have been discussed previously. A few items require further discussion.

Air-powered instrumentation has become popular with neurosurgeons over the years since the first Hall air drill was developed. Modifications of the original instrument continue today. These instruments decrease open wound time and anesthesia time for the patient and conserve energy for the surgeon.

The basic air driver has been adapted by means of special attachments for neurosurgery. Because improvements and new developments in air-powered instruments are ongoing, specific instructions for use and care of such equipment should be obtained from the manufacturer at the time of purchase. Basic information is included here.

The Air Drill 100 (Fig. 22-29) has replaced the Surgairtome or Hall II air drill for precision cutting, shaping, and repair of bone. Its use increases the ease of bone work and reduces operating time. Compressed nitrogen is the power source, as with other air-powered equipment. The Air Drill 100 can be used to widen the graft area in anterior fusions and to unroof the auditory canal in eighth cranial nerve surgery. For use in less accessible areas, such as the sphenoi-

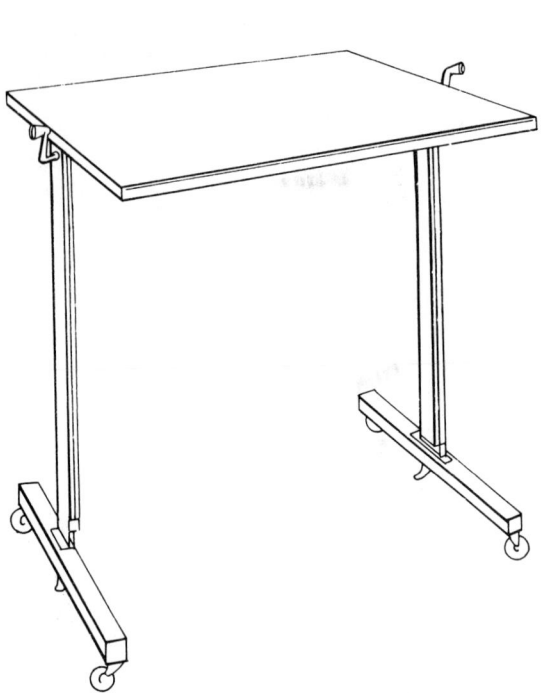

FIG. 22-27   Mayfield overhead instrument table.

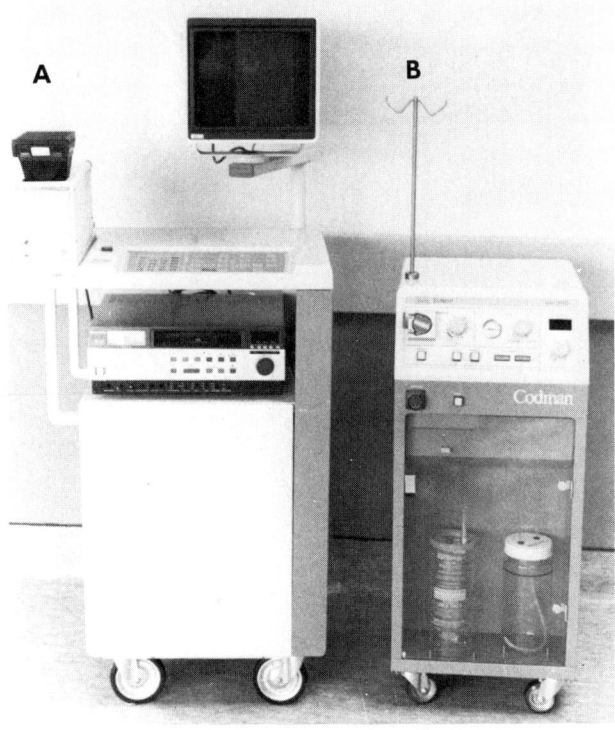

FIG. 22-28   **A,** Intraoperative ultrasound. **B,** Ultrasonic aspirator.

Courtesy Codman & Shurtleff, Inc., Randolph, Mass.

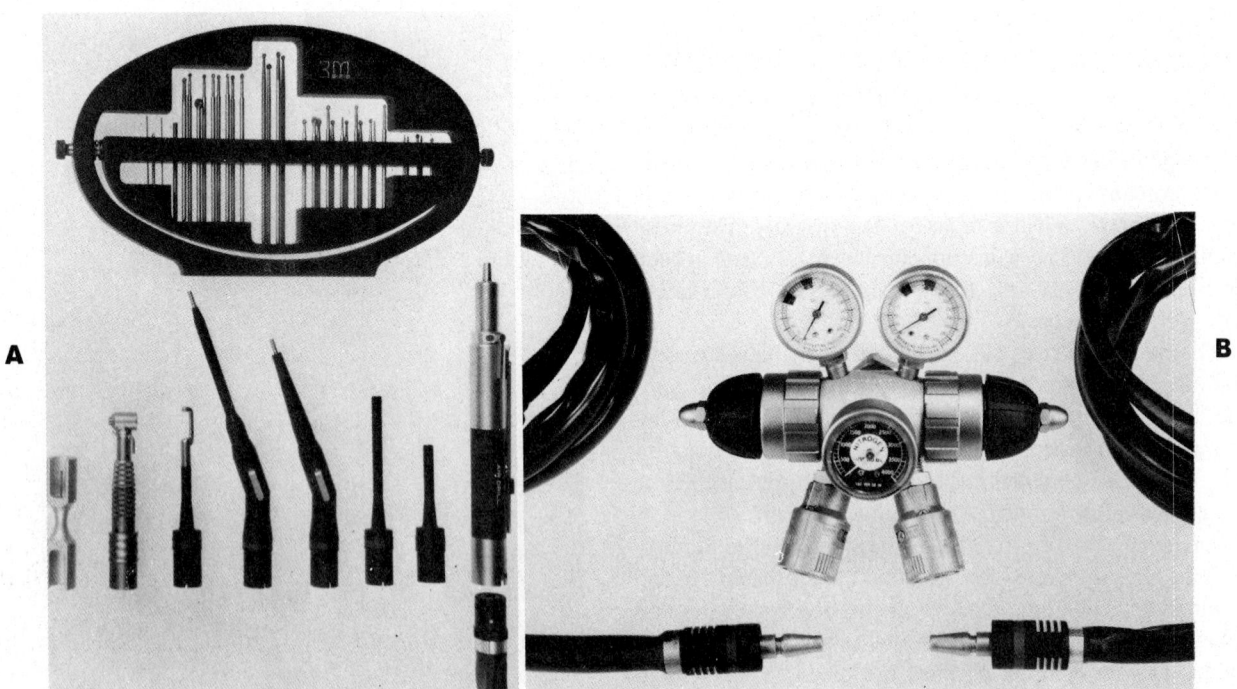

FIG. 22-29   **A,** Air Drill 100 with attachments. **B,** Dual nitrogen regulator.

Courtesy 3M Co., St. Paul, Minn.

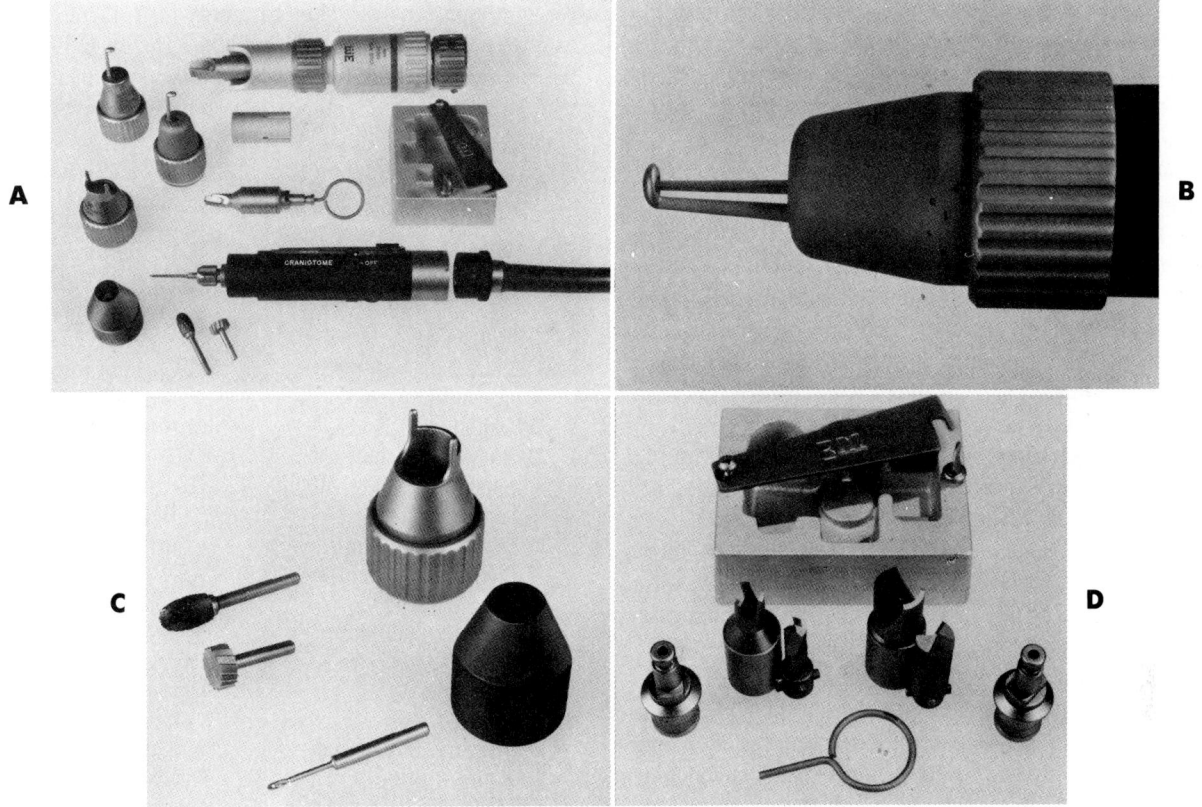

FIG. 22-30 **A,** Craniotome C-100 with attachments. **B,** Craniotome with neuroblade. **C,** Cranioplasty
and wire-pass attachments. **D,** Skull perforators.
Courtesy 3M Co., St. Paul, Minn.

dal sinus, pituitary fossa, and vertebral bodies, 20-degree
and 90-degree angle attachments are available. A range of
burrs and guards is available.

The Craniotome C-100 (Fig. 22-30) is the newest adaptation of the original Hall Neurairtome. A perforator drive
attachment reduces the speed to 1000 rpm for drilling burr
holes. Both 12-mm and 7-mm perforators are available in
disposable and reusable forms. The perforator driver attachment can be removed and a saw blade and dura guard attached to adapt the instrument for cutting a craniotomy bone
flap. The saw blade is interchangeable with a wire-pass drill
bit for drilling holes and placing wires, when a bone flap is
to be wired in place. A cranioplasty burr and skull contour
burr, as well as guards for each type of burr, are available.

Electrically powered instruments were popular and
widely used before the introduction of the air-powered models. Some surgeons prefer power drills such as the Light-
Veley or the Codman-Shurtleff drills with a Smith perforator.

Another versatile pneumatic tool is the Midas Rex instrument (see Chapter 21). The variety of disposable cutting tools of this foot-controlled instrument and its attachments provides the neurosurgeon with a wide capability in
bone cutting, including small rectangular holes in place of

burr holes; bone flaps of any size and shaping; and unroof-
ing areas such as the sphenoid wing. Additionally, large
craniotomy flaps can be turned with only a single burr hole.
Manufacturer's precautions and instructions must be followed.

The operating microscope (see Chapter 17) has revolutionized neurosurgery, making possible procedures never
done before and making other neurosurgical procedures on
vessels, such as aneurysm surgery, and surgery on nerves
more precise and therefore more successful.

The lens system for neurosurgery and the angle of the
microscope are different from those used in otologic surgery. If a microscope is shared by neurologic and otologic
services, the perioperative nurse must be able to adapt the
microscope for use in neurosurgery by attachment of the
appropriate pieces, and the surgeon must check it for focal
length and focus before scrubbing. Disposable drapes are
available for the microscope, as are assistant and observer
lenses. Cameras and closed-circuit television monitors are
also available for use with the operating microscope, if the
situation warrants such sophisticated equipment.

The routine use of video cameras, recorders, and television monitors, if available, is invaluable to teach staff and
enhance interest and understanding of the surgical proce-

dure by perioperative nurses who are otherwise unable to visualize the surgeon's actions directly. By viewing the operative field through the monitor, the experienced scrub nurse will be able to anticipate the neurosurgeon's next move, and will therefore provide better assistance.

Many surgeons routinely use the carbon dioxide (CO_2) laser for precise dissection and hemostasis. The laser produces a concentrated infrared energy beam, generated by CO_2, that can be precisely focused on any point at which it is aimed. The beam, which is made visible by a superimposed red aiming light, causes flash vaporization of cellular water at 100° C. Advantages of the laser include improved hemostasis and healing with decreased tissue trauma, swelling, and risk of metastasis.

The KTP laser also has proven to be a valuable tool for the neurosurgeon. Postoperative morbidity is minimal. The laser is especially advantageous in microvascular surgery and is used to occlude vessels less than 0.5 mm in diameter in operations for aneurysms and arteriovenous malformations, as well as to remove tumors with minimal or no damage to surrounding structures. Tissue damage depends on amounts of energy generated and exposure duration.

Precautions include the need to wear protective glasses or plastic goggles, specific to the laser being used, to prevent accidental damage to eyes of personnel in the room and the need to keep all cottonoid, sponge, and towel materials thoroughly damp to prevent fire that could result from contact between a dry combustible material and the beam. The CO_2 and other gas sources must be checked before use to ensure adequate supply for the procedure. Nonflammable anesthetic agents must be used. Smoke evacuators should be available to remove the smoke generated.

Direct image intensification is essential for an increasing number of neurosurgical procedures, such as placement of nerve stimulator electrodes in brain or spinal areas and stereotaxic procedures. If possible, a C-arm and monitor should be available in the operating room. Otherwise these procedures can be done in the radiology department. Procedures requiring use of the CT scan can also be done in the radiology department.

Choice of instrumentation for a given neurosurgical procedure is largely controlled by the surgeon or, in some operating rooms, by the chief of the department. Exactly what the neurosurgeon needs for a specific procedure is highly individual. Factors that influence the choices include training, experience, type of setting in which the surgery is performed, pathologic condition of the patient, surgical approach planned, and equipment available.

Some hospitals provide a full range of highly specialized neurosurgical instrumentation; some supply only instruments that can be used in orthopedic, otologic, and nasal surgery as well as in neurosurgery. Many neurosurgeons in private practice carry some or all of their own special instruments from hospital to hospital.

Usually several instruments can be used to perform one function. The choice depends on what is available and the surgeon's preference. Therefore only instrument types and examples of each type are listed here. The exact instrument list for any neurosurgeon for each procedure must be written by the perioperative nurse in collaboration with that surgeon.

Basic instruments include the following list (specific names in parentheses are examples):

- 1 Hudson brace (or craniotome) with burrs and perforators)
- 1 Drill guide
- 1 Hand drill with drill bits and key
- 2 Cranial saw handles
- 2 Cranial saw guides (Cushing, Bailey, Poppen)
- 6 Cranial saws (Gigli, Tyler)
- 2 Double-action rongeurs, 9¾ inches (Stille gooseneck, Leksell)
- 2 Double-action rongeurs, 6¾ inches (Zaufel-Janse, Beyer, Fulton)
- 2 Single-action rongeurs (Adson, Stookey, Lempert)
- 2 Cloward punches, 40 degree, 5 mm and 3 mm
- 1 Raney punch
- 1 Kerrison ronguer, 5 mm
- 5 Penfield dissectors, nos. 1, 2, 3, 4, and 5
- 5 Bone curettes, nos. 0, 00, 1, 3, and 4
- 2 Four-prong rake retractors, dull
- 2 Cushing subtemporal decompression retractors
- 4 Self-retaining retractors, dull, 8 inches (Cone, Weitlaner, Anderson-Adson)
- 1 Jansen mastoid retractor
- 36 Scalp clips (Adson, Raney, Michel)
- 2 Scalp clip appliers for the specific clip used
- 1 Scalp clip remover (Adson, Michel)
- 4 Bayonet forceps, smooth, 7¼ inches
- 2 Tissue forceps with teeth, 6 inches
- 2 Cushing forceps, smooth, 7 inches
- 2 Cushing forceps with teeth, 7 inches
- 2 Adson tissue forceps, 5 inches
- 18 Towel clamps, Backhaus type, 3½ inches
- 18 Halsted mosquito hemostats, 12 curved and 6 straight
- 36 Hemostatic scalp forceps (Dandy, Crile, Kolodney, Kelly)
- 10 Rochester-Pean forceps
- 4 Kocher forceps, straight, 6 inches
- 12 Towel clamps, Peers type
- 6 Fishhook retractors
- 4 Periosteal elevators (Cushing, Adson, Langenbeck)
- 1 Dura separator (Sachs, Frazier, Hoen)
- 1 Adson elevator, no. 3
- 1 Cushing periosteal elevator (joker)
- 2 Freer dissectors (Olivecrona, Woodson)
- 4 Ventricular needles with obturators, 3½ inches (Cone, Seletz, Scott)
- 1 Brain-aspirating needle with cannula
- 1 Aneurysm needle
- 2 Brain spoons, 1 small and 1 large (Cushing)
- 6 Suction tips, 2 each large, medium, and small (Frazier, Bucy, Sachs, Cone, Adson)
- 2 Suction tubings
- 1 Electrosurgical pencil with spatula and needlepoint tip

6 Gerald bayonet forceps: 2 each fine with teeth; fine, smooth; and heavy with teeth

6 Davis brain retractors, 2 each narrow, medium, and wide

4 Clip appliers, 2 each medium and small (Hemoclips, Ligaclips, McKenzie)

4 Clip cartridges, 2 each medium and small

1 Clip rack

2 Alligator clip appliers (Penfield, Samuels-Weck)

1 Stainless steel metric ruler

2 Dura hooks, 6 inches

6 Needle holders: 2 each fine, 7½ inches; fine, 6 inches; and heavy, 7¼ inches

3 Adson (tonsil) hemostatic forceps, straight, 7¼ inches

3 Nerve hooks, 7¾ inches, 1 each small, medium, and large

3 Copper pituitary spoons, 1 each small, medium, and large (Cushing)

1 Self-retaining brain retractor with assorted blades (Leyla-Yasargil, Edinborough, DeMartel, Hamby, Greenberg)

6 Knife handles, 2 each nos. 3, 4, and 7

1 Mayo scissors, curved, 7 inches

2 Metzenbaum scissors, 5 and 7 inches

5 Alligator pituitary/disk rongeurs with assorted cup sizes

1 Bipolar electrosurgical forceps and cord

3 Irrigating syringes (Asepto, ear bulb)

6 Syringes, 10 ml, 2 each plain tip, Luer-Lok, and control grip

1 DeVilbiss bone-cutting instruments with 2 blades

The foregoing instrument list is very basic and compiled to help a perioperative nurse in a general hospital rather than a perioperative nurse in a large neurosurgical center. A hospital with an active neurosurgical service has its own basic craniotomy instrument list. The perioperative nurse should use that list and add the special preferences of a given neurosurgeon.

In addition to the basic types of instruments essential for supratenorial craniotomy (Figs. 22-31 to 22-34), suture scissors, wire scissors, and 6-inch Russian forceps should be included. A bone punch (Cone or Ingram), a drill guide and dura protector (Adson or Hamlin), a twist drill that fits the Hudson brace or a Raney brace and perforator, hemostatic clips and applicators, trephines, burr hole covers (Silastic, such as the Todd-Crue buttons, or tantalum), Ray pituitary curettes, a Rayport dura knife, pituitary forceps (Adson or D'Errico), Bonney forceps, Penfield watchmaker's forceps, Hartmann forceps, monopolar electrosurgical bayonet forceps (Davis, Raney, Hoen, Jansen), bulldog clamps, angled dura scissors (Taylor, Frazier, DeBakey, Potts-Smith), and myriad other instruments that a given neurosurgeon may desire can be included.

Many neurosurgeons prefer Allis forceps, rather than towel clamps or Peers clamps, to attach suction, electrosurgical pencils, and other devices to the drapes. Allis forceps used for this purpose should not be used for any other surgical procedures. They can be marked for neurosurgery and kept with the special neurosurgical instruments. They will not effectively hold tissue, such as the edge of the small bowel, after continued use on drape materials. Two 10-ml Luer-Lok and two 10-ml plain-tip syringes should be included in every craniotomy setup. Also included should be six to 12 rubber bands, one or two Penrose drains, two medicine cups, suture material and needles of the surgeon's choice, and dressing headrolls (Kling or Kerlix).

Many neurosurgeons use magnifying loupes. They are made on a custom basis and are usually the personal property of the surgeon.

Posterior fossa or infratentorial craniectomy requires the same instrumentation as supratentorial craniotomy, minus saws, saw handles, and saw guides. A cerebellar extension for the Hudson brace must be included, as well as a larger assortment of double-action and Kerrison rongeurs.

Additional instruments required for laminectomy, anterior fusion, surgery of peripheral nerves, microsurgery, and aneurysm surgery are included in the descriptions of the surgical procedures. An example of a back table setup for craniotomy is shown in Fig. 22-35.

EVALUATION

After the surgical procedure is completed, the patient is transported to the PACU. The patient is evaluated for the previously established outcomes. Bony prominences and pressure points are checked for skin integrity. A report along with documentation is given to the PACU nurse. Included are the outcomes from the identified nursing diagnoses. If the outcomes were met, they may be communicated as follows:

- The patient demonstrated a reduction in anxiety, verbalized feeling less anxious, coped with perioperative routines adequately, and verbalized an understanding of the planned procedure(s).
- The patient and/or family verbalized knowledge of diagnostic and surgical procedures and had realistic expectations of tests, routines, and postoperative care.
- The patient maintained effective breathing patterns; ventilation was maintained, arterial blood gases (ABGs) were within normal limits, and breath sounds were bilateral.
- The patient will continue to report a reduction in pain, ask for pain medication, and verbalize relief or absence of pain.
- The patient will exhibit no signs and symptoms of infection; the wound will be clean and well healed.

SURGICAL INTERVENTIONS

It is not possible in this chapter to provide a detailed approach to each neurosurgical procedure. Specific neurosurgical procedures are numerous, and each has a number of modifications or variations. The operating surgeon decides exactly which procedure and what variation will be performed. Basic general approaches, however, are limited

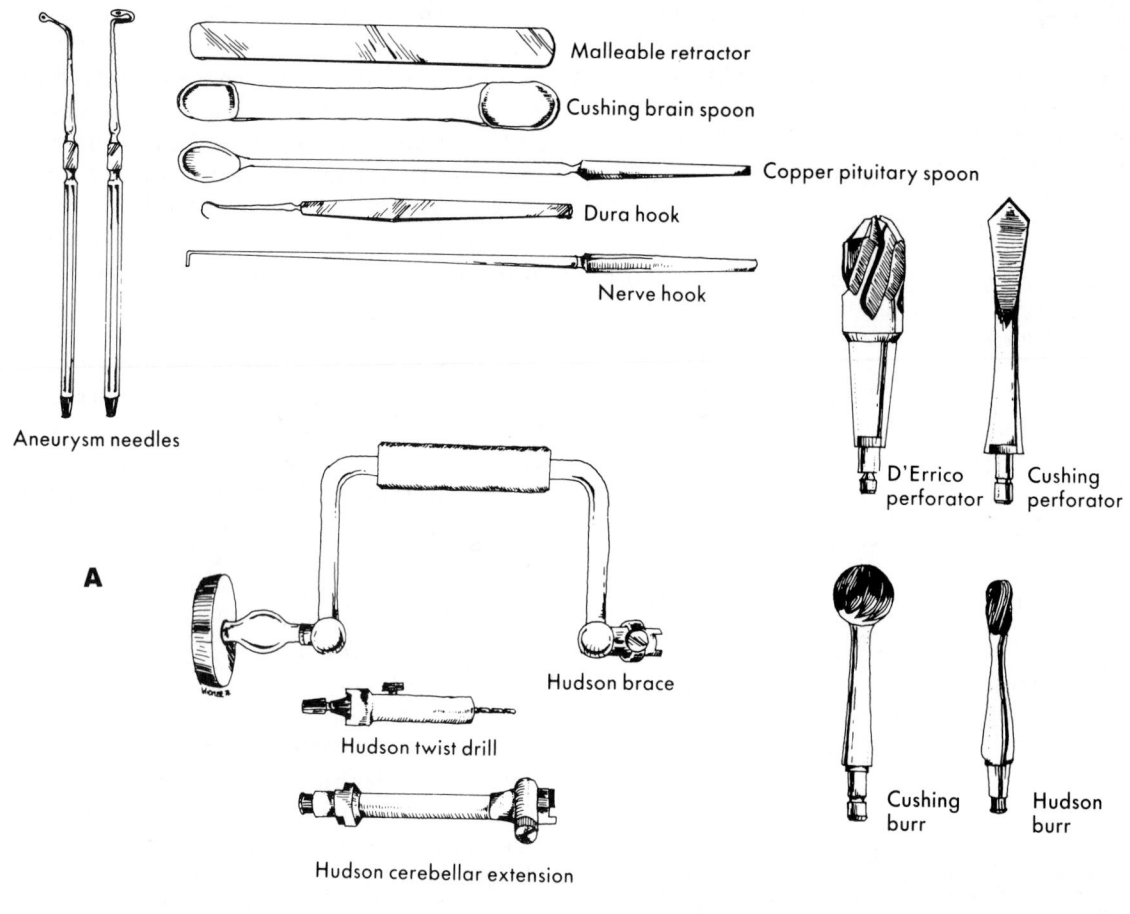

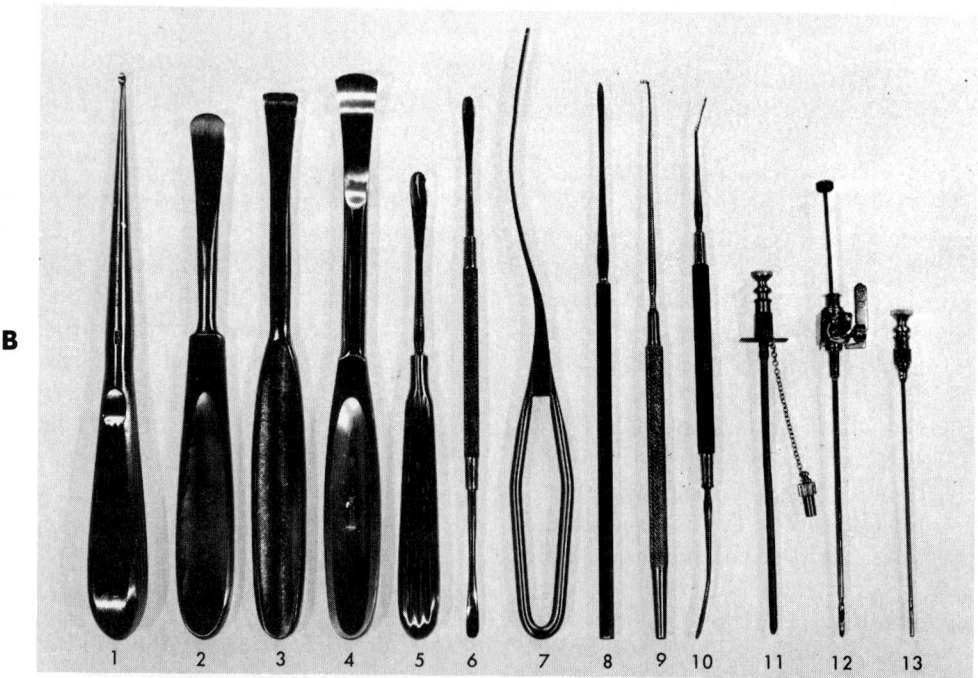

FIG. 22-31 **A,** Some basic instruments for craniotomy. **B,** *1,* Spinal curette, straight; *2,* Cushing periosteal elevator, blunt; *3,* Cushing periosteal elevator, sharp; *4,* Adson periosteal elevator, wide; *5,* Adson elevator no. 3 (joker); *6,* Freer elevator; *7,* Sachs dura separator; *8,* Sunday staphylorrhaphy elevator; *9,* nerve hook; *10,* Olivecrona double-ended dissector; *11,* Scott ventricular cannula; *12,* Seletz ventricular cannula; *13,* Cone ventricular needle.

and can be described in detail. Therefore only a few step-by-step descriptions of basic approaches are presented. The perioperative nurse who is familiar with neurosurgical anatomy and pathologic conditions can learn these basic approaches and adapt them to the specific procedure.

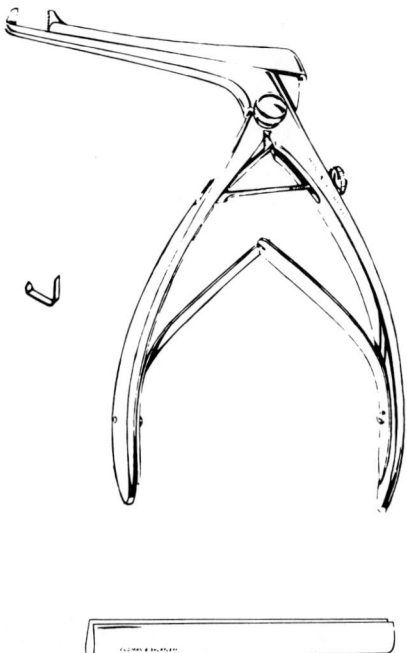

FIG. 22-32 Setup for craniosynostosis may include Ingraham-Fowler tantalum clips. Ingraham-Fowler guillotine applicators, and preformed silicone strip.

Courtesy Codman & Shurtleff, Inc., Randolph, Mass.

HEAD SURGERY
Burr holes

Burr holes are placed to remove a localized fluid collection beneath the dura mater. Fluid not composed of clot can be easily evacuated through a burr hole. Burr holes are also made to tap a lateral ventricle to relieve pressure. Burr holes are used by many surgeons when treating a brain abscess. The abscess may be aspirated, and antibiotics instilled. Other surgeons prefer to treat abscess by craniotomy. Occasionally burr holes are used to locate or drain subdural hematomas. However, a craniectomy is usually necessary to gain adequate exposure in these cases (Fig. 22-36). A burr hole is one of the steps in procedures to shunt ventricular fluid to another body system for absorption or elimination.

Burr holes are placed to introduce air into the lateral ventricles for ventriculography (Fig. 22-37). The air makes the ventricles visible in x-ray studies.

Craniectomy

Craniectomy is the formation of an opening into the skull. This term usually applies when the opening is larger than the average burr hole. A piece of bone is cut with a circular saw that attaches to a Hudson brace. Procedures performed by craniectomy include prefrontal lobotomy, topectomy, cingulotomy, leukotomy, and thalamotomy. Today some of these procedures may be a part of stereotaxic neurosurgery.

Craniotomy

Craniotomy is an incision into the skull to expose and surgically treat intracranial disease.

Procedural considerations. Depending on the location of the pathologic condition, a craniotomy may be frontal,

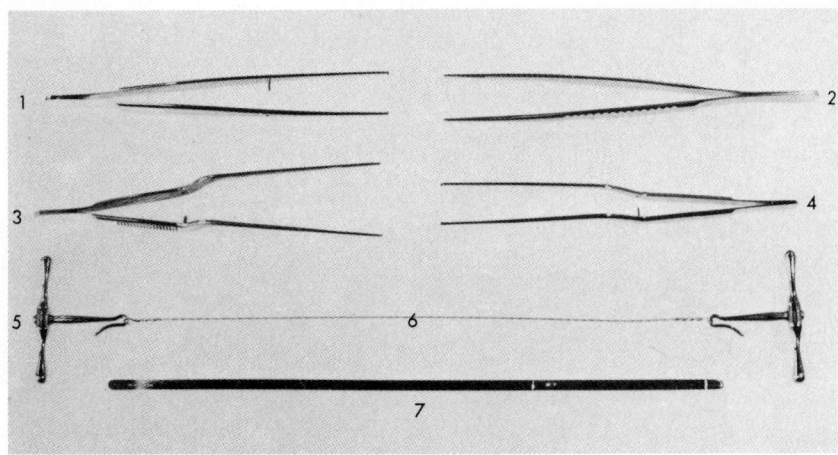

FIG. 22-33 *1*, Cushing tissue forceps; *2*, Cushing dressing forceps; *3*, Cushing bayonet dressing forceps; *4*, Cushing bayonet tissue forceps; *5*, Gigli saw handle; *6*, Gigli saw wire; *7*, Bailey saw guide.

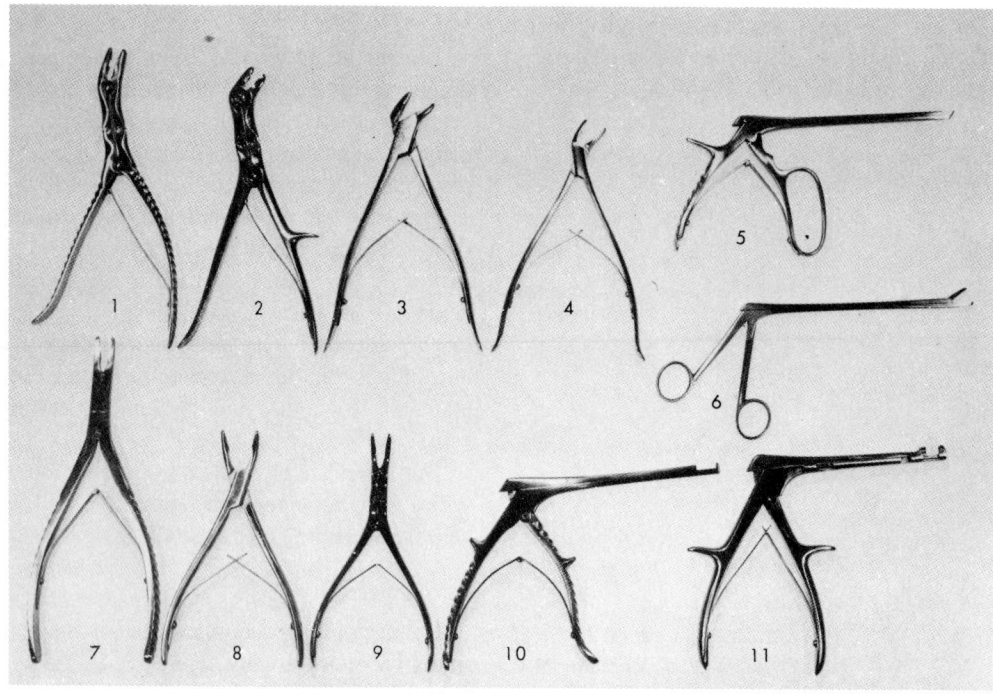

FIG. 22-34   *1,* Leksell rongeur; *2,* Stille gooseneck rongeur; *3,* Bacon rongeur; *4,* Stookey cranial rongeur; *5,* Cloward 40-degree angle punch rongeur; *6,* pituitary disk rongeur; *7,* Fulton rongeur; *8,* Lempert rongeur; *9,* Zaufal-Jansen rongeur; *10,* Kerrison rongeur; *11,* Raney punch.

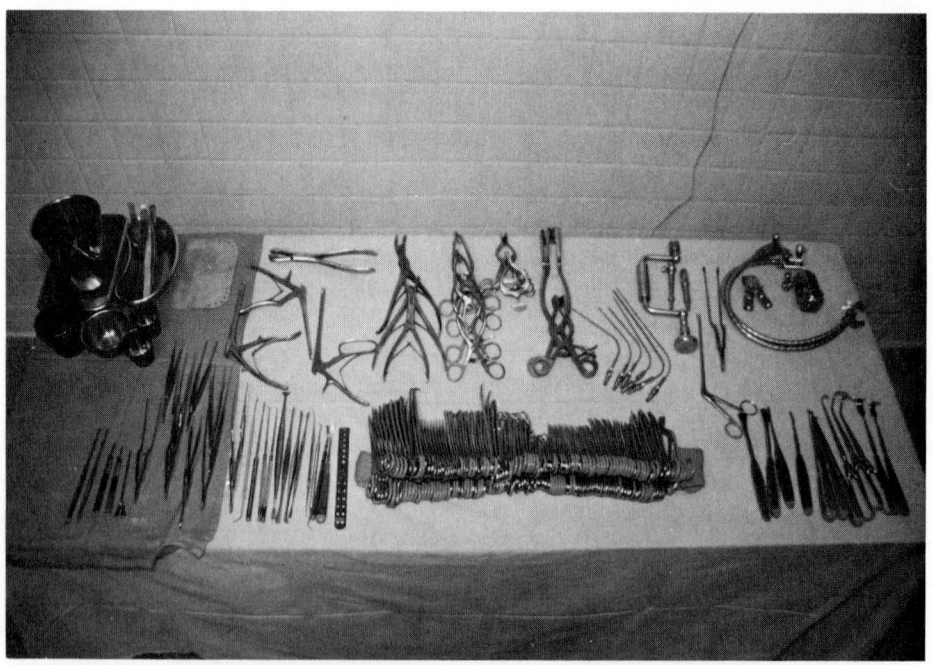

FIG. 22-35   Back table instrument setup for craniotomy.
Courtesy HEALTHSOUTH Medical Center, Richmond, Va.

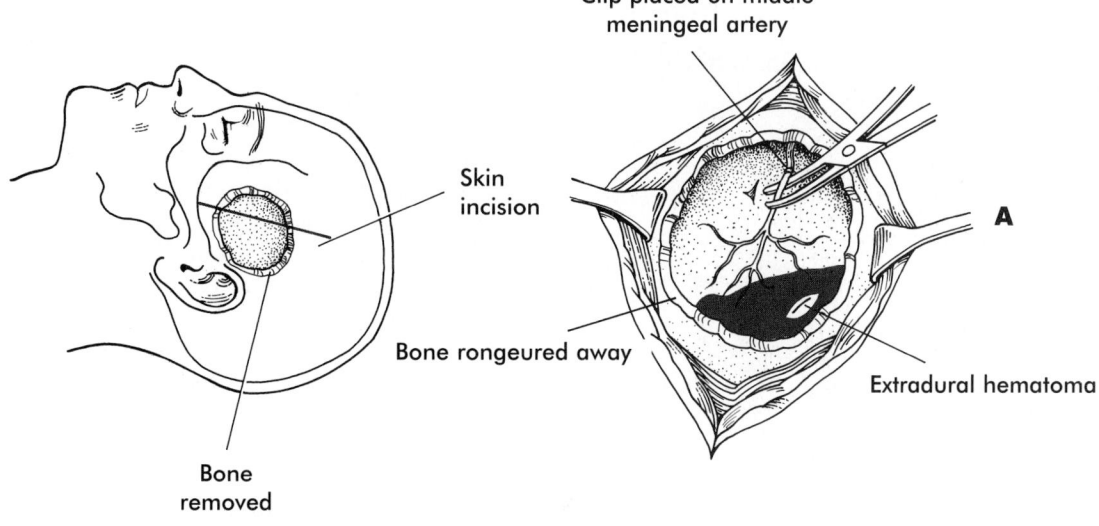

Clip placed on middle
meningeal artery

Skin
incision

Bone rongeured away

Bone
removed

Extradural hematoma

A

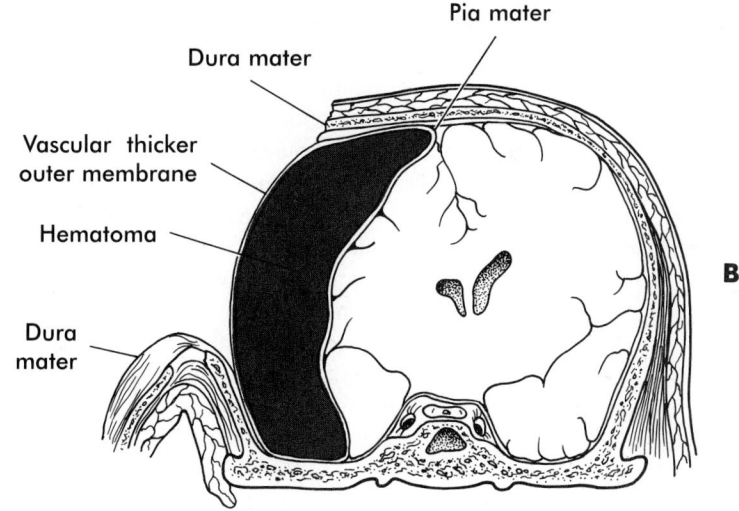

Pia mater

Dura mater

Vascular thicker
outer membrane

Hematoma

Dura
mater

B

FIG. 22-36 **A,** Extradural hematoma. **B,** Subdural hematoma.
From Richards, V. (1956). *Surgery for general practice*. St. Louis: Mosby.

parietal, occipital, temporal, or a combination of two or more of these. When turning a scalp flap for a craniotomy, the surgeon may peel the scalp back off the pericranium; the bone flap is then elevated with the overlying muscles still attached (osteoplastic), or the periosteum may be stripped off the skull prior to turning the bone flap (free flap).

The bone plate may be separated from the soft tissues, removed from the skull, and set aside for replacement at the end of the procedure. It may be placed in an antibiotic solution or an iodophor solution or wrapped in a saline-moistened sponge or one that has been saturated with an antibiotic solution or an iodophor solution. The bone plate is not removed from the sterile field. If it is not replaced, it may be frozen in a sterile container or saved and stored in a marked, unsterile container to use as a template for form-

ing a cranioplastic plate at a later date. The defect can be repaired without use of this template, however. If the bone is not separated from the soft tissues, it is turned back with the temporal muscle and soft tissues.

Operative procedure. After draping and attachment of suction and electrosurgical cords, the procedure is begun.

1. The surgeon and the assistant apply digital pressure over folded 4 × 4 inch radiopaque sponges on both sides of the incision line. The skin and galea are incised in segments, the length of each segment being equal to that over which the finger pressure is applied. The tissue edges are held with 6-inch toothed forceps as scalp clips are placed on the flap edges. Hemostatic clamps are placed on the outside edge of the incision in adults and are grouped in segments and secured to-

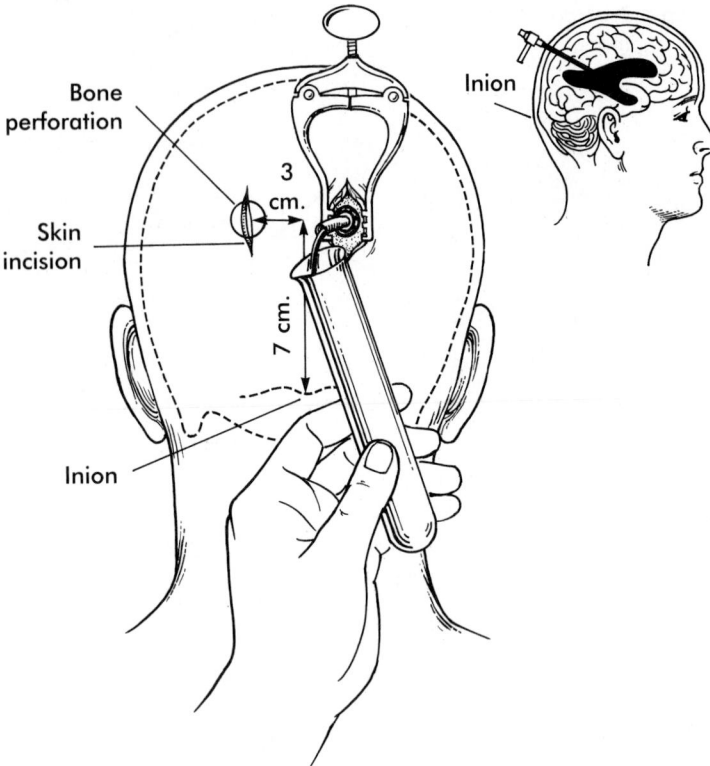

FIG. 22-37   Occipital burr holes for ventriculography.

From Richards, V. (1956). *Surgery for general practice.* St. Louis: Mosby.

gether by rubber bands placed around the handles or by a Penrose drain or open 4 × 4 inch sponge threaded through the handles and tied or clamped together with heavy forceps, such as a Pean (Fig. 22-38). Any remaining active arterial bleeding is controlled by electrocoagulation. If the incision extends into the temporal area, bleeding in the temporal muscle is managed by electrocoagulation, hemostats, tamponade, or suture ligature. Mayo scissors can be used to incise temporal muscle and fascia.

2. The soft tissue is peeled off the periosteum by sharp or blunt dissection or by electrodissection (see Fig. 22-38). The scalp flap is turned back over folded sponges and retracted by use of small towel clamps and rubber bands or muscle hooks on rubber bands. In either case the traction is maintained by securing the rubber band to the drapes with heavy forceps. The flap may be covered with a moist sponge or Telfa strips and a sterile towel. Bleeding is controlled by electrocoagulation.

3. When a free bone flap is planned, the muscle and periosteum are incised. Muscle and periosteum are elevated with the skin-galea flap, turned back, and retracted as a unit, as described previously.

4. The periosteum and muscle are incised with a scalpel or electrosurgical knife except at the inferior margins, which are left intact to preserve blood supply to the bone flap. The periosteum is stripped from the bone at the incision line with a periosteal elevator. Bone wax is used to control bleeding.

5. The scalp edges and muscle are retracted from the bone incision line by a Sachs or Cushing retractor. Two or more burr holes are made with either a hand or power

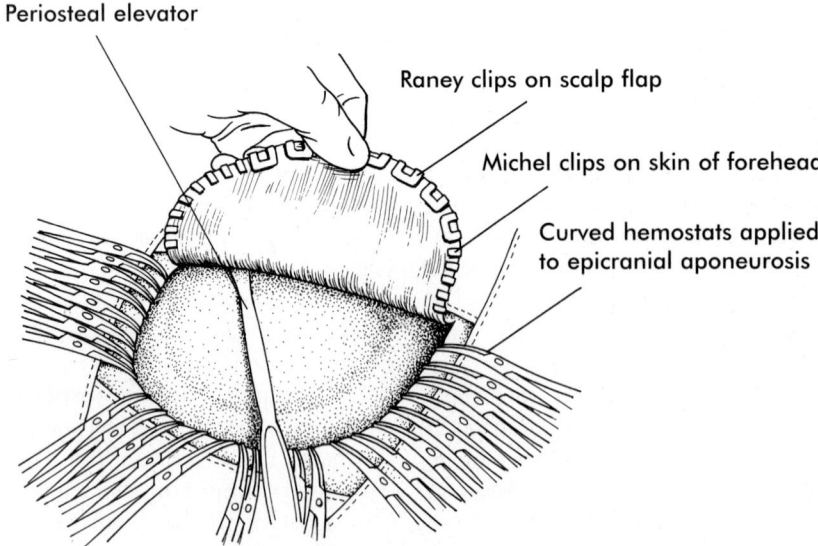

FIG. 22-38   Elevation of scalp flap. Hemostats on outer rim of incision and Raney clips and Michel clips on scalp flap.

From Kempe, L.G. (1968). *Operative neurosurgery* (Vols. 1 & 2). New York: Springer-Verlag.

cranial drill (Figs. 22-39 to 22-41). As each hole is drilled, the assistant must hold the patient's head to diminish the agitation and prevent displacement from the headrest. A great deal of heat is generated by the friction of the perforator or burr against the bone. The scrub nurse or assistant must irrigate the drilling site to counteract the heat and remove bone dust, which collects as the holes are made. Some surgeons prefer that the scrub nurse collect the bone dust for replacement in the burr holes at closure. The dust is placed in a medicine glass and kept moist with a small amount of normal saline solution. A large-gauge suction tip is used to remove both irrigating solution and debris from the field. As the inner table is perforated and the dura exposed, the burr hole may be temporarily tamponaded with bone wax or a cottonoid strip or patty. Each hole is eventually débrided by a no. 0 or 00 bone curette or small periosteal elevator (joker). The dura mater is freed at the margins with a no. 3 Adson elevator, no. 3 Penfield dissector, or right-angle Frazier elevator or

similar instrument. The hole is irrigated and suction applied simultaneously. Active bleeding points in the bone are identified, and bone wax is applied.

6. When all burr holes have been made, the bone flap is cut by sawing between holes after the dura mater has been separated from the bone by a dural separator, such as the Sachs, or by a no. 3 Penfield dissector. Dural separation is done to prevent tearing of the dura mater, especially over venous sinuses. Using a rongeur, the surgeon may cut channels in the two burr holes at the inferior edge of the planned bone flap under the muscle. When the rest of the bone flap has been sawed, this segment can be easily cracked as the bone is elevated and turned back. If the sawing is done by hand, a dural separator is passed from one hole to the next under the bone. A saw guide-passer with a saw attached is passed from one hole to the next in the same manner. The saw is detached from the guide, saw handles are attached to both ends of the saw, and the bone is incised by sawing in a back-and-forth motion. Fric-

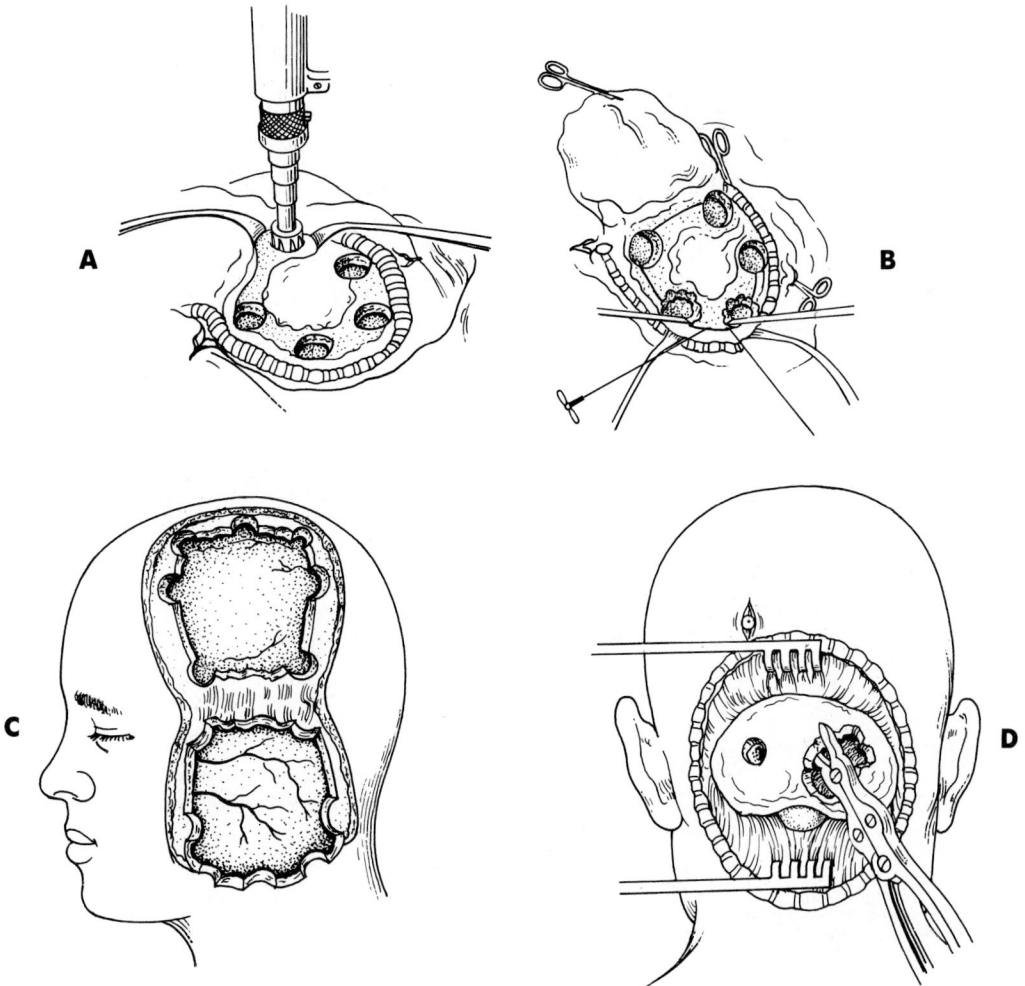

FIG. 22-39 Techniques of cranial surgery. **A,** Drilling burr holes. **B,** Using the Gigli saw. **C,** Bone flap turned down. **D,** Modification for cerebellar craniotomy.

From Barber, J., Stokes, L., & Billings, D. (1977). *Adult and child care* (2nd ed.). St. Louis: Mosby.

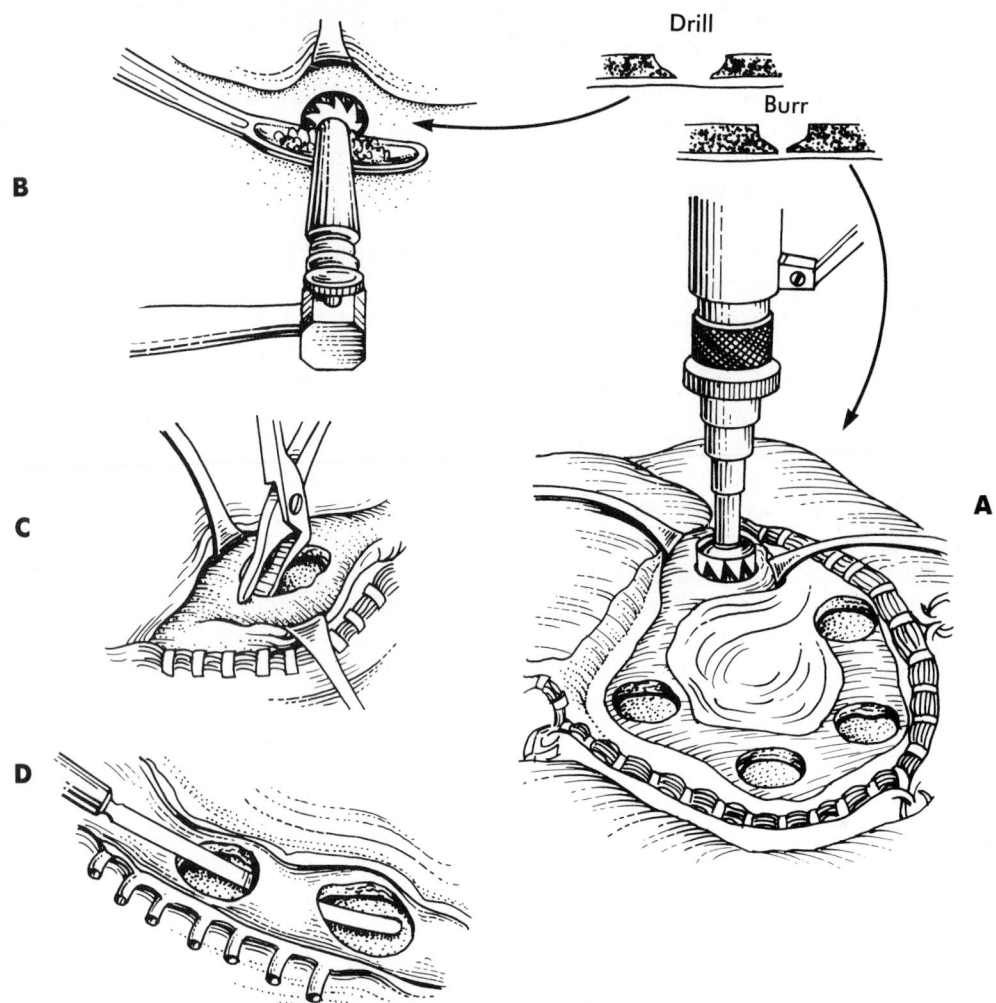

FIG. 22-40 Methods of making osteoplastic flap (craniotomy). **A,** Using electric drill to make burr hole. **B,** Using hand perforator to make burr hole. **C,** Using rongeur to enlarge burr hole. **D,** Separating dura mater from skull.

From Carini, E., & Owens, G. (1974). *Neurological and neurosurgical nursing* (6th ed.). St. Louis: Mosby.

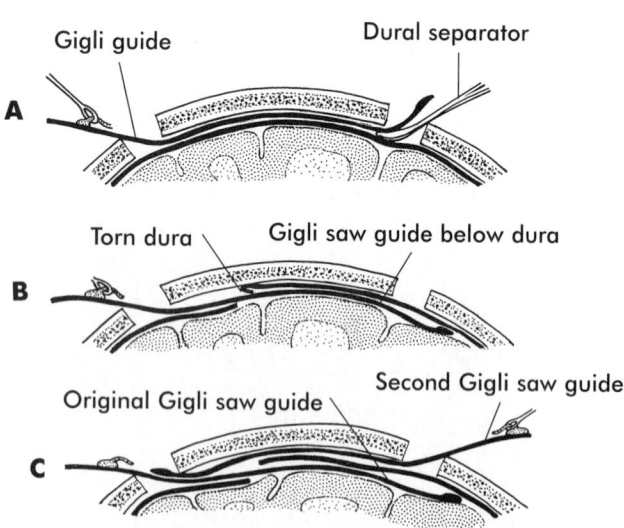

FIG. 22-41 Gigli saw insertion. **A** to **C,** Steps to be taken if Gigli saw tears dura mater.

From Kempe, L.G. (1968). *Operative neurosurgery* (Vols. 1 & 2). New York: Springer-Verlag.

tion generates heat, so irrigation and suction must be used during the process. The procedure is repeated until all segments but the one under the muscle have been cut. Usually a new saw is used each time. An air craniotome or Midas Rex drill can also be used for the opening. Irrigation and suction are required as the bone flap is cut. Soft tissue edges are retracted with Sachs or Cushing retractors.

7. The bone flap with muscle attached is lifted off the dura mater by two periosteal elevators. As it is forced up and back, the bridge of bone under the muscle cracks. Bleeding from the bone is controlled with bone wax. A double-action rongeur is used to remove sharp, irregular edges where the bone cracked. The bone flap is covered with a moist sponge, cottonoid material, or Telfa pads and then a clean sterile towel and is retracted in the same manner as the scalp flap.

8. The dura mater is irrigated. Moist cottonoid strips or patties or Telfa pads may be inserted between the dura mater and bone and folded back to cover the exposed

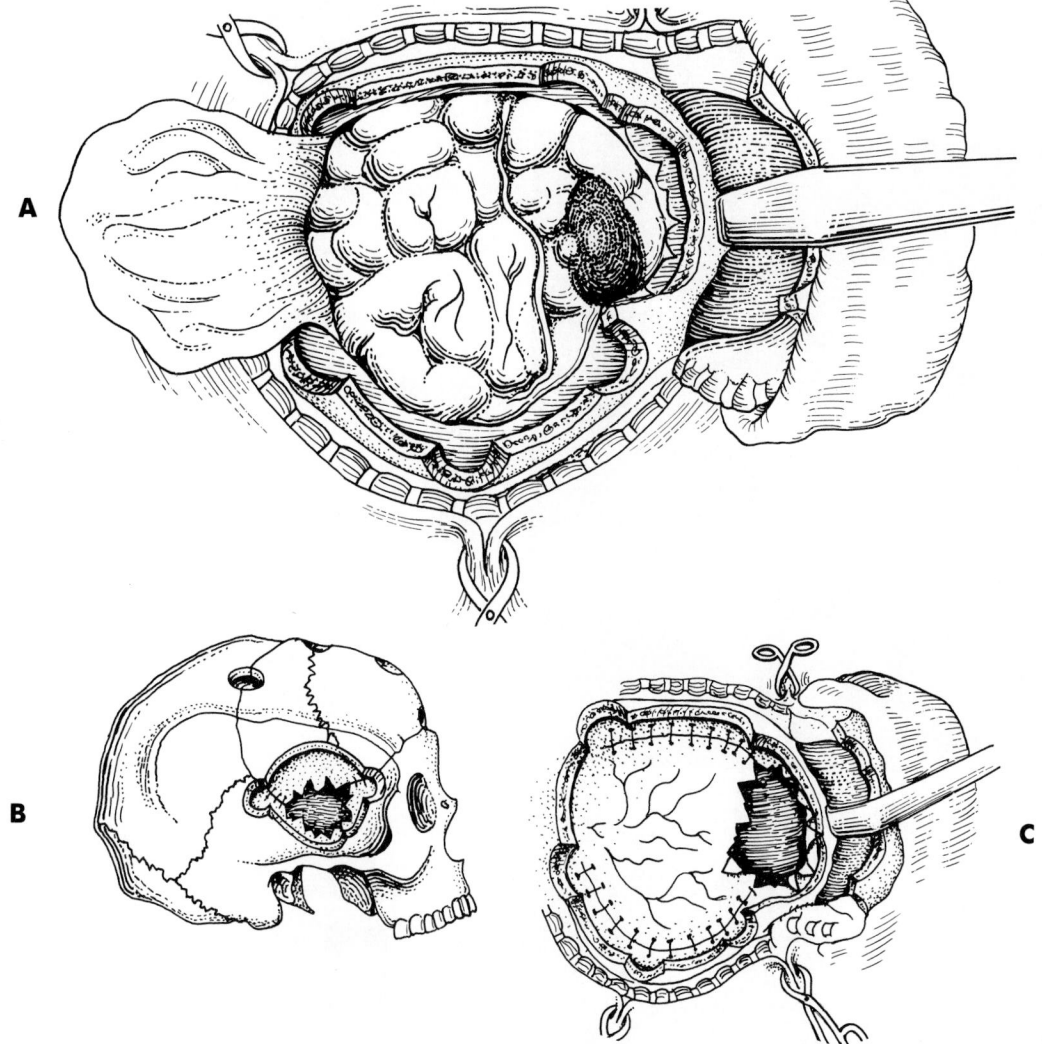

FIG. 22-42 Craniotomy with subtemporal decompression. **A,** Malignant cerebral tumor exposed. **B,** Bony defect. **C,** Dural defect.

From Carini, E., & Owens, G. (1974). *Neurological and neurosurgical nursing* (6th ed.). St. Louis: Mosby.

bone edges. Clean sterile towels may be placed around the operative site.

9. The dura mater is opened (Fig. 22-42). A dura hook may be used to elevate the dura mater from the brain, and a small nick is made in the dura mater with a no. 15 blade on a no. 3 or no. 7 knife handle; or a small opening may be made in the dura mater without elevating it, after which the dural edges are grasped with straight mosquito hemostats or two Adson or Cushing forceps with teeth and are elevated. A narrow, moist cottonoid strip is inserted with smooth forceps (bayonet or Cushing) into the opening to protect the brain as the dura mater is incised and elevated. The dural incision can be made with Metzenbaum scissors, special dura scissors, or a Rayport dura knife. Usually traction sutures are placed at the outer edge of the dura mater and are tagged with small bulldog clamps or mosquito hemostats. Sometimes the tag instruments are attached to the drapes to increase traction and keep tension on them. As the dural veins are approached during dural opening, they are ligated or coagulated before cutting. Ligation is done with hemostatic clips such as Weck Hemoclips, McKenzie clips, or Liga-clips. The brain surface is protected by moist cottonoid strips.

10. The surgeon places cottonoid strips and brain retractors, self-retaining (Fig. 22-43), and manual, appropriately while working toward visualizing the particular pathologic entity.

11. Brain spoons, Cushing pituitary spoons, and Ray curettes, a well as pituitary rongeurs or other tumor forceps, must be available for tumor removal. Also, a selection of dissectors, Cushing and Gerald forceps, and a bipolar coagulation unit are used. Completely filled irrigating syringes and a full range of moist cottonoid patties and strips must be within easy reach of the sur-

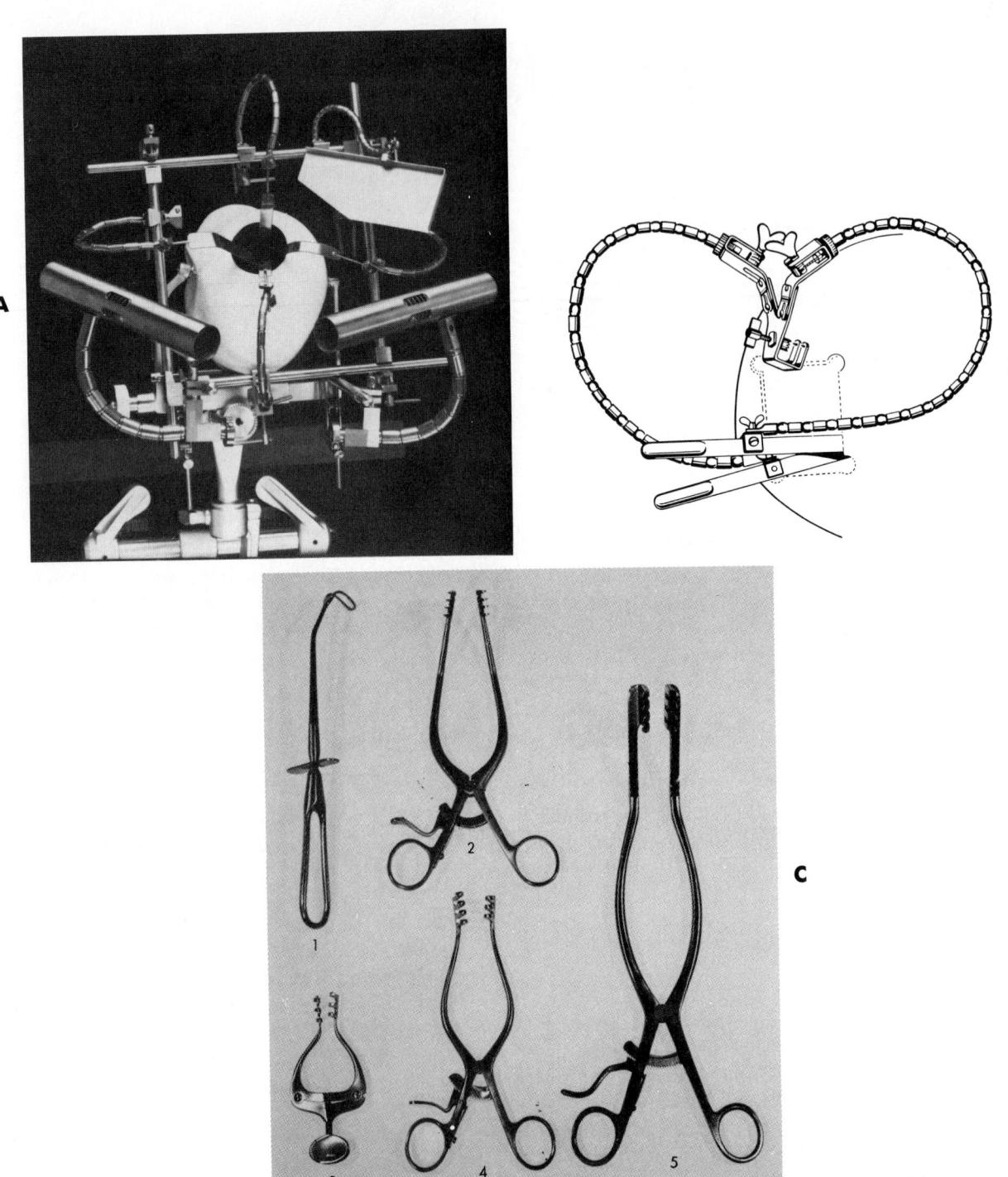

FIG. 22-43 **A,** Greenberg retractor with blades, poles, and adapters. **B,** Leyla-Yasargil self-retaining retractor. **C,** Retractors: *1,* Cushing subtemporal decompression retractor; *2,* Adson cerebellar retractor; *3,* Jansen mastoid retractor; *4,* Weitlaner retractor; *5,* Beckman laminectomy retractor.

A courtesy Codman & Shurtleff, Randolph, Mass.; **B,** courtesy Holco Instrument Corp., New York.

geon and the assistant. Following correction of the pathologic condition and control of bleeding, the brain may be irrigated with an antibiotic solution of the surgeon's choice.

12. The dura mater is usually closed by running or by interrupted sutures of no. 4-0 silk, 4-0 Polyglactin suture, or 4-0 black braided nylon. Under some conditions, dural substitutes may be used. A drain may or may not be used. Epidural tack-up sutures are usually placed around the edge of the craniotomy defect to close the epidural dead space. This is usually done prior to the dural opening.

13. The bone flap may or may not be replaced. If swelling is anticipated, it is usually not replaced. If the flap is free and replaced, holes may be drilled in it and the skull and suture material inserted to secure it in place. Titanium plates and screws are also available for fixation of flaps. The craniotome or Midas Rex can be used for this purpose. During drilling a dura protector is used on the skull side. A brain spoon can serve as a dura protector.

14. Periosteum and muscle are approximated with no. 2-0 or 3-0 Polyglactin synthetic absorbable suture or no. 2-0 or 3-0 silk or Surgilon. The galea is closed with the same sutures as above. Skin closure can be interrupted or continuous and of silk or synthetic suture material, such as nylon, or skin staples.

Craniotomy for cerebrospinal rhinorrhea

Cerebrospinal rhinorrhea is a rupture of the dura mater, with evagination of the torn arachnoid through the dura mater into a hole or fracture in the skull communicating with one of the nasal sinuses or the nasal cavity. This results in leakage of cerebrospinal fluid from the nose. Repairing the defect is necessary to prevent air from being trapped under pressure in the brain and to prevent intracranial infection.

Operative procedure. The procedure is as follows:

1. Usually a bifrontal craniotomy is carried out, and the dura mater is opened. The frontal lobes are elevated until the defect can be visualized. The surgeon may elect to use the microscope.

2. The dura mater is dissected from the orbital and cribriform plates.

3. The defect in the bone is defined, and the bony defect is repaired with a split-thickness graft from the skull or may be filled with methyl methacrylate or covered with tantalum mesh.

4. The dural defect may be closed with sutures, but usually some type of patch is placed over it. A piece of muscle, pericranium, fascia, gelatin foam, silicone sheeting, or freeze-dried dura substitute may be used. These may be sutured or glued. Some surgeons do not fasten the patch into place.

5. The dural incision is sutured, and the wound is closed.

A similar procedure is carried out in the temporal or suboccipital region to repair a defect in cerebrospinal otorrhea.

Craniotomy for intracranial aneurysm

An aneurysm is a vascular dilatation usually caused by a local defect in the vascular wall. Within the cranial cavity an aneurysm may impinge on the third nerve or the optic chiasm. Hemorrhage into the subarachnoid space, causing sudden, severe headache, is generally the first evidence of an intracranial aneurysm.

Modern neurosurgical techniques have made operations on intracranial aneurysms more feasible. Fatal hemorrhage is the greatest hazard of the condition and of the operation. To prevent this, control of blood pressure, as well as vascular supply to the region beyond the limits of the lesion, may be required. Occasionally control of the cerebral circulation at the level of the cervical carotid artery is desired. The artery may be exposed and controlled by means of preplaced ligatures or clamps that can be tightened to occlude the vessel if bleeding occurs at the aneurysm site during the operation. This is a separate preliminary surgical procedure.

Procedural considerations. Aneurysm clips and appliers of the surgeon's choice must be included with the instrumentation. Figs. 22-44 and 22-45 illustrate a few of the clips and appliers available. A minimum of two appliers for each type of clip must be included; both temporary and permanent clips must be available. Temporary clips include Mayfield, McFadden, Drake, Yasargil, Sugita, and Schwartz. Heifetz, Sundt-Kees, Olivecrona, Housepian, Scoville, Yasargil Phynox, and Sugita are types of permanent aneurysm clips. Today most clips have been updated with an alloy that is MRI compatible. Permanent clips can be removed from the vessel if necessary. The clip appliers serve as clip removers.

Aneurysm clips should never be compressed between the fingers. Clips should be compressed only when seated in their appliers. Once a clip has been compressed, it should be discarded. Clips that have been compressed may be sprung and may slip, causing complications such as bleeding or compression of another vessel or a nerve.

The full armamentarium of aneurysm occlusion tools should be available for the surgeon. Besides clips, fast-setting aneuroplastic resinous material, a piece of temporal muscle, ligature carriers, or any other material requested by the surgeon should be in the room and ready to use. Fine silk ligatures and hemostatic clips, with or without bipolar coagulation of the neck of the aneurysm, have also been used successfully.

A basic craniotomy setup is required in addition to the special items mentioned. Supplementary suction must be immediately available on the field to prevent hemorrhage from obscuring the surgeon's vision if the aneurysm dome ruptures during operation and for removing smoke result-

Text continued on p. 908.

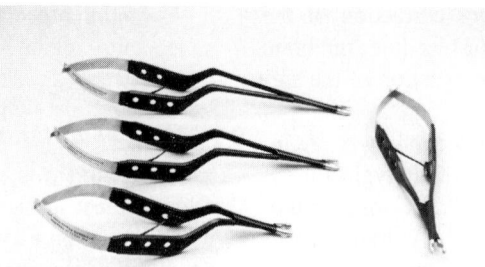

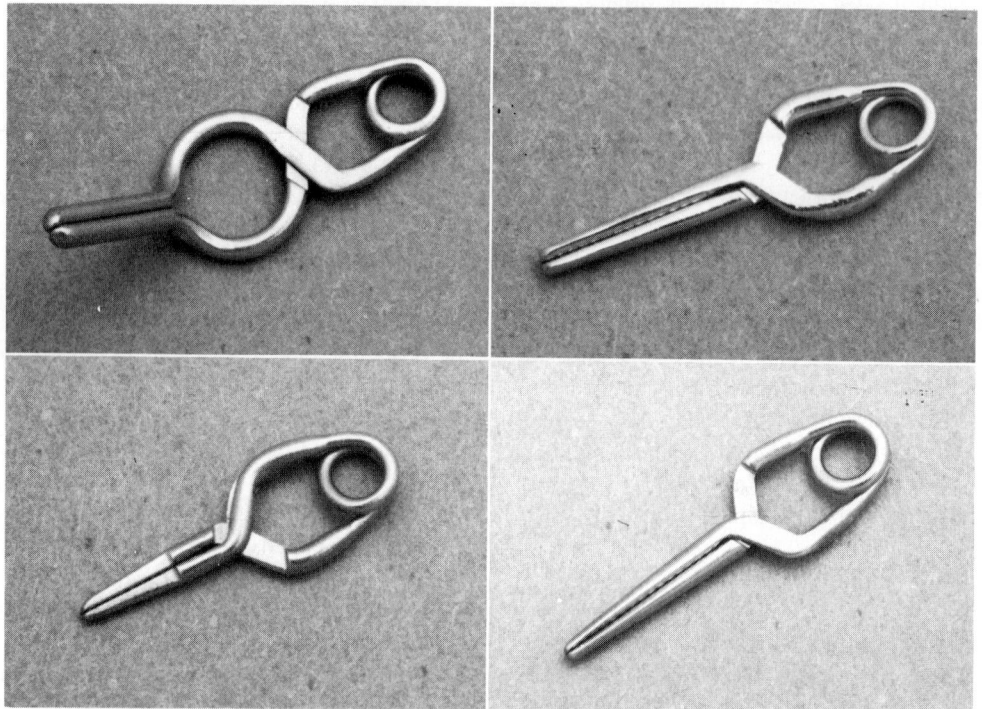

FIG. 22-44   Yasargil microaneurysm, standard aneurysm clips and appliers.
Courtesy Aesculap, Burlingame, Calif.

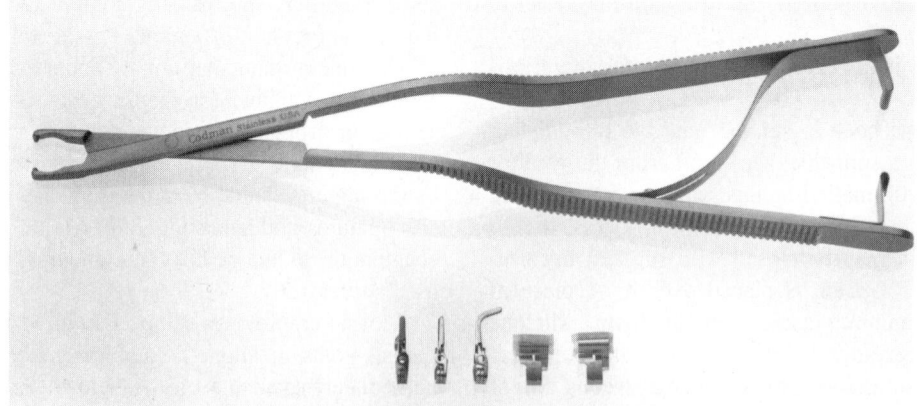

FIG. 22-45   Sundt aneurysm clips and applier.
Courtesy Codman & Shurtleff, Inc., Randolph, Mass.

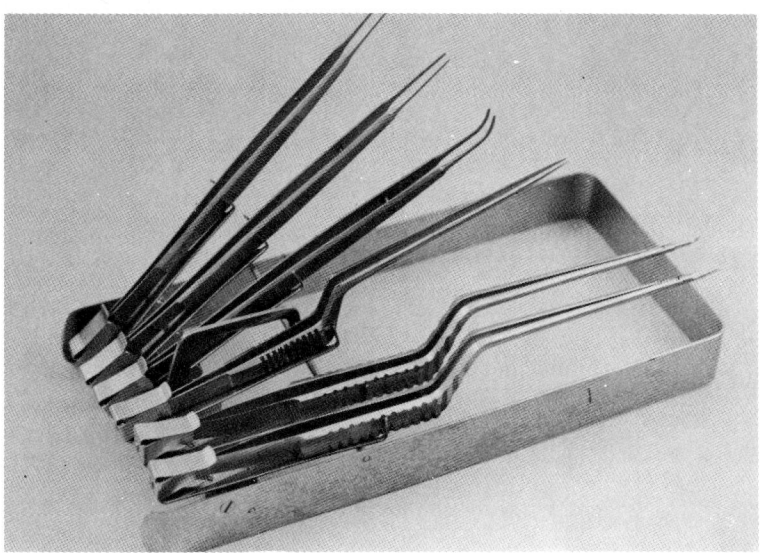

FIG. 22-46 Microscissors and forceps in rack.

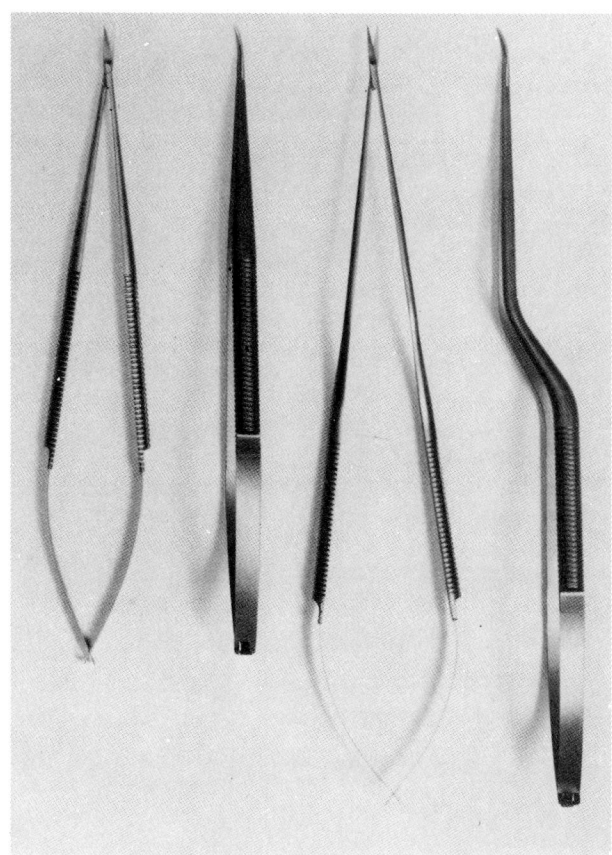

FIG. 22-47 Rhoton titanium microscissors.
Courtesy Codman & Shurtleff, Inc., Randolph, Mass.

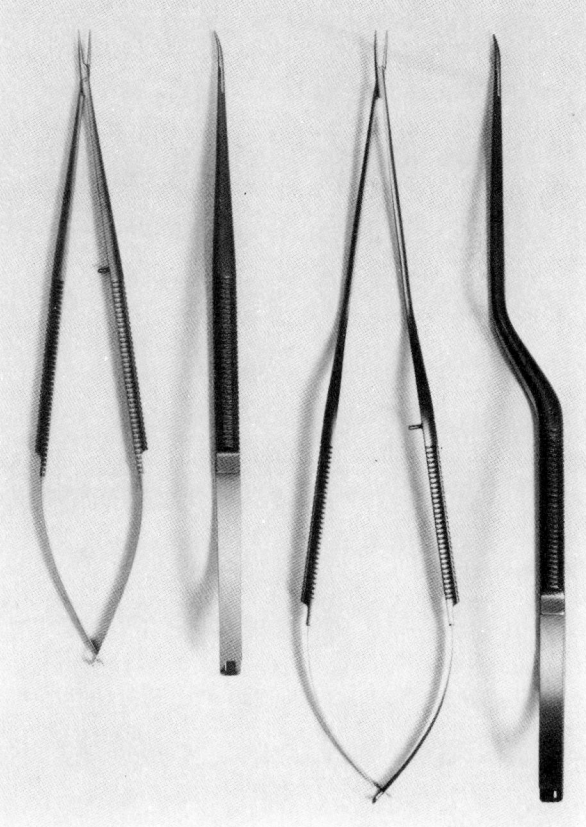

FIG. 22-48 Rhoton microsurgical needle holders.
Courtesy Codman & Shurtleff, Inc., Randolph, Mass.

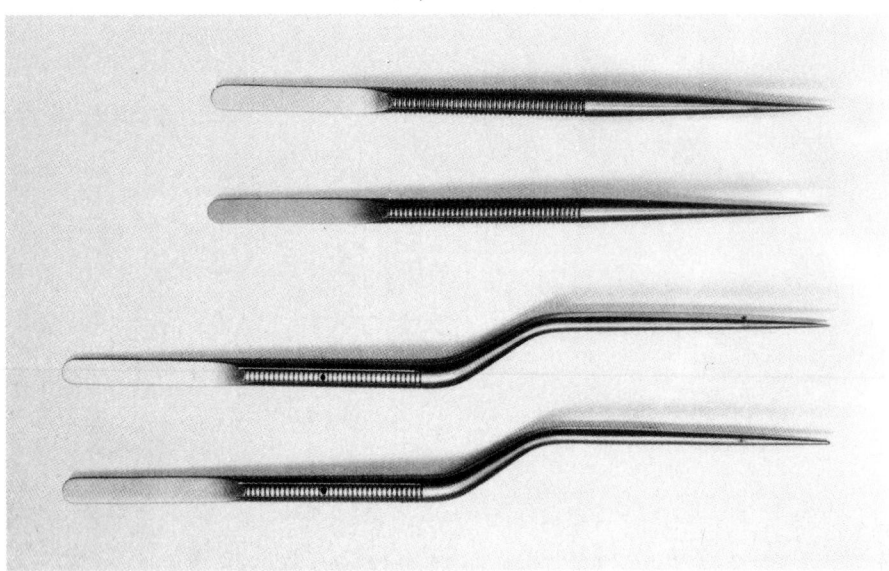

FIG. 22-49   Rhoton microsurgical forceps, straight and bayonet.
Courtesy Codman & Shurtleff, Inc., Randolph, Mass.

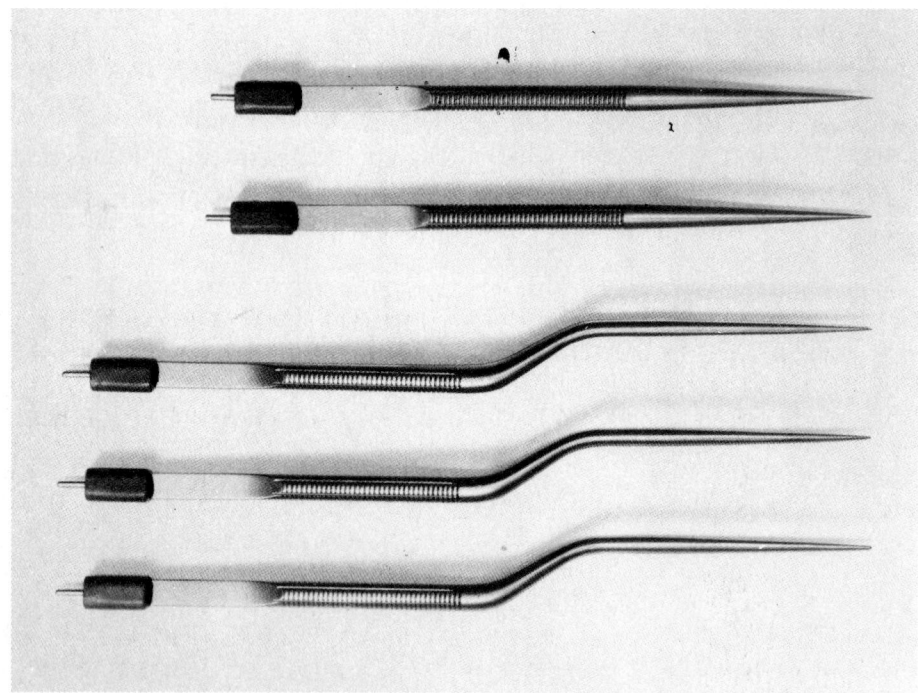

FIG. 22-50   Rhoton microsurgical bipolar forceps, straight and bayonet.
Courtesy Codman & Shurtleff, Inc., Randolph, Mass.

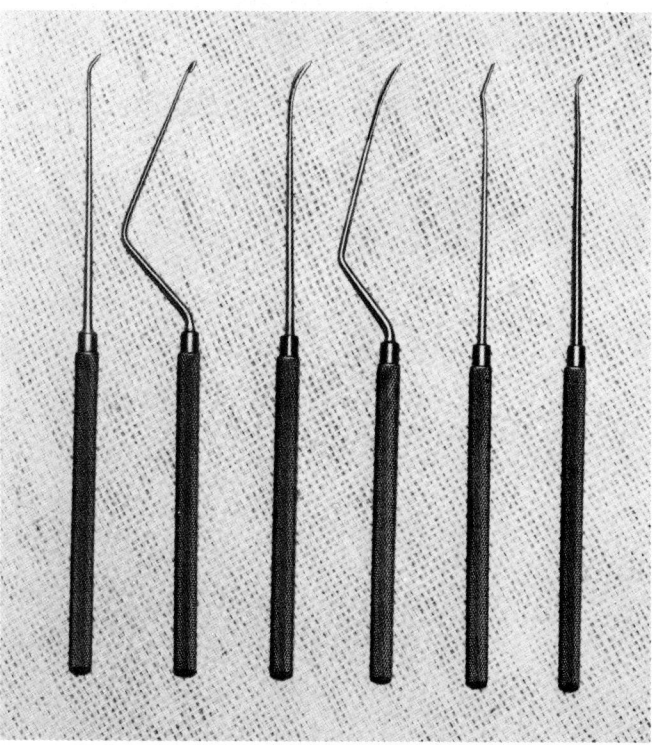

FIG. 22-51   Malis microsurgical instruments. *Left to right,* Semisharp dissector, curette, two elevators, sharp dissector, round dissector.

Courtesy Codman & Shurtleff, Inc., Randolph, Mass.

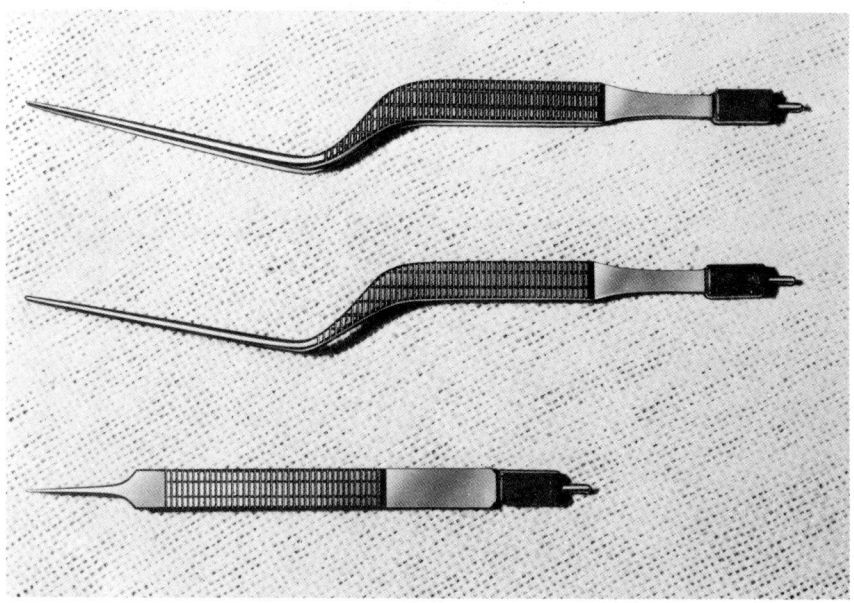

FIG. 22-52   Malis titanium bipolar forceps.

Courtesy Codman & Shurtleff, Inc., Randolph, Mass.

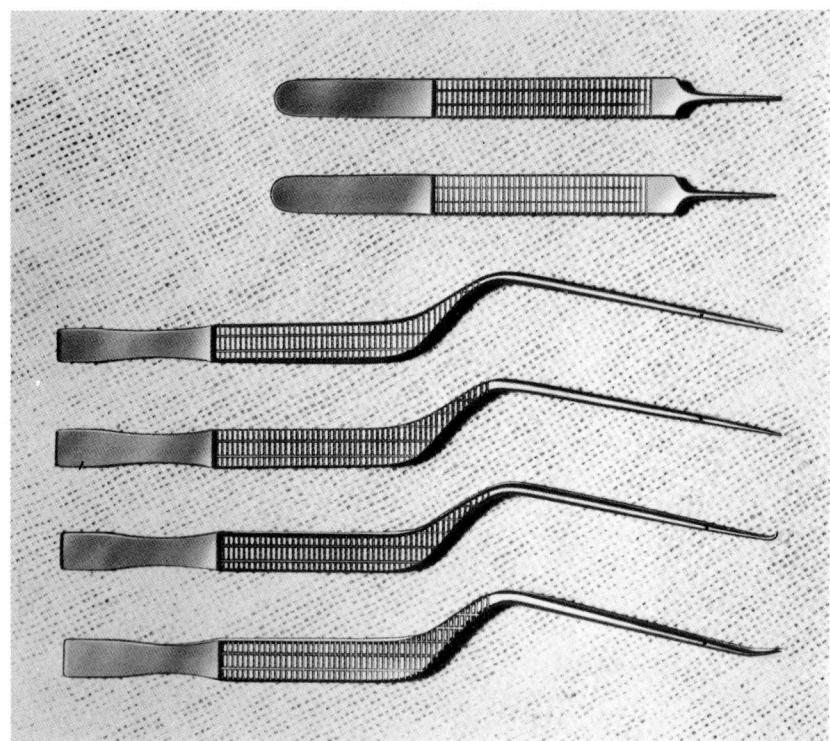

FIG. 22-53 Malis microforceps (titanium), straight and bayonet.
Courtesy Codman & Shurtleff, Inc., Randolph, Mass.

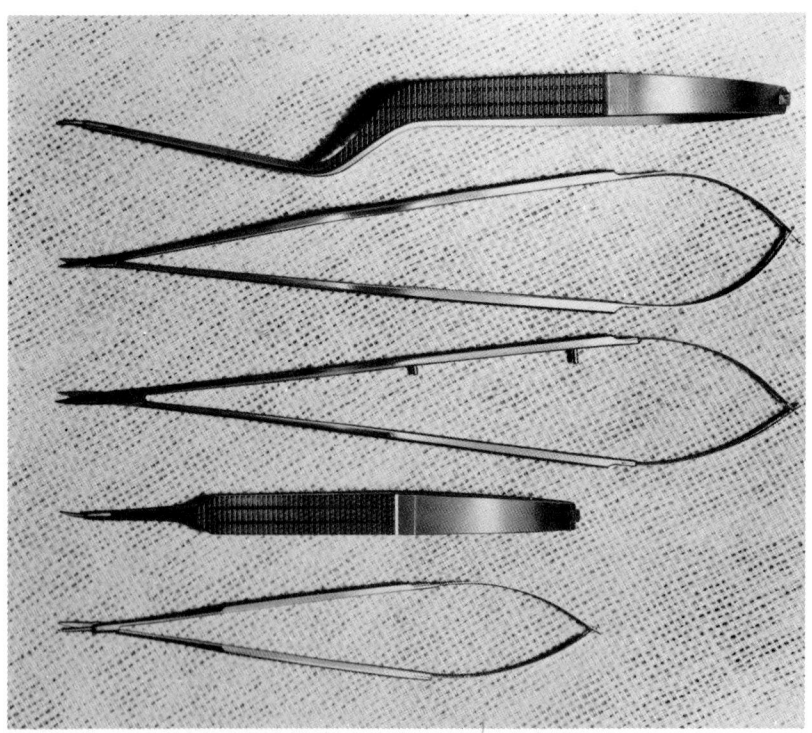

FIG. 22-54 Malis microsurgical scissors.
Courtesy Codman & Shurtleff, Inc., Randolph, Mass.

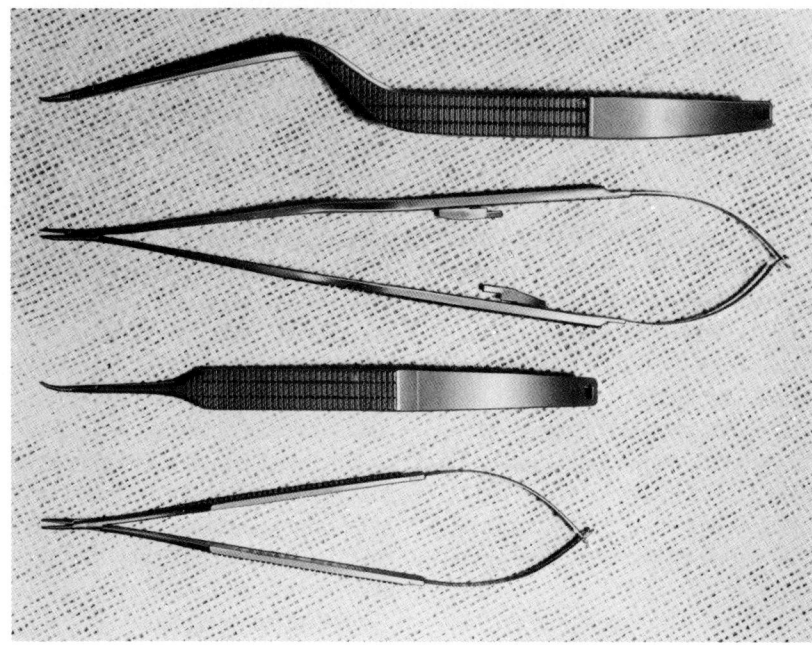

FIG. 22-55 Malis microsurgical needle holders.
Courtesy Codman & Shurtleff, Inc., Randolph, Mass.

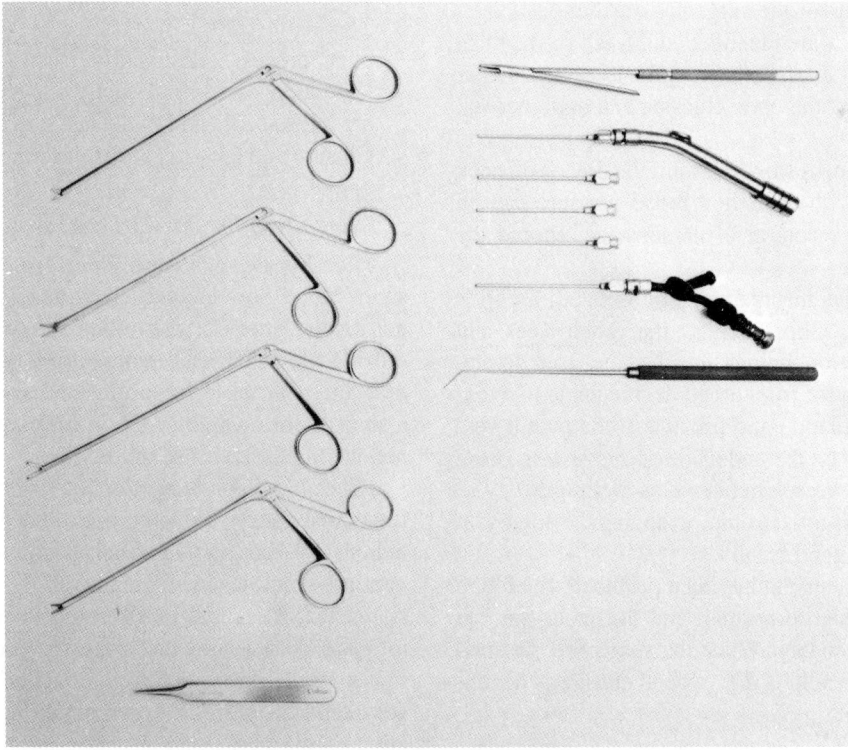

FIG. 22-56 Microinstruments for neurosurgical procedures. *Bottom to top, left,* Forceps, rongeurs, and scissors; *right,* arachnoid knife, Malis suction-coagulation handle and four tips, Cadac microsuction handle and tip, blade breaker and holder.
Courtesy Codman & Shurtleff, Inc., Randolph, Mass.

ing from laser dissection. A cell saver unit should be available for reprocessing of blood for replacement when significant blood loss is expected.

Operative procedure. The procedure is as follows:

1. A frontal, frontotemporal, or bifrontal craniotomy may be done to approach an aneurysm in the area of the circle of Willis. The bifrontal approach requires extra scalp clips and hemostatic forceps. All aneurysm instruments preferred by the surgeon must be included.
2. After the dura mater has been opened, a self-retaining brain retractor is placed, and the optic nerve and subarachnoid cisterns are exposed. The olfactory nerve may be coagulated and divided with a long scissors for better exposure.
3. The operating microscope is positioned. Microinstruments, including a micropolar bayonet, are used (Figs. 22-46 to 22-56).
4. Bridging veins are coagulated with bipolar coagulating forceps. Irrigation, which may be a part of the bipolar unit, is necessary during bipolar coagulation.
5. The covering arachnoidal webs are dissected away with microdissectors, hooks, elevators, scissors, knives, forceps, a micro diamond knife, and an irrigating bipolar.
6. Careful dissection of the arachnoid and clear visualization of the neck of the aneurysm without rupture of the dome are the aims of the surgeon.
7. The parent arteries are identified and freed so they can be occluded with a temporary clip if necessary. Other structures, such as the optic chiasma and optic nerves, are identified.
8. As the surgeon works slowly toward the dome and neck of the aneurysm, the patient's blood pressure can be lowered for easier control of hemorrhage, should the aneurysm rupture.
9a. If the neck of the aneurysm can be isolated, a clip is placed across it. Clips such as the Sundt-Kees and Heifetz have Teflon linings and can be used to approach the aneurysm from a 180-degree angle to avoid excessive manipulation and traction of the parent vessel, if the neck is on the underside of the vessel. These clips support the vessel and serve as a clip graft.
9b. When clipping is not feasible, wrapping the aneurysm with muslin has good results.
10. As soon as the aneurysm has been occluded, the blood pressure is returned to normal, and the aneurysm site is checked for bleeding. When the surgeon is satisfied that the operative field is dry, wound closure is begun.

Craniotomy for arteriovenous malformation

An arteriovenous malformation consists of thin-walled vascular channels that connect arteries and veins without the usual intervening capillaries. These vascular lesions may be microscopic or massive.

Malformations vary widely in size, area of involvement, and structure. Arteriovenous fistulas may be congenital or may result from trauma or disease. Vascular anomalies may also give rise to subarachnoid or intracerebral hemorrhage or may have extensive irritative effects and cause focal or generalized seizures.

These lesions are difficult to treat successfully. Feeding vessels can be clipped with or without partial removal of the lesion. Total removal, when possible, gives best results. Microsurgical techniques and the laser have made total removal without devastating injury to surrounding brain tissue and vessels possible in many cases.

Other methods of treating these malformations have been tried. One successful method has been with the Gamma knife. Only a few health care facilities offer this procedure. Another method is preoperative embolization, which makes dissection much easier.

Operative procedure

1. A supratentorial or infratentorial craniotomy is done, depending on the location of the lesion.
2. The feeding arteries are exposed a distance from the malformation, then traced toward it, and occluded a short distance before they penetrate its substance. This spares as many of the arteries to the brain as possible. The feeding arteries may be occluded by clipping, electrosurgical coagulation, ligation, or laser beam coagulation.
3. The malformation is dissected out with suction and bayonet forceps. Additional vessels are clipped or coagulated along the way. Usually one or more draining veins are left to be ligated as the last step in the removal.
4. Closure and dressing are as described for craniotomy.

Craniotomy for intracranial revascularization

Microbypass technique, developed in 1967, is used to shunt blood flow around an occluded portion of the internal carotid artery or the middle cerebral artery by anastomosing the superficial temporal artery to the middle cerebral artery distal to the occlusion. Today the procedure is also used for revascularization for giant aneurysm, arteriovenous malformations, and tumor.

Procedural considerations. Craniotomy for intracranial revascularization, although brief in description, is long and tedious; 7 hours is not unusual. Positioning is crucial to prevent pressure on superficial nerves, vessels, and vulnerable skin areas. Blood gas monitoring and arterial pressure readings are done routinely during the procedure. An arterial line may be placed before the patient's arrival in the surgery department or as a preliminary procedure in the operating room. Sterile and unsterile probes for the Doppler ultrasonic scanners should be available.

Operative procedure. The procedure occurs in two steps:

1. The *first stage* is reflection of the scalp flap on the operative side to expose the superficial temporal artery for dissection. Care must be taken in placing the hemostatic scalp clips to make sure they are farther apart than usual to prevent compromise of the scalp circulation following diversion of the flow of the temporal artery. Care also must be taken to prevent injury to the temporal artery as the scalp incision is made and the flap reflected.

2. After the superficial temporal artery is identified, the microscope is positioned, and the microinstrumentation is put to use.

3. The portion of the temporal artery to be used is freed but not occluded until the time of anastomosis. It may be supported and covered with Gelfoam or cottonoid material soaked in a papaverine solution. Papaverine helps prevent vessel spasm.

4. The temporal muscle is incised and retracted with fishhook retractors to begin the *second stage* of the procedure.

5. A burr hole is made in the frontotemporal area and enlarged with a rongeur.

6. The dura mater is opened and anchored over the bone edges with silk or black braided nylon sutures. The self-retaining brain retractor is used.

7. The middle cerebral artery is located, and a branch suitable for anastomosis is isolated. Flow is occluded by temporary microvascular clips, such as Heifetz, Sugita, or Yasargil (Fig. 22-57).

8. Flow also is occluded in the superficial temporal artery; the artery is cut, and an end-to-side anastomosis is completed with very fine suture material, such as no. 10-0 monofilament nylon (Fig. 22-58).

9. The temporary microvascular clips are removed. The vessels are observed for patency and flow.

10. The wound is closed, and dressings are applied.

Craniotomy for pituitary tumor (craniopharyngioma, optic glioma, and other suprasellar and parasellar tumors)

Procedural considerations. The setup is as for craniotomy with these additional pituitary instruments:

Ray curettes (ring, sharp)	Angulated suction tips, right and left; large
Spinal needles, no. 22 or 24	and small
Luer-Lok syringe, 10 ml	Curettes, small, nos. 0 through 4-0

Operative procedure. The procedure is as follows:

1. Either a bifrontal or a unilateral incision is made in the frontal or frontotemporal region. Most unilateral approaches are carried out from the right side.

2. Wet brain retractors over moist cottonoids are inserted for exposure of the optic chiasma and the pituitary gland. The frontal and often the temporal lobes are retracted. The olfactory nerve may be coagulated and divided with scissors.

3. A DeMartel, Edinborough, Yasargil, or Greenberg self-retaining retractor is placed to maintain exposure. Aneurysm clips and applicators should be available to con-

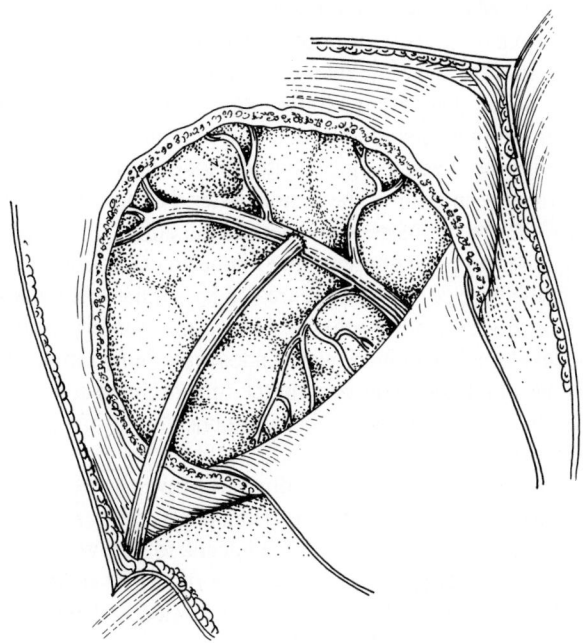

FIG. 22-57 Exposure of middle cerebral artery with clips.
From *Neurosurgery wound closure.* Ethicon, Inc.

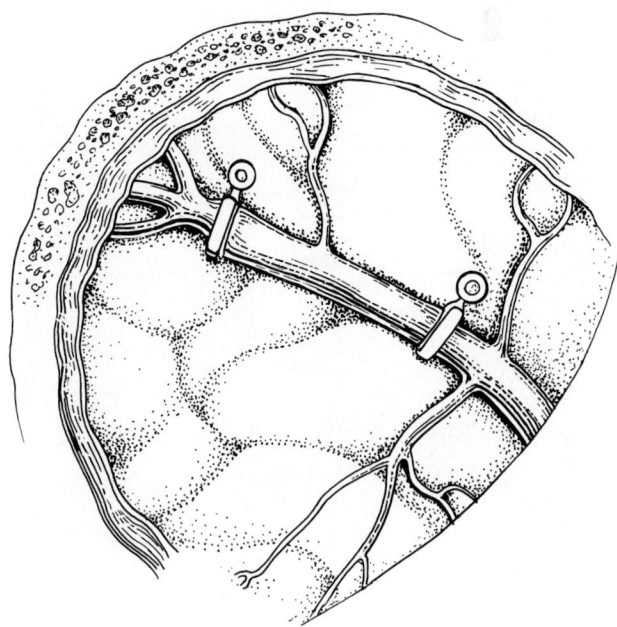

FIG. 22-58 Final anastomosis of superficial temporal artery to middle cerebral artery.

From *Neurosurgery wound closure.* Ethicon, Inc.

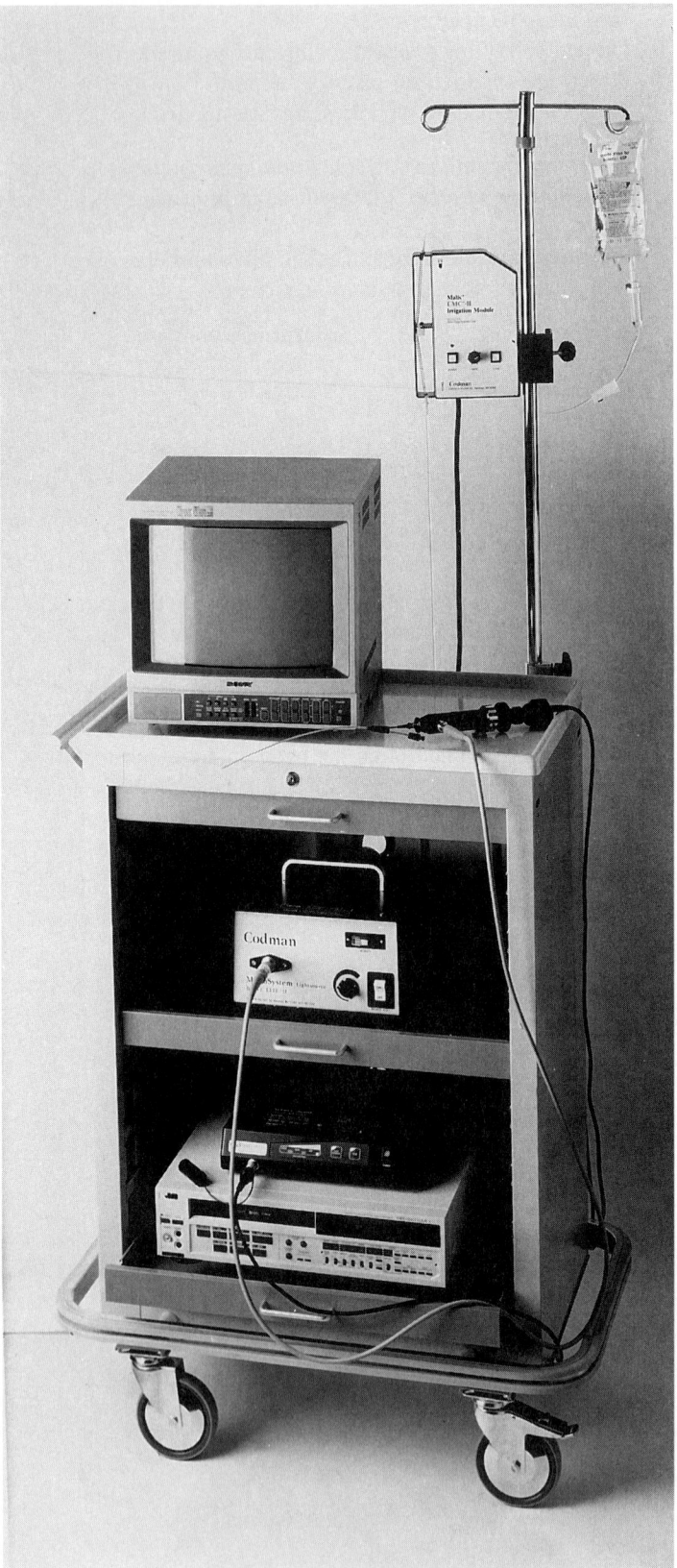

FIG. 22-59 Neuroendoscopy system.
Courtesy Codman & Shurtleff, Inc., Randolph, Mass.

trol unexpected bleeding from major vessels. The microscope may be moved into place.

4. Using a syringe with moistened plunger and a no. 22 or 24 spinal needle, the surgeon attempts to aspirate the contents of the tumor to guard against inadvertently entering an aneurysm or vessel.

5. The tumor capsule is coagulated for hemostasis and incised with a no. 11 blade on a long knife handle. With a pituitary rongeur or cup forceps, the tumor is removed.

6. Small stainless steel, copper, or Ray curettes, as well as suction, may be used during tumor removal.

7. A wide clip may be applied to the stalk of the pituitary, which may then be cut distally. A long angulated scissors is especially helpful for this.

8. If the tumor capsule is to be removed, bayonet forceps, cup forceps, nerve hooks, and suction aid in the dissection.

9. Closure and dressing are as described for craniotomy.

For pituitary adenoma with a prefixed chiasma, the surgeon may elect to remove the anterior wall of the sphenoidal sinus and sella turcica with an air drill to gain access to the tumor.

In the case of craniopharyngioma, extreme caution must be used in removing fluid from the capsule because the fluid is extremely irritating and may cause chemical leptomeningitis. Calcified pieces of tumor are dissected and removed in the same manner as the capsule of a pituitary adenoma. This is an extremely difficult procedure because of deposits on the carotid arteries, the optic nerves, and optic chiasma. The tumor capsule is often left behind on the hypothalamus to avoid striping off blood vessels supplying this structure. Many moist cottonoid strips are used to protect the surrounding areas from the cystic contents.

Suprasellar meningiomas usually arise from the tuberculum sellae just anterior to the optic nerves and chiasma. Tumor removal is similar to that of a pituitary adenoma except that the electrosurgical cutting loop may be used to excavate the interior of the tumor. After the tumor has been removed, the site of its attachment to the dura is thoroughly coagulated to prevent recurrence. Other meningiomas arising at the base of the skull are treated by similar techniques.

Less invasive approaches to intracranial surgery are being developed and performed. Endoscopic intracranial surgery was first addressed around the turn of the century, but recently the technique has been enhanced and has gained popularity among neurosurgeons.

Laser-assisted neuroendoscopy has proven to be a valuable tool in both diagnosis and treatment of central nervous system conditions in and also adjacent to the ventricular system. The neuroendoscope has 3 ports: 1 for viewing, 1 for illumination, and 1 for pulsed irrigation and introduction of a laser fiber (Fig. 22-59).

Neuroendoscopy can be used in diagnosing small seeding tumors, cysts and infectious granulation, which may be seen before detection is made by MRI or CT imaging. Biopsy samples from small tumors can be collected with microforceps introduced through the endoscope. Other applications include the following:

1. Placement of new ventricular shunt catheter
2. Removal of proximal shunt occluded by choroid plexus
3. Choroid coagulation/plexectomy
4. Third ventriculostomy
5. Transseptal fenestration
6. Ventriculocystostomy
7. Tumor biopsy and excision

It is of utmost importance that the perioperative nurse have a systematic method to manage the extensive setup and implementation of neuroendoscopy procedures.

Transsphenoidal hypophysectomy

Endocrine pituitary disorders, such as Cushing's syndrome, acromegaly, malignant exophthalmos, and hypopituitarism resulting from intrasellar tumors, as well as nonpituitary disorders, such as advanced metastatic carcinoma of the breast and prostate, diabetic retinopathy, and uncontrollable severe diabetes, have been successfully treated by transsphenoidal hypophysectomy. Rapid access to the sella turcica is achieved. Complete extracapsular enucleation of the pituitary in cases of hypophysectomy and possible complete removal of small pituitary tumors, with the remaining normal portion of the gland left intact, can be obtained. Patients are relatively free from pain after surgery. No visible scar remains.

Procedural considerations. Transsphenoidal hypophysectomy is performed with the patient under light general endotracheal anesthesia, combined with a local anesthetic. The patient is placed in a semisitting position, with head against the headrest. A portable image intensifier is used. The horizontal beam is centered on the sella turcica. A subnasal midline rhinoseptal approach is used.

The face, mouth, and nasal cavity are prepared with an antiseptic solution. Infiltration of the nasal mucosa and the gingiva with a local anesthetic agent containing 1:2000 epinephrine is helpful in initiating submucosal elevation, as well as diminishing oozing from the mucosa. A sterile adhesive plastic drape is applied to the entire face with additional sterile drapes to ensure a relatively sterile operative field. Sterile sponges or cotton is placed in the patient's mouth so only the upper gum margin is exposed.

A biopsy setup is required, as well as special instruments (Fig. 22-60). The operating microscope is used for the cranial portion of the procedure.

Operative procedure. The procedure is as follows:

1. Using the biopsy setup on a separate small Mayo table,

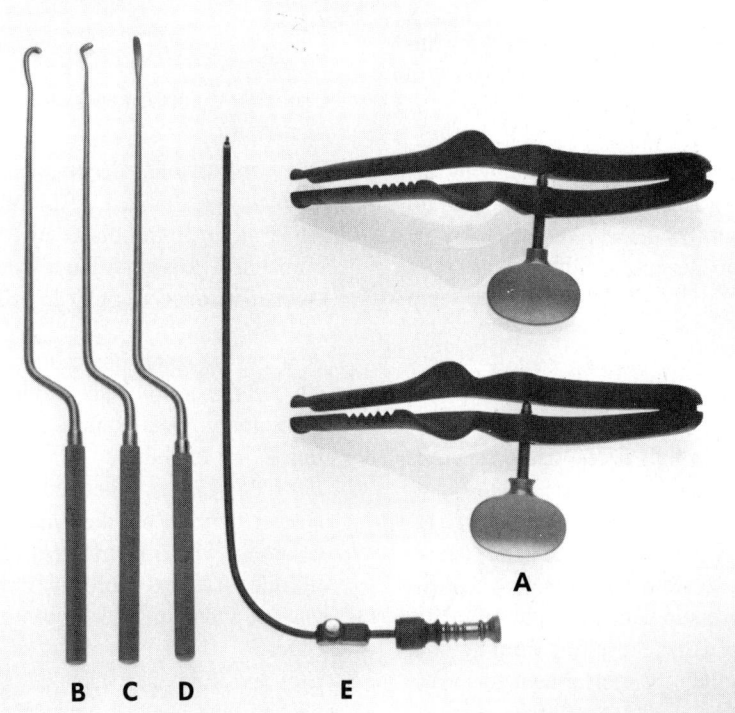

FIG. 22-60 Special instruments for transsphenoidal hypophysectomy. **A,** Hardy's modified Cushing bivalve speculum. **B,** Hardy's enucleator. **C,** Hardy's enucleator. **D,** Hardy's dissector. **E,** Hardy's suction tubes.

Courtesy Codman & Shurtleff, Inc., Randolph, Mass.

the surgeon may take a small piece of muscle from the previously prepared thigh to be used later in the procedure. This is kept in a moist sponge.

2. An incision is made in the middle of the upper gum margin. The soft tissues of the upper lip and nose are elevated from the bone with an elevator, and the nasal septum is exposed. The nasal mucosa is elevated from either side of the nasal septum, which is flanked by the blades of a Cushing bivalved speculum. The inferior third of the anterior cartilaginous septum and osseous vomer are resected, as is the floor of the sphenoidal sinus, exposing the sinus cavity. The floor of the sella turcica can be identified.

3. The floor is opened with a sphenoidal punch, and the dura mater is incised. The hypophyseal cavity should be opened only in patients undergoing surgery for pituitary adenoma. In these patients the gland is explored, and the tumor is identified and removed.

4. The extracapsular cleavage plane is identified, and the superior surface of the pituitary is dissected until the stalk and the diaphragmatic orifice are found. Cotton pledgets are applied for exposure, hemostasis, and protection of structures.

5. The stalk is sectioned low with a sickle knife, and the lateral posterior and inferior surfaces of the pituitary are dissected with an enucleator.

6. The gland is removed in toto, and the sellar cavity may be packed with muscle obtained previously from the thigh to prevent CSF leakage. The floor is reconstructed with cartilage from the nasal septum.

7. Antibiotic powder may be used and nasal packing introduced for 2 days. The gingiva incision is closed with catgut.

Some surgeons prefer to perform this operation by means of a lateral rhinotomy with a transantral-transsphenoidal approach. An ear, nose, and throat (ENT) surgeon may be available to do the initial opening, depending on surgeon preference. If an ENT surgeon does assist, a separate setup is available.

Craniectomy

Craniectomy is incision into the skull and removal of bone by enlarging one or more burr holes, using rongeurs to gain access to the underlying structures.

A craniectomy procedure may be required to remove tumors, hematomas, scars, and infections of the bone. Craniectomy is also indicated as treatment for craniosynostosis in infants and to relieve pressure on the brain from depressed bone or internal hemorrhage resulting from trauma. Today large craniotomies may be performed for acute trauma.

RESEARCH HIGHLIGHT 22-1

Patients with head trauma or bleeding are at high risk for altered cerebral perfusion; as intracranial pressure (ICP) increases, severe neurologic damage and even brain death can occur. Cerebral edema can be managed by both pharmacologic and nonpharmacologic means. Nursing interventions to avoid increases in ICP include maintaining normothermia, maintaining oxygenation and ventilation, and turning and positioning the patient appropriately.

This study focused on the effects of positioning on ICP. Ten patients who experienced either head trauma or neurologic hemorrhage were studied for the effects of four positions—head rotation to the right and left, neck flexion, and neck extension. ICP pressures were measured, and the researchers found that head rotation to the right or left and neck flexion significantly increased ICP in the study subjects. Although the study sample was small, the study design was appropriate. The findings of this study have important applications to perioperative nursing care of the head trauma patient. During patient transfer maneuvers and positioning of the head injury patient, perioperative nurses should strive to maintain a neutral head position, avoiding turning the head and neck flexion.

Williams, A., & Coyne, S. (1993). Effects of neck position on intracranial pressure. *American Journal of Critical Care, 2*(1), 68-71.

Craniectomy with evacuation of epidural or subdural hematoma

Following trauma, decompression of the brain, as well as removal and drainage of blood clots and collections of liquefied blood from outside or beneath the dura mater, is accomplished (Research Highlight 22-1).

Operative procedure. The procedure is as follows:

1. A linear or small horseshoe incision is made over the site of the lesion. The initial procedure is similar to craniotomy. One or more burr holes are made. A bone flap is not turned.

2. If a blood clot or collection of bloody fluid is found outside or beneath the dura mater, the burr hole is further enlarged, with a Kerrison or double-action rongeur, until adequate exposure is obtained. Bone edges are waxed, and cottonoid strips are put in position along the edges.

3. Clot and fluid are evacuated, and hemostasis is accomplished with coagulation or the use of hemostatic clips.

4. In cases of chronic subdural hematoma the inner and outer membranes are stripped and coagulated.

5. The brain is irrigated, using catheters or directly em-

ploying an Asepto or bulb syringe. Large amounts of saline irrigating solution are used until the return appears clear.

6. A silver or a hemostatic clip may be placed on the cortex at the site of a small incision. Another clip is placed on the dura mater. These are tag clips that are visible on postoperative x-ray films to check the bleeding site.

7. A small drain or a polyethylene or red rubber catheter may be inserted subdurally for additional drainage, or a closed drainage system, such as the Jackson-Pratt, may be used through a separate stab wound in the skin posterior to the incision. Additional burr holes are made during the course of the procedure to be sure clots in other areas do not remain undetected and untreated.

Craniectomy for craniosynostosis

Craniectomy for craniosynostosis is performed on infants whose suture lines have closed prematurely. If diagnosis is made shortly after birth, the condition can be corrected by surgically separating the two involved bones and treating the area to prevent resealing until most of the growth of the brain has occurred. The surgeon merely restores the patency of the suture and allows growth of the brain to correct the cosmetic deformity.

Operative procedure. After the scalp incision is made over the appropriate skull suture, the dura mater is stripped off the underside of the skull. A generous strip of the bone edges joining to form the fused suture is then removed with heavy scissors, a craniotome, a rongeur, or a Kerrison punch. The bone edges are waxed. Preformed Silastic sheeting can be inserted over the bone edges bordering the craniectomy and sutured or stapled in place. When sutures are used, holes must be placed in the bone edges bordering the craniectomy before the sheeting is placed.

Suboccipital craniectomy for posterior fossa exploration

Perforation and removal of the posterior occipital bone and exposure of the foramen magnum and arch of the atlas are done to remove a lesion in the posterior fossa (Fig. 22-61).

Procedural considerations. Depending on the type and size of the lesion, the exposure may be unilateral or bilateral. The operation may include the removal of the arch of the atlas. This approach gives the surgeon access to the fourth ventricle, the cerebellum, the brainstem, and the cranial nerves.

The sitting position may be preferred, but the park bench position is also utilized. An extra-high instrument table or two Mayo stands and standing stool are necessary for the nurse.

Operative procedure. The procedure is as follows:

1. Prior to the initial surgical incision, an occipital burr hole is done for placement of a ventricular catheter. This can be done as a separate procedure or concurrently with the procedure.

2. The incision may be made from mastoid tip to mastoid tip, in an arch curving upward 2 cm above the external occipital protuberance.

3. Scalp bleeding is controlled, and the skin flap is retracted with the Weitlaner retractors.

4. A periosteal elevator is used to free the muscles, which are then divided with an electrosurgical blade, using cutting current. The incision is deepened. A self-retaining retractor is used. The laminae of the first two or three cervical vertebrae may be exposed.

5. One or more holes are drilled in the occipital bone. If a Hudson brace is used, the cerebellar extension is attached. The Midas Rex or Anspach drill is very beneficial for this approach because it reduces the time needed to make the opening.

6. The dura matter is stripped from the bone. A double-action rongeur, Raney punch, Kerrison punch, or Leksell rongeur is used to enlarge the hole and smooth the edges.

7. Osseous and cerebellar venous bleeding is controlled at each step with bone wax, Gelfoam, and electrocoagulation to prevent air embolism.

8. The dura mater is opened. A small brain spoon or cottonoid strip is used to protect the brain as the initial nick is extended with scalpel or scissors. The dural incision is continued until the cerebellar hemispheres, the vermis, and the tonsils can be visualized. Hemostatic clips are used on the dura mater as necessary. Dural traction sutures are placed.

9. The cisterna magna is opened, emptied of spinal fluid, and protected with a cottonoid strip.

10. The cerebellar hemispheres are inspected. Bleeding is controlled with the bipolar coagulator. A needle may be introduced through a small coagulated incision in the cerebellar hemisphere in an attempt to palpate or tap a deep lesion.

11. Brain retractors over cottonoid strips are placed for exposure. The handle of the retractor must be kept dry to avoid slippage in the surgeon's hand. However, the inserted edge should be wet to prevent damage or tears in the brain surface. These retractors may be positioned in areas that control respiration or other vital functions, so every effort must be made to avoid jarring these instruments in the operative field. When the pathologic entity is identified, a self-retaining retractor may be placed.

12. Long bayonet forceps, bayonet cup forceps, pituitary forceps, suction, and the electrosurgical loop tips may be used to remove the lesion. Clips may be used to aid in hemostasis. A nerve stimulator may be used to identify cranial nerves; evoked potentials for brainstem monitoring are becoming routine.

13. After the lesion has been removed and bleeding controlled, further checking for adequate hemostasis is required. Venous pressure in the patient's head is increased by the anesthesiologist.

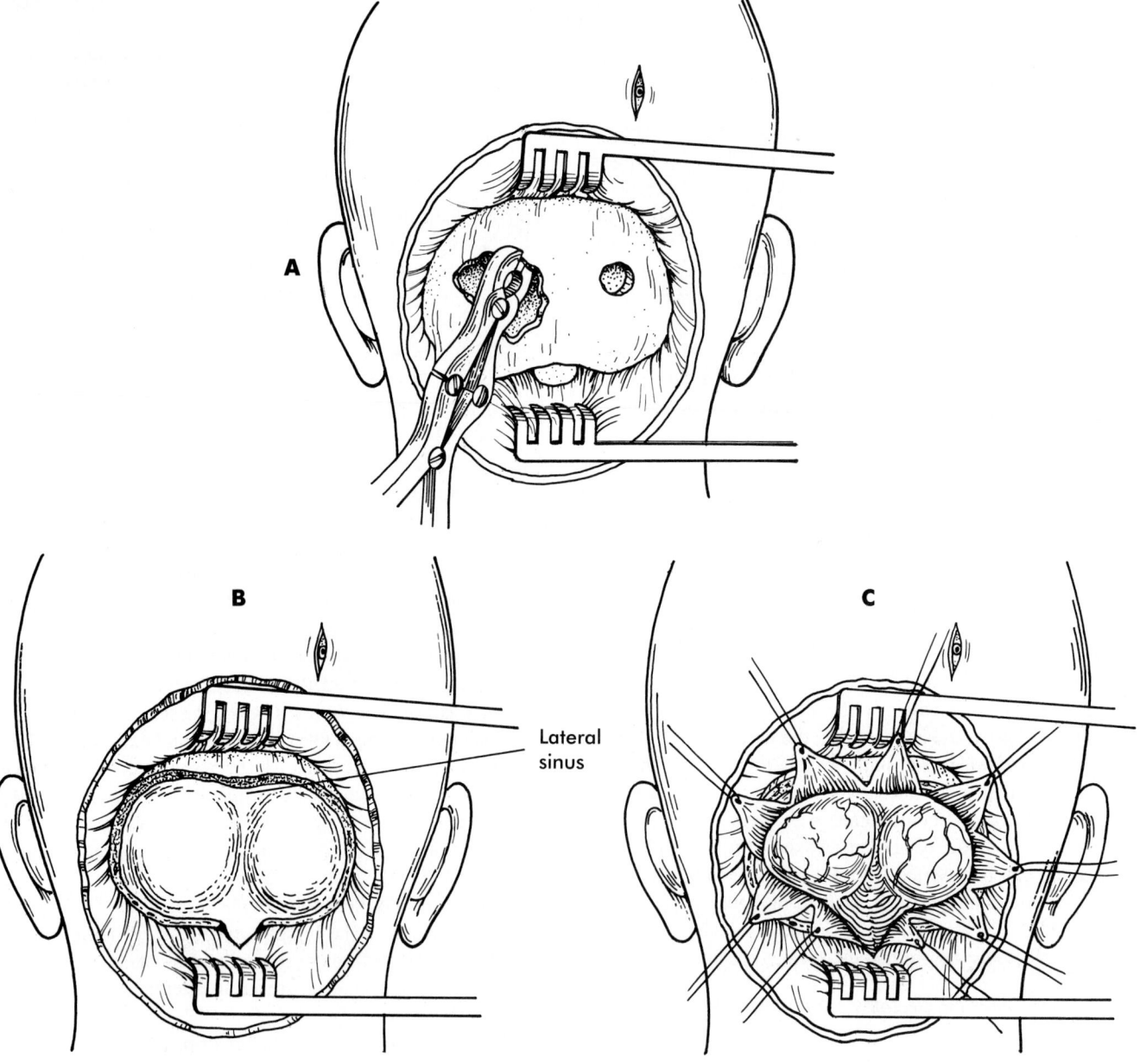

FIG. 22-61   Suboccipital craniectomy. **A,** Craniectomy being performed. **B,** Dura mater exposed. **C,** Dura mater incised and cerebellum exposed.

From Sachs, E. (1949). *Diagnosis and treatment of brain tumors and the care of the neurosurgical patient* (2nd ed.). St. Louis: Mosby.

14. The dura mater may be partially or completely closed. The muscle, fascia, and skin are closed. A dressing is applied.
15. The patient must remain anesthetized until the supine position is achieved and the prongs of the headrest are removed. Particular attention must be given to the patient's head when removing these prongs to prevent tearing the scalp or damaging the eyes.

Subtemporal craniectomy for trigeminal exploration/rhizotomy

Trigeminal neuralgia (tic douloureux, fifth cranial nerve pain) is a condition characterized by brief, repeated attacks of excruciating pain in the face. Temporary relief of trigeminal neuralgia may be obtained by interruption of branches of the nerve divisions (ophthalmic, maxillary, and mandibular) by means of alcohol injection or surgical sectioning. This approach may also be used for exploration for trigeminal neuromas.

Procedural considerations. The patient may be placed in the supine or sitting position, depending on the surgeon's preference.

Operative procedure. The procedure is as follows:

1. A vertical temporal incision extending from the zygomatic process and through the temporal muscles and periosteum is made.
2. The soft tissue is freed from the bone with a periosteal elevator. The bone exposure is maintained with a self-retaining retractor.
3. A burr hole is made. The dura mater is freed from the underside of the temporal bone.
4. The burr hole is enlarged, with a double-action rongeur, to a diameter of about 2½ inches.
5. With a moist brain retractor, the dura mater overlying the temporal lobe is retracted upward. By means of blunt dissection with cottonoids held in bayonet forceps, the dura mater is elevated from the bony floor of the middle fossa.
6. The brain retractor is replaced by a self-retaining brain retractor placed deeper into the wound to hold up the temporal lobe and dura mater. The microscope provides light as well as magnification.
7. As the dura mater is elevated, the middle meningeal artery is seen as it leaves the foramen spinosum to join the dura mater. It is coagulated with bipolar bayonet forceps and may be clipped before being divided. A cottonoid or wax plug is packed into the foramen spinosum.
8. Additional blunt dissection uncovers the mandibular division of the trigeminal nerve and finally the trigeminal (gasserian) ganglion within its own dural sheath (dura propria). Bleeding is controlled with cottonoids and a hemostatic material such as Gelfoam and thrombin.
9. Some surgeons terminate the procedure after stripping the ganglion and its dura mater from that of the overlying temporal lobe. (The ganglion may be injected with saline solution, and the dura mater may be split.)
10. If a root section is to be performed, a no. 11 blade on a long knife handle is used to make an incision into the lateral rim of the dura propria. The sensory and motor roots of the nerve are defined with a fine nerve hook. The mandibular and maxillary sections of the root are usually divided. These are elevated with a nerve hook and divided with fine scissors or a fine blade. The ophthalmic portion of the root is spared, as is the motor root.
11. Absolute alcohol may be injected into the affected divisions of the nerve just distal to the ganglion.
12. Saline solution is injected into the dura mater overlying the temporal lobe to distend it.
13. The incision is closed, and dressings are applied.

Suboccipital craniectomy and decompression for trigeminal rhizotomy

Some surgeons prefer to section the posterior root of the trigeminal nerve by the suboccipital route.

Procedural considerations. The position of the patient for suboccipital craniectomy is sitting, prone, or semilateral. To be prepared, the perioperative nurse must know during the planning phase (usually the day before the procedure is scheduled) which position the surgeon plans to use.

Operative procedure. The procedure is as follows:

1. The incision is made vertically behind the mastoid process. A trephine or burr hole is made and enlarged with a rongeur.
2. The dura mater is opened. The cisterna magna is pierced to empty the CSF and permit backward retraction of the cerebellum. A brain spoon, brain spatula, or lighted retractor over moist strips of cottonoid is used to gently lift the cerebellar hemisphere. The eighth nerve is readily seen. The fifth nerve is approached by opening the arachnoid of the cisterna pontis and suctioning out the fluid. Veins are protected and bleeding controlled by pressure over cottonoid strips.
3. The nerve and the vessels around it are identified. The nerve is decompressed by coagulating the vessel over the nerve or separating the vessel from the nerve with a Teflon pledget. The microscope facilitates microvascular decompression. The motor root medial and anterior to the sensory root is preserved.
4. The wound is closed.

Suboccipital craniectomy and glossopharyngeal nerve section

Posterior fossa exploration for glossopharyngeal neuralgia is occasionally necessary. The same posterior fossa approach is used as for trigeminal neuralgia. The cerebellar hemisphere of the affected side is gently elevated upward and toward the midline. The ninth, tenth, and eleventh nerves are identified and defined with bayonet forceps, nerve hooks, and fine dissectors. The ninth nerve and a portion of the tenth are consecutively elevated with a nerve hook and divided with a fine-tipped scissors.

Suboccipital craniectomy for acoustic neuroma

Usually the acoustic neuroma arises from the vestibular portion of the eighth cranial nerve within the auditory meatus. It is desirable, although not always possible, to remove the complete tumor without damage to the facial nerve.

Operative procedure. The procedure is as follows:

1. The posterior fossa approach may be used. A unilateral straight paramedian incision is made.
2. The cerebellum is retracted gently upward with brain re-

tractors and is cushioned with moist cottonoids. The lower cranial nerves are defined with a nerve or aneurysm hook. A cottonoid is placed over these nerves to protect them. Veins draining the tumor into the superior petrosal sinus are identified and either clipped or coagulated and cut.

3. The tumor is excavated and resected by methods similar to those employed to remove a pituitary adenoma.
4. A nerve stimulator may be used to identify the facial nerve. Use of the operating microscope is advantageous because of the many nerves and vessels in the area.
5. A high-speed air drill may be used to unroof the auditory canal and expose the remaining tumor. Constant irrigation is mandatory during drilling.

Very small tumors confined to the auditory canal may be approached by drilling directly through the temporal bone to open the auditory canal within the bone and avoid the posterior fossa.

Suboccipital craniectomy for Ménière's disease

Ménière's disease is characterized by recurrent explosive attacks of vertigo associated with nausea, vomiting, tinnitus, and progressive deafness. It is usually unilateral. The cause is obscure, and in intractable cases surgical section or partial section of the eighth nerve (acoustic) may be performed for relief. However, surgery is not often performed for Ménière's disease.

Operative procedure. The procedure is as follows:

1. The cerebellum is approached through a lateral vertical incision behind the ear. The cerebellum on the affected side is retracted.
2. The eighth nerve is exposed with bayonet forceps and gentle manipulation. The nerve is freed from the arachnoid of the lateral cistern. It is separated from the underlying structures with a blunt nerve hook. Care is taken to prevent traction on the nearby seventh nerve (facial).
3. With fine scissors the vestibular fibers in the anterior half of the nerve are divided over a nerve hook. If the patient has useful hearing, the posterior auditory branches are preserved. Tinnitus may be relieved by section of the anterior fibers of the auditory portion of the nerve.
4. The dura mater and wound are closed.

Cranioplasty

Cranioplasty is performed for repair of a skull defect resulting from trauma, malformation, or a surgical procedure. Cranial defects covered by muscular areas need not be repaired. The purposes of cranioplasty are to relieve headache, vertigo, fear of injury, and local tenderness or throbbing; to prevent secondary injury to the underlying brain; and for cosmetic effect.

Procedural considerations. Many materials have been used to repair skull defects, including bone and cartilage, celluloid, metals such as Vitallium and tantalum, and synthetic resins such as methyl methacrylate and silicone rubber. All involve technical problems. The use of commercially prepared cranioplastic synthetics that supply the needed chemicals and mixing containers has simplified the procedures of shaping and molding the prosthesis. Sometimes heavy wire mesh is cut to the shape of the defect, and the methyl methacrylate is molded over the mesh.

Operative procedure. The procedure is as follows:

1. A scalp flap is turned, and the bony defect is exposed.
2. The edges of the defect are trimmed, and a ledge is formed to seat the prosthesis.
3. After the bone defect has been prepared so it is slightly saucerized, the methyl methacrylate is mixed by adding one volume of liquid monomer to one volume of the powdered polymer. When this has formed a doughy mass, it is dropped into a sterile polyethylene bag. The soft plastic is then rolled on a flat surface into the desired shape, leaving the thickness to the approximate depth of the skull edges. A sterile test tube, syringe barrel, or other round object can be used, although a stainless steel roller is preferred because of its weight and ease of use.
4. The soft cranioplastic material in the bag is placed over the skull defect and, through light pressing with the ends of the fingers, is fitted into the missing skull area. The plastic bag is stretched by assistants as the surgeon molds the plate into the defect and forms an overlapping bevel edge. This overlapping fringe keeps the plate from falling inside the skull, as does the skull saucerization.
5. When the heat of the chemical reactions begins, the plate is lifted out of the bony wound and removed from the polyethylene bag. Cool saline should be used on the flap while the exothermic reaction takes place.
6. When cool enough to handle, the excess material is trimmed away with bone rongeurs or cut with a saw and placed in the cranial defect.
7. A sterile carborundum wheel attached to the electrical bone saw or craniotome is used to smooth the rough spots and bevel the edges so the plate will blend gradually with the skull.
8. Mixing and fitting the plate take about 7 minutes, as does hardening. Sutures may be used to hold the plate in place, generally at three or more points.

Microneurosurgery

Adaptation of the operating microscope for neurosurgery has resulted in improvement of many neurosurgical procedures and made new procedures possible. For years neurosurgeons have worn magnifying loupes to see small structures. Loupes usually have a magnification of 2 or 2.8. The microscope has a variety of magnifications ranging from 6 to 40, providing flexibility and precision. The coaxial illumination overcomes the difficulties of lighting neurosurgical wounds.

Use of the microscope restricts the surgeon's field of vision and mobility; therefore the scrub nurse must be proficient. The operative field, unless video monitoring is available, cannot be seen. The scrub nurse must understand the surgical procedure, know the anatomy, know the names and uses of all the microinstruments, and be able to place each instrument in the surgeon's hand without delay so the surgeon will be able to use the instrument without readjusting it. The scrub nurse must make it possible for the surgeon to perform the operation without looking away from the operating field. Instruments must be kept free from blood and tissue during use because the microscope also magnifies debris on the instruments, occluding the structure the surgeon is about to approach. The perioperative nursing team must understand the degree of stress these difficult procedures place on the neurosurgeon.

Microneurosurgical instruments are expensive and delicate. Instructions for handling, cleaning, sterilizing, and storing these instruments should be followed. An instrument that is sprung, bent, dulled, hooked, or in any way damaged must never be handed to a surgeon for use but must be repaired or replaced.

Existing microsurgical instruments have been modified and adapted to the requirements of neurosurgery. These instruments often possess the following characteristics: bayonet shape, so the surgeon's hand remains outside the line of vision and the beam of the microscope light; finely sprung and fluted grip; long length for access to deep structures; and slender and delicate tips that take up as little space as possible.

Very fine microsutures are available. The neurosurgeon may want to open the suture pack and ready the suture for use. However, the scrub nurse should be able to open and handle a delicate suture without damaging it. Each time the surgeon must look away and then back to the surgical field, open wound time and anesthesia time are increased while the surgeon becomes reoriented to the field. Therefore the assistance the scrub nurse gives the surgeon saves time and directly benefits the patient.

Microsurgical techniques have been applied to cranial, spinal, and peripheral nerve operations. Perhaps microneurovascular surgery is the area in which the most progress has been made. However, patient outcomes following microsurgical procedures on cranial nerves, spinal nerves, and cord tumors and especially for repair of peripheral nerve injuries have been enhanced.

Some procedures in which microsurgery is of value are posterior fossa explorations, especially for tumors of the fourth ventricle or cerebellopontine angle; translabyrinthine and transpetrosal removal of small acoustic neuromas, with resulting preservation of the facial nerve; and transsphenoidal hypophysectomy and transsphenoidal operations for small intracranial tumors, such as pituitary adenomas or even craniopharyngiomas. Transclival operations are also performed. Small vessel endarterectomy, cerebral arterial bypass, cerebral aneurysm surgery, and excision of arteriovenous malformations are done under the microscope. Microsurgery also has advantages in the treatment of tumors and arteriovenous malformations of the spinal cord.

Stereotaxic procedures

The use of complex mechanisms to locate and destroy target structures in the brain is known as stereotactics. Predetermined anatomic landmarks are used as guides. Special head-fixation devices have been developed by surgeons and engineers for use with radiography, fluoroscopy, CT scans, and MRI to permit accurate placement of a probe directed at the target area. Stereotaxic procedures can also be done on the spinal cord. Common target areas for the stereotaxic approach include tumors, the basal ganglia, the thalamus, the hypophysis, aneurysms, and anterolateral spinal tracts. Target areas undergo biopsy or are destroyed by chemical or mechanical means or electrically stimulated to control intractable pain. Stereotaxic procedures are also done to place electrodes in various regions of the brain to determine the site of origin of seizures. Lesions in target areas are made to perform biopsies and remove tumors, alleviate pain, abolish movement disorders, change endocrine balance to reverse such conditions as retinopathy, acromegaly, and endocrine-sensitive cancers, and obliterate aneurysms.

Operative procedure. The patient's head is placed in the stereotaxic frame and the patient is taken to the MRI or CT room, where the target is located and computer coordinates are determined. The computer then determines target trajectory. The patient is then taken to the operating room, and the stereotaxic procedure with precise coordinates is performed. The probe is checked by the same method after it is believed to rest on target (Fig. 22-62).

Hollow cannulas, coagulating electrodes, cryosurgical probes, wire loops, and other lesion-producing or biopsy instruments have been introduced for the destruction of areas in the brain. Temporary and permanent nerve-stimulator electrodes are also introduced to augment the pain-control function of the central nervous system. These instruments are introduced through a burr hole or twist-drill hole in the skull.

Continuing advancements in technology allow for the use of the laser with stereotaxic equipment, and endoscopic equipment. The numerous stereotaxic frames available include the BRW, CRW, Leksell, Patel, Pelorsus, and Reichert Mundinger.

Surgery of the globus pallidus, basal ganglia, and thalamus

Pallidotomy is incision into the globus pallidus, usually by electrosurgery. *Chemopallidectomy* is introduction of a sclerosing solution through a rigid catheter or cannula to produce a lesion. *Thalamotomy* is incision into the thalamus. *Chemothalamectomy* is creation of a lesion in the region of the ventrolateral nucleus of the thalamus by means of a chemical solution such as alcohol with iophendylate.

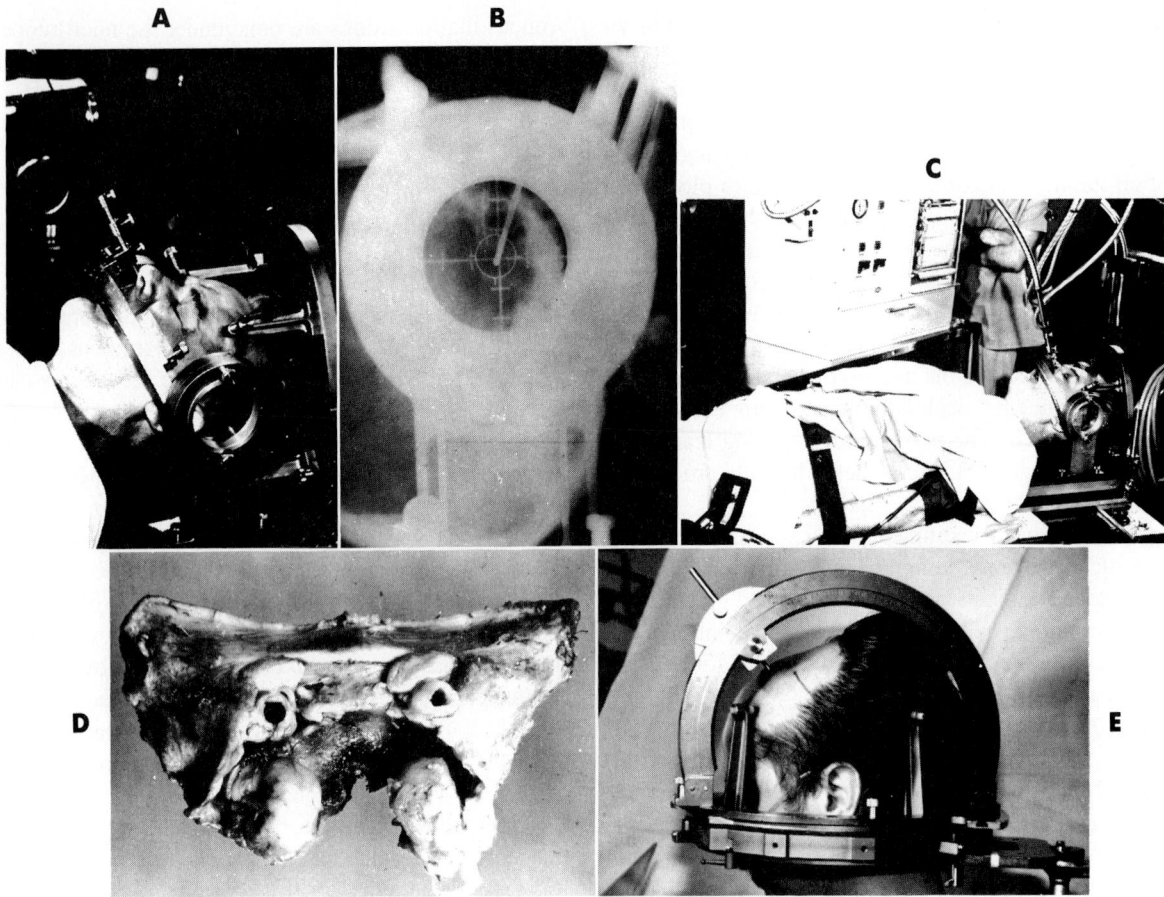

FIG. 22-62   Stereotaxic procedure. **A,** Patient's head is fixed to stereotaxic unit. Twist drill is inserted into anterior wall of sphenoidal sinus by way of left nostril into nasopharynx. **B,** Lateral x-ray film demonstrating freezing unit properly placed in target area (pituitary gland). Circle and cross-hairs are positioned at target points before insertion of cannula. **C,** Cannula in patient's left nostril is attached to freezing unit on table. X-ray equipment is seen in upper left background. Since procedure is performed with patient under local anesthesia, body straps are used to immobilize patient. **D,** Sella turcica viewed from above, demonstrating bone perforation at base through which cannula was inserted. To either side of sella turcica, internal carotid arteries are seen (*below,* siphon; *above,* with open lumen, cranial extension). Above sectioned arteries, optic nerves are seen passing into orbits. **E,** BRW stereotaxic frame.

A to D from Conway-Rutkowski, B.L. (1982). *Carini and Owens' neurological and neurosurgical nursing* (8th ed.). St. Louis: Mosby; **E,** courtesy Radionics, Inc., Burlington, Mass.

This approach is still effective but not done as much as in the past. Surgical intervention is intended to interrupt the nerve pathways and alleviate the crippling locomotor symptoms of persistent, intractable tremor or rigidity associated with multiple sclerosis, severe brain trauma, Parkinson's disease, and various types of cerebellar degeneration. Studies are being conducted on fetal pituitary allografts and transcortical intraventricular adrenal medullary grafting in the treatment of Parkinson's disease. Some new treatment frontiers pose difficult ethical questions for neuroscience research; these will be an ongoing dilemma in the development of new treatment protocols. Operations of this type are also performed on the thalamus in an attempt to relieve pain.

Procedural considerations. The patient must be conscious and cooperative to permit careful examination and observation of response to the procedure and the effects of the symptoms. Local anesthesia is used. The patient may be in a supine or semisitting position.

Operative procedure. The procedure is as follows:

1. The patient's head is positioned and secured in the stereotaxic frame.
2. A skin incision and burr hole are completed as for ventriculography.

3. It may be necessary to take ventriculograms (however, CT and MRI scans have essentially replaced ventriculograms) in addition to viewing the position of the cannulas or needles.
4. When the correct position has been achieved, tests or reversible lesions may be attempted. The patient's response is observed. Finally, the definitive lesion is created at the selected site by means of electrosurgery, chemical solutions, or a cryogenic unit.
5. The dura mater and incision are closed.

Cryosurgery

Cryosurgery is the use of subfreezing temperatures in the treatment of disease to create a lesion. It is used in neurosurgery for transsphenoidal destruction of the pituitary gland in patients with acromegaly, diabetic retinopathy, and metastatic breast carcinoma. It can also be used for the destruction of the posterior portion of the thalamus for the treatment of Parkinson's disease or other involuntary movement disorders.

Transsphenoidal cryosurgery of the pituitary gland

Transsphenoidal cryosurgery is of special benefit to the patient suffering from metastatic carcinoma of the breast. These patients are most likely to respond if they have benefited from previous hormonal therapy or oophorectomy. In the patient with diabetic retinopathy, transsphenoidal cryosurgery is indicated when further laser beam coagulation of retinal lesions is considered useless. With acromegaly, if optic nerve or chiasma compression is present, a craniotomy is usually necessary.

Patients may undergo retrograde jugular venography before surgery to outline the cavernous sinuses and carotid arteries. Patients with tumors must also have contrast CT scanning.

The advantages of transsphenoidal cryosurgery follow:

1. Candidates in poor physical condition tolerate this procedure better than a craniotomy because it is less traumatic. Local rather than general anesthesia may be used.
2. Mortality and morbidity rates are low.
3. Complete destruction can be achieved with fair certainty in neoplastic glands and good certainty in normal glands.

Procedural considerations. Surgery is performed with fluoroscopic control. The patient is under local anesthesia supplemented with neuroleptanalgesia. Transtracheal anesthesia is used before insertion of an endotracheal tube for maintenance of a patent airway during the procedure. The patient is instructed to answer questions with hand signals.
Operative procedure. The procedure is as follows:

1. A topical local anesthetic administered with cotton applicators and 1% lidocaine injections through long needles is used to anesthetize the nasal and nasopharyngeal mucosa.
2. The head is placed in the stereotaxic head holder and fixed after injection of local anesthetic in the skin at the points of fixation.
3. Preliminary x-ray films of the skull are taken to be sure that proper positioning has been achieved.
4. A guide is introduced, and a hole is drilled into the sphenoidal sinus and the floor of the sella turcica through the nasal vault. The guide is positioned fluoroscopically.
5. A cryoprobe is introduced through the guide into the pituitary gland, and its position is confirmed with x-ray films. The temperature of the probe is lowered to $-18°$ to $-19°$ C for 12 to 15 minutes. The probe can be used to feel the exact location of the dura mater surrounding the pituitary gland laterally and the diaphragm of the sella turcica superiorly.
6. The probe may be introduced to several depths of penetration into the sella turcica and additional lesions made. Additional holes may be drilled for further lesions.
7. The probe is withdrawn, and the nasal vault is inspected for bleeding. It can be packed with nasal packing. Antibiotics can be instilled before packing.

Patients are kept supine for 2 to 3 days and placed on a regimen of prophylactic antibiotics and cortisone replacement. Complications are meningitis secondary to CSF leakage, extraocular palsy, damage to the optic nerve, and injury to cranial vessels such as the carotid and cavernous sinus. These can be prevented by an accurate preoperative evaluation and precise probe placement during surgery.

Shunt operations

Hydrocephalus is a pathologic condition in which there is an increase in the amount of CSF in the cranial cavity because of excessive production of, inadequate absorption of, or an obstruction that interferes with the flow of the fluid through the ventricular system.

Noncommunicating, or internal, hydrocephalus results from obstruction within the ventricular system. Ventricular fluid does not communicate with subarachnoid fluid.

Communicating, or external, hydrocephalus results from an obstruction outside the ventricular system. All the ventricles are enlarged, and ventricular and subarachnoid fluids freely communicate. Normal pressure hydrocephalus results from malabsorption of CSF.

Currently the two most widely used methods to divert excessive CSF from ventricles to other body cavities from which it can be absorbed are ventriculoatrial (ventriculocardiac) and ventriculoperitoneal shunts. A catheter is inserted into the ventricular system (usually a lateral ventricle) and connected to a distal catheter that is placed in the right atrium of the heart or the peritoneal cavity (Fig. 22-63). Ventriculoatrial shunts are not used as much as in the past but are still a good alternative for treatment of CSF conditions.

A valve system is used to direct the flow of CSF and regulate the ventricular fluid pressure by opening within a preset range and draining the excess fluid into the atrium or peritoneum. The valve system may be a separate unit, for example, the Holter valve, or Hakim or Denver system. The unit may be placed between the ventricular and distal catheters under the scalp just behind the ear (Fig. 22-64) or may be incorporated into the distal catheter (Fig. 22-65).

Usually a reservoir is inserted into the system between the ventricular catheter and the valve. The reservoir is also placed under the scalp just behind the ear or in a burr hole that was made to tap the lateral ventricle. The reservoir can be punctured through the scalp with a 25- or 26-gauge Huber needle to irrigate and clear an obstruction in the ventricular catheter, to introduce a contrast medium for an x-ray check of patency, to inject medication into the ventricle, or to serve as a flushing device when digital compression is applied (Fig. 22-66). Currently, the Ommaya reservoir is being utilized for the introduction of chemotherapeutic agents and for drainage of cystic brain tumors.

The valve assembly must be checked for patency and pressure before implantation. Each manufacturer provides specific instructions, which must be followed. As with all implantable devices, the shunt assembly must be kept free

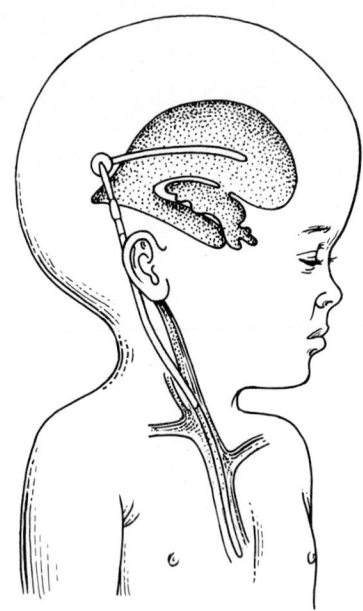

FIG. 22-63   Placement of ventriculoatrial shunt.
From *Neurosurgery wound closure*. Ethicon, Inc.

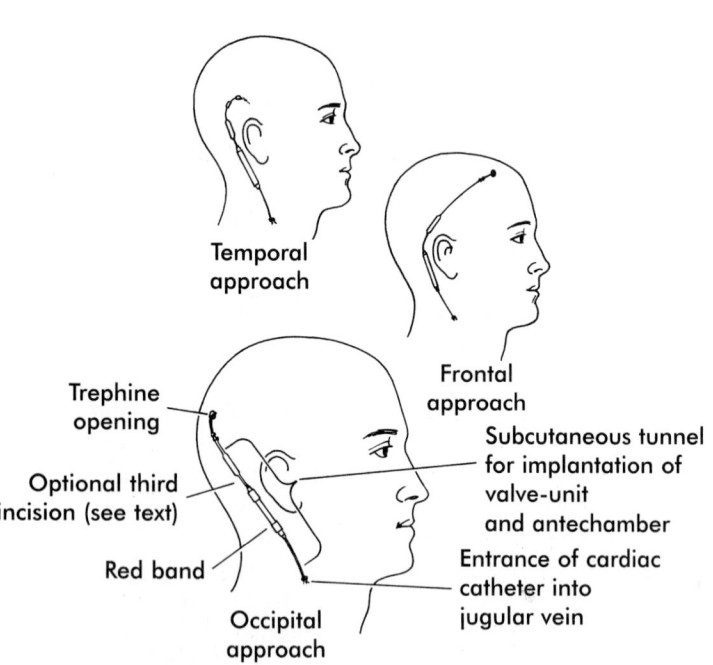

FIG. 22-64   Placement of Hakim ventriculoatrial shunt.
Courtesy Cordis Corp., Miami.

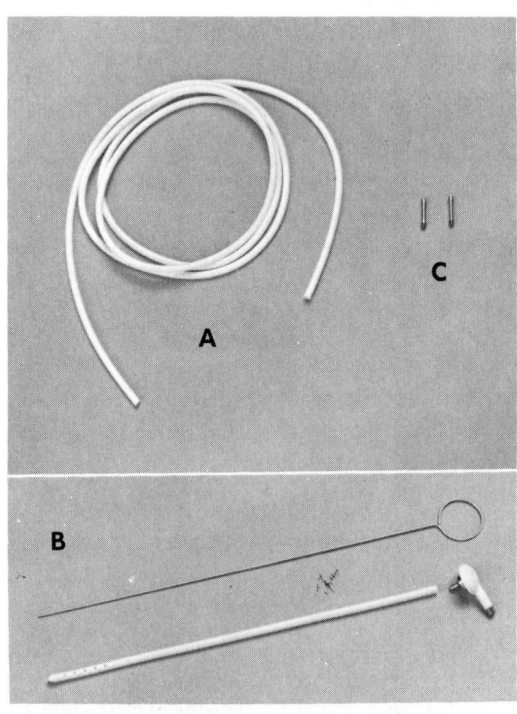

FIG. 22-65   Shunt is made from silicone tubing of special formula and consists of three parts. **A,** Peritoneal catheter. **B,** Ventricular with side perforations. **C,** Connector. Materials used in shunt can be sterilized in autoclave.
Courtesy Codman & Shurtleff, Inc., Randolph, Mass.

from lint, glove powder, and other potential foreign bodies that could cause a reaction in the patient's tissues.

Neurosurgeons and engineers frequently modify and improve shunt assemblies.

Valves are manufactured with pressure ranges of high, medium, low, and extra low. Slit-valve catheters have three pressure ranges: high, medium, and low. All shunt systems and parts can be purchased sterile.

Other procedures that are sometimes done to correct hydrocephalus include cauterization of the choroid plexus of the lateral ventricles by placing a lensed ventriculoscope or laser into the ventricle through a burr hole to visualize and destroy the production site of CSF; lumbar subarachnoid shunt, in which a laminectomy is done and the CSF is diverted into the peritoneal cavity; and ventriculocisternostomy, or Torkildsen procedure, in which a catheter is placed to shunt fluid from a lateral ventricle to the cisterna magna (Fig. 22-67). Endoscopic third ventriculostomy fenestrating the floor of the third ventricle into the cistern space is an excellent procedure for communicating hydrocephalus.

Ventriculoatrial shunt

Procedural considerations. Insertion of a ventriculoatrial shunt is carried out with the patient in a modified supine position. The head is usually slightly elevated and turned to the left and may be supported on a doughnut. An x-ray film of the chest is taken to validate correct placement of the distal catheter, or the catheter can be placed under direct-vision fluoroscopy with the image intensifier.

Operative procedure. When the distal slit-valve catheter is used, an incision is made in the neck to isolate the facial or the internal or external jugular vein. The atrial (distal) catheter is filled with normal saline solution, clamped with a bulldog clamp to prevent air from entering the circulatory system, and threaded into the right atrium through the isolated vein. Most catheters have a radiopaque tip for easy identification of placement during radiography. The catheter should lie at the T6 or T7 level.

Access is gained to the right lateral ventricle through a burr hole or twist-drill hole. The ventricular catheter is placed and connected to a reservoir. A tunnel is made under the skin from the burr hole to the neck incision with uterine packing forceps or a special tunneling device appropriate for the specific assembly being used. The atrial catheter is pulled through the tunnel to the burr hole and connected to the reservoir.

When a separate valve, such as the Holter, is used, the ventricular part of the procedure is carried out first. A special valve introducer and tube passer have been designed for use with the Holter assembly.

A single-catheter shunt system without a reservoir is also available. The distal end is a slit valve, and the proximal end is a ventricular catheter.

Ventriculoperitoneal shunts

The ventricular portion of this procedure is the same as for ventriculoatrial shunts. The distal catheter is much longer and is threaded from the ventricular puncture site under the scalp and superficial tissues of the neck, chest, and abdomen to the abdominal incision. The tip of the distal catheter may be placed under the liver.

Some precautions that must be taken during the valve implant procedures include the following:

1. Trapping of air in the valve assembly unit should be prevented.
2. Storage fluid surrounding the valve should be removed, pumped out of the valve, and replaced with Ringer's solution.
3. Extreme care should be used in handling the unit. It

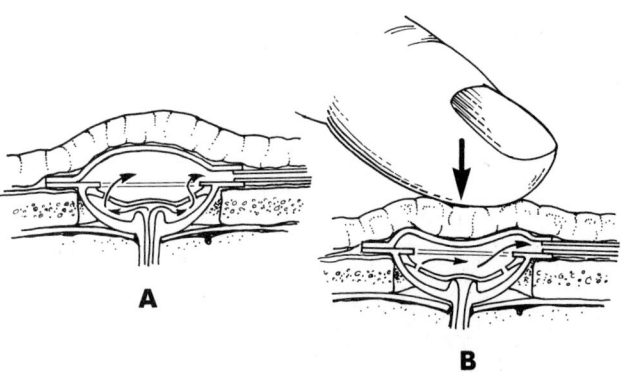

FIG. 22-66   Pudenz valve flushing device for ventricular shunts. **A,** Flanged silicone capsule and diaphragm valve shaped to fit into burr hole in skull. **B,** Pressure on capsule closes ventricular inlet and flushes shunt tube.

Courtesy Codman & Shurtleff, Inc., Randolph, Mass.

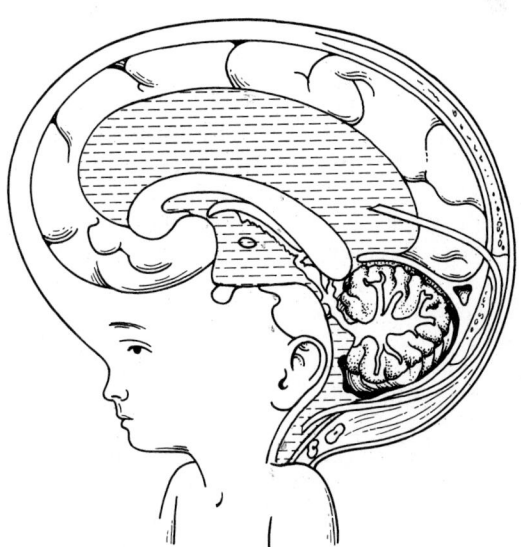

FIG. 22-67   Torkildsen operation (ventriculocisternostomy) showing catheter in place: one end in occipital horn of lateral ventricle, the other in cisterna magna.

From Conway-Rutkowski, B.L. (1982). *Carini and Owens' neurological and neurosurgical nursing* (8th ed.). St. Louis: Mosby.

should never be placed on gauze or linen, to avoid lint or other foreign body. *The unit is always placed in a basin, and should also be kept covered.*

4. Lubricants should never be used on the unit. The patient's body fluid adequately lubricates the device.
5. The valve must be properly oriented. It permits only one-way passage of fluid.
6. The valve system must not be pumped excessively immediately after surgery. This can cause too rapid a fluid loss, leading to a rapid decrease in ventricular size. This is poorly tolerated and may lead to subdural hemorrhage.

Frequently, shunts must be revised. Some shunts become obstructed. Others become disconnected or malfunction mechanically in some way. The growth of infants and children may require revision of distal tubings.

BACK SURGERY
Laminectomy

Laminectomy is removal of one or more of the vertebral laminae to expose the spinal canal. Laminectomy, hemilaminectomy, and interlaminar approach are performed to reach the spinal cord and its adjacent structures to treat compression fracture, dislocation, herniated nucleus pulposus, and cord tumor, as well as for spinal cord stimulation and insertion of infusion pumps for pain control. Section of the spinal nerves, including cordotomy and rhizotomy, requires similar surgical exposure. Laminectomy is also done to insert subarachnoid shunts for hydrocephalus or pseudotumor cerebri.

Procedural considerations. Laminectomy can be done with the patient in the prone, lateral, knee-chest, or sitting position. It is performed on the cervical, thoracic, or lumbar spine.

Laminectomy instruments include the basic neurosurgical set and the following:

2 Straight pituitary rongeurs, large and small	1 Horsley bone cutter, large 10½ inches
2 Angled pituitary rongeurs, large and small	2 Spurling-Kerrison laminectomy rongeurs, downbiting, 3 and 5 mm
1 Tower back retractor with blades	2 Schlesinger cervical punches, thin-lipped rongeur, 3 and 5 mm
1 Scoville hemilaminectomy retractor	2 Love nerve root retractors
4 Beckman-Adson self-retaining laminectomy retractors, sharp, 12 inches, 2 regular and 2 large	2 Angled curettes, nos. 3 and 4
4 Key periosteal elevators, ¼, ½, ¾, and 1 inch	2 Diamond-jawed needle holders, 9 inches
	6 Cone ring curettes
	5 Scoville curettes, no. 1, 3, 4, 5, and 6
2 Adson self-retaining cerebellum retractors, angled	1 Penfield no. 4
	2 Freer dissectors
	1 Murphy ball probe

Operative procedures
Laminectomy for herniated disk (nucleus pulposus)

1. A midline vertical or transverse incision is made at the operative site.
2. Hemostatic forceps may be placed on the underside of the skin edge and everted for hemostasis. Deeper vessels are usually electrocoagulated.
3. Two self-retaining retractors (Cone, Weitlaner, or Adson) are inserted for exposure.
4. The fascia is incised in the midline with Mayo scissors, electrosurgical cutting tip, or a scalpel.
5. One side of the spinous processes is exposed by sharp dissection.
6. The paraspinous muscles and periosteum are stripped off the laminae with a knife and sharp periosteal elevators. Cutting current dissection with the electrosurgical unit may be used.
7. As each area is stripped, a gauze sponge is packed around the bony structures with a periosteal elevator to aid in blunt dissection and to tamponade bleeding. The paraspinous muscles are dissected from all the laminae (Fig. 22-68). In disk surgery this may be done only on one side, the side of the lesion.
8. A laminectomy retractor is then placed in position. Ei-

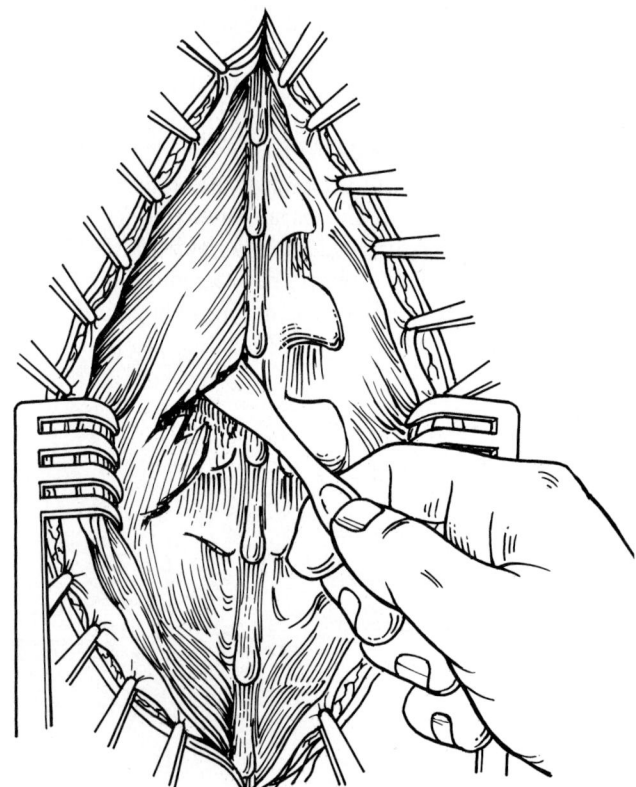

FIG. 22-68 Laminectomy: exposing vertebrae by dissecting muscle away from spine.

From Sachs, E. (1949). *Diagnosis and treatment of brain tumors and the care of the neurosurgical patient* (2nd ed.). St. Louis: Mosby.

ther a Scoville (a blade on the tissue side and a slightly shorter hook on the bone side), Tower, or Beckman-Adson retractor can be used.

9. Cottonoid strips or patties are placed in the extremes of the field for hemostasis.

10. The edges of the laminae overlying the interspace with the herniated disk are defined with a curette. A partial hemilaminectomy of these laminal edges extending out into the lateral gutter of the spinal canal is performed with a Schwartz-Kerrison rongeur. The bone edges are waxed.

11. The flaval ligament is grasped with vascular bayonet forceps with teeth, and a no. 15 blade on a no. 7 knife handle is used to incise it as close to the midline as possible. Cottonoid strips or patties are passed through this incision to protect the underlying dura, and a window is cut in the flaval ligament with a no. 15 blade on a no. 7 knife handle (Fig. 22-69).

12. Additional ligaments out in the lateral gutter of the spinal canal may be removed with a large curette or a Cloward punch after first protecting the dural sac and nerve root with a cottonoid.

13. A dural elevator and a Love or copper nerve root retractor are used to retract the nerve root and dural sac to expose the disk space.

14. Epidural veins are controlled by packing with narrow cottonoid strips and if necessary by careful coagulation with a bipolar bayonet.

15. Any herniated fragment of disk is removed with a pituitary rongeur.

16. After coagulation of its surface, an opening is cut into the posterior aspect of the interspace with a no. 11 or 15 blade on a no. 7 knife handle.

17. Pituitary rongeurs, straight and angled, narrow and wide, are used to remove the disk material from the interspace.

18. Straight and angled Scoville and ring curettes help to further clean out the interspace. Disk material so loosened is removed with the pituitary rongeurs.

19. The area is irrigated with Ringer's or normal saline solution, and the interspace is explored with a suction tip.

20. The nerve roots and extradural space are explored with a blunt nerve hook.

21. If no further specimen is obtained, hemostasis is secured with cottonoid strips or patties. If possible, neither gelatin sponge nor gauze nor other hemostatic material is used.

22. The cottonoid strips are removed from the epidural space, the bed is unflexed, and the area is further irrigated. A change of position sometimes causes more disk material to protrude, and the interspace is reexposed with a nerve root retractor to rule out this possibility.

23. All cottonoid strips and patties and retractors are removed, and the wound is closed.

For cervical or thoracic disks, only the protruding fragment is removed and limited if any exploration of the interspace is performed. This is because attempts of adequate interspace exploration require retraction of the dural sac, which contains the spinal cord at these levels. Such retraction would result in cord injury and paralysis. For thoracic disk a costotransversectomy or transthoracic approach is used.

Laminectomy for spinal cord tumors

1. The fascial incision is made in the midline, both sides of the spinous processes are dissected out, and the paraspinous muscles are taken down bilaterally, one side at a time.

2. One or more double-bladed Scoville or Beckman-Adson self-retaining retractors are placed to maintain the bony exposure.

3. A midline laminectomy is performed, with the spinous processes excised with a Horsley bone cutter. Various rongeurs (such as Leksell, double-ction, Cloward) are used to remove the laminae after defining the edges with a curette. The Midas Rex drill may also be used. The bone edges are waxed.

4. The remaining flaval ligament is removed with scissors, scalpel, and Kerrison or Cloward rongeurs. Epidural fat is electrocoagulated and if necessary removed with dissecting scissors, so the dura mater is exposed fully.

5. A wide moist cottonoid is placed over the superficial soft tissues and muscle down to the bone bordering the exposed dura mater. This provides additional hemostasis.

6. The dura mater is elevated with a small hook and nicked with a no. 15 knife blade. A grooved director is inserted beneath the dura mater, and the dural incision is extended over it, using long forceps and fine scissors. Alternatively, the incision may be lengthened by pulling apart the two edges of the dural incision with bayonet forceps or by pushing at the ends of this incision with the edge of a dural elevator. Traction sutures of no. 4-0 silk or nylon on dura needles are placed in the dural edges, and the cord is exposed (Fig. 22-70).

7. The cord is explored for the pathologic area. Aspiration through a no. 22 needle on a plain-tipped syringe may be carried out. The tumor may be encountered extradurally or intradurally. Whenever possible, the tumor mass is dissected free and removed by suction, dissecting scissors, the cutting electrosurgical forceps, cottonoid, small (pituitary) scoops, curettes, pituitary rongeurs, or an ultrasonic aspirator. Intraoperative ultrasound may also be used to locate intraaxial tumors or cyst cavities. Bleeding is controlled with a moist cottonoid, hemostatic clips, gelatin gauze, and topical hemostatics. Bipolar coagulation is used around the nerves and spinal cord. The spinal subarachnoid space may be explored with a small rubber catheter to detect blockage.

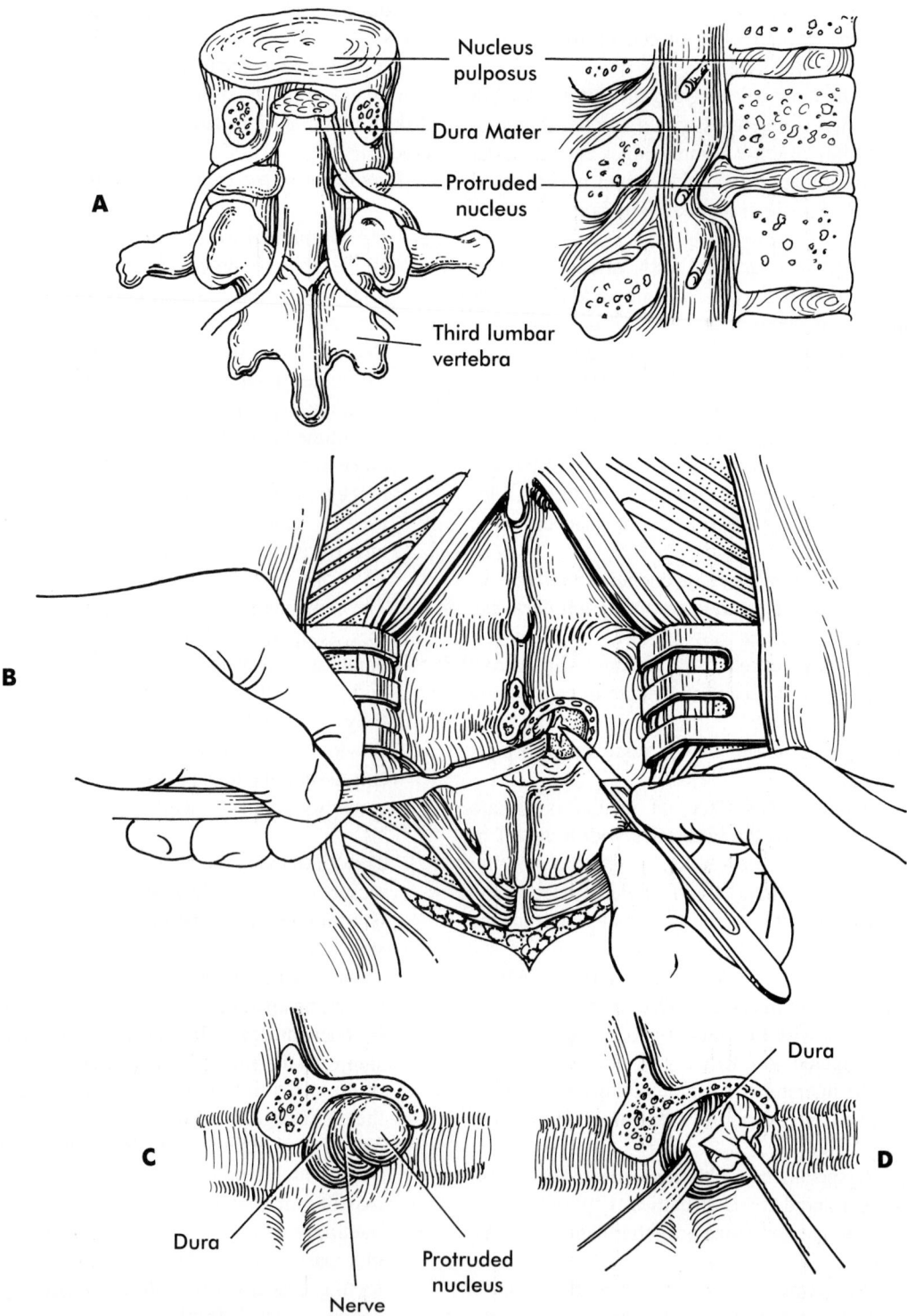

FIG. 22-69 **A,** Normal and herniated nucleus pulposus (disk). **B,** Window has been made in lamina, and ligament has been incised to expose underlying dura mater and nerve root. **C,** Relationship of dura mater, nerve root, and protruded nucleus pulposus (disk). **D,** Retraction of nerve root over dura mater and removal of disk.

From Carini, E., & Owens, G. (1974). *Neurological and neurosurgical nursing* (6th ed.). St. Louis: Mosby.

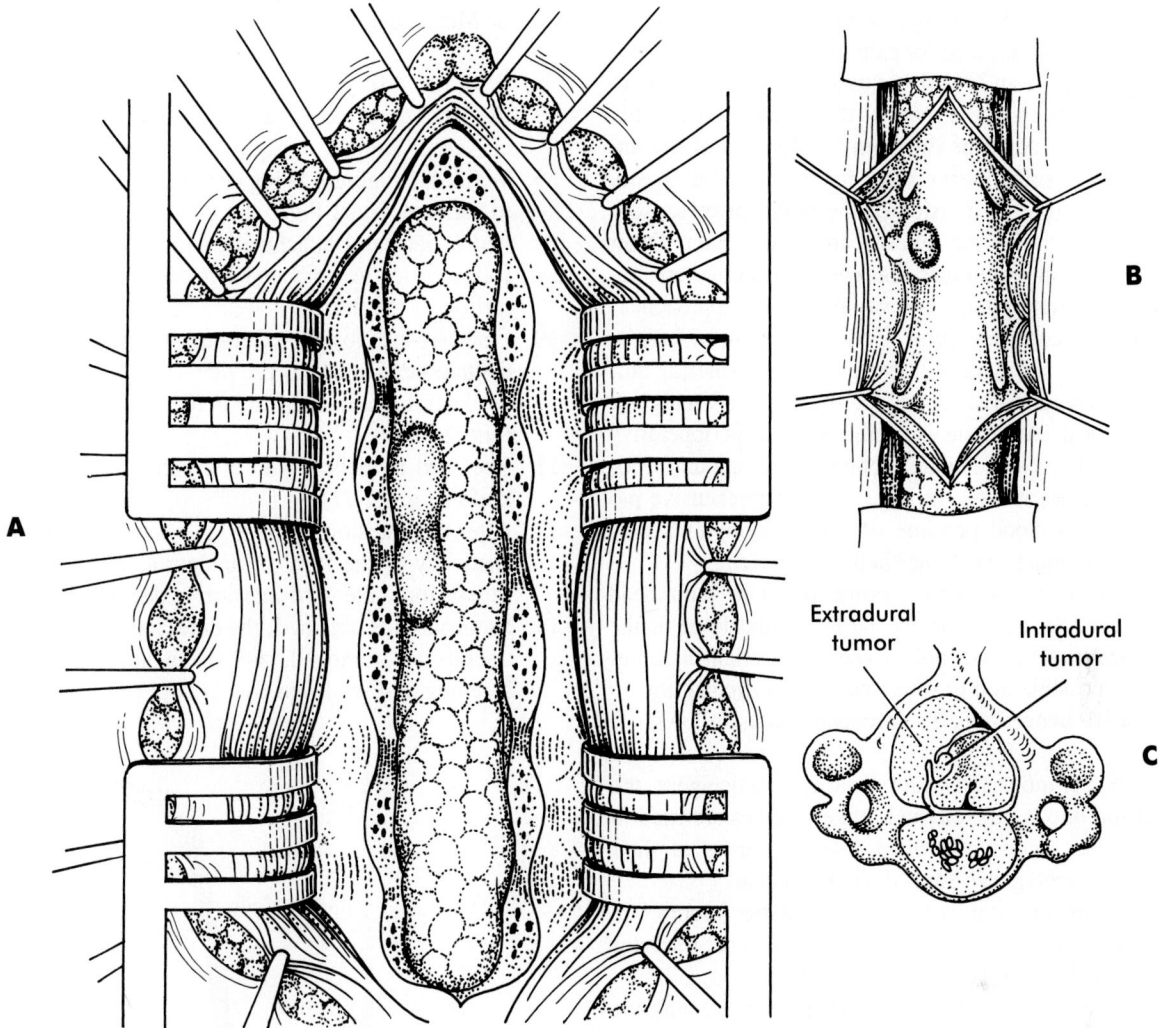

FIG. 22-70 **A,** Laminectomy completed: dura mater and tumor exposed. **B,** Dura mater incised and retracted, revealing pia arachnoid over spinal cord and part of tumor. **C,** Diagram of cross-section of tumor site and location of extradural and intradural pathologic areas.

From Carini, E., & Owens, G. (1974). *Neurological and neurosurgical nursing* (6th ed.). St. Louis: Mosby.

8. The wound is irrigated with normal saline or Ringer's solution, Asepto syringes, and suction.
9. Hemostasis is obtained; the dura mater is closed with a no. 4-0 or 5-0 silk, 4-0 black braided nylon, or 4-0 Polyglactin suture.
10. The incision is checked for further bleeding, and the paraspinous muscles are approximated with no. 0 Polyglactin synthetic absorbable suture or no. 2-0 silk. The remainder of the wound is closed.

In the case of extradural tumors, intradural exploration may be omitted. The operating microscope may be used, especially on intradural tumors and vascular anomalies. The laser also may be used and should be available, along with the intraoperative ultrasound and ultrasonic aspiration.

Laminectomy for meningocele. Malformations such as meningoceles are usually congenital. They are a threat to the life of a newborn infant because the defect may predispose to infection or spinal cord damage. Defects of the cord and spinal nerves are often associated with the condition. There also may be spina bifida, a congenital defect resulting from incomplete closure of the vertebral canal.

Operation for repair of meningocele is directed at preserving intact the neural elements involved and at closing the cutaneous, muscular, and dural defects.

For surgery on infants, small hemostats, retractors, and other instruments are provided. Large bone-cutting instruments may be omitted. The nerve stimulator may be needed.

Cervical cordotomy (Schwartz technique, thoracic cordotomy, rhizotomy)

Cervical cordotomy is division of the spinothalamic tract for the treatment of intractable pain. Pain management techniques, epidural administration of opiates, or percutaneous cordotomy may be initiated for pain management. High cervical cordotomy is an effective surgical procedure. Rhizotomy is interruption of the roots of the spinal nerves within the spinal canal. Anterior rhizotomy is division of the anterior or motor spinal nerve roots for the relief of spasm; posterior rhizotomy is division of the posterior or sensory spinal nerve roots for the relief of intractable pain. Other pain management techniques that can be effective are implantable morphine pumps and variable block approaches.

Procedural considerations. Cervical cordotomy may be performed with the patient under general anesthesia, but, to permit intraoperative testing of the level of analgesia achieved, local anesthesia is preferred. The perioperative nurse should keep an accurate account of the amount of local anesthetic agent used. In a very ill or apprehensive patient, a drop in blood pressure or cardiac symptoms may develop if too much local anesthetic is injected.

The patient is placed in a prone position, with head slightly flexed to a level below the horizontal level of the cervical spine. It is essential to keep the patient as comfortable as possible and to offer reassurance frequently.

Operative procedure. The procedure is as follows:

1. The skin is infiltrated with a local anesthetic agent, the incision line is marked, and longer needles are used to block the second and third cervical nerves at their points of emergence from the spinal canal.
2. A midline incision is used. Hemostatic forceps are placed to control bleeding, and the Weitlaner retractor is inserted for exposure.
3. Using the electrosurgical unit (cutting current) with the spatula blade, the surgeon separates the muscles from one side of the arches and laminae of the first and second cervical vertebrae. An angled periosteal elevator may be used for further dissection. A gauze sponge may be packed into the wound to enhance the dissection as well as to aid hemostasis.
4. A Scoville hemilaminectomy retractor with short hooks and longer blade is inserted between the midline structures and the reflected paraspinous muscles. The flexion of the head is increased when the retractor is inserted.
5. The Schwartz self-retaining retractor (modified Gelpi) is placed, with the multitoothed end in the occipital bone and the sharp point penetrating the spinous process of C2 to widen the interlaminar space between C1 and C2 vertebrae. (For additional exposure it may be necessary to remove some of the laminae with a Kerrison rongeur.)
6. Large, moist cottonoid strips are placed over the superficial tissues and muscle down to the bone bordering the exposed dura mater.
7. With the use of a dural hook, the dural incision is made with a no. 7 knife handle and a no. 15 blade. Vascular

or Metzenbaum scissors are used to lengthen the incision.

8. With no. 4-0, silk stay sutures on an ophthalmic needle, the dural edges are retracted and secured with curved or straight mosquito hemostats.
9. While suctioning is being performed on cottonoid strips to remove spinal fluid, the dentate ligament is identified at its dural attachment with bayonet forceps and followed to the cord and left attached to prevent distortion of the cord.
10. Fine bayonet forceps (Gerald) are used to elevate the dentate attachment to provide visualization of the anterolateral quadrant of the cord and the anterior nerve rootlets.
11. The cord is incised with a slightly curved cordotomy knife (Fig. 22-71).
12. After the incision is made, the patient is checked for adequacy of the level of analgesia. If the level is not satisfactory, the cord incision is deepened.
13. Hemostasis is obtained, the dural incision is closed, retractors are removed, and the wound is checked for bleeding and is closed.

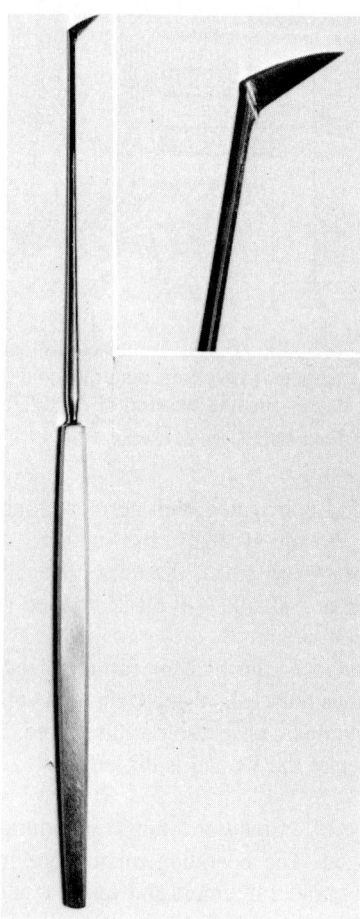

FIG. 22-71   Schwartz cordotomy knife.

Courtesy K. Cramer Lewis, Department of Illustrations, Washington University School of Medicine, St. Louis.

As technology improves, the laser is being utilized in performing this procedure. This procedure can also be done percutaneously in radiology.

For *bilateral cordotomy,* the muscles are separated from both sides of the arches and laminae of the vertebrae. A double-bladed Scoville retractor is used, and the Schwartz retractor (modified Gelpi) is placed according to the side of the cord being approached. The cordotomy is performed on one side and then on the other. With bilateral high cervical cordotomy, falls in blood pressure and respiratory difficulty may occur.

High thoracic cordotomy is performed unilaterally or bilaterally in a similar manner, but a hemilaminectomy or total laminectomy at two levels must usually be performed to gain adequate exposure. The lateral or prone position may be used.

Rhizotomy is performed through a similar exposure with the appropriate nerve roots dissected free of any large radicular vessels, held up with a nerve hook, crushed with a hemostatic forceps, and divided with fine-tipped scissors. A silver clip may be placed on the distal ends of the roots before division. This aids in hemostasis and permits subsequent radiologic visualization of the extent and precise level of the root section (Fig. 22-72).

Removal of anterior cervical disk with fusion (Cloward technique)

This procedure is done to relieve pain in the neck, shoulder, and arm caused by cervical spondylosis or a herniated disk. It entails removal of the disk and fusion of the vertebral bodies. Bone dowels for the fusion are obtained from the patient's iliac crest or from a bone bank.

Procedural considerations. The patient is placed in the supine position, with the head turned very slightly to the left and with the right hip elevated for exposure of the iliac crest (if the bone dowel is to be taken from the iliac crest). The basic minor dissecting set is used, plus the following instruments (Fig. 22-73).

2 Cloward self-retaining retractors, 1 large and 1 small, with assorted blades (with and without teeth)	2 Cloward hand retractors
4 Drill guards (various sizes), cervical drill, and dowel cutters	2 Cloward vertebral spreaders, 1 regular and 1 self-retaining
1 Cloward bone graft holder	1 Mallet
1 Cloward bone graft impactor, double-ended	2 Adson cerebellum retractors, angled
	3 Cloward rongeurs, 2, 3, and 5 mm
	Spinal fusion curettes, straight and angulated, nos. 0, 00, and 3-0

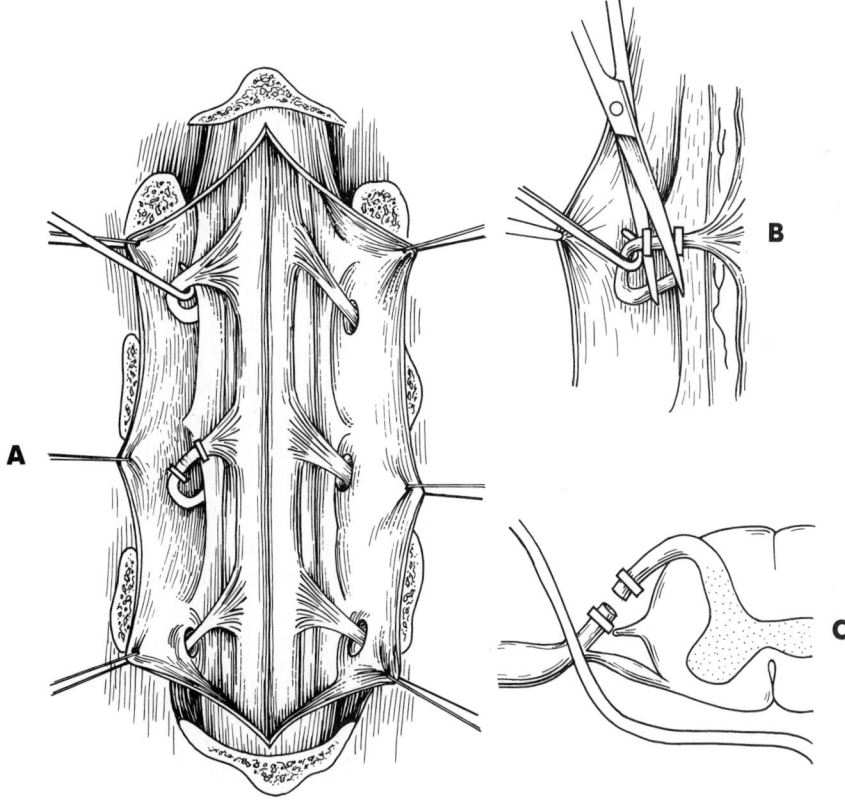

FIG. 22-72   Posterior rhizotomy after laminectomy. **A,** Spinal cord and roots exposed. **B,** Posterior root identified. **C,** Cross-section of spinal cord and divided posterior root.

From Carini, E., & Owens, G. (1974). *Neurological and neurosurgical nursing* (6th ed.). St. Louis: Mosby.

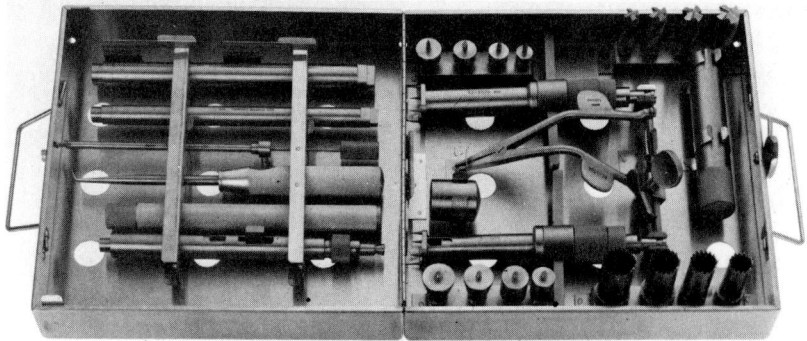

FIG. 22-73   Instruments for anterior cervical disk removal with fusion. *Left side,* Cloward dowel cutter shaft, dowel ejector, osteophyte elevator, depth gauge, guard guide (large, small). *Right side, bottom to top,* Dowel ejector pins, dowel cutter pins, cervical drill guards (small and large), drill guard cap, drill shaft, cervical drills, crossbar handle, dowel cutter shaft guard, vertebra spreader, and spanner wrench.
Courtesy Codman & Shurtleff, Inc., Randolph, Mass.

Operative procedure. The procedure is as follows:

1. A transverse skin incision is made on one side of the neck (usually the right) directly over the involved disk space; curved mosquito hemostats or Michel clips are placed on the skin edges for hemostasis.
2. A Weitlaner retractor is placed, and the platysma muscle is divided with Metzenbaum scissors and tissue forceps with teeth or with the electrosurgical cutting blade.
3. The medial edge of the sternocleidomastoid muscle is defined with the scissors by blunt and sharp dissection.
4. A vertical plane of dissection between the carotid sheath laterally and the trachea and esophagus medially is created by blunt finger dissection. This plane is held open with Cloward hand retractors, Meyerding finger retractors, or U.S. Army retractors.
5. The anterior surface of the spine is identified, and the long muscles of the neck are peeled off the anterior surface of the spine with periosteal elevators. Bleeders are coagulated with a dural elevator or bayonet forceps.
6. A 20-gauge spinal needle is inserted a short distance into the disk space, and a lateral x-ray film is taken to determine the level of the exposure. At this time a C-arm may be brought in to give instantaneous localization of the desired level.
7. While x-ray films are being developed, the neck incision is covered, an incision is made over the iliac crest, and straight hemostats are applied and retracted.
8. Soft tissue is dissected until the crest is reached, using Mayo scissors, tissue forceps, electrosurgical cutting blade, and Richardson retractors for exposure.
9. A Hudson brace with the Cloward Dowel cutter is used to remove the bone graft. (Care must be exercised to use dowel cutter, Cloward guide, and cervical drill guards matched for size.) The dowel should have cortex at both ends. The dowel hole is inspected and

waxed if needed. The incision is packed with gauze sponges and covered.
10. The Cloward self-retaining retractors (two long and two short blades) are inserted into the neck incision. The right blade should be slightly longer than the left. Care is used to protect the carotid artery and the esophagus. A combination of sharp and dull blades is used to acquire the best retraction. If a toothed blade is used, the teeth are carefully hooked beneath the long muscle of the neck.
11. A no. 15 or 11 blade on a no. 7 knife handle is used to cut into the disk space; a fine pituitary rongeur is used to remove the disk material, which is saved and weighed as a specimen. A vertebral spreader is inserted into the vertebral space to widen the area, and further disk material is removed with the rongeur or small curettes (angled or straight, nos. 0 to 4-0) until the entire surface of both vertebrae are clean. A Surgairtome with small burr may also be used.
12. The Cloward bone guide is inserted into the disk space to measure its depth.
13. After the drill guard is adjusted so the drill can protrude no farther than the measured depth of the interspace, the cervical drill guard is inserted around the disk space, with the aid of a mallet, until the points catch the vertebral bodies above and below the interspace.
14. After the guard is in place, the vertebral spreader is removed or spread to a more limited degree.
15. The Cloward drill on a Hudson brace is inserted into the guard, and the hole is drilled. (The bone dust on the drill point is inspected and saved in a medicine glass.) Cottonoid strips or topical hemostatics are used for active bleeders. Bone wax should not be used on the walls of the disk hole. Thrombin-soaked cottonoid pledgets may help control bleeding.

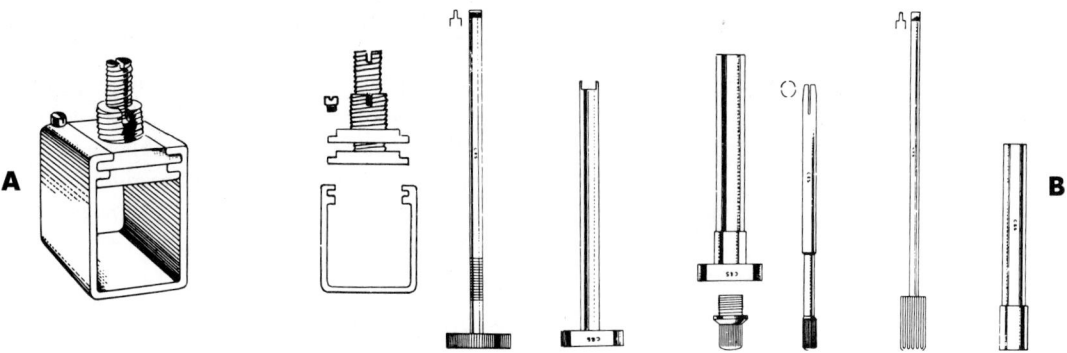

FIG. 22-74 **A,** Selverstone carotid artery clamp. **B,** Selverstone carotid artery clamp accessories.
Courtesy Codman & Shurtleff, Inc., Randolph, Mass.

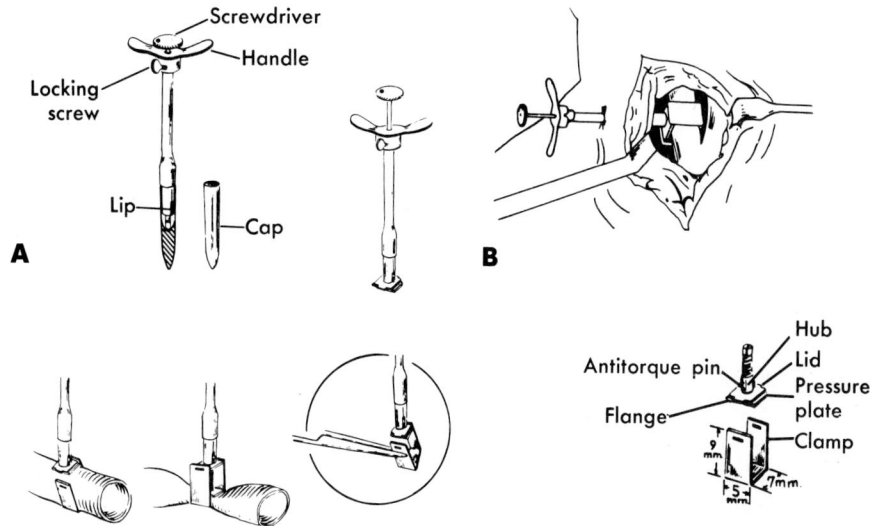

FIG. 22-75 Crutchfield carotid artery clamp. **A,** Control assembly. **B,** Clamp assembly.
Courtesy Codman & Shurtleff, Inc., Randolph, Mass.

16. The bottom of the hole is checked for further disk or cartilaginous material, which is removed. The guide may be removed and replaced, and drilling may be done several times until the desired depth is reached. The drill and guide are then removed.

17. Further bone is removed by use of the Cloward cervical punch or curettes until complete anterior decompression of the nerve root or dural sac is obtained. Nerve hooks may be used here for demonstration of adequate dissection. The Air Drill 100 or Midas Rex may also be used.

18. The depth of the hole is measured and compared with the dowel. The dowel may be trimmed with a drill, rongeur, or rasp. The shaped dowel attached to the impactor is inserted into the hole and tapped into place. The double-edged impactor is used to drive the dowel in deeper if necessary. The spreader is removed, and bone dust may be applied.

19. Hemostasis is obtained and the wound irrigated; the vertebral spreader and retractors are removed, and both incisions are closed.

Other instrumentation designs and techniques have been developed for the anterior approach to cervical disk disease. The perioperative nurse needs to be aware of these to accommodate the neurosurgeon's preference.

CAROTID SURGERY OF THE NECK
Carotid artery ligation

Carotid artery ligation is performed to occlude the internal carotid artery. It may be done to control anticipated hemorrhage during intracranial surgery for vascular anomalies. A permanent occlusion may be necessary for the control of intracranial hemorrhage or small, repeated strokes from an intracranial lesion.

Procedural considerations. Special clamps, such as the Selverstone (Fig. 22-74), Selibi, and Crutchfield carotid artery clamps (Fig. 22-75) are available for gradual occlusion of the artery. Occlusion may protect the patient from debilitating or fatal intracranial hemorrhage from aneurysm and may be used to treat carotid-cavernous fistula. Only a basic minor instrument set is used.

Operative procedure. The procedure is as follows:

1. The skin is incised, and a Weitlaner retractor is inserted for exposure.
2. The carotid artery is freed. A small Penrose tubing, umbilical tape, or vessel loop is passed around the vessel for retraction.
3a. *For temporary control* of the carotid artery (during procedures for very large aneurysms or arteriovenous anomalies): an umbilical tape is passed around the vessel and fixed, using the Roper-Rumel tourniquet in such a manner that occlusion can be accomplished immediately if necessary.
3b. *For permanent occlusion:* two heavy silk ligatures are used, and the artery may be divided between ligatures. Transfixing suture ligatures may be used as well if the artery is divided.
3c. *For gradual occlusion:*
   a. A carotid clamp, such as the Selverstone, Selibi, or Crutchfield, is placed in position around the artery.
   b. A small stab wound is made adjacent to the incision.
   c. The control assembly with cap is passed through the stab wound. By loosening the locking screw and pressing down on the screwdriver, the operator can remove the cap.
   d. The control assembly is snapped on the lid of the clamp, and with a hemostatic forceps holding the clamp, each flange is gently forced into position.
   e. Using the dot on the screwdriver as an indicator, the number of turns for complete occlusion is noted. The clamp is then unscrewed a measured number of turns, and the screwdriver is locked. The control assembly is capped and left in place, protruding through the stab wound.
4. The incision is closed, and a dressing is applied.

After the procedure the carotid artery clamp accessories are packaged and sterilized. They are kept at the patient's bedside for daily adjustments and returned to the operating room or central service for resterilization after each use. They must be returned to the patient's bedside as soon as possible to be available if the patient cannot tolerate the occlusion and the clamp must be opened immediately.

Carotid surgery for carotid-cavernous fistula

Ligation of the common carotid artery is one mode of surgical treatment for a carotid-cavernous fistula. Another form of surgical treatment is to embolize the fistula. In either case, internal carotid ligation is usually done after satisfactory placement of the embolus. In some cases a frontotemporal craniotomy is also performed, and the internal carotid artery clipped intracranially as well. Interventional

radiology can also perform super selective anterior balloon occlusions.

Endarterectomy is another procedure involving the cerebral circulation, although not directly involving the brain and cranial nerves (see Chapter 25). Endarterectomy consists of exposing the carotid artery in the neck at the site of occlusion, incising the vessel, and removing the associated sclerotic tissue. Electroencephalographic (EEG) or evoked response monitoring may be used intraoperatively.

PERIPHERAL NERVE SURGERY
Sympathectomy

Sympathectomy is excision of a portion of the sympathetic division of the autonomic nervous system. Most sympathectomies are performed on the paravertebral chain and are named for the region resected, for example, cervical, thoracolumbar, and lumbar. The periarterial sympathectomy, vagotomy, and presacral neurectomy are other procedures that are occasionally performed on the autonomic system.

The principal diseases treated by sympathectomy are vascular disorders of the extremities and intractable pain from certain nerve injuries, chronic abdominal conditions, and hyperhidrosis.

Procedural considerations. The position of the patient depends on the region to be resected. Basic dissecting instruments and the microscope are used. For *retropleural and transthoracic approaches,* rib resecting instruments are added (Fig. 22-76). For *thoracic and lumbar approaches,* the following are added:

2 Volkman rake retractors, large, eight-pronged, blunt	2 Richardson retractors, large
3 Malleable copper retractors	2 Weinberg retractors, large
2 Deaver retractors	2 Harrington retractors
	2 Beckman retractors

For the *thoracic approach,* Beckman or Scoville laminectomy retractors are added. For the *abdominal approach,* Balfour self-retaining retractors are added.

Cervicothoracic sympathectomy (dorsal)

Dorsal sympathectomy entails removal of the cervicothoracic chain, often from the fourth cervical to the third thoracic ganglion. Sympathetic denervation of the upper extremities and heart may be accomplished by cervicothoracic sympathectomy. The vasospastic phenomenon of Raynaud's disease is relieved by this procedure. It also may be beneficial in relieving intractable angina pectoris.

Procedural considerations. For the anterior approach, both the laminectomy set and rib instruments are used, plus deep retractors and a nerve stimulator. The setup for the posterior approach is as for the anterior approach, plus rib-resecting instruments, periosteal elevators, small rib retractors, a firm rubber pad, and OR bed attachments for the posterolateral position.

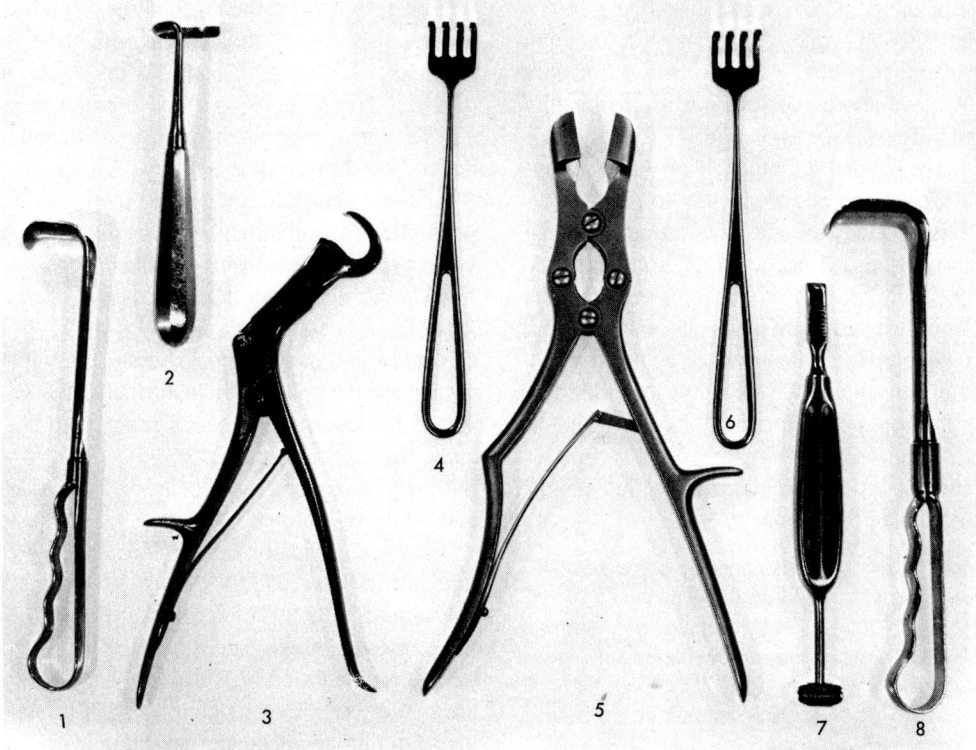

FIG. 22-76   Instruments for rib resection. *1,* Richardson retractor; *2,* Doyen rib raspatory; *3,* Stille rib shears; *4,* blunt rake retractors; *5,* Sauerbruch rib rongeur; *6,* blunt rake retractor; *7,* Alexander costal periosteotome; *8,* Richardson retractor.

Operative procedure
Anterior approach

1. The patient is placed in a supine position with the head rotated to the opposite side, as in mastoidectomy (see Chapter 18). General endotracheal anesthesia is necessary because there is a possibility of puncturing the pleura.
2. A transverse incision is made one fingerbreadth above the clavicle, the clavicular head of the sternocleidomastoid muscle is severed, and the deep cervical fascia is divided.
3. The phrenic nerve and the jugular vein are protected, and the anterior scalene muscle is divided to expose and isolate the underlying subclavian artery. The thyroid axis, one of its branches, is ligated and divided.
4. The stellate ganglion, deep against the vertebral body, is brought into view and lifted on a nerve hook. The sympathetic chain is traced upward to the middle cervical ganglion and divided. Deep dissection behind the pleura exposes the upper thoracic ganglia, which are removed to below the third thoracic ganglion. Clips may be placed on the sympathetic nerves before their division.
5. The wound is closed according to the surgeon's preference.

Posterior approach

1. The patient is placed in the lateral position, and a paravertebral incision is centered over the third rib. The trapezius muscle is divided, and the rhomboid is split in line with its fibers. The third and fourth ribs are isolated extrapleurally, and the posterior 4 to 5 cm is resected. The transverse processes may be removed to provide better exposure.
2. The sympathetic trunk, which lies on the anterolateral aspect of the vertebral body, is reached by carefully reflecting the pleura. The trunk is picked up on a nerve hook, traced up and down, and removed, usually from the stellate ganglion to the fourth thoracic ganglion. Clips may be applied to the nerve before severing the fibers.
3. A firm rubber tube may be left in the wound during closure. Suctioning apparatus is applied to this tube as the last deep fascial suture is drawn tight; all air is aspirated, and the tube is quickly withdrawn.
4. The subcutaneous tissue and skin edges are closed.

Nerve repairs

Peripheral nerve injuries are the most common indication for this surgery. Nerve tumors are rare in comparison. During wartime, injuries of nerves assume particular importance because of their frequency and disabling results.

When the continuity of a nerve is destroyed, function distal to the site of injury is lost. Recovery will occur only if regeneration of nerve axons take place from the healthy proximal segments. These axons must grow down the axis cylinders of the nerve beyond the injury if they are to reinnervate their end organs and allow function to return.

When a nerve is divided, the cut ends retract, become scarred, and form neuromas. Regenerating axons from the proximal segment cannot bridge such a gap or penetrate the scar tissue. An unobstructed path down the axis cylinder must be made available if nerves are ever again to move muscles or transmit sensation. All procedures are directed toward obtaining the best possible conditions for regeneration.

Procedural considerations. A basic dissecting instrument set is used, plus the following:

Nerve stimulator
Jeweler's nerve forceps
Microsutures
Loupes
Operating microscope
Intraoperative EMG recorder
Microforceps
Microscissors

Microneedle holders
Microdissectors
Tongue blades
Sterile double-edged razor blades (can be ethylene oxide sterilized in their paper wrappers)

For lesser procedures such as spinal-accessory-facial anastomosis in the neck, division of the volar carpal ligament for median nerve compression at the wrist, or repair of a small digital nerve, suitable modification may be made.

The positioning, skin prep, and draping of the patient depend on the site of the injury. A large area is prepped.

General anesthesia is usually preferred, with the patient positioned for maximum accessibility to the injured nerve. Exposure must be adequate because considerable mobilization of the nerve is often necessary. A dry field may be achieved by using a tourniquet on the involved extremity.

Operative procedure. The site of injury is explored, with careful attention to hemostasis. Nerve ends are dissected from surrounding scar tissue, and neuromas are excised. Moist umbilical tapes, vessel loops, or Penrose tubing may be passed about the nerve to handle it more easily and with less trauma.

The nerve repair (anastomosis) is made with multiple fine sutures placed only through the nerve sheath or epineurium (Fig. 22-77). Tension at the suture line is eliminated by maneuvers such as freeing up a long length of nerve on either side of the point of injury, transposition of the nerve to shorten its course, appropriate positioning of the extremity with plaster splinting during the postoperative period, and, rarely, use of a nerve graft. Some sur-

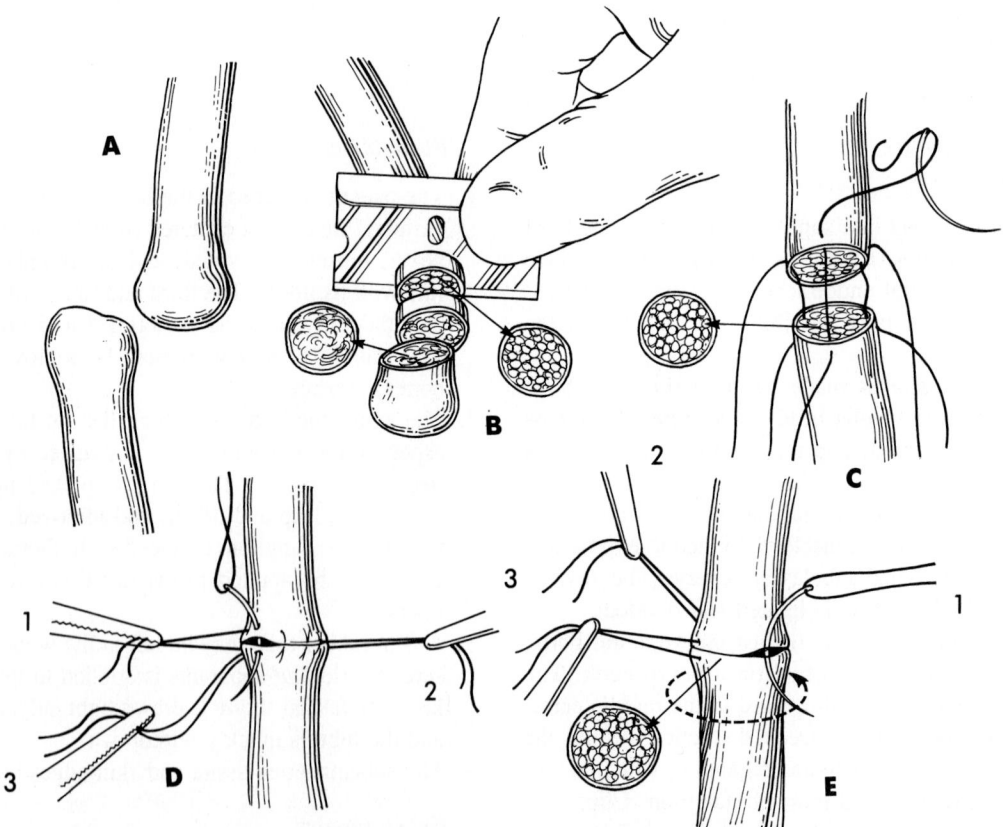

FIG. 22-77   Nerve repair. **A,** Divided nerve with neuroma. **B,** Serial resection of neuroma to healthy nerve fibers. **C,** Placement of sutures in epineurium. **D** and **E,** Approximation and tying of sutures.

From Sachs, E. (1949). *Diagnosis and treatment of brain tumors and care of the neurosurgical patient* (2nd ed.). St. Louis: Mosby.

geons apply a cuff of inert material such as silicone about the anastomosis.

Hypoglossal facial nerve anastomosis

Hypoglossal facial nerve anastomosis is performed to restore function to an injured facial nerve. With certain lesions in the posterior fossa and during some procedures on the posterior fossa, the facial nerve may be damaged.

Operative procedure. An incision is made over the anterior edge of the sternocleidomastoid muscle, extending from the mastoid process downward for a distance of approximately 11 to 12 cm. The fascia and muscles are divided, and further dissection is carried out until the hypoglossal nerve is exposed and divided distally. The facial nerve is exposed and divided close to its exit from the stylomastoid foramen deep to the front of the mastoid process. The proximal end of the hypoglossal nerve is anastomosed to the distal end of the facial nerve with fine arterial or nerve sutures, and the wound is closed.

Occasionally a surgeon uses the accessory or even the phrenic nerve instead of the hypoglossal. Microsurgical techniques and instruments are used.

Carpal tunnel syndrome

Carpal tunnel syndrome is a condition of the hand in which the median nerve is compressed by the transverse carpal ligament or by displacement of the lunate bone or a volar carpal ganglion. Decompression of the nerve is done by removing part of the roof of the fibrous sheath of the ligament or the offending bone or ganglion. Another excellent option for decompression is the scoping procedure, which is gaining popularity in some areas of the country.

Procedural considerations. The patient is placed in the supine position with the operative arm extended on a hand table or armboard. Local, regional, or general anesthesia may be used.

Operative procedure. The procedure is as follows:

1. A longitudinal skin incision is made in the thenar palm crease. This runs perpendicular to and stops at the most distal transverse skin crease in the wrist. This incision generally suffices but may be extended into an L or a T.
2. A Weitlaner, mastoid, or self-retaining spring-action retractor is placed.
3. The fibers of the carpal ligament are divided transversely in blunt fashion at the most proximal point of exposure. A hemostat is introduced through this opening in the ligament, pointed distally, and spread. This protects the underlying median nerve. The ligament is divided between the jaws of the hemostat with Mayo or plastic Metzenbaum scissors.
4. The incision is closed with fine sutures, and a bulky dressing is applied, with the fingers visible.

Ulnar nerve transposition at the elbow

Because of traumatic or anatomic problems, the ulnar nerve may be predisposed to irritation resulting in chronic discomfort. In such instances the position of the nerve can be changed to provide protection and comfort.

Procedural considerations. The patient is placed in the supine position. The arm may be supported in a functional position, with Webril and elastic bandages to attach it to the anesthesia screen, or it may be left free for the surgeon to manipulate during the procedure. The inner, posterior aspect of the upper and lower arm must be exposed for the operation.

Operative procedure. A long incision is made, and the nerve is dissected free from the surrounding soft tissues with Metzenbaum scissors and hemostatic forceps. Moist umbilical tapes, vessel loops, or Penrose tubing is passed around the freed segment of the nerve to aid in handling it for further dissection until a satisfactory length of nerve has been freed from above to below the elbow. The muscle and fascia entered by the nerve at each end of the field may be slit with scissors to prevent tethering and kinking at these points after the nerve has been transposed. A fascial flap overlying the medial epicondyle of the humerus is cut and elevated, and the nerve is transposed beneath it. The fascia is then loosely reapproximated to the fascial edge remaining on the epicondyle with no. 3-0 silk or no. 2-0 Polyglactin synthetic absorbable suture. The wound is closed in layers.

An alternative procedure, medial epicondylectomy is sometimes performed. In this case the nerve is not dissected out, but the medial epicondyle of the humerus is removed with a rongeur and the residual bone is waxed. The fascia and muscle tending to tether or kink the nerve, particularly distally, may be slit with scissors, as in the transposition procedure.

BIBLIOGRAPHY

Barker, E. (1994). *Neuroscience nursing.* St. Louis: Mosby.

Barraquer J. (1980). The history of the microscope in ocular surgery. *Journal of Microsurgery 1,* 288.

Bradley, W., & Crowell, R. (1993). *Yearbook of neurology and neurosurgery.* St. Louis: Mosby.

Carpenter, M.B. (1983). *Human neuroanatomy* (7th ed.). Baltimore: Williams & Wilkins.

Cottrell, J., & Turndorf, H. (1986). *Anesthesia and neurosurgery* (2nd ed.). St. Louis: Mosby.

Eliasson, S.G., et al. (1984). *Neurological pathophysiology* (2nd ed.). New York: Oxford University Press.

Fode, N.C. (1990). Carotid endarterectomy: Nursing care and controversies. *Journal of Neuroscience Nursing, (22)*1, 25.

Guyton, A.C. (1981). *Basic human neurophysiology* (3rd ed.). Philadelphia: W.B. Saunders.

Head, J.M. (1990). Multilevel spine fractures. *Journal of Neuroscience Nursing, (22)*6.

Hickey, J. (1986). *The clinical practice of neurological and neurosurgical nursing* (2nd ed.). Philadelphia: J.B. Lippincott.

Kershner, D.D., & Claussen, J.A. (1986). Craniofacial reconstruction. *AORN Journal 44,* 554.

Lenzi, G.L., & Pantano, P. (1984). Symposium on neuroimaging. In *Neurologic Clinics.* Philadelphia: W.B. Saunders.

Long, D.M. (1992). Current therapy in neurological surgery (3rd ed.). St. Louis: Mosby.

Manwaring, K., & Crone, K. (1992). *Neuroendoscopy* (Vol. 1). New York: Mary Ann Liebert Co.

Mitchell, S., & Yates, R. (1985). Extracranial-intracranial bypass surgery. *Journal of Neurosurgery Nursing, 17,* 5.

Netter, F.H. (1983). *Nervous system.* New York: Ciba Pharmaceutical.

Nolte, J. (1993). *The human brain: An introduction to its functional anatomy* (3rd ed.). St. Louis: Mosby.

Nucleotome surgical protocol. (1987). San Leandro, CA: Surgical Dynamics.

Pincus, J.H., & Tucker, G.J. (1985). *Behavioral neurology* (2nd ed.). New York: Oxford University Press.

Poletti, C., & Ojemann, R. (1985). *Stereo atlas of operative microneurosurgery.* St. Louis: Mosby.

Rand, R. (1985). *Microneurosurgery* (3rd ed.). St. Louis: Mosby.

Ricci, M. (1984). Core curriculum for neuroscience nursing (Vols. I & II). Park Ridge, IL: American Association of Neuroscience Nurses.

Scheithauer, B.W., et al. (1986). Pathology of invasive pituitary tumors with special reference to functional classification. *Journal of Neurosurgery, 65,* 733.

Shillito, J., & Matson, D.D. (1982). An atlas of pediatric neurosurgical operations. Philadelphia: W.B. Saunders.

Smith-Rooker, J.L., Garrett, A., & Hodges, L.C. (1993). Case management of the patient with pituitary tumor. *MEDSURG Nursing, 2*(4), 265-274.

Spera-Ahearn, M. (1990). Cerebral angioplasty: A new treatment for vasospasm secondary to subarachnoid hemorrhage. *Journal of Neuroscience Nursing, 22,* 5.

Sugita, K. (1985). *Microneurosurgical atlas.* New York: Springer-Verlag.

Sundt, T. (Ed). (1989). *Journal of Neurosurgery 71*(4).

Thibodeau, G.A., and Patton, K.T. (1994). *Anthony's textbook of anatomy and physiology* (4th ed.). 1, St. Louis: Mosby.

Vaiden, R., & White, W. (1987). Arteriovenous malformation of the brain. *AORN Journal, 46*(1).

Vogt, G., Miller, M., & Esluer, M. (1985). *Mosby's manual of neurological care.* St. Louis: Mosby.

White, A., Rothman, R., & Ray, C. (1987). *Lumbar spine surgery.* St. Louis: Mosby.

Willis, D., & Harbit, M.D. (1990). Transcatheter arterial embolization of cerebral arteriovenous malformations. *Journal of Neuroscience Nursing, 22*(5).

Wilson, C.B. (1984). A decade of pituitary microsurgery: The Herbert Olivecrona lecture. *Journal of Neurosurgery, 61,* 814.

23

PLASTIC AND RECONSTRUCTIVE SURGERY

KATHERINE J. DONAHOE

Patients who experience plastic and reconstructive surgery have the dual concern of restoration of a normal appearance as well as the desire to achieve cosmetic improvement, hence the term *esthetic surgery*. The field of plastic and reconstructive surgery has experienced rapid advancement in recent years. Patients who require emergency surgery as well as those undergoing elective cosmetic procedures have benefited from innovative and unique technologies and techniques. Experimental reconstructive techniques continue to be developed to afford potential new reconstructive options. Perioperative nurses have the opportunity to become partners in this pioneering field of plastic and reconstructive surgery as it continues to expand.

The word *plastic* is derived from the Greek *plastikos*, which means to mold, form, or contour. Plastic surgery deals with the healing, reconstruction, restoration of function, and correction of disfigurement or scarring resulting from trauma or acquired or congenital defects. Plastic and reconstructive surgery has the goal of restoring normal function and appearance and thus contributing to the patient's body image, self-esteem, and quality of life. Psychosocial integrity is often interwoven with the person's perception of his or her physical appearance. It has been suggested that cosmetic surgery improves body image as well as self-esteem, which is important to physical health. The effects of aging, cosmetically displeasing to some people, may seriously affect their self-images; feelings of unattractiveness may diminish self-esteem and contribute to a negative body image. The perioperative nurse caring for the patient undergoing cosmetic plastic surgery and reconstruction needs to possess creativity, curiosity, insight, and an understanding of the human psyche. Because of its relationship to psychosocial integrity, plastic surgery has been called the surgery of the psyche.

Plastic and reconstructive surgery is not limited either to a single anatomic or biologic system or to a single operative technique. Rather, it relies on the basic techniques of surgery and a view of the patient as a whole biopsycho-social being. Only the anatomy of the hand is discussed in detail in this chapter (see the hand surgery section). Other anatomic relationships are described elsewhere in this book.

A wide variety of operations are standard parts of plastic and reconstructive surgery. The advancement of microsurgical techniques has expanded the repertoire of the surgeon to include sophisticated procedures in replantation of limbs and digits, microvascular free flaps, and the like to restore and retain functional use of esthetic configuration. Breast augmentation, reconstruction, and reduction are included in this chapter. Tissue expanders are discussed with breast reconstruction, although they may be used in other areas of reconstruction. Recession and advancement of the mandible and maxilla and the treatment of hypertelorism and Crouzon's syndrome are included to demonstrate the perioperative nursing challenge of collaborating with a multidisciplinary health care team. The esthetic problems, varieties of congenital and acquired defects, diversity of operative techniques, and the psychologic responses of patients offer unique learning experiences and challenges for providing perioperative nursing care.

PERIOPERATIVE NURSING CONSIDERATIONS

The nursing process is a deliberate, systematic method of individualizing nursing care. Through the nursing process the perioperative nurse is able to focus on unique responses of the patient to the planned surgical intervention. Each step of the nursing process is sequential in that the steps that follow it depend on information gathered and conclusions reached in each successive step. It is an ongoing, dynamic process responsive to both the individual patient and changes within that patient's status.

ASSESSMENT

During assessment the perioperative nurse gathers and analyzes data and information that lead to the identification of actual or high risk health problems or nursing diagnoses. The emphasis of this data collection is on preoperative, intraoperative, and postoperative events. In general, the perioperative nurse is concerned with the patient's ability to communicate, religious or cultural preferences, current health problems, risk factors, knowledge level, mobility limitations, skin integrity, sensory/perceptual status, emotional status, and overall physical condition (Seifert and Rothrock, 1989). Preoperative and postoperative visits by the perioperative nurse provide a sound basis for better understanding the patient, assessing his or her problems, and planning care that meets individual needs. Preoperative education helps to alleviate much of the fear and anxiety usually associated with a surgical intervention. Patients undergoing reconstructive plastic surgery often are experiencing a disturbance in their body image. The procedure may be elective or urgent as a result of trauma. The perioperative nurse must assess the patient for both physical and psychologic impacts from reconstructive and aesthetic surgery and incorporate patient findings into a plan of care.

NURSING DIAGNOSIS

Nursing diagnoses that relate to the patient undergoing plastic and reconstructive surgery might include the following:

- Body image disturbance
- Anxiety related to surgical intervention or outcome
- Knowledge deficit related to perioperative events
- High risk for injury related to surgical positioning
- High risk for altered tissue perfusion related to surgical intervention

OUTCOME IDENTIFICATION

Nursing diagnoses lead to the formulation of desired or expected patient outcomes. These are desirable and measurable patient states, including biologic or physiologic states, psychologic, cultural, and spiritual aspects, and the knowledge or skills related to these states. As such, the patient outcome indicates progress toward or resolution of the nursing diagnosis (McFarland and McFarlane, 1993). For the selected nursing diagnoses, the outcomes might be stated as:

- The patient will acknowledge feelings about altered structure/function.
- The patient's anxiety will be reduced.
- The patient will verbalize an understanding of the sequence of perioperative events.
- The patient will be free from injury related to the surgical position.
- The patient's tissue perfusion will be maintained and/or restored.

PLANNING

Once nursing diagnoses and desired outcomes are identified, the plan of care is designed for the specific patient.

Planning involves setting priorities, identifying nursing interventions, and documenting the nursing care plan. Perioperative nurses often begin the early stages of planning as they are admitting the patient to the surgical suite. While assessing the patient, the nurse may also be planning possible nursing interventions for identified patient problems. A Sample Care Plan for the patient undergoing plastic and reconstructive surgery might be as shown on pp. 937-938.

IMPLEMENTATION

The planning and implementation phases of perioperative patient care are closely interrelated. Implementing a plan of care in the operating room involves gathering required patient care items, providing antimicrobial skin antisepsis, creating and maintaining a sterile field, initiating counts of surgical items, properly disposing of surgical specimens, classifying the patient's wound, dispensing medications, monitoring the patient, and collaborating with other members of the health care team to ensure a safe, efficient environment and outcome for the patient.

Preoperative skin preparation

Most surgical interventions require that the operative site and adjacent areas be cleansed before surgery. This treatment is prescribed by the physician and often carried out by the patient. Special attention is given to the fingernails for patients undergoing hand surgery; to hair for surgery of the head, face, or neck, and to oral hygiene for surgery in or near the mouth. The perioperative nurse should verify with the patient that the prescribed regimens have been carried out. The operative site should be inspected for any rashes, bruises, or other skin conditions. Shaving is avoided, if possible, as it creates an access for the entry of bacteria into the operative site. The eyebrows and eyelashes, in particular, are left intact to preserve facial appearance and expression. Either a povidone-iodine solution, an iodine-alcohol mixture, chlorhexidine, or Septisol may be selected for antimicrobial skin preparation. The use of chlorhexidine should be avoided around the ears and eyes; it has been reported to cause increased intraocular pressure, resulting in blindness.

Positioning and draping

The OR bed must be positioned so that remaining space in the room can comfortably accommodate anesthetic equipment, members of the surgical team, instrument tables, and any adjunct equipment (hand table, drills, microscope, laser) to be used. The patient is carefully positioned on the OR bed so that all operative sites may be appropriately exposed and the airway is easily observable and accessible.

Correct draping procedures depend on the location of the operative site or sites. Disposable drapes (see Chapter 3) are often used because of their barrier qualities, ease of handling and storage, and versatility in adapting to a variety of plastic surgery procedures. However, choosing single-

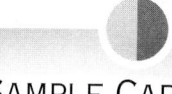

SAMPLE CARE PLAN

NURSING DIAGNOSIS: Body image disturbance
OUTCOME: The patient will acknowledge feelings about altered structure/function.
INTERVENTIONS:

Assist patient to identify and express feelings and perception of physical deformity.

Provide environment (privacy, supportive listening) conducive to expression of feelings.

Help patient identify expectations regarding surgical correction and anticipated changes in body structure/function.

Determine whether expectations are realistic; clarify unrealistic expectations or misconceptions.

Convey sense of respect for abilities/strengths in coping with problems/concerns.

Refer the patient to other health professionals (clergy, social worker, psychiatric liaison) as appropriate.

NURSING DIAGNOSIS: Anxiety related to surgical intervention, outcome
OUTCOME: The patient's anxiety will be reduced.
INTERVENTIONS:

Broadly classify the patient's anxiety (mild, moderate, severe).

Introduce self and other members of the surgical team.

Determine the patient's normal coping patterns.

Communicate with the patient in a calm, unhurried, confident manner.

Encourage the patient to ventilate feelings and concerns.

Reduce distracting stimuli in the perioperative environment.

If the patient is awake, provide reassurance and information about the progress of the surgery.

Provide comfort measures (for example, warm blankets, soft music that the patient prefers).

Use touch as appropriate (for example, softly stroke hand).

Encourage and assist the patient to use personally effective coping strategies (for example, meditation, guided imagery, relaxation).

NURSING DIAGNOSIS: Knowledge deficit related to perioperative events
OUTCOME: The patient will verbalize an understanding of the sequence of perioperative events.
INTERVENTIONS:

Verify surgical consent with operating room schedule and patient's statement of planned surgery.

Solicit the patient's questions; answer or refer questions as appropriate.

Explain the sequence of perioperative events and their purpose, as appropriate (such as holding area, operating room attire, insertion of lines and attachment of monitoring devices, type of anesthesia, postoperative recovery unit and protocols).

Provide sensory (what the patient will hear and feel) as well as factual information.

Whenever possible, provide printed material to reinforce patient education (preoperative routines, explanations of surgical intervention, discharge instructions).

NURSING DIAGNOSIS: High risk for injury related to surgical positioning
OUTCOME: The patient will be free from injury related to the surgical position.
INTERVENTIONS:

Determine whether the patient has any mobility limitations; adapt surgical position accordingly.

When possible, have patient assume surgical position prior to induction of general anesthesia; note areas of discomfort and adapt position accordingly.

Secure the patient to the OR bed; reapply restraints following positional change.

Note the patient's nutritional status, body height and weight, skin integrity, and adequacy of protective tissue at dependent pressure sites.

Apply protective padding to OR bed, dependent pressure sites, and vulnerable neurovascular bundles.

Prevent the compression of body parts against one another (such as crossed legs), the hard surface of the OR bed, positioning accessories.

Maintain the patient in good body alignment; reassess body alignment following positional changes.

Keep sheets under patient dry and wrinkle free.

Provide adequate assistance to safely transfer the patient to and from the OR bed.

Continued.

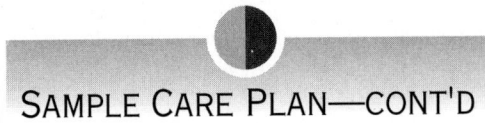

SAMPLE CARE PLAN—CONT'D

NURSING DIAGNOSIS: High risk for altered tissue perfusion related to surgical intervention (microvascular surgery, grafts)

OUTCOME: The patient's tissue perfusion will be maintained and/or restored.

INTERVENTIONS:

Note any sensory/perceptual alterations in the affected body part; document them.

Maintain body temperature with thermia unit, reflective blankets, and the like.

Warm intravenous fluids, blood and blood products, and irrigating fluids.

Increase the temperature in the operating room as indicated.

Monitor the patient's core temperature.

Provide intraoperative medications as prescribed for local irrigation (for example, heparinized saline); label all medications on the sterile field and document their administration.

Monitor tissue perfusion (for example, Doppler ultrasound) as prescribed and flap ischemic time; record results.

Note any swelling, change in color or temperature, or drainage from graft sites prior to discharge from the operating room.

Provide warm blankets for the patient at the conclusion of the surgical procedure.

---

use disposable drapes or reusable drapes must be balanced with environmental concerns about resource use and waste disposal. Analyses tracking each system's cradle-to-grave impact on resource use, energy consumption, and contribution to the waste system should be reviewed by perioperative nurses as they participate in selection and use of single-use or reusable draping systems for the plastic and reconstructive surgery patient (AORN, 1994).

Two of the most frequently used draping techniques in plastic surgery are the head drape and the hand drape. Both of these draping techniques have the goal of providing maximum mobility of the operative part. The *head drape* includes a fluid-resistant drape that encircles the head and the addition of a drape to cover the remainder of the body. The following techniques represent methods of obtaining maximum accessibility and sterile coverage for facial surgery.

1. A barrier sheet, folded in half, and two towels are placed beneath the patient's head with the towels uppermost. The folded barrier sheet covers the headrest or head portion of the OR bed. One towel is brought around the patient's head on each side to cover all hair, leaving the entire face (and ears, as necessary) exposed; the towel is then secured with towel clamps. For craniofacial procedures a towel folded lengthwise in quarters may be placed under the head to assist with moving the head from side to side. Two additional towels are then placed diagonally across the neck just under the chin and secured to each other in the middle over the neck on each side to the towel around the head with towel clamps.

A full sheet is then added to cover the patient from neck to feet (Fig. 23-1).

2. The head portion of the drape is placed as described above. A split, or U, drape is added to cover the patient from neck to feet.

The *hand drape,* described below, can be applied to either upper or lower extremities, as required by the surgical procedure. A commercially prepared extremity drape that has an aperture incorporated into the drape may be substituted for the procedure described in steps 3 to 5.

Before a hand drape is begun, a pneumatic tourniquet cuff is often applied to the upper arm over padding. The patient is supine on the OR bed, with the affected arm extended and supported on a hand table. While an assistant holds the patient's arm with both hands around the tourniquet cuff, the skin preparation solution is applied from fingertips to tourniquet cuff. Care is taken to keep the cuff dry and free of solution.

The following comprises the hand drape (Fig. 23-2):

1. Two folded barrier sheets are used to cover the hand table. The first sheet is placed with the folded edge nearest the patient (thus forming a cuff) and lies directly beneath the tourniquet.

2. Double-thickness, 4-inch stockinette is used to cover the extremity, and the edge is rolled over the tourniquet.

3. The upper arm and upper half of the body are covered by a folded sheet, with the folded edge placed across the part of the stockinette that covers the tourniquet cuff.

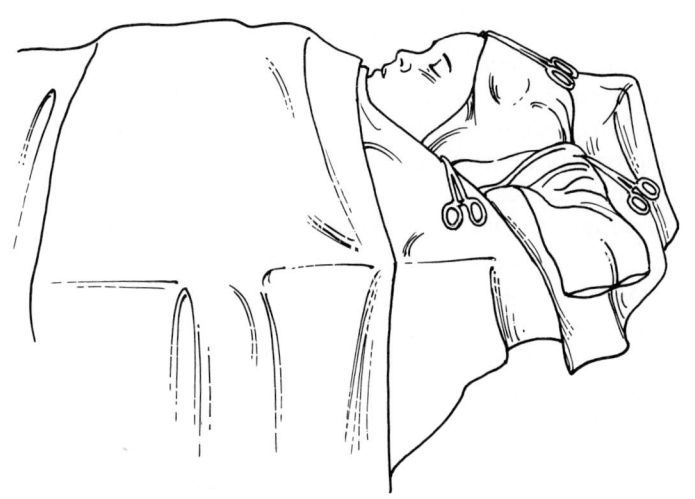

FIG. 23-1   Head drape.

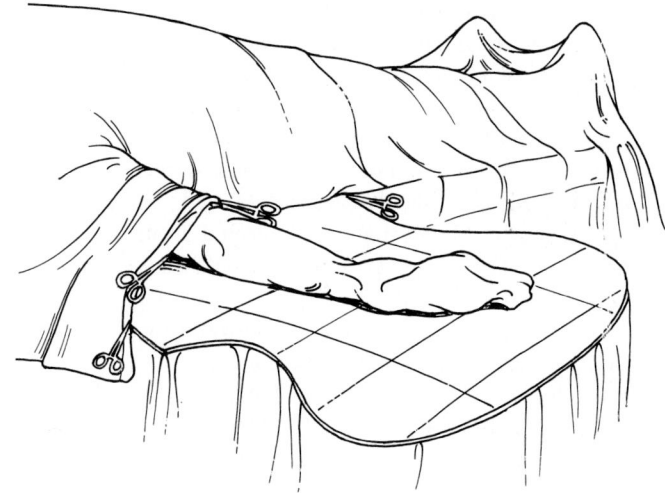

FIG. 23-2   Hand drape.

4. A small towel clamp that grasps the edge of the folded top sheet, the stockinette, and the edge of the cuff of the bottom sheet is placed on each side of the arm. This excludes the tourniquet cuff from the sterile field.

5. The remainder of the body is covered with one or two additional sheets.

Dressings

Dressings are an essential part of the operative procedure in plastic surgery and may contribute to the ultimate outcome of the surgical intervention. Dressings are usually applied while the patient is still anesthetized. In general, the dressing should accomplish the following five goals: (1) immobilize the part, (2) apply even pressure over the wound, (3) collect drainage, (4) provide comfort for the patient, and (5) protect the wound.

Pressure dressings are essential in the elimination of dead space, the prevention of hematoma formation, and the prevention of third spacing associated with liposuction and reconstructive procedures involving transfer of large muscle or tissue flaps. In some cases pressure can be achieved by the use of catheters or drains placed within the operative site and connected to closed-wound suction devices, such as a Hemovac or Jackson-Pratt. In smaller wounds a butterfly cannula may be inserted into the operative site, with the needle end placed in a red top tube.

The perioperative nurse should have the following general dressing supplies available in sterile form:

Nonadherent gauze (for example, Betadine gauze, Adaptic, NuGauze, Xeroform, Biobrane, Scarlet Red)	Petrolatum gauze, ½ inch (used for nasal packing) Telfa Fine mesh gauze Interface

Gauze dressing sponges, 4 × 4 inches, 2 × 2 inches Abdominal pads (most commonly used is 5 × 8 inches) Cotton sheets and balls Webril	Kling, Kerlix fluff, and Kerlix gauze rolls (2, 4, and 6 inches wide) Steri-Strips, flesh colored and regular (⅛, ¼, ½, and 1 inch wide)

Also required are:

Tape (adhesive, plain and waterproof, paper, silk, and foam) Ace bandages	Benzoin spray or swab Coban Plaster supplies (as required for postoperative immobilization)

Anesthesia

Many plastic surgery interventions are performed after the administration of local, topical, or regional anesthesia accompanied by intravenous sedation administered by either an anesthesia staff member or the perioperative nurse. An anesthetic history should be obtained by the anesthesia provider and documented in the patient record. Local anesthetics can cause allergic reaction, cardiovascular, central nervous system, and respiratory depression, or toxicity. Agents used to induce analgesia, such as fentanyl and droperidol, can cause respiratory depression, bradycardia, bronchoconstriction, hypotension, laryngospasm, and hallucinations (Foss and Feistritzer, 1993). Institutional policy and procedures for monitoring the patient by the perioperative nurse should indicate criteria for patient selection, monitoring responsibilities and documentation requirements, frequency of recording monitored data, medications that can be administered by the perioperative nurse, and perioperative nurse credentialing requirements (such as Advanced Cardiac Life Support training).

All patients should have an intravenous line in place and appropriate monitors attached, including a blood pressure cuff, cardiac monitor leads, and a pulse oximeter (see Chapter 6). Emergency drugs, oxygen, and resuscitation equipment should be available before the administration of the anesthetic and/or sedation. All medications, including those on the sterile field, should be clearly labeled with drug name and strength. Medications administered from the sterile field or by the perioperative nurse should be appropriately documented in the patient record.

Patients receiving local anesthesia with or without sedation must have baseline data recorded on admission to the operating room and at prescribed intervals thereafter (for example, every 5 minutes during intravenous sedation; every 15 minutes during local anesthesia unaccompanied by sedation). The perioperative nurse who is monitoring the patient and/or administering the intravenous sedation should have no additional responsibilities such as circulating; attention should be focused on monitoring patient response to drug therapy.

Drugs most frequently administered for *local* anesthesia are lidocaine (Xylocaine) 0.5%, 1%, and 2%, and bupivacaine (Marcaine) 0.25%, 0.5%, and 0.75%. These drugs block the generation and conduction of impulses through nerve fibers. The patient's vital signs and state of consciousness should be closely monitored; early signs of central nervous system (CNS) toxicity include restlessness, numbness or tingling of the mouth, and lightheadedness (Benson and Conte, 1989). CNS stimulation may be followed by CNS depression; the patient may become drowsy or unconscious and hypotensive and demonstrate bradycardia and arrhythmias on the ECG monitor. Before administration of these drugs the perioperative nurse should review the patient record and query the patient regarding hepatic impairment, cardiac or endocrine disease, and history of drug allergy.

Local anesthetics may be combined with epinephrine to slow vascular absorption at the site of injection, prolong the duration of anesthesia, and decrease bleeding in the operative field.

Owing to its vasoconstrictive properties, epinephrine is contraindicated in surgery where it may compromise blood supply in an area with already decreased vascularity; in regional anesthesia, including digital nerve blocks; in patients with hypertension or cardiac arrhythmias; and for patients receiving monoamine oxidase (MAO) inhibitors. The volatile anesthetics, halothane and enflurane, potentiate myocardial sensitivity to circulating catecholamines. Therefore, the anesthesiologist must be alerted prior to the injection of local anesthetics with epinephrine.

Drugs used for *topical* anesthesia include cocaine 4% and tetracaine (Pontocaine) 2%. With topical anesthesia the agent is applied or sprayed to the surface as a solution. It is useful for certain plastic surgery procedures on the ear and nose; it is suitable for use on mucous membranes but not unbroken skin. Tetracaine has a duration of 1 to 3 hours.

Cocaine, a vasoconstrictor, is a short-acting local anesthetic with a duration of 1 to 2 hours.

Drugs commonly prescribed for sedation accompanying the administration of local anesthesia include diazepam (Valium), midazolam (Versed), fentanyl (Sublimaze), and meperidine (Demerol). *Diazepam* is a CNS depressant; it provides sedation, light anesthesia, and anterograde amnesia during the surgical intervention (Benson and Conte, 1989). The CNS side effects are dose related; transient drowsiness, dizziness, ataxia, fatigue, and confusion may be observed. Apnea may occur, especially in the elderly surgical patient. Diazepam is contraindicated in any patient with respiratory depression or hypersensitivity. Intravenous diazepam should be administered slowly to avoid irritation, swelling, venous thrombosis, or phlebitis at the injection site. *Midazolam* is shorter acting than diazepam and less likely to cause pain or tissue irritation at the injection site. Its primary adverse reaction is respiratory depression; appropriate dosage and careful monitoring are essential with this agent. Elderly patients are particularly sensitive to midazolam-induced respiratory depression, which may be delayed for many hours. *Fentanyl* is a potent synthetic narcotic analgesic, altering the perception of and response to pain. The patient must be closely observed for respiratory depression, depressed cough reflex, and skeletal muscle rigidity. Fentanyl must be administered slowly to avoid intercostal muscle rigidity. Extreme response may require the administration of a muscle relaxant and respiratory resuscitation. *Meperidine* produces analgesia as well as sedation. The patient should be closely observed for respiratory depression, hypotension, dizziness, and nausea. Narcotics, including meperidine, should not be administered to patients taking tricyclics or MAO inhibitors (within 14 days of MAO inhibitor use). Unpredictable and sometimes fatal complications such as cardiovascular collapse, seizures, and death may occur.

Implant materials

During surgical reconstruction autogenous (autologous) tissue may be taken from one part of the patient's body and replanted in another part. This tissue has always been considered the most desirable implantation material. Homologous tissue is taken from the same species. Alloplastic materials are inert foreign substances that are readily available, leave no donor defect, are biodegradable, and do not undergo resorption. Implant materials should be noncarcinogenic, nontoxic, nonallergenic, nonimmunogenic, mechanically reliable, capable of resisting strain, biocompatible, sterilizable, and capable of being shaped into a desired shape or form.

Silicone-filled implants (for breast, chin, and testicular uses) have been voluntarily removed from the market by the manufacturer as a result of the Food and Drug Administration (FDA) investigations that occurred in 1992. The correlation between silicone and breast cancer detection,

---

☼

The FDA and its Center for Devices and Radiological Health are responsible for developing and implementing national programs to protect the public health. As part of the FDA responsibility, it aims to ensure the safety, effectiveness, and proper labeling of medical devices. In 1988 the FDA classified all silicone gel–filled breast implants as class III (includes devices that are either life sustaining or life supporting, are implanted in the body, or present potential unreasonable risk of illness or injury; they must have accepted premarket approval applications). In 1991 all manufacturers of silicone gel–filled breast implants were required to submit scientific data demonstrating that their device was safe and effective. In 1992 the FDA issued its decision that applications for silicone gel–filled breast implants would be denied for augmentation purposes. Under certain circumstances the FDA would allow availability for reconstructive purposes. Protocols were established allowing women requiring reconstruction to use silicone gel–filled breast implants if they agreed to participate in clinical studies and were carefully monitored for the future. As part of the protocol, the physician had to certify that saline-filled implants were not a satisfactory alternative for the woman.

In 1993 the FDA published a proposed regulation to require manufacturers to file a premarket approval application for silicone breast prostheses filled with saline. The FDA listed nine risk factors it believes are associated with silicone inflatable breast prostheses: fibrous capsular contracture, deflation, infection, interference with early tumor detection, human carcinogenicity, human teratogenicity, adverse immunologic effects and/or connective tissue disorders, calcification, and biologic effects of silica. Review of this device is ongoing.

Perioperative nurses need to counsel patients who have questions about breast implants. For those women with silicone gel–filled breast implants, monthly breast self-exam should be conducted; yearly mammograms with Eklund views should be administered (the mammogram technician should be informed that the woman has an implant); annual follow-up should be scheduled with the plastic surgeon. Any trauma to the breast, as well as symptoms of persistent burning, change in breast size, shape, or texture, should be reported to the surgeon; these may lead to or indicate implant rupture. Although the FDA does not recommend removal of implants in women who are not experiencing problems, perioperative nurses may be involved in caring for a woman who has opted for gel implant removal, with or without an exchange of the gel-filled implant for a saline-filled implant. These patients are usually extremely anxious; when the implant is not replaced, both physical and psychologic effects must be incorporated as part of the process of planning patient care.

Stombler, R.E. (1993). Breast implants and the FDA: Past, present, and future. *ACS Bulletin, 78*(6), 11-15.

---

connective tissue disorders, and autoimmune disorders has yet to be substantiated. The impact of these investigations with regard to saline-filled silicone shell implants has yet to be determined. Investigations of the use of silicone as an option for implant material are still being conducted (Research Highlight 23-1).

Other implant materials used in plastic surgery include plastics such as Dacron and Marlex, biologic materials such as collagen, metals such as stainless steel, Vitallium, titanium, and tantalum, and ceramics.

The perioperative nurse must exercise care when handling materials for implantation. Implant materials generally are prepackaged and sterile. They must be meticulously handled to prevent contamination. Powder must be wiped from surgical gloves and the implant inspected for any defects and placed on a lint-free surface. Breast prostheses and tissue expanders should be placed in a container with sterile saline or antibiotic solution on the sterile field. If the expander or implant needs to be sterilized, the manufacturer's directions must be followed. A basic procedure is as follows. The perioperative nurse should put on gloves (oil from the skin may cause an inflammatory response), wash the expander or implant in a pure soap (such as Ivory), and rinse it with distilled water. Then 10 ml of normal saline should be placed in the outer lumen with the fill tube of the expander. This tube should be kept in place during sterilization to allow for the exchange of pressures during the sterilization process. The expander or implant should then be placed on a lint-free surface and sterilized according to manufacturer's instructions. The expander or implant should be rinsed thoroughly with normal saline before implantation in the patient. Tissue expanders and implants should not be resterilized with ethylene oxide.

Special mechanical devices

Many special mechanical devices are used in plastic surgery. The perioperative nurse must be familiar with the operation and safety requirements of all equipment used. The manufacturer's instructions for proper sterilization methods and for special care after use must be followed. Each piece of equipment must be kept in working order. The following types of mechanical devices are used in plastic surgery.

Dermatomes

Used for removing split-thickness skin grafts from donor sites, dermatomes are of three basic types: knife, drum, and motor driven.

1. Knife dermatomes
   a. Ferris-Smith (Fig. 23-3)—grafts obtained in freehand manner; sterile blades supplied by manufacturer
   b. Humby or Watson—has adjustable roller to control thickness of graft
   c. Weck (Fig. 23-4)—uses straight razor blades with interchangeable guards (0.008, 0.010, and 0.012 inch) to obtain small grafts; also used for débridement of burn wounds
2. Drum-type dermatomes—operate on the principle of fixing outer surface of skin to half of a metal drum and then moving rotating blade back and forth close to surface of the drum to obtain split-thickness skin graft
   a. Reese (Fig. 23-5)—tape containing adhesive is fixed to drum; dermatome cement is applied to

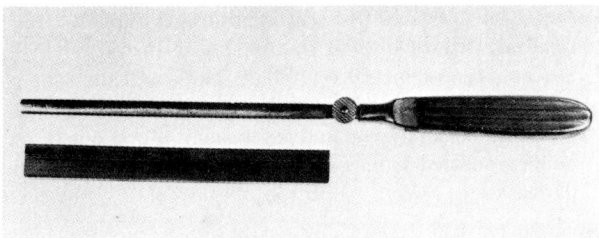

FIG. 23-3 Ferris-Smith knife dermatome handle and blade (straight razor).

skin in thin layer and allowed to dry for 3 minutes; distance between blade and drum (thickness of graft) is adjusted by inserting shim (0.008 to 0.034 inch) adjacent to blade in carrying arm; sterile dermatome tapes, cement, and blades available from manufacturer
3. Motor-driven dermatomes—graft obtained with knife blade that moves back and forth like the blade of a hair cutter; power supplied by electricity or compressed gas; long sterile cable serves as drive shaft and runs between dermatome and its power source; motor activated by foot pedal or hand control
   a. Zimmer dermatome—motor located in the handle, sterile blades provided by the manufacturer; consists of four templates (vary in sizes from 1 to 4 inches, determined by the size of graft needed) and one screwdriver that secures template on top of the blade; depth of graft desired can be determined by a calibrated lever on the handle
   b. Brown air dermatome (Fig. 23-6)—usually powered by compressed air; sterile blades provided by the manufacturer; blade is secured in the handle with a specially designed wrench; depth of the graft can be determined by adjusting the calibrating knobs on the handle; can be steam sterilized
   c. Padgett dermatome—motor is located in the handle; dermatome may be nitrogen powered or electric; if the dermatome is driven by electricity, it is to be sterilized by ethylene oxide only; sterile blades are also available from the company, and different size templates are included; calibration is accomplished by adjusting the knob on the head of the dermatome

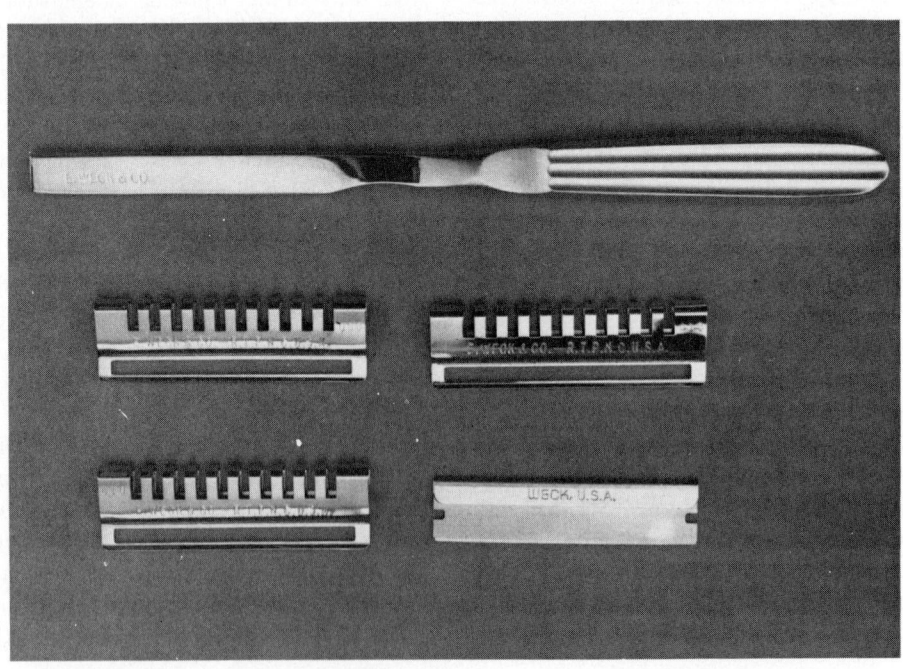

FIG. 23-4 Weck dermatome handle, guards, and blade (straight razor).

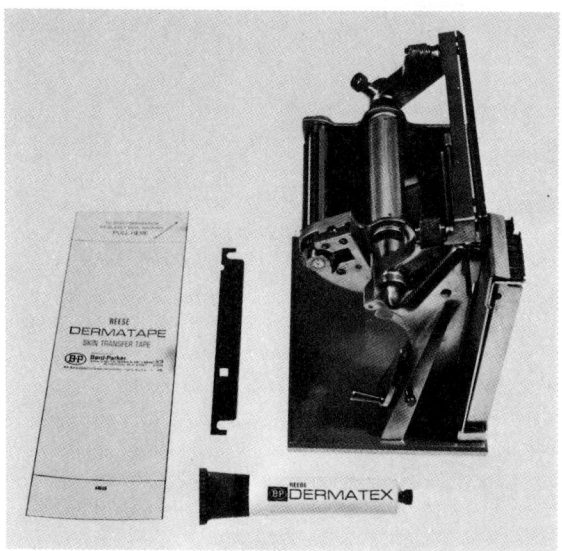

FIG. 23-5 Reese dermatome on stand, with tape, blade, and glue; shims are stored at lower right of dermatome stand.

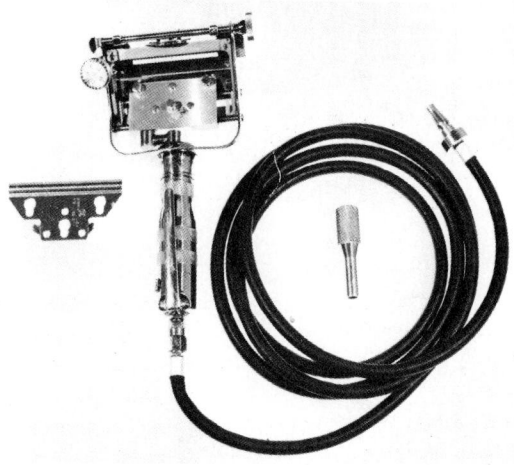

FIG. 23-6 Brown air dermatome and hose assembly with blade and check for securing blade.

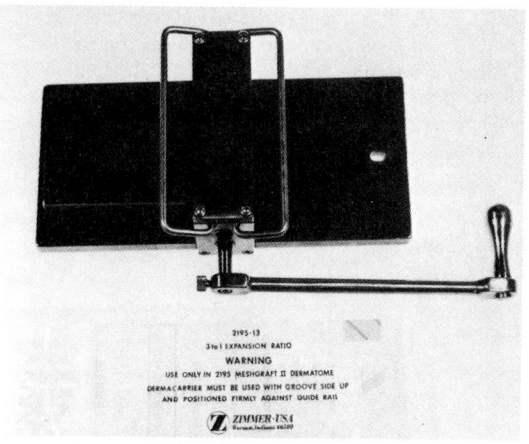

FIG. 23-7 Zimmer mesh graft II dermatome and dermacarrier with 3:1 skin expansion ratio.

Insertion of the knife blade and guards of shims with any dermatome is often done by the surgeon. It is also the surgeon's responsibility to make the final blade adjustment and alignment and to remove the knife blade after obtaining a graft and before any instrument cleansing procedures are begun by perioperative personnel. The blade should be disposed of in an appropriate puncture-resistant container.

Skin meshers

There are several types of skin meshers available (Fig. 23-7), each designed to produce multiple uniform slits in a skin graft, approximately 0.05 inch apart, which allow for the expansion of multiple apertures in graft drainage. The graft is placed on the carrier and passed through the mesher. Sterile carriers for meshers are supplied by manufacturer. They are usually available in several sizes, which determine the expansion ratio of the skin graft (3:1 and 1.5:1 ratios are most commonly used).

Pneumatic-powered instruments (Fig. 23-8, *A* to *D*)

Pneumatic-powered instruments use an inert, nonflammable, and explosion-free compressed gas as their power source. The motor may be activated by a foot pedal or hand control.

The various attachments may be gas or steam sterilized, as recommended by the manufacturer (*not* immersed in liquid). The following attachments are used in plastic surgery:

Kirschner wire driver and bone drill	Roto osteotome, straight
Oscillating saw	Derma-Tattoo (used with reciprocating saw handpiece)
Reciprocating saw	
Sagittal saw	Dermabrader

The Hall II air drill (Fig. 23-8, *E*) is pneumatic powered; the motor is activated by a pedal or a handpiece. Burrs and drill points of varied sizes are available for precision cutting and shaping of bone or for drilling holes in bone for wire passing. The drill may be steam or gas sterilized (*not* immersed in liquid).

A pneumatic tourniquet with an inflatable cuff is used with most hand surgery procedures as well as in other upper and lower extremity surgical interventions. The tourniquet is described on p. 986 in the hand surgery section of this chapter (see also Chapter 21).

Bipolar coagulation unit

The bipolar coagulation unit is described in Chapter 22.

Fiberoptic instruments (Fig. 23-9)

The light source is described in Chapter 24. Fiberoptic instrument attachments used in plastic surgery include a headlight for rhinoplasties, augmentation mammoplasties, and other procedures; a mammary retractor for augmentation mammoplasties; a rhytidectomy retractor; and a Dingman mouth gag attachment for cleft palate repairs.

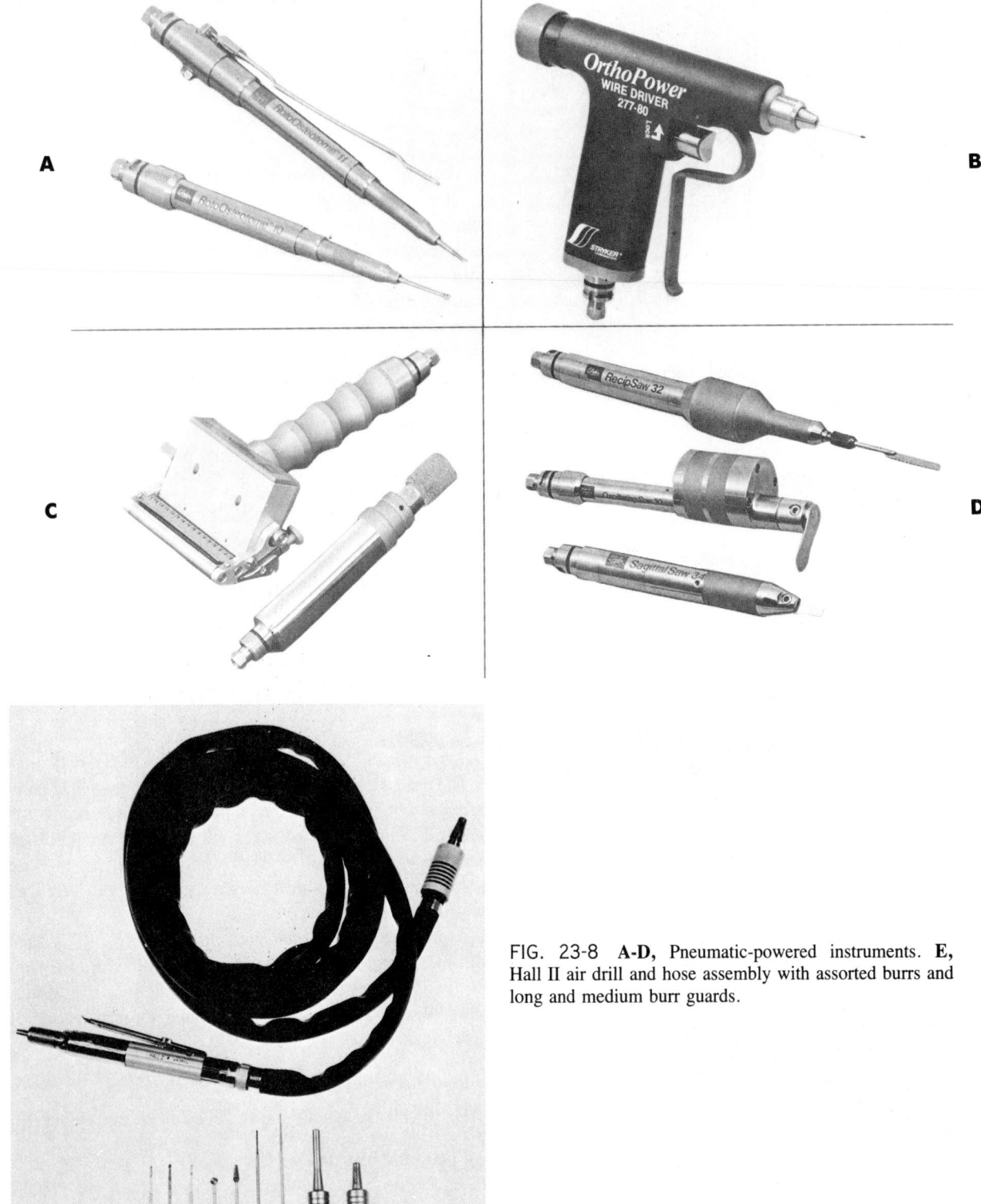

A

B

C

D

E

FIG. 23-8 **A-D,** Pneumatic-powered instruments. **E,** Hall II air drill and hose assembly with assorted burrs and long and medium burr guards.

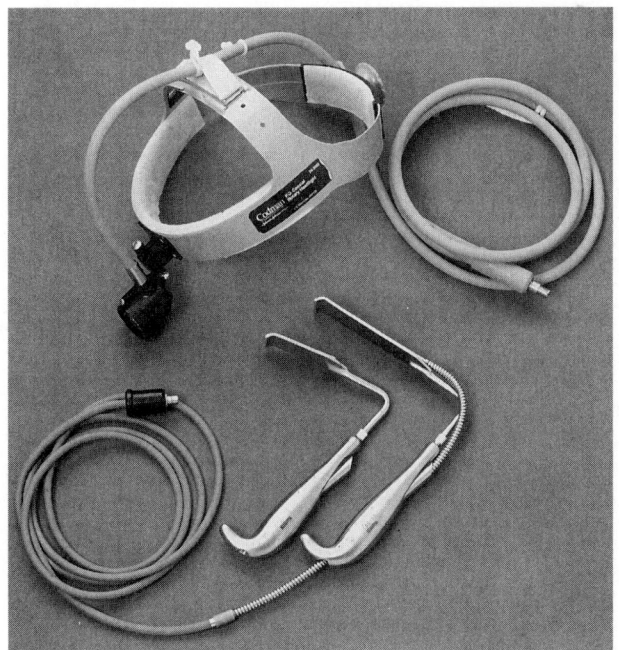

FIG. 23-9   Fiberoptic equipment: headlight, mammary retractors, and cord.

Loupes (Fig. 23-10)

Loupes are magnifying lenses used for microvascular surgery and nerve repairs.

Woods lamp (Fig. 23-11)

The Woods lamp is an ultraviolet light used in determining viability of skin flaps in a darkened room after intravenous injection of 20 ml of 5% sodium fluorescein.

Electrosurgical unit

The electrosurgical unit and safety features are described in Chapter 2.

Microscope

The microscope is frequently used in nerve repairs and microsurgical anastomoses. Chapter 17 provides a full description of operating microscopes.

Instrumentation

Three types of sterile basic instrument trays are kept available in the plastic surgery operating room. With modification by addition of instruments for specific operations, these trays suffice for all plastic surgery operations.

Plastic local instrument set (Fig. 23-12)

Cutting instruments

2 Knife handles, no. 3, with blades, no. 15 or 10
1 Stevens tenotomy scissors, curved
2 Iris scissors, 1 curved and 1 straight

1 Metzenbaum scissors, curved, 5¼ inches
1 Joseph dissecting scissors, curved, 5¾ inches

Holding instruments

1 Sponge-holding forceps, straight, 7 inches
10 Towel clamps, 3 inches
2 Adson tissue forceps, 2 × 1-inch teeth
1 Adson dressing forceps

1 Brown-Adson tissue forceps
1 Dressing forceps, 5 inches
2 Allis forceps
2 Skin hooks, double, 10 mm
2 Skin hooks, double, 2 to 3 mm

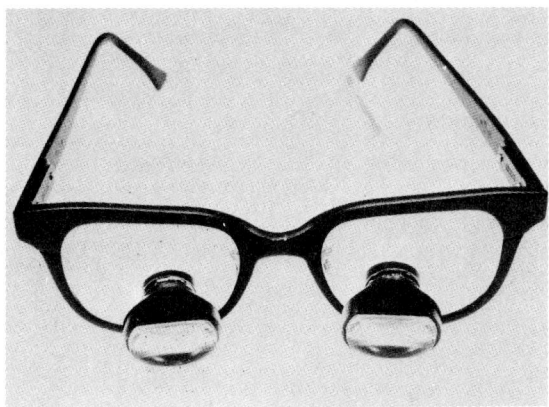

FIG. 23-10   Loupes, used for magnification.

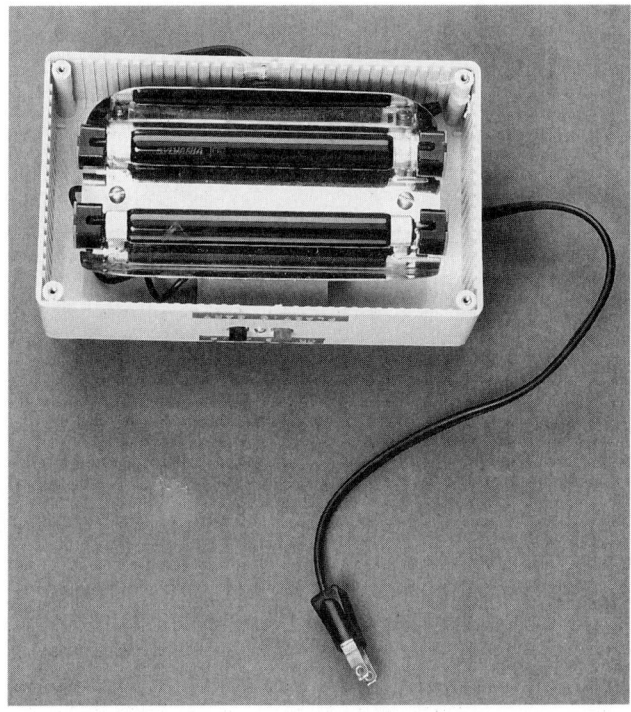

FIG. 23-11   Woods lamp and cord assembly.

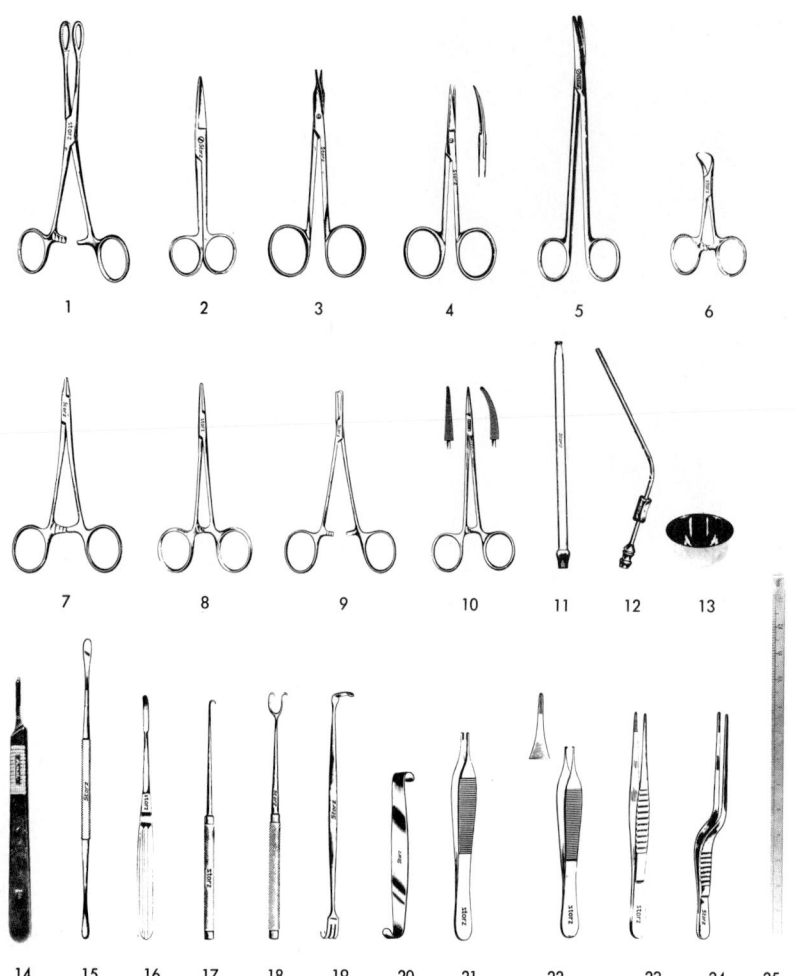

FIG. 23-12   Plastic local instrument set. *1*, Sponge-holding forceps; *2*, Brown dissecting scissors; *3*, Stevens tenotomy scissors; *4*, straight and curved iris scissors; *5*, Metzenbaum scissors; *6*, towel clamp; *7*, Brown needle holder; *8*, Webster needle holder; *9*, straight mosquito hemostat with teeth; *10*, straight and curved mosquito hemostats; *11*, Anthony suction tip; *12*, Frazier-Ferguson suction tip; *13*, small bowl; *14*, Bard-Parker knife handle no. 3; *15*, Freer septal elevator; *16*, Joseph periosteal elevator; *17*, single skin hook; *18*, double skin hook; *19*, Senn-Kanavel retractor; *20*, S-shaped retractor; *21*, Brown-Adson tissue forceps; *22*, Adson tissue and dressing forceps; *23*, dressing forceps; *24*, bayonet dressing forceps; *25*, ruler.

Clamping instruments

12 Mosquito hemostats, curved, 5¼ inches

6 Mosquito hemostats, straight, 5 inches

Exposing instruments

2 S-shaped retractors
2 Senn-Kanavel retractors

Suturing instruments

2 Brown needle holders, 6¾ inches

2 Webster needle holders

Accessory items

1 Joseph periosteal elevator
1 Freer septal elevator
2 Frazier-Ferguson suction tips, nos. 7 and 9
1 Ruler

1 Bowl, small
1 Luer-Lok syringe, 10 ml
2 Needles, 25 and 30 gauge
2 Medicine cups

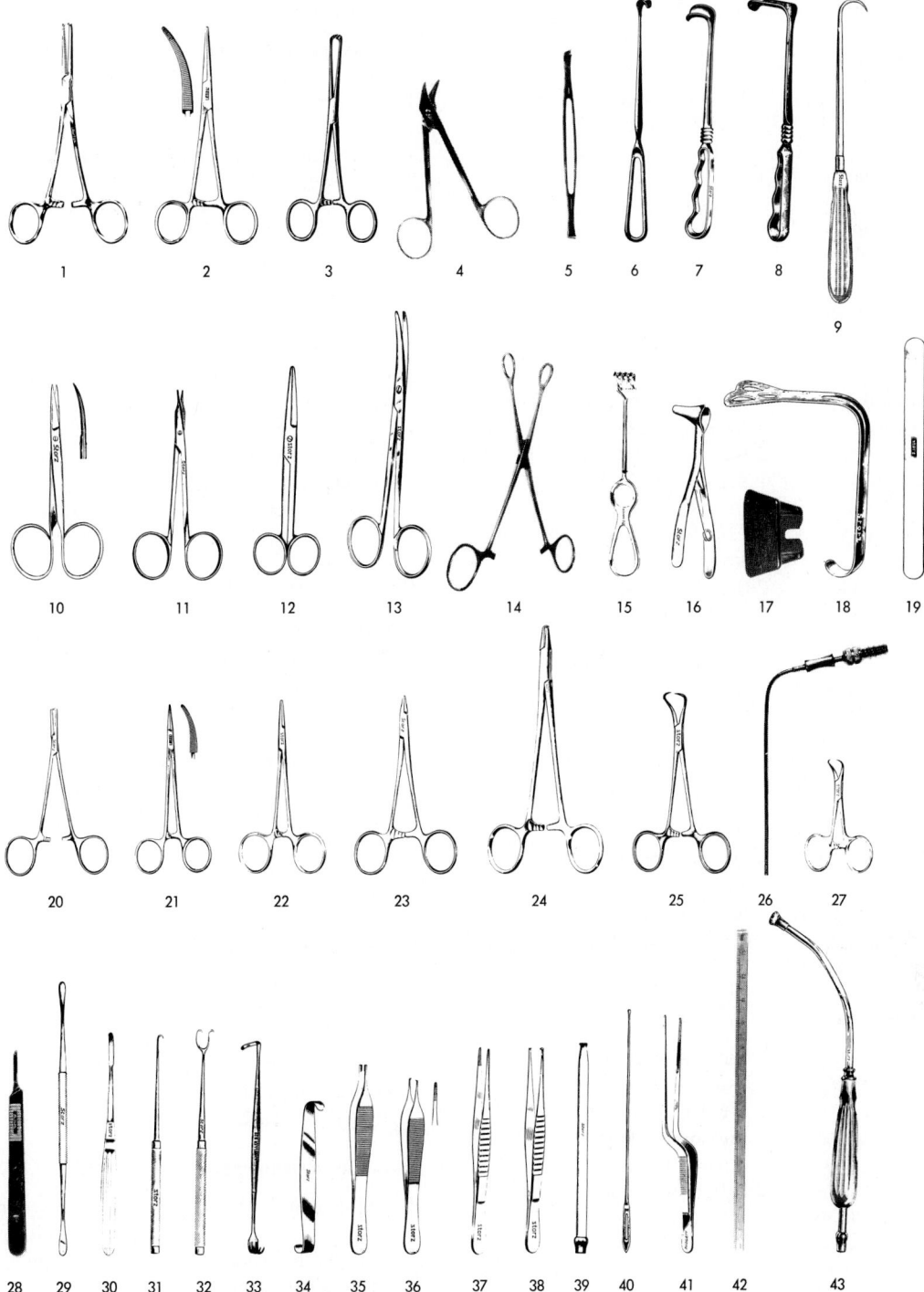

FIG. 23-13 Basic plastic instrument set. *1*, Ochsner forceps; *2*, straight and curved Kelly hemostats; *3*, Allis forceps; *4*, wire suture scissors; *5*, Army-Navy retractor; *6*, Cushing vein retractor; *7 and 8*, Richardson retractors; *9*, jaw hook; *10*, straight and curved iris scissors; *11*, Stevens tenotomy scissors; *12*, straight Mayo scissors; *13*, curved Metzenbaum scissors; *14*, sponge-holding forceps; *15*, rake retractor with blunt prongs; *16*, nasal speculum; *17*, bite block; *18*, Weider tongue depressor; *19*, ribbon malleable retractor; *20*, Halsted forceps with teeth; *21*, straight and curved mosquito hemostats; *22*, Webster needle holder; *23*, Brown needle holder; *24*, Mayo-Hegar needle holder; *25*, large towel clamp; *26*, Frazier-Ferguson suction tip; *27*, small towel clamp; *28*, Bard-Parker knife handle no. 3; *29*, Freer septal elevator; *30*, Joseph periosteal elevator; *31*, single skin hook; *32*, double skin hook; *33*, Senn-Kanavel retractor; *34*, S-shaped retractor; *35*, Brown-Adson tissue forceps; *36*, Adson tissue and dressing forceps; *37*, dressing forceps; *38*, tissue forceps with teeth; *39*, Anthony suction tip; *40*, silver probe; *41*, bayonet dressing forceps; *42*, ruler; *43*, Yankauer suction tube.

Basic plastic instrument set (Fig. 23-13)

Cutting instruments

3 Knife handles, no. 3, with blades, nos. 10 or 15
1 Knife handle, no. 3 long
1 Stevens tenotomy scissors, curved
2 Iris scissors, 1 each curved and straight

2 Metzenbaum scissors, curved: 1 each 5¼ inches and 8 inches
1 Mayo scissors, straight, 6 inches
1 Wire suture scissors, 4¾ inches
1 Kaye dissecting scissors

Holding instruments

1 Sponge-holding forceps, straight, 7 inches
10 Towel clamps, 3 inches
4 Towel clamps, 5¼ inches
2 Adson tissue forceps, 2 × 1-inch teeth, fine
1 Adson dressing forceps
2 Brown-Adson tissue forceps
1 Dressing forceps, 5 inches

1 Tissue forceps with teeth, 5 inches
2 Bayonet dressing forceps: 1 each 5 and 7 inches
4 Allis forceps, 6 inches
2 Skin hooks, single
2 Skin hooks, double, 10 mm
2 Skin hooks, double, 2 to 3 mm

Clamping instruments

24 Mosquito hemostats, curved, 5¼ inches
12 Halsted forceps with teeth, straight, 5 inches

4 Ochsner forceps, 6½ inches
4 Kelly hemostats, curved, 5½ inches

Exposing instruments

2 S-shaped retractors
2 Cushing vein retractors
2 Army-Navy retractors
2 Rake retractors, four blunt prongs
5 Ribbon malleable retractors, assorted widths (4 to 7 inches)

6 Richardson retractors, assorted
2 Weider tongue depressors, 1 large and 1 small
2 Deaver retractors

Suturing instruments

2 Webster needle holders
2 Brown needle holders, 6¾ inches

2 Mayo-Hegar needle holders, 8 inches

Accessory items

1 Joseph periosteal elevator
1 Freer septal elevator
1 Ruler
1 Silver probe, 6 inches
2 Nasal specula, 1 short and 1 long
1 Jaw hook

2 Bite blocks, 1 large and 1 small
2 Anthony suction tips
3 Frazier-Ferguson suction tips, nos. 7, 9, and 11
1 Yankauer suction tube

Plastic hand instrument set (Fig. 23-14)

Cutting instruments

3 Knife handles, no. 3, with blades, no. 15
1 Stevens tenotomy scissors, curved
1 Metzenbaum scissors, curved, 5¼ inches
1 Iris scissors, straight

1 Mayo scissors, straight, 6 inches
Bone-cutting forceps, 1 angular and 1 straight, 7 inches
1 Wire suture scissors, 4¾ inches

Holding instruments

2 Sponge-holding forceps, straight, 7 inches
2 Towel clamps, 5¼ inches
10 Towel clamps, 3 inches
2 Adson tissue forceps, 2 × 1-inch teeth
2 Adson dressing forceps

2 Brown-Adson tissue forceps
1 Tissue forceps with teeth, 5 inches
2 Allis forceps, 6 inches
2 Skin hooks, single
2 Skin hooks, double, 10 mm
2 Skin hooks, double, 2 to 3 mm

Clamping instruments

6 Hartmann mosquito hemostats, curved
12 Mosquito hemostats, curved, 5¼ inches
2 Mosquito hemostats, straight, 5¼ inches

2 Kelly hemostats, curved, 5½ inches
2 Ochsner forceps, 6½ inches

Exposing instruments

6 Senn-Kanavel retractors
2 S-shaped retractors
2 Cushing vein retractors

2 Army-Navy retractors
2 Rake retractors, four blunt prongs

Suturing instruments

3 Webster needle holders

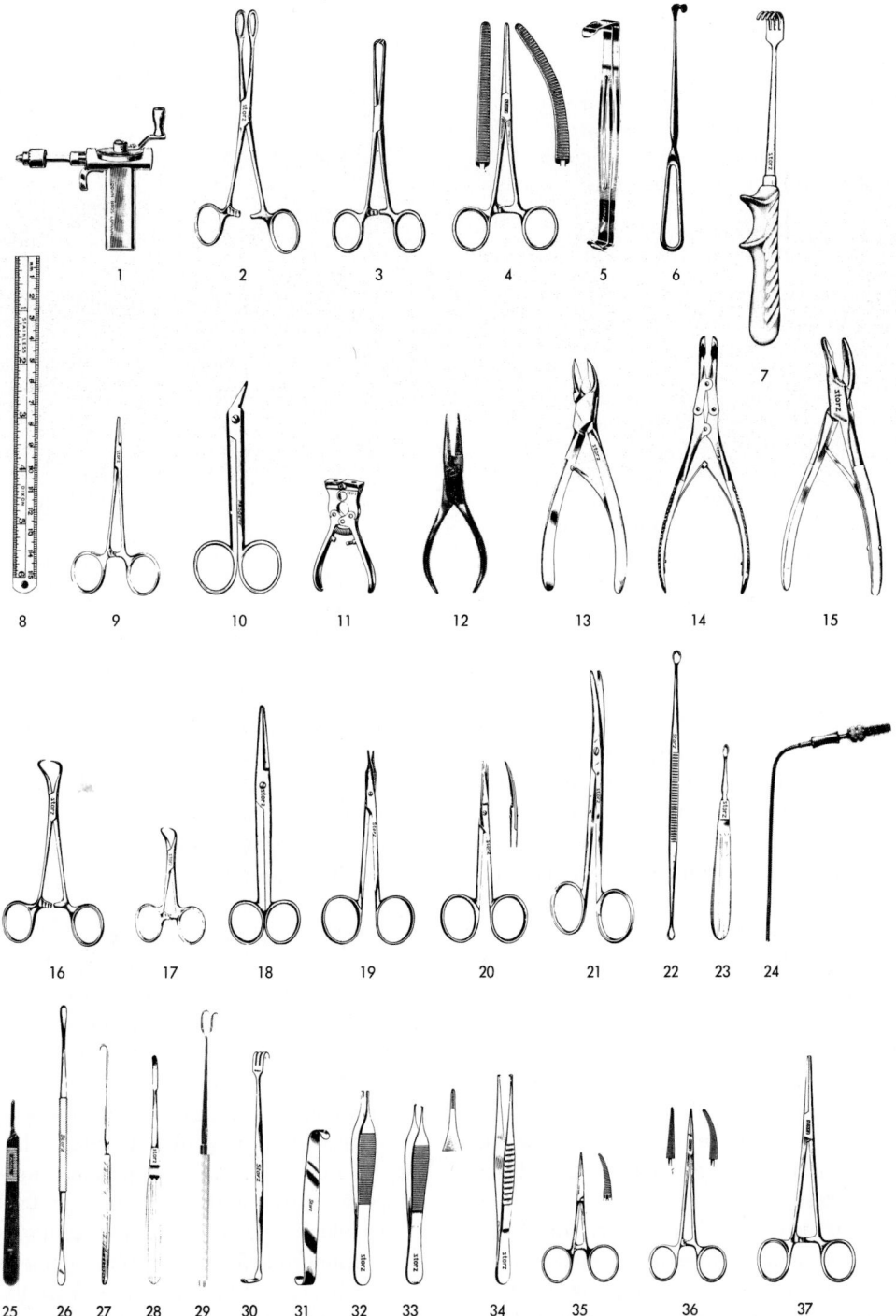

FIG. 23-14 Plastic hand instrument set. *1*, Bunnell hand drill; *2*, sponge-holding forceps; *3*, Allis forceps; *4*, straight and curved Kelly hemostats; *5*, Army-Navy retractors; *6*, Cushing vein retractor; *7*, rake retractor with blunt prongs; *8*, ruler; *9*, Webster needle holder; *10*, wire suture scissors; *11*, Kirschner wire cutter; *12*, needle-nose pliers; *13*, bone-cutting forceps; *14*, Ruskin rongeur; *15*, Lempert rongeur; *16*, large towel clamp; *17*, small towel clamp; *18*, straight Mayo scissors; *19*, Stevens tenotomy scissors; *20*, straight and curved iris scissors; *21*, curved Metzenbaum scissors; *22* and *23*, curettes; *24*, Frazier-Ferguson suction tip; *25*, Bard-Parker knife handle no. 3; *26*, Freer septal elevator; *27*, single skin hook; *28*, Joseph periosteal elevator; *29*, double skin hook; *30*, Senn-Kanavel retractor; *31*, S-shaped retractor; *32*, Brown-Adson tissue forceps; *33*, Adson tissue and dressing forceps; *34*, tissue forceps with teeth; *35*, straight and curved Hartmann mosquito hemostats; *36*, straight and curved mosquito hemostats; *37*, Ochsner forceps.

Accessory items

1 Joseph periosteal elevator	Ruskin rongeurs, 1 large and 1 small
1 Freer septal elevator	1 Lempert rongeur
1 Ruler	1 Set Kirschner wires
1 Bunnell hand drill	1 Kirschner wire cutter
2 Needle-nose pliers, 6¼ inches	Curettes, assorted
2 Frazier-Ferguson suction tips, nos. 7 and 9	

Special supplies

In addition to the basic instrument sets, the following sterile supplies are available at all times and are added to instrument sets for nearly all procedures:

Marking pen	X-ray film, unexposed (for pattern making)
Epinephrine 1:200,00 for injection	Electrosurgical unit
Local anesthetic of choice	

EVALUATION

During the surgical intervention, the perioperative nurse is constantly evaluating the patient's response to nursing interventions, anesthesia, and the surgery itself. Progress or lack of progress toward the identified patient outcomes is constantly monitored. The results of this monitoring enable the perioperative nurse to reassess the patient, reorder priorities of patient care, establish new patient outcomes, and revise the perioperative care plan.

At the conclusion of the surgical intervention the perioperative nurse reviews whether identified patient outcomes have been achieved. The patient's skin integrity is assessed; dressings are applied and their integrity established before discharge from the operating room. Any drains or tubes incorporated in the dressing should be noted. Infusion sites are inspected, and the type of infusing solution, flow rate, and amount infused are noted in the patient record. Documentation of local anesthetics, sedation, or other medications received by the patient is similarly performed. The patient's response during the perioperative period is noted; any unusual or untoward responses are reported to the nurse in the discharge unit. The transport vehicle is obtained; any special equipment needed during patient transport is also obtained and checked for proper functioning. Warm blankets may be provided, and the patient is gently moved to the transport vehicle. The patient who is recovering from general anesthesia is placed in a safe position on the vehicle; the awake patient should be assisted to a position of comfort.

The perioperative nurse should give the report to the nurse in the discharge unit. Areas requiring ongoing patient observation should be noted in this report; the patient's preoperative, intraoperative, and immediate postoperative status is reported also. Using the Sample Care Plan introduced earlier in this chapter, the perioperative nurse may give part of the report based on patient outcomes. If they were achieved, they may be stated as follows:

- The patient acknowledged feelings about altered body structure/function
- The patient's anxiety was reduced.
- The patient verbalized an understanding of perioperative events.
- The patient was free from injury related to the surgical position.
- Tissue perfusion at the graft and surgical site was maintained and/or restored.

SURGICAL INTERVENTIONS
REPLACEMENT OF LOST TISSUE (SKIN GRAFT)
Free skin graft

Skin grafting provides an effective way to cover a wound if vascularity is adequate, infection is absent, and hemostasis is achieved. Skin from the donor site is detached from its blood supply and placed in the recipient site, where it develops a new blood supply from the base of the wound. Color match, contour, and durability of the graft are all considerations in selection of an appropriate donor area.

Skin grafts can be either split-thickness or full-thickness grafts (Fig. 23-15). A split-thickness (or partial-thickness) skin graft contains epidermis and only a portion of the dermis of the donor site; it varies from a thin graft to a thick graft. Although this type of graft becomes vascularized more rapidly and the donor site heals more rapidly than a full-thickness graft, it may exhibit postgraft contraction, be minimally resistant to surface trauma, and look the least like normal skin in texture, suppleness, pore pattern, hair growth, and other characteristics (Vasconez and Vasconez, 1988). A split-thickness skin graft (STSG) may be meshed; meshed grafts can expand to many times their normal size. Meshing allows the graft to be placed on an irregular recipient area; however, its appearance may be esthetically undesirable. A full-thickness skin graft (FTSG) contains both epidermis and dermis; any remaining subcutaneous tissue is trimmed before the FTSG is applied to the graft site. The advantages of this type of graft are that it causes minimal contracture, can be used in areas of flexion, has a greater ability to withstand trauma, can add tissue where there has been a loss or padding is required, and is esthetically more acceptable than an STSG. The donor site can be closed primarily, leaving a minimal defect. Other types of grafts that are available are bone, cartilage, nerve, tendon, and autologous fat grafts. Referred to as composite grafts, these are also free tissue grafts that must reestablish vascularity in the recipient area.

The donor site for an STSG heals by regeneration of epithelium from dermal elements that remain intact. Therefore only a dressing is placed over this donor site. Because

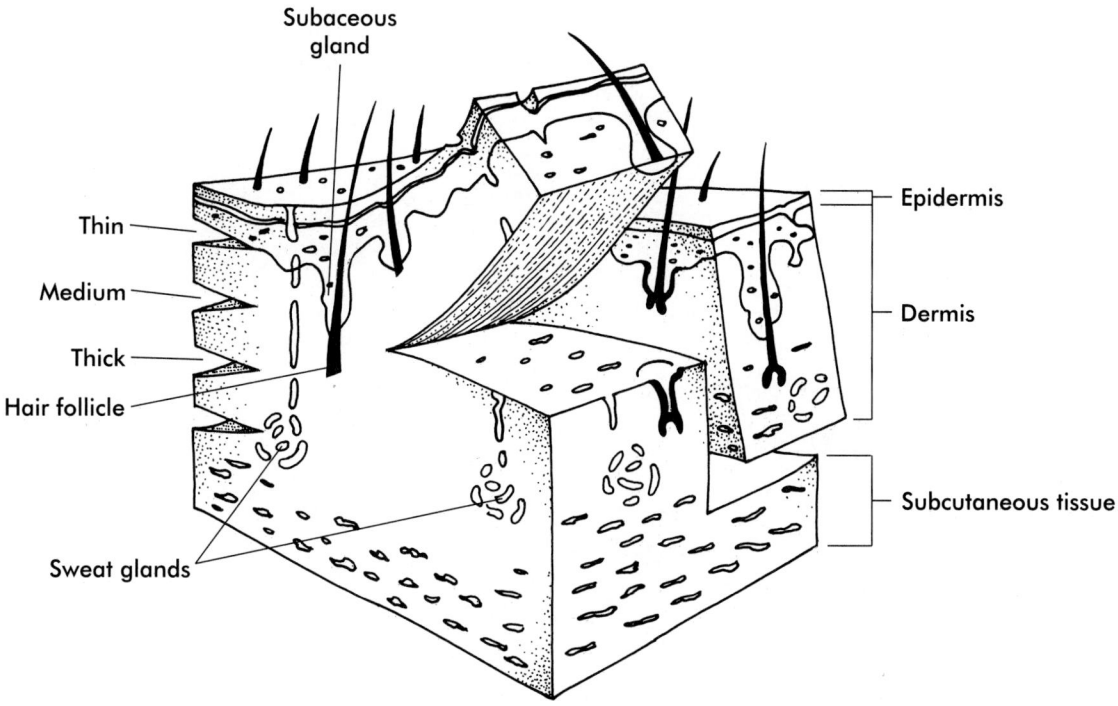

FIG. 23-15   Split-thickness and full-thickness skin grafts.

no dermal elements remain when an FTSG is taken, this donor site does not heal spontaneously. It heals only if another layer of skin is placed over it, either by suturing the wound edges of the donor site together or by applying an STSG over it. A scar remains at the donor site of a skin graft. Therefore donor sites that are covered by clothing are generally chosen.

For a graft to survive the vascularity of the recipient area must be adequate, contact between the graft and recipient bed must be maintained, and the graft-bed unit must be adequately immobilized.

Color, temperature, signs of infection, blanching of the skin, pain and discomfort, edema, vasoconstriction, and venous congestion should be noted and any change reported to the surgeon. Documentation of any changes should be made. If the patient is discharged to home following surgery, patient and family education should include reportable signs and symptoms of potential complications.

A stent or tie-over dressing is often placed over a skin graft (Fig. 23-16). This exerts even pressure, ensuring good contact between graft and recipient site. It also eliminates potential shearing forces at the graft–recipient site interface that might disrupt new blood vessels growing into the graft.

Procedural considerations. A plastic local instrument set is required, plus a dermatome of choice, a skin mesher, a marking pen, and unexposed x-ray film.

The patient is positioned so that both donor and recipient sites are well exposed. Both areas are prepped and draped to maintain adequate exposure and mobility, as required.

Operative procedure

1. The recipient site is prepared as necessary. This step may involve excision of a benign or malignant skin tumor, débridement of an open wound, or release of a scar contracture.
2. Careful planning and marking before harvesting the graft from the recipient site are essential. When feasible, a pattern of the recipient site is made with unexposed x-ray film. This pattern is transferred to the donor site and outlined with a marking pen.
3. STSGs are harvested with a Weck knife or dermatome of the surgeon's choice.
4. Moist sponges soaked in 20 mg Neo-Synephrine per 1000 ml normal saline may be applied to the donor sites to aid hemostasis. A small amount of methylene blue should be placed in the solution of Neo-Synephrine as a marker to identify it from other solutions on the sterile field. Topical thrombin may also be used to aid in hemostasis. It comes prepackaged and ready to attach to the sprayer. Topical thrombin is for *topical* use only and not for injection. These sponges are removed, and the donor site is covered with Biobrane or Opsite.

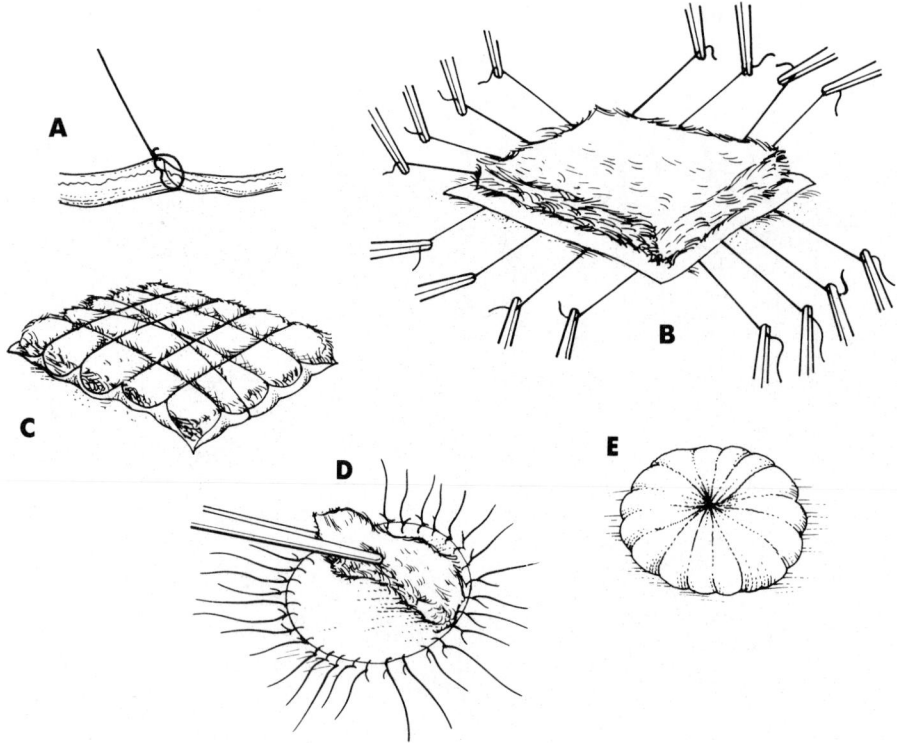

FIG. 23-16 **A,** Method of fixation of skin graft to edges of wound. **B,** Nonadherent dressing is applied over skin graft, and on this a generous pad of acrylic fiber. **C,** Long ends of suture are tied over fiber to produce area of pressure between graft and base. **D,** Similar dressing is applied to circular graft. **E,** Long suture ends are tied over circular graft (often called "stent" dressing).

5. If the graft is to be meshed, it is now applied to specifically supplied carriers for use with certain skin meshers.

6. A graft that is not immediately applied to the recipient site dries quickly, particularly a meshed graft. Therefore grafts should be kept in moist gauze sponges contained in a small basin to prevent inadvertent loss of the graft. Meshed skin should not be removed from its carrier until it is applied directly to the recipient site.

7. Whether applied as a sheet or meshed, STSG may be sutured or stapled with a skin stapler. Nonadherent gauze is usually applied as the first layer of dressing over a graft. Moist dressings should be applied to all meshed grafts to prevent desiccation and loss of the graft.

8. Fat adherent to the graft is trimmed. The graft is applied to the recipient site and usually sutured at the edges, and these sutures are left long to tie over a stent dressing. Blood clots beneath the graft are removed by saline irrigation before the dressing is applied.

Preservation of skin grafts

A skin graft may be harvested but not used immediately. Skin can be obtained from the patient on whom it is to be grafted (autograft) or from a donor (allograft). Skin that is obtained for future grafting must be preserved and stored in a safe, controlled environment until it is used.

Setup

The setup should include the skin specimen and the following items:

Sterile 3-inch rolled gauze	Adhesive tape for sealing and labeling container
Basin with isotonic solution	
Sterile container with screw cap	

Operative procedure

1. The skin should be kept on the instrument table until it is ready for storage.
2. The skin must be kept moist with an isotonic solution such as balanced salt solution or saline at all times.
3. The skin is gently flattened, smoothed out, and placed on a piece of roller gauze moistened with the isotonic solution, with its external surface facing downward.
4. The scrub nurse rolls the gauze and skin loosely, places the roll in the sterile container, and secures the cap.
5. The circulating nurse labels the jar with the donor's name and hospital number, location of donor site, date of collection, and size of graft.
6. If the surgeon anticipates using the preserved skin within 14 days, it may be stored in a refrigerator at between 1° and 10° C (34° and 50° F) until it is used. An alterna-

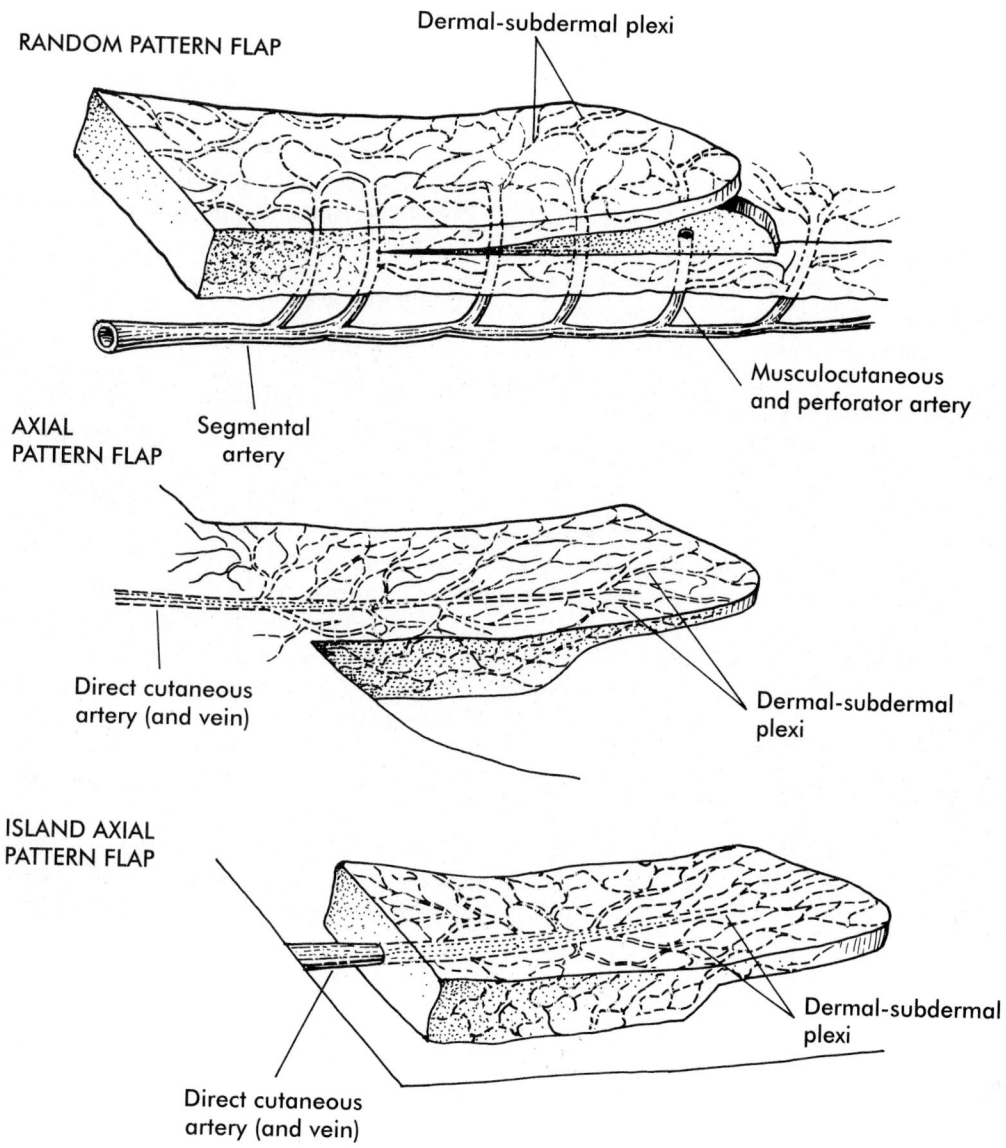

FIG. 23-17 Types of flaps.

tive method is to place the skin in a tissue medium such as McCoy's; the tissue may then be stored in a refrigerator at between 1° and 10° C (34° and 50° F) for 30 days until it is used.

7. If the surgeon does not anticipate using the skin within 14 days, it can be maintained by one of several long-term storage methods. One method is to place the skin in a cryoprotectant (such as ethylene glycol) for 1 to 2 hours at 4° C (39° F), then gradually cool the skin to −70° C (−94° F), and store in a liquid nitrogen freezer.

Flaps

The term *flap* refers to tissue that is detached from one area of the body and transferred to the recipient area with either part or all of its original blood supply intact or reestablished (Fig. 23-17). The base or pedicle of the flap is that portion through which the blood supply enters or exits. Because flaps carry their own blood supply, they are usually used to cover recipient sites that have poor vascularity and full-thickness tissue loss. Flaps are used for reconstruction or wound closure. They are useful for covering exposed bone, tendon, or nerve. They may be used if operating through the wound may be necessary at a later date to repair underlying structures. Flaps containing skin and subcutaneous tissue retain more properties of normal skin and shrink less than skin grafts. Flaps, however, have some disadvantages, such as bulky appearance, failure to match tissue of the recipient site in texture or color, and the possibility of requiring multiple operations and prolonged hospitalization.

Flaps may be classified according to blood supply. *Random pattern* flaps consist of skin and subcutaneous tissue vascularized by random perforators with limited length-to-width ratio. *Axial pattern* flaps have a well-defined arteriovenous supply along the long axis; they can be comparatively long in relation to width. Flaps may also be classified according to position or how they are rotated after elevation. *Advancement* flaps are cut and advanced to reconstruct a nearby defect. *Transposition* flaps are advanced along an axis that forms an angle to the flap's original position. *Rotation* flaps are similar to transposition flaps but are semicircular and rotate along a greater axis. *Island* flaps of isolated sections of skin and subcutaneous tissue are tunneled beneath the skin to new sites. *Pedicle* flaps were the forerunners of *muscle* and *musculocutaneous* flaps. These consist of skin and underlying muscle; they are very mobile and can be rotated into distant defects. *Free* flaps are actually a form of tissue transplantation. Using microsurgical techniques, a defined amount of skin, muscle, or bone can be isolated, detached, and reattached to recipient vessels near the new site. The vascular pedicle may contain functional nerves, yielding sensory flaps to provide protective sensation or motor flaps to restore function. Bone and joints may be transplanted as free flaps, as in the case of toe-to-thumb transfers.

Procedural considerations. A basic plastic instrument set is required, plus the following:

Electrosurgical unit   Marking pen
Extra hemostats   X-ray film, unexposed
Dermatome of choice   Skin mesher

Positioning, prepping, and draping of the patient are carried out to maintain adequate exposure and mobility of both the flap donor and recipient sites.

Operative procedure

1. The recipient site is prepared in the same manner as for a skin graft.
2. When feasible, a pattern of the recipient site is made and transferred to the donor area.
3. The flap is incised, elevated, and transferred to the recipient site. The edges of the flap are sutured to the periphery of the recipient site.
4. The flap donor site is repaired by approximating the skin edges directly or by covering the defect with a skin graft or another flap.
5. Drains are usually placed under flaps.
6. Dressings are applied with particular attention to immobilization of the flap, which may require stockinette, padding, or plaster of Paris.
7. When a pedicle flap is divided, the surgeon may want to check the adequacy of circulation within the flap.

Checking can be done by placing rubber-shod clamps across the base of the pedicle and injecting 20 ml of 5% sodium fluorescein intravenously. After 10 minutes have elapsed, all lights in the operating room are turned off, and a Woods lamp is held over the flap to determine the presence or absence of fluorescence within the flap. Fluorescein may be injected locally for the same purpose.

Composite graft

Composite grafts are composed of compound tissues that are completely separated from the blood supply of the donor site and transplanted to another area of the body. The survival of a composite graft depends on ingrowth of new blood vessels from the recipient site around the periphery of the graft. Therefore, composite grafts are usually small so that no portion of the graft is greater than 1 cm from its periphery. An example of compound tissues used as composite grafts is hair transplants, composed of skin, fat, and hair follicles, which are used to treat male pattern baldness.

Procedural considerations. A plastic local instrument set is required, plus the following:

Marking pen   X-ray film, unexposed

Positioning, prepping, and draping of the patient are such that adequate exposure of both donor and recipient sites is maintained.

Operative procedure

1. The recipient site is prepared by excising tissue, such as a scar or a benign or malignant skin lesion.
2. When feasible, a pattern of the recipient site is made and transferred to the donor site.
3. The composite graft is excised. The donor site is either closed by approximating its skin edges or left unsutured (such as in hair transplant donor sites).
4. Meanwhile, the composite graft is kept in a moist sponge until it is sutured to the edges of the recipient site.
5. Dressings of choice are applied to the composite graft and donor site.

BREAST RECONSTRUCTION

The loss of a breast due to cancer may have a devastating affect on many women. Breasts are symbolic of a woman's femininity and sexuality. They are also functionally necessary for nurturing children. Change in body image resulting from mastectomy is one of the most difficult psychologic aspects of breast reconstruction. The patient must realize that following reconstructive surgery she will not be the same as her preoperative state. The breast will resemble a mound and will be as symmetric as possible to the contralateral side.

Breast reconstruction can be performed immediately following mastectomy or delayed. The patient's condition and preference dictate this decision.

Contraindications to breast reconstruction may include metastasis to major organs such as liver, bone, or lung. The use of chemotherapy and radiation does not preclude reconstruction but may delay it somewhat due to the healing processes.

Reconstruction of the breast can be accomplished in three ways: available tissue and an implant, tissue expanders, and flaps. Use of available tissue is the easiest procedure; however, insufficient tissue remains after mastectomy in numerous patients. When sufficient tissue exists, an implant of the appropriate size is placed under the remaining skin flap and/or muscle, and the contralateral side is adjusted accordingly by either a reduction mammaplasty or mastopexy to achieve symmetry.

Breast reconstruction using tissue expanders

Tissue expansion is a means of stretching normal tissue adjacent to a defect to mechanically create redundancy of normal tissue to correct the defect. For breast reconstruction the expander is basically the same shape as a breast prosthesis. The expander may have a metal-backed, self-sealing silicone valve at its dome or a small, dome-shaped reservoir that is positioned subcutaneously at a distance from the expander but connected to it. In either case, weekly percutaneous injections of normal saline are placed in the expander until the tissue has reached the desired maximum stretch, usually based on a 3:1 ratio. When the desired stretch has been accomplished, the temporary tissue expander is removed and a permanent implant placed.

A combination tissue expander and permanent prosthesis is also available. The procedure of expansion is the same as with a temporary tissue expander; however, when the tissue has reached desired maximum expansion, a portion of the saline fill is removed to achieve a size and "drooping" of the reconstructed breast comparable to the contralateral breast.

Procedural considerations. A basic plastic instrument set is used. The round breast-shape expander is supplied in a sterile package from the manufacturer and is available in multiple sizes (Fig. 23-18). The care of the tissue expander is the same as for other implantable devices. The patient is positioned supine with the arms extended on armboards. Prepping and draping are carried out in the routine manner to expose both breasts.

Operative procedure

1. A submuscular pocket is created for the temporary expander. In addition, a tunnel and pocket are created at an adjacent site from the main sac for the placement of the injection dome and the connecting tube.
2. The tissue expander is tested before insertion for watertight integrity.
3. The expander is then inserted, the reservoir positioned subcutaneously and connected, the wound closed, and the expander filled with sterile saline solution until blanching of the skin is achieved. The amount is recorded on the patient record. Instillation of 3 to 5 ml of methylene blue into the expander can help to identify the proper location of the fill tube postoperatively.
4. Additional inflation of the tissue expander usually begins 2 to 3 weeks after initial placement and thereafter on an average of every 7 days. The time from implant insertion until complete fill varies according to the desired maximum stretch.
5. After the desired expansion has occurred, the temporary expander is exchanged for a permanent prosthesis.

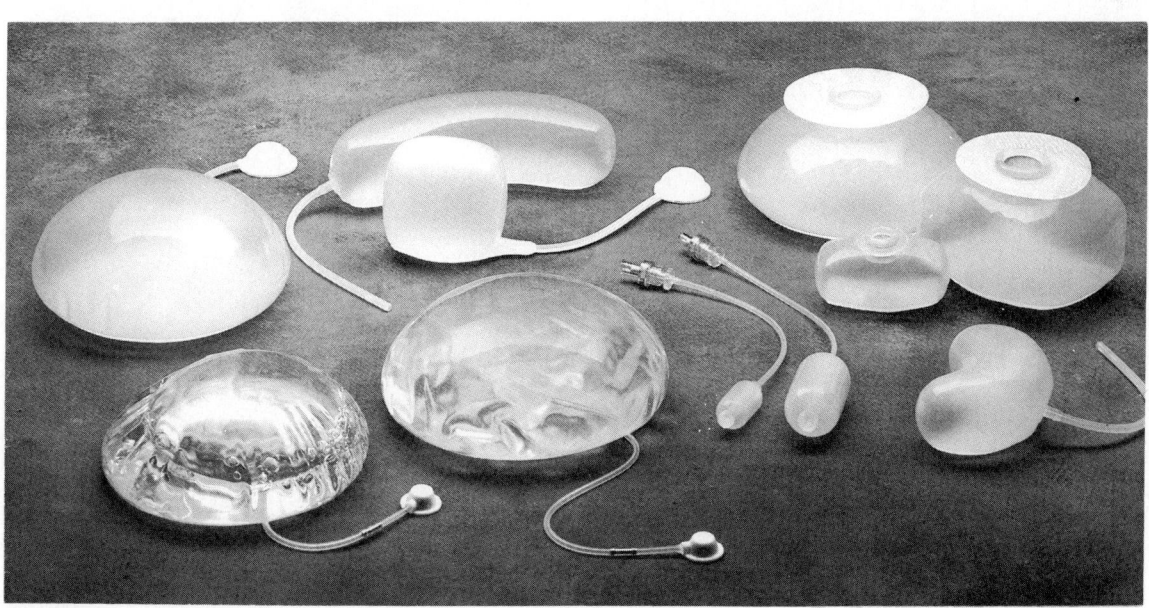

FIG. 23-18   Tissue expanders.

Breast reconstruction using myocutaneous flaps

The latissimus dorsi myocutaneous flap is a single-stage reconstruction of the breast following mastectomy. It is used when significant tissue deficiency occurs following a radical or modified radical mastectomy. The latissimus dorsi muscle is a wide muscle extending over the midthoracic portion of the back and inserting into the humerus; its blood supply comes from the thoracodorsal artery and perforators from the upper lumbar arteries and the intercostal vessels. This rich vascularity allows the surgeon flexibility in orienting and positioning the flap to the pattern of the deficit on the anterior chest wall. Latissimus dorsi flaps for breast reconstruction may be used in conjunction with an internal breast prosthesis, with or without adjustment in the size of the contralateral breast.

Procedural considerations. The skin island and area of dissection for the latissimus dorsi flap are drawn on the patient's back before prepping and draping (Fig. 23-19).

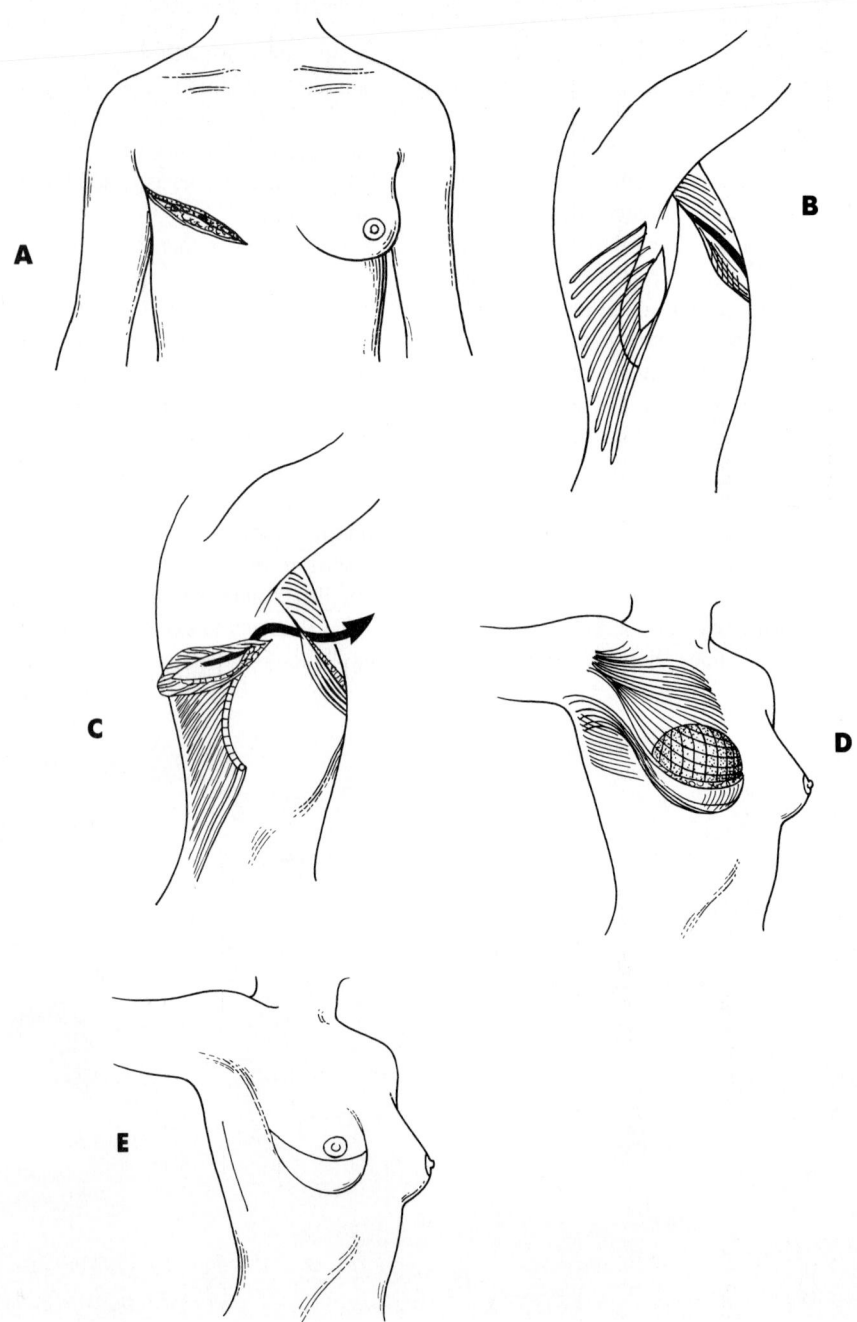

FIG. 23-19   Latissimus dorsi flap for reconstruction following mastectomy (see text for procedure).

The patient is placed in a lateral position with the arm on the operative side extended and elevated on a sling support. Pressure points are protected by the use of pillows and sheet rolls, and the patient is stabilized. The patient is prepped and draped, exposing the affected breast area and muscle.

A basic plastic instrument set is used, plus long Metzenbaum scissors, long DeBakey forceps, Deaver retractors, Freeman areolar markers, lighted breast retractors or a headlight, and a second electrosurgical unit.

Two surgical teams work simultaneously, one freeing the muscle flap and the other preparing the recipient site.

Operative procedure

1. Initially the island of skin is incised transversely across the back, with care being taken so that the scar will be covered by a bra or bathing suit.
2. The muscle is then freed from the overlying skin by undermining so that part or all of the muscle may be mobilized.
3. The skin island and the muscle are then tunneled through the axilla to the chest wall (Fig. 23-19, C). The insertion of the muscle on the humerus and accompanying blood vessels are left undisturbed. The latissimus dorsi muscle fills the space left by the missing pectoralis muscle.
4. The island of skin is oriented to the recipient site, and both are sutured into place (Fig. 23-19, D).
5. A saline-filled implant is placed under the muscle before suturing to reconstruct the breast mound.
6. The wound is drained by closed wound suction catheters.
7. The nipple-areola complex may also be reconstructed by sharing the nipple on the unaffected side or by using groin or auricular tissue. It can be done at the time of reconstruction or at a later date as a minor procedure under local anesthesia (Fig. 23-19, E).

Trans-rectus abdominis myocutaneous (TRAM) flap

The TRAM is a single-stage reconstruction of a postmastectomy breast with the transverse rectus abdominis muscle. This flap gives the patient and plastic surgeon an alternative to the latissimus dorsi flap by taking the excess tissue from the lower abdomen to construct the breast, usually without the need for an implant (Fig. 23-20).

Procedural considerations. Markings on the patient are made preoperatively with the patient in an upright position. A basic plastic instrument set is used as for the latissimus dorsi flap. The patient is positioned supine with arms extended on armboards. Positioning the patient for this procedure is particularly difficult because of the need to promote closure of the abdominal wound, support circulation to the flap, and protect the patient from injury. The OR bed is often flexed; additional padding of the lower extremities may be required. The chest and abdomen are prepped and draped simultaneously.

Operative procedure

1. The skin from the mastectomy scar is excised.
2. The transverse rectus abdominis muscle is dissected and tunneled subcutaneously to the midline.
3. The flap is brought to the chest wall and fixed medially; the thinnest portion of the flap is superior and medial, and the thickest portion is inferior and lateral.
4. Because of the amount of tissue available, an implant is often unnecessary.

There are alternative approaches to the TRAM flap. With the pedicle approach the TRAM is elevated on a vascular pedicle and rotated into place. With the free approach the TRAM is separated from the superior epigastric vessels and anastomosed to the vessels of the chest. A supercharged flap involves elevating the TRAM on its vascular pedicle, rotating it into position on the chest, and anastomosing vessels to augment blood supply to the flap. With the free or supercharged TRAM the microscope, Woods lamp, and loupes need to be available.

Nipple reconstruction

This procedure may be done at the time of the original reconstruction, but most surgeons feel they have a better result if it is done as a secondary procedure after the reconstruction has healed and symmetry is achieved. Tissue may be harvested from the groin, auricular area, or contralateral nipple. Tattooing may complete the reconstruction.

Augmentation mammoplasty

Breast augmentation is done for hypomastia, to correct breast asymmetry, and to recreate the breast after mastectomy. A saline-filled prosthesis is inserted to enlarge or form the breast mound. Placing the implant under the pectoralis muscle also contributes to softness (Fig. 23-21).

Procedural considerations. A basic plastic instrument set is used, plus lighted fiberoptic retractors. The breast implants are packaged in sterile containers from the manufacturer and given to the scrub nurse when breast size is determined. The patient is placed in a supine position. The arms may be extended on armboards to approximately 60 degrees. Alternatively, the hands may be placed over the lower abdomen, the elbows protected with foam padding, and the arms gently secured with adhesive tape to the OR bed. Prepping and draping are carried out in the routine manner to expose the operative site.

Operative procedure. Augmentation mammoplasty is done through areolar, inframammary, or axillary incisions. Either the underlying breast tissue or the pectoralis muscle from the chest wall is elevated. A pocket is dissected and the implant placed in the pocket. Electrocoagulation is used to achieve hemostasis. The pocket may be irrigated with an antibiotic solution before placement of the implant. The wound is closed in layers and a light gauze dressing applied. A bra or an Ace wrap may be used for support.

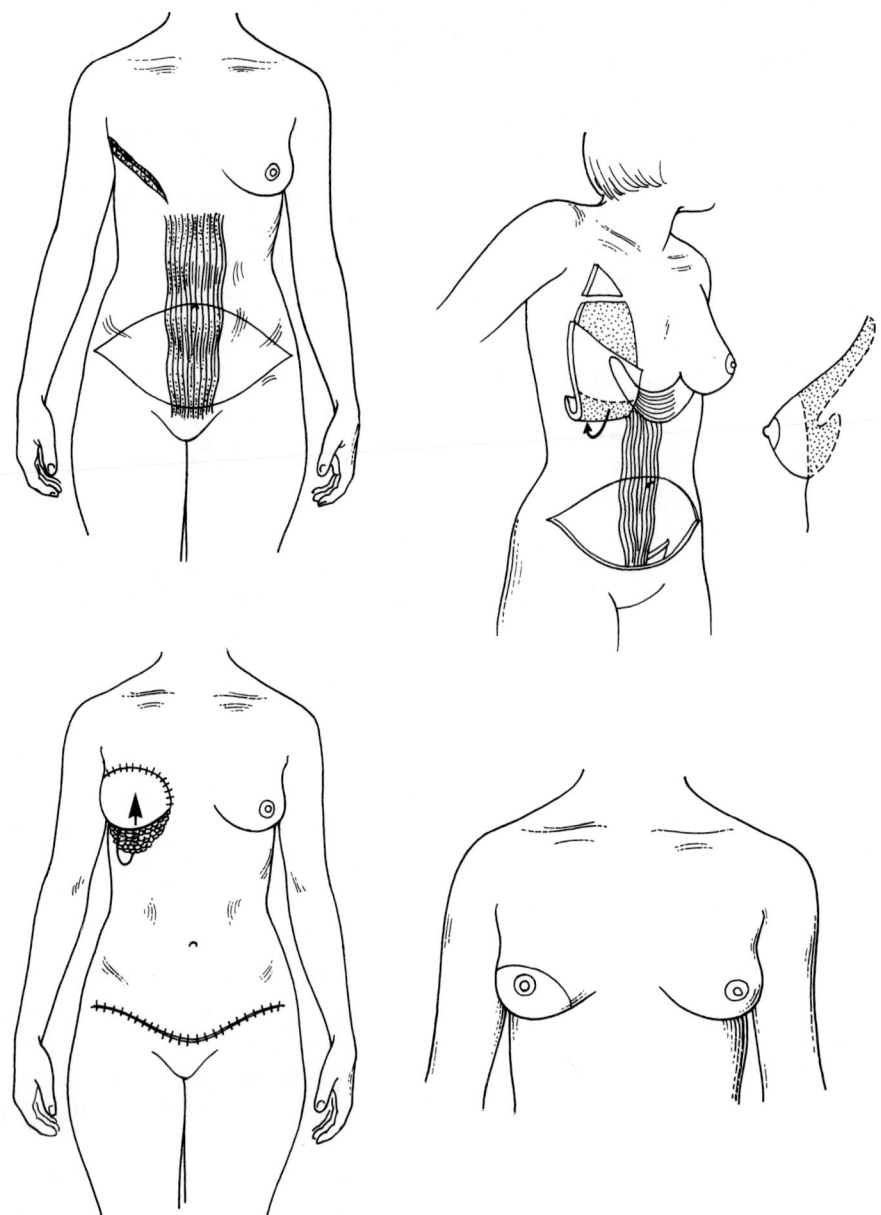

FIG. 23-20 TRAM flap for postmastectomy breast.

Reduction mammoplasty

Reduction mammoplasty is indicated for the patient with gigantomastia or macromastia resulting in back pain, intertrigo, or deep grooving in the shoulders from the weight of the breasts or to achieve symmetry following surgery on the contralateral side following a mastectomy. Excessive breast tissue and its overlying skin is excised, with reconstruction of the breast contour, size, shape, and symmetry (Fig. 23-22). Preoperatively the patient needs to be aware that the scars will be visible and that she may have a slight degree of asymmetry. Autologous blood should be available and the patient typed and cross-matched before undergoing anesthesia.

Procedural considerations. A basic plastic instrument set is used, plus the following:

"Cookie cutter" areola marker	Marking pen
	Tape measure
Skin stapler	2 closed wound suction
Electrosurgical unit	systems

A scale for weighing specimens should also be available, and tissue from each side should be carefully weighed and marked appropriately.

The patient is placed in a supine position with arms slightly extended on padded armboards. The hips should be positioned at the break in the OR bed so that the patient

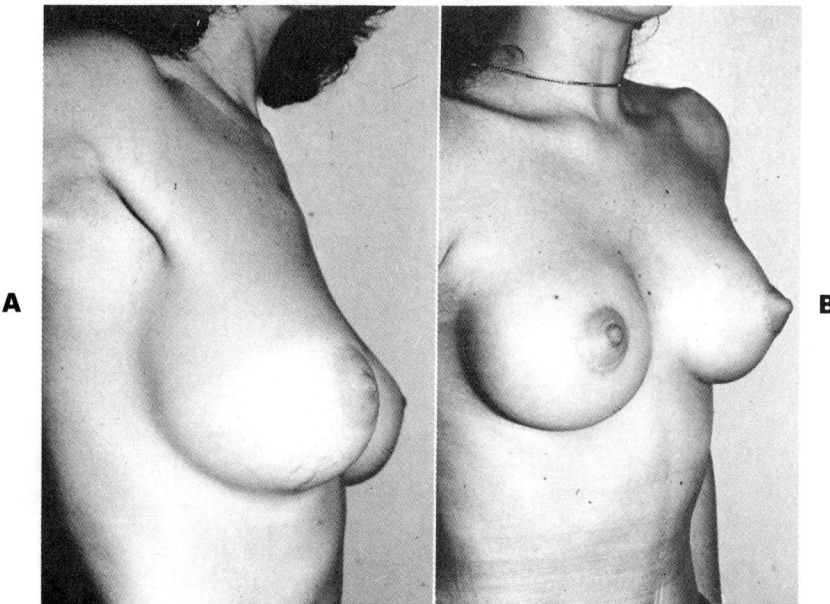

FIG. 23-21 **A,** Augmentation mammoplasty implant under muscle. **B,** Implant under breast tissue.

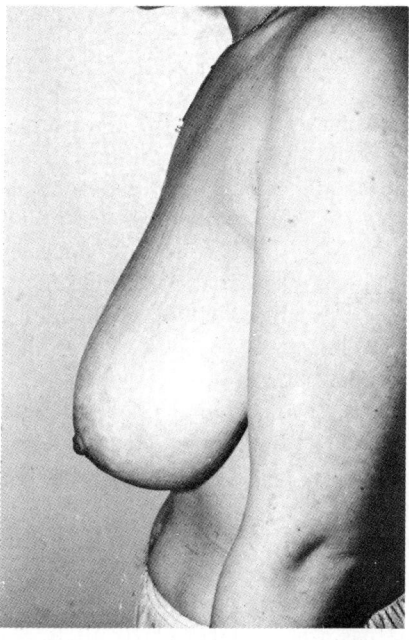

FIG. 23-22 Patient with pendulous breasts before reduction mammoplasty.

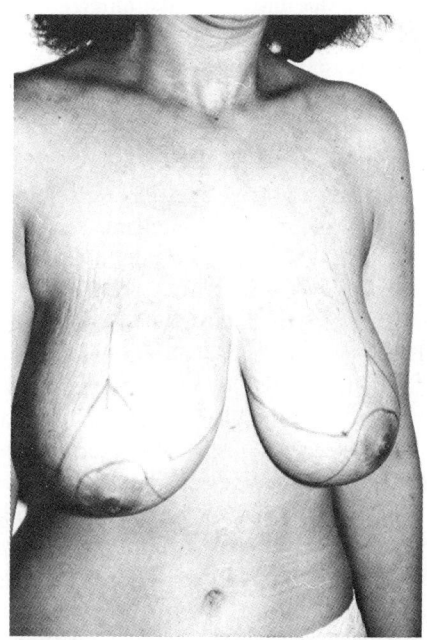

FIG. 23-23 Area of excision marked before surgery.

may be raised to a sitting position if necessary. Standard prepping and draping are done. Care should be taken not to remove the preoperative markings.

Operative procedure

1. The skin to be excised, as well as the new site for the nipple, is marked (Fig. 23-23).

2. The skin between the new and the old nipple sites is incised and removed, the nipple remaining attached to the underlying breast tissue. On patients with very large breasts the nipples are removed and then reapplied as free grafts when the reduction is complete.

3. The redundant segment of breast tissue inferior to the nipple is excised through an inverted-T incision. Tissue

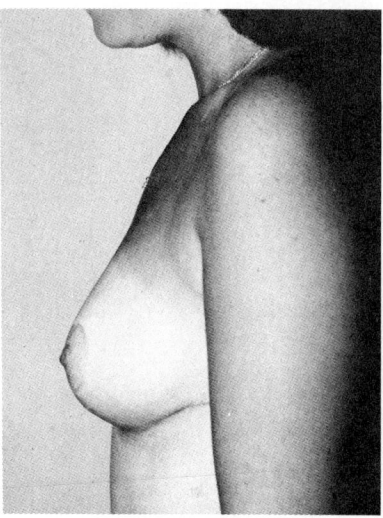
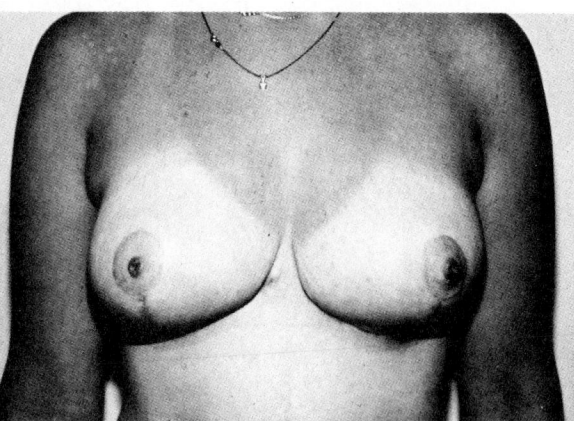

FIG. 23-24 Postoperative reduction mammoplasty.

from each breast is measured and kept separately.

4. The nipple and adjacent tissue are mobilized and sutured in place.
5. The medial and lateral skin edges are approximated in a vertical suture line inferior to the nipple.
6. The inframammary elliptical incision is trimmed and closed transversely (Fig. 23-24). Closed wound suction catheters may be placed. The wound is dressed.

Reduction for gynecomastia

Gynecomastia is a relatively common pathologic condition that consists of bilateral or unilateral enlargement of the male breast. It occurs primarily during puberty or after the age of 40. Although it may be produced by a variety of diseases, it is usually related to excessive hormone production or alterations in hormonal balance. It may also be seen in elderly men and in men following excessive use of marijuana. All subareolar fibroglandular tissue is removed, and the resultant defect is surgically reconstructed. The patient may be positioned in a supine position or semi-Fowler's position, according to the surgeon's preference. Supplies and equipment needed are the same as for a simple mastectomy, plus a basic plastic instrument set. Because suction-assisted lipectomy (SAL) may be used for contouring, suction cannulas, associated supplies, and an aspirator should also be available.

Operative procedure

1. A periareolar incision is made. Through this incision the fibrous and ductal attachments of the underlying glandular tissue to the nipple are divided.
2. A cuff of fatty tissue is left attached to the underlying nipple surface to protect the blood supply.
3. The breast tissue mass is then gently dissected. Carrying the dissection to the pectoralis fascia is usually necessary to remove the entire mass.
4. Hemostasis is carefully achieved.

5. When all subcutaneous tissue has been mobilized, a three-layer closure is carried out. A small drain may be inserted to prevent hematoma formation. A firm pressure dressing is applied.

CORRECTION OF CONGENITAL DEFORMITIES
Cleft lip repair

The normal upper lip is composed of skin, underlying orbicularis oris muscle, and mucosa. Two skin ridges near the midline outline the central philtrum of the lip. The vermilion (red portion of the lip) peaks at the philtral ridge on each side and gently curves downward as it reaches the midline to form the Cupid's bow. A deficiency in tissue (skin, muscle, and mucosa) along one or both sides of the upper lip, or rarely in the midline, results in a cleft at the site of this deficiency. The deficiency of tissue present with a cleft lip results in distortion of the Cupid's bow, absence of one or both philtral ridges, and distortion of the lower portion of the nose. Cleft lip is usually associated with a notch or cleft of the underlying alveolus and a cleft of the palate.

Cleft lip repair is most often performed when the infant is about 3 months of age. Timing of the repair follows the "rule of tens": the infant is 10 weeks of age, weighs 10 pounds, and has a hemoglobin of 10. Early surgical correction aids in feeding and infant-parent bonding. Lip repair is directed toward rearrangement of existing tissues to approximate the normal lip as closely as possible (Fig. 23-25). Some consideration may also be given to correcting the nasal deformity at the time of cleft lip repair.

Procedural considerations. A plastic local instrument set is required, plus the following special instruments (Fig. 23-26):

2 Brown lip clamps   2 Skin hooks, double, 5
2 Calipers   mm
1 Fomon retractor

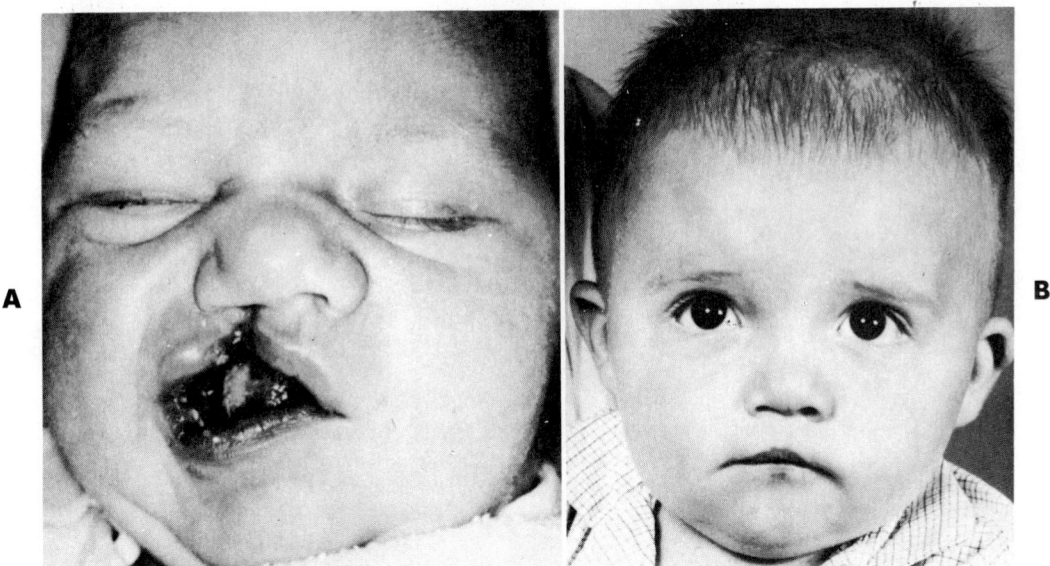

FIG. 23-25 **A,** Infant with complete unilateral cleft of lip. **B,** Repair 1 year later.

Beaver scalpel handles
  and blades, no. 64
  and no. 65
Logan's bow
2 Knife blades, no. 11
1 Needle, 25 gauge, on
  straight hemostat
Marking pen

2 Cotton-tipped applica-
  tor sticks
1 Tongue depressor,
  disposable
Methylene blue
Epinephrine 1:200,000
  (for injection)

The patient is placed in the supine position, with the head at the edge of one end of the OR bed. The face is prepped and the head drape is used. The surgeon may stand or sit at the patient's side or just above the patient's head during the operation.

Operative procedure. Many types of cleft lip repair are in common use, one of which is illustrated in Fig. 23-27. The following steps are applicable to all lip repairs:

1. Normal landmarks are identified and marked or tattooed. Precise measurements, using calipers and a ruler, are made so that corresponding points can be marked along the cleft.
2. The lip may be infiltrated with epinephrine 1:200,000, or lip clamps may be used to aid hemostasis.
3. Incisions are made along the markings for the repair.
4. The abnormal musculature is dissected.

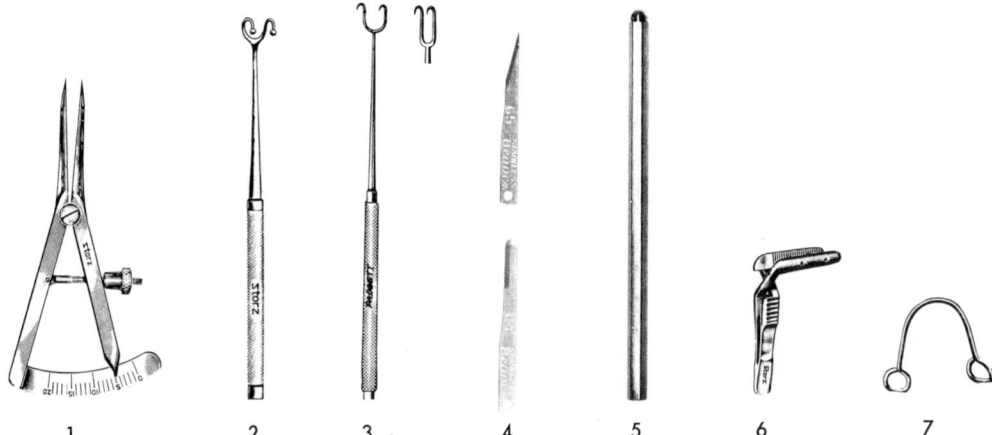

FIG. 23-26 Special instruments for cleft lip repair. *1,* Caliper; *2,* Fomon retractor; *3,* 10-mm and 5-mm double skin hooks; *4,* Beaver scalpel blades nos. 64 and 65; *5,* Beaver scalpel handle; *6,* Brown lip clamp; *7,* Logan's bow.

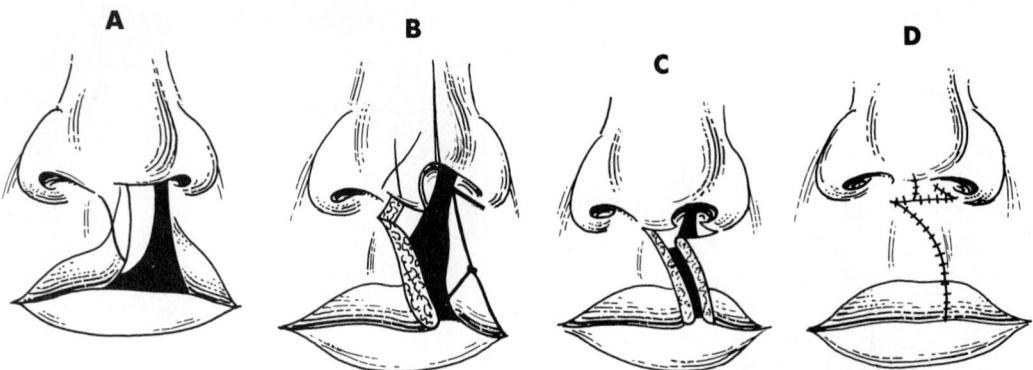

FIG. 23-27 Rotation-advancement method to correct complete unilateral cleft of lip. **A,** Rotation incision marked so Cupid's bow-dimple component *A* will rotate down into normal position; flap *C* will advance into columella and then form nostril sill. **B,** Flap *A* has dropped down, flap *C* has advanced into columella, and flap *B* has been marked. **C,** Flap *B* is being advanced into rotation gap, while skin roll flap is interdigitated at mucocutaneous junction line. **D,** Scar is maneuvered into strategic position where it is hidden at nasal base and floor and philtrum column and interdigitated at mucocutaneous junction.

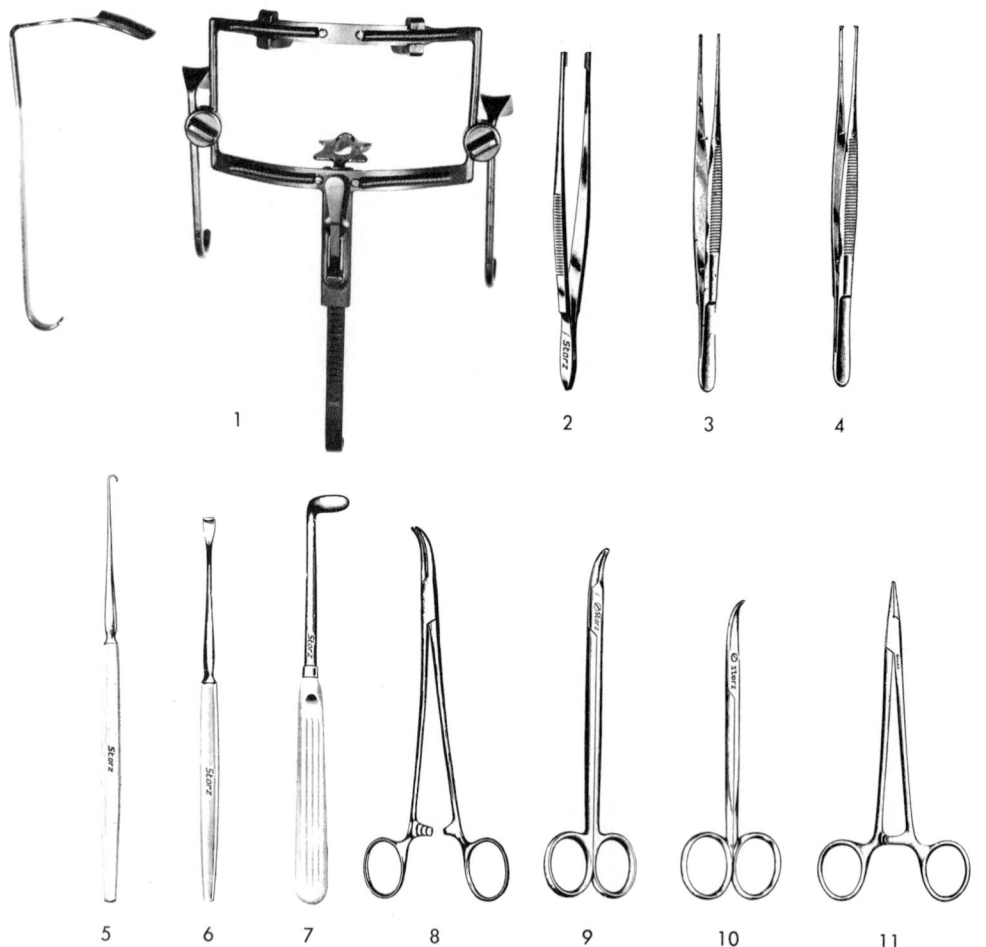

FIG. 23-28 Special instruments for cleft palate repair. *1,* Dingman mouth gag with assorted blades; *2,* Brown forceps; *3,* Cushing dressing forceps; *4,* Cushing tissue forceps; *5,* Blair palate hook; *6,* palate knife; *7,* Blair L-shaped palate elevator; *8,* curved Burlisher clamp; *9,* long Fomon lower lateral scissors; *10,* short Fomon lower lateral scissors; *11,* Crile-Wood needle holder.

5. Additional dissection along the maxilla and nose may be performed.
6. Closure is done in three layers: muscle, skin, and mucosa. Steri-strips may be used.
7. A Logan's bow is applied to the cheeks with tape strips. Elbow restraints are placed.

Cleft palate repair

The palate is made up of the bony or hard palate anteriorly and the soft palate posteriorly. The alveolus borders the hard palate. A separation or cleft of the palate occurs in the midline and may involve only the soft palate or both hard and soft palates. The alveolus may be cleft on one or both sides.

The major function of the soft palate is to aid in the production of normal speech sounds. An intact hard palate is necessary to prevent escape of air through the nose during speech and to prevent the egress of liquid and food from the nose.

Cleft palate repair is usually performed when the child is 6 months of age and should be achieved before the beginning of speech. Variable factors, including the child's weight and the possibility of other disease processes, can affect the timing of the surgery. The various operations used to achieve surgical closure of the palate all employ tissue adjacent to the cleft (in the form of flaps) and shift it centrally to close the defect.

Procedural considerations. A basic plastic instrument set is required, plus the following special instruments (Fig. 23-28):

1 Dingman mouth gag with assorted blades	2 Cushing tissue forceps, 7 inches
1 Blair palate hook	2 Cushing dressing forceps, 7 inches
2 Palate knives	
2 Blair palate elevators, L-shaped, dull and sharp	1 Brown forceps, 6 inches
2 Burlisher clamps, curved	12 Cottonoids, 1 × 1 inch, with strings
2 Crile-Wood needle holders, 6 inches	Epinephrine 1:200,000 (for injection)
1 Stratte needle holder, delicate	Marking pen
2 Fomon lower lateral scissors, 1 short and 1 long	Bipolar electrosurgical unit
	Volumetric suction bottle

The patient is placed in the supine position, with the head at the edge of one end of the OR bed. The head drape is used. Many surgeons sit just above the patient's head and cradle the head on their lap (with the patient's neck hyperextended).

Operative procedure. One of the most frequently used cleft palate repairs is illustrated in Fig. 23-29. The following steps are common to all palate repairs:

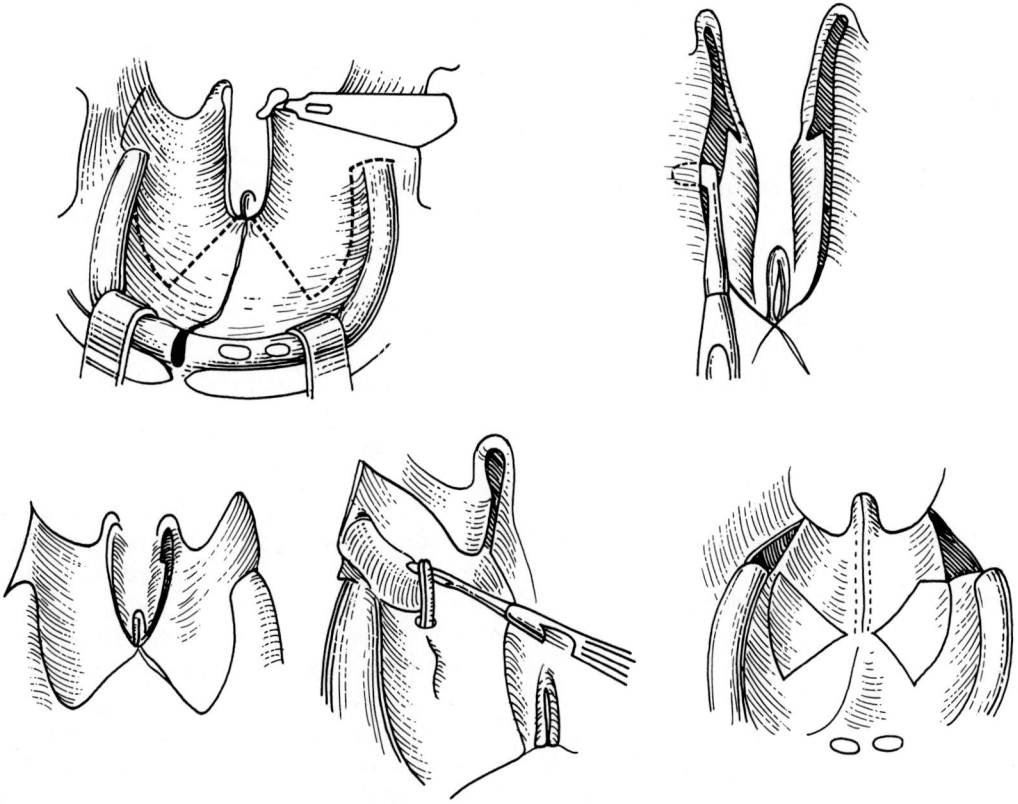

FIG. 23-29 Closure of cleft of soft palate by V-Y(Wardill-Kilner) palatoplasty. A V-shaped incision is made on oral side of palate; mucoperiosteal flaps are elevated on oral and nasal sides, with preservation of blood vessels; Y-shaped closure (in three layers) closes cleft and lengthens palate.

1. The Dingman mouth gag is inserted. Maintenance of the position of the endotracheal tube is crucial at this point.
2. The outlines of the palatal flaps are marked.
3. The palate is injected with epinephrine 1:200,000 for hemostasis.
4. The flaps are incised and elevated.
5. Closure is in three layers: nasal mucosa, muscle, and palatal mucosa.
6. A large horizontal mattress traction suture is placed through the body of the tongue. If the patient experiences upper airway obstruction after extubation, traction is placed on this suture to pull the tongue forward, rather than inserting an airway that might harm the palate repair.

Pharyngeal flap

When abnormal speech (velopharyngeal insufficiency) results despite a cleft palate repair, a secondary surgical procedure may be necessary to improve speech. Typical "cleft palate speech" is characterized primarily by an excess of air escaping through the nose during speech. This hypernasality often results from insufficient bulk or movement of the muscles of the soft palate. To decrease or eliminate this problem, tissue from the pharynx, in the form of a pharyngeal flap, is added to the soft palate. This flap also reduces the size of the opening between the oropharynx and nasopharynx, thus decreasing or eliminating the nasal escape of air during speech.

A pharyngeal flap repair may be done at any age, but most are done before the patient is 14 years old. A pharyngeal flap also may be part of primary cleft palate repair.

Procedural considerations. The same instruments are needed as for cleft palate repair, plus two no. 14 Fr red rubber catheters.

Positioning and draping of the patient are as described for cleft palate repair.

Operative procedure

1. The Dingman mouth gag is inserted.
2. The palate and posterior wall of the pharynx are injected with epinephrine 1:200,000 for hemostasis.
3. The palate is incised, and the pharyngeal flap is incised and elevated.
4. The pharyngeal wall donor site may be sutured or left open.
5. The pharyngeal flap is sutured to the palate, and the palate is closed.
6. A traction suture is placed through the body of the tongue.

Total ear reconstruction

An absent external ear, with either a congenital or traumatic origin, poses to the reconstruction surgical team the dual challenge of being both surgically adept and artistically driven. The patient presents the team with the objective of developing or restoring a part of the appearance that will help with self-esteem and confidence in daily interactions. Emotional support is a key aspect of the plan of care for these patients.

The external ear comprises skin, subcutaneous tissue, and cartilage. The surgical procedure to create an external ear involves the retrieval of rib cartilage, carving of the cartilage, placement of the newly fashioned ear on the side of the patient's head, and skin grafting and dressing the operative sites, while continually assessing and reassessing the preoperative sketches made of the patient's ear with relation to facial structure. This can be accomplished as a one-stage procedure or as a sequence of surgeries. For congenital defects the ideal time for initiating the procedure is between 6 and 10 years of age. In the case of traumatic loss of the external ear (from burns for example), the time is individually determined. The option for the use of tissue expanders has been considered in some cases to stretch the skin surface required to cover the ear.

Procedural considerations. The following instruments are required:

Plastic instrument set (basic)	Local anesthesia with epinephrine 1:200,000
Calipers	
Marking pen	

Total ear reconstruction with autologous rib cartilage retrieval requires the following additional items:

Periosteal elevators: Freer, Key	Clear x-ray films
Rake retractors	Sequential compression boots/antiembolism stockings
Ochsner clamps	
Mallet/osteotomes/ chisels	Foley catheter
Dermatome of choice	Available blood for transfusion
Wire scissors	Gel mattress on OR bed
Unipolar/bipolar ESU	Warming blanket on OR bed
Doppler probe (unsterile with conduction gel for preoperative use and a sterile pencil Doppler with sterile conduction gel for intraoperative use)	

The patient is supine with the arms tucked securely at the sides. Appropriate padding and protection of vulnerable neurovascular bundles and pressure sites are critical. Use of a standard head drape and split drape (or U drape) for the patient's torso allows the team access to the auricular area and chest, respectively. Usually two instrument tables are used with one being designated for the carving of the rib cartilage. Since the procedure is lengthy (6 to 8 hours on the average), comfortable chairs should be provided for the team. Periodic progress of the procedure should be relayed to the patient's family members in the waiting room.

Operative procedure

1. Preoperative sketches of the ear are done with the use of clear x-ray films. Symmetric and anatomic landmarks are vital considerations in the patterns developed for the reconstruction.

2. Assessment of the vascular integrity of the temporoparietal flap is done preoperatively with an unsterile Doppler pencil and conduction gel.

3. The donor skin graft site is identified and prepped with an antimicrobial scrub.

4. When the sketches are complete, the films are sterilized with care not to remove the markings made by the surgeon.

5. The operative side of the head and chest area are prepped and draped in the usual manner.

6. The temporoparietal fascia flap is lifted and a sterile Doppler pencil and sterile conduction gel are used to assess the vascular integrity of the flap.

7. Infiltration of the operative sites with local anesthesia with epinephrine 1:200,000 can be used for hemostasis. Epinephrine in greater dosages (such as 1:100,000) is not recommended for use in the area of the flap due to the possible obliteration of the vascular complexes present.

8. Costocartilage retrieval requires preoperative marking of the patient's chest wall (the area of the sixth, seventh, and eighth ribs). The chest wall is incised and the rib segments are removed with care to preserve the perichondrium. This will encourage bone growth and help to prevent a chest wall defect. The assessment of an intact pleura is critical before closure of the chest. Instillation of saline into the wound is done; if bubbles appear, a chest tube is inserted and attached to a Pleurevac. If bubbles are absent, closure of the wound with the optional injection of local anesthesia to the intercostal areas is performed.

9. While one team closes the chest, another team initiates the carving process, using sterile wood carving tools to accomplish this part of the procedure. The previously marked x-ray films are crucial aids for the artistic abilities of the surgeon. The films are the blueprint for the sculpting phase of the procedure. Surgical wire is used to connect the carved pieces of rib cartilage and shaped to resemble the external ear.

10. A skin graft is taken and the donor site is covered with a dressing of choice.

11. Hemostasis is maintained with the use of electrocoagulation, topical thrombin, and infiltration of local anesthesia with epinephrine.

12. The flap covers the sculpted ear and the skin graft is used to cover any exposed areas (this is a technique used especially with burn patients who have less available skin for coverage).

13. Drainage tubes are placed and attached to closed wound suction, or gauze stents wrapped with nonadherent gauze are sutured in place behind the ear. Soft, bulky dressings are applied to the ear and secured with a head wrap of rolled gauze (such as Kerlix); standard dressings are applied to the chest wall.

Otoplasty

A congenital deformity in which the ear protrudes abnormally from the side of the head is generally the result of an absent or insufficiently pronounced antihelical fold of the external ear. The various methods of otoplasty attempt correction by creating an antihelical fold, which "pins" the ear back against the side of the head (Fig. 23-30).

Protruding ears may be unilateral or bilateral. Otoplasty is usually performed on children just before they start school. It is also performed on adults, in which case either general or local anesthesia may be used.

Procedural considerations. A plastic local instrument set is needed, plus the following:

Calipers	Methylene blue
22-gauge needles or	Marking pen
straight needles	Epinephrine 1:200,000
Cotton-tipped applicator	for injection
sticks	Mineral oil

The patient is placed in the supine position on the OR bed, and a head drape is used, leaving both ears well exposed. The patient's head is turned with the affected ear up and with the lower ear well padded to avoid pressure injury.

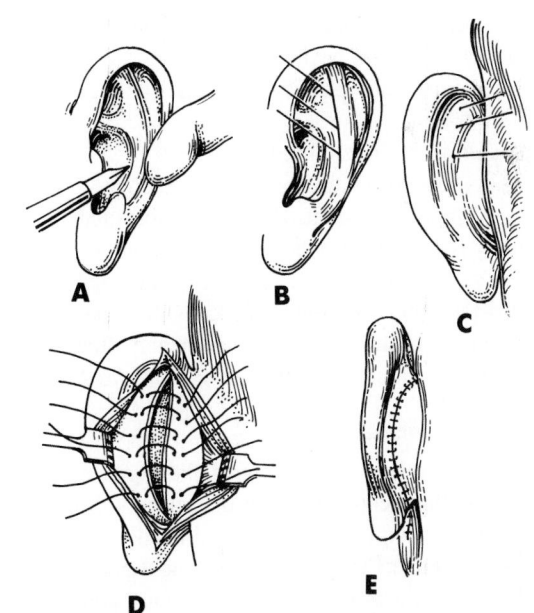

FIG. 23-30 Otoplasty for correction of protruding ears. **A,** Antihelix defined by applying pressure to ear. **B,** Position of antihelical fold marked by passing straight needles through ear. **C,** Needle points visible along posterior surface of ear with ellipse of skin to be excised marked. **D,** Section of ear cartilage incised and scored or excised with sutures placed to hold cartilage back. **E,** Posterior ear incision sutured.

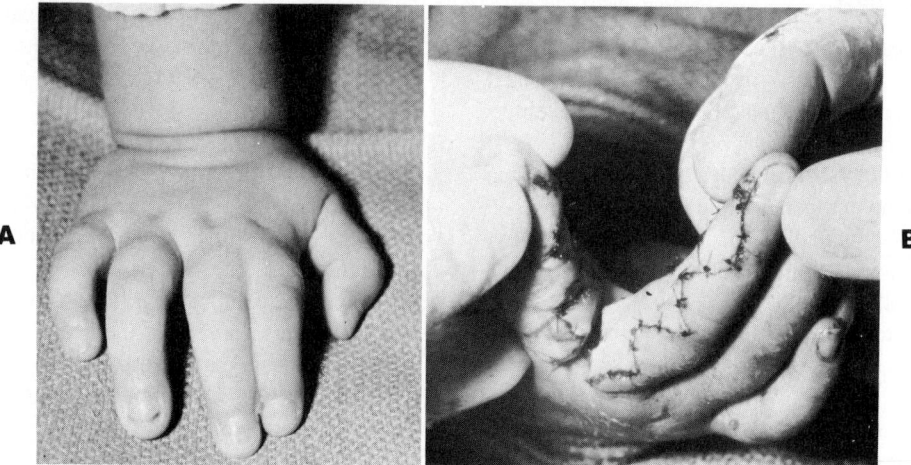

FIG. 23-31   **A,** Syndactyly involving index and long fingers. **B,** Skin web separated; triangular flaps and skin grafts visible along sides of both fingers.

Operative procedure

1. The antihelical fold is created by bending the external ear backward. The position of the antihelical fold is marked by placing 22-gauge or straight needles through the ear from anterior to posterior, applying methylene blue to the tip of the needles, and withdrawing them.
2. An ellipse of skin is excised from the posterior surface of the ear after it has been infiltrated with epinephrine 1:200,000 for hemostasis.
3. The ear cartilage is usually incised near the antihelical fold, and the anterior surface of the cartilage is scored to allow it to bend backward.
4. Sutures are usually placed to hold the cartilage in its new position.
5. The skin incision is closed.
6. A bulky dressing exerting moderate compression on the ears is applied. A nonadherent dressing and fluffs are usually placed behind the ear to avoid pressing the posterior ear surface against the side of the head.
7. A red-top tube with a butterfly cannula makes a convenient drain for the ear reconstruction and allows the subcutaneous pocket to adhere to the framework beneath.

Repair of syndactyly

Syndactyly refers to webbing of the digits of the hand or feet. The most common form of syndactyly is symmetric webbing in two otherwise normal hands. It may, however, be associated with other abnormalities in the hand, such as extra fingers (polydactyly) or bony abnormalities. In syndactyly with normal digits a web of skin joins adjacent fingers (Fig. 23-31, *A*); each finger, however, has its own tendons, vessels, nerves, and bony phalanges. Although the skin web may appear loose, a deficiency in skin is always present when surgical separation is undertaken. Plans for taking a skin graft (usually full thickness) should always be made. Surgical separation of syndactyly is per-

formed at any time after the age of approximately 12 months.

Toe syndactyly is less often treated surgically than finger syndactyly because proper function of the foot does not require fine movements of individual toes. Although the setup and description that follow are for the repair of finger syndactyly, they can also be applied to the repair of toe syndactyly.

Procedural considerations. A plastic local instrument set is required, plus a marking pen, unexposed x-ray film, a pediatric pneumatic tourniquet, and an Esmarch bandage.

The patient is placed in the supine position on the OR bed with the affected arm extended on a hand table. A pediatric pneumatic tourniquet is used. A hand drape is used, and both inguinal areas are prepped and draped (donor sites for FTSGs).

Operative procedure

1. Skin incisions are marked, and the tourniquet is inflated.
2. The skin is incised, and small flaps at the sides of fingers and in the web are elevated.
3. After these flaps have been sutured into position, patterns of areas of absent skin on the sides of fingers are made and transferred to the skin graft donor site.
4. The skin graft is taken, and the donor site wound is dealt with appropriately. If an FTSG is used, it must be defatted before the graft is sutured in place.
5. Skin grafts are sutured to fingers (Fig. 23-31, *B*).
6. Stent dressings are placed over the skin grafts. The entire hand is immobilized in a bulky dressing (see hand surgery section) or in a long-arm plaster cast.

Orbital-craniofacial surgery

A number of congenital anomalies involve the orbital-craniofacial skeleton. These include (1) hypertelorism (Fig. 23-32), in which the distance between the orbits is in-

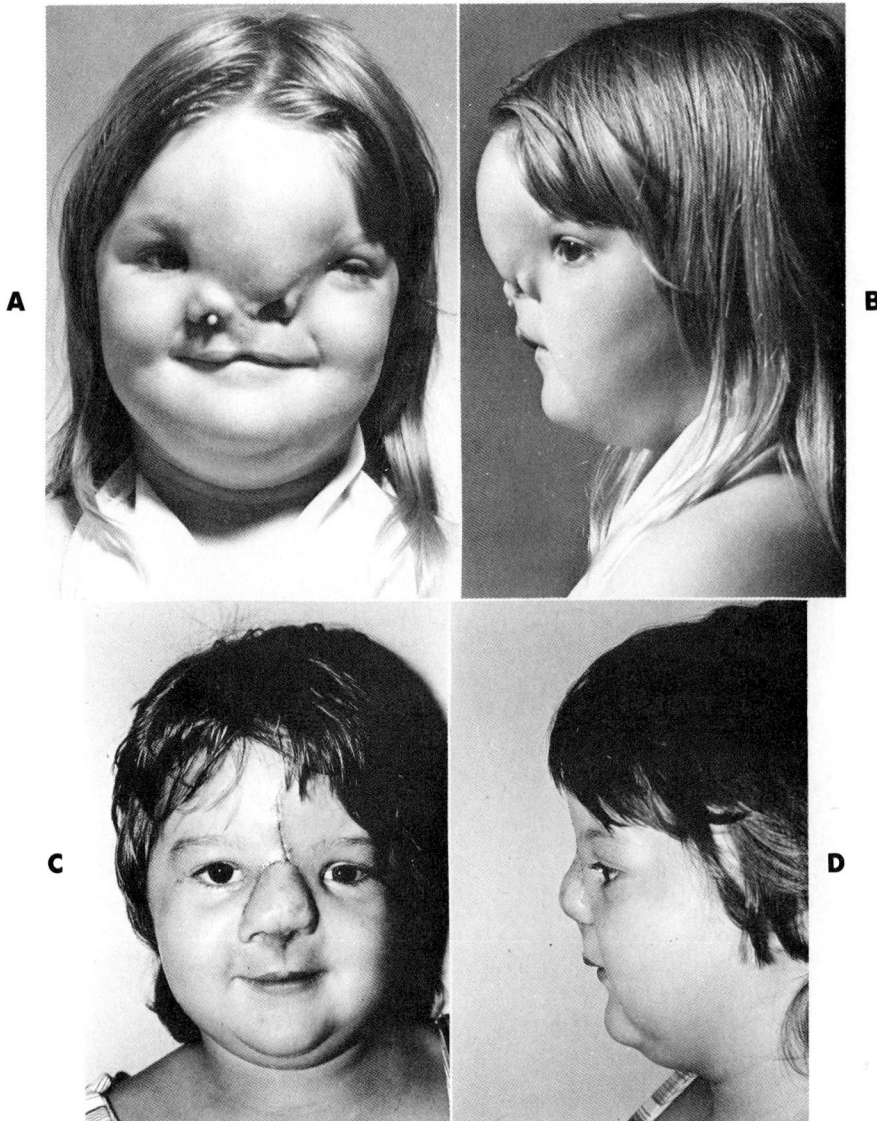

FIG. 23-32 Hypertelorism. **A** and **B,** Before surgery, front and side views. **C** and **D,** After surgery, front and side views.
Courtesy Emory University School of Medicine, Atlanta.

creased; (2) Crouzon's disease (Fig. 23-33), which includes premature closure of the cranial sutures, resulting in an abnormally shaped skull, exophthalmos and hypertelorism, parrot's beak nose, and maxillary hypoplasia; and (3) Apert's syndrome, which includes the same craniofacial deformities as Crouzon's disease plus syndactyly or other hand anomalies. Recent advances in plastic surgery make surgical correction of some of these deformities possible.

Binocular vision is normal in humans. It involves the coordinated use of both eyes to obtain a single mental impression of objects. Binocular vision is usually absent in the craniofacial anomalies because of the increased distance between the orbits. The purpose of orbital-craniofacial surgery is to provide the patient with binocular vision, by moving the orbits closer together, and to provide the patient with

a more acceptable appearance, by moving the bones of the orbital-craniofacial skeleton into a more normal position. Correction of the deformity seen in Crouzon's disease and Apert's syndrome involves a surgically created LeFort III maxillary fracture (see Fig. 23-37).

Although an extracranial approach may be used, an intracranial approach is used in most cases; therefore a neurosurgeon and a plastic surgeon perform these operations through a bifrontal (coronal) craniotomy approach. A tracheostomy may be done before the start of the procedure. Bone grafts from hips or ribs are necessary to augment areas of bone deficit, which result from movement of the craniofacial skeleton.

Procedural considerations. These operations are usually performed on children. They are very extensive proce-

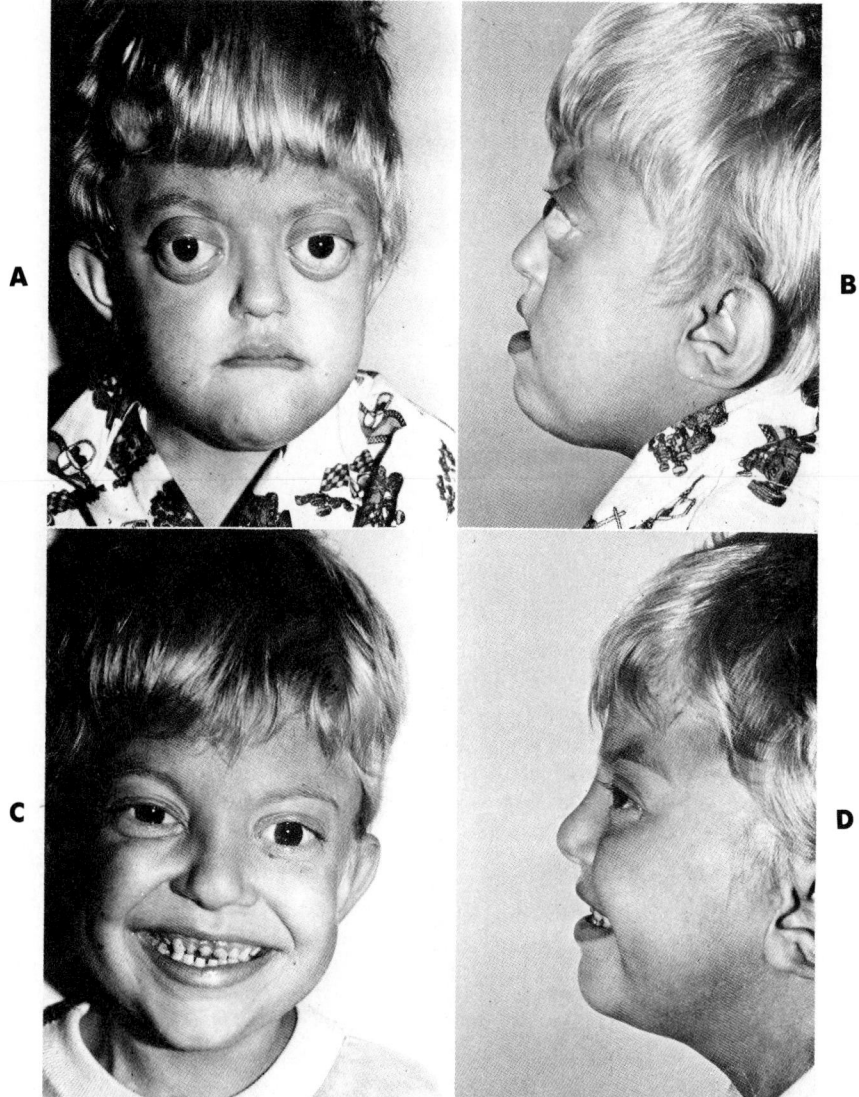

FIG. 23-33   Crouzon's disease. **A** and **B,** Before surgery, front and side views. **C** and **D,** After surgery, front and side views.

Courtesy Emory University School of Medicine, Atlanta.

dures, often lasting 12 to 14 hours. Blood loss is considerable. Postoperative complications, such as cerebral edema or meningitis, can be formidable. The perioperative nurse must pay particular attention to the following important details: (1) insertion of a Foley catheter into the patient's bladder before the operation is started, (2) positioning of the patient on the OR bed so that all bony prominences are well padded, and (3) availability of accurate means for measuring blood loss (usually a volumetric suction bottle and scales for weighing sponges).

A basic plastic instrument set, craniectomy instruments and supplies (see Chapter 23), and tracheostomy instruments and supplies (see Chapter 21) are required, plus the following:

Hall II air drill, Elane, or Midas Rex drill
Oscillating and reciprocating bone saws
6 Osteotomes, assorted sizes, straight and curved
1 Mallet
3 Currettes, assorted
3 Rongeurs, assorted
2 Calipers
1 Brown fascia needle

1 Set coil arch bars
2 Rowe maxillary forceps
2 Polyethylene buttons
2 Foam rubber pads, small
Volumetric suction bottle
Scales for weighing sponges
Marking pen

A separate setup is necessary for obtaining the bone graft. It includes a plastic hand instrument set, plus the following:

1 Weitlaner retractor   1 Mallet
3 Curettes, assorted   Hall II air drill
6 Osteotomes, assorted

The patient is positioned, prepped, and draped as described for a bifrontal craniotomy (see Chapter 22). The entire face is left exposed, however, and may temporarily be covered with a plastic drape until the portion of the operation requiring access to the face is reached. The bone graft donor site is also prepped and draped so that both iliac crests and the lower ribs are exposed.

Operative procedure

1. Tracheostomy, if required, is performed first, followed by application of arch bars, when indicated (as in Crouzon's disease and Apert's syndrome).
2. The bifrontal craniotomy/craniectomy is performed.
3. Orbital osteotomies (Fig. 23-34, *A*) into the anterior cranial fossa are performed bilaterally.

4. Bilateral conjunctival (lower eyelid) and labiogingival sulcus incisions (for Crouzon's disease and Apert's syndrome) are made for other orbital and for maxillary osteotomies.
5. The bones of the orbital-craniofacial region are now moved (Fig. 23-34, *B*), based on measurement of the intercanthal distance (in hypertelorism) or occlusion of the teeth (in Crouzon's disease and Apert's syndrome).
6. Bone grafts may be taken from the calvarium, ribs, or hips to augment areas of bone deficit, which result from movement of the craniofacial skeleton.
7. Bone grafts are fixed in place with interosseous wires and by means of intermaxillary fixation applied to arch bars (for Crouzon's disease and Apert's syndrome) (Fig. 23-34, *C*). Rigid plate and screw fixation is another option.
8. The craniotomy, conjunctival, intraoral, and bone graft donor site incisions are closed.

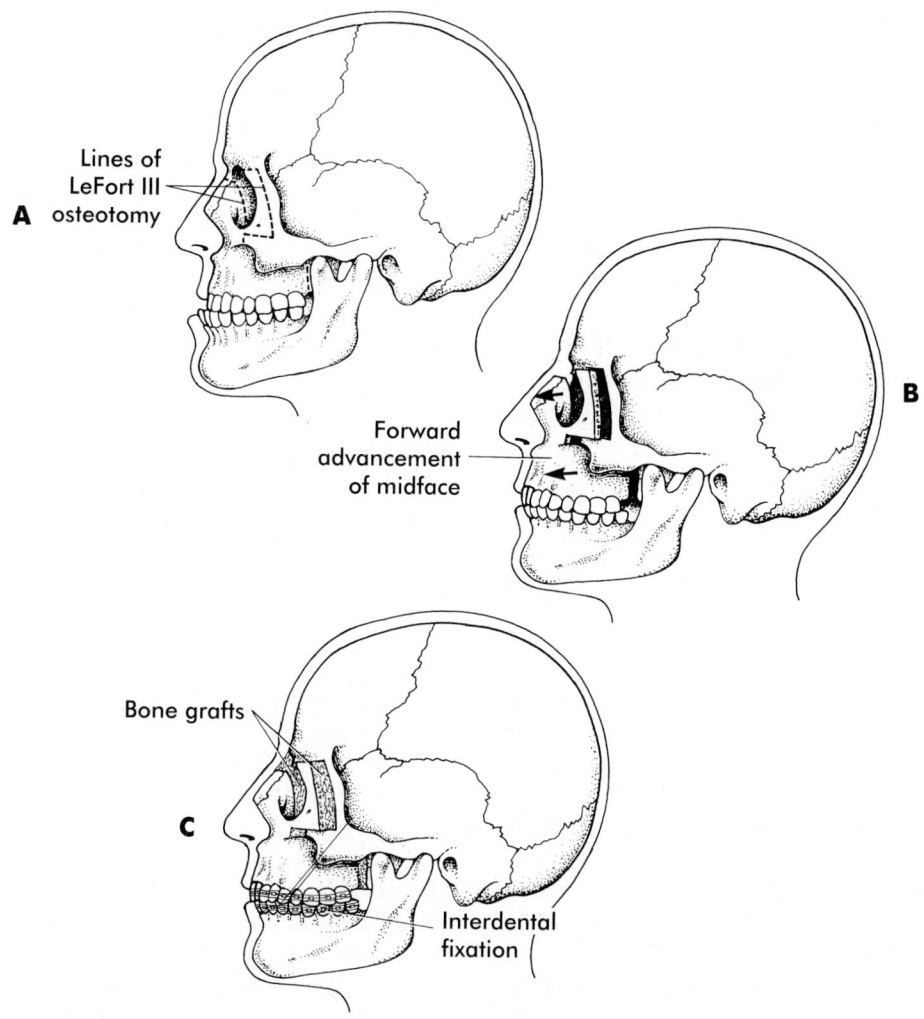

Lines of
LeFort III
A osteotomy

Forward
advancement
of midface

B

Bone grafts

C

Interdental
fixation

FIG. 23-34   Steps in surgical correction of Crouzon's disease deformities.
Courtesy Emory University School of Medicine, Atlanta.

SURGERY FOR MAXILLOFACIAL TRAUMA
Reduction of nasal fracture

Usually a closed reduction of the bony nasal fragments is performed by digital and instrumental manipulation. Occasionally an open reduction with interosseous wire fixation of nasal bone fragments is necessary. A nasal fracture may involve a fracture of the nasal bones or cartilage (including the septum). Closed reduction of a nasal fracture is most often performed under topical and local anesthesia.

Procedural considerations. A plastic local instrument set is required, plus the following:

2 Nasal specula, 1 short and 1 long	4 Metal applicator sticks and wisps of cotton
1 Asch forceps or rubber-shod Kelly hemostat	Topical and local anesthetic agents of choice
1 Brown nasal splint	
Nasal packing of choice	

The patient is placed in the supine position. An intravenous infusion is started and a blood pressure cuff is applied. The head drape is used.

Operative procedure

1. Topical anesthesia for the nasal mucosa and nerve block anesthesia around the nose are administered.
2. Asch forceps are introduced intranasally to elevate the bony fragments, while with digital pressure the surgeon's other hand molds the bones into position.
3. The nasal septum is inspected and realigned with the Asch forceps, if necessary.
4. Bilateral anterior nasal packs are placed.
5. Half-inch tape strips are applied over the skin of the nose, followed by application of the nasal splint and a nasal drip pad.

Reduction of mandibular fractures

The purpose of treatment for a mandibular fracture is to restore the patient's preinjury dental occlusion. With some types of fractures, a closed reduction with immobilization by means of intermaxillary fixation is sufficient for treatment. With a majority of mandibular fractures, however, an open reduction with wire fixation is necessary, plus supplemental intermaxillary fixation to achieve adequate immobilization for healing.

Intermaxillary fixation is most often accomplished by applying arch bars to the maxillary and mandibular teeth. Number 24 stainless steel wires are placed around the necks of the teeth and are ligated around the arch bars to hold the latter in place. Latex bands are attached to the tongs on the maxillary and mandibular arch bars to fix the teeth in occlusion (Fig. 23-35). If the patient is edentulous, arch bars are attached to dentures or specially fabricated dental splints. The dentures or splints are held in place by means of wires placed around the mandible (for the mandibular

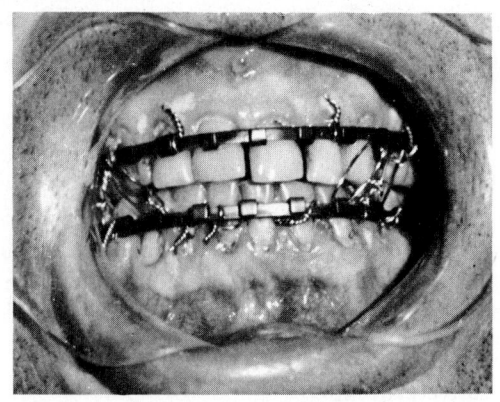

FIG. 23-35 Teeth in occlusion with arch bars in place. Tongs on arch bars will accept latex bands, which maintain occlusion for several weeks (wires around tongs are shown).

arch bar) and through the nasal spine and around the zygomatic arches (for the maxillary arch bar). Scissors or wire cutters must be sent with the patient to PACU to prevent aspiration, should the patient vomit.

Procedural considerations. A basic plastic instrument set, plus the following instruments and supplies, is needed for an open reduction of a fractured mandible:

1 Hall II air drill	Stainless steel wires, nos. 24, 26, and 28
2 Dingman bone-holding forceps (Fig. 23-36)	Electrosurgical unit
1 Concept nerve stimulator	Epinephrine 1:200,000 for injection
1 Marking pen	Rigid fixation system

For the application of arch bars or other types of interdental wiring techniques, a separate Mayo setup with the following instruments and supplies is required:

1 Set coil arch bars and latex bands	2 Weider tongue depressors, large and small
Stainless steel wire, no. 25 or 26	6 Mosquito hemostats, curved, 5¼ inches
2 Mayo-Hegar needle holders, 8 inches	1 Brown fascia needle (if dentures or splints are used)
1 Wire suture scissors, 4¾ inches	1 Drain, small
1 Yankauer suction tube	
1 Freer septal elevator	

If arch bars are applied before the open reduction is performed, this latter setup must be kept completely separate from the instruments used for the open reduction. Because the mouth is a contaminated area, a complete change of gowns, gloves, and drapes is necessary after the intraoral procedure.

The patient is placed in the supine position on the operating room bed. The head drape is used.

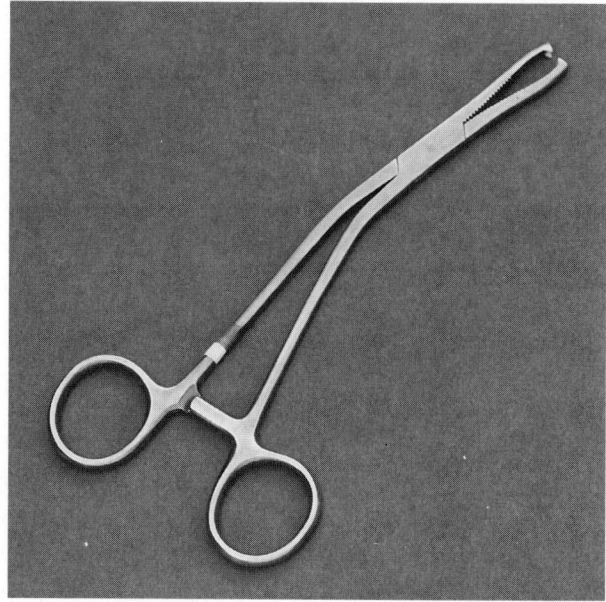

FIG. 23-36   Dingman bone-holding forceps used in reduction of mandibular fractures.

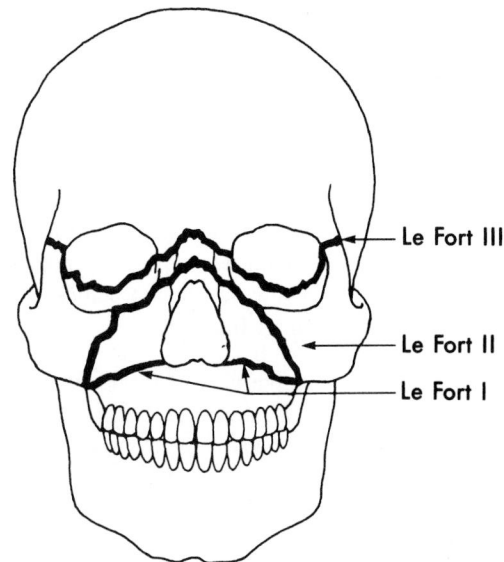

FIG. 23-37   Le Fort's classification of maxillary fractures.
From Neff JA, Kidd PM (1993). *Trauma nursing: The art and science,* St. Louis, Mosby.

Operative procedure

1. Arch bars may be applied before or after the open reduction.
2. A line inferior and parallel to the lower border of the mandible at the fracture site is marked, and the area is infiltrated with epinephrine 1:200,000 for hemostasis.
3. The incision is made so the inferior border of the mandible is exposed. The nerve stimulator may be used to aid in identification of the marginal mandibular branch of the facial nerve in fractures of the posterior body and angle of the mandible.
4. The fracture is reduced by manipulation. Holes are drilled into the mandible on each side of the fracture line with the Hall II air drill, while an assistant holds the reduced fracture with the aid of Dingman bone-holding forceps.
5. Stainless steel wire is inserted through the holes and twisted tightly to secure the fracture fragments in anatomic alignment.
6. In the event that rigid fixation is desired with the use of plates and screws, the appropriate drill bit, tap, and depth gauge are chosen. With these items the proper size prosthesis is placed and the fracture is approximated, aligned, and placed in anatomic position.
7. A small drain is usually placed in the wound, and the wound is closed in layers (periosteum, platysma muscle, and skin).
8. The latex bands may be applied to the arch bars at this time but more frequently are applied later, after the patient is fully awake and reactive.
9. A moderate compression dressing is applied to cover the submandibular wound and drain.

Reduction of maxillary fractures

Maxillary fractures are usually classified as follows: (1) Lefort I, or transverse maxillary fracture; (2) LeFort II, or pyramidal maxillary fracture, and (3) LeFort III, or craniofacial disjunction, which includes fractures of both zygomas and the nose. A maxillary fracture produces malocclusion, as does a mandibular fracture. In addition, depending on the severity of the fracture, it may produce considerable deformity of the middle of the face, usually perceived as a flattening or smashed-in appearance (Fig. 23-37).

Closed reduction with intermaxillary fixation suffices for treatment of LeFort I and some LeFort II fractures. The more severe LeFort II and all LeFort III fractures require open reduction in addition to intermaxillary fixation.

Procedural considerations. The basic plastic instrument set is required, plus the following:

Hall II air drill or Elane drill	Small foam rubber pad
Stainless steel wires, nos. 25, 26, and 28	Marking pen
Rowe maxillary forceps, right and left	Electrosurgical unit
Brown fascia needle	Epinephrine 1:200,000 for injection
Polyethylene buttons	Periosteal elevators
	Rigid fixation system

A separate Mayo setup for the application of arch bars is required, as described for reduction of mandibular fractures.

The patient is placed in the supine position on the OR bed. The head drape is used.

Operative procedure. Arch bars are applied before or after the open reduction, or they may be the only mode of treatment in closed reduction. In addition to ligating the maxillary arch bar to the teeth, it must also be suspended from stable bones superior to the fractured maxilla (which is unstable). In LeFort I fractures suspension may be around both zygomatic arches via passage of percutaneous wires. In LeFort II and III fractures suspension wires are placed through holes drilled bilaterally in the zygomatic process of the frontal bone. This requires incisions in both lateral eyebrow areas. The following description pertains to open reduction of LeFort II and III fractures.

1. After injection of epinephrine 1:200,000 for hemostasis, bilateral incisions are made to expose the infraorbital rims and frontozygomatic suture lines.
2. The Rowe maxillary forceps are applied intranasally and intraorally to disimpact and reduce the maxilla.
3. Holes are drilled into bone on each side of fracture lines along the infraorbital rim (and frontozygomatic area for LeFort III fractures, after reducing the zygomatic fractures).
4. Stainless steel wires are passed through these holes and twisted down tightly to maintain the reduction.
5. Suspension wires are passed from the eyebrow incisions, behind the zygomatic arches, into the mouth with the Brown fascia needle. A pullout wire is looped through each suspension wire within the eyebrow incision, brought out through the skin near the hairline, and tied down over a polyethylene button and foam rubber padding. Self-tapping screws, mini-compression plates, and bone grafts may also be used, based on the surgeon's preference.
6. Incisions are closed.
7. When indicated, reduction of a nasal fracture is then performed.

Reduction of zygomatic fractures

Fractures of the zygoma (the cheek or malar bone) are corrected by either closed or open reduction. The two most common types of zygomatic fractures are depressed fractures of the arch and separation at or near the zygomaticofrontal, zygomaticomaxillary, and zygomaticotemporal suture lines, which constitutes a *trimalar* fracture. Although fractures of the zygoma can interfere with the ability to open and close the mouth properly, their chief consequence is a flattening of the cheek on the involved side, which results from a depressed trimalar or zygomatic arch fracture. Treatment is directed toward elevating the depressed fracture and maintaining the reduction. Closed reduction is the procedure used for treatment of zygomatic arch fractures, whereas most trimalar fractures are reduced by means of open reduction with internal fixation.

Procedural considerations. A plastic local instrument set, a Suraci zygoma hook-elevator, and a jaw hook are required for a closed reduction. A basic plastic instrument set, plus the following instruments and supplies, is required for an open reduction:

Hall II air drill	K-wire driver with set
Stainless steel wires,	of assorted Kirschner
nos. 26, 28, and 30	wires and sterile cork
1 Suraci zygoma hook-	(optional)
elevator	Marking pen
1 Jaw hook	Epinephrine 1:200,000
1 Kerrison rongeur	for injection
2 Blair retractors	Mini-plating rigid fixa-
Bipolar electrosurgical	tion set
unit	

The patient is placed in the supine position on the operating room bed. The head drape is used.

Operative procedure. Closed reduction is performed by elevating the depressed fracture with a percutaneous bone hook. Stabilization of a trimalar fracture may then be achieved by inserting a transantral Kirschner wire from the fractures, side to the normal side.

The technique of open reduction of a trimalar fracture is as follows:

1. Incisions are marked along the lateral eyebrow and lower eyelid over the zygomaticofrontal suture line and zygomaticomaxillary suture line (infraorbital rim) fractures, respectively.
2. After incision with epinephrine 1:200,000 for hemostasis, incisions are made down to bone, and suture lines are identified and exposed.
3. The depressed zygoma is elevated with a Kelly hemostat or periosteal elevator placed behind the body of the zygoma through the lateral eyebrow incision. Bone hooks placed percutaneously or at the fracture sites may be used instead.
4. Holes are drilled in bone on each side of the fracture lines. Stainless steel wires are passed through the hole and twisted down tightly to maintain the reduction. (Reduction and stabilization of two of the three fractures are sufficient.)
5. An alternative method of stabilization of the fractures is interosseous wiring of the zygomaticofrontal fracture and placement of a transmural Kirschner wire.
6. Incisions are closed.
7. An eye-patch dressing may be applied.

Reduction of orbital floor fractures

The orbital floor is the eggshell-thin bone on which the eye and periorbital tissues rest. It separates the orbit from the maxillary antrum. Orbital floor fractures usually occur in combination with fractures of the infraorbital rim (maxillary and zygomatic fractures). An isolated depressed orbital floor fracture with an intact infraorbital rim is called a blowout fracture.

Symptoms of orbital floor fractures are diplopia and en-

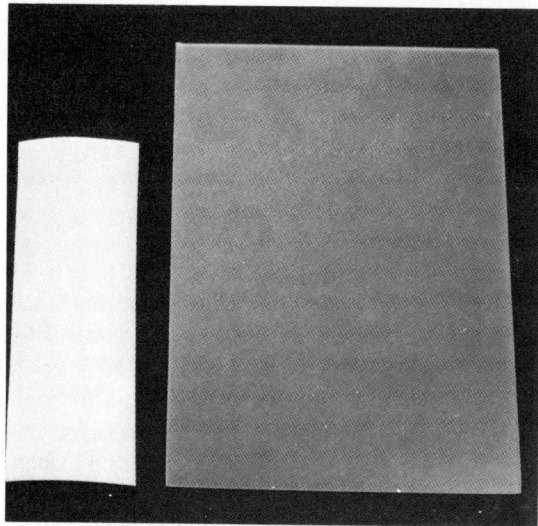

FIG. 23-38   Sheets of alloplastic implant material: *left,* Teflon; *right,* Silastic. Small segments are cut to fit for reconstruction of fractured orbital floor.

ophthalmos. Diplopia is caused by entrapment of periorbital fat and extraocular muscles in the fracture line, which restricts movement of the eyeball. Enophthalmos usually results from a fracture extensive enough to allow herniation of periorbital fat into the maxillary antrum, which gives the eye a sunken appearance. Treatment is directed toward relief of these symptoms.

Because the orbital floor is so thin, comminuted fractures occur frequently and segments of bone may be irretrievably lost into the maxillary antrum. If the floor cannot be reconstructed by elevating the bony fragments, its integrity must be restored with an implant (cartilage graft, bone graft, or alloplastic material).

Procedural considerations. A basic plastic instrument set is required, plus the following:

2 Blair retractors	Bipolar electrosurgical
Hall II air drill	unit
Alloplastic material of	Epinephrine 1:200,000
choice (Teflon or Si-	for injection
lastic sheet) (Fig. 23-	Rigid fixation system
38)	
Marking pen	

In addition, instruments and supplies listed for reduction of maxillary and zygomatic fractures may also be needed because orbital floor fractures often occur in combination with these fractures.

The patient is placed in the supine position on the OR bed. The head drape is used.

Operative procedure

1. A lower eyelid incision is marked and the eyelid injected

with epinephrine 1:200,000 for hemostasis and incised down to the infraorbital rim.
2. Periosteum is elevated from the infraorbital rim and orbital floor.
3. The fracture is identified, and any entrapped periorbital tissues are reduced by gentle traction.
4. Continuity of the orbital floor is reestablished by reducing the fracture, replacing any bone chips if possible, or inserting an autogenous graft or alloplastic implant.
5. The orbital floor implant is secured anteriorly to the infraorbital rim with a suture after a hole has been drilled in the bone.
6. The incision is closed in one layer (skin).
7. An eye-patch dressing may be applied.

ELECTIVE ORTHOGNATHIC SURGERY

A large number of patients are afflicted with either acquired or congenital facial defects that affect the maxilla and/or mandible. The condition of many of these patients can be improved dramatically with orthodontic care: however, many also require surgical rearrangement of the maxilla or mandible.

Psychosocial and functional deficits are related to abnormalities of the maxilla and mandible. Surgical correction of these defects can improve the quality of life for these patients. Surgery is usually delayed until an adequate number of permanent teeth are in place for postoperative immobilization. Proper preoperative planning is of great importance to these patients.

Operative procedure

1. Arch bars are applied for postoperative immobilization.
2. Intraoral incisions provide exposure.
3. The maxilla or mandible is cut as indicated by the preoperative workup.
4. Bone is advanced or set back to a predetermined position.
5. Bones are wired in place with grafts in defects as needed.

SURGERY FOR ACUTE BURNS

A majority of burns result from exposure to high temperatures, which injures the skin. Thermal skin injury may be caused by flame, scald, or direct contact with a hot object. Similar destruction of skin can result from contact with chemicals such as acid or alkali or contact with an electrical current. The latter, however, often involves extensive destruction of the underlying tissue and physiologic systems in addition to the skin.

Intact skin provides protection against the environment for all underlying tissues and organs. It aids in heat regulation, prevents water loss, and is the major barrier against bacterial invasion. Burn patients are therefore some of the most acutely ill patients brought to the operating room. The greater the degree of injury to the skin, expressed in percent of total body surface area (TBSA) and depth of burn, the more severe the injury. The most common method of measuring TBSA is by employing the rule of nines, in which the body is divided into areas equal to multiples of 9 (Box 23-1).

Partial-thickness (first- and second-degree) burns heal by regeneration of skin from dermal elements that remain intact. Full-thickness (third degree) burns require skin grafting to heal because no dermal elements remain intact. Both partial- and full-thickness burns may require débridement of necrotic tissue (eschar) before healing can occur by skin regeneration or grafting. Allograft may be used to cover the burned area during the initial healing process. However, the allograft must be carefully tested for immune deficiency diseases. Xenograft (for example, pig skin) may also be used for covering the burned area.

Procedural considerations. The essentials of skin grafting are discussed in the section on free skin grafts. This section therefore deals only with the procedure for débridement of burn wounds.

A basic plastic instrument set is required, plus a knife dermatome, an electrosurgical unit, topical thrombin solution, a pneumatic tourniquet for isolated extremity burns, and a topical antimicrobial agent of choice.

Because most burn wounds become infected within a few days, burns are contaminated, and appropriate operating room procedures are followed.

Most burn patients arrive in the operating room with dressings covering their wounds. These are removed after the patient has been anesthetized, to minimize pain and loss of body heat through the open burn wounds. The temperature in the operating room should be constantly monitored so that the patient's normal body temperature is maintained. The loss of heat from the body is increased by the lack of intact skin caused by a burn.

Operative procedure

1a. Nonviable tissue is excised down to underlying muscle fascia.

1b. An alternative method is tangential excision of the burn wound, which is performed with a knife dermatome. This type of excision is usually carried down only to subcutaneous fat, rather than to fascia.

2. Hemostasis is obtained with electrocoagulation or use of topical thrombin solution.

3. Dressings saturated with the topical antimicrobial agent of choice are applied.

Although skin grafting may be done at the time of wound débridement, it is usually performed several days later in burns that are extensive.

Cultured epithelial autografting (CEA)

In the event that the patient has been massively burned (greater than 90% of the body surface) or has a wound that would be open 21 days after injury, the need for coverage is critical. A skin biopsy (about the size of a postage stamp) is taken from the axilla, groin, postauricular area, and the sole of the foot. These areas, even in the situations of massive burn injuries, are sometimes available. The biopsy is then sent to a specific technologic laboratory where the full-thickness biopsy is placed in a specially developed culture medium, maintained nutritionally, and allowed to grow. Through the course of 21 days, and fastidious care of the cultured skin by the technology lab, the patient's wounds can be expected to be covered.

Procedural considerations. The previously described considerations for acute burn surgery can be followed. The cultured skin, when ready to be placed on the patient, is transported to the institution in a box that maintains a controlled atmosphere. The cultured skin, placed in individual plastic containers in the atmosphere-controlled box, is positioned on the patient's wound, stapled in place with nylon netting, and the dressings applied. Documentation of the number of cultured skin pieces as well as their location is done by use of photography and notation on the patient's record.

Operative procedure

1. The dressings, Biobrane, or pig skin (if applicable) is removed to expose the burn wound.

2. The cultured skin is applied.

3. The cultured skin is secured with nylon netting, which is stapled in place.

4. Hemostasis is achieved with electrocoagulation and topical hemostatic solutions.

5. The wound is dressed using large pieces of flat gauze, Webril, and Kling wrap.

ESTHETIC SURGERY

Esthetic surgery is usually performed with the patient under local anesthesia with sedation. The perioperative nurse must be prepared to monitor the patient during the procedure. Baseline vital signs should be recorded on the operating room record. A blood pressure cuff, pulse oximeter, and cardiac monitor electrodes should be placed. Intrave-

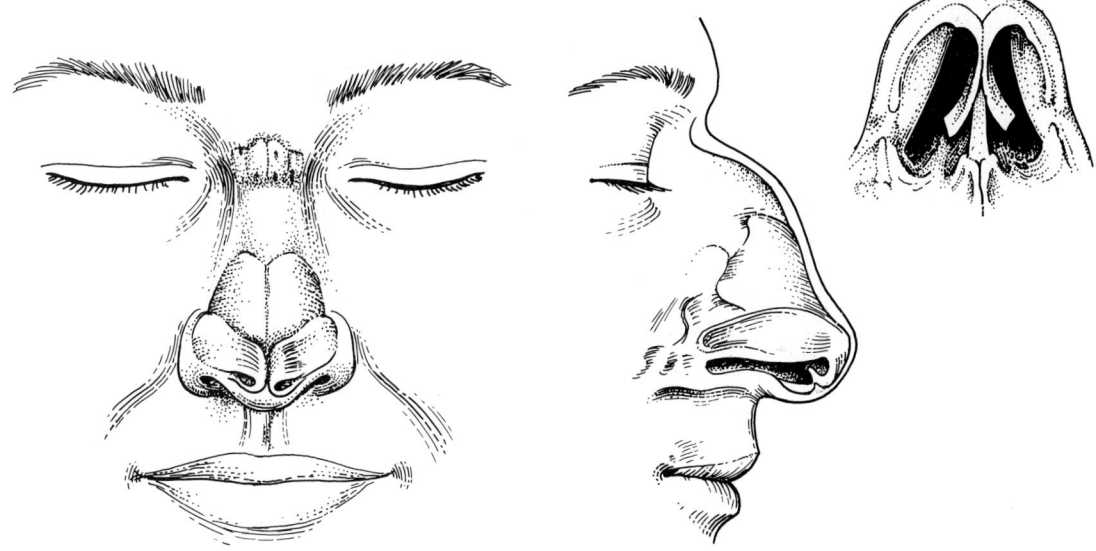

FIG. 23-39   Skeleton of abnormal nose with soft tissues superimposed.

nous fluids should be started. The operating room should be kept quiet and patient privacy protected. Care should be taken to avoid conversation that could be misinterpreted by the patient.

Rhinoplasty

Deformities of the external nose and nasal septum may be congenital or secondary to previous trauma (Fig. 23-39). The goal of rhinoplasty is to improve the appearance of the external nose. This is accomplished by reshaping the underlying framework of the nose, which allows the overlying skin and subcutaneous tissue to redrape over the new framework. Reshaping the nasal skeleton usually includes rasping down of a dorsal hump, partial excision of lateral and alar cartilages, shortening of the septum, and osteotomy of nasal bones. A procedure to alter the nasal septum, *septoplasty* or *submucous resection* (SMR), often accompanies rhinoplasty.

The goal of SMR is to improve the nasal airway by resecting a segment of septal cartilage. Septoplasty reshapes the existing septal cartilage; it may aid in altering the appearance of the nose or in improving the airway.

Rhinoplasty is performed through incisions made inside the nose; it therefore leaves no visible scars. Small external incisions at the alar bases and near the nasal bridge are also used to narrow the nose.

Procedural considerations. A plastic local instrument set is required, plus the following special instruments (Fig. 23-40):

1 Jansen-Middleton septal forceps	1 Formon retractor
4 Metal applicators and wisps of cotton	3 Pituitary rongeurs, assorted sizes, straight and upturned
1 Aufricht nasal retractor	1 Nasal scissors, angled

1 Kazanjian nasal forceps	1 Mallet
1 Fomon lower lateral scissors	1 Brown nasal rasp (upward stroke)
2 Joseph button-end knives, straight and angular	1 Maltz nasal rasp (downward stroke)
1 Ballenger swivel knife, straight	1 Diamond rasp (optional)
2 Joseph saws, 1 right and 1 left	Fomon rasp
2 Chisels, 2 mm and 4 mm	Aufricht rasp
	Silver osteotomes
1 Cinelli double-guarded osteotome, straight	1 Nasal septum forceps (for SMR)
	Brown nasal splint
2 Guarded chisels, straight, right and left	Nasal packing
	Fiberoptic light source and headlight (optional)

Rhinoplasty may be performed with the patient under local anesthesia. A separate local anesthetic setup should contain the following:

Bayonet forceps	Needles, 30 gauge and 25 gauge × 1½ inches
Sponges	
Local anesthetic of choice, topical and local	Petrolatum gauze for nasal packing
Syringe, 10 ml	Atomizer (optional)

Intravenous fluids are started, and a blood pressure cuff, pulse oximeter, and cardiac monitor electrodes are placed. Allergies are screened for and baseline vital signs obtained before initiation of local anesthesia.

From this setup (before scrubbing), the surgeon can do the preliminary nasal preparation, inject the local anesthetic, and pack the nose with gauze or cotton soaked in

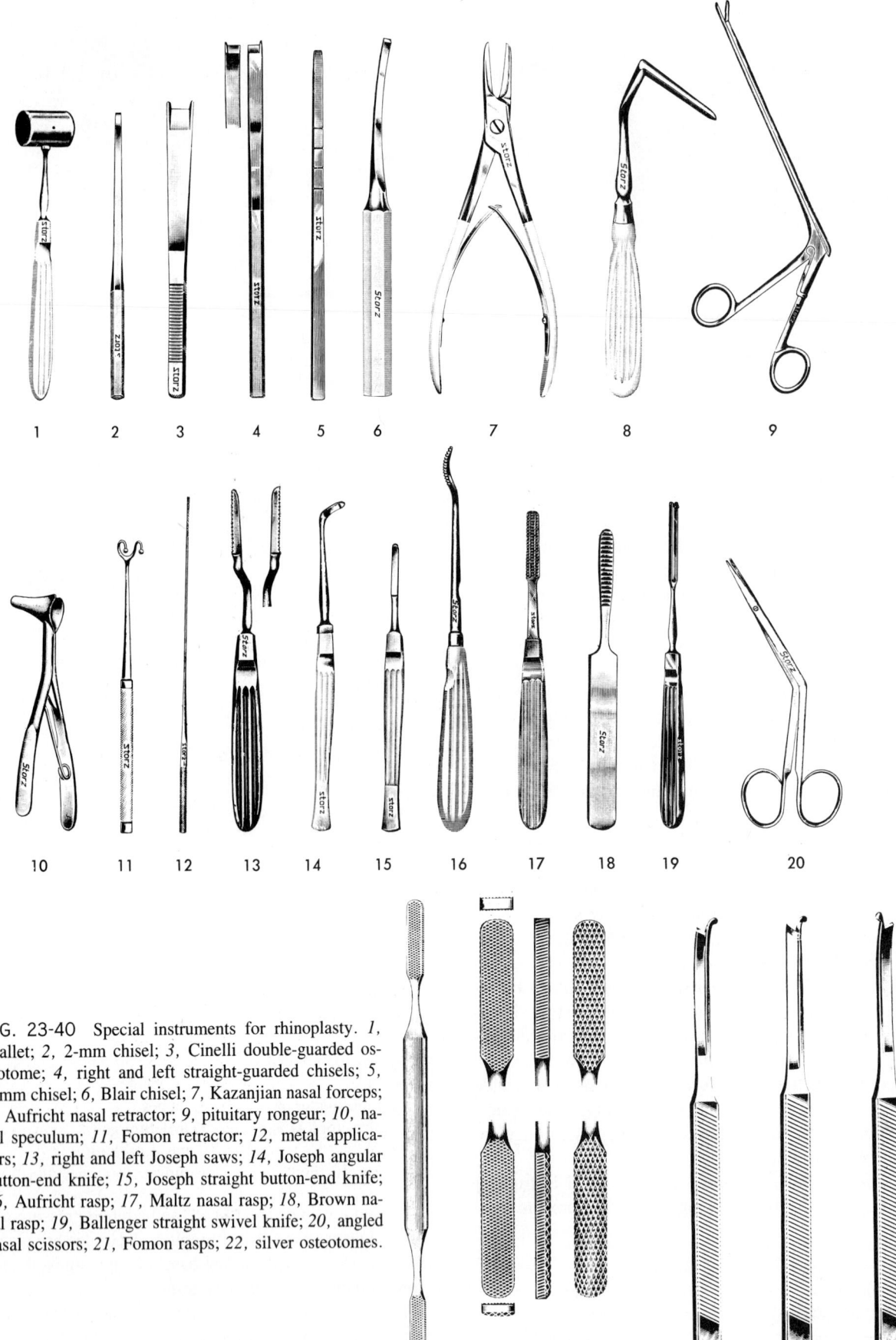

FIG. 23-40 Special instruments for rhinoplasty. *1*, Mallet; *2*, 2-mm chisel; *3*, Cinelli double-guarded osteotome; *4*, right and left straight-guarded chisels; *5*, 4-mm chisel; *6*, Blair chisel; *7*, Kazanjian nasal forceps; *8*, Aufricht nasal retractor; *9*, pituitary rongeur; *10*, nasal speculum; *11*, Fomon retractor; *12*, metal applicators; *13*, right and left Joseph saws; *14*, Joseph angular button-end knife; *15*, Joseph straight button-end knife; *16*, Aufricht rasp; *17*, Maltz nasal rasp; *18*, Brown nasal rasp; *19*, Ballenger straight swivel knife; *20*, angled nasal scissors; *21*, Fomon rasps; *22*, silver osteotomes.

4% cocaine solution. With this procedure the local anesthesia can take effect while the surgeon is scrubbing.

The patient is placed in the supine position on the OR bed. The face is prepped and an ophthalmic ointment may be placed in the eyes to diminish the potential for irritation. The head drape is used. The surgeon may use a headlight while performing the operation.

Operative procedure

1. Topical and local anesthetics are administered by the surgeon. The topical anesthetic is applied with applicator sticks or an atomizer.
2. Intranasal incisions are made, and the skin and soft tissues of the nose are elevated from the underlying nasal bones and cartilage.
3. The tip of the nose is reshaped by excising portions of the alar and lateral cartilages on each side.
4. The nasal dorsum (hump) is reduced by removing portions of the bone and septum.
5. The nasal bridge is narrowed by means of medial and lateral osteotomies of the nasal bones.
6. The intranasal incisions are sutured.
7. Bilateral anterior nasal packs are inserted, and a nasal splint and drip pad (moustache dressing) applied. Cool compresses may be immediately applied to decrease swelling and bruising.

If an SMR is performed at the time of rhinoplasty, it usually immediately precedes step 2. Septoplasty may be performed at any time during the operative procedure.

Blepharoplasty

The aging process causes a sagging or relaxation of eyelid skin and the orbital septum. As the latter becomes weaker, it allows periorbital fat to bulge. These changes are perceived as baggy eyelids, which give the patient a chronically tired appearance. The goal of blepharoplasty is to improve the patient's appearance.

Loose skin and protruding periorbital fat of the upper and lower eyelids is removed. The upper eyelid skin can be so redundant that it encroaches on the patient's field of vision. Blepharoplasty is often performed with rhytidectomy.

Procedural considerations. A plastic local instrument set is required, as well as two Blair retractors, a bipolar or monopolar electrosurgical unit, a marking pen, and a local anesthetic.

Blepharoplasty is usually performed with the patient under local anesthesia with sedation. Intravenous fluids are started, and a blood pressure cuff, pulse oximeter, and cardiac monitor electrodes are applied. Allergies are screened for and baseline vital signs recorded.

The patient is placed in the supine position on the OR bed. The face is prepped and the head drape is used.

Operative procedure (Fig. 23-41)

1. The local anesthetic is injected after the incision lines have been marked bilaterally.
2. An ellipse of excess skin is excised from the upper eyelids.
3. After a strip of the orbicularis oculi muscle and orbital septum is incised or removed, protruding periorbital fat is excised and coagulated.
4. The upper eyelid incisions are sutured in one layer.
5. The lower eyelid incisions are made close to the ciliary margin or through a transconjunctival approach when only fat is to be excised.
6. A skin flap or skin-muscle flap is elevated away from the orbicularis oculi muscle.

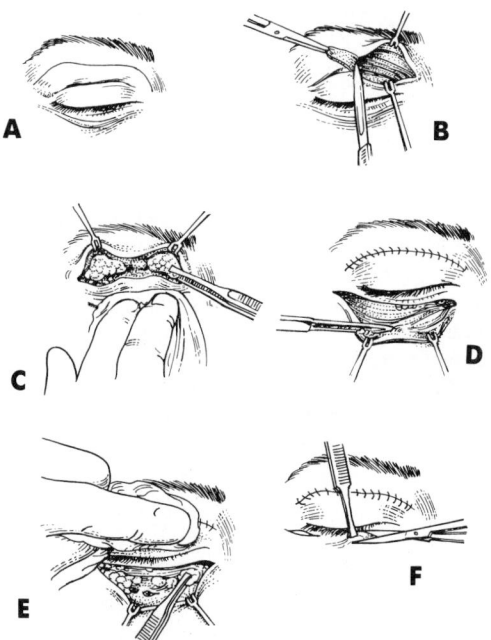

FIG. 23-41 Blepharoplasty for baggy eyelids. **A,** Areas of proposed skin excision marked with methylene blue or marking pen. **B,** Strip of skin excised from upper lid; fat pad shining through orbital fascia and orbicular muscle of eye. **C,** Orbital fascia opened in two places (medially and laterally). Pressure on eyeball causes fat pads to bugle. They are eased out meticulously. **D,** Upper lid incision sutured with continuous no. 6-0 silk. Orbicular muscle fibers are separated from skin. **E,** Orbital fascia opened; fat pads bulge because of digital pressure and are teased out meticulously. **F,** Skin tailored to fit and sutured.

7. Protruding periorbital fat is excised from beneath the orbicularis muscle.
8. The skin flaps are draped over the lower eyelids, and any excess skin is excised. Removal of too much skin from the lower eyelid can cause an ectropion.
9. The lower eyelid incisions are sutured in one layer.
10. Finely crushed ice on moist gauze 4 × 4 pads is applied to the eyes.

Rhytidectomy (facelift)

As the aging process progresses, the skin of the face and neck becomes loose and redundant. This is particularly noticeable in the "jowl" areas and just beneath the chin. A rhytidectomy is designed to improve the patient's appearance by removing some of the excess skin and sometimes the excess fat of the neck. Rather than excising the redundant skin directly, incisions adjacent to or within hairlines are used so that the scars are virtually indiscernible.

Procedural considerations. A basic plastic instrument set is required, plus the following:

1 Gorney or Kaye facelift scissors	Rhytidectomy retractor (optional)
2 Deaver retractors, 1 inch	Metzenbaum scissors, long
2 Army-Navy retractors	Marking pen
2 Cushing tissue forceps, 7 inches	Bipolar electrosurgical unit
2 Brown-Adson forceps	Fiberoptic light source
2 Cushing dressing forceps, 7 inches	Local anesthetic agent of choice
6 Burlisher clamps, curved	Skin stapler

A rhytidectomy may be performed with local anesthesia with sedation or using general anesthesia. Intravenous fluids are started, and a blood pressure cuff, pulse oximeter, and cardiac monitor leads applied. The patient is placed in the supine position on the OR bed. The hair and face are prepped and the head drape is used. Minimal or no hair is shaved.

Operative procedure (Figs. 23-42 and 23-43)

1. Bilateral incision lines are marked—from the temporal scalp, in front of the ear in a natural skin wrinkle line, around the earlobe, onto the posterior surface of the ear, and into the occipital scalp.
2. The incision lines, both temples, cheeks, upper neck, and the submental area are injected with the local anesthetic agent.
3. After the incisions are made, large flaps of skin and subcutaneous tissue are elevated from the face and upper third of the neck, meeting in the midline in the submental area and exposing the SMAS (superficial muscular aponeurotic system) and platysma. The SMAS and platysma are tightened, trimmed, and sutured behind and above the ears.
4. The edges of the flap are grasped with Allis forceps, and superior and posterior traction is placed on the flaps. The excess fat is removed, the platysma is plicated in the midline, and the neck is contoured. Suction may be used for the contouring.
5. Excess skin at the flap edges is excised, which pulls tight the tissue in the previously redundant areas.
6. Drains, if used, are inserted.
7. Incisions are closed in one or two layers.
8. A moderate pressure dressing is applied.

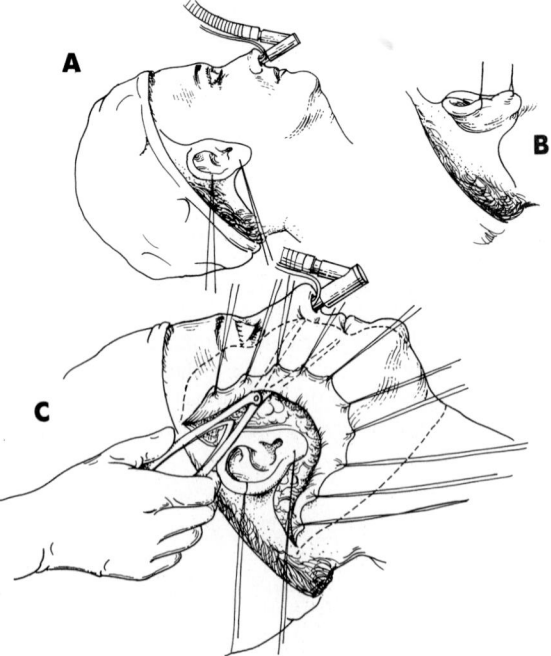

FIG. 23-42 Rhytidectomy: line of incision and undermining. **A,** Traction sutures of no. 4-0 silk placed in auricle; temporal incision curved posteriorly for better support of upward pull. **B,** Incision carried under earlobe and then curved posteriorly upward and then caudad toward midline. **C,** Skin undermined almost to nasolabial fold, to area of mental foramen, and to midline of neck as far down as thyroid cartilage. Care is taken to avoid injury to submandibular branches of facial nerve and facial artery.

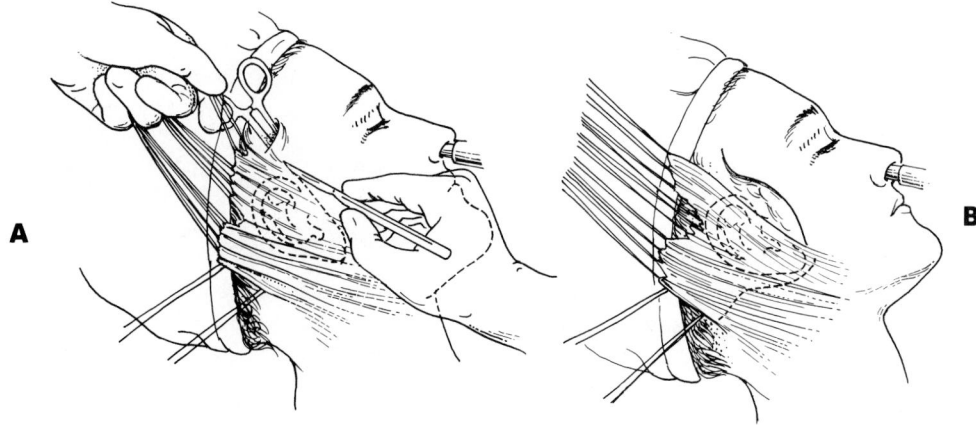

FIG. 23-43   Rhytidectomy: removal of superfluous skin. **A,** Skin drawn upward to proper degree of tension and incision made along posterior margin of clamp. **B,** Incision continued upward around posterior margin of auricle and then backward to excise skin specimen.

Dermabrasion

Sanding or planing of the skin is done primarily to smooth scars and surface irregularities of the skin. Dermabrasion is most commonly performed to improve the appearance of facial scars, especially the irregular scars resulting from acne vulgaris. It may also be used for the removal of foreign body tattoos. It is less successfully used for removal of professional body tattoos and to smooth fine wrinkle lines of the face.

The goal in treating irregular surfaces with dermabrasion is to sand or plane down the high points of elevations so that the low ones appear less deep. Dermabrasion removes epidermis and a portion of the dermis of the skin. Healing occurs from residual dermal elements, as in partial-thickness burns or split-thickness skin graft donor sites.

Procedural considerations. Instrumentation includes a plastic local instrument set, dermabrader, marking pen, and protective goggles.

The operation may be performed with the patient under general or local anesthesia. The patient is positioned and draped so that the area to be dermabraded is well exposed.

Operative procedure

1. The bases of pitted scars and depressions are marked.
2. The skin is planed with the dermabrader.
3. A single layer of the dressing of choice is applied to the dermabraded area.

Scar revision

This involves the rearranging or reshaping of the existing scar by means of a scar revision procedure so that the scar is not as noticeable. The simplest form of scar revision is excision of an existing scar and simple resuturing of the wound. This may improve scars that are wide.

The Z-plasty is the most widely used method of scar revision. It breaks up linear scars, rearranging them so that the central member of the Z lies in the same direction as a natural skin line. Scars that are parallel to skin lines are less noticeable than scars that are perpendicular to skin lines. A contracted scar line also can be lengthened to a limited extent with a Z-plasty.

Procedural considerations. A plastic local instrument set and a marking pen are required.

The operation may be performed under local or general anesthesia. The patient is positioned, prepped, and draped so the scar that is to be revised is well exposed.

Operative procedure

1. The pattern for the planned revision is marked.
2. The scar is excised.
3. The surrounding tissue is undermined and the wound edges approximated according to the surgeon's markings.
4. Dressings may or may not be applied.

Abdominoplasty

Abdominoplasty is particularly useful in improving the appearance (and to a certain extent, function) of persons who have lost a great deal of weight. Obesity produces distention and stretching of the skin of the abdomen. Although weight loss reduces the volume of the underlying fat, it does not produce concomitant reduction in the excess surface area of the overlying skin, resulting from destruction or insufficiency of elastic fibers in the skin. The stretched skin remains as an apron that hangs from the lower abdomen, sometimes as far as the knees. The rectus abdominis fascia is also stretched in obese patients, and weight loss does not restore its integrity.

Abdominoplasty is usually performed to remove redundant skin and fat of the lower abdomen; it also repairs any laxity of the rectus muscle.

Procedural considerations. A basic plastic instrument set is required, as well as extra retractors and clamping instruments, an electrosurgical unit, and a marking pen. Antiembolism hose are usually in place or applied in the operating room.

The patient is placed in the supine position, with slight flexion at the hips. Draping is such that the entire abdomen, lower costal margins, upper thighs, and both anterior iliac spines are exposed.

Operative procedure

1. A low, transverse abdominal incision across both inguinal areas laterally and the superior border of the mons pubis in the midline is marked and incised down to fascia.
2. A large flap of skin and subcutaneous tissue is elevated away from the fascia of the anterior abdominal wall.
3. The umbilicus is left in its normal position.
4. The abdominal flap is elevated further until the xiphoid process of the sternum and the lower costal margins are reached.
5. If diastasis of the rectus abdominis fascia is present, plication is performed from the xiphoid process to the mons pubis.
6. The flap of abdominal skin and subcutaneous tissue is pulled inferiorly, and excess tissue is excised.
7. A small incision is made in the midline of the flap to accommodate the umbilicus, which is then sutured peripherally to the flap.
8. Drains may or may not be used, followed by closure of the lower abdominal incision in two layers.
9. Postoperatively the patient is placed in the hospital bed in high Fowler's position.

Suction lipectomy

In this body-contouring technique, a slender cannula is inserted into the subcutaneous layer and fat is aspirated by vacuum. Suction lipectomy may be used for body contouring on the buttocks, flanks, abdomen, thighs, upper arms, knees, ankles, and chin. Suction lipectomy is not a substitute for weight loss, and it is not a cure for obesity. Plastic surgeons prefer to do this procedure on relatively young patients, those under the age of 40, because the skin of younger patients readily contracts to the newly contoured frame. The procedure may be done in a hospital or an ambulatory surgery facility.

Immediate preoperative preparation includes asking the patient to stand while the area of deformity is outlined. Two lines are usually drawn on the skin surface, one delineating the major area of defect, the other placed a short distance outside the first area. These lines make it easier for the plastic surgeon to make a smooth transition toward the normal tissue by adjusting the amount of fat removed from

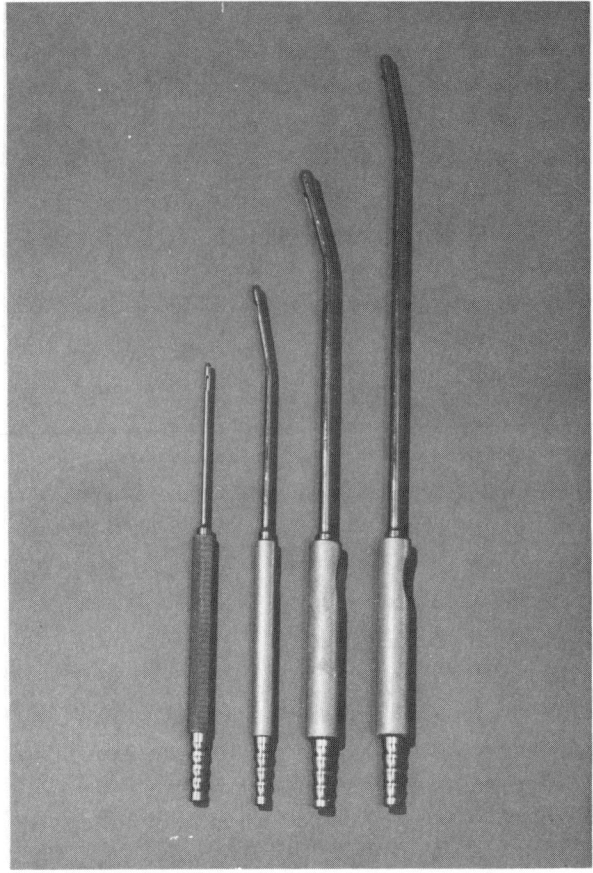

FIG. 23-44   Suction lipectomy curettes.

the center to the periphery of the deformity. The patient may remain standing and be prepped circumferentially with a spray bottle of warm iodophor solution. Care should be taken to protect the patient's privacy.

Procedural considerations. A plastic local instrument set is used. A general anesthetic is administered.

Operative procedure

1. A small incision from ½- to 1-inch long is made in the area closest to the deformity that can best be concealed.
2. A suction curette or blunt cannula (Fig. 23-44) is inserted through the incision.
3. The curette is attached to a firm suction tubing and connected to the aspirating (suction) unit (Fig. 23-45).
4. The high vacuum pressure created by the unit causes the fat cells to emulsify so that they can be suctioned through the vacuum opening near the rounded tip of the curette.
5. The incision is closed by one or two sutures, and a bulky pressure dressing is applied to the area.
6. Compression garments may be applied to maintain even pressure. Taping may also be used, based on the surgeon's preference.

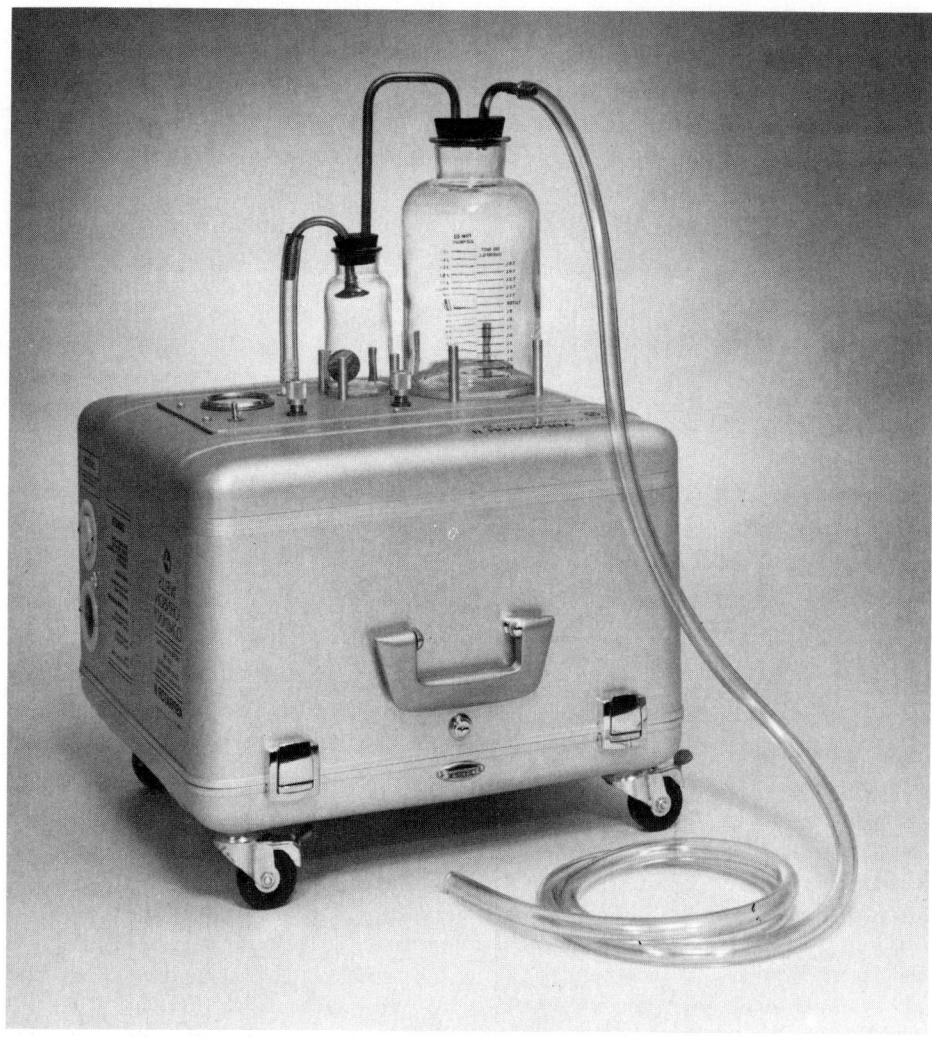

FIG. 23-45   Suction lipectomy vacuum machine and tubing.

TREATMENT OF PRESSURE ULCERS

Pressure ulcers result from prolonged compression of soft tissues overlying bony prominences. However, whether excessive pressure is sufficient to create an ulcer depends on the intensity and duration of the pressure as well as tissue tolerance. Other factors that contribute to pressure ulcer development are shearing force, friction, and nutritional debilitation. The most common sites of pressure ulcers are the sacrum (23%), the ischium (24%), the trochanter (15%), the malleolus (7%), and the heel (8%) (Bryant, 1992). Surgical interventions for pressure ulcers are usually based upon ulcer staging (also referred to as grading). In stage I the ulcer involves the epidermis and has soft tissue swelling that is irregular and ill defined; heat and erythema at the ulcer site are characteristic. A stage II ulcer involves the epidermis and dermis, but not subcutaneous fat. Stage III ulcers show full-thickness skin loss with injury to underlying tissue layers and may contain necrotic

material. Thorough débridement is performed and intravenous antibiotic therapy is instituted. Although débrided stage III ulcers often heal on their own, surgical excision and closure may be done to prevent a lengthy spontaneous closure that may result in a weak, unstable scar, with resultant recurrence. Stage IV ulcers are the deepest, requiring more radical débridement. Adequate soft tissue cover may be obtained by either split-thickness or full-thickness skin grafting or tissue flaps. Tissue expansion may be utilized where there is not enough tissue adjacent to the ulcer site to provide flap coverage.

An alternative to the standard surgical approach is the use of the carbon dioxide laser (Research Highlight 23-2). The laser offers the advantage of minimizing blood loss and possibly reducing infection rates in the presence of gross contamination.

Although many techniques and flaps are surgical options, basic principles apply to all pressure ulcer closure

BOX 23-2

Basic Principles of Pressure Ulcer Closure

1. The patient is positioned on the OR bed to mimic the position of maximal tension on the flap. This prevents wound dehiscence secondary to tension upon patient positioning postoperatively.
2. Perioperative prophylactic antibiotic therapy specific to wound culture is in order. Forty-eight hours of intravenous therapy is required. Although some authors have found quantitative cultures helpful, most have not found them necessary. Even in patients with a radiologic diagnosis of osteomyelitis additional antibiotic therapy is not needed because all involved bone should be excised at the time of closure.
3. Ostectomy of bony prominence is necessary to increase the surface area upon which the patient rests. Total ischiectomy is no longer favored because the weight redistribution results in ulcers on the opposite side or on the perineum.
4. The entire ulcer is excised in pseudotumor fashion, leaving only healthy, unscarred tissue. This also removes the contaminated granulation tissue, thereby decreasing postoperative infection rates.
5. Incisions are planned to allow for possible recurrences in the same or a different location. Since recurrences are common, the surgeon must be sure that planned incisions do not violate potential future flaps.
6. Incisions are planned to avoid suture lines over bony prominences. Scar tissue directly over a bony prominence predisposes the patient to future pressure ulceration.
7. The defect resulting from excision is filled with healthy, unscarred, well-vascularized tissue. This filling-in prevents seroma formation and allows for rapid wound healing.
8. A closed drainage system is used to prevent seroma formation. Drainage can be significant in the early postoperative period. Drainage systems can be discontinued when drainage is minimal (usually 5 to 7 days).
9. Postoperatively the patient is placed in a prone position or on a specialty bed, which provides pressure relief and eliminates shear (such as an air-fluidized bed). A period of 3 weeks prone or in a specialty bed is a minimum requirement.
10. Mobility is gradually increased beginning week 3 postoperatively with careful monitoring of skin and suture lines.
11. Skin grafts are not used to close pressure ulcers because they are usually not durable enough in the long term.

From Bryant, R.A. (1992). *Acute and chronic wounds: Nursing management.* St. Louis: Mosby.

RESEARCH HIGHLIGHT 23-2

In this study 13 patients with stage IV sacral and ischial pressure ulcers underwent excision of the ulcer and immediate flap coverage with a gluteus maximus myocutaneous rotational flap using the CO_2 laser. At surgery the pressure sore was packed with a methylene blue–stained sponge to assist in identifying the ulcer margins. The ulcer and bursa were excised down to viable tissue with the laser. An osteotomy was done when indicated. The rotational flap was demarcated and the skin and subcutaneous tissue incised with the laser. The remainder of the procedure was performed with standard instruments. The mean age within the study group was 65 years; the majority of the patients were septic, malnourished, and debilitated, and four were paraplegic. All patients were treated with perioperative antibiotic therapy and placed on Clinitron or Klin-Air beds postoperatively. Final success rates were 85% for complete flap healing. Postoperative hospitalization averaged 17 days.

Zaccaria, A., Gudicello, F., Dudick, S., & Vozos, F.J. (1993). Treatment of stage IV pressure sores using the carbon dioxide laser. *Contemporary Surgery for Residents, 1*(4), 7-11.

procedures; these are presented in Box 23-2. The following procedure is for an adjacent flap.

Procedural considerations. A basic plastic instrument set is required, plus the following:

Osteotomes, assorted sizes, straight and curved	Duckbill rongeur
	Bone wax
	Dermatome of choice
Mallet	Electrosurgical unit
Gigli saw and handle	Marking pen
Curettes, assorted	Closed wound drainage system
Key periosteal elevator	

The patient is positioned and draped so that the pressure sore, adjacent flap donor site, and a skin graft donor site are well exposed.

Operative procedure

1. The area to be excised and the local flap are outlined.
2. The ulcer is excised along with the underlying bony prominence.
3. Large suction catheters are placed into the defect left by excision of the ulcer and beneath the flap.
4. The flap is sutured in place.
5. An STSG is usually used to resurface the flap donor site.
6. A stent dressing is placed over the skin graft, and gauze dressings or a plastic spray dressing are applied over the suture lines of the flap.

GENDER REASSIGNMENT

Transsexualism defines the condition in which an individual with chromosomes and internal and external organs normal to one sex identifies psychologically and socially with attributes of the opposite sex. Reassignment of sex by means of surgery is the last step to be taken in treatment of transsexuals. It is performed only after the patient has been treated with hormones of the opposite sex, has experienced a period of cross-gender living, and has had intensive psychiatric evaluation. Most institutions performing this type of surgery have gender-identity teams who evaluate and treat transsexuals. These teams usually include a variety of professionals: psychiatrist, psychologist, endocrinologist, plastic surgeon, urologist, gynecologist, and social worker.

The surgical techniques for assignment of male to female are technically easier. A breast augmentation may be performed if hormone therapy has not sufficiently changed breast size. Construction of the neovagina includes radical penectomy, bilateral orchiectomy, urethroplasty, perineal dissection, creation of a neovaginal vault, vaginoplasty, and vulvoplasty.

The surgical technique for female to male is technically more difficult and requires multiple surgical procedures. Considerations that must be addressed are twofold: a neophallus that will allow the patient to stand to void must be constructed, as well as a phallus that will permit stimula-tion of a sexual partner during intercourse. This may require a radial artery forearm free flap with a later-stage surgical insertion of a prosthesis for "stiffening."

HAND SURGERY

Plastic surgery of the hand is directed toward restoration of function. It deals with the treatment of acute injuries, as well as reconstruction in established deformities. A systematic surgical approach for the restoration of hand function includes (1) replacement of lost tissue covering; (2) restoration of bony architecture; (3) repair of severed nerves; (4) restoration of the motor unit, either by tendon repair, tendon graft, or tendon transfer; and (5) replantation of severed digits.

Surgical anatomy

The functional unit in hand surgery consists of the hand, digits, wrist, and forearm. Each of these structures has a *radial* and an *ulnar* side, as determined by its position in relation to the radius and ulna of the forearm, rather than a lateral and medial side. Each also has a *dorsal* and *volar*, or *palmar,* surface. To avoid confusion, the digits of the hand are referred to as the thumb and the index, long, ring, and little fingers.

The skeletal framework of the hand and wrist consists of three distinct parts: (1) the metacarpals, or bones of the

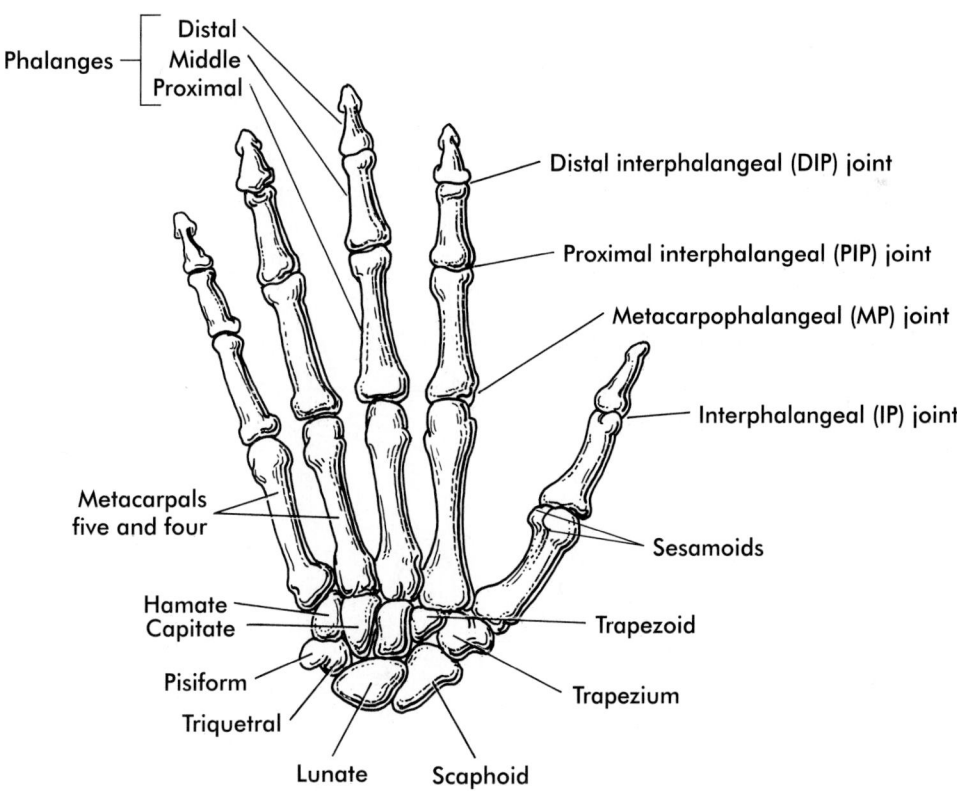

FIG. 23-46 Skeleton of wrist and hand, palmar view.

From Hollinshead, W.H.: *Anatomy for surgeons.* Vol. 3. The back and limb, ed. 2, New York, 1969, Harper & Row, Publishers.

hand; (2) the phalanges, or bones of the digits; and (3) the carpals, or bones of the wrist (Fig. 23-46). The five metacarpals articulate distally with the proximal phalanges of each digit at the metacorpophalangeal (MP) joints. The two bones of the thumb are the proximal phalanx and the distal phalanx, which articulate at the interphalangeal (IP) joint. Each of the four fingers contains three bones: a proximal phalanx, a middle phalanx, and a distal phalanx. Each finger therefore has three joints: (1) the metacarpophalangeal joint, (2) the proximal interphalangeal (PIP) joint between the proximal and middle phalanges, and (3) the distal interphalangeal (DIP) joint between the middle and distal phalanges.

The carpus (wrist) consists of eight bones arranged in two rows. The proximal row includes the scaphoid (navicular), lunate, triquetrum, and pisiform. The distal row includes the trapezium (greater multiangular), trapezoid (lesser multiangular), capitate, and hamate. The metacarpals articulate proximally with the distal row of carpal bones. The proximal row of carpal bones articulates with the radius and ulna of the forearm.

Motion of the thumb and fingers is achieved through the action of muscles intrinsic and extrinsic to the hand. The intrinsic muscles are those whose muscle bellies lie within the hand: (1) the interosseous and lumbrical muscles of the hand, which flex the MP joints while extending the PIP and

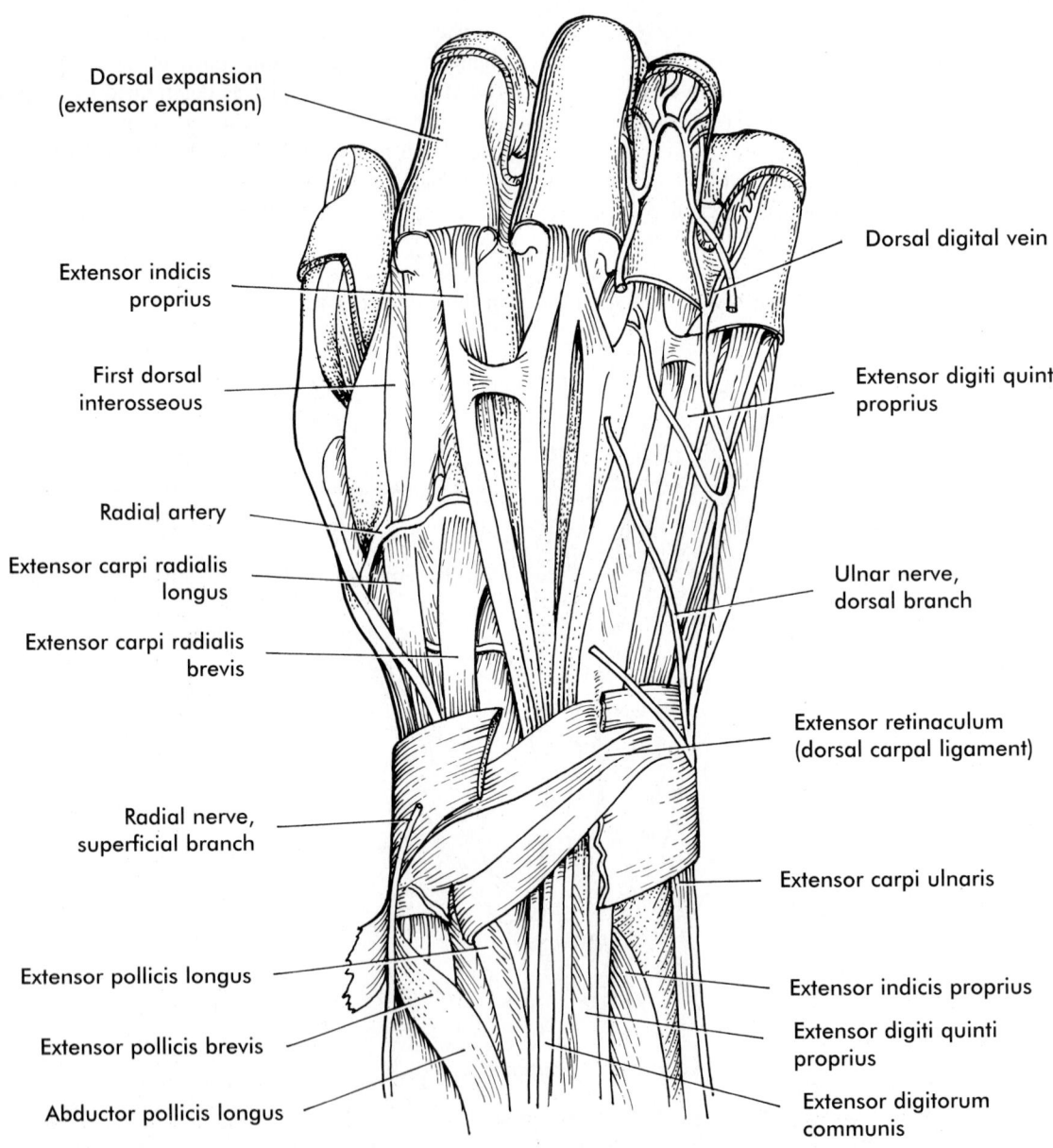

Dorsal expansion
(extensor expansion)

Extensor indicis
proprius

First dorsal
interosseous

Radial artery

Extensor carpi radialis
longus

Extensor carpi radialis
brevis

Radial nerve,
superficial branch

Extensor pollicis longus

Extensor pollicis brevis

Abductor pollicis longus

Dorsal digital vein

Extensor digiti quinti
proprius

Ulnar nerve,
dorsal branch

Extensor retinaculum
(dorsal carpal ligament)

Extensor carpi ulnaris

Extensor indicis proprius

Extensor digiti quinti
proprius

Extensor digitorum
communis

FIG. 23-47   Dorsum of hand and wrist; finger and long thumb extensor tendons pass under extensor retinaculum at wrist.

DIP joints and permit spreading and approximation of the fingers; (2) the muscles of the thenar eminence, which aid in adduction, abduction, flexion, and opposition of the thumb; and (3) the muscles of the hypothenar eminence, which aid in abduction, flexion, and opposition of the little finger.

The extrinsic muscles are so called because the muscle bellies are located in the forearm while the tendons pass into the hand, dorsally beneath the extensor retinaculum (Fig. 23-47), and volarly beneath the flexor retinaculum (Fig. 23-48) at the wrist, to insert on the phalanges of the thumb and fingers. The dorsal group consists of the extensor tendons, which extend the finger MP joints and the thumb MP and IP joints. The volar group consists of the flexor tendons, one for the thumb and two to each finger. The paired finger flexors are the superficial (sublimis) flexor tendons, which flex the PIP joints, and the deep (profundus) flexor tendons, which flex the DIP joints. In addition to the finger and thumb flexors and extensors, other muscles of the forearm have tendinous insertions that work to abduct the thumb and flex and extend the wrist.

Although hand movements are achieved by the action of various muscles and their tendons, muscle function depends on adequate innervation of the muscle belly. The motor nerves of the hand are (1) the radial nerve to the extensors, (2) the median nerve to a majority of the flexor tendons and

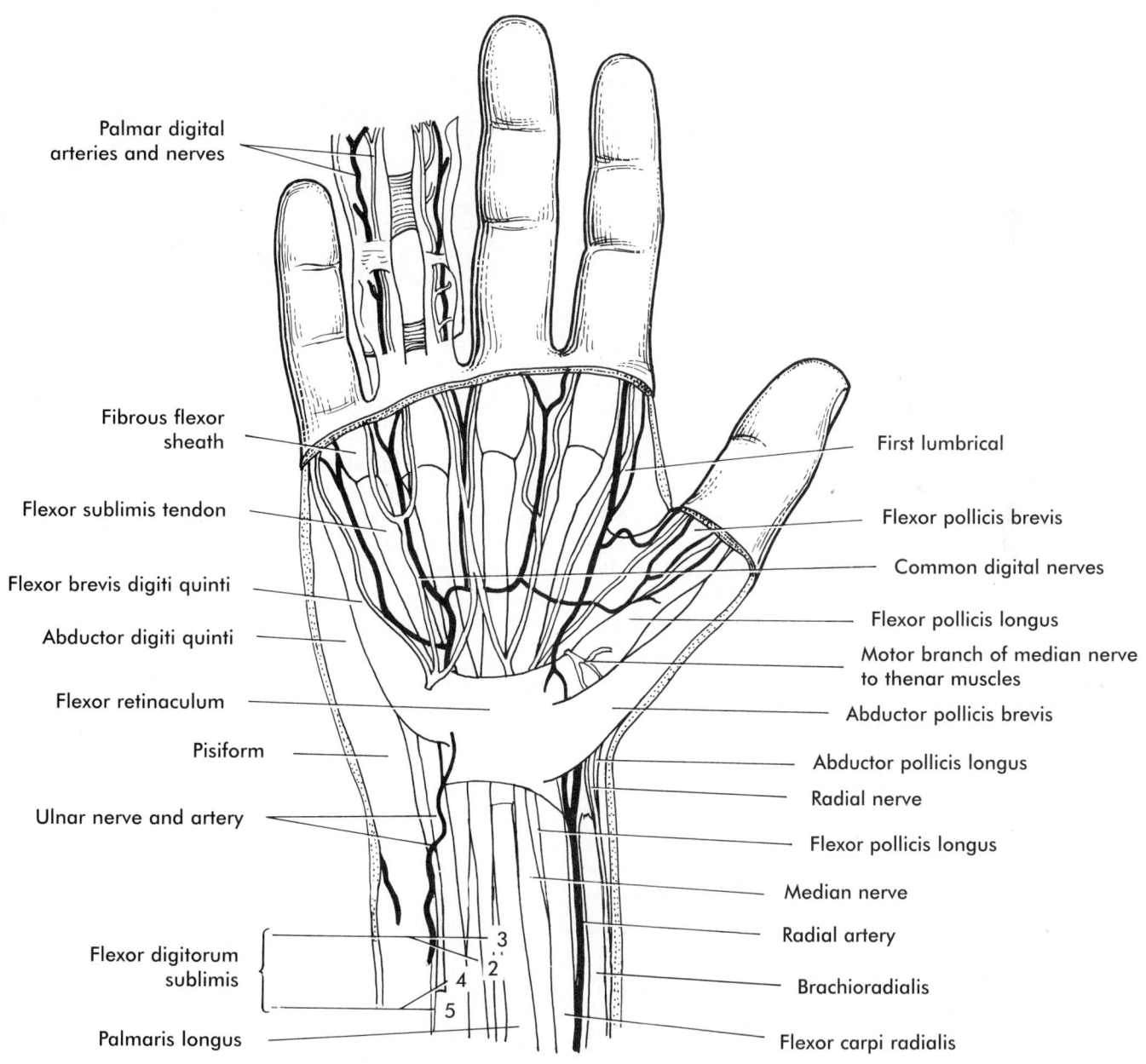

FIG. 23-48 Volar (palmar) surface of hand and wrist; median nerve, finger, and long thumb flexor tendons pass beneath flexor retinaculum (transverse carpal ligament) at wrist.

a few intrinsic muscles, and (3) the ulnar nerve to a majority of the intrinsic muscles and remaining flexors.

Sensation in the hand is provided by the same three nerves: (1) the radial nerve supplies the dorsal radial hand and fingers; (2) the median nerve, the volar (palmar) radial hand and digits (thumb, index, long, and radial side of the ring finger); and (3) the ulnar nerve, the remaining dorsal and volar ulnar hand and fingers. As the terminal sensory branches of the median and ulnar nerves enter the thumb and fingers, they are called digital nerves (see Fig. 23-48).

The principal blood supply for the hand is from the radial and ulnar arteries that form a superficial and deep palmar arch in the hand, giving off terminal branches to both sides of each digit, called digital arteries after they enter the fingers and thumb. A rich network of dorsal veins serves to return blood from the hand.

A minimum of skin and subcutaneous tissue covers the dorsum of the hand and digits. The skin covering the volar (palmar) surface is anchored to underlying fascia in areas of skin folds. Because of these fascial attachments, the skin and subcutaneous fat pads of the volar (palmar) surface do not move about during flexion and grasping of an object. The palmar fascia is a thick fibrous structure overlying the blood vessels, tendons, and nerves in the palm of the hand, to which skin is anchored, principally at the palmar skin creases. The palmar fascia sends extensions into each digit.

Special equipment
Tourniquet

Because it renders the operative field relatively bloodless, a tourniquet is almost essential in dealing with the complex, delicate, and vital structures within the hand. The tourniquet may be the pneumatic type, inflated with compressed gas, the pressure of which can be determined with an accurate gauge. Each tourniquet must be checked at regular intervals against a tourniquet test gauge (Fig. 23-49) or a mercury manometer to maintain the accuracy of its gauge. Electrically powered tourniquets are also available; these units have self-testing mechanisms and continuous readouts of tourniquet time and pressure. The tourniquet can be a dangerous device when not in good working order and when improperly used.

The arm cuff of the tourniquet should be smooth and broad so pressure is distributed evenly over a wide area. Sheet cotton (Webril) or a tourniquet cover may be wrapped smoothly around the limb where the tourniquet will be applied. It should be placed as far proximally on the arm as possible, where a greater amount of soft tissue provides padding for underlying nerves and blood vessels as they are compressed against bone when the tourniquet cuff is inflated. There should be no kinking of the tubing between the cuff and gas-regulating mechanism. To prevent a chemical burn, antimicrobial solutions used for skin preparation should not be allowed to run beneath the tourniquet cuff.

The arm is exsanguinated by progressively wrapping the arm from fingertips to tourniquet cuff (distal to proximal) with a 3-inch Esmarch rubber bandage. The tourniquet is

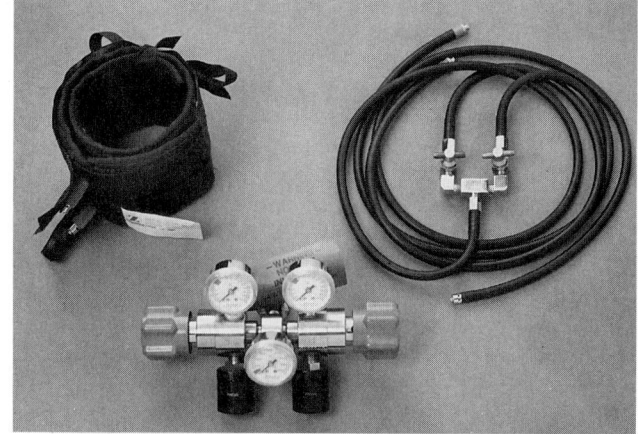

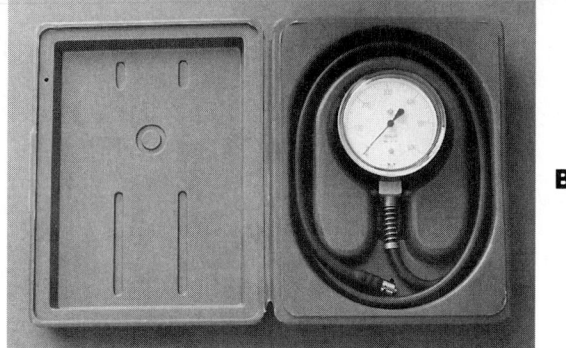

FIG. 23-49 Dual tourniquet cuff set for use with regional intravenous anesthesia. **A,** Dual cuff, dual control valves with tubing, and tourniquet pressure gauge (in mm Hg). **B,** Tourniquet test gauge.

quickly inflated to prevent filling superficial veins before occlusion of the arterial blood flow. The Esmarch bandage is removed after inflation of the tourniquet cuff. The amount of pressure used to inflate the tourniquet depends on the size of the extremity and the patient's age and systolic blood pressure.

Tourniquet time should be kept to a minimum. Times of inflation and deflation should be recorded. After completion of the surgical maneuver that required use of the tourniquet, deflation of the cuff should be accompanied by total removal of the tourniquet cuff from the arm. If the cuff is left on the arm after being deflated, it may cause some obstruction to the return of venous blood, which is perceived as increased bleeding at the operative site.

Boyes-Parker hand operating table (Fig. 23-50)

The hand table is used for most hand operations. Adjustable legs allow fitting to any standard operating room bed level. The legs also provide maximum stability of the operative field. The surgeon and assistants sit during the operation. A stainless steel pan with drain and plug may be placed in the hand table to facilitate irrigation of wounds.

Pulsatile irrigation

When the situation arises that a wound must be copiously irrigated, an electrically powered pulsatile irrigation

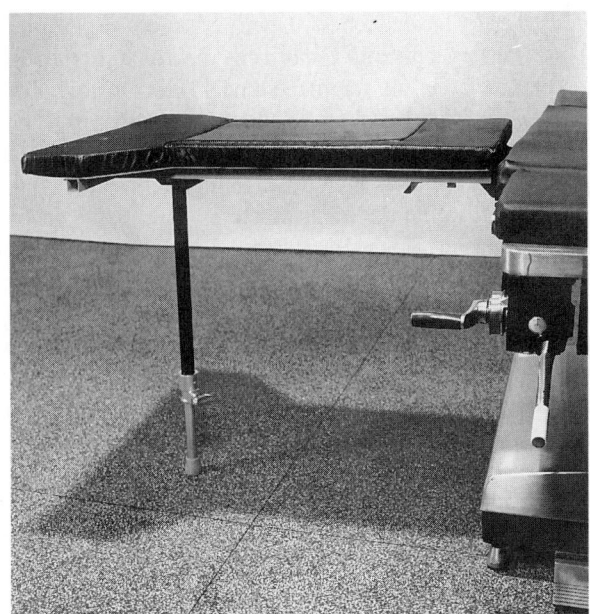

FIG. 23-50 Boyes-Parker hand operating table. Central segment slides out so stainless steel pan can be inserted during wound irrigation.

system can be employed. These systems are packaged in sterile, disposable kits, including pistol grip handles, assorted size irrigation tips, splash shields, spiked tubing for the solutions, and suction tubings. Antibiotics can be added to the irrigation solutions according to physician preference. Protective barriers should be used by the perioperative team to prevent splash exposure.

Intravenous regional anesthesia

Intravenous regional anesthesia (see Chapter 6) is often used for hand operations and may be administered by the surgeon or an anesthesiologist. A pneumatic tourniquet with a double cuff plus dual control valves and tubing (Fig. 23-49) is used. A butterfly needle is inserted into a vein of the affected extremity and secured with tape. The position of the needle within the vein is verified by irrigating with sterile saline solution in a 10-ml syringe, which is left attached to the tubing of the butterfly needle. An Esmarch bandage is used to exsanguinate the extremity and the *proximal* cuff of the tourniquet is inflated. After removal of the Esmarch bandage, 0.5% lidocaine is injected intravenously through the butterfly needle (usual dosage is 3 mg/kg of body weight, not exceeding a total dose of 250 mg). The butterfly needle is removed, and pressure is applied at the venipuncture site for several minutes. Prepping and draping of the patient usually follow.

The advantage of a tourniquet with a double cuff is as follows: When the patient experiences moderate discomfort from the proximal cuff pressure (approximately 30 minutes after inflation of the cuff), the *distal* cuff may be inflated. The distal cuff lies over an anesthetized area on

the arm, and the patient's discomfort should be reduced. After inflation of the distal cuff, the proximal cuff is deflated.

Dressings and immobilization

Basic conditions for good wound healing after hand surgery are immobilization and elevation. Adequate immobilization achieves support and splinting to protect against both active and passive motion. With most hand operations, because of many closely related movements, immobilizing the entire hand, fingers, wrist, and distal two thirds of the forearm is usually necessary. This immobilization is often maintained for 3 or 4 weeks after surgery. Application of the means of immobilization must therefore be performed with care while the patient is still anesthetized. Although plaster of Paris may be used to achieve immobilization, many surgeons prefer a soft, bulky hand dressing. Steps in the application of a hand dressing are as follows:

1. An assistant supports the hand, which is elevated by flexing the elbow and resting it on the hand table.
2. Nonadherent gauze is applied over incisions.
3. Gauze dressing sponges in thin layers are placed between the fingers to prevent maceration. These sponges must be uniform thickness from proximal to distal to prevent pressure on digital blood vessels.
4. A thicker layer of gauze is placed between the thumb and index finger to prevent an adduction contracture of the thumb. In addition to abduction, the thumb is also rotated into opposition as the dressing is applied.
5. Mechanic's waste or acrylic fiber is placed in the palm of the hand for bulk so that it can support the PIP and DIP joints of the fingers in extension. It may also be added to the thumb-index finger web space to maintain thumb abduction.
6. Folded abdominal pads are placed vertically across the dorsal and volar surfaces of the wrist for support.
7. Two Kling gauze rolls are wrapped around the hand and forearm so that the MP joints are in approximately 90 degrees flexion, the PIP and DIP joints are extended, the thumb is in abduction and opposition, and the wrist is in a neutral position. All fingertips must be exposed to permit inspection for determining viability.
8. Inch-wide strips of adhesive tape are applied vertically over the dressing (to avoid constricting bands).

Surgical interventions
Treatment of fractures

Fractures within the scope of hand surgery may involve the phalanges in the fingers, the metacarpals in the hand, and the carpals in the wrist. The basis for treatment of any fracture is reduction of the fracture and immobilization until healing occurs.

Reduction of a fracture may be closed or open. Closed reduction is performed by manipulating the fracture fragments beneath intact skin and subcutaneous tissue. X-ray

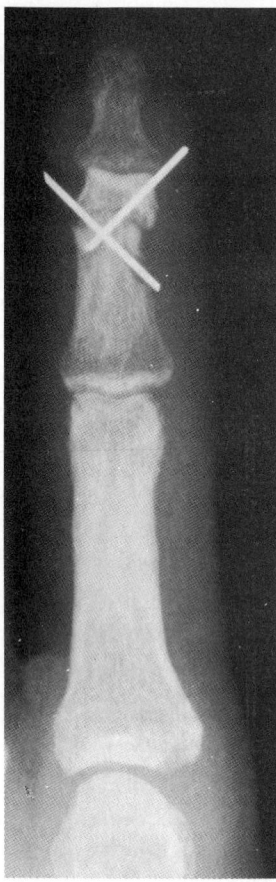

FIG. 23-51 Radiograph shows fracture of middle phalanx of index finger following open reduction, with internal fixation by means of crossed Kirschner wires across fracture site.

studies verify the reduction. Open reduction is performed by making an incision, visualizing the fracture site, and then manipulating the fragments under direct vision. X-ray films are usually also obtained after open reduction.

Immobilization of a fracture may be external or internal. External methods include splinting and casting. Internal immobilization in hand fractures is usually accomplished by inserting Kirschner wires (Fig. 23-51). This may be the sole method by which a reduction can be stabilized. It has the additional advantage of allowing motion in a maximum number of hand joints while immobilizing only the injured part, thus preventing unnecessary joint stiffness.

Procedural considerations. A plastic hand instrument set, a Kirschner wire driver, an Esmarch bandage, and a marking pen are required.

The patient is placed in the supine position on the OR bed, with the arm extended on a hand table. The hand drape is used.

Operative procedure (open reduction, internal fixation)

1. The incision is marked.
2. The pneumatic tourniquet is inflated after exsanguination.
3. The incision is made, and the fracture is exposed.
4. The fracture is reduced by manipulating the fragments digitally or instrumentally under direct vision.
5. While an assistant holds the reduced fracture, Kirschner wires are driven into bone, usually across the fracture site. (Miniscrews and plates may also be used as internal fixation.)
6. After x-ray films are obtained to verify the fracture re-

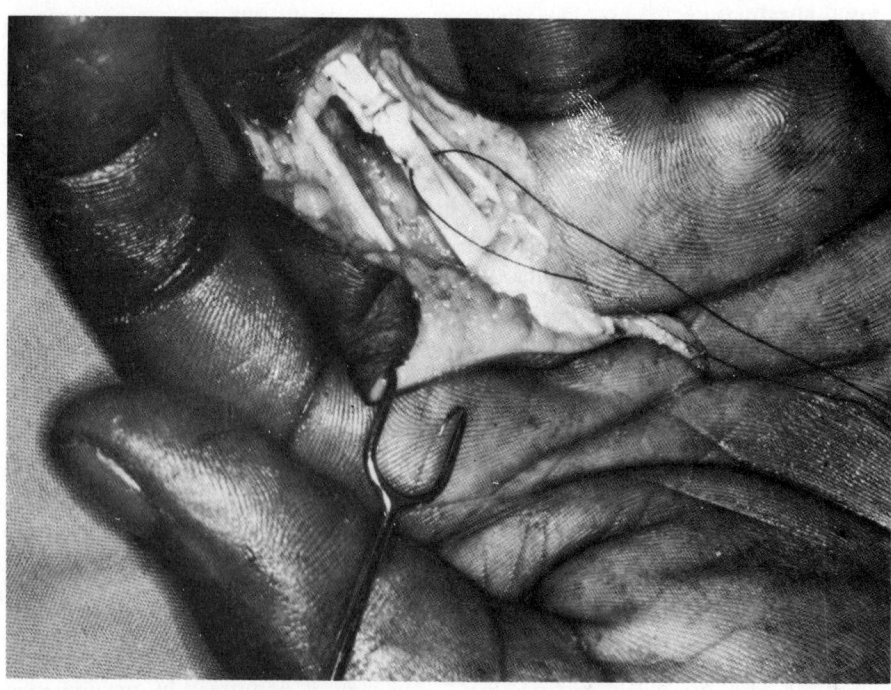

FIG. 23-52 Primary repair of flexor profundus tendon of long finger in distal palm.

duction and immobilization, the Kirschner wires are cut off so that the ends are buried beneath skin or with a short segment protruding through skin. This segment is twisted down with needle-nose pliers. (Fluoroscopy is also a frequently used option for these procedures.)

7. The incision is sutured in one layer (skin).
8. A hand dressing is applied.

Tendon repair

When continuity of a tendon is interrupted by avulsion or laceration, a specific active movement of one or more joints of the hand is lost. The treatment is tendon repair. Primary flexor or extensor tendon repair is usually performed at the time of injury or within several hours of the acute injury. When adequate tendon length is present on each side of the laceration, repair is performed by suturing the tendon ends together (Fig. 23-52). When the laceration is near the bony insertion of the tendon, the distal tendon segment is too short to permit adequate purchase for a suture. In this case tendon repair is performed by reinserting the proximal end of the tendon into bone.

Procedural considerations. A plastic hand instrument set, an Esmarch bandage, a marking pen, and no. 3-0 or 4-0, double-armed, nonabsorbable suture on Keith needles are required.

The patient is placed in the supine position on the OR bed, with the arm extended on a hand table. The hand drape is used.

Operative procedure

1. The skin laceration is usually enlarged to permit adequate exposure of the tendon laceration, after the skin extensions for the laceration are marked and the tourniquet is inflated.
2. An additional incision in the hand or wrist or both may be necessary to identify the retracted proximal tendon end.
3. The tendon is repaired by placing a no. 3-0 or 4-0, double-armed, nonabsorbable suture through the tendon ends and approximating the ends. A pullout suture may or may not be placed through the tendon suture.
4. If the repair involves reinsertion of the tendon into bone, a small bone flap is raised, a straight Keith needle is drilled through the bone with the hand drill, and the suture ends from the tendon are passed through the bone and are tied down over a foam-rubber padding and a polyethylene button.
5. Incisions are closed in one layer.
6. A hand dressing is applied.

Flexor tendon graft

A graft is used to restore function when the original tendon is incapable of so doing because of a large gap between ends of a lacerated tendon or because of a failed primary tendon repair. Although extensor tendon grafts are possible, the vast majority of free tendon grafts are flexor profundus and flexor pollicis longus tendon grafts. A gap large

enough to preclude approximation by direct suturing of the tendon ends results from loss of a segment of tendon at the time of injury or from shortening of the proximal tendon end if too much time has elapsed since the original injury. A failed primary tendon repair is usually caused by scar tissue that inhibits adequate tendon gliding. Tendon gliding must be sufficient to produce appropriate joint movement when the muscle belly of the tendon contracts. If a great deal of scar tissue is present in the tendon bed, a free tendon graft also may fail to glide sufficiently to produce adequate joint movement. In this case a rod may be inserted into the tendon bed. The scar tissue that forms around the rod creates a pseudosheath through which a tendon graft is placed 6 to 8 weeks later. The pseudosheath often permits better tendon gliding.

The most commonly used donor tendon for a free graft is the palmaris longus tendon in the wrist and forearm. The plantaris tendon in the leg is also frequently used. Toe extensor tendons are used less commonly.

Procedural considerations. A plastic hand instrument set is required, plus the following special instruments (Fig. 23-53):

1 Brand tendon stripper	1 Foam rubber pad, small
1 Sanders-Brown fascia needle	1 No. 4 Lane needle, taper cut point
1 Silver probe, 9 inches	1 Esmarch bandage
1 Hegar dilator, no. 6, with hole	Marking pen
1 Freer septal elevator with hole	Double-armed nonabsorbable suture, no. 3-0 or 4-0
1 Keith needle, straight	Tendon rod, 3 mm (optional)
1 Polyethylene button	
1 Goniometer	

The patient is placed in the supine position on the OR bed, with the arm extended on a hand table. The hand drape is used. If the plantaris tendon or a toe extensor tendon is to be used as the donor tendon, the lower extremity also must be prepped and draped. Use of a pneumatic tourniquet on the leg is optional.

Operative procedure

1. After marking incisions and inflating the pneumatic tourniquet, the surgeon makes a distal incision to expose the insertion of the flexor profundus tendon into the distal phalanx, and a proximal incision is made in the hand or wrist or both.
2. Scar tissue in the tendon bed is excised.
3. If the flexor tendon bed is not deemed suitable for a tendon graft, a rod is inserted and sutured distally to the profundus tendon remnant attached to the distal phalanx (Fig. 23-54).
4. If the tendon bed is suitable or a rod has previously been inserted, a free tendon graft is obtained with the Brand tendon stripper.
5. Approximation of the proximal tendon end and graft is performed in the palm or wrist.

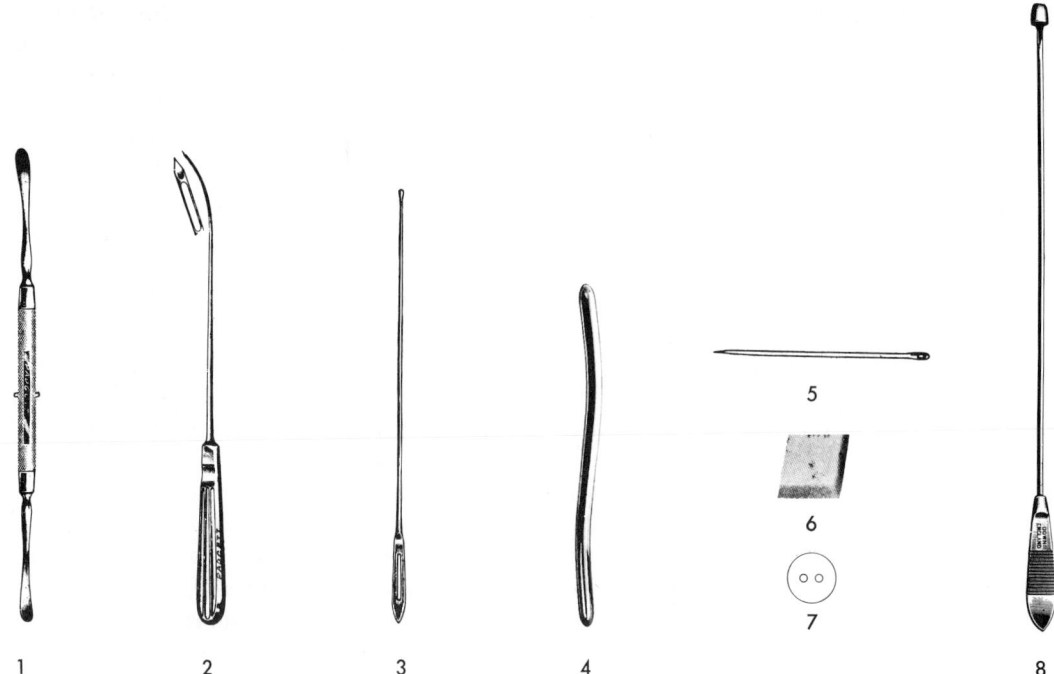

FIG. 23-53   Special instruments for flexor tendon graft. *1*, Freer septal elevator (with hole); *2*, Sanders-Brown fascia needle; *3*, silver probe; *4*, no. 6 Hegar dilator (with hole); *5*, Keith needle; *6*, foam rubber; *7*, polyethylene button; *8*, Brand tendon stripper.

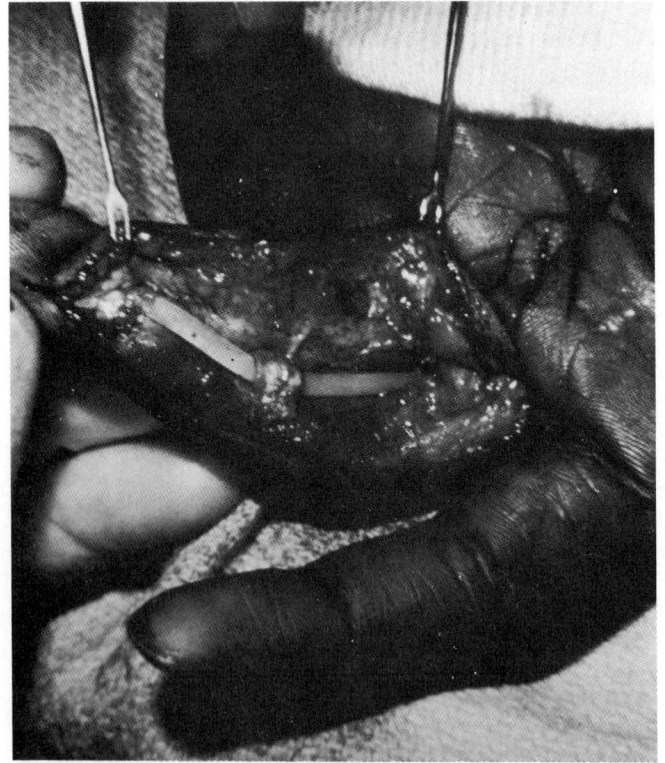

FIG. 23-54   Silicone rod placed into profundus tendon bed of long finger in preparation for flexor tendon grafting.

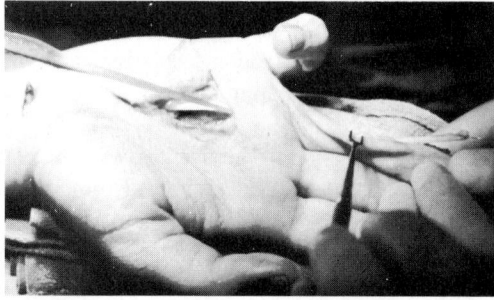

FIG. 23-55   Flexor tendon graft being threaded through profundus tendon bed of ring finger from palm to distal phalanx. Palmaris longus tendon has been obtained with Brand tendon stripper through small wrist incision.

6. The graft is threaded through the tendon bed to the distal phalanx (Fig. 23-55), where it is inserted as described in step 4 of tendon repair, after the tension of the graft has been carefully adjusted.
7. The incisions are closed in one layer.
8. A hand dressing is applied.

Peripheral nerve repair and grafting

Nerve repair is done by direct approximation of nerve or severed nerve ends or by means of a nerve graft to at-

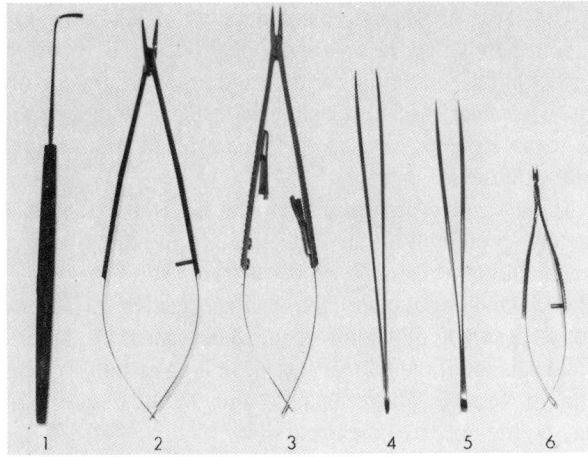

FIG. 23-56 Special instruments for nerve repair and grafting. *1*, von Graefe muscle hook; *2*, Castroviejo needle holder without lock; *3*, Castroviejo needle holder with lock; *4* and *5*, jeweler's forceps; *6*, Castroviejo-Vannas scissors.

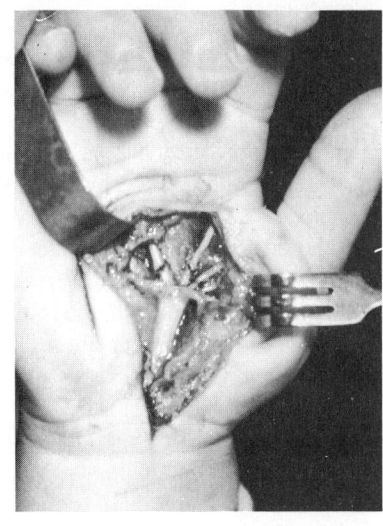

FIG. 23-57 Severed branches of median nerve have been reapproximated with fine sutures.

tempt to restore continuity of a nerve in the hand, wrist, or forearm and regain sensation or motor function.

Procedural considerations. A plastic hand instrument set is required, plus the following special instruments (Fig. 23-56):

1 Jeweler's forceps	Nerve hook (von Graefe
1 Castroviejo-Vannas	muscle hook)
scissors, curved	Nerve stimulator
2 Castroviejo needle	Esmarch bandage
holders, straight, with	Marking pen
and without lock	Loupes or operating
Razor blade	microscope

The patient is placed in the supine position on the OR bed, with the arm extended on a hand table. The hand drape is used. If a nerve graft is to be used, a lower extremity is also prepped and draped. Use of a pneumatic tourniquet on the leg is optional.

Operative procedure

1. After incisions are marked and the tourniquet is inflated, the proximal and distal nerve ends are exposed.
2. Devitalized nerve tissue or scar at the severed nerve ends is resected sharply with a razor blade, back to normal nerve tissue, where individual nerve bundles can be visualized.
3. With the aid of loupes or the operating microscope, individual nerve bundles are approximated (Fig. 23-57) with a fine, nonabsorbable suture (usually no. 7-0 to 10-0 nylon).
4. If a nerve graft is used, it is obtained through a series of short transverse incisions or one long vertical incision along the posterolateral aspect of the leg. Ap-

proximation of the nerve bundles between the graft and proximal and distal nerve ends is performed as in step 3.
5. The incisions are sutured, and dressings are applied. The hand dressing is applied so tension at the site of repair is prevented.

Implant arthroplasty

Destruction of the cartilage that forms the articular surface of a joint results in stiffness and pain during movement of the joint. Traumatic arthritis and rheumatoid arthritis are the most common causes of destruction of articular joint surfaces. Excision of the diseased joint surface affords relief of pain and improves joint motion. Insertion of an implant is an adjunct to resection arthroplasty. The implant serves as a dynamic joint spacer, not a joint prosthesis. In severe cases custom total joint prostheses may be used.

The most commonly used implants in hand surgery are flexible implants made of Silastic. Flexible implants available for arthroplasty within the scope of hand surgery are finger joints (for MP and PIP Joints), wristjoint, carpal trapezium, unate, and navicular(scaphoid).

Procedural considerations. A plastic and instrument set is required, plus the following:

Alloplastic rasps	Alloplastic implant of
Oscillating bone saw	choice with sizer
Hall II drill with Swan-	Esmarch bandage
son burrs	Marking pen

The patient is placed in the supine position on the OR bed, with the arm extended on a hand table. The hand drape is used.

Operative procedure

1. After the incision line is marked and the pneumatic tourniquet is inflated, the involved joint is exposed through an appropriate incision.
2. In finger joint resection arthroplasty, the joint surfaces are excised together with comprehensive soft tissue release of the joint capsule. In resection arthroplasty of a carpal bone, the involved bone is completely excised.
3. In finger joint arthroplasty, the medullary canals of the two adjacent bones are reamed with the Hall II drill with Swanson burrs. In carpal bone implant resection arthroplasty, holes are reamed in one appropriate adjacent bone.
4. The two stems of a finger or wrist joint implant or the single stem of a carpal bone implant is seated in adjacent bones.
5. Soft tissues of the joint capsule (ligaments, tendons) are repaired.
6. The skin incisions are closed.
7. A hand dressing is applied.

Palmar fasciectomy

Dupuytren's contracture is a progressive disease involving the palmar fascia and the digital extensions of the palmar fascia. It usually begins with a small nodular thickening in the palm, most frequently in line with the ring finger. With progression of the disease, additional nodules appear, usually with skin adherent to them. Subsequent contracted longitudinal bands of palmar fascia may appear beneath the skin. When the digital extensions of the palmar fascia become involved in the disease process, flexion contractures of the finger MP and PIP joints result.

The cause of Dupuytren's contracture is unknown. One or both hands may be involved. The disease may also be present in the foot in the form of nodules and cords involving the plantar fascia. It does not result in contracture of the toes, however, because the plantar fascia has no digital (toe) extensions.

Surgery is the preferred treatment for Dupuytren's contracture, preferably at an early stage in the disease before irreparable joint damage occurs as the result of prolonged fixed flexion contracture. Surgical procedures include fasciotomy (simple division of contracted bands) or partial or total excision of the palmar fascia. In long-standing disease with irreversible joint changes, amputation of the finger may be the only treatment possible.

Procedural considerations. A plastic hand instrument set is required, plus an Esmarch bandage and a marking pen.

The patient is placed in the supine position on the OR bed, with the arm extended on a hand table. The hand drape is used.

Operative procedure (Fig. 23-58)

1. Incision lines are marked, often with several Z-plasties to lengthen the involved skin of the finger and palm (as for scar revision).
2. The tourniquet is inflated.
3. After incisions are made, flaps of skin and subcutaneous tissue are carefully elevated to preserve their blood supply, exposing the fibrotic palmar fascia and its digital extensions.
4. Part or all of the palmar fascia and digital extensions is excised.

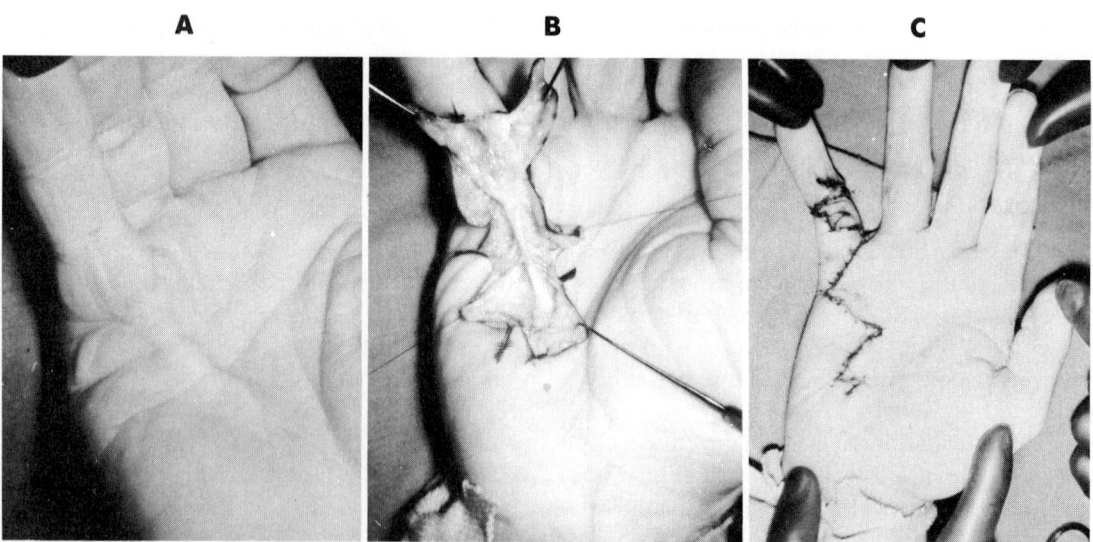

A **B** **C**

FIG. 23-58   Dupuytren's contracture involving palmar fascia and its digital extensions into little finger. **A,** Cord and nodules in palm with mild flexion contracture of little finger. **B,** Contracted band of palmar fascia exposed. **C,** Wound closure with multiple Z-plasties to lengthen contracted skin.

5. The tourniquet is usually released before skin closure so that hemostasis can be obtained.
6. Incisions are sutured. A shortage of skin is sometimes noted at this point, in which case coverage by means of an FTSG is required.
7. If skin grafts are used, they are stented, and then a hand dressing is applied.

Carpal tunnel release

The transverse carpal ligament is incised or excised, with or without synovectomy, to relieve the symptom complex produced by compression of the median nerve within the carpal canal at the wrist. The carpal tunnel is located along the volar surface of the wrist. Its rigid boundaries consist of carpal bones along three sides and the transverse carpal ligament along the fourth (volar) side. The median nerve, superficial and deep finger flexors, and the long thumb flexor tendon all pass through the carpal tunnel before entering the hand. Any condition that decreases the size of the canal, such as fracture of a carpal bone, or increases its volume, such as the hypertrophic synovitis of rheumatoid arthritis, may cause pressure on the median nerve with resultant symptoms of carpal tunnel syndrome. However, in a majority of cases the cause of carpal tunnel syndrome is unknown.

The symptoms of median nerve compression at the wrist are usually pain and paresthesia in the thumb, the index finger, the long finger, and the radial half of the ring finger. Long-standing median nerve compression may result in hand weakness and thenar muscle atrophy. The condition may be unilateral or bilateral.

The procedure to release carpal ligament structures has included the use of endoscopic equipment. The necessary equipment includes video camera, monitor, telescopic lenses, probes, fiberoptic light cords, fiberoptic light source, and small sheaths or obturators. The same considerations with regard to use of the tourniquet as well as draping and prepping routines remain.

Procedural considerations. A plastic hand instrument set is required, plus an Esmarch bandage and a marking pen.

The patient is placed in the supine position on the OR bed, with the arm extended on a hand table. The hand and forearm are prepped to the elbow. The hand drape is used. The operation may be performed with the patient under general, axillary block, or intravenous regional anesthesia.

Operative procedure
Carpal tunnel release

1. After appropriate skin marking and inflation of the pneumatic tourniquet, an incision is made across the volar wrist surface and base of the palm for adequate exposure of the transverse carpal ligament.
2. The transverse carpal ligament is incised along its entire length. A segment of it may be excised.

3. Synovectomy of structures within the carpal canal may or may not be performed.
4. The incision is closed in one layer.
5. A hand dressing is applied.

Endoscopic carpal tunnel release

1. After appropriate skin marking and inflation of the pneumatic tourniquet, an incision is made in the wrist flexion crease. With care, an appropriate size sheath and trocar are inserted and placement of the lens is done by attaching the light cord to the telescope and handing off to the circulator the other end of the cord to be placed in the light source. The camera is placed on the eyepiece of the lens, and the appropriate end of the camera cord is placed into the outlet on the video system.
2. With the use of probes and endoscopic knives, the release is completed with the use of the video monitor.
3. The procedure is completed with steps 4 and 5 as described above.

MICROSURGERY

Reconstructive microsurgery involves the use of an operating microscope and special instruments to reconstruct or replant tissue lost through injury or disease. Today's skilled microsurgeons can successfully anastomose the ends of a vessel measuring less than 1 mm in diameter. The success of microsurgery depends on several factors: (1) the individual and collective experiences of the surgical team and the members' ability to work together, relieving each other as necessary during long operations; (2) the surgeon's knowledge of the physiology of the microcirculation; (3) many hours of practice in the laboratory by the surgical team; and (4) the availability of proper microscopes (Fig. 23-59), microvascular instruments (Fig. 23-60), and microvascular suture.

Replantation of amputated body part

Replantation is an attempt to reattach a completely amputated digit or body part. Revascularization is the procedure performed on incomplete amputations, when the part remains attached to the body by skin, artery, vein, or nerve. Good candidates for replantation are those with the following amputations: (1) thumb, (2) multiple digits (Fig. 23-61) (3) through the palm, (4) wrist or forearm, (5) elbow and above the elbow, and (6) almost any body part of a child.

The success of digital replantation depends primarily on the microsurgical repair of one digital artery and two digital veins. Replantation of an amputated part is ideally performed within 4 to 6 hours after injury, but success has been reported up to 24 hours after injury if the amputated part has been cooled. Proper care of the amputated body part(s) is vital to successful replantation (Fig. 23-62). The ultimate aim of replantation is the restitution of function beyond that provided by a prosthesis.

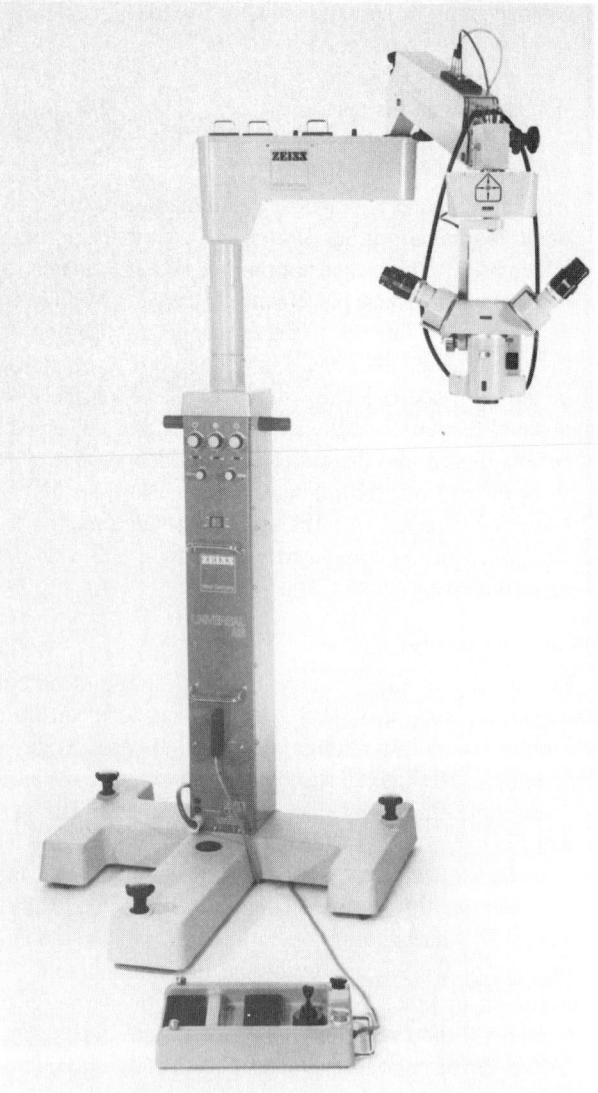

FIG. 23-59   Zeiss OPMI-6 operating microscope.

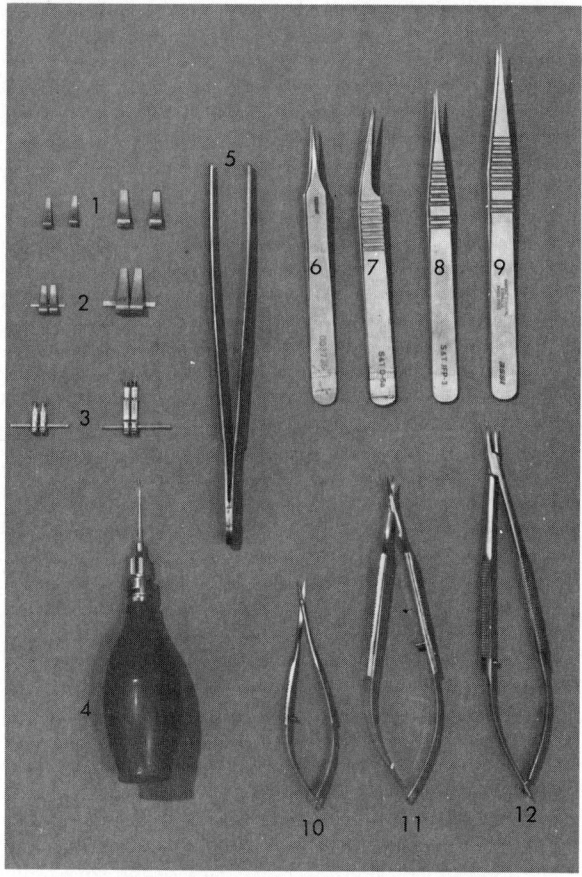

FIG. 23-60 Microvascular instruments. *1,* Single vessel clamps; *2,* approximator clamps; *3,* nerve approximator clamps; *4,* BishopHarmon irrigating bulb and cannula tip; *5,* clamp-applying forceps; *6,* jeweler's forceps; *7,* Acland vessel dilator; *8* and *9,* Pierse tissue forceps; *10,* Vannas scissors; *11,* Castroviejo-Vannas scissors; *12,* Barraquer needle holder.

Procedural considerations. A regional anesthesia is usually given to replantation patients. Because of the length of these surgeries (12 to 16 hours), positioning is important. The OR bed and armboards should be carefully padded with egg crate foam or a gel-filled mattress to support the supine patient. The surgeon may prefer the room temperature to be between 75° and 80° F before the patient arrives because the warm room will reduce vasoconstriction in the extremities. A K-thermia blanket may be placed between the sheet and the mattress of the OR bed to keep the patient's body temperature between 98.6° and 101° F. The surgeon usually brings the amputated part to the operating room before the patient arrives to ensure ample time for preparation of the amputated part for replantation.

Instrumentation includes a plastic hand instrument set,

microvascular instruments, a Kirschner wire driver, Kirschner wires, an operating microscope, and a bipolar electrosurgical unit.

A pneumatic tourniquet cuff is placed on the patient's upper arm, and a hand drape is used.

Operative procedure

1. Bone ends are shortened to eliminate tension on vascular anastomoses to be done later; the bone is stabilized by means of internal fixation with Kirschner wires.
2. Flexor and extensor tendon repairs are usually performed next.
3. The digital nerves are repaired with the aid of loupes or the operating microscope.
4. With microsurgical instruments and techniques, two dig-

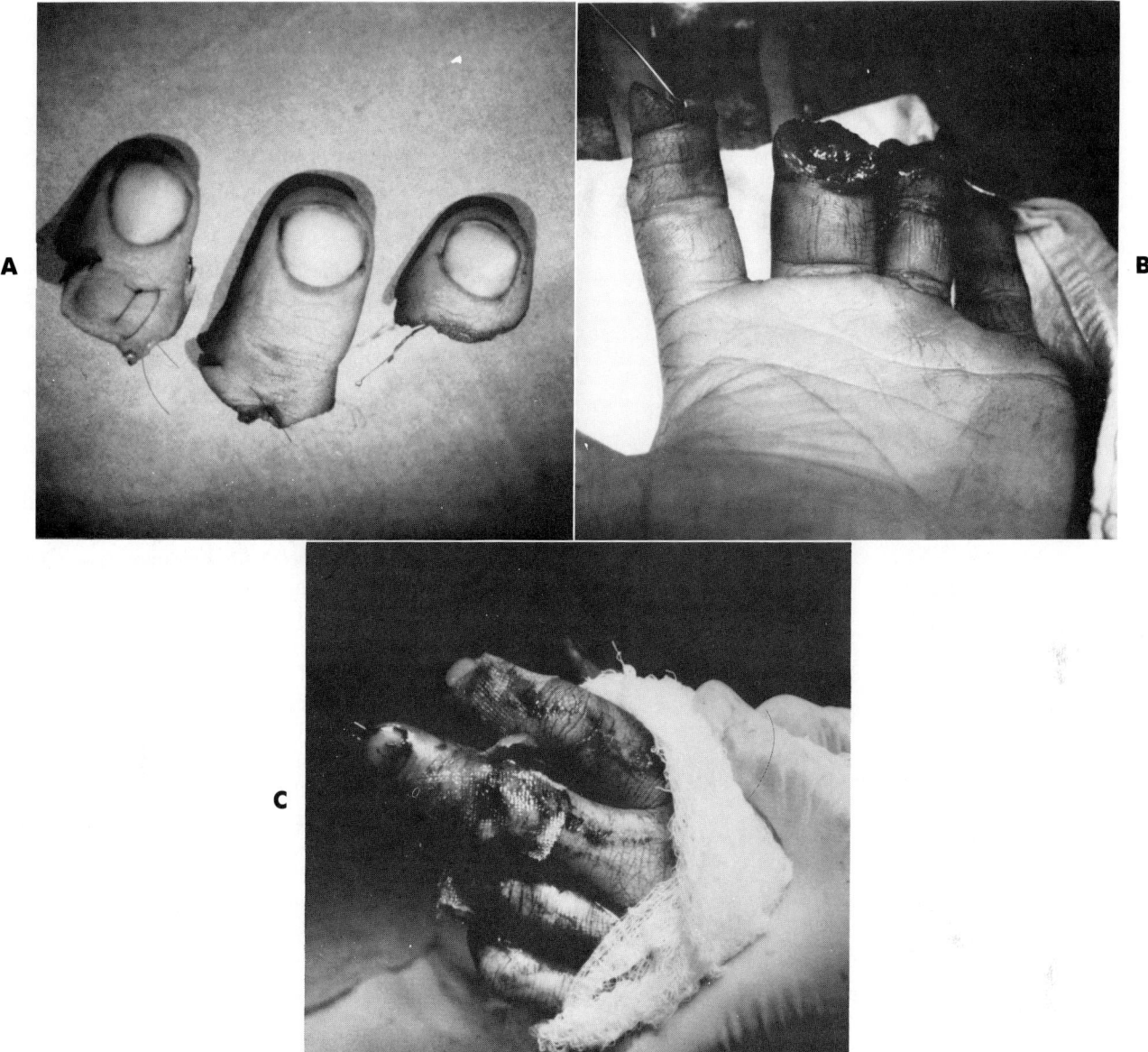

FIG. 23-61 **A,** Complete amputation of three digits from hand. **B,** Hand after amputation. **C,** Reattachment of three completely amputated digits to the hand.

ital veins are repaired, followed by repair of one digital artery. If ischemic time has been prolonged, digital vessel repair may precede repair of tendons and nerves.
5. The skin is sutured.
6. A bulky supportive hand dressing is applied.

Toe-to-hand transfer

This reconstructive procedure involves surgical removal of a single or multiple toes and anastomosing of the vessels of the toes to those on the hand to restore finger and thumb functions. It is lengthy surgery (12 to 16 hours), en-

tailing a two-team approach, one at the foot for toe removal and one at the recipient site, the hand.

Procedural considerations. The patient is placed in the supine position on the OR bed. The patient is placed on an anticoagulation regimen during the anastomosis procedure. Two tourniquets are needed, one on the thigh of the operative foot and one on the operative arm. Both extremities are separately prepped and draped. Instrumentation includes a plastic hand set, microvascular instruments, power Kirschner wire driver, and Kirschner wires. Additional equipment includes the operating microscope, two tourniquet power sources, two bipolar electrosurgical units, marking pen, and Esmarch bandage.

Operative procedure

1. The surgeon preparing the hand determines adequate blood flow and vessel location on the thumb or finger site (Fig. 23-63, *A*). This may prevent a needless amputation of the toe.
2. Appropriate skin flaps are incised to expose the veins on the dorsum of the hand and clamped with microvessel clips.
3. The radial artery or branches are dissected out and prepared for anastomosis.
4. The flexor and extensor pollicis longus tendons are located and transfixed.
5. The bone at the base of the thumb is prepared for the toe.
6. The nerves to the thumb are dissected out with adequate length for suturing without tension.
7. The toe is circumscribed with a racquet-shaped incision (Fig. 23-63, *B*), and the veins are isolated through the dorsal aspect and clamped with micro-vessel clips.
8. The extensor tendon is dissected proximally and transsected over the base of the metatarsal.
9. The dorsalis pedis artery is dissected to the digital vessels with ligation of all branches of that vessel to prepare for the anastomosis.
10. On the plantar surface the digital nerves and flexor tendons are transsected at levels of adequate length for anastomosis (Fig. 23-63, *C*).
11. The toe is transsected at the level previously determined for adequate length of the thumb.
12. The toe vessels are anastomosed microsurgically to the thumb vessels. The toe is attached to the thumb area by Kirschner wires (Fig. 23-63, *D*).

An esthetic and functionally effective hand can be achieved through this procedure (Fig. 23-63, *E*).

Free jejunal tissue transfer

Reconstructive problems in patients undergoing laryngectomy and upper cervical esophagectomy can be adequately solved by free jejunal transfer. Modern microsurgical techniques greatly improve the success rate. Free jejunal transfers have proved beneficial:

1. In patients with massive resection of the laryngopharynx when resection may extend into the oropharynx or even the lower nasopharynx and encompass a large portion of the cervical esophagus
2. In patients with radiation failure in whom laryngopharyngoesophagectomy is required
3. In patients with secondary reconstruction of the hypopharynx or cervical esophagus in whom other methods have failed because of flap necrosis or radiation

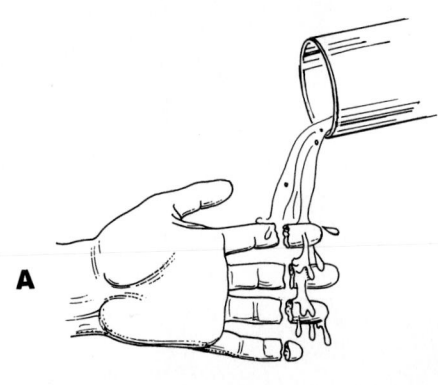

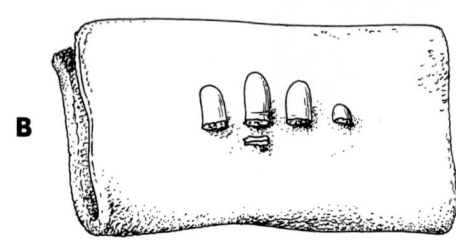

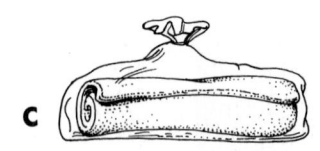

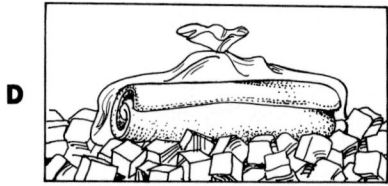

FIG. 23-62 All severed body parts should be sought, including small pieces of mangled tissue. The following steps should be performed: **A**, Rinse; **B**, wrap in moist towel; **C**, place towel in clean plastic bag and seal; **D**, cool on ice. The iced bag should be sent to the replantation center with the patient.

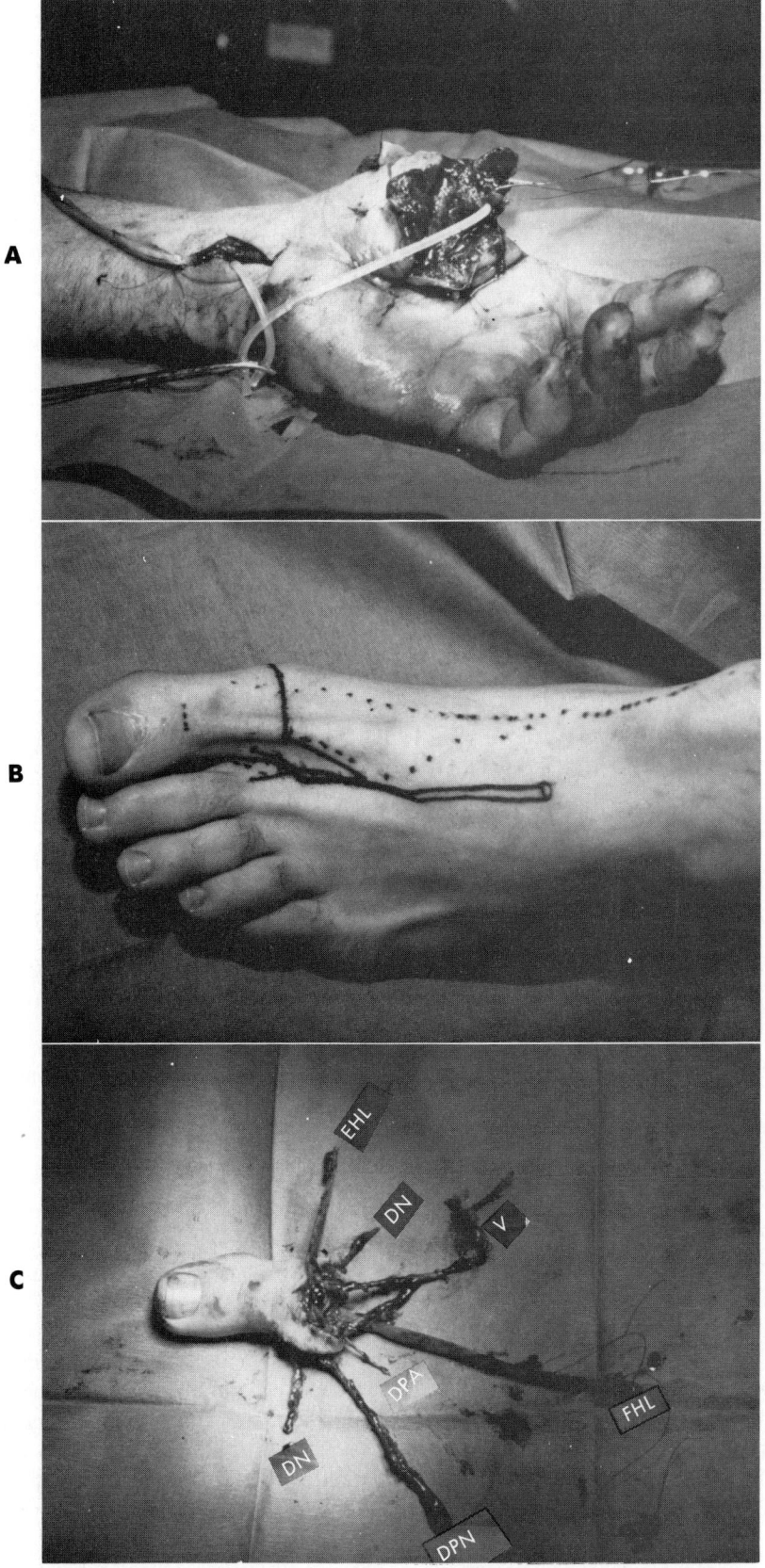

FIG. 23-63   **A,** Preparation of thumb site. **B,** Marking of toe. **C,** Identification of vessels. *DN,* Digital nerve; *DPN,* dorsalis pedis nerve; *DPA,* dorsalis pedis artery; *EHL,* extensor hallucis longus tendon; *FHL,* flexor hallucis longus tendon; *V,* vein.   *Continued.*

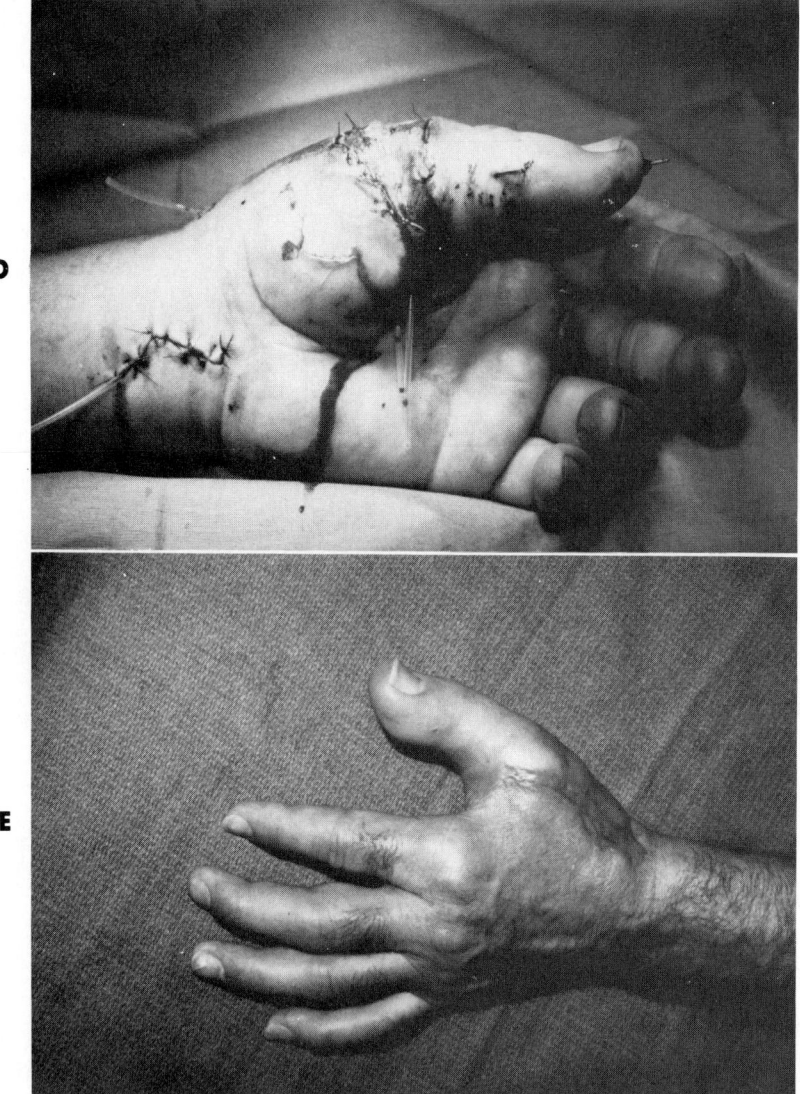

FIG. 23-63, CONT'D   **D,** Attachment of toe to thumb. **E,** Postoperative view of toe-to-thumb transfer.

4. In patients in whom primary pharyngoesophageal radiation has resulted in hypopharyngeal stricture unresponsive to dilation
5. In isolated cases in which a large area of oral lining is lost

Procedural considerations. The patient is positioned, prepped, and draped for laryngectomy with the abdomen exposed. The abdomen is covered with sterile towels during laryngectomy. When laryngectomy is completed, all instruments and drapes are discarded after the wound has been covered with sterile towels. The patient is again prepped and draped for the free tissue graft.

The basic plastic instrument set is used, plus abdominal instruments for the graft and microsurgical and vascular instruments for the graft anastomosis. The operating microscope or loupes may be used for preparation of the graft and graft placement.

Operative procedure. A two-team approach is used. Neck dissection is carried out, at which time donor vessels are identified and preserved. The abdomen is opened, and the ligament of Treitz located. A suitable segment is identified in the first 2 feet of jejunum with a single dominant vascular pedicle. The segment with its pedicle is resected, and bowel continuity reestablished. The abdomen is closed as the microsurgeon prepares the bowel vessel for anastomosis. The donor-recipient vessels in the neck are prepared, using the microscope. The proximal bowel anastomosis is made, followed by the vascular anastomosis. When the microvascular clamps are removed, pulsation of the mesenteric vessels and peristalsis should begin. The distal bowel anastomosis is then done. The neck is closed, leaving a small Silastic window over the jejunal segment to allow for close, postoperative observation of the transplant.

REFERENCES

Benson, D.S., & Conte, R.R. (1989) *89/90 Nursing Meds.* Norwalk: Appleton & Lange.

Bryant, R.A. (1992). *Acute and chronic wounds: Nursing management.* St. Louis: Mosby.

Foss, J., & Feistritzer, N. (1993). Perioperative care of the trauma patient. In J.E. Neff and P.S. Kidd (editors), *Trauma nursing: The art and science.* St. Louis: Mosby.

McFarland, G.K., & McFarlane, E.A. (1993). *Nursing diagnosis and intervention.* St. Louis: Mosby.

Environmental safety in the practice setting. (1994). *AORN* Standards and recommended practices for perioperative nursing, Denver, The Association.

Seifert, P.C., & Rothrock, J.C. (1989). Perioperative assessment tool. In C.E. Guzzita et al. (Eds.), *Clinical assessment tools for use with nursing diagnoses.* St. Louis: Mosby.

Vasconez, L.O., & Vasconez, H.C. (1988). Plastic and reconstructive surgery. In L. Way (Ed.), *Current surgical diagnosis and treatment.* Norwalk, Conn: Appleton & Lange.

BIBLIOGRAPHY

Agee, J.M. (1992). Endoscopic release of the carpal tunnel: A randomized prospective multicenter study. *Journal of Hand Surgery,* 17A: 987-995.

American Society of Plastic and Reconstructive Surgeons. (1983). Background information on suction lipectomy, developed for the media, *Plastic Surgery News,* 8(1), 12.

American Society of Plastic and Reconstructive Surgical Nurses, Inc. (1989). *Core curriculum for plastic and reconstructive surgical nursing.* Pitman, N.J.: Anthony J. Jannetti.

American Society of Plastic and Reconstructive Surgical Nurses. (1993). Straight talk about breast implants: Your guide. Pitman, N.J.: The Society.

AORN. (1994). *AORN standards and recommended practices for perioperative nursing.* Denver: The Association.

Balch, C.M., Singletary, S.E., & Bland, K.I. (1993). Clinical decision making in early breast cancer. *Annals of Surgery,* 217(3), 207-225.

Baptist, G. (1985). Perioperative nursing roles. *Plastic Surgical Nursing,* 5, 86.

Black, J. (1985). Nursing process for the craniofacial surgical patient. *Plastic Surg Nursing,* 5, 18.

Bostwick, J. (1985). Breast reconstruction following mastectomy. *Contemporary Surgery,* 27; 15.

Chang, W.H. (1989). *Fundamentals of plastic and reconstructive surgery.* Baltimore: Williams & Wilkins.

Cohen, B., & Aaronson, S. (1983). Free tissue transfer. *AORN Journal,* 38, 602.

Converse, J.M. (1983). *Reconstructive plastic surgery: Principles and procedures in corrective reconstruction and transplantation.* (4th ed.) Philadelphia: W.B. Saunders.

Fisher, J.C. (1992). The silicone controversy: When will science prevail? *New England Journal of Medicine,* 326, 1696-1698.

Gasparotti, M., Lewis, C.M., & Toledo, L.S. (1993). *Superficial liposculpture: Manual of technique.* New York: Springer-Verlag.

Goin, J., & Goin, M. (1981). *Changing the body: Psychological effects of plastic surgery.* Baltimore; Williams & Wilkins.

Goodman, T. (1989). *Core curriculum for plastic and reconstructive surgical nursing.* Pitman, N.J.: Anthony Jannetti.

Grabb, W.X., & Smith, J.W. (editors). (1980). *Plastic surgery: A concise guide to clinical practice* (3rd ed.). Boston: Little, Brown.

Grazer, F.M., & Klingbeil, R. (editors). (1980). *Body image: A surgical perspective.* St. Louis: Mosby.

Grossman, J.A. (1986). Abdominoplasty: Indications and technique. *AORN Journal,* 44, 582.

Gulanick, M. et al. (1986). *Nursing care plans.* St. Louis: Mosby.

Harbal, M.B., et al. (1984). *Advances in plastic and reconstructive surgery.* Chicago: Year Book Medical Publishers.

Hester, R., et al. (1980). Reconstruction of cervical esophgus, hypopharynx and oral cavity using free jejunal transfer. *American Journal of Surgery,* 140, 487.

Hollinshead, W.H. (1982). Anatomy for surgeons (Vol.3). (3rd ed.). New York: Harper & Row.

Holloway, N.M. (1988). Medical surgical care plans. Springhouse, Pa: Springhouse.

Horton, C.E. (1980). *Plastic and reconstructive surgery of the genital area.* Boston: Little, Brown.

Jacobs, S., & Stoldt, L. (1984). Replantation for traumatic amputations. *AORN Journal* 39, 956.

Kaye, B., & Gradinger, G. (Eds.). (1984). *Symposium on problems and complications in aesthetic plastic surgery of the face.* St. Louis: Mosby.

Kendall, F. (1993). Documenting local anesthesia patient care. *AORN Journal,* 58(4), 715-719.

Kutz, J., Thomson, C., & Klein, H. (1979). Toe-to-hand transfers. In American Academy of OrthopedicSurgeons. *Symposium on microsurgery: Practical use in orthopaedics.* St. Louis: Mosby.

Leber, D.C. (1992). *Textbook of plastic, maxillofacial, and reconstructive surgery.* Baltimore: Williams & Wilkins.

Lindquist, J. (1982). Psychological aspects of microsurgical replantation. *Plastic Surgical Nursing,* 2, 65.

Mangan, M.)1984). Patient education with tissue expanders. *Plastic Surgical Nursing* 6, 76.

Markland, A. (1984). Nursing care of the suction lipectomy patient. *Plastic Surgical Nursing,* 4, 44.

Mathes, S.J., & Nahai, F. (1982). *Clinical atlas of muscle and musculocutaneous flaps.* St. Louis: Mosby.

McClain, L. (1992). Counseling the woman with breast implants. *Plastic Surgical Nursing,* 12(2), 61-62, 70.

Milford, L. (1982). *The hand* (2nd ed.). St. Louis: Mosby.

Moncada, G. (1985). Special nursing considerations for the craniofacial patient. *Plastic Surgical Nursing* 5, 14.

Moncada, G.A. (1990). Plastic and reconstructive surgery. In J. Rothrock (editor), *Perioperative care planning.* St. Louis: Mosby.

Monitoring the patient receiving IV conscious sedation. (1993). *AORN Journal,* 57(4), 978-983.

Morgan, R.F. (1991). Plastic surgery. *ACS Bulletin,* 76(1), 43-46.

National Institutes of Health. (1992). *NIH consensus statement on diagnosis and treatment of early melanoma.* Bethesda, Md: NIH.

Nora, P.F. (1990). *Operative surgery: Principles and techniques.* Philadelphia: W.B. Saunders.

Rees, T.D. (1980). *Aesthetic plastic surgery.* Philadelphia, W.B. Saunders.

Tessier, P. (1981). *Plastic surgery of the orbit and eyelids.* New York: Masson.

Watson, D., & Kaempf, G. (1991). *Monitoring the patient receiving local anesthesia* (2nd ed.). Denver: Association of Operating Room Nurses, Inc.

Woods, J. (1984). Current state of the art in breast reconstruction. *Plastic Surgical Nursing,* 4, 85.

Woodward, J.R., & Cleveland, R. (1982). Application of Horton-Devine principles to the repair of hypospadium. *Journal of Urology, 127,* 1155.

24

THORACIC SURGERY

B R E N D A   G R E G O R Y   D A W E S

A s early as 1499 an unsucessful excision of a hernia-tion of the lung was recorded. Until the 1880s the only thoracic procedures performed were for drain-age of empyema and of lung abscess or treatment of chest wounds. The physiologic impact on the lungs and perceived difficulty entering the chest resulted in hesistancy to per-form thoracic procedures. The first purposeful resection of a part of the lung for traumatic injury was reported by Mil-ton Antony in 1823. In 1861 the French surgeon Pean re-moved part of a lung for tumor; the procedure wasn't re-ported until 1895.

Treatment of tuberculosis (TB), which has been at-tempted for centuries, also provided reasons for develop-ments in thoracic procedures. Thoracoplasty became widely used as a means of collapsing the lungs for treatment of TB followed by other forms of treatment. In 1913 Jacobeus began to divide adhesions with a cautery passed through one cannula, while through the other he passed a cystoscope-like instrument he called a thoracoscope. In the 1920s student textbooks contained only a short paragraph on cancer of the lung. In 1907 an article was published de-scribing surgical techniques for access to the thoracic cav-ity. From that time until the first successful pneumeonec-tomy in 1933 there were many attempts to remove carcino-mas with limited success.

During the past 50 years the understanding of pathophys-iology and improved techniques has expanded the field of thoracic surgery. The thoracic speciality extends beyond the surgical arena into infectious disease, trauma, and oncol-ogy. Improved technology has improved the recovery rate for patients experiencing thoracic diseases. As the ability to treat improves, the responsibilities of the perioperative nurse have expanded, resulting in accomplishments throughout the years that have provided an extensive knowl-edge base and specialized perioperative practitioners.

SURGICAL ANATOMY

The skeletal framework of the thorax is formed anteri-orly by the sternum and costal cartilages, laterally by the 12 pairs of ribs, and posteriorly by the 12 thoracic verte-brae (Figs. 24-1 and 24-2). This airtight compartment is en-closed in the root of the neck by Sibson's fascia and is sep-arated from the abdomen by the diaphragm.

The sternum forms the anterior thoracic wall in the mid-line. It consists of three parts: (1) the upper part, or manu-brium; (2) the body, or gladiolus; and (3) the lower carti-lage, or xiphoid process. The manubrium articulates with the clavicles and the first two ribs on each side; the gladi-olus articulates with the remaining true ribs by separate cos-tal cartilages; and the xiphoid fuses with the gladiolus in early development and is attached to the diaphragm by the substernal ligament (Figs. 24-1 and 24-3).

Normally, the lateral walls of the thorax are formed by the 12 pairs of ribs. Posteriorly each pair of ribs articulates with its corresponding thoracic vertebrae (see Fig. 24-2). Anteriorly the first seven ribs articulate with the sternum. The eighth, ninth, and tenth ribs articulate with the costal cartilages of the rib above; however, the eleventh and twelfth are not fixed to the costal arch (see Fig. 24-1).

The muscles of each hemithorax (Figs. 24-3 and 24-4) include the 11 external and 11 internal intercostal muscles, which fill the spaces between the ribs. An intercostal ar-tery, vein, and nerve accompany each intercostal muscle. The arteries communicate with the internal thoracic artery anteriorly and arise from the aorta posteriorly. The inter-costal veins follow the course of the arteries and commu-nicate with the mammary veins anteriorly and with the azy-gos and hemiazygos veins posteriorly.

During surgery great care is taken to prevent injury to the intercostal nerve, which passes forward and alongside the posterior intercostal artery and which shares with the superior branch of the artery the intercostal groove on the inferior edge of the corresponding rib. When the nerve must be disturbed, an anesthetic agent may be injected to pre-vent postoperative pain.

The thoracic outlet is a junction bound by the manubrium anteriorly and by the first ribs anterolaterally and posteri-orly by the first thoracic vertebrae and posterior angles of the first ribs of the space. The great vessels of the head,

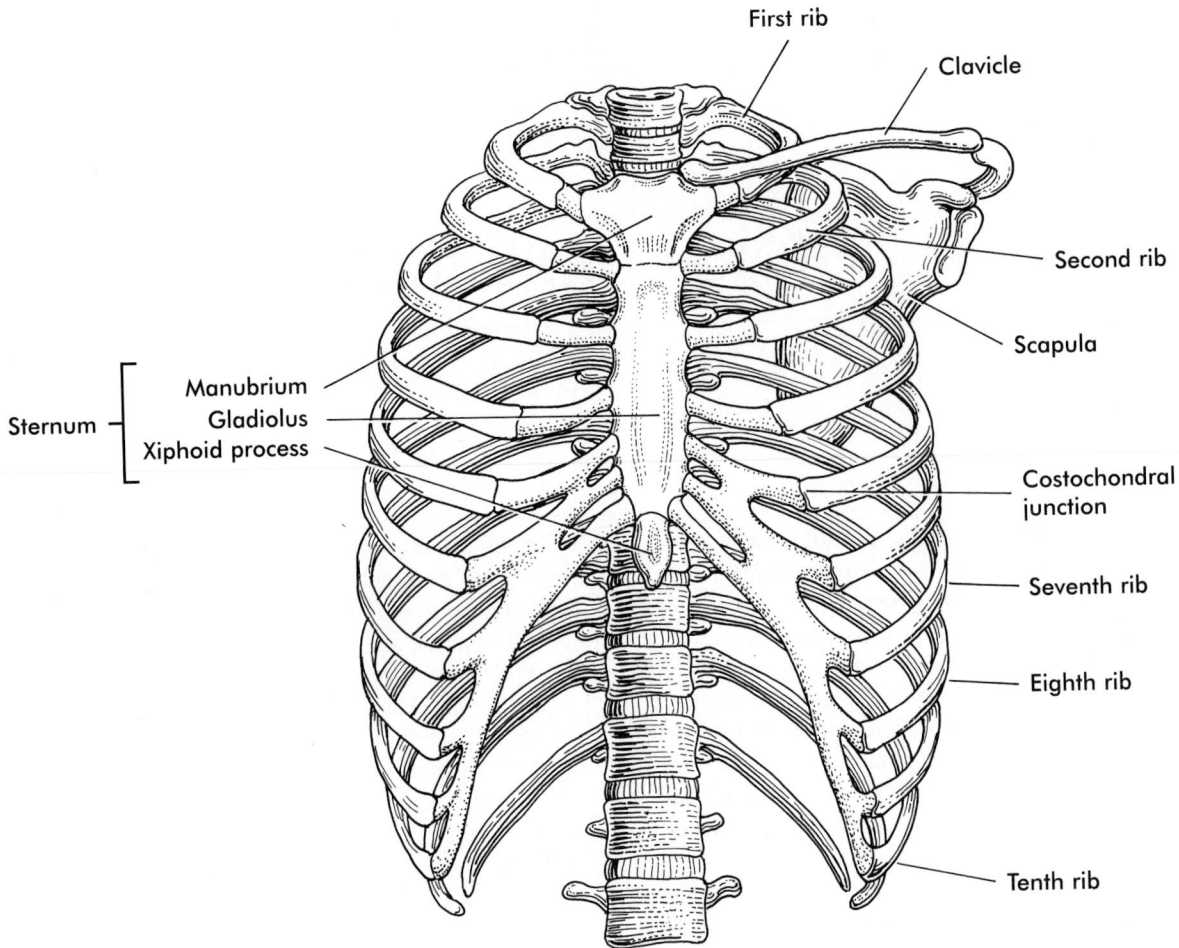

First rib

Clavicle

Second rib

Scapula

Sternum { Manubrium
            Gladiolus
            Xiphoid process

Costochondral
junction

Seventh rib

Eighth rib

Tenth rib

FIG. 24-1   Bony thorax.

neck, and arm pass through this space. Compression of these structures causes thoracic outlet syndrome.

The chest cavity is subdivided into the right and left pleural cavities, which contain the lungs, separated by the mediastinum, which lies medially between the two pleural membranes. The parietal pleura, the membrane that lines the inner surface of each hemithorax, is adjacent to the inner surfaces of the ribs posteriorly and the mediastinum medially and covers the surface of the diaphragm except at the central portion. Part of the parietal membrane is reflected back at the root of each lung to form a sac around it. This reflection is called the visceral pleura. A serous secretion, pleural fluid provides lubrication between these two membranes to minimize friction. Approximately 0.1 to 0.2 ml/kg body weight of fluid exists in the pleural space.

The lungs are the essential organs of respiration. The base of each lung rests on the diaphragm, whereas its apex (upper end) projects into the base of the neck at a level above the first rib. The bronchus, the nerves, the lymphatics, and the pulmonary and bronchial vessels enter and leave the lung on the mediastinal surface in a structure known as the hilum, or root, of the lung. Deep fissures divide the spongy, porous lung into lobes. The primary bronchi divide, then subdivide in each lobe and eventually be-

come bronchioles. The right lung has an upper, middle, and lower lobe; the left lung has only an upper and lower lobe (Fig. 24-5). However, the lungs are similar in that each is composed of 10 major segments. Each segment extends to the pleural surface, expanding in volume from its center to its peripheral edges. Each segment also has its own bronchus and branches of the pulmonary artery and vein.

The bronchial arteries, arising from the aorta, supply nourishment to the lungs. They vary in their number and course. The arrangement may include two branches to the left lung and one branch to the right lung, which later branches into two, or there may be one or two branches for each lung. The pulmonary arteries carry the blood to the pulmonary parenchyma, and the pulmonary veins transport the oxygenated blood to the left atrium.

The nerves of the lungs are a part of the autonomic nervous system (see Chapter 22). They regulate constriction and relaxation of the bronchi and of the blood vessels within the lungs.

Although the thoracic cavity is an airtight space, the lungs inspire outside air through the nasal passages, trachea, and bronchi. The main function of the lungs is to exchange carbon dioxide for oxygen. Normally, as the thorax expands, the lungs also expand as air is drawn in; dur-

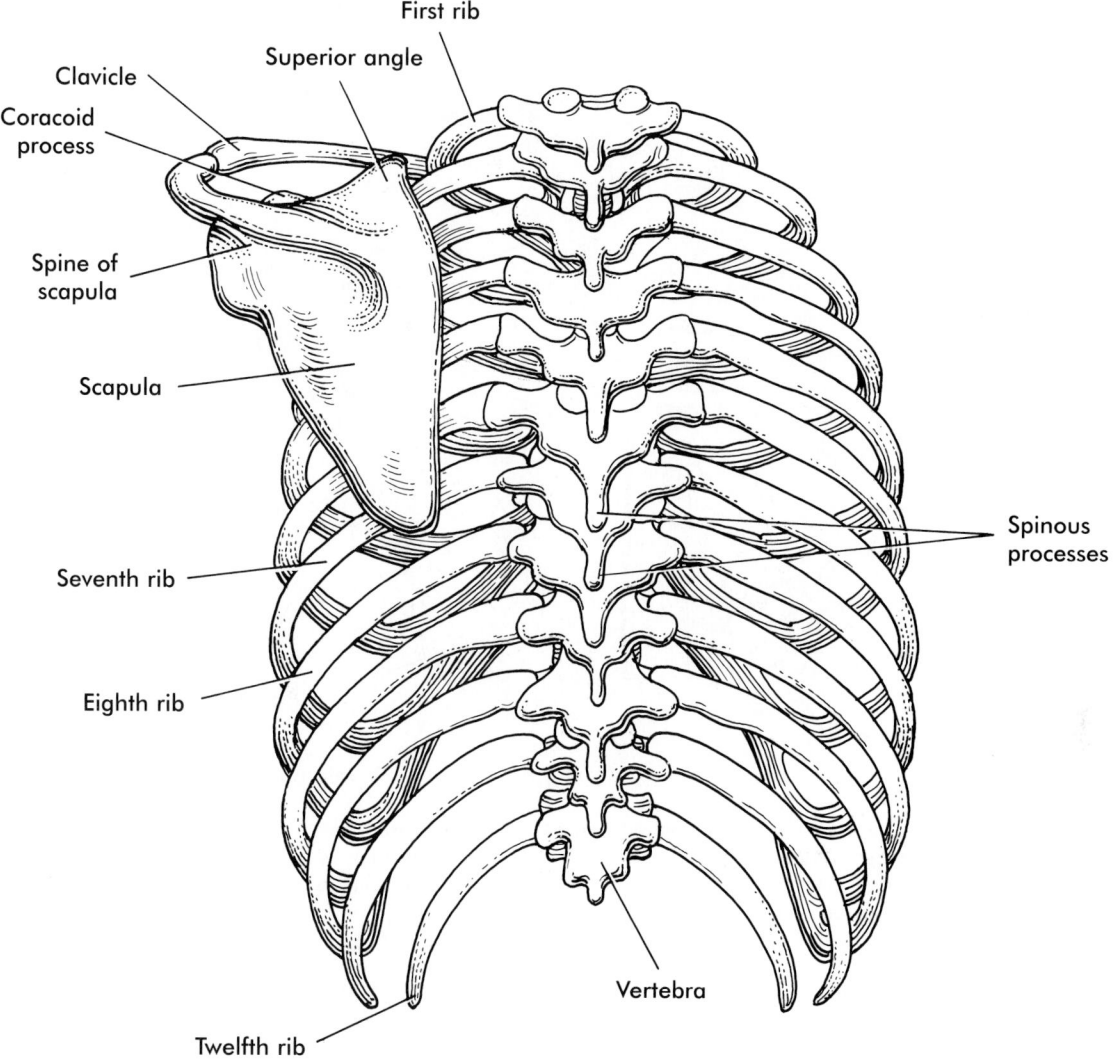

FIG. 24-2 Posterior view of bony thorax.

ing expiration the thorax relaxes, and the lungs passively contract as air is forced out. Inspiration normally takes place when the intrathoracic pressure is slightly below atmospheric pressure (76 cm Hg or 760 mm Hg) and when a partial vacuum exists between the parietal and visceral pleural (intrathoracic) surfaces. As the muscles of inspiration contract to enlarge the chest cage, the lungs passively follow the diaphragm and chest wall because of decreased intrathoracic pressure. The acts of inspiration and expiration are the result of air moving in and out of the lung, causing pressure to equalize with that of the atmosphere at the end of expiration (Fig. 24-6).

The normal intrapleural pressure varies from -9 to -12 cm H_2O during inspiration and from about -3 to -6 cm H_2O during expiration. The greatest amount of air that can be expired after a maximum inspiration is termed the *vital capacity* and the volume of gas remaining in the lungs after maximal expiration is *residual volume*. Size, age, gender, and pulmonary disease of the patient influence vital capacity. Any condition that interferes with the normally negative intrapleural pressure affects respiratory function.

PERIOPERATIVE NURSING CONSIDERATIONS

ASSESSMENT

During assessment the perioperative nurse gathers information (patient data) that is important to planning patient care. Signs and symptoms demonstrated by the patient are confirmed by the perioperative nurse during admission to the operating room, typically in the holding area. The perioperative nurse may begin data collection through a review of the patient's medical record, including results of the history, physical examination, laboratory results, other diagnostic workups, and the nursing history and assessment. It is valuable to assess the patient's understanding of the disease process and of the anticipated procedure. It is also important to assess emotional status, since patients may be asymptomatic, which creates an atmosphere for denial. A focused assessment of the respiratory system should be included during the physical assessment. The nurse questions the patient or otherwise confirms the presence of an

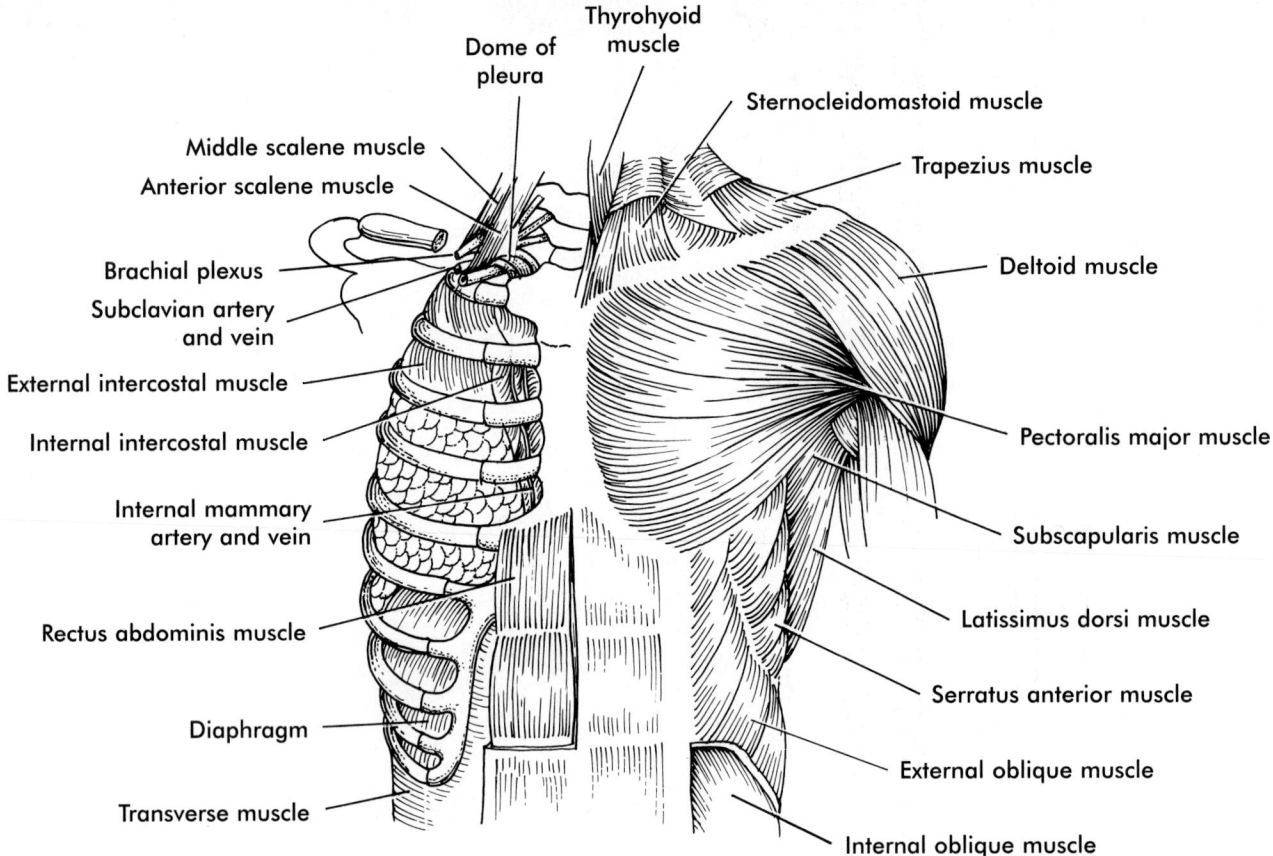

FIG. 24-3 Anterior view of thorax and contiguous portions of base of neck and anterior abdominal wall. *Right half,* Superficial layer of muscles and fascia; *left half,* relations of deep muscles of neck and abdomen to rib cage, intercostal muscles, diaphragm, and internal mammary vessels; relations of muscles, nerves, and vessels with first rib; and anterior relations of lung.

Labels (Fig. 24-3):
- Dome of pleura
- Thyrohyoid muscle
- Sternocleidomastoid muscle
- Middle scalene muscle
- Anterior scalene muscle
- Trapezius muscle
- Brachial plexus
- Deltoid muscle
- Subclavian artery and vein
- External intercostal muscle
- Internal intercostal muscle
- Pectoralis major muscle
- Internal mammary artery and vein
- Subscapularis muscle
- Latissimus dorsi muscle
- Rectus abdominis muscle
- Serratus anterior muscle
- Diaphragm
- External oblique muscle
- Transverse muscle
- Internal oblique muscle

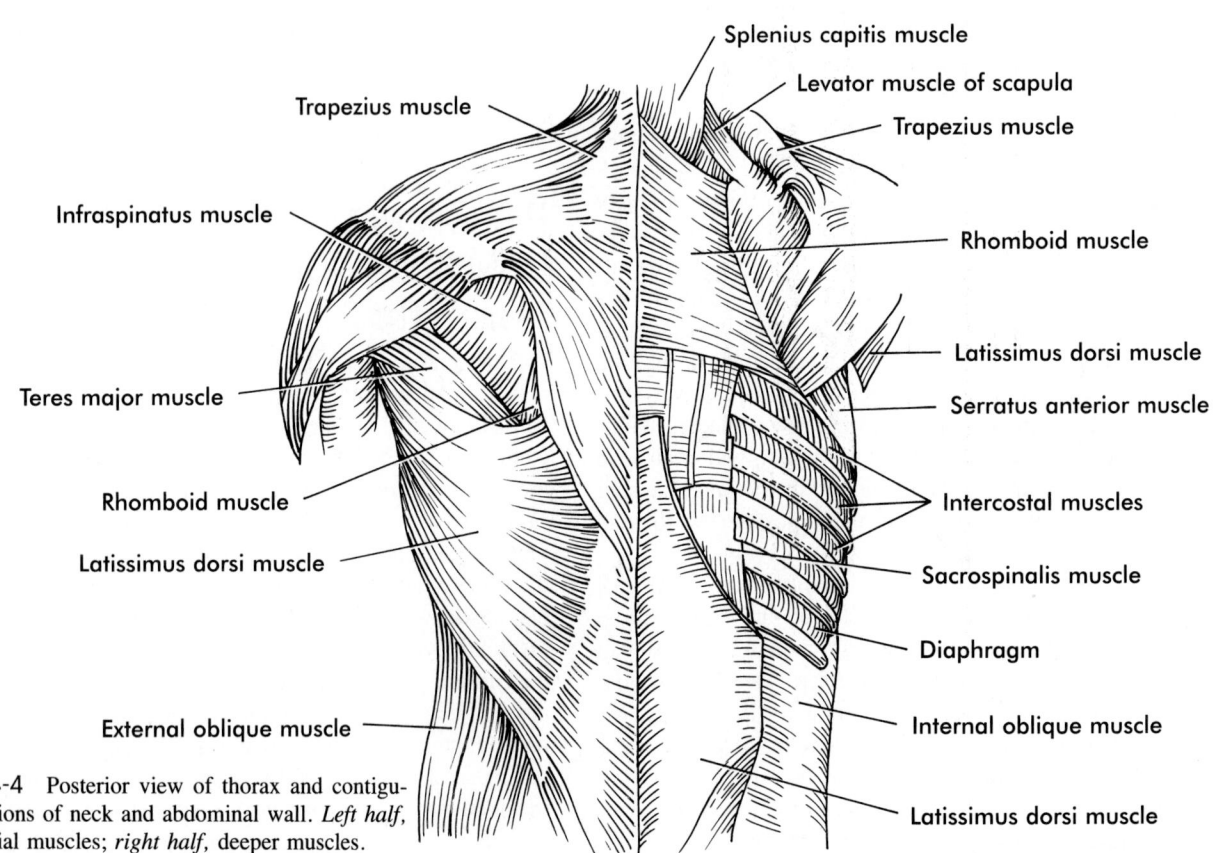

FIG. 24-4 Posterior view of thorax and contiguous portions of neck and abdominal wall. *Left half,* Superficial muscles; *right half,* deeper muscles.

Labels (Fig. 24-4):
- Splenius capitis muscle
- Levator muscle of scapula
- Trapezius muscle
- Trapezius muscle
- Infraspinatus muscle
- Rhomboid muscle
- Latissimus dorsi muscle
- Serratus anterior muscle
- Teres major muscle
- Intercostal muscles
- Rhomboid muscle
- Sacrospinalis muscle
- Latissimus dorsi muscle
- Diaphragm
- External oblique muscle
- Internal oblique muscle
- Latissimus dorsi muscle

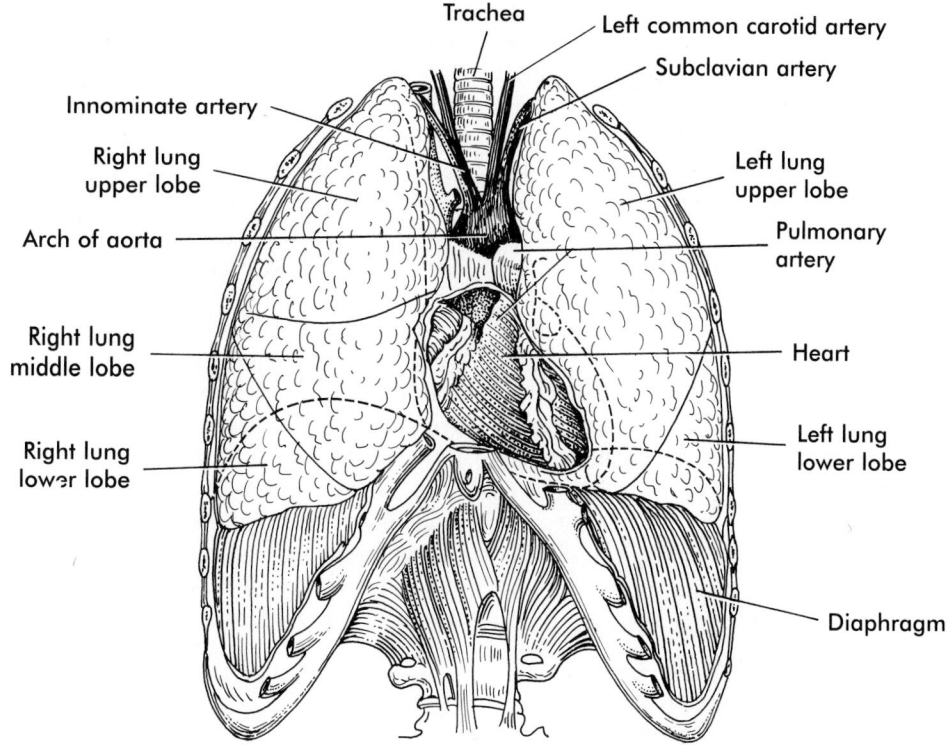

FIG. 24-5 Organs of thoracic cavity. Part of pericardium has been removed to expose heart.

From Schottelius, B.A., & Schottelius, D.D. (1978). *Textbook of physiology* (18th ed.). St. Louis: Mosby.

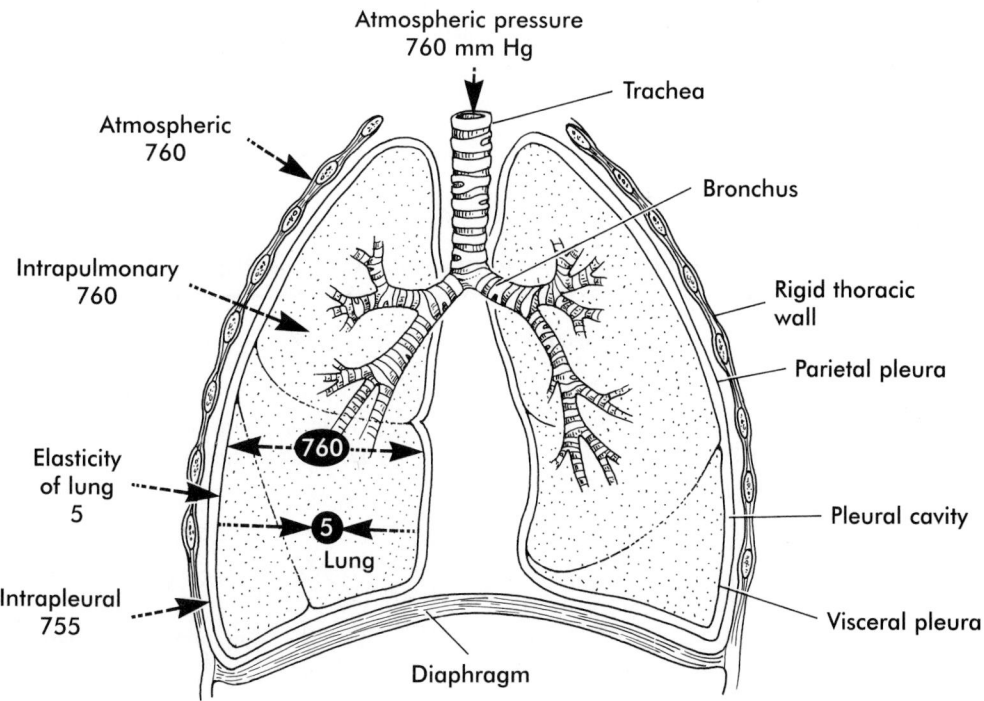

FIG. 24-6 Thoracic cavity structures showing intrapulmonary and intrapleural pressures with chest wall in resting position.

From Schottelius, B.A., & Schottelius, D.D. (1978). *Textbook of physiology* (18th ed.). St. Louis: Mosby.

increased cough, increase in sputum production, recurrent hemoptysis, malaise, shortness of breath, substernal chest discomfort, weight loss, poor appetite, adequacy of nutrition, and hypoxia. The results of the physical examination of the chest should be reviewed; the perioperative nurse may auscultate the chest and confirm the presence of crackles or wheezes on inspiration or expiration.

The review of diagnostic and laboratory tests includes the chest x-ray, sputum analysis confirmed during bronchoscopy, cytology reports, and pulmonary function studies. The chest x-ray will be needed in the operating room (Research Highlight 24-1). This film outlines the lesion, if any is present, and defines its shape and space-occupying nature (tracheal shift). The presence of air in the hilar region, pleural effusion, or atelectasis may also be confirmed by

radiologic evidence. Sputum analysis for culture and sensitivity may alert the perioperative nurse to an infectious process; cytology may confirm a malignancy. The patient may have already undergone diagnostic bronchoscopy or mediastinoscopy; if so, the results should be reviewed for acid fast bacillus smear, culture, bronchial washing, and biopsy results. Computed tomography (CT) scans of the chest, as well as the brain, liver, and abdomen, may reveal the presence or absence of metastasis, pleural calcification, thickening, or plaque; radioisotope scans may have been done for similar reasons. Magnetic resonance imaging (MRI) detects vascular relationships to masses or vascular lesions. The results of pulmonary function tests and arterial blood gases should be reviewed (Table 24-1). Ventilation and perfusion studies show the distribution of each function in the lung. These results assist the perioperative nurse in collaborating with the surgical team to maintain effective gas exchange during the surgical intervention. The results are also valuable in predicting postoperative respiratory function and metabolic responses. Patients hospitalized for surgery related to carcinoma may have received chemotherapy or radiation therapy prior to surgery; assessment of the skin and the patient's general condition is important in preventing perioperative complications.

Following a general and focused review of the patient's medical record and patient interview, the perioperative nurse formulates nursing diagnoses. These statements reflect actual or high-risk problems in which the perioperative nurse will intervene, either independently or collaboratively with the surgical team. Nursing diagnoses should be individualized and prioritized for each patient.

☆

RESEARCH HIGHLIGHT 24-1

Conventional radiographic examination remains an indispensible means of determining chest lesions. One sixth of all inpatient plain chest films contain diagnostic information of therapeutic value. Approximately 10% of all radiographically recognized carcinoma diagnosed through screening programs is found at stage I; during this stage, chances for survival are excellent.

Mendelson, D.S., et al. (1987). Preoperative chest radiography: Value as a baseline exam for comparison. *Radiology, 165*(2), 341-343.

TABLE 24-1

Normal Results of Laboratory Studies for Assessment of Patients Undergoing Thoracic Procedures

Test	Normal results	Purpose
PULMONARY FUNCTION TESTS		
Vital capacity (VC)	>4 L	Detect abnormalities in respiratory function
Maximum voluntary ventilation (MVV)	>80 L/min	Determine extent of pulmonary abnormality
Maximum midexpiratory flow (MMF)	>2 L/sec	
Forced expiratory flow	>32 L	
Forced expiratory flow, 1 sec (FEV1)	>71 L	
PERFUSION STUDIES—ARTERIAL BLOOD GASES		
pH	7.35-7.45	Indicate respiratory and metabolic disturbances
P_{CO_2}	35-45	
HCO_3	21-28	
P_{O_2}	80-100	
O_2 saturation	95%-100%	

NURSING DIAGNOSIS

Nursing diagnoses related to the care of patients undergoing thoracic surgery might include the following:

- High risk for impaired gas exchange related to the surgical intervention
- High risk for impaired skin integrity related to surgical positioning, length of the surgical intervention, and/or the use of chemical antimicrobial agents on the skin
- High risk for injury related to positioning, use of equipment, and length of the surgical intervention
- High risk for fluid volume excess related to decreased surface area of the lung for perfusion and administration of IV fluids during surgery
- High risk for infection related to inadequate secondary defenses (presence of existing disease process) and surgical disruption of tissues

OUTCOME IDENTIFICATION

Outcomes identified for the selected nursing diagnosis could be stated as:

- The patient will experience adequate gas exchange during the surgical procedure.
- The patient's skin integrity will be maintained.
- The patient will be free from injury.
- The patient will maintain appropriate fluid balance.
- The patient will be free from infection.

PLANNING

A Sample Care Plan for a patient undergoing thoracic surgery is included on p. 1008.

IMPLEMENTATION

During implementation of the plan of care the perioperative nurse is concerned with both preparatory patient considerations (such as positioning, presurgical diagnostic interventions, draping) and the requirements of the surgical intervention (medications, instruments, equipment, and supplies). These patient care needs are coordinated with the other nursing interventions identified in the specific patient care plan.

Endoscopy

Endoscopy is use of a scope for visualization. Thoracic endoscopy includes use of the bronchoscope, mediastinoscope, or thoracoscope.

Medications

Topical, local, monitored anesthesia care (MAC) or general anesthesia may be used. The topical (or local) anesthetic setup should include the following:

Headlight	Medication cups
Laryngeal mirrors, various sizes	Emesis basin
Lingual spatula	Basin, small, with very warm water
Sprays with straight and curved cannulas and anesthetic drugs, as ordered	Luer-Lok syringe, 10 ml, and needles, 20 and 22 gauge, for transtracheal injection
Laryngeal syringe with straight and curved cannulas	Gauze sponges, 4 × 4 inches
Jackson cross-action forceps	Box paper tissues
Schindler pharyngeal anesthetizer, if desired	Adjustable stretcher Footstool

The anesthetic drugs frequently used are lidocaine (Xylocaine), procaine (Novocain), and tetracaine (Pontocaine, Cetacaine) with or without epinephrine (Table 24-2). Pauses of 3 to 4 minutes are taken between applications of the anesthetic agent to the tongue, palate, and pharynx, and then to the larynx and to the trachea. The anesthetic agent is applied by means of a spray or laryngeal syringe with a straight or curved cannula.

Some physicians prefer to have the patient sit upright and gargle with the topical anesthetic mixture, rinse it around in the mouth, and then expectorate it, thereby producing a partial anesthesia of the buccal mucosa and pharynx.

For direct bronchoscopy a long metal cannula attached to a syringe is generally used to apply the anesthetic agent to the surface of the vocal cords; then the agent is injected

---

TABLE 24-2

Medications used as Anesthetic for Bronchoscopy

Medication	Purpose	Side effects	Dosage
Lidocaine HCl (Xylocaine)	Topical anesthetic	Swelling, burning, irritation, rash, edema	Varies (1-2 oz)
Procaine (Novocain)	Local anesthetic	Anxiety, restlessness, loss of consciousness, drowsiness, rash, blurred vision, status asthmaticus, respiratory arrest	Varies (10 ml)
Tetracaine/tetracaine HCl (Cetacaine, Pontocaine)	Control of gagging	Rash, irritation, sensitization	Varies (1 oz)

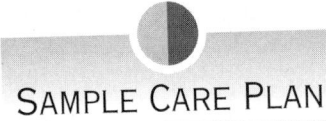

NURSING DIAGNOSIS: High risk for impaired gas exchange related to surgical intervention

OUTCOME: The patient will experience adequate gas exchange during the surgical procedure.

INTERVENTIONS:

Determine the preoperative status of gas exchange by laboratory results and assessing the patient; report deviations of studies.

Obtain chest x-rays for the intraoperative period.

Obtain the double-lumen endotracheal tube with a soft, inflatable cuff.

Obtain humidifier for ventilator gases.

Obtain equipment for and monitor arterial blood gases (ABGs).

Obtain equipment for and assist with patient preparation for hemodynamic monitoring: ECG, CO_2 analyzer, pulse oximeter, arterial pressure, central venous pressure; evaluate results provided by these monitoring devices during procedure.

Obtain equipment for temperature monitoring; monitor temperature during procedure.

Obtain thermal blanket and place on OR bed; check equipment prior to procedure; monitor during procedure.

Place ECG monitoring pads; monitor for arrhythmias.

Position the patient to provide access to the endotracheal tube, enable efficient ventilatory function, and prevent injury.

Obtain and label specimens (ABG, blood count) to be sent to laboratory; evaluate results of tests and report abnormal values.

NURSING DIAGNOSIS: High risk for impaired skin integrity related to position, length of surgical intervention and/or use of chemical antimicrobial agents on the skin

OUTCOME: The patient's skin integrity will be maintained.

INTERVENTIONS:

Note skin integrity preoperatively.

Determine presence of preexisting conditions that could compromise skin integrity (age, obesity, diabetes, allergies, radiation therapy).

Pad the OR bed.

Apply principles of positioning for efficient circulatory function for lateral or supine position during the procedure; protect vulnerable neurovascular bundles. Identify and pad pressure sites:

1. Lateral position: ear, acromion process, iliac crest, greater trochanter, medial and lateral condyles, malleolus

2. Supine position: occiput, scapula, olecranon, sacrum, ischial tuberosity, calcaneus

Stabilize the patient in lateral position on the OR bed; check for tape sensitivity if adhesive tape is used.

If hair is removed from the operative site, use clippers or a depilatory (check patient sensitivity); shave the patient with wet shave if a razor must be used.

Prevent pooling of skin preparation solutions at the bedline, site of ECG electrodes, or electrosurgical dispersive pad.

Monitor temperature of thermal unit during the procedure.

Note skin integrity postoperatively; compare to preoperative status.

NURSING DIAGNOSIS: High risk for injury related to positioning, use of equipment, and length of surgical intervention

OUTCOME: The patient will be free from injury.

INTERVENTIONS:

Test equipment prior to procedure.

Position the patient in the best possible body alignment to allow visualization of the operative field.

1. Assess for preexisting conditions (joint implants, arthritis, restricted movement).

2. Stabilize the patient in lateral position (beanbag, sandbag, soft shoulder roll, pillows between knees).

3. Flex the upper arm slightly (not exceeding 90-degree extension) above the head on a raised padded armboard or supported on padding.

4. Use adequate number of individuals to position the patient for the lateral position.

Consider principles of placement when placing the electrosurgical dispersive pad; shave the area if necessary.

Decrease surgical time by anticipating needs of the patient and surgical team; use instruments and equipment properly.

SAMPLE CARE PLAN—CONT'D

Be familiar with the surgical intervention and its planned execution.

Complete sponge, sharp, and instrument counts.

Secure tubing from urinary and chest catheters; maintain tubing patency.

NURSING DIAGNOSIS: High risk for fluid volume excess related to decreased surface area of the lung for perfusion and administration of IV fluids during surgery

OUTCOME: The patient will maintain appropriate fluid balance.

INTERVENTIONS:

Insert indwelling urinary catheter; use aseptic technique.

Position drainage bag off floor, where it is readily observable.

Monitor urinary output hourly during the procedure; report output less than 30 ml per hour.

Provide access for administration of IV fluids; assist with administration and insertion of lines.

Monitor results of hemodynamic parameters; report appropriately.

Monitor blood loss during the procedure; report appropriately.

Provide blood (including autologous) or blood products for fluid replacement; assist in replacement therapy and patient monitoring.

Observe for symptoms of shock (hypotension, abnormal ECG); report symptoms and initiate corrective nursing actions.

Observe for symptoms of excess blood loss (rapid, weak pulse, rapid respirations, cool, moist skin, and early, slight rise in blood pressure); report symptoms and initiate corrective nursing actions.

Observe for symptoms of fluid excess (tachycardia, increased blood pressure); report symptoms and initiate corrective nursing actions.

Have available and administer furosemide (Lasix) and other diuretic agents as prescribed; monitor for therapeutic results.

NURSING DIAGNOSIS: High risk for infection related to inadequate secondary defenses (presence of existing disease process) and surgical disruption of tissues

OUTCOME: The patient will be free from infection.

INTERVENTIONS:

Create and maintain a sterile field.

Wear proper operating room attire.

Utilize aseptic technique when opening supplies, moving about the sterile field, completing skin preparation, catheterizing the patient, and inserting intravenous lines.

Complete skin preparation at the incision site and point of insertion of monitoring lines to decrease microbial contamination.

Monitor traffic patterns; limit the number of individuals entering and leaving the operating room.

Administer antibiotic of choice for irrigation and intravenous administration; check for patient allergies; record all medications administered by the perioperative nurse or from the sterile field.

Decrease surgical time by anticipating patient needs.

Monitor sterile technique of team members; initiate corrective action for breaks in technique.

Obtain appropriate suture; consider whether patient is obese, malnourished, or presents with symptoms of a secondary disease process when selecting suture.

---

through the anesthetized glottis into the trachea. This act causes the patient to produce a sharp, sudden cough.

For intrabronchial anesthesia a portion of the anesthetic agent is introduced through the bronchoscope.

Refer to Chapter 6 for perioperative nursing considerations when monitoring the patient receiving local or monitored anesthesia care.

Draping

Aseptic technique is used during an endoscopy. The principles of draping for other procedures are followed (see Chapter 3).

Instrumentation

Instruments are designed for direct inspection and observation of the larynx, trachea, bronchi, or mediastinum;

to remove secretions; to obtain washings or tissue for bacterial and cytologic studies, or to remove tissue. They are also designed to remove foreign bodies.

Bronchoscope. The standard bronchoscope is a rigid speculum for visualizing the tracheobronchial tree. The rigid bronchoscope might be selected for biopsy of a large central mass, removal of a foreign object, or to provide a mechanism for hemorrhage control during biopsy of a vascular mass. The rigid bronchoscope remains the instrument of choice for removal of foreign bodies in infants and children. A fiberoptic light carrier is inserted into the bronchoscope to illuminate the distal opening. A side channel has been incorporated into the bronchoscope to permit aeration of the lungs with oxygen or anesthetic gases (Fig. 24-7). An additional device, the Sanders Venturi system, which is available to the anesthesiologist, provides adequate patient observation and ventilation during bronchoscopies and laryngoscopies. Fiberoptic telescopes permit visualization of the upper, middle, and lower lobe bronchi. They can be passed in patients with jaw deformity or rigid cervical spine with less difficulty than the rigid scope. Flexible fiberoptic bronchoscopes are being used with increased frequency, as is video endoscopy.

Mediastinoscope. The mediastinoscope is used to view lymph nodes or masses in the superior mediastinum. The instrument is a hollow tube with a fiberoptic light carrier (Fig. 24-8). A fiberoptic illuminator with a light intensity dial provides power and control of illumination (Fig. 24-9).

Thoracoscope. The thoracoscope is the endoscopic approach to visualization of the thoracic cavity for diagnosis of pleural or disease or treatment of conditions, eliminating the need for a thoracotomy incision.

Lasers. The Nd:YAG or CO_2 laser might be used for treating tracheobronchial lesions, using a bronchoscope. Obstruction of the mainstem bronchus and trachea caused by benign and malignant lesions can effectively be treated (Research Highlight 24-2). Use of laser equipment requires a thorough understanding of the equipment, responsibilities, and the procedure (see Chapter 31).

Light carriers, cord, and illuminator. Each standard scope requires a fiberoptic light carrier, cord, and illuminator. Duplicates of each, along with the appropriate replacement light bulbs for the illuminator, should be available for immediate use. The light source (Figs. 24-9 and 24-10) should be tested periodically and also immediately before use.

Sponge carriers and sponges. The metal sponge carrier (Fig. 24-11) consists of two parts: an inner rod, which has two jaws protruding from its distal end, and an outer band, which is screwed down on the inner rod so a sponge can be held securely within the jaws. Small gauze sponges are used to keep the field dry, remove secretions, and apply a topical anesthetic agent.

Specimen collectors. Cytologic specimen collectors, such as the Clerf (Fig. 24-11) or Lukens, are used to hold secretions as they are obtained.

Aspirators. Aspirating tubes of different lengths and designs (Fig. 24-11) are used to remove secretions and collect material for microscopic examination and cultures. The

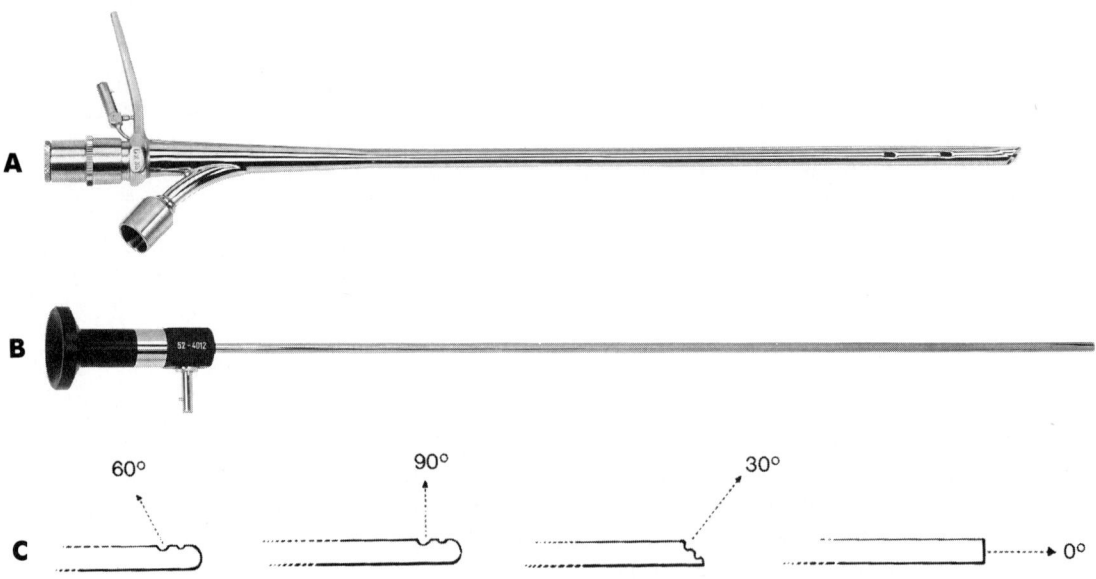

FIG. 24-7   Instruments for bronchoscopy. **A,** Holinger ventilating fiberoptic bronchoscope. **B,** Fiberoptic light carrier. **C,** Fiberoptic bronchoscopic telescopes: *a,* forward oblique 60 degree; *b,* lateral 90 degree; *c,* right angle 30 degree; *d,* forward 0 degree.

Courtesy Pilling Co., Fort Washington, Pa.

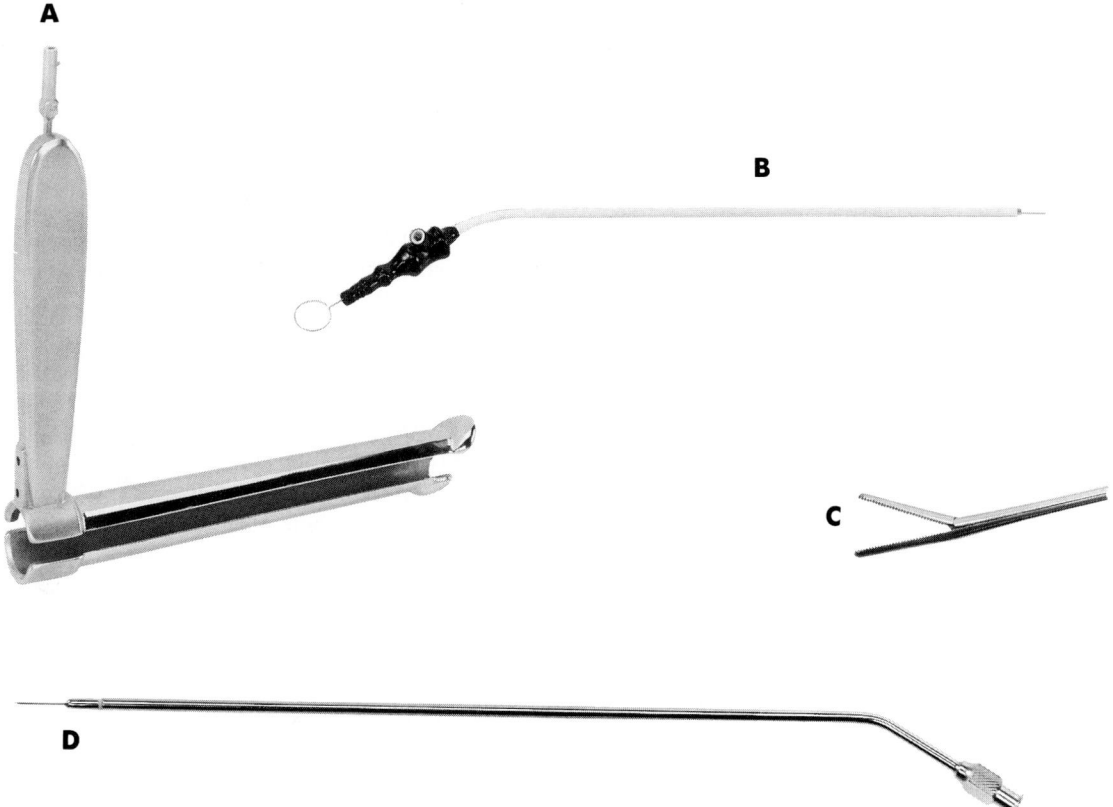

FIG. 24-8 Instruments for mediastinoscopy. **A,** Carlens mediastinoscope. **B,** Insulated suction tube. **C,** Jackson laryngeal forceps. **D,** Aspirating needle.

Courtesy Pilling Co., Fort Washington, Pa.

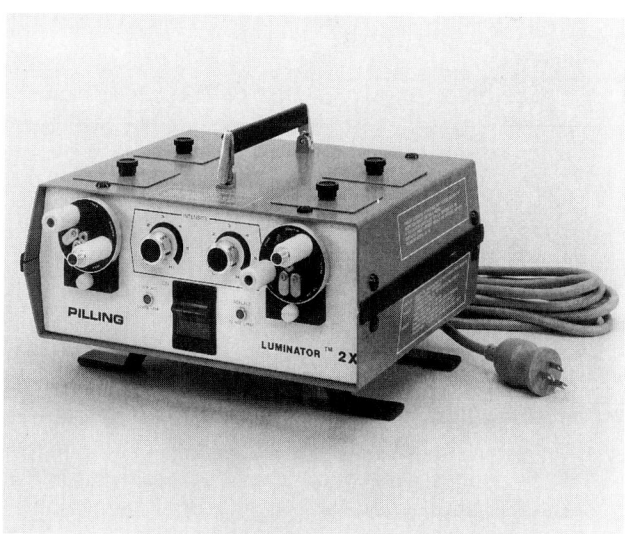

FIG. 24-9 Fiberoptic illuminator with multipurpose adaptor that accepts several types of fiberoptic light cords.

Courtesy Pilling Co., Washington, PA.

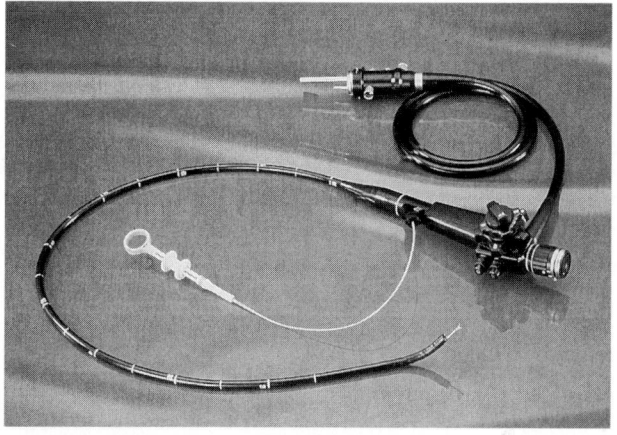

FIG. 24-10 Cold light source with flexible endoscope.

Courtesy Olympus, New Hyde Park, NY.

☀
RESEARCH HIGHLIGHT 24-2

The first report of the application of a laser in treatment of tracheobronchial lesions was in 1974, using a CO_2 laser with a rigid bronchoscope to treat tracheal papilloma. Certain studies, each using a different laser type, classified treatment as effective if general palliation in patients with severe ventilatory disturbance was accomplished. Patients treated by complete resection were compared with patients treated palliatively. A significant difference was found in survival associated with the number of metastases. Studies have resulted in descriptive indications for use of the laser for inoperable malignant tumors located in the trachea or mainstem bronchus that can cause dyspnea. Also, inoperable tumors with uncertain prognosis, such as carcinoids, adenoid cystic carcinoma, and benign tumors with extrabronchial involvement, can be treated.

Martini, N., & Vogt-Moykopf, I. (1989). *Thoracic surgery: Frontiers and uncommon neoplasms.* St. Louis: Mosby.

straight aspirating tube with one or two openings at the distal end is used to remove material from the pharynx, larynx, and esophagus. The curved aspirating tube with a flexible tip is used to remove secretions from the upper and dorsal orifices of the bronchi.

Forceps. Various types of forceps are designed to remove foreign bodies or tissues for histologic study. In bronchoscopy biting tip forceps may be used to secure tissue for study. Forceps with jaws that veer laterally at about a 45-degree angle from the instrument's axis permit visualization during the biopsy maneuver. Bronchoesophageal forceps (Fig. 24-12) consist of a stylet, a cannula with a handle, a screw, a locknut, and a set screw. Forceps for laryngeal and bronchial regions are designed to remove tissue specimens.

Handling, terminal disinfection, and care

Handling of instruments. To ensure long life of the optical system of endoscopes, each instrument should be kept straight at all times when not in use. Flexible endoscopes should never be severely bent.

Only the instrument manufacturer should replace a scope part. When a telescope is sent for repair, it must be properly packed in a padded instrument case and placed within a padded carton to ensure protection of the lens system during transportation. A direct blow can break the objective window or lenses of telescopic endoscopes. The junction of the flexible and rigid portions of the scope is the most vulnerable point.

During use the patient might bite down while the flexible portion of the scope is being passed. A specially designed mouthpiece may be used to prevent damage to the scope. The sheath covering the flexible part may become perforated after contact. When a new covering is needed, the instrument should be sent to the manufacturer.

Preparing endoscopes for terminal storage. The manufacturer's procedures for cleaning, terminally disinfecting, and terminally sterilizing flexible or rigid endoscopes should be followed. Usually, the flexible and rigid scopes can be cleaned with soap and water. A soft brush designed to clean the lumen is used for rigid scopes. Both types can then be soaked in activated glutaraldehyde or an iodophor concentrate germicide and thoroughly rinsed and dried

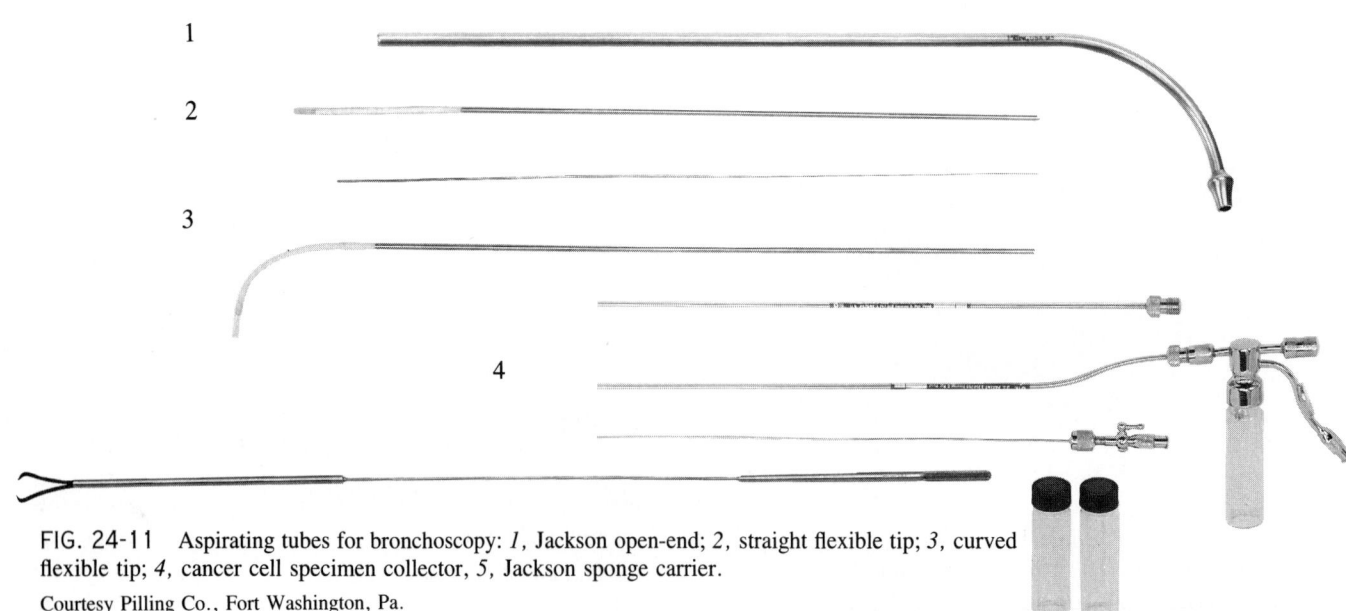

FIG. 24-11   Aspirating tubes for bronchoscopy: *1,* Jackson open-end; *2,* straight flexible tip; *3,* curved flexible tip; *4,* cancer cell specimen collector, *5,* Jackson sponge carrier.

Courtesy Pilling Co., Fort Washington, Pa.

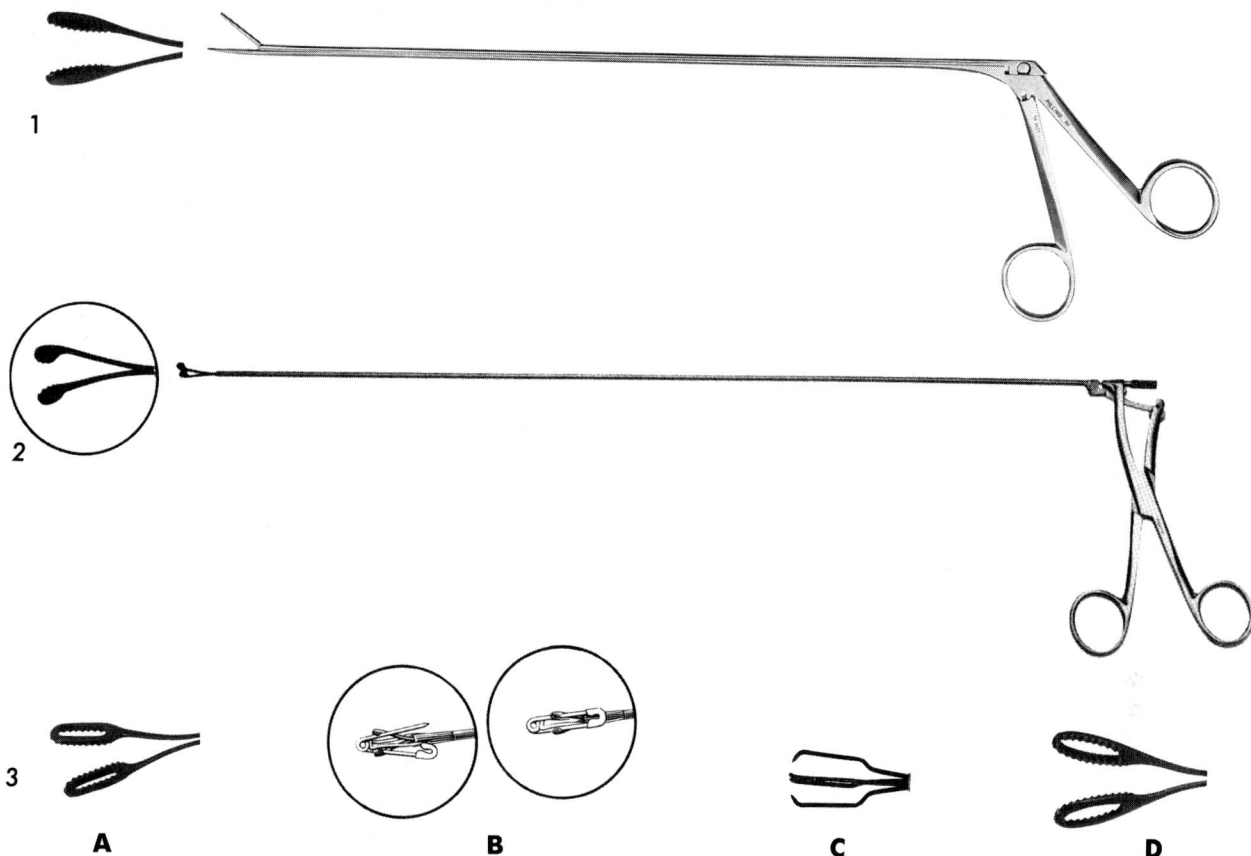

FIG. 24-12   Forceps for bronchoscopy. *1,* Jackson forward grasping forceps with serrated, cupped jaws; *2,* Jackson side-curved grasping forceps; *3,* forceps for foreign body removal: **A,** Jackson fenestrated peanut-grasping forceps, **B,** Clerf-Arrowsmith safety pin closer, **C,** Gordon bead grasping forceps, **D,** Jackson fenestrated meat-grasping forceps.

Courtesy Pilling Co., Fort Washington, Pa.

before storage. If feasible, they can be sterilized according to the manufacturer's recommendations. In some facilities specially designed washers, and in some cases sterilizers, may be available for terminal processing of endoscopes.

Cleaning a telescopic endoscope. The scope is held vertically by its ocular end and is wiped repeatedly with downward strokes, using gauze sponges or a soft brush saturated with surgical soap and water. Special attention is given to surface joints and crevices that may retain mucus. The scope is then dried thoroughly with clean gauze sponges.

Optical telescopes should never undergo boiling or steam sterilization. Sterilizing agents must be recommended for use by the manufacturer. High-level disinfection is achieved by use of a noncorrosive microbicidal solution.

Cleaning aspirating tubes and sponge carriers. These instruments are cleaned and flushed with soap and water and are sterilized by steam or gas. Special care must be given to spiral-tipped aspirators. All bent or broken-tipped aspirators should be sent to the manufacturer for repair.

The sponge carrier collar must be unscrewed before it is cleaned. After sterilization the threads of the carrier are oiled. The carrier is reassembled and stored lying straight.

Cleaning forceps. The forceps may be placed in an ultrasonic cleaner. After cleaning, each forceps is taken apart, one at a time, by unscrewing the nut and removing the stylet. All parts are examined carefully, and noncorrosive solvent oil is applied to the joint of the forceps. Each forceps is reassembled and the action tested; then it is stored lying straight with jaws open. Forceps in good condition should have (1) jaws close together in parallel position; (2) handles touching slightly when the jaws are closed; (3) jaws merging into the cannula when the forcep is closed and protruding widely without expanding the spring when it is open; (4) the end nut, located in the stylet, in place; (5) the side screw tight; and (6) the distal end and jaws' edges smooth on finger examination.

Setting and testing the illumination. To test the fiberoptic light carrier and telescope, the instrument should be held vertically by the ocular end. The endoscope should always be tested immediately before passage into the patient. The light intensity dial should be set at the proper level, as specified by the manufacturer. The light source should be switched on and off to test its function.

Postprocedure concerns

Patient safety during and following endoscopy under topical, local anesthesia or monitored anesthesia care is a concern due to medications administered. The gag reflex may not return for 2 to 3 hours. The patient may be positioned on the side or with the head of the bed elevated to promote drainage of secretions. The patient should be restricted from any oral intake until the gag reflex has returned. During bronchoscopy, particularly with a rigid bronchoscope, teeth could be loosened or oral structures damaged. The lips, teeth, and oral mucosa should be examined to ensure undisturbed integrity. Patients are also anxious to know the results of the procedure and benefit from the nurse's openness and willingness to discuss feelings and perceptions.

Thoracotomy
Positioning

Thoracotomies can be performed with the patient in one of three common positions. The type of position is determined by the operative procedure planned. The three basic approaches are (1) posterolateral thoracotomy, (2) anterolateral thoracotomy (Fig. 24-13), and (3) median sternotomy (Research Highlight 24-3). The prone position can also provide access in some procedures.

Draping

The drapes may be a fenestrated sheet or single sheets surrounding the incision site. A magnetic pad may be placed on the drapes below the incision site when the pa-

---

RESEARCH HIGHLIGHT 24-3

Median sternotomy or lateral thoracotomy are the select approaches for patients undergoing thoracic procedures. A median sternotomy exposure can be extended by performing an anterior thoracotomy if deemed necessary during the procedure. Advantages of median sternotomy over lateral thoracotomy are lower postoperative pain, stress, and morbidity, less restriction and smaller reduction of postoperative pulmonary reserve, and shorter postoperative hospital stays. Lateral thoracotomy remains indicated in surgery for metastases in unilateral tumors, large tumors, and tumors infiltrating the posterior mediastinum or posterior chest wall.

Martini, N., & Vogt-Moykopf, I. (1989). *Thoracic surgery: Frontiers and uncommon neoplasms.* St. Louis: Mosby.

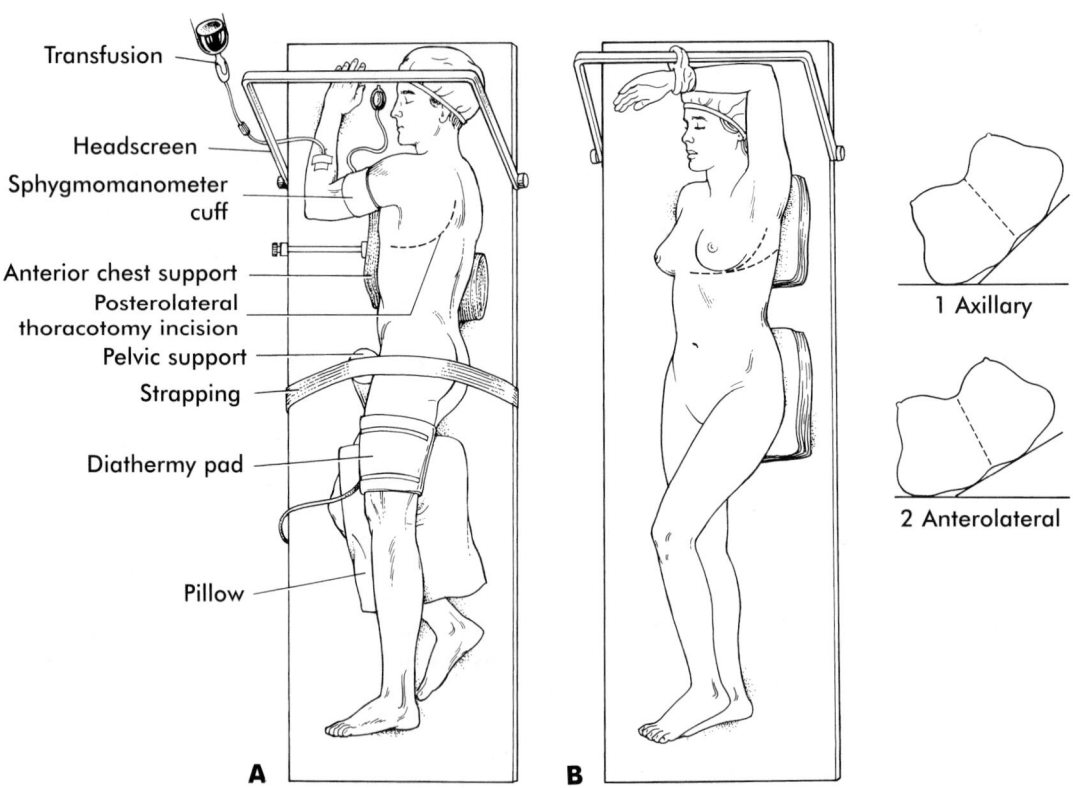

FIG. 24-13   Positions for thoracotomy incisions. **A,** Lateral position for posterolateral incision. **B,** Semilateral position for axillary or anterolateral position.

tient is placed in lateral position to prevent instruments from falling from the field.

Instrumentation

Instrumentation for thoracic surgery includes the laparotomy instrument set (see Chapter 10), plus the following specialty items (Figs. 24-14 and 24-15).

Cutting instruments

2 Nelson scissors, curved, 10 inches (Fig. 24-14)
1 Potts tenotomy scissors, 7½ inches
1 Potts dissecting scissors, angulated 60 degree, 7½ inches
1 Wire cutter

Holding instruments

14 Backhaus towel clamps, 5 inches
2 Potts-Smith vascular forceps, smooth, 7 inches
2 Potts-Smith vascular forceps, fine-toothed, 7 inches
6 Rumel thoracic clamps, 9 inches (Fig. 24-14)
4 Duval lung-grasping forceps (Fig. 24-14)
1 Semb forceps, 9¼ inches

Clamping instruments

6 Right-angled clamps, assorted lengths and angulations
4 Sarot or Less bronchus clamps, right and left (Fig. 24-14)

Vascular instruments

2 Crafoord coarctation clamps
4 Patent ductus clamps, 2 angulated and 2 straight
2 Satinsky clamps
2 Cooley clamps

Bone instruments
(Fig. 24-15)

1 Alexander periosteotome
1 Overholt elevator

2 Doyen rib raspatories and elevators, 1 right and 1 left
1 Liston-Stille bone-cutting forceps
1 Bethune rib shears
1 Sauerbruch rib rongeur, double-action, square jaw
1 Stille-Luer bone rongeur, multiple action

Median sternotomy instruments

1 Sternal saw (Fig. 24-15)
1 Lebsche sternal knife (Fig. 24-15)
1 Mallet
1 Sternal spreader
1 Sternal approximator
2 Bone tenacula, single-hook
1 Bone punch or awl with fenestrated tip

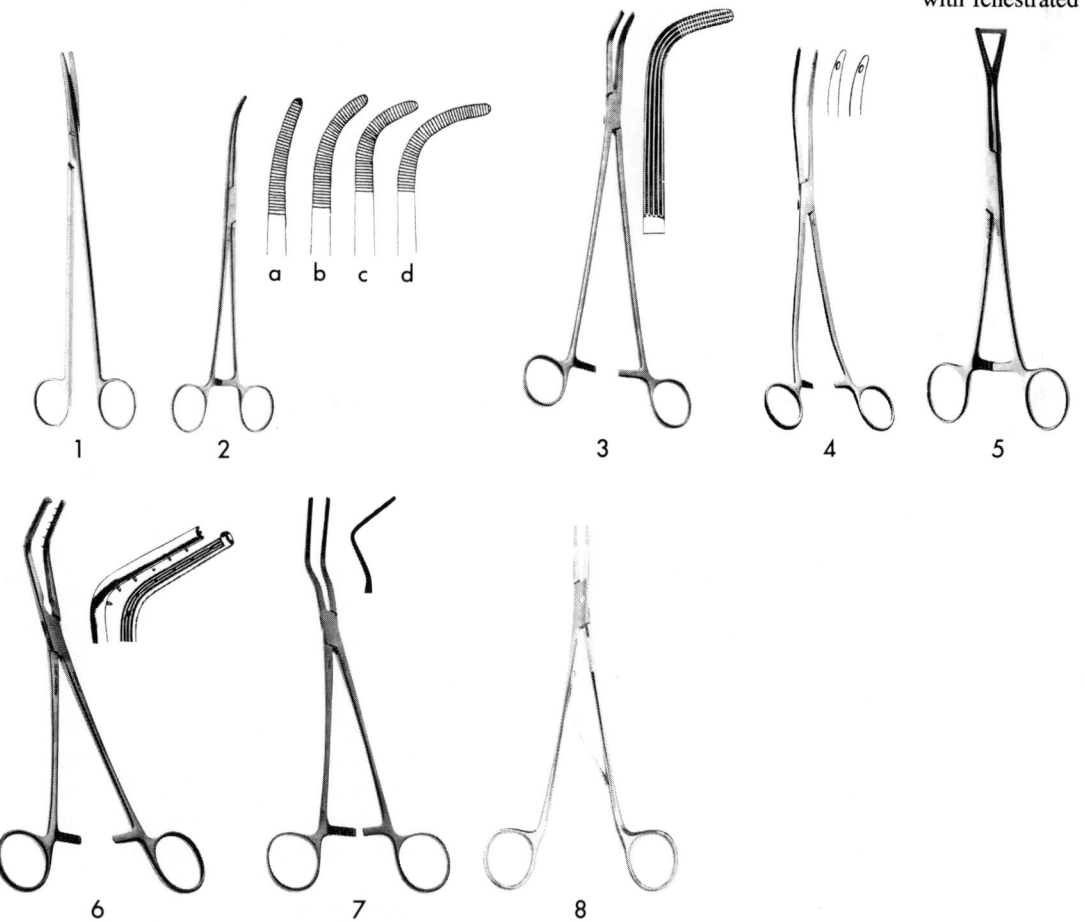

FIG. 24-14 Instruments for lobectomy and pneumonectomy. *1,* Nelson scissors; *2,* Rumel thoracic clamps, *a* to *d; 3,* Harrington forceps; *4,* Willauer-Allis thoracic tissue forceps; *5,* Duval lung-grasping forceps; *6,* Sarot bronchus clamp; *7,* Lees bronchus clamp; *8,* hemoclip appliers.

1 through *7* courtesy Codman & Shurtleff, Inc., Randolph, Mass.; *8* courtesy Zimmer, Inc., Warsaw, Ind.

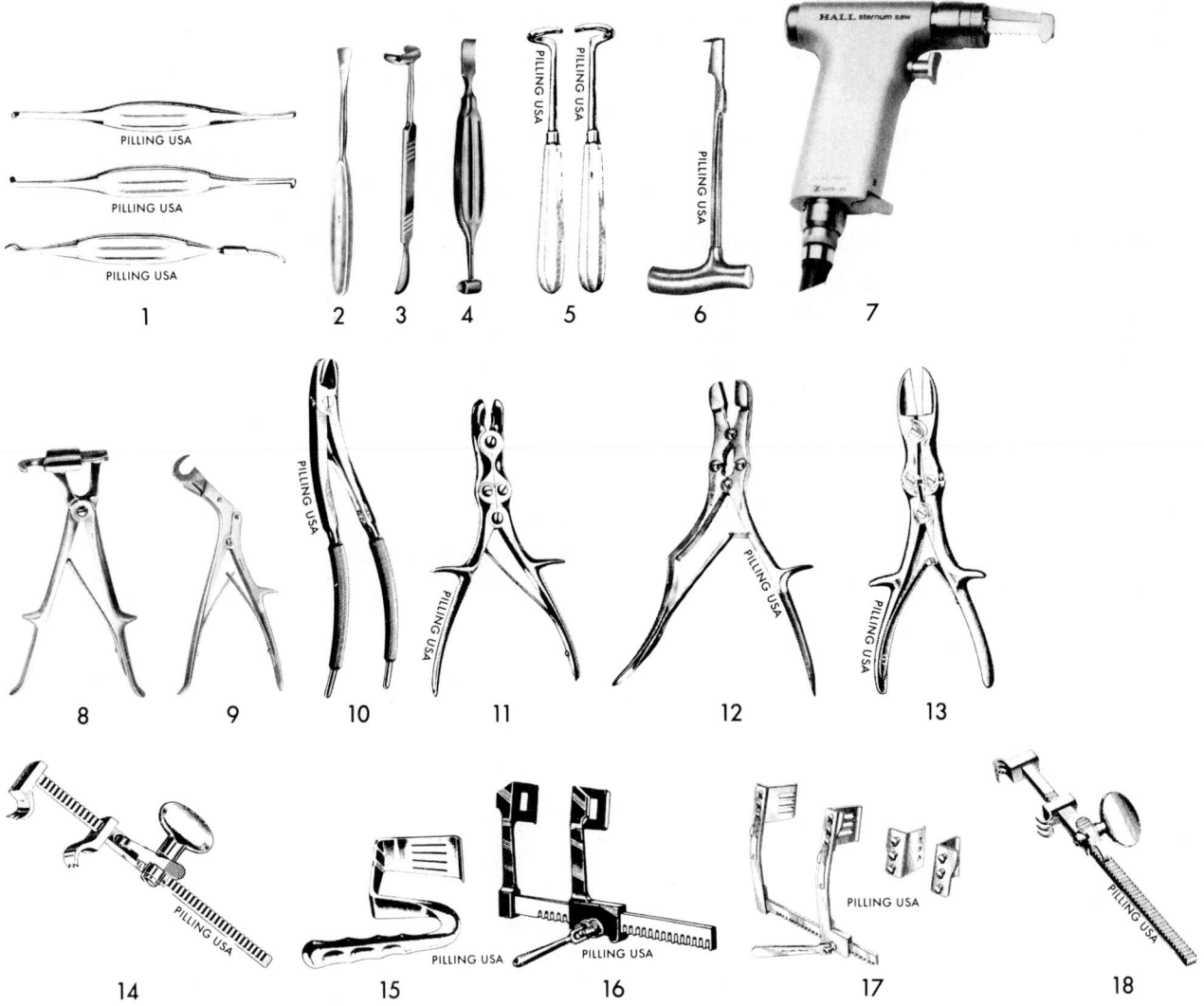

FIG. 24-15   Instruments for thoracotomy. *1*, Overholt elevators, nos. 1, 2, and 3; *2*, Langenbeck periosteal elevator; *3* Matson rib elevator and stripper; *4*, Alexander costal periosteotome; *5*, Doyen rib raspatories, right and left; *6*, Lebsche sternal knife; *7*, sternal saw; *8*, Sauerbruch rib shear; *9*, Giertz (first rib)
rib guillotine; *10*, Bethune rib shears; *11*, Stille-Luer bone rongeur; *12*, Sauerbruch rib rongeur; *13*,
Stille-Liston bone-cutting forceps, straight; *14*, Bailey rib spreader; *15*, Davidson scapula retractor; *16*,
Finochietto rib retractor; *17*, Burford rib retractor with two sets detachable blades; *18*, Bailey rib retractor.

Retractors

2 Volkmann rake retrac-
tors, blunt, six or
eight pronged
2 Kelly retractors, large
1 Burford-Finochietto
rib retractor with 2
sets blades (Fig. 24-
15).
3 Finochietto retractors,
assorted sizes (Fig.
24-15)
2 Bailey rib contractors
(Fig. 24-15)
1 Davidson scapula re-
tractor (Fig. 24-15)

Suturing instruments

6 Sarot needle holders,
10 inches and 12
inches
4 Hemoclip appliers
Bronchus or thoracic
stapler

Accessory items

Electrosurgical unit
2 Disposable chest cath-
eters, selected sizes
(with appropriate con-
nectors)
1 Bone wax
2 Asepto syringes

1 Water-seal drainage
system (Fig. 24-16,
A, B)

2 Suction tubings,
6-foot lengths
6 Pieces umbilical tape,
18 inches

Perioperative nursing staff should determine the thoracic
surgery arrangement of items on the instrument table and
Mayo stand; this arrangement should be an effective standard method that applies principles of work simplification
and thorough knowledge of procedures.

Chest drainage systems

In the presence of restrictive and obstructive pulmonary
disease, the lung may not fully expand or contract,
causing a reduction in alveolar ventilation with resultant
hypoxia. Other conditions that interfere with respiratory

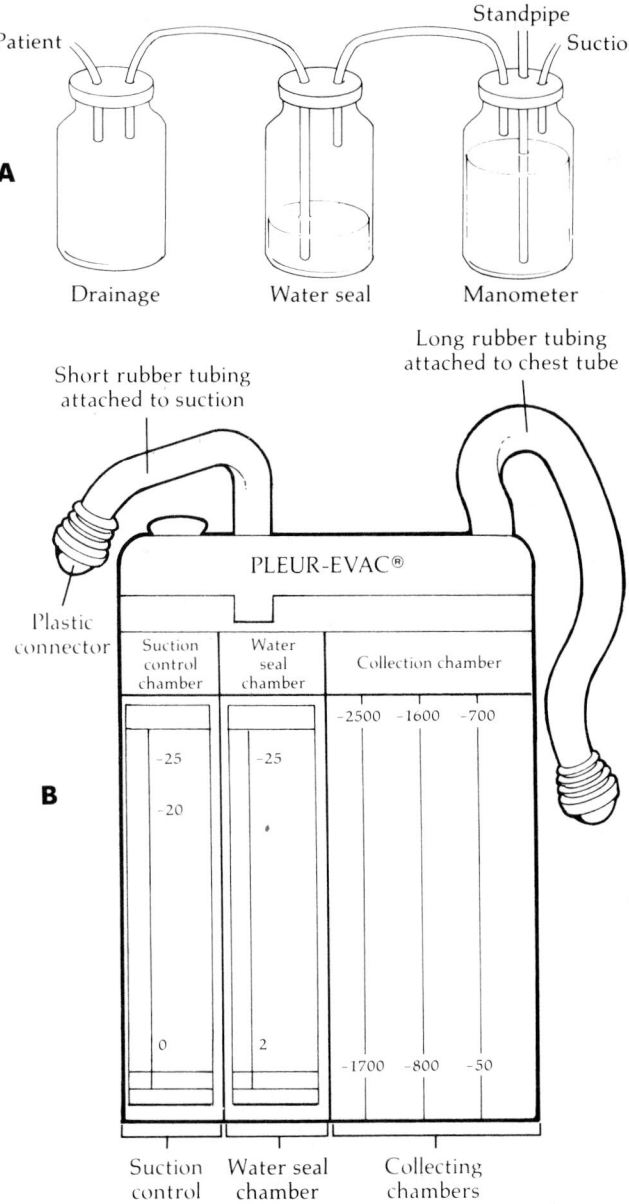

FIG. 24-16 **A,** Method of draining pleural space, using triple-bottle system as model. **B,** Commercial chest drainage system.

From Thompson, J.M., McFarland, G.K., Hirsch, J.E., and Tucker, S.M. (1993) *Mosby's clinical nursing* (3rd ed.). St. Louis: Mosby.

the chest wall. When the pleural space is filled with air, reducing the negative pressure, the lung collapses. This action may cause complete collapse if the pressure within the intrathoracic (pleural) space becomes positive.

A diminished negative pressure or occurrence of actual positive pressure in one pleural space may cause the mediastinum or trachea to shift toward the opposite side. When this happens, not only does the affected lung collapse because of a positive pressure in the pleural space, but the function of the lung on the opposite side may also be impaired as a result of compression by the shifted mediastinum. Tension pneumothorax can produce serious effects as air continues to escape from the lung into the intrapleural space. The air is unable to return to the bronchi to be exhaled, thereby increasing the intrapleural pressure. When a large opening in the chest wall allows direct communication of the pleural space with atmospheric pressure, it may cause death if the mediastinum becomes mobile. The exposure of the pleural space to atmospheric pressure collapses the affected lung. The positive pressure is also transmitted to the mediastinum, which in turn shifts toward the opposite side and may cause the opposite lung to collapse.

Paradoxic motion of the chest results from severe instability of the chest wall because of multiple and often bilateral rib fractures; with inspiration, partial collapse of the thoracic space occurs. The blunt injury that caused the multiple rib fractures also causes severe contusion of the lung itself. This contusion contributes to impairment of lung function by affecting gas exchange, which may result in severe, life-threatening hypoxia.

One or more chest catheters (tubes) may be inserted for postoperative closed chest drainage. The chest tubes provide a conduit for drainage of air, blood, and other fluid from the intrapleural or mediastinal space and reestablishment of negative pressure in the intrapleural space. Drainage systems use three mechanisms to drain fluid and air from the pleural cavity: positive expiratory pressure, gravity, and suction. The chest tubes are connected to a sterile water-seal or gravity drainage system. Water-seal suction may be necessary when a persistent air leak cannot be controlled by drainage alone. Historically, a two- or three-bottle system was used to accomplish this. Several compact, disposable units are available that function like the three-bottle system; these units are preferable because they are easier and safer to use. The principles of operation remain the same and can be described more easily by using the bottle system model (see Fig. 24-16, *A*). The first bottle collects the drainage from the intrapleural space, the second bottle provides the water seal, and the third provides the suction control determined by the level of water. The disposable units have three or four compartments for drainage, water seal, and suction (see Fig. 24-16, *B*).

If two chest tubes are inserted, they may be attached by a Y connector to a single drainage unit or attached individually to two separate units. All connections should be

function are mucus, a foreign body in a bronchus, closed pneumothorax (simple and tension types), open pneumothorax, hemothorax, and multiple rib injuries that produce paradoxic motion of the thoracic cage, or flail chest (Fig. 24-17).

The normal function of the lungs is caused by elasticity and negative intrapleural pressure. Collapse of the normal lung follows any condition that reduces or eliminates the negative intrapleural pressure if the lung is not adherent to

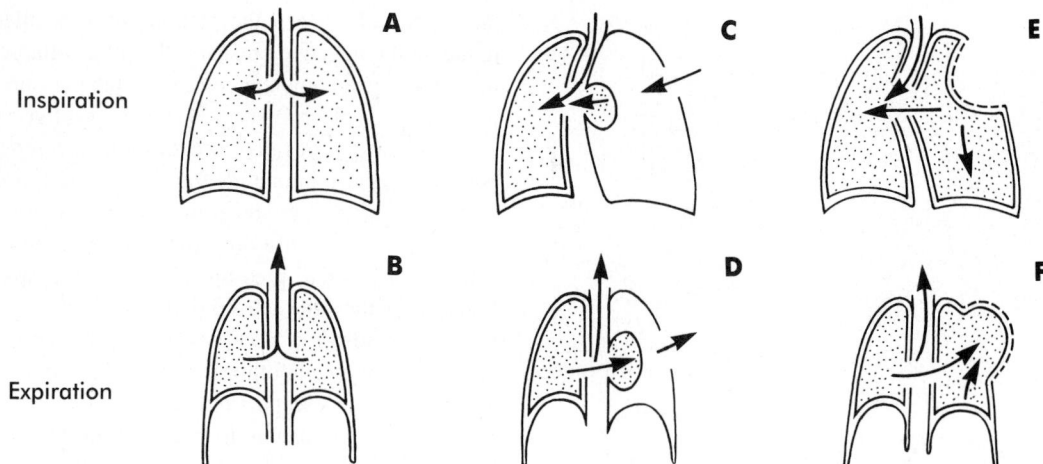

Inspiration

Expiration

FIG. 24-17   Pathophysiology of severe chest injuries. **A** and **B,** Normal physiology of inspiration and expiration. **C** and **D,** Open (sucking) wound of thorax. On inspiration, air at atmospheric pressure rushes in through defect **(C),** collapsing lung. Next, positive pressure causes mediastinum to shift, compressing opposite lung. On expiration **(D)** air from lung on uninjured side reenters collapsed lung and is rebreathed in next inspiration. Impaired cardiopulmonary function in presence of sucking wound of chest is caused by (1) collapse of lung on injured side; (2) partial collapse of opposite lung; (3) increased functional dead space caused by rebreathing of unoxygenated air from collapsed lung; and (4) diminished venous return to right side of heart. **E** and **F,** Primary effect of paradoxical motion resulting from flail or stove-in chest is diminution of pulmonary ventilation and extensive rebreathing from one lung to the other. Venous return to right side of heart is impaired. Appropriate treatment requires intubation of trachea and use of volume-limited ventilator.

From Johnson, J., & Kirby, C.K. (1970). *Surgery of the chest* (4th ed.). Chicago: Year Book Medical Publishers.

banded or otherwise secured to ensure an intact system (Fig. 24-18). The drainage system must be sterile and maintained in a position lower than the patient's body to prevent air and fluid from reentering the chest cavity. Chest tubes are generally removed within 5 to 7 days.

Monitoring

During a thoracotomy the patient requires constant monitoring of laboratory results (ABGs), temperature, blood loss, and urine output. The results are communicated with other team members for continuity of care.

Blood replacement

A procedure requiring extensive tissue dissection and removal in a highly vascular area could result in the need for replacement of blood during or following the procedure. A patient may have autologous blood ordered; however, the diagnosis may prohibit patient donation of his or her own blood. The blood type and amount of blood ordered before the procedure should be noted and its availability determined. During the procedure, every effort should be made to control and monitor bleeding. If blood collection or reinfusion systems are used, manufacturer's instructions and institutional protocols should be followed.

Postprocedure concerns

Patients are transferred to the PACU using care not to dislodge the chest tube, urinary catheter, or monitoring equipment. The endotracheal tube may remain in place to

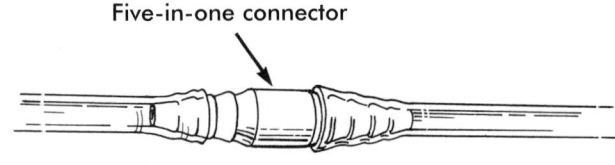

Five-in-one connector

Incorrect: Complete wrapping

Parnham band or

Correct: Tape strips

FIG. 24-18   Method of securing chest tubes after connection to water-seal drainage system.

maintain an adequate air exchange. Air exchange and effective ventilation are two immediate needs of the patient after thoracotomy. Functional capacity may be altered due to muscle injury and pain. A postprocedure epidural catheter with monitoring or injection of Marcaine at the completion of closure for pain management should improve the comfort level of the patient as postoperative activities are encouraged. Patients are often anxious about their limitations, the environment, and the results of the procedure. They benefit from information shared and from being allowed to discuss their feelings and needs. Family members should be informed of the status of the patient following the procedure.

Documentation

Documentation of perioperative care includes assessment of the patient upon admission to the operating room, nursing interventions, and postoperative evaluation. Documentation for a patient undergoing a thoracotomy specifically addresses positioning aids, position of the patient, medications administered, results of laboratory tests completed, equipment used, such as a thermal blanket, urine output, blood replacement, insertion of chest tubes and drainage systems, and postoperative evaluation of skin integrity.

Discharge information

The patient is discharged from the operating room to the PACU following thoracotomy. The report to the PACU nurse is often a collaborative effort of the nurse and anesthesiologist. The perioperative nurse reports the patient's preoperative status, including anxiety level and understanding of the procedure, to assist the PACU nurse in meeting the emotional needs of the patient. A description of the position of the patient during the procedure provides criteria for assessment and evaluation of mobility. Results of immediate postoperative assessment including skin integrity, location and type of dressing applied, location and type of drains, blood loss, fluid replacement, medications administered, and laboratory results obtained during the procedure are reported as a baseline for assessment in the PACU. The PACU nurse must be informed of the procedure completed, particularly if it varies from the anticipated procedure. The perioperative care plan should be reviewed and patient outcomes reported.

EVALUATION

As part of the care planning process, the perioperative nursing goals are evaluated. They may be restated as brief outcomes. For the goals identified for the patient undergoing thoracic surgery, they would be:

- The patient's gas exchange was unimpaired; ventilation/perfusion ratios were adequate as evidenced by laboratory results and vital signs within normal limits; skin, nailbeds, and mucosa were pink; lung fields were clear bilaterally; and chest excursion was normal.

- The patient's skin integrity was maintained; reddened or discolored skin and other signs of altered tissue perfusion were not present.
- The patient sustained no injury from the surgical position; postoperative pain and discomfort unrelated to preoperative conditions or the surgical incision were not present.
- Fluid balance was maintained; there were no fluid excesses or deficits; mental orientation was consistent with preoperative level; serum electrolytes and arterial blood gases were within normal limits and urinary output was stable.
- The patient will not experience a postoperative wound infection; the incision site will remain approximated and dry, without redness, drainage, or undue tenderness. (This is a long-term goal, and its evaluation will require the collaboration of the nurse in the patient care unit.)

SURGICAL INTERVENTIONS
ENDOSCOPY (DIAGNOSTIC OR THERAPEUTIC)

Endoscopy refers to examination of hollow body organs or cavities with instruments that permit visual inspection of their contents and walls. The endoscopic procedures pertinent to thoracic surgery are bronchoscopy, mediastinoscopy, and thoracoscopy. Each endoscopist has preferences regarding the type of endoscope, positioning of the patient, type of anesthetic, and equipment. Invasive diagnostic or therapeutic measures enhance the decision to pursue surgical intervention by providing information related to the disease process, including histology, location of the lesion, and lesion extent. Therapeutic endoscopy provides treatment by removal of the lesion or foreign body.

Standard bronchoscopy using rigid bronchoscope

Standard bronchoscopy is the direct visualization of the mucosa of the trachea, the main bronchi and their openings, and most of the segmental bronchi and includes removal of material for microscopic study if necessary.

Bronchoscopy is an integral part of the examination of patients with pulmonary symptoms such as persistent cough or wheezing, hemoptysis, obstruction, and abnormal roentgenographic changes. Common causes of bleeding (hemoptysis) are bronchiectasis, carcinoma, and tuberculosis. Congenital anomalies and suspected presence of a foreign body, especially in infants and children, are responsible for emergency examination of the respiratory tract.

Bronchoscopy is done to determine the presence of a lesion in the tracheobronchial passages, to identify and localize that lesion accurately, and to observe periodically the effects of therapy. In suspected carcinoma the aspirated secretions obtained by bronchoscopy may contain malignant cells.

Procedural considerations. Bronchoscopy on an adult patient may be completed with the patient under local anesthesia or monitored anesthesia care; a child usually receives general anesthesia. The adult patient receiving local anesthesia may experience discomfort and anxiety. To reduce anxiety, personnel should be introduced, intraoperative activities explained, and reassurance provided to the patient. The oral structures, including the teeth and lips, should be assessed for integrity. Loose teeth may require removal before or during the procedure.

Intravenous sedatives or analgesics may be administered during the procedure. See Chapter 6 for perioperative nursing considerations when monitoring the patient receiving local or monitored anesthesia care.

The patient may be positioned either in supine position, with the shoulders elevated on a small roll or a sandbag to gently extend the head and neck, or in the sitting position. The setup includes the following:

Bronchoscope (see Fig. 24-7)	Forceps, desired types (see Fig. 24-12)
Telescopes, desired types	Bronchial spray and cannula
Fiberoptic light cords	Lubricant (water soluble)
Fiberoptic light source	
Suction tubing	Topical anesthesia set, if desired
Aspirating tubes (see Fig. 24-11)	Emesis basin
Specimen collectors (see Fig. 24-11)	Gauze sponges
Sponge carriers (see Fig. 24-11)	Basin with sterile saline solution

The bronchoscopist risks contamination in the presence of communicable diseases. For this reason the endoscopist and assistants should wear face masks and eyeglasses, goggles, or a transparent shield attached to a headband. With increasing numbers of patients with tuberculosis, particulate respirators are recommended as protective devices. Aseptic technique is used to prevent cross-contamination.

Operative procedure (Fig. 24-19)

1. The head is placed in position for visualization of the bronchus, to the left when the right main bronchi are inspected, and to the right when the left bronchi are inspected. The head is lowered for inspection of the middle lobe.
2. The bronchoscope is inserted over the surface of the tongue, usually through the right corner of the mouth. The patient's lip is retracted from the upper teeth with a finger of the endoscopist's left hand. The epiglottis is identified and elevated with the tip of the bronchoscope.
3. The distal end of the scope is passed through the true vocal cords of the larynx, and the upper tracheal rings are viewed. A small amount of anesthetic solution may be sprayed through the tube on the carina of the trachea and into the bronchus with the bronchial atomizer or spray. The patient's head is moved to the left to obtain a view of the right bronchi. The right-angle telescope is inserted with the light adjusted into the bronchoscope. The optical system should be kept free from precipitated moisture.

4. The segmental bronchial orifices of the upper right lobe bronchi are viewed and the telescope removed. Suction and aspirating tubes are introduced to clear the field of vision.
5. The middle lobe branches are inspected by inserting an oblique 45-degree angle telescope or right-angle telescope and advancing it. The patient's head is lowered to view the right middle lobe or turned to the right to view the left main bronchus.
6. Secretions are aspirated for study. Forceps for biopsy are inserted if desired; foreign bodies are removed with forceps.
7. The bronchoscope is removed. The patient's face is cleansed. If able, the patient is encouraged to sit on the edge of the OR bed before transfer to the stretcher. An emesis basin and sponges should be provided for the patient's use. Assistance and support should be provided to the patient to prevent a fall.

Bronchoscopy using flexible bronchoscope

Flexible bronchoscopy is done to view structures that cannot be observed with a rigid scope. Flexible bronchoscopy may be performed in addition to a standard rigid bronchoscopy or as an independent procedure. If performed separately, the patient may remain on the transporting stretcher during the procedure. The bronchoscopy is completed for the same reasons as a rigid bronchoscopy.

Procedural considerations. Patient considerations are as described for rigid bronchoscopy. The setup for flexible bronchoscopy includes the following:

Flexible bronchoscope	Suction tubing with collection tube attached to collect wash specimen
Fiberoptic light source	
Flexible biopsy forceps	
Flexible brush (optional); if used, slides and alcohol are necessary to collect specimen	Lubricant (water soluble)
	Gauze sponges
Specimen collectors	Basin with sterile saline solution
Syringe for wash	

Operative procedure

1. The lubricated bronchoscope is passed through the adapter on the endotracheal tube, which is held secure by the anesthesiologist.
2. The suction tube is positioned with the specimen collector attached for collection of bronchial washings. When indicated, the suction tubing is connected to the bronchoscope; the container for collection is held securely in an upright position to prevent loss of the specimen through the suction.
3. Approximately 5 ml of saline solution is injected into the channel. Suction is quickly reapplied. This procedure may be repeated.
4. Following completion of the procedure, specimen containers are labeled and sent to the laboratory.

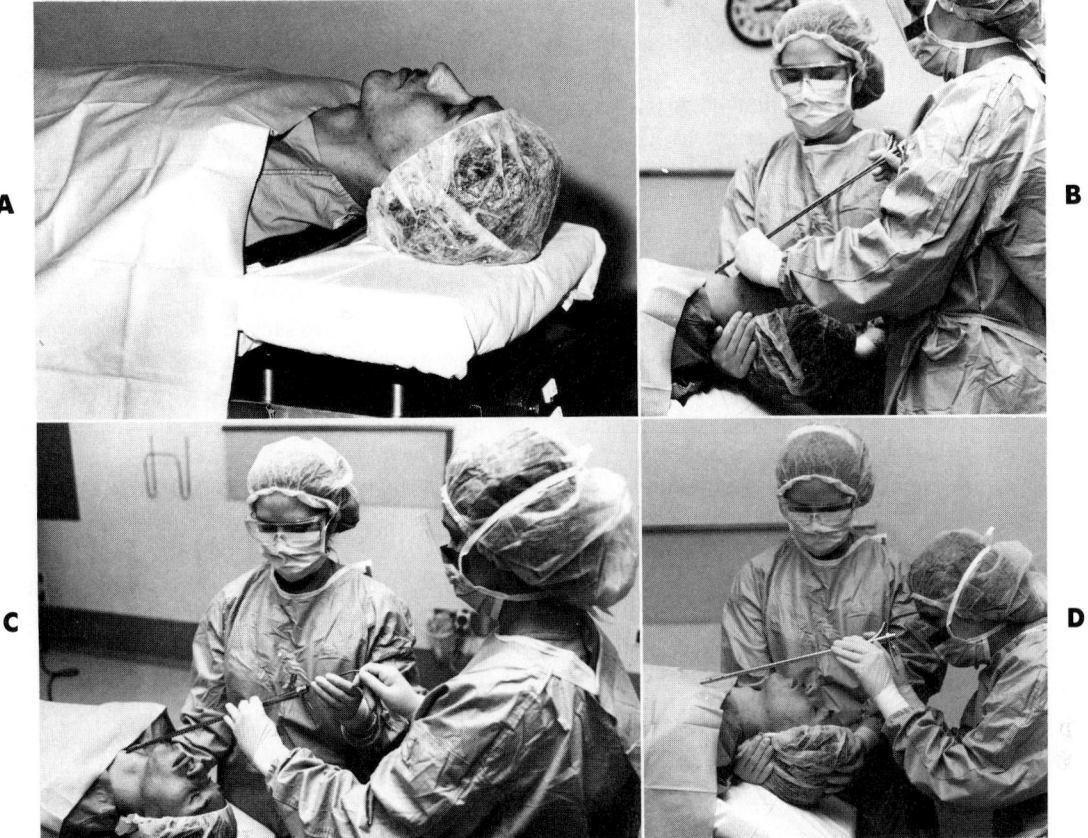

FIG. 24-19 **A,** Patient positioned with shoulder at table break for bronchoscopy. A shoulder roll or sandbag can be placed beneath the patient's shoulders. **B,** Initial position with head held high and supported. **C,** Assistance is provided as the forceps or suction is guided while the head is supported. **D,** Position assumed as the endoscope is inserted; the head will be raised or lowered as the anatomy is viewed.

Mediastinoscopy

Mediastinoscopy is the direct visualization and possible biopsy of lymph nodes or tumors at the tracheobronchial junction, under the carina of the trachea, or on the upper lobe bronchi or subdivisions. Mediastinoscopy may precede an exploratory thoracotomy in known cases of lung carcinoma. Patients with positive findings may be treated with radiation or chemotherapy, as indicated.

Procedural considerations. The setup for mediastinoscopy includes the following:

Minor set of instruments	Suction tubing
Mediastinoscopes, desired type	Aspirating tubes
	Biopsy forceps
Fiberoptic light cords	Electrosurgical unit
Fiberoptic light source	Endocardiac needle, 20 gauge, 8 inches

The patient is placed under endotracheal anesthesia and positioned as for a tracheostomy (see Chapter 20).

Operative procedure

1. A short (approximately 2 cm) transverse incision is made above the suprasternal notch and the pretracheal fascia exposed.
2. The pretracheal fascia is incised.
3. Tunneling is accomplished alongside the trachea by blunt (digital) dissection into the mediastinum.
4. The mediastinoscope is introduced under direct vision deep to the fascial plane and advanced along the side of the trachea toward the mediastinum.
5. The scope is manipulated to visualize the tracheal bifurcation, bronchi, aortic arch, and associated lymph nodes.
6. Lymph nodal tissue is located for biopsy and aspirated with a small-gauge needle and syringe for positive identification of a nonvascular structure.
7. Biopsy forceps are inserted through the scope and a tissue specimen excised. Pressure can be applied to the excision site with a bronchus sponge on a holder. The mediastinum is reinspected for bleeding.
8. The mediastinoscope is withdrawn.
9. Subcutaneous tissue is sutured with absorbable sutures. The skin is approximated and sutured with ligature on a cutting needle.
10. A small dressing is applied.

Thoracoscopy

Thoracoscopy is indicated for diagnosis of pleural disease or treatment of pleural conditions such as cysts, blebs and effusions. Pleurodesis with instillation of talc (Research Highlight 24-4), tetracycline, or other treatment can be accomplished through the thoracoscope. It can also be performed for biopsy of mediastinal masses, to perform wedge resections, pericardectomy, and cervical sympathectomy, to obtain hemostasis, and to evacuate blood clots or divide adhesions. Advantages of thoracoscopy include reduced morbidity through use of small puncture incisions, requiring less time for patient recovery and rehabilitation.

Procedural considerations. Endoscopic instrumentation and equipment are used for a thoracoscopy as follows:

Blunt graspers	Endoscopic soft tissue
Dissectors	instruments (scissors,
Suture ligator	hemostats, suction
Scissors	tips, retractors)
Suction coagulator	Video equipment (tele-
Light cord for lens	vision monitors, vid-
10-mm 0-degree lens	eocassette recorder,
10-mm 30-degree lens	printer, light source
5-mm 0-degree lens	for camera and lens,
Camera	slave television moni-
	tor)
	Insufflator

The patient is positioned supine, semilateral or lateral, depending on the anatomic structures involved.

Operative procedure

1. A 2- to 3-cm incision is made between the fifth and seventh intercostal spaces for insertion of the 10-mm or 12-mm trocar. The 0-degree lens is inserted to view the site to determine the approach.

2. If the procedure can be completed per thoracoscopy, puncture sites are made for insertion of trocars to allow instrument manipulation. The size of trocar and types of instruments depend on the diagnosis.

3. A chest tube is inserted through one of the surgical puncture sites and secured to the skin.

LUNG SURGERY

Pneumonectomy

Pneumonectomy is removal of an entire lung, usually to treat malignant neoplasms (Research Highlight 24-5). Other reasons for removal include an extensive unilateral bronchiectasis involving the greater part of one lung, drainage of an extensive chronic pulmonary abscess involving portions of one or more lobes, selected benign tumors, and treatment of any extensive unilateral lesion. Other resections are often combined with pneumonectomy, such as resection of mediastinal lymph nodes, resections of portions of the chest wall or diaphragm, and removal of parietal pleura.

Procedural considerations. The basic thoracic instrumentation is used. The patient is placed in the lateral position for a posterolateral incision.

Operative procedure

1. The skin, subcutaneous tissue, and muscle are incised using scalpel, suction, and electrodissection. Hemostasis is attained. If a rib is to be excised, the procedure discussed later is implemented.

2. The ribs and tissue are protected with moist sponges; the rib retractor is placed (Fig. 24-20) and opened slowly.

3. The lung is mobilized by freeing peripheral adhesions and dividing the pulmonary ligament. Dissection to the hilum of the involved lobe is carried out.

RESEARCH HIGHLIGHT 24-4

Pleural effusions are a significant cause of morbidity, particularly in patients with advanced cancer. Studies show that from 28% to 61% of effusions seen are malignant. Treatment ranges from observation to pleurectomy. The objective of treatment is to relieve distressing symptoms caused by the effusion, to prevent further fluid reaccumulation, and to restore a functioning pulmonary status. Iodized talc, instilled through a tube thoracostomy or thoracoscope can be used for treatment of recurrent pleural effusion. The efficacy of iodized talc pleurodesis has been evaluated. Results indicated the intrapleural instillation of iodized talc is an adequate and effective treatment for control of neoplastic or benign pleural effusion.

Webb, W.R., et al. (1992). Iodized talc pleurodesis for the treatment of pleural effusions. *Journal of Thoracic and Cardiovascular Surgery, 103*(5), 881-886.

RESEARCH HIGHLIGHT 24-5

Surgical treatment of pulmonary metastases is regarded now as an established procedure, with increasing acceptance in the last 10 to 20 years. Research shows that 95% of the cases of untreated carcinoma have a 1 year mortality and an 8% to 10% overall 5-year survival. With curative resection 5-year survival is 36% overall and 10-year survival is 14% overall. In primary tumors with caval drainage the lung is the first and most frequent site of distant metastasis. The lung is the most frequent site of metastatic spread (30%) in patients who die of malignancy. The lungs are also the sole site in more than 90% of the cases for metastatic spread of osteosarcomas and soft tissue sarcoma.

Roth, J.A. (1985). Treatment of metastatic cancer to the lung. In V.T. DeVita, J.R.S. Hellman, & S.A. Rosenberg (Eds.). *Cancer: principles and practice of oncology* (2nd ed.). Philadelphia: J.B. Lippincott.

4. The superior pulmonary vein is gently retracted and the pulmonary artery dissected.

5. The branches of the pulmonary artery and vein of the involved lobe are clamped, doubly ligated, and divided with fine right-angled vascular clamps, scissors, and nonabsorbable suture.

6. The inferior pulmonary vein is exposed by incising the hilar pleura and retracting the lung anteriorly. The inferior pulmonary vein is clamped, doubly ligated, and divided.

7. The bronchus clamp is applied and the bronchus near the tracheal bifurcation is divided. The stump is closed with atraumatic nonabsorbable mattress sutures or bronchus staples. If staples are applied, the scalpel is used to complete division of the bronchus. The lung is removed from the chest.

8. The pleural space is irrigated with normal saline to check for hemostasis and air leaks during positive pressure inspiration.

9. A pleural flap is created and sutured over the bronchial stump. Other methods of securing the bronchus might be used.

10. Hemostasis is ensured in the pleural space.

11. Chest tubes are inserted (28 to 30 Fr) in the pleural space and brought through a stable wound at the eighth or ninth interspace near the anterior axillary line (Fig. 24-21). An upper tube is inserted through a second stab wound if indicated to evaluate leaking air. The tubes are secured with heavy sutures and connected to water-seal drainage following closure of the pleural space.

12. The rib approximator (Fig. 24-22) is placed and closure begun with interrupted suture.

13. The muscle, subcutaneous tissue, and skin are closed. Drains are anchored to the chest wall with suture.

14. The dressing is applied.

15. Chest tube connections are secured with Parham bands or tape (see Fig. 24-18) and labeled (anterior/posterior).

Lobectomy (left upper)

Lobectomy is excision of one or more lobes of the lung. It is performed to remove metastatic involvement when the tumor is peripherally located and hilar nodes are not involved. Other conditions affecting the lung and resulting in lobectomy might be bronchiectasis, giant emphysematous blebs or bullae, large centrally located benign tumor, fungal infections, and congenital anomalies. Lesser consideration is given for lobectomy of the middle lobe due to bronchial division involvement.

Procedural considerations. The basic thoracic instrumentation is used. The patient is placed in a lateral position for posterolateral incision; the supine position may be used for upper and middle lobe resections. The procedure varies with the specific lobe to be removed due to anatomic structure.

Operative procedure

1. The skin, subcutaneous tissue, and muscle are incised using scalpel, suction, and electrodissection. Hemostasis is attained. If a rib is to be excised, the procedure already discussed is implemented.

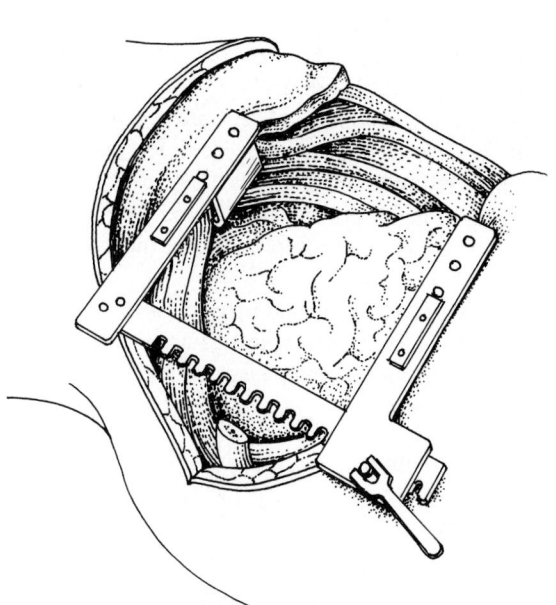

FIG. 24-20   Rib retractor placed for thoracotomy.

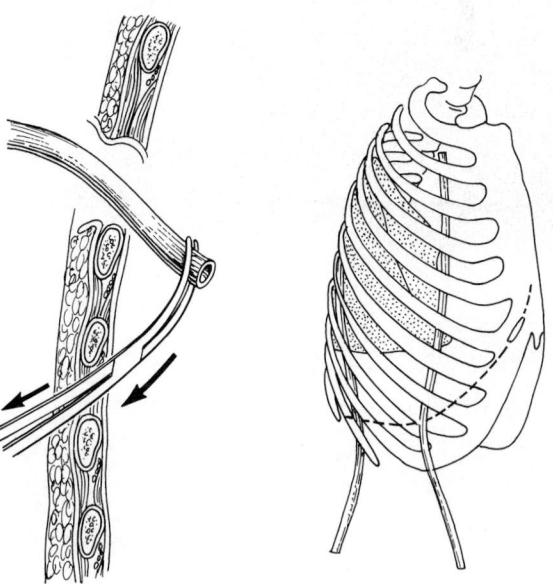

FIG. 24-21   Introduction of chest drainage tube through a stab wound; placement of apical and basal drainage tubes following upper and middle lobectomy.

2. The ribs and tissue are protected with sponges. The rib retractor is placed and opened slowly.
3. The pleura is entered, and peripheral adhesions are freed with scissors, blunt dissection, or a sponge on a sponge-holding forcep.
4. The hilar pleura is incised and separated.
5. The branches of the pulmonary artery(s) and vein(s) are isolated, clamped, double ligated, and divided with fine, right-angled vascular clamps, scissors, and nonabsorbable suture.
6. The main trunk of the pulmonary artery is identified as is the fissure between the lobes.
7. The bronchus clamp is applied. The remaining lung is inflated to identify the line of demarcation. The bronchus is divided with a scalpel or heavy scissors.
8. Bronchial secretions are suctioned.
9. The bronchus is closed with atraumatic, nonabsorbable mattress sutures or bronchus staples. If staples are applied, the scalpel is used to complete division of the bronchus.
10. Incomplete fissures are divided between hemostats with fine Metzenbaum scissors. Edges may be sutured closed.
11. A pleural flap is created and sutured over the bronchial stump. Other methods of securing the bronchus might be used.
12. The pleural cavity is thoroughly irrigated with normal saline and hemostasis is ensured. The remaining lobes are inflated to check for air leaks and the degree of expansion of the remaining lobes is assessed.
13. The procedure is completed as for a pneumonectomy (steps 11 to 14).

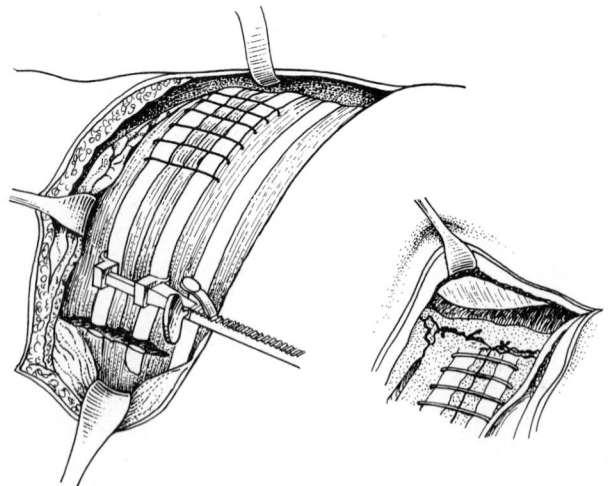

FIG. 24-22 Rib approximator placed for closure of incision. Heavy-gauge suture used for closure of ribs.

Segmental resection

Segmental resection is removal of one or more anatomic subdivisions of the pulmonary lobe. It conserves healthy, functioning pulmonary tissue by sparing remaining segments. Segmental resection is indicated for any benign lesion with segmental distribution or diseased tissue affecting only one segment of the lung with compromised cardiorespiratory reserve. The most common cause for removal is bronchiectasis. Other conditions requiring removal include chronic, localized inflammation and congenital cysts or blebs.

Procedural considerations. The basic thoracotomy instrumentation is used. The patient is placed in lateral position for an incision appropriate for the area removed.

Operative procedure

1. The skin, subcutaneous tissue, and muscle are incised with scalpel, suction, and electrodissection.
2. The parietal pleura is incised with a scalpel and scissors. Adhesions are divided with sharp or blunt dissection.
3. The segmental artery is identified to provide accurate identification of the bronchus of the diseased segment.
4. The segmental pulmonary vein and branches are ligated.
5. The bronchus is clamped with the bronchus clamp and the remaining lung is inflated. The intersegmental boundary is confirmed and proper placement of the clamp is ensured.
6. The visceral pleura is incised around the diseased segment, beginning anterior to the hilum and progressing toward the periphery. Exposure is facilitated with malleable or other type of retractors. The intersegmental vessels are clamped with thoracic hemostats and ligated.
7. The segmental bronchus is transsected. The stump is closed with atraumatic, nonabsorbable mattress sutures or bronchus staples (Fig. 24-23).
8. Dissection is continued to separate segmental surfaces, and vessels are ligated as needed. The segment of the lung is removed.
9. A pleural flap is created and sutured over the bronchial stump. Other methods of securing the bronchus may be used.
10. The lung is reinflated and irrigated with normal saline. Bleeding is controlled with ligature or hemoclips.
11. The procedure is completed as for pneumonectomy (steps 11 to 14).

Wedge resection

Wedge resection is removal of a wedge-shaped section of parenchyma that includes the identified lesion, without regard for intersegmental planes. The resection is used for removal of small, peripherally located benign primary tumor, peripherally located inflammatory disease, and biopsy in chronic diffuse lung disease.

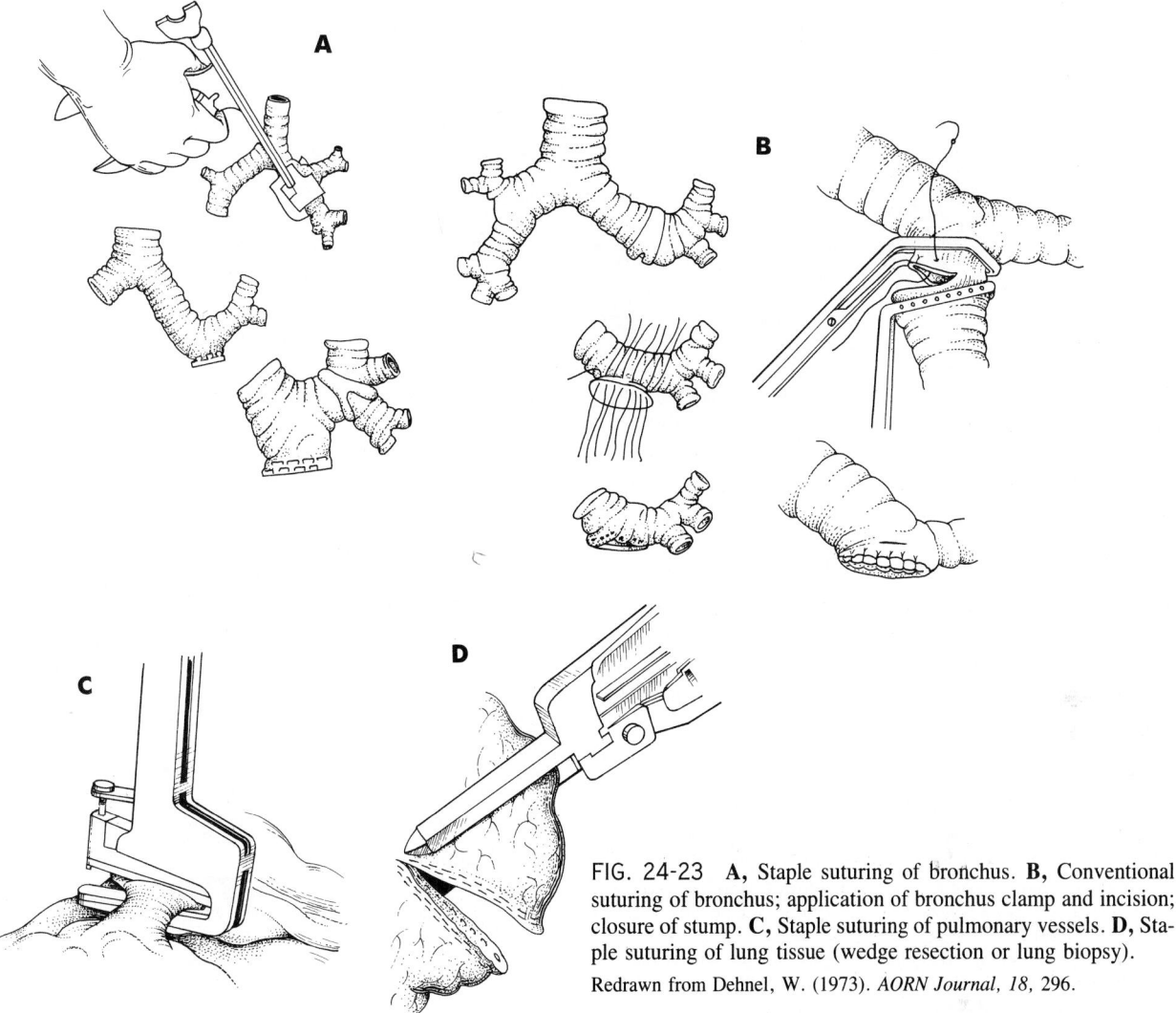

FIG. 24-23 **A,** Staple suturing of bronchus. **B,** Conventional suturing of bronchus; application of bronchus clamp and incision; closure of stump. **C,** Staple suturing of pulmonary vessels. **D,** Staple suturing of lung tissue (wedge resection or lung biopsy).

Redrawn from Dehnel, W. (1973). *AORN Journal, 18,* 296.

Procedural considerations. Thoracic instrumentation is used. The patient is positioned to allow access to the operative site, with consideration of the area of lung to be removed.

Operative procedure

1. The skin, subcutaneous tissue, and muscle are incised using a scalpel, suction, and electrodissection.
2. The rib retractor is placed.
3. Bleeding is controlled, and small bronchi are secured with clamps and ligature. Large bronchi are ligated or sutured to prevent persistent air leak.
4. The wedge is outlined for excision, with a margin of normal tissue left, using one of the following techniques.
   a. Long hemostatic clamps are applied in three rows to outline the wedge. Excision is accomplished with a scalpel. The tissue is sutured with a running absorbable suture behind the clamps before removal. The edges of the tissue are oversewn with a continuous or interrupted suture (Fig. 24-24).

   b. The lobe is grasped with a lung clamp and the thoracic stapling instrument applied to the parenchymal portion of the lung. Staples are applied and the wedge excised with the scalpel. Staples are reapplied to the opposite side of the lesion adjoining the staple lines.
5. The specimen is removed. Air leaks are checked by irrigating. Bleeding is controlled with ligation or hemoclips.
6. The procedure is completed as for pneumonectomy (steps 11 to 14).

Lung biopsy

Lung biopsy is resection of a small portion of the lung for diagnosis. The biopsy allows removal of relatively large specimens for microscopic examination of the lung tissue. Indications include failure of closed methods (needle biopsy) for diagnosis, and the presence of small localized lesions that can be removed by biopsy.

Procedural considerations. The basic instrument setup and the following instruments are used:

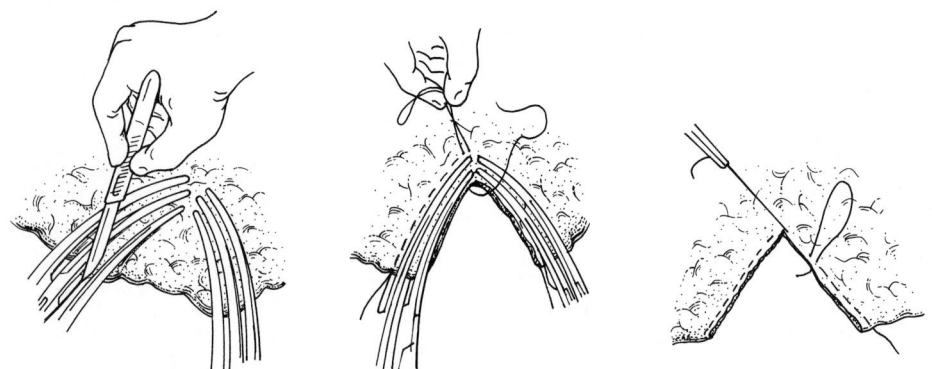

FIG. 24-24   Wedge resection. Clamps applied to edge of lung tissue to be excised with scalpel and sutured with a running suture and oversewn.

1 Dissecting scissors
4 Duval lung-grasping
  forceps
1 Rib retractor, small

The patient is positioned in a semilateral position for anterolateral incision.

Operative procedure

1. A short incision (approximately 5 cm) is made at the fifth intercostal space.
2. The pleural is incised; the ribs are retracted.
3. The lung is secured and pulled out the opening with the Duval lung clamp.
4. Samples from one or more segments of the lung are taken for biopsy with application of a Satinsky clamp or application of staples with a stapling device. The tissue to be removed is excised with a scalpel. Following application of the clamp, tissue edges are approximated with absorbable suture.
5. Bleeding is controlled by applying a moist sponge at the incision site. The area is irrigated and inspected for air leaks.
6. The chest tube (28 to 30 Fr) is inserted and connected to suction.
7. The incision is closed; the chest tube is anchored to the chest wall.
8. The dressing is applied.

Decortication

Decortication of the lung is removal of fibrinous deposit or restrictive membrane on the visceral and parietal pleura that interferes with pulmonary ventilatory function. The procedure results in blood loss and trauma and should be used only if the underlying lung is healthy. The objective is to return the lung to near normal function.

Procedural considerations. The basic thoracic instrumentation is used. The patient is placed in a lateral position for a posterolateral incision.

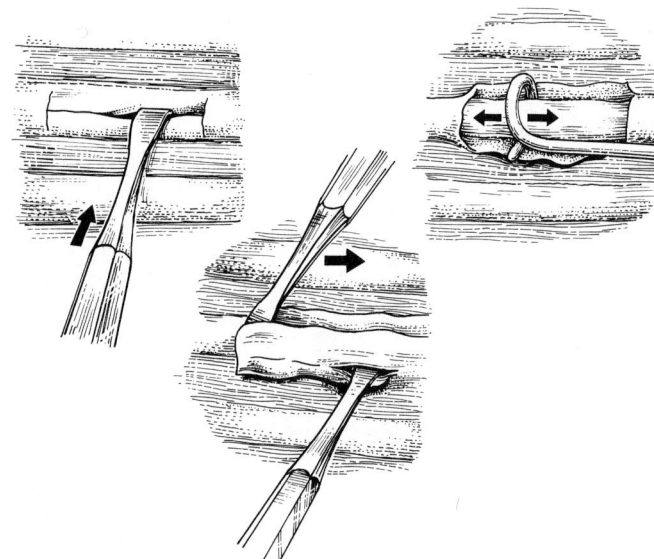

FIG. 24-25   Separation of muscles of rib with a periosteal elevator and rib stripper.

Operative procedure

1. The skin, subcutaneous tissue, and muscle are incised with the scalpel, suction, and electrodissection.
2. A rib, usually the fifth or sixth (Fig. 24-25), is stripped and resected.
3. The ribs and tissue are protected with moist sponges. The rib retractor is placed and slowly opened.
4. Parietal adhesions are divided to the margins of the lung, mediastinal surface, and pericardium with thoracic scissors, forceps, and a moist sponge on sponge-holding forceps.
5. The fibrous membrane is incised and separated from the visceral pleura by using blunt and sharp dissection and by handling the tissues gently (Fig. 24-26).
6. The procedure is completed as for pneumonectomy (steps 11 to 14).

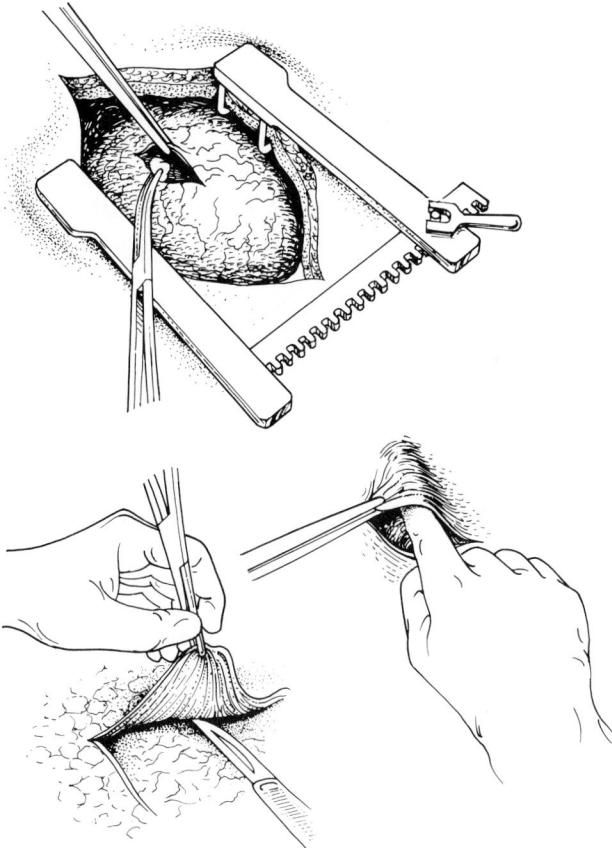

FIG. 24-26 Decortication. Methods of separating fibrous membrane from visceral pleura.

Drainage of empyema

Drainage of empyema is treatment for purulent effusion associated with acute or chronic infection. Empyema must be drained to prevent fibrothorax and further treatment with decortication. Acute empyema could be the result of lung abscess, pneumonia, or infection after thoracotomy. The procedure can be accomplished with the patient receiving local anesthesia when the infection is not extensive. Prolonged intrapleural infection results in chronic empyema,

which can create additional complications such as mediastinal shift, difficulty in swallowing, respiratory limitations, erosion into the bronchus, and deformity of the chest. Sclerosing therapy may be instilled to promote mesothelial inflammation and fibrosis. The agent used must have the least toxicity and best patient tolerance. Medications used might include bleomycin sulfate (Blenoxane) (60 to 90 mg), uracil mustard (nitrogen mustard), or a combination of thiotepa and fluorouracil (5-FU) (Table 24-3).

Procedural considerations. If the patient is anesthetized, the basic thoracic instrumentation is used. The patient is placed in a lateral position for an anterolateral incision. The chest cavity is irrigated profusely during and upon completion of the procedure.

Operative procedure

1. The skin and tissues are incised with a scalpel to expose the affected area of the lung. Suction is used to prevent spillage of drainage from the chest.
2. The pleural space is obliterated and an inflammatory response created by stripping the parietal pleura from the visceral pleura by sharp or blunt dissection and by inserting a catheter and instilling a sclerosing substance.
3. The incision site is closed as for other thoracotomy procedures.
4. A dressing is applied.

Open thoracostomy (partial rib resection)

Partial rib resection is removal of a portion of selected rib(s) through an open thoracostomy incision to allow healing and reinflation of an infected lung. The procedure is performed for treatment of chronic empyemic lesions to establish a mechanism for continuous drainage.

Procedural considerations. The basic thoracic instrument set and bone-cutting instruments are used. The patient is placed in a lateral position for a posterolateral incision. The surgical procedure can be completed with the patient under local anesthesia.

Operative procedure

1. The skin, subcutaneous tissue, and muscle are incised using scalpel, suction, and electrodissection.

TABLE 24-3

Antineoplastic Medications Administered for Sclerosing Therapy

Medication	Dosage	Side effects
Bleomycin sulfate (Blenoxane)	60-90 mg	Nausea, vomiting, anorexia, weight loss, rash, alopecia, fibrosis, pneumonitis, pulmonary toxicity, fever, chills
Uracil mustard (nitrogen mustard)	None recommended topically	Thrombocytopenia, leukopenia, anemia, nausea, amenorrhea, azoospermia, vomiting, diarrhea, alopecia, pruritus, rash
Thiotepa	10-15 mg	Dizziness, nausea, vomiting, anorexia, hematuria, amenorrhea, azoospermia
Fluorouracil (5-FU)	None recommended	Thrombocytopenia, leukopenia, anemia, myelosuppression, amenorrhea, hemorrhage, renal failure, rash, fever, lethargy, malaise

2. The rib is resected.
3. The pleura is incised. Suction is used to control anticipated drainage.
4. Aerobic and anaerobic swabs for culture and sensitivity are obtained.
5. The chest cavity is irrigated.
6. A large chest tube is inserted through the pleural opening.
7. The incision is closed or packed open (depending on the extent of disease process).
8. The chest tube is secured with a suture of heavy-gauge material on a cutting needle by passing through the incision and tying around the tube.
9. The chest tube is connected to a water-seal drainage system, and connections are secured.
10. A dressing is applied. An increased number of layers of dressing to absorb drainage may be necessary.

Closed thoracostomy (intercostal drainage)

Closed thoracostomy is insertion of a chest catheter through an intercostal space for establishment of closed drainage. The procedure provides continuous aspiration of air, blood, or infectious fluid from the pleural cavity. Indications are treatment of spontaneous pneumothorax, traumatic hemothorax, pleural effusion, and acute empyema. If the pleural effusion is malignant, an appropriate sclerosing agent (doxycycline, bleomycin) is required.

Procedural considerations. The basic instrument set is used, with the following instrumentation added:

1 Local anesthesia set including syringes, needles, and anesthetic	1 Luer-Lok syringe, 30 ml
	2 Aspirating needles, 16 gauge, 3½ inches
2 Disposable chest catheters	2 Culture tubes
	1 Water-seal drainage system

The patient is placed in a lateral or sitting position (see Chapter 4). The procedure might not take place in an operating room setting.

Operative procedure

1. The correct depth of insertion is gauged; the catheter is marked.
2. The operative site is anesthetized. An aspirating needle attached to a syringe is introduced into the chest cavity to verify presence of purulent drainage, air, or blood.
3. The skin is incised and a clamp introduced through the incision into the intercostal space and pleural cavity.
4. A catheter that fits the incision site without space around the circumference is inserted. The catheter is clamped to prevent egress of air as it is inserted in the cavity.
5. The incision site is sutured and the catheter secured.
6. The catheter is attached to water-seal drainage and the tubing secured. The clamp is removed.
7. A dressing is applied.

Decompression for thoracic outlet syndrome

Thoracic outlet syndrome is a compression of subclavian vessels and brachial plexus at the superior aperture of the thorax. The cause of compression is usually the first rib, either due to a congenital deformity or a traumatic injury resulting in anatomic changes. Symptoms depend on whether nerves, blood vessels, or both are compressed at the thoracic outlet. Decompression results in partial or entire removal of the rib.

Procedural considerations. Soft tissue and bone instrumentation is used. The patient is positioned in a lateral decubitus position.

Operative procedure

1. The skin and subcutaneous tissue are incised with the scalpel, using suction and electrodissection. Soft tissue dissection continues to identify the neurovascular bundle.
2. The first rib is meticulously dissected subperiosteally using the periosteal elevator and/or rib elevator and stripper and/or rib raspatories, avoiding undue traction in the brachial plexus and damage to the subclavian artery or vein.
3. A wedge is taken from the midportion, or the rib is removed in its entirety using the rib shears.
4. A drain is placed and the incision closed.
5. A dressing is applied.

Excision of mediastinal lesion

This procedure entails the removal of a lesion from the mediastinum, which is divided into superior, anterior, middle, and posterior sections. A mediastinoscopy could determine the diagnosis of an anterior mediastinal lesion. Indications for excision of a mediastinal lesion include cystic hygroma, thymoma, lymphoma, and neurogenic tumor.

Procedural considerations. The thoracic instrumentation is used. A procedure on the superior mediastinum might require use of thyroid instruments (see Chapter 15). The patient is in a supine position for a median sternotomy incision (lateral position alternatively may be used).

Operative procedure (for thymoma)

1. The skin and subcutaneous tissue are incised with the scalpel, using suction, and electrodissection.
2. The sternum is transsected with a power saw or sternal knife. Bleeding is controlled at the bone edges with bone wax (Fig. 24-27).
3. The thymus gland is dissected; vessels are clamped, ligated, and divided. The gland is removed.
4. The incision is closed. The sternum is reapproximated and closed with heavy wire. The skin is sutured closed.
5. A dressing is applied.

Correction of pectus excavatum

Pectus excavatum (funnel chest) is a visually obvious defect of the sternum, seen as a deep depression on the chest wall due to posterior displacement of the sternum (Fig. 24-

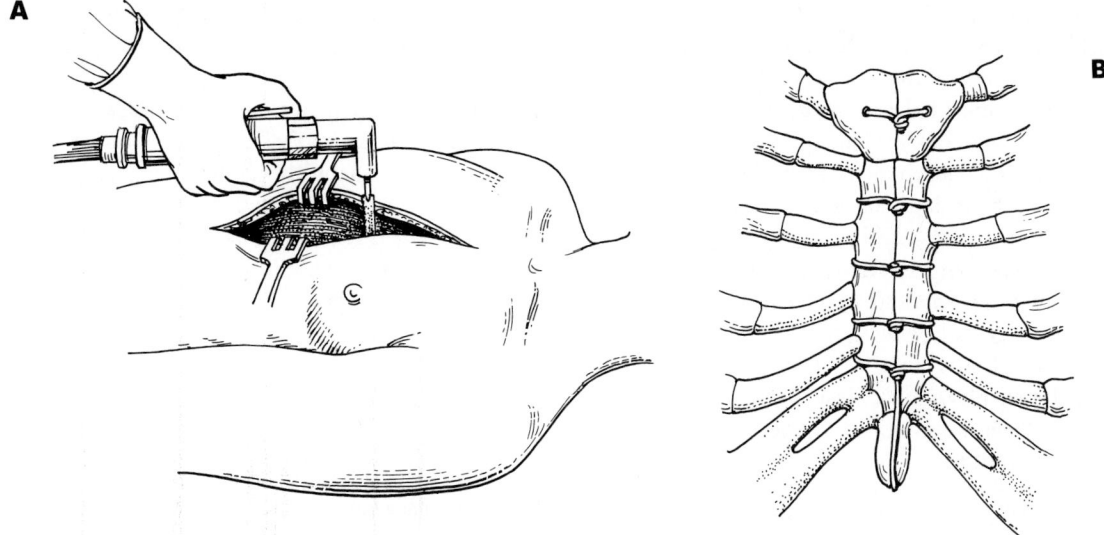

FIG. 24-27 Median sternotomy. **A,** Incision with power saw. **B,** Closure with heavy-gauge wire.

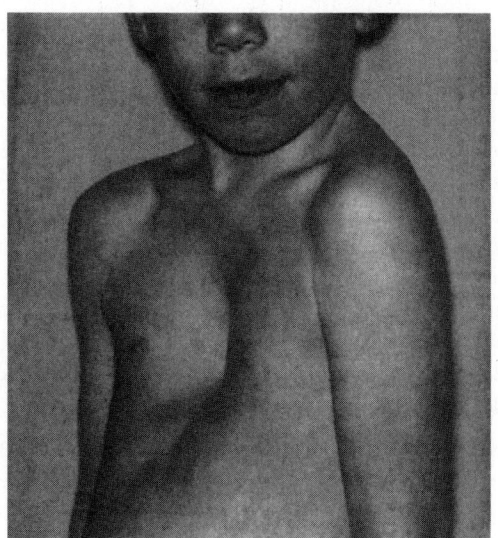

FIG. 24-28 Patient with pectus excavatum.

28). It is usually associated with kyphosis. The defect may be asymmetric, most often deeper on the right side, with sternal angulation. In a majority of cases surgical treatment is cosmetic; impaired cardiorespiratory function has been demonstrated in a few cases. The procedure is most commonly performed at ages 10 to 16, when children become embarrassed to undress in front of peers. Rigid fixation has become a choice for correction of the defect wherein a metal retaining strut is added to gain chest wall stability and prevent recurrence. This strut must be removed 1 or 2 years later (Cohn, Doty, and McElvein, 1993). Other treatments may cosmetically correct the situation short term but result in progressive retraction of the sternum.

Procedural considerations. The thoracic instrument set is used. Instruments for lung resection and long instruments are not necessary. The following are added:

2 Gigli saws and handles	2 Bone hooks
	2 Bone-holding forceps
Osteotomes or chisel	Fixation rod

The patient is positioned supine with a portion of the upper chest elevated on a soft roll or sheets. The incision is a median sternotomy or a bilateral inframammary incision.

Operative procedure

1. A vertical midline incision is made from the level of the manubrium to the point below the xiphisternum.
2. A pectoral muscle flap is raised and origins of the pectoral muscles are detached from the sternum and costal cartilages. The origins of the rectus abdominis muscles are dissected off the lower end of the sternum and costal margins.
3. The deformed costal cartilages are removed completely, preserving the perichondrium.
4. The lower end of the sternum is elevated and mediastinal structures and pleura dissected free.
5. A transverse osteotomy is made through the anterior cortex of the sternum. The sternum is elevated and the fixation rod is placed behind the sternum at the level of the anterior end of the fourth rib. Sutures are used to fixate the bar and adjacent rib.
6. A vacuum drain is passed into the anterior mediastinal space. The rectus muscles are sutured back to the perichondrium and to the lower end of the sternum.

Correction of pectus carinatum

This condition, also known as pigeon chest, frequently results in asymmetric features resulting in several conditions, including a transverse ridge at the level of the manubrium involving a forward projection of the sternum and costal cartilages, a vertical ridge affecting the lower half of the sternum, retraction of the anterior third of the lower ribs, scoliosis resulting in one smaller hemithorax, rotation of the sternum and/or a deep depression affecting the second and third costal cartilages on one side. This is caused by a deformity of the costal cartilages on either side of the sternum. In severe pectus carinatum good stability and chest wall contours may be achieved by complete mobilization of the anterior chest wall with sternal division and costal cartilage resection, followed by repair of the chest wall.

Procedural considerations. The thoracic instruments are used. The patient is positioned supine.

Operative procedure

1. A midline incision from below the suprasternal notch to below the xiphisternum is made. The pectoral and rectus muscles are dissected off the sternum and deformed costal cartilages.
2. A simple deformity may be corrected by removal of the sternal prominence with an osteotome and shaving of the costal cartilages.
3. If the sternum is rotated, a transverse osteotomy at the level of the highest resected costal cartilage is completed. The sternum is divided transversely and rotated into a slightly overcorrected position.
4. Two drill holes are made with an awl about 1 cm from each side of the cut margin. The two halves of the sternum are united with nylon sutures passed through the drill holes.
5. Elevation of the ribs may be necessary by passing a series of heavy sutures around the anterior ends of the lower ribs and securing them to the ribs above.
6. A vacuum drain is inserted. The rectus muscles are reattached to the sternum, perichondrium, and pectoral muscles.
7. A dressing is applied.

Lung transplant

Since the mid-1980s there has been expanded experience with both single-lung transplant (SLT) and double-lung transplant (DLT). For selected patients with progressive end-stage pulmonary disease for whom there are no treatment alternatives, lung transplant involves the allografting of one or both lungs from a cadaver or brain-dead donor. One-year survival rates for SLT range from 69% to 90%. Although there is increasing success with surgical technique, it is anticipated that future application of lung transplant techniques will be limited by donor supply. As the field of lung transplantation continues to evolve, questions regarding quality of life following transplant, and whether the single or double procedure is best in the long run for patients with chronic obstructive lung disease and primary pulmonary hypertension, will need to be answered. Major issues include the shortage of suitable donors, improved

methods for early detection of chronic rejection, and improved immunosuppressive agents and regimens (Cooper, 1993).

Lung transplant requires that the institution have both a transplant team and experience with solid organ transplant in general and rehabilitative pulmonary disease (DATTA, 1993). The United Network for Organ Sharing recommends, as of 1991, the following institutional resources for a lung transplant program:

- A lung transplant team with expertise in complex thoracic surgical problems; individuals having prior experience with clinical LT are desirable
- A pulmonary medicine section with individuals who have expertise in managing chronic lung disease and in pulmonary rehabilitation; an institutional program in pulmonary rehabilitation and in prevention of chronic lung disease is desirable
- Institutional experience with solid organ transplantation in general is essential; this implies the presence and active participation of experts in infectious disease, clinical immunology, and psychiatry and an a appropriate nursing unit for the care of lung transplant recipients
- Staff with experience in complex cardiac surgery; the presence of staff with experience in cardiac transplantation or cardiopulmonary transplantation is desirable
- An intensive care unit with expertise in managing postoperative general thoracic surgical patients, including immunosuppressed patients and their pulmonary problems; the capability for extracorporeal membrane oxygenation treatments is desirable
- At least two clinically experienced thoracic anesthesiologists assigned to the lung transplant program

Procedural considerations. Selection of the donor, recipients, lung preservation, and administration of anesthetic are considerations in this procedure. The nursing care plan is modified considerably for each patient, since nursing personnel are caring for two patients with different needs. The positioning will vary for the techniques being employed. The instrumentation is as that used for a thoracotomy.

Operative procedures (single-lung transplant)
Donor harvesting

1. The patient is prepped from chin to knees and laterally to the midaxillary line. A median sternotomy incision or thoracotomy incision may be used.
2. The inferior and superior venae cavae are dissected free and heavy silk ties placed around each vessel.
3. The aortic arch is dissected free and ligamentum arteriosum divided. The anterior and inferior margins of the pulmonary artery are separated from the main artery and ascending aorta. Umbilical tapes are placed around the pulmonary artery and aorta. A pursestring suture is placed for infusion of the cardioplegia solution in the heart.

4. The heart is prepared for removal; veins and arteries are separated and the heart removed and placed in cold Collins solution.
5. The lung is dissected free from the mediastinum to the hilum anteriorly, posteriorly to the anterior aorta and hilum.
6. The trachea is stapled shut prior to immersion of the lung in cold Collins solution.

Recipient preparation and transplant

1. The patient is positioned supine and the abdomen is prepped from the nipple line to knees.
2. An upper midline incision is made to expose the greater omentum. The omentum is mobilized and placed in the subxiphoid space. (The omentum is used to wrap around the bronchus to provide additional blood supply and support the anastomosis). This incision is closed. The patient is repositioned lateral.
3. An incision is made for a thoracotomy. The procedure depends on which lung is to be removed. If the right lung is being removed, the pulmonary vein is isolated extrapericardially; the pulmonary artery is isolated as close to the lung as possible.
4. The azygos vein is ligated and divided and the pulmonary artery dissected.
5. If the left lung is being removed, the ligamentum arteriosum is divided.
6. Before occlusion of the pulmonary artery, nitroprusside infusion is initiated and the patient monitored. The pulmonary artery is clamped; if instability occurs, partial femoral arteriovenous bypass is initiated. If the patient remains stable, the pneumonectomy is performed.
7. Pulmonary veins are divided extrapericardially. The first branch of the pulmonary artery and descending branch are separated. Blood supply to the bronchus is preserved by not dissecting tissue around the bronchus.
8. The bronchus is divided and the lung removed. The pericardium is opened around the pulmonary veins to allow room for the atrial clamp.
9. Inferior and superior pulmonary veins are incised and joined.
10. Three anastamoses are completed for a single lung transplant: bronchus to bronchus, pulmonary artery to pulmonary artery, and recipient pulmonary veins to donor atrial cuff.
11. Following anastomoses and restoration of circulation, the lung is fully inflated and observed.
12. A retrosternal tunnel is created to the subxiphoid space and omentum drawn up into the thorax and positioned behind the hilum of the lung. The omentum is wrapped around the bronchial anastomosis and tacked into place.

REFERENCES

Cohn, L.H., Doty, D.B., & McElvein, R.B. (1993). *Decision-making in cardiothoracic surgery*. St. Louis: Mosby.

Cooper, J.D. (1993). Commentary on DATTA lung transplantation assessment. *Abstracts of Clinical Care Guidelines, 5*(4), 11-12.

Diagnostic and therapeutic technology assessment: Lung transplantation. (1993). *Journal of the American Medical Association, 269*(7), 931-936.

BIBLIOGRAPHY

Association of Operating Room Nurses. (1994). *Standards and recommended practices for perioperative nursing*. Denver: AORN.

Baue, A.E. (1991). *Glenn's thoracic and cardiovascular surgery* (Vol. 1) (5th ed.). Norwalk, Conn.: Appleton & Lange.

Cohn, L.H., Doty, D.B., & McElvein, R.B. (1993). Decision-making in cardiothoracic surgery. St. Louis: Mosby.

Cooper, J.D. (1993). Commentary on DATTA lung transplantation assessment. *Abstracts of Clinical Care Guidelines, 5*(4), 11-12.

Davis, J.H. (1987). *Clinical surgery*, (Vol. 2). St. Louis: Mosby.

Deslauriers, J., & Lacquet, L.K. (1990). *Thoracic surgery: Surgical management of pleural diseases*. St. Louis: Mosby.

Diagnostic and therapeutic technology assessment: Lung transplantation. (1993). *Journal of the American Medical Association, 269*(7), 931-936.

Fraulini, K.E. (1987). *After anesthesia: A guide for PACU, ICU and medical surgical nurses*, Norwalk, Conn.: Appleton & Lange.

Golanowski, M. (1989). Thoracoscopy, an endoscopic look into the thorax. *AORN Journal 50*(1), 80-85.

Handelsman, H. (1992). *Single and double lung transplantation. Health technology assessment reports*, No. 5, AHCPR Pub. No. 920-028. Rockville, Md.: Office of Technology Assessment.

Holloway, N.M. (1988). *Nursing the critically ill adult* (3rd ed.). Reading, Mass.: Addison-Wesley.

Kirchner, S.A. (1991). Living related lung transplantation: A new dimension in single lung transplantation. *AORN Journal, 54*(4), 704-714.

Kirk, R.N., & Williamson, R.C.N. (1987) *General surgical operations* (2nd ed.). Edinburgh: Churchill-Livingstone.

Lewis, R. (1993). Video assisted thoracic surgery. In *Chest surgery clinics of North America*. Philadelphia: W.B. Saunders.

LoCicero, J. (1992). Diagnostic procedures for thoracic disease. In *Chest surgery clinics of North America*. Philadelphia: W.B. Saunders.

Martini, N., & Vogt-Moykopf. (1989). *Thoracic surgery: Frontiers and uncommon neoplasms*. St. Louis: Mosby.

Meade, R.H. (1961). *History of thoracic surgery*. Springfield, Ill.: Charles C Thomas.

Melamed, M.R., Flehinger, B.J., Saman, M.B., Heelan, R.T., Perchick, W.A., & Martini, N. (1987). Screening for early lung cancer: Results of the Memorial Sloan Kettering study in New York. *Chest 86*, 44-53.

Pagana, K.D., & Pagana, T.J. (1992). *Mosby's diagnostic and laboratory test references*. St. Louis: Mosby.

Pichlmaier, H., & Schildberg, F.W. (1989). *Thoracic surgery*. New York: Springer-Verlag.

Polomano, R.C., Blumenthal, N.P., & Riegler, F.X. (1993). Interpleural analgesia for the management of postoperative pain. *MEDSURG Nursing 2*(3), 185-190.

Potter, P., & Perry, A.G. (1993). *Fundamentals of nursing: Concepts, process and practice* (2nd ed.). St. Louis: Mosby.

Rothrock, J. (1990). *Perioperative nursing care planning*. St. Louis: Mosby.

Schwartz, S., et al. (1989). *Principles of surgery* (5th ed.). New York: McGraw-Hill.

Skidmore-Roth, L. (1994). *Mosby's nursing drug reference*. St. Louis: Mosby.

Tampinco-Golos, I. (1992). Endoscopic thoracotomy: A new approach to thoracic surgery. *AORN Journal, 55*(5), 1167-1180.

Thermann, M., Loddenkemper, R., & Schroder, L. (1985). Thorascopy: A forgotten procedure? *Endoscopy, 6*(17), 203.

Waldenhausen, J.A., & Pierce, W.S. (1985). *Johnson's surgery of the chest* (5th ed.). Chicago: Year Book Medical Publishers.

Wells, F., & Milstein, B.B. (1990) *Thoracic surgical techniques*. London: Bailliere Tindall.

Welsh, S., Myre, L., & Gatch, G. (1987). Pediatric bronchoscopy, special considerations. *AORN Journal, 46*(5), 864-868.

25

VASCULAR SURGERY

BETH ANN MACVITTIE

The history of vascular surgery can be traced as far back as 600 to 800 BC. During this time an Indian surgeon, Shushruta, not only wrote the first surgical text, but was also the first to control hemorrhage with hemp fiber ties and use boiling oil to cauterize bleeding vessels. Through the years many attempts were made to repair arteries and veins, but these efforts failed because of sepsis and thrombosis. In an attempt to place our current practices in perspective, consider the following examples of important discoveries: Lister's principles of asepsis were not reported until 1867; McLean did not discover heparin until 1916, and even then it was too toxic for clinical use until 1940. Thromboendarterectomy, first performed by DosSantos in 1946, was not adequately refined for widespread use until Fogarty developed the Fogarty embolectomy catheter in 1963; carotid endarterectomy, a common peripheral vascular procedure in the United States today, was first reported by DeBakey in 1953 (Friedman, 1992). Peripheral vascular surgery has developed rapidly since these early discoveries.

Improved patient outcomes are enhanced by the current strides in angiography, great improvements in surgical and anesthesia techniques, and the growth of monitoring and intensive care medicine (Friedman, 1992). Preoperative cardiac assessments and intraoperative cardiac monitoring (pulmonary artery catheters, echocardiography) have increased the safety of invasive procedures. Limb salvage is more aggressive and often delays or prevents limb amputations. Great strides have been made in saving limb function by combining bypass with free flap coverage of large nonhealing foot or leg ulcers. Free flaps are done by the plastic surgeon either simultaneously or soon after arterial reconstruction (see Chapter 23). Blood salvage techniques have expanded with the advent of cell-saving and autotransfusion devices.

Peripheral vascular surgery includes interventions to both the arterial and venous systems of the vasculature, excluding the heart itself (see Chapter 27). Vascular disease takes many forms and can best be organized into acute and chronic venous insufficiency and acute and chronic arterial insufficiency. Peripheral vascular disease (PVD) usually refers to arterial insufficiency attributed to atherosclerosis, which can affect any artery. Although all facets of the etiology of PVD have yet to be elucidated, major risk factors include diabetes mellitus and tobacco use in any form or amount. Minor risk factors include hypertension, genetics or family history, diet, and elevated cholesterol.

In the last decade many new technologies have been introduced. Laser-assisted balloon angioplasty (LABA), to open arterial occlusions, was widely used until clinical results indicated the short-lived patency and often deleterious effects in the small vessels of the leg (Research Highlight 25-1). This technique has essentially been abandoned with the exception of iliac artery angioplasty. This seems to be beneficial for patients who have isolated lesions up to 5 cm long or those at high risk for a more invasive procedure. Early results show that percutaneous balloon angioplasty is as successful without the laser (Self and Seeger, 1992).

Other endovascular procedures recently introduced include angioscopy, mechanical atherectomy, and the placement of intravascular stents. Angioscopy, the endoscopic visualization of vessels, began in the mid-1980s and has developed as catheters and microoptics have advanced (Fogarty, 1991). Not a treatment mode in itself, it may be useful to predict the prognosis of vascular bypass procedures or detect technical problems that lend themselves to correction intraoperatively (White, 1992). Peripheral mechanical atherectomy may be performed percutaneously or via arteriotomy to remove plaque by pulverizing and debulking an atheromatous lesion. Four devices currently have FDA approval. Although touted initially as an alternative to balloon angioplasty, atherectomy has not decreased restenosis rates and therefore has limited application (Ahn, 1992).

A variety of stents or intravascular supports has been developing since the 1960s in an attempt to alleviate the drawbacks of angioplasty—elastic recoil and intimal dissection. Only the Palmaz balloon expandable stent is FDA approved for selected use in the iliac arteries (Katzen and Becker, 1992).

RESEARCH HIGHLIGHT 25-1

The use of lasers in the treatment of vascular disease was the subject of an international conference where researchers from various countries presented their study results. Since balloon angioplasty is not appropriate for all patients, study of various lasers and other techniques for treating peripheral vascular disease continues. Thermal lasers (argon) may cause some damage in vessel walls with the hot-tip technique. Excimer lasers, which emit a high-energy ultraviolet beam that is rapidly pulsed and vaporizes tissue with a photochemical effect, leave a clean surface and little or no damage in vessel walls. Excimer laser recanalization in one study was performed with patients who had claudication, pain at rest, or gangrene caused by femoropopliteal occlusion. The procedure was successful in 64% of the patients, but heavy calcified plaques could not be ablated with the short, ultraviolet pulses of the excimer laser. In another study excimer laser angioplasty in 13 patients showed average stenosis of 86% before treatment, 61% following the laser procedure, and 30% following subsequent balloon angioplasty.

Other studies using intravascular ultrasound to recanalize peripheral vessels and to monitor recanalization techniques are ongoing. Perioperative nurses in the future will be increasingly involved with various types of angioscopy, ranging from intravascular imaging to ultrasound and fiberoptic angioscopy. This will require ongoing education in laser use, ultrasonic equipment, computer skills, new angioscope systems, and new atherectomy catheter systems. Expected technologic advances will continue to challenge perioperative nurses' need for new knowledge and skills during implementation of nursing care for vascular surgery patients.

Cruz, L. (1990). Use of lasers in vascular disease discussed at international conference. *AORN Journal,* *51*(5), 1160-1172.

SURGICAL ANATOMY

Basic knowledge of anatomy is essential for all phases of the care of the vascular patient (Fig. 25-1). Arteries and veins have three layers: (1) tunica intima, innermost; (2) tunica media, muscular middle; and (3) tunica adventitia, fibrous outer.

Arteries differ from veins in function and slightly in structure. Structurally arteries have a thicker muscle layer and more elastic fibers and therefore are thicker walled than veins. The properties of elasticity and distensibility enable the vessels to compensate for changes in blood pressure and volume. Because of the thicker muscle layer, severed arteries are capable of contracting and constricting enough to stop hemorrhage. Veins are more fragile and, whether traumatic or iatrogenic, venous bleeding can be difficult to con-trol. Another difference is the presence of semilunar intimal folds or valves in veins, which prevent backflow.

Veins and arteries are nourished by a tiny network of vessels, the vasa vasorum, as well as from the intraluminal blood flow. Both are regulated by the autonomic nervous system with veins having fewer nerve fibers. The two systems are connected: with the exception of the pulmonary artery, arteries, carrying oxygenated blood, branch into smaller arteries, then arterioles, then capillaries to venules to veins. The work of exchanging nutrients and metabolic wastes is done at the capillary level.

Blood flow is a complex process dependent on many factors. Blood flow that travels parallel to the vessel wall, relatively undisturbed, is referred to as *laminar*. When flow is disrupted by an obstruction, stenosis, curve, or bifurcation, the particle motion is referred to as *turbulent*. Turbulence may be evidenced by the presence of a bruit, by auscultation, or a characteristic Doppler signal. Flow depends on blood viscosity, vessel wall resistance, and the peripheral resistance of the arterioles. There must be a difference in pressures or a pressure gradient to allow blood to flow. The contraction of the left ventricle provides this gradient. The negative pressure created by the relaxed right ventricle assists in venous return by creating a suctioning effect, and the skeletal and visceral muscles help propel venous return toward the heart.

VENOUS DISEASE

Acute venous insufficiency is caused by clot in the deep venous system or deep venous thrombosis (DVT). This can be a diagnosis of DVT, phlebitis, thrombophlebitis, or phlebothrombosis, which merely indicates there is a clot, usually in the lower extremity. Virchow, a pathologist, identified three conditions that give rise to vein clots. Dubbed Virchow's triangle, they are stasis, injury to a vein, and hypercoagulability (Verhaeghe and Verstraete, 1993). The etiology of hypercoagulability is sometimes unknown but seen frequently in postoperative and cancer patients. Cancer patients, because of their hypercoagulable state, are at very high risk of DVT, perhaps as high as 40% (Cohen, Grella, and Citron, 1992). General surgical patients run a 20% to 30% chance of acute venous thrombosis, with orthopedic surgical patients and the elderly at even greater risk (Bright and Georgi, 1992). The patient may be asymptomatic or present with limb swelling, pain, and a skin color change. The danger lies in the potential emboli migrating to the right ventricle and proceeding to the lungs. Pulmonary emboli can be fatal. The incidence of fatal pulmonary emboli has been estimated at 200,000 per year in the United States (Reilly and Salluzo, 1990). The majority of these originate in the lower extremities. The usual treatment is medical: heparin and bed rest. In cases that preclude the use of systemic heparin or in which heparin is ineffective, the surgical insertion of a vena cava filter may be indicated.

Chronic venous insufficiency that produces stasis ulcers from postphlebitic syndrome usually occurs in one leg. The

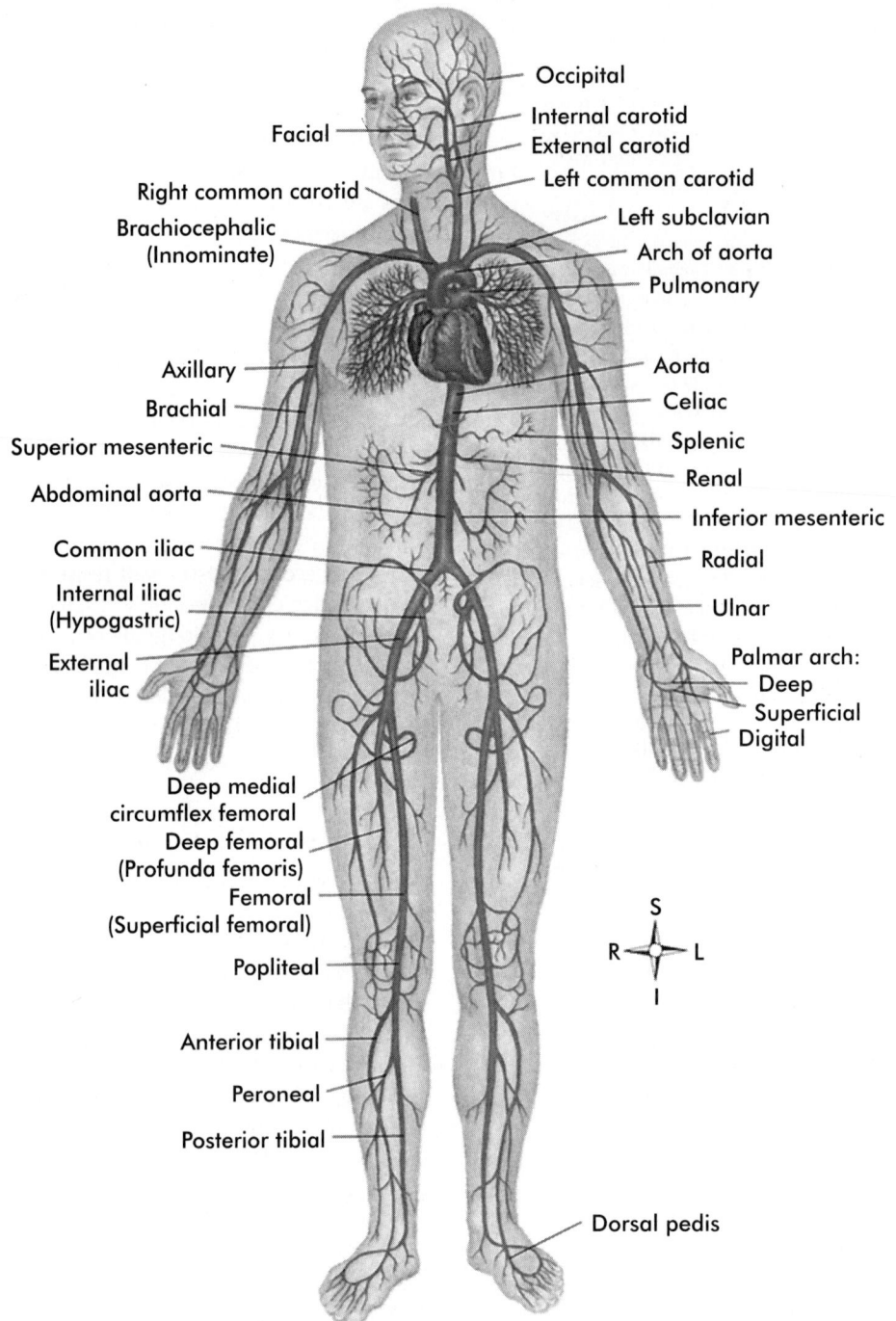

Occipital
Internal carotid
External carotid
Facial
Left common carotid
Right common carotid
Left subclavian
Brachiocephalic
(Innominate)
Arch of aorta
Pulmonary
Axillary
Aorta
Brachial
Celiac
Superior mesenteric
Splenic
Abdominal aorta
Renal
Common iliac
Inferior mesenteric
Internal iliac
(Hypogastric)
Radial
Ulnar
External
iliac
Palmar arch:
Deep
Superficial
Digital
Deep medial
circumflex femoral
Deep femoral
(Profunda femoris)
Femoral
(Superficial femoral)
Popliteal
Anterior tibial
Peroneal
Posterior tibial

Dorsal pedis

FIG. 25-1   Principal arteries of the body.

leg is usually very swollen with a cyclic edema, unlike a leg with lymphedema, which does not change visibly by morning from leg elevation. Stasis ulcers and hyperpigmentation usually are found above the medial malleolus on the leg. The condition is caused by incompetent valves, and the usual management is to apply 20 to 30 mm Hg of external pressure via special pressure stockings. Surgical intervention, valvuloplasty, or valve transposition is occasionally performed but has had limited success (Eriksson, 1990).

ARTERIAL DISEASE

Arterial insufficiency may be acute, as in embolic disease, or chronic, as in atherosclerosis. Atherosclerosis and aneurysmal disease are of prime concern to the vascular surgeon. Emboli may arise from the heart, as in atrial fibrillation, but occasionally result after myocardial infarction (MI). Atherosclerotic plaque can also break loose from other areas and result in an acute arterial blockage. Patients usually present with the onset of the five *Ps:* sudden severe pain, pulselessness, paresthesia, paralysis, and pallor of an extremity (Procter et al., 1992). Heparin is the mainstay to prevent the enlargement of emboli to allow time for collateral blood flow to develop. However, in the threatened limb there are basically two options: surgical removal of the clot (embolectomy) or chemical removal with the use of a thrombolytic drug. If the limb reaches the point where the muscle is rigid, then the limb is not salvageable and amputation is a life-saving procedure (Cambria, 1989).

Chronic arterial insufficiency occurs due to the deposition of calcium and cholesterol within the wall of the artery. *Arteriosclerosis* is a natural part of the aging process whereby the arteries lose their full elasticity. This should not be confused with *atherosclerosis obliterans*, which is a pathologic process that affects the intimal layer of the artery with the buildup of a fibrous plaque of lipids that can calcify and necrose. Atherosclerosis is the most common cause of occlusive disease; the probable mechanism may be initial damage to the intima and subsequent activation and aggregation of the body's platelets. Inflammation follows with the deposition of lipoproteins forming an atheroma. Calcification of this lesion leads to the development of an atherosclerotic plaque. The process is gradual, and a localized lesion is usually indicative of systemic disease. The body develops a network of collateral vessels as an adaptive mechanism to supply the tissues with oxygenated blood.

Many theories have been postulated to explain the process of atherogenesis. The inflammatory process of intimal injury, as described above, seems to be the current and most widely accepted hypothesis. Smoking has a definite link to atherogenesis, but whether this is due to an immunologic response or a direct toxic reaction has yet to be proven. Some research implicates hypertension as a cause, whereas others identify it as a result. Besides the smoker, the diabetic patient is also prone to PVD. Many mechanisms contribute to atherogenesis in the diabetic; hyperglycemia alters the platelet function and could increase thrombosis, and insulin triggers increased smooth muscle cholesterol synthesis (Clement and Verhaeghe, 1993). Most of the vascular surgeon's practice revolves around the results of this type of chronic arterial insufficiency and aneurysmal disease.

Aneurysms are dilatations of artery walls and may be dissecting (a tear allows blood between vessel layers) or false—pseudoaneurysms (a tear goes through all layers). They occur most frequently in the abdominal aorta but are also found in the thoracic aorta, and iliac, femoral, and popliteal arteries. More men than women are affected, and aneurysmal disease tends to be a disease of older patients. Frequently discovered on routine physical exam, they are often asymptomatic unless they are large enough to impinge upon a nerve or until they rupture (Bright and Georgi, 1992).

Abdominal aortic aneurysms occur primarily below the renal arteries. An aneurysm involves intimal damage of the aorta and weakening of the media or elastic portion of the arterial wall. Gradually the vessel wall in the damaged area expands, and atheroma develops within the aneurysm sac.

An abdominal aortic aneurysm has minimal symptoms and is generally discovered on routine history and physical examination. Mortality is low with elective resection of the aneurysm. Dissection and rupture of the aneurysm dramatically increase operative mortality.

The initial symptom of vascular disease in the aortoiliac vessels and distal arteries is *intermittent claudication*. The term claudication is derived from the Latin word *claudicare*, which means to limp. This is the most common symptom of lower extremity PVD (Procter et al., 1992). This symptom occurs distal to the arterial obstruction and occurs with exercise. The increased muscle demand for oxygen with exercise cannot be met distal to the arterial obstruction. Anaerobic metabolism occurs, and muscle cramping develops. As soon as the patient stops walking, the cramps disappear. Surgery is not usually performed for claudication unless it is unusually disabling. The second symptom, rest pain, develops as the vascular disease progresses. Rest pain occurs without exercise and is a constant discomfort, often aggravated at night. The body is now unable to meet the oxygen needs of distal tissues even at rest (Procter et al., 1992). Rest pain may be somewhat relieved by lowering the legs off the bed. Gravity assists in increasing the tissue perfusion and oxygen supply to decrease the pain (Bright and Georgi, 1992). Unless the vascular disease is corrected, nonhealing ulcers and gangrene can develop. Gangrene occurs when the arterial vessels are unable to meet the oxygen needs of distal tissues even at complete rest.

Vascular lesions in the carotid artery occur primarily at the bifurcation of the common carotid artery into the internal and external carotid artery. The internal carotid artery supplies the brain with its oxygen needs. Obstruction in this arterial vessel leads to cerebrovascular insufficiency. Clinical conditions that generally indicate the need for a carotid endarterectomy are transient cerebral ischemia, asymptomatic severe stenoses, and stable strokes.

PERIOPERATIVE NURSING CONSIDERATIONS

ASSESSMENT

A preoperative assessment is necessary for an adequate understanding of the patient's disease, the patient's response, and the proposed surgical procedure. Knowledge of vascular disease and its progression assists the perioperative nurse in performing a comprehensive assessment and developing a plan of care for patients undergoing surgical procedures involving the aortoiliac, femoral, popliteal, and carotid arteries.

The perioperative nurse should assess the patient for the development and extent of vascular symptoms. Medical conditions, including cardiac, renal, pulmonary, coagulation status, and allergies, must be assessed to ensure that the patient can tolerate a possible angiogram, since contrast is toxic, and increased fluid volumes if angioscopy is planned. This is a shared responsibility of the nursing, surgical, and anesthesia team members. The patient's nutritional status, use of alcohol and cigarettes, and the existence of any skin lesions should also be identified. Preoperative location, grading, and marking of distal peripheral pulses can assist the nurse with intraoperative assessment of tissue perfusion. After reviewing the results of the patient's physical examination, the perioperative nurse should verify signs and symptoms of vascular disease that need to be considered during intraoperative care. Muscle and skin atrophy, the presence of tissue ulceration or necrosis, pain, neurovascular status, skin color and temperature, and other integumentary changes should be noted. Elderly, cachetic, and obese patients are at increased risk for pressure injuries.

Assess the patient's mental status, and determine their level of understanding and their emotional response to the surgery. Vascular patients usually have systemic disease, and fear of a stroke (carotid endarterectomy), amputation (ischemic limb), or other complications may be realistic concerns. A skin assessment should include notation of color, integrity, pain, and pulses. Look for any musculoskeletal problems that could preclude patients moving themselves to the OR bed, any weaknesses that may have resulted from a stroke, or that would modify the positioning for surgery. Reinforcement or correction of misunderstandings is possible only if the nurse identifies the patient's current level of knowledge. Identification of the patient's fears and concerns helps the nurse with planning appropriate nursing interventions. In addition, the patient should be able to identify the location and nature of the surgical procedure.

Vascular surgery can be lengthy. Attention to the maintenance of the patient's tissue and skin integrity as well as body temperature is important. Assess the patient's extremities for color, temperature, and strength of pedal pulses during the surgical procedure. This assessment evaluates tissue perfusion distal to the arterial obstruction. When the perioperative nurse knows such assessment will be required, it should be performed during the initial preparation of the patient to provide for baseline comparisons. Invasive diagnostic tests are performed preoperatively to identify the extent and location of the patient's peripheral vascular disease. The introduction of contrast media through a catheter into the arterial or venous system of the patient facilitates this visualization. Angiography also involves the injection of contrast media into the patient's arterial system and the taking of serial radiographic pictures of the movement of the dye through the arteries (Fig. 25-2). Digital subtraction angiography is one such technique, using a computer to make the image along with contrast media. Usually the left side of the film shows the bone for orientation and the right side subtracts out the density of the bone and soft tissue to allow a clearer view of the vessels (Fig. 25-3). These arteriograms should be available in the operating room for the surgical team's reference throughout the surgical procedure.

NURSING DIAGNOSIS

Nursing diagnoses related to the care of patients undergoing vascular surgery might include the following:

- Anxiety related to surgical intervention and its outcomes
- High risk for altered body temperature (hypothermia) related to surgical exposure and anesthesia
- High risk for fluid volume deficit related to loss of body fluids
- High risk for impaired skin integrity and altered tissue perfusion related to surgical positioning, diagnosis, and vascular clamping

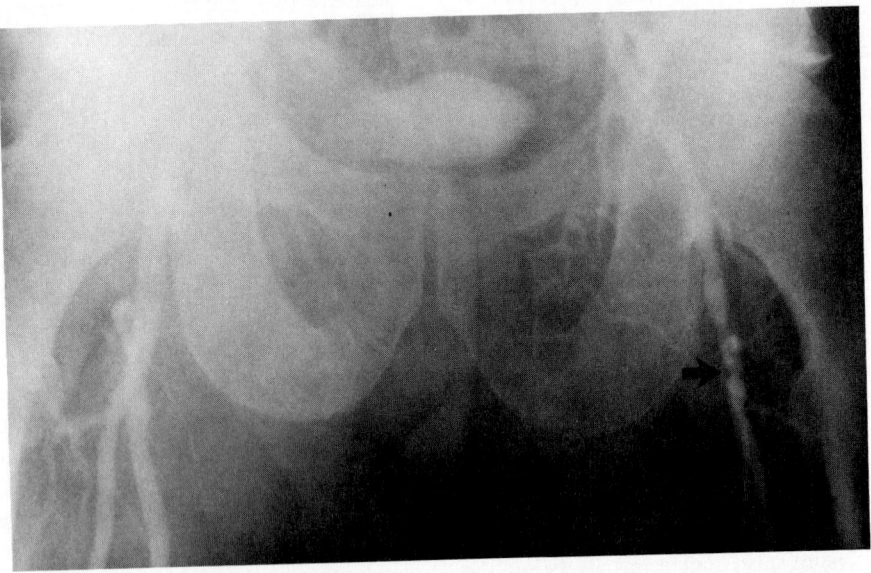

FIG. 25-2　Femoral angiogram. *Arrow* indicates stenosis of the left femoral artery.

Courtesy The Genesee Hospital, Rochester, N.Y.

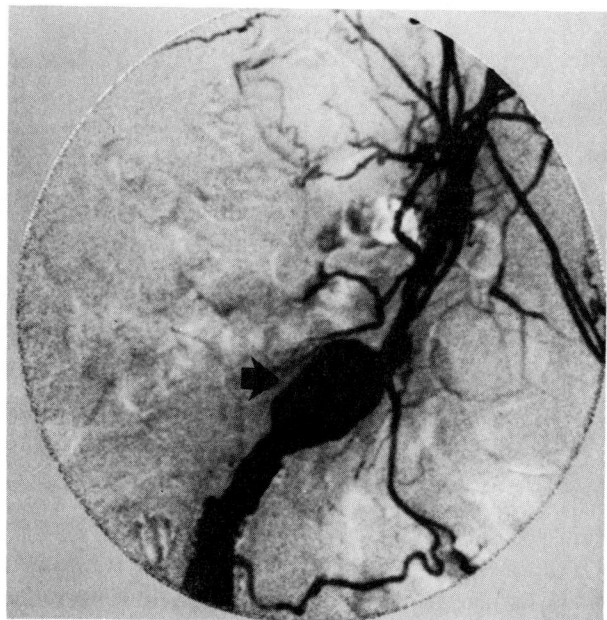

FIG. 25-3 Digital subtraction angiogram. *Arrow* indicates right iliac aneurysm.

Courtesy The Genesee Hospital, Rochester, N.Y.

Based on the perioperative nurse's assessment, the identification and prioritization of nursing diagnoses aid in the development of an individualized plan of care.

OUTCOME IDENTIFICATION

Outcomes identified for the selected nursing diagnoses could be stated as:

- The patient will have all questions answered. The patient will verbalize decreased anxiety and understanding of surgical procedure and perioperative routines. The patient will exhibit increased relaxation as shown by facial expression and/or other body language.
- The patient's body temperature will remain within normal limits as evidenced by postoperative temperature equitable to preoperative level and absence of postoperative shivering.
- Fluid balance will be maintained as evidenced by postoperative pulses equitable to preoperative level, hourly urine output of at least 30 ml, and good skin turgor.
- Skin integrity will be maintained. Skin temperature and color will be within normal limits. No pressure lesions will be in evidence, and the electrosurgical return electrode site will be intact.

PLANNING

Some of the outcomes will have been achieved at the end of the intraoperative phase. Others require ongoing evaluation during the postoperative phase. Because perioperative nursing practice is collaborative, the perioperative nurse develops a plan of care that extends from the admission to the surgical suite through safe recovery from surgery. Some patient goals are measured immediately upon discharge from the operating room; others require the collaboration of the PACU or unit nurse for final evaluation. The perioperative nurse thus develops and contributes to a comprehensive, holistic plan of patient care. Such planning provides evidence of quality patient care and provides a mechanism of communication and continuity of care with other health care professionals.

Before the patient is brought into the operating room, the perioperative nurse should procure the necessary medical and surgical supplies and equipment for the intended surgical intervention. The results of any preoperative tests, such as x-rays, should be obtained. If intraoperative arteriograms are anticipated to visualize or document arterial patency, an appropriate OR bed with x-ray capabilities should be used. The perioperative nurse needs to coordinate the availability of x-ray personnel with the surgical procedure. Appropriate contrast media, catheters, and impermeable sterile x-ray covers must be available. Radiation-protection devices, such as lead aprons and shields, should also be used for the patient, when possible, and for the surgical team members. A Sample Care Plan for the patient undergoing vascular surgery, utilizing the suggested nursing diagnoses, is shown.

IMPLEMENTATION

Intraoperative monitoring

Intraoperative monitoring for vascular patients consists of the basic ECG, pulse oximeter, and blood pressure cuff. For patients undergoing saphenous vein stripping or amputation, these are usually adequate. For lengthy procedures, as in arterial bypass or reconstruction, an arterial line is usually placed percutaneously in the radial artery. This is kept open by a heparin drip, attached to a transducer, and a waveform monitor reads out the systolic and diastolic pressures. The monitor also calculates the mean arterial pressure (MAP), which aids in the evaluation of the perfusion of systemic and cardiac circulation. This arterial line also allows easy access for collecting specimens for arterial blood gas analysis. The ECG and direct arterial lines are used for monitoring and assessment. Continuous assessment of the patient's arterial pressure is a critical part of the surgical procedure. Pulmonary capillary wedge pressure as an index of left atrial pressure (LAP) may be monitored depending on the patient's physiologic status. A general anesthetic may be administered and the patient intubated; local or regional anesthesia may also be used, depending on the surgical intervention. Epidural catheters are placed to provide intraoperative anesthesia that can be augmented to accommodate increased surgical time as opposed to a spinal that provides a finite period of anesthesia. Epidural catheters may be left in place postoperatively for pain management as well. Because many patients undergoing vascular surgery have generalized atherosclerotic disease, the perioperative nurse should be constantly alert for cardiac ar-

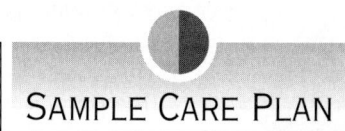

SAMPLE CARE PLAN

NURSING DIAGNOSIS: Anxiety related to the surgical intervention and its outcomes
OUTCOME: Patient will verbalize decreased anxiety.
INTERVENTIONS:

Include the family, significant other, or both, in explanations of perioperative routines.

Allow time for patient's questions; provide explanations or make appropriate referral.

Note verbal and nonverbal indications of anxiety; assist the patient with anxiety-reducing techniques such as rhythmic breathing and relaxation.

Encourage ventilation of concerns and fears.

Provide emotional support and supportive nursing measures (for example, touch).

Demonstrate warmth, calmness, and acceptance of the patient's anxiety.

Maintain a quiet environment.

Document patient's reactions.

NURSING DIAGNOSIS: High risk for altered body temperature (hypothermia) related to surgical exposure and anesthesia
OUTCOME: The patient's body temperature will remain within normal limits during the intraoperative phase.
INTERVENTIONS:

Limit the patient's physical exposure; expose only those body surfaces required for skin preparation.

Cover the patient's head with a blanket or cap.

Use warmed skin preparation solutions (as applicable to agent being used).

Place a warming device (such as a padded hyperthermia blanket) on the OR bed.

Provide the anesthesiologist with a fluid warmer.

Monitor the patient's temperature.

Use warm saline for irrigation.

Provide warm blankets at the end of the surgical procedure.

NURSING DIAGNOSIS: High risk for fluid volume deficit related to loss of body fluids
OUTCOME: The patient will maintain fluid balance.
INTERVENTIONS:

Determine the availability of replacement blood and/or blood products.

Assist with the insertion of intravenous lines and fluid replacement therapy. Keep IV lines patent.

Estimate blood loss on sponges and drapes.

Initiate autotransfusion or utilization of cell-saver as required.

Record the amount of irrigation used.

Document the contents of the suction canisters.

Monitor and document hourly urine output; communicate results of all outcome measurements.

Monitor vital signs and oxygen saturation; assist with the collection and interpretation of intraoperative blood analyses.

NURSING DIAGNOSIS: High risk for impaired skin integrity and altered tissue perfusion related to surgical positioning, diagnosis, and arterial clamping
OUTCOME: The patient will maintain skin integrity and tissue perfusion.
INTERVENTIONS:

Document the patient's preoperative skin condition and tissue perfusion.

Position the patient on a cushioning device (gel-filled or eggcrate mattress) on the operating room bed.

Keep OR bed sheets dry and wrinkle free.

Pad all bony prominences.

Maintain body alignment.

Place restraining straps snugly but not tightly.

Protect vulnerable neurovascular bundles from compression.

Check and record tissue perfusion (color, temperature, pulses) as required.

Elevate drapes off the patient's toes; use appropriate positioning accessories.

Reassess and document the patient's postoperative skin condition and tissue perfusion.

rhythmias and blood pressure changes. Acid-base balance and pulmonary gas exchange may be assessed from the blood gas analysis (Atkinson, 1992).

A central venous pressure catheter (CVP) or various types of pulmonary artery catheters may be inserted, usually via the right internal jugular vein. The CVP line allows assessment of blood volume and vascular tone. The more sophisticated pulmonary artery catheters (such as the Swan-Ganz) can monitor cardiac output, fluid balance, and the cardiac response to drugs (Guzzetta and Dossey, 1992). These would be used for aortic surgery or patients with cardiac disease.

The carotid endarterectomy patient can be monitored with electroencephalography (EEG). This allows immediate observation of slowing of the brain waves due to cerebral ischemia or reduced perfusion. The surgeon may elect to place a temporary shunt in the artery if this occurs during clamping. This could reduce the chances of perioperative stroke.

Transesophageal echocardiography may be used to noninvasively monitor the heart during aortic surgery. The device looks similar to a bronchoscope and can be passed down the esophagus to provide an ultrasonic image. The cardiac structures, blood flow, wall motion, and great vessels can be observed (Canobbio, 1990). The equipment is very expensive and requires highly skilled personnel and thus may not be available in many settings. However, it can detect cardiac changes of impending MI before other monitoring modalities (Docker et al., 1992) and could be important to evaluate the effect of aortic cross clamping in aortic surgery.

Positioning

Positioning of the patient undergoing vascular surgery is of particular importance because of restricted circulation distal to the area of arterial obstruction and a generalized state of poor circulation. Particular care must be exercised in positioning elderly patients (see Chapter 29). Awareness of joint range of motion limitations due to immobility or joint surgery is critical even for a procedure as routine as Foley catheter insertion. Again, preoperative assessment can prevent injury and decrease operative time. Whenever possible, have patients demonstrate the ability to assume the position for the proposed procedure while they are awake and can provide feedback.

A footboard may be applied to the OR bed to prevent the weight of drapes resting on the patient's lower extremities. For a carotid endarterectomy the patient's head may be supported on a head support. A roll may be placed between the scapulae. For surgical procedures involving a lower extremity, the patient's thigh may be externally rotated and abducted with the knee flexed. A small bolster may be used under the knee to support the patient's leg. Proper skeletal alignment during surgery prevents injury to the neuromuscular system. Attention to the skin overlying bony prominences, especially the heels, sacrum, and el-

bows, and the use of proper supports and pads prevent injury to the patient. Owing to the lengthy nature of these procedures, an eggcrate mattress or gel-filled pad can be placed on the OR bed to help prevent patient injury. For the same reasons, members of the scrubbed team should also be cognizant of heavy instruments and drapes resting on the patient's body and take measures to avoid pressure injuries.

Skin preparation and draping

Skin preparation for vascular surgery may be extensive. For abdominal aortic surgery the patient's skin is prepared from the nipple line to the midthigh area. For peripheral vascular surgery on the extremities the patient is prepped from the umbilicus to the feet. The patient's legs are prepared circumferentially. For carotid surgery the patient is prepped from the ear and chin on the affected side to below the clavicle. Draping should permit the surgeon free access to involved areas. For example, abdominal surgery may also require exposure of the groin region for possible exploration of the femoral arteries. A femoral-popliteal bypass on one leg may require access to the other leg for harvesting of the saphenous vein. Impervious drapes should be used to prevent contamination of the surgical field from blood and irrigation fluids.

Monitoring urinary output

A urinary catheter should be inserted, especially if the proposed procedure involves the renal arteries or clamping the aorta above the renal arteries, if considerable blood loss is anticipated, if the planned procedure time is lengthy, or whenever spinal or epidural anesthesia is used because they delay the patient's ability to void voluntarily. Urinary catheterization facilitates accurate hourly measurements of urine during and after the surgical procedure and assists in the assessment of renal perfusion and fluid status.

Medications and solutions

Medications and solutions on the sterile field should always be labeled. Heparin is the most common drug used in vascular surgery. It may be given as an IV bolus to systemically anticoagulate the patient. When administered parenterally, it has an immediate onset of action and peaks in minutes. It has a 2- to 6-hour duration. Because it is metabolized in the liver and excreted by the kidneys, the effects of heparin may be prolonged in patients with liver and renal disease. The anticoagulant effects may be monitored by measuring the activated partial thromboplastin time (APTT) or partial thromboplastin time (PTT) (Baer and Williams, 1992). Patients are anticoagulated just prior to the placement of a vascular clamp to prevent a thromboembolic event. Systemic heparin may or may not need to be reversed at the end of the surgical procedure. Monitoring the activated clotting time (ACT) intraoperatively provides useful data for judging the need for reversal or additional heparin.

Heparin is reversed by protamine sulfate. Protamine sulfate is derived from fish semen, and hypersensitivity to fish may trigger an allergic reaction. There is also an increased incidence of severe hypersensitivity to protamine in insulin-dependent patients taking NPH insulin (Guzzetta and Dossey, 1992). One milligram of protamine neutralizes 100 mg of heparin. The dosage should be calculated to offset half of the last dose of heparin (Clark, Queener, and Karb, 1990). Protamine must be given slowly, at a maximum of 50 mg in 10 minutes, or it may cause dyspnea, flushing, bradycardia, and severe hypotension. Another reason for monitoring heparin is that protamine, given in the absence of circulating heparin, acts as an anticoagulant and could delay hemostasis intraoperatively (Baer and Williams, 1991).

Heparinized saline solution is used as an irrigation. It may be used to irrigate a blood vessel lumen during surgery, usually after the patient has been given heparin systemically. It is also commonly utilized to flush the lumen of tubes used to shunt blood. The probable mechanism is twofold: by creating a negative charge on the tubing wall and interfering with platelet adherence (Clark, Queener, and Karb, 1990). The strength of the heparin solution varies according to the manufacturer's recommendations for certain implant devices or by surgeon preference. A reasonable range is 250 to 1000 units in 250 ml of normal saline.

There are differing ideas on solutions with which to distend, irrigate, or store vein grafts. Some surgeons prefer a cold solution to decrease the metabolic demands of the vessel, whereas others believe this may lead to spasm. Spasm may be of particular concern in working with the small vessels of the distal leg or foot. Papaverine HCl may be added to a heparinized saline for its direct antispasmodic effect on the smooth muscle of the vessel wall and its vasodilating properties (Govani and Hayes, 1985). A reasonable dosage is 120 mg in 250 ml saline. The pressure of a hand-held syringe to distend vein grafts has been viewed as a potential cause of graft failure or graft stenosis because this causes endothelial damage. Papaverine HCl, as a smooth muscle relaxant, allows distention at a lower pressure and may decrease the risk of injury (Cunningham et al., 1981). Concentrations for infiltration range from 0.05 to 0.6 mg/ml or 12.5 to 150 mg/250 ml of solution. The literature suggests that more studies are needed to determine whether cold (4° C) or warm storage solutions are better and exactly what the ideal vein storage solution is (Stanley et al., 1975).

Blood coagulation is controlled by intravascular and extravascular (intrinsic and extrinsic) mechanisms. Injury to the endothelium, such as trauma or atherosclerosis, can trigger this mechanism (intrinsic). The extrinsic coagulation mechanism is triggered by the insult of surgery to tissue and vessels, which precipitates exposure of tissue thromboplastin, resulting in the formation of a clot (Baer and Williams, 1992).

Topical hemostatic agents may be needed. Absorbable hemostatics are effective by creating an environment that promotes the adhesion of platelets (Clark, Queener, and Karb, 1992). An absorbable gelatin sponge, such as Gelfoam, may be applied to a bleeding surface to provide a matrix into which clots form. It may be applied dry, moistened with saline, or soaked in a topical thrombin/saline solution; 100 to 1000 NIH units of thrombin per milliliter of saline or blood may be applied to control bleeding (Govani and Hayes, 1985).

Infections of prosthetic vascular grafts are rare but are extremely serious. Infection may be life threatening for patients with aortic grafts, or limb-threatening in lower extremity procedures. Protecting the prosthetic graft from contact with the skin is essential to prevent bacterial contamination. Prophylactic antibiotic wound irrigation with a neomycin or kanamycin and cephalothin solution has resulted in a decreased wound infection rate even in the absence of parenteral antibiotic therapy (Sheng and Busuttil, 1991).

Vascular grafts

Vascular grafting materials and techniques are of major importance to the field of vascular surgery for bypass procedures and reconstruction. The understanding, study, and comparison of new prosthetic grafts, the use and preparation of autogenous grafts, and the knowledge of long-term patency rates cannot be overly emphasized.

The arteriotomy of a carotid endarterectomy may be closed primarily or with a patch of either vein or synthetic fabric. In aortic surgery, a straight tube or a bifurcated synthetic graft is used. Dacron (polyester) grafts are the typical choice and have been used successfully for over 35 years (Szilagyi et al., 1986). The large vessels have high flow rates and thus have a low incidence of thrombus formation and excellent graft patency rate (Dzsinich and Gloviczki, 1993).

Prosthetic grafts are nonantigenic; tissue incorporates well, which helps prevent infection, and they generally resist thrombosis. For years knitted polyester grafts were preferred over woven polyester because they were easier to handle, although they had to be preclotted due to their high porosity. Woven grafts are somewhat stronger and bleed less through the fabric interstices but can be more inflexible. Newer grafts have been developed to incorporate the best of both by utilizing a velour polyester. They are also being impregnated with albumin, collagen, or gelatin to provide ease in handling without the need to preclot. Preclotting is usually accomplished by submerging the graft in a basin of blood collected prior to systemic heparinization. This makes the graft impervious by allowing fibrin to fill in the fabric spaces (Atkinson, 1992).

The other popular prosthetic material is polytetrafluoroethylene (PTFE). It is available in straight, tapered, and bifurcated styles of varying lengths and may have external support rings to prevent compression (Atkinson, 1992). These grafts do not stretch, and needle hole bleeding may be troublesome.

Human allografts were tried in the 1950s for aortic replacement but ultimately failed due to thrombosis, calcification, or aneurysm development (Wright et al., 1987). Human umbilical cord vein grafts are commercially available for patients who have no usable veins because of previous bypass procedures, saphenous vein stripping, or poor quality or size. Manufacturer's instruction must be followed to rid the umbilical grafts of preservative (Atkinson, 1992).

Volumes have been written on vascular grafts, and the reader should consider this chapter an introduction only. The American National Standards Institute, the Food and Drug Administration, and the Association for the Advancement of Medical Instrumentation are a few of the organizations active in setting standards and regulating usage and development of grafts. Randomized trials to determine the best grafting choices and techniques require many years of patient follow-up (Wright et al., 1987).

Autogenous vein grafting for infrainguinal bypass is considered the gold standard. Undamaged endothelial cells inhibit the clotting mechanism by the natural release of fibrinolytic substances and plasminogen factors (Atkinson, 1992). Two methods of grafting veins have been extensively studied, and the results are not conclusive that one method is better than the other. These are the in situ graft and the reversed vein graft. The in situ method leaves the vein in its place. Side branches are ligated to prevent arteriovenous fistulas, and the valves that would impede arterial flow are disrupted with instruments specifically designed to cut valves, called valvulotomes (Fig. 25-4) (Goldsmith et al., 1992). Reversal of a vein graft is performed per surgeon preference or when it must be harvested from the contralateral limb. Vein grafts are clearly mandated in the below-knee bypass procedures (Veith et al., 1986). Above-knee bypasses may use PTFE or other synthetic graft for vein sparing or in high-risk patients who may not tolerate the longer vein harvesting or have a life expectancy of less than 3 years (Wright et al., 1987). One 25-year review indicated that the medically compromised patient may actually benefit most from bypass procedures to salvage threatened limbs. It appeared that patients who had reconstructive surgery had lower mortality rates, spent fewer days in the hospital, ambulated more successfully, and had an increased survival rate (Ouriel, Fiore, and Geary, 1980) (Research Highlight 25-2). According to Stanley et al. (1991), damage that contributes to graft failure may be caused by the so-called atraumatic clamps used. Rubber, plastic, or hydrostatic jaw clamps are best for protecting vein grafts from injury. Distal bypasses, particularly those in diabetic patients, are more successful today due to improved tissue handling. The use of the pneumatic tourniquet as an alternative to clamping the vessels may improve results. Although there is an increased awareness of this among vascular surgeons, no randomized study has been undertaken to verify this (Green, 1993). The tourniquet is most advantageous when used in the calcified vessels that are typical of diabetic patients (Bernhard, Boren, and Towne, 1980).

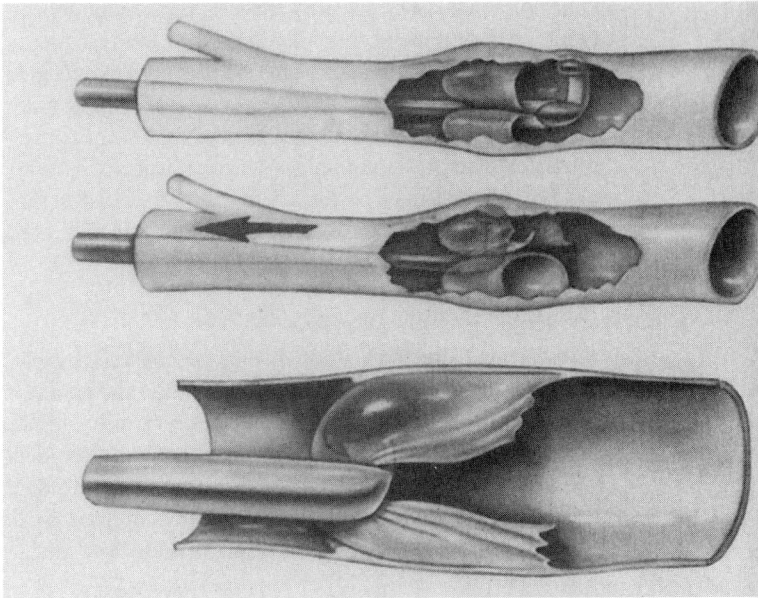

FIG. 25-4   Valve incision with valvulotome.

Sutures

Most vascular sutures are made of synthetic, nonabsorbable materials such as Dacron, polyester, PTFE, and polypropylene. Vascular sutures have swaged-on needles of various sizes and are available in sizes 0 to 8-0. The suture may be single armed or double armed (that is, a needle on

---

⚛ RESEARCH HIGHLIGHT 25-2

In the 1990s vascular surgeons are able to preserve limbs that, in the past, would have required amputation due to far-advanced peripheral occlusive artery disease. Recent studies have shown that, with the use of autogenous vein grafts, either reversed or in situ, continuous graft patency can be expected for approximately 80% at the 5-year interval in both femoropopliteal and femoral-infrapopliteal bypasses with a corresponding 5-year limb salvage rate in excess of 85%. It appears that prosthetic bypasses, preferred by some surgeons for femoral above-knee popliteal reconstructions, have inferior results to autogenous methods in reconstruction extending to below-knee bypasses. Adding to this issue is the continued controversy over comparisons of long-term patency in Dacron versus PTFE bypasses. In the future, perioperative nurses can expect additional studies on graft patency as well as studies that apply modern techniques of cell and molecular biology to answering questions regarding myointimal hyperplasia and reperfusion injury. Myointimal hyperplasia is one of the major causes of failure of both prosthetic and vein bypasses in the lower extremity.

Mannick, J.A. (1993). What's new in peripheral vascular surgery. *ACS Bulletin*, 78(3), 27-30.

one or both ends). The size and curve of the needle depend on the vessel and its location. Teflon felt or leftover pieces of graft material (synthetic or vein) may be used as pledgets or buttresses under a suture (Atkinson, 1992). They are used when tissue is friable to keep the suture from tearing through or when an anastomosis leaks and needs a better seal. The pledget may be loaded onto the vascular suture or added by the surgeon to a suture already in use. The pledget remains on the suture line (Fig. 25-5).

Vascular monitoring equipment

Assessing blood flow through diseased vessels by palpation is often difficult. Physical assessment of the patient's hemodynamic status during surgery can be further complicated by spasm of the vessel walls, the cool environment of the operating room, and alterations in blood pressure caused by hemorrhage. Vascular monitoring equipment can be used by the surgeon in the operating room to evaluate tissue perfusion.

A Doppler device uses ultrasonic, high-frequency sound waves to assess the movement of blood through a vessel. The Doppler device is critical when pulses cannot be palpated. When the sound waves encounter dissimilar tissues, such as red blood cells moving through an artery, some of the sound is reflected back to the probe. The pitch of the sound is directly related to the velocity of blood flow. With the use of a coupling gel, the unsterile Doppler probe can be placed on the patient's skin distal to the surgical site. Some probes can be sterilized and used directly in the surgical wound to assess the flow in an arterial graft or determine whether the blood supply to the intestines or other structures is intact after aortic surgery. Besides providing an audible signal, the Doppler instrument can provide a permanent record of the sound if a recorder is attached. The unit is inexpensive and easily transported. Surgical personnel can use the Doppler after minimal training.

An EEG accurately determines reduced cerebral perfusion during a carotid endarterectomy. This enables the surgeon to decide whether to use a temporary shunt in the carotid artery or if the patient can tolerate clamping. Trained personnel are necessary to operate this equipment.

Instrumentation

The most efficient set-up to have is a basic laparotomy set for scissors, clamps, and retractors (see Chapter 5) and a vascular set as the foundation for all vascular procedures.

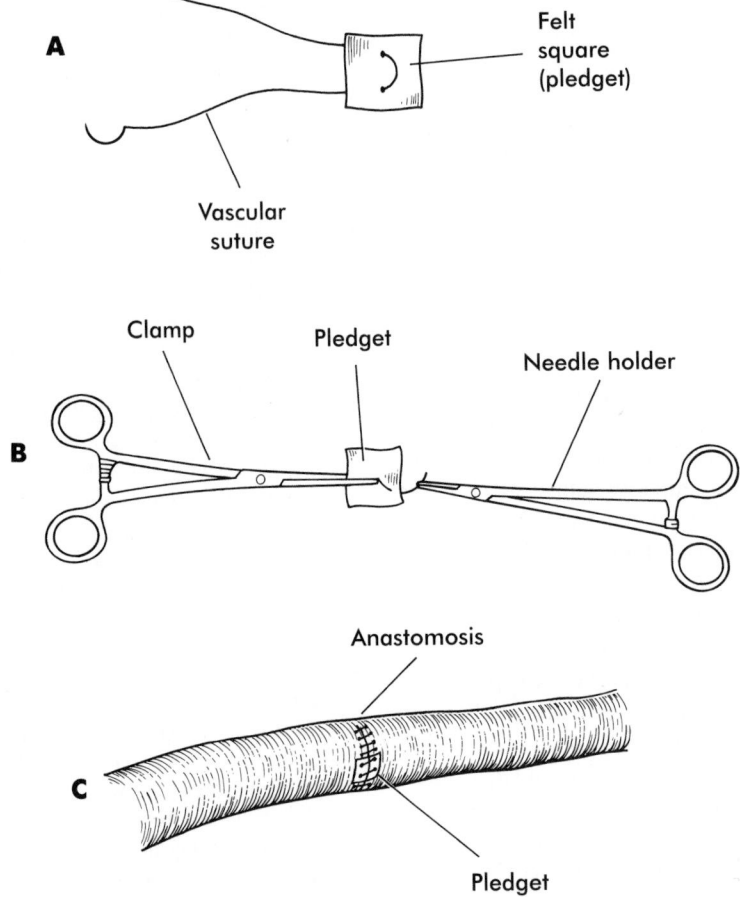

FIG. 25-5 Pledgeted suture. **A,** Double-armed vascular suture prepared with pledget. **B,** Technique for surgeon to add pledget to suture already in use. **C,** Appearance of suture line with pledget in place.

Then add the items specific to each surgical procedure. For abdominal surgery, add a large self-retaining retractor (such as Omni-tract or Bookwalter). Have additional sterile aortic clamps wrapped individually and some long clamps (cystic duct and right angle) and long forceps for larger patients. For peripheral procedures, add a variety of Weitlaner self-retaining retractors. Carotid surgery requires carotid shunt clamps and microforceps for peeling plaque from the artery. The saphenous vein as a graft conduit may be removed and reversed or used in situ. A variety of instruments are available for disrupting the valves to permit arterial flow in the in situ procedure. Amputations do not require vascular instrumentation. A basic minor set and appropriately sized bone instruments are needed.

A basic vascular set might include the following:

Cutting instruments

2 no. 7 knife handles for a no. 15 and no. 11 blade
Potts scissors, different angles
Vascular dissecting scissors, different lengths

Clamping instruments

4 Peripheral DeBakey vascular clamps
4 Aortic occlusion clamps
3 Satinsky or Derra clamps, various sizes
4 Peripheral Fogarty clamps

Suturing instruments

Needle holders (narrow diamond jaw), a variety of lengths
2 Castroviejo needle holders
Mosquito clamps
Bulldog clamps, 4 large and 8 small (variety of types)
2 vein cannulas
Weitlaner retractors, 4 large and 2 small
Tissue occlusion clips and appliers (for example, Hemoclips or Ligaclips)

Holding instruments

2 Potts-Smith tissue forceps
6 DeBakey vascular forceps, 2 long and 4 short
2 microforceps

Bone instruments

Bone cutters
Bone rongeurs
Gigli saw handles, Gigli saw blade
Power saw (optional)
Periosteal elevator
Rasp
Amputation knife

Vessel loops or umbilical tapes
Nerve hook
Submucous elevator

In situ procedure instruments

Vascular dilators
Microvascular scissors
Mills valvulotome
Leather in situ valve cutter kit

Documentation

During the implementation of perioperative nursing care, documentation of patient problems and nursing actions addressing these identified problems is important. Every nursing assessment and intervention should be recorded. Every patient is identified and assessed for allergies; the surgical procedure is verified, and any other interventions performed by the perioperative nurse for patient safety and mandated by institution policy are documented. A brief mental status exam is especially important for vascular patients who are at risk for stroke. For a patient undergoing vascular surgery, possible areas to document include the preoperative and postoperative assessment of the integrity of the patient's skin, the presence or absence of peripheral pulses, the surgical position and positioning devices used, fluid intake and output, and the achievement of patient goals. During surgery various local anesthetic drugs and irrigating solutions, such as thrombin, antibiotics, and heparin solutions may be used. The scrub nurse should label each container with the solution type and strength. The circulating nurse maintains an accurate record of the solutions used and the amounts administered. The type, size, and serial and lot numbers of vascular implants should be documented according to institutional policy and procedure.

EVALUATION

Evaluation is an ongoing process during which the perioperative nurse determines the extent to which the patient goals are met. This phase is continuous throughout implementation of the nursing process. Assessing, observing, and appraising are actions of the perioperative nurse for this phase.

The conclusion of the intraoperative phase is the transfer of the care of the peripheral vascular patient to colleagues in the PACU or the intensive care unit. A nursing report should be given when the perioperative nurse transfers the care of the patient to other individuals. The report should include identification of the patient, the surgical procedure performed, any allergies, and the achievement of patient outcomes. The outcomes may be documented as follows:

- The patient verbalized understanding of the surgical procedure and routines. The patient had no more questions. The patient appeared more calm as evidenced by facial expression and other body language.
- Temperature remained within normal limits.
- Fluid balance was maintained. Intake and output were documented.
- Skin intact, no lesions or reddened areas; skin color, temperature, and turgor adequate.

The care provided in the operating room should complement the patient's care preoperatively and postoperatively.

SURGICAL INTERVENTIONS

ABDOMINAL AORTIC ANEURYSMECTOMY

Abdominal aortic aneurysmectomy is surgical obliteration of the aneurysm, which may or may not include the iliac arteries, with insertion of a synthetic prosthesis to reestablish functional continuity. The majority of abdominal aortic aneurysms begin below the renal arteries, and many extend to involve the bifurcation and common iliac arteries. Severe back pain, along with symptoms of hypotension, shock, and distal vascular insufficiency, usually indicates rupture and represents a true emergency condition. The prime surgical consideration when a rupture occurs is the control of hemorrhage by occluding the aorta proximal to the point of rupture. Abdominal aortic aneurysms (AAAs) are usually asymptomatic and found on routine physical examination. They occur more frequently in men than women. Aneurysmal disease is caused by a disruption of the media, which structurally weakens the aortic wall. Aneurysms occur most often in the abdominal aorta, thoracic aorta, and the popliteal arteries (Atkinson, 1992). Factors that place a patient at greater risk of rupture include an aneurysm diameter of 6 cm or more, chronic obstructive pulmonary disease (COPD), pain, an aneurysm that is a source of distal emboli, one that is associated with sepsis, or one that is enlarging (Hollier and Rutherford, 1989). Risks from AAA surgery include massive hemorrhage, injury to the ureters, renal failure, spinal cord ischemia, and death. Since PVD is systemic, it is not surprising that patients with aneurysms often have concomitant coronary artery disease. Myocardial infarction is the leading cause of death after AAA repair; therefore it is imperative that a patient with cardiac symptoms or ECG abnormalities have a thorough preoperative cardiac assessment (Golden, Whittemore, and Mannick, 1990). Mortality is 2% for elective repair of AAA in an otherwise healthy patient. Death due to rupture is 70% for 7-cm aneurysms, 40% for 6-cm aneurysms, and 20% for 5-cm aneurysms. Death from surgical repair of a ruptured aneurysm is still greater than 50% (DeWeese, 1989).

The nurse must be alert to the fact that, at the time the aortic clamp is released to permit distal flow, declamping shock, or severe hypotension, can occur. This may be due to inadequate volume replacement, the sudden reestablishment of flow to vasodilated distal vessels, potassium, or the release of acidic metabolites. This and hemorrhage have been proposed as causes of renal failure from acute tubular necrosis (Hollier and Rutherford, 1989).

Procedural considerations. The patient is placed in the supine position. The skin is prepped for a midline abdominal incision, and draping is completed to permit access to the groin region for possible exploration of femoral arteries. The pedal pulses should be marked before the beginning of the procedure so they may be located immediately if the surgeon requests a check of the pulses. This assessment of pulses can be done manually or with an ultrasonic instrument (Doppler).

Operative procedure

1. The abdomen is opened through a midline incision (Fig. 25-6, *A*) from the xiphoid process to the symphysis pubis. Hemostasis is accomplished, and exploration is completed as described for laparotomy (see Chapter 10).

2. An abdominal self-retaining retractor is inserted in the wound. If necessary for exposure, a portion of the small bowel can be placed outside the abdomen and covered with moist laparotomy packs.

3. The parietal peritoneum is incised over the aorta and extended superiorly to expose the aneurysm and also inferiorly over the bifurcation and beyond the iliac arteries. Metzenbaum scissors, smooth forceps, and hemostats are used.

4. Careful blunt and sharp dissection is continued to expose the aorta above the aneurysm to permit placement of an aortic clamp. The renal artery and ureters are avoided. The iliac vessels and bifurcation are inspected for evidence of small aneurysms, thrombosis, and calcification.

5. An aortic clamp such as a DeBakey, Fogarty, or Satinsky is applied and closed. Opening of the aneurysm is undertaken with a scalpel or electrosurgical blade and heavy scissors (Fig. 25-6, *B*).

6. The aneurysm is completely opened, and all atheromatous and thrombotic material is removed. The aneurysm walls may be excised but usually are left in place for eventual coverage of the prosthesis. In either case the posterior aspect of the aorta is left intact (Fig. 25-6, *C*). Bleeding is controlled, especially from the lumbar vessels that enter posteriorly.

7. A prosthetic graft of appropriate size is prepared for insertion. If the aneurysm does not involve the aortic bifurcation, a straight tubular graft is used; otherwise a bifurcated or Y-shaped graft is necessary. Preclotting of a knitted graft may be accomplished by immersing the graft in a small quantity of the patient's own blood before systemic heparinization.

8. The aortic cuff is prepared for anastomosis by irrigating it with heparinized saline solution and by removing all fibrotic plaques. One or two vascular sutures (double armed) are used to accomplish the anastomosis by a through-and-through continuous suture (Fig. 25-6, *D*). Additional interrupted sutures may be needed if the anastomosis leaks on completion.

9. The distal vessels are opened and inspected for back-bleeding, and heparinized saline solution may be injected to prevent clotting.

10. Each limb of the graft is anastomosed to the iliac artery, using a smaller vascular suture and similar technique. After the first side of the anastomosis has been completed, blood is permitted to circulate, and the remaining limb of the graft is clamped to prevent leaking during the last part of the anastomosis (Fig. 25-6, *E*).

11. The aneurysm is closed over the graft.

12. The abdominal wound is closed.

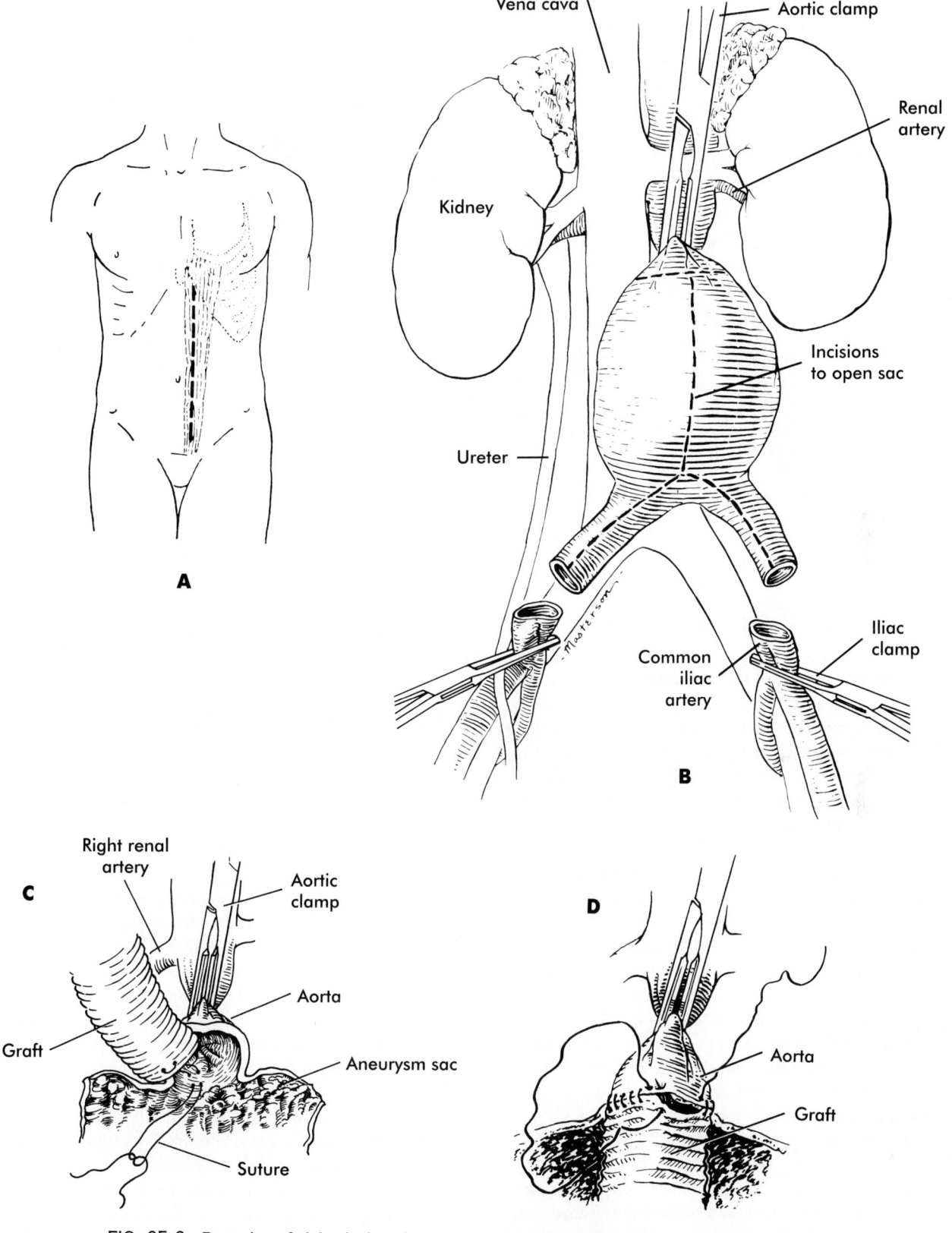

FIG. 25-6 Resection of abdominal aortic aneurysm. **A,** Midline abdominal incision. **B,** Aneurysm sac is opened. **C,** Prosthetic graft is sewn to back wall of aorta, creating a cuff. **D,** Completion of proximal aortic graft anastomosis.

Continued.

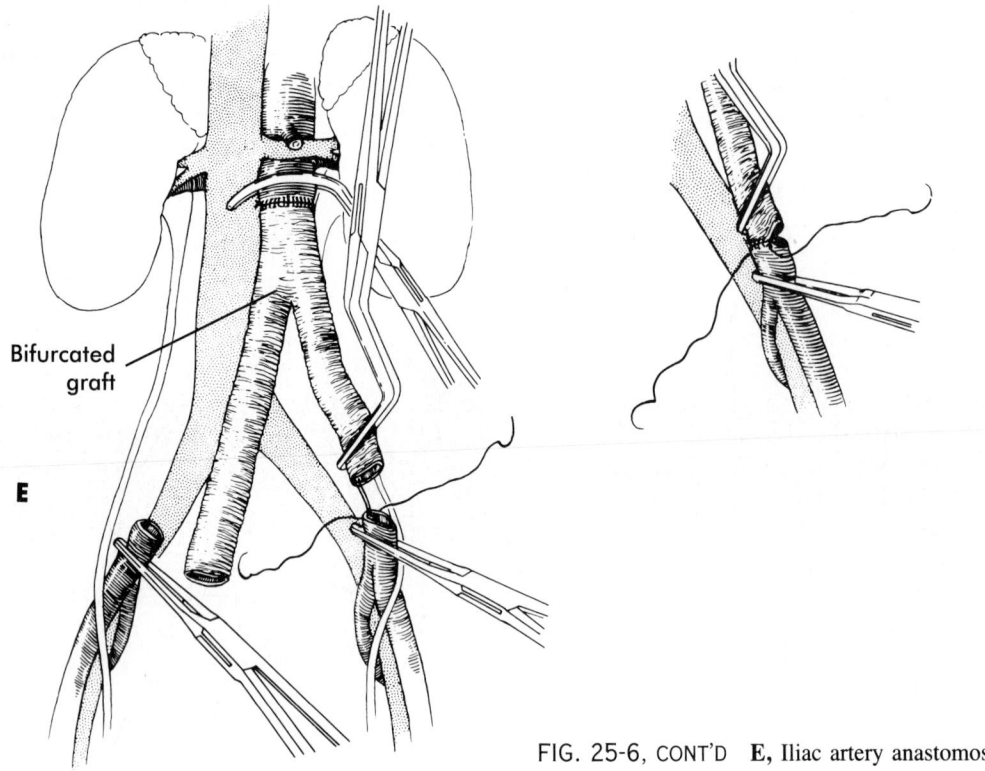

Bifurcated
graft

E

FIG. 25-6, CONT'D   **E,** Iliac artery anastomosis.

FEMOROPOPLITEAL AND FEMOROTIBIAL BYPASS

Femoropopliteal bypass is the restoration of blood flow to the leg with a graft bypassing the occluded section of the femoral artery. The bypass may be a saphenous vein or straight synthetic graft. The patency of an outflow artery must be demonstrated for a successful bypass procedure. If popliteal patency is doubtful, artery exploration is necessary as the first procedure. Involvement of the popliteal artery may necessitate the exposure and use of the tibial vessels for the lower anastomosis. If this occurs, the procedure could require the use of microvascular instruments and technique.

Procedural considerations. The patient is placed in a supine position. The hip is externally rotated and abducted with the knee flexed. Prepping and draping include the entire groin and leg. The instrument setup includes the basic minor and vascular sets plus the following: Gelpi retractors, Garrett or Weitlaner retractors, a tunneler, and supplies and equipment for operative arteriograms.

Operative procedures
Exploration of common femoral artery

1. A vertical incision, extending downward about 3 to 5 inches along the medial aspect of the thigh, is made over the femoral artery below the inguinal area, and a self-retaining retractor is inserted.
2. The common femoral artery is located, the artery is dissected in both directions for complete exposure.

3. Moist umbilical tapes or vessel loops are passed around the common femoral, the superficial femoral, and the deep femoral arteries.

Exploration of above-knee popliteal artery

1. A vertical incision is made along the medial aspect of the lower thigh. If the popliteal artery is diseased, an incision below the knee is necessary to expose the distal popliteal artery.
2. A Weitlaner retractor is used to retract the muscles and expose the artery.
3. The knee is flexed, the popliteal, artery is dissected free, and a moist umbilical tape is passed around the popliteal artery. It may be desirable at this time to perform arteriograms if doubt exists about the patency of the popliteal artery or distal arterial tree.
4. The saphenous vein is exposed by joining the femoral and popliteal incisions the length of the thigh or through multiple short incisions along the medial thigh. If the vein is suitable, the necessary length is resected or prepared for in situ grafting. If a prosthesis is used, the length and size are determined, and the graft may be preclotted as previously described.
5. The saphenous vein is prepared for use by carefully ligating side branches with fine silk. Finally, because of venous valves, the vein is reversed so the end originally in the groin is anastomosed to the popliteal artery.
6. For a synthetic graft, a tunneler is passed beneath the sartorius muscle from the popliteal fossa to the groin.

7. The graft is carefully pulled through the tunnel and positioned to prevent kinks or twists.

8. An incision is made into the femoral artery with a no. 11 knife blade and extended with Potts angulated scissors.

9. The graft is anastomosed to the artery with fine vascular sutures.

10. The knee is flexed and vascular clamps are placed on the popliteal artery at the site of the distal anastomosis.

11. An incision is made into the popliteal artery as explained for the femoral arteriotomy.

12. The graft is sutured to the popliteal artery (or tibial), and before completion the femoral occluding clamp is momentarily opened to eliminate air and debris.

13. All occluding clamps are removed and the graft is assessed for anastomatic leaks.

14. The incision is closed as described previously.

FEMOROPOPLITEAL BYPASS IN SITU

In situ femoropopliteal bypass is the restoration of blood flow to the leg, bypassing an occluded portion of the femoral artery with a patient's saphenous vein, which remains in place. The procedure includes incising the venous valves and interrupting the venous tributaries. The adequacy of the patient's saphenous vein can be validated before the surgical procedure by an ultrasound duplex scan. Varicose veins or a previous saphenous vein ligation and stripping are contraindications to the procedure. The advantages of a vein bypass procedure include increased graft availability and improved patency. A disadvantage is the time-consuming aspect of this technique. Valves can be incised with microvascular scissors, a Mills valvulotome, or a Leather in situ valve cutter kit. An angioscope may be used to monitor the lysis of valve leaflets.

Operative procedure

1. The procedure is as for femoropopliteal bypass. The groin incision is extended downward over the course of the saphenous vein. A skin bridge may be left between the groin and popliteal incisions.

2. The saphenous vein is exposed and divided at its proximal and distal ends. Venous tributaries are occluded with arterial clips, such as Hemoclips, or fine nonabsorbable sutures.

3. The valvulotome is passed from below to the top, usually through side branches. The valvulotome is used to incise the internal valve (Fig. 25-4). In angioscopically assisted bypass, valve lysis is done under direct vision.

4. The saphenous vein is distended with heparinized saline, papaverine, or heparinized blood to identify any valvular obstruction or open venous tributary. Another pass of the valve cutter alleviates the obstruction. Open branches of the saphenous vein can also be ligated with arterial clips or fine nonabsorbable sutures.

5. The incompetent saphenous vein is used to bypass the occluded segment of the femoral artery (see steps 11 to 14 of the femoropopliteal bypass procedure).

FEMOROFEMORAL BYPASS

Femorofemoral bypass is an extraanatomic bypass that is performed to restore blood flow to one leg when an inflow procedure is necessary but a major aortic procedure is not desired or surgical risks for the patient are high because of a complicated medical condition or technical problems with the procedure (Fig. 25-7). Severe cardiac or pulmonary disease may prevent the patient from undergoing a more extensive procedure. Subcutaneous vascular grafting is an option in these conditions because the procedure bypasses normal vascular anatomy and can be done with the patient under local anesthesia with adjunct sedation. The patient must have one good iliac artery for inflow for a femorofemoral bypass to be considered. Another extraanatomic procedure that can be done in these instances is an axillofemoral bypass involving the subcutaneous placement of a prosthesis from the axillary artery to the femoral artery on the same side (Fig. 25-8).

Procedural considerations. The patient is positioned on the OR bed in a supine position. For a femorofemoral bypass a small pad is placed under each knee. The area prepared for surgery extends from the umbilicus to midthigh. The genitalia are covered with a sterile towel.

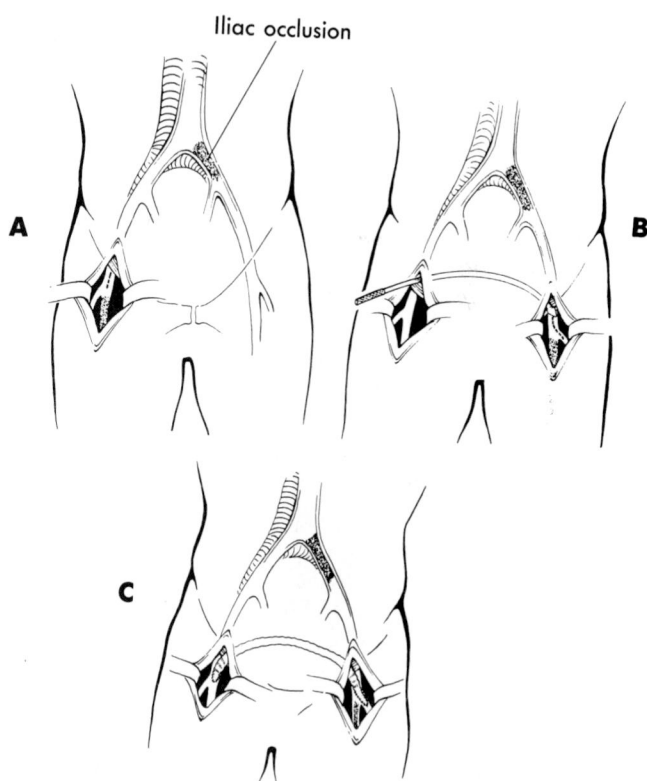

FIG. 25-7 Femorofemoral bypass to restore blood flow to left leg. **A,** Left iliac artery occlusion and right femoral artery exposure. **B,** Exposure of the right and left femoral arteries; tunneling device creating a path for the graft in the subcutaneous tissue. **C,** Femorofemoral bypass graft in place.

From Haimovici, H. (1984). *Vascular surgery: Principles and technique.* Norwalk, Conn.: Appleton-Century-Crofts.

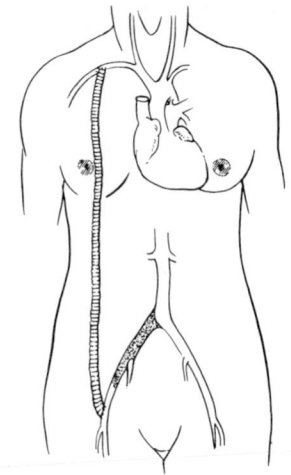

FIG. 25-8 Axillofemoral bypass graft for right iliac artery occlusion.

Operative procedure

1. A longitudinal incision is made over each femoral artery from the inguinal ligament to just below the femoral bifurcation.
2. Each common femoral, superficial femoral, and deep femoral artery is dissected free, mobilized, and secured with umbilical tapes or vessel loops.
3. The graft tunnel between the two femoral arteries is created across the pubic symphysis in the subcutaneous tissue. This tunnel is created with digital dissection, scissors dissection, or the passage of a clamp or tunneler across the preperitoneal space.
4. A Dacron or PTFE vascular graft is passed through the subcutaneous tunnel with care to prevent kinking of the graft.
5. Vascular clamps are placed on the common femoral, superficial femoral, and deep femoral arteries. A longitudinal arteriotomy is made in the common femoral artery.

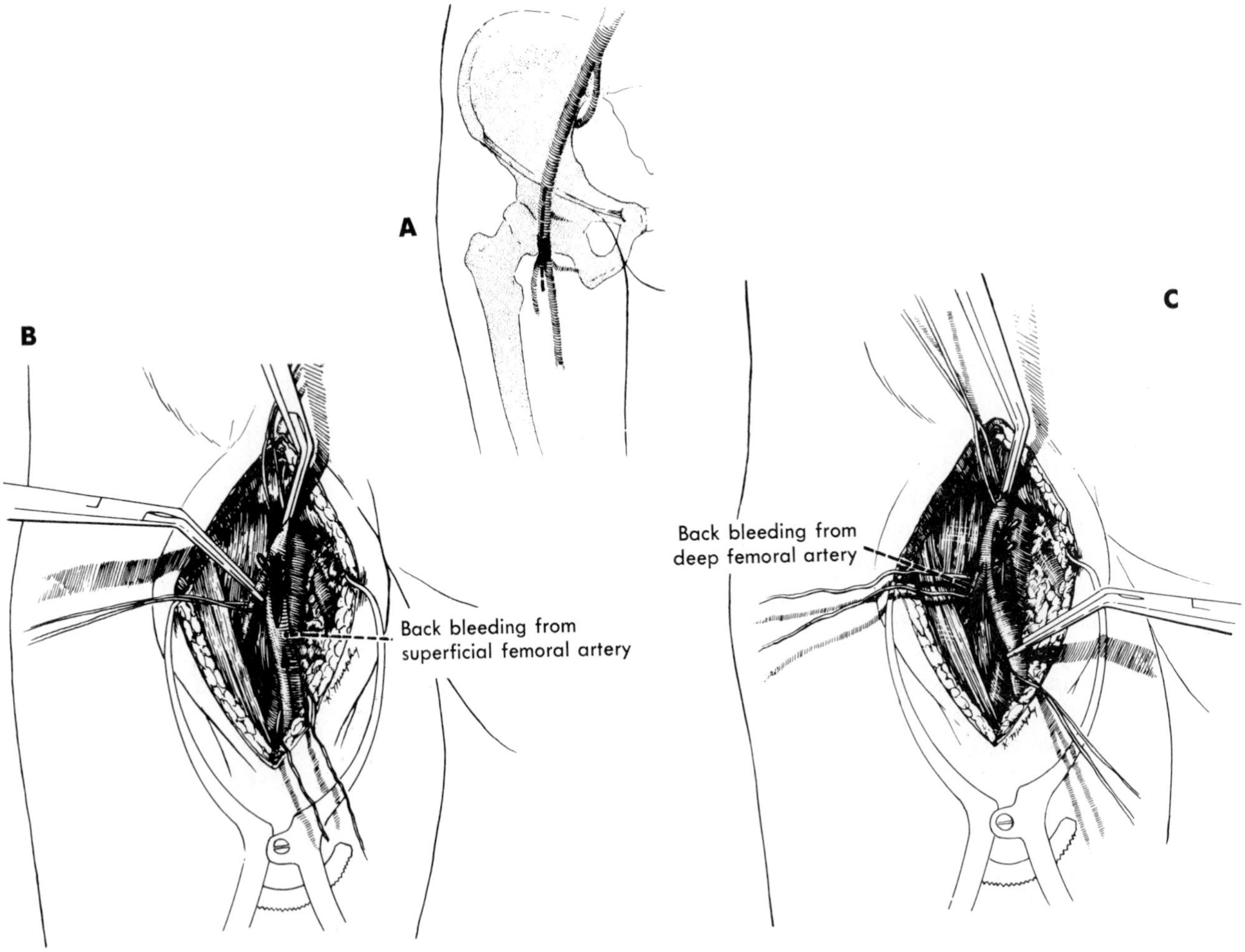

A

B

Back bleeding from
superficial femoral artery

C

Back bleeding from
deep femoral artery

FIG. 25-9 Femoral embolectomy. **A,** Femoral arteriotomy. **B,** Clamp on common femoral and deep femoral (profunda femoris) arteries. Backflow of blood from superficial femoral artery *(SFA)* is checked. **C,** Clamp on common femoral artery and SFA. Backflow of blood from deep femoral artery is checked.

6. An end-to-side anastomosis using nonabsorbable vascular sutures is performed to join the graft with the common femoral artery. A similar anastomosis is done on the other side.
7. After the clamps are released and flow is restored, the patient's pulses are checked; the circulating nurse may be asked to inspect the patient's feet.
8. The femoral incisions are closed.

ARTERIAL EMBOLECTOMY

Arterial embolectomy entails an incision made in the affected artery to remove thromboembolic material (Fig. 25-9) and restore blood flow. Emboli may be clot particles, a foreign body, air, fat, or a tumor that circulates through the bloodstream and becomes lodged as the vessel decreases in size. More often the direct source is a cardiac mural thrombus, associated with cardiac or vascular disease. Pain or numbness distal to the obstruction is the initial symptom, accompanied by other signs of vascular occlusion, such as pallor and absence of pulses.

Procedural considerations. The patient is placed in the supine position, the skin area is prepped, and draping is completed to permit access to the affected area. The instrument setup includes the basic instrument and vascular sets, including Fogarty embolectomy catheters.

Operative procedure

1. The initial incision is completed, and the artery is carefully exposed to permit the application of vascular clamps (see Fig. 25-9, *A* and *B*).
2. An incision is made into the artery with a no. 11 blade and Potts scissors. A Fogarty catheter is carefully inserted beyond the point of clot proximally and distally.

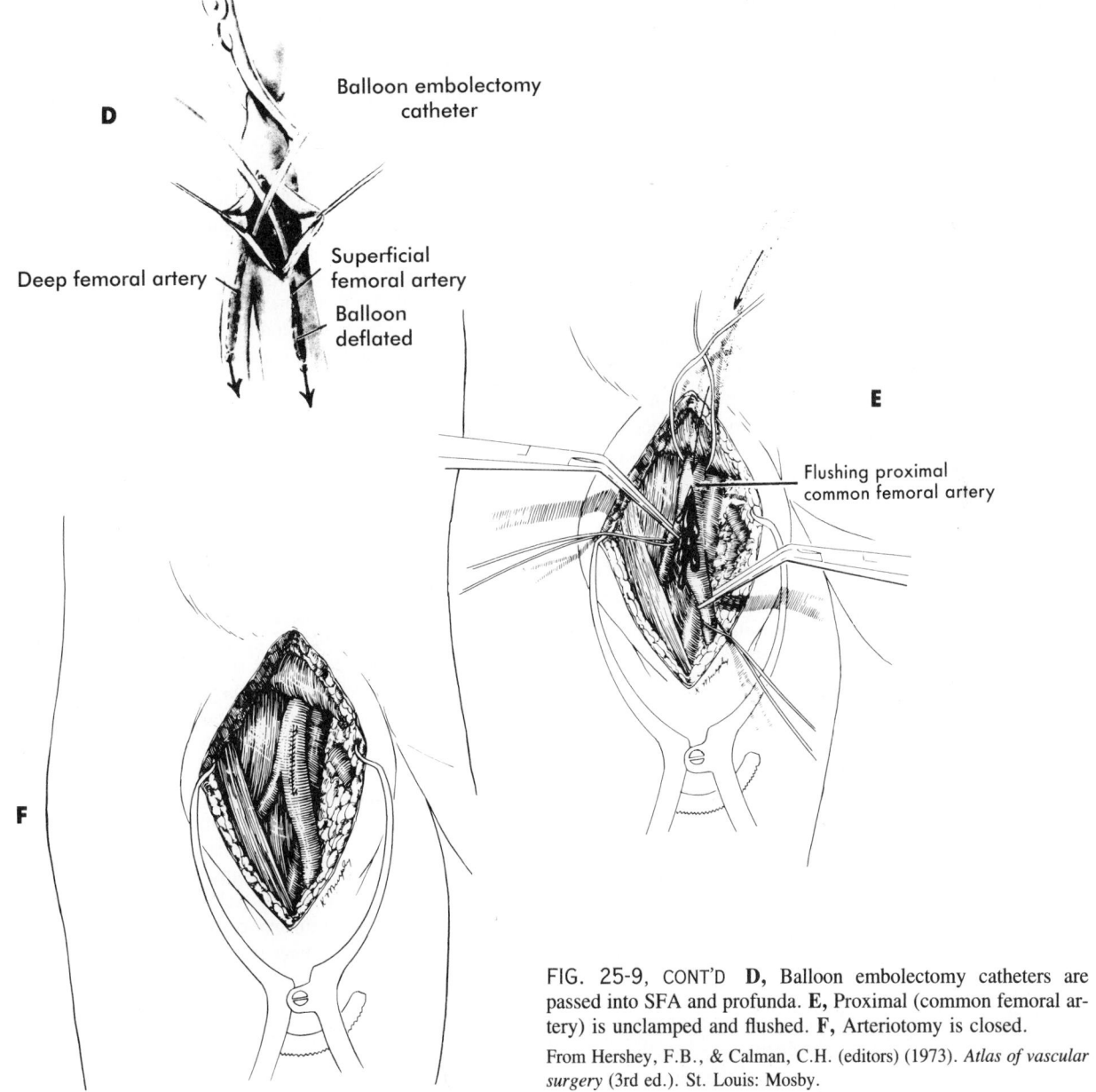

FIG. 25-9, CONT'D **D,** Balloon embolectomy catheters are passed into SFA and profunda. **E,** Proximal (common femoral artery) is unclamped and flushed. **F,** Arteriotomy is closed.

From Hershey, F.B., & Calman, C.H. (editors) (1973). *Atlas of vascular surgery* (3rd ed.). St. Louis: Mosby.

The balloon is inflated, and the catheter is withdrawn along with the detached clot (see Fig. 25-9, *C* and *D*).

3. As backflow is obtained, a vascular clamp is applied below the arteriotomy (see Fig. 25-9, *E*).

4. The artery may be flushed by injection of heparinized saline solution through a small irrigating catheter. Angioscopy or an arteriogram may or may not be requested at this time.

5. The arterial closure is completed with vascular sutures (see Fig. 25-9, *F*). The wound closure is accomplished in the usual manner, and dressings are applied.

CAROTID ENDARTERECTOMY

Carotid endarterectomy is the removal of an atheroma at the carotid artery bifurcation to increase cerebral perfusion and decrease the risk of embolization. Lessening the likelihood of any transient or permanent neurologic deficit is a major concern during a carotid endarterectomy. The use of a temporary carotid artery shunt, such as an Argyle (see Fig. 25-11) or Javid shunt, allows for a continuous blood flow through the carotid artery and to the brain. Some disadvantages in using this temporary device are the additional dissection necessary for its placement and the possibility of dislodging debris when inserting the shunt, as well as a difficult view of the endarterectomy endpoint and increased difficulty in suturing a patch (Research Highlight 25-3).

Two techniques that facilitate continual assessment of cerebral perfusion are cervical block anesthesia and EEG. A conscious patient under cervical block anesthesia can be observed for neurologic deficits encountered during the procedure. In addition, the patient under general anesthesia can be monitored with an EEG. If either method demonstrates reduced cerebral perfusion, the surgeon may decide to use a temporary carotid artery shunt. The shunting device should always be available and sterile at the beginning of the procedure.

Procedural considerations. The patient is placed on the OR bed in a supine position with the head supported on a head support. The head is turned away from the operative side and the neck may be slightly hyperextended. A roll may be placed between the scapulas.

Operative procedure

1. A longitudinal incision is made over the area of the carotid bifurcation. The Weitlaner self-retaining retractor may be placed for exposure (Fig. 25-10).

2. With Metzenbaum scissors the soft tissue is dissected for exposure of the carotid artery and its bifurcation.

3. A moistened umbilical tape or vessel loop is passed around the vessel for ease of handling. The patient is systemically heparinized.

4. The external, common, and internal carotid arteries are clamped.

5. With a no. 11 scalpel blade, an arteriotomy is made over the stenotic area. The incision is lengthened with Potts angulated scissors to expose the full extent of the occluding plaque.

6. With a blunt dissector the plaque or plaques are dissected free from the arterial wall. Heparin solution is used as an irrigant to clean the intima.

❇️
RESEARCH HIGHLIGHT 25-3

Efforts to study quality of clinical care for selected patient populations have become the hallmark of health services research in the 1990s. The appropriateness and outcomes of carotid endarterectomy surgery are the focus of a number of studies. To attempt a correlation between patient risk, appropriateness, and outcomes, two consecutive studies in 1977 and 1984 examined the results of carotid endarterectomy in the same community hospitals. In the first part of the study 11 surgeons performed 228 operations for a combined stroke-plus-death rate of over 21%. In the second series the complication results were much lower, with only 1.6% mortality and 5.4% stroke. More recent randomized trials of carotid endarterectomy among symptomatic and asymptomatic patients indicated that appropriateness for symptomatic patients was high-grade (70% to 99%) ipsilateral carotid stenosis in patients with recent symptoms (within 120 days), age less than 80, and no specific comorbidities such as uncontrolled hypertension, mental incapacity, recent myocardial infarction, clinically important organ dysfunction, or any condition leading the surgeon to suspect a 5-year life expectancy of less than 5 years.

A more recent study attempted to analyze the relationship between surgical volume and quality care. In a small-area analysis of 5657 carotid endarterectomies, the investigators concluded that good results with regard to mortality generally began at about 15 procedures per year. Over half the surgeons in the study had no mortality associated with their patients. The readmission rate for patients in the study was 33%, primarily due to cardiac conditions or vascular disease that was not necessarily of the carotid or cerebral vasculature. Although a limitation of the study was the absence of severity adjustment, the authors recommend that the surgeons without mortality become the benchmark for the best practice. The reason for such outstanding performance should be studied and educational strategies developed to assist all facilities in reaching this level of performance. Perioperative nurses can expect to see more of these types of analyses, exploring links between volume and outcome along with resource utilization. In the future, relationships between these variables may be incorporated into credentialing and the selection of centers of excellence from which managed care groups will elect to purchase surgical services.

Segal, H.E., Rummel, L., & Wu, B. (1993). The utility of PRO data on surgical volume: The example of carotid endarterectomy. *Quality Review Bulletin, 19*(5), 152-157.

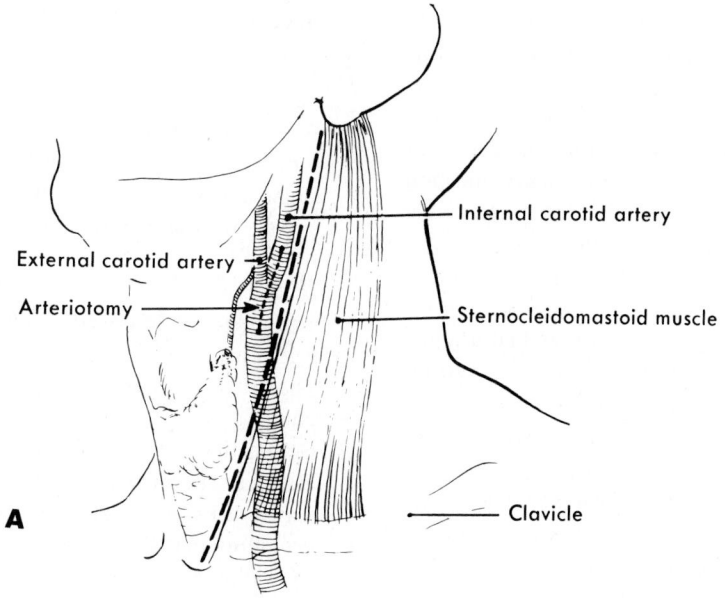

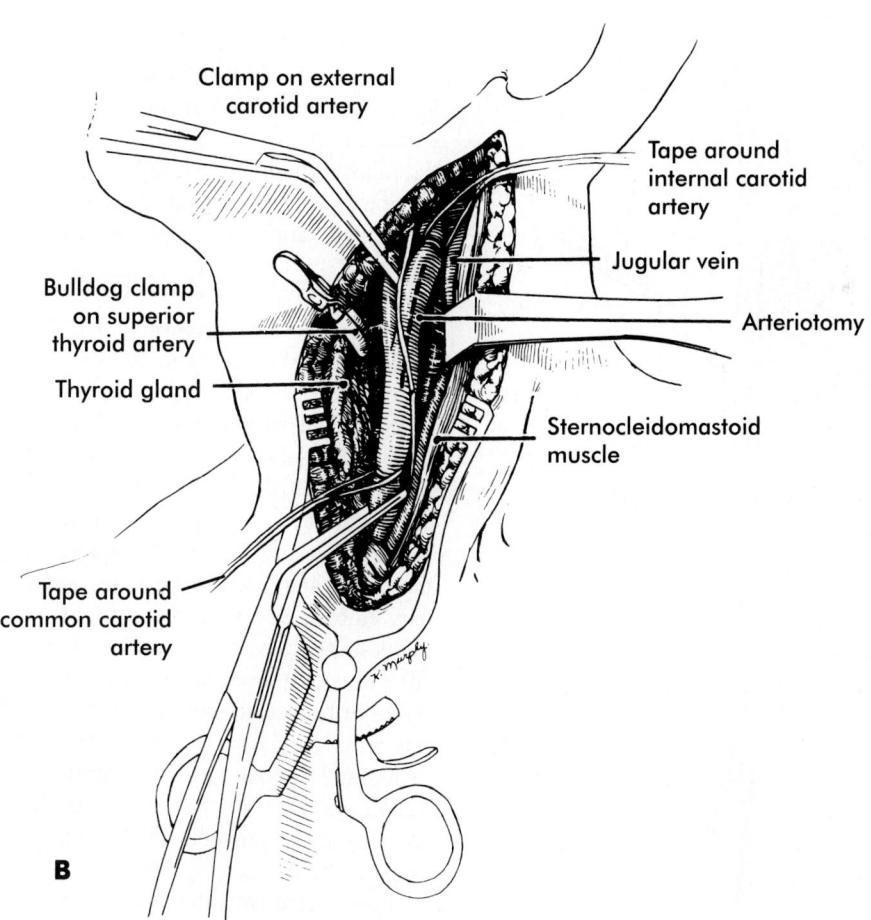

FIG. 25-10 Left carotid endarterectomy. **A,** Incision and anatomy. **B,** Exposure of carotid bifurcation.

From Hershey, F.B., & Calman C.H. (editors). (1973). *Atlas of vascular surgery* (3rd ed.). St. Louis: Mosby.

7. The arteriotomy is closed with fine vascular sutures. A synthetic or autogenous (vein) patch graft may be used to restore the arterial lumen if it is small (Fig. 25-11). Before complete closure, blood flow is temporarily restored through the arteries to wash away any free plaque, air, or thrombi. To do this, the occluding clamps are opened and closed individually, flushing any debris away from the internal carotid artery. The closure of the arteriotomy is completed.

8. The occluding clamps are removed from the external and common carotid arteries; *the internal carotid artery clamp is removed last.* This ensures that any minor debris missed will be flushed harmlessly into the external rather than the internal carotid artery.

9. Additional interrupted sutures may be needed to control leakage.

10. A drain is inserted via a separate stab incision.

11. The wound closure is accomplished in the usual manner, and dressings are applied.

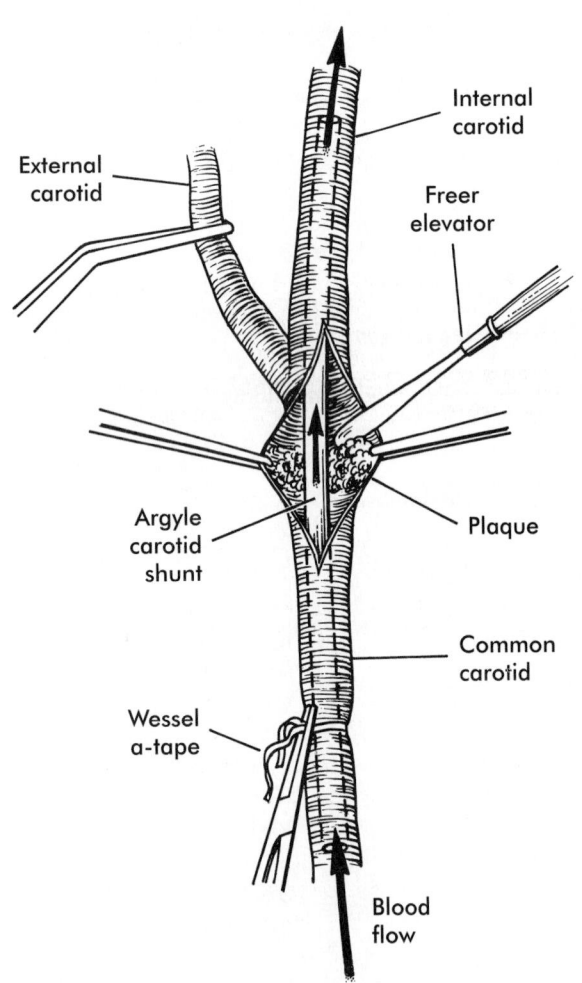

FIG. 25-11 Left carotid endarterectomy. Argyle carotid shunt in place to allow blood flow to brain. Stenotic plaque being removed with Freer elevator.

CAROTID ENDARTERECTOMY WITH SHUNT
Operative procedure

1. The first five steps as described for carotid endarterectomy are followed.

2. A piece of tubing (polyethylene or Silastic) with a suture tied around its center or a commercially prepared shunt device is inserted in the common carotid artery and the internal carotid artery to maintain cerebral blood flow and is held with tourniquets or shunt clamps (Fig. 25-12).

3. The plaque is removed as described for carotid endarterectomy.

4. The arteriotomy is closed with or without a patch (Fig. 25-13).

5. Before the arteriotomy closure is completed, the shunt clamp or tourniquet on the internal carotid artery is released, and the shunt is removed. The external carotid occluding clamp is removed, followed by the common carotid artery clamp, and last the internal carotid artery occluding clamp.

6. The wound is closed in the usual manner.

ARTERIOVENOUS FISTULA

The surgeon may elect to create a direct arteriovenous fistula between the radial artery and the cephalic vein. The dilated vein would then be used for direct cannulation with large-bore needles for hemodialysis. This method is preferable to an external shunt, which carries a high risk of thrombosis and infection. Other alternatives are to use a saphenous vein or a prosthetic graft, such as PTFE to join the brachial artery and cephalic vein.

VENA CAVA FILTER INSERTION

Vena cava filter insertion entails the partial occlusion of the inferior vena cava with an intravascular filter, such as a Greenfield filter, inserted under fluoroscopy with local or monitored anesthesia care. The Greenfield device offers the option of jugular or femoral vein insertion, and the correct kit must be selected. In patients for whom heparin therapy is either contraindicated or not effective, the vena cava filter is the treatment of choice to capture emboli that arise from the pelvis and lower extremities and thus prevent pulmonary emboli. Several types of filters have been used during the past 20 years. The Greenfield filter is the most successful and widely used device, and the mortality and morbidity have been extremely low (Persson, 1989). The device has progressed from the earlier design that required an incision and venotomy to the current percutaneous titanium vena cava filter (Fig. 25-14). The filter maintains a patent vena cava but prevents PE by trapping the emboli at the apex of the device (Fig. 25-15).

Procedural considerations. The patient is placed in the supine position on a radiopaque OR bed to permit fluoroscopic visualization at the level of the renal veins. The head is turned to the left for jugular vein insertion or the groin is

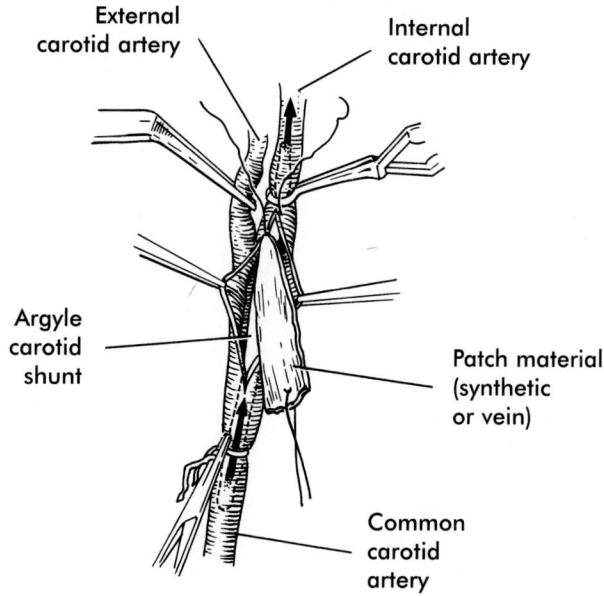

External carotid artery

Internal carotid artery

Argyle carotid shunt

Patch material (synthetic or vein)

Common carotid artery

FIG. 25-12   Left carotid endarterectomy illustrating initial placement and suturing of a patch, synthetic, or vein (shunt is in place).

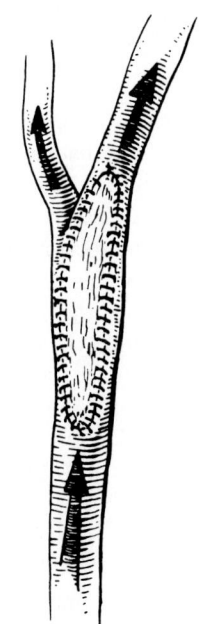

FIG. 25-13   Left carotid endarterectomy: patch sewn in place.

exposed for femoral vein insertion (Fig. 25-16). The right femoral is preferred over the left because the anatomy of the left vein often makes threading the filter more difficult. Local anesthesia, heparinized saline to flush device lumens, and contrast medium should be available. Since this is a percutaneous insertion, no instruments are needed.

Operative procedure for insertion of a femoral Greenfield vena cava filter

1. The right groin area is prepped and draped and infiltrated with local anesthesia.

2. An 18-gauge entry needle is used for right femoral venotomy.

3. The guidewire is inserted and advanced to a level above the renal veins under fluoroscopic guidance.

4. The sheath/dilator is inserted over guidewire (preflush all lumens with heparin solution).

5. The sheath is removed and the introducer catheter is inserted and advanced to the implant site.

6. This catheter carries the preloaded, radiopaque carrier capsule. The sheath is retracted, the filter discharged, and sheath removed.

7. Pressure is applied to the puncture site for approximately 5 minutes or until hemostasis is achieved (Greenfield and Cho, 1990).

HIGH LIGATION OF SAPHENOUS VEINS WITH EXCISION

The saphenous trunk may be ligated and divided with subsequent stripping and excision. A series of cup-shaped valves maintains the venous blood flow in a direction toward the heart. Disease may prevent the normal functioning of these valves, resulting in distention. The veins gradually become dilated. Those in the lower extremities are most frequently affected, particularly the long saphenous vein. The incidence is estimated at 2% in Western populations with women affected two and a half times as often as men. Factors such as age, parity, and occupation may contribute to the problem, but the etiology is still not completely clear (Wilson and Browse, 1993). Dilatation of the saphenous vein produces venous stasis, which may be followed by secondary complications, such as stasis ulcers. Venous obstruction causes an increase in venous pressure, which leads to an increase in capillary pressure. This causes fluid to leak from the capillaries and produce edema (Bright

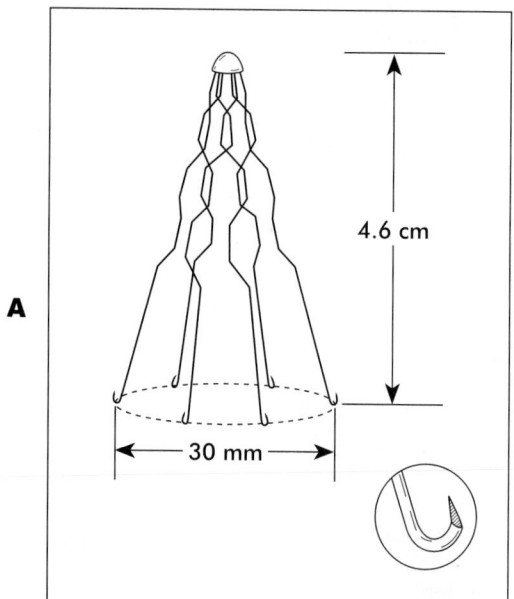 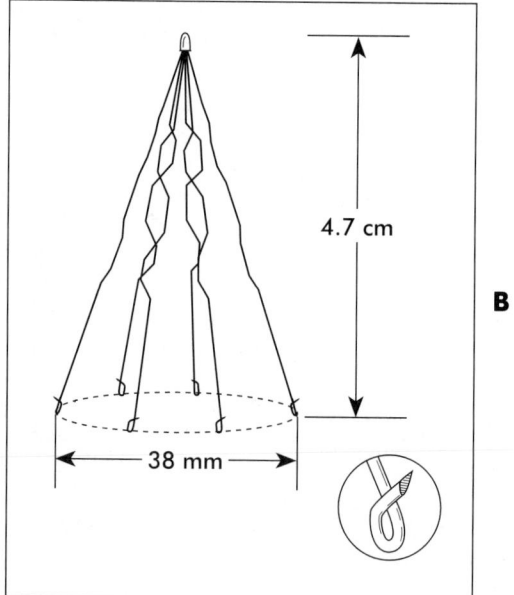

FIG. 25-14   Greenfield vena cava filter. **A,** Older version. **B,** New titanium version for percutaneous insertion.

Courtesy Medi-tech Division of Boston Scientific Corp., Watertown, Mass.

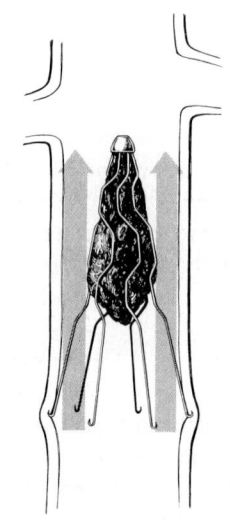

FIG. 25-15   Emboli trapped in Greenfield filter in inferior vena cava.

Courtesy Medi-tech Division of Boston Scientific Corp, Watertown, Mass.

and Georgi, 1992). The objective of surgical intervention is to remove the diseased veins, thus preventing ulceration, secondary edema, pain, and fatigue in the extremity.

Procedural considerations. Before sedation or entrance into the operating room, the patient should stand and the varicose veins should be marked with an indelible marker. This ensures adequate visualization, since the patient is of-ten placed in Trendelenburg position intraoperatively to decrease venous congestion. The patient is placed on the OR bed in a supine position with the legs slightly abducted. Ligation or stripping of the lesser saphenous veins and branches may require placing the patient in the prone position. Drapes are placed to enable flexing and lifting at the knee. Instruments include the basic minor instrument setup (see Chapter 11), plus the following:

Weitlaner self-retaining retractors	Vein strippers with various tips available
Skin hooks	Elastic bandages
Mosquito hemostats	

Operative procedure

1. The incision is made in the upper thigh, parallel to the crease in the groin. Bleeding vessels are clamped and ligated.
2. The saphenous vein is identified and isolated. Margins of the wound are separated with a Weitlaner self-retaining retractor.
3. The saphenous vein branches are doubly ligated with black silk ties or transfixed, clamped, and divided. The proximal stump is dissected upward to the point at which it enters the femoral vein, where it is carefully ligated.
4. If the saphenous vein is to be excised, an incision is made at its distal portion at the ankle, and the vein is identified, ligated, and divided.
5. A vein stripper is inserted and advanced to the proximal end of the vein in the groin, where it is secured with a heavy suture, and the tip is attached.

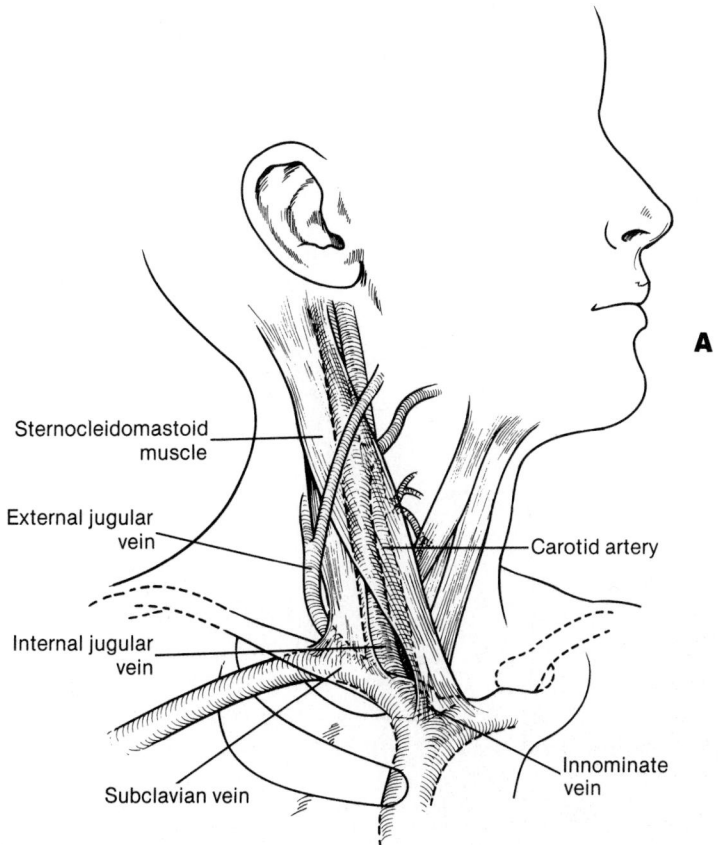

Sternocleidomastoid muscle

External jugular vein

Internal jugular vein

Subclavian vein

Carotid artery

Innominate vein

A

FIG. 25-16   Greenfield vena cava filter insertion. **A,** Anatomy of neck. Vena cava filter insertion may be via the right internal jugular vein or via the right femoral vein.

Continued.

6. As the stripper is pulled up the leg, external compression is applied.
7. Tributaries may be excised through numerous small incisions along the course of the vein.
8. The groin wound is closed in layers and other small incisions are closed with skin sutures or staples. Dressings and circular compression bandages are applied.

AMPUTATION

Amputations may be necessary because of trauma, malignancy, infection, or ischemia.

It is critical to verify the correct limb for this procedure. Since these are often performed with the patient under regional anesthesia, the perioperative nurse must be sure that the patient does not witness the wrapping or transport of the amputated limb. Toe or partial foot amputations may be done in certain instances, but often, a below-knee (BK) or above-knee (AK) amputation is indicated. The level is based on the patient's health, the level of vascularity, and potential for healing and rehabilitation (Atkinson, 1992). Severe infection or toxemia may require amputation as a life-saving procedure. Perioperative mortality is lower for a BK than an AK (8% versus 18%), and full mobility is also better at the BK level (50% versus 25%) (Dormandy,

1993). BK amputations are best done at the junction of the upper and middle third of the lower leg. This allows an immediate postoperative prosthesis, aids in better healing, and may reduce phantom limb pain. AK amputations may be at the middle or lower third of the thigh. Flaps are tailored to provide fascial and skin coverage to cushion the smoothed end of the bone. Meticulous hemostasis and drainage are needed to decrease hematoma formation, since healing is both problematic and critical in these patients. Diabetics are at highest risk for amputation because of their accelerated atherosclerosis, small vessel disease, neuropathies, and decreased ability to fight infection. About 50% of diabetic amputees have the opposite limb amputated within 2 years (La Muraglia, 1989).

Operative procedure

1. The level of amputation is determined and the incision line marked to create a long posterior flap.
2. The incision is made. Muscle and soft tissue are divided. Periosteum is raised with an elevator.
3. Bones are cut, beveled at their anterior aspect, and smoothed with a rougeur and rasp.
4. The wound is irrigated and hemostasis achieved.
5. A drain is inserted.

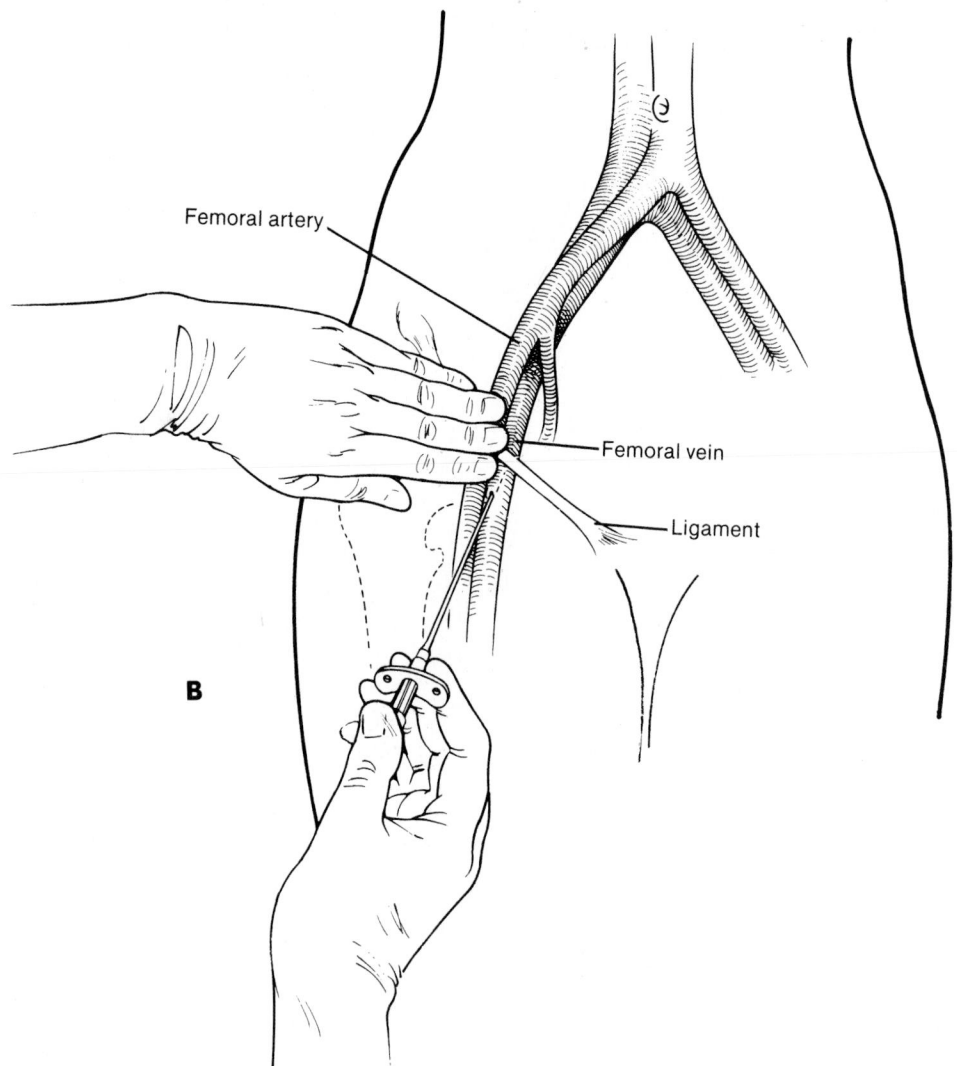

Femoral artery

Femoral vein

Ligament

B

FIG. 25-16, CONT'D **B,** Left femoral vein is possible but more difficult.

6. Fascia is closed with interrupted sutures.
7. Skin is approximated and closed with interrupted suture or staples.
8. An immediate postoperative stump dressing may be applied (Green and Rob, 1985).

REFERENCES

Ahn, S.S. (1992) Status of peripheral atherectomy. In S.S. Ahn & J.M. Seeger (Eds.), *The surgical clinics of North America* (vol. 72). Philadelphia: W.B. Saunders.

Atkinson, L.J. (1992). *Berry & Kohn's operating room technique* (7th ed.). St. Louis: Mosby.

Baer, C.L., & Williams, B.B. (1992). *Clinical pharmacology and nursing* (2nd ed.). Springhouse, Pa.: Springhouse Corporation.

Bernard, V., Boren, C., & Towne, J. (1980). Pneumatic tourniquet as a substitute for vascular clamps in distal bypass surgery. *Surgery, 87,* 709.

Bright, L.D., & Georgi, S. (1992). Peripheral vascular disease: Is it venous or arterial? *American Journal of Nursing 92*(9), 34-43.

Cambria, R.P. (1989). Acute lower extremity ischemia. In D.C. Brewster (Ed.), *Common problems in vascular surgery.* Chicago: Year Book Medical Publishers.

Cannobbio, M.M. (1990). Diagnostic procedures. In M.M. Cannobbio (Ed.), *Cardiovascular disorders.* St. Louis: Mosby.

Clark, J.B., Queener, S.F., & Karb, V.B. (1993). *Pharmacological basis of nursing practice (4th ed.).* St Louis: Mosby.

Clement, D.L., & Verhaeghe, R. (1993). Atherosclerosis and other occlusive diseases. In D.L. Clements and J.T. Shepherd (Eds.), *Vascular disease in the limbs: Mechanisms and principles of treatment.* St. Louis: Mosby.

Cohen, J.R., Grella, L., & Citron, M. (1992). Greenfield filter instead of heparin as primary treatment for deep venous thrombosis or pulmonary embolism in patients with cancer. *Cancer, 70*(7), 1993-1996.

Cunningham, J.N., Catinella, F.P., Nathan, I.M., & Spencer, F.C. (1981). Proposed mechanism for early vein graft thrombosis. In T.R. Bushman (Ed.), *Surgical Forum* (vol. 32). American College of Surgeons, Chicago, Ill.

DeWeese, J.D. (1989). The small aortic aneurysm. In D.C. Brewster (Ed.), *Common problems in vascular surgery.* Chicago: Year Book Medical Publishers.

Docker, C.S., Muthusamy, R., Balasundaramy, S., & Duran, C. (1992). Intra-operative echocardiography: An essential tool in cardiac surgery . . . epicardial echocardiography . . . transesophageal echocardiography. *AORN Journal 55*(1), 167, 169-170, 172, 173.

Dormandy, J.A. (1993). Critical leg ischemia. In D.L. Clement and J.T. Shepherd (Eds.), *Vascular diseases in the limbs: Mechanisms and principles of treatment*. St. Louis: Mosby.

Dzsinich, C., & Gloviczki, P. (1993). Principles of vascular surgery. In D.L. Clement and J.T. Shepherd (Eds.), *Vascular diseases in the limbs: Mechanisms and principles of treatment*. St. Louis: Mosby.

Eriksson, I. (1990). Why do so few surgeons perform reconstructive venous surgery? In J.J. Bergen (Ed.), *Year book of vascular surgery 1992*. St. Louis: Mosby.

Fogarty, A.M. (1991). Angioscopy: New developments in vascular surgery. *AORN Journal 53*(3), 725-728.

Friedman, S.G. (1993). *A history of vascular surgery*. New York: Futura.

Golden, M.A., Whittemore, A.D., Donaldson, M.C., & Mannick, J.A. (1990). Selective evaluation and management of coronary artery disease in patients undergoing repair of abdominal aortic aneurysms: a 16 year experience. *Annals of Surgery, 212*(3), 415-423.

Goldsmith, J., Franco, C.D., Farrell, E.A., Kelley, J., & Veith, F.J. (1992). Advances in the surgical treatment of lower extremity vascular disease. *Journal of the American Academy of Physicians Assistants, 4*(6), 481-487.

Govani, L.E., & Hayes, J.E. (1985). *Drugs and nursing implications* (5th ed.). Norwalk, Conn.: Appleton-Century-Crofts.

Green RM: (April 29, 1993) Personal communication.

Green, R.M., & Rob, C.G. (1985). Amputations. In J.A. DeWeese (Ed.), *Rob and Smith's operative surgery: Vascular surgery* (4th ed.). Boston: Butterworth's.

Greenfield, L.J., & Cho, K.J. (Eds.). (1990). *The Greenfield vena cava filter and 12 French introducer systems: Concept and technique*. Boston: Boston Scientific Corporation.

Guzzetta, C.E., & Dossey, B.M. (1992). *Cardiovascular nursing: Holistic practice*. St. Louis: Mosby.

Hollier, L.H., & Rutherford, R.B. (1989). Aorto-renal aortic aneurysms. In R.B. Rutherford (Ed.), *Vascular surgery* (3rd ed.). Philadelphia: W.B. Saunders.

Katzen, B.T., & Becker, G.J. (1992). Intravascular stents: Status of development and clinical application. In S.S. Ahn and J.M. Seeger (Eds.), *The surgical clinics of North America* (Vol. 72). Philadelphia: W.B. Saunders.

La Muraglia, G.M. (1989). Amputation level selection. In D.C. Brewster (Ed.), *Common problems in vascular surgery*. Chicago: Year Book Medical Publishers.

Murray, K.K., & Hawkins, I.F., Jr. (1992). Angioscopy of the lower extremity in atherosclerotic vascular disease, current techniques. In S.S. Ahn and J.M. Seeger (Eds.), *The surgical clinics of North America* (Vol. 72). Philadelphia: W.B. Saunders.

Ouriel, K., Fiore, W.M., & Geary, J.E. (1980). Limb threatening ischemia in the medically compromised patient: Amputation or revascularization? *Surgery 104*(4), 667-671.

Persson, A.V. (1989). Acute deep venous thrombosis. In D.C. Brewster (Ed.), *Common problems in vascular surgery*. Chicago: Year Book Medical Publishers.

Procter, C.D., Sr., Kazmier, F.J., Hollier, L.H., & Ramee, S.R. (1992). Selection of patients for peripheral revascularization surgery. *The Medical Clinics of North America. 76*(5), 1159-1168.

Reilly, K.M., & Salluzzo, R. (1990) Pulmonary embolism. *Resident & Staff Physician, 36*(10), 43-48.

Self, S.B., & Seeger, J.M. (1992). Laser angioplasty. In S.S. Ahn and J.M. Seeger (Eds.), *The Surgical Clinics of North America: Endovascular Surgery* (Vol. 72). Philadelphia: W.B. Saunders.

Sheng, F.C., & Busuttil, R.W. (1991). Antibiotics in vascular surgery. In W.S. Moore (Ed.), *Vascular surgery: A comprehensive review*. Philadelphia: W.B. Saunders.

Stanley, J.C., Lindenauer, S.M., Graham, L.M., Zelenock, G.B., Wakefield, T.W., & Cronenvett, J.L. (1991). Biologic and synthetic vascular grafts. In W.S. Moore (Ed.), *Vascular surgery: A comprehensive review*. Philadelphia: W.B. Saunders.

Stanley, J.C., Sottiurai, V., Fry, R.E., & Fry, W.J. (1975). Comparative evolution of vein graft preparation media: Electron and microscopic studies. *Journal of Surgical Research 18*(3), 235-246.

Szilagyi, D.E., Elliott, J.P., Smith, R.F., Reddy, D.J., & McFarlin, M. (1986). A 30-year study of the reconstructive surgical treatment of aorto-iliac occlusive disease. *Journal of Vascular Surgery, 3*(3), 421-436.

Veith, F.J., Gupta, S.K., Ascer, E., White-Flores, S., Samson R.H., Scher, L.A., Towne, J.B., Bernhard, V.M., Bonier, P., Flinn, W.R., Astelford, P., Yao, J.S.T., & Bergan, J.J. (1986). Six-year prospective multicenter randomized comparison of autologous saphenous vein and expanded polytetrafluoroethylene grafts in infrainguinal arterial reconstructions. *Journal of Vascular Surgery, 3*(1), 104-114.

Verhaeghe, R., & Verstraete, M. (1993). Hemostasis, thrombosis, and anti-thrombotic and thrombolytic therapy. In D.L. Clement and J.T. Shepherd (Eds.), *Vascular diseases in the limbs: Mechanisms and principles of treatment*. St. Louis: Mosby.

White, G.H. (1992). Angioscopy. In S.S. Ahn and J.M. Seeger (Eds.), *The surgical clinics of North America* (Vol. 72). Philadelphia: W.B. Saunders.

Wilson, N.M., & Browse, N.L. (1993). Venous disease. In D.L. Clement and J.T. Shepherd (Eds.), *Vascular diseases in the limbs: Mechanisms and principles of treatment*. St. Louis: Mosby.

Wright, C.B., Dunn, E.J., Ketterhagen, J.P., Callard, G.M., & Flege, J.B., Jr. (1987). The regulatory environment for vascular grafts. In P.N. Sawyer (Ed.), *Modern vascular grafts*. New York: McGraw-Hill.

26

CARDIAC SURGERY

PATRICIA C. SEIFERT

The treatment of acquired heart disease has been positively affected by a greater understanding of the natural history of the disease, more precise diagnostic techniques, improvements in perioperative management, and an expanding array of surgical interventions. These achievements are reflected in new procedures for the treatment of coronary artery disease, valvular dysfunction, thoracic aneurysms, conduction disturbances, and congenital abnormalities. Patients with conditions formerly considered hopeless, such as end-stage ischemic heart disease and idiopathic cardiomyopathy, can benefit from mechanical circulatory assistance and cardiac transplantation. Future trends include refinements in laser technology and implantable biomaterials as well as clinical applications of genetic engineering and heterograft organ replacements.

SURGICAL ANATOMY

The heart (Fig. 26-1) is a four-chambered muscular organ that acts as a power pump for the circulatory system. It is enclosed in a pericardial sac within the mediastinum, which lies between the lungs, posterior to the sternum, and anterior to the vertebrae, esophagus, and the descending portion of the aorta. The diaphragm is positioned below the heart (Fig. 26-2). The cardiac wall is composed of three layers: the epicardium, the outer lining; the myocardium, or muscular layer, which is the important functional layer; and the endocardium, the inner lining (Fig. 26-3). Two thirds of the heart is located to the left of the midline, and the remaining third to the right. Although functionally divided into right and left halves, the heart is rotated to the left, with the right side located anteriorly and the left side relatively posterior.

Each half of the heart contains an upper and lower communicating chamber: the atrium and the ventricle. The right atrium receives desaturated blood from the inferior and superior venae cavae, and from the coronary circulation via the coronary sinus. The left atrium receives oxygenated blood from the lungs via the pulmonary veins. From the atria, blood flows through the atrioventricular valves into the ventricles.

The left ventricle pumps blood into the major vessels of the *systemic circulatory system:* the aorta and its main branches to the head, upper extremities, abdominal organs, and lower extremities. The right and left internal (thoracic) mammary arteries, used as grafts during bypass surgery, branch off the subclavian arteries in the neck and course behind and parallel to the edges of the sternum. The arteries of the circulatory system subdivide into arterioles and eventually into capillaries, where internal respiration and metabolic exchange occur. From the capillary beds, desaturated blood flows into the venules and veins and finally returns to the right atrium.

In the *pulmonary circulatory system,* blood is pumped from the right ventricle through the pulmonary valve into the main pulmonary artery. It divides into the right and left pulmonary arteries, which further subdivide into arterioles and the capillaries of the lungs. External respiration occurs in the capillary beds, where carbon dioxide is exchanged for oxygen. Freshly oxygenated blood from the lungs flows through the pulmonary veins into the left atrium.

The *coronary circulation* (Fig. 26-4) supplies oxygen and nutrients to the myocardium. The heart receives its blood supply from the left and right coronary arteries, which originate in the sinuses of Valsalva behind the cusps of the aortic valve in the ascending aorta. The left main coronary artery divides into the left anterior descending coronary artery and the circumflex coronary artery; along with the right coronary artery, these arteries represent the three main vessels of the coronary arterial system. Depending on the severity of the lesion, atherosclerotic plaques within these arteries jeopardize myocardial blood flow and oxygenation, producing ischemic pain (in many cases) and irreversible damage if untreated.

The main coronary arteries are situated in the epicardium, which facilitates their accessibility during coronary bypass procedures. From these arteries arise the septal perforators and other branches that penetrate the entire myo-

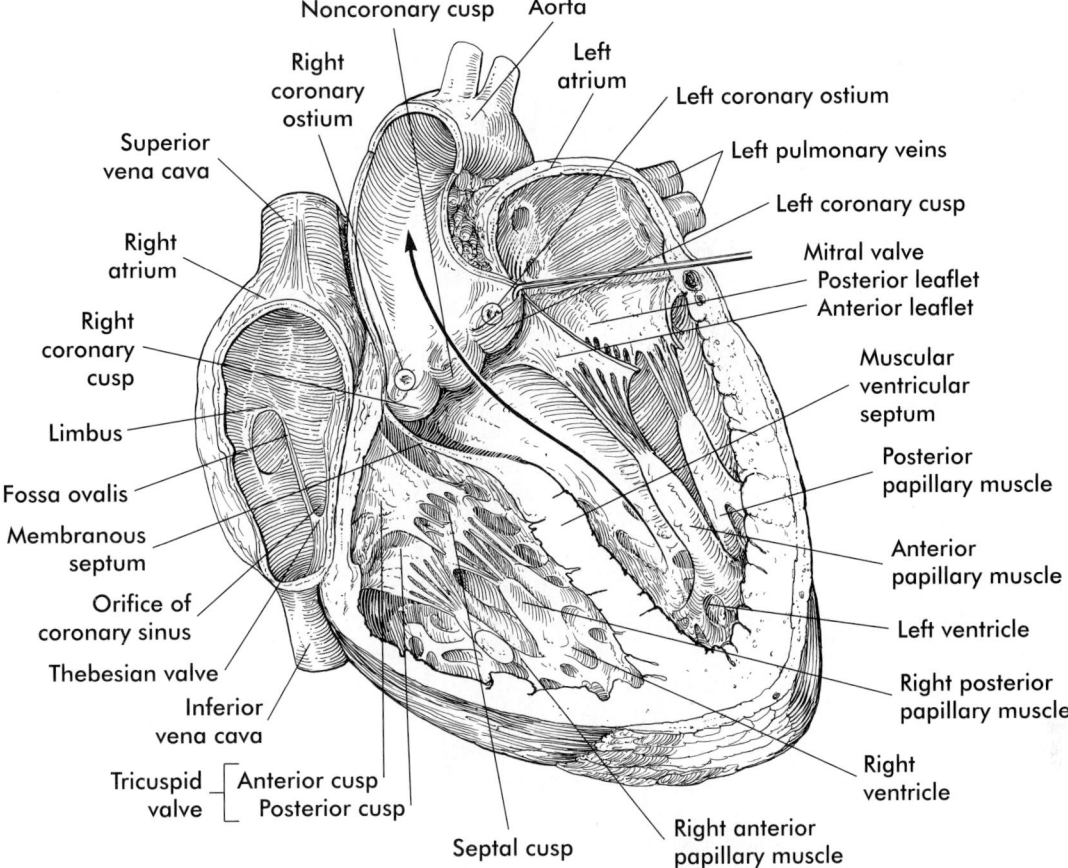

Noncoronary cusp   Aorta
Right
coronary
ostium
Superior
vena cava
Right
atrium
Right
coronary
cusp
Limbus
Fossa ovalis
Membranous
septum
Orifice of
coronary sinus
Thebesian valve
Inferior
vena cava
Tricuspid ⌈ Anterior cusp
valve ⌊ Posterior cusp
Septal cusp

Left
atrium
Left coronary ostium
Left pulmonary veins
Left coronary cusp
Mitral valve
Posterior leaflet
Anterior leaflet
Muscular
ventricular
septum
Posterior
papillary muscle
Anterior
papillary muscle
Left ventricle
Right posterior
papillary muscle
Right
ventricle
Right anterior
papillary muscle

FIG. 26-1   Frontal view of the heart. Systemic venous blood returns to the heart via the inferior and superior venae cavae. It enters the right atrium, flows through the tricuspid valve into the right ventricle, and is ejected through the pulmonic valve (not shown) into the pulmonary circulation. The blood is oxygenated in the lungs and returns to the left atrium through the pulmonary veins. From the left atrium, it flows through the mitral valve into the left ventricle, where it is ejected through the aortic valve into the aorta and the systemic circulation.

Drawing by Peter Stone. From Seifert PC (1994). *Cardiac surgery,* St. Louis, Mosby.

cardium. The cardiac veins empty into the right atrium via the coronary sinus; the thebesian veins, prominent in the walls of the right atrium and the right ventricle, open directly into these chambers.

Nerve impulses to the heart travel from the medulla oblongata (see Chapter 22) along the middle cervical nerve, which is composed of sympathetic fibers, and the vagus nerve, composed of parasympathetic fibers. The sympathetic nerves promote an increase in the force and rate of contraction, and the parasympathetic fibers control the heart rate. Running vertically along the right and left sides of the pericardium are major branches of the phrenic nerve, which innervate the diaphragm and stimulate it to contract. Identifying this nerve is important for protecting the diaphragm in procedures in which the lateral pericardium is incised or excised. Within the myocardium itself, certain areas of tissue are modified to form a *conduction system* (Fig. 26-5).

The process of excitation and contraction originates in the sinoatrial (SA) node, located in the area where the superior vena cava meets the right atrium. The impulse spreads to the atria via the internodal pathways and travels to the atrioventricular (AV) junction (which contains the AV node) located medial to the entrance of the coronary sinus in the right atrium, close to the tricuspid valve. From the AV junction, the impulse spreads to the bundle of His, which extends down the right side of the interventricular septum. The bundle divides into the right and left bundle branches, which terminate in a network of fibers called the Purkinje system. The Purkinje fibers are spread throughout the inner surface of both ventricles and the papillary muscles, which when stimulated produce contraction of the heart muscle. The location of conduction tissue is clinically significant during surgical repair of atrial or ventricular septal defects.

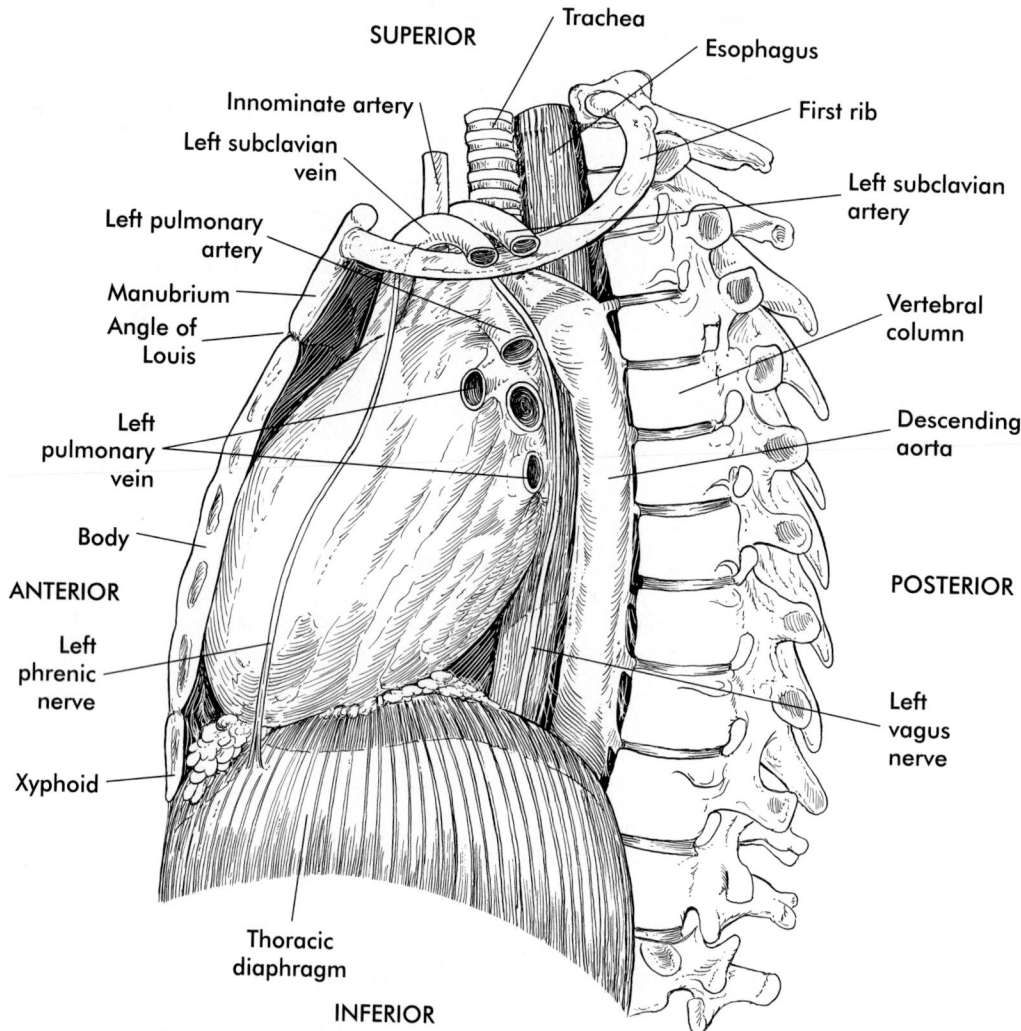

SUPERIOR

Trachea

Esophagus

Innominate artery

First rib

Left subclavian vein

Left subclavian artery

Left pulmonary artery

Manubrium

Vertebral column

Angle of Louis

Left pulmonary vein

Descending aorta

Body

ANTERIOR

POSTERIOR

Left phrenic nerve

Left vagus nerve

Xyphoid

Thoracic diaphragm

INFERIOR

FIG. 26-2 Regions of the mediastinum.

Drawing by Peter Stone. From Seifert PC (1994). *Cardiac surgery,* St. Louis, Mosby.

During myocardial contraction and relaxation, unidirectional blood flow is maintained by the four cardiac valves (Figs. 26-6, 26-7). The atrioventricular valves are located between the atria and the ventricles. The right atrioventricular valve is called the tricuspid valve and contains three leaflets. The left atrioventricular valve, called the mitral valve, consists of two leaflets (Fig. 26-6). Each of these valves is a complex system consisting of a fibrous annulus surrounding the valve orifice, the valve cusps or leaflets, the chordae tendineae, and the papillary muscles, which anchor the valve to the inner ventricular wall (see Fig. 26-1). When the ventricle contracts, these muscles and the chordae tendineae, connected to the valve leaflets, prevent the leaflets from everting into the atrium. All parts of the system must be functioning for the valve to work properly.

The semilunar valves are located at the outlets of the left and right ventricles. These valves are known as the aortic and pulmonic valves, respectively. They are less complex than the atrioventricular valves, and they open and close passively with the cyclic fluctuations in the blood pressure and volume that occur during systole and diastole.

Abnormalities such as stenosis, insufficiency, or a combination of both impair the mechanical function of the valves. Stenosed valves have leaflets that are fibrous and stiff, with uneven and adherent margins. Insufficient or incompetent valves, such as those with leaflet degeneration or perforations, dilated annuli, or ruptured chordae tendineae, produce regurgitation of blood into the originating chamber. These conditions, or a combination of stenosis and insufficiency, strain the myocardium by increasing in-

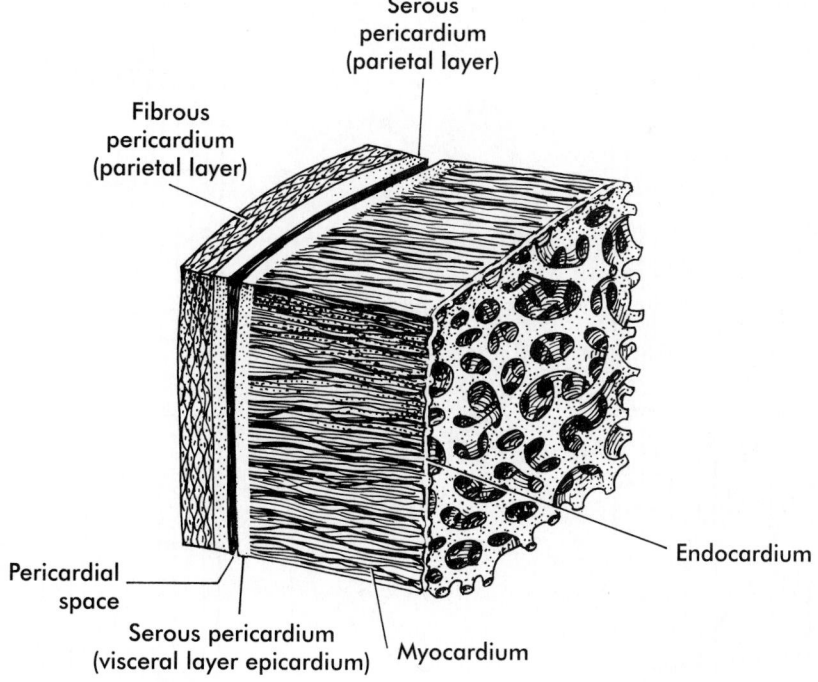

FIG. 26-3 Cross-section of cardiac muscle showing its three layers (endocardium, myocardium, and epicardium) and pericardium.

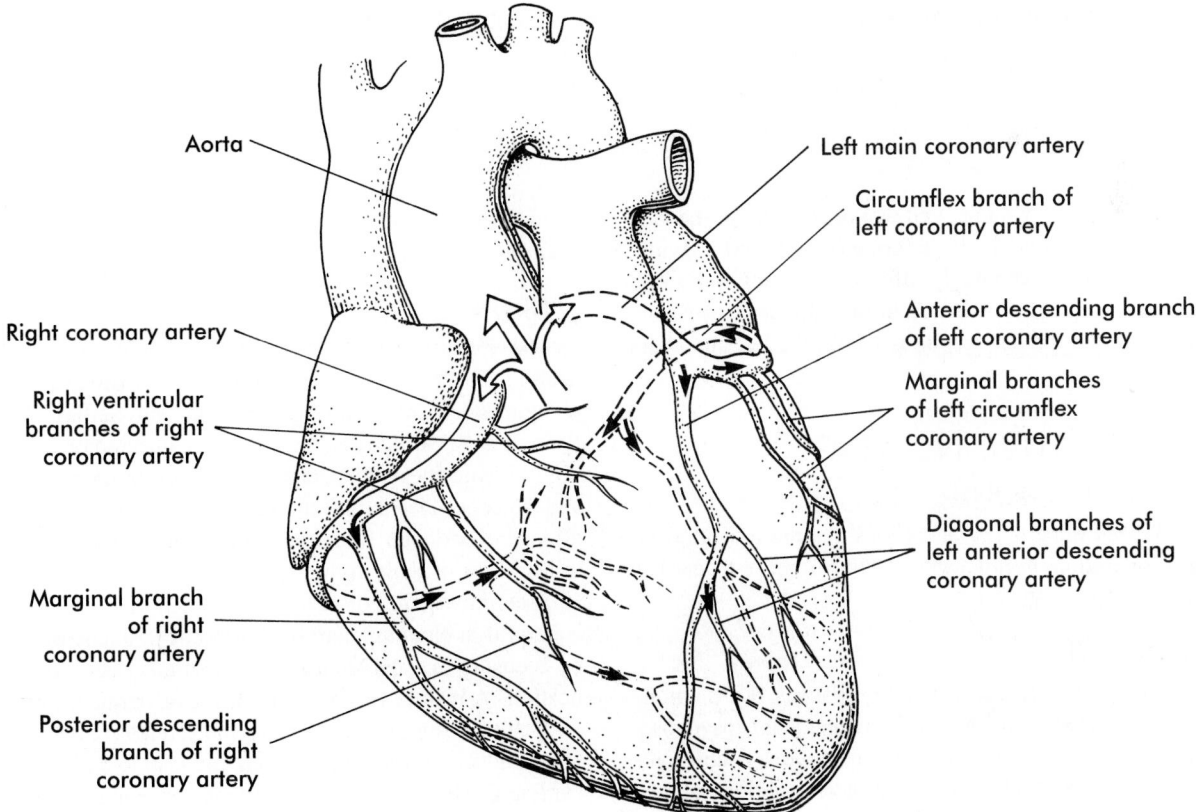

FIG. 26-4 Coronary artery system.

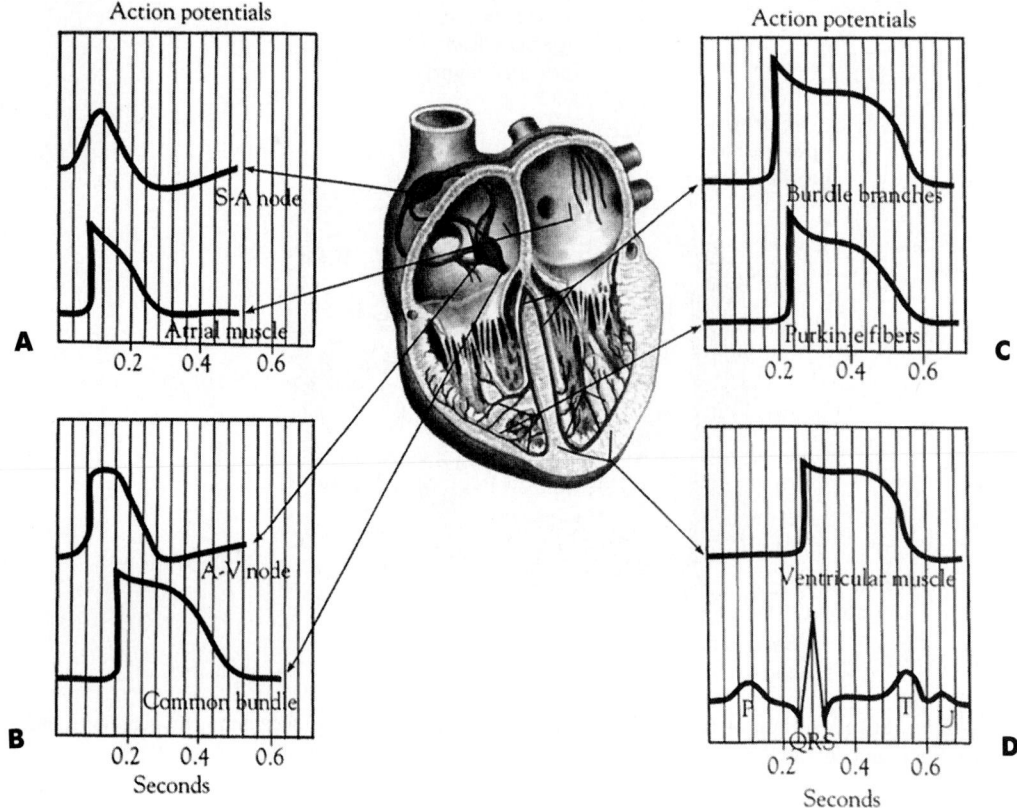

FIG. 26-5   Heart with normal conduction pathways and transmembrane action potential of **A,** Sino-atrial (SA) node. **B,** Atrioventricular (AV) node (AV junction). **C,** Bundle branches. **D,** Ventricular muscle.

From Thompson JM, and others: (1993). *Mosby's clinical nursing,* ed 3, St. Louis, Mosby.

tracardiac pressure, volume, and workload. Any of the four valves may be congenitally deformed. Acquired valvular heart disease most commonly affects the mitral and aortic valves and is thought to be due to the increased stress associated with the higher pressures within the left chambers of the heart.

PERIOPERATIVE NURSING CONSIDERATIONS

Specialized nursing considerations that are indicated for thoracic operations (see Chapter 24) also apply to cardiac surgery.

ASSESSMENT

Because the severity of pathologic changes varies among patients, knowledge of physical derangements, psychosocial concerns, and functional health patterns enables the nurse to plan care and manage the patient perioperatively (Guzzetta and Dossey, 1992). The nursing database should

include the patient's biopsychosocial history, the physical examination, and results from laboratory tests.

History

The history includes information about the patient's health status as well as the response to the disease and the recommended intervention (Guzzetta and Seifert, 1991). Patients with cardiac disease may display symptoms including ischemic chest pain (angina pectoris), fatigue, dyspnea, and syncope. Depending on their severity, these symptoms affect the patient's functional status and ability to engage in activities of daily living (Box 26-1).

A cardiovascular disease risk factor profile (Table 26-1) is helpful in planning care for hospitalization and discharge by focusing on areas that might require further patient education. A history of rheumatic fever or frequent tonsillitis as a child is significant because the sequelae of rheumatic fever and streptococcal infections can lead to damage of the cardiac valves. The presence of diabetes is notable because this disease affects the vascular system and may retard heal-

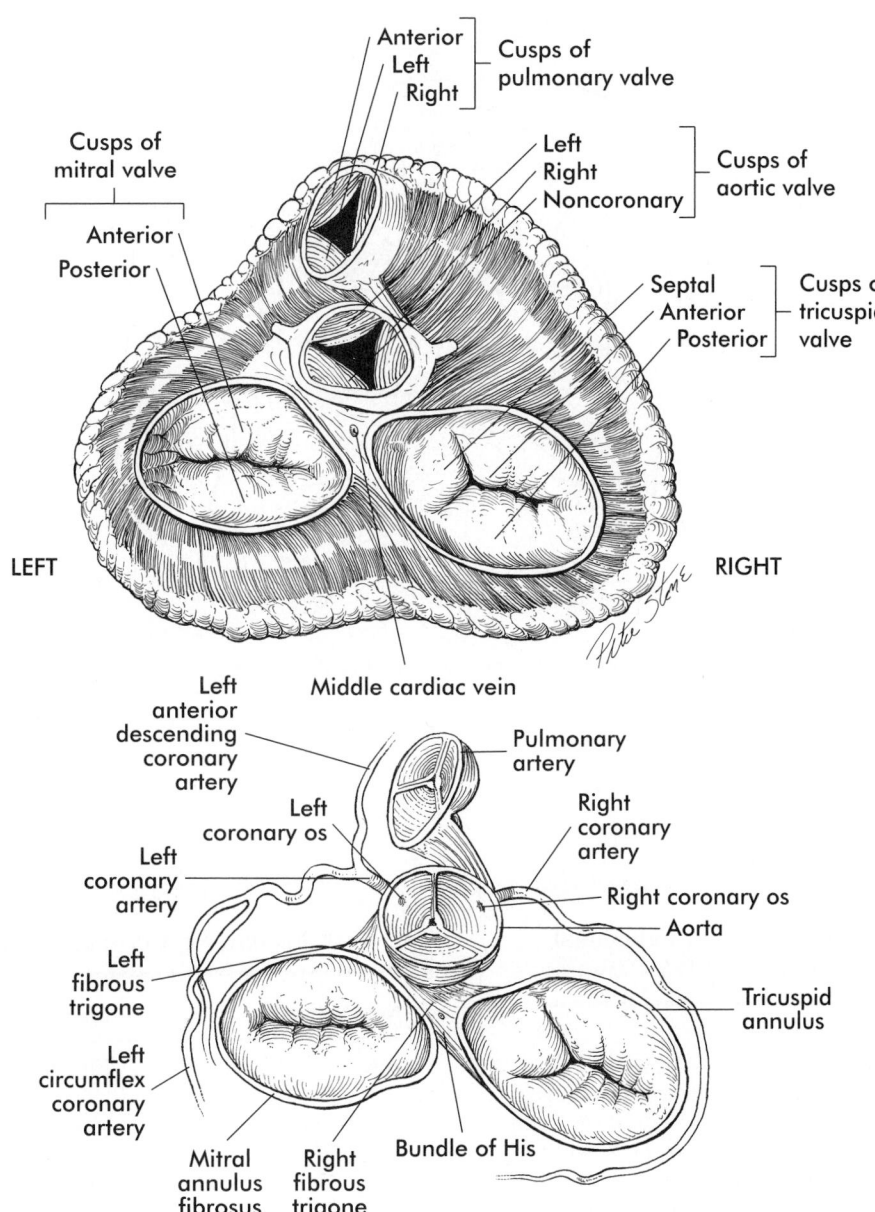

FIG. 26-6　Superior view of cardiac valves. Pulmonary *(top)*, aortic *(middle)*, mitral *(bottom left)*, and tricuspid *(bottom right)*.

Drawing by Peter Stone. From Seifert PC (1994). *Cardiac surgery*, St. Louis, Mosby.

ing and predispose the patient to infection. Hypertension and obesity increase the workload of the heart; obesity may also increase the risk for postoperative infection because adipose tissue is poorly vascularized. Mental stress has been increasingly implicated in the development of myocardial ischemia (Braunwald, 1992).

Risk factors associated with postoperative infection include previous cardiac surgery, duration of surgery and cardiopulmonary bypass, blood transfusion, postoperative blood loss, and length of preoperative hospitalization (Cruse and Foord, 1980).

The patient's knowledge and understanding of the disease process and its effect on his or her functional, physiologic, and psychologic status should also be part of perioperative nursing assessment. The patient's personal strengths, external resources, and coping strategies should be determined. The nurse should note any cultural or religious beliefs that are relevant to perioperative patient care.

Physical examination

The physical assessment provides the perioperative nurse with baseline data and information about potential problems

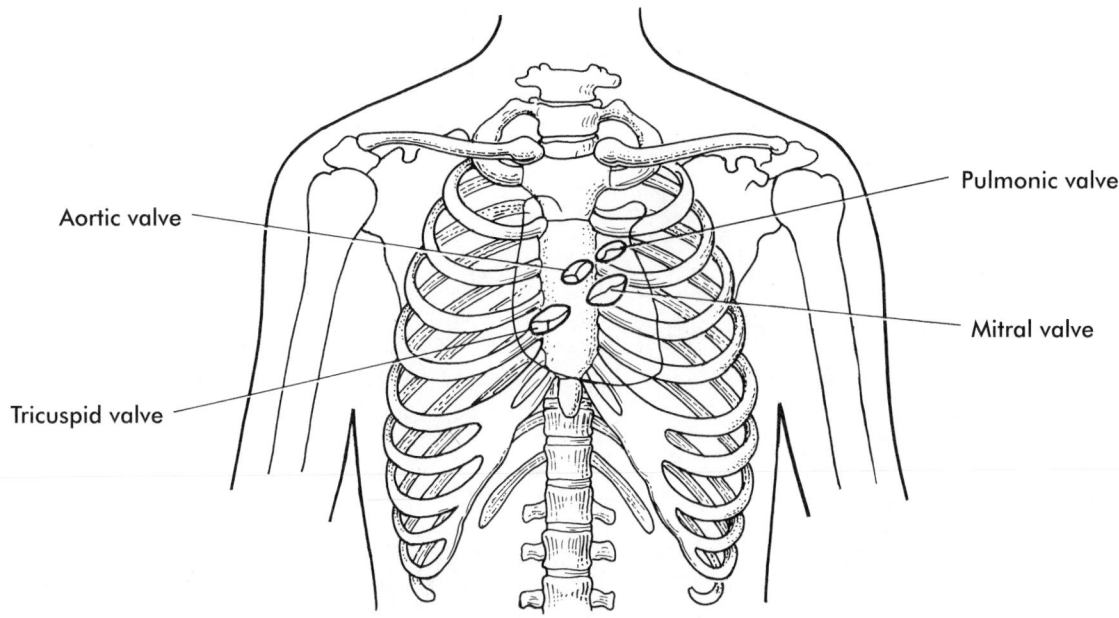

FIG. 26-7   Anatomic position of cardiac valves.

CLASS I

Patients with cardiac disese do not display symptoms of syncope, undue fatigue, dyspnea, or anginal pain with ordinary physical activity.

CLASS II

Patients with cardiac disease are comfortable at rest but display the above symptoms during ordinary physical activity.

CLASS III

Patients with cardiac disease, although comfortable at rest, are markedly limited functionally and display symptoms with less than ordinary exercise.

CLASS IV

Patients with cardiac disease are unable to engage in any physical activity without discomfort and may have symptoms of cardiac insufficiency even at rest.

Adapted from the New York Heart Association (1964). *Diseases of the heart and blood vessels: Nomenclature and criteria for diagnosis* (6th ed.). Boston: Little, Brown.

TABLE 26-1

Risk Factors for Coronary Artery Disease

Nonmodifiable	Modifiable
Age	Elevated serum cholesterol
Sex	Hypertension
Family history	Cigarette smoking
Race	Obesity
	Elevated serum lipids
	Diabetes mellitus
	Psychologic stress
	Personality type

Adapted from Murdaugh, C.L.: (1992). The person with coronary artery disease risk factors. In Guzzetta, C.E. and Dossey B.M. (editors), *Cardiovascular nursing: Holistic practice.* St. Louis: Mosby.

that might require intervention. The appearance of the skin offers clues to the cardiovascular status. Dryness, coolness, diaphoresis, paleness, edema, poor capillary refill, bruising, and petechiae can reflect impaired cardiovascular function. Visual problems and headaches may be related to inadequate cardiac output, atherosclerotic disease, or medications such as digitalis. The presence of chronic or local infection should be identified; if untreated, these may become potential sources of postoperative infection.

Nutritional status is assessed to determine increased risk

for infection, skin breakdown, or other complications.

The patient's level of consciousness, memory, comprehension, and emotional status should be assessed. Confusion, restlessness, slurred speech, numbness, and paralysis can signal impaired perfusion. Their presence preoperatively should be noted by the perioperative nurse.

During respiratory assessment the perioperative nurse should note the use of accessory muscles or nostril flaring and auscultate breath sounds. Adventitious sounds such as crackles and wheezes may point to pulmonary edema. Orthopnea, shortness of breath, or dyspnea may require elevation of the head of the stretcher and assistance during transfer onto the OR bed. If the patient is receiving oxygen, flow rate and method of administration should be noted. Alleviating pain is a prime consideration in the care of the cardiovascular patient because pain is a myocardial stressor. A patient with angina may come to the operating room with nitroglycerin tablets or transdermal patches. Cold also increases the workload of the heart because the shivering that accompanies chilling elevates the metabolic rate; the patient should be kept warm.

Heart sounds, murmurs, and friction rubs provide clues to congenital, ischemic, or valvular heart disease or pericarditis. The patient may complain of palpitations. Apical, radial, and/or femoral pulses also reflect cardiac function; their rate, rhythm, and quality should be determined. The presence of cyanosis or peripheral edema should be noted.

The blood pressure may be high, normal, or low. The hypertensive patient may have left ventricular hypertrophy and the hypotensive patient may display changes in neurologic, gastrointestinal, and renal function. Blood pressures should be checked bilaterally. Unequal pressures in the arms may be a contraindication for the use of the internal mammary artery as a bypass graft on the side of the lower blood pressure, where perfusion may not be optimal. Patients with dissections or aneurysms may have unequal carotid, femoral, brachial, or radial artery blood pressures when the lesion occludes one or more of these vascular branches (Fig. 26-8). Normal changes in the very elderly heart should be differentiated from pathologic conditions (Table 26-2). Because cardiac function affects all of the body's organ systems, assessment of the patient should be comprehensive whenever possible. A thorough assessment also alerts the physician and the nurse to the need for special diagnostic tests and laboratory procedures.

Diagnostic studies

Most patients referred for surgery have had complete clinical evaluations including both invasive and noninvasive studies (Table 26-3). After the history and physical assessment, a resting electrocardiogram (ECG) is ordered. An exercise ECG (stress test) is often performed because ST segment changes indicating myocardial ischemia may be apparent only during or after exercise. In patients with intractable arrhythmias, electrophysiology (EP) studies may be performed to locate the site of irritable atrial or ventricular

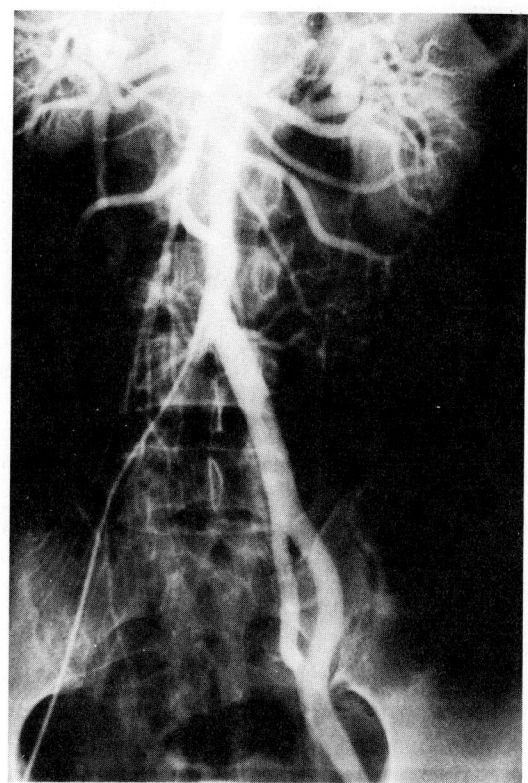

FIG. 26-8 Occluded right iliac and femoral arteries due to compression of the false lumen of dissecting aortic aneurysm against the vessels.

From Seifert PC: Dissecting aortic aneurysms: A problem in Marfan's syndrome, *AORN J.* 43:445, 1986. Reprinted with permission from © The Association of Operating Room Nurses, Inc, 10170 E. Mississippi Avenue, Denver Colo. 80231.

foci that can be surgically ablated or excised or controlled with pharmacologic therapy. EP studies are also performed to determine the need for internal defibrillators or antitachycardia devices.

Chest roentgenography provides information about the size of the cardiac chambers, thoracic aorta, and pulmonary vasculature, as well as the presence of calcium in valves, pericardium, coronary arteries, and aorta (Fig. 26-9). Lateral chest x-ray films of patients with prior sternal operations demonstrate the chest wires and extent of pericardial adhesions (Fig. 26-10). In patients with suspected thoracic aneurysms, arteriography with radiographic dye is performed to determine the size and location of the aneurysm and the site of the intimal tear in dissecting aneurysms (Fig. 26-11). Digital subtraction angiography can provide exceptionally clear images and requires less contrast material.

Echocardiography is a noninvasive test that evaluates both the structure and function of the heart by transmitting sound waves to the heart and measuring those sound waves reflected back to the transducer (Fig. 26-12). They are pro-

---
TABLE 26-2
Physiologic Features of the Very Young and the Very Old (compared with the adult)

Very Young	Very Old	Very Young	Very Old
CARDIOVASCULAR SYSTEM		**RESPIRATORY SYSTEM— cont'd**	
		Higher oxygen consumption	Reduced vital capacity, maximum ventilation volume
Myocardium			
Less contractile tissue	Increased subendocardial fat	Short, narrow airway obstructed easily	
Less compliant	Increased heart weight		
Cardiac output increased by faster heart rate	Reduced resting cardiac output	**RENAL SYSTEM**	
		Glomeruli small and immature	Fewer functional glomeruli
Valves		Tubular concentration of fluids and electrolytes diminished	Reduced renal blood flow and glomerular filtration rate
Less tension created by papillary muscle	Fibrous thickening, calcification of leaflets and annulus	Unable to excrete increased electrolytes and hydrogen ions (acids)	Impaired ability to excrete increased amount of water and electrolytes; reduced ability to secrete hydrogen ions
Coronary arteries			
Rarely, anomalies of coronary arteries	Coronary arteriosclerosis, atherosclerosis; tortuous epicardial arteries	**OTHER**	
		Temperature control	
Conduction system		Immature regulating system; rapid heat loss	Decreased control
Impulse conduction faster	Impulse conduction slower		
		Metabolic rate	
Blood volume		Higher	Lower
Total circulating small amount, volume per kg body weight relatively greater	Reduced plasma volume Reduced blood water content	**Stress response**	
		Decreased phagocytic capability of leukocytes	Limited capability to retain homeostasis
RESPIRATORY SYSTEM		Immature immunoglobulin synthesis	Decreased adrenal activity
Inadequate cough reflex	Decreased ability to eliminate secretions		
Increased chest wall compliance, decreased pulmonary compliance	Increased chest wall rigidity, decreased lung compliance		

Adapted from Fairman, R., Rombeau, J.L. (1988). Physiologic problems in the elderly surgical patient. In T.A. Miller, (editor), *Physiologic basis of modern surgical care*. St. Louis: Mosby; and Hazinski, M.F. (1992). *Nursing care of the critically ill child*, (2nd ed.). St. Louis: Mosby.

cessed by the transducer, which creates visual images of the structure's movements. This test is commonly used to assess ventricular and valvular function before and after surgery and to determine the degree of valvular stenosis or regurgitation. It can also demonstrate a tumor or thrombus in the atrial cavity. Color flow Doppler techniques have greatly enhanced the functional assessment of valvular performance. Transesophageal echocardiography (TEE) is commonly used to evaluate the effectiveness of valve repairs and to diagnose valvular disorders.

Radionuclide imaging is employed to illustrate wall motion and blood flow through the heart and to quantify cardiac function. These noninvasive techniques are generally well tolerated by patients, especially when they may be too unstable to withstand a cardiac catheterization. They may also be used as a complement to catheteriza-

TABLE 26-3

Diagnostic Tests Commonly Performed for Cardiovascular Disorders*

	Coronary artery disease	Valvular heart disease	Conduction disturbance	Thoracic aneurysm	Congenital heart disease (child/adult)
Resting ECG	X	X	X	X	X
Exercise ECG (stress test)	X		X		X
Chest x-ray	X	X	X	X	X
Aortography				X	X
Echocardiogram	X	X	X	X	X
Resting MUGA	X				
Exercise thallium	X				X
Exercise MUGA	X				
CAT scan				X	
PET scan with stress	X				
MRI					X
Electrophysiology			X		
Cardiac catheterization	X	X	X	X	X

Adapted from Sutherland, L.J. (1991). Patient assessment: Diagnostic studies. In Kinney, M.R. et al. (editors), *Comprehensive cardiac care* (7th ed.). St. Louis: Mosby.

*Tests may not be limited to only those disorders designated.

CAT, Computed axial tomography; *ECG*, electrocardiogram; *MRI*, magnetic resonance imaging; *MUGA*, multiple uptake gated acquisition; *PET*, positron emission tomography.

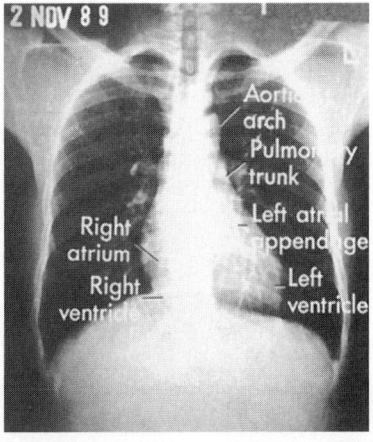

FIG. 26-9   Anteroposterior chest x-ray film (normal).

From Canobbio M. (1990). *Cardiovascular disorders: Mosby's clinical nursing series,* St. Louis, Mosby.

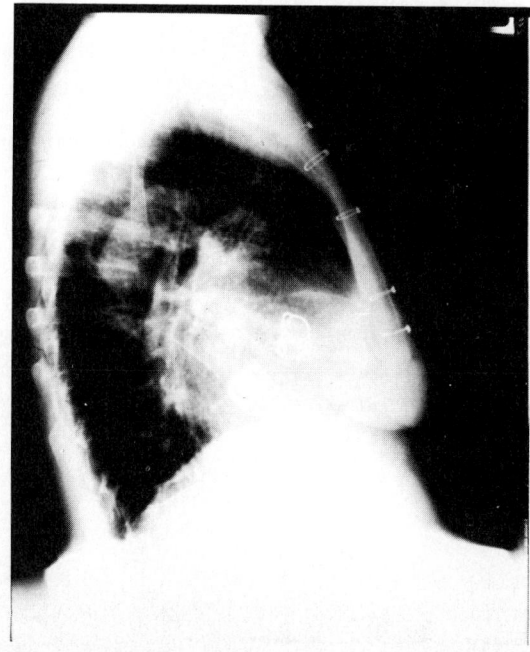

FIG. 26-10   Anterior-posterior chest x-ray film. Note chest wires and pericardial adhesions from previous median sternotomy.

Courtesy Edward A. Lefrak, MD, Annandale, Va.

tion. The most common radionuclide tests are the multiple-gated acquisition (MUGA) scan (also known as blood pool imaging) and exercise thallium perfusion scintigraphy. In the MUGA, multiple images are viewed to evaluate regional and global wall motion of the heart and to determine the ejection fraction (Taubman, 1991). Exercise thallium perfusion scintigraphy provides additional information about the function of the heart in patients with coronary artery disease (CAD) by reflecting deficits in myocardial perfusion at rest and after exercise. The procedure is similar to a MUGA except that there is an exercise portion of the study. Patients unable to exercise may be stressed pharmacologically.

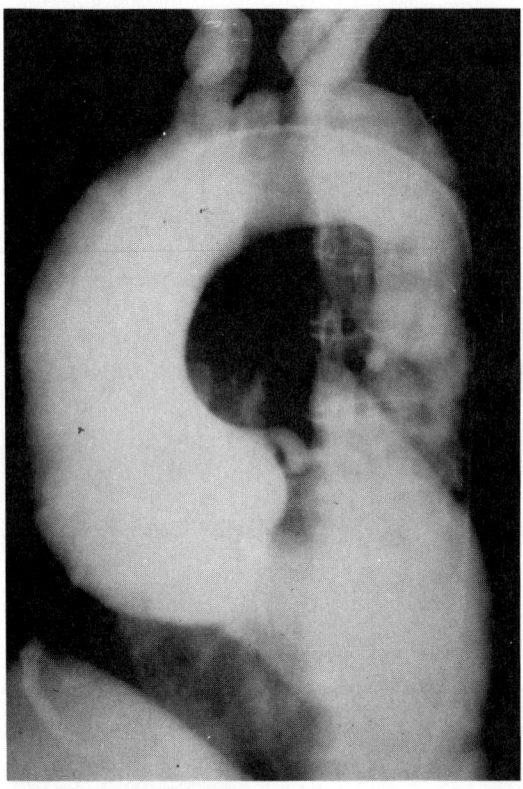

FIG. 26-11 Aortogram of dissecting ascending aortic aneurysm, with aortic insufficiency.

Courtesy Edward A. Lefrak, MD, Annandale, Va.

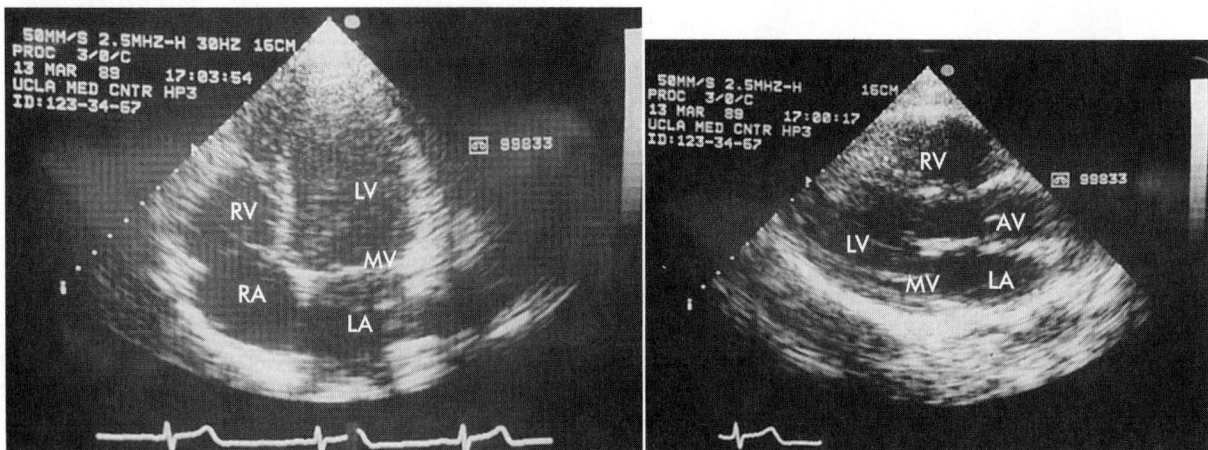

FIG. 26-12 Two-dimensional echocardiography. Note that labels have been added to identify the structures. *RA,* Right atrium; *RV,* right ventricle; *LA,* left atrium; *LV,* left ventricle; *MV,* mitral valve.

From Canobbio MM. (1990) *Cardiovascular disorders: Mosby's clinical nursing series,* St. Louis, Mosby.

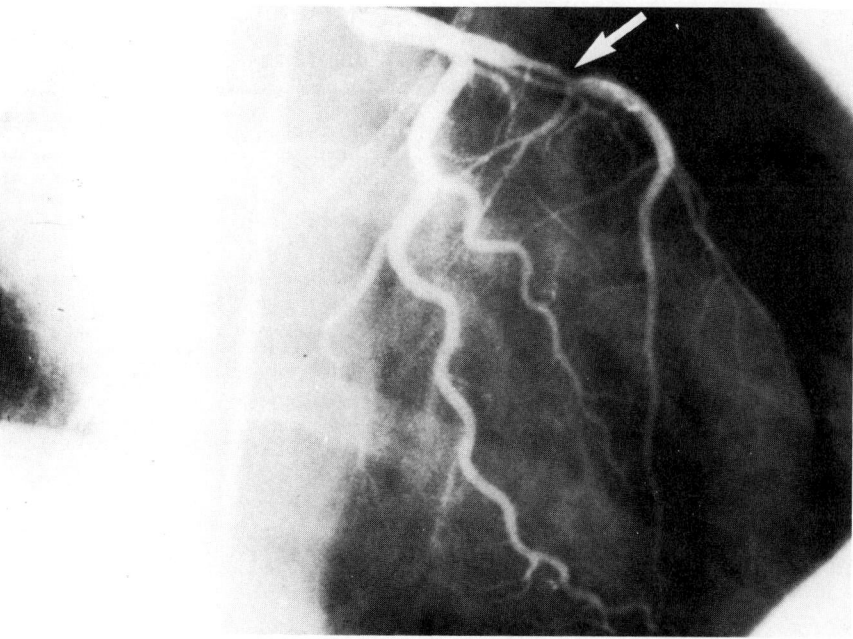

FIG. 26-13   Right anterior oblique (RAO) view of left coronary artery injection demonstrating high-grade stenosis of the left anterior descending coronary artery *(arrow)* at the lead of the first septal perforator.

From Andreoli KG, and others. (1987). *Comprehensive cardiac care,* ed. 6, St. Louis, Mosby.

The integration of computer analysis in imaging techniques has improved quantification of heart disease and refined the diagnostic accuracy of these tests. Computed axial tomography (CAT) scanning provides serial "slices" of the body. This noninvasive technique is useful for assessing the great vessels and other mediastinal structures. Magnetic resonance imaging (MRI) can also be employed to image vascular structures (Kirklin and Barratt-Boyes, 1993).

Cardiac catheterization provides the most definitive information about the extent and location of ischemic, valvular, and congenital heart disease. A radiopaque plastic catheter is inserted retrogradely through the aortic valve into the left side of the heart by a percutaneous puncture or a cutdown to the vessels of the brachial artery (Sones technique) or the femoral artery (Judkins technique). The right side of the heart is approached via a venous route. To perform coronary angiography that demonstrates coronary anatomy, contrast media is injected into the coronary ostia. Obstructions (Fig. 26-13), flow, and distal perfusion can be assessed. Ventriculography illustrates contractile weaknesses of the ventricles as well as shunting and regurgitation of blood. These studies are used to assess the degree of myocardial dysfunction and to plan interventions such as coronary artery bypass grafting, valve repair or replacement, and cardiac transplantation. The cardiologist can compute the orifice of a stenosed valve, or determine the degree of regurgitation of an incompetent valve.

Ventricular, atrial, and pulmonary pressures are recorded and cardiac output and ejection fraction estimated (Box 26-2 and Table 26-4). Oxygen saturation of cardiac chambers and the ratio of pulmonary to systemic blood flow (Q_p/Q_s) are calculated in patients with shunts and congenital or acquired defects. Cinearteriograms record the movement of the heart, and cut films from these cines may be displayed in the operating room during surgery.

The cardiac catheterization laboratory has also become the site for more aggressive interventional therapies related to evolving and acute myocardial infarctions. Coronary thrombolysis with streptokinase and tissue plasminogen activator can dissolve fresh blood clots and reopen, or recanalize, the artery. Percutaneous transluminal coronary angioplasty (PTCA) with or without insertion of intracoronary stents may be performed to dilate the artery. Laser angioplasty and atherectomy to excise intraluminal plaque are becoming more popular. In many instances these interventions may obviate the need for surgical bypass grafting, although restenosis is not uncommon, and eventually the patient may require an operation. Generally, operating room standby is recommended both for PTCA and atherectomy.

EP studies are often performed in the cardiac catheterization laboratory (if a dedicated suite is unavailable). In addition to diagnosing conduction disturbances, EP laboratories may provide therapeutic interventions (such as radiofrequency ablation of accessory pathways seen in Wolff-Parkinson-White syndrome).

TABLE 26-4

Cardiac Catheterization Data

Hemodynamic data		Normal values		
FLOW				
Cardiac output (CO)		4.0-8.0 L/min		
Cardiac index (CI)		2.5-4.0 L/min/m^2		
Ejection fraction (EF)		60%-70%		
Left ventricular end-diastolic volume (LVEDV)		90-180 ml		
Stroke volume (SV)		60-130 ml/beat		
Stroke volume index (SVI)		35-70 ml/beat/m^2		
	SYSTOLIC	**DIASTOLIC**	**MEAN**	
RESISTANCES				
Systemic vascular resistance (SVR)	<20 Wood units			
Total pulmonary resistance	<3.5 Wood units			
Pulmonary vascular resistance (PVR)	<2.0 Wood units			
SHUNTS (Q_P/Q_S)				
Pulmonary flow/systemic flow		1:1		
OXYGEN SATURATIONS				
Venae cavae		70%		
Right atrium		70%		
Right ventricle		70%		
Pulmonary artery		70%		
Pulmonary veins		97%		
Left atrium		97%		
Left ventricle		97%		
Aorta		97%		
VALVE ORIFICES (ADULT)				
Aortic	2-4 cm^2			
Mitral	4-6 cm$_2$			
Tricuspid	10 cm$_2$			

Laboratory tests

Preoperative laboratory tests are used to assess physiologic function (Table 26-5). Hematologic tests include a detailed coagulation profile to uncover hemorrhagic disorders. In patients who have been taking aspirin or dipyridamole, platelet activity has been decreased; this alerts the perioperative nurse to anticipate prolonged bleeding necessitating infusion of this blood product. The patient's blood type is also determined, and the appropriate order placed with the blood bank. Precautions are taken to test the blood for viral contamination and for cold antibodies that could produce agglutination of the patient's blood during surgery when the patient is cooled to hypothermic temperatures.

Liver and kidney function test results may be abnormal in patients with chronic heart failure, possibly owing to congestion related to right heart failure in the former and re-duced blood flow in the latter. Progressive improvement in hepatic and renal function is anticipated with successful operative intervention.

Additional perioperative laboratory examinations may include arterial blood gases and enzyme markers of myocardial damage (such as the creatine-kinase MB isoenzyme, known as MB bands), especially in the presence of persistent angina. Pulmonary function tests are performed to determine baseline data and to plan postoperative care when respiratory function may be impaired owing to the use of extracorporeal circulation and stasis of lung secretions that accompany prolonged surgery.

NURSING DIAGNOSIS

After a comprehensive review of individual patient data, the perioperative nurse identifies relevant nursing diag-

TABLE 26-4

Cardiac Catheterization Data—cont'd

Hemodynamic data	Normal values		
PRESSURES (mm HG)			
Venae cavae			0-5
Right atrium (RA)			2-6
Right ventricle (RV)	20-30	0-5	
Pulmonary artery (PA)	20-30	10-20	
Pulmonary artery wedge pressure (PAWP)			10-15
Left atrium (LA)			4-12
Left ventricle (LV)	120	0-5	4-12
Left ventricular end-diastolic pressure (LVEDP)			5-12
Aorta	120-140	60-80	70-90
Brachial artery	120	70	
Femoral artery	125	75	

ANGIOGRAPHIC DATA	FINDINGS
Coronary arteries	Anatomy/function coronary vascular bed; distal coronary flow; AV fistula; atheroslcerosis; anomalous origin of coronary arteries
Ventriculography	Anatomy/function of ventricles and associated structures; LV aneurysm; congenital abnormalities; valvular stenosis/regurgitation; shunts
Valvular angiography	Intact mitral/tricuspid complex; valvular incompetence/stenosis/regurgitation
Pulmonary angiography	Pulmonary embolism; congenital abnormalities
Aortography	Patency of aortic branches; normal mobility, competence, and anatomy of aortic valve; aneurysms: saccular, fusiform; origin of aortic dissection; shunts or anomalous connections; congenital defect or obstructions

Adapted from Sabiston, D.C., & Spencer, F.C. (1983). *Gibbon's surgery of the chest* (2 V.) (4th ed.). Philadelphia: W.B. Saunders.

noses, from which the perioperative plan for patient care is derived (see Sample Care Plan on pp. 26-15 and 26-16).

For the patient undergoing cardiac surgery, the nursing diagnoses might be as follows:

- Decreased cardiac output related to mechanical factors (altered preload, afterload, contractility, heart rate)
- High risk for infection (wound) related to surgical disruption of tissues
- High risk for injury related to surgical position
- Knowledge deficit related to perioperative events
- High risk for impaired tissue integrity related to cardiopulmonary bypass and hypothermia

OUTCOME IDENTIFICATION

Outcomes for the selected nursing diagnoses might be stated as:

- Patient will demonstrate an adequate cardiac output.
- Patient will be free from wound infection.
- Patient will be free from injury from surgical position.
- Patient will describe perioperative events.
- Patient's tissue integrity will be maintained.

Each additional nursing diagnosis should have a corresponding outcome statement. The outcome should be measurable, with criteria by which to evaluate its achievement. For example, for the outcome "The patient will demonstrate adequate cardiac output," the perioperative nurse might identify criteria such as vital signs and hemodynamic status consistent with or better than preoperative parameters; fluid and electrolyte balance consistent with preoperative levels; absence of rate, rhythm, or conduction defects; absence of iatrogenic injury to the heart; and normal clotting

TABLE 26-5

Laboratory Data

Test	Normal values	Test	Normal values
Arterial blood gases (ABGs)		Creatinine (urine, 24 hour)	
pH	7.38-7.44	Male	20-26 mg/kg/24 hr
Po$_2$	95-100 mm Hg	Female	14-22 mg/kg/24 hr
Pco$_2$	35-40 mm Hg	Electrolytes	
Blood chemistry		Potassium (K)	3.8-5.0 mEq/L
Glucose (fasting)	70-110 mg/100 ml	Sodium (Na)	136-142 mEq/L
Protein (total)	6.8-8.5 g/100 ml	Chloride (Cl)	95-103 mEq/L
Blood urea nitrogen (BUN)	8.0-25 mg/100 ml	Magnesium (Mg)	1.5-2.0 mEq/L
Uric acid	3.0-7.0 mg/100 ml	Lipids	
Cardiac enzymes		Cholesterol	<200 mg/dl
Creatine phosphokinase (CPK)	<70 IU/L	Triglycerides	10-190 mg/dl
		Phospholipids	150-380 mg/dl
CPK-MB (isoenzyme)	0-7 IU/L	Free fatty acids	9.0-15.0 mM/L
Coagulation profile		Liver function	
Platelet count	150,000-400,000/μL	Albumin (serum)	3.5-5.0 g/dl
Prothrombin time (PT)	Depends on thromboplastin reagent used; typically 9.5-12.0 sec	Alkaline phosphatase	20-90 IU/L
		Globulin (serum)	2.3-3.5 g/dl
		Serum bilirubin (total)	0.2-1.4 mg/dl
Thrombin time	Depends on concentration of thrombin reagent used; typically 20-29 sec		
Partial thromboplastin time (PTT)	Depends on phospholipid reagent used; typically 60-85 sec	Pulmonary function (Normal values vary depending on the patient's age, sex, weight, and race. The following are generally calculated.)	
		Residual volume (RV)	
Activated PTT	Depends on activator and phospholipid reagents used; typically 20-35 sec	Tidal volume (TV)	
		Expiratory reserve volume (ERV)	
		Inspiratory reserve volume (IRV)	
Complete blood count (CBC)		Total lung capacity (TLC)	
Hemoglobin (Hgb)		Vital capacity (VC)	
Male	13.5-18.0 g/dl		
Female	12.0-16.0 g/dl	Urinalysis	
Hematocrit (Hct)		Color	Amber, yellow
Male	42%-52%	Clarity	Clear
Female	35%-47%	pH	4.6-8.0
Red blood cells (RBC)		Specific gravity (SG)	1.002-1.035
Male	4.6-6.2 × 10^6/μL	Protein	0.0-8.0 mg/dl
Female	4.2-5.4 × 10^6/μL	Sugar, ketones, RBC, WBC, casts	Negative
White blood cells (WBC)	4.5-11.0 × 10^3/μL		

Adapted from Henry, J.B. (1984). *Todd-Sanford-Davison clinical diagnosis and management by laboratory methods* (17th ed.). Philadelphia: W.B. Saunders.

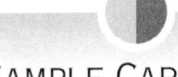

SAMPLE CARE PLAN

NURSING DIAGNOSIS: Decreased cardiac output related to mechanical factors (altered preload, afterload, contractility, heart rate)
EXPECTED OUTCOME: Patient will demonstrate an adequate cardiac output.
INTERVENTIONS:
Check clotting function, coagulation profile, and electrolyte values.
Monitor blood pressures (arterial, CVP, PAWP) and ECG.
Measure and report blood loss (such as suction and sponges).
Maintain adequate supply and assist with administration of replacement blood and/or blood products.
Follow institutional protocol for allergic blood reaction.
Have topical hemostatic agents available.
Have inotropic and antidysrhythmic medications available; assist with administration.
Use autotransfusion system per protocol.
Monitor, report, and record urine output and chest tube drainage; keep tubes and catheters patent.
Have available defibrillator (with appropriate internal and external paddles), fibrillator, external pacemaker, temporary epicardial pacemakers leads, and appropriate ECG cables for cardioversion and intraaortic balloon pump.

NURSING DIAGNOSIS: High risk for wound infection related to surgical disruption of tissues
EXPECTED OUTCOME: Patient will be free from wound infection.
INTERVENTIONS:
Verify that prescribed preoperative prophylactic antibiotic has been administered.
Dress all invasive arterial and venous lines.
Use depilatories or electric clippers to remove hair at the surgical site; avoid razors if possible.
Routinely, prepare anatomic area to knees (or lower if leg vein needed) with antimicrobial antiseptic agent.
Monitor aseptic technique; correct breaks.
Have available prescribed topical antibiotics.
If the OR bed is raised, lowered, or turned from side to side, take measures to maintain sterility of field.
Confine and contain instruments used in groin or leg; change gloves when moving from lower extremities to chest.

Protect sterility of closed urinary drainage system.
Maintain sterility of instrument setup until patient discharged from operating room.
Maintain documentation of all implants.

NURSING DIAGNOSIS: High risk for injury related to surgical position
EXPECTED OUTCOME: Patient will be free from injury due to surgical position.
INTERVENTIONS:
Obtain and prepare appropriate positioning accessories.
Maintain proper body alignment.
Pad and protect vulnerable neurovascular bundles and dependent pressure areas.
Prevent pooling of skin preparation agents at bedlines.
Pad thermia blanket.
Keep all surfaces dry and wrinkle free.
Ensure patency/security of peripheral and central lines, catheters, and electrosurgical dispersive pad on positional changes.
Have adequate personnel to assist with positional changes; lift (do not pull) patient during all positioning maneuvers.
Safely secure patient to OR bed; ensure patient stability.

NURSING DIAGNOSIS: Knowledge deficit related to perioperative events
EXPECTED OUTCOME: Patient will describe perioperative events.
INTERVENTIONS:
Explain/describe the following events:
NPO status
Administration and effects of preoperative medication
Transport to operating room
Holding area
Insertion of peripheral, arterial, and venous lines
Operating room environment (temperature, staff, attire, equipment)
Induction of anesthesia
Skin preparation
Anticipated length of surgery
Surgical intensive care unit and patient status (for example, unable to talk while intubated and plans for alternate methods of communication)

Continued.

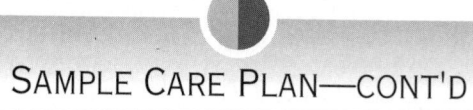

SAMPLE CARE PLAN—CONT'D

INTERVENTIONS—CONT'D

Determine patient's desire for additional knowledge (respect denial).

Answer questions; clarify misperceptions.

Know where family or signficant other will be waiting during surgery; provide communication per institutional protocol.

NURSING DIAGNOSIS: High risk for impaired tissue integrity related to cardiopulmonary bypass or hypothermia

EXPECTED OUTCOME: Patient's tissue integrity will be maintained.

INTERVENTIONS:

Place thermia blanket on OR bed.

Preoperatively, provide warm blankets as required.

Expose only those body areas required for surgical intervention.

Monitor patient's temperature (esophageal, rectal, bladder, and/or ventricular septal).

Adjust room temperature as needed.

Inspect cardiopulmonary bypass lines for patency and presence of particulate matter; alert surgeon as indicated.

Avoid excessive ice particles on heart.

Use solutions of appropriate temperature when irrigating the heart (cold during arrest; warm before and after arrest).

---

parameters. Each of these criteria becomes evidence that the outcome was achieved. When outcomes are evaluated, they should be documented in the perioperative record. Some outcomes will have been achieved at the conclusion of the surgical procedure; others require ongoing evaluation in the postoperative period to be adequately measured. The evaluation section on p. 1093 indicates the requirement for ongoing goal measurement by the use of "will" rather than stating the outcome as having been achieved.

PLANNING

Once the diagnoses and outcomes have been established, a plan of care is devised that will enable the perioperative nurse to achieve the goals that have been set. Patient and family needs, elicited from interviews when possible, should be integrated into the planning. A sample care plan for the patient having cardiac surgery is included; the perioperative nurse will need to identify criteria specific to the patient for each of the stated outcomes.

IMPLEMENTATION

Some considerations, other that those previously mentioned, can be useful in implementing the perioperative plan of care for patients undergoing cardiac surgery.

Special facilities

The operating room must be large enough to accommodate bulky, highly specialized equipment while maintaining aseptic technique. Multiple electrical outlets, auxiliary lighting, and additional suction outlets should be available.

Instrumentation and equipment

The basic setup described for thoracic procedures (see Chapter 24) is used, along with some specialized cardiovascular instruments and equipment.

Vascular clamps, which are designed to occlude blood flow partially or completely, must be maintained in good condition if they are to prevent fracture of the delicate intima of the blood vessels and still retain their specific holding qualities. There are many variations in construction of vascular instruments (see Chapter 25). The jaws may consist of single or double rows of fine, sharp, or blunt teeth or special cross-hatching or longitudinal serrations. The working angles of the clamps also vary. All clamps are designed to hold the vessels securely and without trauma (Fig. 26-14).

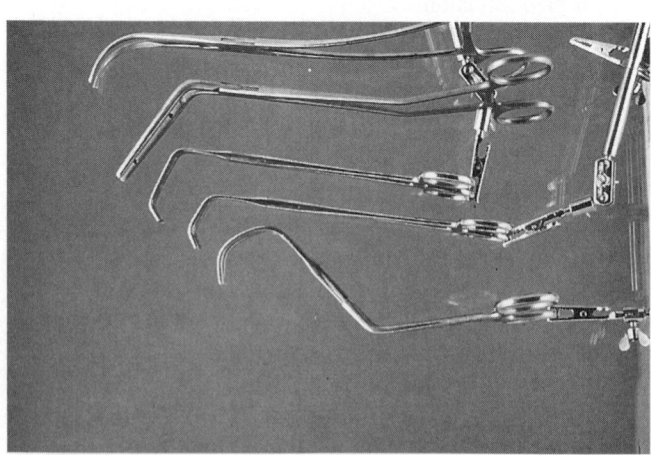

FIG. 26-14   Cardiovascular clamps *(top to bottom):* Semb suture passer, Fogarty cross-clamp (angled, Beck partial occlusion clamp (medium and small), Lambert-Kay partial occlusion clamp.

From Brooks-Tighe S. (1994). *Instrumentation for the operating room,* ed. 4, St. Louis, Mosby.

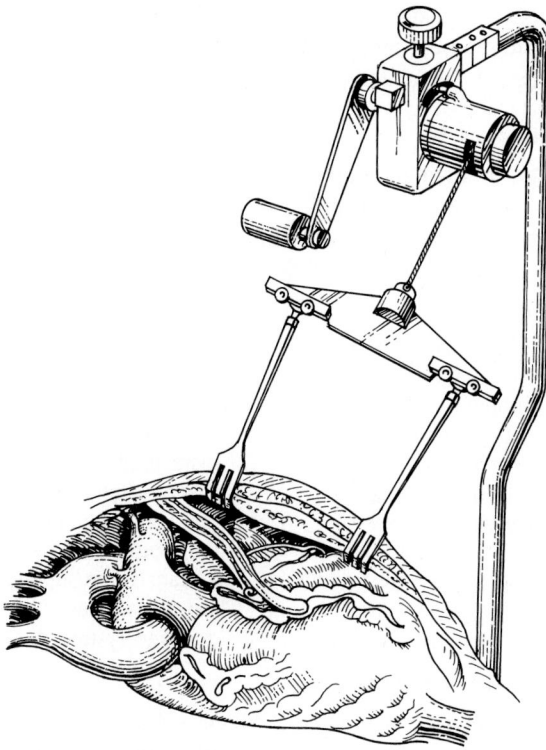

FIG. 26-15 Retractor used to elevate sternal border for exposure of the internal mammary artery.

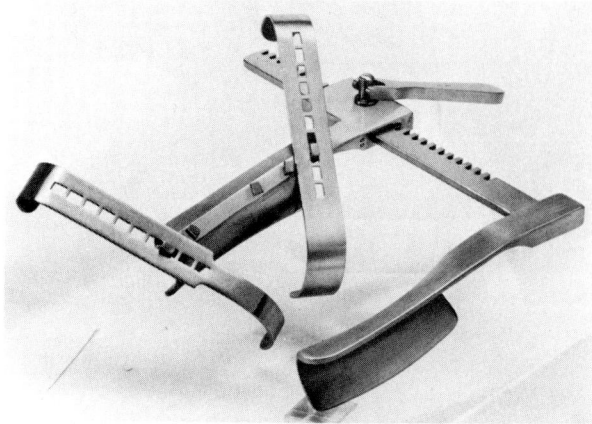

FIG. 26-16 Sternal self-retaining retractor with attachments for left atrial retraction during mitral valve replacement.
Courtesy Pilling Company, Fort Washington, Pa.

A variety of sternal retractors are available to meet specific needs. With the increased use of the internal mammary artery (IMA), exposure of the retrosternal artery bed has been made easier with retractors that elevate the sternal border (Fig. 26-15). Some sternal retractors have attachments that provide improved exposure of the left atrium during mitral valve replacement (Fig. 26-16). Exposure of the left or right atrium, or the aortic root, may also be accomplished with hand-held retractors (Fig. 26-17).

Other equipment commonly used (or available) for cardiac surgery includes the following:

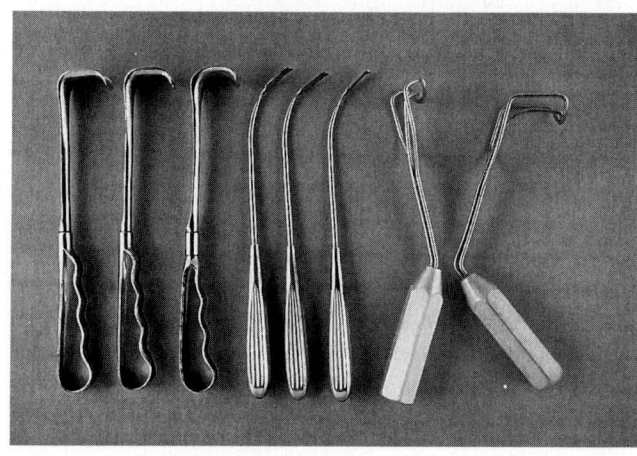

FIG. 26-17 Valve retractors: three aortic valve leaflet retractors *(left),* tricuspid valve retractor, mitral valve retractor *(far right).*
From Brooks-Tighe S. (1994). *Instrumentation for the operating room,* ed. 4, St. Louis, Mosby.

Sternal saw and motor
Autotransfusion system
Electrical fibrillator
DC defibrillator and internal paddles (Fig. 26-18)
External and internal pulse pacemaker generator (single and dual chamber)
Fiberoptic headlight and light source

Epicardial pacemaker leads (temporary and permanent)
Thermia unit
Pump oxygenator
Intraaortic balloon pump
Mechanical assist pumps
Intraoperative mapping, testing equipment for dysrhythmia surgery

Suture materials

A variety of nonabsorbable cardiovascular sutures with atraumatic needles are available from most suture manufac-

turers. Synthetic sutures of Teflon, Dacron, polyester, or polypropylene are usually selected for insertion of prostheses and for vascular anastomoses. Most sutures are double armed with a needle on each end. Because of the number of stitches required for prosthetic valve placement, alternately colored suture may be helpful to avoid confusion. Vessel loops and umbilical tapes are commonly used to identify and to retract blood vessels and other structures. Wire is used to approximate the sternum (Fig. 26-19), with plastic or nylon bands occasionally added to reinforce frag-

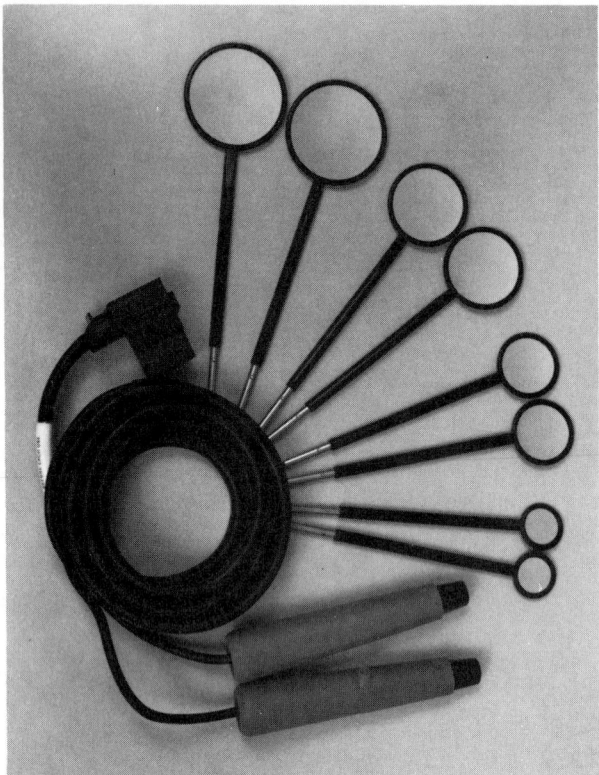

FIG. 26-18   Internal defibrillator paddle tips in assorted sizes, handles, and cord.

Courtesy Hewlett-Packard Company, McMinnville, Oreg.

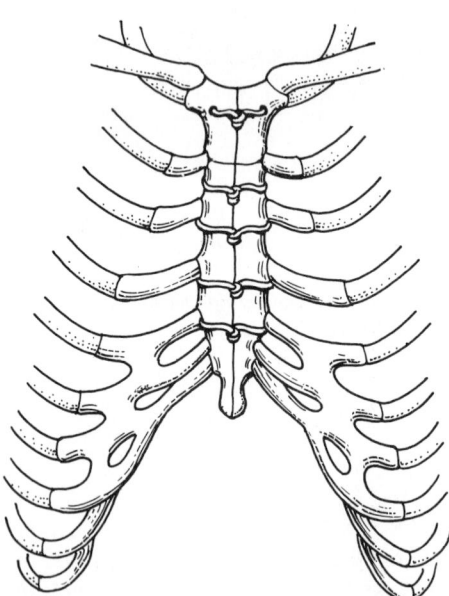

FIG. 26-19   Technique for wire closure of the sternum. In selected patients in whom disruption may be anticipated, for example, obese, elderly individuals with chronic obstructive pulmonary disease, two or more heavy bands of nylon may be passed around the sternum and secured by a twisted stainless steel wire, in addition to the wire sutures.

ile bone. Skin staplers may be used to close skin incisions; a staple remover must accompany the patient to the recovery area if staples have been used to close the chest.

Supplies

The following supplies are generally used in most cardiac procedures. Depending on surgeon preference, other items may be added or substituted.

Rubber-shods	Extra syringes and needles for injections, infusions, and blood samples
Pill sponges	
Various size Silastic or polyvinyl chloride tubing	
Adapters, connectors, stopcocks	Marking pen to identify anastomotic sites and mark grafts
Tourniquet catheters	Irrigation cannulae
Disposable drapes	Disposable vascular (bulldog) clamps
Foot-control and hand-control electrosurgical pencils	Autotransfusion supplies
	Chest tubes, chest drainage system

Prosthetic material

In addition to these general supplies, special supplies are needed for repair or replacement of cardiovascular structures. Intracardiac patches, heart valves, and synthetic grafts should be handled with care to prevent damage or the introduction of foreign materials. Teflon, a fluorocarbon fiber, and Dacron, a polyester fiber, are available in a variety of meshes, fabrics, felts, tapes, and sutures and are also combined with other materials in prosthetic heart valves (Fig. 26-20).

Teflon patches are made in a variety of forms for intra-

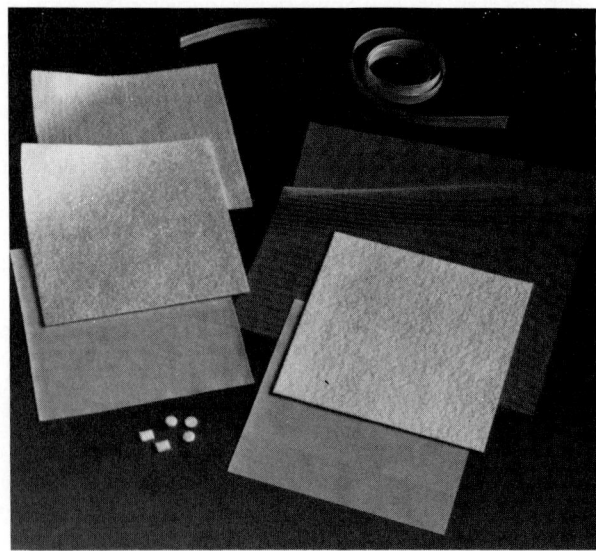

FIG. 26-20   Assorted prosthetic materials to repair intracardiac and extracardiac defects: tapes, Teflon and Dacron patches, and pledgets.

Courtesy Meadox Medicals, Inc., Oakland, N.J.

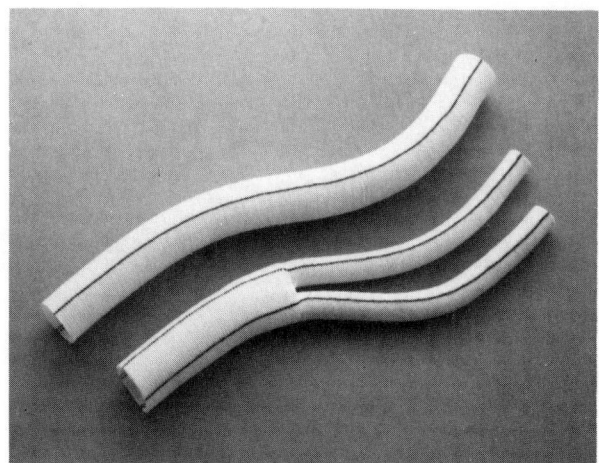

FIG. 26-21   Straight and bifurcated arterial tube grafts.
Courtesy Meadox Medicals, Inc., Oakland, N.J.

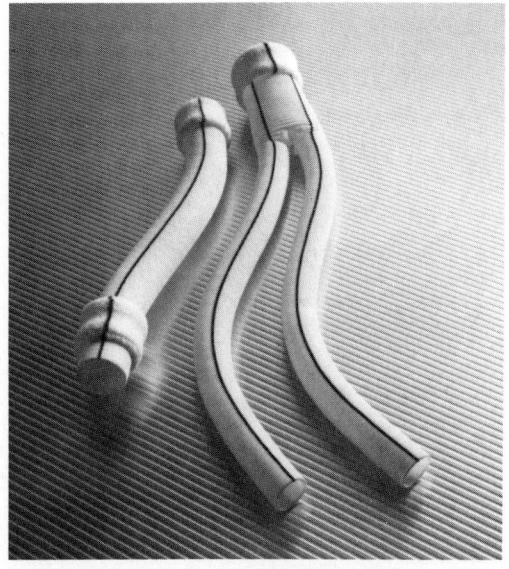

FIG. 26-22   Ringed intraaortic prosthesis, straight and bifurcated, for emergency repair of dissecting aneurysms.
Courtesy Meadox Medicals, Inc, Oakland, N.J.

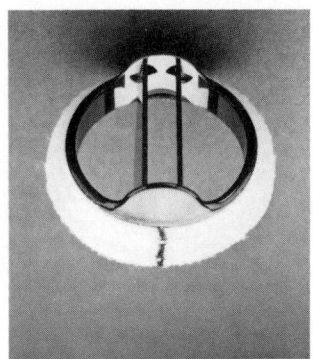

FIG. 26-23   St. Jude Medical bileaflet tilting disc valve prosthesis.
Courtesy St. Jude Medical, Inc., St. Paul, Minn.

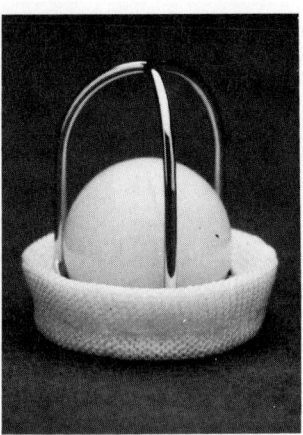

FIG. 26-24   Starr-Edwards ball-cage aortic valve prosthesis.
Courtesy Baxter Healthcare Corp., Edwards CVS Division, Santa Ana, Calif.

cardiac and outflow tract use. Varying degrees of firmness, thickness, and porosity are available for specific uses. Low reactivity, strength retention, and tissue acceptance are important properties to be considered in selecting such patches.

Dacron arterial grafts are usually used in cardiac surgery, although reinforced expanded polytetrafluorethylene (PTFE) is being used with increasing frequency. There are two types of Dacron grafts: knitted and woven. Woven prosthetic grafts are usually employed when the patient has been given heparin because the interstices are tighter and bleeding is usually reduced. Knitted grafts do not fray as readily as woven grafts when cut and they are easier to handle. The grafts are available in sizes suitable for straight arterial grafts, as well as for aortic bifurcated grafts (Fig. 26-21). Newer knitted and woven grafts impregnated with collagen to reduce interstitial bleeding are useful in the thoracic aorta and do not have to be preclotted, even when the patient is fully heparinized for cardiopulmonary bypass.

Tube grafts reinforced at one or both ends with metal rings have been used in surgery for thoracic and abdominal aneurysms; the intraaortic device is anchored in place with nylon tapes tied around the rings. Some surgeons may elect to insert a few interrupted stitches to further secure the prosthesis. If one end of the graft has no ring or the ring has been cut, routine anastomotic techniques are used (Fig. 26-22). Graft sizers are available for these grafts.

Valve prostheses

Valve prostheses are selected according to their hemodynamics, thromboresistance, ease of insertion, anatomic suitability, and patient acceptability (McClung et al., 1983). Most mechanical prostheses employ a ball and cage or tilting disk design. These valves allow complete closure with slight regurgitation to prevent stasis of blood (Figs. 26-23 to 26-25). In addition, porcine heterograft prostheses (Figs. 26-26 to 26-28) are used. The valve consists of

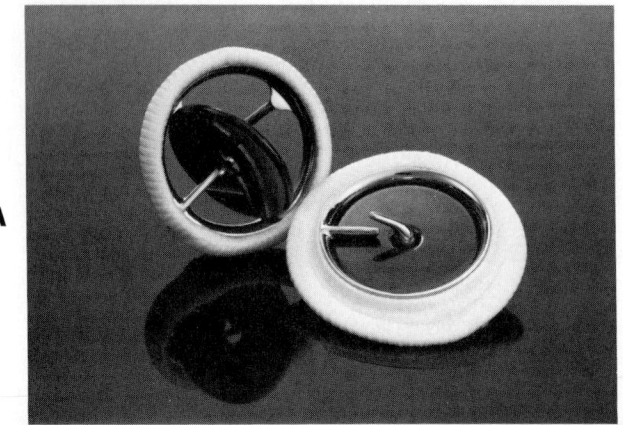

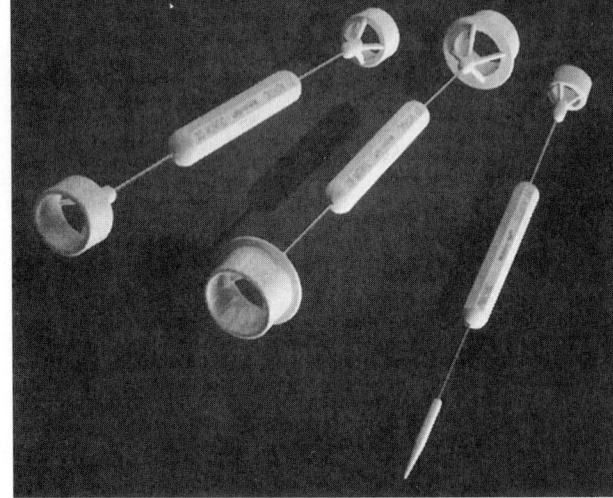

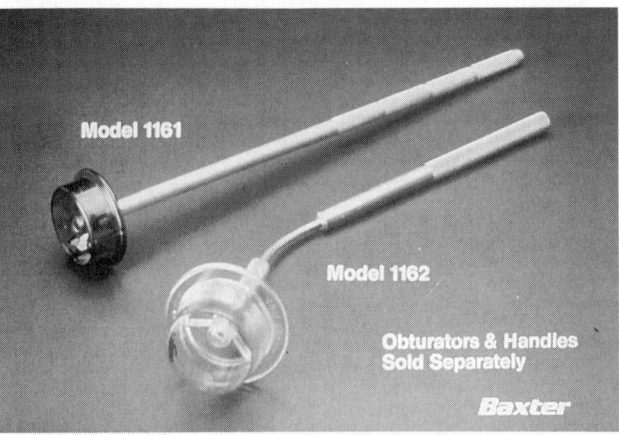

FIG. 26-27 Obturators for Carpentier-Edwards porcine valve prosthesis.

Courtesy Baxter Healthcare Corp., Edwards CVS Division, Santa Ana, Calif.

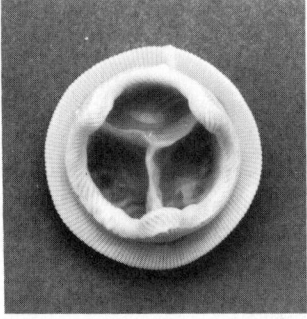

FIG. 26-28 Hancock porcine valve prosthesis.

Courtesy Medtronic, Inc., Minneapolis, Minn.

FIG. 26-25 **A,** Medtronic-Hall tilting disk valve prosthesis. **B,** Double-ended sizing obturators *(left, center)* and probe *(right)* to test leaflet movement.

Courtesy Medtronic, Inc., Minneapolis, Minn.

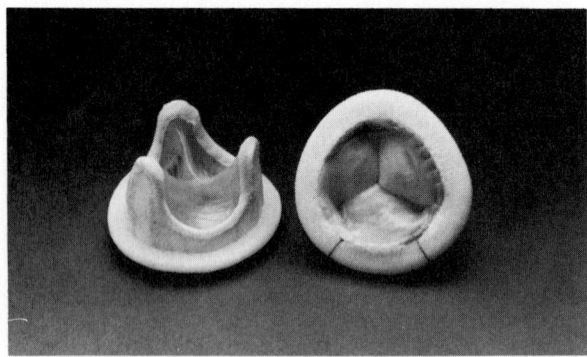

FIG. 26-26 Carpentier-Edwards porcine valve prosthesis.

Courtesy Baxter Healthcare Corp., Edwards CVS Division, Santa Ana, Calif.

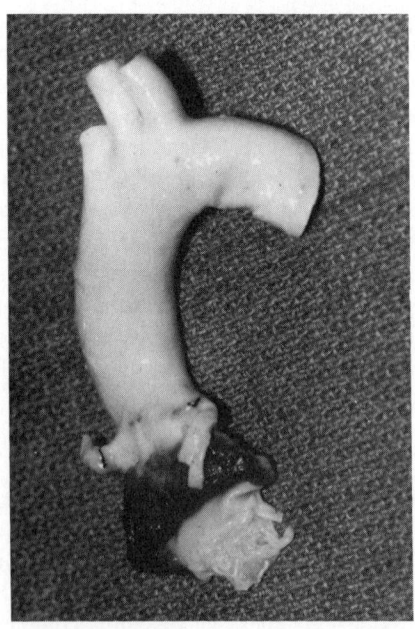

FIG. 26-29 Aortic homograft with aortic valve and arch vessels attached.

Courtesy CryoLife, Inc., Marietta, Ga.

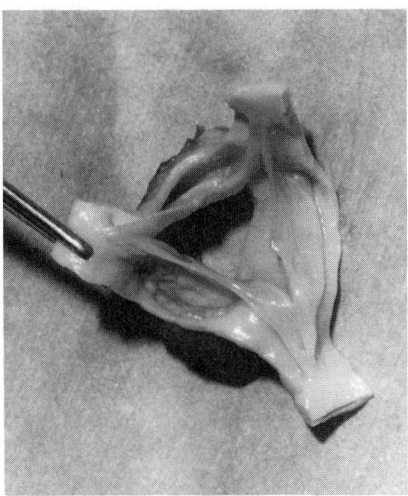

FIG. 26-30   Aortic valve homograft.

Courtesy CryoLife, Inc., Marietta, Ga.

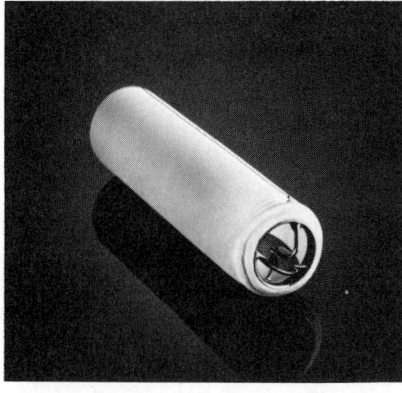

FIG. 26-31   Valved conduit with Medtronic-Hall tilting disk valve prosthesis.

Courtesy Medtronic, Inc., Minneapolis, Minn.

an aortic valve from a pig, which is sutured to a Dacron-covered stent. The advantage of using this valve is that long-term anticoagulants are not necessary in most patients (Edmunds, 1987). Obturators for sizing prosthetic valves as well as valve holders are specific to the prostheses (see Fig. 26-25, *B,* and Fig. 26-27). Table 26-6 compares biologic and mechanical prosthetic heart valves.

Aortic valve allografts (homografts) are used with increasing frequency due to their advantages: little or no risk of thromboembolism, optimal hemodynamic function, no need for anticoagulation drugs, and no risk of sudden catastrophic failure. Moreover, they demonstrate a lower incidence of infective endocarditis than mechanical or biologic valves, and their long-term durability is superior to bioprostheses (Ross, 1991). The entire ascending aorta and valve (Fig. 26-29) or the valve alone (Fig. 26-30) may be inserted. Allografts are cryopreserved and must be thawed in saline according to strict protocol prior to implantation (Lange and Hopkins, 1989).

Conduits consisting of mechanical or biologic aortic valves attached to a tube graft (Fig. 26-31) are used in procedures such as repair of aortic dissections requiring replacement of the aortic valve and ascending aorta. If vein grafts must be inserted into the conduit or if a direct coronary ostial anastomosis is required, an eye cautery is used to make the opening into the graft and at the same time heat-seal the cut edges of the prosthesis. Conduits with biologic valves interposed between tube graft material (Fig. 26-32) may be used when patients are at increased risk for bleeding complications from chronic anticoagulation. Allograft conduits may be used for these procedures as well.

In addition to the use of allografts to avoid the complications associated with prosthetic valve replacement, valve repair rather than replacement is preferred when possible, resulting in greater use of mitral and tricuspid annuloplasty rings (Fig. 26-33) to restore valvular competence (Delouche et al., 1990). Special obturators with a holder are used to size the annulus.

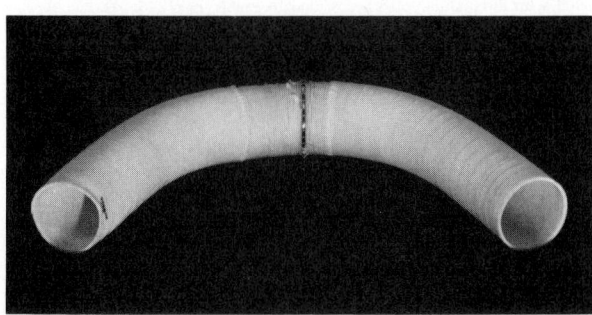

FIG. 26-32   Valved conduit with Hancock porcine valve prosthesis within tube graft.

Courtesy Medtronic, Inc., Minneapolis, Minn.

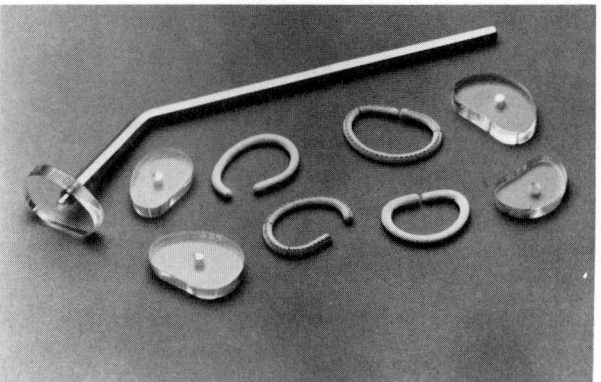

FIG. 26-33   Annuloplasty rings, sizers, and sizer handle. The tricuspid rings are notched to avoid suturing in conduction tissue.

Courtesy Baxter Healthcare Corp., Edwards CVS Division, Santa Ana, Calif.

TABLE 26-6

Commonly Used Mechanical and Biological Valve Prostheses

| | Ball and cage | Tilting disk | |
	Starr-Edwards	Medtronic-Hall, Omniscience	St. Jude Medical
MECHANICAL			
Model/description	6120 mitral; 1260 aortic	Spherical tilting disk	Bileaflet tilting disk
Advantages	Long-term durability	Long-term durability	Long-term durability
	Good hemodynamics	Good hemodynamics in all sizes	Good hemodynamics in all sizes
	Inaudible	Low profile	Low TE rate for a mechanical valve
	Least risk of sudden thrombosis		Low profile
Disadvantages	Anticoagulation required	Anticoagulation required	Anticoagulation strongly recommended
	Higher incidence of TE than disk valves	Sudden thrombosis	Sudden thrombosis
	Suboptimal hemodynamics in small aortic sizes (less than 23 mm)	Noisy	Some noise
		Higher risk of TE in mitral position	Higher risk of TE in mitral position
	High profile not optimal in small LV or aortic root	If Coumadin must be discontinued, there is increased risk of catastrophic thrombosis	If Coumadin must be discontinued, there is increased risk of catastrophic thrombosis
	Higher risk of TE in mitral position		
Special considerations	Sizers and handles specific to prosthesis; must be sterilized	Sizers and handles specific to prosthesis; must be sterilized	Sizers and handles specific to prosthesis; must be sterilized
	Poppet of aortic valve removable to facilitate tying sutures; replaced before aorta closed; mitral poppet not removable		Frequently used in children needing prosthetic valve
	Aortic model has 3 struts; mitral has 4		
Resterilization*	Yes, steam preferred over EO gas	Yes, steam preferred over EO gas	Yes, steam preferred over EO gas

Adapted from Jones, E.L., et al. (1990). Infection, thrombosis, and emboli associated with intracardiac prostheses; and Salzman, E.W., & Ware, J.A. (1990). Thromboembolic complications of cardiac and vascular prostheses. In D.C. Sabiston and F.C. Spencer (Eds.), *Surgery of the chest* (5th ed.). Philadelphia: W.B. Saunders.
*Follow manufacturer's instructions. All prostheses should be stored in a cool, dry, contamination-free area.
TE, thromboembolism; *LV,* left ventricle; *EO,* ethylene oxide; *AVR,* aortic valve replacement.

Safety considerations include storing prosthetic materials in a clean, protected environment and utilizing them according to manufacturers' instructions. Before implantation, biologic valves must be rinsed in three saline baths to remove the glutaraldehyde storage solution. During insertion they should be kept moist with saline. Mechanical valves should be protected from scratching and other injury.

Patient teaching

Patient education and preparation for home care maintenance should begin on the patient's admission. The perioperative nurse acts to reinforce, review, clarify, and add to important information and instructions the patient and family or significant other need in planning for discharge. It should not be assumed that patients undergoing repeat op-

TABLE 26-6

Commonly Used Mechanical and Biological Valve Prostheses—cont'd

	Heterograft		Allograft (Homograft)
	Carpentier-Edwards; Hancock	**Carpentier-Edwards Pericardial Valve**	
BIOLOGICAL			
Model/description	Porcine heterograft (from excised pig aortic valves)	2700 aortic bovine pericardium (cut and shaped into a trileaflet valve)	Aortic valve allograft (cadaver, organ donor, excised cardiomyopathic heart from transplant recipient)
Advantages	Incidence of TE very low; anticoagulation rare after AVR No hemolysis Good hemodynamics Central flow Gradual failure allows elective reoperation	Incidence of TE very low; anticoagulation rare after AVR No hemolysis Good hemodynamics in all sizes Central flow Gradual failure allows elective reoperation Residual gradient minimal	Incidence of TE very low; anticoagulation rare (used mainly for AVR) No hemolysis Excellent hemodynamics, (especially with stentless technique) Central flow Gradual failure allows elective reoperation No residual gradient
Disadvantages	Durability less than 15 years Accelerated fibrocalcific degeneration in children and patients with hypertension or on chronic renal dialysis Suboptimal hemodynamics and residual gradient in smaller sizes (less than 23 mm aorta or 29 mm mitral) May be contraindicated in small, hypertrophied LV	Durability not yet established Available only for AVR Accelerated calcification may be a problem in children, renal patients, or those with hypertension	Limited durability Limited availability
Special considerations	Sizers and handles specific to prosthesis; must be sterilized Prior to insertion, must be rinsed in saline to remove glutaraldehyde storage solution Frequent irrigation recommended to prevent drying Diets low in calcium recommended for children, renal patients	Sizers and handles specific to prosthesis; must be sterilized Prior to insertion, must be rinsed in saline to remove glutaraldehyde storage solution Frequent irrigation recommended to prevent drying Diets low in calcium recommended for children, renal patients Approved for aortic position only	No specific sizers; may use sizers for heterografts Cryopreserved allograft must be thawed per protocol Used for aortic valve replacement; stent attached for use in the mitral and tricuspid position
Resterilization*	Not recommended	Not recommended	Not recommended

⋇

RESEARCH HIGHLIGHT 26-1

Brenner described the perceived learning priorities of patients undergoing repeat coronary artery bypass grafting (CABG) and examined whether reoperative CABG patients' learning priorities were different from those of patients undergoing initial CABG. A 40-item questionnaire developed by the author was given to 36 patients. Subjects were divided into two groups during their postintensive care in a 600-bed community teaching hospital, and again 3 months after discharge. Group 1 (n = 16) underwent reoperation for CABG; Group 2 (n = 20) underwent CABG for the first time.

The major finding was that reoperative patients most frequently rated most items as "very important" to learn about. Reoperative patients demonstrated special interest in knowing who health care workers were and what they were doing to or for the patient. Overall, few of the 40 items were related differently by reoperative and initial CABG patients. Both groups wanted information about areas in which patients could participate in their own care (diet, medications, activity), as well as information about postoperative complications.

An increasing number of patients are undergoing repeat CABG. Perioperative nurses cannot assume that these patients do not have significant learning needs just because they have had previous experience with CABG surgery. The results of Brenner's study suggest that reoperative CABG patients rate learning as very important and that they have learning priorities similar to those of CABG patients undergoing surgery for the first time.

Brenner, A.R. (1993). Patient's learning priorities for reoperative coronary artery bypass surgery. *Journal of Cardiovascular Nursing, 7* (2), 1.

formed consent (and advance directives), laboratory results, diagnostic data, and other pertinent information. Preoperatively, cardiac surgical patients are likely to exhibit more stress and anxiety than other types of patients. Nurses should anticipate and prepare for this reaction because anxiety increases myocardial oxygen consumption. Slogoff and Keats (1989) have demonstrated that postoperative myocardial infarction after coronary bypass was consistently related to the appearance of new myocardial ischemia. Efforts to reduce the family's anxiety level are also important and result in less emotional stress being transmitted to the patient. A peripheral arterial pressure line and venous infusion lines are inserted. A local anesthetic may be used at the insertion sites and a sedative injected intravenously.

Admission to the operating room

Depending on the amount of sedation received preoperatively, the patient may require assistance onto the OR bed. Warm blankets can be provided while the patient is still awake for comfort and to reduce shivering. Padding of the arms, hands, and feet can be performed after application of the pulse oximeter finger cot and while the pressure lines are attached to transducers and the ECG cables are inserted into the monitors.

Anesthesia induction

The choice of anesthetic agent(s) depends on the cardiovascular effects of the anesthetic and the patient's hemodynamics and general health. Because the period of induction is one of the most critical during the procedure, close monitoring of the patient is required, especially for patients with ventricular ischemia from congenital or acquired disease. Anesthetic management focuses on keeping myocardial oxygen demand low and the oxygen supply high (Kaplan, 1993).

Monitoring

Maximal monitoring of hemodynamic and other variables is indicated during cardiac surgery (Table 26-7). After intubation (or before, depending on anesthesia preference), additional pressure lines may be inserted to measure central venous pressure and pulmonary artery pressures. Peripheral and central arterial and venous pressures are usually monitored directly by means of a transducer and oscilloscope. Perioperative nurses may be required to assist with the preparation and placement of central lines; they should observe the ECG monitors for signs of ventricular irritability, such as ectopy or tachycardia, and be prepared to assist with defibrillation of the patient if necessary. If the patient cannot be resuscitated, the chest is opened rapidly and internal cardiac massage is performed.

A urinary drainage catheter is inserted for monitoring renal function, especially during and after cardiopulmonary bypass. It may contain a thermistor temperature probe. Other temperature probes may be placed, usually in the esophagus, nasopharynx, or rectum. Ventricular septal temperatures may be recorded while the patient's heart is ar-

eration have less need for teaching (Research Highlight 26-1). The patient's ability to cough and breathe deeply should be determined; the patient should be taught to use a cough pillow or splinting techniques. Required life-style changes should be reviewed, and the patient's feelings about these modifications elicited. The nurse should verify that the patient knows reportable signs and symptoms associated with the specific procedure and understands prescribed medications, dosages and times, potential side effects, and signs and symptoms. Any misconceptions should be clarified or referred to an appropriate source. The family or significant other's ability and willingness to assist the patient in home care maintenance should be queried; referrals to an agency for assistance at home may be required.

Preinduction care

The patient is brought to the operating room suite, where a preoperative assessment is performed, and the nurse reviews the chart for completion and documentation of in-

TABLE 26-7

Perioperative Patient Monitoring

Monitoring device	Location	Measures
Arterial line	Peripheral Radial artery Central Femoral artery Aorta (with needle attached to pressure tubing, or with sensor in bypass circuit)	Arterial blood pressure (direct)
Blood pressure (B/P) cuff	Arm	Arterial B/P (indirect)
Central venous pressure (CVP) line	Right atrium (RA)	RA pressure (e.g., CVP)
Pulmonary artery (PA) catheter (Swan-Ganz)	RA (proximal port) Right ventricle (RV) (midline port) Distal PA (distal port)	RA pressure (e.g., CVP) RV pressure PA and pulmonary artery wedge pressure (PAWP) Indirect measure of left atrial and left ventricular (LV) pressure Cardiac output
Left atrial (LA) line	Left atrium	LA, LV pressure
Pulse oximeter	Finger	Oxygen saturation of arterial hemoglobin
Urinary drainage catheter	Urinary bladder	Urine output, renal perfusion/ function
Temperature probes	Esophagus Urinary bladder Rectum Ventricular septum Bypass circuit Pulmonary artery catheter	Temperature (core and peripheral)

rested. A pulse oximetry finger cot is attached to measure the level of blood oxygen saturation.

The skin is carefully inspected before ECG and electrosurgical dispersive pads are placed. Bony prominences, such as the coccyx and the back of the head, are padded to prevent pressure necrosis resulting from hypoperfusion and hypothermia during bypass. Because elderly patients are especially vulnerable to skin breakdown, additional precautions to avoid pressure injuries are recommended.

Drugs

Numerous medications are used during cardiac surgery (Table 26-8). They may be stocked by the anesthesia department, perfusionists, or nursing personnel and should be readily available.

Positioning

The supine position provides optimum exposure for the institution of cardiopulmonary bypass and the surgical repair of the heart and great vessels. In addition, there is less respiratory impairment and discomfort with this approach. The arms and hands are padded and placed at the patient's

side. The legs may be slightly everted to provide access to the femoral arteries for insertion of pressure lines or intraaortic balloon pump lines or to excise the saphenous vein. Measures to avoid venous stasis ulcers (especially in the elderly, debilitated, or obese patient) include padding of the coccyx and application of heel protectors. The lateral position (see Chapter 24) may be used in operations on the descending thoracic aorta. The presence of severe mediastinal adhesions may necessitate this approach in some repeat valve operations (Espersen, 1993).

Prepping and draping

For procedures requiring excision of the saphenous vein, the prep extends from the jaw to the toes and includes the anterior chest, abdomen, groin, and legs. The legs and feet are prepped circumferentially and the chest and abdomen from bedline to bedline.

In procedures not requiring saphenous vein excision, the prep extends to the knees to give the surgeon access to the femoral artery and/or saphenous vein, should the need arise. In the lateral position, the patient is prepped anteriorly and posteriorly to the knees.

TABLE 26-8

Medications Used in Adults During Cardiac Surgery

Drug/name	Purpose/description
ANALGESICS AND ANESTHETICS	
Thiopental	Induction, ultrashort-acting barbiturate, intravenous bolus
Fentanyl (Sublimaze)	Synthetic narcotic, intravenous bolus
Sufentanil (Sufenta)	Synthetic narcotic, intravenous bolus
Alfentanil (Alfenta)	Synthetic narcotic, intravenous bolus
Morphine	Narcotic, intravenous bolus
Halothane (Fluothane)	Inhalation anesthetic, maintenance
Enflurane (Ethrane)	Inhalation anesthetic, maintenance
Isoflurane (Forane)	Inhalation anesthetic, maintenance
MUSCLE RELAXANTS	
Vecuronium (Norcuron)	Intubation, maintenance of relaxation
Pancuronium (Pavulon)	Maintenance of relaxation
AMNESIACS	
Midazolam (Versed)	Hypnotic; anxiety-reducing sedative
Scopolamine	Sedative; tranquilizer
CARDIOVASCULAR AGENTS	
Anticholinergics	
Atropine	Decreases vagal tone, treats sinus bradycardia
Glycopyrrolate (Robinul)	Similar to atropine but causes fewer dysrhythmias than atropine
Vasopressors	
Norepinephrine (Levophed)	Increases force and velocity of contraction, increases systemic and pulmonary vascular resistance
Phenylephrine (Neo-Synephrine)	Arteriolar and venous vasoconstriction, increases blood pressure and systemic vascular resistance
Vasodilators	
Nitroglycerine (Tridil)	Dilates coronary arteries, reduces preload
Phentolamine (Regitine)	Decreases systemic and pulmonary vascular resistance
Prostaglandin E_1	Vascular smooth muscle dilator, potent pulmonary vascular dilator; used in patients with severe pulmonary hypertension
Nitroprusside (Nipride)	Arteriolar and venous vasodilatation, reduces preload and afterload
Inotropic Agents	
Amrinone (Inocor)	Increases cardiac output, force, and velocity of contraction
Calcium chloride	In ionized form, increases cardiac output, blood pressure, and contractility
Dopamine (Intropin)	In low doses increases renal and mesenteric perfusion; with moderate doses increases heart rate, contractility, and cardiac output; in higher doses increases systemic and pulmonary vascular resistance
Dobutamine (Dobutrex)	Increases contractility without increase in heart rate; has vasodilatation effect on vascular bed
Ephedrine	Increases contractility, cardiac output, and blood pressure
Epinephrine (Adrenalin)	Increases rate and strength of contraction, blood pressure, (effective bronchodilator)
Isoproterenol (Isuprel)	Increases heart rate, contractility, cardiac output; decreases systemic vascular resistance

Adapted from Larach, D.R. (1990). Cardiovascular drugs. In Hensley, F.A. and Martin, D.E. (editors), *The practice of anesthesia*. Boston: Little, Brown.

TABLE 26-8

Medications Used in Adults During Cardiac Surgery—cont'd

Drug/name	Purpose/description
CARDIOVASCULAR AGENTS—CONT'D	
Antidysrhythmics	
Lidocaine (Xylocaine)	Acts on ventricles, decreases automaticity of ischemic ventricular tissue
Bretylium (Bretylol)	Prolongs duration of action potential and refractory period, useful for ventricular dysrhythmias refractory to therapy
Digoxin (Lanoxin)	Decreases ventricular rate in atrial fibrillation or flutter and other supraventricular dysrhythmias; avoid in patients with Wolff-Parkinson-White syndrome and other accessory atrioventricular pathways
Nifedipine (Procardia)	Calcium channel blocker; reduces coronary artery spasm; produces coronary vasodilatation; extremely light sensitive; must be given PO or via nasal or oral mucosa; antihypertensive
Procainamide (Pronestyl)	Decreases automaticity and conduction in all cardiac tissue (normal and ischemic); stabilizes cellular membranes
Quinidine	Similar to procainamide; atrial and ventricular dysrhythmias
Verapamil (Calan, Isoptin)	Calcium channel blocker used to treat atrial dysrhythmias; slows ventricular rate in atrial fibrillation or flutter; can be given IV
Adenosine	Blocks AV nodal reentry of supraventricular tachycardias (e.g., atrial fibrillation or flutter); given IV (through central line)
Diuretics	
Furosemide (Lasix)	Decreases renal absorption of sodium and chloride; increases excretion of water and electrolytes, especially potassium, sodium, chloride, magnesium, and calcium
Mannitol	Osmotic diuretic; pulls free water out of organs (reducing cerebral edema); protects kidneys
Anticoagulants/coagulants	
Heparin	Systemic anticoagulation during cardiopulmonary bypass (CPB), blocks activation of thrombin (and intrinsic clotting cascade)
Protamine sulfate	Heparin antagonist; NPH insulin–dependent diabetic patients may be at increased risk for protamine reaction
ANTIBIOTICS	
Cephalosporins (Mandol, Ancef, Keflex, Keflin, Cefadyl)	Broad-spectrum prophylaxis
Tobramycin (Nebcin)	Aerobic gram-negative and gram-positive bacteria
Vancomycin	Severe endocarditis
Bacitracin	Topical irrigation
MISCELLANEOUS	
Xylocaine 1% (plain)	Local anesthesia
Papaverine	Reduces arterial spasm (e.g., mammary artery)
Potassium	Replaces electrolyte loss
Sodium bicarbonate	Corrects acidosis
Insulin (NPH, etc.)	Corrects hyperglycemia in diabetic patients
Topical hemostatic agents	Intraoperative control of bleeding

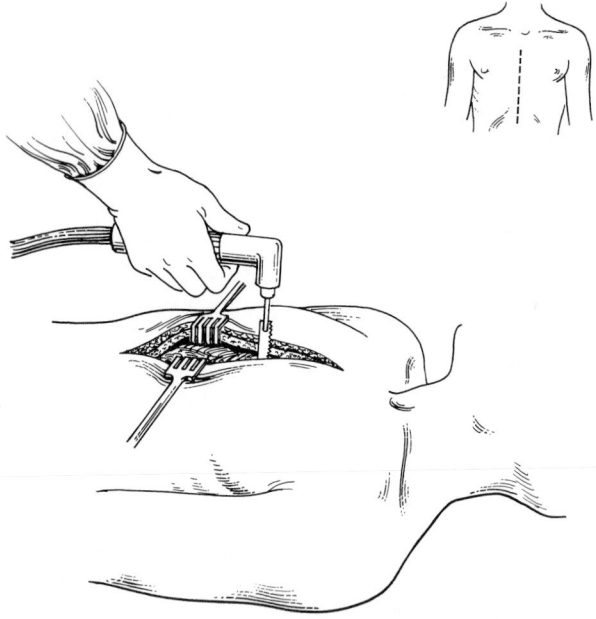

FIG. 26-34   Median sternotomy with sternal saw.

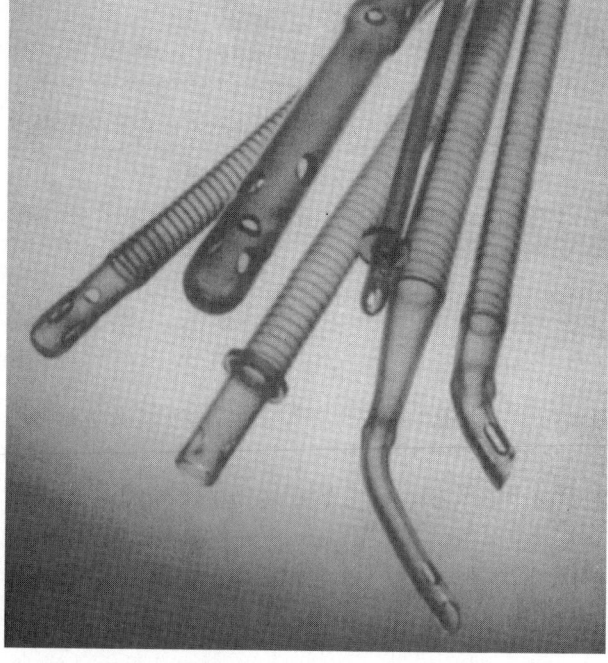

FIG. 26-35   Arterial and venous perfusion cannulas.
Courtesy Bard. Cardiopulmonary Division, Tewksbury, Mass.

After the prep, the patient is draped so that the anterior chest, abdomen, and inguinal area are accessible. The perineum is covered and a towel may be placed across the umbilicus to connect the side drapes. When the saphenous vein is to be excised, both legs remain exposed, with only the feet covered. When draping, the perioperative nurse should consider the placement of bypass lines so that they remain securely attached and do not become contaminated. A small drape or towel may be placed over the groin area when access to it is not immediately necessary. If, later, the femoral artery needs to be accessed, the drape can be discarded.

Median sternotomy

The skin incision extends from the sternal notch to the linea alba below the xiphoid process (Fig. 26-34). The sternum is divided with a saw, and a sternal retractor inserted. If the internal mammary artery and/or the saphenous vein will be used, they are made available at this time. The pericardium is incised and retracted with sutures.

In repeat sternotomies adhesions from a previous cardiac operation must be dissected. The sternum may be split with a vibrating saw and the retrosternal tissue cut free (Regas, 1993). Increased risk of fibrillation from manipulation of the heart, and bleeding and laceration of the ventricle, should alert the perioperative nurse to the possibility of instituting femoral vein–femoral artery bypass (discussed later). If the patient fibrillates during dissection, internal-external paddles may be needed if two internal paddles cannot be inserted into the scarred, adherent pericardium. An external paddle is placed behind the patient prior to the prep; one internal paddle is placed on the anterior surface

of the heart, and the patient is defibrillated. Occasionally, two internal paddles can be used if the pleura is opened; one paddle tip is inserted through the pleural opening and placed against the heart, and the second positioned on top of the heart.

Anterior-posterior and lateral chest x-ray films are useful to determine the extent of retrosternal adhesions and to count the number of chest wires for removal (see Fig. 26-10). On occasion a patient presents for repeat mitral valve surgery. If the initial operation was performed through a thoracotomy incision, sternal adhesions may be minimal or nonexistent, and the special precautions associated with repeat sternotomy may not be necessary.

Cardiopulmonary bypass

The temporary substitution of a pump oxygenator for the heart and lungs provides the surgeon sufficient time to complete complicated and lengthy procedures under direct vision in a relatively dry, motionless field. Systemic venous return to the heart flows by gravity drainage through cannulae (Fig. 26-35) placed in the superior and inferior venae cavae (Fig. 26-36), or through a single cannula in the right atrium (Fig. 26-37) into tubing connected to the bypass machine. Here blood is oxygenated, filtered, warmed or cooled, and pumped back into the systemic circulation through a cannula placed in the ascending aorta or occasionally in the femoral artery (Fig. 26-38). Because blood is oxygenated by the machine, the lungs do not need to function and can be deflated to provide better exposure of the mediastinal structures.

A percutaneous method of instituting cardiopulmonary

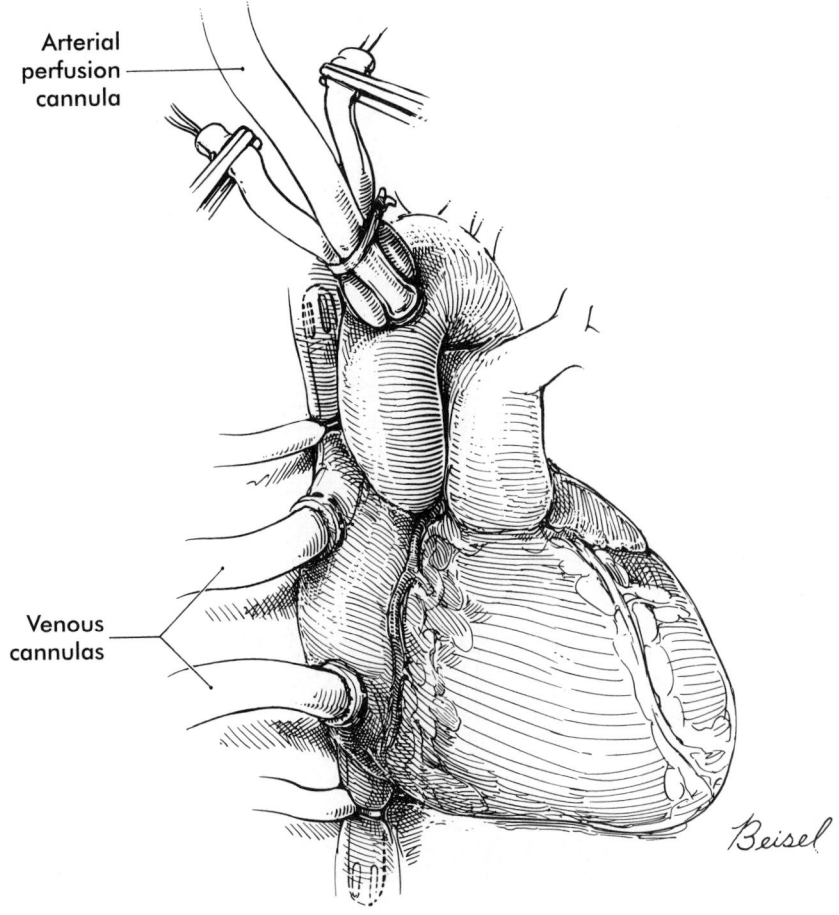

Arterial
perfusion
cannula

Venous
cannulas

Beisel

FIG. 26-36   Bicaval cannulation of the superior and inferior venae cavae; aortic cannulation.
From Waldhausen JA and Pierce WS. (1985). *Johnson's surgery of the chest*, ed. 5, St. Louis, Mosby.

bypass employs thin-walled, wire-reinforced catheters inserted into the femoral artery and veins. It is used in emergency situations in which the environment is not conducive to the more traditional methods, such as the cardiac catheterization laboratory, the intensive care unit, and the emergency department (Phillips et al., 1989). Gravity drainage is impeded by the resistance of the small-bore cannula used in the femoral vein; to overcome this, a centrifugal pump is used to siphon blood to the pump oxygenator.

By diverting blood away from the heart, cardiopulmonary bypass also decompresses the ventricles, thereby reducing myocardial wall tension, a significant determinant of myocardial oxygen demand. This principle is evident when cardiopulmonary bypass or other means of ventricular support are employed to "rest" the heart. Further decompression is achieved by venting the left ventricle to remove air and accumulated thebesian and bronchial venous return, as well as systemic return flowing around the venous cannulas. The venting catheter is inserted into the left ventricle via the right superior pulmonary vein, or, less commonly, through the left ventricular apex. The venting

line is connected to the suction lines of the bypass machine. A small venting catheter is also inserted into the ascending aorta to remove air. Occasionally, a vent is inserted into the pulmonary artery (Fig. 26-39). Extracorporeal membrane oxygenation (ECMO), often used for pulmonary assistance in infants and children with reversible pulmonary insults, can also be used in adults for right ventricular assistance when right heart failure or pulmonary hypertension exists (Bartlett, 1990).

Improvements in filtration methods have substantially reduced the incidence of gaseous and particulate emboli.

Two types of blood oxygenators are available—the membrane (Fig. 26-40) and the bubble. Most often the membrane method is used for gas exchange (that is, removal of carbon dioxide and subsequent oxygenation). With the *membrane method*, oxygen is diffused through a gas-permeable membrane that separates the oxygenating gas and the venous blood. Less commonly, the *bubble method* is employed, whereby oxygen is bubbled through a column of venous blood. Membrane oxygenators are preferred to bubble oxygenators because of better platelet pres-

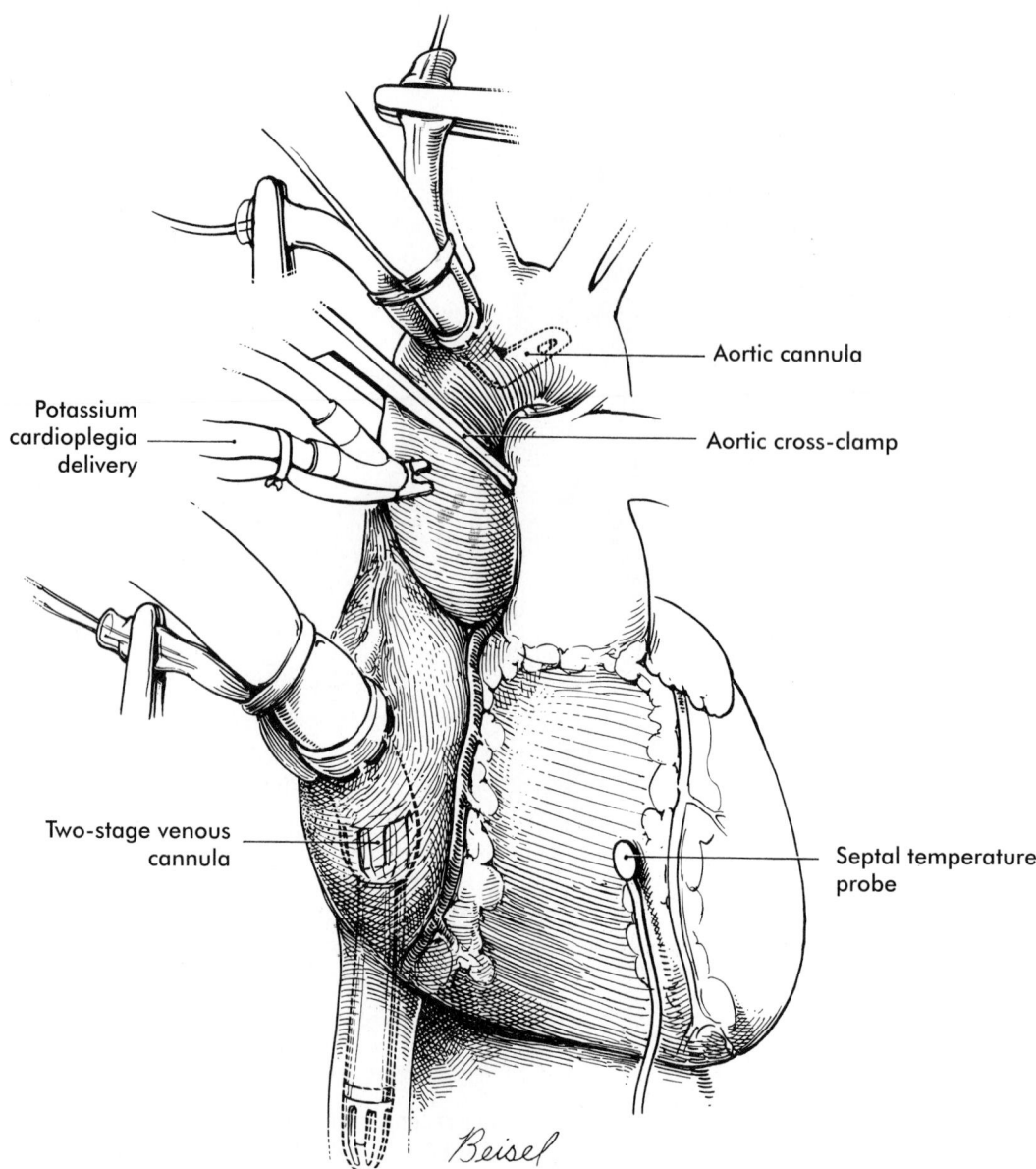

Potassium
cardioplegia
delivery

Aortic cannula

Aortic cross-clamp

Two-stage venous
cannula

Septal temperature
probe

Beisel

FIG. 26-37   Diagram showing aortic and venous cannulae during aortic cross-clamping. Also shown is cardioplegia delivery catheter in the aorta proximal to the cross-clamp and a temperature probe. The single (two-stage) venous cannula has openings in the distal end of the cannula to drain the inferior vena cava; the openings in the midportion of the cannula drain the superior vena cava and the coronary sinus return.

From Waldhausen JA and Pierce WS. (1985). *Johnson's surgery of the chest,* ed. 5, St. Louis, Mosby.

ervation, less use of bank blood, better postoperative renal function, and because they do not employ a direct blood-gas interface, which is inherently destructive to the formed elements of the blood.

The roller pump has important basic features and is commonly used. It propels the blood through flexible plastic (polyvinyl chloride) tubing and, with careful calibration and judicious use, can provide relatively atraumatic blood flow. Arterial blood flow with any roller pump, however, is nonpulsatile and will be manifested by a mean arterial wave

form on the oscilloscope during total cardiopulmonary bypass.

Suction lines are ordinarily used during cardiopulmonary bypass to return lost blood to the venous reservoir and the oxygenator (see Fig. 26-38). These lines usually combine conventional hand-held suction tubes and ventricular decompression lines or sumps (see Fig. 26-39). Before the intitiation of cardiopulmonary bypass, the entire extracorporeal circuit must be primed, or rendered free of air, to prevent air emboli. The priming solution is usually a com-

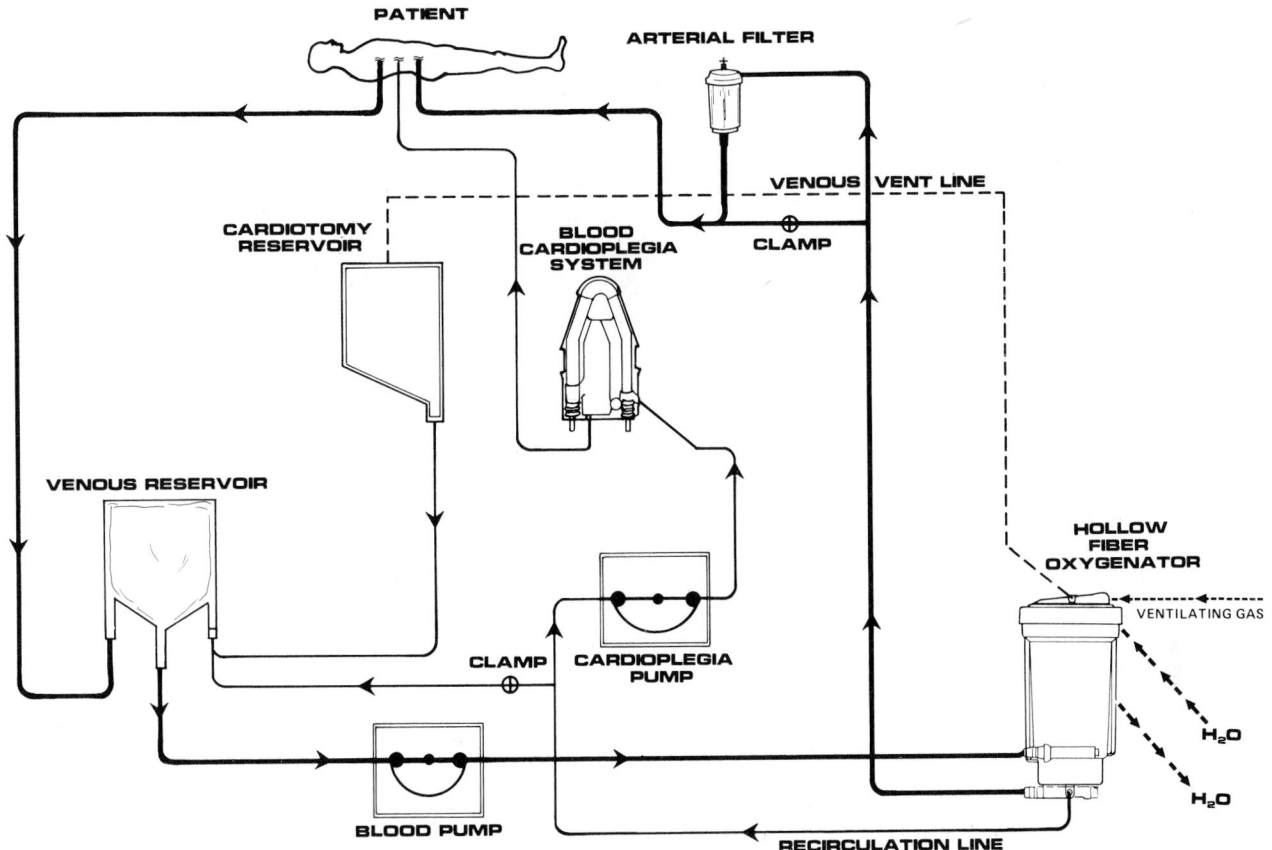

FIG. 26-38 Extracorporeal circuit. This diagram illustrates a typical cardiopulmonary bypass circuit used during cardiac surgery. Venous blood exits the patient and drains by gravity into a venous reservoir. The blood is then pumped into the membrane oxygenator. The oxygenator's heat exchanger controls the temperature of the blood during surgery. The ventilating gas flowing into the oxygenator removes carbon dioxide and adds oxygen to the blood. The oxygenated bloods then flows through the arterial filter and back to the patient. Oxygenated blood is also taken from the oxygenator and mixed with a cardioplegia solution before being pumped through the blood cardioplegia system heat exchanger, where it is cooled. The blood is then periodically infused into the coronary arteries (antegradely or retrogradely) in order to nourish the heart and keep it cooled while it is arrested during the surgical repair.

Courtesy Sorin, Inc., Irvine, Calif.

bination of colloid and crystalloid fluids with a balanced electrolyte component. Most, if not all, institutions today employ the technique of hemodilution, meaning that crystalloid solutions are predominantly used to prime the pump in an attempt to reduce the amount of bank blood being used. It has the advantage of reducing the number of homologous serum reactions and the incidence of hepatitis and human immunodeficiency virus (HIV), as well as providing better perfusion of the capillary beds because of reduced blood viscosity (Bell and Diffee, 1991).

The amount and kind of drugs used in the priming solution vary among institutions, but heparin is routinely added to block clot formation in the bypass circuit. Heparin-coated circuits are also available. Anticoagulation is routinely monitored during bypass, and more heparin is given as

needed. Arterial blood flow rates are estimated according to the patient's height, weight, and body surface area; depending on the arterial and venous pressure values and result of blood gas determinations, flow is adjusted.

Once the patient is on bypass, systemic cooling can be achieved with the heat exchanger incorporated into the oxygenator. When sufficient cooling is achieved (the level of hypothermia depends on the anticipated complexity of the repair and the time required), the repair is performed. The aorta is cross-clamped, and the heart is arrested. Cooling may not be initiated until induced cardiac arrest is achieved to avoid cold contracture, which occasionally develops before the heart stops.

Cardiopulmonary bypass (CPB), although allowing repair of cardiac disorders with relatively low morbidity and

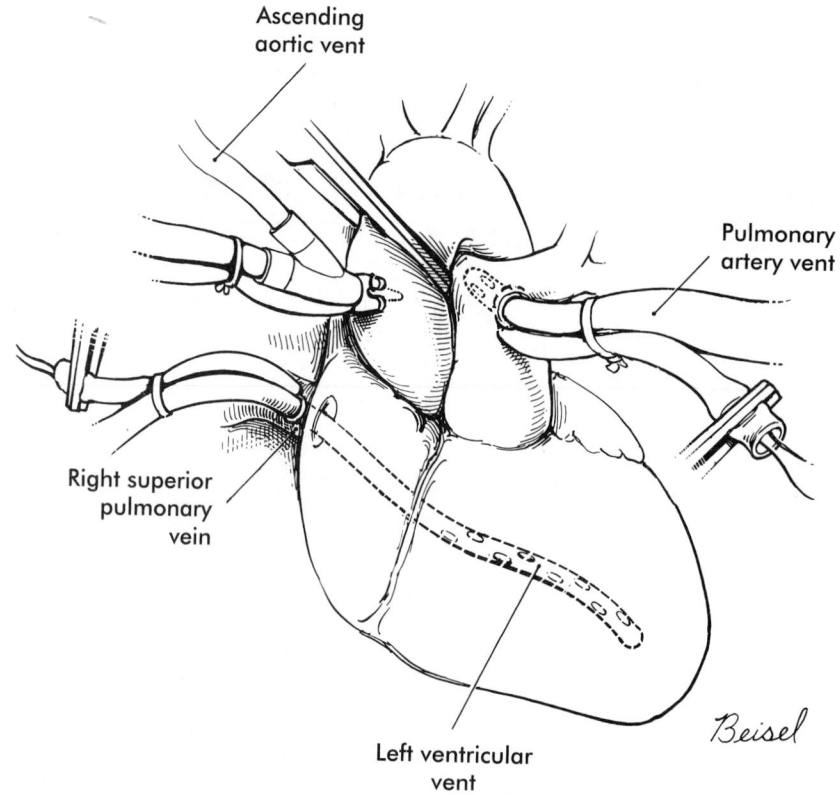

FIG. 26-39   Types of venting catheters.

From Waldhausen JA and Pierce WS. (1985). *Johnson's surgery of the chest*, ed. 5, St. Louis, Mosby.

mortality, is not without adverse physiologic reactions, especially in the very young and the very old. This has been termed *postperfusion syndrome* (Kirklin, 1991) and is evidenced by prolonged pulmonary insufficiency, excessive accumulation of extravascular water, elevated temperature, vasoconstriction, coagulopathy, and variable degrees of organ dysfunction.

The mechanism of injury is thought to be related to the exposure of the blood to the abnormal surfaces of the bypass circuit, hypothermia, and altered blood flow. These can initiate a systemic inflammatory response (complement activation), which releases vasoactive substances (Kirklin et al., 1983). Attempts to minimize the inflammatory reaction have focused on modifying the activation of platelets and blood factors that play a major role in initiating the response (Downing and Edmunds, 1992).

Myocardial protection

Improvement in the results of cardiac surgery are due in great part to progress made in the protection of the myocardium. Circulatory interruptions, ischemia, and hypoperfusion accompanying induced cardiac arrest are necessary to permit the surgeon sufficient time to repair cardiac lesions under direct vision. Unless measures are taken to protect the myocardium during these periods, irreversible damage can result. Protection is achieved by cooling the heart (and the rest of the body) to reduce metabolic demand and

by rapidly arresting the heart so that myocardial energy resources are preserved (Drinkwater et al., 1990).

Hypothermia

Most cardiac surgical procedures performed today employ some degree of hypothermia. In this context, hypothermia is defined as the deliberate reduction of body temperature for therapeutic purposes. A moderate degree of hypothermia, to 28° C (82.4° F), permits reduction of oxygen consumption by 50%. At 20° C (68° F) there is a further reduction of about 25%. Internal cooling is achieved with the heat exchanger of the heart-lung machine. When very cold temperatures (20° C) are employed, additional surface cooling of the head may be used for neurologic protection.

In addition to systemic hypothermia, local hypothermia is used to further cool the heart. The topical application of cold saline or continuous irrigation of the pericardial wall accomplishes this. Insulation pads placed behind the heart can reduce heat conduction from relatively warmer organs. Transmural cooling of the heart is achieved with cardioplegia (discussed later). There are complications associated with the used of hypothermia. Frostbite can occur with surface cooling, during which the patient's head is covered with plastic bags of ice. Wrapping the ears and covering the nose are usually effective in preventing frostbite, and providing additional padding can reduce pressure injuries. Ice chips in pericardial irrigants should be avoided to pre-

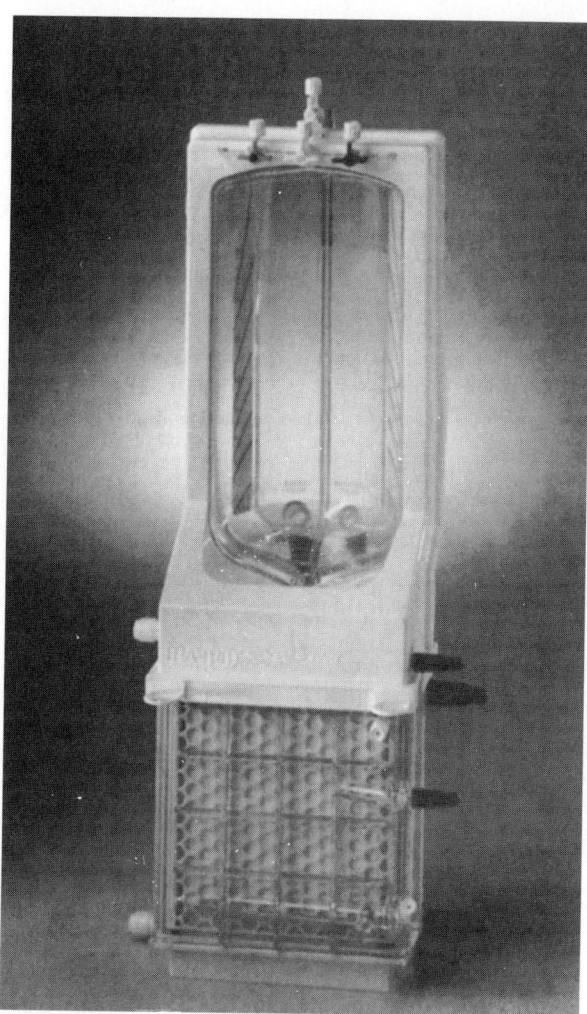

FIG. 26-40 Membrane oxygenator.
Courtesy Bard, Cardiopulmonary Division, Tewksbury, Mass.

vent injury to the phrenic nerve and cardiac tissue (Robicsek et al., 1989).

Ventricular fibrillation can occur during the cooling process. This is usually not a problem when the patient is on cardiopulmonary bypass. It can be a real concern with patients who are undergoing surface cooling before the initiation of bypass. Ventricular fibrillation is unusual at temperatures above 32° C (89.6° F), but it can occur at higher temperatures. Another complication is related to the adverse effect that hypothermia has on coagulation, and this may delay hemostasis after heparin reversal.

Cardioplegic arrest

Rapidly arresting the heart during diastole is beneficial because an arrested heart uses less energy than a fibrillating or beating heart. Cardioplegia with hypothermia reduces energy requirements even further.

Cold cardioplegic arrest is accomplished by infusing the coronary arteries with a 4° to 10° C (39.2° to 50° F) solution containing potassium (2 to 50 mEq/L) and various buff-

ering agents to counteract ischemic acidosis. The use of continuous warm cardioplegia has been advocated to obviate some of the adverse effects of hypothermia and to enhance global delivery of the cardioplegic solution. Because of the technical difficulty associated with a constant flow of cardioplegia obscuring the surgical site, the technique has not gained wide acceptance.

Cardioplegia solution is delivered under pressure to the coronary circulation at frequent intervals to maintain the hypothermic arrest. Potassium is routinely used as the cardioplegic, or paralyzing, agent, causing cardiac arrest by depolarizing the myocardial cell membrane.

The coronary circulation is entered indirectly (see Fig. 26-37) via the aortic root proximal to the aortic cross-clamp. Less commonly, direct cannulation of the coronary ostia is performed. Direct infusion into available vein grafts enhances transmural cooling. Retrograde infusion through the coronary sinus is widely used, especially in the presence of coronary artery obstructions (Drinkwater et al., 1990). When the heart is sufficiently arrested, the ECG reflects a straight line; when electrical activity is noticed on the monitor (fine fibrillation), cardioplegia is reinfused when continued cooling is desired (approximately every 15 to 20 minutes).

During this period the surgical repair is completed. The heart is allowed to rewarm, and the perfusionist rewarms the patient with the oxygenator's heat exchanger. Air is evacuated from the left ventricle. The cross-clamp is removed. The heart should convert spontaneously, but internal defibrillation may be necessary. Temporary epicardial pacing wires may be sutured to the right atrial appendage and the right ventricle, to be used postoperatively for transient dysrhythmias.

When the surgeon is satisfied that the heart is performing adequately, termination of cardiopulmonary bypass is initiated. Venous flow is gradually reduced by clamping the venous line(s), and a commensurate reduction in arterial flow is made by the perfusionist. When heart action is sufficient and systemic and pulmonary blood pressures are stabilized, bypass is terminated and the cannulas removed.

Closing

After hemostasis is achieved, catheters are inserted into the pericardium for mediastinal drainage. If either or both pleura have been entered, chest tubes are inserted as well. The tubes are connected to straight or Y connectors to a water-seal drainage system (see Chapter 24) or an autotransfusion drainage system.

Chest closure in median sternotomy is achieved with wire sutures (see Fig. 26-19). The wire sutures are twisted, cut, and buried into the sternum. The linea alba is closed with nonabsorbable suture. A layer of sutures is placed to approximate the fascia over the sternum and the subcutaneous tissue and skin are closed.

Before transferring the patient, the nurse telephones a report to the recovery area, usually the intensive care unit

---

BOX 26-3

Patient Transfer Report

PROCEDURE (include source of autogenous grafts) _____

MONITORING DEVICES (LOCATION)

CVP _____ ARTERIAL LINE _____ SWAN _____ PERIPHERAL _____

HEMODYNAMICS

B/P _____ PAP _____ PAD _____ PAWP _____ CO _____ CI _____ CVP _____ S_{CO_2} _____

INTRAOPERATIVE OCCURRENCES

BLOOD LOSS _____ URINE _____ DYSRHYTHMIAS _____ BYPASS

PROBLEMS _____ DEFIB X's _____ LO TEMP _____ HI TEMP _____

CROSS-CLAMP TIME _____ PUMP TIME _____

BLOOD: GIVEN _____ AVAILABLE _____ AUTOTRANSFUSION

TOTALS: _____ CC's _____ UNITS

COMPONENTS: FFP _____ PLATELETS _____ CRYO _____

ADDITIONAL ORDERED (TYPE) _____

MEDICATIONS

NEO _____ DOPAMINE _____ DOBUTAMINE _____ LIDOCAINE _____ NITRO _____

LEVOPHED _____ EPINEPHRINE _____ NITROPRUSSIDE _____ INOCOR _____

DDAVP _____ OTHER _____

TUBES/DRAINS: MEDIASTINAL _____ PLEURAL (Rt/Lt) _____

EPICARDIAL LEADS: ATRIAL _____ VENTRICULAR _____

PACING: YES/NO   RATE _____

LABS:

K^+ _____ NA^+ _____ GLU _____ HGB _____ HCT _____

PATIENT CONCERNS _____

_____

ADDITIONAL INFORMATION _____

ICU BED # _____ ETA _____

REPORTED BY _____

To _____ TIME _____

B/P, Blood pressure; *CI*, cardiac index; *CO*, cardiac output; *CRYO*, cryoprecipitate; *CVP*, central venous pressure; *DDAVP*, 1 deamino-8-D-arginine vasopressin (e.g., Desmopressin); *ETA*, estimated time of arrival; *FFP*, fresh frozen plasma; *GLU*, glucose; *HCT*, hematocrit; *HGB*, hemoglobin; K^+, potassium; NA^+, sodium; *NEO*, neosynephrine; *nitro*, nitroglycerine; *PAD*, pulmonary artery diastolic pressure; *PAP*, pulmonary artery pressure; *PAWP*, pulmonary artery wedge pressure; Svo_2 percent saturation of mixed venous blood; *SWAN*, Swan-Ganz (pulmonary artery) catheter.

(ICU). Box 26-3 lists information commonly supplied. In addition, the patient's special concerns and fears as well as significant physiologic alterations should be communicated.

Perioperative documentation follows the standard protocol and should include a complete description of the procedure performed and identification of medications and all implanted material (with lot and serial numbers). Hospital policy should be followed to ensure compliance with the Safe Medical Devices Act.

EVALUATION

Evaluation of perioperative care includes the determination of whether the patient met the outcomes identified in the care plan. Such evaluation assists perioperative nurses in determining if the nursing interventions designed for a specific patient were successful. This type of data collection becomes the basis of the development of future plans of care for similar patients. Evaluation should be documented in the perioperative record. For the nursing diagnoses and the subsequent plan of care presented in this chapter for the cardiac surgery patient, those outcome statements might be as follows:

· The patient demonstrated adequate cardiac output.
· The patient will be free from wound infection.
· The patient was free from injury related to the surgical position.
· The patient described perioperative events.
· The patient's skin integrity was maintained.

SURGICAL INTERVENTIONS

The following section describes operations for acquired forms of heart disease. Unless otherwise noted, they are performed through a median sternotomy incision using aortocaval cardiopulmonary bypass (see Fig. 26-37) and antegrade/retrograde cardioplegia with routine chest drainage and closure as described.

EXTRACORPOREAL CIRCULATION PROCEDURES
Procedure for cannulation

1. A longitudinal pericardial incision is made, and the pericardial edges are retracted by suture to the chest wall.
2. The aorta, if it is to be cannulated for arterial blood return to the patient, is partially dissected from the pulmonary artery. If there are atrial adhesions, these are dissected.
3. Pursestring sutures are placed in the aorta (×2) and right atrium (or both venae cavae) for the eventual placement of the perfusion cannulas. Tourniquets are placed over the suture ends and held with a hemostat.
4. The ascending aorta is cannulated for the arterial blood return. If the aorta is not calcified, a partial occlusion clamp may be used to isolate a segment of the aortic wall. (Calcium may be seen on x-ray and is palpable at

operation.) The wall is incised, the cannula is inserted, and the pursestring suture is firmly secured with the tourniquet. It is important to have the distal end of the cannula clamped before it is inserted into the aorta to prevent back-bleeding from the aorta. The arterial cannulation is generally performed before the caval cannulation so that direct access for blood replacement is available if needed.

5. Venous cannulation: for the venous return to the pump-oxygenator, an incision is made in the right atrial appendage, and the two-stage cannula (see Fig. 26-37) is inserted into the atrium. The distal end of the cannula is placed in the inferior vena cava. The pursestring suture is secured with a tourniquet, and the catheter is permitted to fill partially with blood before being connected to the venous line. When double cannulation is used, a second incision is made in the atrial wall within the pursestring, and the cannulas are placed in the inferior and superior venae cavae (see Fig. 26-36). To force all venous return into the cannulas, umbilical tapes with tourniquets may be placed around each cava and then tightened. This forces all systemic venous return to enter the cannulas, producing total CPB. Coronary sinus venous return from the heart is vented with an intracardiac vent (see Fig. 26-39).
6. In procedures where greater exposure of the right atrium is required (such as tricuspid valve surgery, closure of atrial septal defects in adults), a right-angled cannula may be inserted in the superior vena cava (Fig. 26-41).

Procedure for femoral cutdown for arterial cannulation. To save time, a second team may simultaneously prepare the arterial return site if the femoral artery is selected for cannulation. A vertical or oblique incision is made in the femoral triangle, and the femoral artery is exposed. Umbilical compression tapes are passed around the vessel above and below the proposed arteriotomy. (Two vascular

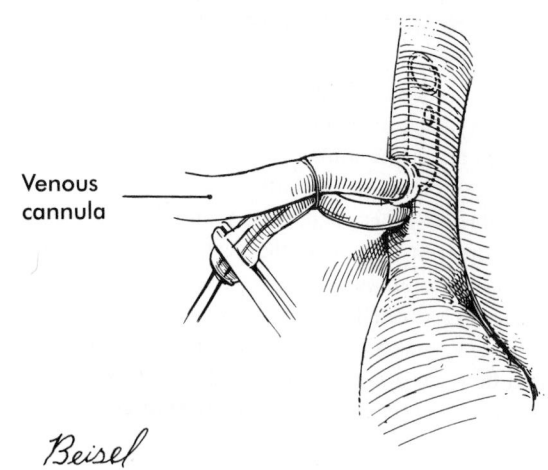

Venous cannula

FIG. 26-41   Right-angle cannula in superior vena cava.
From Waldhausen JA and Pierce WS. (1985). *Johnson's surgery of the chest*, ed. 5, St. Louis, Mosby.

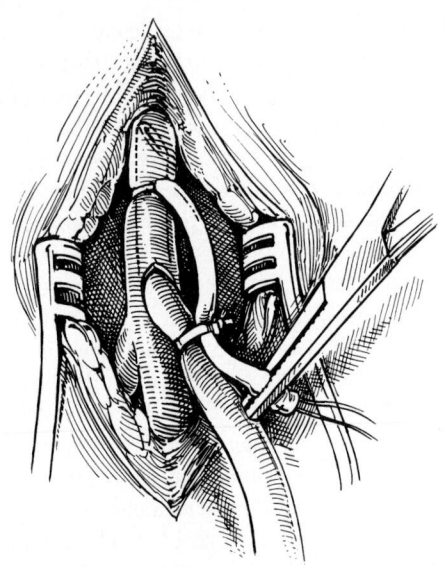

FIG. 26-42 Cannulation of femoral artery.

From Waldhausen JA and Pierce WS. (1985). *Johnson's surgery of the chest*, ed. 5, St. Louis, Mosby.

clamps may also be applied to the vessel.) An incision is made into the vessel, and the perfusion catheter is inserted retrogradely into the artery as the proximal clamp or tourniquet is released. After the cannula is in place, the proximal tourniquet is tightened to prevent bleeding from the arteriotomy. A clamp must be on the distal end of the perfusion cannula before it is inserted into the artery (Fig. 26-42).

Procedure for pump-oxygenator preparation. While the surgical team prepares the cannulations for connection to the pump-oxygenator, the perfusionist tests and completes assemblage of the equipment.

1. Before the incision is made, the tubing is passed to the perfusionist after the proximal ends have been secured to the drapes.
2. After the venous and arterial lines are connected to the pump-oxygenator, blood is pumped through the lines to displace air in the tubing. To prevent air emboli, caution is exercised, particularly as the arterial connection is completed. This connection is usually made under a saline drip, or by having the perfusionist slowly pump priming solution out of the arterial line.
3. When all connections are properly secured and the pump-oxygenator is ready, CPB is begun and the desired flow rate gradually achieved. The perfusion rate is adjusted as necessary during the operation.

Procedure for bypass termination

1. After the intracardiac procedure has been completed, all air is evacuated from the left ventricle. A warm dose of cardioplegia may be given, after which the cross-clamp is removed.

2. Defibrillation is often spontaneous with removal of the aortic cross-clamp and the entry of warm blood into the coronary circulation. If not, electrical defibrillation is necessary. Temporary epicardial pacing wires are attached to the atrium and to the ventricle.
3. Venous flow to the pump is reduced. Arterial flow is also reduced to equal the venous return. When heart action is sufficient and systemic arterial blood pressure is stabilized, venous return is further reduced, and the patient is taken off bypass by clamping all lines and stopping the pump.
4. As the cannulation catheters are removed, the pursestring sutures are tightened and tied. Additional sutures may be required for hemostasis.
5. Chest tubes are inserted into the pericardium (and the pleural cavity if the pleura has been opened).
6. Protamine sulfate, a heparin antagonist, is administered.
7. The pericardium is usually left open so that accumulating drainage does not produce cardiac tamponade.

Closure of femoral incision

1. The femoral catheter is removed, and the arteriotomy is closed with nonabsorbable cardiovascular suture. Compression tapes and bulldog clamps, if used, are removed.
2. The wound is closed with absorbable sutures, and the skin is closed with interrupted or continuous sutures.
3. Dressings are applied to all wounds.

PERICARDIECTOMY

Pericardiectomy is the partial excision of the adhered, thickened fibrotic pericardium to relieve constriction of compressed heart and large blood vessels.

Myocardial contractility is restricted by the adhered portions of the scarred, thickened pericardium. As the pericardial space is obliterated and calcification of the pericardium occurs, the heart is further compressed. Ascites, elevated venous pressure, decreased arterial pressure, edema, and hepatic enlargement result. This condition is usually caused by chronic pericarditis, which may be of tubercular, rheumatic, viral, or neoplastic origin.

Procedural considerations. Occasionally cardiopulmonary bypass may be requested on a standby basis, but usually the supplies and instruments for bypass are not needed.

Operative procedure

1. The lungs are displaced laterally, and the right and left phrenic nerves are identified and carefully protected. The pericardium is incised.
2. The outer thickened pericardium is removed as indicated. Cartilage scissors may be required. The fibrous portions adhering to the atria and ventricles are carefully dissected with dry dissectors and scissors. Caution is exercised to prevent perforation of the atria and right ventricle; thus small areas of adherent pericardium may be retained.
3. Dissection is continued, and the large blood vessels are exposed and freed as indicated.

4. Drainage catheters are placed near the heart or through the pleural spaces. Connections to the water-seal drainage system are established as described in Chapter 24.

SURGERY FOR CORONARY ARTERY DISEASE

Treatment of coronary artery disease includes revascularization of the ischemic myocardium with coronary artery bypass grafting (CABG) using autogenous saphenous vein and the internal (thoracic) mammary artery (IMA) or other conduits, and repair of left ventricular aneurysm. Also included are surgery for ischemia-related disorders: mitral valve regurgitation (MR), dysrhythmias, and ventricular septal defects (VSDs), discussed below. CABG often alleviates angina pectoris, and it prolongs life in patients with left main coronary disease and triple-vessel disease. The IMA demonstrates excellent long-term patency (Loop et al., 1986); the increasing number of reoperations for coronary

---

┌───┐
│   BOX 26-4   │
│   │
│   **Alternative Conduits for Use as Coronary**│
│   **Bypass Grafts**   │
│ ─── │
│   │
│ Gastroepiploic artery   │
│ Inferior epigastric artery   │
│ Splenic artery   │
│ Radial artery   │
│ Lesser saphenous vein   │
│ Cephalic vein   │
│ Basilic vein   │
│ Greater saphenous vein allografts (homografts)│
│ Synthetic grafts (e.g., Dacron, PTFE)   │
│   │
│ Adapted from Glick, D.B., Liddicoat, J.R., & Karp, R.B. (1990). Al-│
│ ternative conduits for coronary artery bypass grafting. In *Advances in*│
│ *cardiac surgery* (Vol. 2). St. Louis: Mosby.│
└───┘

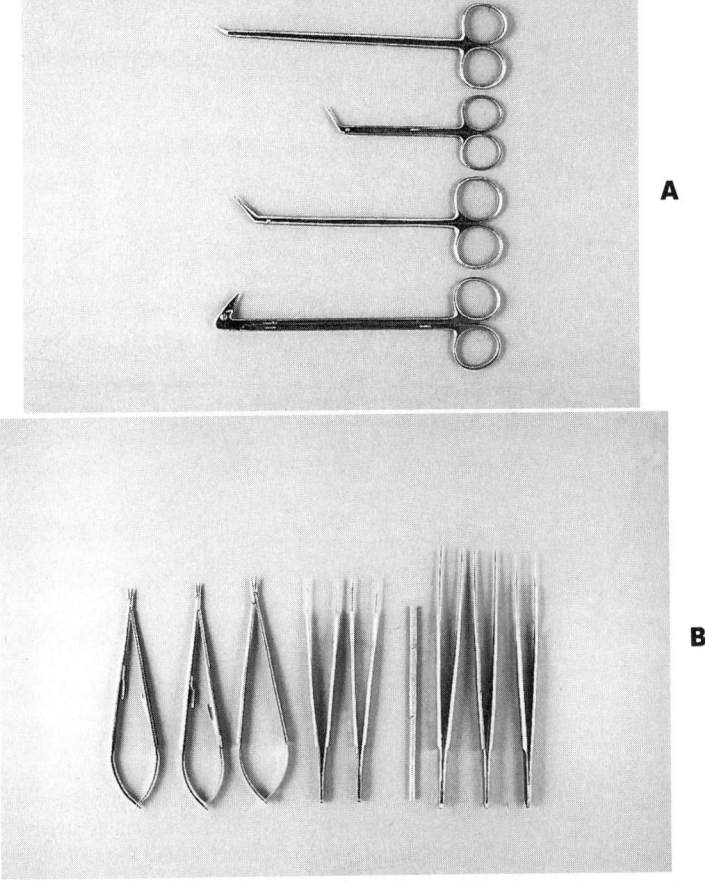

FIG. 26-43 **A,** Potts scissors. **B,** Castroviejo needle holders *(left),* fine forceps, and Beaver knife handle for coronary artery surgery.

From Brooks-Tighe S. (1994). *Instrumentation for the operating room,* ed. 4, St. Louis, Mosby.

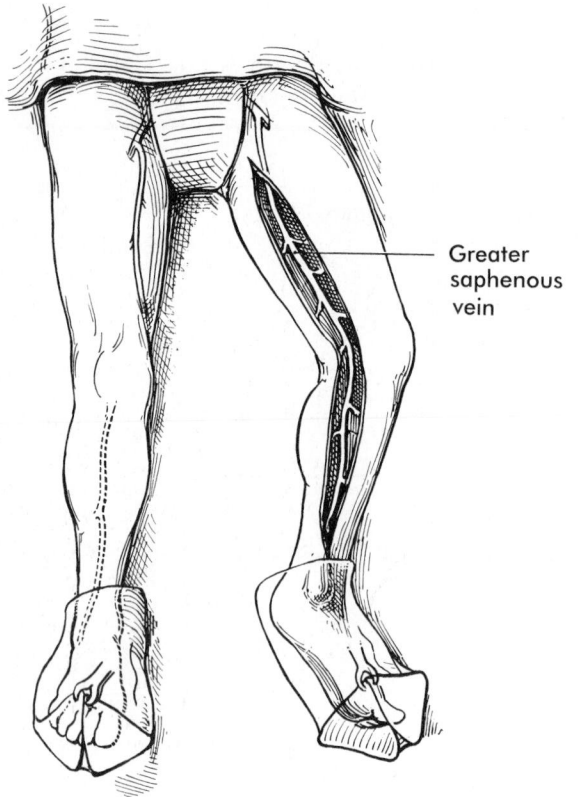

FIG. 26-44   Excision of greater saphenous vein.

From Waldhausen JA and Pierce WS. (1985). *Johnson's surgery of the chest,* ed. 5, St. Louis, Mosby.

artery disease has stimulated the use of alternative conduits (Box 26-4) such as the gastroepiploic artery and the inferior epigastric artery (Lytle et al., 1989; Glick et al., 1990).

Coronary artery instruments (Fig. 26-43) are added to the basic setup for cardiac surgery.

CABG with saphenous vein and IMA
Operative procedure

1. A median sternotomy is performed as described; the necessary length of saphenous vein is harvested from one or both legs (Fig. 26-44), and tributaries are ligated. The distal end of the vein is identified to place the vein in a reversed position so that the semilunar valves do not interfere with the flow of blood. The vein is flushed with heparinized blood or saline and kept moist until needed.

2. The IMA is dissected free from its retrosternal bed (Fig. 26-45). A special retractor, such as the one shown in Fig. 26-15, can be used to expose the IMA until the necessary length is obtained. Clips and electrocoagulation are used for hemostasis. Occasionally, both right and left IMAs are used. (Heparin is given before clamping and cutting arterial grafts to prevent intraluminal thrombosis.)

3. Cardiopulmonary bypass is instituted as previously described. Usually, mild hypothermia is employed. Antegrade/retrograde cardioplegia is infused, after the aorta is cross-clamped.

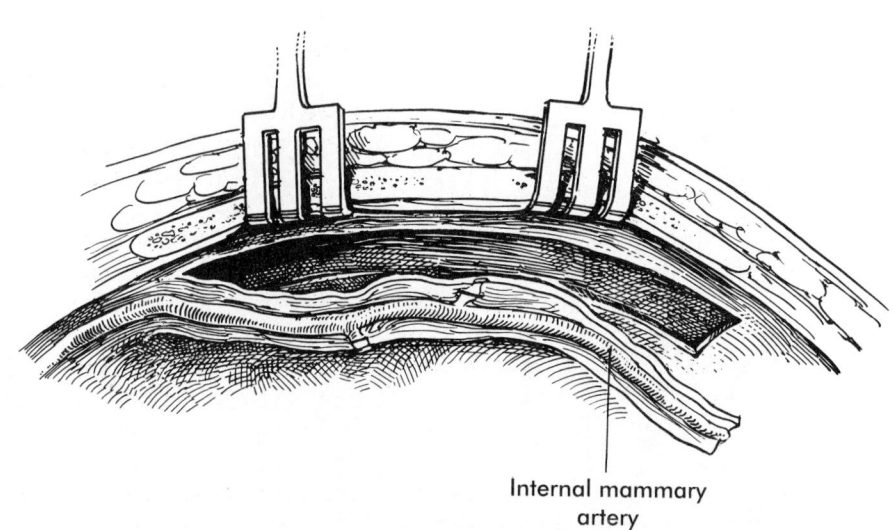

FIG. 26-45   Dissection of internal mammary artery (IMA). Bleeding from side branches is controlled by vascular clips on the IMA side and cautery on the sternal side. Dilute solution of papaverine is sprayed onto, and in the lumen of, the IMA to dilate the artery and reduce muscular spasm. The IMA pedicle may be wrapped in a papaverine-soaked gauze sponge, or placed within the pleural cavity, until needed for anastomosis.

From Waldhausen JA and Pierce WS. (1985). *Johnson's surgery of the chest,* ed. 5, St. Louis, Mosby.

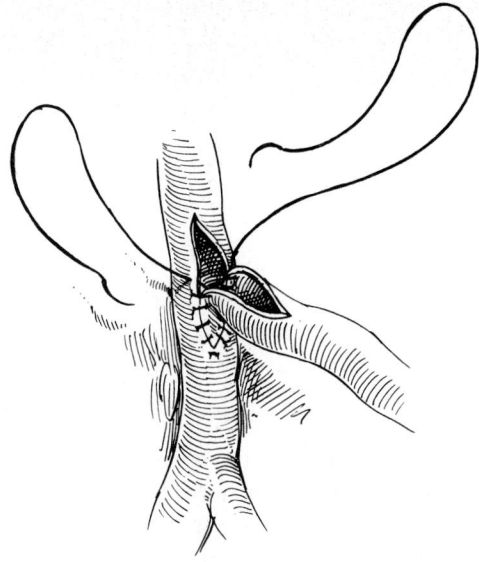

FIG. 26-46   End-to-side coronary anastomosis with vein graft.
From Waldhausen JA and Pierce WS. (1985). *Johnson's surgery of the chest*, ed. 5, St. Louis, Mosby.

4. Coronary anastomoses
   a. The affected coronary artery is identified, and a small incision is made into the coronary artery. The vein is beveled to approximate the incision (side-to-side jump grafts may be performed as well).
   b. The anastomosis is made with fine cardiovascular sutures (Fig. 26-46). Before the anastomosis is completed, the distal coronary artery may be probed to ensure patency.
   c. Steps a and b are repeated for each subsequent anastomosis.
5. The distal anastomosis of the IMA to the coronary artery is done as described for the anastomosis of the saphenous vein graft to the coronary artery. No aortic (proximal) anastomosis is required because the IMA remains intact at its takeoff from the subclavian artery.
6. Aortic anastomoses
   a. Aortic anastomoses may be performed while the aorta is cross-clamped; or the aortic clamp is removed, the heart defibrillated, and the anastomoses completed after each distal (coronary) anastomosis. When the proximal (aortic) anastomoses are performed on a beating heart, the aorta is partially occluded with an angled vascular clamp, such as a Beck or Kay clamp, and a small segment is resected, approximately the diameter of the vein graft. An aortic punch may be used for this (Fig. 26-47).
   b. The vein is anastomosed, end to side, to the aorta with fine vascular sutures. The partial occlusion clamp is removed, allowing the proximal portion of the vein to fill with blood. Needle aspiration of the

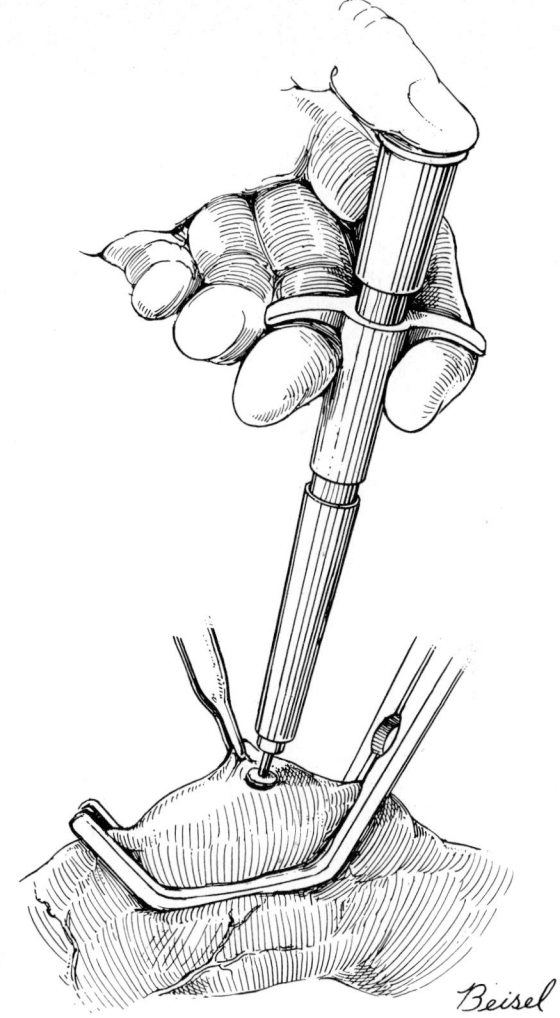

FIG. 26-47   Proximal anastomosis of bypass graft. A partial occlusion clamp isolates the portion of the ascending aorta where the aortotomy is to be made with the punch.
From Waldhausen JA and Pierce WS. (1985). *Johnson's surgery of the chest*, ed. 5, St. Louis, Mosby.

vein graft is performed to prevent air from entering the coronary circulation.
   c. When proximal anastomoses are performed during a single period of cross-clamping, air is aspirated from the grafts before the cross-clamp is removed.
7. The aortic anastomoses of the vein grafts are usually marked with clips or rings for future identification (Fig. 26-48).
8. In patients requiring additional conduits (such as bypass grafts) or in whom arterial grafts are preferred (such as those at high risk for vein graft closure), the gastroepiploic artery may be used (Fig. 26-49). Alternative conduits are listed in Box 26-4.
9. Cardiopulmonary bypass is discontinued, and the sternum is closed.

Ventricular aneurysmectomy

Ventricular aneurysmectomy is the excision of an aneurysmic portion of the left ventricle and reinforcement with synthetic patch material (Fig. 26-50). An aneurysm of the left ventricle occasionally develops after a severe myocardial infarction in which part of the myocardium is replaced

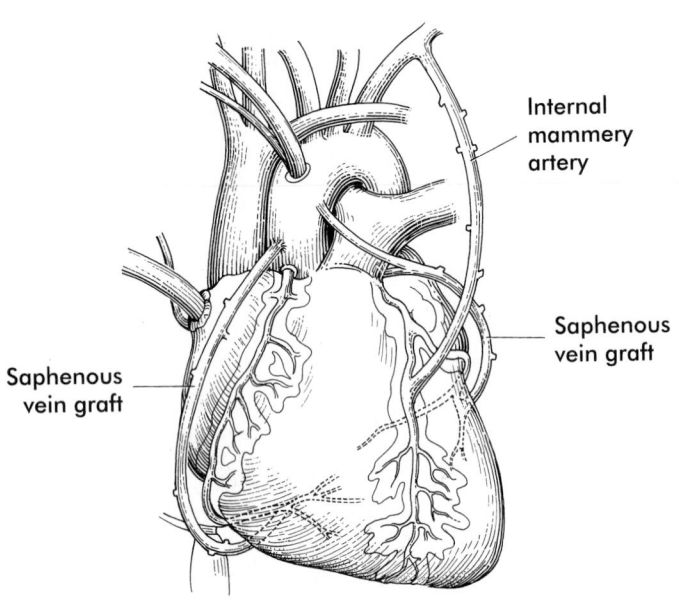

FIG. 26-48   Coronary artery bypass grafts with reversed saphenous vein and the left internal mammary artery.

by thin scar tissue. The scar may stretch as a result of the left ventricular pressure, thus forming an aneurysm. The aneurysm is usually adherent to the pericardium, and it may not be possible to dissect it free until cardiopulmonary bypass has been established.

Procedural considerations. The patient is placed in the supine position. The setup is as described for open heart surgery, plus Teflon felt strips, pledgets, and no. 0 cardiovascular sutures on a large needle. Occasionally, patch closure of the ventriculotomy is performed (endoaneurysmorrhaphy); synthetic patch material and 3-0 or 4-0 polypropylene sutures are used (Cooley, 1989).

Operative procedure

1. A median sternotomy is performed, and cardiopulmonary bypass is begun as described.
2. The scar tissue of the ventricle is excised and any clot removed carefully (Fig. 26-50, *A* and *B*).
3. A cuff of scar tissue is left, through which heavy cardiovascular sutures reinforced with Teflon felt pledgets are passed (Fig. 26-50, *C*).
4. The left ventricle may be vented with an apical catheter; after the ventricle is de-aired, the catheter is removed and closure of the incision completed.

Postinfarction ventricular septal defects (VSDs)

Ventricular septal (or free wall) rupture is a catastrophic complication of myocardial infarction, creating an acute

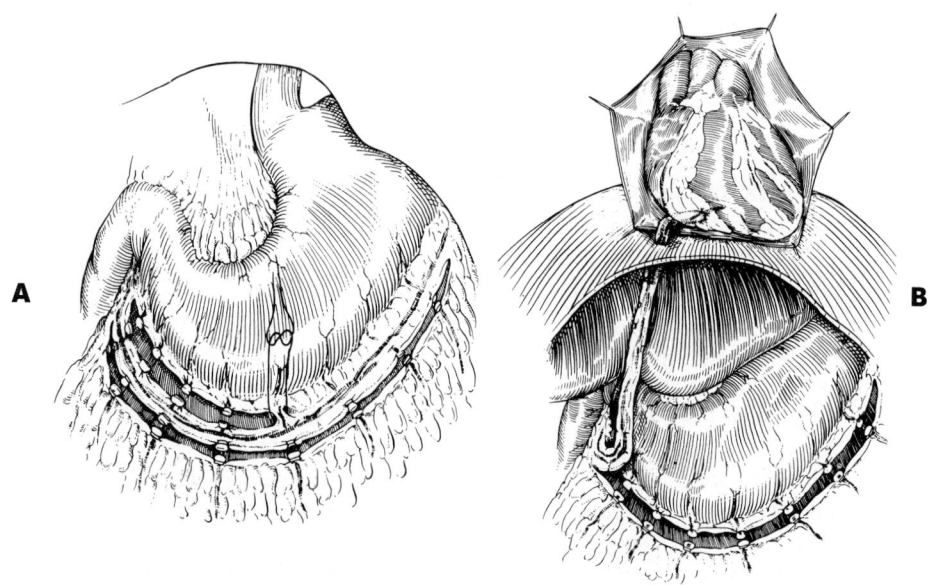

FIG. 26-49   **A,** Branches to the stomach are divided with clamps and ties; omental branches may be divided with a staple gun. The gastroepiploic pedicle is isolated proximal to its origin from the gastroduodenal artery. **B,** The pedicle is brought up into the pericardium and anastomosed to the right coronary artery (shown here). The artery can also be grafted to the distal right and left anterior descending coronary arteries.

From Lytle BW and others. (1989). Coronary artery bypass grafting with the right gastroepiploic artery, *J Thorac Cardiovasc Surg* 97(6):826.

left-to-right shunt and cardiac failure. Emergency surgery is necessary to close the defect with a patch. Surgical technique is similar to that used to close muscular VSDs in the child with congenital VSD (see Chapter 28).

SURGERY FOR THE MITRAL VALVE

Mitral stenosis, the most common acquired valvular lesion, is usually caused by rheumatic fever. The normal opening in the valve is about 5 cm². As the disease progresses, the mitral valve becomes a narrow slit in a fibrotic plaque, severely limiting blood flow into the left ventricle. Mitral stenosis causes a rise in pressure and dilatation of the left atrium. This pressure is transmitted through-

out the pulmonary vascular bed, with subsequent pulmonary hypertension, right ventricular hypertrophy, and possibly tricuspid valve regurgitation.

The major symptoms are dyspnea, fatigue, and orthopnea. Late findings are severe pulmonary congestion and right ventricular failure (Schakenbach, 1987). A characteristic diastolic murmur is heard, and atrial fibrillation is not unusual. An embolism may result from clots in the atrial appendage. Later findings are severe pulmonary congestion and right ventricular failure.

Mitral regurgitation may accompany mitral stenosis or be due to leaflet perforation, annular dilatation, or elongated or ruptured chordae. Ischemic heart disease may produce

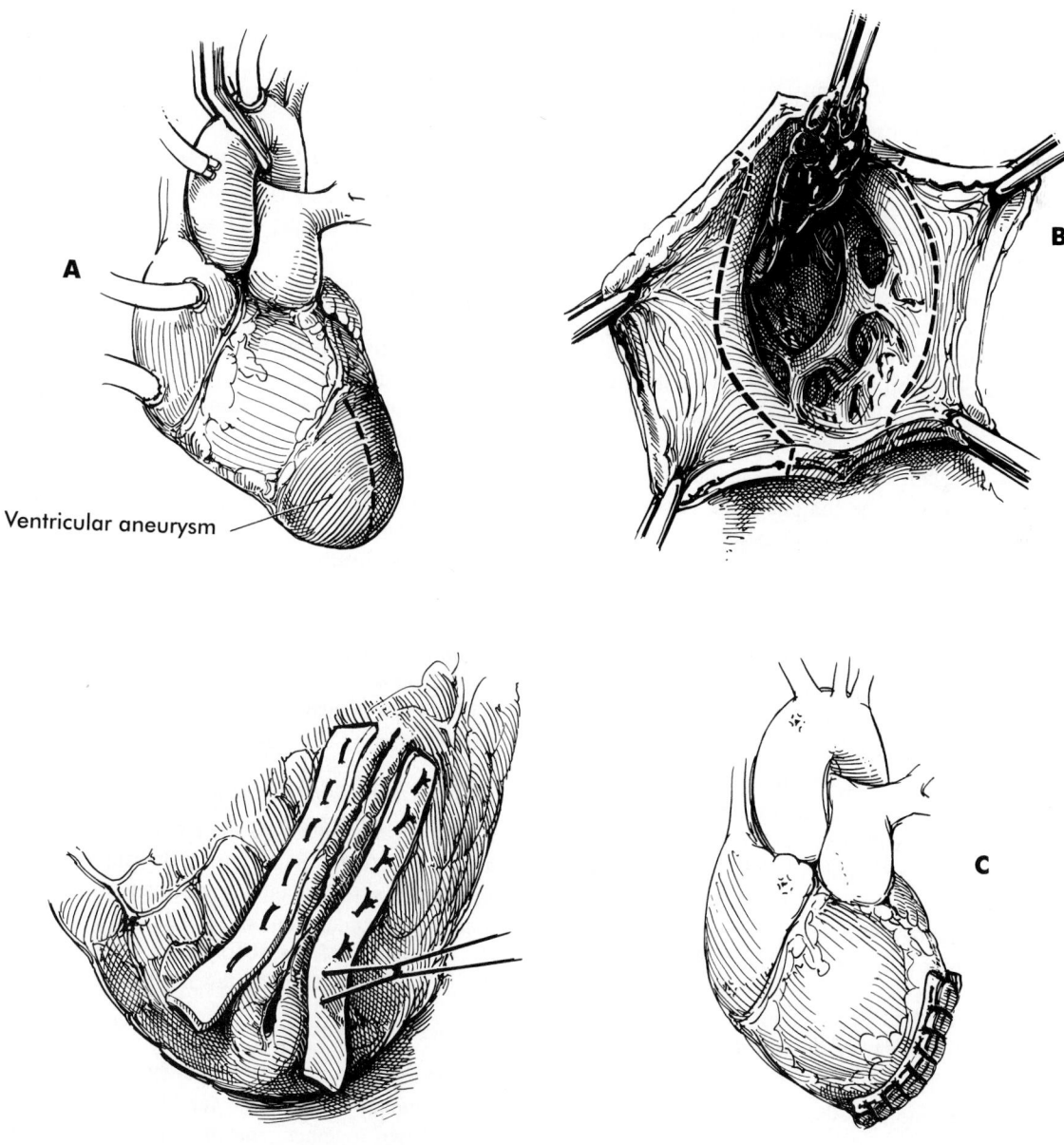

FIG. 26-50 Repair left ventricular aneurysm (see text).
From Waldhausen JA and Pierce WS. (1985). *Johnson's surgery of the chest*, ed. 5, St. Louis, Mosby.

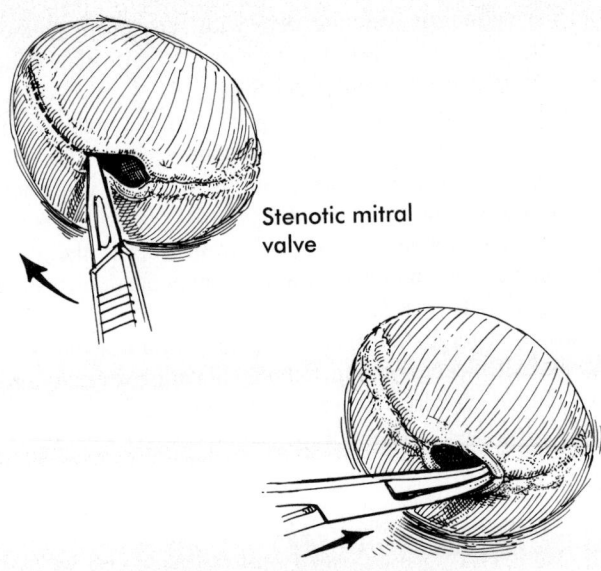

Stenotic mitral valve

FIG. 26-51 Mitral commissurotomy (see text).
From Waldhausen JA and Pierce WS. (1985). *Johnson's surgery of the chest*, ed. 5, St. Louis, Mosby.

papillary muscle dysfunction. Symptoms include those seen with stenosis and with left ventricular dilatation from the increased volume load on the left ventricle.

The surgeon's selection of the procedure (repair or replacement) is determined by the stage of disease, presence or absence of calcification, history of thromboembolism and heart rhythm, ability to tolerate chronic anticoagulation, and any associated pathologic defects.

Reparative procedures that preserve the native valve are widely employed because the complications associated with prosthetic replacement and anticoagulation can be avoided. The technique selected must be tailored to the unique pathophysiologic findings; therefore the surgeon carefully evaluates the leaflets and related structures prior to deciding which operation to perform. Because there is always a possibility that the valve may have to be replaced, instruments (and prostheses) for replacement as well as repairs should be available. Also included are atrial hand-held or self-retaining retractors (see Figs. 26-16 and 26-17), obturators for sizing prosthetic rings and valves (see Figs. 26-25, *B*, and 26-27); sizer or prosthesis handles, and special suture if requested. Bicaval cannulation is used to enhance exposure of the operative field (see Fig. 26-36). Transesophageal echocardiography (TEE) is performed to assess ventricular and valvular function before and after repair.

Mitral valve repairs
Open commissurotomy of the mitral valve for mitral stenosis

Open commissurotomy is the separation of fused, adherent leaflets of the mitral valve under direct vision (Fig. 26-51).

Procedural considerations. The patient is placed in a supine position for a median sternotomy. The setup is as described for open heart procedures, with mitral valve instruments.

Operative procedure

1. A median sternotomy is performed, and bicaval cannulation is performed for cardiopulmonary bypass.
2. The left atrium is incised, and the valve is inspected.
3. Fused leaflets are separated with vascular forceps and scissors and/or a knife (Fig. 26-51). A dilator may be used to enlarge the mitral valve orifice.
4. The valve is again inspected for any resultant insufficiency with a bulb syringe.
5. The left atrium is closed with a continuous cardiovascular suture.
6. TEE can be used to confirm efficacy of the repair after the cross-clamp is removed and the heart resumes beating, and again after bypass is discontinued. TEE can also be used to detect the presence of air within the cardiac chambers.

Mitral annuloplasty for mitral regurgitation

Mitral annuloplasty is the reduction of a dilated annulus using a suture technique or inserting a prosthetic ring (see Fig. 26-33).

Operative procedure

1. The left atrium is incised, and sump suctions are inserted into the atrial cavity to remove blood.
2. The annulus, leaflets, chordae, and the rest of the mitral complex are inspected.
3. If there is generalized annular dilatation, a Carpentier (1983) ring technique is often used. An obturator is used to determine the appropriate size ring (Fig. 26-52, *top*). Interrupted sutures are placed around the circumference of the annulus and then into the ring (Fig. 26-52, *middle*). When the stitches are tied, the excess annular tissue is evenly drawn up against the prosthesis (Fig. 26-52, *bottom*).
4. The valve is inspected for residual insufficiency, and the left atrium is closed.

Mitral valvuloplasty for mitral regurgitation

Mitral valvuloplasty is the repair of the valve leaflets or related structures. Selection of the appropriate repair for perforated or redundant valve leaflets or for shortened or elongated chordae tendineae requires careful assessment and evaluation of the abnormalities present (Delouche et al., 1990; Cosgrove and Stewart, 1989).

Operative procedure

1. Perforated leaflets can be patched with pericardium.
2. Redundant leaflet tissue can be resected. The cut edges are sewn together, and the corresponding annular segment is plicated. An annuloplasty ring also may be inserted as described previously.

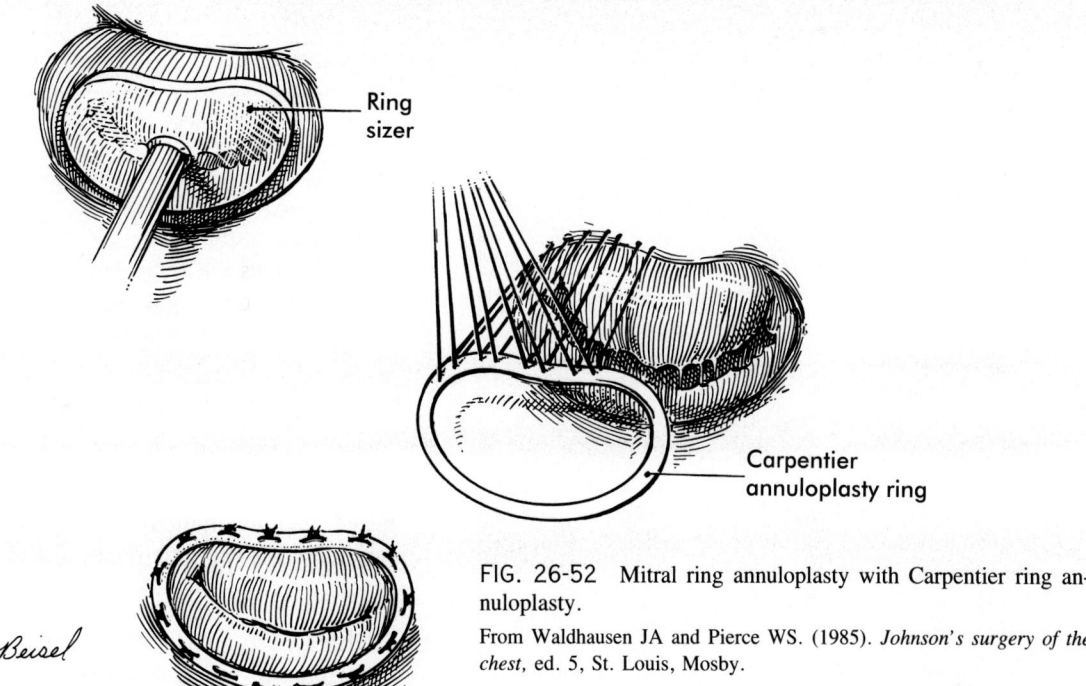

Ring sizer

Carpentier annuloplasty ring

Beisel

FIG. 26-52   Mitral ring annuloplasty with Carpentier ring annuloplasty.

From Waldhausen JA and Pierce WS. (1985). *Johnson's surgery of the chest,* ed. 5, St. Louis, Mosby.

3. Shortened, fused chordae tendineae can be lengthened and mobilized by their division into secondary chordae or by incising the tip of the papillary muscles.
4. Redundant tissue of elongated chordae may be implanted into the papillary muscle head or folded over itself and secured with a suture (Fig. 26-53).
5. TEE is used to assess the repair.

Mitral valve replacement (MVR)

Mitral valve replacement is the excision of the mitral valve leaflets and replacement with a mechanical or biologic prosthesis (see Figs. 26-23 to 26-28). Generally the mural (posterior) leaflet and associated chordae and papillary muscles are retained to maintain ventricular geometry, thereby enhancing ventricular function.

Procedural considerations. Although the surgeon may intend to implant a specific type of prosthesis, patient-related factors (Box 26-5) or prosthetic valve complications (Box 26-6) may modify the plan (Butchart and Bodner, 1992). A complete range of valves should be available, as well as saline to rinse the glutaraldehyde storage solution from biologic prostheses, should they be used. Pledgeted suture of alternating colors is used. Venting catheters and aspirating needles are used to remove air from the heart and ascending aorta. A small dental mirror may be used after a bioprosthesis has been implanted to ensure that sutures are not caught in the subvalvular area.

Operative procedure. Venous drainage cannulae may (Fig. 26-54, *A*) or may not be crossed in the atrium.

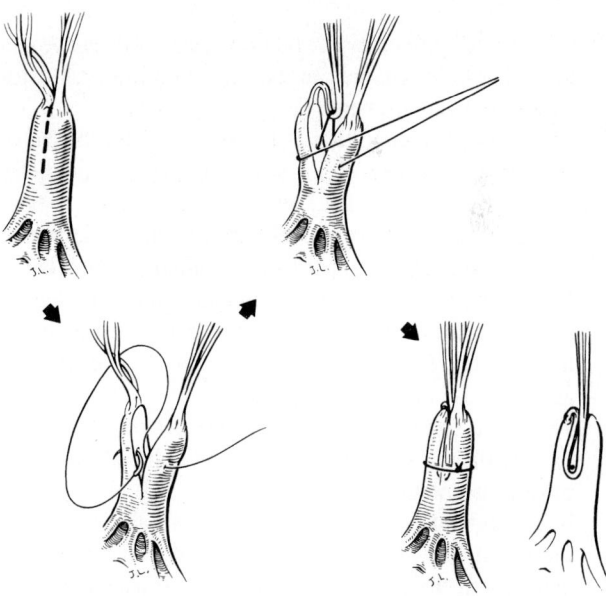

FIG. 26-53   Chordal shortening is accomplished by incising the papillary muscle and burying the chordae in it.

From Cosgrove DM and Stewart WJ. (1989). Mitral valvuloplasty. *Curr Prob Cardiol 14*(7):359.

1. The aorta is cross-clamped with a curved or straight vascular occlusion clamp and cardioplegia infused through the aortic root, or more commonly, retrograde through the coronary sinus.

pleted. It is important to evacuate the air completely before the cross-clamp is removed and the heart resumes beating.

SURGERY FOR THE TRICUSPID VALVE
Tricuspid valve annuloplasty

Tricuspid valve annuloplasty is the reduction of a dilated annulus with a suture technique or a prosthetic ring. Tricuspid valve regurgitation may be caused by bacterial endocarditis (related to the use of nonsterile intravenous drug paraphernalia). It is often the functional result of mitral valve disease. If the tricuspid valve does not regain competence after mitral valve correction or if tricuspid annular dilatation occurs, repairs similar to mitral annuloplasty may be performed. Caution is taken to avoid injury to the atrioventricular (AV) node.

Operative procedure

1. Double venous cannulas are inserted so that they do not cross one another in the right atrium, and occluding tapes are tightened around the cavae and cannulas to prevent venous return from entering the right atrium and obscuring the surgical site. A right-angle venous cannula (see Fig. 26-41) may be placed in the superior vena cava.
2. The right atrium is opened longitudinally to expose the tricuspid valve. Sump suctions are inserted to remove coronary sinus drainage.
3a. In the DeVega technique (Rabago et al, 1980) (Fig. 26-55) a double-armed, felt-pledgeted suture is placed in the valve annulus, beginning at the anteroseptal commissure and continued around to the level of the coronary sinus orifice. The remaining arm of suture is similarly placed. The suture is tied over a pledget with sufficient tension to reduce the annular area to the size desired.
3b. In the Carpentier (1983) technique a prosthetic ring is inserted in a manner similar to mitral valve ring annuloplasty (see Fig. 26-52). To avoid potential injury to the AV node, tricuspid valve rings often have an inter-

2. The left atrium is incised, blood is suctioned away, and the incision is enlarged to expose the mitral valve for subsequent replacement (Fig. 26-54, *A* to *C*).
3. The pathologic condition is determined, and the valve leaflets are excised along with the anterior papillary muscle and chordae tendineae (Fig. 26-54, *D*). Selection of the cutting instrument depends on the degree of calcification present and the method of excision. Rongeurs may be used to débride calcium particles. A small margin of the valve annulus is retained to insert fixation sutures to the valve. The ventricle is inspected, and all loose debris is removed.
4. The valve sizer is used to determine the correct size of the prosthesis, which is delivered to the field. The valve prosthesis holder is attached.
5. Nonabsorbable cardiovascular sutures (about 20) are placed in the retained margin of the valve and then placed into the sewing ring of the prosthesis (Fig. 26-54, *E*).
6. The sutures are held taut (and moistened) as the prosthesis is guided into position and secured, and the sutures are tied and cut.
7. Continuous nonabsorbable sutures are used to close the atriotomy (Fig. 26-54, *F*). The patient is placed in reverse Trendelenburg position and the lungs inflated to remove air from the pulmonary veins and atrium. Air is aspirated from the left ventricle through a hypodermic needle or vent catheter, and the atrial closure is com-

ruption in that portion corresponding to the area of the nodal conduction tissue.

4. Saline may be injected into the ventricle to test the competence of the repair, and TEE also employed.

5. The right atrium is closed with nonabsorbable suture.

SURGERY FOR THE AORTIC VALVE

Aortic stenosis produces obstruction of the left ventricular outflow. Whether caused by rheumatic fever, a congenital bicuspid valve, or calcific degeneration, the fused valve leaflets present an increasing pressure load on the ventricle. To compensate, the ventricle hypertrophies so that it can generate sufficient pressure to eject blood through the narrowed opening. When disease is severe, large pressure gradients are often measured during cardiac catheterization, with differences in systolic pressures between the ventricle and the aorta reaching 50 mm Hg or greater. In the early stages of the disease, a systolic aortic murmur may be heard, but patients are rarely symptomatic; eventually fatigue, exertional dyspnea, angina pectoris, syncope, and congestive heart failure may develop, presenting a grave prognosis. Sudden death is not uncommon.

Balloon valvuloplasty has been performed in elderly patients for whom surgery poses too great a risk (Braunwald, 1992) but valvuloplasty is not without risk (the operating room is often on "standby"). Total valve excision and replacement with a prosthesis (or an allograft) are often necessary.

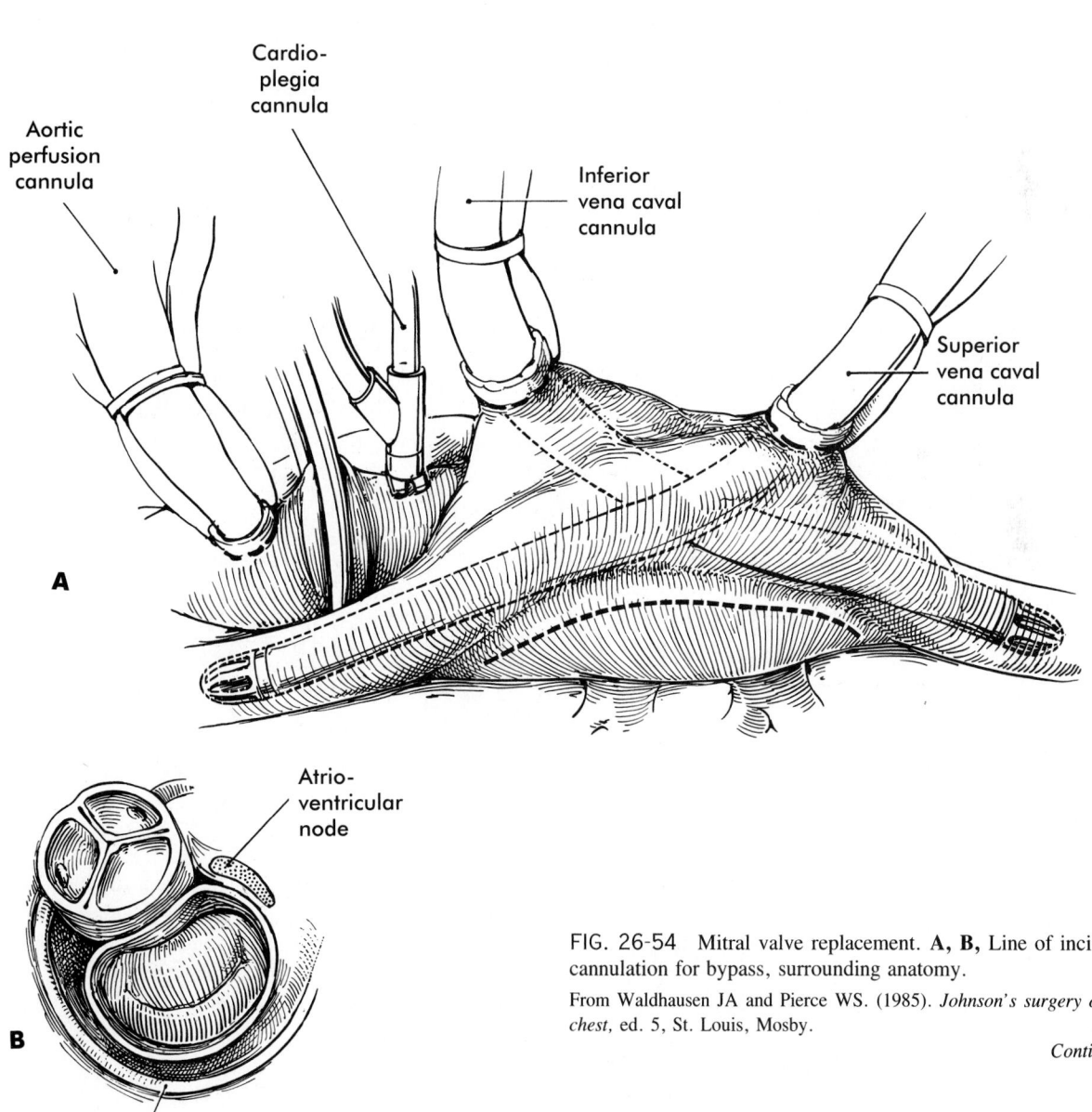

FIG. 26-54 Mitral valve replacement. **A, B,** Line of incision, cannulation for bypass, surrounding anatomy.

From Waldhausen JA and Pierce WS. (1985). *Johnson's surgery of the chest,* ed. 5, St. Louis, Mosby.

Continued.

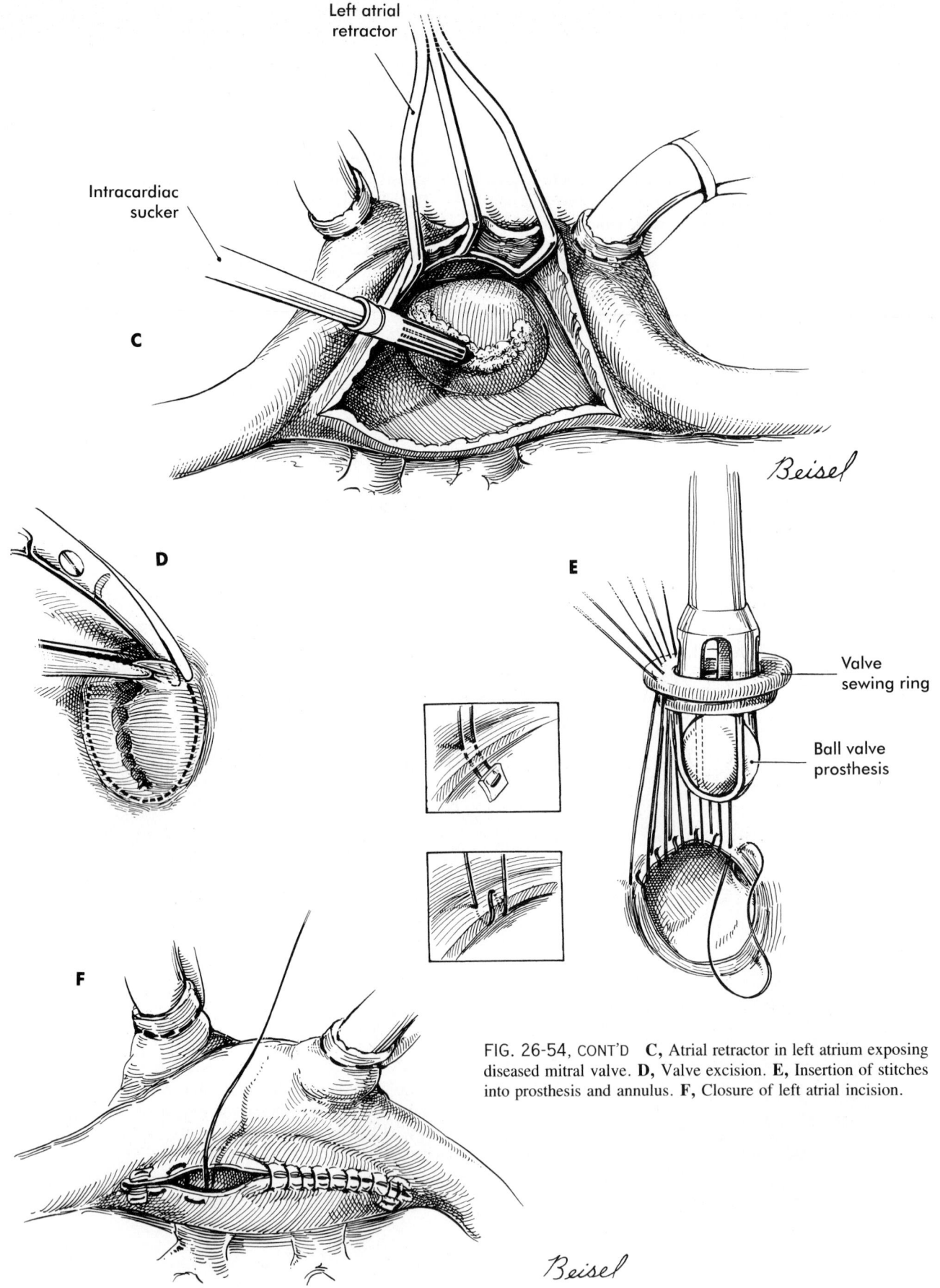

Left atrial
retractor

Intracardiac
sucker

C

Beisel

D

E

Valve
sewing ring

Ball valve
prosthesis

F

FIG. 26-54, CONT'D   **C,** Atrial retractor in left atrium exposing
diseased mitral valve. **D,** Valve excision. **E,** Insertion of stitches
into prosthesis and annulus. **F,** Closure of left atrial incision.

Beisel

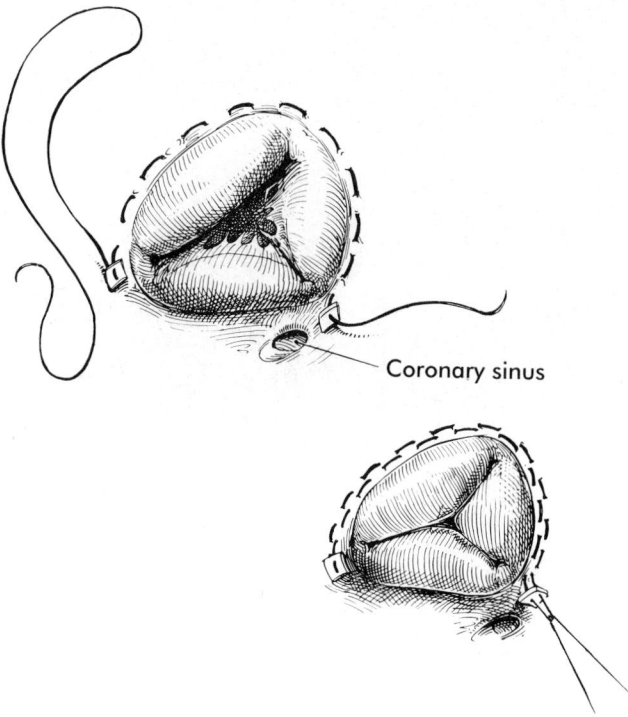

Coronary sinus

FIG. 26-55   DeVega tricuspid annuloplasty.

From Waldhausen JA and Pierce WS. (1985). *Johnson's surgery of the chest*, ed. 5, St. Louis, Mosby.

Diastolic regurgitation of blood into the left ventricle is caused by aortic insufficiency. Rheumatic fever, connective tissue disorders, and infective endocarditis may be responsible. As this volume load increases, the left ventricle compensates by dilatation and, later, hypertrophy. Symptoms of coronary insufficiency, cerebral hypoperfusion, and congestive failure are later findings.

Aortic valve replacement

The aortic valve is excised and replaced with a mechanical or biologic prosthesis or an aortic valve allograft (see Figs. 26-29 and 26-30).

Procedural considerations. To the basic setup are added the following:

Aortic valve instruments
Aortic valves, sizers, and holders
Saline to rinse biologic prostheses or allografts

Coronary artery retrograde infusion cannula and venting catheters

Operative procedure

1. After the institution of CPB, a left ventricular vent is inserted through a stab wound into the right pulmonary vein, and the tip is advanced into the left ventricle (Fig. 26-56, *A*).
2. The aorta is cross-clamped. If aortic insufficiency is present, the initial bolus of cardioplegia is infused retrogradely. If aortic stenosis is present, the initial bolus of cardioplegia may be infused into the aortic root. Once the heart is arrested, the aorta is opened.
3. The native valve is inspected and the extent of the pathologic defect confirmed. If calcium deposits are present, they are débrided with scissors or rongeurs. The valve is carefully excised to avoid injury to the annulus and underlying structures (Fig. 26-56, *B*). Narrow packing may be used in the left ventricle to confine small, loose, calcified fragments that could subsequently embolize. Instruments should be wiped clean frequently.
4. The annulus is sized, the proper prosthesis selected, and a prosthesis holder attached.
5. If a biologic valve is selected, it is delivered to the field and rinsed in saline baths.
5b. If an allograft is used, it is delivered to the field and thawed in saline baths according to protocol.
5c. If a mechanical valve is chosen, it may be placed in an antibiotic solution until inserted. (Antibiotic solutions should not be poured directly onto biologic valves.) Biologic valves should be kept moist with frequent saline irrigation.
6a. The new valve is implanted using a technique similar to that previously described for mitral valve replacement (Fig. 26-56, *D* and *E*).
6b. If the aortic annulus is too small to accept a prosthesis of adequate size, a Konno procedure can be used to enlarge the annulus and proximal portion of the ascending aorta (Waldhausen and Pierce, 1985). A diamond-shaped patch of bovine pericardium or Dacron graft is placed longitudinally in the proximal anterior ascending aorta where the aortic annulus has been cut. The valve prosthesis desired is sutured to the natural annulus and then to the patch. The patch is sutured to the remaining edges of the aortotomy (Fig. 26-57).
7. The aorta is closed with nonabsorbable sutures, and the cross-clamp is removed (Fig. 26-56, *E*).
8. The left side of the heart is de-aired (by vent, by moving the OR bed side to side, or by other maneuvers chosen by the surgeon). The patient is placed in the Trendelenburg position and the lungs inflated. The heart is not allowed to contract and eject blood until the surgeon is satisfied that no air remains within the left ventricle. The heart is defibrillated if it does not resume beating spontaneously.
9. Rewarming of the heart continues, the venting catheter(s) are removed, and the chest is closed in the routine manner.

When *CABG* is to be performed in conjunction with *AVR*, the procedure is done in the following order:

1. The diseased valve is excised, the annulus sized, and the prosthesis selected.
2. Distal coronary anastomoses are performed.
3. The prosthetic valve is inserted.
4. The aorta (or left atrium in MVR) is closed.

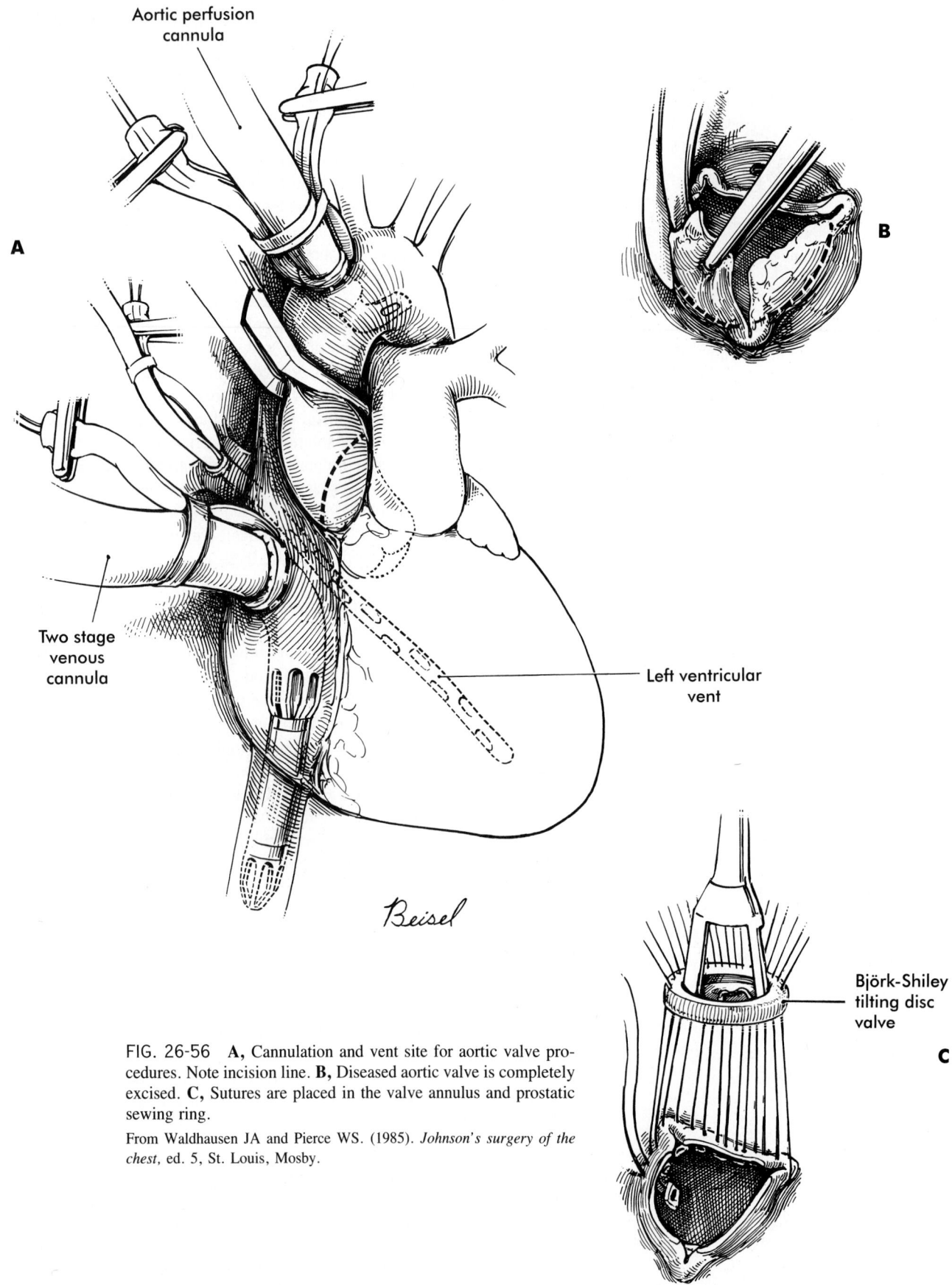

Aortic perfusion
cannula

A

B

Two stage
venous
cannula

Left ventricular
vent

Beisel

Björk-Shiley
tilting disc
valve

C

FIG. 26-56 **A,** Cannulation and vent site for aortic valve procedures. Note incision line. **B,** Diseased aortic valve is completely excised. **C,** Sutures are placed in the valve annulus and prostatic sewing ring.

From Waldhausen JA and Pierce WS. (1985). *Johnson's surgery of the chest,* ed. 5, St. Louis, Mosby.

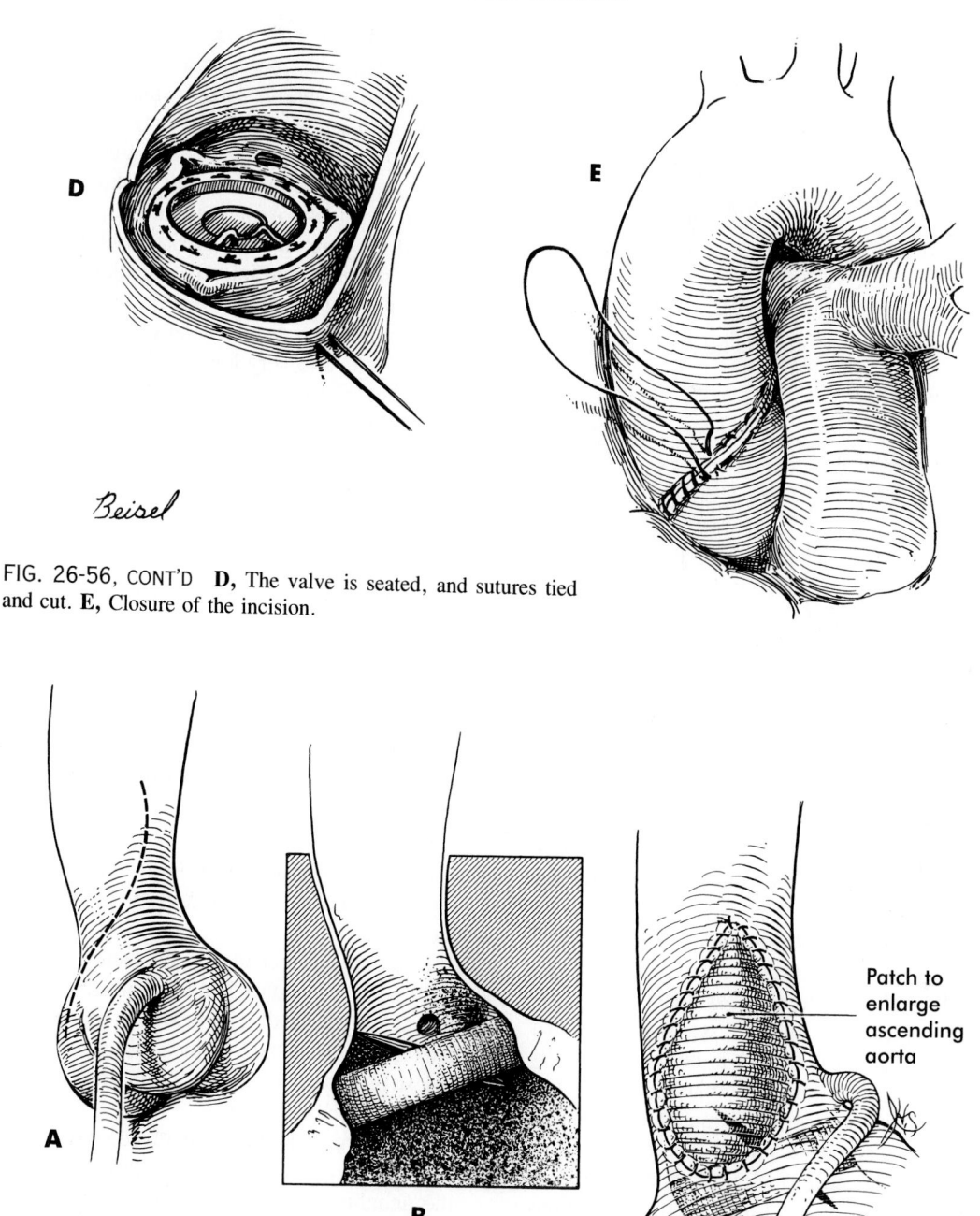

Beisel

FIG. 26-56, CONT'D **D,** The valve is seated, and sutures tied and cut. **E,** Closure of the incision.

Patch to
enlarge
ascending
aorta

FIG. 26-57 Konno technique to enlarge ascending aorta. **A,** Incision. **B,** The aorta above the annulus is too small for a disk (or a ball-cage) valve to open properly. **C,** Patch inserted.
From Waldhausen JA and Pierce WS. (1985). *Johnson's surgery of the chest,* ed. 5, St. Louis, Mosby.

5. The proximal coronary anastomoses are inserted into the aorta, after which the aortic cross-clamp is removed.

When the *aortic and mitral valves are both replaced,* the valves are first excised and the annuli sized. Then the mitral valve is implanted, followed by the aortic valve. The aorta is closed, and after sufficient de-airing of the left ventricle the left atrium is closed.

SURGERY FOR THE THORACIC AORTA

Thoracic aortic aneurysmectomy is excision of an aneurysmal portion of the ascending, arch, or descending thoracic aorta and replacement with a prosthetic graft (see Fig. 26-21), valve-graft conduit (see Fig. 26-31), or intraaortic prosthesis (see Fig. 26-22). Graft material placed in the thoracic aorta is usually preclotted to reduce bleeding, although grafts are available that do not require preclotting. Aneu-

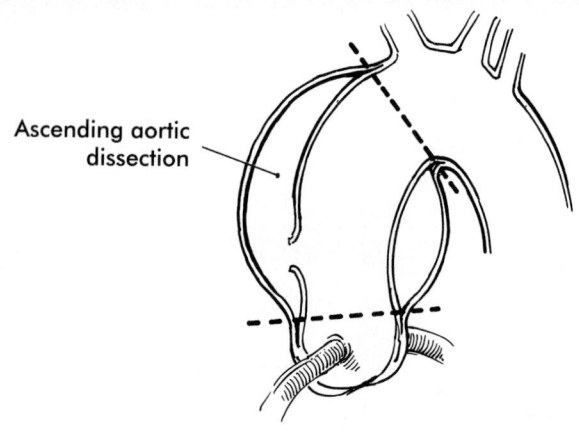

Ascending aortic
dissection

FIG. 26-58   Aortic dissection.

From Waldhausen JA and Pierce WS. (1985). *Johnson's surgery of the chest*, ed. 5, St. Louis, Mosby.

rysms may be caused by atherosclerosis, arteriosclerosis, trauma, infection, or medial degeneration (Crawford, 1990). *Atherosclerosis* is a lesion affecting large and medium arteries, with deposits in the intima of yellowish plaques containing cholesterol, lipoid material, and lipophages. *Arteriosclerosis* is defined as a condition marked by loss of elasticity, thickening, and hardening of the arteries. Further degeneration and destruction may lead to aneurysm formation. Any artery may become involved. Aortic dissection is a unique entity and is related to changes in the medial layer of the artery.

Surgical intervention becomes necessary when presenting symptoms indicate a compromised circulation or danger of rupture; generally, medical management with hypotensive agents to reduce stress on the vessel is the preferred initial treatment until surgical repair can be performed.

Aneurysms can be characterized morphologically as follows: (1) saccular—a sac type of formation with a narrowed neck projecting from the side of the artery and (2) fusiform—a spindle-shaped formation with complete circumferential involvement of the artery. Aortic dissections involve a splitting of the intima of the aorta, permitting blood to pass between the layers of the wall to form a false channel; as the channel extends and enlarges, the blood flow is obstructed (Fig. 26-58).

Procedural considerations. Several methods of surgical treatment are available. In situations where ascending aortic aneurysm or aortic dissection produces annular dilatation with subsequent aortic valve insufficiency, a Bentall-Bono procedure with a valved conduit (see Fig. 26-31) may be performed to replace the aortic valve and the aneurysmal aorta (Fig. 26-59). Retrograde cardioplegia is usually employed, although selective infusion is necessary (Fig. 26-59, *B*). This procedure necessitates reimplanting the right and left coronary ostia into the prosthetic graft. In patients with coronary artery disease, vein grafts may be inserted and anastomosed proximally to the prosthesis.

The type of CPB depends on the location of the aneurysm. Generally the atrium is cannulated for venous return and the femoral artery used for arterial inflow (because the weakened aorta cannot be safely cannulated). Profound hypothermia with circulatory arrest may be needed in particularly complex lesions of the aortic arch where the aneurysm extends into the arch vessels, making placement of a cross-clamp difficult. After the patient has been cooled to the desired temperature, the bypass machine is turned off. When the repair is sufficiently completed, the pump is turned on and the body slowly rewarmed. Because this technique prolongs the procedure and imposes additional risk, the body is cooled to very low temperatures (15° C) to protect the heart and other organ systems (Waldhausen and Pierce, 1985).

In descending thoracic aortic aneurysms, the heart is not arrested; it continues beating to perfuse the upper body. Femoral bypass is instituted to perfuse the kidneys and lower extremities; normothermia is maintained.

Repair of ascending thoracic aortic aneurysm/dissection

Procedural considerations. To the basic setup are added aneurysm instruments. Valve instruments, coronary instruments, and an array of tube grafts, valves, and/or valved conduits should be available. Bicaval cannulation for venous drainage may be performed.

Operative procedure

1. The patient is positioned for a median sternotomy.
2. Cannulation of the right atrium and femoral artery is performed.
3. The sternum is opened and the aneurysm inspected.
4a. If the aortic annulus is not involved, the aneurysm is incised longitudinally, and a woven graft is anastomosed proximally and distally to the healthy aorta (Fig. 26-60). Felt strips incorporated into the anastamosis may be used to bolster friable tissue.
4b. If the aortic annulus is involved, the ascending aorta is incised to the annulus. The leaflets are excised and the annulus measured. The proximal end of a valved conduit is inserted (see Fig. 26-59, *C*). An eye cautery is used to create openings in the graft at the location of the right and left coronary ostia, which are anastomosed to the graft (see Fig. 26-59, *D*). (If the patient has concomitant coronary artery disease, saphenous vein grafts are inserted.) The distal end of the conduit is sutured to healthy aorta, and the aneurysmal remnant is wrapped around the conduit (see Fig. 26-59, *E*).
5. Bypass is discontinued and all incisions closed.

Repair of aortic arch aneurysm

Procedural considerations. Aneurysm instruments and woven grafts are available. If profound hypothermia is to be used, the patient's face and head may be covered with bags of ice at the beginning of the procedure. Precautions to prevent frostbite are instituted. The patient is positioned for a median sternotomy.

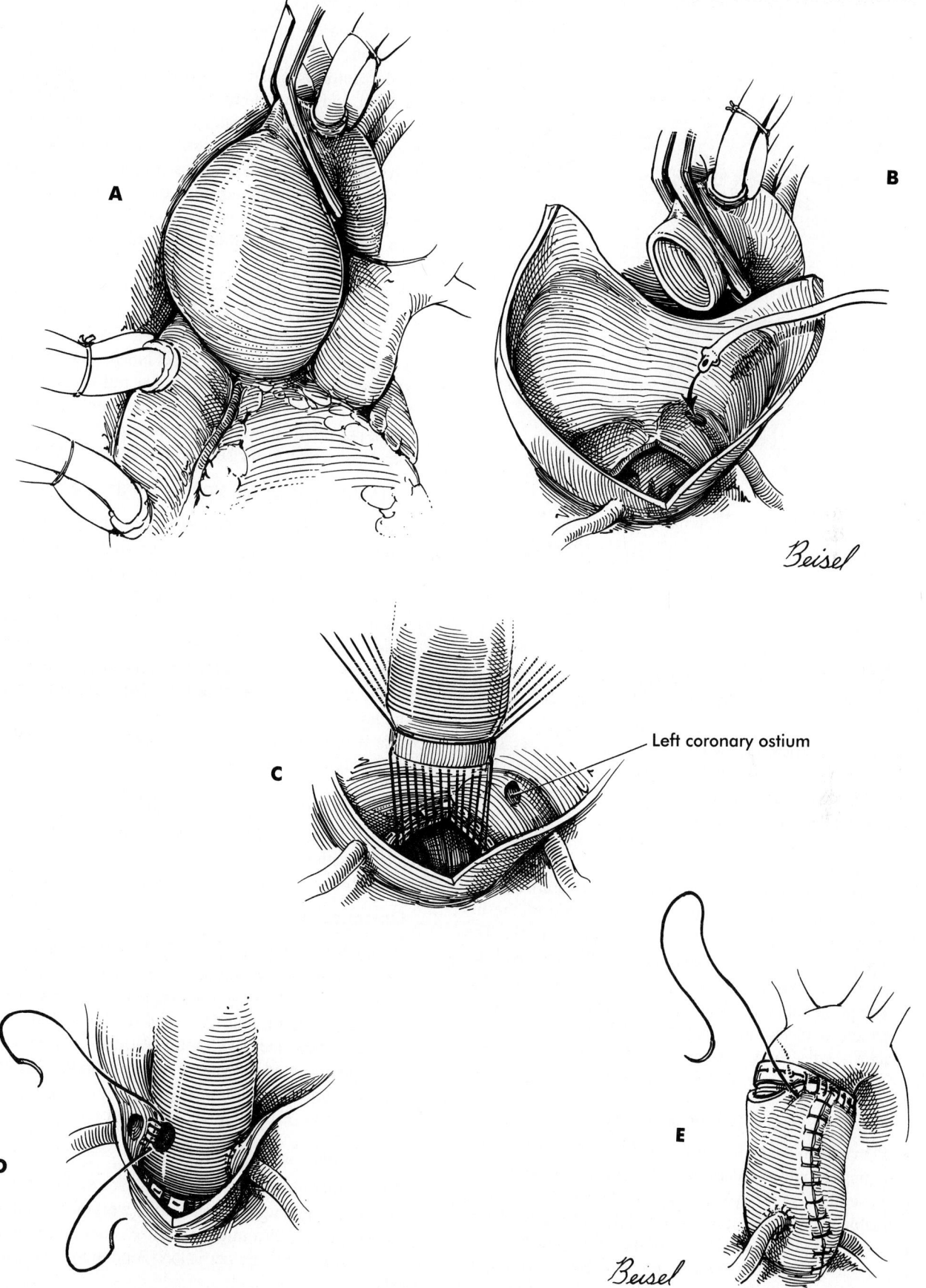

Left coronary ostium

FIG. 26-59   Bentall-Bono procedure (see text).
From Waldhausen JA and Pierce WS. (1985). *Johnson's surgery of the chest*, ed. 5, St. Louis, Mosby.

Operative procedure

1. Cannulation for femoral vein–femoral artery bypass is performed.
2. A thoracotomy incision is made, and the aneurysm is exposed and surrounding structures inspected. (Occasionally the surgeon makes two thoracotomy incisions for better access to and control of the aorta.) Renal involvement is assessed; if indicated, measures to protect the kidneys are instituted (for example, local cooling).
3. Normothermic femoral bypass is initiated.
4. The aneurysm is incised longitudinally, and the aorta is sized.
5a. A woven graft (Fig. 26-62) is inserted, and the aneurysmal remnants are wrapped around the graft.
5b. If an intraaortic prosthesis (see Fig. 26-22) is used, it is inserted into the true aortic lumen and the aorta wrapped around the prosthesis. Dacron tapes are used to encircle the aorta and the proximal and distal rings. The tapes are tied, securing the prosthesis. Stay sutures may be inserted to further secure the prosthesis.

MECHANICAL CIRCULATORY ASSISTANCE

A small percentage of patients cannot be weaned from CPB after open heart operations, even with the use of inotropic and vasodilator drugs. Various mechanical devices are available to support the circulation while the heart recovers or while the patient awaits cardiac transplantation. They include the intraaortic balloon pump (IABP) and the Hemopump. The latter is an axial flow pump inserted retrogradely from the femoral artery into the left ventricle. As the pump rotates, it draws blood from the left ventricle and propels it into the aorta and distal vascular beds, thereby supplementing cardiac output.

Intraaortic balloon pump (IABP)

The IABP is a technique that employs the principle of counterpulsation. It increases the cardiac output and may permit separation of the patient from CPB (Fig. 26-63).

Operative procedure

1. A flexible guidewire is passed through a percutaneous needle into the femoral artery. The needle is removed, and graduated dilators are inserted over the guidewire to dilate the overlying tissue and the artery wall.
2. The IABP catheter (with the furled balloon) is inserted into the artery and advanced to a position just distal to the left subclavian artery.
3. The balloon is unfurled and activated.

Ventricular assist device

Ventricular assist devices (VADs) are designed to augment cardiac output and decrease the workload of the heart by diverting blood from the ventricle to an artificial pump that maintains systemic perfusion (Pennington and Swartz, 1992).

Procedural considerations. If patients cannot be

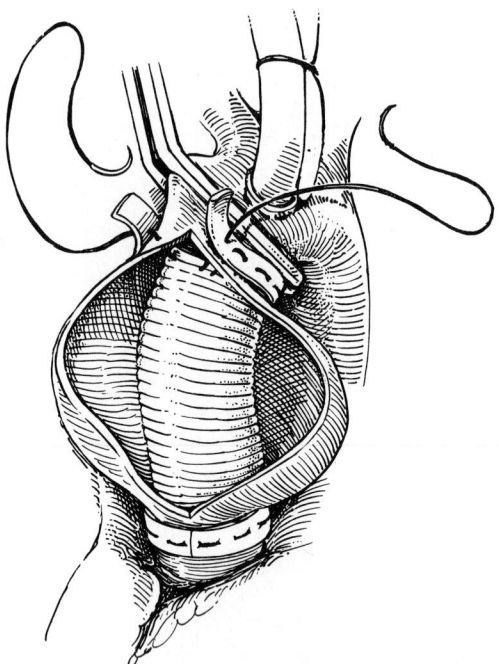

FIG. 26-60 Graft repair of ascending aortic aneurysm.
From Waldhausen JA and Pierce WS. (1985). *Johnson's surgery of the chest*, ed. 5, St. Louis, Mosby.

Operative procedure

1. Cannulation of the right atrium and femoral artery is performed.
2. Once the patient is cooled to the desired temperature, the arch vessels are individually cross-clamped (Fig. 26-61, A and B). (If circulatory arrest is indicated, cross-clamps are not used.) The aneurysm is incised, a tube graft selected, and the anastomosis to the descending aorta performed.
3. An opening is made into the side of the graft and the graft is anastomosed to the common origin of the innominate, left carotid, and left subclavian vessels. The graft is cross-clamped proximally to the arch and de-aired (Fig. 26-61, C).
4. The proximal aorta is anastomosed to the graft while the patient is rewarming. The graft is de-aired and the patient weaned from bypass (Fig. 26-61, D).
5. All incisions are closed.

Repair of descending thoracic aortic aneurysm

Procedural considerations. Thoracotomy instruments and supplies are added to the basic setup; additional long aortic cross-clamps may be needed. Prosthetic grafts are available. The patient is positioned for a left posterolateral thoracotomy. Femoral vein–femoral artery bypass is performed to perfuse the lower body. The heart perfuses the upper body proximal to the aneurysm. Normothermia is maintained.

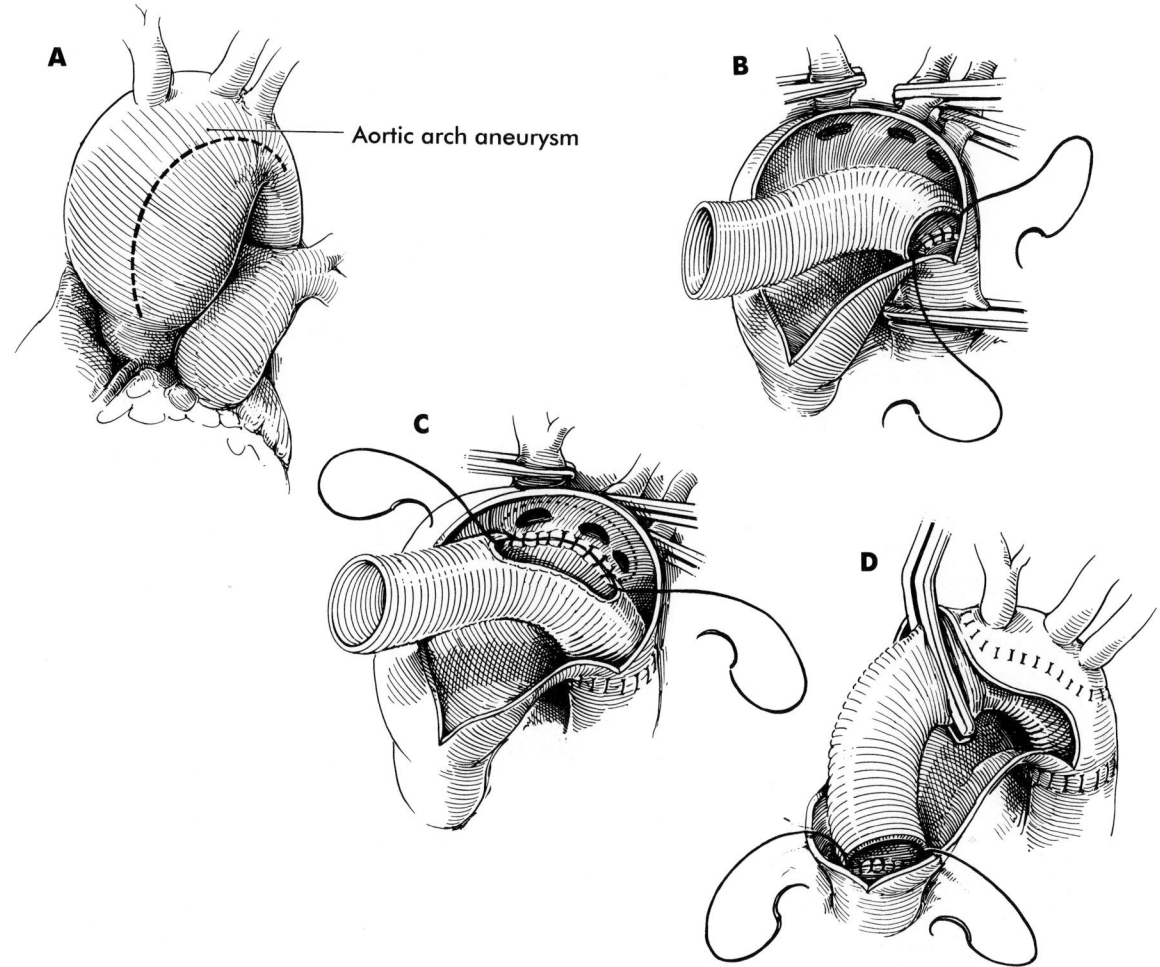

FIG. 26-61   Repair aortic arch aneurysm. **A,** Incision. **B,** Distal anastomosis. **C,** Anastomosis of graft to common origin of arch vessels. **D,** Proximal anastomosis.

From Waldhausen JA and Pierce WS. (1985). *Johnson's surgery of the chest,* ed. 5, St. Louis, Mosby.

weaned from CPB with IAPB, an assist system can be used in some circumstances. Cardiac support devices include external centrifugal pumps (Fig. 26-64) and pneumatic (Fig. 26-65) or electric power internal assist devices. In the device described below, pulsatile flow can be achieved. Bioprosthetic valves are incorporated into the circuit to maintain unidirectional blood flow. Other VADs capable of pulsatile flow include the Abiomed and the Thoratec systems.

Operative procedure (Thermedics Heart Mate left ventricular assist device [LVAD])

1. A median sternotomy and midline laparotomy are made in preparation for placement of ventricular and aortic cannulas and the intraabdominal pump.
2. The right atrium and femoral artery are cannulated for CPB.
3. The graft is preclotted and the valves rinsed. Caution should be used to prevent injury to the graft material and the valves.

4. The pump and fittings are washed and assembled.
5. The pump is placed in the left upper quadrant of the abdomen intraperitoneally, and the drive line is passed through a stab wound in the lower abdomen and connected to the power source.
6. Bypass is instituted.
7. The inlet tube of the pump is passed through an incision in the lateral diaphragm and inserted into the left ventricular apex.
8. The aortic (outflow) graft is anastomosed to the aorta and then to the outflow tube. The pump is filled with blood.
9. The pump, left ventricle, and aorta are de-aired, and the pump is started.
10. All connections are secured.
11. Bypass is discontinued and the cannulas removed. To remove the pump, the patient is returned to the operating room, the sternotomy reopened, and the cannulas removed.

cle to reinforce or partially replace the heart muscle (Chachques et al., 1989; Chiu, 1991).

HEART AND HEART-LUNG TRANSPLANTATION

Heart transplantation (Fig. 26-66)

With the introduction of the immunosuppressive agent cyclosporine A, cardiac transplantation has become a clinically feasible treatment for end-stage heart disease (May and Adams, 1992). Orthotopic transplantation (replacing the heart with another) is most commonly performed, but heterotopic (piggyback) and combined heart-lung procedures are done as well. Important considerations continue to be recipient selection, the immune response, and control of infection (Augustine, 1990).

Procedural considerations. Individual instrument setups are necessary for the donor and the recipient.

Operative procedure

Donor heart. The donor heart is exposed through a median sternotomy. The aorta, pulmonary artery, and venae cavae are dissected. The venae cavae are occluded, the left atrium is opened to decompress the ventricle, and the heart is rapidly cooled and arrested.

The heart is excised by incising the left atrium circumferentially at the level of the pulmonary veins and by severing the aorta and pulmonary artery. The donor heart is immediately placed in cold saline and transported to the site where it will be inserted into the recipient.

Recipient heart. The recipient is placed on bypass with cannulation of the inferior vena cava and the superior vena cava; caval tapes are placed around the cavae. The patient is cooled to approximately 25° C and the caval tapes tightened. The pulmonary trunk and aorta are dissected immediately above their respective semilunar valves; the atria are incised to leave intact portions of the right and left atrial walls and the atrial septum of the recipient. The recipient heart is then removed.

The donor heart is placed in the pericardial well. The interatrial septum and the left and then the right atrial walls are approximated with running cardiovascular sutures (Fig. 26-66, *A* and *B*). The donor and recipient aortas are similarly joined (Fig. 26-66, *C*). Air is removed from the left side of the heart.

The aortic clamp is removed, and a clamp is placed across the donor pulmonary artery. The caval tape is removed, and vigorous ventricular fibrillation of the donor heart commences. Local cooling of the heart is discontinued at this point, and, before the pulmonary artery is sutured, all atrial suture lines are carefully inspected for significant bleeding areas. The pulmonary arteries are united (Fig. 26-66, *D*) and the clamp removed. Defibrillation of the ventricles is usually effected with a single DC shock. A needle vent in the ascending aorta, allows residual air to escape. The patient is then gradually weaned from bypass. Cannulas are removed from the venae cavae and the aorta. The incisions are closed as described previously.

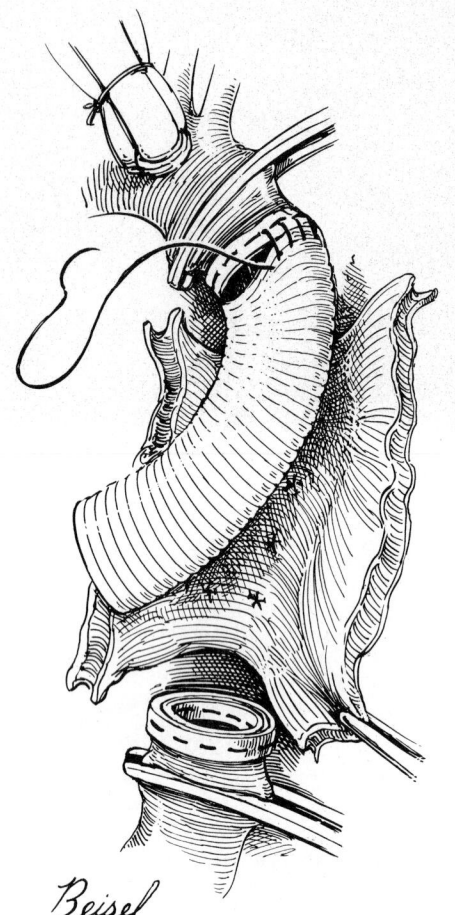

Beisel

FIG. 26-62 Resection and graft replacement for descending thoracic aortic aneurysm.

From Waldhausen JA and Pierce WS. (1985). *Johnson's surgery of the chest,* ed. 5, St. Louis, Mosby.

If a centrifugal pump is used, the left atrium is cannulated for inflow to the pump, and the ascending aorta is cannulated for outflow from the pump. (Prosthetic valves are not required because the rotating pump maintains forward, nonpulsatile blood flow.) These assist devices may be used for right ventricular failure or bilateral ventricular failure as well.

Total artificial heart (TAH)

The total artificial heart has not demonstrated great success as a permanent cardiac replacement, due to thromboembolism and infection. Long-term right and/or left VADs have been increasingly employed as a bridge to cardiac transplantation by supporting the circulation while a suitable donor heart can be found.

Biologic ventricular support

Among the newer trends in providing ventricular support is the use of latissimus dorsi muscle for *cardiomyoplasty*. This technique uses electrostimulated skeletal mus-

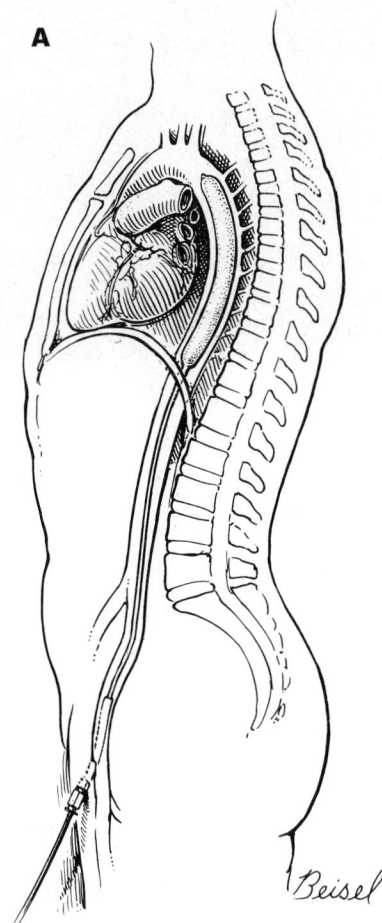

FIG. 26-63 Phases of balloon pumping. **A,** Balloon inflation occurs from closure of aortic valve to end of diastole. Inflation causes retrograde flow of blood in aorta, increasing coronary perfusion pressure without increasing myocardial work or oxygen demand. Inflation also causes antegrade flow, increasing mean arterial pressure, renal flow, and cerebral flow. **B,** Balloon deflation occurs from just before opening of aortic valve to closure of aortic valve. Deflation encourages antegrade flow, decreasing afterload or resistance to left ventricular ejection. Deflation also decreases oxygen required by left ventricle, shortens systolic ejection, and increases stroke volume. **C and D,** When the balloon reinflates, the cycle is repeated.

From Waldhausen JA and Pierce WS. (1985). *Johnson's surgery of the chest,* ed. 5, St. Louis, Mosby.

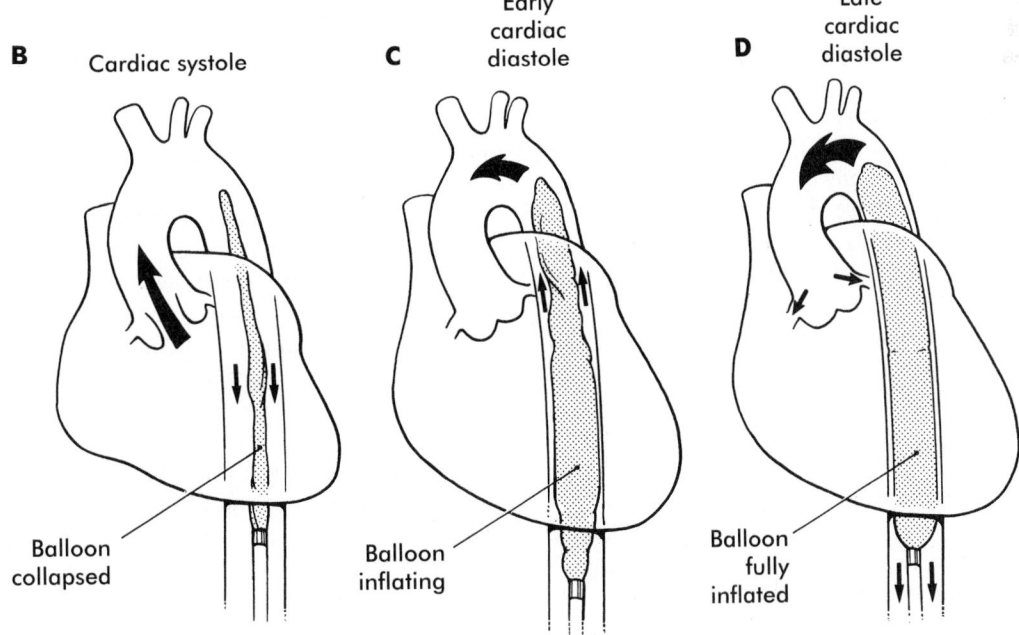

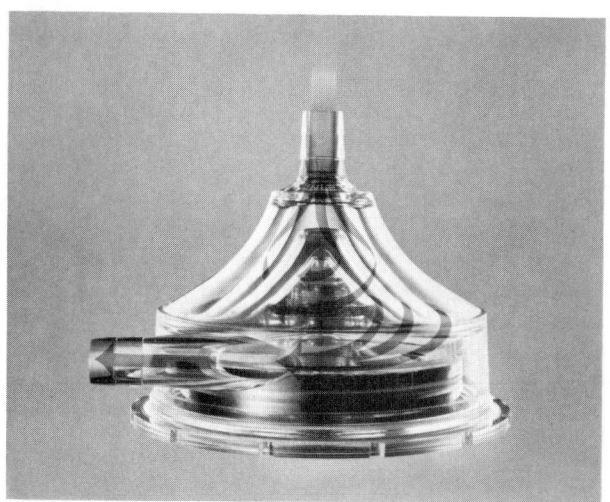

FIG. 26-64   Centrifugal pump. The Bio-Medicus pump can be used for extracorporeal circulation during cardiac surgery or as a ventricular assist device.

Courtesy Medtronic, Inc, 1991.

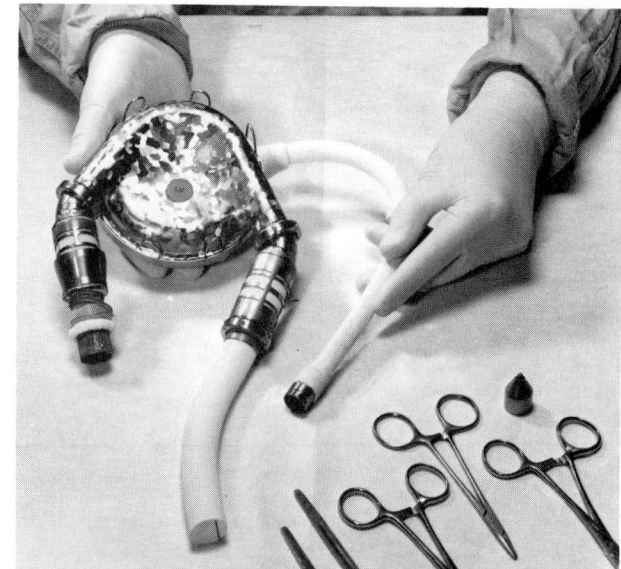

FIG. 26-65   Placement of ventricular assist device. Blood flows from the ventricle into the mechanical ventricle located below the diaphragm and is pumped into the ascending aorta.

Courtesy Thermo Cardiosystems, Inc., Woburn, Mass.

Heart-lung transplantation (Fig. 26-67)

A three-anastomosis technique for combined heart-lung transplantation has been devised. This technique ensures preservation of the donor's sinus node and preservation of the recipient's recurrent laryngeal, vagus, and phrenic nerves (Holmquist and Gamberg, 1992; Ahrens and Powers, 1990).

Operative procedure. The recipient's diseased heart and lungs are excised separately or en bloc, with care taken not to injure the major nerves listed previously. The recipient's right atrium is saved to create a large atrial cuff for attachment to the donor heart. The bronchi are transsected and the stumps clamped to prevent contamination. The trachea is transsected just above the carina. The donor heart and lungs are brought onto the field. The right lung is placed in the right pleural space and the left lung positioned in the left pleural space. The tracheal and the right atrial anastomoses are performed, and rewarming is begun. The aortic anastomosis is performed, the aorta is de-aired, and the cross-clamp is removed.

SURGERY FOR CONDUCTION DISTURBANCES

Disturbances of the conduction system can affect the rate and rhythm of the contracting heart. Surgical techniques have been developed to treat most types of supraventricular dysrhythmias and both ischemic and nonischemic ventricular tachydysrhythmias (Zipes, 1992). Techniques include resection of the myocardial dysrhythmogenic focus, such as subendocardial resection, ablation of abnormal conduction pathways, and the insertion of pacing and antitachycardia devices.

Surgical ablation of accessory pathways

Ablation of accessory conduction pathways is the destruction of these pathways through freezing, radiofrequency, or excision. Patients with Wolff-Parkinson-White syndrome have accessory conduction pathways that bypass the normal AV node—His bundle system. Patients have frequent, recurring, symptomatic tachydysrhythmias that overstimulate the heart and can impair ventricular filling and cardiac output (Regas et al., 1986).

Operative procedure. Before surgery the patient's accessory pathways are mapped in the electrophysiology laboratory to determine the origin of the pathway, its role in the tachydysrhythmia, the existence of additional pathways, and the effects of medication on the dysrhythmia. At operation the surgeon initiates cardiopulmonary bypass and attaches electrodes to each atrium and ventricle. Intraoperative mapping is performed to verify the accessory system. When the pathway is located, the surgeon dissects down to it and ablates the tissue with one of the methods described above. After termination of bypass and the achievement of hemostasis, the chest is closed in the routine fashion.

Surgical treatment of atrial fibrillation has been developed whereby multiple incisions are made in the atria so that the electrical impulses (which are unable to cross suture lines) are routed from the sinoatrial node to the atrioventricular node. The incisions are then closed with suture,

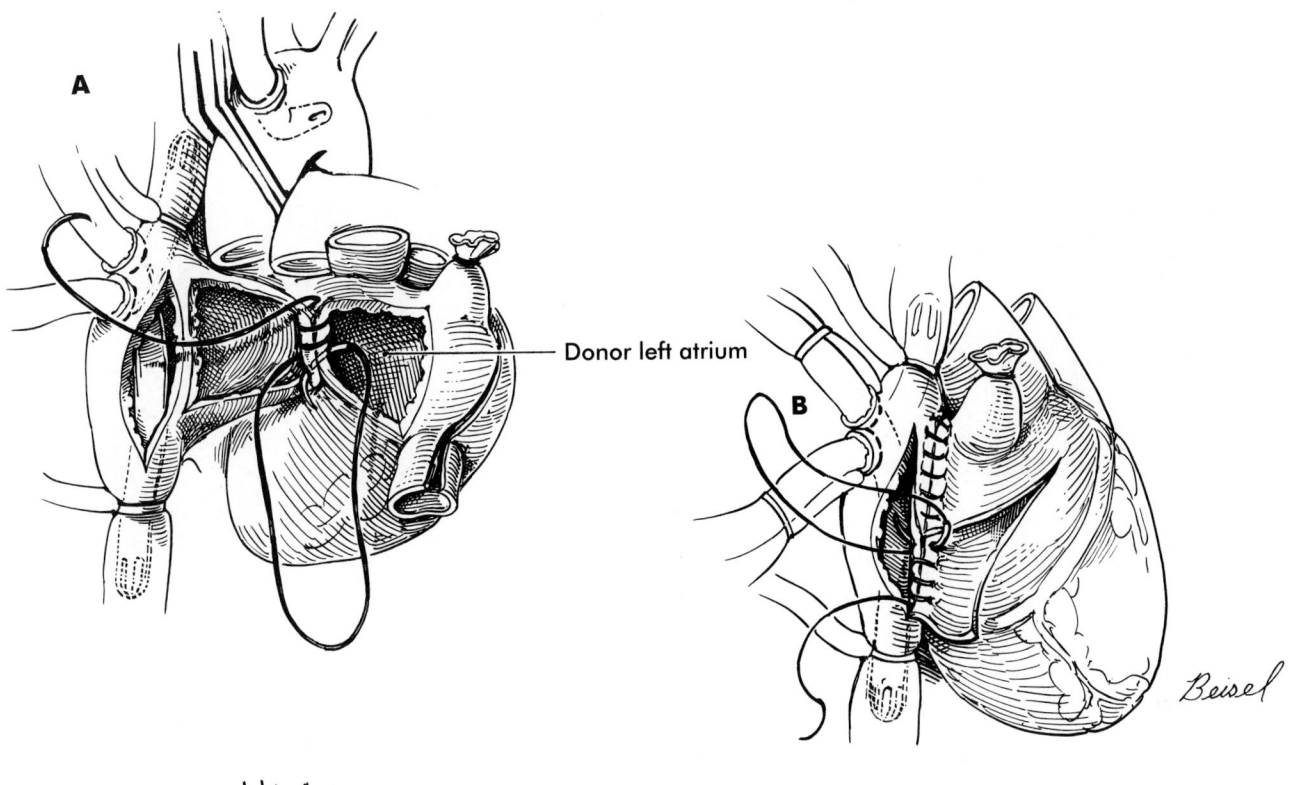

Donor left atrium

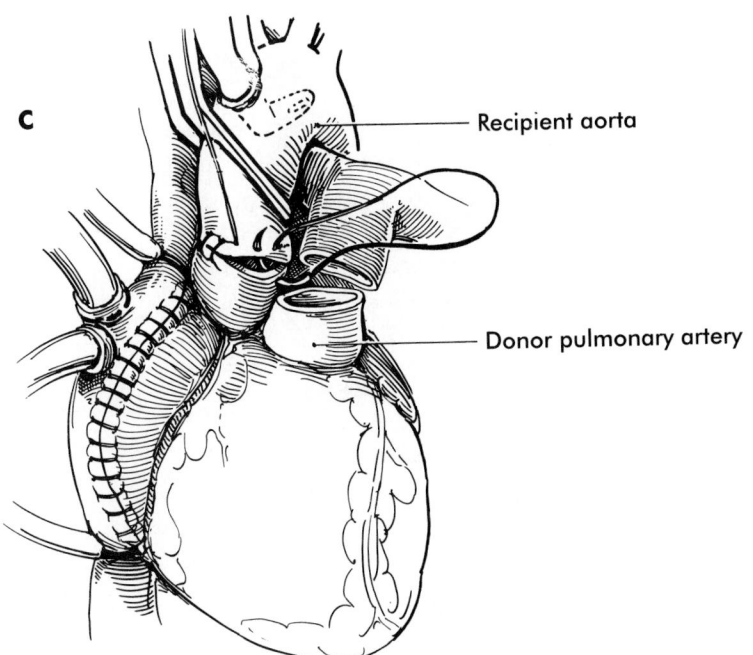

Recipient aorta

Donor pulmonary artery

FIG. 26-66   Heart transplantation. **A,** The recipient and donor left atria are anastomosed. **B,** Anastomosis at the right atria. **C,** Aortic anastomosis. **D,** Pulmonary artery anastomosis.

From Waldhausen JA and Pierce WS. (9185). *Johnson's surgery of the chest,* ed. 5, St. Louis, Mosby.

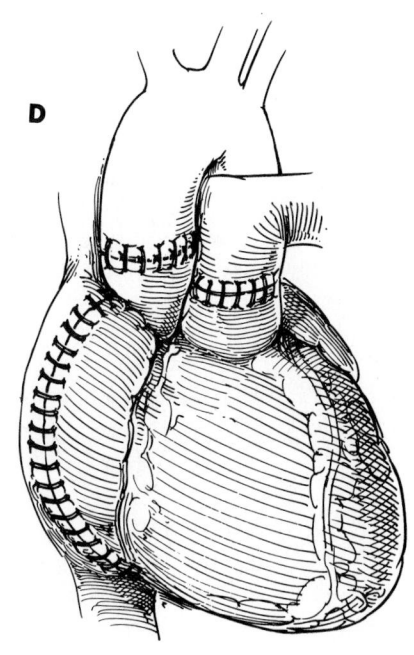

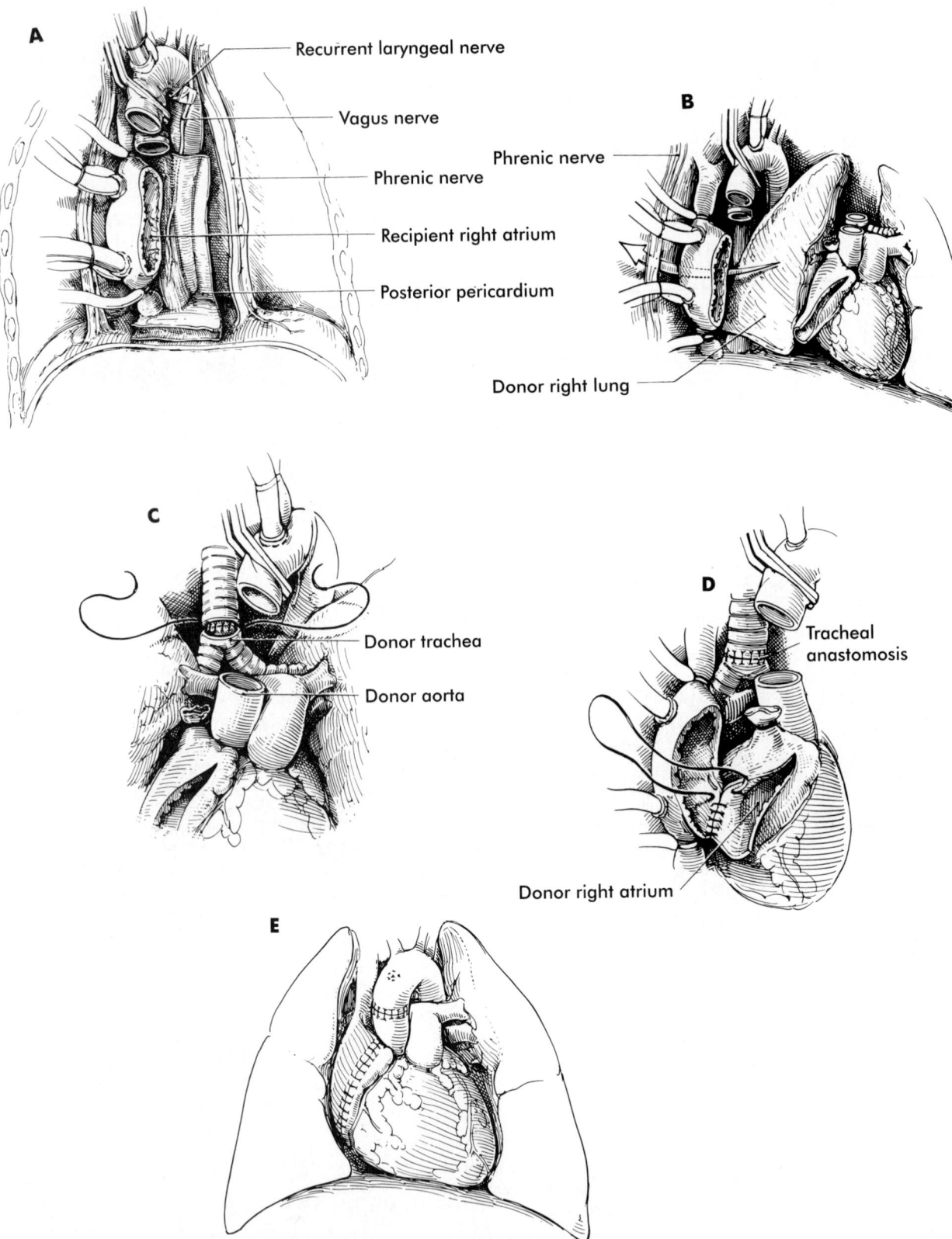

FIG. 26-67 Heart-lung transplantation. **A,** Recipient's heart and lungs are removed. **B,** Donor organs are placed in the field. **C,** Tracheal anastomosis. **D,** Right atrial anastomosis. **E,** Completed procedure. From Waldhausen JA and Pierce WS. (1985). *Johnson's surgery of the chest,* ed. 5, St. Louis, Mosby.

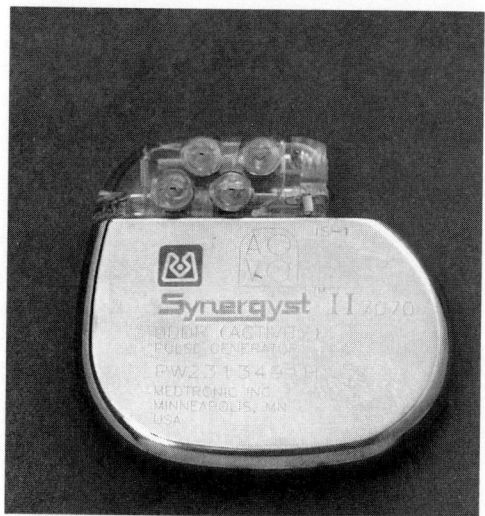

FIG. 26-68   Pacemaker generator.
Courtesy Medtronic, Inc., Minneapolis, Minn.

creating a maze that directs the impulses in the desired direction (Cox et al., 1991).

Insertion of permanent pacemaker

A permanent pacemaker (pulse generator and electrodes) initiates atrial and/or ventricular contraction. Complete heart block and bradyarrhythmias are the most common indications for pacemaker implantation. The development of multiprogramable and physiologic pacemakers (Futterman and Lemberg, 1993) has made possible the treatment of many forms of dysrhythmias and neuroconductive disturbances, as well as tachydysrhythmias (Futterman and Lemberg, 1992). A temporary pacemaker may also be used for acute forms of heart block and dysrhythmias that occasionally occur during and after cardiac surgery.

Two methods of placing electrodes for permanent cardiac pacing include transvenous and epicardial approaches. The transvenous route is most commonly used because it does not require a major thoracotomy or a general anesthetic and is therefore safer for high-risk patients. Permanent epicardial electrodes are often placed during cardiac operations when the chest is opened and the heart is exposed; a subxiphoid approach may be used to place epicardial leads without having to open the sternum.

Pulse generators (Fig. 26-68) are typically powered by lithium, which lasts 5 to 10 years. Life expectancy depends on the amount of power used and the frequency of demand. The generators are classified into three groups: fixed rate (or asynchronous), ventricular demand, and physiologic. The asynchronous was the first type implanted and fires at a fixed rate, independent of the electrical activity of the heart. A major disadvantage of this type of pacing is competition between the heart's intrinsic beat and the paced beat, possibly resulting in ventricular fibrillation if the paced beat occurs during the T wave period of the ECG.

Ventricular demand pacemakers were developed in response to this problem and fire at a fixed rate only if spontaneous ventricular activity fails. Adding a sensing mechanism to the existing stimulating mechanism makes this type of pacing possible. "Physiologic" pacemakers can stimulate both the atria and the ventricles, maintain atrioventricular synchrony, and can enhance cardiac output by as much as 20%. Pacemakers are also capable of adjusting the rate of stimulation in response to increased metabolic activity (such as rate-responsive pacers).

There are two types of electrodes: myocardial (epicardial), which are attached to the heart muscle under direct vision, and endocardial, which are inserted transvenously. The stimulating and sensing electrodes are located at the tip of the lead, which attaches to the pulse generator.

Pacing systems are also available as unipolar or bipolar. A pacemaker with one stimulating electrode at the tip of the lead is unipolar. The electrical current flows between the electrode and the pulse generator. A bipolar pacemaker has two stimulating electrodes at the tip of the lead. Electrical current flows between the two electrodes.

Insertion of transvenous (endocardial) pacing electrodes

Procedural considerations. The patient is placed in the supine position. Continuous ECG monitoring is essential. A defibrillator and emergency drugs should be available because dysrhythmias can occur during catheter insertion. The patient should be made as comfortable as possible because this procedure can sometimes be lengthy and is frequently performed using local or local standby anesthesia (monitored anesthesia care).

Fluoroscopy is required; thus either a portable image intensifier is needed or the procedure is done in the special studies section of the radiology department.

A minor set of instruments is used, plus the following:

2 Vascular forceps	Vascular scissors
2 Vascular needle holders	External pacemaker (for testing) or a pacing system analyzer (PSA)
1 Tunneling instrument (may be sponge-holding forceps or vaginal packing forceps)	Introducer set
Sterile pacemaker, electrodes, and connecting cable (alligator cable)	Screwdriver and other accessory items as needed

Operative procedure (Fig. 26-69)

1. The skin and subcutaneous tissue are infiltrated with a local anesthetic, and the patient is placed in Trendelenburg's position (to engorge the vein for easier access and to avoid air emboli).
2. A skin pocket is made close to the subclavian vein (Fig. 26-69, A). The vessel may be encircled with a heavy suture.

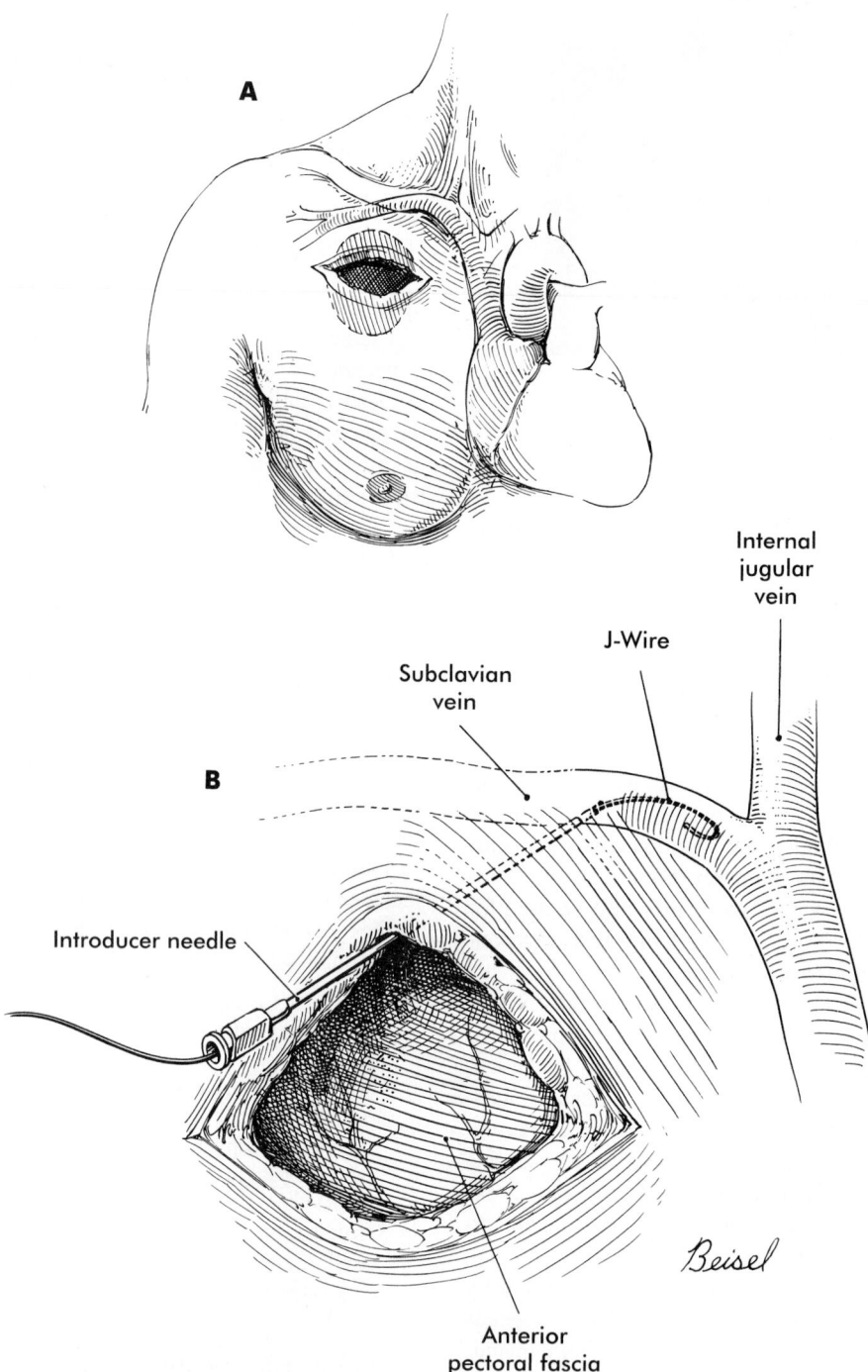

FIG. 26-69   Insertion of transvenous pacemaker (see text).
From Waldhausen JA and Pierce WS. (1985). *Johnson's surgery of the chest,* ed. 5, St. Louis, Mosby.

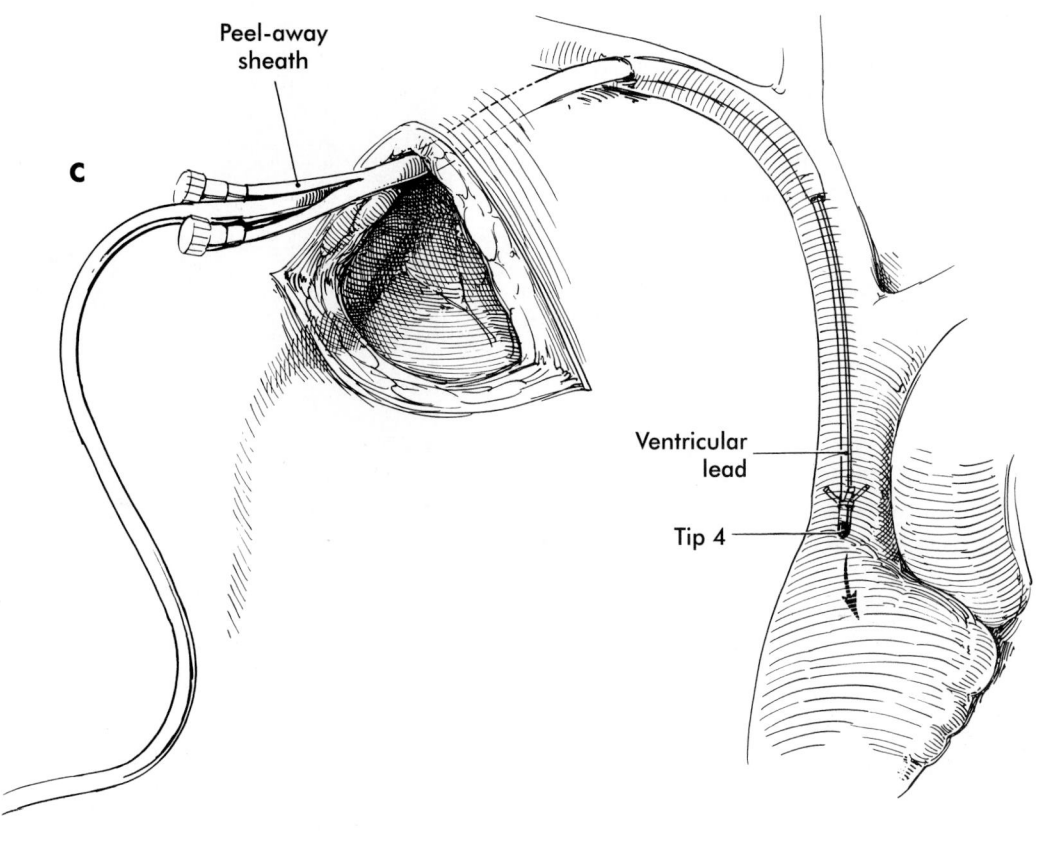

Peel-away sheath

C

Ventricular lead

Tip 4

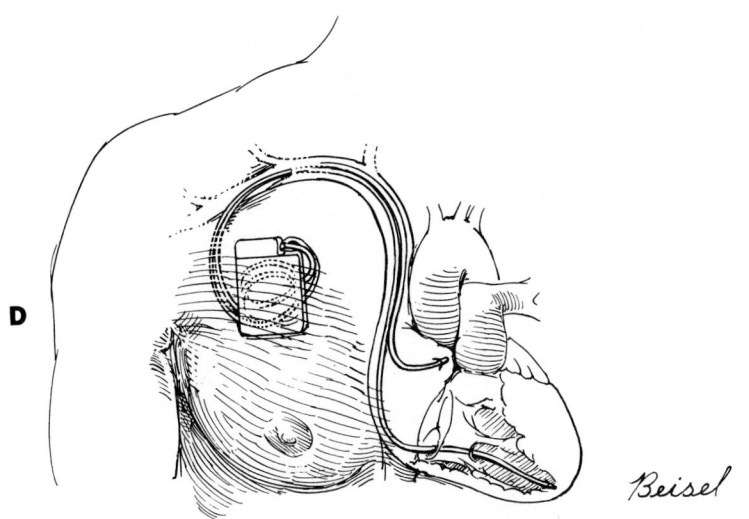

D

Beisel

FIG. 26-69, CONT'D   For legend see opposite page.

3. A venotomy is performed with an introducer needle (Fig. 26-69, *B*), and the pacing electrode is inserted through a dilator sheath, which is withdrawn after the lead insertion (Fig. 26-69, *C*).

4. The electrode is advanced, under direct fluoroscopic vision, into the right atrium, through the tricuspid valve, and into the right ventricle (Fig. 26-69, *D*).

5. The surgeon attempts to entrap the tip of the electrode in the trabeculae carneae of the right ventricular apex to stabilize it. If a dual chamber pacemaker is inserted, the second lead is entrapped in the right atrial appendage (Fig. 26-69, *D*).

6. The electrodes are attached, by appropriate cables, to an external pulse generator or a pacing analyzer for testing (Fig. 26-69, *D*).

7. The electrode is brought down and attached to the pulse generator.

8. The pulse generator is placed in the pocket, and the incision is irrigated with an antibiotic solution. If the pocket must be made farther away from the vein, a tunneling device may be used to thread the electrode to the pocket.

9. The incision(s) is closed in layers with absorbable sutures.

Insertion of myocardial (epicardial) pacing electrodes
Subxiphoid process approach

Procedural considerations. The setup is as described for placement of endocardial electrodes.

Operative procedure

1. If local anesthesia is used, the subxiphoid process and left upper quadrant area are infiltrated with the anesthetic.

2. A small, transverse incision is made below the xiphoid process and is carried down to the linea alba. A tunnel is created under the xiphoid process to the pericardium, which is incised to expose the heart.

3. The pacing electrode, mounted on its carrier, is screwed into the ventricular myocardium, and the carrier is removed.

4. The remainder of the procedure is as described for insertion of the endocardial electrode.

Sternotomy approach
Operative procedure

1. The mediastinum is opened, and an area of myocardium is chosen for placement of the pacing electrodes.

2. The electrode tips are screwed into or are sutured to the myocardium and are attached by an appropriate cable to an external pulse generator or pacing analyzer for testing.

3. The pocket and subcutaneous tunnel are created, as described for insertion of the endocardial electrode.

4. A chest drainage catheter is inserted, and the thoracotomy incision is closed.

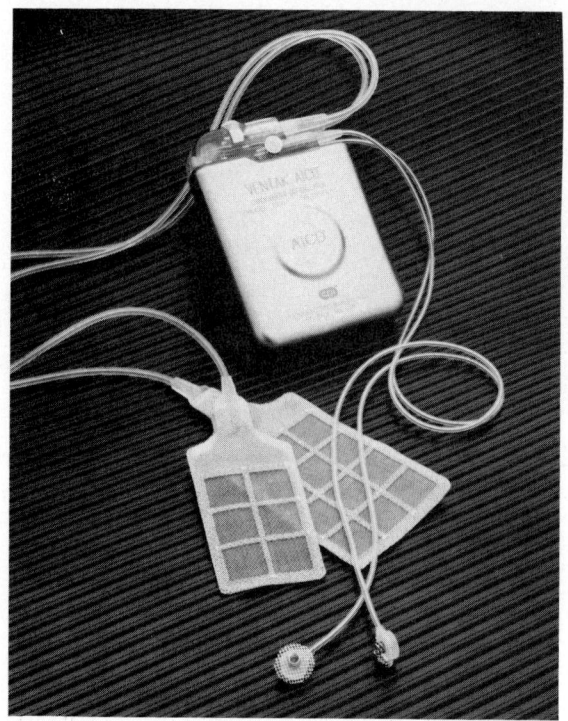

FIG. 26-70 Internal cardioverter defibrillator: generator *(top)*, ventricular patch leads *(middle)*, screw-in sensing leads *(bottom)*. Courtesy CPI, Cardiac Pacemakers, Inc., St. Paul, Minn.

Insertion of implantable cardioverter defibrillator (ICD)

Sudden cardiac death from malignant ventricular dysrhythmias (ventricular fibrillation and ventricular tachycardia) annually strikes more than 450,000 persons in the United States (Mason and McPherson, 1992). Many of these patients cannot be helped by surgery or pharmacologic intervention. The ICD is an electronic device designed to monitor cardiac electrical activity and deliver prompt defibrillatory shocks (Fig. 26-70). The ICD differs from a pacemaker in that the former senses ventricular tachycardia or fibrillation and the latter senses asystole. Newer models are capable of tiered therapy, whereby increasingly stronger impulses are delivered depending on the underlying dysrhythmias. These devises are capable of pacing as well as defibrillating (pacing cardioverter defibrillators [PCDs]). The ICD device consists of a generator, myocardial patches, and sensing electrodes. EP studies are performed before and after insertion to diagnose the dysrhythmia and to evaluate device function, respectively (Zipes, 1992).

Operative procedure. One of three approaches may be selected by the surgeon: a lateral thoracotomy, a subxiphoid, or a median sternotomy incision (Prinkey, 1992). The thoracotomy approach is often used for patients who have mediastinal adhesions from previous surgery. The subxiphoid approach is indicated when there is no history of cardiac surgery and none is planned. The median sternotomy approach is used when a concomitant cardiac operation is performed. The sensing leads may be inserted via a transvenous or epicardial route to the right ventricle. The ventricular patches are sewn to the epicardium anteriorly and posteriorly. The generator is housed in a subcutaneous pocket near the umbilicus. The free ends of the lead system are tunneled to the generator and inserted. The device is tested, and the incisions are closed.

REFERENCES

Ahdrens, T.S., & Powers, C. (1990). Heart-lung transplantation. In S.L. Smith (Ed.), *Tissue and organ transplantation*. St. Louis: Mosby.

Augustine, S.M. (1990). Nursing care of the heart and heart-lung transplant patient. In W.A. Baumgartner, et al. (editors), *Heart and heart-lung transplantation*. Philadelphia: W.B. Saunders.

Bartlett, R.H. (1990). Extracorporeal life support for cardiopulmonary failure. *Current problems in surgery, 27* (10, 623.

Bell, P.E., & Diffee, G.T. (1991). Cardiopulmonary bypass: Principles, nursing implications. *AORN Journal 53* (6), 1480.

Braunwald, E. (Ed.), (1992). *Heart disease* (4th ed.). Philadelphia: W.B. Saunders.

Butchart, E.G., & Bodnar, E. (editors), (1992). *Thrombosis, embolism and bleeding*. London: ICR Publishers.

Carpentier, A. (1983). Cardiac valve surgery: The French correction. *Journal of Thoracic and Cardiovascular Surgery, 86*, 323.

Chachques, J.C., Grandjean, P.A., & Carpentier, A. (1989). A latissimus dorsi dynamic cardiomyoplasty. *Annals of Thoracic Surgery, 47*, 600.

Chiu, R.C. (1991). Dynamic cardiomyoplasty: An overview. *PACE, 14* (4), 577.

Cooley, D.A. (1989). Ventricular endoaneurysmorrhaphy. *Texas Heart Institute Journal, 16* (2), 72.

Cosgrove, D.M., & Stewart, W.J. (1989). Mitral valvuloplasty. *Current Problems in Cardiology, 14* (7), 359.

Cox, J.L., et al. (1991). Successful surgical treatment of atrial fibrillation: Review and clinical update. *JAMA 266* (14), 1976.

Crawford, E.S. (1990). The diagnosis and management of aortic dissection. *JAMA 264* (9), 2537.

Cruse, P.J., & Foord, R. (1980). The epidemiology of wound infection: A ten-year prospective study of 62,939 wounds. *Surgical Clinics of North America 80*, 27.

Delouche, A., et al. (1990). Valve repair with Carpentier techniques: The second decade. *Journal of Thoracic and Cardiovascular Surgery, 99* (6), 990.

Downing, S.W., & Edmunds, L.H. (1992). Release of vasoactive substances during cardiopulmonary bypass. *Annals of Thoracic Surgery 54*, 1236.

Drinkwater, D.C., Laks, H., & Buckburg, G.D. (1990). A new simplified method of optimizing cardioplegic delivery without right heart isolation: Antegrade/retrograde blood cardioplegia. *Journal of Thoracic and Cardiovascular Surgery, 100*, 56.

Edmunds, L.H. (1987). Thromboembolic and bleeding complications of prosthetic heart valves. *Annals of Thoracic Surgery, 44*, 430.

Espersen, C. (1993). The R.N. first assistant in cardiac surgery. In J.C. Rothrock (Ed.), *The R.N. first assistant: An expanded perioperative role* (2nd ed.). Philadelphia: J.B. Lippincott.

Futterman, L.G., & Lemberg, L. (1992). Pacemaker update: 1992. Part I. General remarks and electrocardiographic assessment of pacemaker function. *American Journal of Critical Care, 1* (3), 118.

Futterman, L.G., & Lemberg, L. (1993). Pacemaker update. Part II. Atrioventricular synchronous and rate-modulated pacemakers. *American Journal of Critical Care, 2* (1), 96.

Glick, D.B., Liddicoat, J.R., & Karp, R.B. (1990). Alternative conduits

for coronary artery bypass grafting. In *Advances in Cardiac Surgery* (Vol 2), St. Louis: Mosby.

Guzzetta, C.E., & Dossey, B.M. (1992). Cardiovascular nursing: Holistic practice. St. Louis: Mosby.

Guzzetta, C.E., & Seifert, P.C. (1991). Cardiovascular assessment. In Kinney, M.R., et al. (Eds.), *Comprehensive cardiac care* (7th ed.). St. Louis: Mosby.

Holmquist, T., & Gamberg, P.L. (1992). Heart and heart-lung transplantation. *Today's OR Nurse, 14* (2), 12.

Kaplan, J.A. (1993). *Cardiac anesthesia* (3rd ed.). Philadelphia: W.B. Saunders.

Kirklin, J.K. (1991). Prospects for understanding and eliminating the deleterious effects of cardiopulmonary bypass. *Annals of Thoracic Surgery, 51*, 529.

Kirklin, J.W., & Barratt-Boyes, B. (1993). *Cardiac surgery* (2nd ed.). New York: Churchill Livingstone.

Kirlin, J.W., et al. (1983). Complement and the damaging effects of cardiopulmonary bypass. *Journal of Thoracic and Cardiovascular Surgery, 86* (6), 845.

Lange, P.L., & Hopkins, R.A. (1989). Allograft valve banking: Techniques and technology. In R.A. Hopkins (Ed.), Cardiac reconstructions with allograft valves. New York: Springer-Verlag.

Loop, F.D., et al. (1986). Influence of the internal mammary artery graft on 10-year survival and other cardiac events. *New England Journal of Medicine, 314*, 1.

Lytle, B.W., et al. (1989). Coronary artery bypass grafting with the right gastroepiploic artery. *Journal of Thoracic and Cardiovascular Surgery, 97* (6), 826.

Mason, P., & McPherson, C. (1992). Implantable cardioverter defibrillator: A review. *Heart & Lung, 21* (2), 141.

May, D., & Adams, R.H. (1992). Management and administration of the operating room during transplantation. *Seminars in Perioperative Nursing, 1* (1), 3.

McClung, J.A., et al. (1983). Prosthetic heart valves: A review. *Progress in Cardiovascular Disease, 26*, 237.

Penington, D.G., & Swartz, M.T. (1992). Assisted circulation and mechanical hearts. In E. Braunwald (Ed.), *Heart disease* (4th ed.). Philadelphia: W.B. Saunders.

Phillips, S.J., et al. (1989). Percutaneous cardiopulmonary bypass: Application and indication for use. *Annals of Thoracic Surgery, 47*, 121.

Prinkey, L.A. (1992). Defibrillation, cardioversion, and the automatic implantable cardioverter defibrillator. In C.E., Guzzetta, and B.M. Dossey, (Eds.), *Cardiovascular nursing: Holistic approach*. St. Louis: Mosby.

Rabago, G., et al. (1980). The new DeVega technique in tricuspid annuloplasty. *Journal of Thoracic and Cardiovascular Surgery, 21*, 231.

Regas, M.L. (1993). Reoperative cardiac surgery. *AORN Journal, 57* (5), 1131.

Regas, M.L., Hill, S.B., Schmidt, C.V. (1986). Wolff-Parkinson-White syndrome: cryosurgical ablation of accessory pathways. *AORN Journal, 44*(5), 742.

Robicsek, F., et al. (1989). Experiments with a bowl of saline: The hidden risk of hypothermic-osmotic damage during topical cardiac cooling. *Journal of Thoracic and Cardiovascular Surgery, 97*, 461.

Ross, D. (1991). Technique of aortic valve replacement with a homograft: Orthotopic replacement. Annals of Thoracic Surgery, 52, 154.

Schakenbach, L.H. (1987). Physiologic dynamics of acquired valvular heart disease. *Journal of Cardiovascular Nursing, 1*, 1.

Slogoff, S., & Keats, A.S. (1984). Randomized trial of primary anesthetic agents on outcome of coronary artery bypass operations. *Anesthesiology, 70*, 179.

Taubman, M.R. (1991). Advances in diagnostic testing. In S. Wingate (Ed.), *Cardiac nursing: A clinical management and patient care resource*. Rockville, MD: Aspen Publishers.

Waldhausen, J.A., & Pierce, W.S. (1985). *Johnson's surgery of the chest* (5th ed.). Chicago: Year Book Medical Publishers.

Zipes, D.P. (1992). Management of cardiac arrhythmias: Pharmacological, electrical, and surgical techniques. In E. Braunwald (Ed.), *Heart disease* (45th ed.). Philadelphia: W.B. Saunders.

BIBLIOGRAPHY

American Nurses' Association Division on Medical-Surgical Nursing Practice and the American Heart Association Council on Cardiovascular Nursing. (1981). *Standards of cardiovascular nursing practice.* Kansas City: The Association.

Canobbio, M.M. (1990). *Cardiovascular disorders.* St. Louis: Mosby.

Crawford, E.S., & Crawford, J.L. (1984). *Diseases of the aorta.* Baltimore: Williams & Wilkins.

Edmunds, L.H., Norwood, W.I., & Low, D.W. (1990). *Atlas of cardiothoracic surgery.* Philadelphia: Lea & Febiger.

Gay, W.A., Jr. (1990). *Atlas of adult cardiac surgery.* New York: Churchill Livingstone.

Roberts, W.C. (1987). *Adult congenital heart disease.* Philadelphia: F.A. Davis.

Seifert, P.C. (1994). *Cardiac surgery.* St Louis: Mosby.

Seifert, P.C. (1990). *Cardiac surgery.* In J.C. Rothrock (editor), *Perioperative nursing care planning.* St. Louis: Mosby.

Seifert, P.C., & Lefrak, E.A. (1984). Atrial septal defect in the adult. *AORN Journal, 39,* 617.

Shumacker H.B. (1992). *The evolution of cardiac surgery.* Bloomington: Indiana University Press.

Waldhausen, J.A., & Orringer, M.B. (1991). *Complications in cardiothoracic surgery.* St. Louis: Mosby.

PART THREE

SPECIAL CONSIDERATIONS

27

AMBULATORY SURGERY

DONNA S. WATSON AND CHERYL A. SANGERMANO

Ambulatory surgery is referred to as early as 3000 BC in writings from Egyptian scrolls. Ambulatory surgery is interwoven within medical and nursing history and is referred to in the Bible and early Indian and Hindu literature. In ancient Greece and Rome homes and temples were sites for worship and healing. During the Middle Ages the Church continued to provide treatment to the needy through church-sponsored hospitals that included both inpatient and outpatient care. The nineteenth century began an age of medical discovery. Great pioneers in health care and infection control included Vesalius, Harvey, Lister, Pasteur, and nursing's Florence Nightingale. Advances during this time for medicine and nursing progressed rapidly. Discoveries influencing medicine and nursing included the development of anesthesia, the germ theory, the delineation of the anatomy and physiology of the human body, bacteriology, and antibiotic therapy. These discoveries had tremendous impact on the care of the surgical patient.

In the United States the initial concept of ambulatory surgery began in 1818 when Massachusetts General Hospital established the first outpatient department. It was not until the 1960s that interest in ambulatory surgery became a reality. In part this was due to new anesthetic agents and techniques that allowed for a more rapid recovery with fewer side effects. Two highly recognized successful ambulatory programs included the Cohen and Dillon hospital-based surgical outpatient program at the University of California, Los Angeles, and the "come and go" surgery unit at George Washington University, Washington, DC.

The first freestanding surgical center that was independently owned and operated was the Phoenix Surgicenter, which was founded by Drs. Wallace Reed and John Ford. Dr. Reed has stated the key concepts for safety in the ambulatory setting include patient selection, types of procedures, anesthesia, careful surgery, well-defined discharge criteria, and appropriate follow-up (Mathias, 1987). The Phoenix Surgicenter quickly became a prototype for other centers across the country and originated many concepts and practices that continue to influence the field of ambulatory surgery today.

Reasons for the resurgence of ambulatory surgery include improved technology in surgical procedures, improved anesthesia technology and agents, and better management in the postoperative phase (Llewellyn, 1991). In addition to increased public awareness and support, ambulatory surgery is proving to be cost effective with third-party payers, Medicare, and Medicaid. Safety and quality of care issues are used as guiding factors to determine appropriateness of the surgical procedure and patient selection. Many procedures that were once considered only appropriate for inpatient treatment are now being performed with great success as ambulatory surgery.

The Association of Operating Room Nurses (AORN) has issued a statement on perioperative nursing practice in ambulatory surgery (Box 27-1). The statement recognizes the significance and importance of a skilled perioperative nurse who is clinically and professionally competent to provide care to the ambulatory surgery patient in a short time frame. The care provided should be "cost-effective, convenient, and efficient." Nursing care should be consistent with established standards of perioperative nursing practice and must include the patient and family/significant others throughout the surgical experience. The AORN recognizes the move from "the highest quality care at any price" toward "the best care at the lowest price" that offers safe, efficient care throughout the patient's surgical experience.

In 1966, Ferguson and Kaplan described the ambulatory patient as

one who does not require hospital in-patient care. This presupposes that the patient is able to walk and travel to his home after his treatment, safely, often without aid from other persons. It should be understood from the first that ambulation should not interfere with or retard the required treatment. Ambulatory care does not necessarily mean care in a private office. It may mean treatment given in an adequately equipped and staffed emergency room, out-patient department, or private office, or even in an operating room, to a patient who can return to his home after his treatment.

Today this definition is still appropriate and adequately describes the ambulatory patient who is discharged with the intention of having postoperative care provided by the patient and family or significant others.

FACILITIES

The types of facilities used for ambulatory surgery include hospital integrated, hospital separated, freestanding, office based, and recovery center. Patient condition and type of procedure assist in determining the most appropriate facility. Questions often asked to determine appropriateness of patient selection and facility include the following (Reiling, 1990):

1. Is the facility equipped to deal with emergency situations related to the surgical procedure, patient condition, and anticipated medications?
2. Can the procedure be performed without hospitalization?
3. Is the risk to the patient minimal if the procedure is performed at the facility?
4. Will extended recovery be necessary?
5. Are quality standards adhered to at the facility?
6. Does the patient need any special care (e.g., equipment) that may not be available at the facility?
7. Do the patient and family/significant others understand and accept the concept of ambulatory surgery?

The concept of ambulatory surgery is for a safe, convenient, and cost-effective surgery to be provided at a facility with the patient discharged to a short-term recovery center or home. The patient should have no unusual problems and the family/significant others should be willing to monitor, provide treatment as necessary, and care for the patient once discharged.

HOSPITAL-INTEGRATED FACILITY

The hospital-integrated facility is the most common system across the country. This setting uses the main operating room suites for all ambulatory surgery patients. However, many hospitals have different preoperative and postoperative areas that are designated specifically for ambulatory surgery patients. Scheduling of ambulatory surgery patients is usually done using the same protocols as for inpatients (i.e., block scheduling or time available). Ambulatory procedures may either be interspersed with inpatient procedures on any given day or done on a day or in an operating room reserved solely for ambulatory patients. The admitting process for these patients may be handled by the hospital's admitting department or by the ambulatory unit itself. In this type of setting family members of both inpatient and ambulatory surgery patients usually share a common waiting area.

In addition to admitting ambulatory surgery patients, hospital-integrated facilities may handle the processing of *day of surgery* patients or *AM admission* patients, who are to be admitted to the hospital following surgery. Preoperative laboratory and diagnostic tests are usually done on an outpatient basis prior to surgery, and these patients are admitted to the hospital following surgery. The length of stay depends on the procedure and appropriate recovery period.

The advantages of a hospital-integrated facility include shared personnel among the different areas, available equipment and supplies, rapid admission to the hospital if necessary, and sharing of cost related to capital budget. However, there is less control of the scheduling and delays due to ambulatory surgical patients potentially following an inpatient procedure or being cancelled in the event of an inpatient surgical emergency.

HOSPITAL-SEPARATED FACILITY

This type of unit is affiliated with the hospital but is a separate ambulatory surgery department with designated preoperative, intraoperative, and postoperative areas. The facility may be located within the hospital complex, adjacent to the hospital, or at a satellite location some distance from the hospital. In contrast to the hospital-integrated facility, the hospital-separated facility has a dedicated staff, equipment, policies and procedures, and postanesthesia recovery care area for the ambulatory surgery patient. The facility is physically and organizationally separate from the hospital's main operating room suites and is exclusive for the ambulatory surgery patient population. Advantages of this type of facility include convenient scheduling, availability of hospital services, easy admission of the patient to the hospital if necessary, less likelihood of delay or cancellation due to scheduling complications, sharing of certain equipment with the main operating room suite, and use for more complicated procedures and high-risk patients.

FREESTANDING FACILITY

The freestanding facility is independently owned and operated and is not hospital affiliated. These facilities are operated on a for-profit basis and may be owned by entrepreneurs, physicians, and nurses. The types of ownership vary and generally include corporate, joint venture, or independent. A growing trend has been for health care corporation chains to own and operate such facilities. These facilities comprise a growing segment of the industry, are conveniently located, and cater to the desires and needs of the patient, while providing safe, quality care that is cost effective (Research Highlight 27-1).

RESEARCH HIGHLIGHT 27-1

The purpose of this study was to determine patient satisfaction of hospital-based versus freestanding facilities. Variables studied included patient satisfaction toward nursing care, the nursing staff, convenience of facility, and cost. Greater patient satisfaction in the freestanding ambulatory surgery was noted in the following areas: care received, ease and convenience of facility, handling of complaints, comfort and design of facility, staff courtesy, and cost.

This information is critical to the competitive environment that exists between hospital-based and freestanding ambulatory surgery facilities. Often marketing efforts are directed toward the physician and not the patient. The influence the patient has over family and friends should not be underestimated in the existing competitive environment.

Pica-Furey, W. (1993). Ambulatory surgery—hospital-based vs freestanding. *AORN Journal*, 57(5), 1119-1127.

OFFICE-BASED FACILITY

The office-based facility is much like a free-standing facility but is operated on a smaller scale. These facilities allow for ambulatory surgery to be provided safely and effectively in a physician's office. These for-profit facilities often have elaborate equipment, specially trained personnel, and an appropriate inventory of supplies and instrumentation. Advantages include more schedule flexibility both for the physician and patient, cost-effectiveness of the procedure, and staff with training specific to the procedures being performed. Limitations include strict patient selection criteria and the lack of a regulating agency to assess and determine that standards of quality are being implemented. The office-based facility specializing in the delivery of a single-specialty surgery may be at risk if reimbursement from third-party payers, Medicare, or Medicaid is dropped or decreased. In addition, patients may be lost to other ambulatory facilities that provide multiple services (Slomski, 1993).

RECOVERY CENTER

The concept of a freestanding facility with an adjacent recovery center is becoming popular in many areas of the country. The recovery center offers an alternative to the patient and family or significant others when skilled nursing care is desired but acute care is unnecessary. The center generally is equipped with private rooms designed with a decor similar to a hotel. A family member or significant other is allowed to stay with the patient if desired. The needs of the patient and visitor are catered to (for example, meals, telephone, television, stereo, minibar).

Llewellyn (1991) described typical admission criteria to a recovery center as the following: anticipated stay less than 72 hours, patient must be able to provide own basic self-care needs, adequate pain management to be achieved within 72 hours, and the patient must have adequate psychomotor and cognitive skills to learn proper self-care techniques for discharge to home. Types of procedures likely to be done in a recovery care center include knee ligament reconstruction, acromioplasty, cholecystectomy, hemorrhoidectomy, and mastectomy (Cruz, 1990).

PATIENT SELECTION

Criteria for appropriate patient selection should be identified. Because surgical intervention in an ambulatory facility does not decrease the chance for potential complications, each patient should be carefully selected. In the past, patients considered appropriate for ambulatory surgery were healthy, young, and had no underlying illness. However, procedures being performed today are more complex and the patients are older and less healthy (Box 27-2).

Those responsible for determining appropriate patient selection include the surgeon, anesthesia personnel, and perioperative nurse. The surgeon is responsible for assessing underlying problems that may lead to unexpected compli-

---

BOX 27-2

Procedures Frequently Performed in Ambulatory Surgery

General surgery
  Breast biopsy
  Hemorrhoidectomy
  Laparoscopic procedures
Gynecology
  Tubal ligation
  Vaginal hysterectomy
  Dilatation and curettage
  Laparoscopy
Ophthalmology
  Cataract extraction
  Keratotomy
Orthopedics
  Arthroscopy
  Tendon release
  Removal of plates, screws
Otolaryngology
  Tonsillectomy
  Adenoidectomy
  Nasal polypectomy
  Myringotomy
  Vocal cord biopsy
Plastic surgery
  Nasal fracture reduction
  Skin graft
  Mammoplasty
  Liposuction
  Blepharoplasty
  Facelift
Urology
  Cystoscopy
  Ureteroscopy
  Vasectomy
  Biopsy
  Circumcision
Dental surgery
  Dental implant
  Extractions
Cardiovascular surgery
  Arteriography
  Cardiac catheterization
Gastroenterology
  Colonoscopy
  Bronchoscopy
  Esophagoscopy

---

and underlying disease processes should be determined inappropriate for ambulatory surgery and scheduled in the main operating room. Anesthesia personnel are responsible for assessing any known or unknown problems related to the chosen anesthetic course. The perioperative nurse is responsible for assessing and evaluating the patient for factors that could lead to potential complications throughout the perioperative period.

A commonly used classification system is that of the American Society of Anesthesiologists (ASA) (see Table 6-2). The surgeon, anesthesia personnel, or perioperative nurse assigns the patient an ASA physical status classification. Patients classified as physical status 1 or 2 are perfect candidates for ambulatory surgery. These patients generally pose no great risk for procedures performed with general or local anesthesia or IV conscious sedation. Patients classified as physical status 3 must be carefully evaluated and determined that no untoward event is likely to occur during the intraoperative and postoperative phases. Any concomitant disease must be well managed before the patient is acceptable for ambulatory surgery. All patients should be monitored appropriately throughout the perioperative period.

ANESTHESIA

Ambulatory surgery is possible in part due to advances of anesthesia and the desire for the ideal agent. Although the ideal agent has yet to be discovered, desirable characteristics of anesthesia for the ambulatory patient include a rapid recovery period and few side effects. The type of anesthesia care delivered to the ambulatory patient is a departure from traditional anesthesia practice due to increasing pressure to discharge the patient in a shorter amount of time.

PREMEDICATION

A premedication may be prescribed to decrease the patient's anxiety and fear toward the scheduled surgery (Table 27-1). Additional advantages for administration of a premedication include analgesia effect, amnesia effect (depending on drug and dosage), and often a decreased incidence of postoperative nausea and vomiting. Following the administration of a premedication the patient is limited to bed. Often the effects of a premedication generate a longer postoperative recovery period for the patient than most ambulatory procedures. For these reasons the use of a premedication is often avoided. However, a patient experiencing anxiety and apprehension should never be denied a premedication if necessary.

GENERAL ANESTHESIA

In the event a procedure requires more than the administration of local anesthesia, general anesthesia is administered by anesthesia personnel. For the ambulatory surgery patient receiving general anesthesia, consideration must be

cations during the procedure. A patient with complex medical conditions unrelated to the procedure may be scheduled at a hospital-affiliated facility versus a freestanding facility because of the potential for specific complications (such as dialysis). Patients with complex medical conditions

TABLE 27-1

Premedications

Medication	Dosage
SEDATIVE	
Diazepam	5-10 mg, IV
Midazolam	0.07-0.08 mg/Kg, IM
	0.5-2.5 mg, IV
Droperidol	5-10 mg, PO
	2.5-10 mg, IV or IM
NARCOTIC	
Meperidine	50-100 mg, IM
Fentanyl	50-100 μg, IV or IM

BOX 27-3

Anesthetic Agents

INDUCTION AGENTS
Thiopental sodium
Methohexital sodium
Etomidate
Ketamine
Midazolam
Propofol

NEUROMUSCULAR BLOCKING AGENTS
Succinylcholine
Mivacurium
Atracurium
Vecuronium
Pancuronium

INHALATION AGENTS
Halothane
Nitrous oxide
Enflurane
Methoxyflurane
Isoflurane
Sevoflurane
Desflurane

BOX 27-4

Local Anesthetic Agents

AMINO AMIDE
Prilocaine
Mepivacaine
Lidocaine
Bupivacaine
Etidocaine
Ropivacaine

AMINO ESTER
Procaine
Chloroprocaine
Cocaine
Tetracaine

given to readiness for timely discharge of the patient. Recently approved agents allow for quick induction, short duration of action, and few effects on the patient's vital signs, and are relatively safe to administer (Box 27-3).

LOCAL ANESTHESIA

Local anesthesia is commonly used for the ambulatory surgery patient. The medication is administered by the physician, and the perioperative nurse is responsible for monitoring the patient throughout the procedure. Local anesthetics are classified as either amino esters or amino amides (Box 27-4). Local anesthetics are chosen by the surgeon based on the desired duration of action, surgery site, and potency potential. Epinephrine may be added to the local anesthesia agent for vasoconstricting properties in the area injected, slower rate of absorption of the local anesthetic agent, and lower incidence of toxicity (Rivellini, 1993). This allows for a longer duration of action for the agent and reduces blood flow to the area injected. The perioperative nurse should monitor the patient for presence of side effects such as central nervous system disturbances, cardiovascular problems, hypersensitivity to medication, and toxic reaction resulting from high levels of the local anesthetic agent.

CONSCIOUS SEDATION

The perioperative nurse is responsible for monitoring and often administering medications to achieve intravenous (IV) conscious sedation (Box 27-5). Conscious sedation is defined as "a condition where the patient exhibits a depressed level of consciousness, but retains the ability to independently and continuously maintain a patent airway and respond appropriately to verbal commands or physical stimulation" (AORN, 1993c). For optimal care of the patient receiving IV conscious sedation the following monitoring parameters should be applied: respiratory rate, oxygen saturation, blood pressure, cardiac rate and rhythm, level of consciousness, and skin condition. Continuous uninter-

rupted monitoring should be provided by the perioperative nurse responsible for the management of the patient receiving IV conscious sedation. The nurse may be requested to divert attention away from the patient, leaving the potential for subtle symptoms of an impending problem to go unobserved. Therefore, a second circulator should be assigned to assume the circulating responsibilities during the procedure.

BOX 27-5

Commonly Administered Agents for IV Conscious Sedation

SEDATIVE-HYPNOTICS

Diazepam
Midazolam
Methohexital sodium
Ketamine
Propofol
Florazepam

NARCOTICS

Fentanyl
Alfentanil
Sufentanil
Butorphanol
Nalbuphine

APPEAL OF AMBULATORY SURGERY

It has been estimated that by the year 2000 over 70% of procedures that would now be done at inpatient hospital facilities will be treated at alternative facilities such as ambulatory surgery facilities, physician offices, and other alternative settings (Michel and Myrick, 1990). With safety, efficiency, and cost-effectiveness well established, third-party payers not only support, but also encourage and in many procedures require the use of ambulatory surgery facilities by their subscribers. As an incentive for use, higher reimbursement for procedures performed at an ambulatory surgery facility is often provided. Government agencies, especially those associated with Medicare and Medicaid, are actively involved in discussion and legislation relating to the balance between acceptable care and decreased cost. Ambulatory care is a focal point and a prime topic of consideration in the health care arena today.

Ambulatory surgery is appealing to the patient and family or significant others because there are fewer disruptions of normal daily activities, less separation from family or significant other, less time away from the workplace, and less worry about financial outlays. The ambulatory surgery patient and family or significant other are active participants in the patient's plan of care.

For health care professionals the advantages of ambulatory surgery are clear. There is convenience and less time away from the office for the surgeon. There is opportunity for anesthesiologists to enter into and specialize in a different arena in which anesthetic agents and techniques are continuously being improved to enhance rapid patient recovery and return to ambulation. There are opportunities for the perioperative nurse to condense and refine nursing skills and to develop nursing practice models that focus on well-

ness, safety, comfort, patient education, and continuity of care. The emphasis on cross-training, productivity, versatility, and independence is appealing to the motivated perioperative nurse practicing in ambulatory surgery. The patient scheduled for ambulatory surgery has fewer preoperative tests and fewer medications and may be active, awake, and involved throughout the entire perioperative period. The chances for an expanded role are numerous for the nurse specializing in the care of the ambulatory surgery patient.

The advent of ambulatory surgery has caused a shift of many traditional beliefs and myths related to care of the surgical patient. Patients must now assume responsibility for their own self-care, and they do so with ease when properly instructed by the perioperative nurse (Lea and Phippen, 1992). The ambulatory surgery patient is mobile soon after surgery and recuperates at home with care provided by the patient and family or significant other. Long and costly hospital stays are unnecessary for the healthy patient scheduled for an uncomplicated surgical procedure.

Ambulatory surgery facilities are small in comparison with the entire organizational structure and makeup of a hospital. However, it is this unique feature that has resulted in the overwhelming success and acceptance of the ambulatory surgery concept. One-stop surgery appeals to the patient who is selected according to preestablished criteria, is well prepared, and is informed about the impending surgical experience. These factors, and a well-educated staff of professionals, allow ambulatory surgery to deliver high-quality patient care.

NURSING CARE FOR THE AMBULATORY PATIENT

Perioperative nursing in the ambulatory surgery setting incorporates all elements of the AORN standards of perioperative nursing (Box 27-6). However, the paradigm from which the perioperative nurse manages care of the ambulatory patient is very different from that of the hospitalized patient. The ambulatory patient is essentially healthy and the time spent in the ambulatory setting is relatively short, ranging from a few hours to 1 day. Therefore the plan of care for the ambulatory surgical patient must be organized and efficient.

Responsibility for most of the preoperative and postoperative care is assumed by the patient and family or significant other. Therefore their education is an integral part of ambulatory surgery and must be fully understood by each. The education process is continuous, begins preoperatively, and proceeds after the patient is discharged. This allows for the caregiver to be prepared for the role once the patient is discharged. The ultimate goal of providing education to the patient and family or significant other is to facilitate adequate preparation for meeting postoperative care needs and seeking additional assistance, if necessary.

AORN Standards of Perioperative Nursing

STANDARDS OF PERIOPERATIVE CLINICAL PRACTICE

Assessment
Diagnosis
Outcome identification
Planning
Implementation
Evaluation

STANDARDS OF PERIOPERATIVE PROFESSIONAL PERFORMANCE

Quality of care
Performance appraisal
Education
Collegiality
Ethics
Collaboration
Research
Resource use

PREOPERATIVE PHASE

The physician and patient determine the appropriateness of surgical intervention at an ambulatory facility. The patient's fears and concerns toward having ambulatory surgery are discussed. Patients should not feel they are receiving a lesser standard of care because the procedure is scheduled at an ambulatory surgery facility.

Preoperative communication with the patient includes patient education and assists in determining an individualized plan of care for discharge planning. The following information is presented to the patient by the perioperative nurse:

1. Time and nature of surgery
2. Location, parking, and suggested time of arrival to the ambulatory surgery center
3. Food and liquid restrictions
4. Suggested clothing for discharge
5. Necessary items to bring (such as glasses, hearing aids)
6. Instructions regarding valuables
7. Identification of responsible adult escort for discharge
8. Who to call for any questions prior to the procedure
9. Necessary insurance papers to bring
10. Resources available in the home

To assist in data collection the patient may be asked health-related questions that describe pertinent physical disabilities, previous surgeries and anesthetics with associated responses, and vital information such as height, weight, allergies, and current medications. This assessment may be completed preoperatively in various ways, including preoperative phone interview (Fig. 27-1), preadmission clinic (Research Highlight 27-2), time of admission to the facility, and written questionnaire. When preadmission information is obtained before the day of surgery, the admitting process is shortened.

The style, decor, ambiance, color, physical arrangement, and traffic flow should be thoughtfully designed and bring to mind the comforts of home, rather than giving the impression of confinement and austerity. Following admission to the facility and correct identification of the patient, the patient and family or significant other should be given an orientation to the facility and explained the expected sequence of events that will follow. The patient then changes into the appropriate surgical attire, and provisions are made for the safekeeping of clothing and any valuables the patient may have brought. The following assessment parameters should be obtained and documented by the perioperative nurse.

Observation and assessment of general physical and psychosocial behavior, sensory-perceptual alterations, emotional status, interaction with family, and compliance with preoperative instructions
Baseline vital signs
Verification of required laboratory values, x-rays, history and physical examination
Administration of preoperative medications as ordered
Assessment of anxiety and apprehension related to impending surgical procedure
Assessment of patient knowledge regarding impending surgical procedure, recovery, and postoperative care
Assessment of patient expectations regarding pain control and management postoperatively
Development of appropriate plan of care (see Fig. 27-1).

An intravenous line may be inserted as ordered. The family or significant other should be permitted to stay with the patient in the preoperative area, and provisions should be made for their comfort. These individuals are an integral part of the patient's well-being and should always be included as part of the patient's surgical experience. Colorful surroundings and the promotion of relaxation through means such as music, television, videos, should be provided.

The patient may walk to the surgical suite or be transported by wheelchair or stretcher. The mode of transportation depends on the patient's abilities, the effects of premedications if administered, and the policies of the facility. The family or significant others are directed to the waiting area, informed of the approximate time for the procedure, and made comfortable with refreshments, reading material, music, or television.

ASC PRE-OP PHONE CALL

Date	Procedure	Office notified of inability to reach patient	Person instructed
Time	Physician	☐ Yes ☐ No ☐ N/A	Relationship

INSTRUCTIONS REVIEWED

Arrival time:_____per   hospital   office
☐ Preferred Name_____
☐ Parking
☐ Responsible adult available for transport to/from
   Hospital and 24 hours after surgery
☐ Insurance Card
☐ No make-up, nail polish, jewelry, valuables or
   alcoholic beverages X 24 hrs. pre-op
☐ Clothing (according to surgery)
☐ NPO after MN. or _____
   (unless otherwise instructed per physician)
☐ Advance Directives (DOS only)
☐ Understanding of surgical procedure_____
   _____
☐ Expected Post-op needs:_____

MEDICAL HISTORY

YES	NO	
☐	☐	Diabetic
☐	☐	Cardiac
☐	☐	Hypertension
☐	☐	Seizures
☐	☐	Disabilities/Limitations
☐	☐	Asthma, COPD, Black Lung
☐	☐	Recent Cold Symptoms
☐	☐	Smoker_____ppd X_____yrs
☐	☐	Anesthesia Complications
☐	☐	Hepatitis

PEDIATRICS

☐	☐	Immunizations Current
☐	☐	Developmental Age Appropriate

CURRENT MEDICATIONS

Comments:

Pre-Op Call Information verified ☐ Yes ☐ No ☐ N/A
Comments:

Signature:

PRE-OPERATIVE ASSESSMENT / CHECKLIST

ALLERGIES/REACTIONS: _____

Date	HT: _____	Vital Signs
Time	WT: _____	B/P_____ T____ P____ R____

CHECK LIST

	Yes	No	N/A
NPO@_____			
H&P			
Surgical Consent Signed (if ordered by Physician)			
Surgical Attire			
ID Band			
Allergy Band			
Addressograph			
Pre-Op ATB'S Ordered			
Voided			
Nursing History Done			

Other Equipment

LAB RESULTS

	On Chart	Obtained	N/A
K+ (if>16 yrs. of age & general anesthesia)			
Glucose (if Diabetic)			
CBC			
HGB (OP only)			
HCG/Serum Urine (If ordered)			
PT/PTT (if ordered)			
ABG'S (if ordered)			
U/A			
T&C/Screen/Hold Clot (if ordered # units_____)			
EKG (>40 yrs. of age)			
Radiology (ordered / brought)			
Other _____			

ABNORMAL RESULTS REPORTED   ☐ N/A
Time: _____ Physician _____
Comments: _____

Time	Pre-Op Medication	Route / Dose	Administered By
	☐ Refer to MAR		

Transport to Pre-Op holding per: ☐ Cart ☐ W/C ☐ Amb ☐ Carried
Signature:

SKIN INTEGRITY
☐ Normal
☐ Red
☐ Edema
☐ Blister
☐ Dry
☐ Ecchymosis
☐

SELF CONCEPT/ COPING
☐ Alert
☐ Calm/Relaxed
☐ Anxiety
   (Mild, Moderate, Severe)
☐ Disoriented
☐ Oriented/But Sedated
☐ Lethargic
☐ Combative
☐ Cultural/Spiritual
   Needs _____
☐

OXYGENATION/ CIRCULATION
☐ Regular
☐ Labored
☐ Assisted
☐ Oxygen
☐

COGNITION/PERCEPTION DEFICITS
☐ None
☐ Blind
☐ Deaf/Hard of Hearing
☐ Mute
☐ Language Barrier
☐

ACTIVITY / REST
☐ Normal   ☐ Limited ROM
☐ Paralysis   ☐ Restraints
☐ Obesity   ☐
☐ Prothesis

SAFETY & SECURITY

ITEMS REMOVED	N/A	FAMILY	OTHER	LOCKER
☐ Contact Lenses				
☐ Eye Glasses				
☐ Dentures/Partials				
☐ Prosthesis				
☐ Hearing Aids				
☐ Jewelry/Hair Pins				
☐ Nail Polish				
☐ Underwear				
☐ W/C, Canes, etc.				
☐				

FIG. 27-1   Preoperative nursing care record.
Courtesy Grant Medical Center, Columbus, Ohio.

| ☐ Refer to current Patient Care Plan | Signature: _____ | Date: _____ |
| ☐ Refer to current Teaching-Learning Flowsheet | Signature: _____ | Date: _____ |

NURSING DIAGNOSIS	INTERVENTIONS	TEACHING METHOD	OUTCOME
☐ High risk for non-compliance related to fear, anxiety or knowledge deficit.	☐ 1) Answer questions about O.R. to allay anxiety and fear, offer reassurance as needed. ☐ 2) Explain reasons for restrictions and importance of compliance with instructions.	☐ Verbal ☐ Written ☐ Demonstrated ☐ Other	Patient will demonstrate compliance with pre-operative instructions. ☐ Met ☐ Not Met
☐ High risk for patient/family/ significant other knowledge deficit related to surgical procedures.	☐ 1) Review with patient/family/significant other their understanding of surgical procedure. ☐ 2) Answer questions about surgical experience and involve physician as needed. ☐ 3) Explain labs, EKG's, meds, IV's, holding area, anesthesia type & effects. ☐ 4) Explain PACU/ASC recovery phase and what to expect. ☐ 5) Allow family/significant other to assist in care.	☐ Verbal ☐ Written ☐ Demonstrated ☐ Other	Patient/family/significant other verbalizes understanding of pre-operative, intra-operative and post-operative activities. ☐ Met ☐ Not Met
☐ High risk for anxiety related to surgical experience.	☐ 1) Identify level of anxiety: MILD MODERATE SEVERE ☐ 2) Explain procedures to reduce fear of unknown. ☐ 3) Allow patient to verbalize fears. ☐ 4) Answer questions and offer support to patient/family/significant other. ☐ 5) Notify anesthesia of greater than or equal to moderate anxiety.	☐ Verbal ☐ Written ☐ Demonstrated ☐ Other	Patient will demonstrate no more than moderate anxiety. Met ☐ Not Met
☐			

COMMENTS: _____

_____

_____

_____

_____

_____

_____

Signature: _____ Date: _____

FIG. 27-1, CONT'D   For legend, see opposite page.

⚘
RESEARCH HIGHLIGHT 27-2

The purpose of this research was to develop a preadmission program that would facilitate the admitting of patients scheduled as AM admission and 1-day surgery. Patients were admitted 60 to 90 minutes before their scheduled procedure. The patient and family or significant others were given preoperative instruction, appropriate lab specimens were collected, and necessary billing information was obtained. Proper consent forms and patient teaching were provided by a perioperative nurse. The surgeon and anesthesiologist were consulted regarding abnormal laboratory values and histories. All patients admitted were contacted with a postoperative visit or telephone call as appropriate.

The preadmission clinic received positive evaluations from both patients and physicians. Approximately 1.5% to 2% of all scheduled procedures resulted in cancellation. The early cancellation was cost-effective because of the reduction in operating room cost and surgical staff time. This allowed for cases to be moved up and prevented unnecessary setup and room charge to the patient. Today it is important to become more efficient while decreasing cost for the facility and patient. The study results provide statistical support of the economic value of establishing a preadmission clinic.

Muldowny, E.H. (1993). Establishing a preadmission clinic. *AORN Journal,* 58(6), 1183-1191.

INTRAOPERATIVE PHASE

Intraoperative nursing care for the ambulatory surgery patient is consistent with the AORN standards and recommended practices utilized for an inpatient. Nursing care and responsibilities include the following:

Identify the patient, introduce self, and review chart.

Report to the physician any relative or absolute contraindications to intraoperative medications that may be used.

Safely transfer the patient to the OR bed.

Properly position patient and maintain correct body alignment.

Assist anesthesia personnel as appropriate.

Administer medications for IV conscious sedation, under the direction of a physician.

Monitor the patient receiving IV conscious sedation and report any changes such as restlessness, cyanosis, pallor, flushing, diaphoresis, nausea, low oxygen saturation, dysrhythmias, and allergic reaction.

Manage nursing care of the patient throughout the surgical intervention; duties are similar to the inpatient setting (that is, scrub, circulator, RN first assistant).

Monitor for safety precautions, aseptic techniques, skin integrity, and fluid and electrolyte balance.

Document plan of care in a contemporaneous manner according to facility policy and procedure (Fig. 27-2).

Maintain AORN standards and recommended practices for the perioperative patient.

It is common practice in ambulatory surgery for the patient to receive IV conscious sedation administered and/or monitored by the perioperative nurse. In addition to the preoperative assessment parameters previously described, the nurse responsible for managing the care of the patient receiving IV conscious sedation during the intraoperative phase should conduct a thorough nursing assessment (Box 27-7). The goal of this assessment is to determine any contraindications to the administration of IV conscious sedation medications and patient appropriateness for nurse management.

The AORN has developed recommended practices that specifically address monitoring parameters applicable to the ambulatory patient in the intraoperative phase. These include "Recommended practices for monitoring the patient receiving intravenous conscious sedation" and "Recommended practices for monitoring the patient receiving local anesthesia" (AORN, 1994). The recommended practices are intended for optimal patient care and should be applied by the perioperative nurse in the ambulatory setting. Other nursing associations have developed and endorsed a position statement circulated by the ANA entitled "Position statement on the role of the RN in the management of patients receiving IV conscious sedation for short-term, diagnostic, therapeutic, or surgical procedures" (AORN, 1992). Controversies and issues continue to exist on the appropriate roles and responsibilities of the nurse managing the care of the patient receiving IV conscious sedation. Policy and procedures should be developed and in place based on guidelines and recommendations set forth by the state board of nursing and national nursing associations.

One nurse should be responsible for monitoring the patient receiving IV conscious sedation (Watson, 1991). This nurse should "have no other responsibilities that would leave the patient unattended or compromise continuous monitoring" (AORN, 1992). The patient's vital signs are monitored by use of electrocardiogram (ECG), pulse oximetry, noninvasive blood pressure monitor, and general observation. The nurse must be familiar with the various types of monitoring equipment and have a basic understanding of ECG interpretation. A second circulator should be assigned to assist with circulating responsibilities during the procedure.

After completion of the surgical procedure, the patient is transferred to the appropriate recovery area. A complete report on the status of the patient, procedure performed, medications administered, dressings, and allergies is communicated to the receiving nurse by the perioperative nurse or anesthesiologist, as appropriate.

BOX 27-7

Nursing Assessment for the Patient Receiving IV Conscious Sedation

1. Does the patient have any history of:
   Seizure disorder?
   Substance abuse?
   Posttraumatic stress syndrome?
   Cardiovascular problems?
   Liver or kidney problems?
   Respiratory problems?
   Thyroid problems?
   Allergies to medications?
2. Has the patient ever had a bad experience in surgery or an outpatient office such as the dental office?
3. What medications is the patient currently taking? When was the last dose? Noted sensitivity to any medication?
4. NPO status?
5. Height and weight?
6. Any known medical condition unrelated to the procedure? Is the condition well controlled?

POSTOPERATIVE PHASE

Ambulatory surgery is followed by a rapid recovery period, which includes two distinct phases. The first phase is emergency from anesthesia, the same for both the inpatient and the ambulatory surgery patient receiving general anesthesia. The second phase allows for readaptation to the environment where the patient is encouraged to sit up, stand, void, and ambulate. Although not always possible, many ambulatory surgery facilities have separate phase one and phase two recovery areas. The area to which the patient is transferred following surgery is determined by the type of anesthesia administered.

Assessment during phase one should be determined and established as a policy and procedure. This will assist staff in utilizing a uniform method of assessing all patients in phase one. The most common assessment parameters include respiration status, circulation status, level of consciousness, skin color, and level of voluntary activity. A variety of scoring systems that are simple to use allow for standardized reporting, such as the Aldrete Score (see Fig. 6-16).

Patients administered local anesthesia without IV conscious sedation are taken directly to the phase two recovery area. The patient is monitored for lightheadedness, dizziness, hemorrhage, nausea, vomiting, significant changes in baseline vital signs, pain management, psychomotor and cognitive function. Methods that may be used to assess psychomotor and cognitive function include paper and pencil test, single reaction time, coordination and attention tests, ability to walk in a straight line, Maddox wing test, flicker fusion test, and psychomotor test.

Postoperative nursing care and responsibilities applicable to both phase one and phase two include the following:

- Assess for inadequate ventilation related to anesthesia or airway obstruction.
- Monitor potential for fluid volume deficit related to anesthesia or hypovolemia.
- Monitor for injury related to emergence delirium.
- Monitor for alteration in comfort related to pain.
- Monitor for nausea and vomiting related to anesthesia and/or surgical procedure.
- Protect areas sensitized by the administration of local anesthetic agent.
- Monitor for alteration in circulation related to surgical procedure and/or dressing/cast.
- Encourage early ambulation and progressive fluid ingestion.
- Document plan of care according to facility policy and procedure (Fig. 27-3).
- Apply appropriate written discharge instructions.

The perioperative nurse documents the care given and progress of the patient throughout the postoperative phase. The patient and family or significant other review the discharge instructions, and when home readiness is determined, the patient is discharged.

DISCHARGE

Changes from the Joint Commission on Accreditation of Healthcare Organizations (JCAHO) allow authorized personnel to discharge patients when criteria are identified. It is unlikely that a physician is available to discharge every ambulatory surgery patient; therefore the authorized person most likely responsible for determining appropriateness of meeting the specified criteria and home readiness is the perioperative nurse. The criteria may be predetermined as a set of standing discharge orders or written separately as an order by the surgeon. Criteria to determine home readiness are intended to meet the needs of the patient, nursing staff, and facility. The following is a common list of discharge criteria that may be applied to the ambulatory surgery patient (Research Highlight 27-3).

Order from the physician
Stable vital signs
No evidence of respiratory depression
Oriented to person, place, and time
Ability to void, as appropriate
Ability to take fluids orally, as appropriate
Ability to dress
Ability to ambulate without assistance
Minimal nausea and vomiting
No excessive pain
No bleeding or excessive drainage
Written discharge instructions: possible complications, activity restrictions, diet, medications, wound care and hygiene, precautions and plan for follow-up care (Fig. 27-4)
Responsible adult escort

Text continued on p. 1141.

INTRAOPERATIVE NURSING NOTES

DATE

ASSESSMENT

SAFETY & SECURITY	SKIN INTEGRITY	SELF CONCEPT / COPING	OXYGENATION / CIRCULATION	COGNITION / PERCEPTION DEFICITS	ACTIVITY / REST
Arrived Holding	☐ Normal	☐ Alert	☐ Regular	☐ None	☐ Normal
NPO @	☐ Red	☐ Oriented, But Sedated	☐ Labored	☐ Blind	☐ Traction
☐ Contacts/Glasses Removed	☐ Edema	☐ Disoriented	☐ Assisted	☐ Deaf / Hard of Hearing	☐ Paralysis
☐ Dentures Removed	☐ Blister	☐ Lethargic	☐ E.T.T./Trach/ Nasal Canula/Mask	☐ Mute	☐ Obesity
☐ Jewelry Removed / Taped	☐ Abrasions	☐ Calm, Relaxed		☐ Language Barrier	☐ Prosthesis
☐ Prosthesis Removed	☐ Ecchymosis	☐ Anxiety (Mild, Moderate, Severe)	☐ Oxygen_____ L/M	☐ Hearing Aide Removed	☐ Limited ROM
☐ Lab Data Within Normal Limits	☐ Drain / Catheter	☐ Combative			☐ Restraints
☐ Abnormal Values / MD Notified	☐	☐	☐	☐	☐
☐ NKA					
☐ Allergic To _____					

☐ Assessment data reviewed and verified from Preoperative Nursing Care form.

Signature _____   Time _____

Preoperative Comments

☐ O₂ Sat   Signature

NURSING DIAGNOSIS	EXPECTED OUTCOMES / EVAL.	YES	NO	N/A	NURSING INTERVENTION / DOCUMENTATION
1. High risk for injury related to inappropriate identification of patient.	Patient will undergo correct procedure performed by correct surgeon.				Verify surgical site with patient
					Verify surgeon with patient
					Verify ID bracelet with patient
					Verify operative procedure with patient
	Outcome achieved				Signature
2. High risk for anxiety related to impending surgery and unknown surroundings.	Patient will experience minimal anxiety while awake in O.R. suite.				Provide quiet, comfortable O.R. atmosphere
					Remain at patient's side until anesthetized
					Explain procedures done in O.R. while patient is awake
	Outcome achieved				
3. High risk for infection related to surgical procedure.	Patient will experience an aseptic environment.				Apply appropriate skin prep
					Monitor and enforce aseptic techinque
					Check flash autoclave graph
					Check indicator strips
	Outcome achieved				

Wound Classification
- ☐ Clean
- ☐ Clean/Contaminated
- ☐ Contaminated
- ☐ Dirty

NURSING DIAGNOSIS	EXPECTED OUTCOMES / EVAL.	YES	NO	N/A	NURSING INTERVENTION / DOCUMENTATION
4. High risk for injury / unplanned break in skin integrity related to: ☐ Position ☐ Chemical ☐ Compression Devices ☐ Tourniquet Cuff ☐ Sequential Stockings ☐ Electro - Surgical Unit	Patient will be free of intraoperative injury as evidenced by no break in skin integrity due to position, chemical agents, compression and / or electrical equipment.				Assess areas at risk related to positioning

Assess areas at risk related to positioning
☐ Lateral ☐ Supine ☐ Jackknife ☐ Prone
☐ Lithotomy ☐ Other

Apply appropriate padding and support devices
☐ Rolls ☐ Support ☐ Pads

Electrosurgical equipment:
- Check pad / cord for expiration date and damage
- Choose a smooth fleshy pad site - avoid bony prominence
- Apply pad to clean dry skin that has minimal amount of hair
- Avoid spilling prep solution on or around pad site
- Reassess system if there are unusual requests for higher power
- Avoid wrinkled or wet sheets under patient
- Inspect tourniquet cuff integrity
- Test tourniquet cuff and tank pressures
- Pad tourniquet site
- Reassess pressure points and ground pad when patient repositioned

Outcome achieved

DOCUMENTATION

☐ Tourniquet No. _____
Cuff up _____
Cuff down _____
Setting _____
☐ K-thermia No. _____
Temperature _____

ELECTROSURGICAL GENERATOR
No. ____ Cut ____ Coag. ____
No. ____ Cut ____ Coag. ____
SCD Settings:
Ankle ____ Calf ____ Thigh ____

FIG. 27-2 Intraoperative nursing notes.
Courtesy Grant Medical Center, Columbus, Ohio.

ITEM LOCATIONS

1) Safety Strap =
2) Bovie Ground ☐
3) Monitor Lead ○
4) Tourniquet +
5) B/P Cuff △
6) Skin Prep ■ ☐ Oral ☐ Vaginal
Prep Solution -
☐ Iodophor ☐ Sol ☐ Gel ☐ Other_____

SKIN INTEGRITY

	BEFORE				AFTER			
	Overall	Prep	Pad	Cuff	Overall	Prep	Pad	Cuff
Normal	☐	☐	☐	☐	☐	☐	☐	☐
Red	☐	☐	☐	☐	☐	☐	☐	☐
Edema	☐	☐	☐	☐	☐	☐	☐	☐
Blister	☐	☐	☐	☐	☐	☐	☐	☐
Abrasions	☐	☐	☐	☐	☐	☐	☐	☐
Ecchymosis	☐	☐	☐	☐	☐	☐	☐	☐

Time	Medication	Route / Dose	Dispensed By	Time	Medication	Route / Dose	Dispensed By

NURSING DIAGNOSIS	EXPECTED OUTCOMES	YES	NO	N/A	NURSING INTERVENTION / DOCUMENTATION
5	High risk for injury related to medication administered from field or directly by nurse.	Patient will receive correct drug in proper dosage and route without allergic reaction.				Check for documented medication allergies / Repeat drug and dose when presenting medication / Medication labels applied to Syringe/Basin / Check expiration date / Document order for medication on order sheet
		Outcome achieved			■	
6	High risk for fluid volume deficit related to surgical process.	Patient's fluid output will be monitored to facilitate volume replacement as needed to maintain fluid electrolyte balance.				Place sponges in clear view of anesthesia / Suction canister contents in view of/or reported to anesthesia / **Drain / Catheter** ☐ Jackson - Pratt ☐ T-Tube / ☐ Reliavac ☐ Sump ☐ N/G / ☐ Chest ☐ Penrose ☐ Foley / ☐ Other Drainage
		Outcome achieved			■	
7	High risk for loss of body heat related to cool room temperature, body exposure, or open wound.	Patient will experience an environment where external factors that can affect the loss of body heat are controlled.				Expose only as much of patient's skin as needed / Maintain warm irrigation solutions on field per procedure / Monitor room temperature / Apply warm blankets after procedure
		Outcome achieved			■	
8	High risk for injury related to retention of foreign body.	Patient will have absence of foreign body upon completion of surgery except when surgical procedure indicates.				Perform and document appropriate counts / Complete and submit implant sheet / Packing - Type _____ / Size ____ Location ____ Number ____
		Outcome achieved			■	
9	High risk for injury related to laser.	Patient will be free from injury as demonstrated by no skin or tissue injuries related to use of laser.				Moist sponges on field / Laser resistant E.T. Tube / Water available in room
		Outcome achieved			■	

Intraoperative Comments

Disposition ☐ PACU ☐ ICU/CCU ☐ Patient Room ☐ Ambulatory ☐ Other **Status** ☐ Alert ☐ Sedated/Drowsy ☐ Agitated ☐ Unresponsive

Transported ☐ Cart ☐ Bed ☐ Wheelchair ☐ Carried ☐ Ambulatory

RN Signature / Initials

LASER DEPT. USE

Laser Type	Power	Time On	Time Off	Exposure Time
Total Energy	Total Spots	☐ Plume Tubing / Filter ☐ Disposable Fiber ☐ Contact Tip		
Signature		☐ Plume in Line ☐ Glasses		

FIG. 27-2, CONT'D For legend, see opposite page.

Ambulatory Surgery Post Operative Record

ASSESSMENT

☐ ASC ☐ Phase II Recovery completed in PACU   Date: _____   Time: _____

Returned from OR/PACU via: ☐ Ambulatory ☐ Wheelchair ☐ Cart   ☐ Carried   Procedure: _____

Vital Signs: BP _____ T _____ P _____ R _____

Anesthesia Type: ☐ Local   ☐ MAC   ☐ General   ☐ Regional   ☐ Spinal/Epidural

Level of Consciousness: ☐ Alert   ☐ Oriented   ☐ Drowsy but arousable   ☐ Other _____

Skin Color/Condition: ☐ Satisfactory ☐ Pale   ☐ Other _____

☐ No Visible non-surgical impairment to skin integrity

RN SIGNATURE: _____   INITIAL: _____

PATIENT CARE PLAN

NURSING DIAGNOSIS	NURSING INTERVENTION/DOCUMENTATION	REASSESSMENT	EXPECTED OUTCOME
☐High risk for fluid volume deficit related to NPO status and loss of body fluid.	ASSESSMENT: ☐ 1) Dressing/Packing: ☐ Dry ☐ Intact Comment: _____ ☐ 2) Drainage/Device: ☐ Small ☐ Moderate ☐ Large ☐ Ice Bag ☐ Other _____ Comment: _____ ☐ 3) Oral Intake: ☐ Nausea ☐ Fluids/Solids Retained Comment: _____ ☐ 4) Output: ☐ Voided ☐ Emesis ☐ Drains ☐ None Comment: _____ ☐ 5) Medications: Time: _____ Name/Dose/Route: _____ ☐ 6) IV: site_____ solution_____ Amt. to count_____	Time _____ ☐ No Change Comment _____ ☐ No Change Comment _____ ☐ No Change Comment _____ ☐ No Change Comment _____ Comment: _____	Fluid volume will be maintained as evidenced by stable vital signs, intake and output. ☐ MET ☐ NOT MET
☐High risk for altered tissue perfusion, peripheal.	NEUROVASCULAR ASSESSMENT: ☐ 1) Edema: ☐ Slight ☐ Moderate ☐ Severe ☐ None ☐ 2) Capillary refill time: _____ ☐ 3) Skin Temperature: ☐ Warm ☐ Cool ☐ Cold ☐ 4) Sensation: ☐ Intact ☐ Numbness/Tingling ☐ 5) Pulses Palpated: _____ ☐ 6) Comfort Measures: ☐ Ice Bag ☐ Elevation Comment: _____	Time _____ ☐ No Change Comment: _____ ☐ No Change Comment: _____ ☐ No Change Comment: _____ ☐ No Change Comment: _____ ☐ No Change Comment: _____ ☐ No Change Comment: _____	Patient experiences no greater than slight edema and capillary refill time ≤3 seconds on discharge. ☐ MET ☐ NOT MET

FIG. 27-3 Ambulatory surgery postoperative record.
Courtesy Grant Medical Center, Columbus, Ohio.

NURSING DIAGNOSIS	NURSING INTERVENTION/DOCUMENTATION	EXPECTED OUTCOME

PATIENT CARE PLAN

☐ Alteration in comfort related to surgical experience.

☐ 1) Assesses discomfort: None   Severe
                            0   1   2   3   4   5
Comment: _____

☐ 2) Comfort Measures Provided: ☐ Warm Blanket ☐ Positioning ☐ Other
Comment: _____

☐ 3) Medications: Time: _____
Name/Dose/Route: _____

☐ 4) Patient verbalizes improved comfort level post-intervention.
Comment: _____

Patient verbalizes no greater than mild discomfort on dischage.

☐ MET

☐ NOT MET

☐ Knowledge deficit of home care related to lack of experience/ instruction.

☐ 1) Home Care Instructions reviewed with patient/family/significant other.
_____

☐ 2) Copy of Home Care Instructions given to patient/family/significant other.
_____

☐ 3) Prescriptions/supplies given to patient/family/significant other: _____

Patient/family/signif-icant other verbalizes understanding of discharge instructions.

☐ MET

☐ NOT MET

☐ Actual/Potential
For _____

☐ MET

☐ NOT MET

Comments:

DISCHARGE

Seen by Dr._____, or ☐ meets discharge criteria   DISCHARGE TIME: _____
TIME: _____ BP _____ T _____ P _____ R _____

Accompanied by: ☐ Family ☐ Other   Discharge via: ☐ W/C ☐ Ambulatory ☐ Cart ☐ Carried

Comments: _____
_____

RN SIGNATURE:_____ INITIAL: _____

POST-OP CALL

POST-OPERATIVE TELEPHONE FOLLOW-UP

Home Care Instructions were adequate and followed: ☐ YES   ☐ NO

Satisfied with nursing care provided: ☐ YES   ☐ NO

Patient voices satisfactory condition: ☐ YES   ☐ NO

☐ No Phone   ☐ Unable to Reach   Comment: _____
_____
_____

DATE: _____   TIME: _____   RN SIGNATURE: _____

FIG. 27-3, CONT'D   For legend, see opposite page.

Home Care Instructions/Surgical Procedures

Medications
- ☐ No medications, including nonprescription medications, unless ordered by the physician for 24 hours.
- ☐ Resume own medications.
- ☐ Prescription given for _____

Wound Care and Hygiene
- ☐ Do not remove dressing.
- ☐ Keep incision dry until _____
- ☐ Remove dressing on _____

Activity
- ☐ No restrictions.
- ☐ Resume normal activities in ☐ 24 hours or ☐ ____ hours.
- ☐ May return to school/work on _____ _____

Diet
- ☐ Drink plenty of liquids and eat a light meal on the day of the surgery, resume regular diet tomorrow.
- ☐ Regular diet.

Anesthesia Precautions
- ☐ No special precautions.
- ☐ Do not operate a vehicle (automobile, bicycle, motorcycle), machinery, or power tools, make any important decisions, or drink any alcoholic beverages for 24 hours.
- ☐ Arrange for a responsible adult to remain with you for 24 hours. You may be drowsy and lightheaded.

You Can Expect
- ☐ Mild pain/slight swelling.
- ☐ Minimal amount of drainage and/or bleeding.

Call Your Doctor for
- ☐ Persistent or heavy bleeding.
- ☐ Temperature above 100 degrees.
- ☐ Redness or pus at the operative site.
- ☐ Severe pain at the operative site.

Additional Instructions
_____
_____
_____
_____

Call your doctor's office as soon as possible for an appointment on _____ / _____ / _____

Physician's Signature _____

Office _____ Home _____

I have received and understand the above instructions _____

Patient, Parent, or Guardian

Nurse's Signature _____ ___ Hospital Contact Number _____

FIG. 27-4 Home care instructions.

Courtesy Grant Medical Center, Columbus, Ohio.

☆
RESEARCH HIGHLIGHT 27-3

The study identified seven categories used by the nurse when determining home readiness following day surgery. The categories were determined by an extensive literature review and a descriptive study examining recovery and patient welfare. The seven categories identified were mental state, mobility, pain, eating and drinking, elimination, information, and social factors. Each category included a comprehensive literature review of research and nursing implications for patient management, as applicable, and was subdivided to include essential and desirable criteria. Determining home readiness is critical to the safety and welfare of the patient. This research can help in deciding essential versus desirable criteria that should be met before discharging the patient who has had day surgery.

Stephenson, M.E. (1990). Discharge criteria in day surgery. *Journal of Advanced Nursing, 15,* 601-613.

The ambulatory surgery patient should be informed that recovery and convalescence are not complete upon discharge. The patient is instructed not to plan to resume usual activities until at least a day following surgery, and often longer. Discharge instructions related to possible complications, activity restrictions, diet, prescriptions, wound care, and plan for follow-up care are reinforced to patient and family. At the time of discharge, all written instructions forms are signed and a copy is given to the patient or family member or significant other. Any additional questions regarding postoperative care are answered.

Upon discharge from the facility, patients may be given a questionnaire to be completed at their convenience. The questionnaire provides the facility feedback about its services, any postoperative complications the patient may experience, and any additional comments or suggestions from the patient. It is one way to measure the quality of services provided by the facility. The perioperative nurse contacts the patient with a follow-up phone call 24 hours after surgery to evaluate recovery, general condition, and to answer any questions regarding care that the patient might have (Young, 1990). The patient is advised to consult the surgeon for any complications related to the surgical procedure. In addition, the perioperative nurse may notify the surgeon regarding the complication. Postoperative calls are an important tool for the ambulatory facility to determine patient satisfaction and effectiveness of care.

CONTINUING EDUCATION AND CONTINUOUS QUALITY IMPROVEMENT

Continuing education and staff development for all staff members must be relevant, ongoing, and documented. Staff should annually attend educational programs on CPR, fire and safety, and infection control practices. Other educational opportunities may include programs related to the latest in technologic advances, new procedures, IV conscious sedation, updated AORN standards and recommended practices, and continuous quality improvement activities. Observation and assessment skills are essential in ambulatory surgery nursing and should be updated periodically.

Quality improvement in conjunction with continuing education promotes high-quality patient care. Standards utilized in quality improvement activities include structure standards (management of the facility), process standards (what the nurse does for the patient), and outcome standards (what the patient can expect from the caregiver). The facility's quality improvement program must identify the scope of service provided and important aspects of care (Box 27-8). For effective monitoring and evaluation of care given, quality improvement activities must identify indicators that will monitor the important aspects of care. Continuous quality improvement activities are an important part of the care delivered in the ambulatory surgery setting.

DOCUMENTATION

Principles of documentation along with legal consideration guide the manager and staff of an ambulatory surgery facility in the development and revision of existing patient records. Many ambulatory facilities develop a separate local anesthesia record that is used with the basic intraoperative nursing record to more accurately record nursing care for the patient receiving local anesthesia or IV conscious sedation (Kendall, 1993). Using the AORN recommended practices for documentation of perioperative nursing care as a guide, the following should be included in patient record forms:

1. Face sheet (such as demographics)
2. Consent for surgical procedure and anesthesia
3. History and physical examination reports
4. Health history
5. Applicable laboratory test results
6. Preoperative and postoperative instruction sheets
7. Preoperative nursing assessment sheet
8. Physician order sheet
9. Anesthesia record
10. Local anesthesia record—nursing
11. Intraoperative record
12. Postoperative record
13. Report of operation
14. Pathology report, when applicable

All forms should be reviewed periodically and revised as needed. Medical record dictums, accreditation standards, regulations, facility policies, and nursing and physician requests should be considered when developing forms for the facility. Criteria for documentation include legal and professional considerations and standards, validation of the

---

BOX 27-8

Quality Assessment and Improvement for the Ambulatory Surgery Patient

---

IMPORTANT ASPECT OF CARE

Preoperative assessment and patient education

INDICATORS

A preoperative nursing assessment is made for each ambulatory surgical patient.

The patient/family/significant other learning needs are identified and recorded.

Discharge instructions are written and reviewed with the patient/family/significant other; demonstration of understanding is documented on the nursing care plan.

IMPORTANT ASPECT OF CARE

Patient safety

INDICATORS

Patient is free from injury related to positioning, extraneous objects, chemical, physical, and electrical hazards.

IMPORTANT ASPECT OF CARE

Discharge planning

INDICATOR

A responsible escort who will accompany the patient when discharged and will be present before the start of surgery.

IMPORTANT ASPECT OF CARE

Skin integrity/infection management

INDICATORS

Skin is assessed preoperatively and postoperatively.

Skin assessment is documented on nursing care plan.

IMPORTANT ASPECT OF CARE

Management of physiologic functions for the patient receiving IV conscious sedation

INDICATORS

Nasal cannula is in place for all patients.

Vital signs are stable throughout the surgical procedure.

Nausea and vomiting are evaluated.

Level of consciousness is continually assessed.

Management of pain is assessed and documented.

IMPORTANT ASPECT OF CARE

Customer satisfaction

INDICATORS

All returned patient questionnaire complaints are recorded, and suggested improvements are noted.

Quarterly patient surveys with comment cards are sent.

IMPORTANT ASPECT OF CARE

Documentation

INDICATORS

Nursing record is completed according to established policy and procedures.

Patient response to IV conscious sedation medications is documented.

Consent form is correctly completed.

Physician orders are documented and signed by the nurse.

---

level of medical and nursing care provided, degree of patient education and understanding, and policies of the institution. Documentation should be concise and appropriate.

POLICIES AND PROCEDURES

The purpose of a policy and procedure manual is to provide a framework for daily operation of a facility. The manual should provide information to the user that describes the expected course of action to be followed. A comprehensive policy and procedure manual is an effective tool for communication, education, and prevention of legal issues if correctly followed. Policies and procedures for the ambulatory surgery facility may differ in form and content from institutional hospital regulations due to governing

body, ownership, medical staff, accrediting and licensing bodies, and management.

The ambulatory surgery facility policy and procedure manual may include, but is not limited to, the following:

Admission of patient to hospital
Admission and scheduling of patients
Ambulatory surgery discharge criteria
Ambulatory surgery patient teaching plan
Anesthesia guidelines
Aseptic practices
Borrowing and lending of equipment and supplies
Cancellation
Chart documentation and requirements
Consent forms: for example, surgery, anesthesia, conscious sedation, blood transfusions, refusal of blood, sterilization

Continuing education
Counts
Disaster plan
Emergency drug/equipment cart
Goals for patient care
Handling and safekeeping of patient valuables
History, physical and preoperative lab studies, and any additional preoperative requirements
Infection control measures
IV conscious sedation
Location, storage, and procurement of medications, supplies, and equipment
Means of securing assistance in an emergency
Medical records
Medical staff privileges and bylaws
Monitoring of patient receiving local anesthesia
Monthly reports
Operational hours
Organization, direction, philosophy, and mission statement
Orientation
Overnight stay program (if applicable)
Patient appointment system
Patient selection criteria
Patient discharge criteria
Patient opinion questionnaire
Patient transportation
Performance evaluation
Postoperative patient procedure
Preadmission procedure
Preoperative assessment
Preoperative patient education/instruction
Preoperative and postoperative transportation
Preoperative telephone interview with patient
Postoperative patient follow-up
Quality improvement plan
Regulations concerning unemancipated minor patients
Safety practices
Scope of service
Social services
Staffing
Surgical authorization
Traffic control
Types of elective procedures

FUTURE TRENDS

Ambulatory surgery will be a driving force in the continuing growth of ambulatory care in the 90s. As the American health care system undergoes changes with health care reform, the ambulatory surgery arena will feel the impact. Key issues in health care reform include access to service, quality of care, and cost containment. Each affects ambulatory surgery facilities, and strategic plans to maintain viability and success in the marketplace will need to be developed.

A driving force in the future of ambulatory surgery is the continued expansion of technology, particularly in minimally invasive surgery. This technology provides the patient with an alternative modality of treatment, and surgery will often be performed outside the operating room in areas such as ancillary departments, mobile services, and physician offices. This will lead to a reshaping of the scope of ambulatory surgery services.

Customer-focused care will be an important component of patient satisfaction for the continued success of ambulatory surgery. The patient's needs and expectations will continue to evolve and must be explored to incorporate participatory care from both the patient and family or significant others. The patient is an integral part of the decision-making process and planning outcome-oriented care.

Expect the future for ambulatory surgery to include increased competition between hospitals and physicians, continued technology explosion, noninvasive diagnostic and therapeutic surgical interventions, focus on service orientation, development of physician/nurse collaborative models, continued emphasis on patient/family/significant other education, increase in managed care, limiting of complex, high-risk procedures, better collaboration with community resources, and alternative delivery sites for care, such as recovery centers, medical motels, and home health care.

The future will produce many changes for ambulatory surgery. These changes will provide challenges and opportunities for health care providers and patients. Ambulatory surgery has been and will continue to be a key force in the delivery of health care services in the future.

SUMMARY

The success and growth of ambulatory surgery will continue to flourish as new technology and health care concepts push forward. Perioperative nursing care is the most constant and pervasive part of ambulatory surgical services. Care that was formerly spread over a period of several days is now completed in a few hours. Perioperative nurses must remain responsive to future health care changes and continue to be a key influence in shaping ambulatory surgical care.

REFERENCES

Association of Operating Room Nurses. (1992). Position statement on the role of the RN in the management of patients receiving IV conscious sedation for short-term therapeutic, diagnostic, or surgical procedures. *AORN Journal, 55*(1), 207.

Association of Operating Room Nurses. (1993a). Position statement on perioperative nursing practice in ambulatory surgery. In *AORN standards and recommended practices for perioperative nursing.* Denver: The Association.

Association of Operating Room Nurses. (1993b). Recommended practices for documentation of perioperative patient care. In *AORN standards and recommended practices for perioperative nursing.* Denver: The Association.

Association of Operating Room Nurses. (1993c). Recommended practices: Monitoring the patient receiving IV conscious sedation. *AORN Journal, 57*(4), 978.

Association of Operating Room Nurses. (1993d). Recommended practices for monitoring the patient receiving local anesthesia. In *AORN standards and recommended practices for perioperative nursing*. Denver: The Association.

Association of Operating Room Nurses. (1994). *AORN standards and recommended practices*. Denver: The Association.

Cruz, L. (1990). Ambulatory surgery—the next decade. *AORN Journal, 51*(1), 241-247.

Ferguson, L.K., & Kaplan, L. (1966). *Surgery of the ambulatory patient*. Philadelphia: J.B. Lippincott.

Kendall, F. (1993). Documenting local anesthesia patient care. *AORN Journal, 58*(4), 715-719.

Lea, S.G., & Phippen, M. (1992). Client education in the ambulatory surgery setting. *Seminars in Perioperative Nursing, 1*(4), 203-223.

Llewellyn, J.G. (1991). Short stay surgery present practices, future trends. *AORN Journal, 53*(5), 1179-1191.

Mathias, J.M. (1987). Ambulatory surgery meeting stresses quality of care. *AORN Journal, 45*(5), 1191-1200.

Michel, L.L., & Myrick, C. (1990). Current and future trends in ambulatory surgery and their impact on nursing practice. *Journal of Post Anesthesia Nursing, 5*(5), 347-349.

Muldowny, E.H. (1993). Establishing a preadmission clinic. *AORN Journal, 58*(6), 1183-1191.

Pica-Furey, W. (1993). Ambulatory surgery—hospital-based vs freestanding. *AORN Journal, 57*(5), 1119-1127.

Reiling, R. (1990). Day surgery and outpatient care. In *American College of Surgeons Care of the Surgical Patient*. Vol. 2 Elective Care. New York: Scientific American, Inc.

Rivellini, D. (1993). Local and regional anesthesia. *Nursing Clinics of North America, 28*(3), 547-572.

Slomski, A.J. (1993). Your own surgery center—still a good idea? *Medical Economics for Surgeons, 12*(10) 26-31.

Stephenson, M.E. (1990). Discharge criteria in day surgery. *Journal of Advanced Nursing, 15*, 601-613.

Watson, D. (1991). Clinical issues: Issues surrounding intravenous conscious sedation. *AORN Journal, 54*(1), 105-107.

Young, C.M. (1990). The postoperative follow-up phone call: An essential part of the ambulatory surgery nurse's job. *Journal of Post Anesthesia Nursing, 5*(4), 273-275.

28

PEDIATRIC SURGERY

LYNN S. HARKINS, CHERYL NYGREN, AND JANE C. ROTHROCK

The highly specialized field of pediatric surgery began its dramatic development in the first half of this century. Prior to this, little distinction was made between the surgical treatment of children and that of adults. Pediatric surgery is now recognized as a separate subspecialty of surgery with board certification status.

The successful and rapid advancements in pediatric surgery can be attributed to improved diagnostic procedures and techniques; better understanding of physiologic, psychologic, and sociologic problems affecting infants, small children, preteens, and adolescents; improvements in newborn intensive care management; increased knowledge about fluid and electrolyte balance, pharmacology, and nutrition and their effects on various pediatric age groups, and the causes and physiology of congenital malformations; improved anesthetic agents and techniques, along with better understanding of their effects on pediatric patients; and improved surgical techniques with more appropriate instrumentation and support equipment and implementation of more effective medical and perioperative nursing care.

The development of high-risk pregnancy centers for mothers with problem pregnancies has resulted in earlier detection of malformations in fetuses as well as of other problems. Earlier detection has led to development of lifesaving operative procedures that can be performed in utero or immediately after delivery.

Current priority research areas in pediatrics include the development of guidelines for management of specific pediatric conditions and development of functional health outcome measures for specific conditions (Child Health Care, 1993). An area of nursing research that is gaining attention is the assessment of postoperative pain in children. As multidimensional pain research instruments are developed, nursing will have more reliable methods to assist children and adolescents with the management of postoperative pain (Research Highlight 28-1). The Agency for Health Care Policy and Research published *Acute Pain Management In Infants, Children, and Adolescents: Operative and Medical Procedures* in 1992. This guideline includes elements of assessing and managing postoperative and procedure-related pain, pain assessment tools, and dosage charts for analgesics. Important elements of these guidelines are presented in Box 28-1.

RESEARCH HIGHLIGHT 28-1

Based on the underlying belief that children and adolescents can describe their pain, and that a developmentally appropriate tool could assist in this process, this research tested the Adolescent Pediatric Pain Tool (APPT) with 65 multiethnic children ranging in ages from 8 to 17 years. All of the children had undergone surgery in one of four acute care hospitals. The range of surgical procedures was wide (orthopedics, abdominal, thoracic, urologic, neurosurgery, and miscellaneous other procedures). The APPT is a one-page, two-sided instrument with a diagram of the body, a word-graphic rating scale, and a pain descriptor list. It measures the dimension, location, and quality of pain. The children completed the tool on the first through fifth postoperative days.

Based on the markings on the body diagram, it was concluded that children are able to consistently report where they hurt. Pain intensity varied, as would be expected, over the postoperative course, with more pain being reported on days 1 and 2. The pain quality scores also decreased over the postoperative course. Words such as "awful," "never goes away," "bad" were used typically on day 1. By day 5 more typical words used were "uncomfortable," "sore," "aching."

The children had no trouble completing the APPT. There was no attempt in this study to correlate the administration of pharmacologic or nonpharmacologic relief, since the primary purpose of the study was to test the research instrument.

Savedra, M.C., Holzemer, W.L., Tesler, M.D., & Wilkie, D.J. (1993). Assessment of postoperative pain in children and adolescents using the Adolescent Pediatric Pain Tool. *Nursing Research, 42*(1), 5.

BOX 28-1

Pain Assessment and Reassessment

PRINCIPLES

- Routine assessment increases the health care professional's knowledge of the child. Knowing the child in turn optimizes the assessment of pain and its subsequent management.
- Children who may have difficulty communicating their pain require particular attention. This includes children who are cognitively impaired, psychotic, or severely emotionally disturbed; children who do not speak English; and children from families where the level of education or cultural background differs significantly from that of the health care team.
- Unexpected intense pain, particularly if sudden or associated with altered vital signs such as hypotension, tachycardia, or fever, should be immediately evaluated, and new diagnoses such as wound dehiscence or infection considered.

PAIN ASSESSMENT PROCEDURES

- Tailor assessment strategies to the child's developmental level and personality style and to the situation.
- Obtain a pain history from the child and/or the parents at the time of admission. Learn what word the child uses for pain (e.g., hurt, boo-boo, owie).
- Elicit from the family culturally determined beliefs about pain and medical care.
- Measure the child's pain using self-report and/or behavioral observation tools. Use tools that have known reliability, validity, and sensitivity and are practical for the provider and simple for the child.
- Use self-report measures whenever possible. Self-report tools are appropriate for most children 4 years and older and provide the most accurate measure of children's pain. Children over the age of 7 or 8 who understand the concept of order and number can use a numerical rating scale or a horizontal word-graphic rating scale. (See sample pain measurement tools at the end of Box.)
- Use behavioral observation with preverbal and nonverbal children and as an adjunct to the self-report measure of an older verbal child. Include factors such as vocalizations, verbalizations, facial expressions, motor responses, body posture, activity, and appearance.
- Interpret behaviors cautiously. Behaviors such as watching television, playing, and sleeping may be strategies for coping with pain. Continued severe pain, depression, fatigue, extreme illness, and the use of sedatives or hypnotics may blunt behaviors. For example, an ill child with severe pain may whimper and lie still rather than cry.
- Use the parent's report of pain when the child is unwilling or unable to give a self-report.
- Use physiologic measures (e.g., heart rate and blood pressure) only as adjuncts to self-report and behavioral observation. They are neither sensitive nor specific as indicators of pain.

POSTOPERATIVE ASSESSMENT

- Assess pain at regular intervals. For example, assessment after major surgery could occur at least every 2 hours for the first 24 hours and every 4 hours thereafter. More frequent assessment is necessary if pain is poorly controlled.
- Interview the child and parent about the pain.
- Assess pain with other routine assessments such as taking vital signs. Document information about the pain and response to intervention on the bedside flow sheet or another easily visible and accessible place.
- Note changes in the child's behavior, appearance, activity level, and vital signs. Changes in these parameters may indicate a change in the pain intensity.
- Before discharge, review with the child and family the interventions used and their efficacy and provide specific discharge instructions.

UNCERTAINTY ABOUT THE PRESENCE AND AMOUNT OF PAIN

- Even after implementing these assessment strategies, health care professionals may be uncertain about the presence and amount of pain, especially in infants or young children. If there is any reason to suspect pain, a diagnostic trial of analgesics is often appropriate.

Acute Pain Management Guideline Panel. (1992). *Acute pain management in infants, children, and adolescents: Operative and medical procedures. Quick reference guide for clinicians.* AHCPR Pub. No. 92-0020. Rockville, Md.: Agency for Health Care Policy and Research, Public Health Service, U.S. Department of Health and Human Services.

WONG-BAKER FACES PAIN RATING SCALE

Explain to the person that each face is for a person who feels happy because he has no pain (hurt) or sad because he has some or a lot of pain. **Face 0** is very happy because he doesn't hurt at all. **Face 1** hurts just a little bit. **Face 2** hurts a little more. **Face 3** hurts even more. **Face 4** hurts a whole lot. **Face 5** hurts as much as you can imagine, although you don't have to be crying to feel this bad. Ask the person to choose the face that best describes how he is feeling. *Recommended for persons age 3 years and older.*

Research reported in Wong, D., & Baker, C. (1988). Pain in children: Comparison of assessment scales. *Pediatric Nursing, 14*(1),9.
This tool may be reproduced for use in the clinical setting.

BOX 28-1

Pain Assessment and Reassessment—cont'd

0   1   2   3   4   5

NUMERIC SCALE FOR PAIN ASSESSMENT

No pain   Worst pain

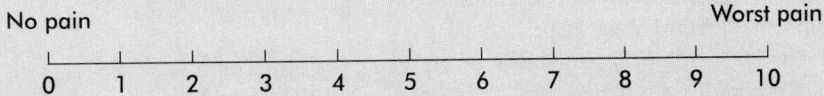

0   1   2   3   4   5   6   7   8   9   10

Explain to child that at one end of the line is a 0, which means that a person feels no pain (hurt). At the other end is a 10, which means the person feels the worst pain imaginable. The numbers 1 to 9 are for a very little pain to a whole lot of pain. Ask child to choose number that best describes own pain.

This tool may be reproduced for use in the clinical setting.
From Wong, D.L. (1993). *Pediatric quick reference*. St. Louis: Mosby.

Most hospitals classify pediatric patients according to the following age groups:

1. Premature infant: less than 37 weeks of gestation
2. Neonate, or newborn: birth to 1 month of age; however, a premature infant may remain in this category until about 3 months of age
3. Infant: up to 1 year of age
4. Toddler: 1 to 3 years of age
5. Preschooler: 3 to 6 years of age
6. School-age child: 6 to 11 years of age
7. Adolescent: 11 to 18 years of age; many hospitals consider 16 years as the upper age limit, with patients over this age considered as adults

Pediatric patients may also be hospitalized in mixed age units or according to clinical specialty.

PERIOPERATIVE NURSING CONSIDERATIONS

ASSESSMENT

The nursing process is the basis for perioperative nursing care of pediatric patients, and the perioperative assessment is the first phase of the nursing process. The goal of a comprehensive nursing assessment is to gather sufficient data to formulate nursing diagnoses from which desired outcomes are identified and care is planned, implemented, and evaluated. The unique aspects of care of the pediatric surgical patient center on the fact that the child is a growing organism. Normally, infants and children have higher metabolic rates and different physiologic makeup than those of adults. Their oxygen, fluid, and caloric requirements are greater; add to these the stress of illness and/or surgery, and these requirements climb even higher. The perioperative nurse must have a good understanding of the normal physical and psychologic parameters for pediatric patients and be able to recognize deviations from these parameters. In addition, the perioperative nurse must be familiar with normal growth and development factors for each age group. During any given day the perioperative nurse may care for all age groups of children—neonates through adolescents.

The preoperative visit is the first step in assessment. For children undergoing an ambulatory surgical procedure, the child and family visit the surgical suite and ambulatory surgical area 1 to 2 weeks prior to surgery, depending on the developmental level of the child. For children who are inpatients, the perioperative nurse may visit the child and family in the unit. First the patient's chart is reviewed with particular attention given to the patient's age and developmental level, the seriousness of the physical condition, size including height and weight, and a review of the current nursing diagnoses and care plan. A discussion with the primary nurse facilitates data collection, assists in providing continuity of care, and provides the perioperative nurse with information regarding preoperative education done thus far.

The perioperative nurse then interviews the child and family. The purpose of the interview is to gather data, educate, and provide emotional support to both patient and family. The focus of this visit is a discussion of the perioperative process, not necessarily to provide preoperative education regarding the surgical procedure. In pediatric centers preoperative education is often the responsibility of the primary nurse, child life therapists, and/or clinical nurse specialists. During the preoperative visit the perioperative nurse discusses how the child progresses through the immediate preoperative, intraoperative, and postoperative phases of care. If any questions do arise concerning the surgical procedure, the family is referred to the surgeon, primary nurse, or anesthesiologist for further clarification or reinforcement of previous teaching. The perioperative nurse may briefly describe the roles of staff members, alleviating anxiety to a certain extent by allowing the parents and child to identify a real person behind the mask, gloves, and gown. The family is informed that the child may bring a favorite security object to the operating room and at what point after the operation the child can see the parents. Teaching is always done within a developmental framework, taking into account the cognitive and psychosocial abilities of the child (Table 28-1). Medical play items, audiovisual aids, puppets, and photographs are all used in the education process.

Assessment continues when the child arrives in the surgical suite. Because the focus of operative preparation is psychologic rather than pharmacologic, the child usually arrives awake and alert. The perioperative nurse performs an abbreviated physical assessment, focusing on vital signs, cardiopulmonary status, integumentary system, nutritional/metabolic status, and psychologic state. The preoperative checklist is completed, which includes positive patient identification, verification of NPO status, a check of any patient allergies and preoperative laboratory data, communication of deviations from normal, noting the presence of an informed consent on the chart, and labeling the child's personal belongings. Throughout this process, the perioperative nurse provides emotional support to the child and family and helps to alleviate fear by administering care with a gentle, calm, trusting approach.

NURSING DIAGNOSIS

At the completion of the assessment phase, the perioperative nurse identifies nursing diagnoses. Five nursing diagnoses that apply to pediatric patients might be as follows:

- Knowledge deficit related to perioperative events
- Ineffective thermoregulation
- High risk for impaired skin integrity
- High risk for fluid volume deficit
- High risk for injury related to use of electrosurgical unit

OUTCOME IDENTIFICATION

Perioperative nursing care is predicated on relevant nursing diagnoses. For each nursing diagnosis a desired outcome is identified. Outcomes should be measurable with criteria by which to judge their attainment. Thus for the desired outcome "The patient and family will demonstrate knowledge of perioperative events and the role of various perioperative team members," measurable criteria such as the child and family's ability to describe preoperative preparation and the perioperative routine on the day of surgery,

the child's ability to locate the planned site of the surgical incision on a doll, and the child's ability to draw a picture of what he or she expects the surgical site to look like postoperatively might be identified.

Outcomes identified for the selected nursing diagnoses for the pediatric patient could be stated as:

- The child and family will demonstrate knowledge of perioperative events and the role of various perioperative team members.
- The child's body temperature will be maintained at an appropriate level during the surgical intervention.
- The child's skin integrity will be maintained.
- The child will remain normovolemic.
- The child will be free from injury.

PLANNING

Assessment data, combined with knowledge of the planned surgical procedure, allow the perioperative nurse to anticipate requirements for surgical positioning, instrumentation, equipment and supplies, medications, and activities necessary to prevent injury to the pediatric patient. Along with information about developmental levels and additional information specific to the individual child's physical and psychosocial status, the perioperative nurse develops a plan for patient care during surgery. For the five nursing diagnoses identified a Sample Care Plan has been developed. For each of the desired outcomes the perioperative nurse needs to identify criteria appropriate to the child and surgical setting. A Sample Care Plan for the pediatric patient might be as shown on pp. 1152-1153.

IMPLEMENTATION

Age-appropriate communication is important in implementing the pediatric nursing care plan. Implementation begins during the perioperative nursing assessment and continues through discharge to the PACU or other area. The toddler often fears parental separation and abandonment; separation or the surgical intervention may be perceived as a form of punishment. Toddlers fear, among other things, strangers, the dark, and machines. They attribute lifelike qualities to inanimate objects, believing that they, like the toddler, have feelings. Thus a blood pressure cuff that squeezes the child's arm may be perceived to be doing so because it is angry with the toddler. Toddlers may also believe that their body is held together by their skin; anything that violates the skin integrity is feared. For this reason plastic bandages are very important.

Toddlers react with the environment using their senses. The perioperative nurse should allow the toddler to touch and play with objects, such as putting a mask on a teddy bear, as appropriate. Sensory information should be provided in a soft, gentle voice: what things will look like and feel like and what the toddler will touch and hear. A security object is extremely comforting. The operating room should be quiet; background noise should be controlled. In-

Text continued on p. 1153.

TABLE 28-1

Features of Development that are Pertinent to Helping Children Deal with Procedures

	Birth to 2 years	2 to 7 years	7 to 12 years	Adolescence
How the child thinks and problem-solves	Sensory-motor experience develops (well-defined and repeated sequences of actions and perceptions). Memory is obvious by 3-4 months and is demonstrated in second year by child's imitations of parents' activities. Between about 18 and 24 months, use of symbols for thought-reasoning-communication appears.	Preoperational stage (thinking is dominated by the child's perceptions rather than logic). Verbally communicated information is increasingly important in learning; exploratory manipulation of objects also helps the child to learn. Child watches, listens, asks questions (why? how?). Child can (a) label (classify) familiar things; perception is often limited to a single, salient feature, making it difficult for child to see things in a context or differentiate unessential from essential properties of an experience; (b) use memory to reconstruct past events; (c) use imagination to deal with events, people, objects; (d) about age 4, begin to infer outcomes; (e) define objects/events in terms of their use/function. Thinking relies on the child's own point of view (egocentricity), since children do not have the capacity to identify a point of view other than their own. As the child gets older, he or she begins to be able to think in terms of quantities (e.g., to recognize variation in quantity; to use numbers to count). Attention is increasingly selective as the child's schema or perceptual sets become more refined.	Concrete operational phase. Child learns from observing/interacting with peers as well as from own experiences. Can use symbols to organize thoughts and represent experience. Features of thinking include increasing capacity to (a) understand viewpoints of others; (b) see the relative nature of things (e.g., this hurts a little; that hurts a lot); (c) use deductive logic in respect to tangible (concrete) experiences (if this, then that); (d) classify things in terms of several characteristics, implying that the child can view things in context, for example, "The shot hurt, but it will make me feel better"; (e) evaluate painful intrusive actions in terms of logical function rather than in terms of punishment; and (f) understand unseen body mechanics/functions. Child can make use of sensory as well as procedural information.	Stage of formal operations. At this point there is use of reason and logical thinking and interest in theoretically possible problems and questions. The adolescent can engage in reflection and think about own thinking and can learn from verbally presented ideas and arguments.

From Redman, B.K. (1993). *The process of patient education.* St. Louis: Mosby.

Continued.

TABLE 28-1

Features of Development that are Pertinent to Helping Children Deal with Procedures—cont'd

	Birth to 2 years	2 to 7 years	7 to 12 years	Adolescence
Major fears and worries	After about 6 months: separation from parents; unfamiliar people/ experiences/places, especially when not accompanied by parent.	Separation from parents; harm to body, including fears of castration after about age 3; punishment for wrongdoing.	Body injury; disability (loss of body functions); loss of control; loss of status.	Uncertainty about selves as persons (especially early and middle adolescence); concern about whether or not body, thoughts, and feelings are "normal."
Understanding cause and effect	By about 3 months, may associate an action with a result. In second year: magical thinking: belief that what is wished for happens.	Beliefs: (a) everything happens by intention; (b) imminent justice—misbehavior is followed by punishment: (c) belief that events that in fact are associated only by happenstance are connected.	Child 6-8: conclusions are based on perceptions. Child 9-12: applies logical operations (deductive thinking) to concrete (immediately experienced) circumstances. Prior to about 9 years, children are likely to view their illness as a consequence of transgressions of rules. (Rules exist in their own right and misdeeds have their own inherent punishment.) Prior to about 9 years, children are likely to believe that illness is caused by germs whose presence is sufficient for illness. At about 9 years, children begin to understand that (a) an illness may have multiple causes; (b) the body's response to an agent or a combination of agents may vary; and (c) host factors interact with agent(s) to cause illness.	Can use formal rule of logic and evidence to assess cause and effect.
Concept of time	By about 3 months, shows anticipation for feedings. Can wait as a consequence of perceiving clues of a familiar and desired activity.	Organized around familiar/routine activities of daily living. By about age 4, has concept of time and day and knows days of week.	Has a concept of the past and future as well as of the present. Can understand time intervals between events and can tell time by a clock. Sense of time is thus more independent of perceptual data, e.g., activities of daily living.	Can synthesize the past, present, and future in thinking.

Intentions, goals, and plans	By about 4 months, may show signs of intention/a sense of making an effort to get a result. In second year, child can make a choice of two options.	About age 4, begins to plan and anticipate actions in the near future; has objectives for activities.	Plans more elaborate projects that involve others to a greater extent.	By midadolescence (about age 15), makes future plans for self. Can think in terms of tasks as well as responsibilities in relation to them.
Handling emotion	By about 7 months, the child cries for attention, help, or when distressed. By about 9 months, begins to express fears (e.g., separation) in play.	Expresses emotion motorically and through play. Learns to label feelings. Needs trusted adult to reassure, set limits, prevent loss of self-control.	Has a greater capacity to express emotion in verbal terms; can describe fears. Can use projective methods to describe fears (e.g., explain how another child might feel or respond in a specific situation).	May use a range of modalities, from relatively sophisticated verbal or written expression to motoric activity and, perhaps, regressed ways of behaving. Thoughts, feelings, and fears may be shared with friends, especially peers.
Relationship with parent/clinicians	Developing a sense of self/others. In latter half of first year, beginning to sustain the memory of parent in parent's absence, at least for a short time. Depends on adult to know child's wants/needs.	Child is likely to have had experience in relating needs and worries to day-care or church school teachers or clinicians. Children may not expect clinicians to perceive/understand how they feel about things until about the age of 10 years.	May test limits set by caretaker/clinician.	By midadolescence, has begun to learn how to negotiate a relationship with a clinician.
Self-evaluation	Feelings about self are derived from feeling tones communicated by others and perceived by the child.	Develops expectations of self; learns to inhibit own actions. Begins to use other children as models.	Evaluates self in terms of performance relative to that of peers and in relation to the set of norms that children believe to be predetermined for them.	May use a set of criteria consciously adopted to evaluate self.

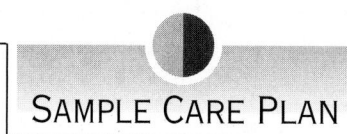

SAMPLE CARE PLAN

NURSING DIAGNOSIS: Knowledge deficit related to perioperative events

OUTCOME: The child and family will demonstrate knowledge of perioperative events and the role of various perioperative team members.

INTERVENTIONS:

Perform preoperative visit and interview; educate the child and family, and provide emotional support.

Utilize audiovisual aids such as photographs, drawings, items for medical play, and/or a tour of the surgical suite.

Provide explanations on the child's level and at the parent's level of understanding.

Refer to nursing and other interdisciplinary team members to review, reinforce, or supplement preoperative education.

NURSING DIAGNOSIS: Ineffective thermoregulation

OUTCOME: The child's body temperature will be maintained at an appropriate level during the surgical intervention.

INTERVENTIONS:

Adjust room temperature approximately an hour before arrival of the child: 26° to 27° C (78.8° to 80.6° F) for infants and newborns; 23° to 24° C (73.4° to 75.2° F) for older children.

Consider wrapping lower extremities in Webril or stockinette and encasing in plastic bag for newborns and infants.

Place hyperthermia blanket on OR bed; adjust blanket temperature to 38° to 40° C (100.4° to 104° F).

Provide radiant heat lamp for use during placement of monitoring lines, induction of anesthesia, positioning, skin preparation, and draping.

Warm blankets, skin preparation solutions, irrigation, and other solutions to body temperature prior to use.

Use warmers during administration of intravenous fluids and blood products; temperature settings should not exceed 38° C (100.4° F).

Monitor body temperature by rectal, esophageal, tympanic membrane, or other automatic temperature-monitoring device.

Document temperature at prescribed intervals; take appropriate action for temperature extremes.

NURSING DIAGNOSIS: High risk for impaired skin integrity

OUTCOME: The child's skin integrity will be maintained.

INTERVENTIONS:

Prevent skin preparation solutions from pooling at bedline or under child.

Utilize body supports that conform to the size of the child (rolled diapers, towels, sheets, flexible sandbags, foam rolls); use inflatable bag or rolled sheet in place of kidney rest; use rolled towel for neck or shoulder elevation or support. Maintain all bed sheets and positioning supports dry and wrinkle free.

Provide infant armboards or use padded tongue depressors to stabilize limbs containing intravenous lines.

Position Mayo stand over child's legs and lower part of OR bed to support weight of drapes off child's body.

Use nonwoven, lightweight drapes (when possible) to reduce drape weight.

Determine any skin sensitivity to adhesive prior to application of self-adhering drapes or adhesive tape.

Have available, and use, nonallergenic or paper tape as indicated.

NURSING DIAGNOSIS: High risk for fluid volume deficit

OUTCOME: The child will remain normovolemic.

INTERVENTIONS:

Maintain and protect patency of intravenous lines.

Review laboratory analyses for results of total blood volume.

Calculate estimated total blood volume using formula of 85 to 90 ml/kg of body weight if total blood volume has not been determined by laboratory tests.

Provide gram scales for weighing sponges discarded from operative field; weigh sponges and report estimated loss.

Provide suction units with reservoirs that measure in 5- to 10-ml increments.

Measure and record quantity of irrigating fluid used.

Provide appropriate amounts of intravenous fluid replacement (such as 250-ml containers).

Measure and record urinary output and output from other drainage tubes.

Send laboratory specimens for analysis as indicated; review results indicating fluid status.

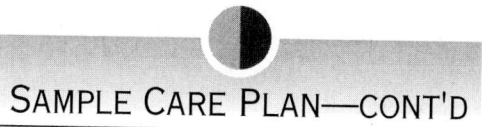

SAMPLE CARE PLAN—CONT'D

NURSING DIAGNOSIS: High risk for injury related to use of electrosurgical unit
OUTCOME: The child will be free from injury.
INTERVENTIONS:
Select appropriate size of adhesive electrosurgery dispersive pad; pad should be able to be molded or contoured to fit application surface yet provide sufficient body mass coverage.
Select pad application site with good tissue mass, as close to operative site as possible; shoulder, but tocks, thigh, or lengthwise on extremity may be selected.
Note condition of skin at dispersive pad placement site prior to placement and on pad removal.
Apply dispersive pad with firm but gentle pressure.
Verify that child is not lying on cord or pad connection.
Protect dispersive pad site from pooling of solutions.
Check dispersive pad contact after any positional changes.

---

struments, which are frightening to the toddler, should be kept from view. The toddler should be brought into the room when everything is ready to allow quick induction of anesthesia.

The preschool and school-age child may still perceive hospitalization or surgery as a punishment; there may be feelings of guilt associated with something the child thinks he or she said or did. Fear of bodily injury and mutilation, loss of control, and the unknown and being left alone characterize these developmental stages. The preschooler benefits from simple and concrete explanations. However, verbal explanations are not enough and pictures, models, actual equipment or play are important. Events should be re-explained as they occur; the perioperative nurse cannot assume the preschooler remembers previous explanations.

The school-age child still fears painful procedures; death may also be a fear at this age. Simple explanations in familiar terms are helpful at this developmental stage; a book or other teaching aid is useful during explanations. This child should be given as many choices as possible (for instance, letting the child decide into which hand the intravenous line will be inserted).

Adolescents may fear peer rejection, disability, loss of a body part, loss of control and status, altered body image, and perhaps death. They need as much privacy as possible, and their attempts to be independent should be respected. The adolescent may not wish to show any fear. Questions might not be asked while the parents are present. The perioperative nurse should provide explanations and answer questions as reasonably and truthfully as possible. If appropriate, some choices should be allowed, such as wearing underwear to the operating room. Patient care procedures that violate privacy, such as hair removal, skin preparation, and insertion of an indwelling urinary catheter, should be conducted after anesthesia is induced.

Key points in providing perioperative care to pediatric patients include never leaving the child unattended, keeping the room quiet during induction, allowing the child to express fear and fearful behaviors (such as crying), using simple words without double meanings, allowing security objects to remain with the child until induction has been completed, and not being dishonest. If the child asks if something will hurt, explain that it will hurt like something they are familiar with (a bee sting, mosquito bite, and so on). The way children fall asleep during induction is likely to be the way they will wake up; thus all attempts should be made to calm and reassure the child. Parents should be alerted to delays in the surgery schedule; in some instances, the child may be sent back to the pediatric unit if surgery is delayed.

Implementing the nursing care plan includes continual assessment and reassessment, as well as the initiation of activities that facilitate the surgical intervention and anticipate patient needs. In addition to positioning, surgical skin preparation, creating and maintaining a sterile field, collecting, dispensing, and recording specimens, administering medications, and providing a safe environment, special instruments and sutures must be provided for the pediatric patient.

Instrumentation

The same types of instruments used in adult surgery are used in pediatric surgery. However, pediatric instruments are usually shorter, have more delicate or less pronounced curves, and are lighter. A complete range of instrument sizes is necessary to make the appropriate size available for each child. Fewer instruments are normally required because incisions in children are shorter and more shallow. Use of basic instrument sets, grouped according to types of surgery performed (for example, minor or major), facilitates instrument counts. These sets are easily adapted to the patient's needs, as well as the surgeon's needs, and eliminate unnecessary instruments from the sterile field.

The following sets are examples of instrumentation used in surgery. The minor set is used for procedures such as inguinal hernia repair or pyloromyotomy. The major set is used for major chest and abdominal cases such as tracheoesophageal fistula (TEF) and diaphragmatic hernia repair, omphalocele repair, and resection and pull-through for Hirschsprung's disease.

Smaller and larger instruments should be packaged separately and dispensed to the surgical field as required.

Minor pediatric instrument set

2 Regular needle holders, 6 inch
1 Fine needle holder, 6 inch
1 Metzenbaum scissors, 7½ inch
1 Metzenbaum scissors, 5½ inch
1 Suture scissors
1 Straight strabismus scissors
1 Curved strabismus scissors
2 Fine mosquito or Halsted hemostats
4 Regular curved mosquito or Halsted hemostats
2 Curved hemostats
2 Babcock forceps

6 Regular straight mosquito or Halsted hemostats
3 Sponge-holding forceps, 9½ inch
6 Towel clamps, 3½ inch
2 Thymus/Lukens retractors
2 Phrenic retractors
2 Cushing vein retractors
2 Richardson retractors, ¾ inch
2 Knife handles, no. 3
2 Adson forceps with teeth
4 Debakey forceps, 6 inch

Major pediatric instrument set

2 Regular needle holders, 7 inch
2 Fine needle holders, 6 inch
1 Regular needle holder, 6 inch
1 Metzenbaum scissors, 7½ inch
1 Metzenbaum scissors, 5½ inch
1 Lincoln scissors
1 Curved Mayo scissors
1 Suture scissors
1 Straight strabismus scissors
1 Curved strabismus scissors
2 Fine curved mosquito or Halsted hemostats
10 Regular curved mosquito or Halsted hemostats

6 Regular straight mosquito or Halsted hemostats
2 Curved hemostats
2 Straight hemostats
6 Pean forceps
2 Allis forceps
4 Babcock forceps
1 Fine Schnidt clamp
3 Regular Schnidt clamps
1 Right-angle clamp, 7 inch
1 Lahey gall duct forceps
3 Sponge-holding forceps, 9½ inch
1 Towel clamp, 3½ inch
2 Army-Navy retractors
2 Thymus/Lukens retractors

2 Phrenic retractors
2 Cushing vein retractors
2 Small Deaver retractors
1 Set of Richardson retractors (2 of each size)
2 Adson forceps with teeth
1 Tissue forceps with teeth
2 Debakey forceps, 6 inch

2 Debakey forceps, 7½ inch
2 Tuttle forceps
1 Knife handle, no. 7
1 Knife handle, no. 3
1 Grooved director
1 Tonsil suction tube
1 Frazier suction tip, no. 11
1 Small Poole suction tube

Sutures

Small sizes of absorbable and nonabsorbable sutures are appropriate for the delicate and fragile tissues of infants and children. Sutures should have attached needles (atraumatic) to reduce tissue damage. The most common sizes are nos. 000 to 5-0 with ½ inch- and ⅜ inch-circle needles. Staples, both pediatric and regular sizes, are often used. Many skin incisions are closed with subcutaneous suture using subcuticular techniques; paper adhesive dressing strips or collodion is then applied.

EVALUATION

The perioperative nurse evaluates care provided throughout the perioperative period. At the conclusion of the surgical intervention, the skin is inspected, especially at dependent pressure points and at the site of the electrosurgical dispersive pad. Inspection is carried out to detect any reddened, irritated areas or evidence of compression injury. The temperature of the skin is noted, as is the core temperature. The cardiopulmonary status is closely monitored as the child emerges from anesthesia; the perioperative nurse assists anesthesia personnel during emergence and protects the child from injury. Dry, warm blankets are provided. Hydration status is determined, replacement fluids administered, and fluid output noted. The child is transferred to and positioned on the PACU stretcher. The airway is protected, as are tubes, drains, and drainage devices.

The perioperative nurse provides an oral report to the nurse in PACU, focusing on the condition of the child, the response to surgery and anesthesia, presence of catheters and drains, the quality and amount of wound drainage, and a description of the dressings applied. Part of this report should focus on the outcomes established in the perioperative care plan. For the care plan presented in this chapter, they might be as follows:

· The child and family demonstrated knowledge of perioperative events and the roles of perioperative team members.
· The child's body temperature was maintained at an appropriate level during the surgical intervention.

- Skin integrity was maintained.
- The child remained normovolemic.
- There was no evidence of injury related to use of the electrosurgical unit.

The perioperative nurse may receive further feedback on the child's progress after the child is discharged from the PACU; this information may be relayed by the surgeon, unit nurse, or clinical nurse specialist. This type of informal feedback helps close the loop of information. It allows the perioperative nurse to informally collect additional data regarding effectiveness of the care plan and provides information about the outcomes of the perioperative care provided.

SURGICAL INTERVENTIONS

Pediatric surgery encompasses all specialties but, in general, can be divided into three major areas: congenital malformations or defects, acquired diseases of infancy and childhood, and trauma. A discussion of pediatric trauma is beyond the scope of this chapter. Several surgical procedures that may be designated pediatric have been presented in previous chapters of this text under particular specialty headings. Surgical interventions presented here include procedures that are commonly and uniquely performed in the area of pediatric general and cardiac surgery.

CORRECTION OF GASTROINTESTINAL DISORDERS

Central venous catheter placement

The exposure and cannulation of a major vessel for the purpose of inserting and positioning a catheter in the vena cava just above the atrium are indicated for infants and children who require total parenteral nutrition (TPN) because feeding through the gastrointestinal (GI) tract is impossible, inadequate, or hazardous. Common conditions necessitating TPN are bowel fistulas, inadequate intestinal length, chronic diarrhea, extensive burns, and multiple trauma. The TPN fluids are delivered through a central venous catheter to avoid peripheral inflammation and thrombosis. Occasionally, a central venous catheter is indicated for infants or children who require chemotherapy, antibiotic therapy, or other long-term IV medical treatment.

The preferred site of placement is the external jugular vein. The internal jugular may be chosen if the external jugular has been used or is too small. From the cannulation site the catheter is tunneled under the skin about 5 to 10 cm. This is done to inhibit contamination of the bloodstream from frequent dressing changes. In cases where the internal or external vein sites are unavailable, the catheter may be placed in the external iliac vein by way of a cutdown in the greater saphenous vein. In these cases the catheter is tunneled out into the abdominal wall.

Procedural considerations. The manufacturer's instructions for handling, preparing, and sterilizing the catheter must be followed. The catheter must not contact linty materials, glove powder, or other foreign matter. Before insertion the catheter is flushed and filled with the infusion solution, special formula, or dextrose 10% in water to prevent air bubbles from entering the circulatory system and to eliminate blood clots in the catheter lumen. The catheter is connected to the pump, and infusion should begin as soon as the catheter is secured. In some instances the catheter is flushed with a dose-dependent (according to the child's size) heparin solution and pump infusion begun in the PACU.

The child is appropriately positioned as dictated by the site chosen for cannulation. The area is prepped and draped.

Operative procedure

1. A transverse incision is made over the lower portion of the medial border of the sternocleidomastoid muscle.
2. The external jugular vein is exposed and prepared for cannulation.
3. Using a long, hollow needle with an obturator (a tendon passer or neurotunneler may be used on a larger child) a subcutaneous tunnel is created, extending from the neck incision to the chest wall medial to the nipple.
4. The obturator is withdrawn, and the catheter is passed through the needle. The needle is removed, and the catheter then lies in the subcutaneous tunnel.
5. The external jugular vein is ligated distally and incised; the catheter is passed into the vein and advanced so that it lies at the point where the superior vena cava enters the atrium.
6. The position of the catheter is then confirmed by radiography in the operating room.
7. The catheter is secured at the exit site on the chest wall with nonabsorbable sutures.
8. Antimicrobial ointment is applied to the exit site, and an occlusive, transparent dressing is placed over this. The catheter is coiled under this dressing to avoid tension on the line and accidental displacement.
9. The infusion pump is connected to the infusing solution before the child is moved from the OR bed.

Repair of atresia of the esophagus

Atresia of the esophagus is repaired through a right retropleural thoracotomy, with closure of the TEF and anastomosis of the segments of the esophagus.

This congenital anomaly may arise between the third and sixth weeks of fetal life. Several types are recognized, the most common being an upper segment of esophagus ending in a blind pouch and a lower segment of esophagus communicating by a fistula with the trachea (esophageal atresia with TEF). Ideally this defect is recognized in the first hours of life, but more often the diagnosis is made in the first 36 to 48 hours of life. Drooling, the need for frequent suctioning, and coughing or cyanosis during oral feeding are the most common presentations (Holder and Manning, 1991). Prompt surgical intervention allows the child to breathe and eat without the danger of aspirating mucus, saliva, feedings, or stomach contents.

Procedural considerations. A gastrostomy may be done first to decompress the air-distended stomach, thus facilitating chest movement and ventilation and preventing reflux of stomach contents into the trachea. The patient is then positioned for a right thoracotomy, prepped and draped. The major instrument set is required, with the addition of the following:

Baby chest retractors	Ligaclips
Baby T-malleables	Cotton tip applicators
Regular malleables	Umbilical tape
Infant malleables	Chest tube (check size)
Senn retractors	Infant Pleurevac
Gemini mixters	Malecot catheter (check
Neuromastoid retractors	size)
Dilators	Fogarty catheters
Vessel loops	Mineral oil

Operative procedure

1. The chest is entered through the fourth intercostal space. Removal of the rib is not necessary (Fig. 28-1, *A*).

2. The pleura is gently dissected off the chest wall (Fig. 28-1, *B*).

3. As the dissection proceeds posteriorly, the azygos vein is encountered, which is reflected inferiorly after dividing its highest intercostal branches to expose the fistula beneath (Fig. 28-1, *C*).

4. Tape or silk is passed under the fistula to apply traction gently (Fig. 28-1, *D*). Dissection of the mediastinum begins with the TEF and distal esophagus. The vagus nerve is an important landmark for the distal esophagus.

5. The fistula is clamped and transsected, leaving a thin cuff of esophageal tissue on the tracheal side to allow closure of the trachea without narrowing it and compromising the lumen of the airway (Fig. 28-1, *E*).

6. To close the fistula, three or four interrupted sutures of 5-0 nonabsorbable suture are used.

7. The upper esophageal pouch is dissected; passage of a nasogastric or replogle tube by the anesthesiologist aids in its identification.

8. The proximal pouch is then identified and dissected as needed to allow it to reach the distal esophageal segment with minimal tension for anastomoses. At this point the surgeon makes the decision to attempt primary anastomosis. If primary anastomosis is impossible, the distal esophagus is closed and tacked high on the prevertebral fascia. Infrequently, the gap between the proximal and distal portions of esophagus is so long that esophageal replacement is required. In these cases the upper pouch is brought out to the neck in the form of a cervical esophagostomy. When the child reaches 1 year of age, esophageal replacement is attempted

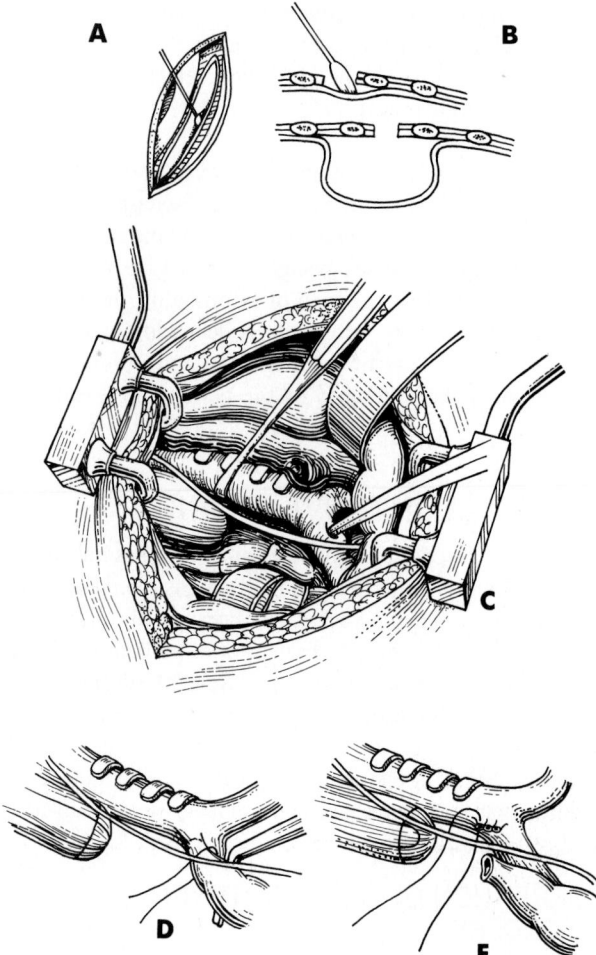

FIG. 28-1   Repair of atresia of the esophagus. **A,** Incision at fourth intercostal space. **B,** Dissection of pleura off chest wall. **C,** Identification and division of azygos vein to expose fistula beneath. **D,** Traction applied to fistula. **E,** Transsection of fistula leaving 3-mm cuff on trachea.

Reprinted with permission from Coran, A.G., et al. (1978). *Surgery of the neonate.* Boston: Little, Brown.

through colon interposition or construction of a reverse gastric tube.

9. Primary anastomosis is performed with 5-0 or 6-0 nonabsorbable suture, taking full-thickness bites along anterior and posterior borders (Fig. 28-2). Some surgeons prefer the Haight or two-layer anastomosis (Fig. 28-3). The inner layer is comprised of the upper pouch mucosa sutured to the full thickness of the distal esophagus. The muscular sleeve of the upper esophagus is then pulled down over the inner anastomosis and sutured to the muscular layer of the inferior esophagus. The incision is irrigated with saline.

10. Some surgeons place a no. 14 or 16 Fr extrapleural chest tube near the anastomosis through a posterior stab wound. It is secured with sutures to prevent it from putting direct pressure on the anastomosis.

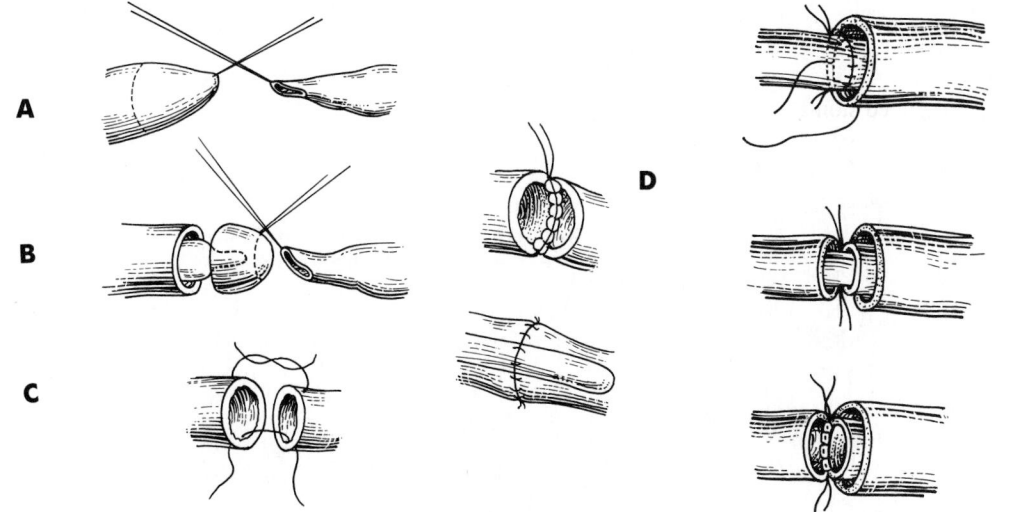

FIG. 28-2 Primary repair of atresia of the esophagus: single layer repair. **A,** Traction applied to proximal and distal esophagus. **B,** Blind proximal pouch transsected. **C,** Full-thickness bites of anterior and posterior borders. **D,** Repair completed with replogle tube in place to allow adequate lumen of esophagus.

Reprinted with permission from Coran, A.G., et al. (1978). *Surgery of the neonate.* Boston: Little, Brown.

FIG. 28-3 Haight anastomosis. Mucosal layer of proximal pouch sutured to full thickness of distal esophagus. Muscular sleeve of upper pouch pulled down over inner anastomosis and sutured to muscle of distal esophagus.

Reprinted with permission from Coran, A.G., et al. (1978). *Surgery of the neonate.* Boston: Little, Brown.

11. Muscle layers are closed with interrupted 5-0 or 6-0 nonabsorbable sutures or continuous 3-0 absorbable suture.
12. Skin is closed with a continuous 5-0 suture, and a collodion dressing or dressing of gauze and tape is applied.
13. The extrapleural chest tube is water sealed, and a chest x-ray is obtained.

Repair of congenital diaphragmatic hernia

A congenital diaphragmatic hernia is repaired by replacement of the displaced viscera into the abdominal cavity with surgical correction of the defect (Fig. 28-4). The conventional surgical repair is through the abdomen. The concurrence of intraabdominal abnormalities is somewhat high in babies with diaphragmatic hernia; therefore treatment is facilitated with an abdominal approach. It is technically easier to extract the viscera from below than to push them out of the thorax. The abnormal intrathoracic intrusion of the abdominal viscera usually causes severe compromise of intrathoracic pulmonary and vascular activities. Therefore urgent restoration of more normal intrathoracic and intraabdominal relationships is the rule in these newborns. The lung may be hypoplastic because of prolonged compression in utero by the displaced abdominal viscera. A residual intrapleural space usually remains for a few days after surgery.

Procedural considerations. A chest tube can be inserted and connected to water-seal drainage. Insertion of a gastrostomy tube minimizes postoperative distention and fa-

cilitates feeding. Direct suturing of the margins of the defect is usually possible. Insertion of a prosthetic Silastic sheeting is occasionally required, and the sheeting should be available.

The major instrument set is required, plus the following:

Medium Ligaclips	Infant Pleurevac (may
Baby malleables	fill to either 3.5 or
Baby Deavers	5 cm of water)
Chest tube (check size)	Red rubber catheter
Umbilical tape	Mineral oil

Have available:

Neuromastoid retractors
Chest retractors
Bone wax
Marlex mesh or Silastic sheet

The infant is positioned supine on a hyperthermia blanket.

Operative procedure

1. A contralateral chest tube may be placed in the anterior axillary line of the second intercostal space to prevent tension pneumothorax during surgery.
2. A subcostal incision going through all muscle layers is made on the side of the defect.
3. The abdominal viscera are withdrawn from the chest and held downward through the abdominal wound. Because abnormalities of abdominal viscera such as malrotation

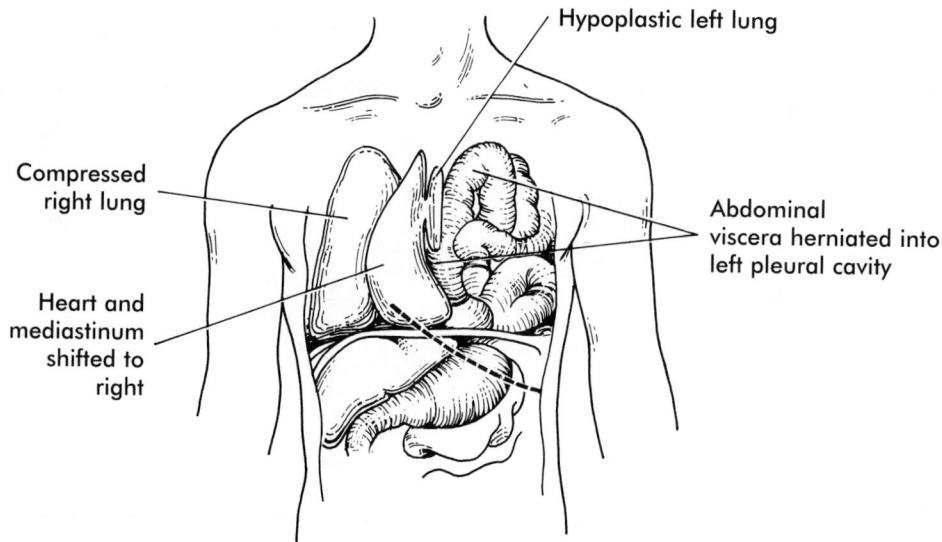

FIG. 28-4　Diaphragmatic hernia.

are associated with diaphragmatic hernia, the surgeon performs careful inspection of the organs at this time. If a malrotation is found, some surgeons prefer to repair it if the clinical condition of the infant allows it.

4. The defect is then carefully inspected, including a search for a hernia sac, which is present in less than 5% of cases. If a sac is identified, it is excised. An ipsilateral chest tube is placed before the diaphragm is closed.

5. The posterior and anterior rims of the diaphragm are identified, and primary closure is performed with mattress sutures of 2-0 nonabsorbable material. If the rim of tissue is too small for mattress sutures, ample sutures of 2-0 or 3-0 nonabsorbable are used. Occasionally, reinforced Silastic sheeting may be needed if sufficient diaphragm is not available for primary closure.

6. Gastrostomy is then performed in most cases.

7. The abdominal wall is then closed. If the musculature cannot accommodate the abdominal viscera, it is left open and skin is closed to leave a ventral hernia. The infant is returned to the operating room within 7 days for repair of the ventral hernia.

Nissen fundoplication

Nissen fundoplication is the wrapping of the fundus of the stomach around the esophagus at the gastroesophageal junction. Nissen fundoplication is indicated for infants and children who suffer from severe gastroesophageal reflux (GER). The cause of GER in these patients is thought to be an inadequate antireflux barrier. The antireflux barrier consists of a combination of anatomic and physiologic factors, including sufficient amount and strength of muscle fibers located in the lower esophageal sphincter, adequate length of the abdominal esophagus, and a high-pressure zone in the lower esophagus. The combination of these fac-

tors forms the antireflux barrier and thus prevents GER. An incompetent antireflux barrier can result in life-threatening complications of GER, including obstructive apnea, aspiration pneumonia, esophagitis, and failure to thrive. The goal of the Nissen fundoplication is to recreate a competent antireflux barrier.

Procedural considerations. The major instrument set is required, plus the following:

Medium Ligaclips	Sterile specimen cup
Drain (¼ inch to ⅜ inch—check size)	Malecot catheter (check size)

Have available:

Deaver retractors	Bookwalter retractor
Long instruments	Maloney dilators (surgeon will place prior to scrubbing)
Iron intern retractor	
Balfour retractor	

The patient is positioned supine. An appropriate size dilator is passed into the esophagus to prevent the wrap from impinging on the lumen of the esophagus (Fig. 28-5).

Operative procedure

1. A left subcostal incision is performed to allow exposure of the lower esophagus to create adequate intraabdominal length.

2. The esophagus is mobilized to create adequate intraabdominal length.

3. The stomach is mobilized to allow loose wrap of the fundus around the esophageal junction; it is used as the lower edge of the wrap.

4. Sutures of 3-0 or 4-0 nonabsorbable are placed through the seromuscular layers of both stomach and esophagus to fix the wrap.

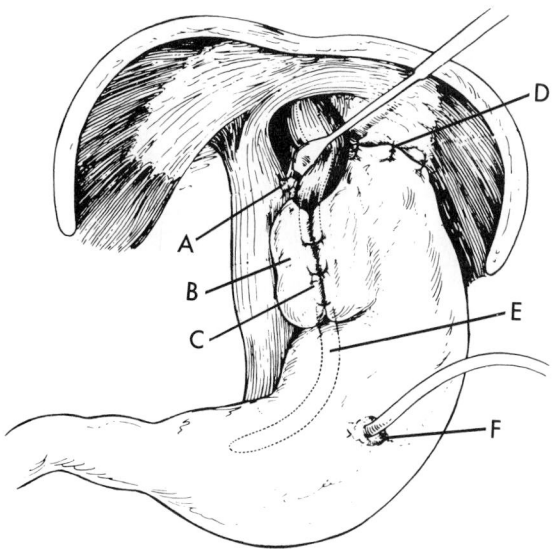

FIG. 28-5 Salient features of Nissen fundoplication in infants. *A,* Crural sutures to reduce hiatus. *B,* Generous loose, adequate tissue in wrap. *C,* Sutures placed through seromuscular depth of both gastric and esophageal walls. *D,* Sutures to fix fundus to diaphragm. *E,* Appropriate-sized mercury-filled dilator to ensure adequate lumen. *F,* Gastrostomy in all infants and whenever there is any question of gastric outlet problems.

From Randolph, J. G. (1985). *Annals of surgery, 198,* 579. Reprinted with permission.

5. Sutures are then placed to tack the fundus to the diaphragm (fundoplication); the posterior fundus is wrapped behind the esophagus and the anterior fundus in front. Two layers of sutures may be used. The first layer passes from the anterior fundus, through the right margin to the posterior fundus. The second layer may be added between the anterior and posterior fundus for additional security (Johnson, 1991).
6. Some surgeons place clips at the level of the gastroesophageal junction and the wrap to aid in follow-up radiographic studies.
7. A gastrostomy is done in most cases.
8. The incision is closed in layers, and a collodion dressing is applied.

Ramstedt-Fredet pyloromyotomy for pyloric stenosis

The Ramstedt-Fredet pyloromyotomy for pyloric stenosis is the incision of the muscles of the pylorus to treat congenital hypertrophy of the pyloric sphincter that is obstructing the stomach. Signs and symptoms of high GI obstruction appear at 2 to 6 weeks of age. The first sign is projectile vomiting that is free of bile. There may be a severe loss of body fluids and electrolyte imbalance, evidenced as hypochloremic, hypokalemic metabolic alkalosis. Once the diagnosis of hypertrophic pyloric stenosis is made, either through physical examination or imaging techniques, surgical correction is planned.

Procedural considerations. The stomach is emptied just before induction of anesthesia, and the nasogastric tube is removed to guard against reflux of gastric contents around the tube during induction. A minor instrument set and a pyloric spreader are used. The patient is prepped in the usual manner.

Operative procedure

1. The abdomen is opened through a right subcostal transverse skin incision. The rectus muscle is retracted or split longitudinally in the middle with spreading clamps, and the peritoneum is opened.
2. After the hypertrophied pylorus is delivered into the wound with a small vein retractor, the prepyloric area is grasped and rotated to expose the anterior superior border of the mass. An incision is made in the serosa on the anterior wall of the pyloric mass from the duodenal junction proximally to a point proximal to the area of hypertrophied muscle (Fig. 28-6, *A*).
3. The circular muscle is spread with the pyloric spreader on the submucosal base, so that all muscle fibers are completely divided (Fig. 28-6, *B*).
4. After completion of the separation the pyloric end of the stomach is returned to the abdomen, and the peritoneum and posterior rectus sheath are closed with a continuous, absorbable no. 3-0 suture. The anterior rectus sheath is closed with a no. 4-0 absorbable suture.
5. The skin is closed with fine subcuticular sutures. Small adhesive strips or collodion is applied as dressing.

EMERGENCY GASTROINTESTINAL PROCEDURES
Gastrostomy

Gastrostomy is establishment of a temporary or permanent channel from the gastric lumen to the skin to permit gastric emptying, liquid feeding, or retrograde dilatation of an esophageal stricture. The procedure may be emergent in nature or performed with other surgical procedures to facilitate care of the infant or child after surgery. Placement of the gastrostomy tube may be through an abdominal incision (described below) or percutaneously using an endoscope and local anesthesia (PEG). For children receiving long-term gastrostomy feedings a skin level device (Button, Gastroport) may be inserted after the gastrostomy is well established. These devices, which protrude slightly from the abdomen, are more cosmetically acceptable and allow more mobility for the child.

Procedural considerations. A minor instrument set is required, plus a mushroom or Malecot catheter (no. 14 or 16 for infants and no. 18, 20, or 22 for older children) and a no. 11 knife blade on a knife handle. Routine prepping is done.

Operative procedure

1. A short incision is made over the outer border of the left rectus muscle (Fig. 28-7, *A*).

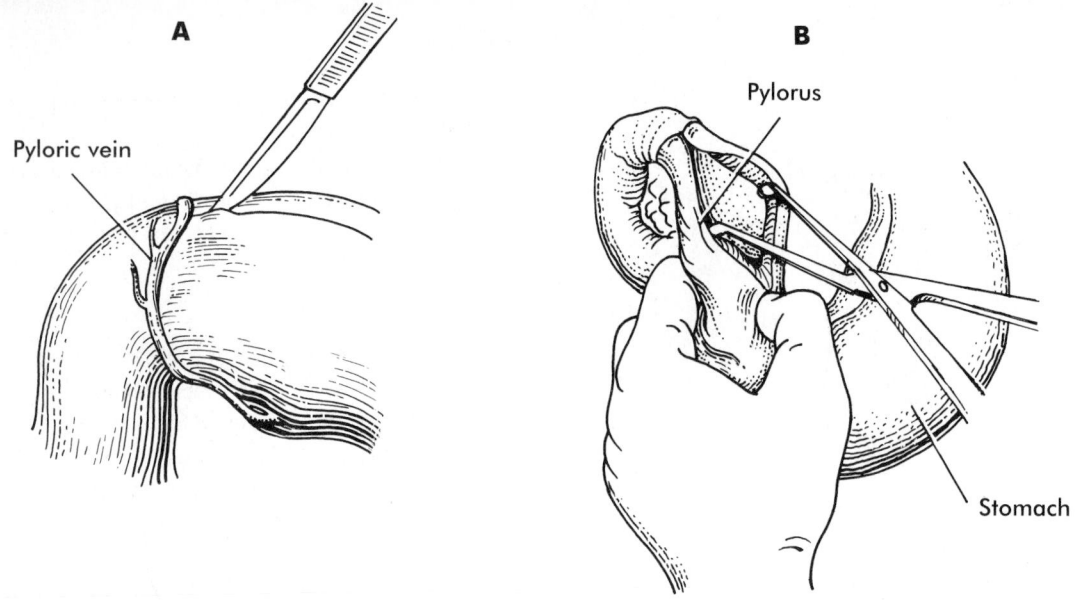

FIG. 28-6 Operative technique for pyloric stenosis.

From Benson, C.D. (1969). Infants' hypertrophic pyloric stenosis. In Mustard, W.T., et al. (editors), *Pediatric surgery* (2nd ed.). Copyright 1969 by Year Book Medical Publishers, Inc., Chicago. Used by permission.

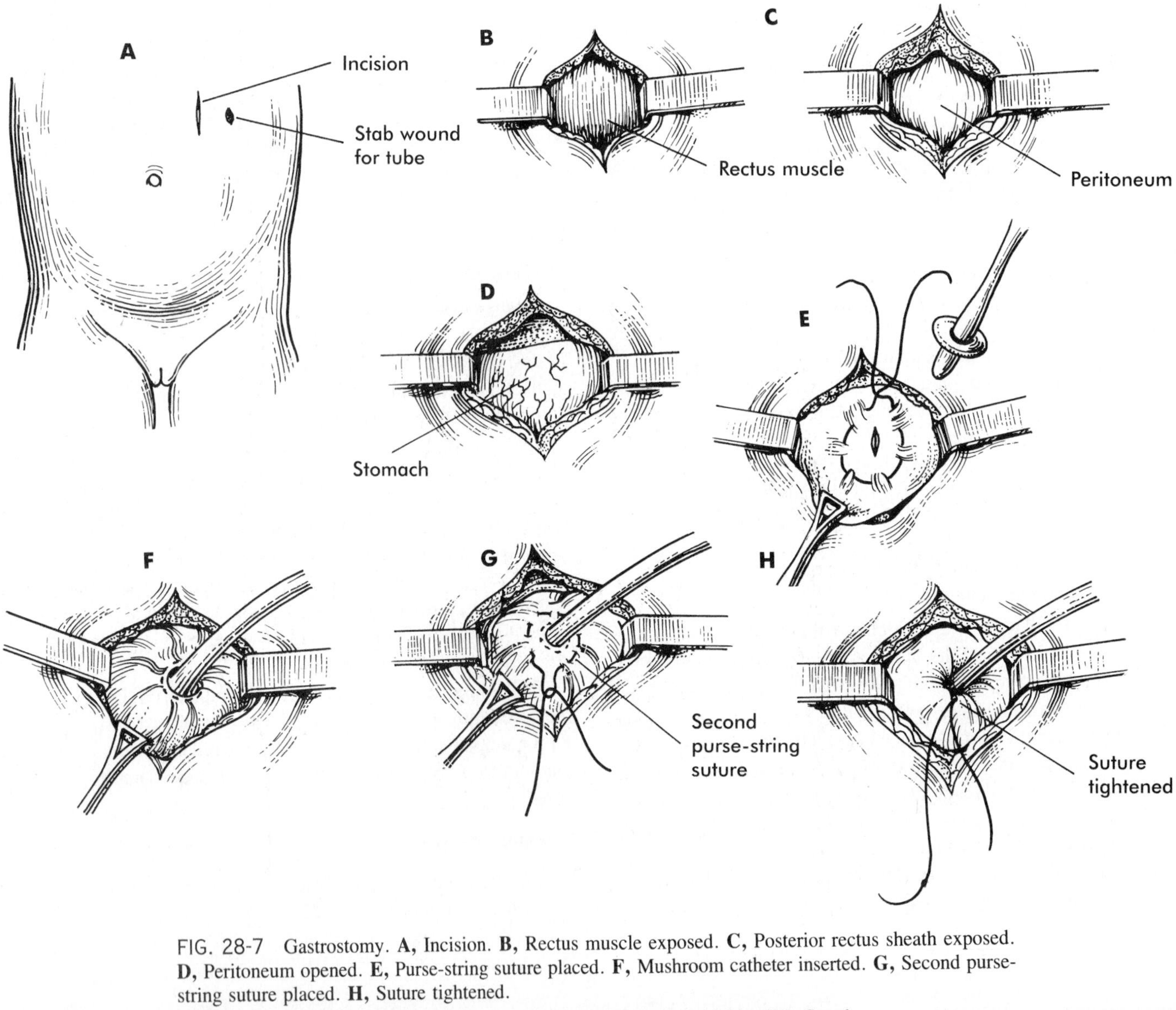

FIG. 28-7 Gastrostomy. **A,** Incision. **B,** Rectus muscle exposed. **C,** Posterior rectus sheath exposed. **D,** Peritoneum opened. **E,** Purse-string suture placed. **F,** Mushroom catheter inserted. **G,** Second purse-string suture placed. **H,** Suture tightened.

Modified from Gross, R.E. (1970). *An atlas of children's surgery*. Philadelphia: W.B. Saunders.

2. The subcutaneous tissues and rectus fascia are exposed with two small retractors (Fig. 28-7, *B*).

3. The anterior rectus fascia is opened, and the rectus muscle is split with clamps, exposing the posterior rectus sheath (Fig. 28-7, *C*).

4. The peritoneum is opened, exposing the liver edge and the greater curvature of the stomach (Fig. 28-7, *D*).

5. The stomach is pulled out through the wound with Babcock forceps. A circular pursestring suture of no. 4-0 nonabsorbable suture is placed; in the center of this a stab wound is made through the gastric wall (Fig. 28-7, *E*).

6. A mushroom catheter, often with the tip cut off, is inserted into the stomach, and the pursestring suture is tied (Fig. 28-7, *F*).

7. A second pursestring suture is placed outside the previous one, and the same needle is then taken through the peritoneum and the posterior rectus fascia to place the stomach against the peritoneum and thus prevent leaks (Fig. 28-7, *G* and *H*).

8. The catheter is brought out through a left lateral stab wound (Fig. 28-7, *A*).

9. The stomach wall adjacent to the gastrostomy site is tacked to the undersurface of the peritoneum with interrupted sutures of 4-0 nonabsorbable.

10. Routine abdominal closure is performed.

Prior to using the gastrostomy tube for feedings, an upper GI study is usually performed to exclude the possibility of distal intestinal atresia (Woolley, 1991).

Omphalocele repair

Omphalocele is the protrusion of abdominal viscera outside the abdomen into a sac of amniotic membrane and peritoneum at the base of the umbilical cord. There is no skin covering.

Omphalocele occurs during the eleventh week of fetal life when the viscera fail to withdraw from the exocoelomic position and occupy the peritoneal cavity. The resulting abdominal wall defect can vary in size from 2 to 15 cm. The sac may contain only a few loops of bowel to nearly all the intestines plus liver and spleen. Associated anomalies include malrotation and abnormal fixation of the bowel.

Since the infant is at risk for hypothermia, hypoglycemia, shock, sepsis, and vascular injury to the bowel, immediate management after birth is necessary (Vegunta et al., 1993). Treatment consists of applying warm saline packs on the sac surface, inserting a nasogastric tube to prevent distention and aspiration, and initiation of intravenous access with fluid resuscitation and antibiotic therapy. Surgical intervention is necessary to prevent rupture of the sac, infection, or both. If intrauterine rupture of the sac has occurred, the newborn is kept warm, the bowel is inspected for perforation and torsion, and moist, warm dressings are applied.

An omphalocele is repaired by replacement of the viscera in the abdominal cavity, with reconstruction of the abdominal wall (Fig. 28-8).

Procedural considerations. Particular attention to maintaining body temperature is essential because of the massive exposed surface area from which body heat can be lost. The use of nitrous oxide as an anesthetic agent is avoided during this procedure because it causes increased gas in the intestine, which in turn makes the reduction of abdominal contents into the peritoneal cavity more difficult. Repeated rectal irrigation with warm saline to evacuate meconium from the bowel may be carried out prior to the

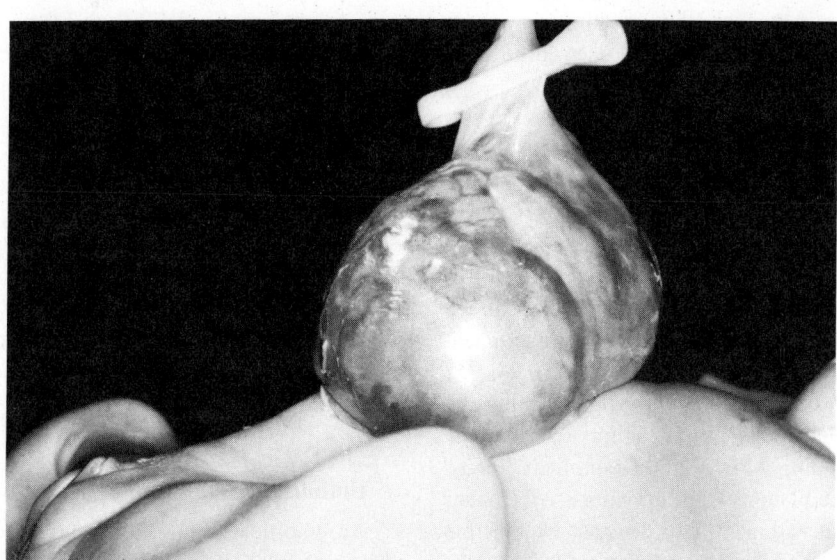

FIG. 28-8 Omphalocele containing liver.

Courtesy John R. Campbell, University of Oregon Health Sciences Center, Portland; from Jensen, M.D., and Bobak, I.M. (1993). *Maternity and gynecologic care: The nurse and the family* (5th ed.). St. Louis: Mosby.

abdominal prep. The major instrument set is required, with the addition of the following:

Baby malleables
Ligaclips
Red rubber catheter

Have available:

Silastic sheeting   Replogle tube
Foley catheter with   Malecot catheter
   urimeter

The infant is positioned supine, and the abdomen, umbilical cord, and sac are gently prepped with a povidone-iodine solution; if the prep solution is warmed, follow manufacturer's directions.

Operative procedure

1. In the presence of small defects, primary closure is attempted. The skin edges are freed, and the sac is excised. Abdominal contents are gently relocated into the peritoneal cavity. The abdominal cavity is closed in layers using 3-0 nonabsorbable suture.

2. In certain cases where the defect is of medium to large size, a primary closure may not be accomplished. In these situations a staged procedure is done utilizing prosthetic reduction. In the first stage the infant is brought to the operating room and positioned and prepped as previously described.

2a. The sac is excised, and the umbilical vein and arteries are ligated.

2b. Gastrostomy may be performed at this time.

2c. A silo is then created with Silastic mesh (Fig. 28-9). The mesh is secured through all layers of the edge of the defect utilizing a continuous locking suture of 2-0 nonabsorbable (Fig. 28-9, *A*). The open end of the silo is closed in the same manner, thus creating a cylinder of mesh extending upward from the abdomen (Fig. 28-9, *B*).

2d. The open end of the cylinder is tied closed with umbilical tape (Fig. 28-9, *C*) or, alternatively, attached to a specifically designed roller clamp.

2e. The mesh silo suture line and edge of the defect are wrapped with Kling dipped in an iodophor solution to prevent infection. The infant is transferred to an open isolette, and the silo is suspended from the top of the isolette. Plastic wrap is applied to the silo to prevent heat loss.

2f. The infant is then transported to the neonatal intensive care unit, where daily reduction of abdominal contents is performed by adding a lower tie of umbilical tape or adjusting the roller clamp. The abdominal viscera are completely reduced within 5 to 10 days, at which time the infant is returned to the operating room for the second stage of repair (Fig. 28-9, *D*).

2g. To avoid an appendectomy in the future on a child with

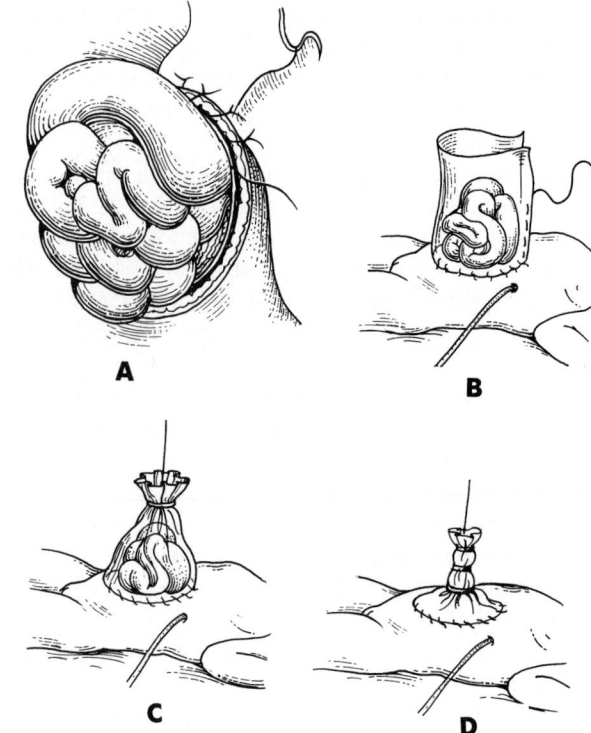

FIG. 28-9   Staged repair of omphalocele. **A,** Silastic mesh secured to all layers of edge of defect. **B,** Silo closed, creating cylinder of mesh. **C,** Open end of silo tied with umbilical tape. **D,** Lower ties of umbilical tape applied to silo to gradually reduce viscera.

Reprinted with permission from Coran, A.G., et al. (1978). *Surgery of the neonate*. Boston: Little, Brown.

a malrotated colon, an appendectomy may be performed at this time.

2h. The silo is removed, and the fascia is closed with interrupted sutures of 2-0 or 3-0 nonabsorbable.

2i. The skin is closed with interrupted 4-0 nonabsorbable suture. In an attempt to create an umbilicus, a purse-string suture is utilized in closing the inferior 2 cm of incision.

3. Another technique for treating large omphaloceles is painting the sac and surrounding skin with a 2% solution of merbromin (Mercurochrome) until an eschar forms to add strength to the sac and resist infection, or the sac may be treated with moist 0.5% silver nitrate dressings. The sac membrane gradually contracts, and skin closes the abdominal wall defect. Later surgery then repairs the abdominal musculature.

REPAIR OF HERNIAS
Umbilical hernia repair

An umbilical hernia, a condition commonly seen in pediatric populations, is corrected by repair of the part of the intestine protruding at the umbilicus. An umbilical hernia is always covered by skin. Small umbilical hernias may be left untreated. They usually close within a few months to a year. If surgical repair is required in a large fascial defect, it may be delayed until the child is at least 2 years of age with some surgeons delaying repair until 4 years of age.

Procedural considerations. Surgical correction of umbilical hernia may be an ambulatory surgical procedure. General anesthesia is used. A minor instrument set is required. The child is prepped as discussed previously. Several variations in technique have been used; an infraumbilical approach is most common and is described below.

Operative procedure

1. An incision is made below the umbilicus through the skin and subcutaneous tissue.
2. Flaps of skin and subcutaneous tissue are mobilized and held back with small retractors to expose the rectus fascia and hernial protrusion.
3. The hernia sac, which is between the rectus muscle sheaths in the midline, is completely freed from all surrounding structures.
4. The hernia sac may be invaginated, dissected free and ligated, or excised.
5. The peritoneum is closed with a continuous suture.
6. The two edges of the rectus fascia are brought together using interrupted no. 3-0 nonabsorbable sutures.
7. Subcuticular closure of the skin with a continuous, fine, absorbable suture is performed, and a pressure dressing is applied.

Inguinal hernia repair

An inguinal hernia is corrected by repairing a protrusion of a hernia sac, containing the intestine, in the inguinal canal. The testis develops high on the posterior wall of the abdomen. It gradually descends into the scrotum. Before the testis enters the inguinal canal, the processus vaginalis projects downward but retains a communication with the peritoneal cavity. The upper part of the processus does not; the remaining sac constitutes an indirect inguinal hernia. In a girl, a similar hernial sac is contiguous with the round ligament.

Procedural considerations. A minor instrument set is used, and routine prepping is done.

Operative procedure

1. An incision is made over the inguinal area in the direction of the skin crease.
2. The subcutaneous tissue is opened, and hemostats are placed on bleeding vessels, which are then ligated or electrocoagulated.
3. Right-angle retractors are placed inferiorly and medially.
4. The external ring is identified, and the external oblique fascia is cleaned and freed with small Metzenbaum scissors.
5. The external oblique fascia is opened with a no. 15

knife blade on a knife handle, and the upper flap is freed. The lower flap is freed to expose the inguinal ligament.

6. Cord structures are opened at the upper end of the cord. Two forceps are used to grasp tissues at the same level and separate them.
7. The hernia sac is grasped with a hemostat, and structures of the cord are peeled downward and away from the sac with forceps until the sac is freed. Care is taken to protect the spermatic cord and major vessels as the sac is freed.
8. After the sac is opened and the surgeon's index finger inserted, the sac is pulled upward. The upward traction is maintained with two or three hemostats.
9. The sac is ligated with no. 3-0 nonabsorbable suture, and excess sac is removed. Repair of the inguinal canal may be done with nonabsorbable sutures.
10. The subcutaneous tissue is closed with interrupted, fine sutures; closure of the skin is with fine, nonabsorbable subcuticular sutures. Collodion or paper adhesive dressing strips are applied.

REPAIR OF OBSTRUCTIVE DISORDERS
Repair of intestinal obstruction

Repair of intestinal obstruction includes (1) untwisting of a volvulus, (2) division of a congenital band, (3) release of an internal hernia, (4) resection of bowel with anastomosis, and (5) creation of an intestinal stoma. Intestinal obstruction is the most frequent GI emergency requiring surgery in the newborn. Early recognition is essential. Surgical intervention is usually within the first few hours after birth; delay may increase the risk.

Intestinal obstruction can occur in the infant for a variety of reasons: atresia, stenosis, congenital aganglionosis, meconium ileus, or malrotation. Lesions characterized by complete obliteration of intestinal lumen are classified as atresia. Those which produce a narrowing or partial obliteration of the lumen are classified as stenosis.

Procedural considerations. The major instrument set and pediatric intestinal instruments are required, plus culture tubes, syringes, and a 25-gauge needle. Routine prepping is done.

Operative procedure

1. The abdomen is opened through an incision appropriate to the exposure of the particular form of obstruction.
2. Exploration and displacement of the intestines to the abdominal wall help determine the obstructive lesion. With atresia or stenosis, the entire bowel must be examined to rule out multiple areas of involvement.
3. Detorsion or reduction of bowel decompression or resection is performed when indicated.

Reduction of intussusception

Intussusception is the telescopic invagination of a portion of intestine into an adjacent part with mechanical and vascular impairment. It is relieved by reduction of invaginated bowel by the hydrostatic pressure of a barium enema or by laparotomy and manual manipulation. Intussusception is the most common cause of intestinal obstruction in the 2-month to 3-year-old age group, and therefore one of the most common surgical emergencies in this age group. A frequent site for intussusception is the ileocecal junction. Intussusception in children is most often idiopathic; other causes may include Meckel's diverticulum, polyps, or hematoma of the bowel. Early diagnosis and reduction are essential to bowel viability.

Procedural considerations. The child is prepped for surgery as described previously. Reduction by barium enema should be attempted only with the full cognizance of the radiologist, surgeon, and pediatrician, with the operating room team on standby. Should reduction not be accomplished, a laparotomy must be done. The major instrument set is used with the addition of pediatric intestinal instruments.

Operative procedure

1. A right lower quadrant transverse or right paramedian incision is made, and the peritoneum is entered (Fig. 28-10, *A*).
2. The cecum and ileum are identified; the intussusception is located and elevated with fingers (Fig. 28-10, *B* and *C*).
3. If there is no evidence of bowel compromise, the bowel immediately distal to the intussusception is occluded with one hand and stripped proximally with the other in an attempt to achieve manual reduction. If the serosa splits during attempted reduction, or if the mass cannot be reduced, bowel resection is done; this may be required in 35% to 41% of children (West, 1991).
4. The abdomen is closed in layers, and the wound is dressed.

Colostomy

Colostomy is the surgical construction of an artificial excretory opening from the colon. Most congenital anomalies that result in colonic obstruction require a temporary colostomy. These include imperforate anus and Hirschsprung's disease. Both conditions ultimately require further pelvic operative procedures, and proper construction of a colostomy is important. In Hirschsprung's disease the colostomy must be placed in a section of bowel containing ganglia.

Procedural considerations. A major instrument set and pediatric intestinal clamps are used. The child is prepped as described previously.

Operative procedure

1. A transverse incision usually is preferred, and the abdomen is entered in the right upper quadrant for a transverse colostomy or the left lower quadrant for a sigmoid colostomy.

2. The loop of colon is freed of peritoneal attachments until it can be brought easily through the abdominal wall without tension.
3. The edges of the mesentery are then sutured to the parietal peritoneum, and the serosa of the colonic loop is sutured with fine absorbable suture materials to the peritoneum and fascia as well as the skin.
4. The colostomy may be sutured immediately. Some surgeons prefer to close the skin under a colostomy loop; others prefer to suture mucosa directly to skin edges. This decision may depend on the location of the colostomy. An important point is that each layer must be securely attached to the serosa of the colon to prevent evisceration and prolapse. The posterior wall of a loop colostomy may be divided by electrosurgery several days after surgery.

CORRECTION OF BILIARY ATRESIA
Hepatic portoenterostomy (Kasai procedure)

The Kasai procedure is the construction of a bile drainage system by utilizing an intestinal conduit. Biliary atresia is a disease that results from nonpatent extrahepatic bile ducts that prevent the drainage of bile from the liver and lead to eventual cirrhosis. The Kasai procedure recreates a drainage system using a limb of intestine. This procedure is indicated in patients with extrahepatic biliary atresia who are under 3 months of age. All atretic segments of the existing bile ducts are removed. An operative cholangiogram and frozen section biopsy of the hepatic duct remnant are prerequisites to the actual procedure.

Procedural considerations. The infant is positioned supine over an x-ray plate. Both a major instrument set and intestinal instruments are required, with the addition of the following:

3-way stopcock	Ligaclips
6 Syringes, 1 each	Umbilical tape
3 ml, 6 ml, 12 ml,	Mineral oil
and 3 TB	Jelco catheters, 18 and
Injectable saline	20 gauge
Hypaque dye (mix half	Sterile light handles or
dye, half saline)	light handle covers
Foley catheter and	Sterile specimen cup
urimeter	Taut cholangiogram
Petri dishes	catheter

Have available:

Deaver retractors	Bowel clamps
Kitner or Cherry dissec-	Headlight
tors	Drain
Carmalt hemostats	Malecot catheter
Kocher forceps	Tru-cut biopsy needle

Operative procedure

1. A right upper quadrant incision is made and the gallbladder is identified.

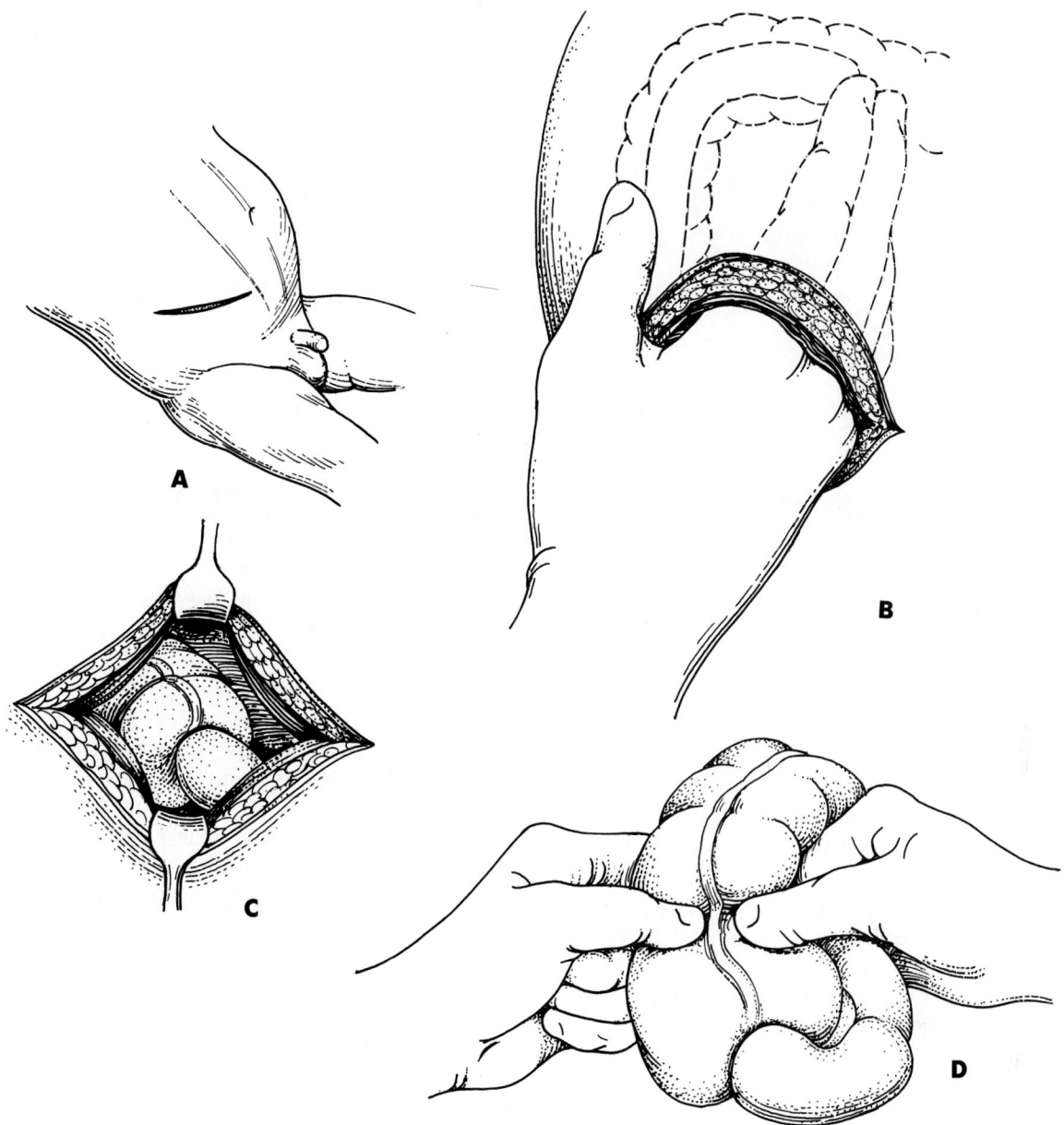

FIG. 28-10 Reduction of intussusception. **A,** Transverse abdominal incision. **B,** Location of intussusception. **C,** Mass delivered into incision. **D,** Milking reduction.
From Lewis, J.E. (1967). *Atlas of infant surgery.* St. Louis: Mosby.

2. A small catheter is placed into the gallbladder and secured with a purse-string suture. Radiopaque dye is instilled into the gallbladder, and an x-ray film is taken. The surgeon notes free flow of bile through the ducts and the duodenum. Occasionally free flow of bile will be seen. These patients are then categorized as having correctable biliary atresia. In such situations a liver biopsy is performed, and the incision is closed. The majority of patients with correctable biliary atresia demonstrate progressive improvement. More commonly, though, there is a very small amount of flow or none at all. In these cases of noncorrectable biliary atresia the Kasai procedure is performed.

3. Because of the high incidence of associated anomalies, a thorough inspection of the intraabdominal organs is then performed.

4. The hepaticoduodenal ligament is explored and all drainage structures are ligated (Fig. 28-11, *A*).

5. The hepatic duct remnant is identified and traced to the liver hilum. The remnant is transsected as high as possible, using frozen section biopsies as a guide. Frozen section biopsies are also obtained at the portahepatis to denote the presence of ductules. Precise identification of this location is essential (Fig. 28-11, *B*).

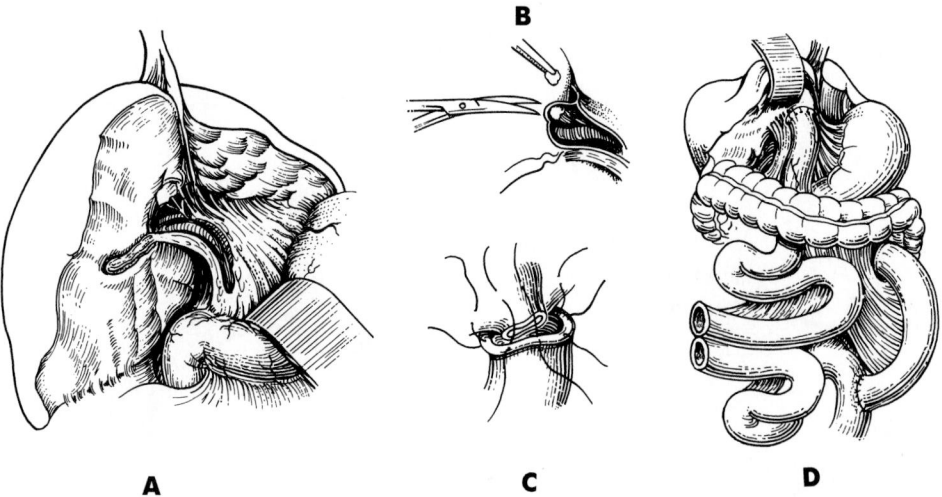

FIG. 28-11 Kasai procedure. **A,** Exploration of hepaticoduodenal ligament and ligation of drainage structures. **B,** Transsection of hepatic duct remnant using frozen section biopsies as a guide. **C,** Anastomosis of jejunal conduit at portahepatis. **D,** Exteriorization of conduit using double-barreled Roux-en-Y approach.

Reprinted with permission from Coran A.G., et al. (1978). *Surgery of the neonate.* Boston: Little, Brown.

6. The proximal jejunum is generally used as the intestinal conduit. A meticulous anastomosis is performed at the portahepatis as previously identified, using a single running layer of absorbable sutures (Fig. 28-11, *C*).
7. The conduit is exteriorized with a double-barreled Roux-en-Y approach (Fig. 28-11, *D*).
8. A liver biopsy is then performed.
9. A drain is placed, and the incision is closed in layers.

The procedure described above is one approach of many. Others include exteriorization of the jejunal conduit as a cutaneous jejunostomy and use of double Roux-en-Y loops, avoiding any need for an enterostomy.

RESECTION OF TUMORS

Nearly two thirds of childhood cancer occurs as solid malignancies. As is always the case, the therapy administered depends on the type of tumor. Examination and judicious investigation of all unusual masses are imperative. Thorough diagnostic workup and prompt definitive treatment may result in cure, even if the tumor is proved malignant. Chemotherapy and radiation therapy are adjuncts to surgical excision of tumors.

Wilms' tumor

Wilms' tumor, also known as nephroblastoma, is the most common intraabdominal childhood tumor. It presents as a painless mass whose enlargement may laterally distend the abdomen.

Procedural considerations. The child is positioned supine with a roll under the affected side. Both chest and abdomen are prepped. Infrequently, the tumor extends into the inferior vena cava as well as the atrium, and in such cases cardiopulmonary bypass should be readily available. Because of the possible need to clamp the inferior vena cava, lines are placed in the arms and neck. Clean gloves and instruments should be available for inspection of the contralateral kidney. Careful attention should be given when handling tumor and lymph nodes to avoid tumor spillage.

Operative procedure. If the tumor is operable, the following aspects are important:

1. The transabdominal approach, which may be extended to a combined transabdominal-transthoracic approach, is used to inspect abdominal contents and clamp the vessels of the renal pedicle before tumor dissection.
2. All suspicious lymph nodes are removed, placed in separate containers, and labeled. If no suspicious nodes are present, biopsy specimens are obtained of those in adjacent areas.
3. The opposite kidney is explored before dissection of the tumor.
4. The extent of the tumor can be marked with hemostatic clips to facilitate radiation therapy.
5. The entire primary tumor is removed if doing so does not place the patient in jeopardy.
6. Any residual tumor is marked with clips.
7. Due to its close proximity to the kidney, the adrenal gland is usually removed.
8. The abdominal cavity and viscera are thoroughly inspected for evidence of tumor extension or metastases. Extensive surgery may include partial colectomy or partial resection of the diaphragm.

Neuroblastoma

Neuroblastoma, one of the most common solid tumors of childhood, is a highly malignant tumor. It arises from neural crest tissue and can develop along any sympathetic ganglion chain, with the most common sites the retroperitoneum and adrenal medulla. The mass is usually firm, irregular, and nontender. It is a silent tumor in its early stages and metastasizes rapidly. Treatment includes an operation to ligate the tumor's blood supply and remove as much of the tumor as possible, as well as chemotherapy and radiation.

Sacrococcygeal teratoma

A sacrococcygeal teratoma is a tumor that originates early in embryonic cell division. The sacrococcygeal area is the most common extragonadal site of teratoma. The tumor presents as a large protuberance rising from the sacrococcygeal area. It may be irregular or symmetric, varies in size, and may be pedunculated.

A sacrococcygeal teratoma is usually resectable in the newborn but may undergo malignant changes if not removed early in life. Tumors resected in the newborn period show microscopic evidence of malignant cells, but surgical cures have been achieved. Early surgical resection is important because these tumors are not sensitive to irradiation and are only temporarily responsive to chemotherapy.

The tumor is in the area of the sacrum and coccyx but may extend into the pelvis or abdomen. Resection is usually feasible by placing the patient in the Kraske (jackknife) position and excising the tumor mass and coccyx en bloc (Fig. 28-12). Infrequently, in cases where the tumor extends high into the pelvis, an abdominal incision may also be required.

PROCEDURES REQUIRING COLOSTOMY

The following procedures require emergent colostomy at the time of presentation. Definitive repair of the anomaly usually occurs at about 1 year of age.

Resection and pull-through for Hirschsprung's disease

Resection and pull-through for Hirschsprung's disease, the definitive surgical procedure, consists of the removal of the aganglionic portion of the bowel and anastomosis of the normal colon to the anus. Hirschsprung's disease is characterized by the absence of ganglion cells in a distal portion of the bowel. The distal colon is more frequently involved, but the disease may encompass the entire colon, with a less favorable prognosis. The absence of ganglion cells results in a lack of peristalsis. The normal proximal colon becomes dilated, and intestinal contents do not pass through the involved segment. The child presents with an abnormally distended abdomen. On barium enema proximal distention of the colon is seen, then a transition zone where the bowel appears funnel shaped, followed by the distal aganglionic segment, which is narrowed. The child

is taken to the operating room for a leveling colostomy. Multiple frozen section biopsies of specimens from the muscularis of the proximal colon are done to determine the presence of ganglion cells. The colostomy is performed at the most distal portion of the colon that contains ganglion cells. Some surgeons prefer a routine right transverse colostomy at this time and delay frozen section biopsies until the time of the definitive procedure. The child is returned to the operating room for definitive repair at 1 year of age, if clinical and nutritional status permits.

Several surgical techniques have been devised. Soave's procedure of endorectal pull-through employs internal bypass of the involved segment. The internal sphincter muscle of the anus is kept intact for continence.

Procedural considerations. The patient is prepped and draped from the nipples down to and including the buttocks, genitals, perineal area, and upper thighs to permit positioning for the perineal stage without redraping. (Before preparation, the rectum may be irrigated with warm saline solution.)

A folded towel is placed under the buttocks. The patient is placed in the supine position with knees bent and legs in a modified ski position (hips and knees flexed) to facilitate abdominal and perineal approaches without redraping. An indwelling catheter is inserted to keep the bladder empty during the operation. The major instrument set, extra towels and gloves, as well as the following are required:

Foley catheter (check size) and urimeter	On second Mayo:
Kitner dissectors (30-60)	Minor set
	6 extra curved mosquito clamps
Small Kocher forceps	Small needle pad
Medium Kocher forceps	2 Tonsil hemostats
2 Syringes, 3 ml	Penrose drain, ¼ inch
1 Syringe, 5 ml	Sterile safety pins
Needle, 25 gauge	Electrosurgical pencil, hand controlled
Injectable saline	Suction
Penrose drain, ¼ inch	Muscle and nerve stimulator
Sterile safety pins	
Large rakes (dull)	
3 Small tonsil suction tubes	
Hegar dilators	

Have available:

Deaver retractors	Salem sump
Long instruments	K-Y Jelly
Gastrointestinal stapling device (GIA)	Red rubber catheter (22 to 24 Fr)
Ligaclips	Mineral oil
Extra no. 15 blades	

Operative procedure

1. A left paramedian incision that includes the sigmoid colonic stoma, if present, is made.
2. The stoma is freed from the abdominal wall, and the left colon is mobilized. (If there is no sigmoid colonic

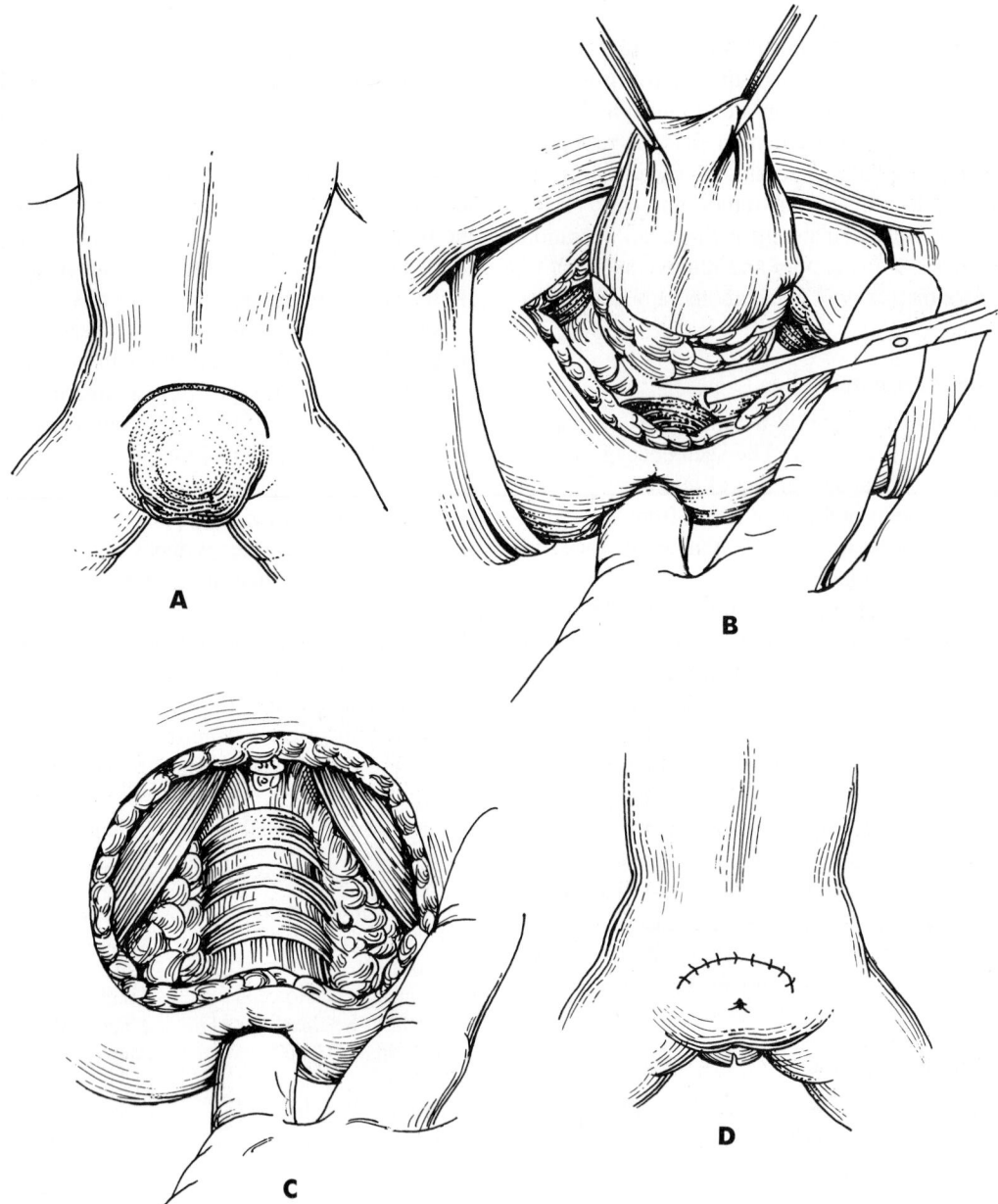

FIG. 28-12   Excision of sacrococcygeal teratoma. **A,** U-shaped incision. **B,** Dissection of teratoma. **C,** Tumor excised while rectum remains intact. **D,** Closed incisional line.

From Lewis, J.E. (1967). *Atlas of infant surgery.* St. Louis: Mosby.

stoma, the extent of aganglionic intestine is established by biopsy and frozen section, and all involved colon is excised. If a stoma is present and the area has already been established as normal, the colon above it constitutes the proximal end of the resection.)

3. The mesocolon and the vessels of the intestine to be resected are divided close to the intestine, with care taken to preserve the blood supply to the rectum (Fig. 28-13, *A*).

4. The mucosal tube is freed from the outer muscular layers by sharp and blunt dissection with Metzenbaum scissors and a gauze-tipped instrument (Fig. 28-13, *B*).

5. A muscular sleeve is transsected, and traction sutures of no. 4-0 nonabsorbable are placed on the distal edge (Fig. 28-13, *C*). The mucosa is stripped down to the anus. The depth of the dissection may be checked by inserting a finger in the anus (Fig. 28-13, *D*).

6. When the mucosa is adequately freed, the perineal phase is started, and the perineal instrument table is used.

7. The anus is dilated and retracted with Allis forceps. A circumferential incision is made, and the mucosal stripping is completed (Fig. 28-13, *E*).

8. The proximal portion of the intestine is pulled through

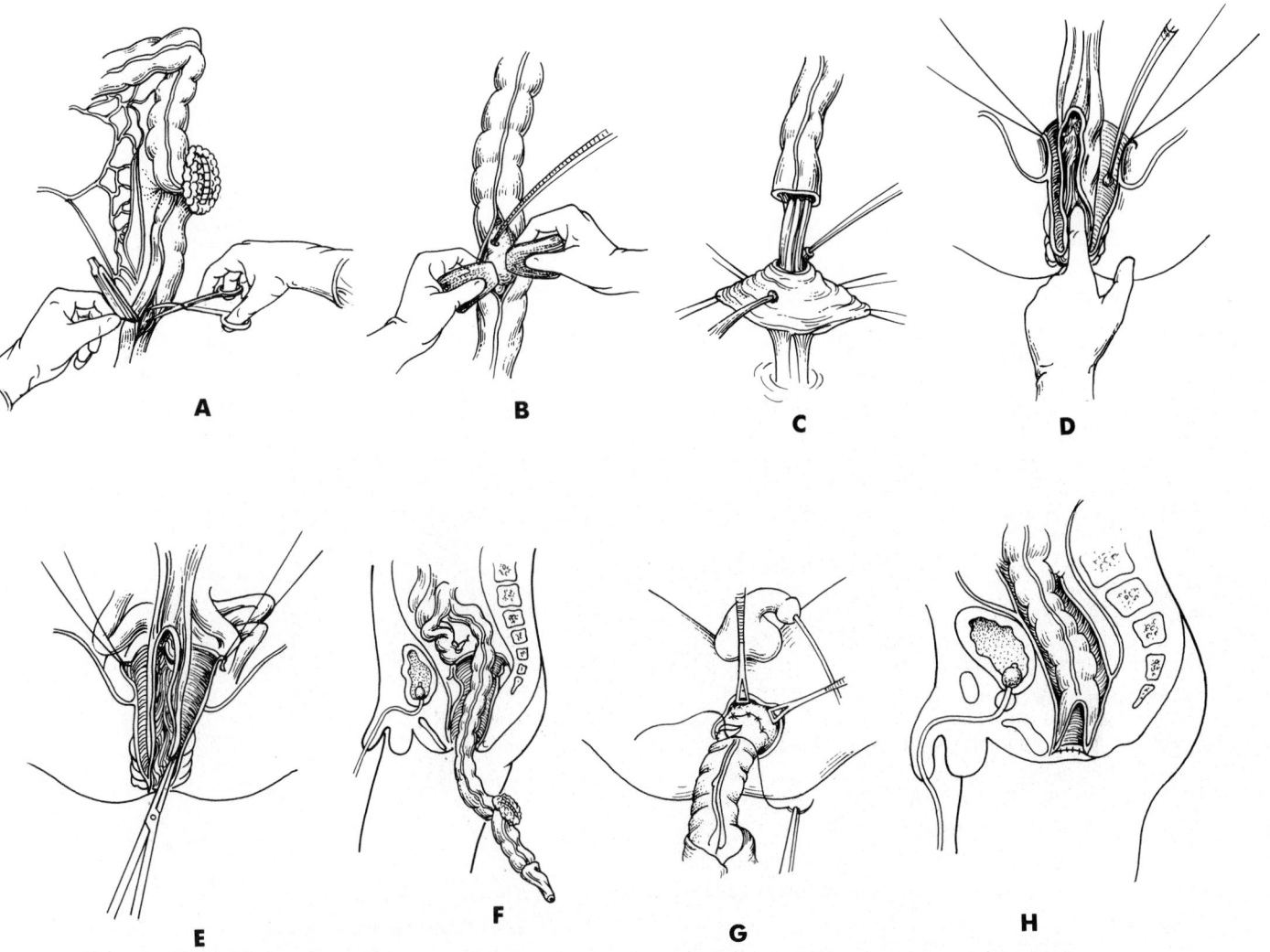

FIG. 28-13   Pull-through for Hirschsprung's disease. **A,** Dissection of mucosal tube begun through longitudinal incision. **B,** Gauze-tipped dissecting instrument used to dissect entire circumference of tube. **C,** Muscular sleeve transsected. **D,** Depth of dissection determined by inserting finger in anus. **E,** Circumferential incision made. **F,** Mucosal tube and proximal portion of colon and stoma pulled through rectal muscular cuff. **G,** Anastomosis performed between all layers of colon and anal mucosa. **H,** Anastomosis completed.

Modified from Boley, S.J. (1968). An endorectal pull-through operation with primary anastomosis for Hirschsprung's disease. *Surgery, Gynecology and Obstetrics, 127*:(2), 353. By permission of *Surgery, Gynecology, and Obstetrics.*

the rectal muscular sleeve and out the anus (Fig. 28-13, *F*). If the portion of colon to be resected is large, it is excised abdominally before the proximal portion of the intestine is pulled through the anus.

9. Absorbable sutures are used to secure the seromuscular layers of the intussuscepted colon to the rectal muscular cuff. The colon is divided into axial or longitudinal quadrants, and an anastomosis is performed with no. 3-0 absorbable sutures (Fig. 28-13, *G*).

10. Gowns and gloves are changed, and abdominal instruments are used. The abdominal phase of the operation is completed by approximating the proximal edge of

the muscular cuff to the seromuscular layer of the colon with nonabsorbable no. 4-0 sutures (Fig. 28-13, *H*). The abdomen is closed in the routine manner, without the use of drains.

REPAIR OF ANORECTAL MALFORMATION
Repair of imperforate anus

An imperforate anus is repaired by establishing colorectoanal continuity through the external anal sphincter and closure of fistulas, if present. Imperforate anus presents in a variety of forms classified as low, intermediate, and high lesions. Girls commonly have low lesions, and boys primarily exhibit high lesions. A covered anus and anovulvar fistula is an example of a low lesion. A high lesion consists of a blind rectal pouch, a "flat bottom," and a posterior urethral fistula or fistula to the bladder. This type is the most prevalent and the most difficult to repair.

Repair of low imperforate anus in a girl: anal transposition

Procedural considerations. The infant is placed in the lithotomy position with the legs extended on skis. A Foley catheter is inserted, and the perineum is prepped and draped. The major instrument set is required, with the addition of the following:

Extra towels	Kitner dissectors
Needle-point electrosurgical tip	Penrose drain, ½ inch
Suction	Sterile rubber bands with small brass
Nasal speculums	safety pins
Small tonsil suction tube	K-Y Jelly
Senn retractors	Hegar dilators
Foley catheter (check size) and urimeter	Vaseline gauze
	Nerve stimulator

Operative procedure

1. An electrical stimulator is applied to define the center of the true anus.
2. Stay sutures are placed in the fistula, and it is excised using an oval incision (Fig. 28-14, *A*).
3. The bowel is dissected free from surrounding structures, with care taken not to damage the vagina (Fig. 28-14, *B*).
4. When the dissection is complete, a vertical midline incision is performed at the opening of the true anus, and the fibers of the external sphincter are identified (Fig. 28-14, *C*).
5. The mobilized rectum is pulled down through the subcutaneous tissue to its new location.
6. The end of the fistula is amputated. With interrupted sutures of 4-0 nonabsorbable, the external sphincter is sutured to the rectal serosa.
7. Using 4-0 absorbable suture, a new anus is constructed with interrupted sutures through all layers (Fig. 28-14, *D*).
8. A drain may or may not be placed in the anterior incision before it is closed in layers with interrupted 4-0 absorbable sutures.
9. A Hegar dilator is used to calibrate the size of the new anus after closure.

Repair of high imperforate anus: the posterior sagittal anorectoplasty

When a high imperforate anal anomaly presents, surgical intervention is indicated within 24 to 48 hours of life. A transverse or sigmoid colostomy is performed to irrigate

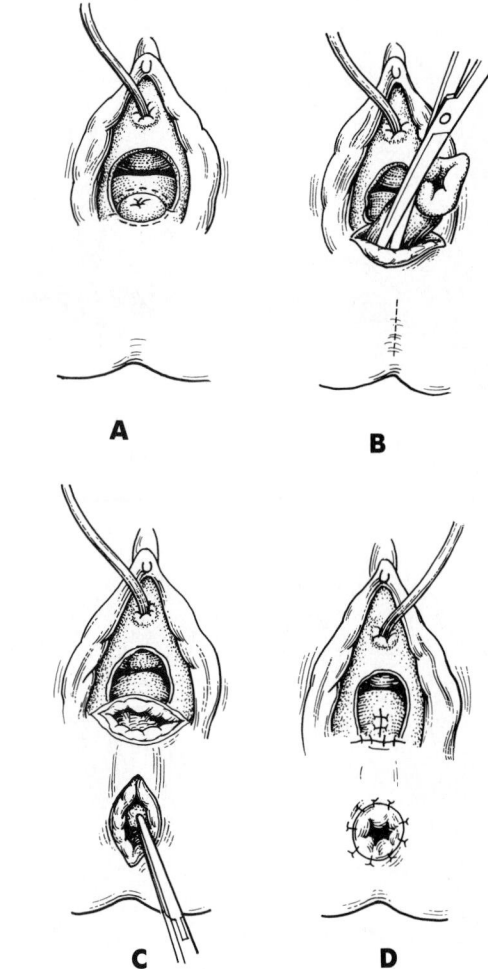

FIG. 28-14   Anal transposition. **A,** Fistula excised using oval incision. **B,** Dissection of bowel from surrounding structures. **C,** Vertical midline incision at site of true anus; identification of external sphincter fibers; mobilized rectum pulled down through subcutaneous tissue to new location. **D,** External sphincter sutured to rectal mucosa; new anus constructed with interrupted sutures through all layers.

Reprinted with permission from Coran, A.G., et al. (1978) *Surgery of the neonate.* Boston: Little, Brown.

the hiatal lumen and to remove meconium plugs while allowing proximal colon function. After the colostomy, further diagnostic studies, such as cystogram and vaginograms are done. The posterior sagittal anorectoplasty (PSARP) is the definitive surgical procedure and is performed when the condition and size of the child permits, usually around 1 year of age.

The PSARP is a highly technical procedure that utilizes electrostimulation throughout and may require position changes (Fig. 28-15).

Procedural considerations. The child is placed in a prone jackknife position with the hips flexed. Adequate padding must be placed under the hips to avoid compres-

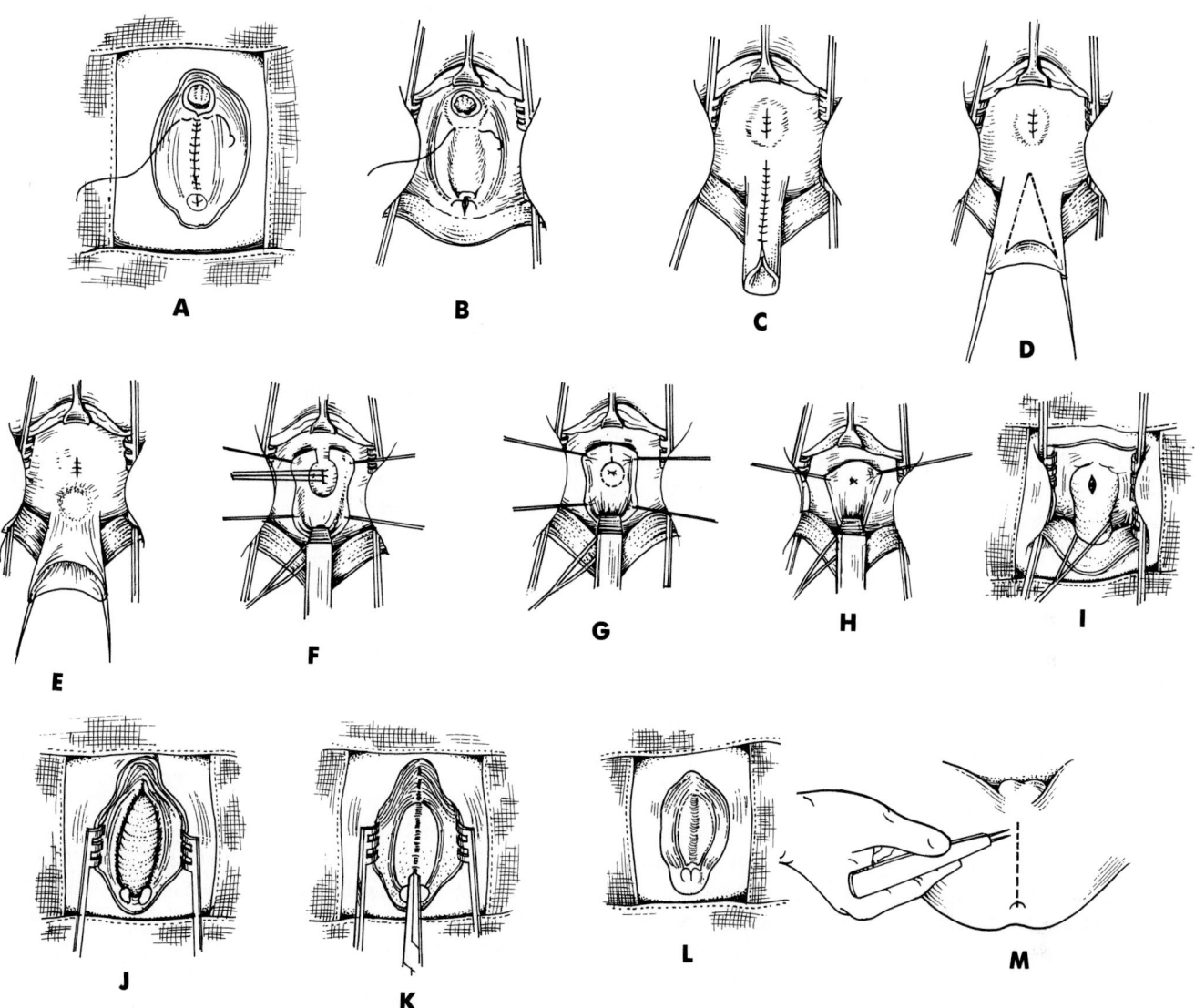

FIG. 28-15 Posterior sagittal anorectoplasty. **A,** Line of incision and electrical stimulation to determine appropriate anal site. **B,** Midsagittal incision through coccyx and external sphincter fibers of anus,
showing striated muscle complex deep to anal site; subcutaneous external sphincter extending about halfway to coccyx; superficial external sphincter inserting on coccyx; levator deeper in midline. **C,** Right-
angled forceps beneath levator ani. **D,** All layers of striated muscle partially retracted laterally exposing
visceral endopelvic fascia. **E,** Sagittal incision in terminal bowel after proximal dissection around rectum
and placement of tape around rectum proximally. **F,** Retracted rectotomy showing fistula site. **G,**
Hemicircumferential incision through mucosa-submucosa for placement of first sutures to close fistula.
H, Completed closure of fistula orifice. **I,** Stippled area where muscular bowel wall is left in place and
clear area above where peritoneum may be encountered. **J,** Extent of anterior wedge resection for tapered repair of rectum *(dotted line).* **K,** Approximation of tapered edges of rectum. **L,** First and deepest
suture for approximation of levators to establish beginning of canal. **M,** After reapproximation of levator
ani to coccyx, interrupted sutures are placed in edges of superficial external sphincter muscle.

From de Vries, P.A. (1984). Posterior sagittal anorectoplasty. In S. Holmann v. Kap-herr (editor), *Anorektale Fehl-
bildungen.* Stuttgart: Gustav Fischer Verlag. Reprinted with permission.

sion injury to the femoral nerves. The major instrument set is required with the addition of the following:

Foley catheter (check size) and urimeter	Mastoid retractors
Catheter tray (disposable)	Senn retractors
Muscle stimulator and probe	Stevens tenotomy scissors
Needle-point electrosurgical tip	Orthopedic saw, instruments
Feeding tubes, 5 Fr and 8 Fr	Marking pen
	Hegar dilators
	K-Y Jelly

Operative procedure

1. The electrostimulator is used to locate the true anus, and a midsagittal incision is made through the skin from the midsacrum to the anterior border of the anal site.
2. Dissection continues through subcutaneous tissue until the external sphincter muscle layers are identified.
3. With electrostimulation, these fibers are dissected midsagittally, exactly in the midline.
4. A midsagittal split of the coccyx is performed, and the striated muscle complex found beneath the coccyx is incised sagittally along with the visceral endopelvic fascia. Electrostimulation is used to aid in identifying muscle complexes.
5. Next the rectal pouch and urethra are identified, and the bowel is incised vertically to expose the fistula.
6. The fistula is closed in layers, first the mucosa with interrupted absorbable sutures and then the muscle layer with 5-0 nonabsorbable sutures.
7. The rectum is then mobilized and tapered to allow its placement within the muscle complexes. Tapering consists of excising a wedge of bowel from either the ventral or dorsal surface. The edges are approximated and the mucosal layer closed with 5-0 absorbable interrupted sutures. The muscularis layer is closed with interrupted 5-0 nonabsorbable sutures.
8. Again using electrostimulation, the tapered rectum is placed deep within the muscle complex. Then 5-0 nonabsorbable sutures are used to reconstruct the muscles. The seromuscular layer of the bowel is incorporated into these sutures to keep it securely positioned within the muscle complex.
9. The external sphincter muscles and coccyx are reapproximated.
10. Excess bowel is trimmed before securing it to the skin edges of the anus.
11. Running absorbable subcuticular sutures are used to close the skin.

In cases of very high rectal pouches and fistulas, an abdominal approach may be required. At this point, after the midsagittal incisions and dissections are completed, a rubber tube is placed through the pelvis with one end in the peri-

---

┌─────────────────────────────────────┐
BOX 28-2

Congenital Heart Disease Classifications*

ACYANOTIC DEFECTS
Atrial septal defect (ASD)
Ventricular septal defect (VSD)
Patent ductus arteriosus (PDA)
Atrioventricular canal (AV canal)
Aortic stenosis (AS)
Pulmonary stenosis (PS)
Coarctation of the aorta
Mitral stenosis (MS)

CYANOTIC DEFECTS
Tetrology of Fallot (TOF)
Pulmonary atresia with intact ventricular septum (PA with IVS)
Tricuspid atresia
Interrupted aortic arch (IAA)
Truncus arteriosus
Total anomalous pulmonary venous return (TAPVR)
Hypoplastic left heart syndrome (HLHS)
Transposition of the great arteries (TGA)
Double outlet right ventricle (DORV)

*Congenital heart disease is often classified according to acyanotic or cyanotic hemodynamics. In general, acyanotic lesions involve increased pulmonary blood flow or obstruction to blood flow from the ventricles. The cyanotic lesions involve decreased pulmonary blood flow or mixed blood flow.
└─────────────────────────────────────┘

toneal cavity and the other through the center of the anus to the skin, where it is temporarily sutured. The child is turned supine, and an abdominal incision is performed. The rectal pouch is mobilized and the fistula closed. The bowel is tapered as described previously, and the terminal portion is attached to the rubber tube, which then is used to pull the rectum through the anal orifice. The bowel is sutured to the muscle complex, and reapproximation of the coccyx and external sphincter muscle is done as described earlier.

SURGERY FOR CONGENITAL HEART DISEASE

Congenital cardiac abnormalities occur in 1% to 2% of live-born infants and are differentiated on the basis of whether they are cyanotic or acyanotic lesions (Box 28-2). The cyanosis-producing abnormalities carry a graver prognosis. Cyanosis is present because of a failure of delivery of pulmonary venous return to the systemic circulation (for example, transposition of the great vessels) or reduction in the volume of pulmonary blood flow (for example, tetralogy of Fallot and tricuspid atresia). The degree of cyanosis is affected by the amount of pulmonary blood flow or the extent of intracardiac mixing of blood through a shunt.

Among the acyanotic group are the obstructive lesions (for example, aortic or pulmonary stenosis and coarctation of the aorta) that place an extra burden on the associated

TABLE 28-2

Distribution of Selected Congenital Heart Defects and Association with Other Conditions

Defect	Percentage of specific defects*	Disorders associated with increased incidence of defect†
Ventricular septal defect	32.1%	Down syndrome Holt-Oram syndrome Fetal alcohol syndrome
Transposition of great arteries	2.6%	Diabetes or prediabetes in mother
Tetralogy of Fallot	3.8%	Down syndrome Fetal alcohol syndrome
Coarctation of aorta	6.7%	Turner syndrome Apert syndrome
Patent ductus arteriosus	8.3%	Rubella syndrome Down syndrome
Hypoplastic left heart syndrome	3.1%	—
Atrioventricular valve defect	3.6%	Down syndrome
Pulmonic stenosis	8.6%	Rubella syndrome Noonan syndrome
Atrial septal defect	7.4%	Noonan syndrome Holt-Oram syndrome Down syndrome Fetal alcohol syndrome
Aortic stenosis	3.8%	Turner syndrome
Truncus arteriosus	1.7%	—

*U.S. multicenter data. From Hoffman, J.I. (1990). Congenital heart disease: Incidence and inheritance. *Pediatric Clinics of North America, 37*(1),31.
†Data from Noonan, J.A. (1978). Association of congenital heart disease with syndromes or other defects. *Pediatric Clinics of North America, 25*(4),797.

ventricle and can lead to heart failure. (Cyanosis may be apparent if the lesion is severe.) Shunt lesions (such as patent ductus arteriosus, ventricular septal defect, and atrial septal defect) increase pulmonary blood flow. If a large shunt is present, congestive heart failure can ensue. Table 28-2 reviews the incidence of common cardiac anomalies and disorders that may be associated with the defect.

Palliative procedures (described later) attempt to increase or decrease pulmonary blood flow or to increase intracardiac mixing of blood.

Repair of atrial septal defect

Congenital defects in the atrial septum are closed, under direct vision, by a simple suture technique or by inserting a synthetic prosthetic patch or pericardial patch. An atrial septal defect (ASD) is a common congenital abnormality, and its classification is based on anatomic location and associated abnormalities (Fig. 28-16).

The ostium secundum defect is located in the superior and central portion of the septum. The ostium primum defect is in the lower portion of the atrial septum and is associated with other defects in the atrioventricular canal,

usually with a cleft of the mitral valve or occasionally of the tricuspid valve. An accompanying ventricular septal defect may also be present. The sinus venosum defect is located at the atriocaval junction and is associated with partial anomalous pulmonary venous return.

An ASD results in a left-to-right atrial shunt that may be well tolerated in early life if the opening is small. However, if the defect is large or of the ostium primum type, with a marked shunting of blood, the workload of the right side of the heart is increased. The right side of the heart and the pulmonary artery and its branches become enlarged. The vascularity of the lung field is increased, with resulting pulmonary hypertension and subsequent failure of the right side of the heart. At this point the shunt may reverse (Fig. 28-17). In early life the patient may be asymptomatic. The initial symptoms may include fatigue, retardation of normal weight gain, and increased susceptibility to respiratory infections. Later symptoms include those of failure of the right side of the heart and cyanosis with a reverse shunt. A systolic murmur is heard with greatest intensity over the base of the heart.

Procedural considerations. The child is placed in the

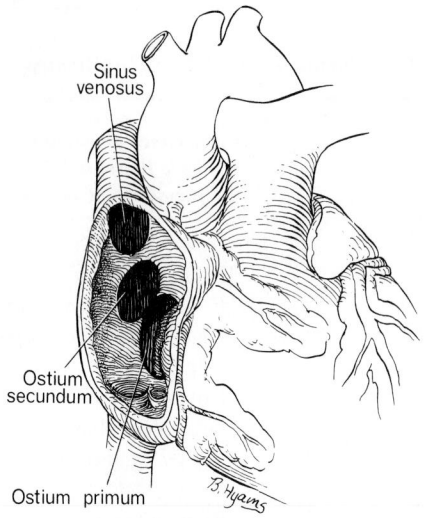

FIG. 28-16   Atrial septal defects are common congenital anomalies occurring in the sinus venosus, ostium secundum, and ostium primum.

From Cooley, D.A., & Norman, J.C. (1975). *Techniques in cardiac surgery*. Houston: Texas Medical Press.

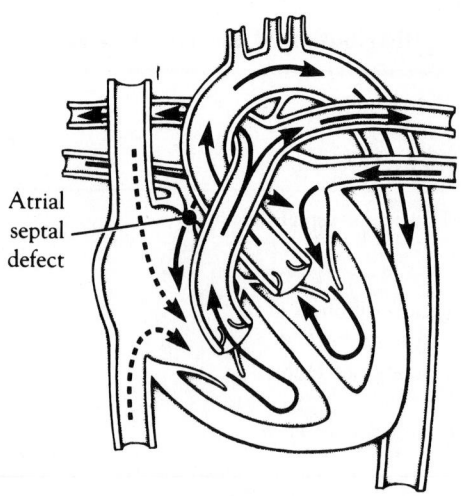

FIG. 28-17   Atrial septal defect.

From Whaley, L.F., & Wong, D.L. (1991). *Nursing care of infants and children* (4th ed.). St. Louis: Mosby.

supine position for a median sternotomy or in a right anterior oblique position for an anterolateral thoracotomy. The instrument setup is as described for basic open heart surgery (see Chapter 26), with consideration given to the age and size of the child, plus intracardiac patch material, 2 × 2 inches or larger.

Operative procedure (Fig. 28-18)

1. A median sternotomy incision is made, and cardiopulmonary bypass is begun as described. (Infrequently, a right anterolateral incision is performed.) There are a number of bypass strategies that can be employed. With bicaval cannulation the child remains on bypass during the repair and blood is directed away from the right atrium through cannulas in the superior and inferior venae cavae. However, in this method the cannulas may obstruct the view of the ASD. With single venous cannulation a cannula is placed in the right atrium and the child remains on bypass during the repair. With this technique the venous line is clamped immediately before the right atrium is incised and pump suctions are placed in the inferior and superior venae cavae during ASD closure. Deep hypothermic circulatory arrest is usually used in more complicated repairs, such as primum ASD or sinus venosum defects associated with anomalous pulmonary venous return.

2. The right atrium is incised and the pathologic defect determined.

3. The defect is closed with a continuous suture, or a patch of pericardium or prosthetic material may be used. By filling the atrium with blood before the atriotomy is completely closed, the surgeon can express air from the atrium. For the ostium primum defect with a cleft mi-

tral valve, repair of the cleft is accomplished by approximation, using interrupted sutures.

Repair of a ventricular septal defect

Under direct vision a congenital defect in the ventricular septum (Fig. 28-19) is closed by a simple suture technique or, in most instances, by inserting a synthetic prosthetic or pericardial patch. One of the most common congenital cardiac anomalies, a ventricular septal defect (VSD) is of little physiologic importance if small. A murmur is evident, but the patient is otherwise asymptomatic, and the heart size is normal. Larger defects with a significant left-to-right shunt, high right ventricular pressure, increased pulmonary blood flow, and enlarged heart are repaired by surgery (Fig. 28-20). If left uncorrected, pulmonary volume overload results in pulmonary hypertension with subsequent reversal of the shunt to right-to-left and in cyanosis.

Operative procedure (Fig. 28-21)

1. A median sternotomy is performed, and cardiopulmonary bypass is begun as described.

2. The location of the defect determines the location of the incision. For membranous and canal defects, an incision is usually made in the right atrium, the atrium is retracted, and the VSD is identified using a pump suction through the tricuspid valve into the right ventricle. For supracrystal VSDs an incision is usually made in the pulmonary artery and may be extended into the right ventricle. A muscular VSD may require an incision in the apex of the heart.

3. A patch is used to close the defect. A continuous 6-0 or 5-0 nonabsorbable suture on a small needle may be used,

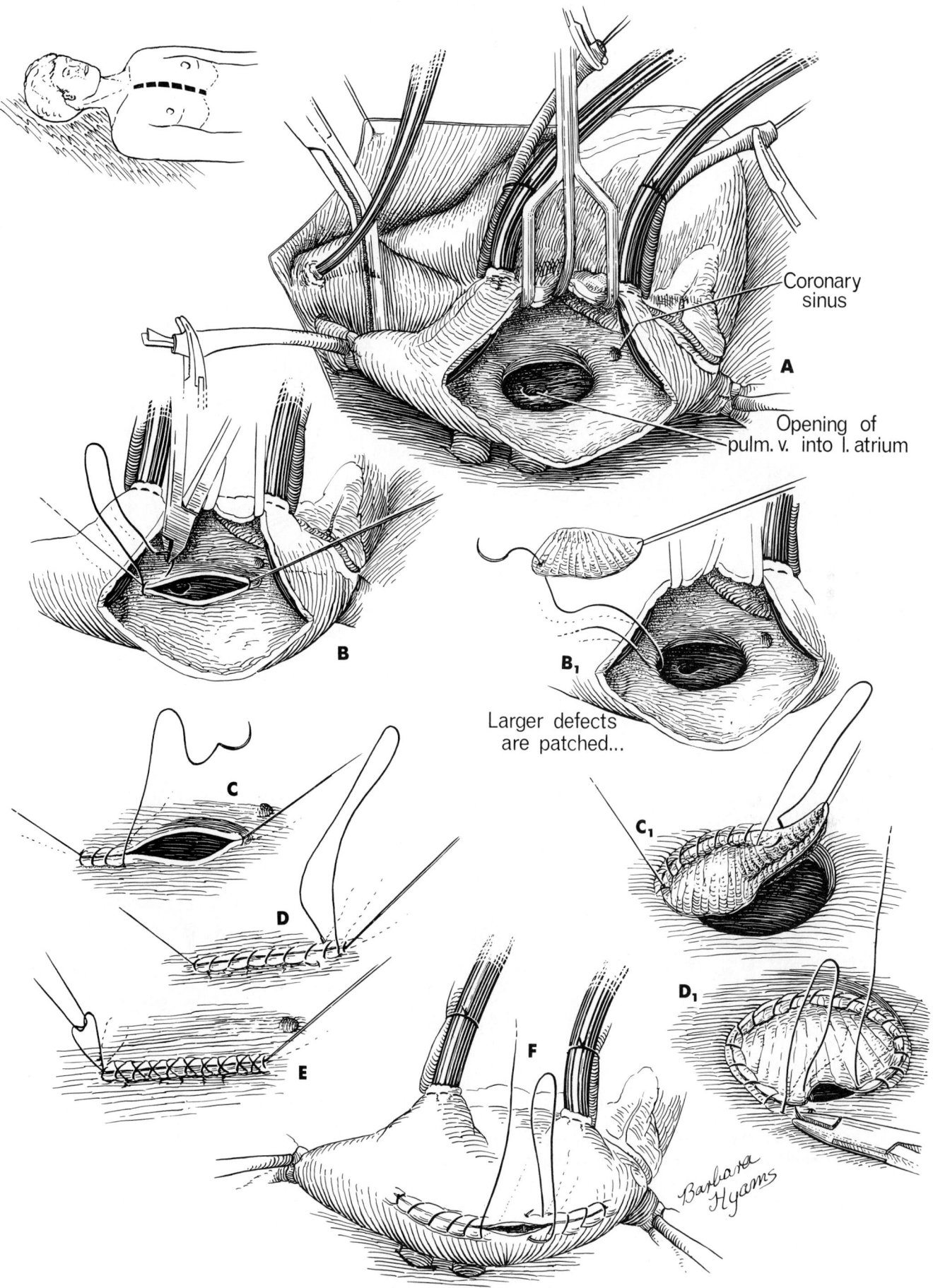

Coronary
sinus

A

Opening of
pulm. v. into l. atrium

B

B₁

Larger defects
are patched...

C

D

C₁

E

D₁

F

Barbara
Hyams

FIG. 28-18   Repair of ostium secundum defect. Patch closures *(B₁ through D₁)* are done for larger defects.

From Cooley, D.A., & Norman, J.C. (1975). *Techniques in cardiac surgery*. Houston: Texas Medical Press.

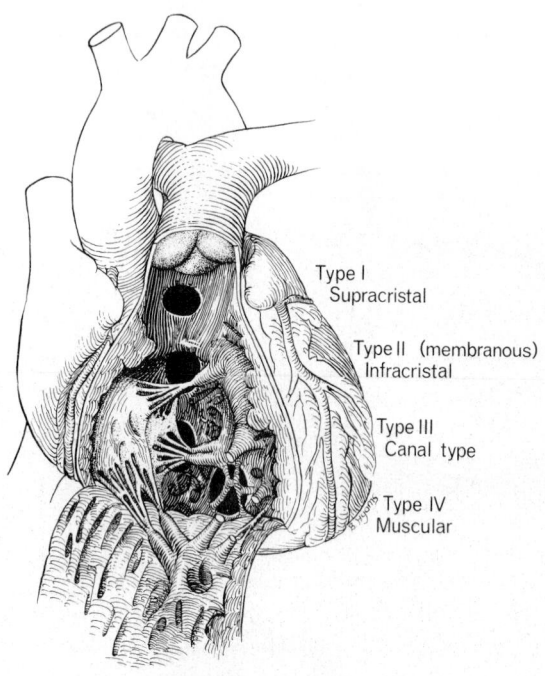

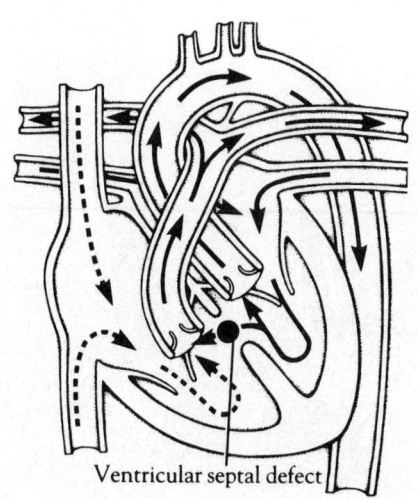

FIG. 28-19 Ventricular septal defects: anatomic classification.

From Cooley, D.A., & Norman, J.C. (1975). *Techniques in cardiac surgery*. Houston: Texas Medical Press.

FIG. 28-20 Ventricular septal defect.

From Whaley, L.F., & Wong, D.L. (1991). *Nursing care of infants and children* (4th ed.). St. Louis: Mosby.

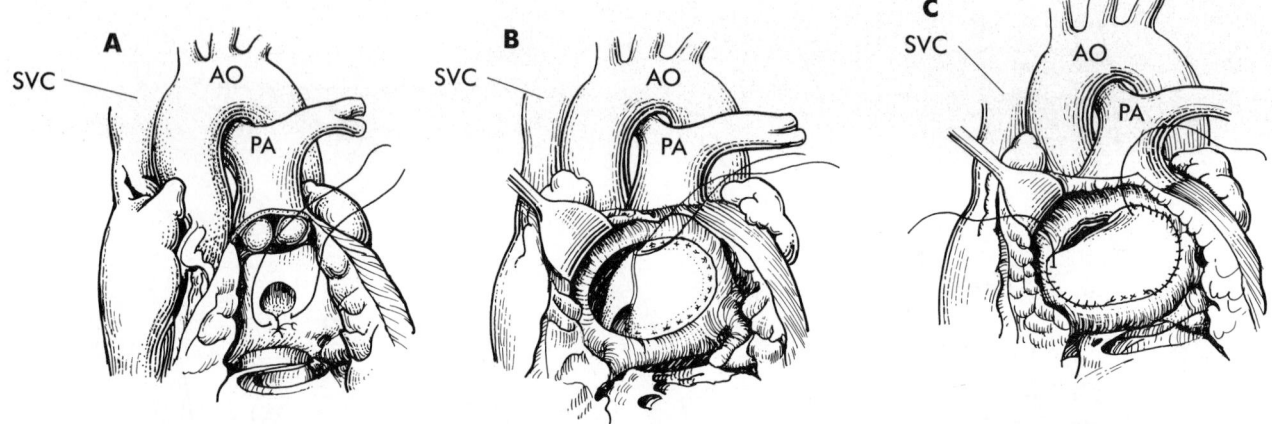

FIG. 28-21 Techniques for closing ventricular septal defects. **A,** Simple interrupted suture may be used if defect is small and has fibrous margins. **B,** Patch closure of ventricular septal defect with interrupted mattress sutures. **C,** Patch closure of ventricular septal defect using interrupted sutures at bottom of defect and continuous suturing technique for remainder of defect.

From Effler, D.B. (1978). *Blades' surgical diseases of the chest* (4th ed.). St. Louis: Mosby.

or an interrupted suture with or without pledgets, to place the patch. Rarely is the defect closed primarily.

4. Cardiopulmonary bypass is discontinued, and the sternum is closed.

Correction of tetralogy of Fallot

Tetralogy of Fallot is the most common congenital cardiac anomaly in the cyanotic group. Cyanosis, as seen in the superficial vessels of the skin, is the result of shunting unoxygenated blood into the systemic circulation. The essential features of this condition are pulmonary stenosis, high ventricular septal defect, and overriding of the septal defect by the aorta, with resulting hypertrophy of the right ventricle—all of which may be subdivided into more complex variations (Fig. 28-22). The infundibular form of pulmonary stenosis is a long, localized constricture in the pulmonary outflow tract of the right ventricle. It is the most common type of this anomaly. Valvular stenosis and infundibular stenosis, however, may occur independently.

In tetralogy of Fallot blood flow into the lungs decreases as a result of pulmonary obstruction, and a right-to-left shunt of venous blood from the right ventricle to the left ventricle and aorta occurs. Symptoms of tetralogy are cyanosis, dyspnea, episodes of acute dyspnea with cyanosis, retarded growth, clubbing of extremities, and reduced exercise tolerance. A systolic murmur and secondary polycythemia are usually present. Cardiac catheterization and angiocardiography aid in determining the diagnosis and plan of surgical treatment.

The selection of a palliative or corrective procedure is based on the age and general condition of the patient and the severity of the pulmonary stenosis. The treatment of choice is primary repair; contraindications for primary repair include anomalous origin of the anterior descending coronary artery and presence of pulmonary atresia.

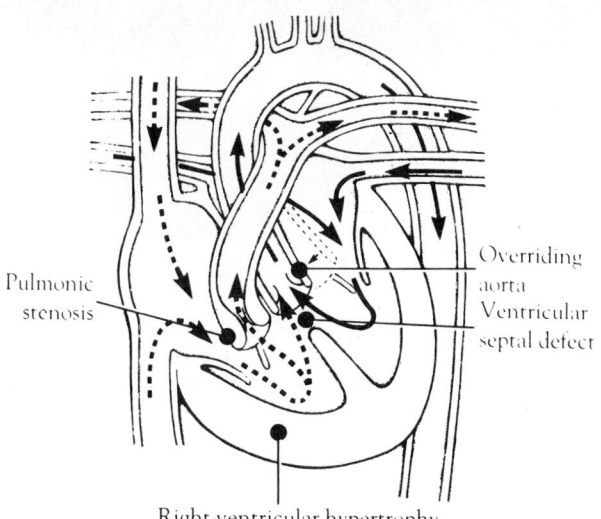

FIG. 28-22 Tetralogy of Fallot.
From Whaley, L.F., & Wong, D.L. (1991). *Nursing care of infants and children* (4th ed.). St. Louis: Mosby.

Open corrective repair

The open corrective repair is done under direct vision and is the complete repair of the infundibular stenosis or pulmonary valve stenosis and closure of the VSD.

Procedural considerations. The child is placed on the OR bed in a supine position. The setup is as described for open heart surgery, with consideration given to the child's age and size. Additional items to be added to the basic open heart setup include the following:

1 Intracardiac patch, 2 × 2 inches
1 Outflow cardiac patch, 2 × 2 inches
1 Felt patch, 4 × 4 inches

Operative procedure

1. A median sternotomy is performed, and cardiopulmonary bypass with hypothermia is begun as described.
2. A vertical ventriculotomy over the infundibular area is performed (Fig. 28-23).
3. The ventricular septal defect is identified. Closure requires an intracardiac patch in almost all instances. This can be of a synthetic material or a piece of pericardium.
4. Interrupted or continuous cardiovascular sutures are placed in the septum with caution because of the danger of suturing a branch of the neuroconductive system.
5. The hypertrophied infundibular muscle is excised, as completely as possible, from the right ventricular outflow tract. If the pulmonic valve is stenosed, the fused commissures are incised.
6. An estimate is made about whether the right ventricle can be closed primarily or whether a patch is necessary. If the pulmonic stenosis cannot be relieved adequately by valvulotomy and infundibulectomy, an outflow patch of synthetic material or pulmonary homograft tissue may be needed to enlarge the outflow tract. If the pulmonary artery or valve annulus is quite small, it may be necessary to extend the patch across the valve ring to the proximal portion of the pulmonary artery.
7. Cardiopulmonary bypass is discontinued, and the sternum is closed.

Operation for tricuspid atresia

Absence of communication between the right atrium and right ventricle is always accompanied by a second defect, an ASD, or a patent foramen ovale. Other abnormalities are also present in tricuspid atresia (Fig. 28-24). The infant displays cyanosis, periods of dyspnea, easy fatigability, and growth retardation. Congestive failure progresses rapidly.

Palliative operations consist of the Blalock-Hanlon procedure (see Fig. 28-39, *C*), which enlarges the ASD, or anastomotic procedures for shunting the circulation to relieve the cyanosis, including the Blalock-Taussig, Potts-Smith, and Glenn procedures, described later. Alternatively, a Fontan procedure may be performed, described later in this chapter.

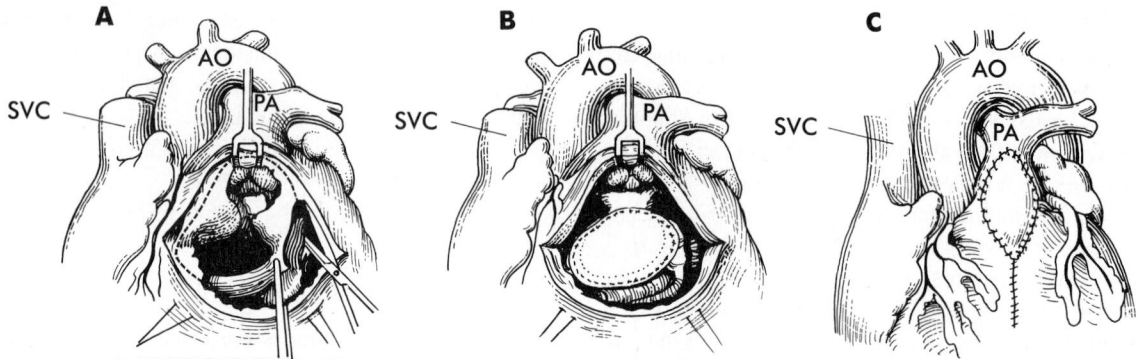

FIG. 28-23 Operation for correction of tetralogy of Fallot. **A,** Infundibulectomy or removal of outflow tract obstruction to right ventricle by sharp dissection. **B,** Closure of ventricular septal defect. **C,** If pulmonary annulus is too narrow, or if infundibulectomy does not open outflow obstruction adequately, patch in outflow tract may be necessary.

From Effler, D.B. (1978). *Blades' surgical diseases of the chest* (4th ed.). St. Louis: Mosby.

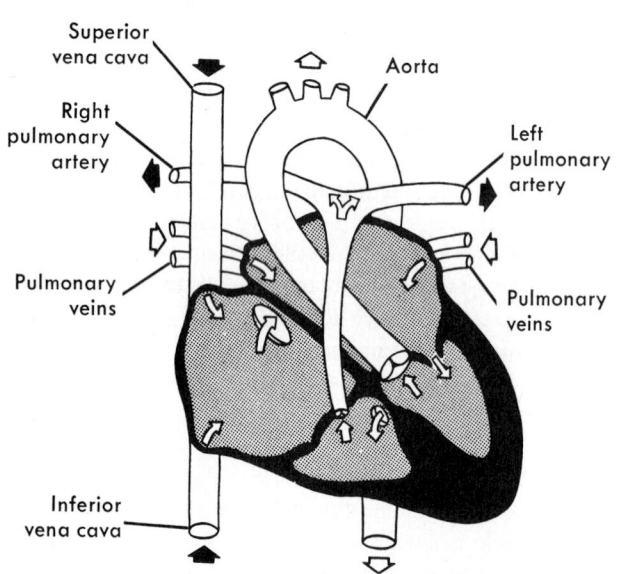

FIG. 28-24 Tricuspid atresia is characterized by small right ventricle, large left ventricle, and diminished pulmonary circulation. Atrial septal or other congenital defect is necessary to sustain life.

From Nursing Education Service. (1970). *General signs and symptoms of congenital heart abnormalities.* © Ross Laboratories, Columbus, Ohio.

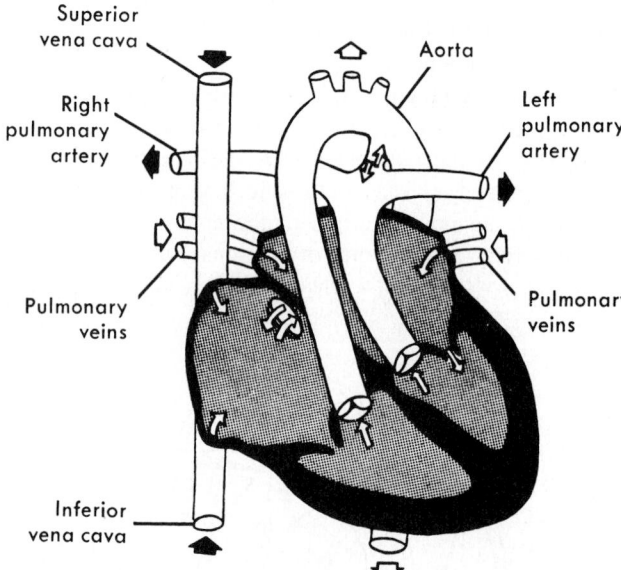

FIG. 28-25 Complete transposition of great vessels produces two separate circulations. Since aorta originates from right ventricle and pulmonary artery from left ventricle, abnormal communication between two chambers must be present to sustain life.

From Nursing Education Service. (1970). *General signs and symptoms of congenital heart abnormalities.* © Ross Laboratories, Columbus, Ohio.

Operations for transposition of the great arteries

In the anomaly in which the aorta arises from the right ventricle and the pulmonary artery from the left ventricle, circulation is reversed (Fig. 28-25). However, to sustain life, there must be a communication between the two sides of the heart or major vessels: a patent foramen ovale, patent ductus arteriosus, ASD, VSD, or partial transposition of the pulmonary veins, which permits oxygenated blood to enter the systemic circulation.

The newborn with this condition is cyanotic at birth and becomes severely incapacitated, with an enlarged heart that rapidly increases in size and progresses to congestive failure.

Palliative procedures that tend to improve intracardiac mixing, thereby increasing the oxygen content of the systemic blood, are done to sustain life until the infant has attained sufficient growth to tolerate a long corrective procedure. Palliative procedures include the Blalock-Hanlon procedure and the Rashkind atrial septostomy (see Fig. 28-39, *C*).

Corrective procedures include the atrial switch, the Senning atrial switch, and the Mustard and the Rastelli procedures. For each procedure described, the child is placed on the OR bed in a supine position. The setup is as described for open heart surgery, with consideration given to the age and size of the patient.

Arterial switch procedure

Anatomic repair of the transposition is performed by switching the pulmonary artery to the right ventricle and the aorta to the left ventricle. Use of a prosthetic graft is avoided. The left ventricle must have developed sufficient contractile force to maintain systemic pressure once the procedure is completed. It occurs in patients with VSD and reversible hypertension; in patients without these defects, pulmonary artery banding (see Fig. 28-39, *B*) is first performed to strengthen the left ventricle. Transfer of the coronary arteries must be accomplished without kinking, torsion, or tension.

Operative procedure (Fig. 28-26)

1. Median sternotomy and CPB are performed as described.
2. The aorta is dissected away from the main and branch pulmonary arteries.
3. The coronary arteries are inspected, and the site for their transfer into the pulmonary artery is marked.
4. The aorta is cross-clamped and transsected above the sinuses and aortic valve; the pulmonary artery is transsected above the pulmonic valve.
5. The orifices of the coronary arteries with a rim of adjacent aortic wall are excised.
6. The corresponding sinuses of the pulmonary arteries are incised where previously marked. The cuff and coronary artery are then sutured into place. Care is taken not to kink the coronary arteries.

7. The distal pulmonary artery is brought anterior to the aorta. The distal aorta is anastomosed to the proximal pulmonary artery.
8. Bovine or homograft pericardium may be used to enlarge the aorta and patch the defects created by the excision of the coronary ostia.

Senning procedure

This alternative inflow procedure redirects venous flow. The Senning operation is sometimes preferred to the Mustard procedure (described later) because it is technically easier to perform and does not require the use of a patch that can eventually cause venous obstruction.

Operative procedure (Fig. 28-27)

1. A median sternotomy is made and CPB instituted.
2. A right atrial incision is made longitudinally, extending to the insertion of the eustachian valve at the orifice of the inferior vena cava.
3. A lateral atrial septal flap is made and sutured above the left pulmonary veins.
4. The new systemic venous atrium is completed by suturing the edge of the original right atrial incision to the remnant of atrial septum between the mitral and tricuspid valves. This step creates a tube of right atrium containing the venae cavae at each end.
5. Pulmonary venous blood flows around this tube from an opening in front of the right pulmonary veins to the tricuspid valve.

Mustard procedure

Under direct vision the Mustard procedure excises the remaining segments of the atrial septum; a pericardial or synthetic patch is sutured in place in the atrial cavities creating a baffle so that the venous inflow is reversed. This permits the pulmonary venous return to be redirected into the right ventricle and the systemic venous return to be redirected into the left ventricle (Fig. 28-28). Previous creation of an ASD may serve as a first stage for this procedure. Pericardium or synthetic patch is used as a baffle. Patients with an intact ventricular septum are candidates for an atrial switch type of operation.

Operative procedure

1. A median sternotomy incision is completed as described.
2. A section of pericardium 2 × 3 inches is excised and placed in a heparin solution (Fig. 28-28, *A*).
3. Extracorporeal circulation is established as previously described.
4. A curved incision is made in the wall of the right atrium (Fig. 28-28, *B*).
5. The entire atrial septum is excised. The orifice of the coronary sinus is enlarged (Fig. 28-28, *C*).
6. A double-armed suture is placed three fifths of the way along the long margin of the pericardial graft.

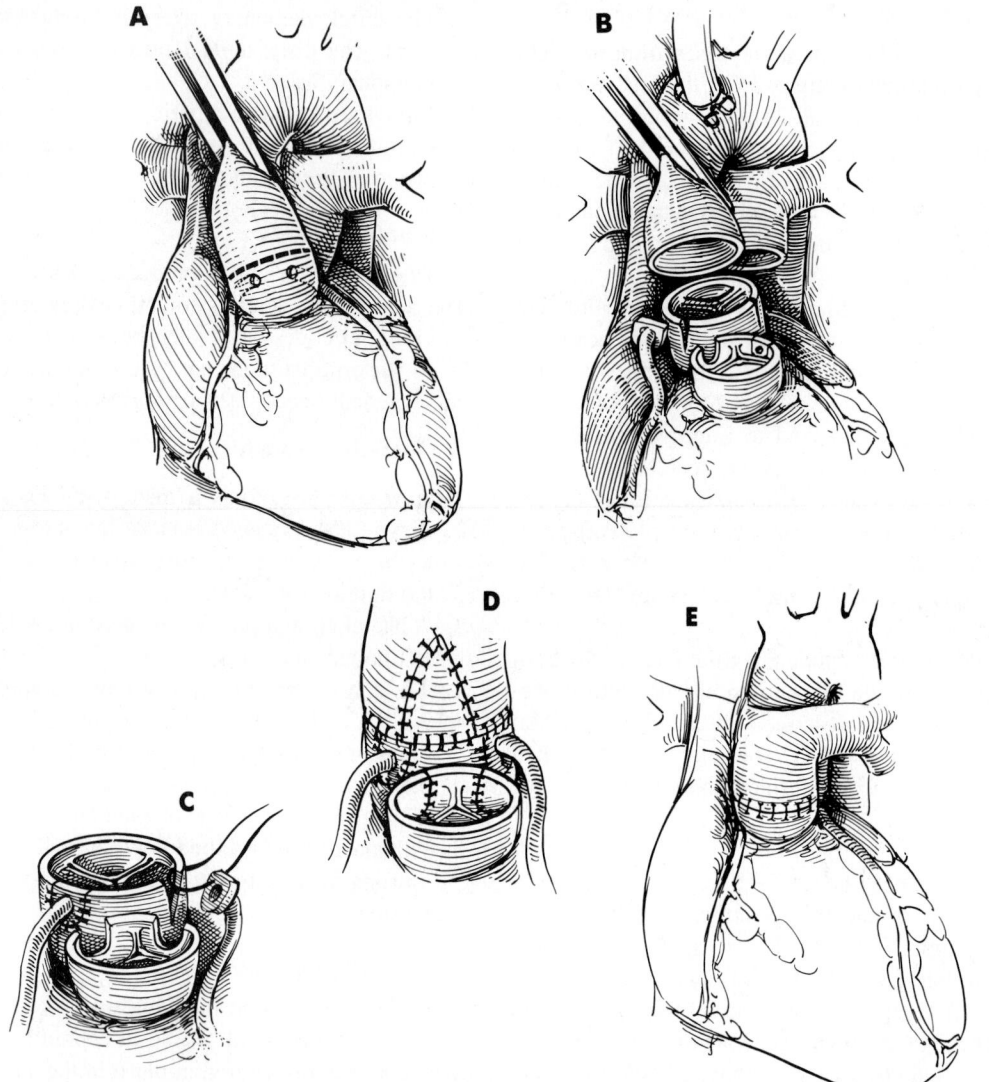

FIG. 28-26 Arterial switch operation for transposition of great arteries. **A** and **B,** Aorta and pulmonary artery are transsected. **C,** Coronary arteries are transposed to proximal pulmonary artery cuff. **D,** Distal aorta is anastomosed to proximal pulmonary artery (patch enlargement may be required). **E,** Distal pulmonary artery is brought anterior to aorta and sutured to proximal aortic stump.

From Waldhausen, J.A., & Pierce, W.S. (1985). *Johnson's surgery of the chest* (5th ed.). Chicago: Year Book Medical Publishers.

7. The pericardial graft or synthetic intracardiac patch is sutured in place, excluding the coronary sinus and the left atrial appendage (Fig. 28-28, *C* and *D*).
8. An additional section of pericardium or synthetic patch is placed in the wall of the right atrium that enlarges the new left atrium.
9. Extracorporeal circulation is discontinued, and closures are completed.

Rastelli procedure

In patients with VSD and subpulmonary stenosis the atrial switch operations have not demonstrated favorable results. The Rastelli procedure is an anatomic correction that has the advantage of converting the left ventricle to the systemic pumping chamber. Either a valved conduit or an aortic valve homograft may be used to connect the right ventricle and the pulmonary artery.

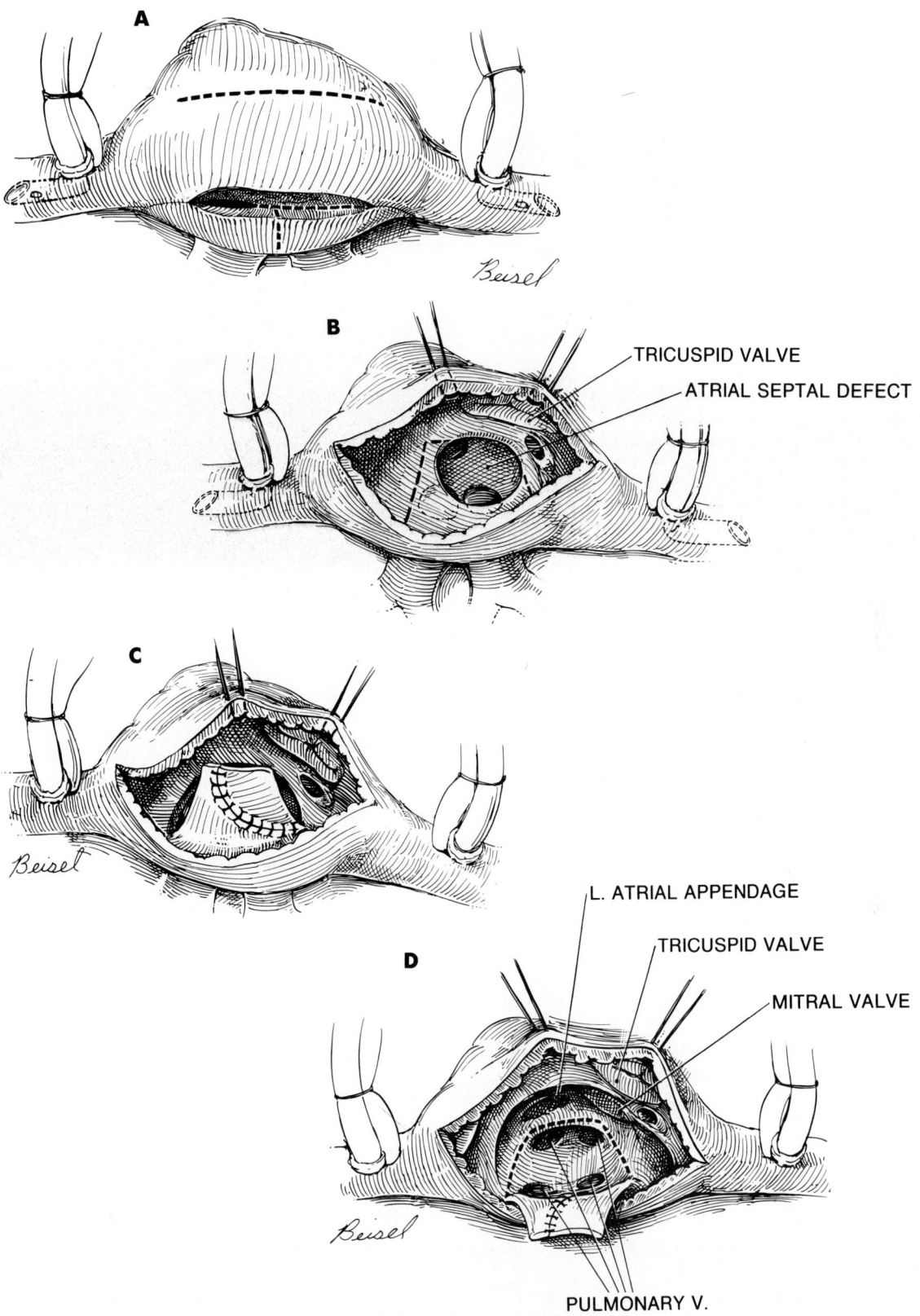

FIG. 28-27 Senning procedure for transposition of great arteries. **A,** Right atrial incision extended to eustachian valve at orifice of inferior vena cava. **B** and **C,** Septal flap is developed and piece of pericardium sutured in area of absent septum secundum. **D,** Flap is sutured around left pulmonary vein orifices.

Continued.

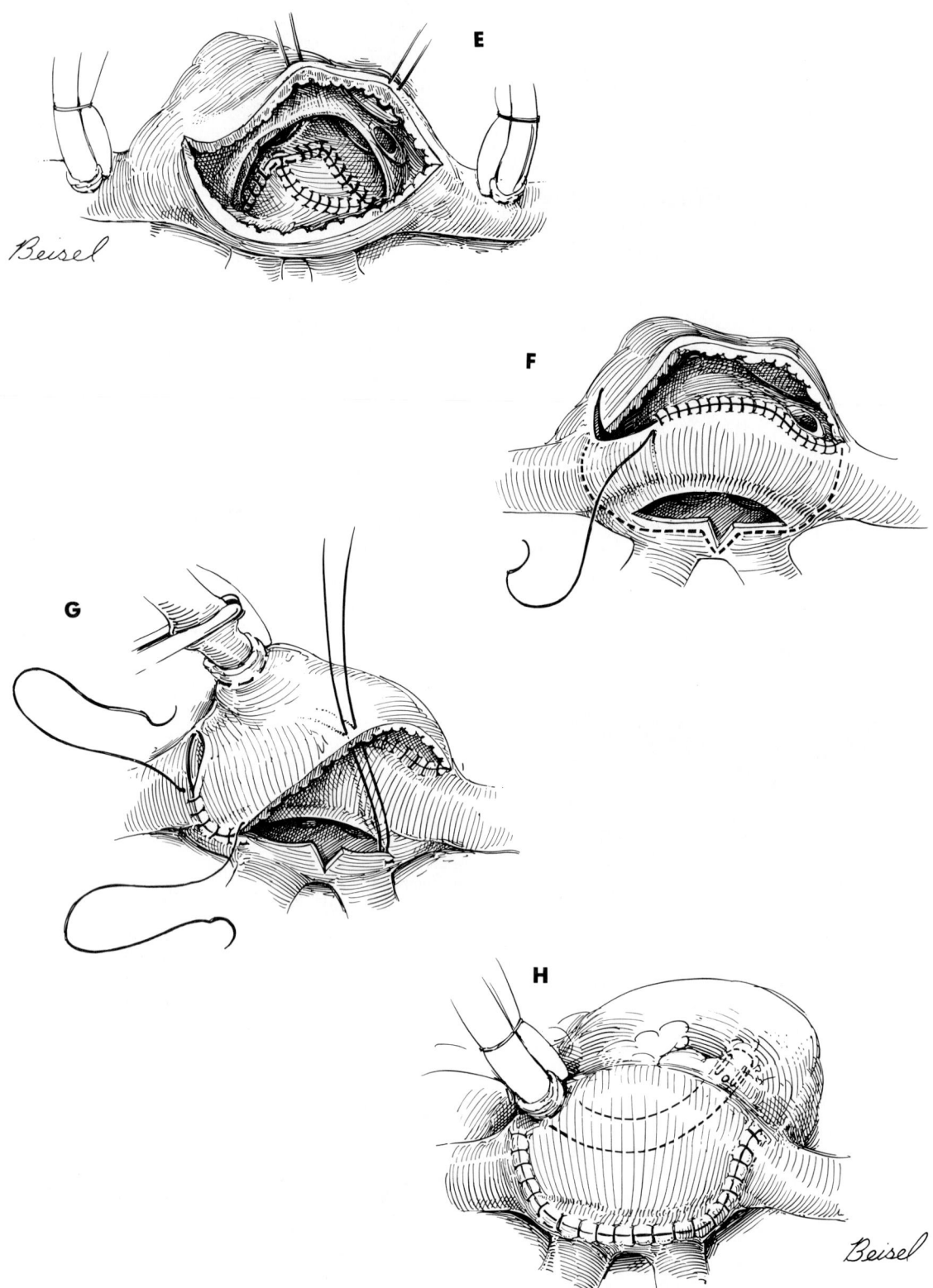

FIG. 28-27, CONT'D   **E,** Ends are carried toward base on both sides of flap. **F,** Left atrial wall is incised and free edge of right atrium is sutured to remnant of atrial septum and eustachian tube. **G** and **H,** Atrial flap is sutured across venae cavae so as not to constrict them.

From Waldhausen, J.A., & Pierce, W.S. (1985). *Johnson's surgery of the chest* (5th ed.). Chicago: Year Book Medical Publishers.

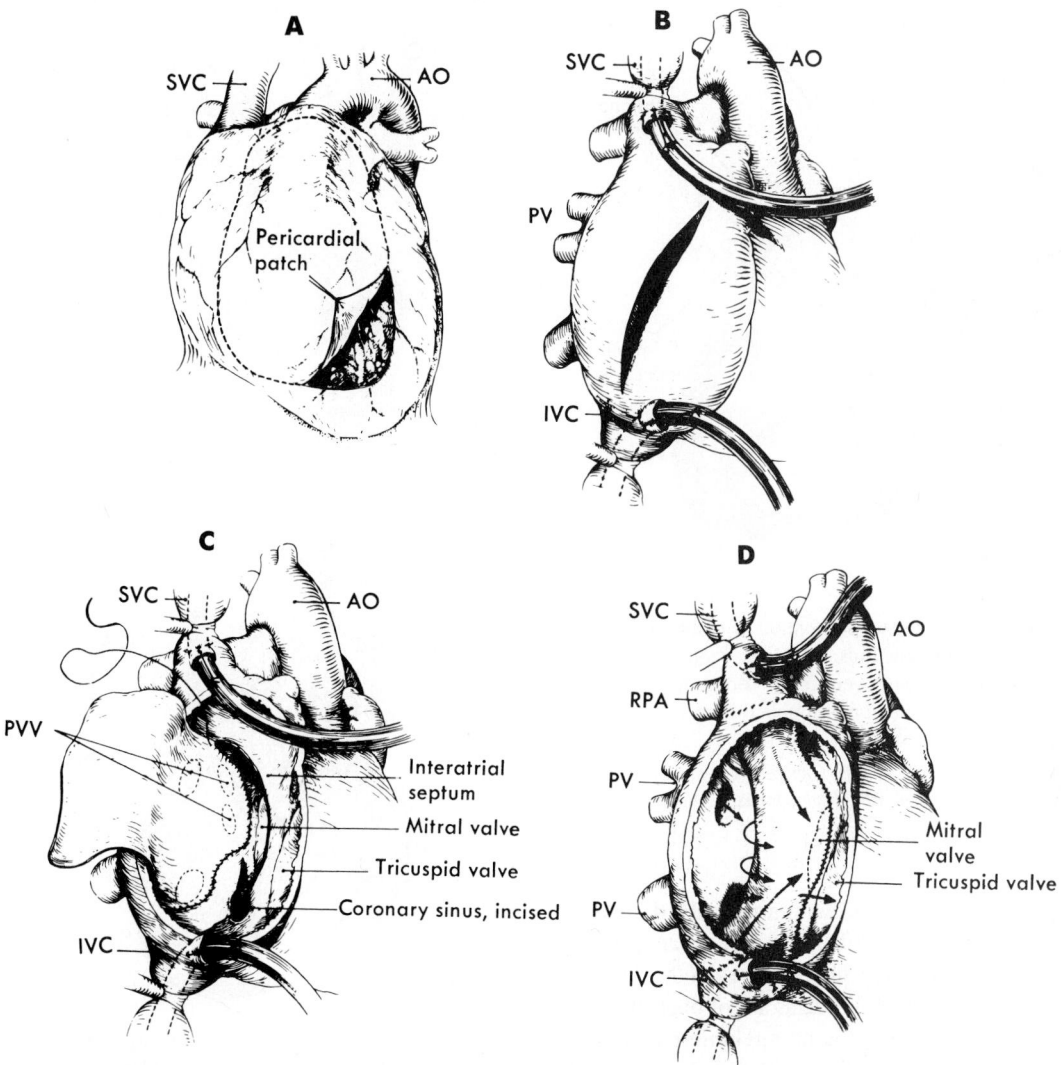

FIG. 28-28 Mustard procedure. **A,** Rectangular patch of pericardium or synthetic material is harvested with its long axis vertically. Length is from diaphragm to reflection onto aorta. Width leaves one comfortably away from phrenic nerves. **B,** Caval cannulas are inserted at junction of venae cavae and right atrium. Superior part of atriotomy goes toward atrial appendage. **C,** Patch is sutured between pulmonary veins and mitral valve, dividing atrial septal defect in half. Incising coronary sinus will commit coronary sinus flow into new systemic venous atrium. **D,** Completed repair. Vena cava flow is now directed to mitral valve, and pulmonary venous blood to tricuspid valve. *SVC,* Superior vena cava; *AO,* aorta; *PV,* pulmonary vein; *IVC,* inferior vena cava; *PVV,* pulmonary veins; *RPA,* right pulmonary artery.

Operative procedure

1. Median sternotomy and CPB are instituted.
2. The pulmonary artery is divided, and the proximal stump oversewn.
3. The right ventricle is incised high in the outflow tract.
4. A tunnel is created using Dacron prosthetic material to direct blood through the VSD into the aorta.
5. An outflow conduit is placed between the right ventricle and distal pulmonary artery.

Repair of truncus arteriosus

Truncus arteriosus is a retention of the embryologic bulbar trunk. It results from failure of normal septation of this trunk into an aorta and pulmonary artery. In this anomaly a single great vessel leaves the base of the heart through a single semilunar valve. This vessel is situated just above the VSD and receives blood from both ventricles. It gives rise to the coronary arteries and supplies the entire pulmonary and systemic circulations (Fig. 28-29).

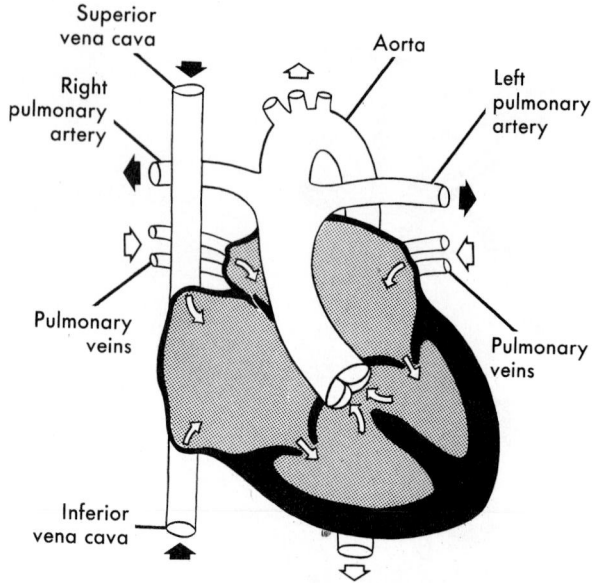

FIG. 28-29 Truncus arteriosus is retention of embryologic bulbar trunk. This single arterial trunk overrides ventricles and receives blood from them through ventricular septal defect. Entire pulmonary and systemic circulation is supplied from this common arterial trunk.

From Nursing Education Service. (1970). *General signs and symptoms of congenital heart abnormalities.* © Ross Laboratories, Columbus, Ohio.

Correction is quite successful with a nonvalved conduit of polytetrafluoroethylene (PTFE). The left atrial appendage is opened and used as the floor of the conduit with a patch of pulmonary homograft tissue as a roof over the conduit. With this technique there is no circumferential conduit to replace and no further surgery is required as the child grows. Small (12- or 14-mm) extracardiac valved conduits may also be used to create a main pulmonary artery; in this instance replacement of the conduit will be required two or three times as the child grows.

Infants who do not undergo repair show severe congestive heart failure with cyanosis and failure to thrive.

Procedural considerations. The child is placed in the supine position. The basic setup for a sternotomy is used, with consideration given to the child's age and size. Depending on the corrective approach selected, a valved conduit, intracardiac patch material, 2 × 2 inches, and a ½ × 4 inch strip of Teflon felt may be required.

Operative procedure

1. A median sternotomy is performed, and cardiopulmonary bypass is begun as previously described.
2. A cross-clamp is placed on the aorta, the pulmonary artery is excised from the aorta, and the aortic defect is closed with a double layer of continuous cardiovascular suture. The cross-clamp is removed.
3. A right ventriculotomy is made and the VSD repaired (Fig. 28-30, *A*).

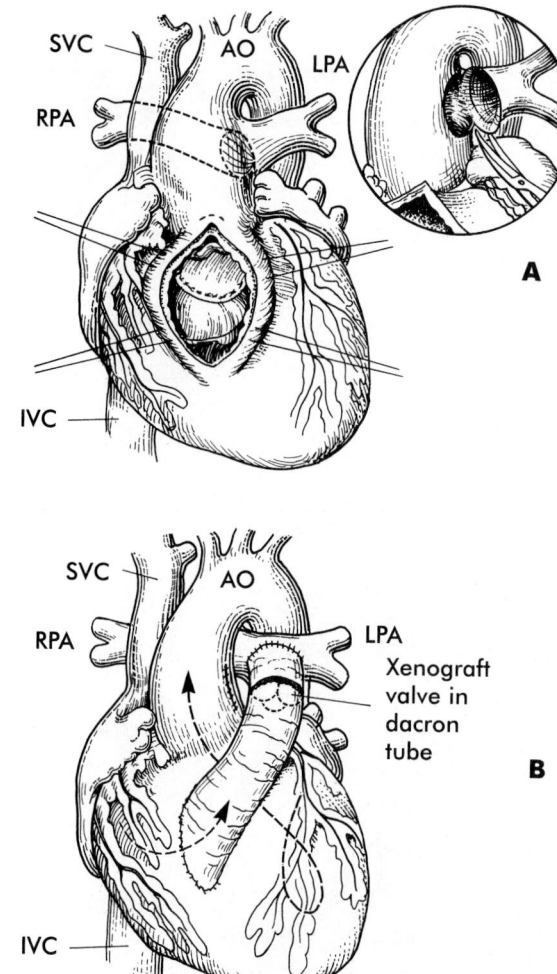

FIG. 28-30 Repair of truncus arteriosus. **A,** Ventricular septal defect has been closed with patch, and left ventricle is committed to aorta. Only outlet for right ventricle is ventriculotomy. *Inset* shows pulmonary artery of this type II lesion being disconnected from truncus. **B,** Completed repair has valve in Dacron graft connecting ventriculotomy site and pulmonary artery.

From Effler, D.B. (1978). *Blades' surgical diseases of the chest* (4th ed.). St. Louis: Mosby.

4a. If a valved conduit is used, the distal end is anastomosed to the pulmonary artery.
4b. The proximal end of the valved conduit is anastomosed to the right ventriculotomy using a Teflon felt buttress, which prevents sutures from cutting through the ventricular wall and enhances hemostasis (Fig. 28-30, *B*).
5. CPB is discontinued, and chest closure is completed.

Open valvulotomy and infundibular resection for pulmonary stenosis

Open valvulotomy is the separation of the stenosed leaflets under direct vision; infundibular resection for pulmonary stenosis is excision of the hypertrophied infundibulum.

Procedural considerations. The child is placed in the

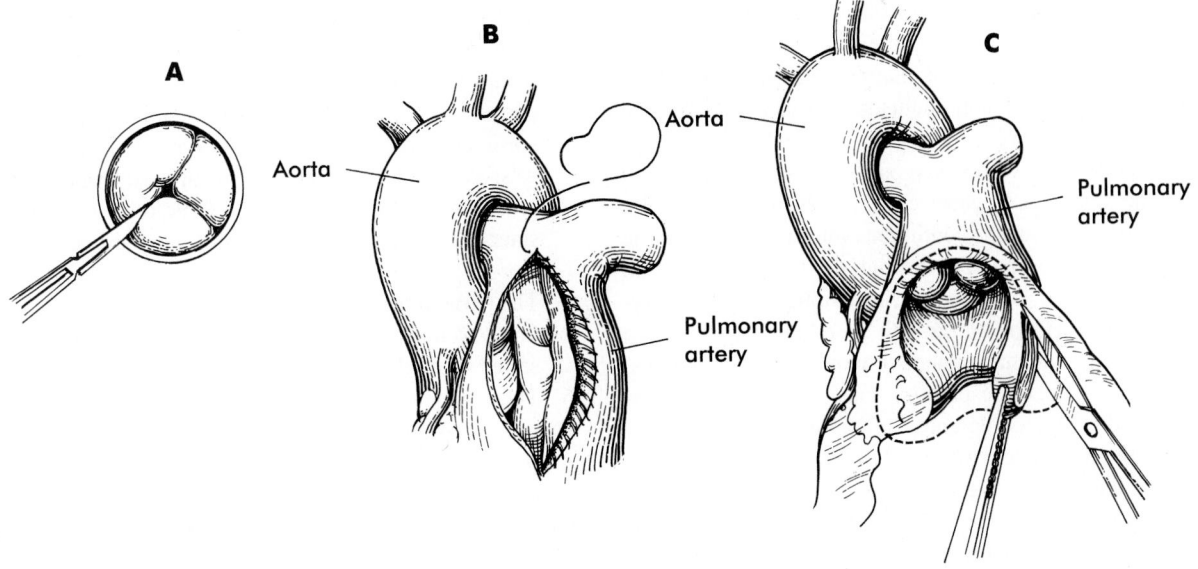

FIG. 28-31 **A,** Commissurotomy of stenotic valve. Knife is used, and care is taken to incise exactly on commissures. **B,** Diamond-shaped patch being used to enlarge pulmonary outflow tract and pulmonary valve annulus. If vertical pulmonary artery incision is made directly through anterior commissure of valve, three valve cusps remain intact, and some valve competence is retained. **C,** Excision of obstructing infundibular tissue.

From Effler, D.B. (1978). *Blades' surgical diseases of the chest* (4th ed.). St. Louis: Mosby.

supine position. The basic setup for a sternotomy is used, with consideration given to the child's age and size.

Operative procedure

1. A median sternotomy is performed, and the cannulations are made for CPB as previously described.
2a. For open valvulotomy the pulmonary artery is opened longitudinally, and the stenotic valve is incised with a scalpel or scissors (Fig. 28-31).
2b. For infundibular resection, the outflow tract of the right ventricle is opened, and the resection is performed, as described for tetralogy of Fallot.

Other procedures. Some surgeons use a valved conduit for the more severe forms of pulmonary stenosis and atresia. The Rastelli procedure (described previously) may be used to suture the conduit to the right ventricle and to the pulmonary artery, thus bypassing the atretic valve.

Closure of patent ductus arteriosus

Closure of the patent ductus arteriosus, an abnormal communication between the aorta and pulmonary artery, is achieved by suture ligation or by division of the ductus. The patent ductus arteriosus is an important fetal vascular communication whereby blood is shunted from the pulmonary artery into the aorta during intrauterine life. During fetal life the lungs are inactive, and the blood is oxygenated in the placenta. Normally the muscular coats of the ductus begin to contract soon after birth; the lumen is subsequently obliterated and blood flow through the shunt ceases.

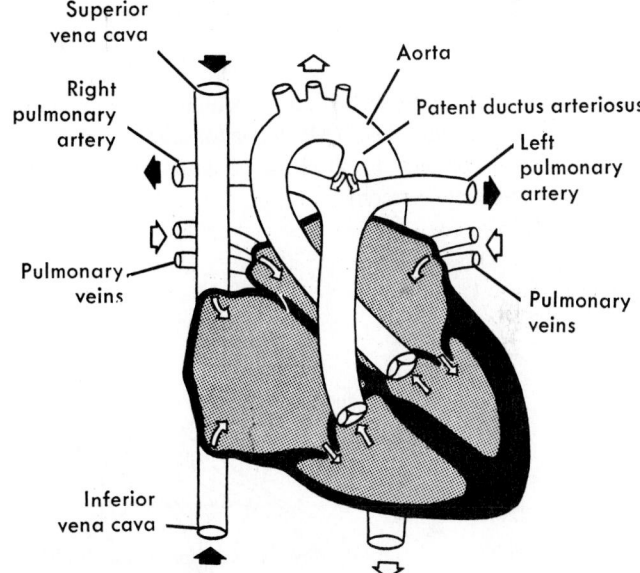

FIG. 28-32 Patent ductus arteriosus. Ductus fails to close after birth.

From Nursing Education Service. (1970). *General signs and symptoms of congenital heart abnormalities.* © Ross Laboratories, Columbus, Ohio.

When the ductus remains patent after birth (Fig. 28-32), it creates a shunt from the aorta through the ductus into the pulmonary circulation. This increases the work of the heart and causes subsequent enlargement and hypertrophy of the left atrium and ventricle. However, when persistent patency of the ductus is associated with other malformations such as tetralogy of Fallot and extreme stenosis of the pulmonary orifice, it is a means of maintaining life. Surgery is not performed if the patent ductus arteriosus is serving in a compensatory capacity.

Many children have few symptoms because of the small size of the shunt. A frequent clinical sign associated with this condition is a harsh, continuous murmur. Because the blood is oxygenated passing through the shunt, there is no cyanosis, clubbing, or reduction in peripheral arterial oxygen saturation. However, growth is retarded in children who have a large ductus. Other symptoms may include dyspnea, frequent upper respiratory tract infections, palpitation, limited exercise tolerance, and cardiac failure.

Procedural considerations. For newborn infants the surgeon and anesthesiologist may elect to perform this procedure in the intensive care nursery bed because the operation is a short one. The infant is placed in a right lateral position. The setup is as described, without items for CPB, but with special patent ductus clamps. Generally a left posterolateral approach is used; in some cases, however, a left anterolateral approach is used.

Operative procedure

1. The incision is carried through the muscles over the fourth interspace. The chest wall is entered through the third or fourth intercostal space, using items as described for thoracotomy (see Chapter 24). The wound edges are protected and retracted with a Finochietto rib spreader.
2. The pleura is incised with Metzenbaum scissors, and the left lung is protected and retracted with a moist pack and a malleable retractor.

3. The mediastinal pleura is opened between the phrenic and vagus nerves over the region of the ductus. The pleura is retracted by insertion of stay sutures. The recurrent laryngeal nerve is identified and protected. The aortic arch and pulmonary artery are dissected with fine scissors and dry dissectors. Fine arterial branches are divided and ligated with curved Crile or mosquito hemostats and nonabsorbable ligatures and cardiac suture ligatures.
4. The parietal pleura overlying the ductus is dissected with fine vascular forceps and scissors. Stay sutures are inserted to facilitate retraction.
5. The adventitial layer of the ductus is dissected free. A small portion of the obscure posterior ductus is carefully freed to admit a right-angle clamp. Tapes are passed around the aorta and below the ductus.
6a. For the suture-ligation method (Fig. 28-33) two ligatures are placed around the ductus, one near the aorta and the other near the pulmonary artery side, both of which are tied in place. Between these two ligatures two transfixion sutures are inserted.
6b. For the division of the ductus method the patent ductus clamps are applied as close to the aorta and pulmonary artery as possible. The ductus is divided halfway through and partially sutured with mattress cardiovascular sutures and continued back over the free edge with an over-and-over whip suture. After both openings are sutured, a sponge is held on the area for compression while the patent ductus clamps are removed.
7. The mediastinal pleura is closed with interrupted sutures. The lung is reexpanded, and a chest catheter is

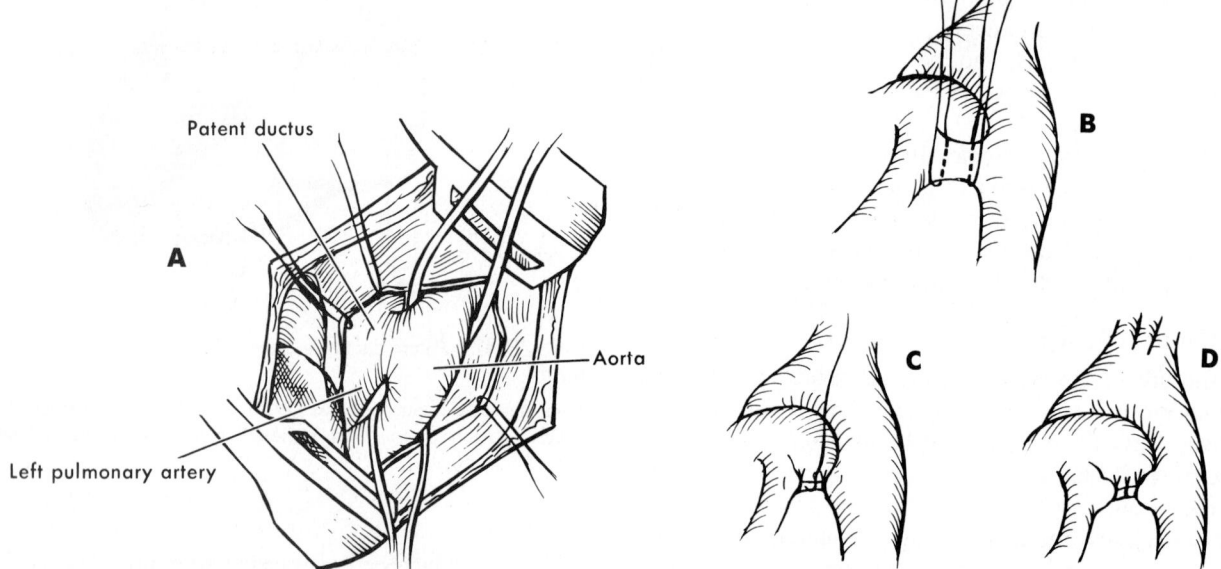

FIG. 28-33   Suture ligation of patent ductus arteriosus. **A,** Potts-Smith aortic clamp and ductus clamp in place. **B,** Ductus arteriosus partially divided. **C,** Closure of ductus arteriosus begun before division completed to permit better control of bleeding should one clamp slip. **D,** Clamps removed showing completed suture lines.

inserted to establish closed drainage. In newborns reexpansion of the lung may be accomplished by gradual withdrawal of a catheter during closure; no chest drainage tube is required unless there is oozing.

8. The chest wall is closed in layers, and dressings are applied.

Repair of coarctation of the aorta

Coarctation of the aorta (Fig. 28-34) is repaired by excising a constricted segment of the aorta, plus an end-to-end anastomosis—with or without a graft—to reestablish continuity. In some instances a woven Dacron or PTFE patch may be used to enlarge the aortic diameter at the site of the coarctation, or a subclavian flap is used.

The lesion that narrows or constricts the lumen of the aorta may be classified as infantile or adult. In the infantile type the constriction is long and usually located in the aortic arch proximal to the junction of the aorta and ductus arteriosus. The ductus usually remains patent and may be associated with other cardiac defects. In the adult type the coarctation consists of a constricted area at or just distal to the junction of the aorta and left subclavian artery and the ductus, which is generally closed. This type is compatible with life for a considerable period.

Coarctation of the aorta is a fairly common congenital malformation, and the adult patient suffers from hypertension and complains of dyspnea, palpitation, vertigo, headache, epistaxis, and weakness. However, when the aorta is almost obstructed, hypertension is manifested in the upper

part of the body with hypotension in the lower extremities. With hypertension above the constriction the collateral blood supply, which unites the blood vessels of the shoulder, the upper extremities, and the lower extremities, increases markedly. In so doing the intercostal vessels dilate, allowing their branches to carry blood from the subclavian arteries downward. Occasionally the vessels erode the lower margins of the ribs.

Procedural considerations. The child is placed in the right lateral position. Instrumentation is as described for basic cardiac surgery, plus Teflon or Dacron woven or knitted vascular prostheses in assorted sizes, to be used as necessary when primary anastomosis is not possible. Items for CPB are not needed.

Operative procedure (Fig. 28-35)

1. A left posterolateral incision is carried through the chest wall, as described for thoracotomy. As previously stated, the collateral blood vessels are somewhat enlarged, and bleeding may be profuse. Sponges may be weighed to determine accurate blood replacement, depending on the preference of the anesthesia provider. A Burford or Finochietto retractor is used.

2. The pleura is incised and the lung is retracted. The mediastinal pleura is incised over the constricted portion of the aorta, and the edges are sutured to the chest wall.

3. Careful dissection with fine vascular forceps and dry dissectors is continued to mobilize the aorta and the surrounding intercostal vessels. The laryngeal nerve is identified and protected. The ductus arteriosus is ligated and divided between ductus clamps.

4a. For patch repair the curved or angled vascular clamps are applied, and a longitudinal aortotomy is performed with a no. 11 knife blade, a Potts scissors, and vascular forceps.

4b. A piece of graft material is inserted, large enough to widen the aorta, using a continuous cardiovascular suture.

4c. The clamps are removed, one at a time, as described in step 5c.

5a. For resection with graft replacement (Fig. 28-35, *C*) the curved or angled vascular clamps are applied, and the constricted segment is divided between them. A second set of clamps may be applied above and below, as a safety factor, in fashioning the cuffs for reapproximation.

5b. End-to-end anastomosis is accomplished with a continuous, everting mattress technique for the posterior wall and interrupted, everting mattress sutures for the anterior row. If the stricture is long, a synthetic aortic prosthesis is used to bridge the defect, or a gusset type of patch is used to enlarge the defect.

5c. The clamps are released slowly, the distal one first and then the proximal one. The blood pressure is noted at this time. Removal of clamps is not completed until the blood pressure is stabilized.

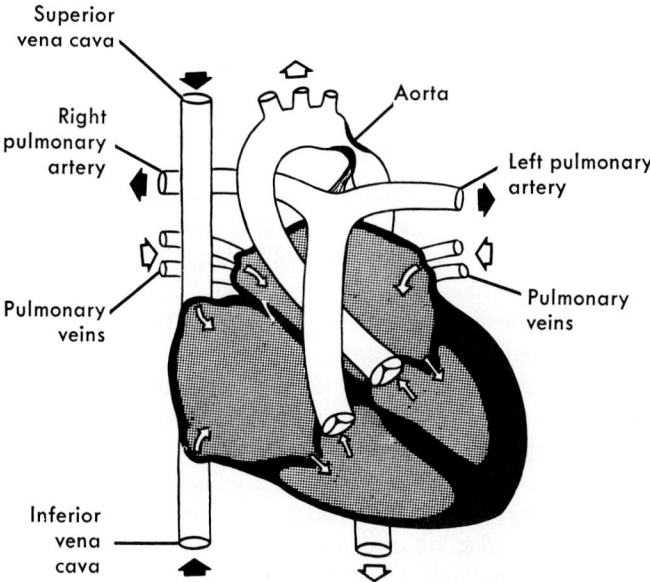

FIG. 28-34　Coarctation of aorta is characterized by narrow aortic lumen and exists as preductal or postductal obstruction, depending on position of obstruction in relation to ductus arteriosus.

From Nursing Education Service. (1970). *General signs and symptoms of congenital heart abnormalities.* © Ross Laboratories, Columbus, Ohio.

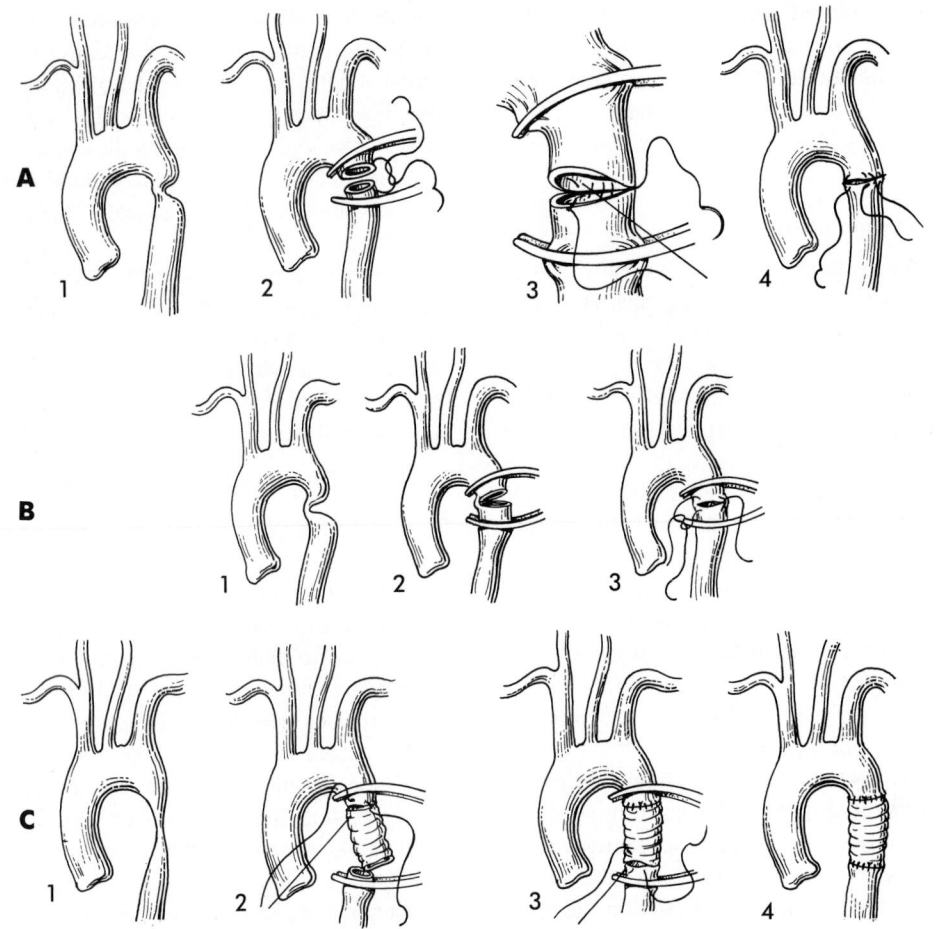

FIG. 28-35   Diagrams showing coarctation of aorta: types with methods of correction. **A,** Short, narrow obstruction and steps in end-to-end anastomosis. **B,** Wedge excision with partial anastomosis completed. **C,** Segmental excision with graft replacement.

From Blades, B. (editor), *Surgical diseases of the chest* (3rd ed.). St. Louis: Mosby.

6a. For subclavian flap repairs (Fig. 28-36) the aorta above and below the patent ductus is dissected out, as is the subclavian artery. The subclavian artery is ligated at the origin of the vertebral artery, which is also ligated.

6b. The aorta is incised distal to the area of narrowing, through the coarctation to the subclavian artery.

6c. The aorta is opened and the coarctation excised.

6d. The tip of the subclavian flap is brought down into the aorta and sutured with absorbable running sutures or nonabsorbable interrupted sutures.

6e. The reverse subclavian flap procedure (Fig. 28-37) is used in infants with coarctation of the aortic arch. The subclavian artery is ligated and transsected at the origin of the vertebral artery. An incision is made in the aorta through the coarctation and into the subclavian artery. The subclavian flap is then sewn into the incision as in steps b through d above.

7. The parietal pleura is closed, leaving a small opening at the lower point. Closed drainage is established, and the chest wall is closed in layers. A dressing is applied.

Pulmonary artery banding

Pulmonary artery banding is the constriction of the pulmonary artery to reduce its diameter, thereby decreasing pulmonary blood flow (see Fig. 28-39, *B*).

An infant with an enlarged heart in intractable failure and a large left-to-right shunt may be treated effectively by a palliative pulmonary artery banding operation. This procedure is designed to reduce the flow of blood through the pulmonary artery to approximately one half to one third of the existing rate. A tape is looped about the artery and secured in place by a simple suture technique. Pressures are measured by direct needle puncture and before and after banding. A reduction of the distal pulmonary artery pressure by 50% to 70% is sought. Repair of the interventricular septal defect may be postponed until the child has been clinically stabilized and can withstand an open heart procedure.

Procedural considerations. The child is placed in the left lateral position if an anterolateral incision is to be used or in the supine position if a median sternotomy is to

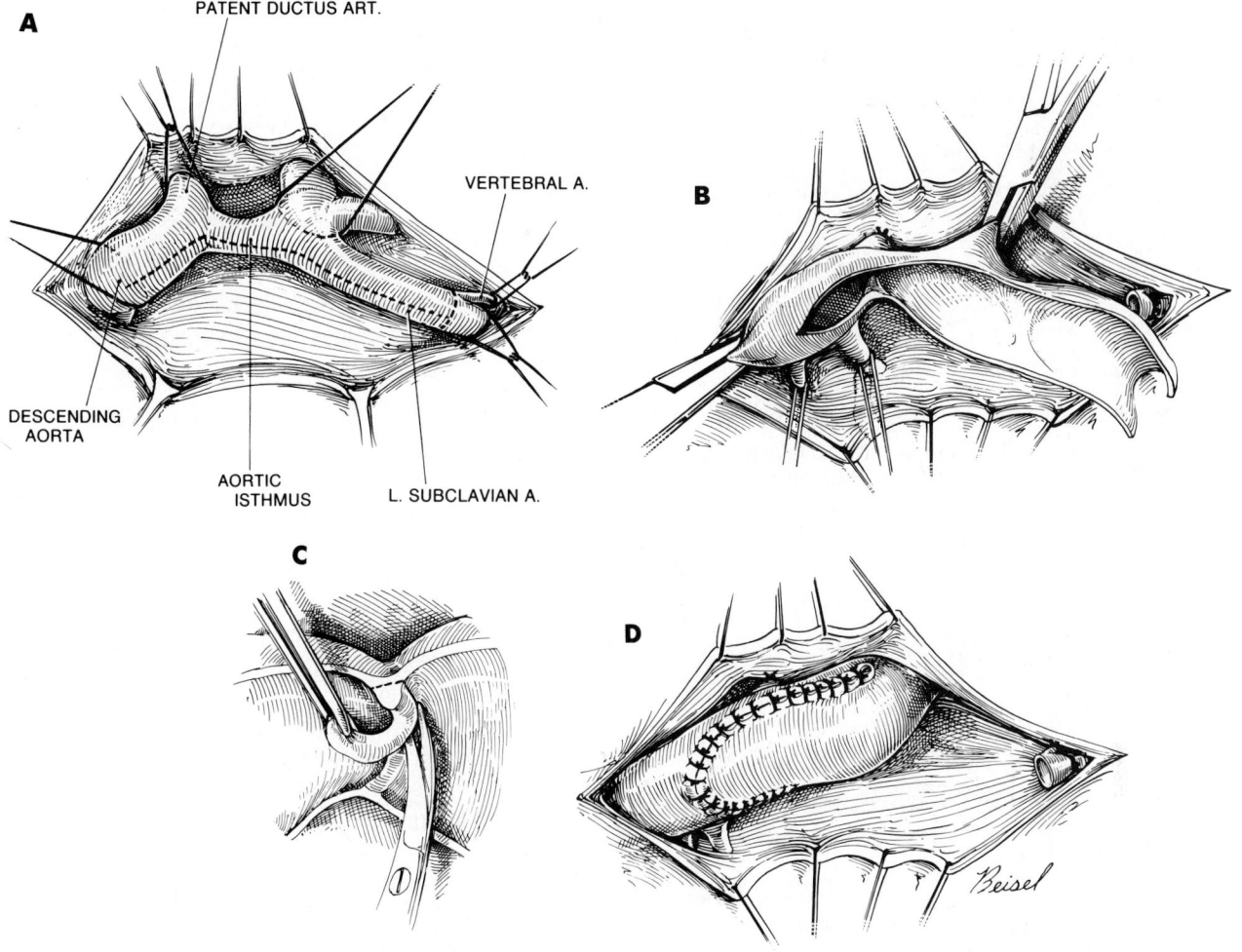

FIG. 28-36   Subclavian flap procedure for coarctation of the aorta. **A,** Retraction stitches around transverse arch, descending aorta, and left subclavian artery; patent ductus arteriosus is ligated. **B,** Aorta incised. **C,** Coarctation shelf removed. **D,** Subclavian flap anastomosed to descending aorta.

From Waldhausen, J.A., & Pierce, W.S. (1985). *Johnson's surgery of the chest* (5th ed.). Chicago: Year Book Medical Publishers.

be used. Eight-inch pieces of various width tapes (surgeon's preference), with appropriate sizes for children, are used.

Repair of hypoplastic left heart syndrome
(Fig. 28-38)

Hypoplastic left heart syndrome (HLHS) is the fourth most common congenital heart defect presenting in infancy. HLHS describes a spectrum of congenital cardiac malformations that have in common underdevelopment of the left-sided heart structures, which include aortic valve atresia and stenosis with associated hypoplasia or absence of the left ventricle. The ascending aorta and arch are usually only a few millimeters in diameter and are functionally a branch of the ductus arteriosus–thoracic aorta continuum with blood flowing retrograde through the aortic arch and into the small ascending aorta to the coronary arteries (Fig. 28-

38). There is also mitral valve atresia or stenosis present (Jacobs and Norwood, 1992).

Since patency of the ductus arteriosus is needed for systemic circulation, children are maintained on an infusion of prostaglandin before surgical intervention. If left untreated, a majority of these neonates will die within the first month of life; without surgical intervention the disease is fatal.

It was not until the development of the Fontan procedure, a surgical correction for another form of single ventricle—tricuspid atresia—that long-term survival in patients with HLHS was considered possible. However, due to the neonate's high pulmonary vascular resistance, the Fontan procedure is not a surgical option in the newborn period. A palliative repair (stage I) was developed in the late 1970s by Norwood to prepare the heart for the Fontan procedure.

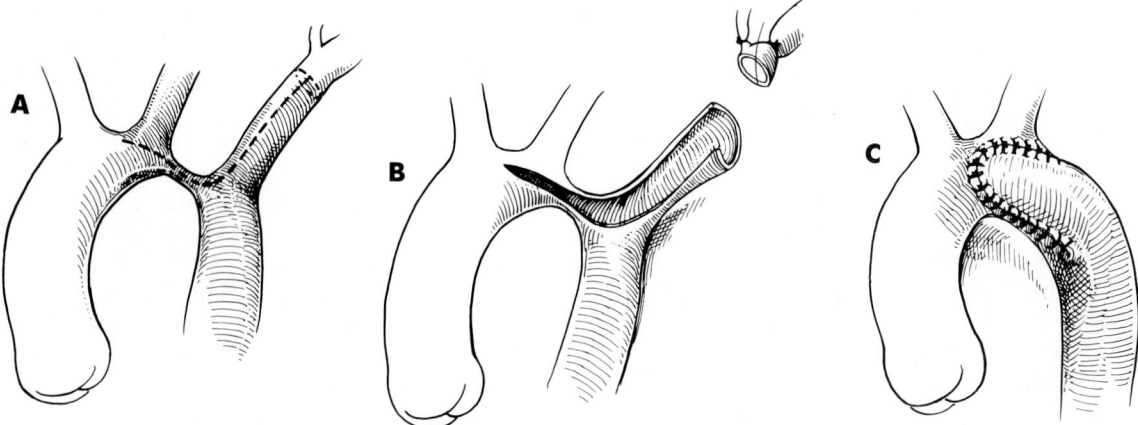

FIG. 28-37   Reverse subclavian flap procedure for coarctation of aorta. **A,** Coarctation of aortic arch (left subclavian artery is ligated and transsected). **B,** Aortic incision. **C,** Subclavian flap sewn to aorta.

From Waldhausen, J.A., & Pierce, W.S. (1985). *Johnson's surgery of the chest* (5th ed.). Chicago: Year Book Medical Publishers.

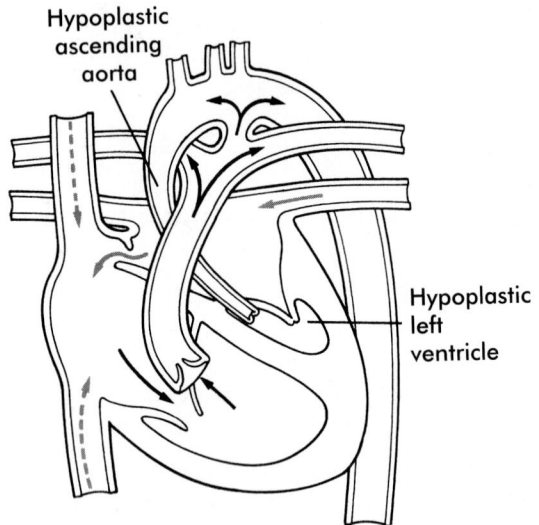

FIG. 28-38   Hypoplastic left heart syndrome (HLHS). *Gray arrows,* Saturated blood; *broken arrows,* desaturated blood; *black arrows,* mixed blood.

From Whaley, L.F., & Wong, D.L. (1991). *Nursing care of infants and children* (4th ed.). St. Louis: Mosby.

Two surgical options for patients with HLHS exist: a series of reconstructive procedures or a heart transplant. The series of reconstructive procedures usually involves three stages. Stage I is performed during the newborn period. The goals of stage I are to (1) maintain systemic perfusion, (2) preserve the function of the only ventricle, and (3) allow normal maturation of the pulmonary ventricle. The first goal is met by creating an unobstructed communication between the right ventricle and the systemic circulation. This is accomplished by transsecting the main pulmonary artery and

creating a neoaorta from the main pulmonary artery, native aorta, and pulmonary homograft tissue. The other two goals are met by creating a right modified Blalock-Taussig (BT) shunt and a nonrestrictive interatrial communication. These measures allow for adequate pulmonary blood flow and for the pulmonary vascular resistance to decrease as the child grows while limiting the volume interposed on the single ventricle.

The modified Fontan procedure was initially performed at approximately 18 months of age. However, since 1989 a staged approach to the Fontan procedure has been undertaken to minimize the impact of rapid changes in ventricular geometry and diastolic function that can be associated with a primary Fontan procedure and to attempt to reduce the postoperative complications of effusions associated with it. In the stage II procedure—hemi-Fontan—SVC blood flow is directed to the lungs and IVC blood flow continues to flow to the right ventricle. The third and final stage, the modified Fontan procedure, separates the systemic and pulmonary circulations.

Procedural considerations. Additional items for the open heart setup include the following:

Stage I

PTFE tube graft, 4 mm
Pulmonary homograft tissue

Stage II

Oscillating saw
Pulmonary homograft tissue

Stage III

Oscillating saw
PTFE tube graft, 10 mm

Operative procedures
Stage I (Fontan procedure)

1. A median sternotomy is performed. The aortic cannula is placed in the main pulmonary artery rather than the diminutive aorta, and the venous cannula is placed in the right atrium. CPB is instituted, and the right and left pulmonary arteries are immediately occluded with tourniquets to force the blood through the ductus arteriosus to the systemic circulation.
2. When deep hypothermic circulatory arrest is about to be instituted, the innominate and left carotid arteries are occluded with tourniquets. The venous and aortic cannulas are removed.
3. The septum primum is excised through the venous cannulation site; occasionally a right atriotomy is necessary to facilitate the atrial septectomy.
4. The main pulmonary artery is transsected immediately before the takeoff of the right and left pulmonary arteries.
5. The distal pulmonary artery is closed with a small patch of homograft tissue.
6. The ductus arteriosus is then exposed and closed using a 2-0 Tevdek tie. The tie is left long to better expose the thoracic aorta. The ductus is transsected.
7. At the point where the ductus was attached to the aorta, the thoracic aorta is opened 1 to 2 cm, and the aortic arch and ascending aorta are opened to a point adjacent to the main pulmonary artery.
8. A gusset of homograft tissue is joined to the aorta starting at the thoracic end, and the pulmonary artery is incorporated at the proximal end of the ascending aorta. A continuous monofilament stitch is used. Occasionally interrupted sutures are used to attach the main pulmonary artery to the aorta.
9. To perform an RBT shunt, the innominate artery is cross-clamped and incised, and a 4-mm PTFE tube graft is interposed.
10. CPB is instituted, and the pulmonary end of the shunt is performed by incising the pulmonary artery and interposing the distal end of the tube graft.
11. Immediately after the shunt is completed the shunt must be occluded with a bulldog clamp until termination of bypass.

Stage II (hemi-Fontan)

1. Since these patients have had previous surgery, an oscillating saw is used for the median sternotomy.
2. The aorta, right atrium, and RBT shunt are exposed.
3. CPB is instituted, and the shunt is immediately occluded with a clip.
4. The branch pulmonary arteries are exposed.
5. Deep hypothermic circulatory arrest is instituted.
6. An incision is made in the confluence of the pulmonary arteries, extending to the pericardial reflections.
7. An incision is made in the dome of the right atrium, extending to the SVC.

8. The pulmonary artery is then anastomosed to the SVC–right atrial junction.
9. The pulmonary arteries are augmented with a gusset of homograft tissue, incorporating part of this tissue intraatrially as a dam between the common atrium and the caval-pulmonary anastomosis.
10. CPB is reinstituted until the patient is normothermic. CPB is discontinued and chest closure is completed.

Stage III (modified Fontan procedure)

1. Repeat step 1 of stage II (hemi-Fontan).
2. The aorta and right atrium are exposed.
3. CPB is instituted.
4. Deep hypothermic circulatory arrest is instituted.
5. A lateral incision is made in the right atrium.
6. A 10-mm PTFE tube graft is cut in half lengthwise and is placed intraatrially by suturing the inferior end of the graft around the orifice of the IVC and up the right lateral free wall of the right atrium to the superior dome of the right atrium. This creates a tunnel in which the inferior blood flow is directed to the pulmonary arteries. The superior caval blood flow was directed to the pulmonary arteries during the stage II repair. (Variations on this procedure may be performed, such as excluding a hepatic vein and making small openings in the PTFE tube graft.)
7. The atria are closed and CPB is reinstituted until the patient is normothermic. CPB is discontinued and chest closure is completed.

Shunt for palliation

The shunt for palliation is one of several palliative procedures designed to divert poorly oxygenated blood from one of the major arteries back through one of the pulmonary arteries to the lungs for reoxygenation, thereby increasing the total blood flow in the pulmonary circulation.

Shunt procedures that increase pulmonary flow are described in Fig. 28-39, along with procedures to reduce pulmonary blood flow (pulmonary artery banding) and to increase intracardiac mixing of blood (Blalock-Hanlon ASD and Rashkind septostomy). The Blalock-Taussig procedure consists of an end-to-side anastomosis between the proximal end of the subclavian and pulmonary arteries. The procedure is performed on the side opposite the aortic arch. This shunt may be dismantled or ligated if a future operation for full correction is anticipated; however, the shunt has a tendency to decrease in size as the child grows. Currently the most commonly used form of shunt is a modification of the Blalock-Taussig in which a PTFE graft is used to connect pulmonary and systemic vasculature. It connects the subclavian artery to the ipsilateral pulmonary artery or the innominate artery to the right pulmonary artery. Occasionally a central shunt is used in which the PTFE graft connects the aorta and main pulmonary artery.

The Potts-Smith and Waterston procedures involve direct anastomosis of the aorta to the pulmonary arteries.

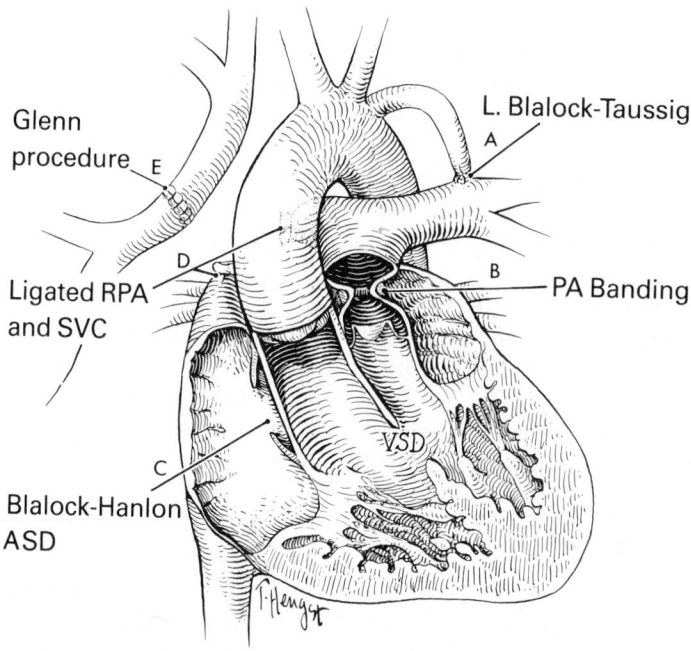

FIG. 28-39   Palliative procedures for congenital cardiac anomalies. *A,* Left Blalock-Taussig subclavian to pulmonary artery shunt applicable for tetralogy of Fallot and also for other congenital anomalies associated with insufficient pulmonary arterial flow. (Modification of Blalock-Taussig procedure consists of interposing PTFE graft between left subclavian artery and pulmonary artery, thereby preserving subclavian artery.) *B,* Pulmonary artery banding used for anomalies associated with excessive pulmonary blood flow due to large intracardiac left-to-right shunt. These include ventricular septal defect, truncus arteriosus, and others. *C,* Blalock-Hanlon creation of interatrial septal defect used predominantly for transposition of great vessels but also for anomalies such as mitral or tricuspid atresia in which large opening is advantageous to reduce intraatrial pressure. Dilatation of patent foramen ovale may be done with balloon-tipped catheter (Rashkind technique). *D* and *E,* Glenn procedure is used primarily for tricuspid atresia but is also used for transposition of great vessels. In *D* superior vena cava is anastomosed to right pulmonary artery to direct approximately 35% of systemic venous return to right lung for oxygenation. This technique cannot be used if pulmonary vascular resistance is elevated, as often occurs in transposition. Glenn procedure *(E)* is usually performed by implanting distal end of pulmonary artery into side of superior vena cava. Cava is then ligated at atriocaval junction. Ligation of azygos vein may enhance flow through cavopulmonary anastomosis but may also increase pressure in veins draining upper half of body. Techniques of delayed azygos ligation have been described in infants and children.

From Cooley, D.A. (1984). *Techniques in cardiac surgery* (2nd ed.). Philadelphia: W.B. Saunders.

These are rarely performed due to the potential for deformity of the pulmonary arteries, producing excessive pulmonary blood flow and congestive heart failure (Sade, 1992).

The Glenn procedure consists of anastomosis of the SVC to the right pulmonary artery. This operation is employed infrequently in the treatment of tetralogy of Fallot (Fig. 28-39, *E*).

Procedural considerations. The child is placed in a position that is specific for each procedure (supine or right or left lateral). Instruments are as previously described for open heart surgery, plus the following, with appropriate sizes for infants and children:

2 Potts-Smith aortic occlusion clamps	2 Hendrin ductus clamps
2 Johns Hopkins modified Potts clamps	2 Cooley anastomosis clamps

Operative procedures

Blalock-Taussig procedure (Fig. 28-39, *A*)

1. An anterolateral incision is made from the sternal margin to the midaxillary line. The chest cavity is opened and the lung retracted, as described previously.

2. The mediastinal pleura is incised and retracted with a stay suture.

3. The pulmonary artery is dissected from the surround-

ing tissue, with vascular forceps, dry dissector sponges, and Metzenbaum scissors. As the artery and branches are mobilized, heavy ligatures, moistened umbilical tapes, or fine silicone tubing is placed about them.

4. Branches of the vagus nerve are protected and retracted.

5. The subclavian artery is dissected completely from its origin to where it produces the internal mammary and costocervical branches. Its distal end is marked with a silk suture.

6. The subclavian artery is occluded with a vascular clamp, a ligature is placed at the distal segment, and the vessel is divided.

7. The pulmonary artery is occluded temporarily with a curved vascular clamp.

8. An incision of sufficient size to accommodate the subclavian artery is made with a scalpel with a no. 11 knife blade and Potts scissors.

9. An end-to-side anastomosis is completed with cardiovascular suture.

10. The clamps are released, and the suture line is inspected for hemostasis.

11. The mediastinal pleura is closed.

12. Closed chest drainage is established, and the chest wound is closed.

Potts-Smith procedure

1. A left posterolateral incision is made in the fourth intercostal space.

2. The pulmonary artery is dissected from its surrounding tissue, and the descending aorta is mobilized. Occluding tapes and Blalock or Potts-Smith clamps are applied.

3. A longitudinal incision is made in each artery, and a side-to-side anastomosis is completed with cardiovascular sutures.

4. The pulmonary artery is released, and the suture line is inspected for hemostasis.

5. The aortic clamps are then removed.

Waterston procedure

1. A right anterolateral incision is made in the fourth interspace. The pericardium is opened, and the ascending aorta is exposed.

2. The right pulmonary artery is dissected as it passes beneath the ascending aorta.

3. A heavy suture is passed around the right pulmonary artery and is used to occlude the artery temporarily. A curved vascular clamp is placed so one blade is behind the pulmonary artery and the other occludes a posterolateral portion of the ascending aorta.

4. On closure of the clamp, both the right pulmonary artery and a posterior portion of the ascending aorta are occluded.

5. Parallel incisions are made in the aorta and the right pulmonary artery.

6. An anastomosis is then made between the ascending aorta and right pulmonary artery.

Cardiac extracorporeal membrane oxygenation (ECMO)

Following the initial successful use of ECMO for neonates in the 1970s, the evolution of protocols and multicenter studies have led to newer techniques such as extracorporeal CO_2 removal (ECCO$_2$R), intravascular oxygenation (IVOX), mobile ECMO (MECMO), and ECMO for cardiac support. ECMO may be instituted for patients failing to wean from CPB, for severe left ventricular failure, treatment of hypercontractile right ventricle associated with reduced stroke volume, or with neonates with cardiac defects that are diagnosed as correctable when the neonate cannot be stabilized before cardiac catheterization or surgery (Faulkner, 1993). Although it is now performed only in established ECMO centers, the ongoing research and development of new circuits and pumps may in the future allow successful support of premature infants and pediatric trauma patients.

REFERENCES

Child health care. (1993). AAP Research Update, a publication of the American Academy of Pediatrics, No. 9.

Faulkner, S.C. (1993). *ECMO in the 90's.* Paper presented at the VIth Annual Meeting, Cardiac Surgery: Current Issues, November 18-20, 1993, St. Thomas, U.S. Virgin Islands.

Holder, T.M., & Manning, P.B. (1991). Esophageal atresia with tracheoesophageal fistula. In Grosfeld, J.L. (editor), *Common problems in pediatric surgery.* St. Louis: Mosby.

Jacobs, M.L., & Norwood, W.I. (1992). *Pediatric cardiac surgery.* Boston: Butterworth-Heinemann.

Johnson, D.G. (1991). Gastroesophageal reflux. In Grosfeld, J.L. (editor), *Common problems in pediatric surgery.* St. Louis: Mosby.

Sade, R.M. (1992). Surgical options in univentricular atrioventricular connection. In Jacobs, M.L. and Norwood, W.I. (editors), *Pediatric cardiac surgery.* Boston: Butterworth-Heinemann.

West, K.W. (1991). Intussusception. In Grosfeld, J.L. (editor), *Common problems in pediatric surgery.* St. Louis: Mosby.

Woolley, M.M. (1991). Type A esophageal atresia. In Grosfeld, J.L. (editor), *Common problems in pediatric surgery.* St. Louis: Mosby.

Vegunta, R.K., Cooney, D.E., & Cooney, D.R. (1993). Surgical management of abdominal wall defects in infants. *AORN Journal, 58*(1), 53.

BIBLIOGRAPHY

Ackley, B.J., & Ladwig, G.B. (1993). *Nursing diagnosis handbook.* St. Louis: Mosby.

Arensman, R.M., & Cornish, J.D. (1993). *Extracorporeal life support.* Boston: Blackwell Scientific Publications.

Atkinson, L.J. (1992). *Berry and Kohn's operating room technique* (7th ed.). St. Louis: Mosby.

Bandelow, L.R., Best-Devenish, P., & Heffron, T.G. (1993). Living related liver transplants: A solution to donor shortage in pediatric patients. *AORN Journal, 58*(1), 258.

Barber, G. (1990). Hypoplastic left heart syndrome. In Garson, A., Bricker, J.T., & McNamara, D.G. (editors), *The science and practice of pediatric cardiology.* Philadelphia: Lea & Febiger.

Chapman, R.A., & Bartlett, R.H. (1993). *Extracorporeal life support for adult and pediatric patients.* Ann Arbor: University of Michigan Medical Center.

Hatch, E.I., & Baxter, R. (1987). Surgical options in the management of large omphaloceles. *American Journal of Surgery, 153,* 449.

Hazinski, M.F. (1992). *Nursing care of the critically ill child.* St. Louis: Mosby.

Jarvis, C. (1992). Developmental tasks across the life cycle. In *Physical examination and health assessment.* Philadelphia: W.B. Saunders.

Joy, C. (1990). Pediatric surgery. In Rothrock, J.C. (editor), *Perioperative nursing care planning.* St. Louis: Mosby.

McFarland, G.K., & McFarland, E.A. (1993). *Nursing diagnosis and intervention.* St. Louis: Mosby.

Nicols, D.E., & Cameron, D.E. (1993). *Critical heart disease in children.* St. Louis: Mosby.

Pena, A. (1988). Surgical management of anorectal malformations: a unified concept. *Pediatric Surgical Institute, 3,* 82.

Rushton, C.H. (1988). The surgical neonate: principles of nursing management. *Pediatric Nursing 14,* 141.

Sinacore, J., Rosser, J.C., & Boeckman, C.R. (1993). Pediatric laparoscopic cholecystectomy: A case study. *AORN Journal, 58*(1), 64.

Smallwood, S.B. (1988). Preparing children for surgery through play. *AORN Journal, 47*(1), 177.

Stockman, J.A. (1993). *Year book of pediatrics.* St. Louis: Mosby.

Ward, H.C., & Brereton, R.J. (1988). Cervical repair of esophageal atresia. *Journal of Pediatric Surgery, 23,* 802.

Whaley, L.F., & Wong, D.J. (1991). *Nursing care of infants and children* (4th ed.). St. Louis: Mosby.

Wilkins, S., & Pena, A. (1988). The role of colostomy in anorectal malformations. *Pediatric Surgical Institute, 3,* 105.

29

GERIATRIC SURGERY

PATRICIA FELICE MECKES

A s a biologic process, aging has changed little in the last 300 years. We age neither faster nor slower than we did in Colonial America, and our maximum life span has not changed substantially. Essentially, we will enjoy a period of sustained but undramatic growth in the elderly population for the next 20 years. Beginning in the year 2010, however, with the aging of the "Baby Boomers," the gerontology boom will emerge, whether we're prepared for it or not.

The older population, which includes those 65 and older, numbered 31.8 million in 1991 and represented 12.6% of the United States population. The number of older Americans increased by 6.1 million or 24% since 1980, compared with an increase of 9% for the under-65 population. By 2030 there will be about 66 million older persons, which represents twice their number in 1990. In 1990 persons reaching age 65 could expect to live an additional 17.3 years (19.0 years for women and 15.3 for men). If current fertility and immigration levels remain stable, the only age groups to experience significant growth in the next century will be those past 55. In 1991 the 65 to 74 age group (18.3 million) was eight times larger than it was in 1900, the 75 to 84 age group (10.3 million) was 13 times larger, and the 85+ group (3.2 million) was 25 times larger (AARP, 1992).

Now surpassing the 80 to 85 age group, the 100+ elderly are the fastest-growing age group among the over-65 United States population. The Census Bureau, generally conservative in its estimates of the aged population thus far, now predicts an astonishing 1 million American centenarians by the year 2050 and close to 2 million of them by 2080. Advances in health care and the treatment and prevention of disease may mean that the average percentage of centenarians within each generation—currently about 1%—could increase to 2% or more in future years (Brandt, 1988).

Translating these demographics into health care trends produces even more startling implications for perioperative care. As a result of the "graying" of America, the health care business will never be the same. Most older persons have at least one chronic condition; many have multiple conditions. In 1990 the most frequently occurring conditions for the noninstitutionalized elderly were arthritis, 47%; hypertension, 37%; hearing impairments, 32%; heart disease, 29%; orthopedic impairments, 17%; cataracts and sinusitis, 15% each; and diabetes and tinnitus, 9%. Of all hospital stays in 1990, older people accounted for 34% of them and 45% of all days of care in hospitals. By 2000 the figure will rise to 58%. The average length of hospital stay for older people was 8.7 days, as compared with 5.3 days for those under 65 years of age. However, the average length of stay for older adults decreased 5.5 days since 1968 and 2 days since 1980 (AARP, 1992).

Of all persons age 60 and over, 50% will require surgery before they die, and those over 75 will require one third more surgery than all other age groups. Before discharge, older adults in acute care hospitals will require surgical intervention 40% more often than any other age group. Despite recent advances in surgery, anesthesia, and perioperative care the hazards of surgery in elderly patients are greater than in younger individuals (see Research Highlight 29-1).

.ᵕ.
RESEARCH HIGHLIGHT 29-1

Gross and Kammerer (1990) reported overall mortality as 1% in patients less than 65 years old, 5% to 10% in 65- to 80-year-olds, and 10% in patients older than 80. Surgical procedures with substantial high risk in elderly patients are emergency surgery, abdominal and thoracic procedures, neurosurgery, and radical neck dissection.

Postoperative mortality was attributed to cardiac disease in 12% to 32%, pulmonary complications in 28% to 62%, sepsis in 15% to 28%, cancer in 6% to 18%, and renal failure in 3% to 8%.

Gross, R.F., & Kammerer, W.S. (1990). Special topics. In W.S. Kammerer and R.D. Grass (Eds.), *Medical consultation: The internist of surgical, obstetric, & psychiatric services.* (2nd ed.). Baltimore: Williams & Wilkins.

This dramatic growth in elderly (over 65) and aged (over 85) surgical patients punctuates the necessity for perioperative nurses to recognize the special needs of these patients. Understanding how normal aging changes and chronic disease affect the successful outcome of any surgical procedure is of utmost importance and is therefore the emphasis of this chapter.

PERIOPERATIVE NURSING CONSIDERATIONS

PRELIMINARY EVALUATION

Before an elderly patient actually arrives in the operating room for surgery, many preliminary decisions are made by the physician to determine whether the benefit of surgery outweighs potential risks. In the not too distant past the attitude of some surgeons was to avoid surgery in geriatric patients until all nonsurgical modalities were exhausted. Because surgical morbidity and mortality increase with age, the surgeon's reluctance is understandable. Overall surgical mortality ranges from 3.9% to 14.1%, increases to 11% to 21% in major procedures, and is greatest in patients undergoing abdominal and thoracic surgery (Ewen and Keating, 1990). Coexisting medical disease, particularly of the cardiorespiratory system, puts the patient at great risk of mortality. However, most surgeons agree that age alone is not a contraindication to surgery. In fact, studies confirm that even the very old can have successful positive surgical outcomes (Research Highlight 29-2). More recently attitudes have changed toward a more aggressive approach and a belief that surgical risk can be substantially reduced by careful evaluation preoperatively.

Surgical decision making in the elderly is a difficult task. A frequent mistake is to compare the risk in elderly patients with that of younger patients. What should be considered more often is the risk of not operating (Cohen, 1990). The decision for surgery is within the purview of the physician, but nurses should be aware of its implications. Important factors that need to be evaluated are (1) life expectancy versus the natural course of the disease, (2) independence versus dependence, (3) motivation, and (4) risk of nonoperative management versus surgical risks (Ferris, 1976).

1. *Life expectancy versus natural course of disease*. If the patient has surpassed the expected norm for number of years of survival (persons reaching age 65 in 1990 had a life expectancy of 19.0 years for women and 15.3 years for men), surgical intervention may not be appropriate if the course of the disease is poor. Conversely, if the patient has several years of life expectancy left and is likely to outlive the condition with minimal morbidity, surgical treatment may be the treatment of choice.

2. *Independence versus dependence*. The patient's right to self-determination and making health care decisions should always be considered. The need for in-

---

☆

RESEARCH HIGHLIGHT 29-2

Schrader and co-workers (1991) reviewed the results of surgery in 46 patients over the age of 90. These patients had undergone 51 surgical procedures, none of which included invasive monitoring. There were 18 general surgical procedures, 30 orthopedic procedures, and three other unidentified surgeries.

Forty-three procedures were performed with the patient under general anesthesia and seven were done using spinal anesthesia. The 30-day mortality in this very elderly group was a remarkable 0%, and only one major complication within 48 hours after surgery occurred.

Hasting and colleagues (1989) studied 795 patients over 90 years old and compared their long-term survival from surgery with an age-matched population. There was an initial fall in survival, but in 2 to 5 years a crossing of survival lines between the two groups occurred, indicating that the surgical population had an increase in survival in the long term.

Schrader, L.L., McMillan, M.A., & Watson, C.B. (1991). Is routine preoperative hemodynamic evaluation of nonagenarians necessary? *Journal of the American Geriatric Society, 39,* 1.

Hasting, M.P., Warner, M.A., & Lobdell, C.M. (1989). Outcomes of surgery in patients 90 years of age and older. *JAMA, 261,* 1909.

---

dependence is of utmost importance to elderly persons, and they are far more interested in maintaining health than longevity. Complications of surgery are not well tolerated by the elderly and can quickly develop into life-threatening situations. If surgical intervention will further incapacitate an already debilitated individual, alternative treatment should be considered. However, if surgery will help to alleviate debilitating conditions and improve or maintain independence, it should be considered an appropriate modality of care.

3. *Motivation*. Evaluation of the elderly patient's level of motivation must be considered when surgery is planned. Many elderly patients are reluctant to undergo surgery. They are concerned that the surgery will not improve their quality of life and that it will make them more dependent on others or destine them to a life in a care facility. In addition, they do not want to withstand the pain, discomfort, and rigors of surgery and the recuperative period necessary to treat a condition that might not really bother them very much. This lack of motivation will have a negative impact on the results of the surgery. Patients who show a strong sense of determination in doing all that is necessary to get well and stay well are more likely candidates for surgery than those who believe illness

is a prelude to death. Obviously the outcome of surgery is enhanced if the patient is motivated to have a positive result.

4. *Risk of nonoperative management versus surgical risks.* Making a decision between the risks of nonoperative management and surgical intervention is particularly difficult with elderly patients. Mortality rates for emergency surgery in elderly patients are double that of elective surgery. Surgical and anesthetic risk increase in proportion to the emergent nature of the patient's condition. When an acute emergency condition taxes an already overburdened physiologic state, the chances of survival are less likely. The elderly patient's family is not consoled in knowing that the surgical procedure was successful even though their loved one died. To increase the chances of survival from a surgical procedure, the elderly person must be in optimum condition, and adequate preoperative assessment and preparation must precede an elective procedure.

Another important consideration relates to the extent of surgical treatment. The decision for the extent of surgery relies heavily on the patient's physical status at the time of surgery and how extensively the disease has progressed. The surgeon may justify a radical procedure or decide to use nonsurgical management if it will enhance the elderly person's life.

ASSESSMENT

In elderly persons a preoperative medical assessment is conducted mainly to determine present physiologic functioning. Application of these findings identifies operative risk, minimizes postoperative complications, and establishes the presence and status of any concomitant disease process that could negatively affect the outcome of the surgery. The preoperative nursing assessment is conducted to plan patient care throughout the perioperative period. In particular, assessment data are used to establish presurgical baseline data so that health status changes, primarily during the intraoperative and postoperative periods, are more readily recognized.

Using chronologic age as a valid predictor of a patient's response to surgery is not advisable. A person of 75 can be in better physical and mental condition for surgery than a much younger person. Using biologic age as a measurement criterion is much more reliable. Establishing biologic age, however, becomes the greatest challenge. Chronic conditions may interfere with the elderly person's ability to distinguish between recent and long-standing ailments. Therefore the preoperative interview, especially in elderly persons, should be conducted in a quiet, relaxed environment with as few distractions as possible. The elderly person should be allowed to respond to each question independently without prompting from a spouse or other family members unless absolutely necessary (Fig. 29-1). This helps to maintain the patient's dignity, independence,

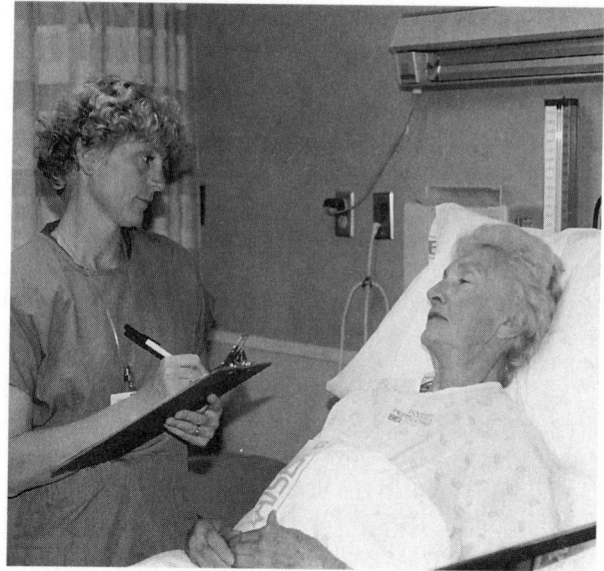

FIG. 29-1   Allowing elderly person to respond to questions independently, without prompting from family members, helps maintain patient's dignity and control.

and control, which are extremely important to the older adult.

Normal age-related changes

In general, the aging process imposes a decline in organ functions, altered responses to pain and temperature, alterations in pharmacokinetics, and atypical signs and symptoms of disease, all of which may vary from one elderly person to the next. Having a clear understanding of normal age changes helps to establish appropriate nursing diagnoses and care plan development. The following review of systems focuses on age-specific changes of particular importance to perioperative care planning.

Physiologic changes

Integumentary system. The skin loses elasticity and subcutaneous fat and becomes more prone to shear force and pressure injury. Because of the thinness of the skin and small vessel fragility, bruising is quite common. The skin tends to be dry and lacks turgor, which may or may not be attributed to dehydration. The vascular system of the skin has nutritional and protective roles. It is necessary for body heat regulation; provides defenses against microbial and physical damage; provides nutrient supply to the avascular epidermis; and promotes wound healing. All of these roles are extremely important for a patient undergoing surgical intervention. However, papillary capillaries, responsible for epidermal nourishment and heat dissipation, degenerate with aging. What is left is only the horizontal arteriovenous plexus lying beneath the skin surface. This progressive impairment of vascular circulation and tissue nutrition and the loss of subcutaneous tissue predispose to a feeling of cold, especially in cool environments like the operating room. Therefore the ability to maintain thermoregulation is compromised in the elderly and must be controlled through external measures.

Respiratory system. Lungs lose elasticity, which contributes to an increase in functional residual capacity, residual volume, and dead space. Calcification of costal cartilages, dorsal kyphosis, and osteoporosis result in a rigid chest wall. Muscles responsible for inhalation and exhalation may be weakened, resulting in a diminished ability to increase and decrease the size of the thoracic cavity. All these changes contribute to a minimal tidal exchange, which makes the elderly patient more susceptible to pulmonary complications.

Cardiovascular system. A 35% decrease in coronary artery blood flow is more likely in elderly persons. Because of a shift in blood flow, there is a greater decrease in circulation to the kidneys and liver than to the brain and heart. Blood pressure rises as a result of increased arterial resistance. When the elderly person is at rest, the heart rate remains approximately the same as that of a younger person. However, the older heart requires a longer recovery time after each beat, which means that it reacts poorly to stress and anxiety-produced tachycardia. In general, the capacity of the cardiovascular system to tolerate and buffer insults is limited.

Digestive system. The secretion of salivary and digestive glands decreases, mucus becomes thicker, and saliva becomes more alkaline. Decrease in peristalsis and a reduction of gastric motility—results of muscle tone loss—cause a delay in stomach emptying. The absorption of drugs is affected because of a reduction of blood flow to abdominal viscera, hydrochloric acid, and delayed gastric emptying. Decrease of total body water and plasma volume results in a smaller volume of distribution for water-soluble drugs. Lean body mass decreases and the percentage of body fat increases, which increase the volume of distribution and storage of lipophilic drugs such as diazepam and lidocaine (Galazka, 1988). These factors are of particular importance for assessing the patient's response to preoperative, anesthetic, and postoperative medications.

Urinary system. Nephrons decrease in function with age, so by age 75 a person has probably lost a third to a half of original nephron function. Elasticity and tone are lost in the ureters, bladder, and urethra, which leads to incomplete emptying of the bladder. Benign prostatic hypertrophy is almost universal; it is found in 70% of elderly male patients. Difficulty in voiding and retention are common with this condition. Total bladder capacity also declines, so elderly persons experience a more frequent and urgent need to urinate. Because blood flow to the kidneys is decreased, elimination of drugs through these organs is affected. The danger lies in the possible cumulative and adverse effects of drugs. Close observation and consideration of the impact of age-related changes on the kidneys are extremely important during the perioperative period. During this part of the patient's hospital stay the greatest number

and variety of drugs are given, increasing the chances for adverse and consequential results.

Musculoskeletal system. A significant change in the elderly person's skeleton is the loss of bone mass, which contributes to skeletal instability and makes fractures of the hip and vertebrae very common. Curvature of the spine and arthritis of the joints are also commonplace. Back pain is related to dehydration and decreased flexibility of the vertebral disks. Poor posture tends to be proportional to the degree of back pain experienced and may greatly compromise internal organ function. Joint range of motion is impaired to varying degrees and may affect surgical positioning.

Nervous system. Although not functionally significant, a steady loss of neurons begins at about age 25. Inappropriate or slow response to stimuli is primarily a result of a decrease in some organ systems' ability to send reliable messages to the brain and spinal cord. Nerve cells are particularly sensitive to lack of oxygen. Because elderly persons may have, in varying degrees, cerebral arteriosclerosis and atherosclerosis, decreased blood flow and nervous system deficits such as insomnia, irritability, visual motor deficits, and memory loss are not uncommon. Other neurologic changes significant to perioperative care include a loss of position sense in the toes, decreased tactile sense, and to some extent an increased tolerance to pain. In addition, benign hypothermia (temperature below 98.6° F) is a common problem in the elderly. In the operating room maintaining balance between heat gain (metabolic production, muscular contraction, and hot ambient temperature) and heat loss (radiation, convection, evaporation, ventilation, cold fluid infusion, blood loss, antithermoregulatory drugs, and impaired heat production) is difficult at best in older surgical patients.

Sensory changes. Sensory changes in vision, hearing, and cognition may have an impact on the patient's response to care. Farsightedness, or presbyopia, is a result of the lens becoming more rigid and less pliable. Consequently visual acuity and accommodation are decreased. Color perception changes, due to a yellowing of the lens, make distinguishing blue, green, and purple more difficult for the elderly person. Of particular importance in the operating room is an awareness of the older person's difficulty in adapting to changes in light. Moving patients from a dimly lit holding area to the bright lights of the operating room can cause momentary "blindness."

Presbycusis, or loss of hearing sensitivity, is irreversible, bilateral, and primarily sensorineural, although metabolic and mechanical causes are also possible. It is the most frequent cause of hearing loss in the geriatric patient. Hearing loss, which appears to be greater in men than women, is mostly within the higher frequencies (above 1000 Hz). In addition, cerumen thickens and the eardrum becomes less pliable, which also contribute to diminished hearing. Often geriatric patients are labeled confused or senile because they respond inappropriately to questions they did not hear or describe what they see inaccurately because of poor vision.

Psychologic changes

Physiologic and psychologic stress may result in confusion in the geriatric patient, which is analogous to convulsions in the pediatric patient. In the elderly, mental change can be a warning of some underlying problem. Confusion should therefore not be dismissed as an expected behavior of the geriatric patient who is, after all, "just senile." The most important assessment factor is determining whether the confusion is chronic or acute. Chronic conditions such as depression and Alzheimer's disease can make communication with the patient difficult. Depending on the stage of disease, patients may or may not be able to understand explanations. Family members are the best resource in determining the patient's ability to comprehend and respond to questions and instructions. Behavioral changes such as aggressiveness, agitation, and paranoia are not uncommon. Soft restraints may be necessary during local procedures in the operating room to ensure patient safety. Taking the time to talk slowly, being deliberate in movements, getting to know the patient, and developing a trusting relationship before surgery can help to lessen the patient's anxiety and control the combative outbursts that occur in some Alzheimer patients.

Acute confusional states in the elderly can be precipitated by any number of conditions (Evans and Kenny, 1993). Some of the most common causes are embolus or thrombosis, cardiac arrhythmia, diabetes, anemia, hemorrhage, B_{12} deficiency, infection, tranquilizers, sedatives, cardiovascular drugs (diuretics, antihypertensives, and digitalis), fecal impaction, urinary bladder distention, dehydration, and electrolyte imbalance. Even the disruption of relocation into the hospital, which brings the patient into an unfamiliar environment, can cause acute confusion, particularly during the postoperative period. Validation of the patient's previous mental state with a relative or significant other can help to determine if the onset occurred since hospitalization.

Routine laboratory and diagnostic tests

The physiologic changes of aging do not significantly alter the diagnostic values of complete blood count (CBC), urinalysis, and blood chemistries; therefore, abnormalities should be evaluated. The chest x-ray may reveal increased anteroposterior diameter, osteopenia, and degenerative joint disease. The heart size should appear normal, even in the elderly. Cardiomegaly can contribute to postoperative complications and should be evaluated. The ECG may show P wave notching, ST depression, and T wave flattening or inversion. An increase in bundle branch block, hemiblock, and first-degree block may also be noted, largely as a result of degenerative disease of the conduction system. Other diagnostic tests that are considered important for elderly surgical patients are hemoglobin or hematocrit, creatinine, BUN, glucose, and arterial blood gases. Serum electrolytes are evaluated because they demonstrate underlying disease and increased risk. In particular they should be evaluated when patients are taking diuretics because muscle relaxants, mechanical ventilation, and IV fluids can exacerbate an electrolyte disturbance (Fagraeus and Katz, 1990).

Because most elderly patients take several medications, assessing their drug history is important. Digoxin and nitroglycerin may be stopped during the perioperative period, whereas diuretics and antihypertensives may be taken as needed but not used routinely during the postoperative period. Any patient who had been receiving steroids within the previous 12 months should receive parenteral steroids starting the evening before surgery and continuing through the initial postoperative course.

Control of diabetes is often difficult during the perioperative period. For patients taking oral hypoglycemics the medication is stopped and serum glucose and urinary sugar closely monitored. Long-acting parenteral insulin is discontinued, and regular insulin is given during the preoperative period. Patients who are fasting the morning of surgery should have an IV inserted with 5% dextrose and water and receive half their usual morning dose of insulin. Thereafter, until the patient assumes a normal diet, serum glucose levels and urine fractionals are covered as necessary with insulin.

Additional assessment data

Another very important but often overlooked area of assessment is dental evaluation. The condition of the patient's temporomandibular joint and the presence of mouth pathology including loose teeth and dentures can make the difference between a smooth and safe anesthetic and a disaster. Mouth pathology, like any number of physiologic, psychologic, or social factors, can affect the nutritional condition of the patient. Many elderly persons simply do not care to eat because of ill-fitting dentures or poor dentition.

Life changes can also affect the nutritional state. Of particular importance are the losses endured with aging such as the loss of one's spouse, family, or friends through death or relocation; loss of a prior standard of living through retirement; and loss of physical or mental well-being. These changes can affect older persons to the point that they either cannot afford to buy nutritious foods or lose the ability or interest to prepare food. The ultimate effect, among other things, is a nutritionally debilitated patient. Any nutritional deficits should be corrected before surgery because the success of the operative procedure, the rate of wound healing, and the length of hospital stay are directly related to the nutritional state.

Determination of operative risk

After assessment of the patient, any number of medical conditions may be identified that can add to the patient's operative risk (Box 29-1). Additional risk factors identified by Cohen (1990) include age over 75, impaired mobility, aortic stenosis, cirrhosis, and chronic renal failure. Surgical procedures, including cardiac, abdominal, thoracic, and multioperations performed on an emergency basis, signifi-

---

BOX 29-1

Risk Factors for Surgery in Elderly Patients

GENERAL

Dehydration

Anemia

Malignancy

Recent stroke

Acute confusion, depression, dementia, pseudodementia

CARDIOVASCULAR

Recent myocardial infarction

Unstable arrhythmias

Decompensated congestive heart failure

Unstable angina

Uncontrolled hypertension

PULMONARY

Infection

Decompensated chronic obstructive lung disease

Smoking

GASTROINTESTINAL/NUTRITIONAL

Active peptic ulcer disease

Hepatic insufficiency

Severe malnutrition

ENDOCRINE

Adrenal insufficiency

Hypothyroidism or hyperthyroidism

Uncontrolled diabetes

GENITOURINARY

Infection

Obstruction

From Barry, P.P. (1987). Primary care evaluation of the elderly for elective surgery. *Geriatrics, 42,*77. Copyright © 1987 by Geriatrics. Reprinted by permission.

Class 2: Mild to moderate systemic disturbance from the condition requiring surgery or other processes

Class 3: Severe systemic disturbances

Class 4: Severe systemic disturbances of a life-threatening nature that may or may not be correctable with surgery

Class 5: The patient is in serious condition with little chance of survival

In general, patients 80 years old and older are considered class 2 and are considered at higher risk based solely on their age (Galazka, 1988).

NURSING DIAGNOSES

In evaluating, synthesizing, and prioritizing the data collected during the preoperative assessment, the perioperative nurse can formulate nursing diagnoses that will form the basis of the plan of care.

Nursing diagnoses related to the care of geriatric surgical patients might include the following:

· High risk for infection

· High risk for fluid volume deficit

· Ineffective thermoregulation

· High risk for impaired skin integrity

· Sensory/perceptual alterations (visual and/or auditory)

OUTCOME IDENTIFICATION

Outcomes identified for the selected nursing diagnoses could be stated as:

· The patient will be free from infection throughout the postoperative period.

· The patient will maintain adequate fluid volume levels intraoperatively and postoperatively.

· The patient will maintain normothermia $\pm 1°$ F throughout the perioperative period.

· The patient will maintain skin integrity intraoperatively.

· The patient will accurately perceive and interpret environmental and sensory stimuli throughout the perioperative period.

PLANNING

As a result of anatomic and physiologic effects of aging, geriatric patients have, in varying degrees, general decline in organ function and an altered ability to recover from stressful events. In addition to normal age changes, many older adults suffer from one or more chronic conditions that influence the risk of surgery. Successful surgical outcomes in the geriatric patient depend upon elective versus emergency surgical procedures, optimum physical condition of the patient, thorough preoperative assessment, close intraoperative and postoperative monitoring, and preventive measures to decrease the likelihood of complications.

A typical care plan for a geriatric surgical patient follows.

---

cantly increase operative risk. Whenever possible, medical conditions are treated before surgery. Sometimes correction is not possible, and the risk of forestalling surgery outweighs any other medical problem. The determination of operative risk for the patient is generally based on the physical status scale of the American Society of Anesthesiologists (Dripps et al., 1988). Although the actual classification of the patient is done by the anesthesiologist or anesthetist, noting the parameters from which a decision is made is important.

Class 1: No evidence of physiologic, biochemical, or psychiatric disturbance; the condition necessitating surgery is not systemic

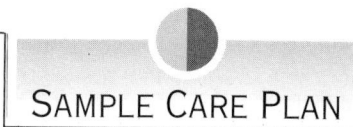

SAMPLE CARE PLAN

NURSING DIAGNOSIS: High risk for wound infection related to intraoperative procedures and length of surgery secondary to age-associated reduction in efficiency of the antigen-antibody reaction and endocrine function
OUTCOME: Patient will be free from infection throughout the postoperative period.
INTERVENTIONS:
Monitor for breaks in aseptic technique throughout the procedure.
Take corrective action for breaks in techniques immediately.
Perform preoperative skin preparation using appropriate technique as defined by AORN recommended practices and hospital policy.
Restrict traffic within the operating room.
Keep doors closed during surgical procedures.
Check equipment and assemble all supplies before surgery to prevent intraoperative delays.
Confine and contain contaminants.
Ensure availability of antibiotics as needed.

NURSING DIAGNOSIS: High risk for fluid volume deficit related to NPO status and intraoperative blood and body fluid losses secondary to age-associated decreases in total body water and plasma volume
OUTCOME: Patient will maintain adequate fluid volume levels intraoperatively and postoperatively.
INTERVENTIONS:
Monitor and record intraoperative intake and output.
Provide visualization of sponges and suction canister.
Closely monitor blood versus irrigation fluid amounts in suction bottle.
Ensure visualization of the urine drainage bag.
Ensure availability of blood replacement as needed.
Ensure availability of IV fluids as needed.
Report intake and output to PACU nurse.

NURSING DIAGNOSIS: Ineffective thermoregulation related to poikilothermy secondary to age-associated physiologic decompensation
OUTCOME: Patient will maintain normothermia $\pm 1°$ F throughout the perioperative period.

INTERVENTIONS:
Use warm blankets during transport to operating room and replenish as needed throughout the perioperative period.
Place warmed sheet on OR bed before patient transfer.
Use hyperthermia blanket beneath patient for lengthy procedures; begin warming prior to patient's arrival in operating room.
Maintain room temperature at comfortable levels.
Monitor patient for fluctuations in temperature.
Provide additional head covering (cloth, plastic, or reflective) during surgical procedure.
Prevent overexposure of patient.
Use warmed irrigation and prep (as recommended by manufacturer) solutions.
Use warmed prep solutions.
Administer warmed blood and blood products and IV fluids at room temperature.
Administer warmed irrigation fluids.
Remove wet linens before transport to PACU.

NURSING DIAGNOSIS: High risk for impairment of skin integrity related to surgical positioning secondary to alterations in skin turgor, sensation, peripheral tissue perfusion, and skeletal prominence
OUTCOME: Patient will maintain skin integrity intraoperatively.
INTERVENTIONS:
Assess potential pressure areas before anesthesia and positioning.
Avoid shearing forces by utilizing a four-person lift when transferring patient to or from the OR bed.
Place safety strap above the knees; prevent undue pressure on the popliteal space and heels.
Provide pillows and other padding devices during positioning to protect potential pressure areas.
Maintain body alignment within restrictions imposed by musculoskeletal age-related changes.
Prevent wrinkling of linen under the patient or positioning devices.
Place electrosurgical dispersive pad in the most appropriate area while avoiding bony prominences.
Avoid pooling of solutions under the patient.
Apply tape sparingly to prevent skin injury during removal.

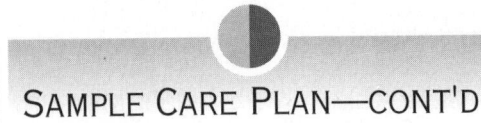

SAMPLE CARE PLAN—CONT'D

NURSING DIAGNOSIS: Sensory/perceptual alterations: visual and/or auditory related to removal of eyeglasses and/or hearing aid in the operating room secondary to age-associated changes in sensory organs

OUTCOME: Patient will accurately perceive and interpret environmental and sensory stimuli throughout the perioperative period.

INTERVENTIONS:

Remove operating room mask to introduce self and explain procedures prior to surgery.

Ask the patient to state his or her name and continue to call the patient by stated name.

Attract the patient's attention before speaking.

Face the patient directly when speaking.

Speak slowly and distinctly in a low-pitched, clear voice.

Use gestures to supplement words.

Write instructions as needed to clarify information.

Allow ample time for patient to ask questions.

Prepare patient for changes in light intensity.

Assist patient with transfers and mobility.

Inform patient before positioning or procedures done before anesthesia.

IMPLEMENTATION

Perioperative geriatric patient care is very similar to the care provided to younger adults. However, modifications are made that consider age-specific differences between the two groups. The perioperative nurse who recognizes the special needs of the elderly patient during this perhaps most critical period of hospitalization helps to enhance the course of surgical intervention and postoperative recovery.

Preoperative education

The preoperative interview is an opportune time to evaluate the patient's psychosocial status and educational needs. As previously mentioned, the motivation of the patient can have an effect on operative risk and successful surgical outcomes. Awareness of psychologic and emotional status is closely aligned with evaluation of physiologic status. Many times the patient's concerns are focused on spouse or other family members rather than on the impending surgery. An unexpected hospitalization can be very disruptive to an elderly patient who perhaps was the sole caretaker of an ill spouse, a parent, or even a pet. The worry of how that individual or pet will be cared for can have an effect on the surgical outcome. In addition, the concern for quality of life and the fear of institutionalization after surgery can be extremely upsetting. Utilizing the assistance of the discharge planner or case manager to arrange for resources may help to allay the patient's concerns.

Family members who are present should be included in the preoperative educational session when teaching the patient about perioperative routines. Ensuring that postoperative routines such as turning, coughing, deep breathing, and leg exercises are understood and performed correctly is especially important. Having backup support from a family member helps to produce successful outcomes.

Education should be conducted at a time when the patient is at rest rather than during preoperative preparations. Too much stimuli from outside sources can interfere with the patient's ability to concentrate and motivation to learn. Giving the patient postoperative instructions in written form also helps to ensure successful outcomes. The written instructions should be modified for elderly patients whose vision may be impaired. Using large type on colored paper of warm tones (yellow, tan) makes them easier to read. The instructions can then be used as an immediate reference, allowing elderly persons to maintain some control over their own care without continually having to ask for help from others. Patients should, however, be made aware that assistance is available when needed.

Sensory deficits occurring either as a result of age-related changes or merely because eyeglasses and hearing aids are removed can make communication with geriatric patients more difficult. In addition, if preoperative medications have not been adjusted in smaller dosages for the older adult, cognitive impairment may result, thus giving the nurse the impression that the patient is senile. Unresponsive or uncooperative behavior is therefore expected and ignored. As discussed earlier, acute confusion in the elderly is the most important indicator of possible underlying conditions that could seriously and adversely affect surgical intervention and outcomes.

The nurse should take advantage of the time spent in preoperative holding, the presurgical care unit, or the surgical corridor to introduce herself or himself and explain events to follow. Because a surgical mask is generally not required in these areas, this time is opportune for talking with the older adult and thus facilitating better communication. Once the patient is taken into the operating room, reassuring touch and remaining close to the patient, particularly during anesthesia induction, can help to allay anxiety (Fig. 29-2).

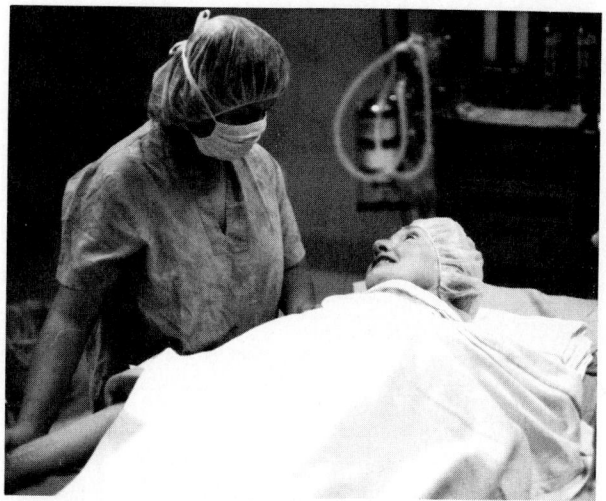

FIG. 29-2 Perioperative nurse's presence and reassuring touch help to allay patient's anxiety before anesthesia induction.

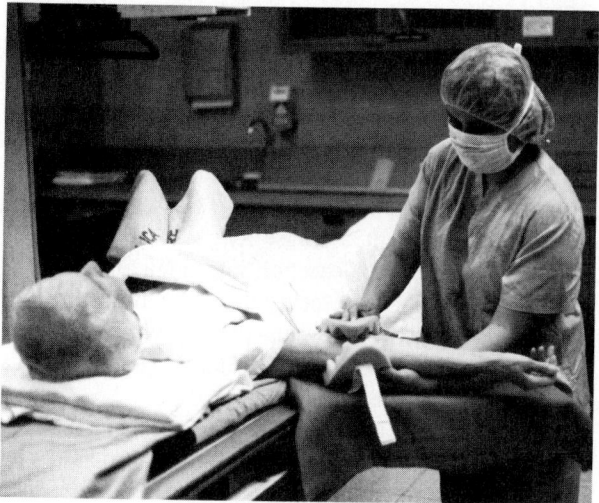

FIG. 29-3 Pillows or padding devices aid patient comfort and prevent residual pain or injury postoperatively.

Anesthesia induction

Geriatric patients frequently have changes in airway anatomy that make appropriate ventilation difficult. Changes in facial contour from sunken cheeks or lack of dentition result in an inadequately fitting anesthesia mask. Keeping dentures in place often offsets this problem; however, if intubation is planned, dentures are usually removed. The joints of the head and neck may exhibit limited range of motion, making intubation more difficult in the elderly. Assessment of these potential problems before anesthesia facilitates a smooth induction period.

The choice of anesthesia in the elderly patient depends upon physiologic status, length of the operative procedure, and preference of the anesthesiologist or anesthetist. Accurate predictions of how the elderly patient will respond to drugs or anesthesia are difficult to make because of decrease in systems function. Older patients have both an altered pharmacodynamic (relation between plasma concentration and drug effect) and pharmacokinetic (distribution and elimination of drugs) response to drugs. This is important in understanding the increased incidence of side effects. Minimal blood levels of a drug may produce undesired side effects before therapeutic levels are reached. Likewise reduced liver and kidney function, altered body composition, decreased albumin, and decreased cardiac output all modify the aged person's ability to eliminate drugs from the body (Fagraeus and Katz, 1990). The nurse should be prepared to respond quickly in assisting the anesthesiologist or anesthetist to stabilize the patient when adverse reactions occur.

Positioning

Protection of skin integrity is of utmost importance. Loss of subcutaneous fat, poor skin turgor, and tissue fragility can all potentiate a postoperative skin problem. Aging changes in the skin accentuate bony prominences and decrease in range of motion make positioning one of the most

important considerations of care. Elderly patients should be lifted into position, rather than slid or dragged, to prevent shearing injuries.

Often, because of musculoskeletal deformity, elderly patients cannot fully extend the spine, neck, or upper and lower extremities. Using pillows or padding devices to compensate for these skeletal changes not only makes the patient more comfortable during the procedure but also prevents residual pain or injury postoperatively (Fig. 29-3). Depending on the situation, positioning the patient before anesthesia induction may be best so that the patient can direct positioning efforts in regard to comfort.

Skin preparation

Temperature fluctuations are common in the elderly due to impaired thermoregulation. Warming devices are highly recommended, particularly when a lengthy surgical procedure is expected. Prepping solutions should be carefully chosen to prevent skin irritation and warmed (if recommended by the manufacturer) to help decrease hypothermic effects. Ensuring that the patient is not lying in prep solution or on wet linens also helps to reduce skin injury and inadvertent lowering of body temperature.

As the body is exposed to cold temperatures, blood is shunted away from peripheral body parts to the head. Because the head lacks fat depots and vasoconstriction capabilities, heat loss from the head can be as much as 25% to 60% of total body heat loss (Evans and Kenny, 1993). Elderly patients should therefore have some form of head covering to prevent the ill effects of hypothermia.

Aseptic techniques and safety measures

Age-related decline in the immune system and some age-associated diseases have a detrimental effect on the aging body's ability to appropriately respond to infectious agents. In the lungs, the cough reflex and ciliary action weaken specialized defense mechanisms against foreign body invasion. Incomplete emptying of the bladder can cause urinary tract infection. Immobility and drug therapy can alter flora in the intestines and make the body more vulnerable to infectious organisms. Because infection and delayed healing of wounds are poorly tolerated and often fatal in the debilitated elderly patient, strict adherence to aseptic technique is extremely important. Because length of surgical procedure is related to incidence of infection, ensuring that needed supplies and equipment are readily available is important. This practice prevents unnecessary delays, decreases surgical exposure and also the length of time the elderly patient is under anesthesia.

Fluctuations in fluid volume are common in the geriatric patient. Volume deficits occur as a natural course of aging, whereas volume excess can occur from intraoperative fluid replacement. Careful measurement of intake and output is essential. Closely monitoring sponges, suction bottle contents, and urinary drainage also helps to prevent potentially fatal complications.

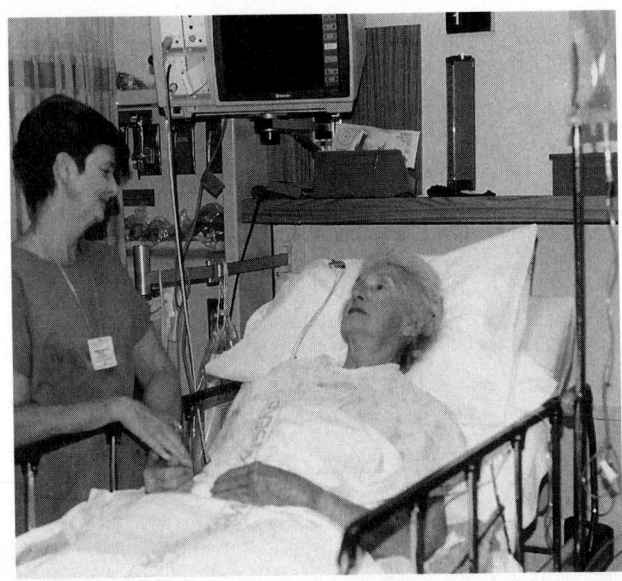

FIG. 29-4   Explanations to elderly patient before any procedure enhance cooperation.

EVALUATION

Before transporting the patient to the PACU, the perioperative nurse should assess the care provided intraoperatively by evaluating expected versus actual outcomes. Specific outcome criteria established for each nursing diagnosis provide the basis for evaluation of care.

The skin is examined for signs of injury, particularly over bony prominences and under the electrosurgical dispersive pad. To prevent skin injury postoperatively, wet linens from beneath the patient are removed, and the patient is carefully lifted from the OR bed to the PACU stretcher. Anticipated frequency of dressing change, such as in a draining wound, should govern the method used to secure the dressing. A minimal amount of tape should be used because its removal can cause additional skin trauma. Depending on the wound site, rolled gauze over the primary dressing may be better so that tape does not have to be applied directly to the skin. Another alternative is Montgomery straps. For smaller wounds the least possible amount of hypoallergenic tape should be used. Because infection is poorly tolerated, the choice of dressing should maximize wound protection while being the least irritating to the skin.

In collaboration with the anesthesiologist or anesthetist, an assessment of intake and output is completed and recorded. Because of the consequences of postoperative dehydration or fluid volume overload in the elderly patient, fluids are increased or decreased accordingly. Blood loss is carefully evaluated, recorded, and reported. The wound is closely observed for bleeding before dressing application and postoperatively because the elderly person's ability to recover from hemorrhage and shock is extremely poor.

Evaluation of body temperature is particularly important in the elderly because postoperative hypothermia is quite common and can precipitate agitation and confusion. To prevent any adverse response, the patient should be covered with warmed blankets throughout the recovery period.

As previously discussed, the elderly patient responds poorly to infectious agents. Monitoring the patient frequently for potential sources of contamination is extremely important because physical reserves following surgery are greatly reduced. Special attention to sterile and clean procedures and frequent handwashing can make the difference between an uneventful surgical outcome and one fraught with complications.

Depending on the patient's level of consciousness, explanation should be given about the impending transfer to PACU as a form of reality orientation. As appropriate, the patient should be introduced to the PACU nurse and told what to expect in the unit. Explanations should always precede any procedure. Often the elderly person is reluctant to cooperate simply because no one has taken the time to explain what is going to happen (Fig. 29-4).

Because of the relatively fine line between stability and the development of postoperative complications, the elderly patient's response to surgery must be closely evaluated. Verbal communication between the perioperative and PACU nurses should include any pertinent preoperative and intraoperative information that could affect postoperative care outcomes, including sensory limitations, intake and output; allergies, type and location of catheters, drains, packing, and implantable devices, anesthesia and medications received, and any unusual occurrences that could affect the patient's recovery (Fig. 29-5).

Documentation of outcome evaluation can be phrased as follows:

• The patient's skin integrity was maintained, free from redness, bruises, and abrasions; patient reports no pain or impairment of the skin or joint mobility.
• The patient's fluid balance was maintained; urinary

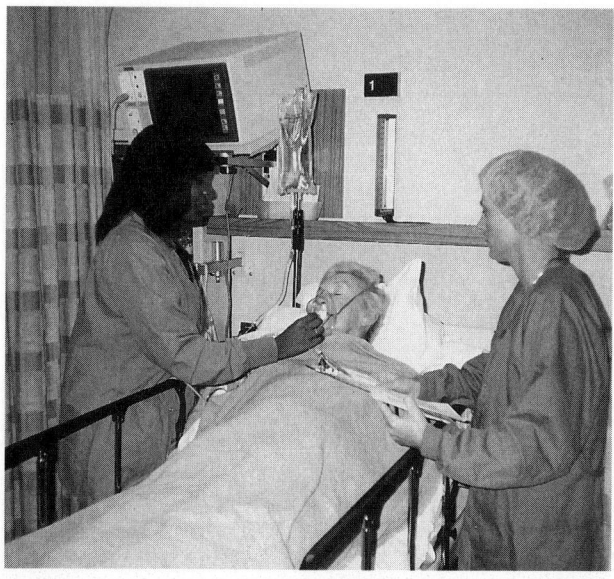

FIG. 29-5 Pertinent information that could affect postoperative care outcomes is communicated to PACU nurse.

output was within normal limits; patient's skin had good turgor, and vital signs were stable.
- The patient's temperature was ±1° F of normal range; skin was warm to touch, and patient verbalized comfort.
- The patient exhibited no signs of infection on postoperative evaluation in the surgical unit; wound was free from redness and swelling; lab values and vital signs were within normal limits.
- The patient accurately perceived and interpreted environmental stimuli, expressed and demonstrated understanding of procedures, and responded appropriately to auditory and verbal stimuli.

SURGICAL INTERVENTIONS

Unlike the pediatric patient, surgery in the elderly does not include special instruments, equipment, or drapes that are made for the geriatric patient exclusively. Surgical procedures that can be considered classically geriatric are governed more by pathology than by anatomy because the spectrum of diseases in the geriatric population is quite different from that in younger adults.

Throughout the remainder of this chapter, surgical procedures that are commonly seen in geriatric patients are discussed briefly. Reference is made to other sections of the text for a more in-depth description of the technical aspects of the procedures.

COMMON SURGICAL PROCEDURES IN GERIATRIC PATIENTS

A survey of the top 25 most frequently performed surgeries in the United States (*Healthweek,* 1989) included all age groups; 25% of those surgeries were performed on pa-

tients 60 years of age and over (Table 29-1). Of the 13 surgeries performed most often in the 60+ age group, the most common was transurethral prostatectomy at 91%, followed by knee replacement (86%), open reduction and internal fixation of fractured femur (83%), bone marrow biopsy (65%), unilateral simple mastectomy (62%), combined right and left heart catheterization (55%), cystoscopy (54%), balloon angioplasty (54%), venous catheterization (52%), left cardiac catheterization (52%), inguinal hernia repair (47%), wound debridement (45%), and total cholecystectomy (37%).

Looking at procedures done only in geriatric patients, Keating (1987) reported on surgical diseases and procedures most commonly affecting patients 65 years and older (Box 29-2). Additions in Keating's list not previously reported by *Healthweek* include cataract with intraocular lens, pacemaker implants, above- and below-knee amputations and amputations of the toes, thoracentesis, transurethral resection of bladder lesion, laparotomy for gastrointestinal and genitourinary conditions, sympathectomy, permanent tracheostomy, total hip replacement, and repair and plastic operations on bones except facial.

ABDOMINAL SURGERY

Accurate diagnosis of abdominal disease is important in the elderly to plan timely and appropriate operations. However, clinical signs of abdominal disease such as tenderness, pain, muscle rigidity, and fever are frequently less obvious in elderly patients. The common use of nonsteroid antiinflammatory drugs (NSAIDs) may mask symptoms or even predispose elderly patients to acute abdominal disease.

Surgery on the biliary tract constitutes the majority of abdominal procedures and surgical mortality in the aged. One third of emergency abdominal surgeries in patients over 70 are for biliary disease (Burns and Parikh, 1990). Most often, operations are performed for complications of calculus disease and less often for malignant obstruction of the bile ducts. The incidence of gallstones increases with age. In females the incidence rises from 5% at age 20, to 25% at age 60, and 35% at age 80.

Acute cholecystitis should be treated by cholecystectomy. Conservative treatment of an acute condition followed by interval cholecystectomy is not advisable because elderly men are prone to perforation of an acutely inflamed gallbladder, and the mortality rate is 15% to 25%. All biliary surgery in patients 70 and older should be done with antibiotic prophylaxis. See Chapter 11 for an in-depth description of operations of the biliary tract.

Upper gastrointestinal tract bleeding corresponds with higher mortality in geriatric patients particularly if the bleeding is from a gastric ulcer. The incidence of gastric ulcer increases with age. Diagnosis is established in more than 90% of cases by gastroscopic biopsy (Burns and Parikh, 1990). Some ulcers get very large and quickly extend outside the stomach into the liver and pancreas. Bleeding gastric ulcers are best treated by gastric resection. In poor risk patients suture plication with vagotomy and py-

TABLE 29-1

Top 25 Most Frequently Performed Surgeries*

| Rank | Procedure | Total* | By age group | | | | Payment | | Average stay (days) | Percent mortality† |
			0-17	18-39	40-59	60+	Medicare and Medicaid	Other		
1	Cervical caesarean section	895,574	30,661	852,020	12,893	0	168,922	726,652	4.7	<0.1
2	Total cholecystectomy (gallbladder removal)	515,358	4,525	159,203	162,290	189,340	185,660	329,698	7.1	0.8
3	Abdominal hysterectomy	441,191	126	178,808	216,896	45,361	58,762	382,429	5.3	0.1
4	Left cardiac catheterization	391,889	677	18,000	167,549	205,663	160,941	230,948	4.4	0.8
5	Transurethral prostatectomy	327,184	269	427	27,095	299,393	247,017	80,167	6.2	0.5
6	Repair of obstetric laceration	325,039	13,530	307,655	3,854	0	66,744	258,295	2.2	0
7	Appendectomy	269,851	89,466	124,581	36,264	19,540	31,637	238,214	4.7	0.1
8	Intervertebral disk excision	233,757	1,041	89,173	101,878	41,665	33,140	200,617	6.6	0.1
9	Forceps delivery with episiotomy	220,552	12,249	206,680	1,623	0	30,961	189,591	2.6	0
10	Wound debridement (removal of foreign material)	167,540	14,451	43,701	33,625	75,763	85,233	82,307	14.3	5.9
11	Contrast myelogram	165,167	1,120	57,496	66,834	39,717	35,688	129,479	3.8	0.7
12	Open reduction of fracture with internal fixation (femur)	159,099	3,496	11,365	11,938	132,300	124,393	34,706	14.4	3.7
13	Balloon angioplasty	156,347	107	5,385	66,639	84,216	60,645	95,702	5.4	1.1
14	Combined right/left heart catheterization	149,640	10,034	7,952	48,954	82,700	71,876	77,764	5.1	1.6
15	Vaginal hysterectomy	149,142	59	61,897	55,891	31,295	29,470	119,672	4.4	<0.1
16	Cystoscopy (examination of bladder with cystoscope)	142,412	3,014	26,506	35,709	77,183	75,065	67,347	7.5	1.7
17	Venous catheter	130,760	9,543	20,150	32,722	68,345	73,640	57,120	13.6	20.8
18	Unilateral simple mastectomy	121,581	125	7,556	38,974	74,926	59,465	62,116	5.1	0.1
19	Knee replacement	110,459	231	1,190	13,920	95,118	81,029	29,430	11.1	0.2
20	Vacuum extraction with episiotomy	109,163	5,345	102,853	965	0	13,269	95,894	2.5	<0.1
21	Dilatation and curettage, postdelivery	107,066	6,352	97,494	3,220	0	18,505	88,561	1.6	0
22	Open reduction of fracture with internal fixation (tibia/fibula)	103,957	8,226	42,221	29,525	23,985	21,950	82,007	5.8	0.1
23	Repair of inguinal hernia	95,012	8,781	19,767	21,735	44,729	37,393	57,619	2.6	0.2
24	Bone marrow biopsy	93,845	5,765	11,189	16,043	60,848	60,221	33,624	12.1	7.7
25	Tonsillectomy/ adenoidectomy	93,198	88,381	4,589	168	60	10,562	82,636	1.2	0

From *Healthweek,* November 1989, p. 59.

*U.S. short-term, general, nonfederal hospitals, 1988; principal procedures only.

†Patients may have died of causes related to their initial hospitalization rather than as a result of surgery.

loroplasty can lessen the operative risk. Elderly patients tolerate a surgical procedure better than prolonged or recurrent bleeding. See Chapter 10 for an in-depth description of ulcer surgery.

HERNIA

The elective repair of inguinal and femoral hernias is strongly advised due to the risk of incarceration with subsequent emergency operation. As with other emergency procedures in the elderly, mortality rates are 7.5% as compared with 1.37% for elective procedures. The operation can be performed as an ambulatory procedure, and local anesthesia provides a very satisfactory alternative to general or spinal anesthesia. General or spinal anesthesia is not

believed to be necessary and may predispose the elderly patient to significant cardiopulmonary and urologic complications. Decisions for local versus spinal or general anesthesia are made based on the patient's overall physiologic status and surgical risk.

In elderly men the coexistence of inguinal hernia and prostatism is fairly common. Depending on the size of the prostate, the hernioplasty should be postponed until after the prostate surgery.

Not unusual in the aged are large neglected scrotal hernias. The repair of these hernias is not routine in that the abdominal wall defect may be so large that primary repair cannot take place without tension. Synthetic abdominal wall replacements are helpful in management of such large hernias. The repair of huge scrotal hernias can have a tremendous impact on the personality of the geriatric patient, who is much relieved after removal of what can be considered an accessory appendage that is offensive, difficult to clean, and often an impedance to daily activities. See Chapter 12 for an in-depth description of herniorrhaphy.

GENITOURINARY SURGERY

The predominant reason for urologic surgery in elderly men is benign prostatic hypertrophy (BPH). Indications for prostatectomy are obstructive signs and symptoms that are persistent and progressive, such as urinary retention, bilateral hydroureteronephrosis, compromised renal function, gross hematuria, recurrent urinary tract infections, and bladder calculi (Van Arsdalen, 1990). BPH may be silent or have minimal symptoms in the presence of severe bladder decompensation. Prostate surgery, especially transurethral resection of the prostate (TURP), is relatively safe and generally well tolerated. TURP is indicated if the surgeon feels that total resection can be accomplished in 1 hour and there is no bladder disease or impairment to urethral access. Suprapubic prostatectomy, a transvesical adenoma enucleation, is the preferred method when the adenoma weighs over 60 g or when a stone, diverticulum, or other bladder condition must be treated concurrently (Wheatley, 1988).

Other indications for suprapubic resection are unsuitability of the patient for lithotomy position, a severe stricture of the posterior urethra, or a small bladder capacity. Complications can include pulmonary embolism, but this potential can be minimized by early postoperative ambulation. Sudden dilution of blood from bladder irrigation may occur after TURP and cause hyponatremia and hypotension requiring prompt reversal (Keating, 1987). See Chapter 14 for an in-depth description of prostate surgery.

OPHTHALMIC SURGERY

Given a long life span, undergoing eye surgery (most commonly for cataracts) is more likely than other surgical procedures. Most ophthalmic procedures are minimally invasive and have a high success rate. Because elderly patients may have concurrent systemic disease, even a low-stress procedure should not be treated lightly. Elderly patients may be confused, uncooperative or have hearing problems that may make it impossible to follow directions. In addition, they may have significant musculoskeletal disease and be unable to lie still for 2 to 3 hours. Patients with chronic lung disease lying in the supine position may experience coughing, which can increase intraocular pressure and jeopardize the surgery.

Cataract surgery is among the most common and successful of all surgical procedures. The majority of these cases are performed in an ambulatory setting with patients returning home the day of surgery. The vast majority of eye surgery patients make the decision to have the procedure done after months of deliberation and slow, progressive loss of vision. The overall mortality risk is low, ranging from 0.06% to 0.3%, and doesn't change much whether local or general anesthesia is used (Adler and Kountz, 1990). Nearly a million cataract operations are performed in the United States each year, and more than 90% of patients regain the potential for full visual acuity (Kozarsky and Cavanagh, 1988). Intraocular lenses can be safely implanted in the majority of patients. Microsurgical wound closure ensures a secure incision that allows immediate ambulation. The surgical stress is considered so low and visual rehabilitation so rapid that severe visual impairment is considered a reasonable indication to perform surgery even if the elderly patient is debilitated. See Chapter 17 for an in-depth description of cataract surgery.

ORTHOPEDIC SURGERY

Osteoporosis is the most obvious skeletal change that occurs with advancing age. It leads to susceptibility to fracture, which doubles every 5 years after the age of 50 (Ochs, 1990). An approximate loss of 40% of the mineral content of the bone must be present before detectable change is evident on x-ray. To some degree osteoporosis is related to a lessening of physical activity, but it is also related to lessened hormonal secretion. Thus postmenopausal women are more prone to develop the condition and therefore more likely to sustain a hip fracture.

Age-related changes in bone increase the incidence of displaced femoral and intertrochanteric fractures of the upper femur. Because the usual cause of death in patients with upper femur fracture is pulmonary embolus, surgery is designed to relieve the severe pain, allow movement in and out of bed, and return the patient to his or her former environment as quickly as possible with minimal debilitation.

A displaced femoral neck fracture must be surgically repaired or healing will not occur. In elderly patients, 70 and older, prosthetic replacement is usually done because it allows for early ambulation and will last throughout the remaining years of the patient's life. Intertrochanteric and subtrochanteric fractures are best treated with internal fixation. These methods also allow for early mobility (Whitesides, 1988).

Degenerative joint disease (osteoarthritis) and inflammatory polyarticular disease (rheumatoid arthritis) are the primary indications for total joint replacement in the hip and knee (DeAndrade, 1988). In these patients pain that disrupts normal daily activities and interrupts sleep is the major reason for surgery regardless of the patient's age. Usually these procedures are elective and patients have better functional status and a higher bone mass than those with hip fracture. These factors increase the success of the prosthesis (Ochs, 1990). See Chapter 21 for an in-depth description of hip and knee surgery.

CARDIOVASCULAR SURGERY

Cardiovascular disease remains the number one cause of death in the elderly. Of 500,000 persons dying of heart disease in 1992, about 340,000 were 65 years or older (*JAMA*, 1992). It is estimated that 55% of men and 45% of women aged 65 or older have heart disease. In men 65+ years it is estimated that 20% have ischemic heart disease, 10% have hypertensive heart disease, 7% have combined ischemic and hypertensive disease, and 4% have valvular disease. Elderly women have slightly different but very similar cardiovascular disease; 14% have hypertensive heart disease, 12% have ischemic disease, 7% have combined hypertensive and ischemic disease, and 6% have valvular disease (Weitz, 1990).

Coronary bypass surgery is performed in increasing numbers of patients over 65 with an operative mortality of 3% to 6%. Elective peripheral vascular reconstructive procedures are also encouraged in the geriatric patient. Patients older than 80 are reported to have had as little as 5.5% hospital mortality and a 13.8% complication rate in various vascular procedures, including cerebrovascular reconstruction, aortic aneurysms, grafts of upper and lower extremity vessels, and embolectomy in acute arterial occlusion.

In another group of 80-year-olds undergoing elective aortic aneurysmectomy, the patients' mortality rate was reported to be only 4.7%, and 86% of the patients were reported to have quality of life equal to or better than preoperative status. The facts that 25% of abdominal aortic aneurysms 4 to 7 cm in diameter do rupture and that the operative mortality rate for ruptured aneurysm is about 40% provide a strong argument for elective surgery in carefully screened and prepared elderly patients. See Chapters 25 and 26 for a more in-depth description of vascular and cardiac surgery.

ADDITIONAL CONSIDERATIONS

Every surgical procedure carries with it a certain amount of risk no matter what the age of the patient. As discussed previously, the physiologic deficits of aging increase surgical risk in the aged patient. Procedures that are performed in the thorax or the peritoneal cavity are considered of high mortality risk. Procedures of moderate risk include vascular and hip procedures, and low-risk procedures include prostatectomy and mastectomy. However, any procedure, even those considered low risk, can have poor outcomes, depending on the patient's overall condition.

No particular surgical technique is applicable to elderly patients. As described by Vowles (1979), careful assessment, good preoperative preparation, skillful anesthesia, gentle handling of tissues, and the necessary care to get it right the first time and thus avoid complications and the need for secondary operations are the steps most likely to lead to success.

REFERENCES

Adler, A.G., & Kountz, D.S. (1990). Eye surgery in the elderly. *Clinics in Geriatric Medicine, 6* (3), 659-667.

American Association of Retired Persons (AARP). (1992). *A profile of older americans*. Washington DC: The Association.

Brandt, E. (1988, October). To cherish life. *Parade Magazine*, p. 4.

Burns, G.P., & Parikh, S.R. (1990). Abdominal surgery in the elderly patient. *Clinics in Geriatric Medicine, 6* (3), 589-607.

Cohen, M.M. (1990). Perioperative responsibilities of the surgeon. *Clinics in Geriatric Medicine, 6* (3), 469-480.

DeAndrade, J.R. (1988). Total hip joint replacement. In M.F. Lubin, H.K. Walker, and R.B. Smith (Eds.), *Medical management of the surgical patient* (2nd ed.). Boston: Butterworths.

Dripps, R.D., Eckenhoff, J.E., & Vandam, L.D. (1988). *Introduction to anesthesia: The principles of safe practice* (7th ed.). Philadelphia: W.B. Saunders.

Evans, C., & Kenny, P. (1993, April). Postoperative confusion in the elderly. *Nurseweek, 6*(4), 30-31.

Ewen, E.F., & Keating, H.J. (1990). Alternatives to major surgery in the high-risk elderly. *Clinics in Geriatric Medicine, 6* (3), 481-492.

Fagraeus, L., & Katz, S.M. (1990) Anesthetic considerations for geriatric patients. *Clinics in Geriatric Medicine, 6* (3), 499-510.

Ferris, P. (1976) Surgical management of the elderly. *Hospital Practice, 11*, 65.

Galazka, S.S. (1988). Preoperative evaluation of the elderly surgical patient. *Journal of Family Practice, 27*, 622.

Gross, R.F., & Kammerer, W.S. (1990). Special topics. In W.S. Kammerer & R.D. Grass (Eds.), *Medical consultation: The internist of surgical, obstetric, and psychiatric services* (2nd ed.). Baltimore: Williams & Wilkins.

Guidelines for cardiopulmonary resuscitation and emergency care: Recomendations of the 1992 National Conference. *The Journal of the American Medical Association, 268*(16), 2174.

Hasting, M.P., Warner, M.A. & Lobdell, C.M. (1989). Outcomes of surgery in patients 90 years of age and older. *JAMA, 261*, 1909-1915.

Keating, H.J. (1987). Preoperative considerations in the geriatric patient. *Medical Clinics of North America, 71*, 569.

Kozarsky, A.M., & Cavanagh, H.D. (1988) Cataract surgery. In M.F. Lubin, H.K. Walker, & R.B. Smith (Eds.), *Medical management of the surgical patient* (2nd ed.). Boston: Butterworths.

Ochs, M. (1990). Surgical management of the hip in the elderly patient. *Clinics in Geriatric Medicine, 6*(3), 571-587.

Schrader, L.L., McMillin, M.A., & Watson, C.B. (1991) Is routine preoperative hemodynamic evaluation of nonogenerians necessary? *Journal of the American Geriatric Society, 39*, 1-5.

Top 25 most frequently performed surgeries. (1989, November) *Healthweek*, p. 59.

Van Arsdalen, K.N. (1990). Prostate surgery. *Clinics in Geriatric Medicine, 6*(3), 609-631.

Vowles, K.D.J. (1979). *Surgical problems in the aged*. Bristol: John Wright & Sons.

Weitz, H.H. (1990). Noncardiac surgery in the elderly patient with cardiovascular disease. *Clinics in Geriatric Medicine, 6*(3), 511-529.

Wheatley, J.K. (1988). Transurethral resection of the prostate. In M.F. Lubin, H.K. Walker, & R.B. Smith (Eds.), *Medical management of the surgical patient* (2nd ed.). Boston: Butterworths.

Whitesides, T.E., (1988). Surgery for hip fractures. In M.F. Lubin, H.K. Walker, & R.B. Smith (Eds.), *Medical management of the surgical patient* (2nd ed.). Boston: Butterworths.

BIBLIOGRAPHY

Arron, M.J., Martin, G.J., & Webster, J.R. (1992). Perioperative care of the elderly. *Comprehensive Therapy, 18*(11), 4-10.

Barry, P.P. (1987). Primary care evaluation of the elderly for elective surgery. *Geriatrics, 42*, 77.

Beck, L.H. (1990). Perioperative renal, fluid, and electrolyte management. *Clinics in Geriatric Medicine, 6*(3), 557-569.

Cataract Guideline Panel. (1992). *Management of functional impairment due to cataract in the adult: Clinical practice guideline*. AHCPR Pub. No. 930542. Rockville, Md.: Agency for Health Care Policy and Research, Public Health Service, U.S. Department of Health and Human Services.

Cavalier, T.A., Chopra, A., & Bryman, P.N. (1992). When outside the norm is normal: Interpreting lab data in the aged. *Geriatrics, 47*(5), 66-70.

D'Antonio, M.D. (1993, March). The new generation gap. *Los Angeles Times Magazine*, pp. 16-20, 46-48.

Dellasega, C., & Burgunder C. (1991, June). Perioperative nursing care for the elderly surgical patient. *Today's OR Nurse, 13*(6), 12-17.

Gawlinski, A., & Jensen, G.A. (1991). The complications of cardiovascular aging. *American Journal of Nursing, 91*(11), 26-30.

Interpretation of abnormal laboratory values in older adults. Part I. (1993). *Journal of Gerontological Nursing, 19*(1), 39-45.

Interpretation of abnormal laboratory values in older adults. Part II. (1993). *Journal of Gerontological Nursing, 19*(2), 35-40.

Kapp, M.B. (1990). Informed, assisted, delegated consent for elderly patients. *AORN Journal, 52*, 857-862.

Kenne, A. (1991). Perioperative assessment and nursing implications for the elderly. *Plastic Surgical Nursing, 11*(4), 143-150.

Kjernik, D.K., & Weisensee, M.G. (1992). Empowering older people is a perioperative nursing challenge. *AORN Journal, 55*(4), 1086-1089.

Lieber, C.P., Seinje, U.L., & Sataloff, D.M. (1990). Choosing the site of surgery: An overview of ambulatory surgery in geriatric patients. *Clinics in Geriatric Medicine, 6*(3), 493-497.

Maddox, G.L. (1991, Winter). Aging with a difference. *Generations*, pp. 7-10.

Malasanos, L., Barkauskas, V., & Stoltenberg-Allen, D. (1990). Assessment of the aging client. In L. Malasanos, V. Barkauskas, & D. Stoltenberg-Allen (Eds.), *Health assessment* (4th ed.). St. Louis: Mosby.

Merli, G.J. (1990). Prophylaxis for deep vein thrombosis and pulmonary embolism in the geriatric patient undergoing surgery. *Clinics in Geriatric Medicine, 6*(3), 531-542.

Reiss, R., Deutsch, A., & Nudelman, I. (1992). Surgical problems in octogenarians: Epidemiological analysis of 1,083 consecutive admissions. *World Journal of Surgery, 16*, 1017-1021.

Suter-Gut, D., Metcalf, A.M., Donnelly, M.A., & Smith, I.M. (1990). Post-discharge care planning and rehabilitation of the elderly surgical patient. *Clinics in Geriatric Medicine, 6*(3), 669-683.

Tavani, C.A. (1990). Perioperative psychiatric considerations in the elderly. *Clinics in Geriatric Medicine, 6*(3), 543-556.

Wang-Cheng, R., & Cheng, E.Y. (1990, February). Is your patient too old for surgery? *Senior Patient*, pp. 24-30.

30

TRAUMA SURGERY

ANTOINETTE KANNE LEDBETTER

Trauma is ranked as the foremost health care problem in the United States today. It accounts for the cause of death in more than 140,000 Americans per year (Lopez-Viego, 1994). Injury, resulting from trauma, is the leading cause of death for people 44 years or less, with men having a greater risk of fatality than women. Whether the injury is a result of a car accident, violence, crime, or work-related injury, trauma occurs unplanned and without warning. It can strike at any moment, which is why trauma can pose the greatest challenge to the perioperative nurse.

Historically, the potential for injury has existed since human existence. Most of the major advances in care of the critically injured have been accomplished through experience in the military. Clearly, the shorter the response time, the greater the survival rate for casualties. This was demonstrated by the success of the Mobile Army Surgical Hospitals (MASH), which brought the necessary supplies, equipment, and personnel closer to the battlefields and consequently improved patient outcomes.

Eventually this concept was applied to the civilian population and is most commonly referred to as the "golden hour" of trauma care. More specifically, the golden hour refers to the time immediately after the injury when rapid and definitive interventions can be most effective in reduction of morbidity and mortality (Sheehy, 1994).

Death as a result of trauma may occur in three phases (Trunkey, 1983). The first phase occurs immediately after the injury. This accounts for about 50% of the deaths due to trauma and is usually a result of lacerations to the heart or aorta or brainstem injury. These patients rarely survive and die at the scene. The second phase of deaths occurs within the first 1 to 2 hours after the injury, representing about 30% of the total fatalities. These patients have lacerations to the spleen, liver, lung, or other organs, which result in significant blood loss. This is the group in which definitive trauma care may have the largest effect (the golden hour). The third phase of deaths occurs days to weeks after the injury, often during the intensive care phase, and is usually caused by complications or a failure of multiple organ systems (Neff, 1993) (Fig. 30-1). In other words, time is of the essence in providing definitive care to the critically injured.

A significant number of deaths can be prevented if there is provision for rapid transport from the accident scene to a facility equipped to provide resuscitation and treatment in an efficient and timely manner. This concept is reflected in the national development of the Emergency Medical Services (EMS) system. Facilities and resources are allocated to provide specific interventions for a group of patients. For instance, in the trauma system facilities that meet certain criteria to accommodate the specialized needs of the critically injured patient are designated as trauma centers. Transfer and triage protocols that allow for a trauma patient to reach the appropriate facility with the least out of hospital time possible are established. In some areas this may be accomplished by a helicopter with a specially trained flight crew or through the use of ground transport via an ALS ambulance team (Fig. 30-2).

Trauma centers are designated by four specific levels of care that can be provided. A level I trauma center is committed to provision of qualified personnel on a 24-hour basis as well as technologic equipment necessary for rapid diagnosis and treatment. A level II center has the ability to treat the seriously injured, but most often lacks some of the specialized clinicians and resources required for the level I designation. A level III trauma center may be a community hospital in an area that does not have a level I or level II facility. A Level IV trauma center has the ability to provide advanced trauma life support before patient transfer. These facilities may be located in rural areas with limited access and may be a clinic or a hospital. Consequently, the tiering of the trauma system allows injured patients to be stabilized and transferred according to preestablished protocols that allow for the most efficient access to definitive care (American College of Surgeons, 1993).

A level I trauma facility is the receiving institution for severely injured patients in the region. In rural areas there can be a long transport time in the absence of helicopter availability. Therefore time is of the essence. A level II facility may also provide surgical intervention if resources

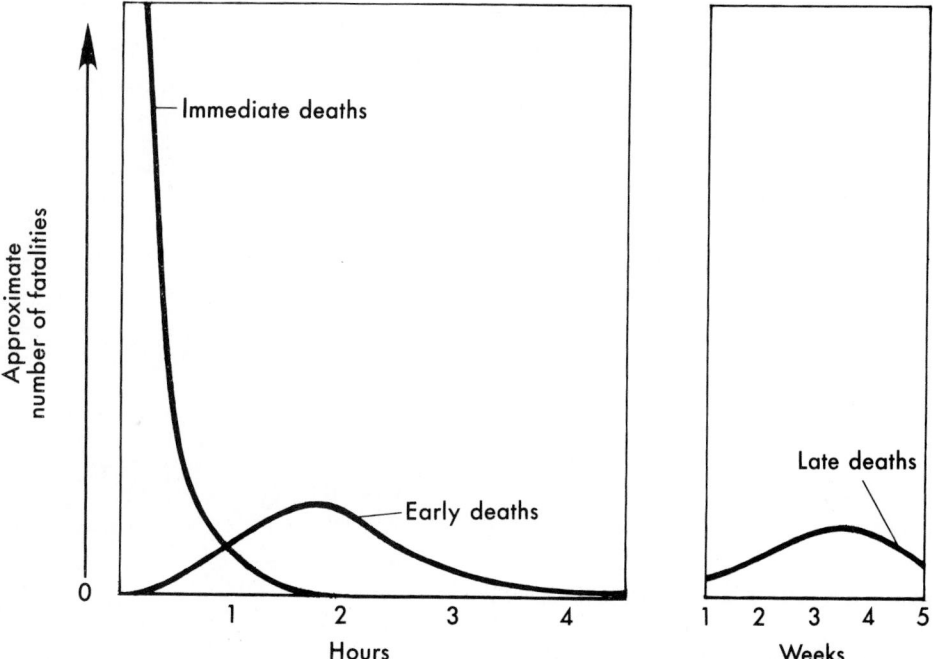

FIG. 30-1   Distribution of fatalities caused by trauma as function of time after injury. Note that trimodal distribution occurs: 50% of deaths occur in first phase (immediate deaths), 30% of deaths occur in second phase (early deaths), and 20% of deaths occur in third phase (late deaths).
From Neff JA, Kidd PS: *Trauma Nursing: The Art and Science,* St. Louis, 1993, Mosby.

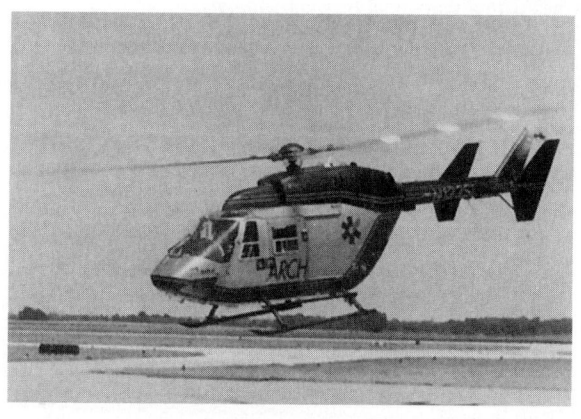

FIG. 30-2   Rotary-wing aircraft.
From Sanders MJ: *Mosby's Paramedic Textbook,* St. Louis, 1994, Mosby.

match the patient need or if the critical nature of the injury dictates immediate intervention before transfer to a major trauma facility.

Trauma patients require immediate access to the operating room 24 hours a day, 365 days a year. Some patients with an isolated system injury may be classified as urgent to allow for triage of several trauma victims at the same time. The elective surgery schedule may need to be interrupted to expedite care for the trauma patient. Such scheduling policies and procedures should be established collaboratively by the departments of surgery, trauma, anesthesia, and perioperative nursing services. Consequently the perioperative nurse should be familiar with supplies and equipment located in the operating room designated for trauma or in the operating rooms most frequently used for these patients.

PERIOPERATIVE NURSING CONSIDERATIONS

PRELIMINARY EVALUATION: MECHANISM OF INJURY

Trauma can occur at any time, and most often it is the on-call perioperative nursing team who cares for these patients requiring surgical intervention. In contrast to the elective procedure, little information is known about these patients, and preparation time is often minutes at the most. A working knowledge of the mechanism of injury is essential to assist the perioperative nurse in rapid assessment of the patient soon to arrive.

Mechanism of injury (MOI), or kinematics, involves the action of forces on the human body and their effects. Knowing the forces applied provides invaluable information in evaluation of the patient and injuries that may be present. Upon initial evaluation of the trauma patient at the scene of the injury, careful observations are made by the first responding EMS team. For instance, position of the passenger in a car, whether the person was the driver, whether the person was seated in the back seat or front seat, estimated velocity of the vehicle, location of impact, and use of seat belt or air bag are all pieces of information to iden-

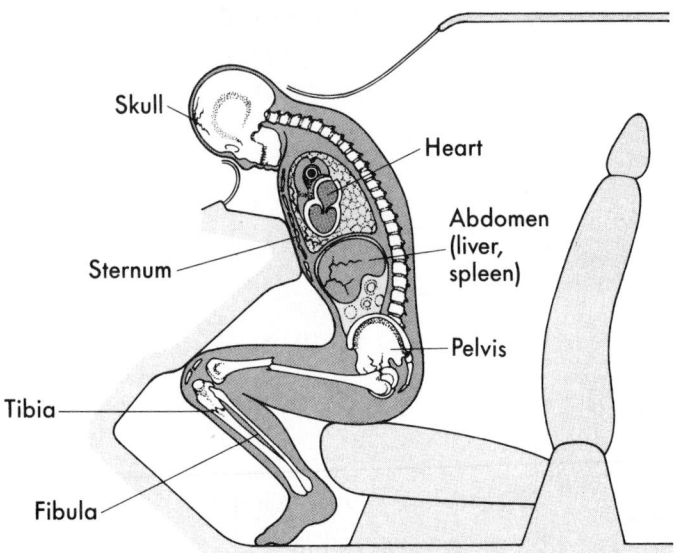

FIG. 30-3   Potential injury sites of unrestrained passenger in front seat.

From Neff JA, Kidd PS: *Trauma Nursing: The Art and Science*, St. Louis, 1993, Mosby.

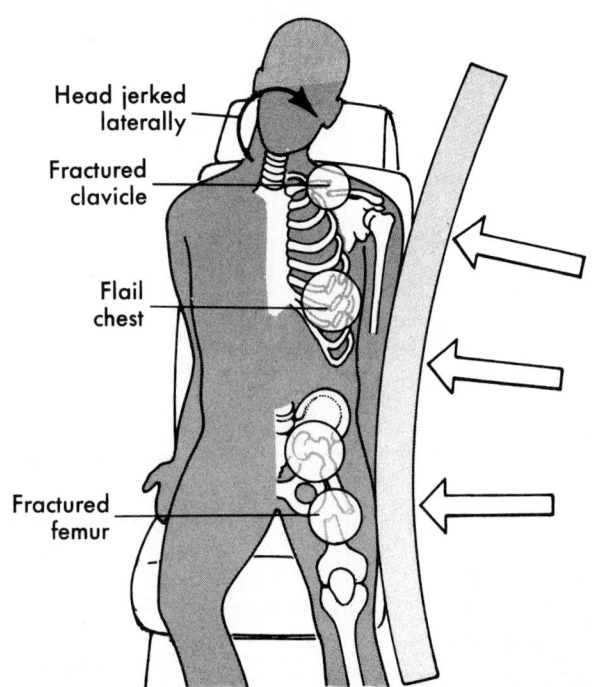

FIG. 30-4   Potential injury sites in lateral-impact collision. Note that injury is still possible in lateral crash, even with airbag inflation, because airbags were designed specifically for frontal crashes. However, injuries are usually fewer in lateral-impact crashes *with* airbag inflation than *without*.

From Neff JA, Kidd PS: *Trauma Nursing: The Art and Science*, St. Louis, 1993, Mosby.

tify the potential injuries of the patient (Fig. 30-3). After addressing the immediate threats to life, the MOI can provide valuable clues as to potential injuries (Fig. 30-4). This systematic approach can reduce morbidity and mortality (Box 30-1).

The MOI is a product of the type of injuring force and the resulting tissue response. The velocity of the collision, shape of the object, and the tissue's flexibility are all influential in the magnitude of the injury sustained. For example, long bone tissue has little or no flexibility. A strong collision involving a long bone most often results in a fracture of some type (Fig. 30-5). This is a tissue deformity greater than the tissue's ability to recover. In contrast, soft tissue injury from a colliding force may result in a contusion, a localized bruising, since this tissue has greater flexibility.

Blunt trauma is injury resulting from a combination of forces, such as acceleration, deceleration, shearing, and compression. It may be more life threatening than penetrating trauma because diagnosis is more difficult when injuries are less obvious. Examples of blunt trauma include motor vehicle crashes (MVCs), falls, contact sports injuries, and aggravated assault. The spleen is the most common abdominal organ injured. Head, spinal, thoracic, and skeletal system injuries can also occur.

Acceleration and deceleration injuries occur most frequently in blunt trauma. A ruptured thoracic aorta is an example of an injury that occurs as a result of these types of forces. In an MVC the large vessels are stopped or decelerated rapidly, resulting in vessel damage caused by stretching that exceeds its elastic ability. This affects the aorta at the ligamentum arteriosum, the anatomic point where it is

---

BOX 30-1

Predictable Injuries in MVCs

UNRESTRAINED DRIVER
Head injuries
Facial injuries
Fractured larynx
Fractured sternum
Cardiac contusion
Lacerated liver or spleen
Lacerated great vessels
Fractured patella and femur
Fractured clavicle

RESTRAINED DRIVER
Caused by lap restraint
   Pelvic injuries
   Spleen, liver, and pancreas injuries
Caused by shoulder restraint
   Cervical fractures
   Rupture of mitral valve or diaphragm

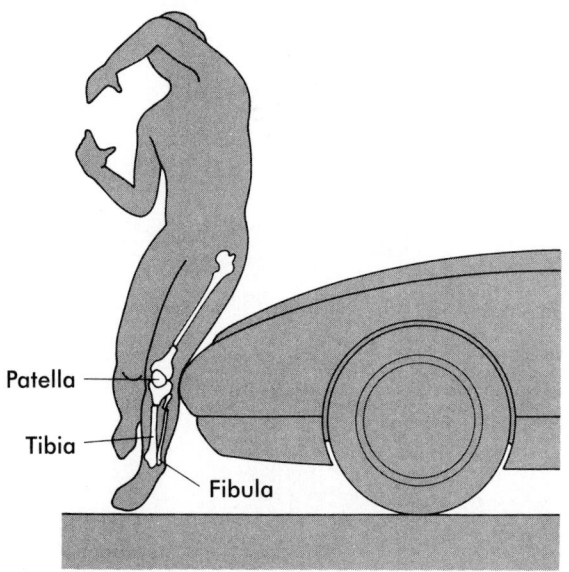

Patella

Tibia

Fibula

FIG. 30-5 Potential primary injury sites of adult pedestrian.
From Neff JA, Kidd PS: *Trauma Nursing: The Art and Science,* St. Louis, 1993, Mosby.

affixed tightly to the chest wall, just below the origin of the subclavian artery. This shearing below the attachment site causes a rupture as the aorta continues to move in a forward motion after the chest wall motion has stopped.

MVCs account for approximately 50% of blunt trauma (Lopez-Viego, 1994). During an MVC, three collisions occur. The first collision is that of a car into another object. The second collision is that of the occupant's body with the vehicle's interior. The third collision happens when an internal body structure hits a rigid bony surface. A coup-contrecoup injury of the brain, for example, is the result of an acceleration force to one area of the brain and a deceleration force to an opposite area.

Falls also contribute highly to the cause of traumatic death in the United States (Cardonna, 1994). Injuries are most commonly associated in children experiencing falls greater than twice their height. In adults, falls greater than 10 to 15 feet are usually accompanied by significant injury. Deceleration forces in falls produce forces of stretching, shearing, and compression. Consequently, aortic injuries are also suspect in this group of patients. Skeletal injuries occur as well, due to the compressive forces present.

Penetrating trauma is a result of the passage of a foreign object through tissue. The degree or extent of tissue injury is a function of the energy that is dissipated to the tissue and the surrounding areas. The anatomic structures most often injured include the liver, intestines, and vascular system. Extent of the injury includes the nature of the foreign object, such as bullet caliber, size of knife, distance from the weapon, structures penetrated, and amount of energy dissipated to the structures.

The velocity of a bullet is responsible for the degree of injury or cavitation to the tissue. A low-velocity bullet is

one that travels at a lower speed (1000 feet per second or less) and has little disruptive effect other than the bullet tract and immediate surrounding area. A high-velocity or military type weapon fires a bullet traveling at a greater speed (3000 feet per second or greater) and causes significantly more damage and tissue destruction, since the bullet tract involves more extensive surrounding tissue (Fig. 30-6). Distance from the weapon also influences the degree of injury, since the velocity is greatest when the bullet leaves the weapon and decreases as it travels. Type of bullet (such as shotgun shells with multiple pellets and hollow point bullets, which mushroom on impact) influences the degree of injury. Commonly the entrance wound is smaller than the exit wound due to the dissipation of energy, but an exit wound may not always be present. If the bullet completely fragments or is lodged in a structure internally, there will not be an exit wound. Depending on the position of the bullet and any resultant injury it may cause, bullets are not always removed.

Stab and impalement wounds are considered to be low-velocity wounds. The associated injuries usually correspond to the path of the penetrating object. Factors such as width and length, of the object assist in identification of potential injuries. A single injury site may penetrate several different organs or cavities. Penetrating injuries located at or below the nipple line may cause both chest and abdominal injuries. This is due to the diaphragmatic excursion that occurs with inspiration and expiration.

Impaled objects are not removed at the scene or in the emergency room. The impaled object provides a tamponade effect to injured blood vessels and is removed only when the ability to control potential bleeding from those vessels is present. Wound débridement may also be necessary. These objects are removed in an operating room where the needed supplies and instrumentation are present.

Injuries may also result from explosions and are related to the effects of the blast. Fragments may become high-velocity missiles, and shock waves can also produce tissue disruption. Traumatic amputations are also possible. Thermal and electrical tissue damage may occur from an explosion or as a sole mechanism of injury. These patients are usually resuscitated and require operative intervention for débridement on a nonemergent basis, unless the injury is limb or life threatening.

Injuries can be scored objectively according to the severity. This scoring system assists medical personnel in more effective triage and provides a universal method of communication between facilities, departments, and nursing personnel. The revised trauma score (RTS) (Champion et al., 1989) incorporates physiologic criteria including head injury severity (Glascow Coma Scale). The scale ranges from 0 to 12. An RTS of 11 or less at initial triage is usually an indication for transfer to a trauma center (Table 30-1).

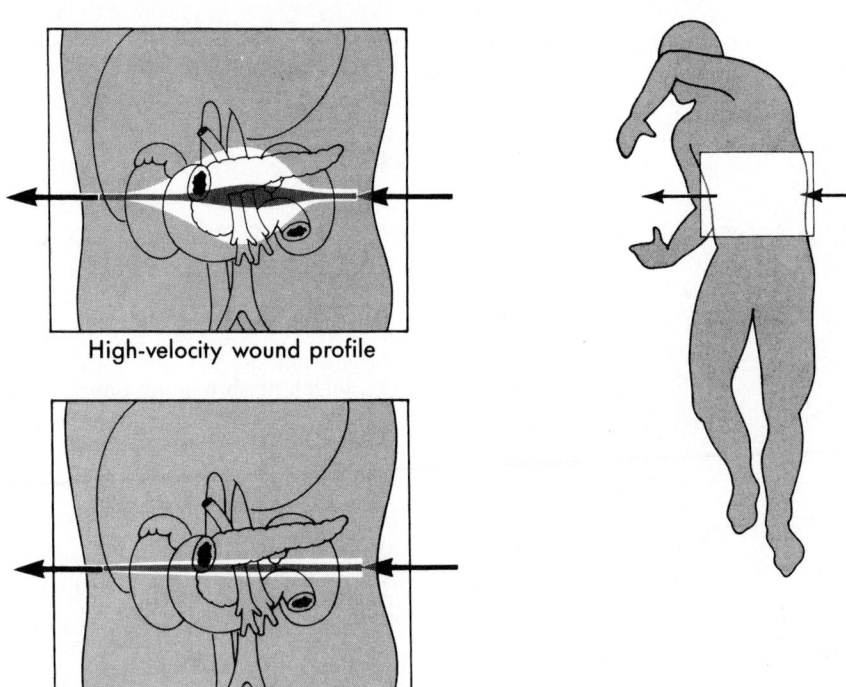

FIG. 30-6   Potential injury path of high- and low-velocity bullets.

From Neff JA, Kidd PS: *Trauma Nursing: The Art and Science,* St. Louis, 1993, Mosby.

ASSESSMENT

The resuscitative process begins upon arrival of emergency personnel to the scene and ends when the patient has been stabilized, received definitive care, and undergone a complete and thorough physical exam for determination of all injuries sustained. Upon arrival at the emergency department, the trauma team initiates a primary survey. This is a logical, orderly process of patient assessment of potential life threats. These assessment activities are based on established protocols defined by the trauma service. Utilizing the acronym ABCDE, assessment of *a*irway (with cervical spine precautions), *b*reathing, *c*irculation, *d*isability or brief

neuro exam, and *e*xposure (to reveal all life-threatening injuries) is accomplished. During this time the trauma surgeon or emergency department physician and trauma team are identifying life threats that are present and correcting them as they are discovered before progressing to the next part of the exam (American College of Surgeons, 1990). For instance, a patient may have a penetrating wound with evisceration of abdominal contents. However, the obvious is ignored until the trauma team is assured of a patent airway, cervical spine precautions have been implemented, and an effective breathing pattern exists. An evisceration needs to be corrected, but an inadequate airway is an immediate life threat and assumes primary priority.

After completion of the primary survey and correction of any immediate life threats, the secondary survey is completed. The purpose of the secondary survey is to identify all injuries present. Sometimes this second survey may be completed by the perioperative nurse, the postanesthesia recovery nurse, or the critical care nurse. A patient requiring immediate surgery is transported to the operating room, undergoes surgical intervention, and then is transferred to the PACU or ICU, depending on patient condition. This survey is a more in-depth exam of the patient from head to toe, including a back exam. The entire body is palpated to reveal any other sites of injury. All vital signs are obtained, including a rectal temperature, unless contraindicated.

A brief history is obtained from family or significant other when possible. This history is referred to as the AMPLE history and may be obtained even after the patient is

---

TABLE 30-1

Revised Trauma Score

Glasgow Coma Scale	Systolic blood pressure	Respiratory rate	Coded value
13-15	>89	10-29	= 4
9-12	76-89	7-29	= 3
6-8	50-75	6-9	= 2
4-5	1-49	1-5	= 1
3	0	0	= 0
Range 12 to 0			

From Champion, H.R., et al. (1989). *Journal of Trauma,* 29(5), 624.

transferred to the operating room by the emergency department personnel. The history includes: *a*llergies, *m*edications, *p*ast medical history, *l*ast meal, *l*ast menstrual period (if appropriate), and *e*vents or *e*nvironment leading to the accident or injury (American College of Surgeons, 1990). If obtained after the initiation of surgery, it is important to communicate the history to the surgeon and the anesthesia team.

ROUTINE LABORATORY TESTS

During the resuscitation phase two large-bore IVs (16-gauge or larger) are initiated and blood is drawn. Certain laboratory tests are usually performed. These include complete blood count (CBC), prothrombin time (PT), activated partial thromboplastin time (APTT), hemoglobin/hematocrit (H/H), blood alcohol level (BAL), toxicology screen, a type and screen, and a serum electrolyte panel (Box 30-2). The results of the laboratory studies, as applicable to the patient, should be reviewed and communicated as appropriate. Abnormal clotting studies are of obvious significance in this patient population. These results may be due to anticoagulant medication the patient is taking or the effects of profound hypothermia. H/H values are also important to note. Caution is advised in evaluating an H/H drawn in the emergency department. There can be a significant time delay between bleeding and a drop in H/H (Sheehy, 1994). Frequently, abnormal values in the blunt trauma patient alert the team to the possibility of internal bleeding. BAL also assists the trauma team in their evaluation. If the level is significantly high, the physical exam and patient response may be unreliable. In addition, the neurologic status of these patients is very difficult to assess.

A blood type and screen allows the blood bank to decrease time in obtaining a cross-match if needed later. Most trauma centers have several units of type O negative blood (universal donor) available in the event that a blood transfusion is required before a type and cross-match can be performed. Initially, trauma patients are resuscitated with crystalloid solutions such as lactated Ringer's or normal saline. If a patient presents in a hypotensive state, 2 L of warmed crystalloids may be given as a fluid challenge (State of Illinois Trauma Nurse Specialist Course, 1990). If the patient's blood pressure responds, diagnostic exam continues. However, if the hypotension returns, blood may be initiated and the patient transported immediately to the operating room for exploratory surgery.

If indicated by the injury, an arterial blood gas (ABG) measurement is also taken (Box 30-3). This test provides an accurate assessment of the ventilatory status of the patient and also evaluates resuscitative airway and breathing interventions. Metabolic acidosis or a large base deficit, with all other causes ruled out, may be indicative of internal bleeding.

Often during resuscitation a Foley catheter is inserted. After insertion, urine is obtained for a urinalysis and urine drug screen (Box 30-4). The identification of specific drugs in the urine may assist in further diagnosis and treatment.

The urine will also be dipsticked to determine the presence of red blood cells. Depending on the amount of hematuria present, there may be a renal contusion or other renal injury.

The perioperative nurse may be asked to insert an indwelling urethral catheter in the operating room. The urinary meatus should be inspected for the presence of blood before insertion. If blood is noted, the surgeon should be notified. The patient may have a ruptured bladder, an injury that is commonly associated with a pelvic fracture. The surgeon at this point may wish to perform a retrograde urethrogram to examine the bladder and urethra for the presence of tears or disruption.

DIAGNOSTIC PROCEDURES
Radiology

Depending on the trauma center protocol, a blunt trauma radiographic series is part of the resuscitative phase. This minimally includes a lateral view of the cervical spine and an anteroposterior (AP) view of the chest. In addition, lateral thoracic and lumbar spine films are taken and an AP of the pelvis. Any area with deformity, swelling, or pain may also be radiographed. Trauma patients are always treated as if they have a cervical spine injury until proven otherwise. *Adequate spine films for clearance of the cervical spine from injury are imperative.*

If the resources are available, trauma center protocol may also include computerized axial tomography (CAT scan), as a diagnostic or screening tool. Depending on the MOI, for instance a fall, a CAT scan of the head and abdomen may be performed. Since injuries in blunt trauma are very difficult to diagnose, the CAT scan is frequently taken before patient transfer to the operating room. A high index of suspicion is maintained for other injuries until proven otherwise. Bowel injuries may be missed during initial scanning. A CAT scan of the brain revealing an injury incompatible with life may alter the course of definitive treatment for a patient.

An arteriogram may be indicated in diagnosis of vascular injuries. If the patient is hemodynamically stable, this test is of great value in determining the extent of the injury. It is particularly beneficial in the diagnosis of a ruptured thoracic aorta, in which extravasation of the dye at the area of aortic fixation to the chest wall is noted. Other uses include evaluation of penetrating wounds, especially in the extremity. Vessel injury can be noted and the need for surgical intervention accomplished.

Other diagnostic tests

Cardiac monitoring is also a component of the initial phase of trauma care. Particularly important in blunt trauma, early detection of ventricular arrhythmias may be indicative of a myocardial contusion or bruising of the heart. An electrocardiogram (ECG) is obtained when indicated by the mechanism of injury or patient symptoms. Undiagnosed heart disease, as evidenced by an abnormal ECG, is noteworthy in a patient requiring operative intervention.

BOX 30-2

Normal Laboratory Values: Blood and Serum Electrolytes

RED BLOOD CELLS (RBCS, ERYTHROCYTES)

RBC values vary, depending on the age, sex, and geographic location (in relation to sea level) of the patient.

Normal values

Neonates (up to 2 months)	4.4-5.8 million/μl
Infants (over 2 months)	3-3.8 million/μl
Children (>1 year)	4.6-4.8 million/μl
Adults	
Males	4.5-6.3 million/μl
Females	4.2-5.4 million/μl
Pregnant females	Elevated

Abnormal values	**Probable cause**
↑	• Dehydration
↓	• Hypovolemia
	• Fluid overload (dilutional)

WHITE BLOOD CELLS (WBCS, LEUKOCYTES)

A white blood cell count is obtained to identify the presence of an infection.

Normal values

4100-10,900/μl (elevated in pregnancy)

Abnormal value	**Probable cause**
>10,900/μl	• Infection/inflammation
	• Tissue necrosis
	• Immunocompromise

HEMATOCRIT (HCT)

A hematocrit value is obtained to determine the percentage of red blood cells in whole blood.

Normal values

Neonate	55%-68%
7-day infant	47%-65%
1-month infant	37%-49%
3-month infant	30%-36%
1-year-old	29%-41%
10-year-old	36%-40%
Adult:	
Male	42%-54%
Female	35%-46%
Pregnant female	Elevated

Abnormal values in trauma	
↓	• Hemodilution
	From compensated hypovolemia
	From excessive volume replacement
↑	• Hemoconcentration

Note: When blood is lost acutely, the amount of hematocrit lost is in the same ratio as that of whole blood. Therefore the percentage of hematocrit in a whole blood sample would remain normal. It is only after hemodilution occurs (from shock compensation or crystalloid replacement) that hematocrit drops.

BOX 30-2

Normal Laboratory Values: Blood and Serum Electrolytes—cont'd

HEMOGLOBIN (HGB)

Hemoglobin value is obtained to measure the amount of hemoglobin in whole blood. The amount of hemoglobin determines the oxygen-carrying capacity of blood.

Normal values

Neonate	17-22 g/dl
1-week infant	15-20 g/dl
1-month infant	11-15 g/dl
Child	11-13 g/dl
Adult	
Male	14-18 g/dl
Female	12.4-14.9 g/dl
Pregnant female	Elevated
Elderly female	11.7-13.8 g/dl

Abnormal values in trauma	**Possible cause**
↓	Hemorrhage

Note: When whole blood is lost acutely, the amount of hemoglobin that is lost is proportionate. It is only after hemodilution occurs (as a result of shock compensation or crystalloid volume replacement) that hemoglobin drops.

PLATELETS (THROMBOCYTES)

A platelet count is obtained to test the amount of platelet function. Platelets play an essential role in coagulation. Particularly in trauma, platelets are essential to hemostasis when vascular trauma occurs.

Normal values

130,000-370,000/mm^3

Abnormal values	**Probable causes**
↑	• Splenectomy
	• Living at high altitude
	• Hemorrhage
↓	• Disseminated intravascular coagulation (DIC)

COAGULATION STUDIES: PROTHROMBIN TIME (PT/PROTIME)

A prothrombin time is evaluated in trauma patients to measure clotting time (caused by factors V, VII, and X, fibrinogen, and prothrombin). This is important in determining the blood's ability to clot.

Normal values

Males	9.6-11.8 sec
Females	9.5-11.3 sec

Abnormal values	**Probable cause**
↑	Deficiency of factors V, VII, X, fibrin, or prothrombin; 2.5 × normal values means that there is an abnormal bleeding tendency

Note: There may be prolonged clotting times in the presence of excessive alcohol ingestion or the use of anabolic steroids. Clotting times decrease with the use of antihistamines and diuretics.

COAGULATION STUDIES: ACTIVATED PARTIAL THROMBOPLASTIN TIME (APTT)

An APTT is obtained to screen for problems with intrinsic clotting factors (except factors VII and XIII). It can also be used to monitor the effectiveness of anticoagulation with heparin. This laboratory test measures the amount of time it takes for fibrin to form a clot. In the trauma patient, it is used to determine the patient's tendency to bleed.

Continued.

BOX 30-2

Normal Laboratory Values: Blood and Serum Electrolytes—cont'd

---

Normal values

25-36 seconds for the clot to form (after the clinical reagent
  is added)

Abnormal values	**Probable cause**
>36 seconds	• Intrinsic factor deficiency

Note: Be sure to fill the lab tube, because the tube contains anticoagulant and the ratio of blood to anticoagulant may be
  altered, causing a false prolonged clotting time if the tube is not filled.

SERUM ELECTROLYTES: SODIUM (NA)

Sodium is one of the two major extracellular cations. It is the major cause of osmotic pressure in extracellular fluid. Sodium also plays a major part in both acid-base balance and neuromuscular function.

Normal value

135-145 mEq/L

Abnormal values	**Possible causes**
>145 mEq/L (hypernatremia)	• ↓ Fluid intake/fluid loss
	• ↑ Sodium intake
<135 mEq/dl	• ↓ Sodium intake
	• ↑ Sodium loss

SERUM ELECTROLYTES: POTASSIUM (K⁺)

Because potassium is one of the two major cellular cations, it is essential for the maintenance of cellular osmosis. It plays
  a major role in the electrical conductivity of both cardiac and skeletal muscle. In addition potassium plays a major role
  in both acid-base balance and kidney function.

Normal value

3.8-5.5 mEq/L

Abnormal values	**Possible causes**
>5.5 mEq/L (hyperkalemia)	• Major burns
	• Renal failure
	• Major crush injuries
<3.8 mEq/L (hypokalemia)	• Hypovolemia

SERUM ELECTROLYTES: CHLORIDES (CL)

Measurement of serum chlorides is important for the assessment of acid-base status. Chloride is a major extracellular anion that plays a role in the maintenance of oncotic pressure and, thus, blood volume and arterial pressure.

Normal value

100-108 mEq/L

Abnormal values	**Possible causes**
>108 mEq/L (hyperchloremia)	• Dehydration
	• Renal failure
	• CNS trauma with central neurogenic breathing
<100 mEq/L (hypochloremia)	• Excess vomiting
	• Excess gastric suctioning

BOX 30-3

Normal Laboratory Values: Arterial Blood Gases

NORMAL VALUES

Pa_{O_2}	Amount of oxygen in arterial blood	80-100 mm Hg
Pa_{CO_2}	Pressure of carbon dioxide in arterial blood and a measurement of how well the lungs are getting rid of carbon dioxide (CO_2 is controlled by the lungs)	35-45 mm Hg
pH	Acidity or alkalinity of arterial blood; a measurement of hydrogen ion concentration	7.35-7.45
HCO_3	Amount of bicarbonate in arterial blood; it is controlled by the kidneys	22-26 mEq/L
O_2 saturation	Percentage of hemoglobin that is carrying oxygen	94%-100%

ABNORMAL VALUES | | **POSSIBLE CAUSE**

Pa_{O_2}	<50 mm Hg	Hypoxia
pH	<7.35	Acidosis
	>7.45	Alkalosis
Pa_{CO_2}	>45 mm Hg	Hypoventilation/CO_2 retention by the lungs
HCO_3	<22 mEq/L	Renal excretion of too much bicarbonate
	>26 mEq/L	Renal retention of too much bicarbonate

Diagnostic peritoneal lavage (DPL) can often be performed to determine the presence of abdominal injury. This diagnostic tool is of particular benefit when evaluation of the abdomen is difficult, such as when the patient is intoxicated, unconscious, or hemodynamically unstable. However, the presence of retroperitoneal blood may be missed. DPLs can be performed in the emergency department, operating room, postanesthesia recovery room, or the ICU (Fig. 30-7). It may be performed closed or open, based on established protocols, with the exception of the pregnant or obese patient and the patient with a pelvic fracture. If any of these factors are present, an open procedure is performed (Cardonna, 1994). Before the DPL an indwelling urethral catheter and nasogastric tube are placed to decompress the bladder and stomach, respectively, to avoid injury. In the presence of facial fractures the nasogastric tube is placed orally. A local anesthetic is injected just below the umbilicus and a long trocar needle or catheter over stylet is inserted and syringe attached. If 10 ml of frank red blood are withdrawn, the tap is considered positive. Otherwise, 1 L of warmed normal saline or lactated Ringer's solution is infused with a pressure bag or by gravity drainage, into the abdomen. The liter bag is then inverted, the fluid is allowed to return by gravity, and a sample of the fluid is sent to the laboratory for analysis. The presence of food particles, greater than 100,000 red blood cells, greater than 5000

white blood cells, and amylase greater than serum amylase are considered positive results (Lopez-Viego, 1994). A positive result is indicative of an injury necessitating surgical intervention.

Internal compartment pressures may be measured in the patient with an injury to the extremity. Swelling of the muscles below the fascia covering may compromise circulation and result in the eventual loss of the extremity due to tissue necrosis. This is known as compartment syndrome. Compartment pressures are measured by the use of a manometer/stopcock/syringe (Fig. 30-8) or a commercial compartment measuring device (Fig. 30-9). Normal compartmental pressures are less than 20mm. Pressures greater than 30 mm require a fasciotomy. Symptoms include severe pain, paresthesias and decrease in motor movement in the involved extremity (Table 30-2).

ADMISSION ASSESSMENT

The first opportunity for the perioperative nurse to obtain information concerning the trauma patient may be as the patient arrives in the operating room area for surgical intervention. If the patient's condition permits, the perioperative nurse should obtain a precise but brief report from the emergency department nurse containing the following information: MOI, an AMPLE history (if available), condition upon arrival (level of consciousness), availability of

BOX 30-4

Normal Laboratory Values: Urinalysis (UA)

A urinalysis is done to check for injury to the genitourinary system and for the presence of specific diseases.

NORMAL VALUES

Color	Yellow-straw
Appearance	Clear
Specific gravity	1.005-1.020
pH	4.5-8.0
Protein	Negative
Glucose	Negative
Ketones	Negative
Microscopic	
RBCs	0-3/hpf
WBCs	0-4/hpf
Epithelial cells	Few
Casts	0
Crystals	Few
Bacteria	0
Yeast	0
Parasites	0

ABNORMAL VALUES		**IN TRAUMA, MAY INDICATE**
Color	Dark or red	• Presence of blood
Appearance	Dark or red	• Presence of blood
Specific gravity	>1.020	• Shock
pH	Alkaline >8.0	• Alkalosis
	Acidic <4.5	• Acidosis
Glucose	Present	• Diabetes
		• Increased intracranial pressure
Protein	Present	• Renal failure
Ketone	Present	• Diabetes
		• Diarrhea/vomiting
Microscopic		
RBCs	3/hpf	• Kidney, ureteral, bladder trauma
WBCs	4/hpf	• Urinary tract infection
Epithelial cells	↑	• Renal tubular necrosis
Casts	↑	• Glomerular capsule trauma
Bacteria ⎫		• Abnormalities not usually seen in
Yeast ⎬		early trauma
Parasites ⎭		

hpf, High-power field.

blood products, spine clearance, injuries present and any other pertinent information (such as family present, completion of secondary survey). If the injury is life or limb threatening, implied surgical consent is assumed (that is, if the patient were able, consent would be given).

Additional data are collected as the perioperative nurse accompanies the patient to the operating room. The status of the airway, as well as breathing patterns and circulatory condition, can be observed. The emergency department record also provides information concerning amount and type of IV fluid received, vital signs, core temperature, and laboratory and diagnostics performed. A quick visual survey of the patient when preparing for the procedure enables the perioperative nurse to identify other sites of injury that might require attention.

The patient's psychologic status can also be assessed. If the patient is awake, the perioperative nurse is challenged to allay fear and anxiety. The trauma patient has endured a

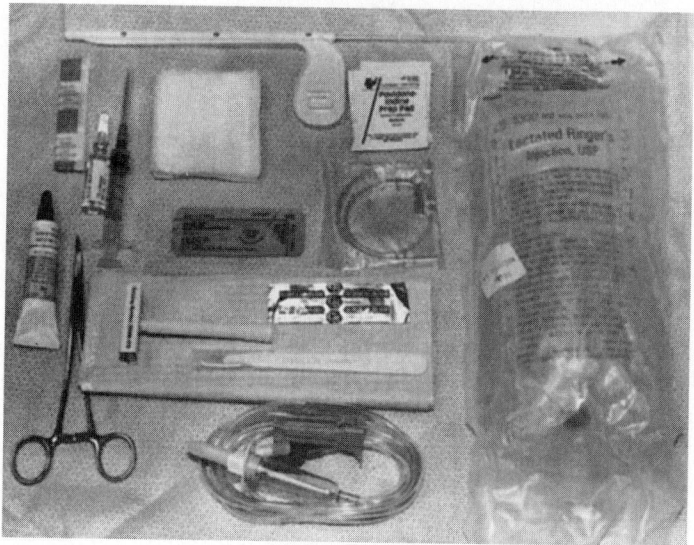

FIG. 30-7   Basic equipment for peritoneal lavage.

From Sheehy SB, Marvin JA, Jimmerson CL: *Manual of Clinical Trauma Care: The First Hour,* ed 2, St. Louis, 1994, Mosby.

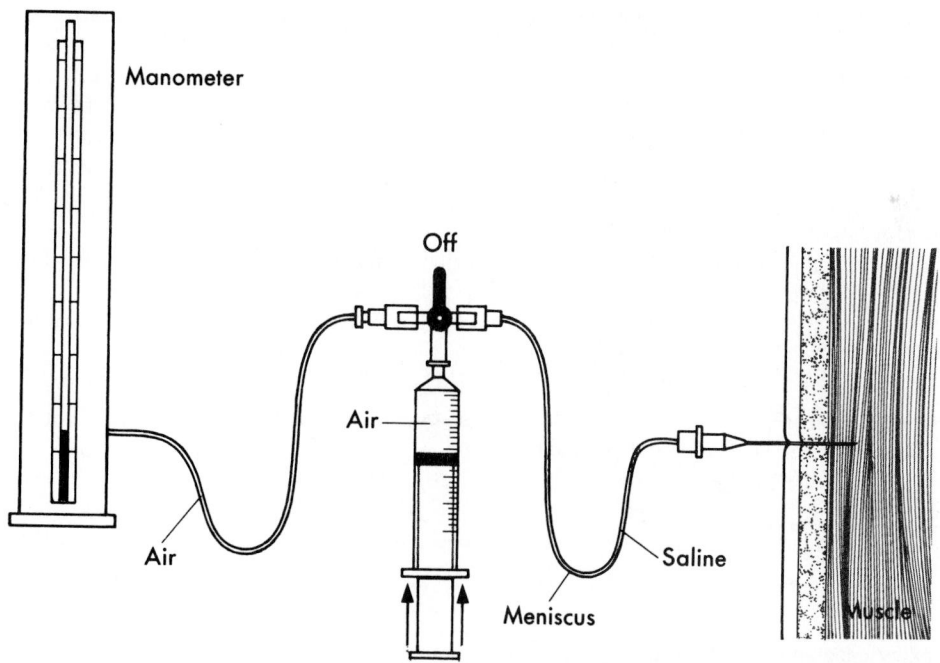

FIG. 30-8   Whitesides technique of tissue pressure measurement. Tubing is fitted to mercury manometer tubing and side port. Needle is inserted into muscle through skin, subcutaneous tissue, and fascia.

From "Acute Onset of Compartment Syndrome" by B.M. Kuska, 1982, *Journal of Emergency Nursing,* 8(2), p. 78.

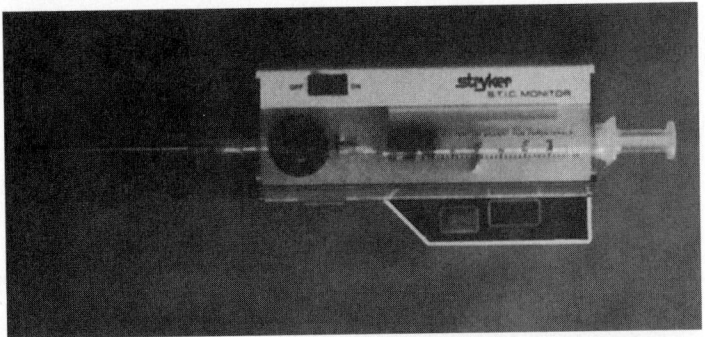

FIG. 30-9   Stryker Solid-State Transducer Intra Compartmental (S.T.I.C.) Pressure Monitor System.
Courtesy Stryker, Inc., Kalamazoo, MI.

TABLE 30-2

Signs and Symptoms Associated with Compartmental Syndromes

Compartment	Location of sensory changes	Movement weakened	Painful passive movement	Location of pain/tenseness
LOWER LEG				
Anterior	First web space	Toe extension	Toe flexion	Along lateral side of anterior tibia
Lateral	Dorsum (top) of foot	Foot eversion	Foot inversion	Lateral lower leg
Superficial posterior	None	Foot plantar flexion	Foot dorsiflexion	Calf
Deep posterior	Sole of foot	Toe flexion	Toe extension	Deep calf—palpable between Achilles tendon and medial malleoli
FOREARM				
Volar	Volar (palmar) aspect of fingers	Wrist and finger flexion	Wrist and finger extension	Volar forearm
Dorsal	None	Wrist and finger extension	Wrist and finger flexion	Dorsal forearm
HAND				
Intraosseus	None	Finger adduction and abduction	Finger adduction and abduction	Between metacarpals on dorsum of hand

Adapted from Matsen, F.A. (1975). Compartmental syndromes: A unified concept. *Clinical Orthopaedics and Related Research, 113*, 10.

---

very frightening experience and is in need of support. The perioperative nurse is often the best member of the surgical team to communicate with the patient and explain the interventions occurring before anesthesia induction. A touch or handhold is an important aspect of this communication process.

NURSING DIAGNOSES

Nursing diagnoses related to the care of many trauma patients might include the following:

- Anxiety related to recent traumatic injury
- Fluid volume deficit related to the excessive blood loss and/or decreased plasma volume
- Potential for infection related to presence of traumatized tissue and increased environmental exposure and contamination
- High risk for aspiration related to reduced level of consciousness
- Acute pain related to traumatic injury

OUTCOME IDENTIFICATION

Outcomes for the selected nursing diagnoses could be stated as:

- The patient will demonstrate decreased level of anxiety as evidenced by: less apprehension, ability to maintain eye contact, decreased quivering voice, ability to follow directions, even though anxiety persists.
- The patient will be afebrile with BP and pulse within normal limits for the patient, will have a H/H within normal limits postoperatively, and will have a balanced intake and output.
- The patient is free from signs and symptoms of infection postoperatively.
- The patient will be free from signs and symptoms of aspiration pneumonia.

- The patient reports relief from acute pain when analgesia is utilized.

PLANNING

Due to the unexpected nature of trauma, planning perioperative care is of the utmost importance. Utilizing a knowledge of kinematics, the perioperative nurse can optimize the minimal preparation time available. A high index of suspicion is maintained for potentially related injuries until the injury is ruled out. Consequently equipment, instruments, and supplies that have a high probability of use must be immediately available. Autotransfusion or cell-saving devices should also be considered during patient care preparation.

A typical care plan for a trauma patient follows.

SAMPLE CARE PLAN

NURSING DIAGNOSIS: Anxiety related to recent traumatic injury

EXPECTED OUTCOME: The patient will demonstrate decreased level of anxiety as evidenced by: less apprehension, ability to maintain eye contact, decreased quivering voice ability to follow directions, even though anxiety persists.

INTERVENTIONS:

Monitor level of anxiety by assessing the patient's state of alertness, ability to comprehend, and ability to follow directions.

Help patient to focus on the present situation to assist in identifying coping mechanisms to decrease anxiety.

Reassure patient during interactions by touch and empathetic verbal and nonverbal exchanges.

Reduce excessive stimulation by maintaining a calm and safe environment.

Explain environment to the patient and what to expect to assist in reduction of anxiety.

Instruct patient to take slow, deep breaths and utilize deep breathing techniques as necessary.

NURSING DIAGNOSIS: Fluid volume deficit related to excessive blood loss and/or decreased plasma volume

EXPECTED OUTCOME:

The patient will be afebrile with BP and pulse within normal limits for patient.

The patient will have an H/H within normal limits postoperatively, and will have a balanced intake and output.

INTERVENTIONS:

Assist in accurate monitoring of intake and output during the surgical procedure.

Monitor and report blood loss intraoperatively.

Assist in monitoring fluid volume status by completion of intraoperative labwork: H/H, serum electrolytes, BUN, and creatinine.

Consider autotransfusion or cell-saving devices when patient injuries are suspected or excessive preoperative blood loss is present. Assist with placement of invasive monitoring lines (arterial, CVP) and required fluid volume replacement therapy.

NURSING DIAGNOSIS: Potential for infection related to presence of traumatized tissue and increased environmental exposure and contamination

EXPECTED OUTCOME: The patient is free from signs and symptoms of infection postoperatively.

Continued.

SAMPLE CARE PLAN—CONT'D

INTERVENTIONS:
Preoperatively, assess the wound and identify presence of risk factors or environmental contamination.
Determine and document the appropriate wound classification.
Consider utilization of pressurized wound irrigation for wounds contaminated with debris.
Maintain a sterile environment.
Administer antibiotics as ordered.

NURSING DIAGNOSIS: High risk for aspiration related to reduced level of consciousness
EXPECTED OUTCOME: The patient will be free from signs and symptoms of aspiration pneumonia.
INTERVENTIONS:
Ensure operation of suction apparatus preoperatively.
Have suction canister and Yankauer suction tip available at bedside during anesthesia induction and postoperatively.
Provide cricoid pressure, under direction of the anesthesia team, during induction until correct intubation is confirmed and endotracheal tube cuff is inflated.

Assist with placement of nasogastric tube.

NURSING DIAGNOSIS: Acute pain related to traumatic injury
EXPECTED OUTCOME: The patient reports reasonable relief from acute pain when analgesia is utilized.
INTERVENTIONS:
Collaborate with anesthetist/surgeon on pain management to increase patient's level of comfort, if condition permits.
Assess nonverbal cues regarding level of pain and discomfort.
Provide care in a supportive manner.
Convey acceptance of patient's report of discomfort by a willingness to provide comfort measures.
Reassure patient in a quiet, calming manner.
Use a visual or numerical scale to assess change in discomfort.

IMPLEMENTATION

Multiple operative procedures

Depending on the severity of the injuries, the multiple trauma patient may require a number of surgical interventions. Some of these procedures may be performed simultaneously. This is determined through a collaborative effort among the trauma surgeon, anesthesiologist, specialty surgeons, and the perioperative nurse. If a patient has sustained severe head and abdominal trauma, the neurosurgeon will need to place an intracranial pressure monitoring device into the head for purposes of intracranial pressure monitoring. However, the exploratory laparotomy is also emergently indicated. Consequently the severe condition of the patient may require performance of both these procedures at the same time.

Multiple procedures, either simultaneously or in succession, require a great deal of preparation by the perioperative nurse and the trauma team. Order of procedures is determined by the presence or absence of potential life threats. The usual order of priority is chest, abdomen, head, and extremities. However, this priority must be determined for each individual patient situation.

Performance of simultaneous procedures should be encouraged when physically possible. Anesthesia time is decreased for the critically ill patient, and definitive surgical interventions are accomplished more rapidly.

Increased risk of infection

Many trauma patients suffer wounds that are contaminated with roadside debris, dirt, grass, or automobile parts. Other patients perforate a full stomach and release food particles into the peritoneum increasing risk of peritonitis. Consequently, these patients are at a very high risk for infection. Sterile technique may be compromised secondary only to immediate life threat. Pouring of povidone-iodine solution across the surgical site may be the only surgical skin preparation allowed when an immediate life threat exists.

Wounds may be grossly decontaminated prior to the surgical prep. Sterile scrub brushes or a mechanical irrigation-under-pressure device may be utilized preoperatively and intraoperatively. Care must be exercised to remove as much contamination as possible, without creating further damage to the wound or body part.

Traffic in the operating room should be limited to essential personnel. Often a broadcast on the radio or television will precipitate a parade of curious staff members. Increased traffic in the room increases chances for contamination to an already compromised patient, as well as potentially interfering with expedient care.

Procedure preparation

Most level I trauma centers have a designated trauma operating room that contains all equipment and supplies potentially needed for trauma patients. Many hospitals maintain an emergency abdominal procedure set, craniotomy procedure set, and chest procedure set either within the operating room suite sterile supply area or immediately available in the central supply department. This streamlines preparation for the surgical procedure and allows for the possibility of rapid preparation in those instances where the patient bypasses the emergency room upon arrival and is transported directly to the operating room suite.

Once the perioperative nurse is notified of the surgical procedure, operating room determination is made in consultation with the anesthesia staff and surgeon. Considerations include:

- Equipment required by the surgeon(s) to perform the surgical procedure
- Room availability
- Room size (equipment, staff, and multiple procedures)
- Need for additional staff
- Capability for autotransfusion or cell-saver
- Availability of emergency procedure supplies (including power equipment)
- Selection of OR bed

Additional diagnostic procedures are often required during multiple trauma procedures. A fluoroscopic electric OR bed provides increased flexibility in patient management. The bed can be rotated on its base to facilitate two teams operating at once. The fluoroscopic capabilities allow for additional radiographs and arteriograms as needed. The bed should easily transform into different positions such as lithotomy or lateral rotation. Although this bed is not required for trauma surgery, it may be considered a necessary adjunct to surgical trauma care. If a fluoroscopic bed is not available, consideration for performance of radiologic diagnostic procedures intraoperatively must be considered.

Before transfer of the patient to the OR bed, the perioperative nurse must ascertain if the spinal column has been cleared by the trauma surgeon or attending physician as free from injury. If the spine has not been cleared, the surgeon must be consulted prior to removal of the patient from the backboard. Logrolling technique must be utilized in transfer of the patient from the cart to the OR bed. This necessitates a minimum of four people, positioned on either side and one each at the head and foot of the transfer cart. The person at the head of the patient is deemed in charge. This person maintains manual in-line cervical spine immobiliza-

tion at all times and counts out loud before the rolling and transfer of the patient. The nose of the patient is kept in line with the umbilicus and feet as the patient is rolled as one unit, avoiding any twisting of the spinal column. Even if the spine is cleared, remember that initial radiographs are examined rapidly during initial evaluation, and a very subtle injury to the vertebrae may be overlooked. Therefore use of log-rolling technique during all patient transfers is advocated.

Positioning of the patient is based on the surgical approach. This is of the greatest consequence concerning chest and orthopedic procedures. Ascertaining the location of the wound, anterior or posterior, and type of operative procedure dictates the patient position. For example, an aortic injury may be approached through a thoracotomy incision or a median sternotomy. The thoracotomy requires lateral positioning devices and the sternotomy necessitates a supine position.

If several procedures are being performed, positioning may change intraoperatively. Changing the anesthetized patient's position is accomplished under the supervision of the anesthesia team. The patient is moved slowly, allowing for assessment of vital sign changes in response to the position movement. All precautions regarding positioning are reexecuted with special attention provided to the electrosurgical grounding pad. This pad may loosen during patient repositioning and may require replacement to ensure adequate pad contact.

Established sponge, instrument, and sharp count policies should address surgical procedures of an emergent nature within the institution. Every attempt is made to verify appropriate numbers of counted items, without compromising the timeliness of intervention in a life-threatening situation. If a preprocedural count is not performed, the perioperative nurse must document the occurrence and rationale utilized in accordance with established hospital policies and procedures. Some institutions require a radiograph postoperatively to examine the patient for the presence of a retained object.

In the presence of clotting difficulties or specific types of organ injuries with continuous oozing of blood, the surgeon may elect to pack the surgical site with laparotomy sponges and close the patient as a temporary measure. After a period of 24 to 48 hours, the patient returns to the operating room for removal of the laparotomy sponges and primary closure, if possible. In such instances the perioperative nurse must document and record accurately the number of sponges utilized for packing. When the sponges are removed, the exact number is verified and the sponges are isolated and contained in accordance with established hospital policy and procedure.

Autotransfusion

In this era of blood-borne disease, and considering the high blood loss associated with traumatic injuries, autotransfusion has become a vital asset in trauma care. Preoperative blood loss that is associated with a hemothorax is collected in a designated chest drainage device for reinfusion within 4 hours to avoid bacterial contamination. Intraoperative blood loss is collected, filtered, and reinfused to the patient. This provides immediate volume replacement, decreases the amount of bank blood used, and negates the possibility of transfusion reactions or risk of the spread of infectious disease.

The autotransfusion device or cell-saver requires some specialized training for operation. Institutional policies vary regarding appropriate personnel designated for operation of the equipment. Capabilities for autotransfusion should be considered during procedure preparation, since additional qualified personnel may be required.

During cell-saver use the sterile scrub team member squeezes out additional blood and fluid from saturated sponges before discarding them from the surgical field. The cell-saver suction is used whenever possible to maximize the amount of blood salvaged. However, care must be taken to ensure that the blood collected in the cell-saver is free from contamination. For instance, if the abdomen is contaminated with free food particles or colonic perforation is present, the blood cannot be used. Similarly, once antibiotic irrigation is initiated, the cell-saver is not utilized.

Evidence preservation

If the injury to the patient is a result of a violent crime, attention must be given to preservation of evidence during the course of patient care. Physical evidence (bullets, bags of powder, weapons, pills, and other foreign objects), trace evidence (hair and fibers), biologic evidence (body fluids and blood), and clothing are considered types of evidence to be preserved (Baulch and Hall, 1991). Specific procedures on handling of evidence may differ by institution and law enforcement agencies.

Clothing must be handled properly. When clothing is removed from the patient, cut along the seams or around the bullet or stab wound holes. The shape of the hole may help in identification of the weapon used. A clean white sheet may be placed on the floor and clothing placed on it to collect potential evidence. The sheet is folded up and given to law enforcement personnel. Clothing is placed in paper bags and labeled appropriately. Plastic bags trap moisture and may facilitate growth of mold, which could destroy evidence. The transfer cart sheet should also be handled in a similar manner, since evidence may be present. Descriptions of wound appearances, body markings consistent with gang or cult activity, and statements from the patient must be accurately recorded.

The chain of custody for all evidence is followed, including clothing. This process allows for identification of all people handling the evidence. Documentation must verify that the evidence has been in secure possession at all times. All evidence discovered must be recorded as to site of origin and when and to whom it was given. A system of documentation using receipts or a specific form should be established to ensure appropriate compliance.

Gunpowder residues, tissue, hair, or other valuable information may be present on the hands of a trauma patient. This evidence can be preserved by placing the patient's hands in a paper bag and securing with tape. Washing the hands should be avoided. If the patient survives the injury, this may not be feasible.

Bullets and retained implements offer valuable evidence as well in identifying the assailant. The weapon firing the bullet and the bullet itself can be linked together by the specific grooves and markings placed on the bullet by the gun barrel when fired. Most bullets are composed of soft lead, and handling with metal instruments can interfere with the markings. Therefore the use of metal instruments in the handling of bullets is avoided (Neff, 1993). Once a bullet is removed, it should be placed in dry, clean gauze into a plastic specimen container and passed off the sterile field to the circulator. The container is labeled appropriately. Following the chain of custody procedures, the circulator should dispose of the bullet according to established institutional policies. Some of the newer exploding types of bullets can offer a risk to perioperative team members during wound exploration. Care should be exercised to avoid sterile glove tears and personal injury, since these types of bullets are extremely sharp.

Deep vein thrombosis prophylaxis

Due to the prolonged immobilization anticipated for the trauma patient, prevention of deep vein thrombosis is an important concern. Placement of sequential compression devices preoperatively is ideal. These pneumatic compression devices are believed to decrease the possibility of deep vein thrombosis, and their effect is optimized when applied before surgical intervention. Preoperative placement is subject to the physician's preference; clinical research regard-

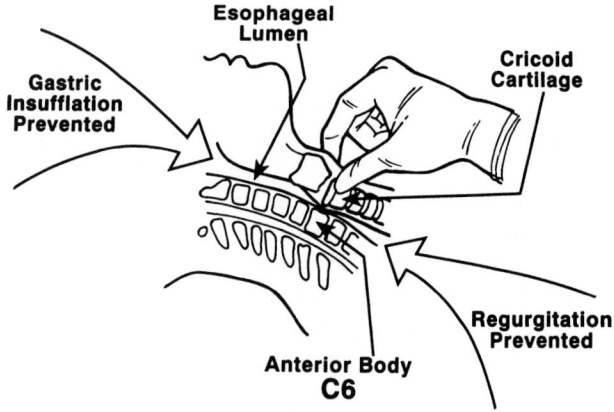

FIG. 30-10 Application of cricoid pressure. Thumb and forefinger are used to depress cricoid cartilage, causing it to impinge on lumen of esophagus, and sealing it closed against anterior body of C-6. As a result, gastric insufflation secondary to positive-pressure ventilation (bag-valve-mask apparatus) from above, as well as regurgitation of stomach contents from below, is largely prevented.

From Grande CM: *Textbook of Trauma Anesthesia and Critical Care*, St. Louis, 1993, Mosby.

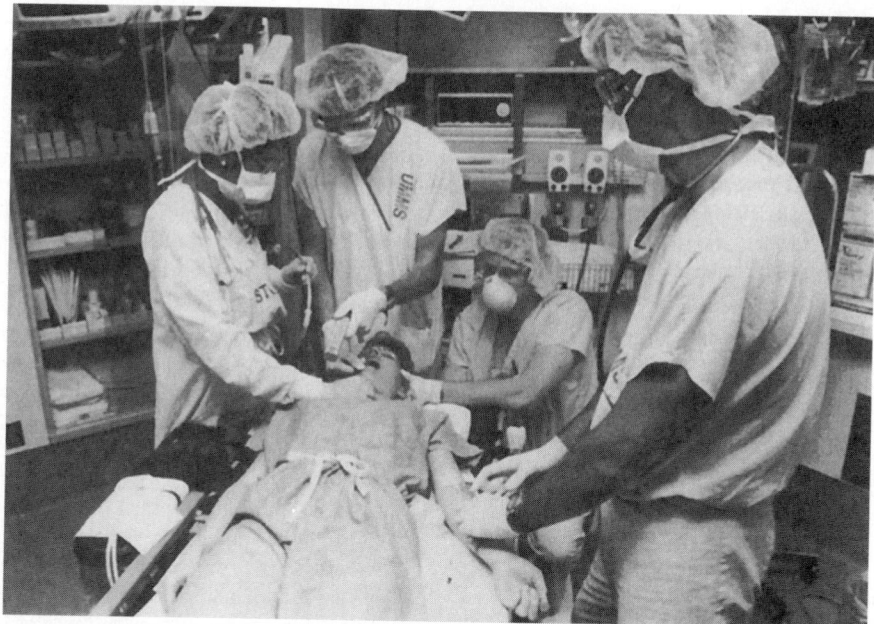

FIG. 30-11 Technique of oral intubation performed by four-person team using laryngoscopy and "manual-in-line axial traction" in emergency trauma patient. Individual on left applies cricoid pressure (while also identifying landmarks for a cricothyroidotomy if it becomes necessary) and holds endotracheal tube ready. At center, intubator opens patient's mouth with right hand and holds laryngoscope with left hand. On right, assistant (ideally, the neurosurgical consultant) uses both hands to stabilize head and neck. Note that anterior portion of cervical collar has been removed. Fourth person is responsible for administering intravenous induction agents.

From Criswell JC, Parr MJA: *Emergency airway management in trauma patients with cervical spine injury,* presented at 5th Annual Trauma Anesthesia and Critical Care Symposium, Amsterdam, June 1992.

ing similar devices and demonstrated product effectiveness is ongoing.

Anesthesia implications

Depending on institutional protocol, the anesthesia team may be directly involved in resuscitation of the trauma patient immediately after arrival at the emergency department. The anesthesia member maintains the airway inclusive of intubation, if necessary. In addition, some interventions are performed in the emergency department of a trauma center. These interventions vary from insertion of an intracranial pressure monitor to an emergent exploratory thoracotomy.

However, if diagnostic evaluation can be accomplished without intubation and sedation, the patient may arrive at the operating room awake. A trauma patient is assumed to have a full stomach. Thus these patients are at high risk for aspiration and resultant pneumonia. Under the direction of the attending anesthesia team member, cricoid pressure is provided by the perioperative nurse (Fig. 30-10). This pressure is maintained over the cricoid area until the cuff on the endotracheal tube is inflated and tube placement is verified. This type of intubation is often referred to as a *crash induction* and is used in the presence of a hiatal hernia or when NPO status is uncertain.

In addition, the patient may require intubation for protection of the airway, prior to radiologic examination of the cervical spine. If the cervical spine is not cleared or if the radiographic screening exam is not performed before intu-

bation, endotracheal intubation is done maintaining cervical spine precautions (that is, in-line intubation) (Fig. 30-11). Hyperextension of the neck is avoided, since an injury to the cervical spine is always presumed until proven otherwise in the trauma setting. This type of intubation procedure requires a person to be positioned at the head of the patient, whose *only* responsibility is to maintain the head in midline position during the intubation procedure.

In injuries of the face, where midface fractures are present, nasal intubation and nasogastric tube placement are avoided. Documented tube placement in the brain through a fracture of the cribriform plate is a well-known complication. In these instances oral endotracheal intubation is the technique of choice. Stomach decompression will be achieved by placement of the gastric tube orally. An awake oral intubation is often necessitated because anesthesia and muscle relaxants can result in the loss of any remaining airway in the presence of facial trauma.

Large-bore IV tubing used in conjunction with rapid fluid warmers may be employed in the emergency department. These fluid warmers can deliver high volumes of crystalloid solution at body temperature (Fig. 30-12). Use of the fluid warmer may continue during the intraoperative phase to facilitate volume replacement.

Hypothermia

The trauma patient may suffer from prolonged environmental exposure and be subject to a decrease in core tem-

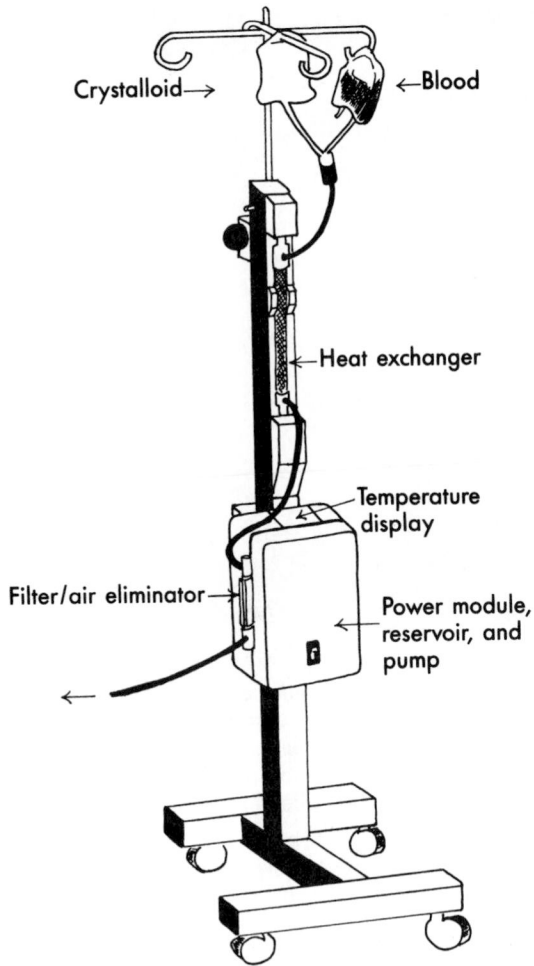

FIG. 30-12   Level I System 250 fluid warmer unit.
From Neff JA, Kidd PS: *Trauma Nursing: The Art and Science,* St. Louis, 1993, Mosby.

⋆̣⋆
RESEARCH HIGHLIGHT 30-1

Gregory et al. conducted a study on the occurrence and location of hypothermia in the trauma patient requiring surgical intervention; 100 trauma patients were included in the study, which spanned 12 months. Core temperatures were recorded within 10 minutes of arrival to the Emergency Department (ED) and postoperatively. Hypothermia was defined as a temperature less than 36° C, with severe hypothermia defined as temperatures less than or equal to 34° C. Forty-two patients (57%) became hypothermic between the time of injury and the end of the surgical procedure. Eight of these patients were reported to suffer severe hypothermia. Of the patients, 92% lost temperature in the ED, and 46% left the ED hypothermic. It was noted that patients arriving in the OR hypothermic had a more severe injury (lower trauma score), arrived in the ED colder, and received more fluids. Upon analysis of data, severity of injury correlated significantly with severity of hypothermia. No relationship was found concerning the time of year and incidence of hypothermia. The authors concluded that the severity of injury is a major risk factor in the development of hypothermia in the trauma patient. Heat loss during the prehospital and ED courses of treatment in these patients was noted to be significant. Infusion of cold IV fluids was also related. Recommendations from the study include warming of prehospital and ED fluids, use of a warming blankets, and limiting the time and amount of skin exposure. Once heat is lost, it is difficult to regain in the absence of active rewarming measures.

Gregory, J., et al. (1991). Incidence and timing of hypothermia in trauma patients undergoing operations. *The Journal of Trauma, 31*(6).

perature (Research Highlight 30-1). Immersion victims or patients whose accident occurred several hours before discovery may be hypothermic despite the ambient temperature. The perioperative nurse needs to be aware of several effects on the body when hypothermia is present. For purposes of definition, generalized hypothermia is considered to be present when the core temperature is below 35° C. These patients are subject to prolonged bleeding and clotting times. Coagulopathies of this sort become clinically significant in a multiple trauma patient undergoing surgical intervention. Viscosity of the blood is also increased. Thrombocytopenia and decreased platelet counts have also been noted. Additional information concerning hypothermia is discussed in a later section of this chapter.

The pediatric patient

Fluid resuscitation of the pediatric patient is based upon body weight as well as medications. Body size of the patient determines the instrumentation sets required. Pediatric trauma instruments, including vascular clamps, retrac-

tors, and suture supplies, should be available. Creative problem solving may be required of the perioperative nurse in adaptation of feeding tubes, drains, and other equipment.

Maintenance of body temperature is of utmost concern in the pediatric population, and undue skin exposure should be avoided. Fluids for irrigation and IV infusion are warmed. Whenever possible, room temperature is elevated and a head covering of stockinette or other suitable material is used to prevent heat loss.

Blunt injury and falls are the most common mechanisms of injury in the child, including pedestrian–motor vehicle accidents (Cardonna, 1994). Due to the pliable nature of the skeletal system, if broken bones are present, a severe force of injury must be assumed. Neurologic injuries are the most common in children, but a high index of suspicion is maintained for other severe injuries. As children have a much smaller reserve than adults, once a decline in vital functions is noted, demise is rapid (Tables 30-3 and 30-4; Boxes 30-5 and 30-6).

TABLE 30-3

Sizes for Pediatric Airway Equipment

Age	Laryngoscope	Endotracheal tube size	Suction catheter (French)
Infant (Birth-12 months)	Miller 0-1	2.5-4.5 (uncuffed)	5-8
		4.5 (uncuffed)	8
Toddler (1-3 years)	Miller 2		
	Flagg 2		
Preschool-age child (4-5 years)	Miller 2	5.0 (uncuffed)	10
	Flagg 2		
School-age child (6-12 years)	Miller 2	5.5-7.0 (uncuffed to the age of 8)	10-12
	MacIntosh 2		
Adolescent (13-20 years)	MacIntosh 3	7.0-8.0 (cuffed)	12
	Miller 3		

Adapted from Chameides, L. (Ed.). (1988). *Textbook of pediatric advanced life support.* Dallas: American Heart Association.

TABLE 30-4

Normal Respiration and Heart Rates for the Pediatric Patient

Age	Respiration (breaths/minute)	Heart (beats/minute)
Infant (birth-12 months)	30-60	120-160
Toddler (1-3 years)	25-40	90-140
Preschool-age child (4-6 years)	22-34	80-110
School-age child (6-12 years)	18-30	75-100
Adolescent (13-18 years)	12-20	60-100

BOX 30-5

Specific Differences Between the Adult and Pediatric Trauma Patient

- Growth, development, and psychologic skills vary with age.
- Children have smaller airways with more soft tissue and a narrowing of the cricoid cartilage. The openings of the trachea and esophagus are closer together, which can make intubation more difficult.
- Children have faster respiratory rates and become hypoxic more quickly.
- The temperature control mechanism is immature in infants and small children.
- Children are easily dehydrated.
- Children have faster heart rates.
- Young children's extremities are likely to appear mottled. This may be a response to cold. Capillary refill may be a better indicator of circulatory status in the child.

A cuffless endotracheal tube is used in infants and children. The size can be approximated by noting the width of the fifth digit of the hand. IV access is often difficult in the pediatric patient, and an intraosseous line may be initiated in the emergency department. These lines are inserted by using an intraosseous needle or bone marrow aspirate needle and are placed slightly below the knee on the anterior aspect of the tibia at a 90-degree angle (Fig. 30-13). Stabilization of the line may be difficult, but the line can remain for up to 24 hours and provides rapid access when other routes are too time consuming or difficult to access.

Pregnancy

The normal physiologic changes that occur during pregnancy increase the challenge of evaluation and treatment when these individuals are victims of trauma. It is most important to remember that two patients are being treated. The

BOX 30-6

Estimating Blood Pressure for the Pediatric Patient

Systolic BP (mm Hg) = (2 × Age in years) + 80
Diastolic BP (mm Hg) = ⅔ systolic

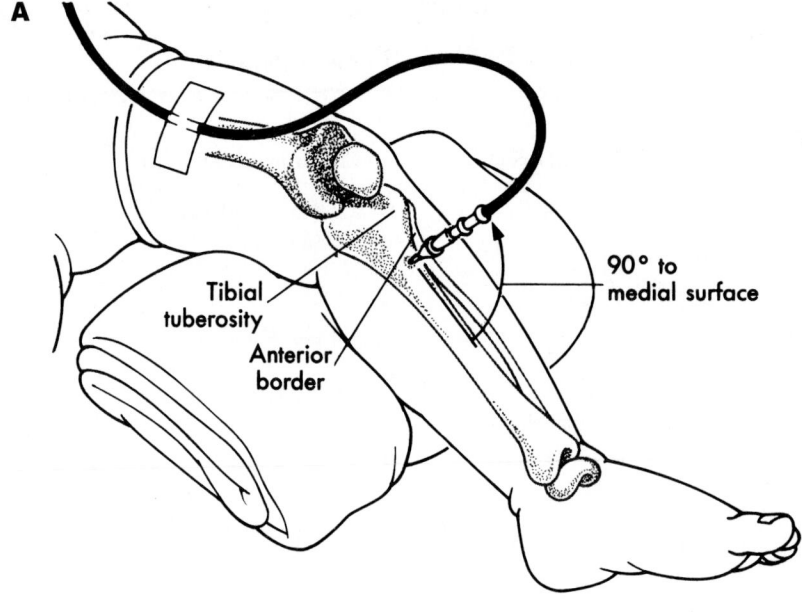

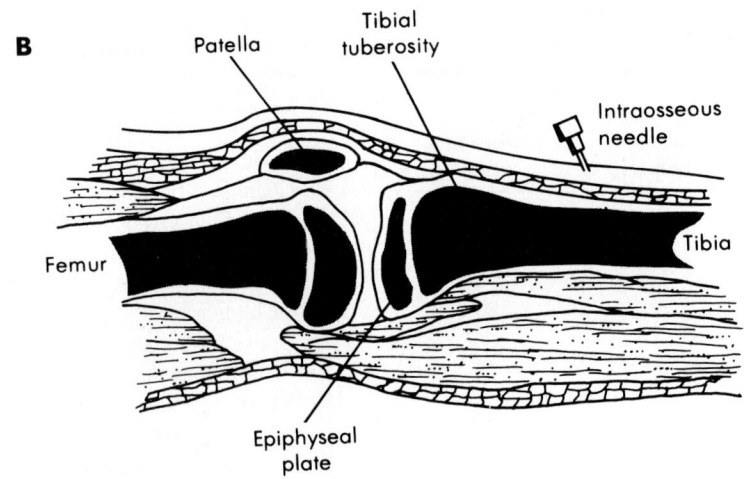

FIG. 30-13 **A,** Intraosseous infusion technique. **B,** Insertion.

Note. A, Redrawn from *Pediatric Advanced Life Support* (p. 44) by L. Chameides (Ed.), 1988, Dallas: American Heart Association. **B,** From *Emergency pediatrics: A guide to ambulatory care* (3rd ed.) by R.M. Barkin and P. Rosen, 1990, St. Louis: Mosby-Year Book, Inc.

key to resuscitation of the fetus is to resuscitate the mother. One of the first physiologic changes to note is that the pregnant trauma patient has a much larger circulatory volume. The cardiac output may be increased by as much as 40%. Oxygen requirements are increased. Heart rate increases over the prepregnant state (Table 30-5). It becomes obvious that the usual clinical indicators of hypovolemic shock are unreliable in the pregnant trauma patient (Table 30-6). It is imperative that the pregnant trauma victim be assumed to be in shock until proven otherwise. Early aggressive treatment is a must. The uterus is enlarged and no longer a pelvic organ, and it elevates the bladder out of the pelvis as well. Supine position for the pregnant patient can result

in a decrease in cardiac output as a result of compression of the inferior vena cava. By term, there can be as much as 30% reduction of cardiac output as a result of compression on the inferior vena cava (Cardonna, 1994). Consequently, patients who are 20 weeks or more into their pregnancy should be placed in the left lateral decubitus position to avoid a hypotensive episode. If this is not possible, manual displacement of the uterus by lateral abdominal pressure should be attempted.

The pregnant trauma patient and fetus are treated as one during the resuscitative phase. The best chance of maintaining the viability of the fetus is in expedient treatment of the mother. Ultrasound studies are conducted to deter-

---

TABLE 30-5

Central Hemodynamic Changes

	Nonpregnant	Pregnant
Cardiac output (L/min)	4.3 ± 0.9	6.2 ± 1.0
Heart rate (beats/min)	71 ± 10.0	83 ± 10.0
Systemic vascular resistance (dyne $\times$ cm $\times$ sec^{-5})	1530 ± 520	1210 ± 266
Pulmonary vascular resistance (dyne $\times$ cm $\times$ sec^{-5})	119 ± 47.0	78 ± 22
Colloid oncotic pressure (mm Hg)	20.8 ± 1.0	18.0 ± 1.5
Colloid oncotic pressure/pulmonary capillary wedge pressure (mm Hg)	14.5 ± 2.5	10.5 ± 2.7
Mean arterial pressure (mm Hg)	86.4 ± 7.5	90.3 ± 5.8
Pulmonary capillary wedge pressure (mm Hg)	6.3 ± 2.1	7.5 ± 1.8
Central venous pressure (mm Hg)	3.7 ± 2.6	3.6 ± 2.5
Left ventricular stroke	41 ± 8	48 ± 6

From Clark, S., Cotton, O., Lee, W., et al. (1989). Central hemodynamic assessment of normal term pregnancy. *American Journal of Obstetrics and Gynecology*, 161, 1439-1442.

TABLE 30-6

Signs of Hypovolemic Shock in Pregnancy

Circulating blood volume deficit	Early (20%)	Late (25%)
Pulse	<100 beats per minute	>100 beats per minute
Respiratory rate	12-20 per minute	>20 per minute
Blood pressure	Normal	Hypotensive
Skin perfusion	Warm, dry skin	Cool, ashen skin
Capillary refill	<2 seconds	>2 seconds
Level of consciousness	Alert	Agitated, lethargic
Urine output	>30-50 ml/hr	<30-50 ml/hr
Fetal heart rate*	High; low, with late decelerations	High, low, absent, late decelerations

*Fetal heart rate normally 120-160 beats per minute.

---

mine viability of the fetus when possible. In the event of a ruptured uterus, a cesarean section and hysterectomy may be required, if the fetus is viable. Neonatal resuscitation is of the utmost importance immediately on delivery of the fetus.

Fetuses of pregnant patients requiring surgery require fetal assessment intraoperatively. Any fetal movement should be noted. In addition, fetal monitoring is continuous. This is inclusive of fetal heart rate and uterine contractions. Fetal monitoring provides information on the condition of the fetus and response to uterine contractions, if present. Fetal heart rate can usually be obtained after 10 weeks of gestation. Personnel qualified in the interpretation of fetal heart rate patterns must be present. This expertise may be provided by the obstetric nursing staff.

Perimortem (postmortem) cesarean section may be performed in the event of the sudden death of the mother and presence of a viable fetus. The fetus can survive approxi-

mately 10 minutes of anoxia without severe side effects (Neff, 1993). An emergency cesarean section may also alter the maternal outcome favorably by improving the hemodynamic state in a clinically dead patient.

Emergency department (ED) interventions

If a patient has had very recent loss of vital signs, either on route to the hospital or upon arrival at the ED, the trauma surgeon may elect to perform an emergency thoracotomy in the ED. A left-sided approach is usually performed, since this allows rapid access to the heart for external cardiac massage and exposure of the great vessels for clamping in the event of severe blood loss. The incision can be extended to the right side by cutting across the sternum. This procedure can be used to gain control in hemorrhage of the great vessels, to access the heart, or in a grave situation as a final effort to save a life (Fig. 30-14). The procedure is utilized more often in penetrating injuries where a laceration

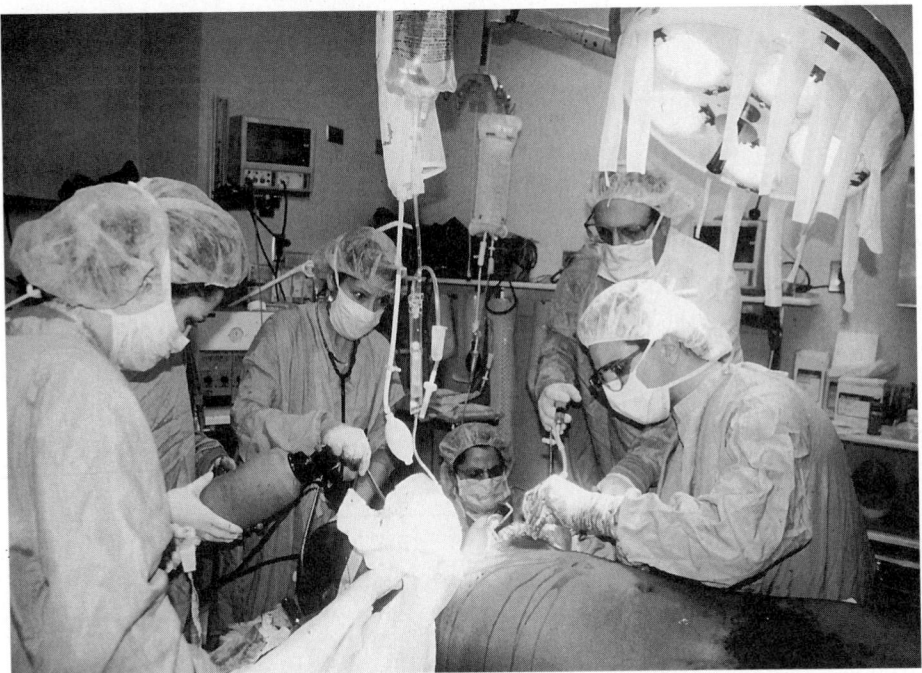

FIG. 30-14   Patient undergoing emergency department exploratory thoracotomy.

to a ventricle or other potentially treatable, life-threatening injury may be present.

Because of the knowledge of surgical instrumentation held by the perioperative nurse, assistance in this procedure in the ED is often required of the perioperative team. Rapid access to the heart and great vessels is the goal. The patient is transported to the operating room suite for additional interventions once hemorrhage control is established.

In a similar fashion an exploratory laparotomy can be initiated in the ED to control abdominal hemorrhage, especially when a splenic rupture is suspected and the patient is severely compromised.

If all other techniques of airway access are unsuccessful, a cricothyrotomy is performed. A vertical incision is made through the skin and the cricothyroid membrane is incised. A pediatric size endotracheal or tracheostomy tube can be inserted through the membrane to create an airway. In the event a tube is not immediately available, a large-bore needle can be inserted into the membrane and the catheter left in place. This provides a temporary airway access measure but is inadequate to ventilate the patient without a jet oscillating ventilator.

Successive surgical interventions

Often the multiple trauma patient requires a multitude of surgical procedures, either specialty related or as a step-wise progression in the primary treatment of the initial injury. Acalculous cholecystitis is often a secondary complication of the trauma patient's postoperative course, which requires cholecystectomy. Secondary wound closures, dé-bridements, and fixation of initially undiscovered fractures comprise the majority of follow-up procedures. Initially the trauma patient is critically ill and requires intensive care facilities. When surgery is scheduled, the perioperative nurse may need additional assistance in transport of the patient, and transport monitoring of the ECG, arterial line, and blood pressure is performed. Oxygen and mechanical ventilation with Ambu bag are necessary for the intubated patient.

Additional opportunities for intervention are afforded the perioperative nurse, since the patient might undergo several surgical procedures during a week. Increased familiarity with the patient's needs, as well as the ability to monitor the patient's recovery progress, is possible.

EVALUATION

The evaluation of the patient should reflect the effectiveness of the interventions. Did the patient remain free from ontoward complications? Was there progress toward the expected outcomes as described in the perioperative care plan? The following are examples of evaluation statements in relation to the sample care plan.

- The patient demonstrates decreased level of anxiety as evidenced by: less apprehension, ability to maintain eye contact, decreased quivering voice, ability to follow directions, even though anxiety persists.
- The patient is afebrile with BP and pulse within normal limits for patient, has an H/H within normal limits postoperatively, and has a balanced intake and output postoperatively.
- The patient is free from signs and symptoms of infection postoperatively.

- The patient is free from signs and symptoms of aspiration pneumonia.
- The patient reports relief from acute pain when analgesia is utilized.

Upon completion of the procedure(s) the perioperative nurse is afforded an opportunity to further assess the trauma patient, as well as evaluate the plan of care implemented. If the patient has sustained numerous injuries and remains critically injured, the PACU may be bypassed and the patient transferred directly to the ICU. The perioperative nurse should accompany the patient, along with the anesthesia team, to the ICU. Once the anesthesia report is given, the perioperative nurse can provide a wealth of information to the critical care nurse. At this point, family members may have been contacted or are present, allowing more specific medical history information to be obtained. However, the mechanism of injury and events surrounding the accident are still significant. A high index of suspicion remains during postoperative care of the patient sustaining multiple injuries. Attention can be diverted from a less significant injury in the presence of a highly visible or obvious trauma. Once the obvious trauma undergoes intervention, pain or discomfort from other injuries becomes more apparent. In the care of a patient with neurologic deficit, physical assessment and continued evaluation are essential because patient self-report is nonexistent.

Status of progress in the secondary survey should also be reported. Any additional labwork or interventions that have yet to be completed should be discussed. It is imperative in a thorough examination to view the back of the patient in an effort to locate all injuries.

Additional diagnostic procedures may be required after completion of the surgical procedure if the patient's condition is stable. The perioperative nurse may be requested to accompany the patient to diagnostics with the anesthesia team. In addition, respiratory care may assist in patient transport and maintenance of the airway.

CRITICAL INCIDENT STRESS DEBRIEFING

Unfortunately, some trauma injuries result in death. This can be particularly difficult for the perioperative team, since most surgical interventions are of a curative or restorative nature. In many emergency medical systems a critical incident stress debriefing team exists. It is composed of specially trained volunteers who are also professionals in the health care field. Police officers, firefighters, paramedics, ED nurses, and ICU nurses can comprise the team. In the event of a particularly tragic death of a patient, the team can be contacted and a meeting with that patient's care providers is arranged. The benefit of this team is enhanced when intervention is timely. Opportunity for the patient care members to discuss their feelings and emotions is provided and encouraged, as each provider discusses personal participation in care of the patient. Critical incident stress debriefing teams are very successful and can provide a healthy professional growth from what is otherwise a tragedy.

SURGICAL INTERVENTIONS

INJURIES OF THE HEAD AND SPINAL COLUMN

Trauma to the head is responsible for half of all trauma deaths. Brain injury occurs either as a direct result of the trauma to the tissue or as a complication. Often forces of energy from the impact are tolerated by the rigid skull, but the soft tissue of the brain is traumatized. This results in formation of subdural, epidural, or intracerebral hematomas (Fig. 30-15). In addition, cerebral swelling can result in herniation of the brain despite treatment (Fig. 30-16).

A baseline neurologic exam is of extreme importance. The pupils are examined and the presence or absence of posturing is noted. The Glasgow Coma Scale (Box 30-7) provides a universally accepted mechanism to assess the baseline for the trauma team. But in the presence of alcohol, a pediatric patient, or drug intoxication the scale cannot be used. For patients with a score of less than or equal to 8, intubation with hyperventilation is the immediate treatment of choice. In the highly combative patient, intubation may also be performed to allow adequate assessment of the extent of injury.

Hyperventilation is very effective in decreasing intracranial pressure during initial management of the patient. An osmotic diuretic, such as mannitol, can be used if the patient is not severely hypotensive. The diuresis assists in

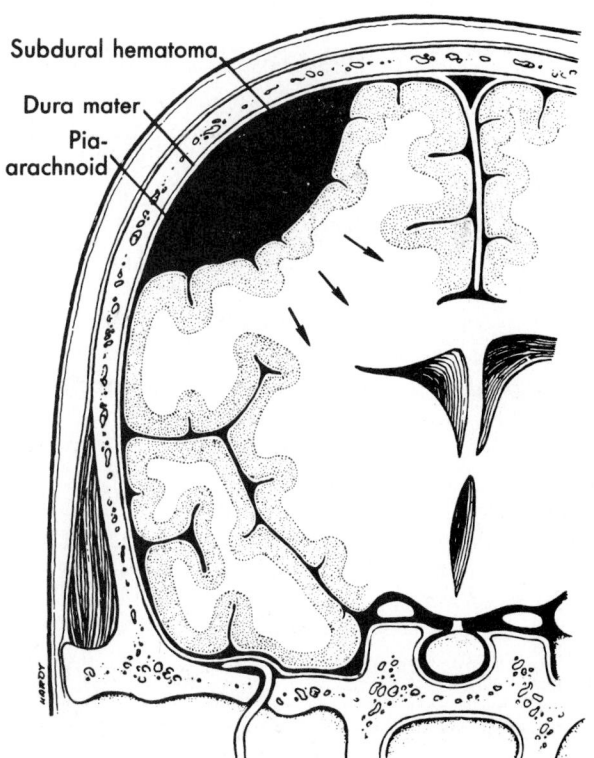

Subdural hematoma

Dura mater

Pia-arachnoid

FIG. 30-15 Subdural hematoma causing increased intracranial pressure with shifting of tissue.

From *The Practice of emergency care* (2nd ed.) (p. 331) by J.H. Cosgriff, Jr., and D.L. Anderson, 1984, Philadelphia.

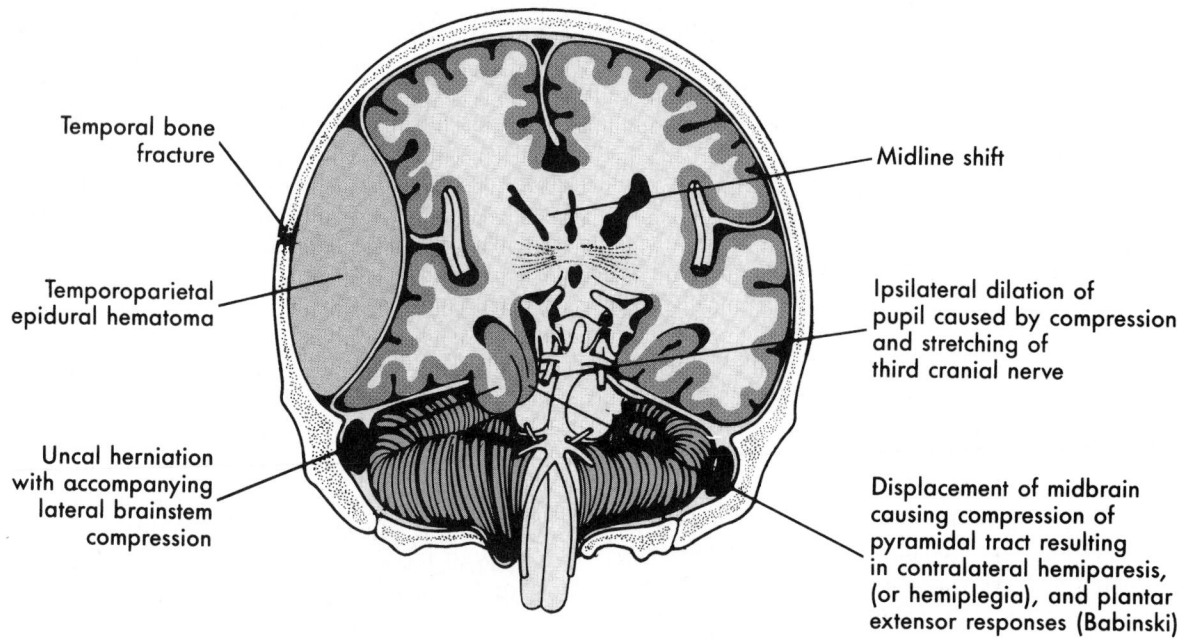

FIG. 30-16 Cross section showing herniation of lower portion of temporal lobe (uncas) through tentorium caused by temporoparietal epidural hematoma. Herniation may occur also in cerebellum. Note mass effect and midline shift.

Note. Redrawn from *Advanced Concepts in Clinical Nursing* (2nd ed.) by K.C. Kintzel (Ed.), 1977, Philadelphia: J.B. Lippincott.

BOX 30-7

The Glasgow Coma Scale (GCS)*

Subscale	Description	Score
Eye opening	Spontaneously	4
	To speech	3
	To pain	2
	Do not open	1
Best verbal response	Oriented	5
	Confused	4
	Inappropriate speech	3
	Unintelligible speech	2
	No verbalization	1
Best motor response	Obeys command	6
	Localizes pain	5
	Withdraws from pain	4
	Abnormal flexion	3
	Abnormal extension	2
	No motor response	1

*Best total score = 15; E4, V5, M6. Worst score = 3.

Skull fractures usually do not require operative intervention when there is no displacement and the fracture is linear. Depressed fractures or the presence of bone in the brain frequently requires elevation and débridement (Fig. 30-17). Hematoma evacuation is based on the location of the hematoma, size, and number present. Before a craniotomy or burr hole is performed, the CT scan, the neurologic status of the patient, morbidity/mortality associated with the procedure, other injuries present, and any underlying medical problems if known are evaluated. An intracranial pressure monitor may be placed in the patient who is at risk for increased intracranial pressure. At some institutions this procedure is performed in the trauma room of the emergency department or in the ICU. The perioperative team may be asked to assist with the procedure wherever it is done. Specific discussion of the neurosurgical procedures is found in Chapter 22.

In the trauma patient the spinal cord is always considered to be injured until proven otherwise. The patient with a cervical spine injury at or near C3 to C5 is at great risk for respiratory difficulties, since this is the area of diaphragmatic innervation. There is also the possibility of swelling above the area of injury, and the perioperative nurse should be alert for the potential of respiratory distress even if not initially present. A 24-hour dose of methylprednisolone (Solu-Medrol), calculated by body weight, is thought to decrease initial cord swelling.

lowering the intracranial pressure. Elevation of the head of the bed at 30 degrees and keeping the head midline (to promote venous drainage) can also be beneficial.

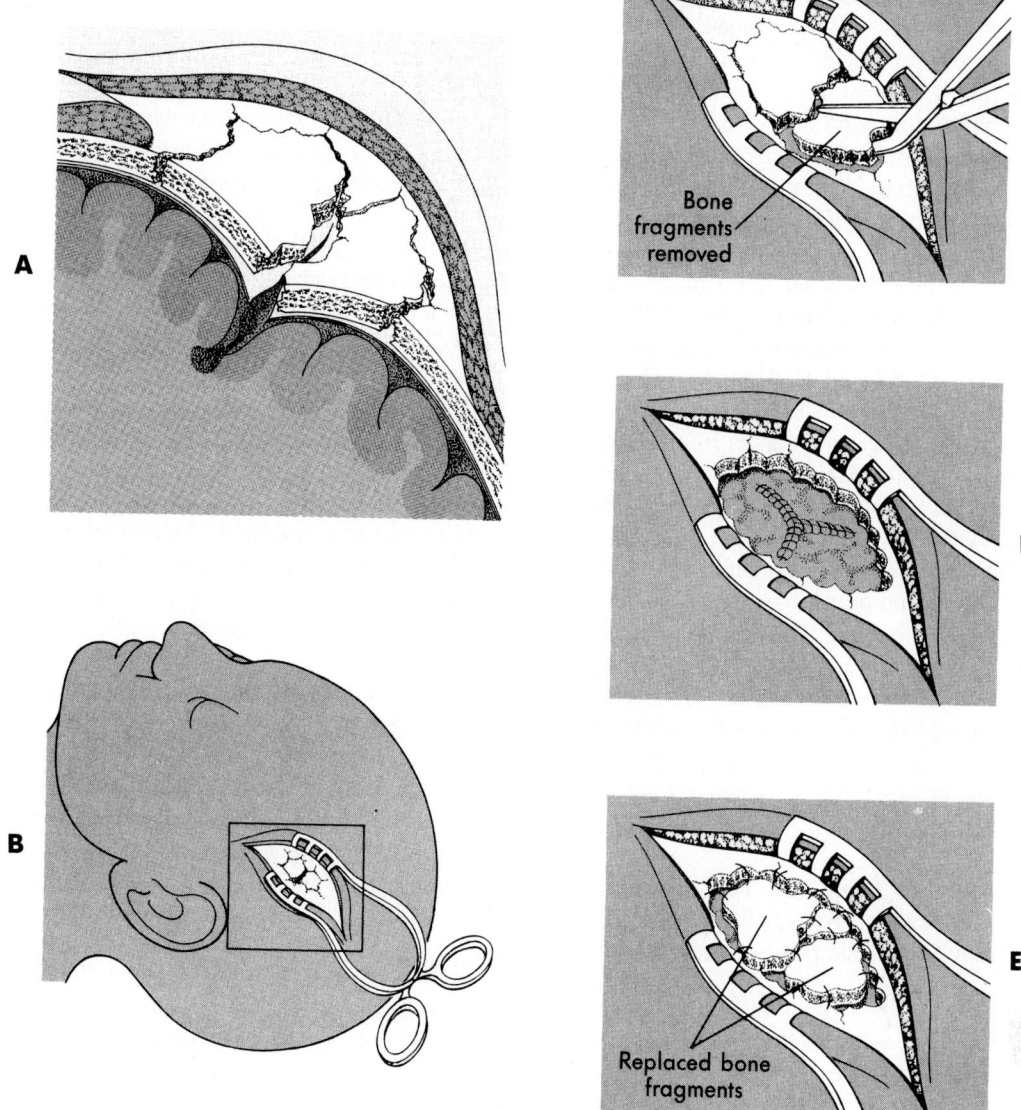

FIG. 30-17 Treatment of compound depressed fracture of skull. **A,** Depressed skull fracture and scalp injury. **B,** Incision to expose fracture and remove devitalized scalp. **C,** removal of impacted bone by burr hole to locate and identify normal dura, followed by resection of bone fragments. **D,** Watertight closure of dura afterbrain debridement. **E,** Replacement and fixation of bone fragments.

Note. Redrawn from Diagnosis and treatment of head injury (pp. 2017-2148) by D.P. Becker, G.F. Gade, H.F. Young, and T.F. Fewerman. In *Neurological surgery* (3rd ed.) by J.R. Youman (Ed.), 1990, Philadelphia: W.B. Saunders.

The hallmark indicators of possible cord injury are absence of rectal tone and bradycardia in the presence of hypotension. The body's normal response is to increase heart rate in the presence of decreased blood flow or hypotension. These responses are not present in injury of the spinal cord, and bradycardia results.

Injuries involving the spinal cord can range from complete transsection, without hope of recovery, to a contusion of the cord. Fractures or dislocation of the vertebra can result in the protrusion of small pieces into the spinal canal. This is known as a burst fracture. Several vertebrae may be fractured or have fractured components. Generally, in compression fractures, if loss of vertebral height is greater than 20%, surgical treatment may be indicated. Bracing can be considered an option if the compression is less than 20% and no neurologic symptoms are present.

Treatment of spinal column fractures can involve surgery. Stabilization of the fracture may be necessary, depending on the severity of the injury. For cervical spine fractures traction may be used initially to reduce the fracture followed by surgical intervention as soon as patient condition permits. Internal fixation devices are discussed in Chapter 26.

INJURIES OF THE FACE

Motor vehicle crashes account for about 60% of maxillofacial injuries (Lopez-Viego, 1994). Mandibular fractures alone are highly associated with assault as the MOI. In the patient who presents with facial injury, the airway must be secured. This requires removing any items that pose the threat of aspiration in addition to ensuring patency. If a midface fracture is present, nasogastric tube placement and nasotracheal intubation are avoided. A tracheostomy may need to be performed before initiation of the operative procedure. Control of scalp or facial hemorrhage can be achieved through a pressure dressing until surgical intervention is possible, since exsanguination can occur. Treatment of the fracture may be delayed until the immediate life threats have been successfully managed. Goals of operative intervention are to reduce and immobilize the fracture, prevent infection, and restore facial cosmesis and function.

Facial fractures can be categorized into Le Fort I, II, or III (Fig. 30-18). A Le Fort I fracture is the most common maxillary fracture. It involves a horizontal interruption of the anterior and lateral wall of the maxillary sinus. Le Fort II is a pyramidal fracture along the maxilla and lacrimal bones and through the infraorbital rim. Le Fort III is otherwise known as craniofacial dysjunction. The midface is completely disengaged from the cranial base, resulting from a fracture across the frontomaxillary sutures. Specific information regarding these injuries is located in Chapter 23.

INJURIES OF THE EYE

Injuries to the eye can result from blunt or penetrating types of trauma. Penetrating objects in the globe are stabilized and not removed until the patient is in the operating room. These injuries threaten loss of vision due to the injury itself, inflammation, or infection. Blunt injury to the eye can result in hematomas and accompanying fractures. A blow-out fracture is the result of a blunt force to the eye that pushes soft tissue through the thin bony orbital floor. The patient has recession of the eye into the orbit and loses the ability to gaze upward. Surgical repair is often indicated. For further information see Chapter 17.

INJURIES OF THE NECK

Injury to the neck and soft tissue structures is most commonly a result of penetrating trauma. The neck can be divided into three zones with respect to injury and consequence. Zone I is the base of the neck below the clavicles. Anatomic structures located in this region are the great vessels and aortic arch, the innominate veins, trachea, esophagus, and lungs. Zone II is the area in the middle of the neck between the clavicles and the mandible. Structures located in this area include the carotid artery, internal jugular vein, trachea, and esophagus. Zone III is located between the angle of the mandible and the base of the skull. The primary target of evaluation in these injuries is vascular structures.

Zone II injuries may necessitate an otolaryngology specialist. Penetrating injuries to the larynx and trachea can be primarily repaired. Blunt force to the larynx can result in a fracture and impose immediate airway obstruction. These patients require immediate tracheostomy followed by repair of the fracture when it is unstable or displaced. Specific information concerning these procedures is located in Chapter 20.

INJURIES OF THE CHEST AND HEART

Trauma to the chest area is the primary cause of death in 25% of trauma victims (Cardonna, 1994). Blunt trauma is most often associated with high-speed motor vehicle accidents. Penetrating trauma is on the rise with an increase in violent crimes. Penetrating injuries at or immediately below the nipple line or level of the scapular tips is evaluated for both chest and abdominal involvement. Diaphragmatic injury is also a possibility.

Deceleration injury, such as with a fall or striking the steering wheel in a motor vehicle accident, may cause contusions of the chest wall, rib or sternal fractures, cardiac or pulmonary contusions, or rupture of the aorta and other major vessels. Rib fractures are also associated with a hemothorax or pneumothorax. If there is respiratory distress and diminished breath sounds, a chest tube is indicated immediately. An autotransfusion chest drainage device should be considered. Chest tube output must be closely monitored intraoperatively, since accumulation of 1000 to 1500 ml of blood is an indication for chest exploration. Penetrating wounds, either as a result of gunshot or stab injuries, may cause hemothoraces and pneumothoraces as well. Lacerations or perforation of the lung, heart, great vessels, trachea, esophagus, and bronchus are possible.

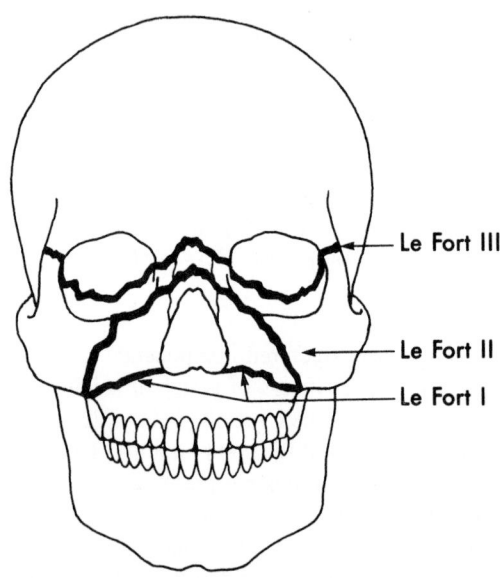

FIG. 30-18 Le Fort's classification of maxillary fractures.

From Neff JA, Kidd PS: *Trauma nursing: The art and science*, St. Louis, 1993, Mosby.

Myocardial contusion usually involves the right ventricle and can be evidenced by dysrhythmias upon patient arrival or shortly thereafter. The patient is monitored on a telemetry unit and surgical intervention is not required. Rupture of a heart valve can occur, depending on which part of the cardiac cycle the heart is in at the time of contusion. If valve rupture has occurred, then surgical repair is necessary. Heart sounds should be evaluated during the secondary survey to document the presence or absence of murmurs. Heart valve rupture can occur as a late complication of myocardial contusion. Pericardiocentesis is performed for signs and symptoms of pericardial tamponade (Fig. 30-19). These include jugular venous distention, muffled heart sounds, and a narrowing pulse pressure. Patients may present to the operating room for a pericardial window either emergently or during the recovery phase.

An emergency thoracotomy may be indicated in the patient with penetrating trauma to the chest in full arrest or pulseless electrical activity on ECG. If a laceration to the heart is suspected and the patient is rapidly deteriorating, a thoracotomy may be performed in the ED (Fig. 30-20). The laceration may be primarily repaired and the patient taken to the operating room for irrigation, débridement of wounds, and closure. Otherwise, surgical intervention is initiated in the operating room. Wounds located across the mediastinum accompanied by hemodynamic instability or massive penetrating lung injuries require surgical intervention. Disruption of the trachea, bronchus, or esophagus is also an indication. Rupture of the thoracic aorta is another injury requiring an operation and includes the use of extracorporeal bypass. This injury is an obvious life threat but may be difficult to diagnose. An arch aortogram is indi-

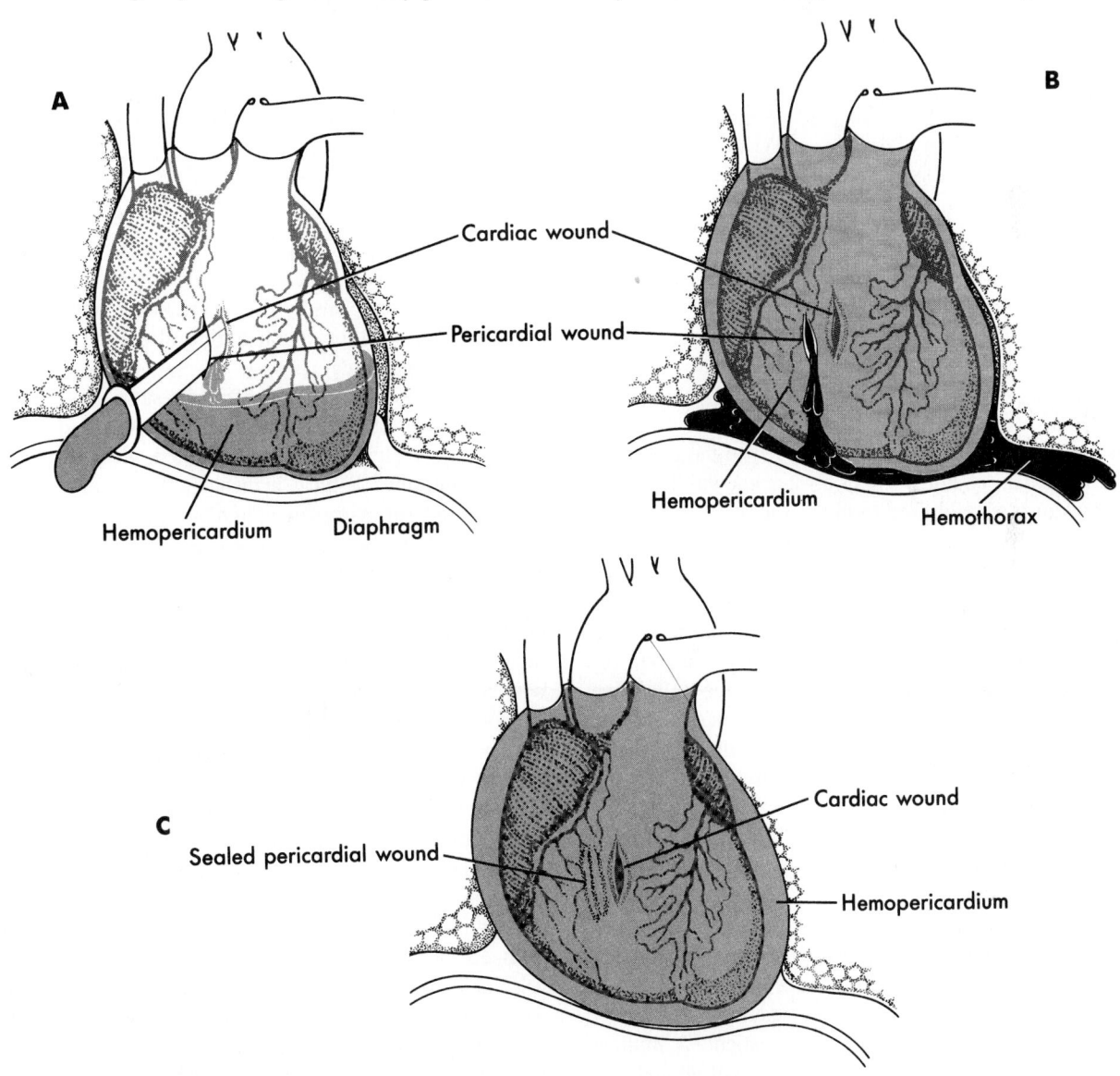

FIG. 30-19 **A,** Cardiac injury with pericardial disruption. **B,** Bleeding from heart through pericardial tear into pleural space. **C,** Self sealing of pericardial wound resulting in pericardial tamponade.

From Neff JA, Kidd PS: *Trauma nursing: The art and science,* St. Louis, 1993, Mosby.

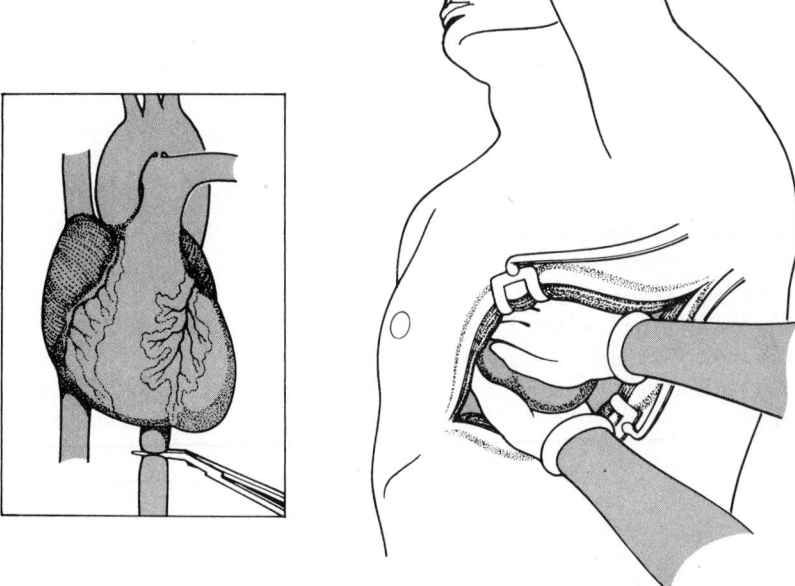

FIG. 30-20   Emergency left thoracotomy site with internal cardiac massage. Descending aorta is shown cross-clamped with vascular clamp.

From Neff JA, Kidd PS: *Trauma nursing: The art and science*, St. Louis, 1993, Mosby.

cated in patients with significant mechanism to cause such an injury. This injury is associated with first rib or sternal fractures. Chapters 24 and 26 provide additional information on associated surgical procedures.

INJURIES OF THE ABDOMEN

When the trauma patient is transferred to the operating room, the extent of injury is not always known. The perioperative nurse should prep from the suprasternal notch to the midthigh area. This allows for rapid access to the chest to clamp the aorta should massive hemorrhage control be indicated, as well as exposure of the femoral arteries for potential cannulation and access to the thigh for harvesting of a saphenous vein. The spleen is the most common organ injured in blunt trauma, and the liver, due to its large size, is the most common organ injured in penetrating trauma. Initial efforts were aimed at performing splenectomy with splenic injury. However, research has shown the role of the spleen in the body's defense against infection. Therefore every effort is made to control hemorrhage in the spleen and avoid its removal. Injury to the spleen occurs with deceleration injuries resulting in fracture of the organ due to its multiple fixation points. Rupture of the spleen can be immediate or delayed. Splenic lacerations are treated conservatively by close monitoring and bed rest or may be treated operatively if necessary. Treatment is determined by the condition of the spleen and of the patient. A midline incision is used, which allows for exposure of all abdominal contents. Splenorrhaphy, which is the placement of an absorbable polyglycolic acid mesh around the spleen, is utilized in capsular tears (Fig. 30-21). Topical hemostatic

agents are also used with success, as well as suturing and argon laser in some instances. A laceration involving the splenic hilum or complete shattering of the organ usually results in splenectomy.

Liver injury is managed in much the same way. Conservative treatment is indicated in minor capsular and subcapsular injuries. This can be accomplished with bed rest and close monitoring. Topical hemostatic agents and suturing are techniques of management in minor injuries. Fibrin glue is also used in some institutions as a topical hemostatic agent. More severe injuries with active expanding hematomas or lobe disruption may necessitate hepatic resection or ligation of associated vasculature. With massive hemorrhage, control of bleeding is the utmost concern. Packing with laparotomy sponges may be indicated along with manual compression of the organ if intraoperative hypotension become severe (Fig. 30-22). A pressure dressing of absorbable mesh laparotomy sponges may be applied and the wound closed temporarily until associated coagulopathies, hypothermia, and hemodynamic instability can be corrected. The patient is returned to the operating room usually within 24 to 72 hours postoperatively, or when condition permits, for further exploration and removal of the sponges.

Injuries to the gastrointestinal system are also associated with abdominal trauma. Bowel injuries may be missed on abdominal CT scan during the initial diagnostic period. Any perforation of the gastrointestinal tract carries with it a chance for peritonitis and sepsis. In the event of a penetrating injury, the trajectory of the missile or the implement is examined and organs within the area are considered po-

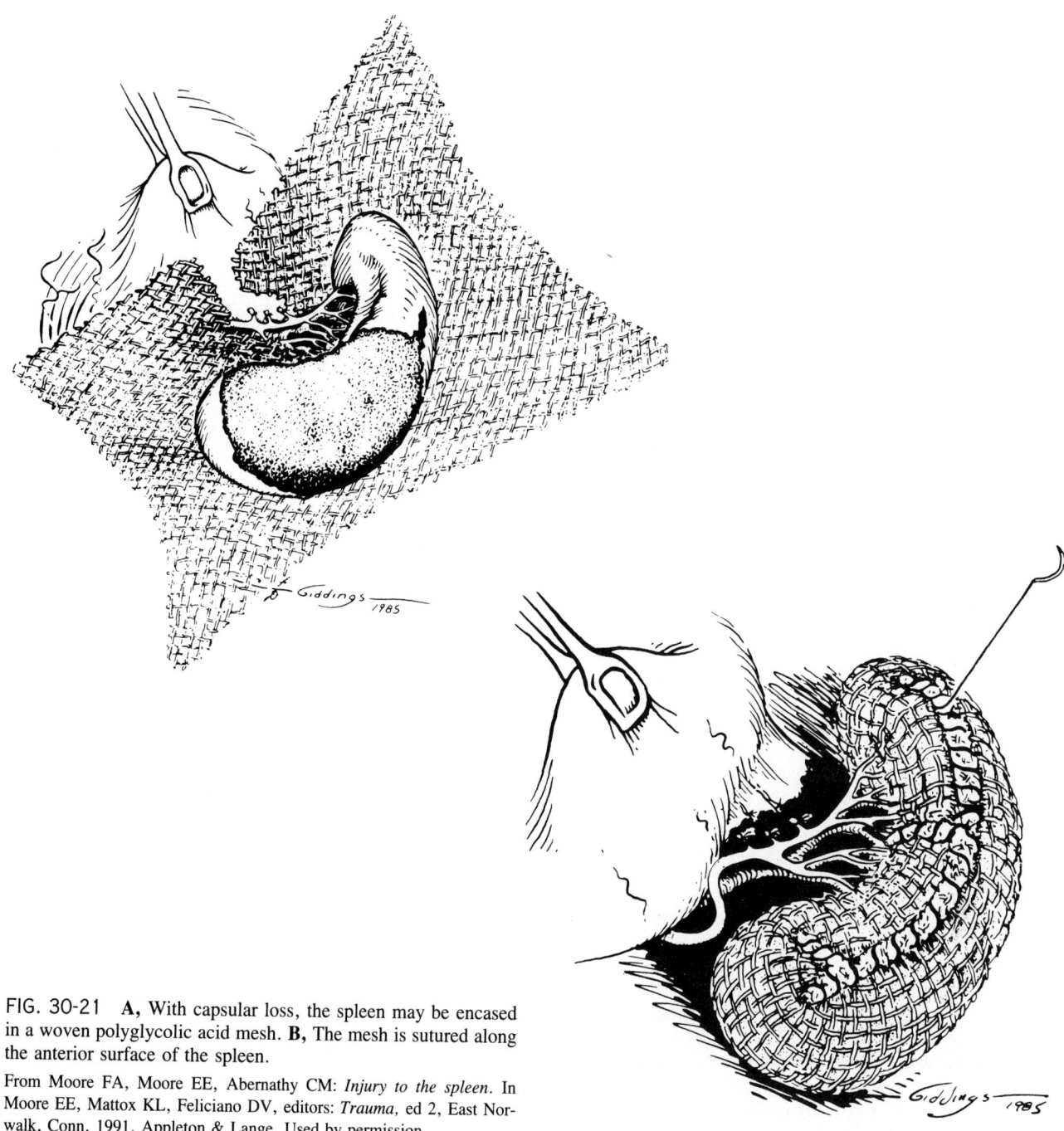

FIG. 30-21 **A,** With capsular loss, the spleen may be encased in a woven polyglycolic acid mesh. **B,** The mesh is sutured along the anterior surface of the spleen.

From Moore FA, Moore EE, Abernathy CM: *Injury to the spleen.* In Moore EE, Mattox KL, Feliciano DV, editors: *Trauma,* ed 2, East Norwalk, Conn, 1991, Appleton & Lange. Used by permission.

tentially injured. Exploration is indicated, and the components of the gastrointestinal system are thoroughly examined for any perforations, contusion, hemorrhage, or compromise of vasculature, such as a mesenteric hematoma. Once the injury is identified, suturing, stapling, or segmental excision may be indicated. Further information on these procedures is in Chapter 10.

Diagnostic laparoscopy is being used increasingly for di-

rect visualization of abdominal organs to diminish the need for a negative exploratory laparotomy (Research Highlight 30-2). This procedure allows the surgeon to more effectively evaluate for the presence of injury and develop an appropriate plan of treatment in the stable patient. Some interventions may also be performed via the laparoscope, thus avoiding the more invasive laparotomy. Further indications for this procedure in the trauma setting are being evaluated.

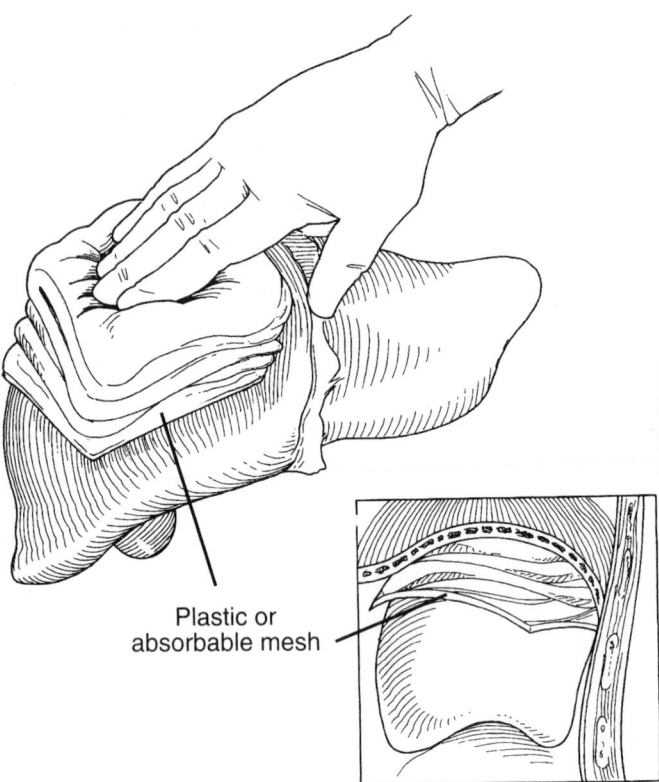

Plastic or
absorbable mesh

FIG. 30-22   Perihepatic packing using a folded Steri-Drape and
laparotomy pads.

From Feliciano DV, et al: Packing for control of hepatic hemorrhage, *J
Trauma* 26:738-743. Used with permission.

RESEARCH HIGHLIGHT 30-2

**Ivatury, Simon, and Stahl conducted a follow-up
study on the role of laparoscopy in penetrating
abdominal trauma. One hundred stable patients with
penetrating wounds were studied in an effort to
validate the diagnostic accuracy of laparoscopy in this
patient population. Fifty-seven patients had
penetration of the peritoneum and were noted to have
hemoperitoneum, solid organ injury, or diaphragmatic
laceration as well. Fifty-four underwent laparotomy
and had confirmation of the diagnoses during
laparoscopy. The authors concluded that the major
role of this procedure in penetrating trauma is in
prevention of unnecessary laparotomy in tangential
stab and gunshot wounds where the complete extent of
injury is unclear. Evaluation of the diaphragm is
achieved in the presence of thoracoabdominal wounds.
Hollow viscus injuries should not be excluded on the
basis of laparoscopy. Future studies were
recommended to investigate the use of therapeutic
laparoscopy.**

Ivatury, R., Simon, R., & Stahl, W. (1993). A critical
evaluation of laparoscopy in penetrating abdominal
trauma. *The Journal of Trauma, 34*(6).

INJURIES OF THE GENITOURINARY SYSTEM

Laceration of the kidney, a retroperitoneal structure, is
closely associated with fracture of the ribs and transverse
vertebral processes. Since the organ is retroperitoneal, the
presence of bleeding may not be noted on diagnostic peritoneal lavage. Renal contusions often produce hematuria.
Gross clots may also be seen in more serious injury, but it
should be noted that hematuria is not present in a complete
avulsion injury. Management of renal contusions can be
conservative with monitoring of hematuria. Lacerations involving the collecting system, severe crush injuries, or
pedicle injuries necessitate surgical intervention. Nephrectomy may be indicated with severe injury of the pedicle or
massive hemorrhage.

Rupture of the bladder and urethral injury are most often associated with pelvic fractures. Both blunt and penetrating trauma are causative factors. The type of bladder injury is a direct result of the amount of urine present in the
bladder at the time of injury. Blunt forces applied to a full
bladder result in an intraperitoneal rupture. This type of rupture is closely associated with alcohol consumption because
of alcohol's diuretic effect. Pelvic fracture is associated
with an extraperitoneal bladder rupture. Most often these
patients present with gross hematuria. A small extraperitoneal rupture may be managed by urinary catheter drainage.
A large extraperitoneal rupture and intraperitoneal rupture

require surgical intervention. A suprapubic cystostomy tube is placed and the bladder is repaired. Pelvic fracture reduction and fixation are also performed.

Urethral injuries require exploration and primary repair. These types of injuries are more common in the male. A fall or straddle type of injury is usually responsible. This injury is detected by the presence of blood at the urinary meatus. In these instances an indwelling urethral catheter should not be inserted. Blood at the urinary meatus may be indicative of a tear in the anterior urethra. A retrograde urethrogram may be performed to evaluate for extravasation of urine and potential injury. Chapter 14 provides additional information on urologic procedures.

SKELETAL INJURIES

Trauma to the skeletal system usually results in contusion or fracture. After stabilization of the patient, any body part that is distorted, edematous, painful, or highly suspicious for fracture or dislocation is radiographed. Treatment of fractures is aimed at restoring function with a minimum of complications. Immobilization of fractures can be accomplished by casting, bracing, splinting, and application of traction or hardware fixation. Femur fractures in particular can be associated with a high risk of hemorrhage and require traction before surgical repair. Closed and open reductions, application of internal and external fixators, and some types of traction may be performed in the operating room. The perioperative nurse involved in care of the trauma patient must have a working knowledge of the orthopedic specialty. Fractures must be repaired in a timely manner to avoid untoward complications; however, immediate life threats are corrected first. Open fractures are at an increased risk of infection. Chapter 21 contains information on the surgical procedures utilized in fracture management.

Pelvic fractures may pose an additional challenge to the perioperative team. Fractures within the pelvic ring are associated with hemorrhage and shock. Systemic peripheral vascular resistance is increased. A tamponade effect may be provided to blood vessels that are disrupted due to the pelvic fracture. Pneumatic antishock garment or PASG trousers provide stabilization of the fracture and also can possibly reduce associated hemorrhage when applied to the patient before arrival at the hospital (Fig. 30-23). However, much controversy exists concerning their use and possible complications. Once applied, the patient may be transported to the operating room with the trousers still inflated. The perioperative nurse must be familiar with deflation procedures. The attending anesthesia member directs deflation in collaboration with the surgeon. Blood pressure and other vital signs are closely monitored. The abdominal compartment is deflated first. Deflation continues slowly while IV fluids are infused to maintain blood pressure. A 5 mm Hg drop in blood pressure requires fluid resuscitation of approximately 200 ml before deflation of the next compartment. If the patient remains stable, each leg compartment

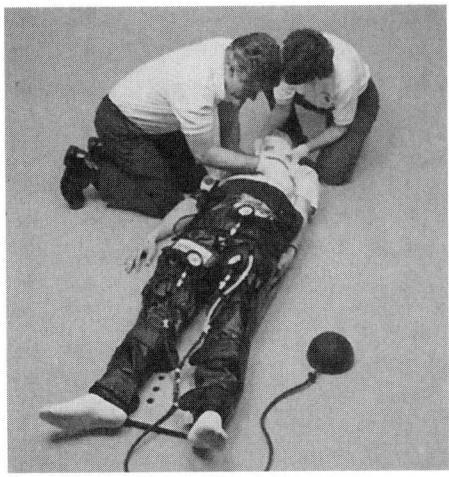

FIG. 30-23   After PASG positioning, the Velcro straps are securely fastened.
From Sanders MJ: *Mosby's paramedic textbook,* St. Louis, 1994, Mosby.

is deflated slowly, one at a time. Severe hemorrhage associated with the fracture may be controlled by arterial embolization performed in the radiology department if surgical intervention must be delayed. Fixation of the fracture ultimately provides hemorrhage control.

Soft tissue injuries of an extremity are subject to compartment syndrome. This is a result of swelling of the soft tissues and muscles encased in the fascia. With a significant amount of swelling, pain is increased and the surrounding circulation may be compromised. The patient may experience a decrease in motor and sensory function. This injury must be treated surgically by performance of a fasciotomy. Incising the fascia allows space for tissue swelling. Several days later, the patient returns to the operating room for closure, which may require skin grafting for complete coverage.

HYPOTHERMIA

Hypothermia can be classified into three types. *Mild hypothermia* is a core temperature between 32 and 35° C. These patients may appear gray and are cool to the touch. Some alterations in level of consciousness can be present. Treatment is aimed at passively rewarming the patient by providing warm fluids, blankets, and allowing shivering to occur to generate body heat. *Moderate hypothermia* is characterized as core temperatures between 28 and 32° C. Warmed fluids are given IV and also by gastric/peritoneal lavage. A warming blanket may also be initiated. Immersion in a Hubbard tank filled with warm water has also been successful. An irritable myocardium may cause dysrhythmias to be present. Shivering may or may not be present. *Severe hypothermia* is diagnosed in the patient with a temperature below 28° C. Heart rate and respiratory rate are greatly decreased. This patient is comatose, often appears dead, and requires active rewarming processes. It is advisable to warm the core first to avoid complications associated with rewarming. This can best be accomplished by core heating via cardiopulmonary bypass, which directly warms internal vital organs, including the heart. The patient should be handled gently during transfers to avoid further tissue injury and stimulation of an irritable myocardium (Cardonna, 1994).

It should be noted that severe cases of hypothermia mimic death, and no patient can be pronounced dead until he or she is warm and dead. Resuscitation measures are ceased if the patient is rewarmed to at least 35° C and cardiac functions are still nonexistent.

THERMAL INJURIES

Heat and cold exposure injuries require prompt initial management in the ED setting. Some institutions transfer pediatric burn patients and severely burned adult patients to a burn center for treatment once the patient is stabilized. In addition to treatment of the site of injury to decrease further tissue damage, fluid management is of the utmost importance in these patients. After hemodynamic stabilization of the patient, burn and frostbite wounds usually require a series of débridement. These patients may have multiple surgical débridement procedures before skin grafting and cosmetic interventions. Restoration of function is important. Circumferential burns may restrict the neurovascular structures during eschar formation. Chest burns with eschar may restrict movement of the chest wall and ventilatory function. An escharotomy may be performed. This is incising of the eschar to alleviate the constriction. If necessary, this procedure may be performed at the bedside and the perioperative team may be asked to assist.

ORGAN/TISSUE PROCUREMENT

As previously noted, trauma primarily affects young people. In the event that resuscitation efforts or surgical interventions are not successful, the patient may be declared dead. Depending on the cause of death and preexisting medical conditions, the patient may be an organ donor candidate. Both federal and state laws mandate that local organ procurement facilities are notified of potential donors and that families are informed that organ donation exists as an option. Organ donation agencies can be contacted early and will assist in assessing the potential donor as well as providing a protocol for donor management once the patient is declared dead. Definition of brain death is not uniform throughout the country. The perioperative nurse should be familiar with the state's definition of brain death and the institution's criteria for the declaration. Once a patient is declared dead and becomes a potential organ donor, all financial costs acquired from that point are not incurred by the patient's family. The patient is not disfigured in any way that will interfere with bereavement rituals.

Patients up to the age of 70 may be considered potential organ donors. Exclusion criteria include the presence of IV drug abuse, preexisting untreated infection, malignancy (exclusive of brain tumor), and active tuberculosis (Cardonna, 1994).

A transplant coordinator assists in managing the organ donor patient in the ICU setting until the procurement teams arrive. The perioperative nurse must prepare for the organ procurement procedure. The harvesting of organs and tissue may take several hours and additional members of the perioperative team. Different organ procurement agencies will provide a surgical team, but additional scrub and circulating personnel are needed. The transplant coordinators actively seek tissue and organ recipients during the harvest procedure. Most organ transplant agencies contact the institution and provide follow-up information regarding the ultimate success of the transplant procedures and information about the recipients.

The heart is removed first, followed by the lungs, pancreas, liver, and kidneys. Tissue dissection is performed in such a manner as to allow for optimal organ transplantation. Sterile technique remains important. In addition, traffic control is of concern during these procedures. Any nonessential personnel should be limited. Bone, skin, and corneas can also be removed. Some procurement agencies remove bone and corneas in the morgue, rather than in the operating room.

SUMMARY

Nowhere is the team concept more important than in the provision of definitive care to the multiple trauma patient. The perioperative nurse is a vital member of the trauma team. Through the application of principles of trauma care as outlined in this chapter, perioperative nurses can significantly contribute to positive outcomes for trauma patients.

REFERENCES

Cardona, V.D., et al. (1994). *Trauma nursing* (2nd ed.) Philadelphia: W. B. Saunders.

Champion, W.S., et al. (1989). A revision of the trauma score. *The Journal of Trauma, 29*(5), 624.

Committee on Trauma (1990). *Advanced trauma life support program.* Chicago: American College of Surgeons.

Lopez-Viego, M.A. (Ed.). (1994). *The parkland trauma handbook.* St. Louis: Mosby.

Neff, J.A., and Kidd, P.S. (1993). *Trauma nursing: The art and science.* St. Louis: Mosby.

State of Illinois Trauma Nurse Specialist Course Manual. (1990).

Trunkey, D. (1983). Trauma. *Scientific American, 249,* 28-35.

BIBLIOGRAPHY

Clark, S. et al. (1989). Central hemodynamic assessment of normal term pregnancy. *American Journal of Obstetrics and Gynecology, 161,* 1439-1442.

Feliciano, D.V. (1990). Packing for control of hepatic hemorrhage. *The Journal of Trauma, 26*(6), 738-743.

Grande, C. (Ed.). (1993). *Textbook of trauma, anesthesia, and critical care.* St. Louis: Mosby.

Kim, M.J., McFarland, G.K., & McLane, A.M. (1991). *Pocket guide to nursing diagnoses* (4th ed.). St. Louis: Mosby.

Kuska, B.M. (1982). Acute onset of compartment syndrome. *Journal of Emergency Nursing, 8*(2), 78.

Lederer, J.R., Marculescu, G.L., Mocnik, B., & Sealey, N. (1991). *Care planning pocket guide.* Reading: Addison-Wesley Nursing.

Matsen, F.A. (1975). Compartment syndromes: A unified concept. *Clinical Orthopedics and Related Research, 113,* 10.

Maull, K.I. (Ed.). (1993). *Advances in trauma and critical care.* St. Louis: Mosby.

Moore, F.A., et al. (1991). *Trauma* (2nd ed.). Norwalk, CT: Appleton & Lange.

Najarian, J.S., & Delaney, J.P. (Eds.). (1992). *Progress in trauma and critical care surgery.* St. Louis: Mosby.

Rosen, P., & Barkin, R. (Eds.). (1992). *Emergency medicine: Concepts and clinical practice* (3rd ed.). St. Louis: Mosby.

Sheehy, S.B. (1992). *Emergency nursing: Principles and practice* (3rd ed.). St. Louis: Mosby.

Sheehy, S.B., & Jimmerson, C.L. (1994). *Manual of clinical trauma care* (2nd ed.). St. Louis: Mosby.

Trunkey, D., & Lewis, F. (1991). *Current therapy of trauma* (3rd ed.). Philadelphia: B.C. Decker.

31

LASERS

KAY A. BALL

Perioperative nursing, perhaps more than any other nursing specialty, has been tremendously affected by the technologic explosion of the past several decades. Nurses practicing in surgical environments during the last 25 to 30 years have witnessed and participated in a great number of changes in procedure techniques, instrumentation, and equipment used during these advancements in surgery. Throughout this transition the primary concern of perioperative nurses has been the care, comfort, and safety of patients encountering surgical intervention. Continual developments in technology have, however, forced perioperative nurses to improve their organizational skills and mechanical aptitudes to cope competently with the maze of sophisticated and often complex devices used, while still ensuring high-quality perioperative patient care.

One of the health care revolutions that has occurred in the last three decades is the birth and evolution of an amazing tool called the *laser*. The perioperative nurse of the 1990s must be keenly aware of the expanded responsibilities associated with laser applications. The laser has radically changed surgery by making possible less invasive procedures, thus decreasing inpatient hospitalization, diminishing postoperative complications, and saving health care dollars.

LASER BIOPHYSICS

HISTORICAL PERSPECTIVE

During the early 1900s Albert Einstein first described the theory that involved the stimulation of matter to cause the release of energy. In 1958 Schawlow and Townes used this concept of stimulated emission to develop the principle of laser, which is an acronym for *l*ight *a*mplification by the *s*timulated *e*mission of *r*adiation.

In 1962 Theodore Maiman developed the first laser for medicine and surgery using a ruby crystal. The ruby laser was utilized for dermatologic applications and for retinal photocoagulation in patients with diabetic retinopathy. It was not very efficient, however. Other lasers, such as the argon, carbon dioxide, Nd:YAG, holmium, and diode lasers, have been developed and are now being used in many surgical disciplines. New lasers, such as the excimer and free electron lasers, continue to be investigated and refined for clinical use. Advancements in laser technology have provided the physician with a precision tool for cutting, coagulating, vaporizing, and welding tissue during surgical intervention.

PRINCIPLES OF LIGHT

Laser is an acronym that describes a process in which light energy is produced. This term also refers to the device that generates the laser energy.

Light is a form of electromagnetic energy that can be graphically illustrated on a continuum known as the electromagnetic spectrum (Fig. 31-1). The unit of measurement that delineates the continuum is called a wavelength, which is the distance between two successive peaks of a wave. Wavelength determines color and is usually measured in nanometers (10^{-9} m) or microns (1000 nm). The various wavelengths of laser energy extend from the shorter waves in the ultraviolet area to the longer waves in the infrared region along this perpetual line. The visible laser wavelengths occupy only a small portion of this continuum. The radiation of laser technology is nonionizing in that it does not present the hazard of cellular DNA disruption through continual tissue exposure. Therefore pregnant women can work with lasers, since laser energy does not produce harmful ionizing radiation.

Briefly, the laser functions in the following way. A negatively charged electron orbits a positively charged nucleus while the atom is in its ground or resting state, which is at its lowest possible level of energy. An outside source of energy can excite the atom and cause an electron to jump to a higher, less stable, orbit. The electron almost immediately returns to its stable orbit, and the atom resumes its normal resting state. As this process occurs, a tiny bundle of surplus energy called a photon is spontaneously emitted. If the photon is close to another atom still in the excited state, it then interacts with this atom. The photon triggers the excited second atom to return to its resting state, and in this process another photon of laser light is emitted. These two photons of identical energy then travel together.

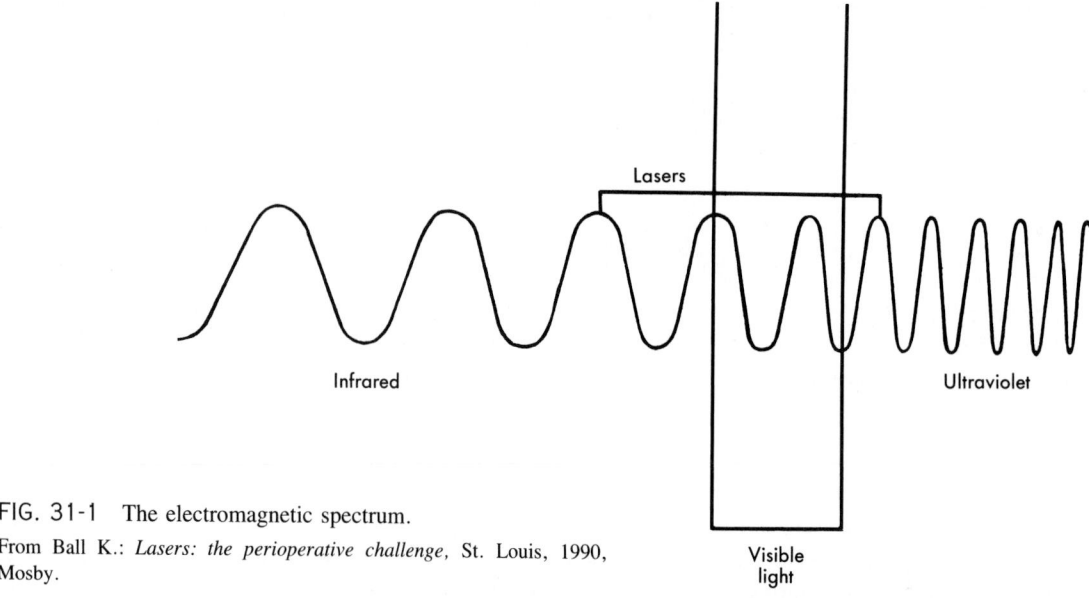

FIG. 31-1   The electromagnetic spectrum.
From Ball K.: *Lasers: the perioperative challenge,* St. Louis, 1990, Mosby.

Thus the process of stimulated emission has occurred and laser energy has been initially formed (Fig. 31-2).

This activity occurs in the resonating chamber of the laser, where the lasing medium is contained. The name of the laser is usually derived from the actual medium that causes the lasing action. The photons that are generated during the stimulated emission process are reflected back and forth between mirrors at each end of the resonating chamber as the process is amplified, until the number of excited atoms surpasses the number of resting atoms. This is known as population inversion. One of the mirrors in the chamber is partially reflective and, when activated, allows a stream of laser photons to escape the unit. These photons are then introduced to the target area via a specific delivery system.

CHARACTERISTICS OF LASER LIGHT

Three distinct characteristics distinguish laser light from ordinary light. Laser light is monochromatic, collimated, and coherent.

Monochromatic light is composed of photons of the same wavelength or color. In contrast, ordinary light consists of many different colors or wavelengths.

A collimated laser beam consists of waves parallel to each other that do not diverge significantly, thus minimizing any loss of power. When a collimated beam is passed through a lens, the light is focused into a tiny spot that tremendously concentrates the energy. In comparison, the light waves from a flashlight are not parallel and lose intensity as they travel away from the source. A lens cannot easily focus these noncollimated waves to concentrate the light into a small area.

Laser light is coherent—all the waves are orderly and in phase with each other as they travel in the same direction. All peaks and troughs of the waves are opposite each other in both time and space. This property provides an ad-

ditive effect that gives the laser beam power. Ordinary light is incoherent, since the waves radiate away from the source without being in phase or in an orderly pattern.

LASER POWER

The power, or energy, of a laser beam is measured in watts. One of the most critical factors in laser application is the concept of power density, or irradiance of the beam. Power density is the amount of power that is concentrated within an area and is described by the following formula:

$$\text{Power density} = \frac{\text{Watts}}{\text{Spot size (cm}^2)}$$

The spot size of the laser beam can be controlled by passing the beam through a special lens that causes the beam to converge. The focal configuration of the lens determines at what distance from the lens the beam will be most intense; this is called the focal point. If the beam is defocused into a larger spot size, the laser energy is spread over a greater area, thus decreasing the intensity or power density of the beam. In contrast, a small spot size of the beam concentrates the power into a smaller area, thus increasing the intensity or power density of the beam. When the power density is increased, the beam has the potential for causing a greater depth of penetration into the tissue.

A joule is the unit of measurement used to describe the total energy used. A joule is expressed by the power multiplied by the time duration of beam exposure. Fluence is a term that involves the power and duration of exposure of the beam and measures the specific amount of energy that is delivered to the tissue. The following equation calculates the fluence:

$$\text{Fluence} = \frac{\text{Watts} \times \text{Duration time}}{\text{Spot size (cm}^2)}$$

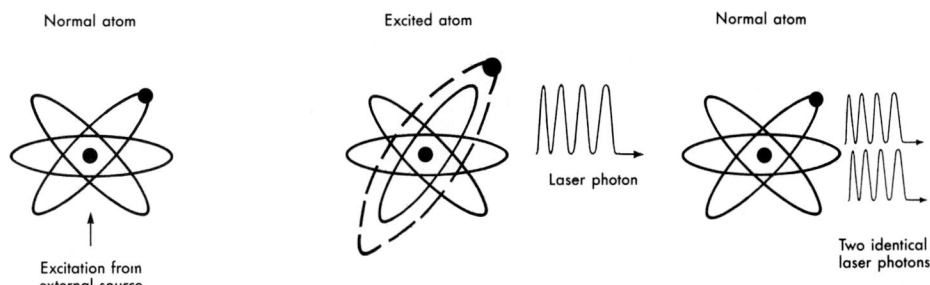

FIG. 31-2 Laser energy is produced when an external source excites the atom to emit a photon spontaneously. This photon can then "stimulate" the emission of two identical photons.

From Ball K.: *Lasers: the perioperative challenge,* St. Louis, 1990, Mosby.

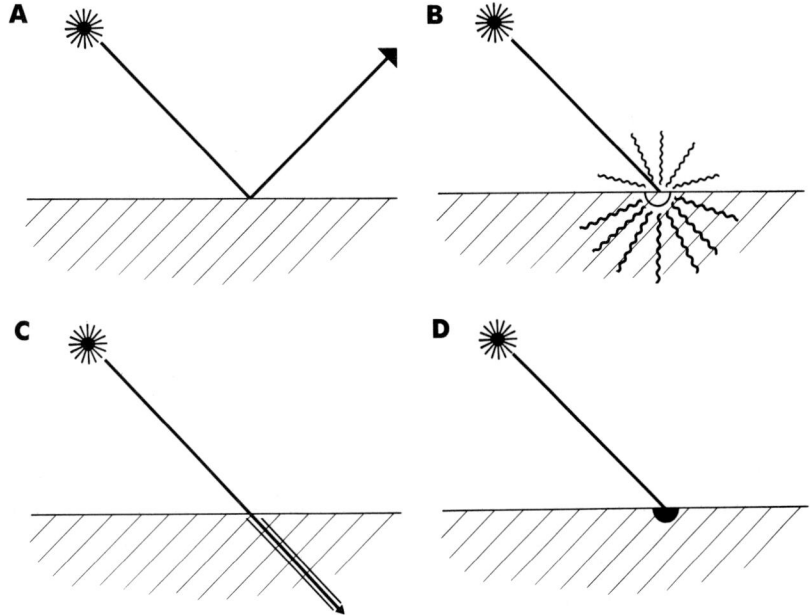

FIG. 31-3 Laser tissue interaction: reflection, scattering, transmission, absorption.

From Ball K.: *Lasers: the perioperative challenge,* St. Louis, 1990, Mosby.

The transverse electromagnetic mode (TEM) determines the precision of the beam by the distribution of the power over the spot area. The most precise or fundamental mode. TEMoo, evenly distributes the power over an area, with the most concentrated energy in the center and with the intensity of the beam decreasing toward the periphery.

TISSUE INTERACTION

When laser energy is delivered to the target area, four different interactions can occur: reflection, scattering, transmission, or absorption (Fig. 31-3). The extent of the reaction of the beam on the target depends on the laser wavelength, power settings, spot size, length of time the beam is in contact with the tissue, and the characteristics of the tissue.

Reflection of the laser beam occurs when the direction of the beam is changed after it contacts an area. Specular reflection occurs when the angle of the incoming light is equal to the angle of the reflected light. Laser light can be intentionally reflected in this manner off a reflective mirror to contact hard-to-reach areas. This type of reflection can also pose safety problems by inadvertently striking untargeted areas if it is not controlled at all times.

Scattering of the laser light occurs when the beam spreads over a large area as the tissue causes the beam to disperse. The intensity of the beam is decreased as the waves travel in different directions. The neodymium: yttrium-aluminum-garnet (Nd:YAG) laser beam can backscatter up an endoscope and possibly cause damage to the end of the scope, the optics, or the operator's eye.

Transmission of the laser beam occurs when the beam passes through fluids or tissue without thermally affecting the area. For example, the argon beam can be transmitted through the clear fluids and structures of the eye to the retina and cause thermal photocoagulation. The cornea, lens, and vitreous are unaffected by the transmission of the beam.

Absorption of the laser light results when the tissue is altered from the impact of the beam. This reaction is usually thermal but can sometimes be acoustic. The consistency, color, and water content of the target tissue often determine the rate of absorption of the laser energy. The laser wavelength also affects the absorption of the beam. Certain laser light, such as that from the argon laser, is highly absorbed by pigmented tissues. The carbon dioxide (CO_2) laser, however, is independent of color-selective absorption. The CO_2 laser light is absorbed superficially by tissue to a shallow depth of approximately 0.1 to 0.2 mm, whereas the holmium laser beam is absorbed to about 0.4 to 0.6 mm. Argon laser light is readily absorbed by pigmented tissue to a depth of approximately 1 to 2 mm, whereas that of the noncontact Nd:YAG laser beam is more readily absorbed by darkened tissue to a depth of 3 to 5 mm.

Tissue reaction becomes more pronounced as the temperature of the impact area increases (Table 31-1). During this thermal reaction the laser energy is absorbed, causing the cellular water to be heated. Intracellular protein is destroyed; as the temperature rises, the water inside the cell turns to steam. Eventually the membrane ruptures from increased pressure, spewing cellular debris and plume (smoke) from the tissue. The surrounding tissue is also heated because it borders the impact site. The degree of adjacent tissue damage depends on the duration of the laser beam exposure that causes the thermal injury.

LASER SYSTEMS

New laser systems are being introduced into health care regularly. Constant efforts by researchers and physicians to explore the use of different wavelengths are changing surgical approaches in a variety of specialties. Table 31-2 describes some of the more popular lasers used in medicine and surgery today.

PARTS OF A LASER SYSTEM

The five major components of a laser system are the laser head, excitation source, ancillary components, control panel, and delivery system. When a laser malfunctions, an organized investigation of each of these parts (Fig. 31-4) can usually determine the source of the problem.

The laser head, or resonating chamber, is the part where the laser energy is generated and amplified. The laser head contains the active medium or substance that actually produces the photons that generate the laser light. The active medium can be a gas (CO_2 or argon), a solid (Nd:YAG), a liquid (tunable dye), or a semiconductor crystal (diode).

The excitation source supplies the energy to excite the active medium in the laser head. Different sources include flash lamps, electricity, radio waves, battery, chemicals, and other laser systems. For example, the CO_2 laser gas is excited by electrical current or radio waves, and the Nd:YAG laser crystal is excited by flash lamps.

The ancillary components are the other laser parts that are needed to help produce the laser energy. A cooling system maintains the appropriate temperature of the laser head to keep the unit from overheating. Usually lasers are either

---

TABLE 31-1

Tissue Changes with Temperature Increases

Temperature	Visual change	Biologic change
37°-60° C	No visual change	Warming, welding
60°-65° C	Blanching	Coagulation
65°-90° C	White/grey	Protein denaturization
90°-100° C	Puckering	Drying
100° C	Smoke plume	Vaporization, carbonization

From Ball, K. (1990). *Lasers: the perioperative challenge*, St. Louis: Mosby.

TABLE 31-2

Description of Laser Color and Wavelength

Laser	Color	Wavelength (nm)
Excimer	Ultraviolet	
ArF		193
KrCl		222
KrF		248
XeCl		308
XeF		351
Helium-cadmium		325
Argon	Blue	488
	Green	515
Frequency-doubled YAG (KTP)	Green	532
Krypton	Green	531
	Yellow	568
	Red	647
Dye laser	Variable with dyes	
	Red	632
	Yellow	577-585
Gold vapor	Red	628
Helium neon	Red	632
Ruby	Deep red	694
Nd:YAG	Infrared	1064
		1318
Holmium-YAG	Infrared	2100
Erbium-YAG	Infrared	2900
Carbon dioxide	Infrared	10,600

From Ball, K. (1990). *Lasers: the perioperative challenge*, St. Louis: Mosby.

air cooled or water cooled. A vacuum pump may be required in a CO_2 laser to pull the gas mixture from an external cylinder into the laser head for laser light production.

The control panel consists of the board that regulates the delivery of laser energy. Various power settings, modes, time durations, and other parameters can be selected as desired. Many laser panels are now computerized, allowing the laser to be quickly and accurately controlled. Wireless control modules have been developed that can be placed in a sterile plastic bag so that the surgical team can control the laser from the operating field. The laser team should be exceedingly familiar with the operation of the laser control panel or module.

The delivery system of the laser is the device or accessory that actually conducts the laser energy from the laser head to the target area. CO_2 laser energy is usually delivered to the tissue through an articulated arm with a series of special mirrors at each joint. Argon and Nd:YAG lasers deliver energy through a fiber system. Advancements in laser technology are refining delivery systems to make them more adaptable, convenient, and user friendly.

CARBON DIOXIDE (CO_2) LASER

The CO_2 laser is versatile and widely used. Its wavelength of 10,600 nm is located in the infrared region of the electromagnetic spectrum. Because this light is invisible, a visible helium neon laser beam is usually transmitted coaxially with the CO_2 laser energy to serve as an aiming beam.

The CO_2 laser is characterized by its superficial tissue interaction (0.1 to 0.2 mm), since the beam is highly absorbed by water. The degree of tissue response is related to the amount of heat buildup from the absorption. There-

fore, the longer the CO_2 beam is in contact with the tissue, as with other laser wavelengths, the more destruction is noted and a greater depth of penetration can be achieved. The tissue reaction is quite visible and has been described as "what you see is what you get." The CO_2 beam is independent of color selectivity, meaning that lighter tissue absorbs the beam as readily as darker tissue.

Currently two types of CO_2 lasers are available that use electricity or radio waves as the excitation source. The free-flowing CO_2 laser system requires an external cylinder of a special laser gas mixture of carbon dioxide, helium, and nitrogen. The concentrations of these gases must be specific to the particular laser unit so that the laser operates properly. The gas is pulled into the laser head by a vacuum pump, laser energy is generated, and then harmless disassociated by-products are discharged from the unit. The laser gas cylinder is replaced when empty.

The other type of CO_2 laser is the sealed-tube system, which contains the special mixture of carbon dioxide, helium, and nitrogen within a tube that is sealed. A catalyst is added to the tube that causes regeneration of the mixture so that lasing action can be produced again. The shelf life (functional period) of this type of tube is usually from 1 to 4 years. At the end of this time the tube can be reprocessed by the manufacturer to replace the special gas and catalyst mixture.

With both types of CO_2 lasers the laser beam is delivered to the target area through a hollow tube called an articulated arm. Mirrors are positioned within the arm to reflect the laser energy forward. Because the helium-neon aiming beam runs coaxially with the CO_2 beam, care must be taken when moving the laser so that the mirrors are not jarred out of alignment.

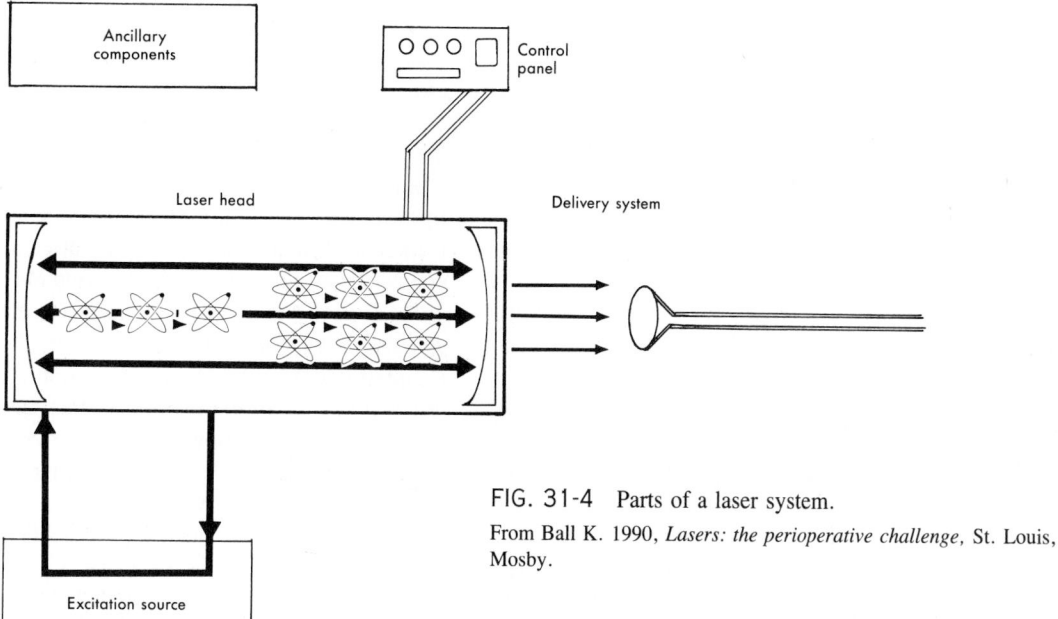

FIG. 31-4 Parts of a laser system.

From Ball K. 1990, *Lasers: the perioperative challenge*, St. Louis, Mosby.

The articulated arm can be attached to a microscope or a special handpiece. A lens system within these attachments causes the beam to converge at a certain point called the focal point. A special coating on the lens maintains the beam's integrity and intensity and must be cared for carefully so that the coating is not disrupted. The manufacturer's instructions that provide information on the appropriate lens care must be followed closely. At the lens focal point the beam is most intense, because all the energy is concentrated into a very small spot. The size of the spot can be changed by focusing or defocusing the lens to allow the spot to become larger or smaller. Sometimes tubing is connected to the handpiece or microscope adapter to conduct a purge gas or compressed air that blows the laser smoke away, thus keeping the lens cool and free from debris.

The CO_2 laser beam can also be conducted through a hollow flexible tube that allows the energy to "wiggle" down its path by being reflected off the surface of the inner lumen. Because of this reflection, some of the power of the beam is lost as it exits this delivery device. Solid fibers are currently being developed that will conduct the CO_2 wavelength to the target site.

The CO_2 laser energy can be delivered to tissue in a variety of modes. The continuous mode allows the laser energy to be delivered continuously as long as the foot pedal is depressed. The timed mode delivers the energy either one pulse at a time or in a repeat manner that specifically controls the duration of exposure. The superpulse mode delivers the energy in an extremely quick sequence of interrupted pulses that may appear to be a continuous mode. The energy may peak from 5 to 10 times higher than the desired wattage, but the duration of exposure is extremely limited, thus providing great precision. This type of interaction allows the adjacent tissue to cool so that tissue destruction is minimized.

ARGON LASER

The argon laser is another popular laser system. This laser produces an intense, visible blue-green light of approximately 488 and 515 nm, respectively. In clinical applications this combination of light wavelengths allows more complete tissue absorption. The depth of penetration is usually 1 to 2 mm. The aiming system is low-power argon laser energy because the beam is visible.

The argon energy is highly absorbed by hemoglobin, melanin, and other similar pigmentation and is less absorbed by lighter tissue. The absorbed laser energy is then converted to heat to cause coagulation or vaporization. Because of the high color selectivity of the beam, adjacent tissue injury is reduced significantly when the laser is being used on a localized pigmented area.

The argon wavelength is transmitted through clear fluids and structures. The argon laser energy is delivered to the target area through a fiber system. The fiber can be attached to a slit lamp, microscope, or handpiece, depending on the surgical approach. Because the argon light

diverges 10 to 14 degrees when exiting the fiber, the size of the spot can be altered by changing the distance of the fiber tip to the tissue. Special handpieces that contain an internal lens can be adjusted to change the spot size of the beam.

ND:YAG LASER

The neodymium:yttrium-aluminum-garnet (Nd:YAG) laser wavelength is in the infrared region of the electromagnetic spectrum at approximately 1064 nm. This invisible wave is usually accompanied by a visible helium-neon beam or other colored light, such as white light, to provide an aiming source. The Nd:YAG laser has a solid crystal of yttrium-aluminum-garnet that is doped with neodymium, which produces the lasing energy when exposed to bright flash lamps.

The Nd:YAG wavelength, like the argon wavelength, is transmitted through clear fluids and structures and is more highly absorbed by darker tissue. This laser light tends to scatter within the tissue and cause thermal damage to approximately 5 mm. Tissue absorption produces a homogeneous coagulative effect as tissue is heated to the point of coagulation without vaporization occurring. The Nd:YAG beam can easily backscatter, posing an eye safety concern when used through an endoscope.

The Nd:YAG energy is delivered to the tissue through a fiber system. The core fiber, usually made of quartz, is surrounded by a Teflon silicone coating or cladding that keeps the light in. This is known as a bare fiber. If the bare fiber is encased by a catheter sheath, then a purge gas, air, or fluid can be conducted down the length of the fiber. This purge is used to cool the fiber tip and keep debris from accumulating.

The Nd:YAG laser wavelength can be delivered to the tissue in a noncontact mode, meaning that the fiber does not touch the tissue.

Nd:YAG laser energy can also be delivered to the tissue using the contact method. A synthetic sapphire contact probe or scalpel can be attached to the end of a fiber with a special connector to deliver the Nd:YAG energy directly to the tissue in a more concentrated manner. The depth of penetration then is limited to less than 1 mm. These contact tips are available in a variety of geometric configurations. Depending on the desired tissue effects, the appropriate contact tip is chosen. A scalpel is used to cut, and a rounded probe is used to vaporize. A flat probe may be used to coagulate tissue. The end of the quartz fiber may also be sculpted into a geometric configuration that can be used in direct contact with the tissue. Contact technology provides precision, since the power output of the beam is confined to a very small area. It causes less thermal buildup so that adjacent tissue is relatively unaffected. The beam does not scatter as readily as the free Nd:YAG energy, and less plume is generated.

Another Nd:YAG wavelength being investigated is in the 1318-nm range. This laser causes minimal heat dissipation and allows greater cutting precision.

Besides the continuous-mode Nd:YAG laser, a special pulsed-mode Nd:YAG laser for ophthalmologic applications delivers the energy to the tissue in extremely short pulsations of nanoseconds. This laser works with an acoustic effect instead of a thermal effect. For example, a clouded membrane behind an artificial lens implant can be ruptured quickly and painlessly with this Nd:YAG laser beam through the production of an acoustic effect at the target site.

The frequency-doubled YAG laser is also popular in health care today. An Nd:YAG beam of 1064 nm is passed through a potassium-titanyl-phosphate (KTP) crystal to produce an intense green laser light of 532 nm. This process of delivering the Nd:YAG incident beam of 1064 nm through the KTP crystal shortens the wavelength in half, to 532 nm, while doubling the beam's frequency. The emergent beam then is visible. If the original Nd:YAG beam is once again desired, the crystal is rotated out of the way by pressing a button on the control panel.

The 532-nm wavelength responds to tissue in the same manner as the argon beam. It is very color selective and is highly absorbed by hemoglobin, melanin, and other similar pigmentations. The beam is conducted to tissue via a fiber, and this wavelength can also be transmitted through clear solutions and structures. The depth of penetration is approximately 1 to 2 mm.

HOLMIUM:YAG LASER

Another YAG laser that has been widely accepted into the surgical arena today is the holmium:YAG laser. The YAG crystal is doped with holmium, which is a rare earth element. This laser produces a wavelength of 2100 nm and is delivered to the tissue in a quick pulsed mode. The holmium wavelength is absorbed intensely by water so the depth of penetration is limited to approximately 0.4 to 0.6 mm. It has many of the same benefits of CO_2 laser technology in that it can ablate tissue very precisely but it can also be conducted to the target via a flexible fiber. This wavelength can be delivered to tissues in a fluid environment, since it produces a vapor bubble that transmits the laser energy. If the fiber is held almost in contact or directly in contact with the tissue, cutting occurs. If sculpting or ablating is needed, the fiber is held at a distance of approximately 2 mm from the target. Adjacent tissue is left significantly unharmed, thus enhancing the precision of this wavelength.

OTHER LASER SYSTEMS

The *tunable dye laser* allows the operator to dial in the desired wavelength within a limited range, such as 400 to 1000 nm. By changing dyes or other certain parameters, the wavelength can be changed. Tunable dye lasers produce a range of colors by exposing a liquid dye to an intense light source, such as an argon laser beam. The dye then absorbs the laser light and fluoresces over a broad spectrum of colors. By using special crystal prisms, diffraction gratings, or birefringent filters

within the laser, a specific wavelength can be produced.

This laser has become very popular in treating pigmented dermatologic conditions. A yellow laser beam can be generated at 585 nm that is readily absorbed by hemoglobin and less absorbed by the epidermal melanin, thus leading to less scarring. The tunable dye lasers have been refined to provide very quick pulsations in milliseconds that allow increased power to be used. Less adjacent tissue damage is realized with the shorter durations of exposure, and greater tissue response occurs through the increased wattage used. Advancements to produce an array of different wavelengths with a variety of pulsation modes are continually being developed to successfully treat dermatologic conditions.

The *excimer laser* derives its name through the use of an active medium that is an excited dimer. This laser is also known as a rare gas–halide laser in that it combines a rare gas with a halide, usually a halide-oxide or a halide-halide dimer. The dimeric media are excited to emit the laser energy. Depending on the chemical composition of the active medium, a variety of the shorter ultraviolet wavelengths can be produced. Four of the most popular wavelengths are argon fluoride (ArF) at 193 nm, krypton fluoride (KrF) at 248 nm, xenon chloride (XeCl) at 308 nm, and xenon fluoride (XeFl) at 351 nm. One of the hazards of the excimer laser is that these gases are extremely toxic; therefore appropriate laser housings and exhausts must be employed. Some excimer lasers are quite large, so more floor space should be planned for.

Excimer lasers are popular for their significant ablative capabilities. The beam penetrates less than 1 μm into the tissue and disassociates the molecular bonds of the cells. There is no significant damage to the adjacent tissue because the beam provides a sharp, clean cutting action at the target site without any thermal damage. Therefore this laser has been used very successfully to sculpt corneas for refractive purposes and to ablate plaque in arteries. Other applications continue to be developed and researched for FDA approval.

Diode lasers, since they are extremely compact and reliable, are being used in a number of consumer products, such as video disk players and computers. This technology is now being used for surgical lasers with approximately 30 W of output in the 750 to 950-nm range. With the efficiency, small size, and reliability of these systems, increasing medical applications can be anticipated in the near future. With the advent of the high-power semiconductor diode lasers in the gallium-arsenide family (840 to 910 nm), smaller laser photocoagulators for ophthalmic applications have been developed. This laser energy can be delivered directly to the tissue through a fiber or can be attached to an existing slit lamp microscope. Other clinical applications are being explored that will allow this type of laser to be used in place of other wavelengths, such as the Nd:YAG laser.

As technology continues to advance, laser wavelengths are being combined into one unit so that a selection of wavelengths, such as the Nd:YAG or holmium:YAG can easily be used during a procedure. The delivery systems must be compatible for this type of setup. A variety of wavelengths are being developed as other active media are being explored. New delivery systems are being perfected as different material combinations are being discovered that will more efficiently conduct the laser energy to the tissue.

BENEFITS OF LASER TECHNOLOGY

Laser technology continues to evolve as more surgical applications are developed. Once controversial, the laser has now become a respected and valued medical device that is revolutionizing surgery. As physicians become more adept in laser applications, utilization continues to grow. The laser has fostered the development of new minimally invasive procedures and endoscopic techniques. The true potential of the laser has yet to be realized as health care practitioners explore different applications of laser technology. The following list describes some of the advantages that have been associated with laser technology, depending upon the procedure performed.

- Seals small blood vessels (less intraoperative and post-operative blood loss).
- Seals lymphatics (decreases postoperative edema and the chance of spread of malignant cells in the lymphatic system).
- Seals nerve endings (on selective procedures, to decrease postoperative pain).
- Sterilizes tissue (from the heat generated at the laser tissue impact site).
- Decreases postoperative stenosis (by decreasing the amount of scarring that could lead to stenosis).
- Produces minimal tissue damage (from precision of the laser beam).
- Reduces operative and anesthesia time.
- Allows shift to more ambulatory surgery procedures.
- Allows more use of local anesthesia instead of general anesthesia.
- Provides quicker recovery and return to daily activities.

As new laser technology is introduced and refined, perioperative nurses have the responsibility of expanding their knowledge base by keeping current with the safety requirements and operation of these systems. Laser technology is a challenge to the perioperative nurse's professional growth. It offers the opportunity to develop creative methods of perioperative nursing practice to deliver high-quality patient care during laser procedures. The full potential of laser use is still being realized, and the perioperative nurse continues to have an instrumental role in the development of this technology in the 1990s.

SAFETY

Because laser systems are capable of concentrating high amounts of energy within very small areas, they present po-

tential hazards. Safe and appropriate use of the laser during surgical intervention is the responsibility of the entire health care team. Each member must be acutely aware of the many controls needed to prevent accidental injury. Often the laser team member is given the responsibility and authority to shut down the laser system if safety policies are not being followed.

The laser is a class III medical device that is subdivided into four subclasses. The lasers designated as subclass III and IV have the potential to cause injury. Some of the ophthalmic Nd:YAG lasers that cause an acoustic instead of a thermal reaction are classified in the subclass III category and can cause injury with sustained interaction. Most of the lasers used in surgical applications today are known as subclass IV lasers and can cause thermal reactions that can lead to fire, skin burns, and optical damage by either direct or scattered radiation. Specific safety precautions must be followed to prevent injury from these laser systems.

Many agencies are beginning to address the regulation of laser safety. Health care facilities must develop safety protocols in anticipation of mandates by these regulatory agencies as the technology advances and grows.

The American National Standards Institute (ANSI), a nongovernmental organization of experts, published the ANSI Z136.1 standards in 1973 as safety guidelines for laser use in warfare, industry, and health care. In 1988 ANSI Z136.3 standards were established to provide specific recommendations for laser use in health care environments. The appendix of ANSI Z136.3 discusses a consensus on laser safety in each of the special areas of medicine and surgery. These standards are reviewed periodically and revised as surgical trends continue to change. It is recommended that both ANSI standards be acquired for reference, since the Z136.3 document often refers to the Z136.1 publication.

Other guidelines have been suggested by the Center for Devices and Radiological Health (CDRH), Association of Operating Room Nurses (AORN), American Society for Laser Medicine and Surgery (ASLMS), Laser Institute of America (LIA), Food and Drug Administration (FDA), Occupational Safety and Health Administration (OSHA), and individual state and local regulatory bodies.

Hospitals and other health care delivery facilities need to formulate laser safety policies and procedures using these groups of experts as resources. In the development of safety guidelines for a facility, protocols should individually address situations without being too general or too specific. A policy or procedure must be general enough to address the need but not so detailed that the surgical team cannot follow it. Facilities must realize that they can be held liable for following their own safety policies and procedures. Therefore basic inservice education on the written laser policies and procedures for all personnel in the surgical environment (including orderlies and housekeeping personnel) should be mandatory. National standards and guidelines are currently being developed as the technology continues to grow and mature.

EYE PROTECTION

Because the eye is extremely sensitive to laser radiation, great care must be taken to protect the eyes during laser intervention. Even low levels of laser radiation can lead to permanent optical damage. The area of possible ophthalmologic injury depends on the type of wavelength. The CO_2 laser can damage the cornea, since this beam is readily absorbed by the surface cells. Immediate pain is associated with this injury. The argon and Nd:YAG laser beams, in contrast, are transmitted through the clear optical structures and fluids and can be refocused by the lens of the eye. The intensity of the beam after refocusing can permanently damage the retina. Sometimes pain is not even felt during this destruction (Fig. 31-5).

Adequate eye protection requires understanding the two concepts of maximum permissible exposure (MPE) and nominal hazard zone (NHZ). According to the ANSI Z136.3 standards the MPE is the level of laser radiation to which a person may be exposed without hazardous effects to the eye or skin. The MPE levels are determined by considering the laser wavelength, power, exposure time, and pulse repetition.

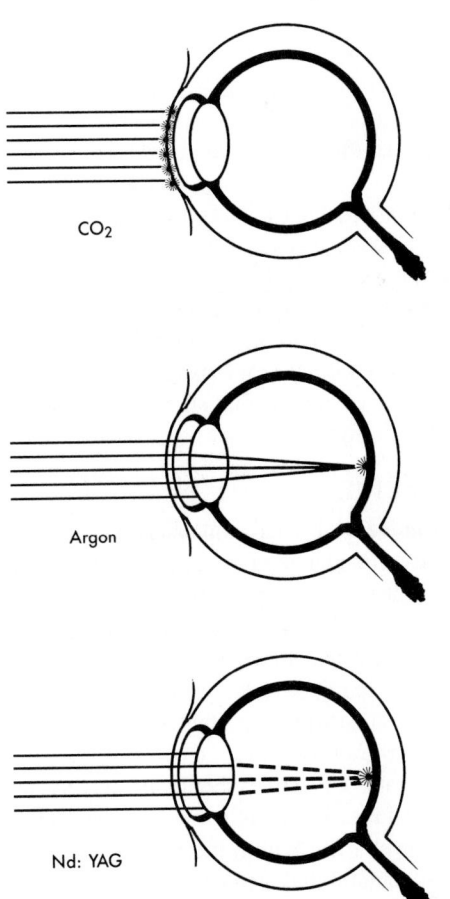

CO₂

Argon

Nd: YAG

FIG. 31-5   The CO_2 laser beam can damage the cornea; the argon and Nd:YAG beams can injure the retina.

From Ball K. 1990, *Lasers: the perioperative challenge,* St. Louis, Mosby.

The NHZ is the space where the level of the direct, reflected, or scattered radiation during normal laser operation exceeds the MPE; therefore eye, skin, and fire safety precautions must be followed while within this hazard zone. The NHZ can be calculated mathematically to determine the distance from the laser beam emission in which the beam can cause skin and eye damage. Since the power, operating modes, and other parameters are changed frequently during a procedure, this calculation would also change. Therefore the area inside the surgical room is usually considered to be within the NHZ so that consistency and simplicity can be maintained when lasers are used in health care.

Recommendations suggest that protective goggles, glasses, and endoscope lens covers should be inscribed with the appropriate filtering capabilities and adequate optical densities for the specific wavelength being used. For example, a pair of Nd:YAG goggles may be inscribed "1064 nm, optical density 4." The optical density of the lens is the ability of the lens material to absorb a specific wavelength. The darker lens shades do not necessarily have higher optical density or give more protection. Technology has introduced lighter lens shades with high optical densities that provide adequate safety. The perioperative nurse must ensure that eyewear is properly labeled, handled, and stored so that hazards are minimized and scratching and damage are avoided.

During surgical procedures utilizing multiple wavelengths protective eyewear must be changed as the wavelengths are changed. There are some types of eyewear that protect against a limited range of wavelengths. If the range is expanded to block a greater variety of wavelengths, then the eyewear is more difficult to see through.

Controversy exists as to the appropriateness of using one's own prescription glasses to serve as CO_2 laser eye protection when the wearer is not in the immediate vicinity of the laser beam emission (such as the circulating nurse). Prescription eyeglasses do not have the wavelength protection inscribed on them and have not been tested to note the protective ability of the lens; therefore adequate protection cannot be guaranteed. Opponents state that the NHZ is so limited when the CO_2 beam is passed through the focusing lens that those persons who are not close to the laser emission port are not at a high risk for eye damage. Facilities must address this controversial issue and develop a policy for the surgical team to follow. Contact lenses and half glasses definitely do not offer adequate protection against CO_2 laser energy.

During a microscopic procedure the optics of the microscope provide eye protection against CO_2 laser energy. But when other wavelengths are used, such as argon or Nd:YAG, an automatic lens shutter can be connected to the microscope head. During the laser activation the shutter allows a lens filter to drop in place to provide a shield from any laser backscatter. When this device is attached to the microscope head, any observer tube being used must also be placed above the filter so that all portal optics have protection provided.

A lens filter can be placed over the eyepiece of a rigid or flexible endoscope. The lens must offer the appropriate protection for the specific laser being used. Guidelines suggest that the other surgical team members also wear eye protection, even though the laser energy appears to be confined within an enclosed cavity. Optical injury is always possible if a fiber or articulated arm becomes separated from the endoscope while the laser is being activated or if a fiber is fractured and the beam escapes at that fracture site.

The ANSI standards recommend that a baseline eye examination, noting visual acuity and retinal health, be performed on those health care professionals who routinely work with laser systems. Another eye examination can be performed after any ophthalmic accident or upon termination of employment. The baseline exam then provides a foundation for comparison with abnormal findings from subsequent examinations. This preventive procedure protects the facility from a potential worker's compensation claim for retinal damage from incidental beam reflection, should the problem occur. Some facilities have opted not to follow this rather expensive and difficult to monitor guideline because they strictly enforce their eye safety policy, thus minimizing the chance of any ophthalmic accidents.

The patient's eyes must be protected during laser intervention. When general anesthesia is used, patients should have their eyes covered with wet gauze, eye pads, or a towel; the eyes should be taped closed. If awake or under local anesthesia, the patient should wear appropriate eye protection. Explanations should be provided to the patient regarding this safety action. If the laser is to be used in the immediate vicinity of the eye, such as to lighten a port wine stain on the eyelid, a special laser eye shield can be placed on the surface of the eye after instillation of a drop of an ophthalmic local anesthetic. Box 31-1 summarizes actions to promote eye safety during laser surgery.

CONTROLLED ACCESS

Inadvertent access to rooms where laser treatments are being performed should be prevented. Laser warning signs must be placed at all entrances to the treatment area so that access is granted only to those individuals who have been appropriately education in laser safety. The word *Danger* and the universally accepted laser symbol should be present on any laser warning sign to indicate the possibility of hazards. Laser signs should be removed when the procedure has been completed.

Windows and ports into rooms where lasers are utilized must be covered with the appropriate protection for the specific laser being used. The CO_2 laser beam is stopped by clear glass or Plexiglas panels, but the argon and Nd:YAG laser wavelengths can be transmitted through this glass. Therefore the windows and ports must be covered with a blocking barrier that stops the transmission of specific wavelengths.

The laser key must not be left in the laser during storage. The key should be available only to authorized per-

BOX 31-1

Guide to Eye Safety during Laser Surgery

- Ensure that everyone in the laser room is wearing the appropriate eye protection before activating the laser. The eyewear should have the laser wavelength protection and optical density of the lens material inscribed on it.
- A special lens cover can be placed over the eyepiece of an endoscope to protect the physician's eye from laser backscatter. Remember that the physician's other eye will be unprotected.
- Everyone in the laser room should wear eye protection during laser endoscopic procedures.
- An automatic lens shutter can be connected to a microscope head to provide eye protection for persons viewing the procedure through the microscope.
- When general anesthesia is used, cover the patient's closed eyes with moistened gauze pads. When the patient is awake, place the appropriate glasses or goggles on the patient. Explain the need for eye protection to the patient.
- During laser surgery near the eye, a special laser eye shield may be placed directly on the anesthetized eye surface.
- Ensure that the appropriate protective eyewear is available at all entrances to the laser room for anyone entering the area.
- When storing protective eyewear, guard against scratches and mishandling. Scratches on the lenses may decrease their effectiveness.

sonnel who have the appropriate education and training to operate the laser. Laser keys can be stored in the narcotics cabinet or in a special key lockbox to control access. Box 31-2 summarizes actions that should be initiated to control access to laser rooms.

FIRE SAFETY

An awareness of laser biophysics and tissue interaction is necessary to understand the actions needed to prevent laser fires. A fire can be started by a reflected beam as easily as from a direct impact. The laser team must be able to respond quickly if a fire occurs. Immediate action is the key to minimize injury to the patient and the surgical team. Box 31-3 summarizes important measures to support fire safety during laser surgery.

Sterile water or saline should be readily available to douse a small fire. A halon fire extinguisher should be available to control a fire within the laser system. This fire extinguisher contains halogenated hydrocarbons that do not produce a residue that could harm the internal delicate components of the laser. Halon is known to destroy the ozone layer so its use has become controversial. In contrast, a CO_2 fire extinguisher can cause thermal damage to the laser components from the extremely cold temperature of the residue

BOX 31-2

Guide to Controlled Access during Laser Surgery

- Hang laser warning signs at all entrances to the laser room to prevent unauthorized persons from entering.
- The warning sign should include *Danger* and the universal laser symbol.
- Cover windows or ports with the appropriate protection for the specific laser wavelength being used.
- Do not store the laser key in the laser. The laser key must be available only to authorized persons.

BOX 31-3

Guide to Fire Safety during Laser Surgery

- Sterile water or saline should be immediately available to douse a small fire near or on the patient.
- A halon fire extinguisher should be available in the department in case the laser catches on fire.
- Do not place fluids or solutions on the laser unit. Protect the laser system from spillage or splatter that could cause short-circuiting and fire.
- Do not place dry combustibles in the vicinity of the laser impact site. Use wet towels, nonflammable drapes, or special laser retardant materials near the laser target area. Moisten dry drapes and sponges with sterile saline or water to prevent ignition. Constantly monitor the moisture level throughout the procedure.
- Do not use flammable materials near the laser impact site.
- Utilize nonreflective instrumentation in or near the laser tissue impact site to decrease accidental direct reflection of the laser beam. Cover larger instruments, such as retractors, with wet sponges or towels to protect against reflection.
- Do not prep with flammable skin preparations, such as alcohol.
- A wet pack may be inserted into the rectum as a tamponade to prevent methane gas from escaping into the surgical area. A cleansing bowel prep before surgery will also decrease this risk.
- Use a specially prepared or a commercially manufactured laser endotracheal tube or wrap during laser procedures of the oropharynx. An unprotected PVC endotracheal tube can readily be ignited from an inadvertent laser beam impact. Inflate the endotracheal tube cuff with a solution to provide a heat sink if the cuff is penetrated by the laser beam. Protect the endotracheal tube cuff with wet gauze sponges.
- Place the laser in the standby mode when not in use.
- Identify the laser foot pedal to avoid accidental activation.

that is emitted. A dry chemical fire extinguisher is not appropriate, since it discharges a fine dust that damages the optics and circuitry of the laser system, and this dust is difficult to remove from the surgical environment.

During the surgical intervention combustibles, such as sponges or towels, near the laser tissue impact site should be kept wet to prevent ignition. The surgical team should constantly monitor the moisture level of the sponges and other materials to prevent drying that could eventually support a fire.

Flammable draping material can be easily ignited by a laser beam. Some water-repellent drapes and other laser-safe materials are able to withstand laser impact, and thus the flammability of the material is decreased. If the restrictions of draping material or any other supplies are questionable, the item can be tested for flammability in the manufacturer's or researcher's laboratory. The laser beam can be directed to the item using different power settings to determine any limitations before clinical use. Water should be immediately available during these experiments.

Instrumentation used in the immediate vicinity of the laser tissue impact site should be nonreflective to decrease the chance of the laser beam bouncing off the surface and accidentally impacting another area. The laser beam can easily be reflected off shiny instrument surfaces and can cause skin or eye injury or ignite flammable materials. An instrument may be ebonized by coating the instrument with a special substance (usually black) to decrease reflectivity. Many companies offer this service at a low cost. The instrument should be inspected regularly to ensure the integrity of the coating. Any scratched surface or area where the ebonization has worn off should be recoated as necessary.

An instrument may also be anodized or surfaced with a matte finish to decrease reflectivity. Other coatings and surfaces are being introduced that cause the laser light to scatter and diffuse upon impact. Larger retractors can be covered with wet sponges or towels so that the laser beam cannot accidentally be reflected off the shiny surface.

Other instrumentation may be used to provide a backstop for the laser energy to decrease adjacent tissue damage and the chance of fire. Titanium rods are effective backstops and can be reprocessed easily. Quartz rods are often used as backstops for the CO_2 laser beam, but the argon and Nd:YAG beams may be transmitted through them. Glass rods must never be used with a CO_2 laser because the glass material heats and shatters after continuous impact by the laser beam. Teflon backstops should not be used because they can melt when heated and produce toxic fumes. Wet sponges can also be used as backstop material.

Special laser mirrors have been introduced that directly reflect the beam onto a hard-to-reach area. Mirrors may be made of rhodium or stainless steel. Glass-surface mirrors do not withstand laser impact and will heat and shatter instead. Using a laser mirror requires skill, since the beam must be focused on the target area and not on the mirror to deliver the full impact of the laser energy. A laser beam that is misdirected off a mirror can easily cause a fire.

Flammable skin preparations should not be used for laser procedures. During skin cleansing the prep solution can pool underneath a patient, and ethanol vapors from alcohol-based preparations can become trapped beneath the drapes. The volatility of these vapors increases the risk of a surgical drape fire. Iodophor or any other tinted prep solution should be rinsed before using argon or Nd:YAG lasers, since the tint may unexpectedly increase laser absorption.

When a laser is used in the rectal area, a wet pack may be used to tamponade the methane gas that could enter the surgical area and cause an explosion. The wet sponges used for the pack must be counted so that the packing is not inadvertently left in place after the surgery is completed. A cleansing bowel preparation before surgery also helps to decrease this potential hazard.

Airway explosion caused by the laser beam igniting the endotracheal tube can cause a potentially lethal accident for the patient. A polyvinylchloride endotracheal tube is highly flammable, especially as a high concentration of oxygen flows through it during anesthesia administration. Specific laser-retardant endotracheal tubes, special endotracheal tube protective wraps, or foil-wrapped red rubber endotracheal tubes should be used during oral, tracheal, or esophageal laser procedures that require general anesthesia. The laser power limitations of a commercially prepared endotracheal tube or wrap must be followed closely to ensure proper performance of the protective material. The cuff of the endotracheal tube should be inflated with sterile saline to provide a heat sink and retard a fire if it is perforated by the laser beam. Saline may be tinted with methylene blue to immediately note cuff rupture. A protocol should be developed that describes the emergency procedure needed to control an endotracheal fire. Immediate considerations include the following:

1. Remove the flaming endotracheal tube and instruments. Stop the flow of oxygen by pinching the oxygen tube or shutting off the supply valve.
2. Reintubate immediately to prevent laryngospasm.
3. Inspect the mouth, oral cavity, and bronchial tree.

Jet ventilation may also be used during a laser microlaryngoscopy. A jet ventilator is a mechanical ventilation unit that delivers the anesthetic gases through a small metal needle used in conjunction with a rigid laryngoscope. Under pressurization the jet ventilator is set to deliver a determined amount of anesthesia gas while setting the rate, psi, and percent of inspiratory time. The needle is positioned between the vocal cords on the side opposite the lesion. The needle extends into the trachea so that the proper amount of anesthesia gas can be delivered easily. After the surgery, the patient may be intubated to maintain an open airway if postoperative edema or tracheal spasm is anticipated.

ENDOSCOPE SAFETY

Special precautions should be followed when using the laser during an endoscopic procedure. When a laser fiber is introduced through the biopsy port of a flexible or rigid endoscope, the operator must view the tip of the fiber be-

fore activating the laser. If the end of the fiber is still within the sheath of the endoscope and the laser is fired, the heat from the laser energy will quickly damage the optics and channel of the endoscope.

When a "bare" fiber is placed down the biopsy channel of a flexible endoscope, the sharp tip can possibly tear the inside lumen of the channel. A length of medical grade tubing can be placed over the fiber with the tip recessed within the sheath. The entire unit is then passed through the endoscope. Once the end of the tubing is observed, the medical grade tubing is withdrawn sufficiently to expose the end of the fiber. This procedure effectively protects the inside lumen of the endoscope channel.

SMOKE EVACUATION

Smoke evacuation and odor control must be adequate whenever plume is generated, whether it is from the laser, electrosurgical unit, or other surgical devices being used (Research Highlight 31-1). Research has conclusively determined that the size of the particulate matter in surgical smoke is extremely small and that this plume could coat lung alveoli if inhaled over time. Controversy exists today as to the viability of surgical plume, and more research is needed to conclusively prove the potential of transmitting infectious diseases through inhaling the smoke. Surgical plume contains carbonized particles, water, cellular debris, trace amounts of acrolein, benzene, formaldehyde and other elements, and an offensive odor; therefore adequate smoke evacuation is necessary to remove these contaminants from the air. Small amounts of generated plume can be evacuated through a special in-line suction filter positioned between the wall outlet and the suction canister. If the amount of plume is greater, an individual smoke evacuation unit that can filter particulate matter as small as 0.1 μm should be used. Smoke evacuator filters should be changed regularly as specified by the manufacturer.

Contamination by the surgical plume and tissue splatter is also decreased when the surgical team wears gloves, gowns, and masks. High-filtration masks that filter particulate matter of at least 0.3 μm should be used. A standard surgical mask usually filters particulate matter that is 5 μm.

The key to adequate smoke evacuation and elimination of inhalation hazards is to evacuate the plume at the laser-tissue impact site. Constant vigilance is mandatory to ensure that the smoke evacuation wand or suction device is very close to the laser target. Research continues in this area to develop devices to control the plume so that the surgical team and the patient are not subjected to inhalation contaminants and offensive odors. Box 31-4 summarizes important measures for smoke evacuation during laser surgery.

OTHER SAFETY MEASURES

Foot pedals can also present safety problems if mistakenly activated. Technology has given the physician more pedals to control devices and instrumentation in today's surgical environment. The number of foot pedals placed on the floor for the physician can often be confusing and can easily lead to accidents. The laser pedal should be clearly

BOX 31-4

Guide to Smoke Evacuation during Laser Surgery

- Use the appropriate smoke evacuation system for the amount of plume generated. Never use a nonfiltered in-line suction system to remove surgical smoke.
- Change the smoke evacuation filter(s) as often as recommended.
- Maintain the smoke tube or evacuation device as close as possible to the laser-tissue impact site.
- Wear high-filtration surgical masks that provide adequate filtration (capable of filtering 0.3 or 0.1 μm particular matter) when surgical plume is generated.

RESEARCH HIGHLIGHT 31-1

A research study on the hazards of surgical smoke was conducted by Barry L. Wenig MD, Kerstin M. Stenson MD, Bruce M. Wenig MD, and Diana Tracey, BS in 1992. Laboratory rats were exposed to laser as well as electrocautery plume for a designated period of time. The rats were divided into three groups. The first group was exposed to the plume generated by using the contact Nd:YAG laser on pigskin for two minutes followed by two minutes of rest. This was repeated four times during 4 days. The second group was exposed to the plume generated by using noncontact Nd:YAG laser energy for four minutes followed by two minutes rest. Four sessions were conducted on each of 7 days. The third group was exposed to electrocautery plume for a total of 14 days with time sequences like the second group. All of the rats were then euthanized and the cardiorespiratory systems were removed for examination. The specimens showed signs of harmful smoke effects on the lungs, including muscular hypertrophy of the vessel walls, emphysematous changes, and alveolar congestions. The control rats, who were not subjected to the smoke, revealed normal lung parenchyma. There was no significant specimens differences in the length of exposure time or the difference in surgical tools (laser vs. electrocautery).

In conclusion, the plume generated from an electrocautery device is just as hazardous as the laser and must be evacuated. This study and other previous research strongly support the use of an effective smoke evacuator to protect the patient and the surgical team during any procedure that produces smoke.

Wenig, BL; Stenson, KM; Wenig, BM; & Tracey, D. (1993). Effects of plume produced by the Nd:YAG laser and electrocautery on the respiratory system, *Lasers in Surgery and Medicine, 13*:242-245.

identified for the physician and should be used by only the physician who is actually delivering the laser energy to the target area.

Laser team members should appreciate the potential for electrical hazards because the laser is a high-voltage piece of equipment. Water and other solutions should not be placed on the laser unit, and the components of the laser should be protected against spillage or splatter that could cause short-circuiting. The outside housing of the laser should never be removed by unauthorized personnel, since the potential for electrical shock or electrocution is high.

Transportation hazards are always a potential threat because some of the laser systems are quite heavy. When these units need to be moved from one area to another, proper body mechanics must be employed to prevent injury to the transporter. The laser should never be bumped against a wall because the internal components can be damaged or thrown out of alignment.

DOCUMENTATION

Complete and accurate documentation that notes the safety parameters followed during a laser procedure is critical. Documenting laser safety is important for medicolegal reasons, as for any potentially hazardous piece of equipment. Documentation can be on a laser log form or as part of the existing intraoperative nursing notes. Either record should be placed on the patient's chart so that safety activities that were performed can be recorded.

A special laser log can be designed to be a permanent part of the patient's record and could include information such as the laser used, power, pulse duration, and other laser parameters. The use of smoke evacuation, fibers, and contact tips should also be documented, especially if specific charges for these items are made. Sometimes the reimburser will challenge the payment of an item if its use is not documented on the patient's record. A sample laser log is shown in Box 31-5.

ROLE OF THE LASER TEAM MEMBER

As the popularity of laser technology continues to grow, the role of the laser team member becomes increasingly important. The backbone of a progressive and successful laser program is the enthusiastic and dedicated laser team. Expanded responsibilities are being assumed by the laser team member to provide consistency and promote a safe environment for the patient and the surgical team. Some of the roles of the laser team member may include becoming the laser safety officer, serving on the laser committee, becoming actively involved with laser procurement, and promoting the laser program through marketing.

COMPOSITION OF THE LASER TEAM

According to ANSI Z136.3 standards the laser safety officer (LSO) is the individual who has the responsibility to determine laser hazards and monitor and enforce laser safety. This person is usually a nurse but can be a technician, physician, or researcher. The LSO investigates laser accidents and reports safety infractions to the laser committee for evaluation and resolution.

Interpretations of the ANSI Z136.3 standards defining the role of the LSO note that each health care facility should designate one individual to assume these responsibilities. Other laser team members are guided by the LSO to ensure that consistency and safe laser practices are being maintained within the laser program.

The LSO is also responsible to ensure that the other laser team members have received adequate and appropriate laser education and practical experience. Laser training for the LSO and the laser team member involves attendance at an educational offering that focuses on laser physics, tis-

sue interaction, safety, and clinical application. The laser team member is the generalist who must understand laser applications in all specialty areas. Unlike physicians who focus on their own specialty, the laser team member must be able to provide support during all types of laser procedures. This expertise level is achieved by constant review of the literature to understand new techniques and developments.

The LSO oversees and coordinates the responsibilities of the other laser team members. Consistency within the laser program to provide cohesiveness among the team is critical to ensure satisfaction and success. Some of the expanded responsibilities that the LSO may authorize the laser team member to fulfill are listed below:

Set up and test fire the laser system
Operate the laser control panel
Place the laser on standby when it is not actually being used to prevent accidental and uncontrolled laser firing
Perform preventive maintenance and minor troubleshooting on the laser
Monitor and enforce laser safety according to written policies and procedures
Participate in quality management activities
Report to the LSO any infractions of the written policies
Document the laser procedure, laser charges, and laser service
Inventory and maintain laser supplies and accessories
Attend laser committee meetings when requested
Assist with patient education
Help monitor physician credentialing
Stay abreast of laser technology by attending continuing education conferences or reading laser publications
Actively assist with laser system evaluations when a new laser is needed
Act as the laser resource person for the surgical team
Make suggestions to enhance the laser program
Assist with a laser marketing program to increase visibility and utilization

Perioperative nurses who are part of the laser team are often involved with patient education. The perioperative nurse reinforces what the physician has described to the patient before the laser procedure. When told that surgery is needed, the patient is often anxious because of the unknown. When it is mentioned that laser surgery is needed, the anxiety may be compounded because the patient is confronted with two alarming unknowns. Many patients develop an uneasiness about laser procedures based on information from science fiction movies, talk shows, and other such sources. The patient should always have the opportunity to discuss the laser procedure to allay any worries. After the physician has explained the procedure and has had the surgical consent form signed, the perioperative nurse may provide additional information if the patient has any further questions about laser technology. Ideally, the con-

---

BOX 31-5

Sample Laser Log

Date _____ O.R. Room No. ____

PATIENT INFORMATION
Name _____ Patient ID No. _____
Zip Code _____ Sex: M F Age _____

Status: IP   OP

Insurance _____

SURGERY INFORMATION
Physician _____ Anesthesia: General Local

Procedure _____

LASER INFORMATION
Laser _____ Wavelength _____

Power _____ Duration _____

Total spots _____ Total energy _____

Laser time on _____ Laser time off _____
    Total laser time _____

Laser riber _____

Contact tip _____

Smoke evacuation _____

Comments: _____
_____
_____
_____

Laser team member _____

sent form should reflect that the laser will be used during the surgical experience. Some physicians have noted that the laser is merely a tool used during the surgical intervention and do not feel the need to list the laser use on the consent form.

An adequate amount of time should be allotted for patient questions before the procedure. If local anesthesia is used, the patient should understand what to anticipate during the surgery, what sounds or odors will be present, why eye protection is needed, and what the patient's role is during the procedure. If the patient understands the application, the role of the laser, and his or her responsibility during and after the procedure, the perioperative nurse can expect better compliance and diminished anxiety in the patient.

Discharge instructions are required for any ambulatory procedure; therefore laser discharge instructions may be preprinted for each surgical application. These written instructions should be reviewed and given to the patient upon discharge. A follow-up phone call helps the perioperative nurse evaluate the care delivered during the laser intervention and the patient's compliance with the postoperative instructions.

Sometimes the perioperative nurse is placed in a compromising position by being expected to circulate during the surgical procedure and also operate the laser. This nurse then has the tremendous responsibility of being accountable for two critical roles in the operating room, and the risk of a laser incident is increased. In the traditional setting one nurse circulates while another nurse or a technician, who is part of the laser team, operates the laser. The health care facility must determine what procedures require more staffing to handle each perioperative nursing role.

Documentation is a critical responsibility of the laser team member. Laser utilization must be documented on the patient's chart according to the facility's specific protocols.

A biomedical laser technician may be included as part of the laser team as the number of laser systems increases. If only a few lasers are in the program, a service contract may be purchased after the warranty period has expired on the laser. As the number of laser systems grows, however, the economic rationale to add the position of biomedical laser technician may be justified. This person usually has attended a training school or program on laser and optics technology. The addition of this position allows preventive maintenance to be performed on a regular basis and laser malfunctions to be addressed immediately.

LASER COMMITTEE

Any facility that uses laser technology should form a laser committee. The laser committee can initially be part of the surgical committee but eventually, as the program expands, it should become an independent committee in the health care facility. Membership on this committee includes but is not limited to a representative from administration, physicians from different specialty areas, laser team members, operating room director, facility risk manager, librar-

ian, and a public relations or marketing representative. Others can be invited to attend as mandated by the agenda of each meeting. Meetings should be held regularly (at least quarterly or monthly) and may be open to anyone interested in the laser program to encourage participation by more people.

A major purpose of the laser committee is to provide guidance to the laser program so that laser technology is expanded and enhanced to benefit patients. The success of the laser program is usually in direct response to the activities of the laser committee. The laser team member plays an important role by serving on the laser committee and implementing these activities and other proposed suggestions. Feasibility studies should be conducted regularly to note physicians' needs and interests. For example, if another laser system is to be purchased, a survey should be sent to physicians to note preferences and forecast usage. Potential volume and revenue can then be projected to justify the procurement of a specific laser system. The utilization trends of the laser program can note the need to expand into a local anesthesia laser center or determine the support from different specialty areas. The laser team member can help conduct these surveys and verbalize any trends they notice happening or interests physicians have expressed to them.

The laser committee is responsible for developing a physician credentialing policy that the laser team members help to enforce. The specific laser credentialing protocol is determined by each facility because no national regulations have mandated a ruling. Recommendations of ANSI and the ASLMS suggest that a physician receive information about laser physics, safety, tissue interaction, and clinical application. Laser technology is beginning to be introduced in medical schools as part of the student's initial education process. Currently many specialty laser courses are available for practicing physicians to attend. Usually a facility requires that the physician attend a course with hands-on experience and then have a preceptor (one who is already credentialed to use the laser) oversee one or more laser procedures to document the physician's safe and appropriate use of the laser. The physician's credentialing is sometimes reviewed by the specialty department and then is approved by the governing board of the hospital. Written credentialing approval should be kept on record in the physician's file in the medical staff office. The laser committee also should address a credentialing protocol for residents who want to become involved with laser technology. Written guidelines should be established to allow a resident to participate in clinical laser applications. Usually a resident must attend a laser course or participate in a laser educational session so that laser biophysics and safety are thoroughly understood before the resident is allowed to assist with a laser procedure.

Because laser technology is continually changing, an annual credentialing review process may be developed by the laser committee. This process involves determining the number of laser procedures that each credentialed physician has performed within a certain time period. Because laser use requires skill, a physician who uses the laser infrequently may need a refresher course or a preceptorship to decrease the chance of any problems. Sometimes an annual credentialing review determines why a physician is using the laser at another facility more often. This information can be used to help market the laser program to encourage more physician participation.

The laser team member should have immediate access to the list of laser credentialed physicians that notes what wavelength the physician can use and if a preceptorship is needed. This information should also be available in the surgery scheduling office. If a physician needs to have a preceptor, then the laser team member can make sure that a preceptor form or special documentation sheet is available for completion when the preceptorship occurs. The laser committee may want to review this documentation too before it is placed on file in the medical staff or credentialing office.

The laser team member is a vital participant in the task of formulating safety policies and procedures by the laser committee. Written guidelines must be developed within a laser program to provide consistency. These rules must be readily available to and openly communicated by the laser team so that compliance can be consistently enforced. Often the laser committee gives the laser team members the responsibility and authority to shut down a laser system if written safety policies are not being followed. Safety policies and procedures should be reviewed annually for appropriateness and should reflect the standard of care followed during laser procedures.

LASER PROCUREMENT

The laser team member is often involved in the procurement of a laser system. Careful planning is required to procure a laser system, since these highly technologic pieces of equipment can be very expensive. Procuring a laser system is a three-phase process involving justification, evaluation, and acquisition.

The justification phase is usually conducted by the laser committee with the help of the laser team members. This process determines if there is an actual need for the laser system. A justification survey is sent to physicians who might use the system. The written responses are tallied to decide need and interest.

After the determination has been made that a system is needed, then the evaluation process begins. Several of the leading laser companies are invited to participate in this process. A comparison sheet can be developed to note the features of the different laser systems. The advantages and disadvantages are thoroughly examined for each unit. Often lasers are brought into the hospital for a clinical trial period. The laser team members need to help organize and control this evaluation because the cost to the manufacturer or distributor to provide this service can become very expensive. After the planned evaluation of the various units, the opinions of physicians and laser team members are con-

sidered in open discussions. Some factors for deciding which system to buy can involve the laser warranty package, cost of service contracts, service response time, availability of the laser system and accessories, cost of laser supplies, FDA approved procedures, future laser applications, ongoing research and development, the cost of the system, and the education included with the purchase. Usually a laser is purchased that will address the needs of more than one specialty area to ensure utilization after the laser is procured. A well-planned evaluation of the different laser systems will help determine which laser is most appropriate so that future utilization will be guaranteed.

The acquisition phase is usually the responsibility of the financial department after the decision has been made as to which laser will be procured. Several methods, including outright purchase, leasing, developing a foundation, and promoting donations, can be used to procure a laser system.

The outright purchase method of laser procurement offers immediate possession of the laser unit. The laser can be purchased from capital equipment funds and then a tangible asset is immediately realized. Monthly budgeting for cash expenditures is not necessary because one lump sum is used to buy the system. Two disadvantages of this method are loss of potential investment monies and early outdating of an owned, highly technologic piece of equipment.

Because laser technology continues to change at a rapid pace, ownership of the laser system may not be desirable. Leasing the laser is an option that can be designed to spread the payment of over time. Usually a laser is leased for 3 to 5 years. At the end of the lease, a buy-out option can be arranged. Laser leases are offered by the manufacturer, the distributor, or a third-party financier who is in the business of leasing medical equipment. Some manufacturers even lease the laser system per each use, but there is often difficulty in tracking the utilization. Whichever leasing agreement is used, the facility should scrutinize the leasing contract carefully.

A limited partnership may be formed by physicians to purchase the laser if the hospital is unable or unwilling to purchase or lease the system. The physician group can then set up a fee schedule for the hospital to repay the group as the laser is used. This method of procurement ensures that the physicians use the laser because the investors have a vested interest in its use. As tax laws and regulations are introduced, physicians must be aware of changes concerning physician limited partnerships that own equipment that will generate revenue and also be used in their practices.

Donations can also be used to help procedure a laser system. If a hospital is a nonprofit organization, the donations may be tax deductible. Benevolent gifts and fund-raising events can defray the cost of expensive laser systems. Because laser technology is considered futuristic and has been shown to benefit patients, community organizations and individuals are usually eager to donate funds to help medical advancement in their community.

Whenever an order is placed for a laser, plans must be

made to accommodate the system when it arrives. Special water or electrical hookups that may be required should be installed before the system is delivered so that it can be used immediately. If a hospital is not prepared for the laser when it arrives, the warranty period begins before the laser is used, and the period of return on investment for the laser is prolonged.

If the health care facility is not able to actually purchase or lease a laser, then the services of a laser rental company may be investigated. These mobile laser businesses have become very popular over the past several years since some hospitals or clinics are unable and/or unwilling to assume the financial responsibility of a laser system. Some of these companies also provide the services of a laser team member as part of the leasing plan. The facility should develop a policy to address the responsibilities of these laser team members whose services have been purchased.

The laser team member may also be involved with exploring the economical viability of a laser program. The laser team member may be asked to determine the cost of performing a laser procedure, including tallying all direct and indirect expenses. Patient charges may be based on this vital information. Laser charges have been developed based on a per laser use basis or per time basis. Some hospitals have absorbed the laser charge into bundled surgical charges and then only submit a charge for the use of the extra disposables, such as a laser fiber or smoke evacuation tubing. This type of system encourages more use of laser technology in that the patient is not directly charged for the use of the laser itself.

Determining the amount of reimbursement for different laser procedures helps the laser team member ascertain how quickly a return on investment for the laser system can be expected. Because laser technology can be expensive, the amount that is reimbursed often decides the growth of the laser program. The cost to perform the laser procedure should be less than the reimbursed amount.

Laser technology has decreased hospitalization for some procedures and has even converted inpatient surgeries to ambulatory status. The trends in laser usage have helped to decrease the health care dollars spent as less invasive procedures are introduced, fewer complications are realized, and fewer ancillary supplies are needed.

When the amount of reimbursement is compared to the costs of performing a procedure, profitability can be determined. Cost containment measures can be encouraged to decrease the expense related to each procedure. Cost containment requires the continuing efforts of the laser team members and everyone else involved in surgery. Awareness of the actual expense related to the laser system or special supplies, coupled with an understanding of the amount of reimbursement, can help the laser team manage costs through creative implementation and administration.

MARKETING

Assisting with marketing can be an exciting responsibility for the laser team member. Many times a carefully

planned laser program is implemented and does not begin to grow because a marketing plan to encourage utilization has not been shared with the laser team members or physicians. The "dusty laser syndrome" occurs as large amounts of money are expended to meet the needs of the laser program, but due to the lack of marketing and interest the laser is not being used. Physicians become distressed because they have no patients on whom to use the laser, the administration becomes disappointed because the return on investment is not happening, and the laser team members are discouraged because their special laser training is not being employed. The missing link is a marketing program to promote the laser to the community and to referring physicians.

A well-planned marketing program begins with an external assessment to analyze the laser market within a geographic area. This assessment should document historical trends of laser technology, potential clinical applications of the laser, community needs, and competition in the area. An internal assessment determines physician interest in the laser, the knowledge and willingness of referring physicians to send patients to specialists who use the laser, and the support and experience of a qualified laser team. After a comprehensive review, the determination of where the laser program can fit into the overall marketplace and into local competition can be made. Opportunities for the laser program can be highlighted, and threats to the program can also be disclosed.

The laser team member can help develop the marketing plan by actively participating in defining the objectives of the laser program. These objectives must be measurable so that the degree of achievement can be evaluated. The objectives should be formed through the coordinated efforts of not only the laser team members but anyone who is involved with the laser program. The finalized written objectives should be communicated openly so that everyone is working toward the same goals. When the laser team members and others are involved with this phase of marketing, ownership in the program is widely felt and commitment is fostered.

The target audience for laser marketing must be determined so that the marketing plan is designed specifically to reach this group. Usually marketing programs designate the patient as the primary target audience, with referring physicians as the secondary group.

In formulating the plan of action for the marketing program, characteristics of the laser program should be designed to reflect the uniqueness of the services that are offered. Also, budgetary commitments to marketing efforts should be resolved early so that financial limitations can be initially realized and the best marketing can be achieved for the money to be spent.

Implementing a marketing plan for a laser program can be accomplished through advertising, personal selling, sales promotion, and publicity. A combination of these methods is usually the most cost-effective manner to promote a laser program.

An advertising campaign usually is most successful if the primary emphasis is on the benefits of laser surgery and the secondary emphasis is on the laser program itself. The consumer needs to hear or read of the advantages and benefits of laser technology before getting involved with the services of a specific laser program. The consumer must believe in the product before the service will be used. The various media available to advertise a laser program include newsprint, radio, television, billboards, and direct mail. The laser team member can be very actively involved with the personal selling of the laser services through speaking engagements and personal contacts with physicians. The laser team member can also assist with promoting the publicity of the laser program by helping to develop news releases to the media, manning a laser booth display at a health fair, and distributing informational brochures that carry the message about the laser program.

Any marketing program should be evaluated regularly to determine the results and the continuity of the marketing activities. The success of each endeavor should be documented so that strengths and weaknesses are noted. Alterations to a marketing plan should be expected as the laser program grows and changes. Successful marketing depends on the financial commitment from administration and the energies of the laser team member and physicians.

BIBLIOGRAPHY

Achauer, B.M., Vander Kam, V.M. & Berns, M.W. (1992). *Lasers in plastic surgery and dermatology*. New York: Thieme Medical Publishers.

American National Standards Institute, Inc. (1988) *American national standard for the safe use of lasers in health care facilities*, ANSI Z136.3. New York: The Institute.

Ball, K. (1990). *Lasers: the perioperative challenge*. St. Louis: Mosby.

Dubuque, S. (Aug. 27, 1988). *Advertising a laser program*. New York: Clinical Laser Management Postconference.

Fuller, T.A. (1993). *Thermal surgical lasers, a technical monograph*. Oaks, Pa.: Surgical Laser Technologies.

Garden, J.M., et al. (1988). Papillomaviris in the vapor of carbon dioxide laser–treated verrucae. *JAMA, 8*, 1199.

Joffe, S.N. & Oguro, Y. (eds.). (1988). *Advances in Nd:YAG laser surgery*. New York: Springer-Verlag.

Joint Commission on Accreditation of Healthcare Organizations. (1994). *Accreditation manual for hospitals*. Chicago: The Commission.

Lobraico, R.V., Schifano, M.J., & Brader, K.R. (1988, Fall). A retrospective study on the hazards of the carbon dioxide laser plume. *Journal of Laser Applications*, p. 6.

Mechenbier, J. (1992, February). Jet ventilator in microlaryngoscopy reduces anesthesia risks. *Clinical Laser Monthly*.

Pfister, J.I., Kneedler, J.A. & Purcell, S.K. (1988). *The nursing spectrum of lasers*. Denver: Education Design.

Sliney, D.H. (1993). *Medical lasers and their safe use*. New York: Springer-Verlag.

Wright, V.C. & Fisher, J.C. (1993). *Laser surgery in gynecology*. Philadelphia: W.B. Saunders.

32

ENDOSCOPIC SURGERY

CYNTHIA A. BRAY

Endoscopy, the examination of hollow organs of the body by means of an endoscope, has been practiced for several centuries. Although primitive, the first use of reflected light for inspection of the uterine cervix is credited to Abulkasim (936-1013), an Arabian physician. From this new conquest came instrumentation to examine the nasal sinuses and urinary bladder. Of primary concern during this initial era of endoscopy was the thermal tissue injury caused by intense heat emitted by the light sources utilized. Incandescent lighting was eventually incorporated into the tips of certain endoscopes (such as cystoscopes and ureteroscopes) that could be cooled by continuous irrigation. Modifications allowed for examination of the nasal sinuses, larynx, bronchus, and sigmoid colon. Procedures, however, were restricted to those performed through endoscopic placement in *external* body orifices.

In 1910 Jacobaeus, a Swedish physician, first reported using a cystoscope to examine the peritoneal cavity (Zucker, 1991). Only *diagnostic* capability was realized; pneumoperitoneum was yet to be developed. Thus numerous complications were associated with these brave attempts. Commonly reported were injuries to bowel and vascular structures, complications which today, although not unknown, are quite uncommon. In an attempt to reduce morbidity Decker (1946) introduced the cul-de-sac approach to pelvic endoscopy (culdoscopy). Instead of inserting the scope through the abdomen, he did so through the cul-de-sac. During this era the importance of introducing air into the abdomen was recognized. Knee-chest and Trendelenburg positions were used. Air introduction was enhanced by use of a syringe and needle.

It was not until 1964 that an automatic insufflation device was developed by the German surgeon Kurt Semm (Semm, 1982). Laparoscopy was still considered to be blind surgery and because of this did not gain rapid popularity in either North America or Europe. During this decade two other developments enhanced the endoscopic revolution. In 1966 the rod-lens system was designed by the British optical physicist Hopkins, which improved brightness and clarity. Fiberoptic (cold) light sources were also introduced,

which even further reduced the risk of visceral and bowel burns.

In the late 1970s to early 1980s endoscopic surgery moved from the category of diagnostic to that of operative. Kurt Semm termed his pioneering work *pelviscopy*. His work led to many technologic advances in instrumentation, equipment, and technique. Diagnostic and operative laparoscopy was becoming the technique of choice for gynecologists throughout the world. Endoscopic procedures were also increasing for urologists, internists, and otorhinolaryngologists. In the 1970s orthopedic surgeons began to appreciate the concept of arthroscopy.

It was not until the 1980s that the laparoscope was introduced in general surgery. General surgeons were familiar with laparoscopy, since many were consulted to assist gynecologists when evaluating right lower quadrant pain in young patients. The evolutionary process enabled surgeons to perform their own laparoscopic procedures for diagnosis of acute appendicitis.

In the late 1980s the "laparoscopy revolution" began in the United States. As surgeons and perioperative nurses were scrambling for knowledge and information, industry was desperately trying to accommodate the rapid change from open surgical procedures to that of the newer concept of minimally invasive surgery (Table 32-1). For the perioperative nurse came increased opportunity for growth; new equipment, instrumentation, surgical approaches, patient education, and professional self-satisfaction resulted despite initial frustration. Reports indicate that by 1992 more than 2 million endoscopic procedures had been performed in the United States.

VIDEO THEORY

A basic medical video system includes the scope, light cable, light source, camera head, camera cord, camera-scope coupler, camera controller, and video monitor. Additional peripheral equipment is also necessary for specific surgical procedures and is discussed later.

A video system takes light energy from a beginning

TABLE 32-1

Advantages of Minimally Invasive Surgery Over Open Surgery

Minimally invasive	Open
Ambulatory or short hospital stay	Hospital admission
Short postoperative recuperation	4- to 6-week recuperation
Reduced postoperative pain; reduced need for pain medications	Postoperative pain related to surgical site; more analgesics
Earlier return to normal life-style	Return to normal life-style varies with recuperation period

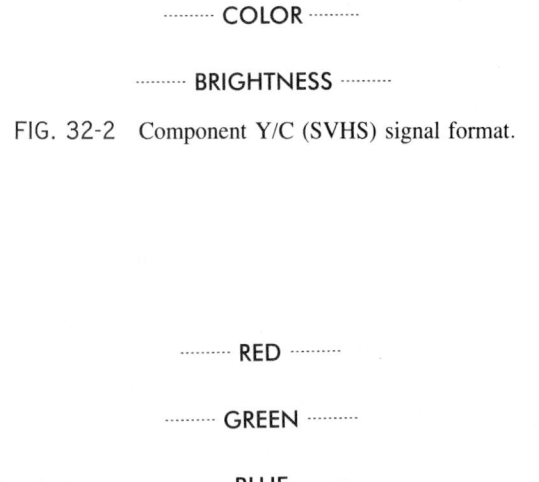

FIG. 32-2   Component Y/C (SVHS) signal format.

FIG. 32-3   Component RGB signal format. Brightness is generated as percentage of three primary colors.

source, converts it into electrical energy, and then back into light energy to achieve a picture. The camera head contains a sensor, which is light sensitive. The sensor used today is a solid state unit, or chip, called a *charged coupled device* (CCD); it produces the unprocessed video signal. The CCD has replaced the outdated vacuum tubes and, as a result, offers greater sensitivity and resolution. The CCD is made up of small picture elements called pixels, which in the presence of light become conductive and in the absence of light remain nonconductive. Each pixel is capable of sensing either red, blue, or green light. The picture is then transformed into a matrix made up of the conductive and nonconductive pixels. This matrix is scanned at a rate of 525 lines per frame, 30 frames per second, generating a signal frequency. The scanning rate is standardized by the National Television Systems Committee (NTSC). The picture is then reproduced at its terminal destination.

The NTSC is the standard video format in the United States, Canada, Japan, and most of South America and Asia. It was established to be used for broadcast purposes. A *format* is the way electronic camera signals carry brightness and color information. The three most commonly used formats are the composite, Y/C, and RGB. The standard format is termed *composite* because it carries both color and brightness on the same signal (Fig. 32-1). The advantage is that it *is* standard. The disadvantage is that when both color and brightness information are combined on one signal, cross-talk or interference between the two can result in increased video noise (disturbance).

Another commonly available signal transmission method is Y/C. *Y* stands for the brightness signal and *C* for the color signal. Video information is carried on two different sig-

nals and is commonly referred to as super VHS (S-VHS) (Fig. 32-2). This transmission method does not have cross-talk problems and produces sharper pictures with higher resolution on both video recorders and hard copy producers. These systems require more expensive monitors and recorders. Another disadvantage is that color and brightness travel at different speeds and, over longer cord distances, may be out of synchronization, requiring extra electronic circuitry.

The third commonly used video format, RGB, also a component system, separates video information into red, green, and blue signals and carries each separately (Fig. 32-3). Brightness is generated as a percentage of the three colors (30% red, 59% green, 11% blue). Advantages of this format include less noise interference, resulting in sharper pictures with distinct color separation. It is the format of choice for computer interfacing, which is rapidly becoming significant. Some RGB components are extremely expensive, and the three signals must be synchronized.

Several cameras are available with all three formats, which allow for flexibility. One must keep in mind, however, that accompanying equipment must be compatible with the camera's format. For example, for the Y/C or RGB camera format to be advantageous, the monitor utilized must also be capable of handling these components as well as composite signals. It becomes apparent that system compatibility is crucial. For this reason the composite format is still very desirable.

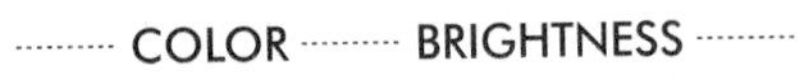

EQUIPMENT

VISUALIZATION SYSTEMS

Endoscopic visualization was once restricted to the operating physician. Microscope adaptation, where appropriate, was added to enhance and magnify anatomic structures and pathology. The teaching side arm provided direct visu-

FIG. 32-1   Standard composite signal format.

alization for the resident and/or perioperative nurse. Often, however, images seen through the side arm were not identical to those seen through the primary optics. The inability to effectively interact with the physician was frustrating and time consuming. In the late 1960s and early 1970s medical video and still cameras were working their way into the marketplace. This allowed for still photography as well as video documentation of select surgical procedures. Tube style cameras were large, bulky, and heavy, leaving much to be desired. Video technology rapidly changed with the introduction of the chip TV camera. Its lightweight, low-profile design triggered the era of video-guided surgery. Cameras that once weighed several pounds now weigh only a few ounces (Fig. 32-4). These rapid developments in video imaging have also resulted in higher resolution monitors. Together this integrated system provides increased assurance of sterility during direct visualization, enhanced participation by assistants, and promotion of accurate assessment and planning by the perioperative nursing staff. Today video technology has found its way into daily health care delivery. All disciplines have been enhanced by its capability.

CAMERA

The video camera represents the optical-electronic interface. A camera cable transfers the signal frequency to a camera controller (processor), which modifies the signal and then transmits the image to a video monitor, recorder, and/or hard copy picture. The camera is the most important component of the video system. Camera options vary according to available technology, specialty, and personal preference. Cameras have either one or three CCDs. Three-chip cameras provide enhanced color and image quality but are larger, can cost up to three times that of a single-chip camera, and are not as light sensitive. Color and the resulting image are enhanced because each chip is dedicated to one of the primary colors: red, green, blue. For this reason they are often used in conjunction with microscopes when the higher magnification requires increased resolution. Newer single-chip cameras are available with digital processing in their control units, which boosts resolution. In essence, this technology incorporates three-chip quality in a single chip. Although the signal processing in the control unit may be digital, the video output from most cameras is an analog signal. Digital processing refers to the way information is delivered through the various components of the control unit. This processing format allows for image enhancement and manipulation of the video image. It also allows multiple video signals to be shown on one monitor as well as electronic zoom capability. Digital processing also provides the user with freeze frame capability when using video printers and when using picture-in-picture systems. The disadvantage of *complete* digital processing of images is the ability to refresh the picture on the monitor in real time. This processing method produces a jumpy, jittery picture. Thus most cameras are currently converting

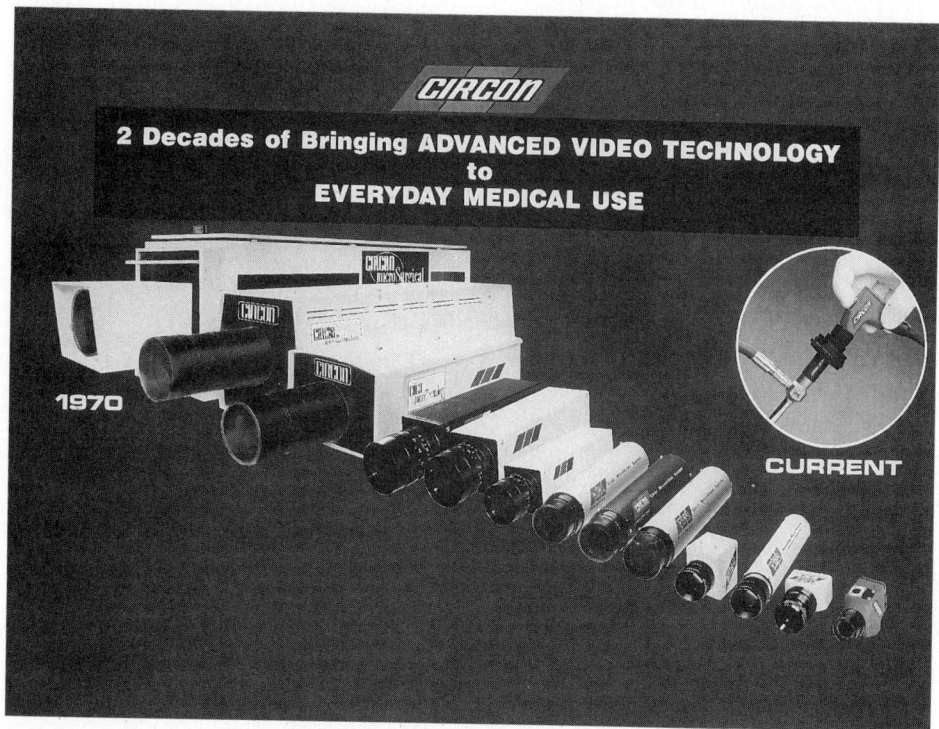

FIG. 32-4 Evolution of medical video cameras.
Courtesy CIRCON ACMI, Santa Barbara, Calif.

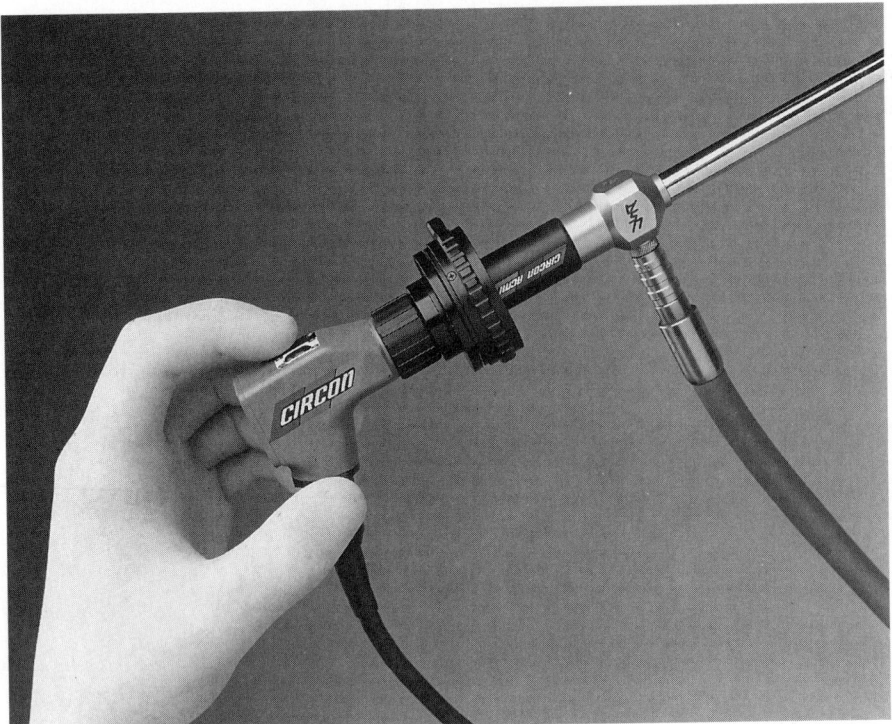

FIG. 32-5   Microdigital I RGB color video camera with fingertip control.
Courtesy CIRCON ACMI, Santa Barbara, Calif.

the digital image back to an analog signal before sending it to the video monitor.

Most cameras feature the ability to adjust to changes in light intensity while in use. This is done by an automatic shutter (iris), which measures the availability of light and adjusts accordingly. Automatic shutter activation also helps reduce glare from reflected light off instrumentation and moist viscera. The ability for continuous variable shutter speeds rather than discrete shutter speeds allows for instruments to be brought into the field without glare while still maintaining adequate illumination of background objects. The shutter's response should be rapid and without perceptible stepping of image intensity.

Camera heads now have buttons to control certain functions. Some of these include white balancing, light sensitivity boosting (ability to provide a brighter picture when the image requires more light, especially when using a scope smaller than 3 mm during sinuscopy), starting and stopping the VCR, and taking hard copy prints. This gives the surgeon control of these functions instead of requesting the circulating nurse to do so each time. The surgeon also has the ability to capture events exactly when they occur (Fig. 32-5).

Remote control hand-held devices are also available for additional functions. These mimic the familiar household VCR remote control. As in the home setting, these devices take time to master. If used routinely, they can become the perioperative nurse's best friend (Fig. 32-6).

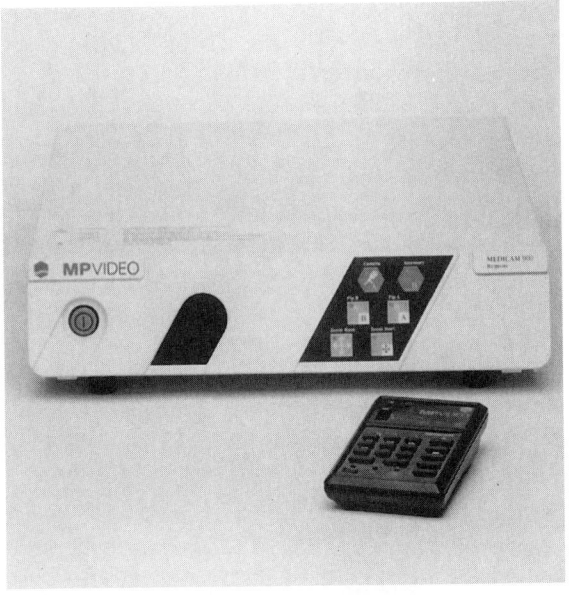

FIG. 32-6   Camera control unit with remote control.
Courtesy MP Video, Hopkinton, Mass.

All cameras have focusing capability at the camera-coupler interface. Some also have zoom capability, allowing for closer visualization of specific structures or pathology. A camera cable connects the camera head to the camera control unit (Fig. 32-7). Most camera malfunctions are cable, not camera, related. For this reason a system that

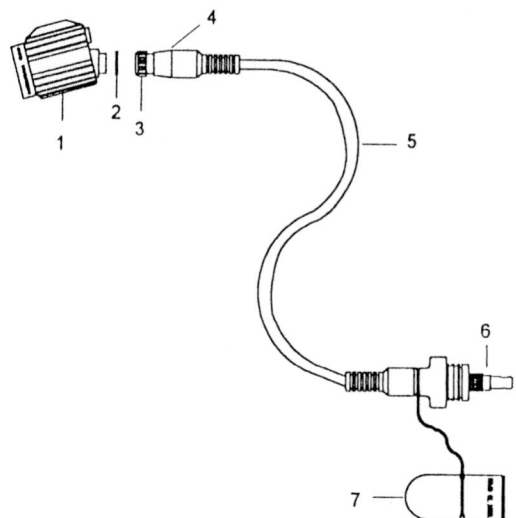

FIG. 32-7 Camera and field-replaceable cable. *1*, Camera head; *2*, O-ring; *3*, knured ring; *4*, cable connector; *5*, replaceable cable; *6*, camera connector; *7*, soak cap.

Courtesy MP Video, Hopkinton, Mass.

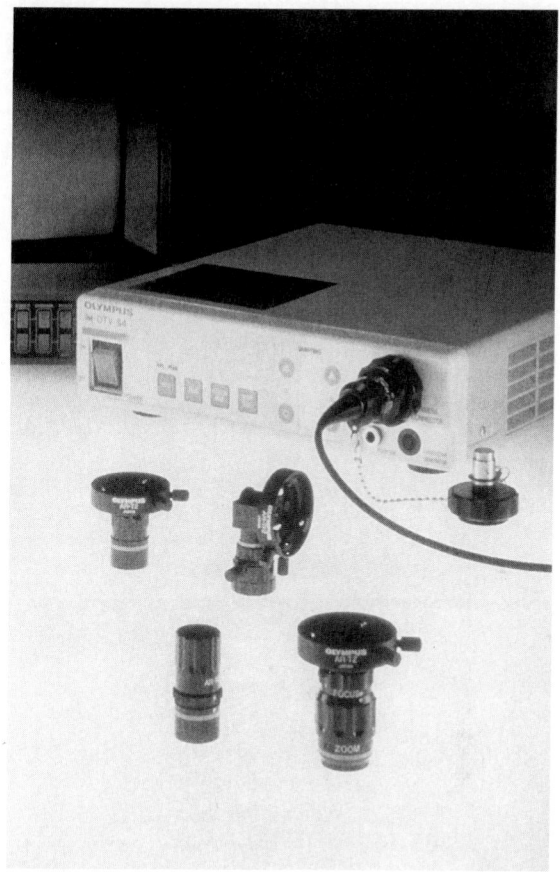

FIG. 32-8 OTV-S4 digital signal processing video camera system with various couplers. Starting upper left and moving clockwise: AR-T2 video coupler; AR-TF2 beamsplitter coupler; AR-TZ zoom video coupler; AR-TD2 direct video coupler.

Courtesy Olympus America, Inc., Lake Success, N.Y.

provides field-replaceable cables is most appealing. Should wires in the cable break, a new cable can be quickly exchanged, reducing downtime from having to ship the camera and cable for repair. Since wires in the flexible cable can break, it must be handled with care. Cables should never be twisted, crimped, or kinked. They should also be long enough to allow sufficient space between the sterile field and the visualization system.

COUPLERS (ADAPTERS)

Endocouplers are optical coupling devices used to connect cameras to various endoscopes. They are usually available in both 28-mm and 35-mm focal lengths and with different optical magnifications.

The specific type of coupler required depends on the type of surgery or diagnostic procedure performed. When viewing only on a monitor, a direct link coupler between the telescope and camera head is required (Fig. 32-8). For the surgeon to look directly through the endoscope and also have monitor viewing capability, a beam splitter coupler is necessary (Fig. 32-9). Beam splitters are often used with flexible endoscopes. There are rotating beam splitters designed for the surgeon who operates in a sitting position. Zoom couplers provide variable focal lengths, usually from 22.5 to 50 mm.

A videoscope is a new design of camera-to-scope connection without the use of a coupler. Since a coupler adds one more link to the chain, it is potentially an area where there is loss of light as well as lens fogging. Connecting the camera and scope with a screw-in design instead of the coupler clamp achieves a tighter fit. This design, however, requires that the camera and scope be bought as a unit; thus there is no interchangeability between systems (Fig. 32-10).

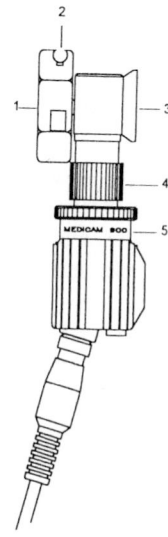

FIG. 32-9 Camera head with beam splitter. *1*, Endoscope attachment; *2*, locking screw; *3*, eyepiece; *4*, focusing mechanism; *5*, C-mount threads.

Courtesy MP Video, Hopkinton, Mass.

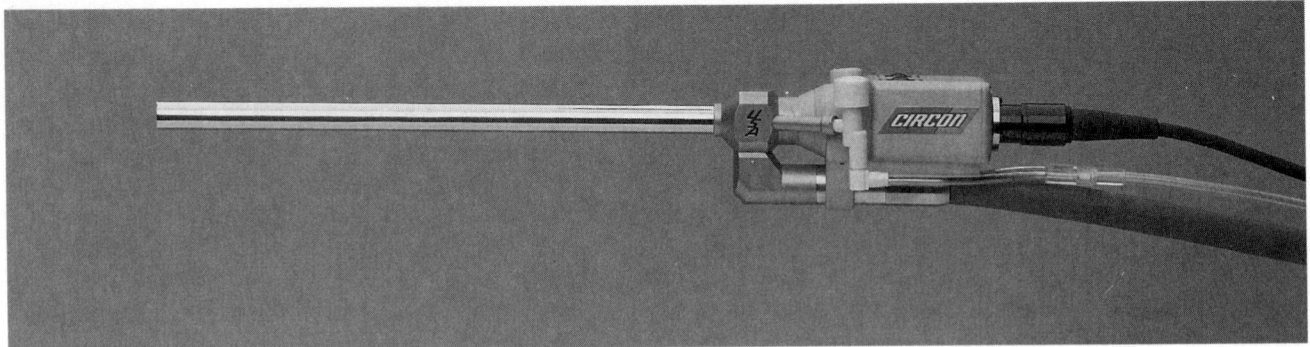

FIG. 32-10   Video hydroscope for laparoscopy and thoracoscopy.
Courtesy CIRCON ACMI, Santa Barbara, Calif.

B

A

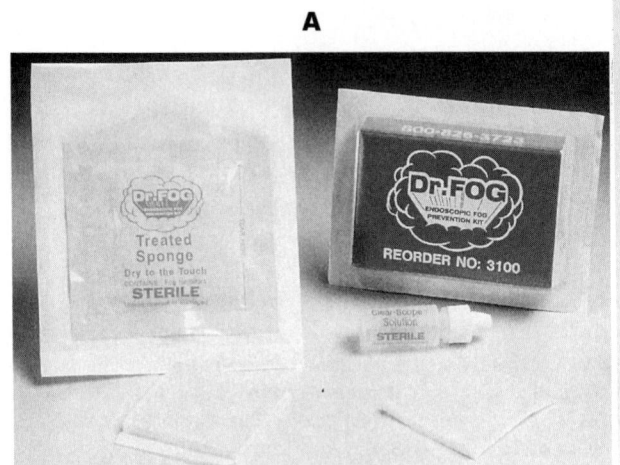
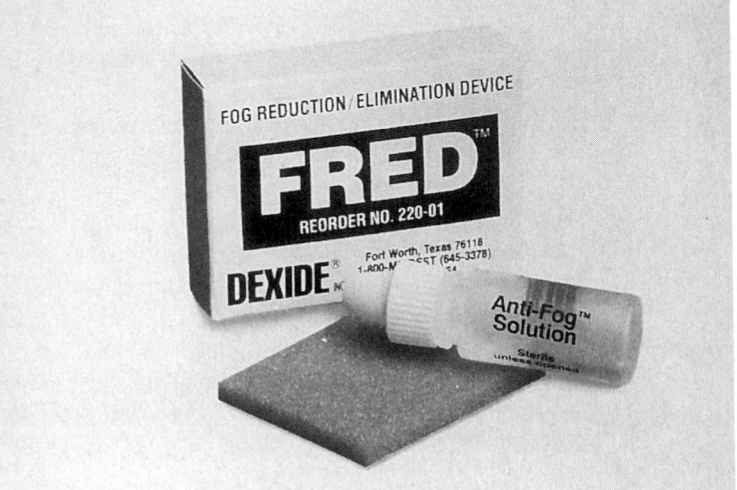

FIG. 32-11   **A,** Dr. Fog sterile endoscopic fog inhibitor. Product is shown in its treated sponge and
liquid forms. **B,** Fred sterile antifog solution and sponge.
A, Courtesy O.R. Concepts, Inc., Burnsville, Minn.; **B,** courtesy Dexide, Inc., Fort Worth, Tex.

It also does not allow for sterile bagging of the camera. Videoscopes can be purchased with optional lens washing and irrigation capability.

Lens fogging can be very frustrating. It occurs because a cool metal scope is introduced into a warm body. Several ways to handle this phenomenon have been developed. The elimination of a coupler has already been discussed. Sterile defogging solutions are available for application to the telescope and coupler lenses (Fig. 32-11). These provide a coating and reduce the incidence of fogging. Other options on the market include O-ring seals at connections, sapphire lenses, and various water seals. Warming of the telescope before insertion may also help reduce fogging. This can be accomplished by wrapping the telescope with lap sponges that have been soaked in warm sterile water. Another method is to utilize a CO_2 insufflator, which warms the gas (if used) before it enters the body. It may be sufficient to change the insufflation site to a secondary port, once initial pneumoperitoneum has been achieved. The sur-

geon may also opt to warm the lens of the telescope by gently touching an intraabdominal structure. This also requires visualization.

ENDOSCOPES

Endoscopes are designed to meet the needs of surgeon and procedure. Since there are unlimited combinations, it is economical to take a multidisciplinary team approach during the selection process. Perhaps this means involvement by the materials manager and hospital purchasing department as well as the OR manager and user surgeon(s). Most endoscope manufacturers allow products to be used on a trial basis. This should be encouraged, since endoscopes are a capital investment. Wherever and whenever a product can have multiple users and uses, the sooner a return on investment can be realized by the institution.

Not all endoscopes can be used for a variety of procedures, since the basic design, size, and capabilities are often limited. Cystoscopes, sinuscopes, ureteroscopes, angio-

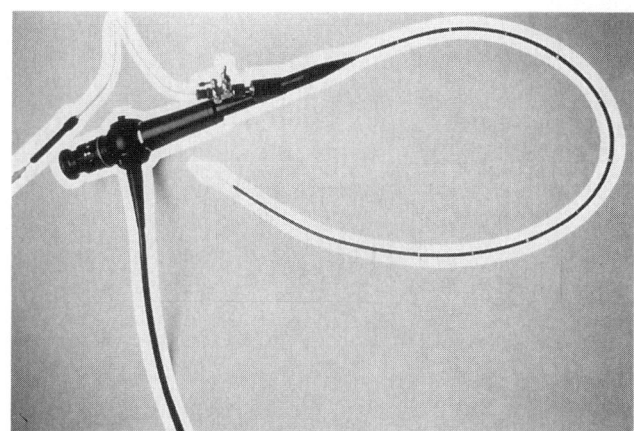

FIG. 32-12 VRF-P2 translaparoscopic choledochoscope.
Courtesy Olympus America, Inc., Lake Success, NY.

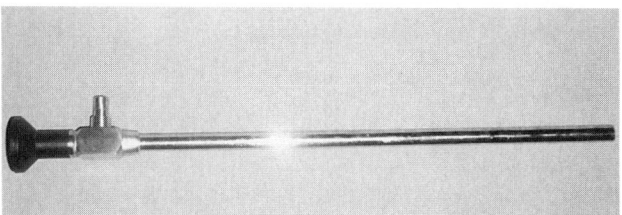

FIG. 32-13 Rigid diagnostic laparoscope.

scopes, and arthroscopes are prime examples. Although an angioscope could be used to view the common duct during a cholecystectomy, it has only diagnostic value unless it has an operating channel. In this case a choledochoscope or flexible pediatric ureteroscope is a better choice.

Endoscopes are rigid, semirigid, or flexible. Flexible scopes include, but are not limited to, angioscopes, bronchoscopes, choledochoscopes, colonoscopes, cystonephroscopes, hysteroscopes, mediastinoscopes, ureteroscopes, and ureteropyeloscopes (Fig. 32-12). Rigid scopes include, but are not limited to, cystoscopes, laparoscopes, sinuscopes, arthroscopes, bronchoscopes, laryngoscopes, and hysteroscopes (Fig. 32-13). As the list depicts, many are manufactured in both rigid and flexible forms. A semirigid scope such as the ureteroscope provides some movement, although it is fairly rigid (Fig. 32-14). The rigid endoscope uses a rod-lens system whereby light is transmitted through quartz rods (optical fibers). These, added to the objective lens and eyepiece mechanism, provide internal visualization.

Endoscopes can be diagnostic or operative. Diagnostic scopes are for observation only and have no operating channels (Fig. 32-14). The system is sealed at both ends. A diagnostic scope can be used, however, when multiple access sites are planned. Operative endoscopes are channeled for irrigating, suctioning, and inserting and connecting

other adjunctive instrumentation. When using a CO_2 laser, gynecologists often use an operating laparoscope. The video camera is attached to the lens of the scope, and the laser is attached to the operating port (Fig. 32-15).

When a surgeon is using KTP or Nd:YAG laser energy, the fibers can be inserted through the operating channel of the endoscope. Since the fibers are flexible, they can pass through either a flexible or rigid scope. When this type of laser wavelength is used in conjunction with video equipment, the camera must be protected from the laser energy. Cameras designed today are built to withstand laser energy, although special filters are installed between the endoscope and the camera coupler to reduce blooming or glare when the laser is activated (Fig. 32-16). This does not eliminate the need for other laser safety measures, such as wavelength-specific protective eyewear.

Endoscopes come in a variety of diameters and lengths, based on specific patient and procedural requirements. Optical capability through a rigid scope can be seen direct (0-degree angle) or angled (30, 70, and 120 degrees). Flexible scopes by their very nature allow for a panoramic view.

As indicated, the purchase of an endoscope is not easy. Time, interdisciplinary collaboration, and trial use before purchase can result in overall satisfaction and system compatibility.

LIGHT SOURCES AND FIBEROPTIC CABLES

As previously discussed, early endoscopic procedures were performed utilizing incandescent light sources. These became very hot and were hazardous to use. With the development of fiberoptics came an entirely new surgical approach. Fiberoptic design offers increased illumination, cold light capability, and a control unit where intensity can be adjusted accordingly and from a distance.

Although the light is referred to as being cold, this means only that the heat is not transmitted throughout the scope and tissue is not damaged. The surgical team must be extremely cautious, however, to keep the ends of the fiberoptic cables out of contact with patient and personnel skin or any flammable material. These ends *are* extremely hot. If the fiberoptic cable is disconnected from the endoscope during surgery, the scrub nurse must ensure that the cable end is held away from drapes or placed on a moist towel to prevent burns and fires.

Light sources should have adjustable brightness modes, both manual and automatic. The automatic mode adjusts brightness according to the video image. If set in this mode, it eliminates the need for the circulating nurse to constantly make the adjustments.

When selecting a light source, certain options should be considered. One that can adapt to several endoscopic systems is desirable, such as one with a universal light cable adaptor, which enhances flexibility and usage (Fig. 32-17). If a previously purchased unit does not provide this feature, universal light cables with an interchangeable light source as well as endoscope adapters are available (Fig. 32-

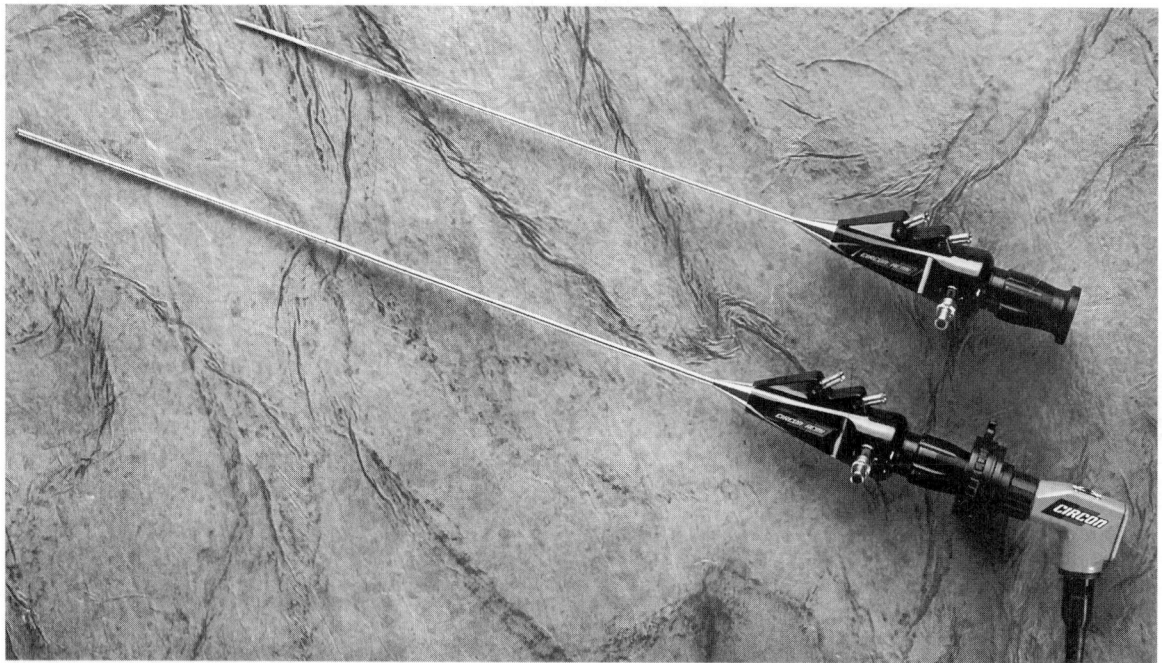

FIG. 32-14   Semirigid ureteroscope with and without video camera connected.
Courtesy CIRCON ACMI, Santa Barbara, Calif.

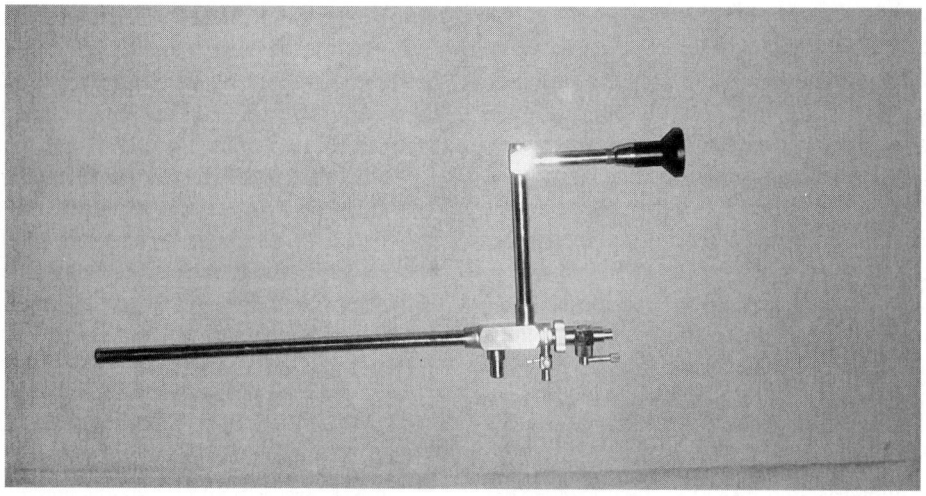

FIG. 32-15   Operative laparoscope.

18). This allows a generic cord to be utilized with most scopes as well as light sources. Light sources must have connection capability with different camera units.

Cables must be handled with extreme care. Fiberoptics consist of hundreds of glass fibers that transmit light. These fibers can be broken if kinked or dropped. Cables should be coiled, not bent, when not in use. After multiple uses,

fibers *do* break. Cables should be checked after each use. To do this, hold one end of the cable toward a bright light and look at the opposite end. Do not test the cable by looking into the end with it attached to the light source. The visible and ultraviolet light produced could be harmful. "Peppering" on the end indicates broken fibers. Once 18% to 20% of the fibers are broken, the cable should be re-

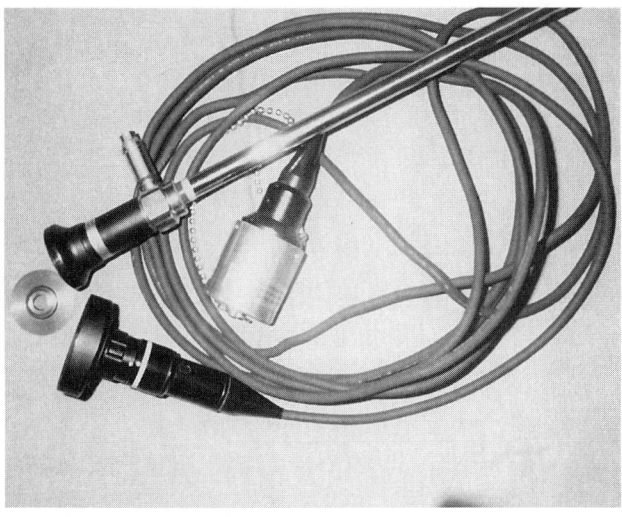

FIG. 32-16 Laparoscope, video camera with endocoupler, and laser filter. The filter is placed between scope and camera to reduce blooming/glare during laser activation.

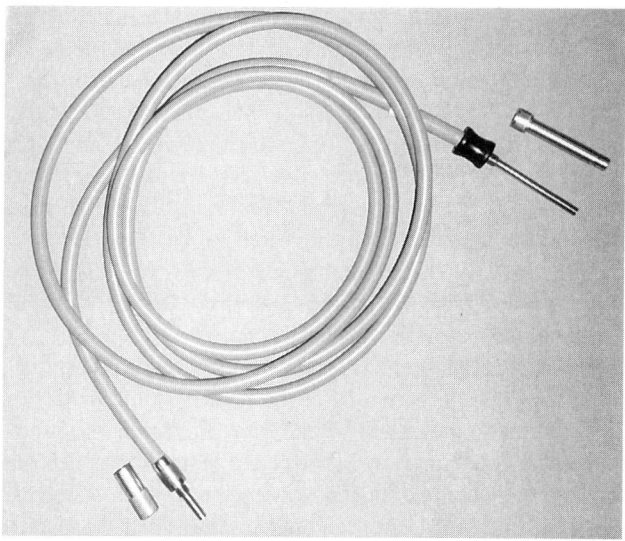

FIG. 32-18 Universal light cable with interchangeable light source as well as endoscope adaptors.

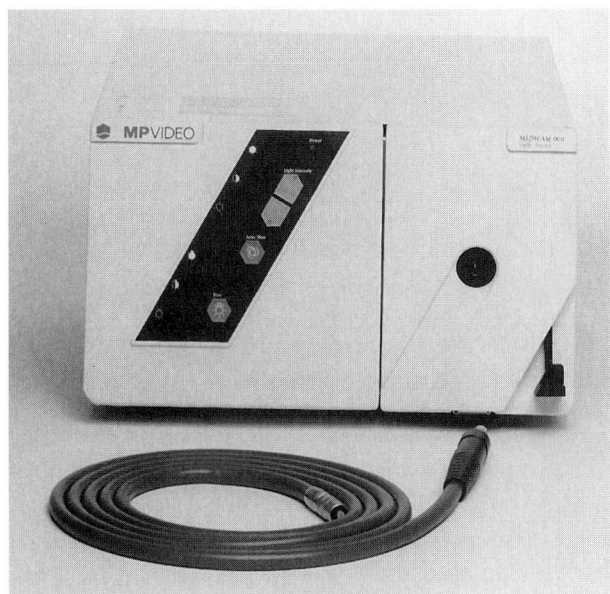

FIG. 32-17 Light source with universal light cable adapter. Courtesy MP Video, Hopkinton, Mass.

placed. Adequate light for visualization will not be transmitted.

Bulbs should require only minimal replacement effort. Most are located in lamp assembly drawers, which are readily accessible. The bulb itself should not have to be touched. Nonmetal handles should be built into the unit for bulb removal when the bulb is hot.

The two specific types of light sources available are xenon and metal halide. Advantages and disadvantages are associated with each. Whiteness of the light is rated about the same. Metal halide bulbs have a shorter life span (about 250 hours) and are less expensive (about $400). Xenon

bulbs cost twice the amount, but last twice as long. Metal halide bulbs are easier to handle as well as to replace and do not require large fans to cool them. Xenon is better for the smaller diameter endoscopes (2 mm or less) because it can focus down to a smaller spot size. Personal preference and condition of use are the parameters for choice. A light source that incorporates a lamp life status testing mode is desirable.

Halogen light sources are also manufactured for office and hospital use. They do not offer the light intensity necessary for endoscopic and video requirements.

Since different light sources produce different colors of light, the camera must be white balanced each time a unit is used. White balancing is merely adjusting the camera to all other optical components (endocoupler, light cable, laparoscope). This is a method for the camera to reference white so that it can properly identify all primary colors. White balancing should be performed only when the scope and light cable are connected and the light source is turned on.

VIDEO MONITORS

High-resolution video monitors represent the end of the chain in endoscopy. They have become the windows of observation during minimally invasive surgery. Monitors should closely match the resolution quality of the camera being used. For example, it is necessary to purchase a high-resolution monitor that meets or exceeds the horizontal resolution specification of the camera used. The camera-monitor system will always have the resolution of the least detailed element. Most monitors outperform the cameras, so discrimination in this purchase is less important. It is often difficult to determine the picture quality of monitors unless they are side by side. It is the picture tube design that alters the picture quality. Monitors must be able to handle the camera/recorder format (Y/C, RGB).

Some monitors are designed primarily for home viewing. These all have softer colors and less sharpness for a warmer picture. Operating room monitors are designed for sharper imagery, increased edge enhancement, increased contrast, and true color reproduction. Video monitors used for endoscopy differ from televisions in that they are capable only of receiving input through direct cables. They cannot receive broadcast signals. Some have the capability of both but are not necessary for the operating room.

Many operative procedures require two video monitors. One is placed on each side of the patient so that both primary surgeon and assistant can view the screen comfortably and simultaneously. The second monitor is called the slave monitor. Abdominal and thoracic procedures are performed in this manner. Certain procedures can be accomplished using only one monitor. Whenever the monitor can be placed in a position of visibility to both surgeon and assistant comfortably, only one is necessary. This is usually the method of choice for urologists, endoscopists, gynecologists, and otorhinolaryngologists. Most general surgeons require only one monitor whenever performing surgery with the endoscope directed toward the patient's feet, (for example, endoscopic herniorrhaphy). Of course, monitor selection, as with most equipment, is based upon personal preference as well as educational training. It is important for the perioperative nurse to be flexible and prepared, either way.

Monitors should be at least 13 inches (diagonal measurement of screen) for good visualization. When the endoscopic revolution began, most institutions purchased 19- or 20-inch main monitors and 13-inch slave monitors. Today many institutions are purchasing only 19- or 20-inch monitors. This increases flexibility in usage as well as excellent visibility from most observational angles and distances.

When using only one monitor and a composite signal, the 75-ohm termination on/off switch must be in the *on* position. When using multiple monitors, the switch on the last monitor in line to receive the video signal should be *on* and all others should be in the *off* position to enhance picture quality. Some monitors are self-terminating and do not have termination switches (Fig. 32-19).

RECORDING SYSTEMS
Video printer

There are additional recording devices that allow for archiving the surgical procedure or selected portions of it. The most commonly used is the video printer, or Mavigraph (Fig. 32-20). It is similar to a Polaroid camera in that it takes still photography instantly. The printer stores the selected image and then reprints it onto special paper. Many units can be programed to print one, four, nine, and even 25 pictures on one piece of 5½ × 8-inch paper in split-screen fashion. Comparisons can be made as pathology changes. Information such as patient name, date, time, and operating surgeon can also be superimposed on top of the print. These prints can be utilized for teaching purposes or remain as a

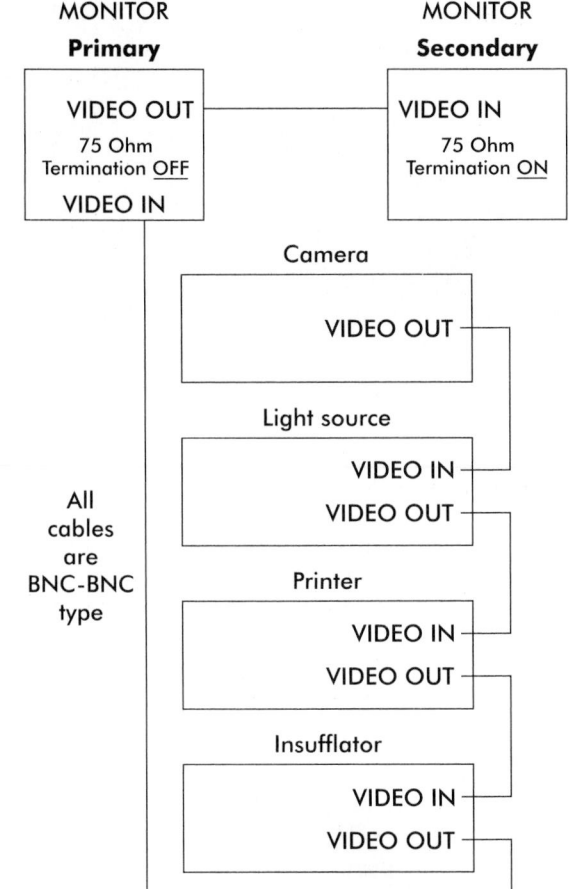

FIG. 32-19   Basic wiring configuration.
Courtesy MP Video, Hopkinton, Mass.

permanent record in the patient's chart. Some patients are quite interested in seeing prints of their "before and after."

Video disk recorder

Video disk recorders are available when considering storage and easy access to information. The disk recorder may very well become the documentation format of the future. To use this format a video printer must also be used, since the images are limited to video.

VCR

The VCR is used when moving image documentation is needed. This is usually required for teaching purposes and is not utilized as often as the printer. Image quality is not as clear when using a commercial VCR. Professional grade VCRs differ in that they do not have tuners and RF converters. Although rarely used, the best quality recorder available is the ¼-inch U-matic cassette recorder. It provides the best resolution available but also has advantages and disadvantages. It is an expensive piece of equipment, but it has low theft incentive because it cannot be used with standard ½-inch VCR tapes. This feature also becomes a deterrent because videos taken in surgery are ¾-inch and usually cannot be reviewed in surgeons' offices or at home. If security and quality resolution are both issues, the best

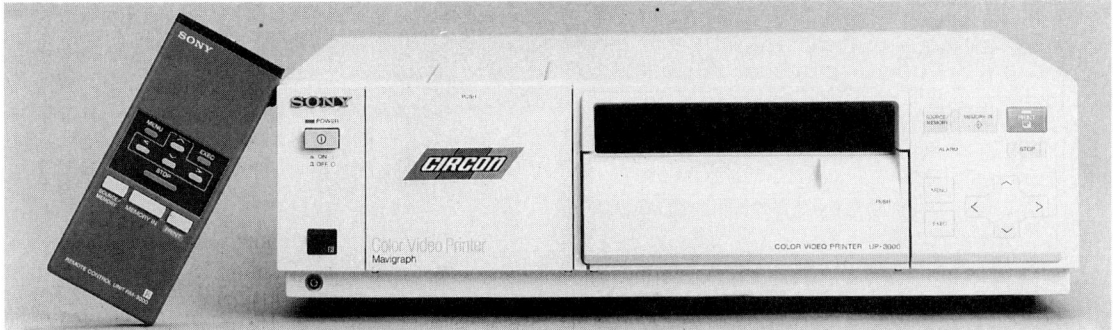

FIG. 32-20   Video printer with remote control.
Courtesy CIRCON ACMI, Santa Barbara, Calif.

VCR is the professional grade ½-inch S-VHS. It costs more but is not subject to theft because it cannot be connected to household televisions. S-VHS recorders have the ability to record in the standard VHS format as well as the S format. When recorded in the S format, tapes can be played back only on an S-compatible VCR.

STORAGE SYSTEMS

Space, storage capability, security, and required components determine the type of video storage cart(s) needed. It is beneficial to purchase a cart that can house multiple components of the video system (Fig. 32-21). This eliminates clutter from multiple smaller carts and tables. It also eliminates the number of cord connections to wall outlets, since most carts have power strips incorporated. *Note:* If the cart has a power strip, there is usually an on/off main switch located near the base. Make sure the switch is *on* or no equipment plugged into the strip will work. Because of the location of the switch, it can easily be turned off during transport and cleaning. Time and embarrassment can be avoided if this is checked before each use.

Articulating arms can be used as monitor mounts. Surgeon preference and room space determine if this option is necessary. If a room has been set aside for endoscopy, the monitor can be suspended from the ceiling on a swivel mount. The mount should be placed in a location where the monitor can be easily and comfortably viewed as well as cleaned.

Carts have either a locked (Fig. 32-22) or open (Fig. 32-23) shelf design. Institutional security will determine this need. Consideration of storage capability, tampering with equipment, and key availability is important. A locked drawer may be an ideal area to store VCR tapes, thermal printing paper, and the computer disk if these options are available. Carts should also be selected for ease in movement, component accessibility, and cleaning. They should include an optional storage bracket for E-cylinders when insufflation is required.

Secondary (slave) monitor carts usually do not contain multiple shelving and cabinet components. If a slave monitor is used, irrigation systems can be placed here, eliminating the need for another table.

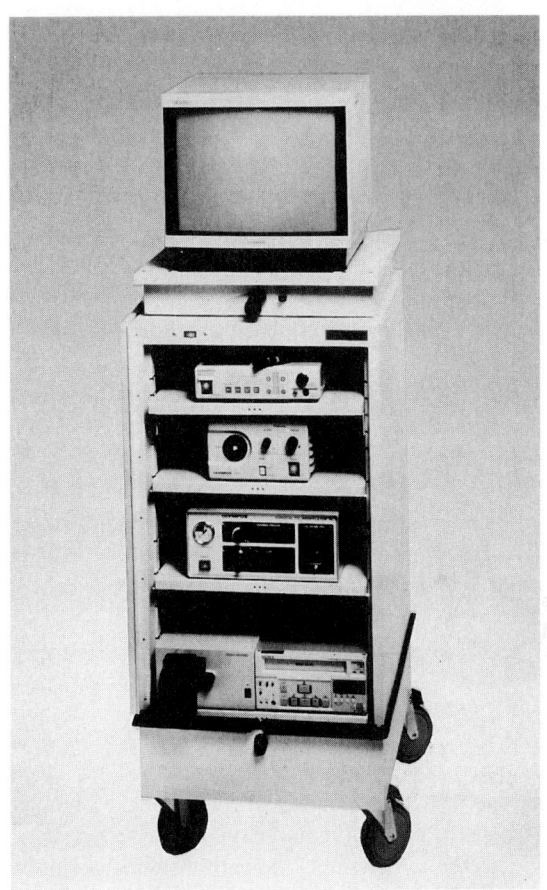

FIG. 32-21   Video laparoscopy cart.
Courtesy Olympus America, Inc., Lake Success, N.Y.

INSUFFLATION

To visualize abdominal (and often thoracic) structures and to operate safely, pneumoperitoneum is created. To do so, a paraumbilical incision is made and an insufflation (Verres) needle (Fig. 32-24) is inserted into the abdomen. Trendelenburg position is selected to reduce risk of visceral perforation. While the surgeon inserts the needle, the patient's abdomen is lifted up by grasping a fold of tissue on

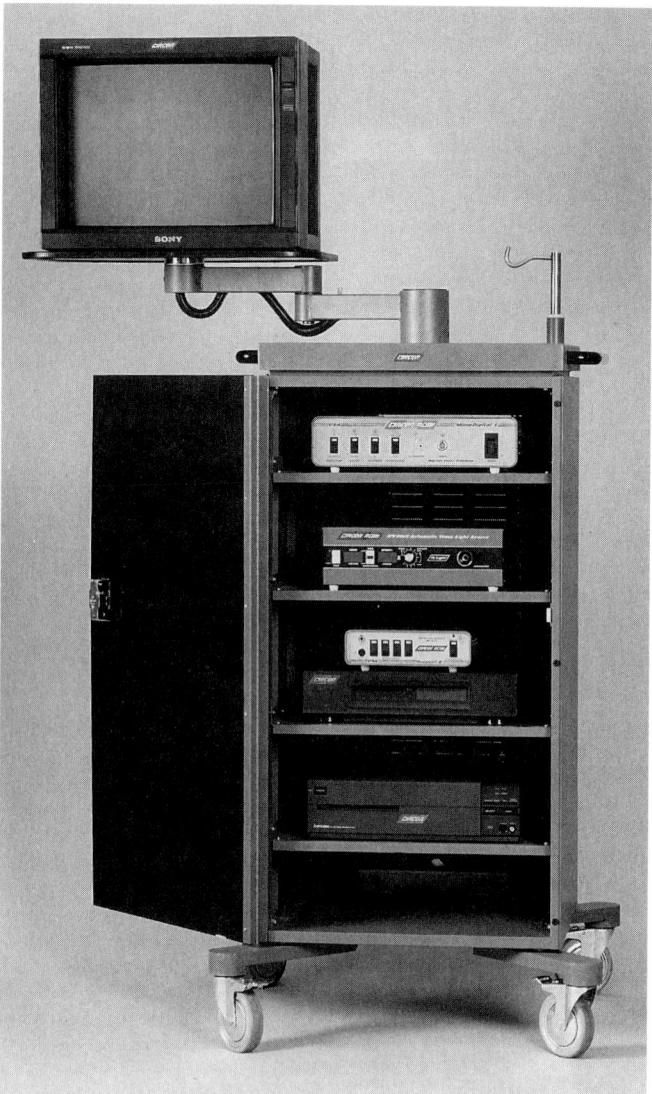

FIG. 32-22   Video storage cart with swivel monitor arm and lockable door.

Courtesy CIRCON ACMI, Santa Barbara, Calif.

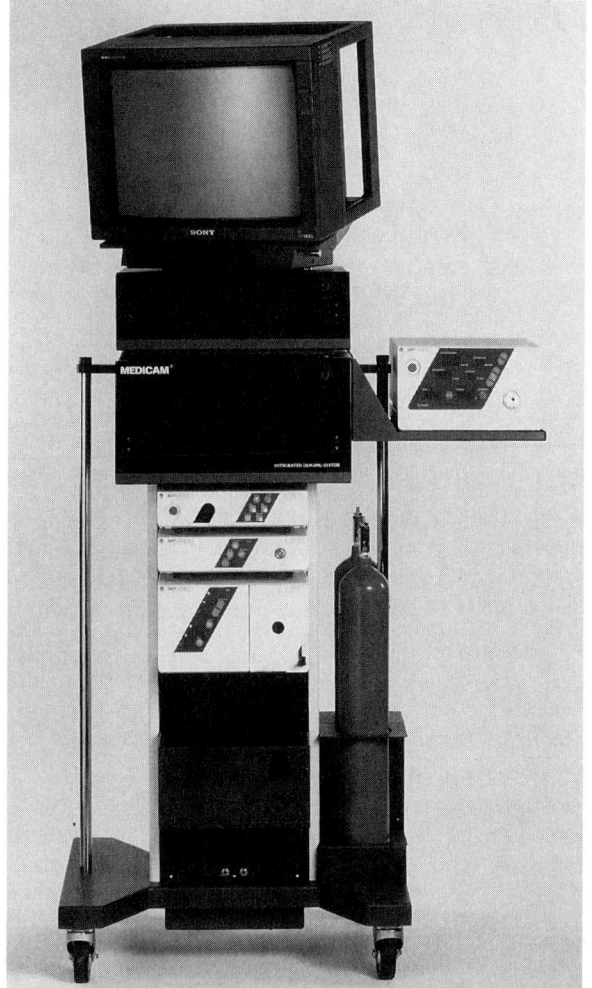

FIG. 32-23   Combination lockable/open video storage cart. Cart also incorporates shelf for insufflator and bracket for CO_2 cylinder.

Courtesy MP Video, Hopkinton, Mass.

either side of the umbilicus. Preoperative patient education should include the possibility of finger pinched bruising at the site where the abdominal tissue is grasped.

The needle safely enters the peritoneum if positioned at a 45-degree angle. Placement is usually confirmed by a negative bowel and blood return on aspiration and saline instillation that meets no resistance. This is a relatively blind procedure, since no scope can be introduced until pneumoperitoneum has been established.

Once needle confirmation is established, the insufflation tubing is connected and the process begun. The peritoneal cavity is filled starting at a low flow rate and then increased to a high flow rate of at least 9 L/minute ideally. Flow rate refers only to how quickly a predetermined intraabdominal pressure can be reached. Intraabdominal pressure is the actual parameter that must be closely monitored and should be maintained between 14 and 16 mm Hg. High flow rates

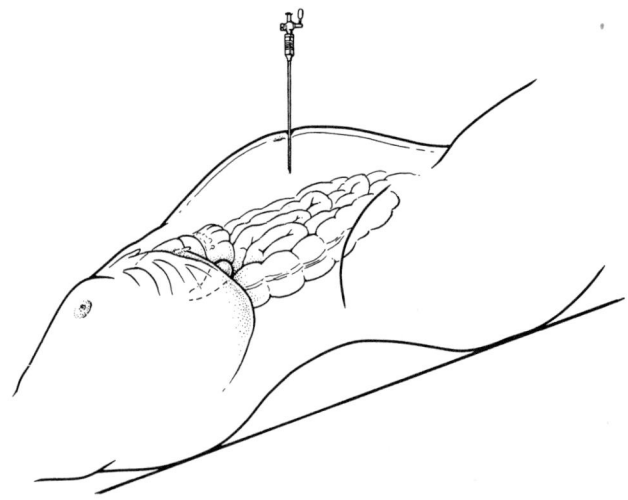

FIG. 32-24   Verres needle insertion into abdomen.

From Ponsky, J. (1992). *Atlas of surgical endoscopy*. St. Louis: Mosby.

are important because during the procedure CO_2 gas can escape. The more quickly it can be replaced, the less time has to be spent waiting for the abdomen to be redistended. CO_2 gas is used for insufflation. In the past, many gases have been used, including air, oxygen, and nitrous oxide. Air and oxygen have been eliminated as choices because of the risk of air embolism. Additionally, oxygen supports combustion, which could be fatal since electrosurgery and often laser energy are used. Nitrous oxide has also been eliminated because of the potential risk of unpredictable, uncontrollable absorption. CO_2 does not support combustion, can be absorbed at rather large volumes per minute without serious side effects, and is also fairly inexpensive.

Selection of an insufflator that can accommodate as high a flow rate as is needed for the specific procedure is important. In the initial phases of the endoscopic revolution flow rates of 6 L/minute were adequate. Today, because of the increased complexity of endoscopic procedures, increased numbers of secondary ports, and longer procedures (due to surgical complexity), pneumoperitoneum must be maintained over longer time frames. This requires flow rates of no less than 9 L/minute. Those delivering 15 to 20 L/minute are much more supportive and effective.

Of even greater concern during the selection process should be the guarantee that an insufflator can and will continuously monitor insufflation pressure, stop the insufflation process once this predetermined set pressure has been reached, and release pressure if there is an inadvertent increase (called "taking a breath"). Intraabdominal pressure can be increased for reasons other than CO_2 insufflation; for example, leaning on the abdomen and additional gas introduction from other sources such as a CO_2 laser can inadvertently increase intraabdominal pressure.

Overpressurization can be extremely hazardous to the patient and must be avoided. Excess pressure can force CO_2 to diffuse into the blood, resulting in hypercarbia. End-tidal CO_2 monitoring becomes a critical assessment parameter to detect increased CO_2 absorption. Excess pressure also increases diaphragmatic pressure, which could result in gastric regurgitation and aspiration of stomach contents. It could also reduce intrathoracic space, resulting in decreased respiratory effort and cardiac output. The phrenic nerve innervates the diaphragm and is responsible for some motor activity associated with respiration. CO_2 gas irritates this nerve, causing postoperative pain in the shoulder and neck. Although a common complaint, excessive pressure could cause tremendous discomfort as well as more severe nerve damage. It is in the best interest of the patient that the perioperative nurse remind the surgeon to press on the patient's abdomen to release as much residual CO_2 gas as possible before removal of the last trochar. Insufflators that automatically vent excessive CO_2 gas into the air provide assurance that many associated complications can be avoided.

A two-way filter should be incorporated into the insufflation tubing. These can be purchased as a disposable unit (Fig. 32-25). It is one disposable feature that many institu-

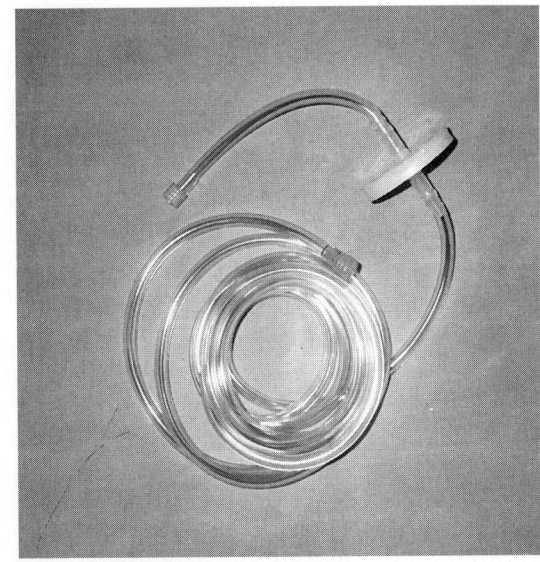

FIG. 32-25   Disposable insufflation tubing with two-way filter.

tions choose to maintain because of the time and energy required to reprocess reusable tubing. The filter provides patient protection from harmful gas tank contamination such as chromium particles (Mackin, 1992). It also provides protection from the colonization of organisms in the insufflator itself. Without a filter, when the insufflator is turned on, organisms such as *Klebsiella, Pseudomonas,* and *Staphylococcus aureus* can be blown into the patient. This could jeopardize the patient's welfare and surgical outcome. It could be deadly for a very ill, elderly, or immunocompromised patient. It is important to adhere to manufacturer's written instructions when implementing CO_2 insufflation (Box 32-1).

An insufflator capable of warning the operative team of insufflation parameters throughout the procedure is highly desirable. If these parameters are then periodically visualized on the monitor, information can be immediately processed and action taken. Alarms that sound when there is

---

BOX 32-1

Steps to Reduce Cross-Contamination of Patient and Insufflator During CO_2 Insufflation Procedures

- Flush insufflator/tubing with CO_2 gas before attaching to patient.
- Use a disposable hydrophobic filter on insufflation tubing. Discard after procedure.
- Disconnect tubing from insufflator *before* turning off, at end of procedure.
- Keep insufflator *elevated* above the patient to prevent fluid back-flow.

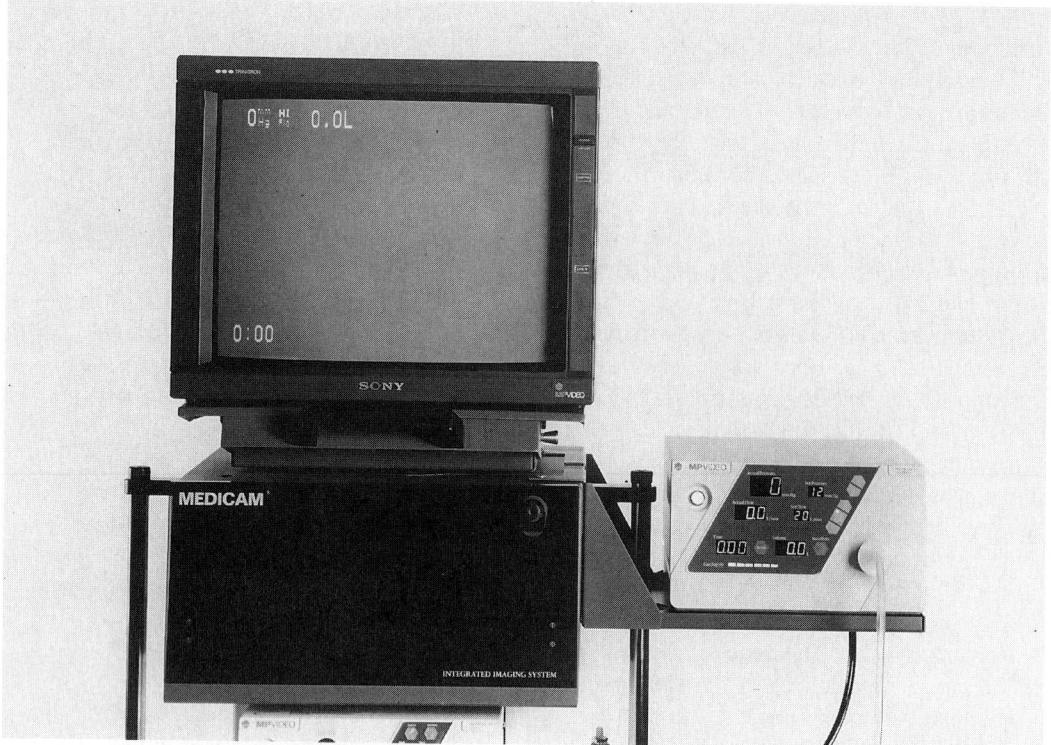

FIG. 32-26 Insufflation parameters visualized on TV monitor can be immediately processed.
Courtesy MP Video, Hopkinton, Mass.

an alteration in predetermined parameters also call attention to the need for immediate intervention (Fig. 32-26), for example, an alarm ringing and a monitor blinking "Gas Supply Low." An alarm sounding when overpressurization occurs from a secondary source (such as leaning on the abdomen) also alerts the team of the need for corrective action.

Insufflators are also available with CO_2 warming devices (Fig. 32-27). Cylinder CO_2 is in liquid form and as it is released it expands into a gas. During this conversion from liquid to gas, energy is lost and the gas becomes colder. The higher the flow, the colder the gas (Ott, 1991). Some warming does occur as the gas travels through the insufflation tubing. Use of cold CO_2 *could* cause a decrease in patient temperature. Although there are many factors that contribute to the reduction of body temperature during endoscopic procedures (such as cold irrigation, room temperature, surface exposure, length of the procedure, patient's age and medical history, anesthetic choice), cold CO_2 represents an additional one. The best way to reduce patient heat loss is to address all the variables and intervene wherever possible (Research Highlight 32-1).

Cold CO_2 also contributes to fogging of telescope lenses. Fogging occurs whenever a cold instrument enters the warm, moist environment of the body. Some methods to reduce this condensation process have been discussed. Moving the insufflation site to a secondary port away from the scope is often sufficient.

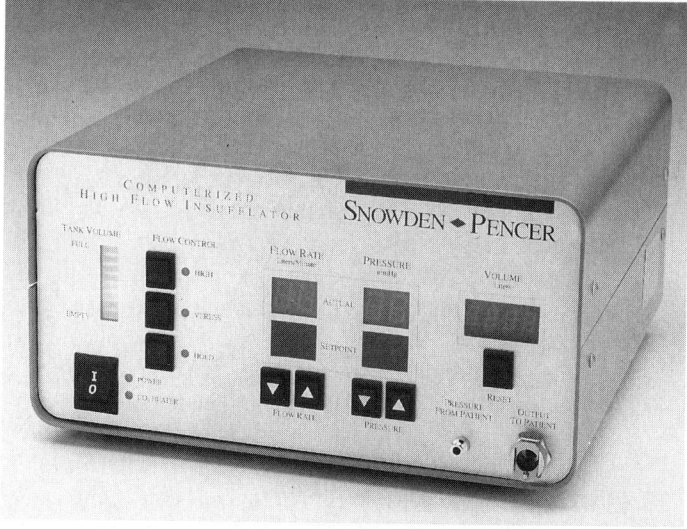

FIG. 32-27 Computerized high-flow insufflator with CO_2 warmer.
Courtesy Snowden-Pencer, Inc., Tucker, Ga.

IRRIGATION

Irrigation is essential during most endoscopic procedures. This is accomplished through irrigating channels built into endoscopes or by irrigating systems inserted through an operating port, cannula, or operative endoscope.

Irrigating fluid can be manually introduced by a syringe and stopcock attached to an irrigation tubing on one end

RESEARCH HIGHLIGHT 32-1

During this study evaluation of core and intraabdominal temperatures of 40 female patients undergoing laparoscopy was performed. Twenty patients had pneumoperitoneum via unheated CO_2. Twenty patients had pneumoperitoneum via CO_2 warmed to 35.0° to 35.5° C before abdominal entry. Temperatures were recorded at timed intervals of CO_2 insufflation. IV solutions were given at room temperature. All patients had endotracheal intubation and the use of a passive heat humidifier in the breathing circuit. Ambient operating room temperature was maintained at a constant level.

Each patient's temperature was recorded preoperatively, intraoperatively at timed intervals, and postoperatively until the findings were within 0.1° C of the original preoperative temperature. A control group of 20 female patients undergoing arthroscopy or breast surgery had preoperative, intraoperative, and postoperative tympanic temperature recordings and core esophageal temperature monitoring.

Intraabdominal temperatures and core esophageal temperatures were equal at the onset of CO_2 pneumoperitoneum in both heated and unheated groups. Intraabdominal and core temperatures were the same when heated CO_2 was used. In the unheated CO_2 group heat loss of 0.3° C per 50 L of consumed CO_2 was noted. Patient PACU temperatures were within 0.1° C of preoperative and intraoperative findings in the warmed group and remained stable during the 30-minute recordings. Temperature stabilization of the unheated group did not always occur with the termination of the surgical procedure.

The temperature of unwarmed CO_2 entering the peritoneum is about 21.1° C. This, in addition to the general anesthetic, length of the surgical procedure, bodily exposure, and room air temperature, can create a potential thermal hazard for patients. The study's findings indicate that warming CO_2 insufflation gas to 30.0° to 30.5° C before it enters the abdominal cavity in conjunction with other measures helps reduce heat loss and maintains a steady core temperature.

Ott, D. (1991). Correction of laparoscopic insufflation hypothermia. *Journal of Laparoendoscopic Surgery, 1*(4), 183-186.

Pumps are available when large quantities of fluid are used and manual operation is cumbersome and time consuming. Pumps are beneficial when irrigation is used for aquadissection. More force can be exerted over longer periods, and pressure is adjustable (Fig. 32-28).

A common pump irrigation system includes the irrigation pump (CO_2 or electric), irrigation bottle caps, irrigation probe with dual trumpet valves, and Y tubing irrigation set. When a CO_2-controlled system is in use, an E-cylinder of CO_2 gas must be attached by means of a tank yoke and input hose. A wrench should always be available to turn off the tank when not in use. It is important to check tank pressure before and after each use.

The pump has an adjustable pressure on/off capability and dual irrigation bottle selection. As one bottle is emptied, a flip of the switch redirects CO_2 flow to the second bottle. Bottles can be replaced as needed. The system operates by the displacement of water or saline with CO_2 gas. The equipment is safe, since no electricity is involved.

Disposable tubing connects each irrigation bottle to the distal irrigation tubing as well as the pump to each irrigation bottle. Caution must be taken when connecting the tubing to the bottles, since sterility of the inner tubing and connections must be maintained throughout the procedure. A clamp is incorporated into the distal tubing leading to the irrigation probe to control flow until attachment takes place. The unit must be in the off mode until all connections have been made. If a connection is made between the CO_2 tank and the pump but not between the irrigation bottle and the distal tubing, fluid can and will be shot across the room.

The distal tubing attaches directly to an irrigation probe. The time and amount of irrigation are controlled by a trumpet valve. Probes are available as reusable, disposable, or a combination of both. All three types incorporate a second trumpet valve for suctioning purposes.

If reusable probes are used, they must be completely disassembled for cleaning and sterilization/disinfection (Fig.

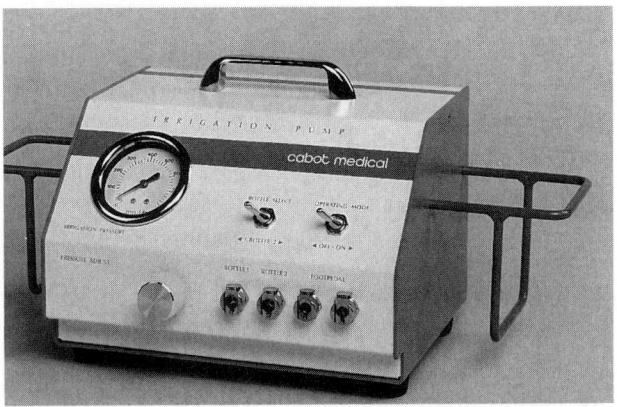

FIG. 32-28 Irrigation pump used for endoscopic surgery. CO_2 gas is used to force fluid throughout system. Side brackets hold sterile irrigation bottles.

Courtesy Cabot Medical Corporation, Langhorne, Pa.

and an irrigation bag and tubing assembly on the other (the original IV pole, Y tubing, and irrigation system). Fluid flows by gravity and is manually forced through the distal tubing. A pressure bag can be used to increase flow, if necessary.

Irrigation through a flexible endoscope is accomplished by a syringe attached to an irrigation port. Fluid travels through a specific channel built into the scope. Rigid scopes such as ureteroscopes, cystoscopes, and hysteroscopes also have this capability, as do operative laparoscopes.

32-29). Each trumpet valve has a spring mechanism (almost like a ballpoint pen). The springs are under pressure when the trumpet valve is inserted. During disassembly it is important to hold one's hand over the valve so that the spring does not eject and become lost or cause eye injury. Protective eyewear should be worn during this process. Extra springs should be available.

Completely disposable units are also available (Fig. 32-30). Some systems incorporate disposable with reusable. Tubing and pistol grip handles containing the trumpet valves are disposable, and the suction/irrigation probes are reusable (Fig. 32-31). The disposable and disposable/reusable units also incorporate electrosurgical capability into the system. This allows the device to be used for three separate functions.

The Nezhat-Dorsey hydrodissection system uses dual 1000-ml bags instead of the bottles. Irrigation bags are spiked with specific tubing, which then attached to the pump. The pump is then attached to the sterile irrigation tubing from the operating room field, per routine. Not only does this system eliminate the need to sterilize the metal umbrella bottle caps, but it also reduces the risk of contamination during connection. Using bag irrigation in place of bottle irrigation further aids in reducing overall cost. Current systems can be equipped with this bottle eliminator capability (Fig. 32-32). Incorporating a disposable reusable approach, the Nezhat-Dorsey pump also uses disposable tubing and handpieces in conjunction with reusable quick-disconnect probe tips (Fig. 32-33).

Irrigation pumps used for arthroscopy are usually electrically controlled. Foot pedal operation is utilized. Dual irrigation bags are attached by Y tubing. If a pump is not used, irrigation tubing is directly attached to the cannula.

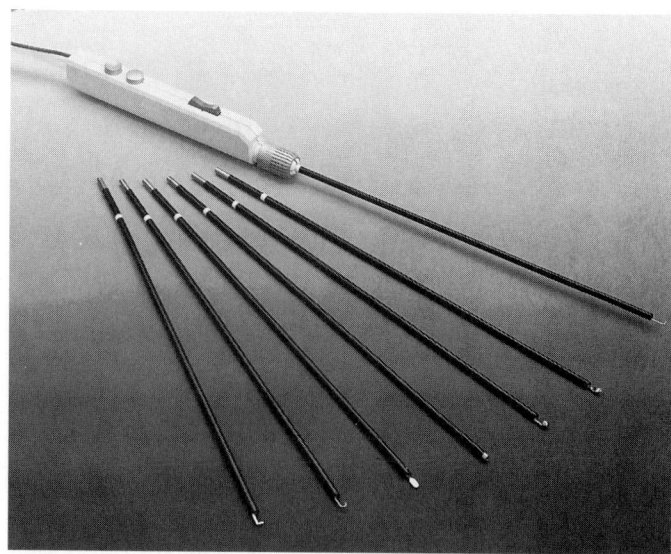

FIG. 32-30 Disposable laparoscopic system with irrigation, suction, and monopolar electrosurgical capability. Electrosurgical probes are available in variety of tips.

Courtesy Valleylab, Inc., Boulder, Colo.

Irrigation fluid depends on surgeon preference. Traditionally, normal saline has been used. Because saline is a conductive fluid, there is concern when monopolar electrosurgery is used. The disadvantage rests with the potentially associated risk from transfer of heat and current to adjacent tissues. Because of this, distilled water should be considered to prevent electrosurgical energy from being transferred to alternate sites whenever excessive monopolar electrosurgery is anticipated. Sorbitol, which is also used as an irrigation medium during hysteroscopy, can be rapidly absorbed into the vascular system, especially during excessive venous bleeding. The patient must be carefully monitored because of the potential for congestive heart failure.

TROCARS AND CANNULAS

When a natural orifice does not exist for diagnostic or operative procedures, one or several can be created. To do so, a trocar and cannula are necessary. Those used for arthroscopy are very small in comparison with those used in the chest or abdomen. The basic principle remains: to provide a mechanism for inserting and removing instrumentation while performing the surgery. The cannula or sheath is inserted into the operative site by using a trocar as an obturator. Once the port of entry has been made, the trocar is removed.

If reusable trocars and cannulas are used, it is of utmost importance to sharpen the trocar tip routinely. On/off stopcock and trumpet valves must be inspected before and after each use to ensure proper functioning. Internal gaskets may need occasional replacement. The trocar and cannula must fit properly and may not always be interchangeable. Care must be taken so that component parts are kept together. They must be disassembled completely for cleaning and sterilization.

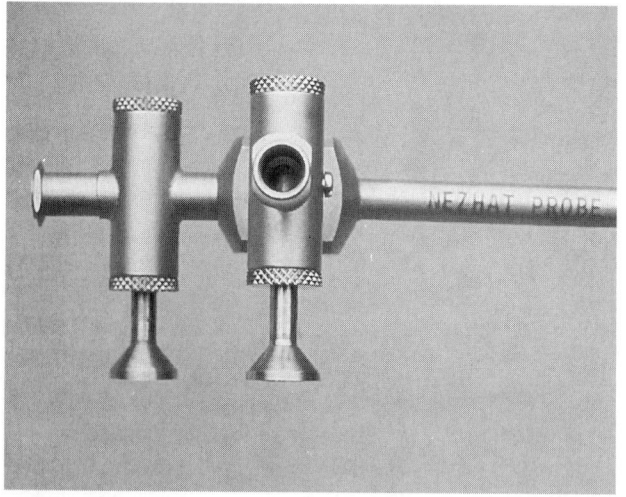

FIG. 32-29 Reusable Nezhat suction-irrigation probe with trumpet valves.

Courtesy Cabot Medical Corporation, Langhorne, Pa.

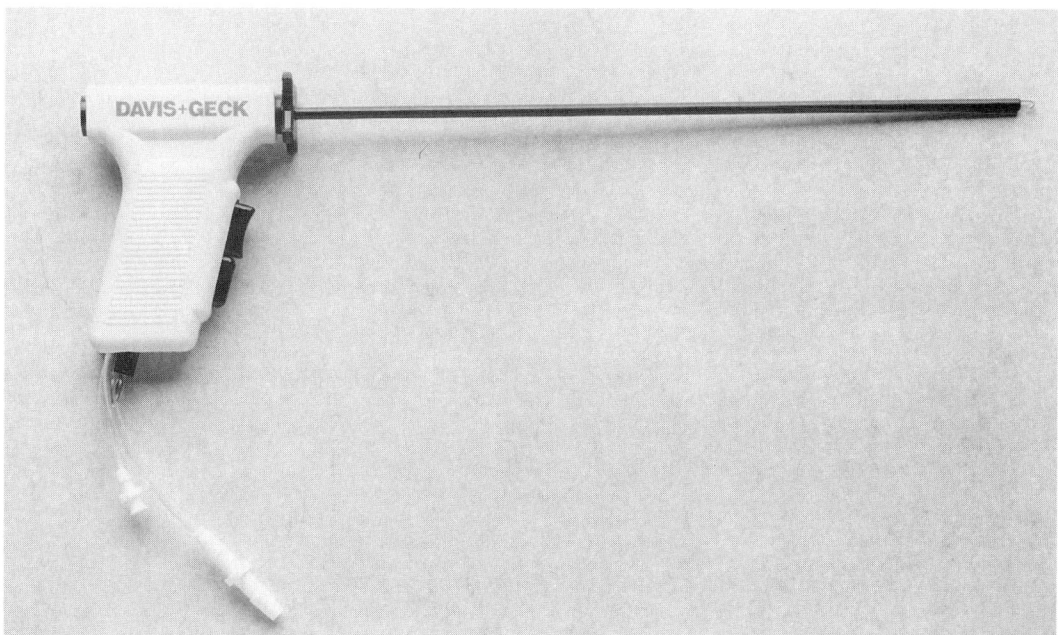

FIG. 32-31 Disposable-reusable suction, irrigation, monopolar electrosurgical system. Handpiece and tubing are disposable. Interchangeable monopolar electrosurgical probes are reusable and are manufactured in variety of tips.

Courtesy Davis & Geck, Danbury, Conn. Other than as explicitly set forth above, Davis & Geck makes no representations or warranties regarding the information supplied.

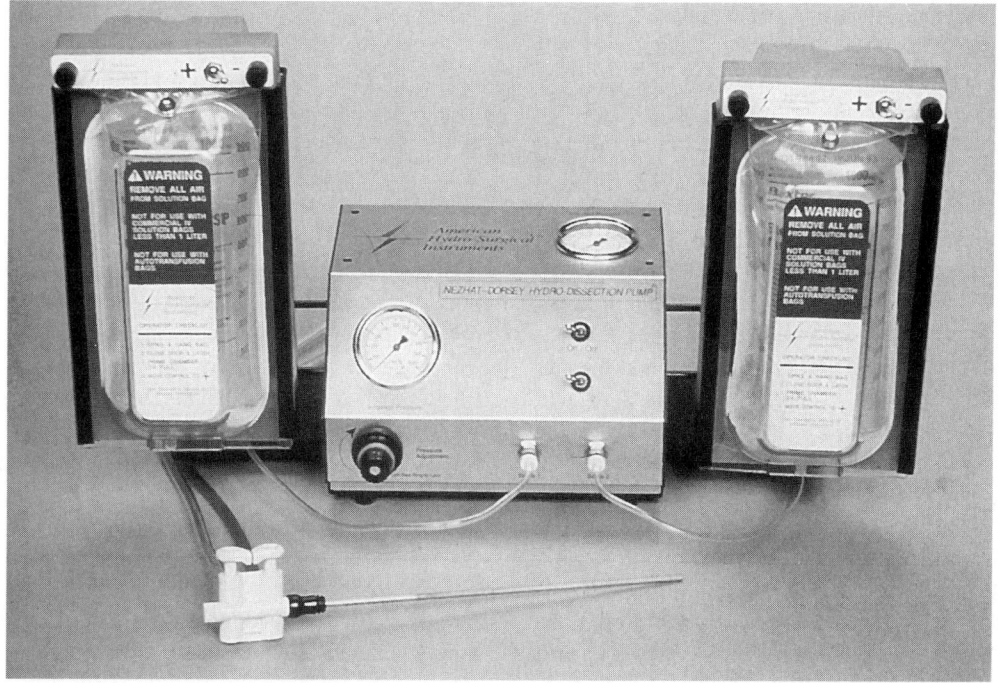

FIG. 32-32 Nezhat-Dorsey irrigation system utilizes bag instead of bottle irrigation, further reducing total cost.

Courtesy American Hydro-Surgical Instruments, Delray Beach, Fla.

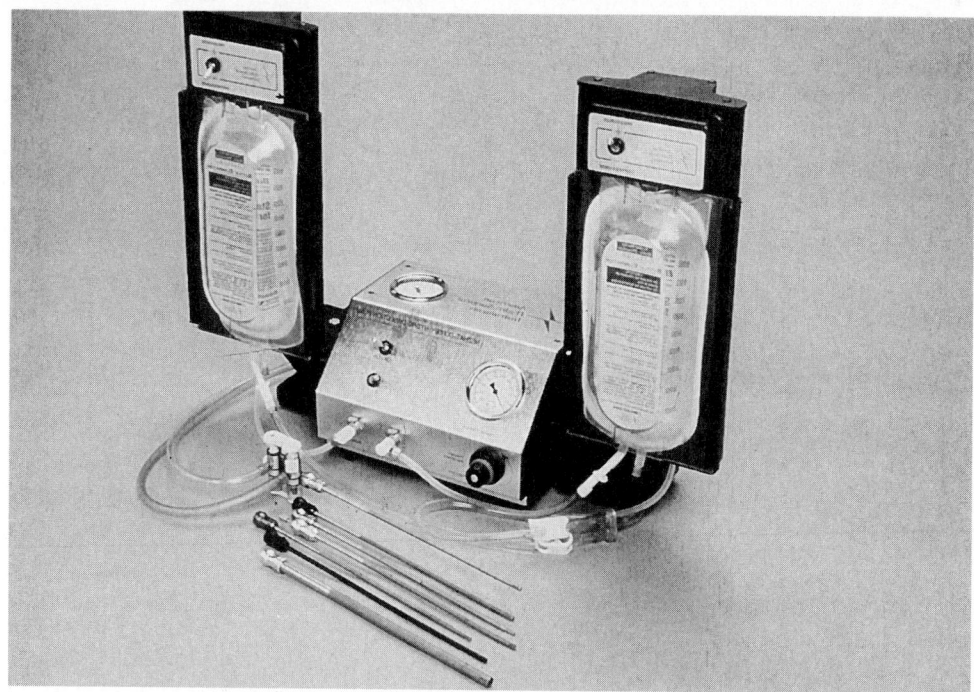

FIG. 32-33 Nezhat-Dorsey disposable irrigation tubing and handpiece, bottle eliminators, and reusable quick-disconnect probes.

Courtesy American Hydro-Surgical Instruments, Delray Beach, Fla.

Disposable systems offer several additional features as well as advantages. The most obvious advantage is that the trocar is always sharp. When multiple ports of the same size are used, the same trocar can be reused (for the same patient). Some manufacturers package one trocar and two sheaths of the same size. Prepackaged procedural kits that offer the same components are also available.

Disposable systems also offer the advantage of siliconized trocar tips as well as safety features once entry has been made. Systems are available that either engage a safety shield to automatically advance over the trocar tip once entry is made or provide retractability of the trocar tip once entry is made (Fig. 32-34). No reusable trocar systems currently have built-in automatic safety shields.

Disposable cannulas also have gripping devices that can reduce the risk of accidental cannula removal during repeated advancement and withdrawal of instrumentation (Fig. 32-35). Grippers are incorporated either into the cannula or as separate entities. Grippers can be used with reusable cannulas as long as the fit is appropriate.

Disposable cannulas have a stopcock assembly for insufflation gas, much the same as the reusable system. One-way flapper valves in disposables provide leak-proof protection and operate automatically for instrument insertion, specimen removal, or rapid desufflation.

The diameter of instrumentation varies with design and use. For this reason various sizes of trocar/cannula systems may be required for one procedure. To increase this flexibility, converters and reducers are used to adapt the size of the instrument (Fig. 32-35). Converters can be separate or

built into the cannula as a diaphragm seal. Both systems are designed to further reduce CO_2 leaks.

Radiolucent disposable systems offer the ability to visualize all pathology without obstruction. This may be critical during an endoscopic cholangiogram. Other times this design may not be necessary. Both reusable and disposable systems come in a variety of diameters and lengths.

Occasionally a procedure is scheduled as an *open* laparoscopy. Patients who have had multiple surgeries or have developed adhesions present an added risk. When a surgeon is unsure of underlying structures, the laparoscopy may be done in an open fashion. A small paraumbilical incision is made and tissues are dissected. Peritoneum is opened and a large blunt tip trocar/sheath assembly is inserted (Fig. 32-36). The sheath is designed to fit snugly against the peritoneum from underneath and skin from above. Stay sutures are used to close any excess incision. Wafer seals (much like colostomy wafers) further reduce loss of CO_2 gas. Pneumoperitoneum is then created. If a reusable system is used, stay sutures are also used to stabilize the system. S-type retractors are usually needed for both (Fig. 32-37).

When extracorporeal surgery must be performed during laparoscopy, an even larger diameter port is used. During certain bowel resections, for example, loops of bowel are brought through the port to be resected or sutured. To enter the chest, shorter blunt trocars are used. Grippers provide stabilization while in the pleural cavity. This type of trocar does not have insufflation ports (Fig. 32-38). If insufflation is required to assist the anesthesiologist in collapsing the lung, regular ports are used.

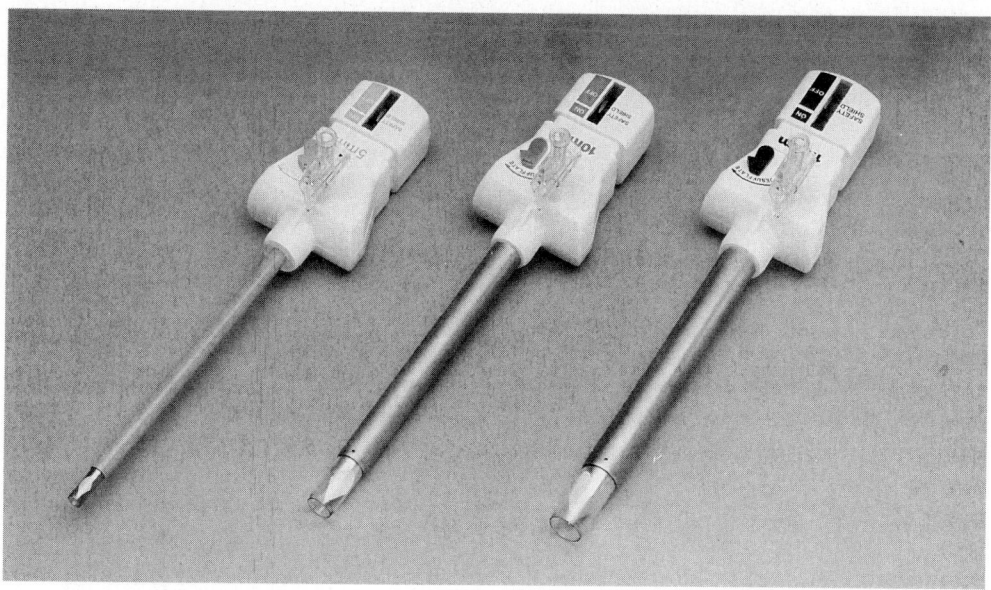

FIG. 32-34   5-mm, 10-mm, and 12-mm disposable trocars with safety shields.

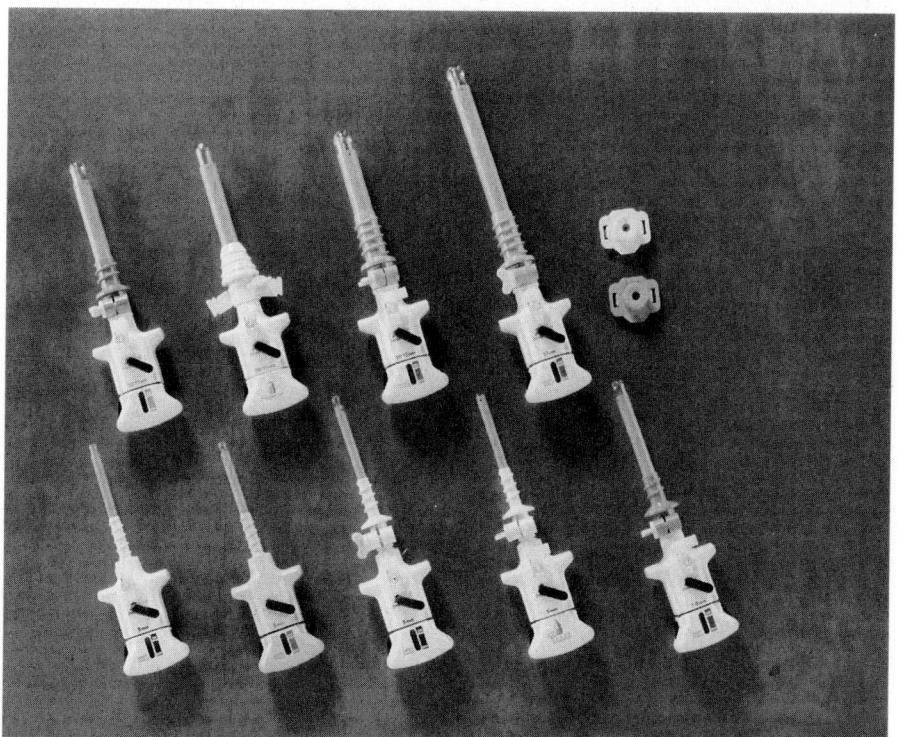

FIG. 32-35   Disposable trocars/cannulas with grippers. Two converters/reducers are also shown.
Courtesy Ethicon Endo-Surgery, Cincinnati, Ohio.

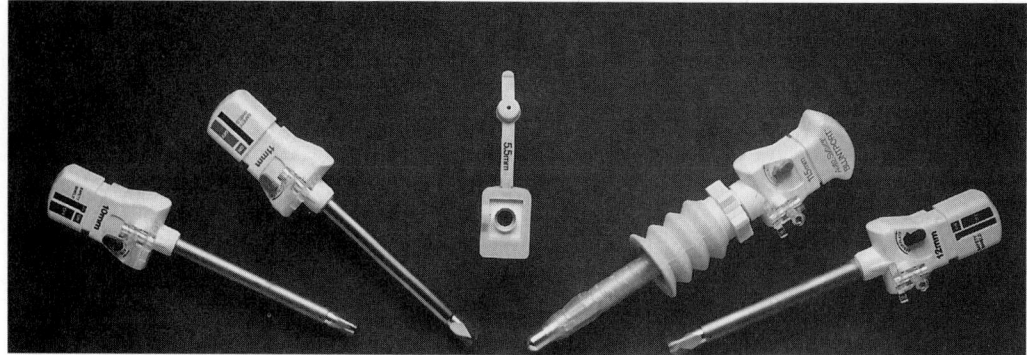

FIG. 32-36   Blunt port/sheath assembly is often used for open laparoscopies *(second from right)*. Sharp trocar/cannula units as well as converter/reducer are also shown.

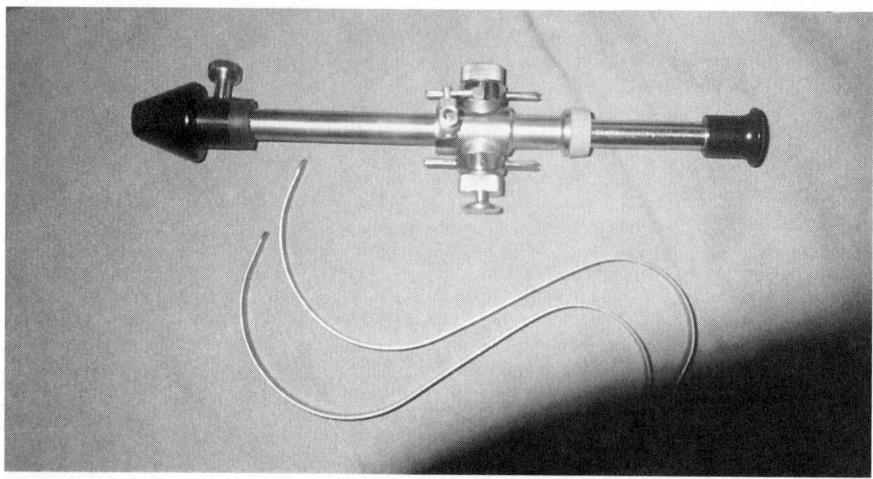

FIG. 32-37   Reusable blunt-tip Hassan type trocar and S retractors.

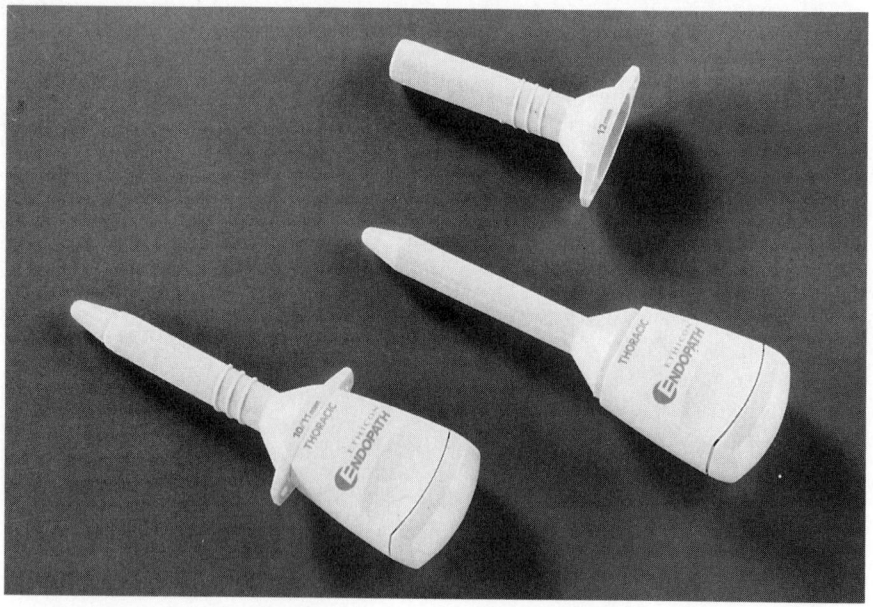

FIG. 32-38   Thoracic blunt trocar and gripper assembly. Notice absence of stopcock insufflation capability.

Courtesy Ethicon Endo-Surgery, Cincinnati, Ohio.

INSTRUMENTATION

Endoscopic instrumentation has been designed to correspond to the surgical site. Length, working end, and hand control are designed with this in mind. Because endoscopic surgical approaches differ from the traditional open-surgical equivalents, modifications of existing instruments were made. Some basic patterns had been used for years. Others were designed to accommodate the new approaches.

It is impossible to describe every system on the market. If equipment exists for an open approach, it more than likely exists for all endoscopic approaches. Instruments used for open arthrotomy were once adapted to arthroscopy. Additionally, what was once used for traditional sinus surgery was modified to enhance functional endoscopic sinus surgery. The impact of this new era in surgery was realized less than a decade ago and already instrument designs are in their third and fourth generations. As surgery becomes more sophisticated, so do the instruments required for successful intervention (Fig. 32-39).

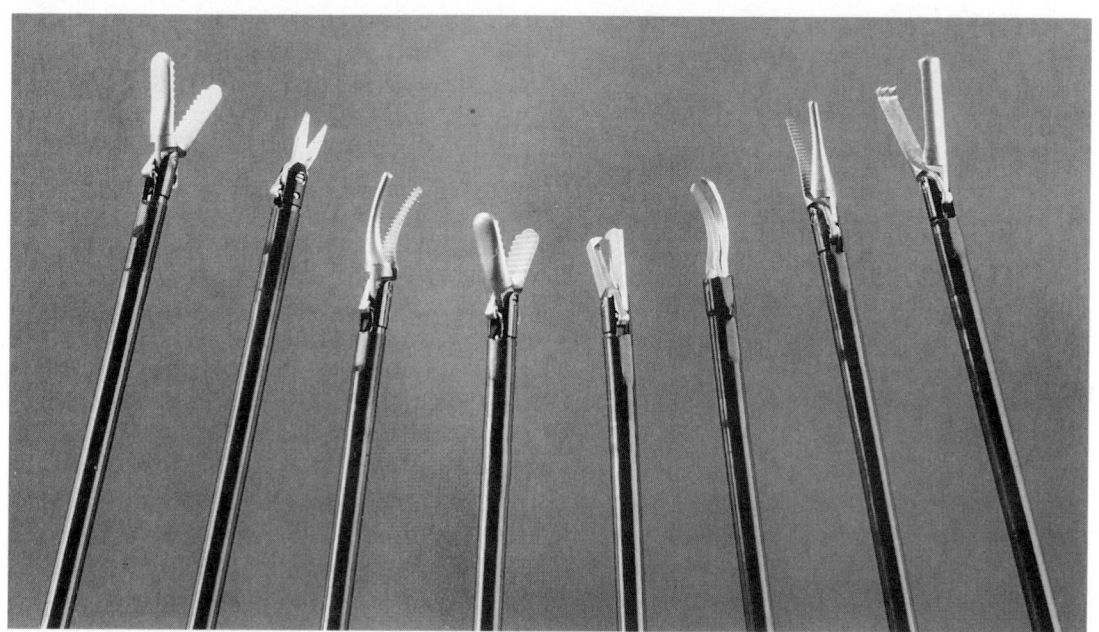

FIG. 32-39 Disposable endoscopic instruments are designed to meet procedural needs during endoscopic surgery.

Courtesy Ethicon Endo-Surgery, Cincinnati, Ohio.

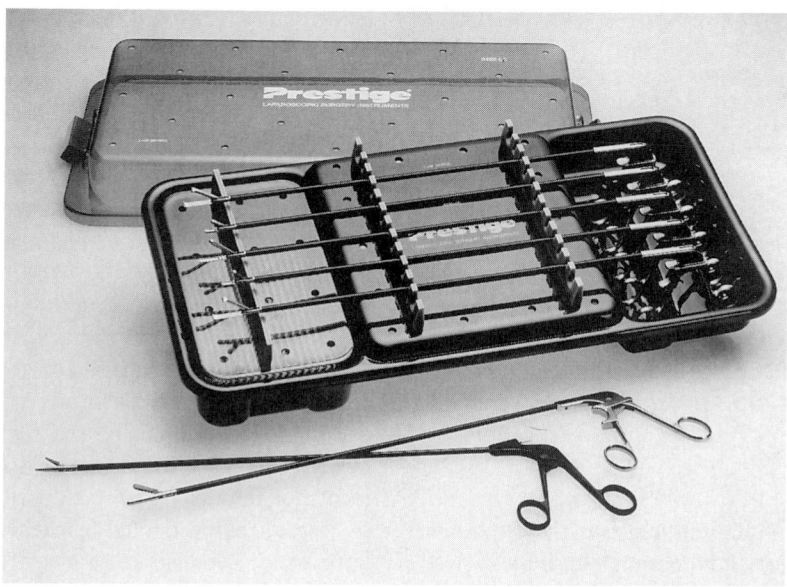

FIG. 32-40 Reusable grasping forceps assembled in their own sterilization tray.

Courtesy Davis & Geck, Danbury, Conn. Other than as explicitly set forth above, Davis & Geck makes no representations or warranties regarding the information supplied.

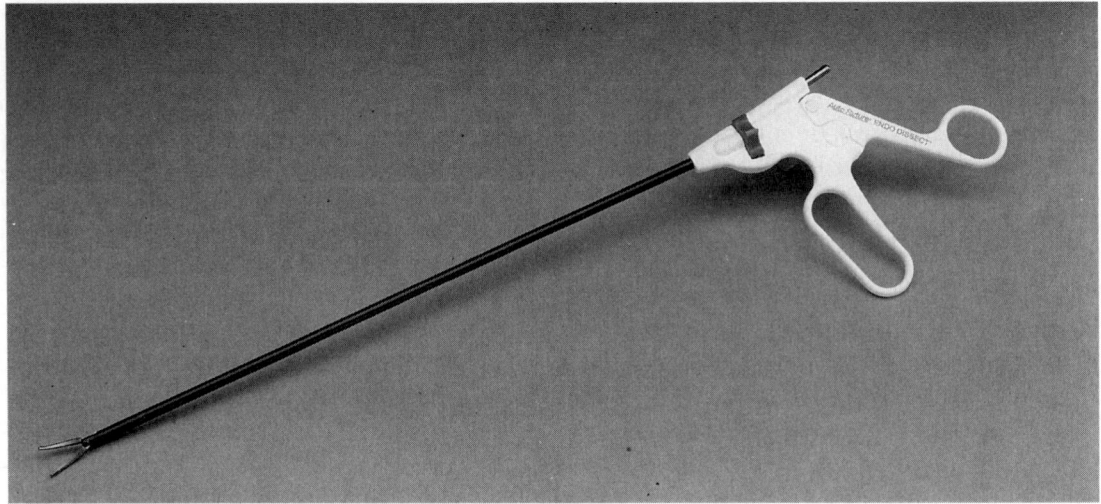

FIG. 32-41   Disposable dissector with swivel design and monopolar electrosurgical capability.

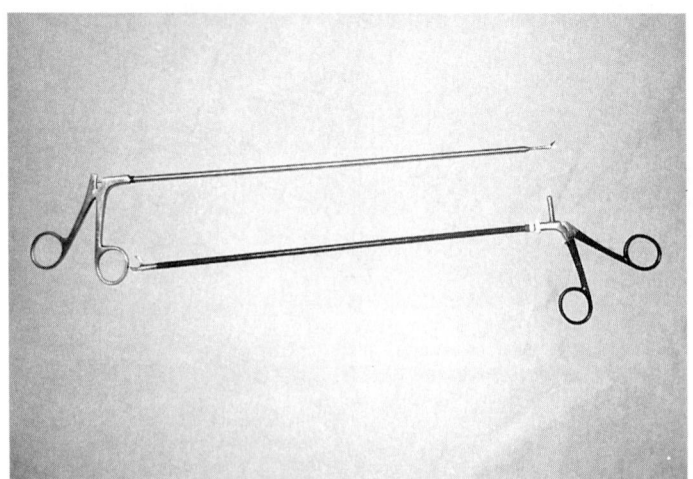

FIG. 32-42   Reusable endoscopic scissors. *Top,* Microscissors. *Bottom,* hook scissors with monopolar electrosurgical capability; shaft and handpiece are insulated.

Forceps and dissectors

Instrument categories are identical to their open procedure counterparts. Forceps and grasping instruments provide for manipulation of tissues (Fig. 32-40). Dissectors are usually finer and can also be used to retract delicate structures. Their primary functions are to separate, spread, and divide tissues (Fig. 32-41). Scissors come in a variety of designs (Fig. 32-42).

Endoscopic clips

One of the most important instruments in the hemostatic category is the clip applier. It represents the safest, easiest, and quickest way to occlude small vessels and structures. Reusable appliers exist, but they must be removed from the cannula each time to be reloaded. This adds time, contributes to loss of pneumoperitoneum (if utilized), and causes frustration when the clip is dislodged upon reinsertion. The automatic feed, reloadable, disposable version remains the ideal (Fig. 32-43).

Endoscopic staplers

Endoscopic stapling devices provide cutting and stapling during endoscopic resections (Figs. 32-44 and Fig. 32-45). Certain structures can be easily resected intracorporeally (such as the ovary and appendix). Others may necessitate extracorporeal resection or reanastomosis. If this occurs, traditional stapling devices are used.

Electrosurgery

Electrosurgical instruments provide cutting and coagulating ability. Current can be provided in either monopolar or bipolar modes. Endoscopic spatulas and hooks are routinely used with monopolar current, but virtually any dissector, blunt grasper, and scissors can be manufactured with this option. When used in this fashion, the instrument's shaft must be insulated (Fig. 32-46). Traumatic injury can occur if instruments are not insulated properly. Instruments should be inspected before and after each use for breaks in insulation.

Capacitive coupling occurs when radio frequency energy (electrosurgical energy) is transferred through *intact* insulation into nearby conductive materials. A common example is when an electrode is activated within a suction irrigator. Induced current on the suction irrigator can cause bowel burns. The use of monopolar electrosurgical instrumentation through *metal* suction irrigators increases the risk of visceral burns through capacitive thermal energy. The laparoscope can also cause alternate site burns if the electrosurgical electrode is used through the scope. Direct coupling can also occur if the active electrosurgical electrode touches another uninsulated, metal instrument; this includes the laparoscope.

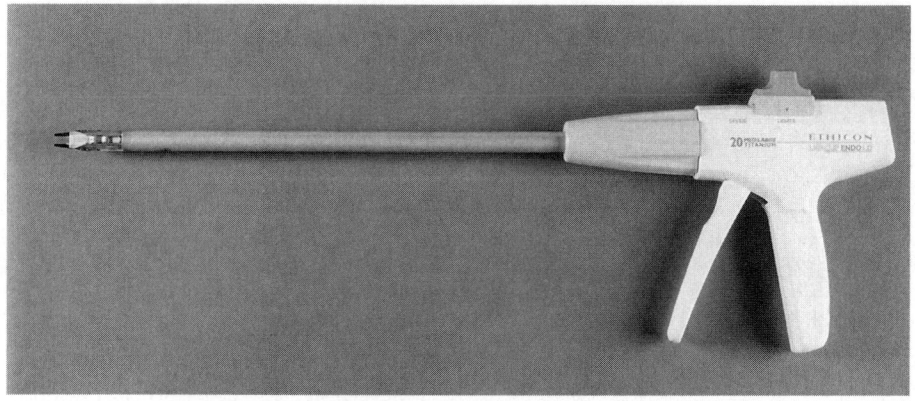

FIG. 32-43   Disposable endoscopic rotating clip applier.
Courtesy Ethicon Endo-Surgery, Cincinnati, Ohio.

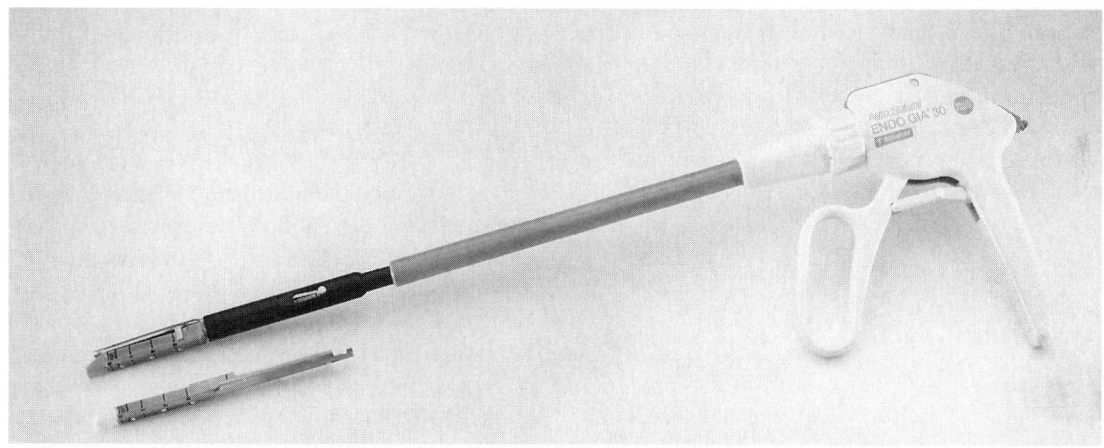

FIG. 32-44   Disposable endoscopic stapling device (Endo GIA 30 and reloading unit).
Copyright © 1993 United States Surgical Corporation. All rights reserved. Reprinted with the permission of United States Surgical Corporation.

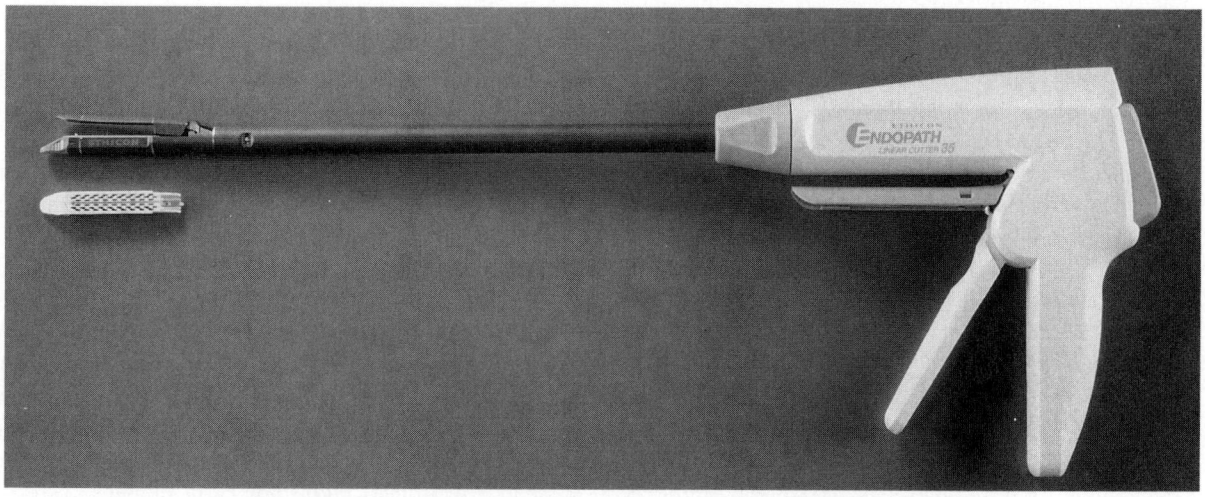

FIG. 32-45   Disposable linear cutter and reloading unit (Endopath ELC 35).
Courtesy Ethicon Endo-Surgery, Cincinnati, Ohio.

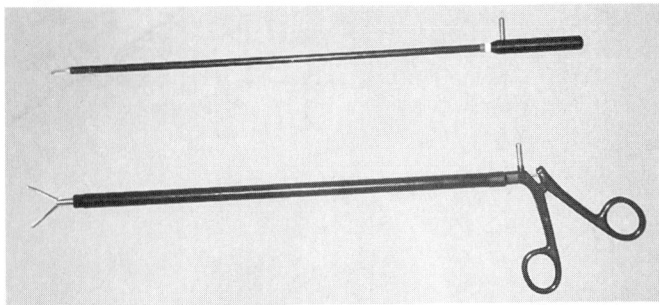

FIG. 32-46 Reusable insulated dissector and spatula.

If insulation is defective, current can escape at the point of defect. Adjacent tissue can be burned, causing unnecessary injury. Inadvertent bowel and vascular injuries can result if sparking occurs during monopolar electrode use. To prevent sparking, current should not be discharged until tissue contact has been made. To protect adjacent tissue and structures, a monopolar hook electrode is often used. The hook allows the surgeon to lift tissue away from any underlying structure before electrosurgical activation.

A bipolar electrosurgical system is also used. Since bipolar current is very precise and travels only between the two poles of the forceps, it is often used in areas where this precision is required. The most widely used is the Kleppinger system (Fig. 32-47).

LAPAROSCOPIC SUTURING AND LIGATION

Endoscopic surgical techniques have challenged traditional suturing and ligation methods; several devices and techniques have been developed for laparoscopic tissue suturing.

When surgical clips cannot be used, a laparoscopic suture may have to be substituted. Conditions that preclude the use of clips include large arteries and edematous or inflamed ducts. Most general surgeons prefer to use nonabsorbable sutures and ligation materials to prevent rapid absorption.

The three basic types of laparoscopic suturing materials are loop ligatures, extracorporeal sutures, and intracorporeal sutures. Preknotted suture loops are used to ligate pedicle tissues. The suture loop is packaged in conjunction with an introducer sleeve, which can be inserted through one of the trocars. The loop is passed over the targeted tissue or pedicle using a grasping forcep to assist. Once the loop is in position, the existing suture knot is pushed down the introducer sleeve until it is cinched tightly around the tissue. The suture is then cut with endoscopic scissors (Fig. 32-48).

Tissue can be approximated intraabdominally by tying the knot extracorporeally (outside the body). To accomplish this, endoscopic swaged sutures are used. The suture is grasped proximal to the needle, and both are inserted through one of the trocars into the abdomen. The needle is then held with the grasper or laparoscopic needle holder and driven through the desired tissue. A second grasper or needle holder inserted through a second trocar is used to assist. The needled end of the suture is pulled through the tissue and out through the trocar. The needle is removed and a knot is tied extracorporeally. The knot is advanced down the trocar and onto the tissue. The suture is cut using laparoscopic scissors (Fig. 32-49). The three types of knots tied extracorporeally are the slip knot, the fisherman's knot, and the surgeon's knot. The surgeon determines which knot is used.

Suture ligature can also be passed through the trocar. The tissue is approximated in the same fashion but tied intracorporeally (inside the abdomen) using grasping forceps and/or laparoscopic needle holders. Some surgeons prefer this simplified technique.

It is important for the perioperative nurse and RN first assistant to become familiar with all three techniques and supplies needed for each. The technique is not only surgeon specific but can be determined by surgical site.

ANESTHETIC CONSIDERATIONS

Although anesthetic technique and delivery are the responsibility of the anesthesia care provider, it is essential for the perioperative nurse to anticipate and appropriately respond to associated risks during endoscopic intervention. Many open surgical procedures, which require lengthy hospitalization and result in substantial postoperative pain, are now performed endoscopically as ambulatory or short-stay surgeries. Postoperative pain has been minimized for most patients. Because of these changes, anesthetic technique has also changed. Today there is an emphasis on minimal anesthesia during surgery. Short-acting drugs are used so that the patient awakens quickly and experiences as few side effects as possible.

The three major goals of the anesthesia care provider remain the same: respiratory stability, appropriate muscle relaxation, and hemodynamic stability. Additionally, during many laparoscopic and pelviscopic procedures it is necessary to control diaphragmatic excursion.

When Trendelenburg position is used, there is an increase in intraabdominal pressure, which can result in respiratory complications including hypoxia. CO_2 absorption from the peritoneal cavity can further aggravate this situation. Reverse Trendelenburg position could result in decreased venous return, cardiac output, and blood pressure. CO_2 insufflation in this position could lead to an increase in total peripheral resistance, especially if intraabdominal pressure is high and the aorta is compressed. The perioperative nurse must be prepared to change the position of the OR bed when necessary and decrease the CO_2 flow rate of the insufflator. The anesthesia care provider may require assistance with medications and extra supplies.

CO_2, highly soluble in blood, does not generally become

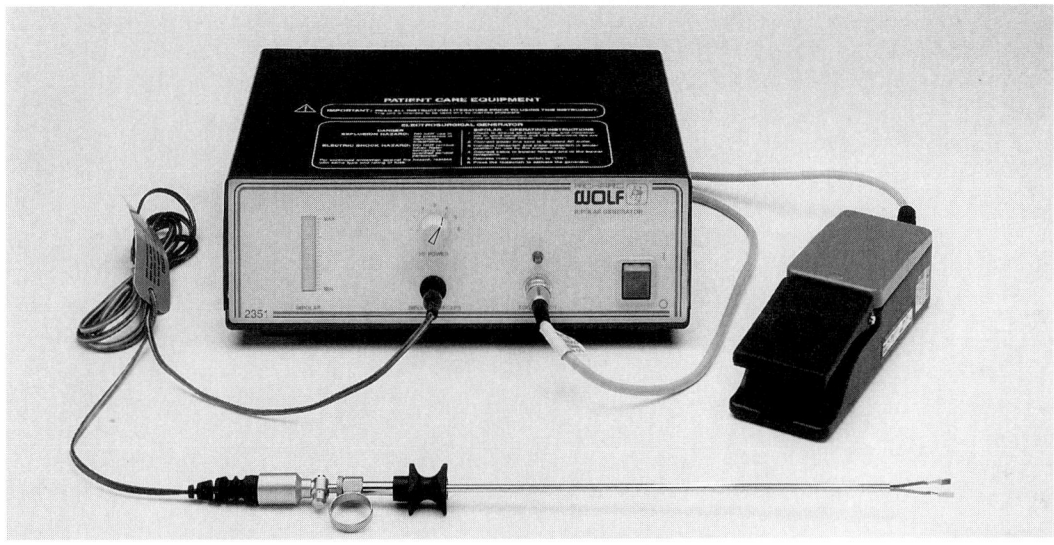

FIG. 32-47   Kleppinger bipolar unit and forceps.

Courtesy Richard Wolf Medical Instruments Corp., Vernon Hills, Ill.

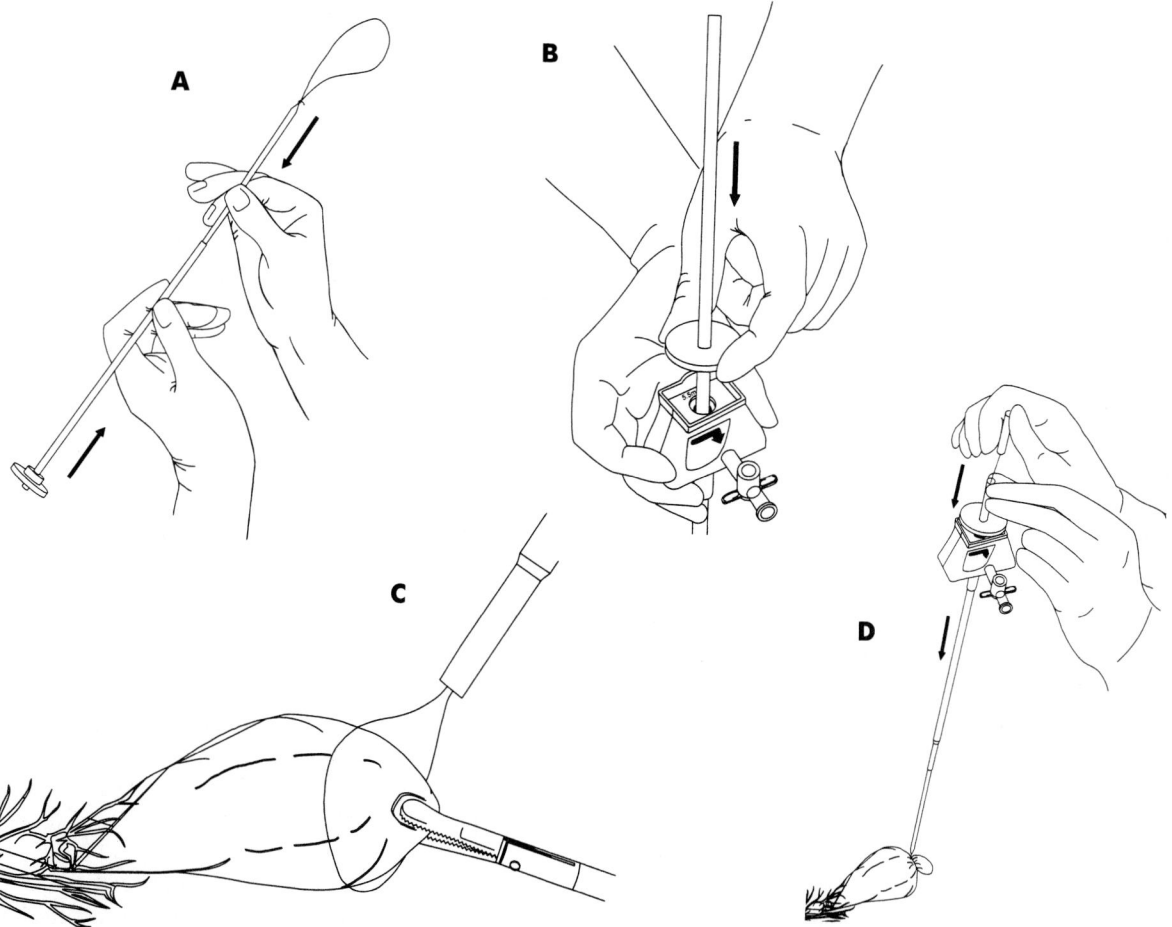

FIG. 32-48   Surgitie ligating loop. **A,** Back load loop into introducer completely. **B,** Insert introducer into trocar, all the way down. **C,** Push suture loop through introducer. Grasp desired tissue with grasping forceps (passed through another trocar) and maneuver loop over tissue. **D,** Push down knot by advancing nylon carrier all the way until knot is cinched. Cut suture.

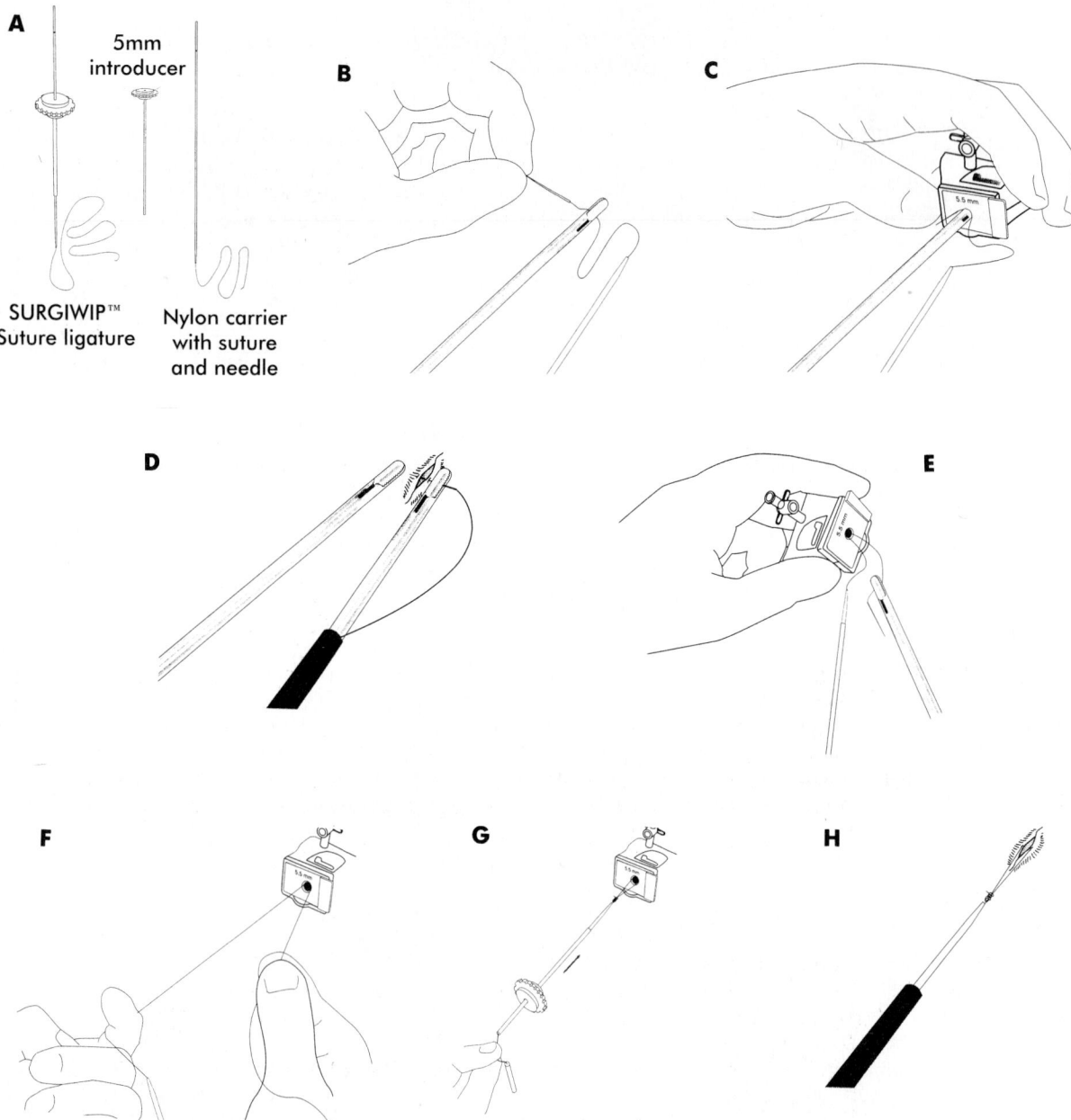

FIG. 32-49 Surgiwip suture ligature application for approximating tissue intraabdominally by extra-corporeal knot tying (outside body). **A,** Component pieces. **B,** Grasp suture behind swage of needle with tissue grasper or needle holder. **C,** Introduce grasper/needle holder and suture through trocar into abdomen. **D,** Drive needle through tissue to be approximated. Place instrument close to center of needle for control. Pull needle through tissue using second grasper (introduced through another trocar). **E,** Regrasp needle behind swage intracorporeally and pull it through and out the same trocar. (Allow for slack of suture to avoid tissue tears.) **F,** Remove needle. Tie fisherman's knot. **G,** Once knot is tied, break end of nylon carrier. **H,** Push knot down with nylon carrier and out onto tissue. Cut suture. For additional suturing, repeat **A** to **H** until tissue is satisfactorily approximated.

a hazard when used during laparoscopic insufflation because it is rapidly absorbed in the splanchnic vascular region. Excessive intraabdominal pressure or any anesthetic technique that reduces splanchnic blood flow, however, could increase the potential for CO_2 gas emboli. This could lead to circulatory collapse. CO_2 could also advance from the heart to the pulmonary circulation, causing acute pulmonary hypertension with right heart failure. If these effects are undetected and CO_2 insufflation continues, cardiac arrest and death could occur.

Signs of CO_2 embolus include sudden fall in blood pressure, dysrhythmia, heart murmurs, cyanosis, pulmonary edema, and an abrupt increase in end-tidal CO_2. If an embolus is suspected, continuous monitoring of heart sounds, blood pressure, and end-tidal CO_2 can help the anesthesia care provider make a rapid diagnosis. Immediate deflation of pneumoperitoneum is necessary. Treatment may include immediate placement of the patient in a left lateral position and aspiration of the CO_2 gas through a central venous catheter. The perioperative nurse should assist in patient repositioning while maintaining sterility of equipment and the surgical field wherever possible. Assistance may be required during central venous catheter placement. Debilitated patients may require preoperative invasive monitoring.

Hypotension can result from excessive bleeding, excess intraabdominal pressure, and hypoxia. CO_2 insufflation rates may have to be reduced. Extra intravenous fluids may be needed.

Hypertension resulting from increased intraabdominal pressure and increased CO_2 gas absorption may also be evidenced. Increased bleeding may result. Again, the perioperative nurse can help by decreasing CO_2 insufflation flow rates; additional hemostatic agents and endoscopic clips may be required.

Gastric reflux is a concern if the patient is obese, a hiatal hernia is present, or excessive pneumoperitoneum occurs. The hiatal hernia could be discovered during the preoperative assessment. A nasogastric or orogastric tube may be inserted after general anesthesia is induced. There will be less postoperative discomfort if an orogastric tube is used. During epidural and regional anesthesia, patients are usually awake, and insertion of a gastric tube may be poorly tolerated. For this reason the tube is not inserted unless gastric distention occurs. The perioperative nurse must be quick to respond if assistance is required during gastric tube insertion.

Intercostal nerve blocks offer surgical pain relief and abdominal muscle relaxation when the patient is awake during surgery. This anesthetic technique requires extreme patient cooperation, since several injections are necessary. The perioperative nurse's role during intercostal nerve block induction is to remain at the patient's side and help to reduce anxiety.

The perioperative nurse's understanding of the potential for associated risk factors along with appropriate nursing interventions can have a significant affect on outcome, producing organization and control from chaos.

SPECIAL NURSING CONSIDERATIONS
EDUCATION AND COORDINATION

As with any new surgical procedure, a learning curve exists for all members of the surgical team. Educational opportunities must be intense initially and must be ongoing so that competencies are maintained. Multidisciplinary inservicing should be provided before the introduction of new products.

The concept of "train the trainer" works very well. An endoscopy nurse who is responsible for the maintenance and coordination of perioperative nursing practice, education, supplies, and equipment related to endoscopic surgery is ideal. This perioperative nurse serves as a clinical expert to enhance the institutional endoscopic program (Fig. 32-50). She or he should be a member of a multidisciplinary team to assess new products, cost effectiveness, and practice patterns (Box 32-2).

A technical video expert is also necessary. The endoscopy nurse can address the video aspects. Having a member of the institutional biomedical department in partnership with the endoscopy nurse is even better. This team approach facilitates coordination, cooperation, and positive outcomes.

CLEANING AND PROCESSING

The cleaning and processing of endoscopic instrumentation and equipment have been under scrutiny and heated debate. Compliance with federal, professional, and regional standards cannot be ignored. High-level (cold soak) disinfection has been the accepted gold standard for endoscopic instrumentation. Today the concern over viruses and microorganisms such as HIV, hepatitis B virus, and tuberculosis, coupled with the need for comparable levels of pa-

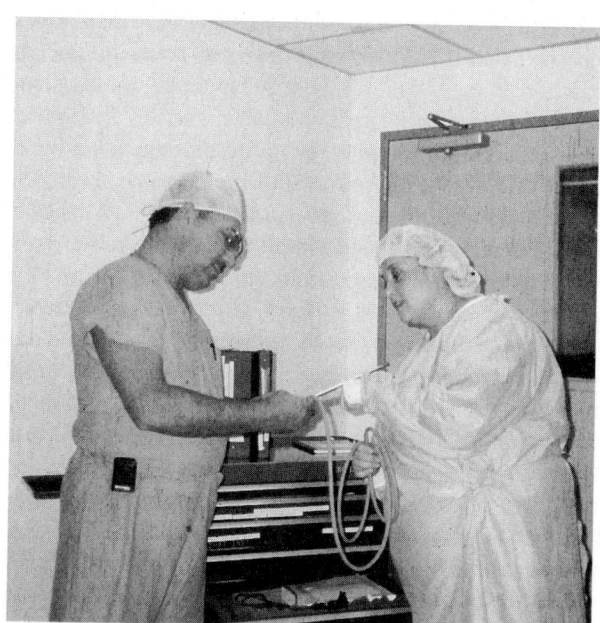

FIG. 32-50 Endoscopy RN and surgeon collaborate on equipment needed for endoscopic surgery.

BOX 32-2

Multidisciplinary Approach to Endoscopic Surgical Evaluation

VIDEO NEEDS: ADMINISTRATION

- Appropriate capital purchase
- Enhanced return on investment
- Adequate warranty
- Rapid service turnaround
- Adaptability to future technology
- Satisfied external and internal customers
- Flexible financing terms

VIDEO NEEDS: PERIOPERATIVE NURSING

- User friendliness
- Consistency and reliability
- Manufacturer's problem-solving capability
- Minimal down-time
- Universal adaptability and compatibility
- Ease in sterilization/disinfection

VIDEO NEEDS: SURGEON

- Clear, crisp picture
- True-to-life color
- Accurate lighting
- Remote control capability
- Reliability
- Lightweight camera
- Adaptability to future technology

tient care, has sent perioperative nurses back to the drawing board.

If we consider the ideal, all instruments and equipment coming in contact with sterile tissues and the vascular system should be sterile. Those coming in contact with mucous membranes or nonintact skin can be high-level disinfected. This can be interpreted to mean sterility is required for all laparoscopy, angioscopy, thoracoscopy, and arthroscopy procedures. Cold soak disinfection may be acceptable for colonoscopy, laryngoscopy, bronchoscopy, cystoscopy, and other diagnostic procedures. The question becomes, "How can we best address current standards and recommendations?"

Institutional policy sets the guidelines from which to work. Provision of comparable levels of care when there are not equal numbers of instruments to match scheduled procedures takes insight and coordination. If sterile instruments are required for a particular endoscopic procedure, sterile instruments must be used for *all* patients undergoing that procedure. Enough instrumentation and equipment must be purchased to accommodate the endoscopic patient volume, or other measures must be implemented.

Sterile camera drapes can be used when there are more procedures than cameras. These drapes cannot be used with the newer one-piece camera/scope models. Cameras can be

ethylene oxide sterilized. Most endoscopes can only be ethylene oxide sterilized. Endoscope prototypes that will withstand steam sterilization are currently being tested. Disposable laparoscopes are available. Instrumentation can be steam sterilized between procedures, if necessary; certain instrumentation is available as disposable.

A sterile processing system that uses peracetic acid provides just-in-time sterile endoscopes, cameras, and instruments. The STERIS system is appropriate for heat-sensitive items that can be cleaned and completely immersed (Research Hightlight 32-2). The processing cycle is less than 30 minutes and is less damaging to delicate instruments than

RESEARCH HIGHLIGHT 32-2

Peracetic acid has been found to be bactericidal at 0.001%, fungicidal at 0.003%, and sporicidal at 0.3%. Although there are no current data to demonstrate how the sterilant actually works, it is believed to function like other peroxides and oxidizing agents through rupture of the cell wall.

The Environmental Protection Agency (EPA) has approved the sterilant, and both the STERIS sterilizer and sterilant are cleared for marketing by the Food and Drug Administration (FDA). The manufacturer has also shown that difficult items with channels are effectively sterilized. Large quantities of spores (10^7) were placed inside scope channels and then subjected to the sterilization process. Rinse cultures produced negative results. More research data to demonstrate the effectiveness of the sterilant in a clinical setting are needed, however. Although spore strips biologically monitor each sterilization cycle, some critics believe that this testing must be done at the most difficult scope areas—inside the channels. To date there is no method for this to be done for *any* sterilization process.

Anticorrosive chemicals are combined with the sterilant because of its corrosive tendency. The system provides a method of sterilizing heat-sensitive *immersible* instruments and equipment rapidly. Processing time varies from 20 to 30 minutes depending on how extensively the water supply must be filtered and on the initial water temperature.

The sterilant can be used only in the STERIS sterilizer and has been found to have advantages for disinfection and sterilization not found in any other agent. It has no harmful decomposition products (by-products), has infinite water solubility, is nonfoaming and fast acting, does not affect glues found in most endoscopes, is cost-effective (approximately $6/cycle), and is environmentally friendly. Two disadvantages are that only items which can be totally immersed can be sterilized, and only one scope or a few instruments can be processed in a cycle.

Crow, S. (1992). Peracetic acid sterilization: A timely development for a busy healthcare industry. *Infection Control and Hospital Epidemiology, 13*(2), 111-113.

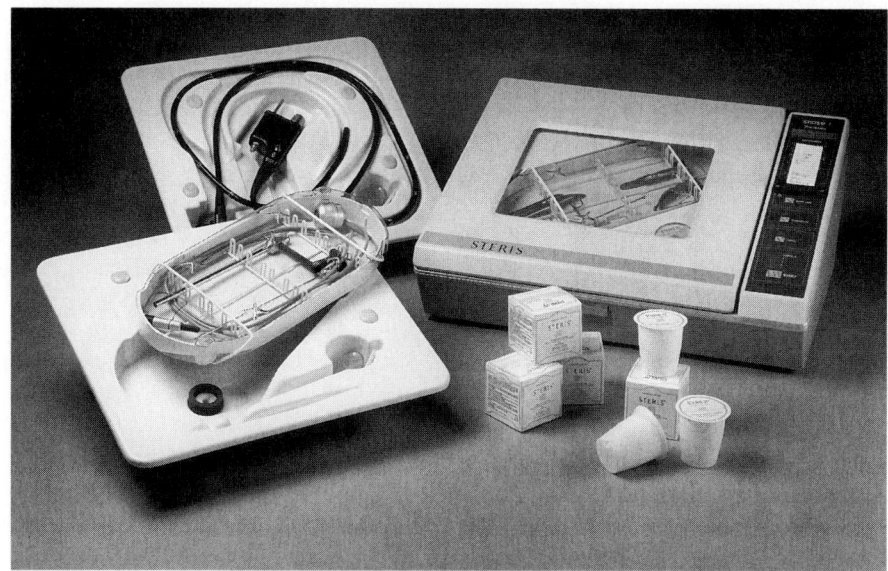

FIG. 32-51   STERIS System I.
Courtesy STERIS Corporation, Mentor, Ohio.

steam. Its compatibility with a wide variety of instruments and equipment as well as the environmental safety of its by-products makes the system valuable. Instruments are placed into removable trays where the solution can reach all surfaces, lumens, and ports. Channeled instruments are also sterilized. Only completely immersible items can be placed into the unit and only one scope and a small amount of instruments can be processed at one time (Fig. 32-51).

Instruments must be clean and free from all bioburden before sterilization or high-level disinfection can be considered. Sterilization and disinfection parameters are based on this assumption. During routine use bioburden accumulates in channels, ports, crevices, and other movable parts of scopes and instruments. Periodically throughout the procedure, gross blood and bioburden should be removed with sterile water by the scrub nurse. Channels should be flushed so that buildup is minimized.

After each procedure all equipment must be decontaminated before reprocessing can occur. Immersible equipment should be cleaned and/or flushed with an enzymatic detergent solution whenever possible. This loosens organic material and makes it easier to remove. Careful rinsing and flushing with copious amounts of water must follow. The process should continue until clean. Manufacturer's written recommendations for cleaning and processing should always be followed. Instruments must be dried before disinfection or sterilization.

The recent introduction of the Endoflush system has brought an economical, practical, and effective way to initially clean reusable channeled instruments. The apparatus, simple to use, provides a method to remove organic debris (Figs. 32-52 and 32-53). Even though instruments have flush ports, debris can become lodged distally. The system simply provides a means to flush in a retrograde fashion, forcing debris out the larger proximal port. Sealed instruments can also be tested for seal integrity using this system.

REUSABLE VERSUS DISPOSABLE EQUIPMENT

The climate surrounding health care has become one of uncertainty and ever-present change. With spiraling costs come new opportunities and challenges for redesign. The directive to "do more with less" has become a way of life. Endoscopy has paved the way for surgical and diagnostic procedures to be performed with reduced patient discomfort and earlier discharge (often the same day). Patients are happier because they can go home and return to normal lifestyles more quickly.

Case management and clinical pathways are important guides to enable a safe, rapid hospital discharge. Hospital administrators and third-party payers are rapidly turning to the concept of cost per discharge. The endoscopic revolution has indeed reduced a patient's length of stay significantly. Operating room expenditures, on the other hand, have increased. Institutional policy may dictate whether reusable or single-use items are chosen. When analyzing the risk/benefit ratio, several issues should be considered.

Many facilities are using a combination of reusable and single-use laparoscopic instruments. Advantages of single-use items include sharpness, reliability related to function, guaranteed sterility, and safety. Indirect advantages include no reprocessing time and effort, no associated repair costs, and the provision of comparable levels of patient care. Upgrade designs are also more easily purchased if they are single-use. Disadvantages may include the need for increased storage space, budgetary implications, and environmental concerns related to biohazardous waste.

Advantages of reusable instruments include less storage space required, a reduced budgetary impact (except for initial purchase), and minimal waste.

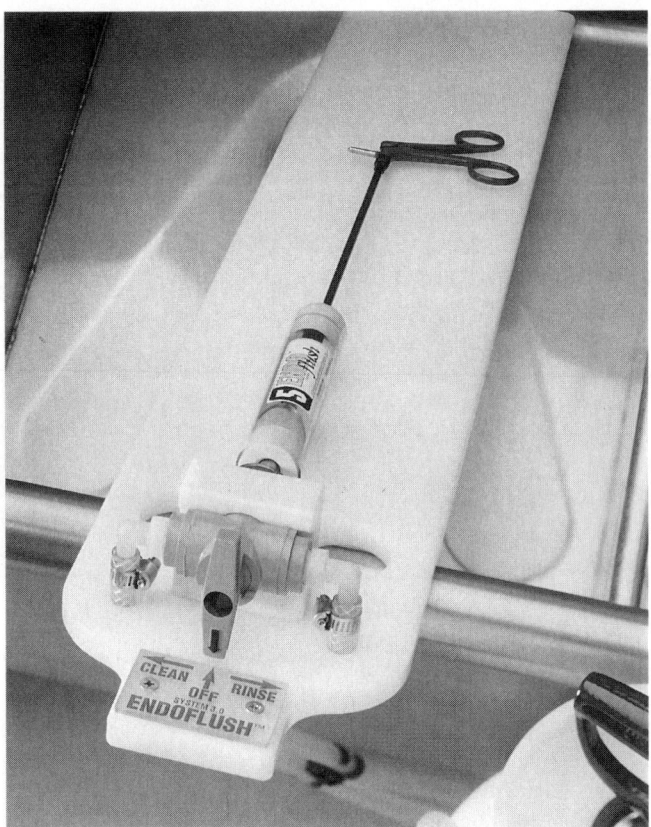

FIG. 32-52 Endoflush endoscopic instrument cleaner—manual.
Courtesy Specialty Medical Systems, Shawnee Mission, Kansas.

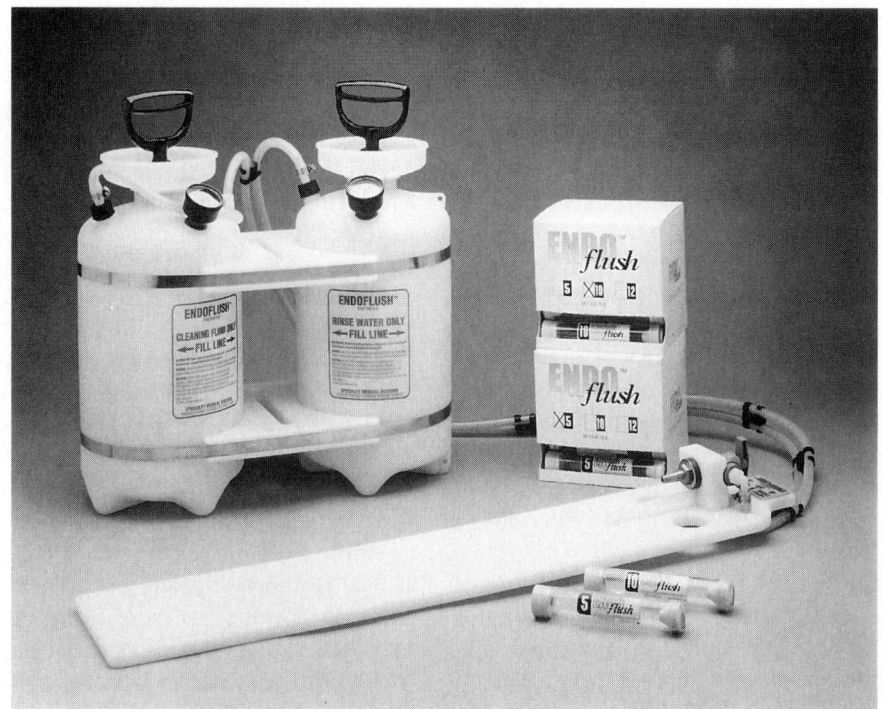

FIG. 32-53 Endoflush endoscopic instrument cleaner—hydraulic.
Courtesy Specialty Medical Systems, Shawnee Mission, Kansas.

With reusables it is important that the decontamination/reprocessing system used is reliable, is compatible with the equipment being processed, and can be monitored for effectiveness. Above all, safe and effective patient outcome should be the criterion against which all else is compared.

It is wise to investigate all avenues before purchase. As perioperative nurses, part of patient advocacy is to evaluate patient care practices, justify products used, and provide a safe environment for patients and personnel. We must be open to suggestion and change, whenever it is practical and economical to do so. This is the time for the entire surgical team and industry to form collaborative relationships that enhance practice and patient outcome. The determination to choose disposable or reusable instrumentation and equipment must be thoroughly evaluated in each individual practice setting and justified accordingly (Research Highlight 32-3).

VIDEO GLOSSARY

auto exposure an electronic circuit built into cameras to electronically (within the camera) eliminate excess light from the picture; sometimes referred to as electronic shutter.

automatic gain control ability to increase or decrease the video output level depending on the average light level of the viewed object.

blooming a glaring effect on the monitor caused by excessive light.

boost the ability to increase the signal strength of the camera. When used under low light conditions, boost provides increased sensitivity.

chromiance defines the video camera's ability to handle the color red, the most difficult color to reproduce. The more accurate the color reproduction, the higher the chromiance.

C-mount standard thread size and diameter for a standard video camera lens.

color bars a test pattern used to adjust controls on the monitor for color, brightness, and contrast.

color reproduction ability of an imaging device to reproduce colors exactly as the human eye perceives them.

composite video output (NTSC) the most commonly used video signal; the typical television video signal.

electronic shutter ability of a camera to freeze image information within fractions of a second (1/60, 1/125, 1/1000, 1/10,000).

footcandle standard measure of luminance; the amount of light emitted by a standard candle at a distance of 1 foot from the frame; 10 lux equals 1 footcandle. The lower the footcandle or lux number, the more sensitive the camera.

light gain another circuit within the camera to electronically amplify the picture to show a brighter image; sometimes referred to as AGC (automatic gain control) or boost circuit.

NTSC National Television Standards Committee; type of television signal used in the United States.

orientation a mark or ridge on the camera head to orient the top portion of the video monitor.

pixel a signal sensor element on a solid state video chip; most solid state chips used in medical videography have about 400,000 pixels on their surface. Each pixel is light sensitive and sees its own small part of the total picture.

RESEARCH HIGHLIGHT 32-3

Findings regarding the economic impact of laparoscopic surgery are presented in this report. Hospital costs, including the cost of equipment and instrumentation for laparoscopic surgery and the costs of four different procedures (laparoscopic cholecystectomy [LC], laparoscopic inguinal herniorrhaphy [LIH], laparoscopic assisted vaginal hysterectomy [LAVH], and thoracoscopic wedge resection [TWR], were examined relative to open versus laparoscopic approaches.

Nine hospitals throughout the United States were used to determine hospital costs. The study showed that laparoscopic approaches are a cost-effective alternative to traditional open surgery. If considering total system costs, each of the four procedures is cost-effective. If only hospital cost is considered, two laparoscopic approaches save money (LC, TWR), one is about equal (LAVH), and one (LIH) is slightly more expensive than its open surgical counterpart.

The study also indicated that single-use laparoscopic instruments can be a cost-effective alternative to reusable instruments. Instrument costs include purchase as well as labor and supply costs needed for cleaning and sterilization, costs for maintenance and repair, as well as disposal. All hospitals surveyed used a mixture of single-use and reusable instrumentation.

Single-use and reusable laparoscopic instruments were very similar in overall cost. Certain factors were hard to quantify. The most significant of these is the effectiveness of the cleaning and sterilization process used. The findings of this study suggest that current procedures used do not ensure that reusable instrumentation is properly cleaned and sterilized 100% of the time. The choice between single-use and reusable laparoscopic instruments revolves around several complex issues. Hospitals need to analyze their specific situations to make informed decisions.

Economic impact of laparoscopic surgery. (1993). Houston: Deloitte & Touche.

resolution an optical device's ability to separate fine detail. Usually expressed in TV lines. Traditionally measured by aiming the camera at a target chart with squares of fine lines. The maximum resolution of the optical device is determined at the point where it begins to blur the lines together. If a box showing 400 lines per inch is still clear with spaces between the lines, the optical device has at least 400 lines per inch resolution.

sensitivity the response to low light levels by a video system.

S-VHS output a signal from the camera that splits the chroma and luminance, allowing for a richer resolution recording.

white balance different light sources produce different temperatures of light, therefore, different colors of light. White balancing adjusts the camera for various sources of light.

REFERENCES

Decker, A. (1946). Pelvic culdoscopy. In J. Meigs and S. Sturgis (Eds.), *Progress in gynecology*. New York: Grune & Stratton.

Mackin, P. (1991). Laparoscopy risks are focus of research. *Laser Nursing, 6*(3), 74-75.

Ott, D. (1991). Correction of laparoscopic insufflation hypothermia. *Journal of Laparoendoscopic Surgery, 1*(4), 183-186.

Semm, K. (1982). Advances in pelviscopic surgery. *Current Problems in Obstetrics and Gynecology, 5*(10), entire issue.

Zucker, K.A. (1991). *Surgical laparoscopy*. St. Louis: Quality Medical Publishing.

BIBLIOGRAPHY

Anderson, B. (1993). Endoscopic carpal tunnel release: A new approach to carpal tunnel syndrome. *AORN Journal, 57*(2), 422-425, 428.

Ayliffe, G., Babb, J., & Bradley, C. (1992). Sterilization of arthroscopes and laparoscopes, *Journal of Hospital Infection, 22*(4), 265-269.

Crow, S. (1992). Peracetic acid sterilization: A timely development for a busy healthcare industry. *Infection Control and Hospital Epidemiology, 13*(2), 111-113.

Deardorf, M. (1990). Increasing multipuncture laparoscopic instrument longevity. *AORN Journal, 54*(2), 357-358, 360.

Dent, T. (1991). Training, credentialing and granting of clinical privileges for laparoscopic general surgery. *American Journal of Surgery, 161,* 399-403.

Eccliston, S. (1992). Laparoscopic cholecystectomy. *Todays OR Nurse, 14*(1), 15-18, 35-36.

Ely, S., & Kron, I. (1993). Thoracoscopic implantation of the implantable cardioverter defibrillator, *Chest, 103*(1), 271-272.

Hales, A. (1989). Arthroscopically assisted anterior cruciate ligament reconstruction. *AORN Journal, 49*(1), 234-255.

Holzman, M., Sharp, K., & Richards, W. (1992). Hypercarbia during carbon dioxide gas insufflation for therapeutic laparoscopy: A note of caution. *Surgical Laparoscopy and Endoscopy, 2*(1), 11-14.

Kaczmarek, R., Moore, R., McCrohan, J., et al. (1992). Multi-state investigation of the actual disinfection/sterilization in health care facilities. *American Journal of Medicine, 92*(3), 257-261.

Matthews, K. (1988). Pelviscopy: An endoscopic alternative to laparotomy. *AORN Journal, 47*(5), 1218-1221, 1224-1229.

Meagher, T. (1992). Videoarthroscopy: A new perioperative challenge. *Todays OR Nurse, 14*(12), 13-18, 25-26.

Nicholson, C., Coleman, C. & Mack, M. (1993). Are you ready for video thoracoscopy? *American Journal of Nursing, 93*(3), 54-57.

O'Connell, W. (1992). Video technology: Basics for perioperative nurses. *AORN Journal, 56*(3), 442-454.

Reddic, E., & Olsen, D. (1989). Laparoscopic laser cholecystectomy: A comparison with mini-lap cholecystectomy. *Surgical Endoscopy, 3,* 131-133.

Reichert, M. (1993). Laparoscopic instruments: Patient care, cost issues. *AORN Journal, 57*(3), 635-662.

Summers, J. (1990). Endoscopes and equality, *Journal of Healthcare and Materials Management, 8*(3), 66-68.

Tampinco-Golos, I. (1992). Endoscopic thoracotomy. *AORN Journal, 55*(5), 1167-1178.

Vesley, D., Norlien, K., Nelson, B., et al. (1992). Significant factors in the disinfection and sterilization of flexible endoscopes. *American Journal of Infection Control, 20*(6), 291-300.

Whelan, J., & Jackson, D. (1992). Videoarthroscopy: Review and state of the art. *Arthroscopy 8*(3), 311-319.

Wolenski, M., Markus, E., & Pelosi, M. (1991). Laparoscopic appendectomy incidental to gynecologic procedures. *Todays OR Nurse, 13*(12), 12-18.

33

CONTEMPORARY ISSUES

DONNA S. WATSON

Excellence has been demonstrated during the past half century by nurses committed to the perioperative patient. This commitment has been enthusiastically shared by nurses with a vision for a future that includes unity in numbers, universal access to health care, active advocacy for the surgical patient, fostering public awareness of perioperative nursing, promoting nursing research, and influencing health care policy at both the federal and state level. The past has greatly influenced what perioperative nursing is today and where it is headed tomorrow.

AGENCY FOR HEALTH CARE POLICY AND RESEARCH

The 1970s brought about drastic changes in the United States health care system. Cost containment was key. Doing business as usual in health care was no longer acceptable. An outgrowth of this philosophy included new payment mechanisms such as prospective payment systems, health maintenance organizations (HMOs), and peer review organizations. These mechanisms, however, offered no answers and seemed to create more problems than they were developed to solve. Thus discontentment with the present health care system, which is considered wasteful and inefficient, continues. It is estimated that 25% of all medical care is unnecessary (Kent, 1992). If controlled, this could translate into saving as much as $18 billion annually.

When compared internationally, the United States ranks as one of the highest for health care cost and one of the lowest for quality care. More than 8 million children in the United States have no insurance, and it is suggested that well over 40% do not receive routine immunizations. Universal access to immunizations for all children continues to be an ongoing debate between state and federal agencies.

In an effort to offset upward spiraling of health care costs and increase the quality, Congress mandated the Omnibus Budget Reconciliation Act of 1989 (Public Law 101-239) to establish the Agency for Health Care Policy and Research (AHCPR). This agency is among eight within the U.S. Department of Health and Human Services Public Health Service (Fig. 33-1). The purpose of the agency "is to enhance the quality, appropriateness, and effectiveness of health care services through a broad program of scientific research and information dissemination" (AHCPR, 1991).

The structure within the agency supports eight organizational units that are involved in carrying out its mission (Fig. 33-2), which is to enhance quality of care by improving knowledge that can be used to meet society's health care needs and expectations.

OFFICE OF THE FORUM FOR QUALITY AND EFFECTIVENESS IN HEALTH CARE

The Office of the Forum for Quality and Effectiveness in Health Care is responsible for the development of performance measures, standards of quality, and review criteria and for updating the clinical guidelines. The office investigates variations and develops guidelines that may reduce clinically significant variations among physicians. For instance, if a diagnostic procedure does not contribute to a beneficial outcome, it may not be recommended for a certain condition. The practitioner may choose to use it anyway, however, if deemed appropriate for that patient. It is estimated that 10% to 30% of health care expenditures can be saved by reducing variations in practice for a given condition (Mitchell and Durenberger, 1990).

The AHCPR definition for clinical guidelines is "systematically developed statements to assist practitioner and patient decisions for appropriate health care for specific clinical circumstances" (Hastings, 1991). Guidelines assist the practitioner managing patient care while allowing both the practitioner and patient alternative choices. Current guideline development for clinical conditions is based on needs and priority areas determined by the Medicare and Medicaid programs.

These government-sponsored guidelines differ from those developed by various associations in that they are multidisciplinary and include input from the consumer. Although the concept of government-sponsored guidelines is

U.S. Department of Health & Human Services
Public Health Service

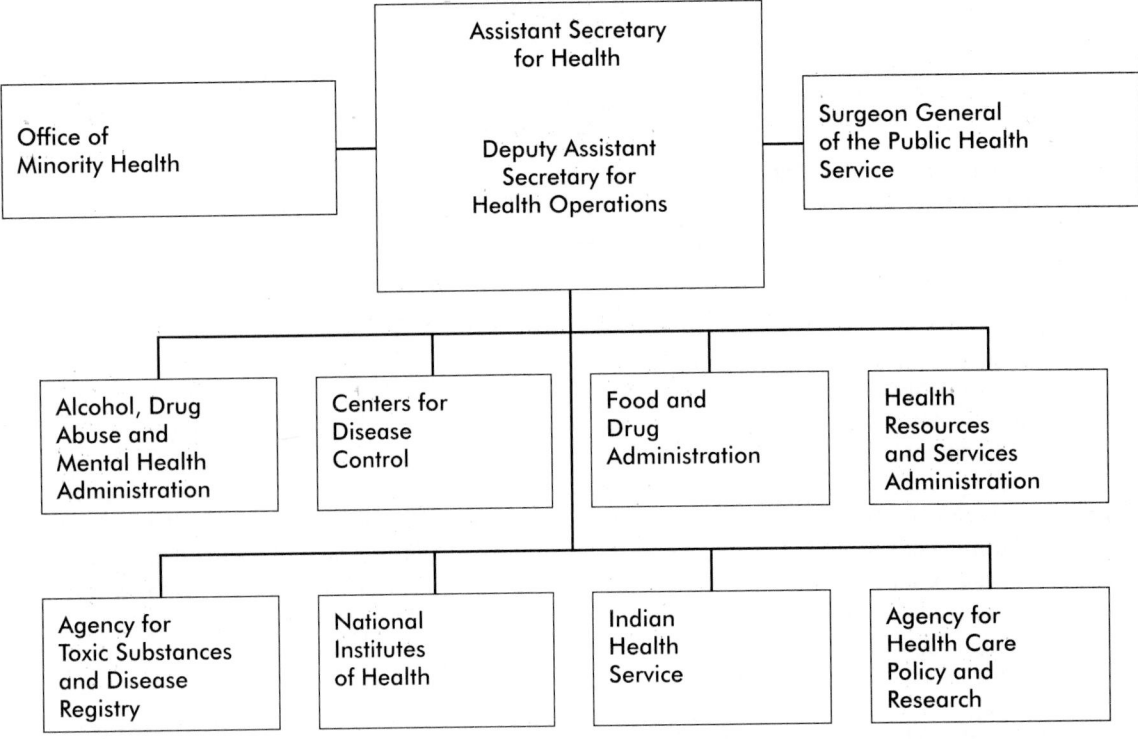

FIG. 33-1   Organizational chart for the U.S. Department of Health and Human Services Public Health Service.

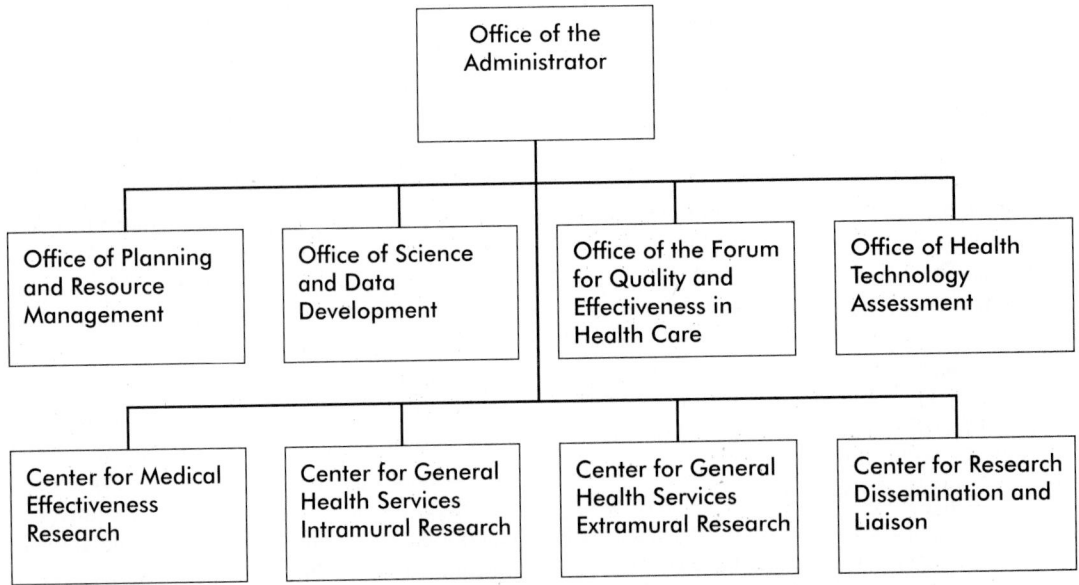

FIG. 33-2   Organizational chart of the Agency for Health Care Policy and Research.

supported by many, there is concern that such guidelines will lead to "cookbook medicine" (Kosterlitz, 1991).

The intent of the guidelines is to provide the practitioner and patient with what is considered appropriate care specific to prevention, diagnosis, treatment, and management of a given clinical condition. Clinical conditions are selected for guideline development based on how frequently the clinical condition occurs, evidence that variation in practice occurs, risk to the population, and cost of treatment.

Once a guideline is developed, the most effective plan of care is described, based on scientific evidence obtained via a comprehensive review of the literature and consensus of the panel's clinical experts and consumer representatives (Research Highlight 33-1). To date, the following guidelines have been developed or are in progress:

- Prediction, prevention, and early treatment of pressure ulcers in adults
- Pain management (see Chapters 8 and 28)
- Urinary incontinence in the adult (see Chapter 13)
- Diagnosis and treatment of depressed outpatients in primary care settings
- Management of functional impairment due to cataract in the adult
- Diagnosis and treatment of benign prostatic hyperplasia
- Sickle cell disease
- Otitis media in children
- Diagnosis and treatment of heart failure secondary to coronary vascular disease
- Poststroke rehabilitation
- HIV-positive asymptomatic patient: evaluation and early intervention
- Management of cancer-related pain
- Treatment of stage II and greater pressure ulcers
- Low back problems
- Screening for Alzheimer's and related dementias
- Quality determinants of mammography

Significant application of the AHCPR pressure ulcer guideline for perioperative patient care has been developed

---
RESEARCH HIGHLIGHT 33-1

Guidelines are "systematically developed statements to assist practitioner and patient decisions for appropriate health care for specific clinical circumstances" (Hastings, 1991). Each guideline is developed by a nonfederal panel of multidisciplinary experts based on an explicit, scientifically based methodology, and expert consensus for proper management of the given clinical condition.

Extensive literature review is conducted to determine and evaluate the empirical evidence. The guidelines are reviewed for validity, reliability, and utility by peers and by field review. Suggested practice is reflective of the knowledge and research at the time of development.

To obtain guideline information, call the AHCPR Clearinghouse toll-free number: 1-800-358-9295; or write to Center for Research Dissemination and Liaison, AHCPR Clearinghouse, P.O. Box 8547, Silver Spring, MD 20907.

(Meeker et al., 1993). One of the first goals of the guideline is to identify at-risk patients. All perioperative patients should be assessed for factors that increase the risk for pressure ulcers. These factors include patients with immobility, limited activity levels, incontinence, inadequate nutrition, altered level of consciousness, and dry, flaky, or scaling skin.

The second goal for patients identified at risk for pressure ulcer development is prevention. A systematic inspection of the skin before positioning the patient should be conducted and documented. The third goal is to prevent adverse effects related to positioning and external forces such as pressure, friction, and shearing. Numerous perioperative nursing interventions are aimed at prevention of pressure ulcers; these include the following:

- Padding and positioning bony prominences to avoid excess pressure and massage
- Cleansing skin to eliminate sources of contamination from fecal or urinary incontinence and chemical sources such as pooling of prep solutions
- Minimizing exposure to cold operating room temperature
- Draping patient in a manner to optimize moisture resistance to avoid pooling of fluids
- Utilizing appropriate personnel to position patient so as to avoid skin injury due to pressure, friction, and shear forces
- Applying protective padding to decrease friction around all pressure areas (such as heels, elbows, occiput, sacrum); doughnut devices should not be used
- Avoiding placing bony prominences (such as ankles and knees) in direct contact with each other
- Avoiding direct pressure on the trochanter when patient is placed in a lateral position, as well as padding knees, feet, dependent ankle, and dependent knee
- Determining patient's risk of pressure ulcer development and utilizing foam, alternating air, gel, or water mattress as procedure permits
- Assessing every patient for postural alignment, distribution of weight, balance, stability, and pressure point relief

The last goal is appropriate education and dissemination of information. Educational programs for preventing pressure ulcers in adults should be structured, organized, and comprehensive. All perioperative staff who assist in transporting, transferring, and positioning the surgical patient should participate. The perioperative nurse can make a major contribution in reducing the incidence of pressure ulcers for the surgical patient at risk.

CENTER FOR MEDICAL EFFECTIVENESS RESEARCH

The Medical Treatment Effectiveness Research Program (MEDTEP) located within the Center for Medical Effectiveness Research is responsible for researching unexplained variations in practice. It also determines the most effective and appropriate plan of care for a given condition. The major functions of MEDTEP include development of medical effectiveness research, development of data bases, and development and dissemination of clinical guidelines. Activities include facilitating and funding extramural research to determine the most effective treatments and patient outcomes. Congressional authorization has allowed for funding of $185 million in 1994.

Patient outcomes research teams (PORTs) collect and analyze existing literature and conduct research on a specific clinical condition. PORT projects are multidiscipline, multisite, and multiyear studies. Studies identify the best approach for clinical management of the condition and how to reduce the use of costly procedures that add no benefit to the final outcome. Some of the conditions and procedures that have been funded for PORTs include low back pain, total knee replacement, acute myocardial infarction, benign prostatic hyperplasia (Research Highlight 33-2) and localized prostate cancer, cataracts, ischemic heart disease, biliary tract disease, hip fracture repair and osteoarthritis, pneumonia, and diabetes. Other PORT research that is not specific to the Medicare population includes studies investigating cesarean delivery, otitis media, dental implants, and lens extraction. About one third of the funding focuses on non-Medicare populations (Salive, Mayfield, and Weisman, 1990).

Once research is completed, MEDTEP is responsible for dissemination of the findings to healthcare providers and the public. Research data collected from PORTs is included in the databases of AHCPR's Office of Science and Data Development and the Center for Research Dissemination and Liaison.

CENTER FOR GENERAL HEALTH SERVICES INTRAMURAL RESEARCH

The Center for General Health Services Intramural Research is responsible for health policy research and analysis of data on issues related to health care use. Most noted is the National Medical Expenditure Survey (NMES), which used a national probability sample to gather data on insurance status, insurance policy variations, and health care use for 35,000 persons. The center also collects and analyzes hospital discharge data on the Provider Studies Program and long-term care. Through this research the center has been effective in influencing federal policies such as the Medicare Catastrophic Coverage Act of 1988.

CENTER FOR GENERAL HEALTH SERVICES EXTRAMURAL RESEARCH

The Center for General Health Services Extramural Research operates three divisions: cost and financing, primary care, and technology and quality assessment. The division of cost and financing is responsible for studying cost and effect issues, productivity, third-party reimbursement, and alternative delivery systems. This division is conducting the AIDs Cost and Services Utilization Survey. The division of primary care supports research on the "organization, delivery, content, processes, practices, and outcomes of primary care" (AHCPR, 1990). Special emphasis is on research of primary care in rural areas and populations such as the elderly, mothers and children, persons with HIV, and disabled persons. The division of technology and quality assessment "supports research examining health care technology, health care information systems, and improvement of health care quality" (AHCPR, 1990). It also supports research to develop criteria to assess health care technology, its effectiveness, and how well the technology may be accepted. Further research in this area may have significant implications in the perioperative arena, where the introduction of new technology is a daily occurrence.

OFFICE OF HEALTH TECHNOLOGY ASSESSMENT

The Office of Health Technology Assessment "evaluates medical technologies, procedures, and services and recommends to Federal health programs whether they should be covered" (AHCPR, 1990). This office makes recommendations to approve or deny approval of a specific technology. Before the final recommendation is made, an extensive literature research is conducted. Then a conclusion on the efficacy and utility of the technology is formulated, and policy recommendations are developed and forwarded to appropriate federal programs.

Technology will always be a significant factor in the perioperative environment. However, as the percentage of

---

RESEARCH HIGHLIGHT 33-2

The AHCPR-funded PORT on benign prostatic hyperplasia treatment has released a 5-year study researching variations in treatment and outcomes. Studies (Wasson et al., 1993; Lu-Yao et al., 1993; Fleming et al., 1993; Whitmore et al., 1993) indicate that radical prostatectomy and radiation therapy have better outcomes on younger males with higher grade tumors. Males 75 years and older have a higher incidence of morbidity and mortality following radical surgical intervention and external radiation. Based on the limited information available, the studies suggested that watchful waiting for patients with well-differentiated tumor grades is as effective as the more aggressive treatment of surgery and radiation. If the limited findings of this PORT project are implemented, the perioperative nurse can anticipate a decrease in the number of radical prostatectomy procedures performed. This should decrease dramatically from the sixfold increase noted in the literature from 1984 to 1990.

the gross national product spent on health care continues to soar, there is increasingly more emphasis on demonstrating that a specific technology is safe and cost-effective. Technology assessment involves obtaining data on the following four aspects: safety, effectiveness, cost benefits, and social impact (Pillar, Jacox, and Redman, 1990). The data are utilized to improve the quality of care and should identify technology that is outdated (Perry, 1987). Although some form of technology assessment has always existed, in recent years there has been increased emphasis due to rising health care costs. The United States government— particularly Medicare administrators, private third-party payers, and proponents of the Prospective Payment System—is concerned about "the value, benefit, and safety of technologies provided to their clients" (Perry, 1987). Thus careful scrutiny of technologies has occurred.

The perioperative nurse is rarely involved in all aspects of technology assessment, yet the nurse is generally the primary operator of the equipment or is required to set it up, maintain it, and troubleshoot in the event of malfunction. It is important to have a perioperative staff nurse involved in technology assessment, and the following questions should be addressed from both nursing and medical perspectives:

Specific to medicine (Perry, 1987)

1. Is the technology safe; do the benefits outweigh the risk?
2. Does it serve the stated purpose?
3. Is the technology a real improvement over other technologies?
4. How can it best be used?
5. What problems does the technology pose for the patient?
6. Is it cost-effective?

Specific to nursing

1. Is there special training required to operate the equipment?
2. How will the technology affect the nursing care provided to the patient?
3. Will it dehumanize care to the patient?
4. Will it affect the staffing pattern?

Once the technology assessment is completed and approved, the nursing department should collaborate with appropriate departments to develop nursing practice guidelines for implementation.

OFFICE OF SCIENCE AND DATA DEVELOPMENT

The Office of Science and Data Development "is responsible for increasing the quality and quantity of data available for health services research, specifically for MEDTEP and patient outcomes research" (AHCPR, 1990). It determines the feasibility of linking private and public patient care data banks to determine the most effective treatment and links to patient outcomes.

CENTER FOR RESEARCH DISSEMINATION AND LIAISON

The Center for Research Dissemination and Liaison is responsible for disseminating publications and information of the agency. Its goal is to make research findings and agency guidelines available to health care providers and consumers.

OFFICE OF PLANNING AND RESOURCE MANAGEMENT

The Office of Planning and Resource Management is responsible for the overall coordination of the eight organizational units within the agency. "The Office coordinates program planning across AHCPR organizational units and monitors ongoing research, demonstration, and evaluation activities of the Agency in relation to changing research priorities" (AHCPR, 1990).

NURSING'S INVOLVEMENT

Initially nursing's role in the agency was minimal. The agency quickly learned, however, what a significant contribution nursing would have in the development of guidelines. From January 31 to February 1, 1990 a nurse adhoc advisory panel was convened to determine what nursing's contribution to the MEDTEP initiative and guideline development would include. The panel consisted of 45 national nursing leaders, clinicians, researchers, educators, and administrators. Three of the clinical conditions that the panel recommended for clinical practice guideline development were selected by the agency for development. Guideline panels that have been chaired or cochaired by a nurse researcher include urinary incontinence in the adult, acute postoperative pain management, and prediction, prevention, and early treatment of pressure sores in adults. To date, all guideline panels have nursing participation in guideline development.

It remains unclear what impact the agency will have on reforming health care in America. There are no mechanisms in place now to force the various disciplines to use the recommendations suggested in the guidelines. It is likely, however, that Medicare, Medicaid, and private insurers will use the guidelines as a determinant of reimbursement for services rendered. It is likely that those services not included in the suggested criteria will be deemed inappropriate and denied reimbursement unless justified.

As an active participant working closely with the Agency, nursing will continue to influence change at the federal level. It is critical for nursing research to demonstrate nursing activities and interventions that make a difference in the outcomes of patient care. Nursing is vital to the reshaping of the health care system. Hernandez and Hastings (1991) emphasize the importance of nursing to the effectiveness initiative and include nursing care, nursing data, and nursing research as critical components. In addition, the American Nurses Association (1990) concurs with the importance of these critical components as evidenced by the suggested responsibilities for specialty nursing practice groups. Specialty nursing practice groups are encouraged to participate in the development of standards of nursing practice, development of a national nursing data bank, and universal nursing practice guidelines. It is suggested that specialty nursing practice groups assume the following (ANA, 1990a):

- Ongoing monitoring of nursing within their specialty area and undertaking activities to promote nursing and quality client care
- Participating in the design of the overall framework for the development of standards of nursing practice, practice guidelines, and databases
- Developing criteria for measurement of standards
- Developing specialty practice guidelines using an agreed-upon framework
- Contributing to and using the national nursing database bank
- Sharing information concerning the ongoing examination of the legal implications of promulgating standards and guidelines for specialty nursing practice
- Conducting research in the specialty area that will contribute to a better understanding of the effectiveness of nursing care

In the future, there may be universal nursing guidelines much like those of the Agency. To gain support, recognition, and respect from other disciplines, this evolutionary process must be based on scientific research and not consensus alone. To meet the needs of the future, nursing must collaborate not only among its specialty organizations, but with sources outside of nursing, such as the Agency, which can influence the future direction of nursing practice.

HEALTH CARE REFORM

Nursing is involved daily with America's crisis in health care. The nurse can easily identify with the patient who is denied access to care and at the same time envision a better future that supports universal access. In retrospect 1993 may be viewed as the "Year of Health Care Reform." President Clinton moved toward health care reform with the establishment of a Task Force on National Health Care Reform and the introduction of several bills. It was estimated that between 34 and 37 million Americans were uninsured in 1993, with more than a fourth of these being children. In addition, approximately 60 million were underinsured in the event of a serious illness. In absence of reform, it was estimated that national health expenditures in the year 2000 will exceed $1.6 trillion, or 16.4% of the gross national product (Sonnefeld et al., 1991).

Some financial policies that have influenced nursing practice include legislation in 1983 that changed Medicare reimbursement from a retrospective cost-based system to a prospective payment system. This system, based on diagnosis related groups (DRGs), established a payment system for Medicare inpatient hospital services before services are provided. It encourages decreased admissions and shorter lengths of stay for patients. Reimbursement is at a fixed rate. If the institutions costs are less than the DRG payment, the institution benefits fiscally.

In 1986 the Physician Payment Review Commission (PPRC) was established by Congress. It advises Congress on what to pay physicians for services rendered to Medicare patients. Nursing closely monitors the activities of the PPRC to determine how physician payment is reviewed and revised and how nursing payment may be developed in the future. The PPRC has recommended the resource based relative value scale (RBRVS) for payment to nonphysician providers who render care to Medicare patients. This system does not pay nonphysician and physician providers equally for like services.

The present payment mechanisms are not effective. It is projected that the Medicare trust fund will be depleted by the year 2005. Private payer insurance companies are indirectly paying for medical care of uninsured people. Insurance rates continue to spiral upward, with no ceiling in sight. The private payer is paying increasingly more. Many businesses have increased co-payments of insurance or completely dropped insurance as an employee benefit because the costs often exceed their profits. It has been projected that, for every car sold in the United States, $1100 is allocated for health insurance. Most state-operated Medicaid programs are on the brink of financial disaster.

As the country attempts to overhaul the health care system for its 260 million citizens, nursing has been visible in making known *Nursing's Agenda for Health Care Reform* (American Nurses Association, 1991a). The key elements suggested in the proposed reform include universal access of a defined set of benefits for all citizens, utilization of managed care systems, development and implementation of clinical practice guidelines, case management for long-term care, health promotion, and greater consumer involvement and responsibility. It suggested utilization of nursing in preventive primary care through increased community care at nontraditional settings such as schools, community centers, places of employment, and individuals' homes. It supported the idea that cost can be controlled if disciplines such as nursing are used in a more resourceful manner.

The profession of nursing is not being used to its fullest potential. Opportunities that allow for greater responsibilities and better use of nursing services include prescriptive authority, which is now in effect in some states, direct reimbursement for nursing services, education of the public in techniques that contribute to promotion of wellness and prevention of illness, and privileges to admit patients to the hospital when designated criteria are met. Nursing has the capability of delivering 60% to 80% of preventive and primary care services, currently provided by physicians, and at a lower cost (Cassetta, 1993). Nursing will continue to emerge as a significant contributor and participant in the reformed health care system. As reform measures are phased in, nursing will keep some of its traditional roles and gain many nontraditional roles.

The roles and responsibilities of the perioperative nurse are certain to be affected by health care reform. Perioperative nursing practice is in a state of change. No longer are the definitions of *scrub nurse* and *circulator* adequate to reflect the actual practices and responsibilities of perioperative nurses. As health care reform moves forward, so will the roles and responsibilities of the perioperative nurse. The future for perioperative nurses might involve new or more significant responsibilities in areas such as pain management, first assisting, case management, utilization review, discharge planning, information systems, environmental waste management, risk management, research, consulting, and policy making (Rothrock and Hixon, 1991). In the future it might be the perioperative nurse who administers specific short-term therapeutic, screening, and diagnostic procedures. Perhaps the future perioperative nurse will routinely repair simple lacerations, administer intravenous conscious sedation throughout the institution, function as the first assistant on all surgical procedures, or accompany the patient home for postoperative care. Although it is uncertain what specific new roles and responsibilities will emerge with the reforming of health care, it is certain that the perioperative nurse of today will readily accept the challenges of tomorrow.

REIMBURSEMENT FOR NURSING SERVICES

The PPRC was formed to analyze physician payment issues and make recommendations regarding reforms in Medicare payment to physicians. At the request of Congress in 1989 the PPRC studied issues of reimbursement for nonphysician assistants (that is, physician assistant, RN first assistant [RNFA], certified surgical technician) during surgery. Issues included "the necessity and appropriateness of using an assistant at surgery, the use of physician and nonphysician assistants, the appropriateness of providing payment and levels of payments, and the effects of the Omnibus Budget Reconciliation Act (OBRA) 1986 on the employment of RNs as assistants at surgery" (Cruz, 1991). Nursing supports the key concept of "same service equals same pay." That is, if a qualified RNFA is able to first assist during a procedure and provide the same service as that of a physician assistant during surgery, the RNFA should receive the same reimbursement. The only nonphysician providers receiving reimbursement for their services in urban areas are physician assistants. In rural areas, the only non-physician providers receiving medicare reimbursement are nurse practitioners, clinical nurse specialists, and midwives.

The PPRC presented three options for paying nonphysician providers: (1) pay for all services rendered by the nonphysician provider; (2) deny payment to any nonphysician provider (such as physician assistants); or (3) maintain the status quo. The PPRC chose to maintain the status quo. There was some discussion to deny payment altogether to any nonphysician provider by excluding the physician assistant, who is entitled to reimbursement privileges under the Omnibus Budget Reconciliation Act (OBRA) of 1986. However, the commission clearly acknowledged the inequity of the present system and suggested additional studies of the issue.

For nurses to be effective in obtaining reimbursement for services, they must be knowledgeable about payment reforms. Markus (1990) presents the following six reasons why payment reforms are important to nursing:

First, the rules are important because they reflect, in a very real sense, the views of insurers and the public about the worth of the services provided by different specialties. Second, payment policies have a direct bearing on the willingness and the ability of patients to obtain services from different types of professionals. Third, payment policies play a major role for salaried workers, since such policies affect the willingness and capacity of hospitals and others to employ health care workers. Fourth, purchaser payment rules will determine the ability of some nursing specialties to practice independently and to receive payments for their services directly, if they choose to do so. Fifth, payment rules are also important because they reflect changing attitudes of lawmakers about other national concerns, e.g., about manpower issues, how medical care should be organized and delivered, and so forth. Lastly, changing Medicare payment policies are critical for the nursing specialties because of the federal government's trend-setting role.

The 1993 AORN House of Delegates approved the revised AORN *Official Statement on RN First Assistants* (Box 33-1). The revised statement reflects necessary changes to allow the RNFA to compete with other nonphysician providers in obtaining reimbursement. Questions previously asked by the PPRC regarding the RNFA role assumption and practice delineation included educational and training requirements, certification requirement, and regional variations in the use of the RNFA (Schlepp, 1990).

In the spring of 1993 the Board of Directors of the National Certification Board, Perioperative Nursing, Inc., administered the first Registered Nurse First Assistant examination allowing for certification. Criteria for eligibility to take the examination include current RN license, current CNOR, and proof of at least 2000 hours of practice as a RNFA of which 500 of those hours must have occurred in the 2 years immediately before taking the exam. The examination tests clinical competencies related to the role of the RNFA.

If nursing is to receive the same fee for the same service, nursing must be prepared to justify and defend the educational and clinical requirements, credentialing mechanisms, and qualifications of the RNFA to meet the expectations of third-party payers.

DECLINING NURSING SHORTAGE

After a decade of what was cited as the worst nursing shortage in history, 1993 witnessed a change in this trend. Over 70% of operating room managers reported no nursing shortage in their operating rooms (*OR Manager*, 1993).

BOX 33-1

AORN Official Statement on RN First Assistants*

PREAMBLE

Perioperative nursing practice has historically included the role of the RN as assistant at surgery. As early as 1980, documents issued by the American College of Surgeons supported the appropriateness for qualified RNs to first assist.

AORN officially recognized this role as a component of perioperative nursing in 1983 and adopted the first Official Statement on RN First Assistants (RNFA) in 1984. Acceptance of this official statement by many state boards of nursing has supported that RNFA behaviors are recognized within the scope of nursing practice.

AORN's official statement delineates the definition, scope of practice, qualifications, educational requirements, and clinical privileges that must be met by the perioperative nurse who practices as an RNFA. AORN further recognizes the need for appropriate compensation/reimbursement to RNs who fulfill this role in providing perioperative patient care.

DEFINITION OF RN FIRST ASSISTANT

The RN first assistant at surgery collaborates with the surgeon in performing a safe operation with optimal outcomes for the patient. The RN first assistant practices perioperative nursing and must have acquired the necessary specific knowledge, skills, and judgment. The RN first assistant practices under the supervision of the surgeon during the intraoperative phase of the perioperative experience. The RN first assistant does not concurrently function as a scrub nurse.

SCOPE OF PRACTICE

The scope of practice of the nurse performing as first assistant is a part of perioperative nursing practice. Perioperative nursing is a specialized area of practice. The activities included in first assisting are further refinements of perioperative nursing practice which are executed within the context of the nursing process. The observable nursing behaviors are based on an extensive body of scientific knowledge. These intraoperative nursing behaviors may include:
- Handling tissue
- Providing exposure
- Using instruments
- Suturing
- Providing hemostasis

These behaviors may vary depending on patient populations, practice environments, services provided, accessibility of human and fiscal resources, institutional policy, and state nurse practice acts.

The decision by an RN to practice as a first assistant must be made voluntarily and deliberately, with an under

standing of the professional accountability that the role entails.

QUALIFICATIONS OF THE RN FIRST ASSISTANT

Qualifications for RN first assistants should include, but not be limited to:
- Certification in perioperative nursing (CNOR)
- Knowledge of surgical anatomy, physiology, and operative technique related to the operative procedures in which the RN assists
- Ability to perform cardiopulmonary resuscitation
- Ability to perform effectively in stressful and emergency situations
- Ability to recognize safety hazards and initiate appropriate preventive and corrective action
- Ability to perform effectively and harmoniously as a member of the operative team
- Ability to demonstrate skill in behaviors unique to the RN first assistant (as defined)
- Meets requirements of statutes, regulations, and institutional policies relevant to RN first assistants

PREPARATION FOR THE RN FIRST ASSISTANT

AORN has stated, "The complexity of knowledge and skill required to effectively care for recipients of operating room nursing services compels nurses to be well educated and to continue their education beyond generic nursing programs."†

Perioperative nurses who wish to practice as RN first assistants must develop a set of cognitive, psychomotor, and affective behaviors that demonstrate accountability and responsibility for identifying and meeting the needs of the recipients of their nursing services.

Development of this set of behaviors begins with and builds upon the education program leading to licensure as an RN, which provides basic knowledge, skills, and attitudes essential to the practice of perioperative nursing. Further preparation for the RN first assistant includes perioperative nursing practice with diversified experience in scrubbing and circulating. This should culminate in the nurse achieving certification as a CNOR. Additional preparation is then acquired through completion of formal education programs including didactic instruction and supervised clinical learning activities.

These programs should consist of curricula that address all of the content areas of the modules in the *Core Curriculum for the RN First Assistant*, take place in institutions approved by The Association of Higher Education (or its equivalent), and award a degree or certificate upon successful program completion.

BOX 33-1

AORN Official Statement on RN First Assistants*—cont'd

ESTABLISHMENT OF CLINICAL PRIVILEGES FOR THE RN FIRST ASSISTANT

To determine if an RN qualifies for clinical privileges as a first assistant, an approval process must be established by the institution in which the individual will practice.

The process of granting clinical privileges should include mechanisms for:

- Assessing individual qualifications for practice
- Assessing continuing proficiency
- Evaluating annual performance
- Assessing compliance with relevant institutional and departmental policies

- Defining lines of accountability
- Retrieving documentation of participation as first assistant
- Establishing systems for peer review

Each RN first assistant demonstrates behaviors that progress on a continuum from basic competency to excellence. Once having met the educational and experiential requirements, the RNFA is encouraged to attain a bachelor of science in nursing degree and to achieve and maintain certification (CRNFA) for this specific role.

Reprinted with permission from the Association of Operating Room Nurses. 1993. AORN Official Statement on RN First Assistants. *AORN Journal*, 57(6), 1319-1321.

*Submitted March 1984; adopted March 1984 by House of Delegates, Atlanta; proposed revision to board submitted September 1992; adopted March 1993 by House of Delegates, Anaheim, Calif.

†Davis, D.L., Kneedler, J.A., & Manuel, B.J. 1978. *Surgical experience: A model for professional nursing practice in the operating room.* Denver: Association of Operating Room Nurses.

Two of the most frequent reasons cited for this sudden change were workplace restructuring and economic reasons (Scott, 1993). In the perioperative setting workplace restructuring has resulted in many institutions moving from a costly all-RN staff to a mixed ratio of RNs, surgical technicians, and LPNs. To support the cost of an all-RN staff, research linking staff mix to patient outcomes is needed.

Perioperative nursing remained in the forefront of anticipated reform by addressing issues of redefinition and reconceptualization of perioperative nursing practice (Rothrock and Hixon, 1991). Although current philosophical roots of perioperative nursing are deeply embedded in the intraoperative phase with emphasis on the traditional roles of circulating and scrubbing, the future will be more broad, and new roles for the perioperative nurse will surface. With the new roles will come new opportunities in settings outside the operating room. Although the perioperative nurse will continue to care for the patient throughout the surgical experience, the specific roles and expectations will evolve to meet the needs of the patient into the next century.

With proper preparation in advance, transition will be less unsettling. It is anticipated that services will move from hospital based to community based. The surgical suite may be a mobile unit that travels from home to home, or may be based as an adjunct facility to a school or employment site. Whatever health care reform presents, perioperative nurses must position themselves to ensure that quality perioperative patient care is managed by those best prepared to deliver safe, efficient, quality care—the perioperative nurse.

MANAGEMENT OF MEDICAL WASTE

Medical waste disposal is increasingly becoming a major issue of health care facilities. As technology has advanced, so has the packaging and use of disposable items. Many institutions prefer disposables over reusables because the product is ensured of sterility and function. In addition, potential exposure to bloodborne pathogens during cleaning is decreased, and overall productivity of the nurse is increased, allowing more time for patient care (Reichert, 1993). The operation of a single surgical suite generates a significant amount of medical waste. There are gloves, gowns, backtable covers, patient drapes, needles and other sharps, sponges, body fluids/secretions, and other items that must be disposed of. This does not include medical waste from the private offices of dentists and physicians. The cumulative effect of disposal is significant, and the effect on the environment is becoming more apparent.

Society has demanded accountability of health care facilities in proper disposal of medical waste. In 1987 the New Jersey shoreline was covered with syringes, bloody vials, and needles from medical waste that had been dumped into the ocean. Beaches were closed, and a public outrage began for more efficient methods of medical waste disposal. The public attention was in part due to the fear and concern of exposure to the human immunideficiency virus (HIV) and to hepatitis B virus (HBV). Management of medical waste quickly became a widespread public concern.

Tracking of medical waste is costly and time consuming. In addition to tracking facilities such as hospitals, private physicians' offices, ambulatory surgery centers, and blood banks, methods would have to be developed to track medical waste related to patient home care, IV drug users, and private clinics.

The 1994 AORN House of Delegates ratified the position statement on "Regulated Medical Waste Definition and Treatment: A Collaborative Document" (AORN, 1994). The collaborative document included representatives from

13 organizations with each recognizing that there is little consensus on an accepted definition and management of regulated medical waste. However, it is generally agreed that medical waste "has the potential to transmit infectious disease" (AORN, 1994, p. 1179). When defining what should be considered medical waste, hospitals should closely evaluate the type of pathogen, transmission, host, and appropriate safe disposal of the waste. *Tracking of medical waste is generated in the United States. . . . STET. . . .*

Medical waste is disposed of by methods such as steam sterilization, thermal inactivation, chemical disinfection, grinding, microwaves, high density lasers, and dumping into landfills. Some companies offer recycling options for their products. One reason for not having a universally accepted treatment requirement for management of medical waste, hospital waste, infectious waste, and regulated medical waste is because of the inconsistencies in definitions. For example, the definition of infectious waste is exactly what is implied: it is medical waste that is considered infectious and may cause disease. It has been estimated that close to 20% of all medical waste can be classified as infectious waste (Fay et al., 1990).

Using the above definition, however, one could interpret infectious waste as any material exposed to blood and body secretions. It could be interpreted to mean that all materials in contact with the patient are infectious waste. Such a misinterpretation would have a significant impact. Not only would the disposal and cost be insurmountable, but the environmental impact would be significant. There are fewer landfills available, and other methods of disposal come with potential hazards to the environment.

Classification and standardization of waste management definitions would eliminate some confusion. Also, there is a lack of regulatory control on proper removal, storage, and disposal of hospital waste. Recommendations vary according to city, state, and federal sources, and there are inconsistencies. Institutions may be fined large amounts when disposal recommendations are not followed.

In the perioperative setting infectious waste will continue to be an issue well into the next decade. The AORN Statement on Protection of the Environment (Box 33-2) supports the ongoing examination of waste management and notes implications specific to perioperative practice and contributions that can be made by the nurse. The AORN Subcommittee on Environmental Issues (Spry et al., 1991) recommended the following activities for the perioperative nurse advocating a cleaner environment:

1. Increase awareness of the problem and become intensely involved with both federal and state regulatory agencies regarding management of medical waste and infectious waste.
2. Become part of the solution. Closely evaluate the products that are to be used in the operating room. Consider using reusable items instead of disposables.
3. Select and evaluate surgical products wisely. The goal is to decrease unnecessary medical waste.
4. Educate colleagues and the general public. Become an advocate for the environment. Many are unaware of the acute problem of medical waste management both on a professional and personal level.

The perioperative nurse must accept the challenge, examine what changes the nurse can initiate, and implement these changes accordingly. Perioperative nurses must be proactive in preserving the environment not only for themselves, but also for future generations.

ETHICAL ISSUES

The nursing profession is involved with ethical decisions related to health care reform; the continuous surge of technology, how it is used, and who benefits from it; and aggressive surgery for the terminally ill. The perioperative nurse is not immune to ethical dilemmas and the impact that ethical decision making has. Ethical decisions are especially critical for the surgical patient who is sedated or unconscious. It is the perioperative nurse who may have to intervene on the patient's behalf when ethical dilemmas arise. Ethical situations specific to the perioperative setting may result from a technical error made by the surgeon, who then requests no documentation be made of the incident; performing surgery on a brain-dead child for the sake of the family; issues of mandatory HIV testing for both the patient and health care worker; having unauthorized persons present in the operating room observing a procedure; suspected drug abuse by one of the team members; operating on the wrong patient or wrong side; rushing "do-not-resuscitate" patients to the recovery area to expire; and unclear criteria for confirming death in a patient.

Perioperative nurses dealing with what is ethically and morally right or wrong should base their decisions and actions in accordance with the *ANA Code for Nurses with In-*

┌─────────────────────────────────┐
BOX 33-2

AORN Statement on Protection of the Environment

AORN recognizes that aspects of perioperative practice result in the generation of medical waste that impacts the environment. The Association strongly supports efforts to improve and preserve the environment through judicious selection, management, and disposal of surgical supplies and through environmentally sound programs of waste management. The Association encourages individual members to participate in research, to promote education, and to dialogue with others for the purpose of developing effective means to reduce the environmental impact of surgical waste.

Reprinted with permission from Association of Operating Room Nurses. 1991. *AORN Journal,* 53(4), 905.
└─────────────────────────────────┘

terpretive Statement—Explications for Perioperative Nursing (Seifert et al., 1993). These professional codes of conduct establish expectations for the perioperative nurse, who is accountable for upholding them and being responsible to the public, health care team members, and the profession of nursing. The following current ethical issues relate to perioperative nursing.

ORGAN PROCUREMENT

Most perioperative nurses have participated in an organ procurement. For many the most difficult time occurs when the organs are procured and the anesthesia machine is turned off. The procurement team goes quickly to implant the organs, anesthesia personnel are gone, and the perioperative nurse is left to prepare the patient for the family. This should not overshadow the opportunities offered to the recipients, but in reality it is a difficult time for the surgical team and especially the perioperative nurse.

Since the 1970s there has been widespread acceptance of guidelines for brain death and criteria that allow the patient to become a candidate as a heart-beating cadaver donor. More recently, because of the increasing need for organs, the University of Pittsburgh Medical Center and the Regional Organ Bank of Illinois are becoming pioneers in new criteria and protocols for organ donors that differ from the traditional method of using brain death as a determinant.

The University of Pittsburgh is using cardiopulmonary status as a determinant for non–heart-beating cadaver donors, for which the timing and place of death are controlled (Youngener and Arnold, 1993). The Pittsburgh protocol involves the family decision of forgoing all life-sustaining treatment. When this decision has been made, consent is obtained from the family. The patient is then transported to the operating room, and the organs are removed immediately after pronouncement of death. It is preferable that the surgical team not be present in the operating room until death has been declared. The certification of death is met when the following criteria have been determined: the patient who is apneic and unresponsive is weaned from the ventilator and may be administered sedatives and narcotics if pain is demonstrated; irreversible cessation of cardiac function must occur (2 minutes of pulselessness), and rigorous documentation accompanies the course of events.

The Regional Organ Bank of Illinois is using a protocol that includes infusing the kidneys with cold preservation solution at the time of uncontrolled death. Death is determined by cardiopulmonary criteria and usually involves patients who have undergone unsuccessful resuscitation or polytrauma. Initially, the center obtained permission before infusing the kidneys with preservation fluid. But due to the high incidence of family refusal, consent is no longer required. By proceeding with methods to preserve the kidneys, the families have more time for a final decision.

Both of these protocols have tremendously complex ethical dilemmas for the medical profession, nursing profession, and society. Although death is a natural occurrence of life, it rarely is easy. What seems to be overlooked with both protocols is the involvement of family at the time of death. With one protocol the patient, in essence, dies without the presence of loved ones. The other involves the intervention of preserving the kidneys without the family's permission. The definition of death and whether death is being hastened for the supply and demand of available organs can be made an issue. In addition, the surgical team may feel they are participating in the termination of life.

As new opportunities arise to meet the endless list of recipients for donated organs, new ethical dilemmas emerge. The professionals, patients, and society will need to discuss these issues and come to a common understanding for application of new criteria and practices for procuring organs from non–heart-beating cadaver donors.

DO-NOT-RESUSCITATE ORDERS

The do-not-resuscitate order "is deemed clinically, ethically, and legally appropriate when resuscitation would be futile and would prolong the patient's death" (Murphy, 1993). It is common practice in the operating room to suspend do-not-resuscitate (DNR) orders when the patient is undergoing a surgical procedure, since surgery on a DNR patient may be performed for a variety of reasons. Most often it is related to an attempt to decrease patient suffering (such as decreasing pain related to an obstruction or pressure from a growing mass). Although surgery is not curative for the terminally ill patient, it may offer an opportunity for an increased level of comfort and may increase the quality of life. Ethically, DNR orders suspended in the operating room could be challenged, based on refusal or lack of recognition by the surgical team to implement a patient's legal right, even if the result is death (Murphy, 1993). At a symposium on the operating room environment (Giordano, 1993) one of the topics of discussion included DNR in the operating room. Institutions are increasingly becoming aware of the ethical inconsistencies that exist when DNR orders are suspended in the operating room.

Many institutions are developing interdisciplinary policies addressing DNR orders specific for the operating room. Developing a policy for patients with advanced directives, such as a living will that includes the patient's desire not to be resuscitated, allows for staff input and discussion on the ethical issues and concerns. Do-not-resuscitate orders are honored throughout an institution's various units. Why should this standard of care be any different for the operating room? Reeder has suggested that a DNR policy should include a clear chain of communication for resolving questions about DNR orders and protocols to assist the surgical team in the event of death of any patient (Giordano, 1993). Today patients are participants in their own care, demanding to be heard and to be the final decision makers.

ALLOCATION OF RESOURCES

With health care reform comes widespread support of universal care for all individuals. There are inequities in the current system, with many individuals being turned away from much needed health care. In New York City a patient may have to wait up to 3 days in the emergency room before a hospital bed becomes available. Twelve other nations have a higher life expectancy than the United States. The United States ranks twenty second for infant mortality. Many believe this is due to the lack of prenatal care (Kennedy, 1991).

As emphasis is placed on preventive medicine, there will continue to be ethical discussions on where to best spend and limit money. The state of Oregon implemented an aggressive approach to its residents by initiating a prioritization of health care services known as the Oregon Plan. In this plan money is funded for treatment based on feasibility and cost. For example, money that was available for coverage of organ transplantation is no longer available; instead it is funneled to allocate more funds for maternity care (Klevit et al., 1991). There have been and will continue to be debate on the ethical issues of such a plan. But with the reforming of health care in America, prioritization of health care services will continue to be a topic of national debate.

Ethics is a fundamental part of nursing. Carper (1978) described the four patterns of knowing for nursing to include: "(1) empirics, the science of nursing, (2) esthetics, the art of nursing; (3) the component of a personal knowledge in nursing and (4) ethics, the component of moral knowledge in nursing." All four patterns are tightly interwoven and provide a foundation for building nursing knowledge. Working through ethical decision making, the perioperative nurse might ask questions such as: What is right about this situation? What is wrong about this situation? How will the situation affect the patient? What is my part in the situation and care of the patient? What is the expected patient outcome?

Although in ethics there are no clear answers, only directions, the perioperative nurse will continue to face ethical dilemmas and must challenge many issues and problems. Of utmost importance, however, is the value and respect for human life, autonomy, and dignity.

OPERATING ROOM RISK MANAGEMENT

In 1992 the Association of Operating Room Nurses published the new *Standards of Perioperative Nursing,* which included *Standards of Clinical Practice* and *Standards of Professional Performance* (AORN, 1992). These standards were developed from the American Nurses Association (1991b) *Standards of Clinical Nursing Practice,* which were published in 1991. During revision of the ANA standards, perioperative nursing representatives provided input regarding the role, nature, and purpose of practice standards. Expectations regarding the promulgation of nursing standards were also shared from the point of view of the perioperative nurse as well as other nursing specialty organizations. The collaborative effort among specialty nursing organizations and the ANA provided a framework for the development of nursing practice standards.

Standards are "authoritative statements by which the nursing profession describes the responsibilities for which its practitioners are accountable" (ANA, 1991b). Simply stated, standards are an expected level of care. They describe a level of competency that is expected to be provided to the patient at all times. In the past, the legal system placed emphasis on the standard of care in a specific community versus nationwide. Today that emphasis has shifted to national standards taking precedence over community standards (Kemmy, 1992). A court of law may use national standards in determining whether reasonable and prudent care was provided.

The profession of nursing is experiencing a tremendous amount of change in the reforming of the health care system. This is evident by the changing nurse practice acts, many of which include specific roles and functions for the RN first assistant, prescriptive authority, and evaluation, diagnosis, and treatment as part of nursing care. Along with the added responsibilities are increased accountability and risk of liability.

Nurses are responsible for maintaining competency through knowledge and skills in their given practice specialty. Knowledge and skills may be enhanced through a variety of educational activities. The nurse must be aware of national standards, guidelines, recommended practices, and the institution's standard of care and follow accordingly; failure could result in legal implications if patient harm occurs. The nurse should know the standards of nursing practice and their proper implementation; attend education activities that will enhance or maintain nursing knowledge; and keep abreast of current issues by reading nursing literature. Standards of nursing practice are integrated into everyday practice and generally are documented as standards of care for the institution.

SUMMARY

The time is right for the profession of nursing to make a significant impact on the delivery of health care in the United States. Contemporary issues related to the reforming of health care, reimbursement for nursing services, medical waste management, ethical dilemmas, appropriate utilization of unlicensed assistive personnel and risk management influence the practice of nursing. As a powerful driving force, nursing will unravel its new roles and responsibilities for the twenty first century. Today's nurses are charting their own course and destiny by building a solid foundation of perioperative nursing knowledge to support the perioperative nurses of tomorrow.

REFERENCES

AHCPR. (1990, September). *AHCPR purpose and programs.* Rockville, Md.: U.S. Department of Health and Human Services.

AHCPR. (1991, May). *Report to Congress: Progress of research on outcomes of health care services and procedures.* Rockville, MD: U.S. Department of Health and Human Services. (AHCPR Pub No. 91-0004).

American Nurses Association. (1991a). *Nursing's agenda for health care reform*. Kansas City: The Association.

American Nurses Association (1991b). *Standards of clinical nursing practice*. Kansas City: The Association.

American Nurses Association. (1990). *Task force on nursing practice standards and guidelines*. Working paper.

Association of Operating Room Nurses. (1994). Business Proceedings: Regulated Medical Waste Definition and Treatment: A Collaborative Document. *AORN Journal* Vol 59, No 6, pages 1176-1183.

Association of Operating Room Nurses. (1992). Standards of perioperative nursing. *AORN Journal, 55*(4), 1047-1056.

Carper, B. (1978). Fundamental patterns of knowing in nursing. *Advanced Nursing Science, 1*(1), 13-23.

Cassetta, R.A. (1993). Opening doors for advanced practice opportunities. *The American Nurse, 25*(6), 18-19.

Cruz, L. (1991). A history of the RN first assistant reimbursement issue. *AORN Journal, 53*(6), 1536-1540.

Fay, M.F., Beck, W.C., Fay, J.M., & Kessinger, M.K. (1990). Medical waste: The growing issues of management and disposal. *AORN Journal, 51*(6), 1493-1508.

Fleming, C., Wasson, J., & Albertsen, P. et al. (1993). A decision analysis of alternative treatment strategies for clinically localized prostate cancer. *Journal of the American Medical Association, 269*(20), 2650-2658.

Giordano, B. (1993). Symposium on the operating room environment. *AORN Journal, 58*, 340-344.

Hastings, K.E. (1991). Legal aspects of the AHCPR pressure ulcer guideline. *Decubitus, 4*(2), 36-38.

Hernadez, G.A., & Hastings K.E. (1991). The effectiveness initiative: Implications for nursing practice and research. *Nursing Outlook, 39*(5), 198-199.

Kemmy, J. (1992). Tailoring national guidelines to fit the needs of individual facilities. *AORN Journal, 55*(3), 872-878.

Kennedy E.M. Health America: Affordable health care for all Americans. Statement on the introduction of Health America, June 6, 1991, Washington, DC.

Kent, C. (1992). Jarrett Clinton: Shaking up medical care. *Journal of American Health Policy, 2*(2), 10-14.

Klevit H.D., Bates A.C., Castanares T., Kirk E.P., Sipes-Metzler P.R., & Wopat R. (1991). Prioritization of health care services. *Archives of Internal Medicine, 151*(5), 912-916.

Kosterlitz, J. (1991). Cookbook medicine. *National Journal, 23*(10), 574-577.

Lu-Yao, G.L., McLerran, D., Wasson, J., & Wennberg, J. (1993). An assessment of radical prostatectomy. *Journal of the American Medical Association, 269*(20), 2633-2636.

Markus, G.R. (1990, March). Medicare payment reforms: Implications for the nursing specialties. *Specialty Nursing Forum, 2*(2), 1, 3-5.

Meeker, M., Carelock, H., Gregory, B., Harvey, C., Rothrock, J., Stone, R., Ward, S., & Applegeet, C. *From guidelines to practice: Interpreting the clinical practice guideline for pressure ulcers in adults for perioperative patient care*. AORN Pre-Congress, February 27, 1993, Anaheim, Calif.

Mitchell, G.J., & Durenberger, D. (1990). Promoting value in health care: The new agency for health care policy and research. *Academic Medicine, 65*(3), 204-205.

Murphy, E. (1993). Do-not-resuscitate orders in the OR. *AORN Journal, 58*(2), 399-401.

Perry, S. (1987). Assessment and management of medical technology in the United States. *International Journal of Technology Assessment in Health Care, 3*, 588-598.

Pillar, B., Jacox, A., & Redman, B. (1990). Technology: Its assessment and nursing. *Nursing Outlook, 38*(1), 16-19.

Reichert, M. (1993). Laparoscopic instruments. *AORN Journal, 57*(3), 637-655.

Rothrock, J., & Hixon, J. (1991). Leaders in perioperative nursing convene to discuss their vision of the future, the specialty, AORN. *AORN Journal, 53*, 312-318.

Salary survey: OR managers see raises slip. (1993). *OR Manager, 9*(9), 1, 6-11.

Salive, M.E., Mayfield, J.A., & Weissman, N.W. (1990). Patient outcomes research teams and the agency for health care policy and research. *Health Services Research, 25*(5), 697-708.

Schlepp, S. (1990). Physician payment reform commission studies assistant at surgery issue; RN first assistants tell their side. *AORN Journal, 52*(2), 223-228.

Scott, K. (1993). RN layoffs of growing concern to ANA. The *American Nurse, 25*(6), 3.

Seifert, P.C., Killen, A.R., Bray, C.A., Hamblet, J.L., King, C.A., Kuhn, J.E., Reeder, J.M., Uruburu, A., Randolph, B.J., & Smith, C.D. (1993). ANA code for nurses with interpretive statements—Explications for perioperative nursing. *AORN Journal, 58*(2), 369-388.

Sonnefeld, S.T., Waldo, D.R., Lemieus, J.A., & McKusick, D.R. (1991). Projections of national health expenditures through the year 2000. *Health Care Financing Review, 13*(1), 1-15.

Spry, C., Botsford, J., Baker, J.D., & Shumaker, R. (1991). A report on infectious and noninfectious surgical waste disposal and its relation to the overall waste problem. *AORN Journal, 53*(4), 905-916.

Wasson J.H., Fleming, C., Bruskewitz, R., et al. (1993, February). The treatment of localized prostate cancer: what are we doing, what do we know, and what should we be doing? *Seminars in Urology, 11*(1), 23-26.

Whitmore, W.F. Jr. (1993). Management of clinically localized prostatic cancer. *Journal of the American Medical Association, 269*(20), 2676-2677.

Youngener, S.J., & Arnold, R.M. (1993). Ethical, psychosocial, and public policy implications of procuring organs from non-heart beating cadaver donors. *Journal of the American Medical Association, 269*(21), 2769-2774.

INDEX